Gammer Dip

3000 M? fug
5.28 03 for Tick
2.64 03 " other insects

Mange & Fungus

Thiobenzole BBZ

Dogs:
10 m/lb.
(60 lb. dog 1 level tsp) used until
hair grows back

If Nausea =
Split dose into b.i.d.

Put powder on Feed

MS Indocin Arthritis
Aramine Shock

**EDITED BY**

# ROBERT W. KIRK, D.V.M.

*Professor of Small Animal Medicine*
*Chairman of the Department of Small Animal Medicine and Surgery*
*Director of the Small Animal Clinic*
*New York State College of Veterinary Medicine*
*Cornell University*
*Ithaca, New York*

**Consulting Editors**

## FREDERICK W. OEHME
*Chemical and Physical Disorders*

## N. EDWARD ROBINSON
*Respiratory Diseases*

## STEPHEN I. ETTINGER
*Cardiovascular Disorders*

## JACK E. HATHAWAY
*Hemolymphatic Disorders and Oncology*

## RICHARD E. W. HALLIWELL
*Dermatologic Diseases*

## STEPHEN I. BISTNER
*Diseases of the Eye*

## FREDRIC L. FRYE
*Diseases of Exotic Animals*

## ALEXANDER DE LAHUNTA
*Neuromuscular Disorders*

## PETER THERAN
*Gastrointestinal Disorders*

## AD RIJNBERK
*Metabolic Disorders*

## CARL A. OSBORNE
*Genitourinary Disorders*

## FREDRIC W. SCOTT
*Infectious Diseases*

# CURRENT VETERINARY THERAPY VI

## SMALL ANIMAL PRACTICE

1977

W. B. SAUNDERS COMPANY · PHILADELPHIA · LONDON · TORONTO

W. B. Saunders Company:  West Washington Square
Philadelphia, PA 19105

1 St. Anne's Road
Eastbourne, East Sussex BN21 3UN, England

1 Goldthorne Avenue
Toronto, Ontario M8Z 5T9, Canada

Listed here is the latest translated edition of this book together with the language of the translation and the publisher.

Spanish (3rd edition)—Editorial Continental, Mexico

Japanese (4th edition)—Ishiyaku Publishers, Inc., Tokyo, Japan

Current Veterinary Therapy                               ISBN 0-7216-5470-3

Last digit is the print number:     9    8    7    6    5    4    3    2    1

# CONTRIBUTORS

GUSTAVO AGUIRRE, V.M.D., Diplomate, American College of Veterinary Ophthalmologists, Assistant Professor of Ophthalmology, School of Veterinary Medicine, University of Pennsylvania, Philadelphia, Pennsylvania.

ROBERT B. ALTMAN, D.V.M., Lecturer, Avian Diseases, University of Pennsylvania, School of Veterinary Medicine; Co-director, A and A Veterinary Hospital, Franklin Square, New York.

WILBUR B. AMAND, V.M.D., Senior Veterinarian/Curator at the Philadelphia Zoological Garden; Adjunct Assistant Professor, School of Veterinary Medicine, University of Pennsylvania; Consultant on Exotic Pets, Veterinary Consultants, Inc., Media, Pennsylvania.

NEIL V. ANDERSON, D.V.M., Ph.D., Diplomate, American College of Veterinary Internal Medicine, Professor, College of Veterinary Medicine, Kansas State University; Comparative Gastroenterologist, Dykstra Veterinary Hospital, Kansas State University, Manhattan, Kansas.

MAX J. G. APPEL, D.V.M., Ph.D., Professor of Veterinary Virology, New York State College of Veterinary Medicine, Cornell University; James A. Baker Institute for Animal Health, Ithaca, New York.

PAUL ARNSTEIN, D.V.M., M.P.H., National Cancer Institute, State of California Department of Health, Berkeley, California.

CARL E. ARONSON, Ph.D., Associate Professor of Pharmacology and Head, Laboratories of Pharmacology, School of Veterinary Medicine, University of Pennsylvania, Philadelphia, Pennsylvania.

CLARKE E. ATKINS, D.V.M., Resident in Medicine, Valley Veterinary Hospital, Walnut Creek, California.

DAMON RIVERS AVERILL, JR., D.V.M., Diplomate, American College of Veterinary Internal Medicine and American College of Veterinary Pathologists, Assistant Professor of Pathology, Harvard Medical School; Assistant Neuropathologist, Children's Hospital Medical Center; Consulting Neurologist, Angell Memorial Animal Hospital, Boston, Massachusetts.

E. MURL BAILEY, JR., D.V.M., M.S., Ph.D., Diplomate, American Board of Veterinary Toxicology, Associate Professor of Toxicology, Department of Veterinary Physiology and Pharmacology, College of Veterinary Medicine, Texas A & M University, College Station, Texas.

HENRY J. BAKER, D.V.M., Diplomate, American College of Laboratory Animal Medicine, Professor of Comparative Medicine, Schools of Medicine and Dentistry, University of Alabama, Birmingham, Alabama.

R. A. BANKOWSKI, D.V.M., Ph.D., Diplomate, American College of Veterinary Microbiologists, Professor of Epidemiology and Preventive Medicine, School of Veterinary Medicine, University of California, Davis, California.

RALPH E. BARRETT, D.V.M., Assistant Professor of Veterinary Medicine, Department of Clinical Medicine and Surgery, College of Veterinary Medicine, Washington State University Small Animal Clinic, Pullman, Washington.

ROY W. BELLHORN, D.V.M., M.Sc. (Ophth.), Diplomate, American College of Veterinary Ophthalmologists, Associate Professor of Ophthalmology, Albert Einstein College of Medicine; Research Associate, Montefiore Hospital and Medical Center, Bronx, New York.

BRUCE E. BELSHAW, D.V.M., Diplomate, American College of Veterinary Pathologists, Small Animal Clinic, State University of Utrecht, The Netherlands.

DAVID A. BEMIS, Ph.D., Postdoctoral Associate, New York State College of Veterinary Medicine, Cornell University; James A. Baker Institute for Animal Health, Ithaca, New York.

JOHN BENTINCK-SMITH, D.V.M., Diplomate, American College of Veterinary Pathologists, Professor of Clinical Pathology, New York State College of Veterinary Medicine, Cornell University, Ithaca, New York.

MICHAEL BERNSTEIN, D.V.M., Director of Clinics, Angell Memorial Animal Hospital, Boston, Massachusetts; Adjunct Assistant Professor of Medicine, Department of Clinical Studies, School of Veterinary Medicine, University of Pennsylvania, Philadelphia, Pennsylvania.

DARRYL N. BIERY, D.V.M., Diplomate, American College of Veterinary Radiology, Associate Professor of Veterinary Radiology, School of Veterinary Medicine, and Associate Professor of Radiological Science, School of Medicine, University of Pennsylvania, Philadelphia, Pennsylvania.

STEPHEN IRA BISTNER, D.V.M., Diplomate, American College of Veterinary Ophthalmologists, Associate Professor of Veterinary Ophthalmology, University of Minnesota, St. Paul, Minnesota.

GARY R. BOLTON, D.V.M., Associate Professor of Small Animal Medicine and Cardiology, New York State College of Veterinary Medicine, Cornell University, Ithaca, New York.

JOSEPH GREGG BORING, D.V.M., M.S., Diplomate, American College of Veterinary Radiology, Assistant Professor of Radiology, School of Veterinary Medicine, Auburn University; Staff Radiologist, Section of Radiology, Auburn, Alabama.

DAVID ERIC BOSTOCK, M.A., Vet. M.B., M.R.C.V.S., University Lecturer in Animal Pathology, Department of Clinical Veterinary Medicine, University of Cambridge, Cambridge, England

KENNETH C. BOVEE, D.V.M., M.Med. Sci., Diplomate, American College of Veterinary Internal Medicine, Associate Professor, Section of Medicine, School of Veterinary Medicine, University of Pennsylvania, Philadelphia, Pennsylvania.

TIMOTHY H. BRASMER, D.V.M., Ph.D., Diplomate, American College of Veterinary Surgeons, Professor, College of Veterinary Medicine, University of Minnesota, St. Paul; Veterinary Teaching Hospitals, University of Minnesota, St. Paul, Minnesota.

EUGENE M. BREZNOCK, D.V.M., M.S., Ph.D., Assistant Professor of Veterinary Surgery, University of California, School of Veterinary Medicine, Davis, California.

ROBERT S. BRODEY, D.V.M., M.Sc. (Surg.), Diplomate, American College of Veterinary Surgeons, Professor of Surgery, School of Veterinary Medicine, University of Pennsylvania; Head, Small Animal Tumor Clinic, Philadelphia, Pennsylvania.

KATHLEEN KEATING BROWN, D.V.M., Lexington Clinic of the Cold Stream Animal Hospital, Pennsylvania.

GARY M. BRYAN, D.V.M., M.S., Diplomate, American College of Veterinary Ophthalmologists; Associate Professor, Department of Veterinary Medicine and Surgery, College of Veterinary Medicine, Washington State University; Staff Ophthalmologist and Director, Washington State University Small Animal Hospital, Pullman, Washington.

JAMES W. BUCHANAN, D.V.M., M.Med. Sci. (Cardiology), Diplomate, American College of Veterinary Internal Medicine, Professor of Medicine, School of Veterinary Medicine, University of Pennsylvania, Philadelphia, Pennsylvania.

WILLIAM B. BUCK, D.V.M., M.S., Diplomate, American Board of Veterinary Toxicology, Chief of Diagnostic Services, Mississippi State University, College of Veterinary Medicine, Mississippi State, Mississippi.

RALPH G. BUCKNER, D.V.M., M.S., Diplomate, American College of Veterinary Internal Medicine, Professor, Veterinary Medicine and Surgery, Oklahoma State University, College of Veterinary Medicine; Small Animal Clinic, Stillwater, Oklahoma.

ROBERT W. BULL, D.V.M., Associate Professor, Department of Small Animal Surgery and Medicine, College of Veterinary Medicine, and Departments of Medicine and Surgery, College of Medicine, Michigan State University, East Lansing, Michigan.

THOMAS JEFFERY BURKE, D.V.M., M.S., Assistant Professor of Veterinary Clinical Medicine, University of Illinois College of Veterinary Medicine, Urbana, Illinois.

COLIN F. BURROWS, B.Vet.Med., M.R.C.V.S., Diplomate, American College of Veterinary Internal Medicine, Associate in Medicine, Pennsylvania Plan Scholar in Gastroenterology, Department of Clinical Studies, School of Veterinary Medicine, University of Pennsylvania; Head, Intensive Care Unit, University of Pennsylvania Veterinary Hospital, Philadelphia, Pennsylvania.

CHARLES C. CAPEN, D.V.M., M.Sc., Ph.D., Diplomate, American College of Veterinary Pathologists, Professor of Pathobiology, College of Veterinary Medicine, and Professor of Endocrinology and Metabolism, College of Medicine, The Ohio State University; Consulting Clinician, The Ohio State University Veterinary Teaching Hospital, Columbus, Ohio.

JACK H. CARLSON, D.V.M., Ph.D., Assistant Professor of Microbiology, College of Veterinary Medicine and Biomedical Sciences, Colorado State University, Fort Collins, Colorado.

LELAND E. CARMICHAEL, D.V.M., Ph.D., Diplomate, American College of Veterinary Microbiologists, John M. Olin Professor of Virology, New York State College of Veterinary Medicine; James A. Baker Institute for Animal Health, Ithaca, New York.

JAMES LAWRENCE CARPENTER, D.V.M., Diplomate, American College of Veterinary Pathologists, Director of Pathology, Angell Memorial Animal Hospital, Boston, Massachusetts.

BILLY R. CLAY, D.V.M., M.S., Diplomate, American Board of Veterinary Toxicology, Assistant Professor of Veterinary Toxicology, Department of Physiological Sciences, College of Veterinary Medicine, Oklahoma State University, Stillwater, Oklahoma.

FRANK HERBERT COMHAIRE, M.D., Lecturer, Department of Internal Medicine, Section of Endocrinology, Faculty of Medicine, State University of Ghent, University Hospital, Ghent, Belgium.

GAYLORD M. CONZELMAN, JR., Ph.D., Associate Professor of Pharmacology, School of Veterinary Medicine, University of California, Davis, California.

GERALD E. COSGROVE, M.D., Pathologist, Biology Division, Oak Ridge National Laboratory, Oak Ridge, Tennessee.

SUSAN M. COTTER, D.V.M., Diplomate, American College of Veterinary Internal Medicine, Staff Member, Angell Memorial Animal Hospital; Research Associate in Oncology, Harvard School of Public Health, Boston, Massachusetts.

LARRY D. COWGILL, D.V.M., Assistant Professor of Medicine, Department of Medicine, School of Veterinary Medicine, University of California, Davis, California.

STANLEY R. CREIGHTON, D.V.M., Staff, Brentwood Pet Clinic, 11718 Olympic Boulevard, West Los Angeles, California.

JOHN F. CUMMINGS, D.V.M., M.S., Ph.D., Associate Professor of Veterinary Anatomy, New York State College of Veterinary Medicine, Cornell University, Ithaca, New York.

MICHAEL G. DEAR, B.Sc., B. Vet. Med., M.R.C.V.S., Richmond, British Columbia, Canada.

JAN J. de BRUYNE, M.S., Clinical Chemist, State University of Utrecht; Small Animal Clinic, State University of Utrecht, Utrecht, The Netherlands.

JAN F. DETRICK, D.V.M., Fort Bragg, California.

M. JOSEPHNE DEUBLER, V.M.D., M.S., Ph.D., Assistant Professor of Pathology in Medicine, School of Veterinary Medicine, University of Pennsylvania, Philadelphia, Pennsylvania.

PAUL F. DICE II, V.M.D., M.S., Diplomate, American College of Veterinary Ophthalmologists, Animal Eye Clinic of Seattle, Seattle, Washington.

ROBERT ARTHUR DIETERICH, D.V.M., Professor of Veterinary Science, University of Alaska, Institute of Arctic Biology; Chairman, Program in Wildlife Diseases and Veterinary Science, Fairbanks, Alaska.

RICHARD T. DIXON, M.V.Sc., M.S., Diplomate, American College of Veterinary Radiology, Consultant in Veterinary Radiology, 1051 Pacific Highway, Pymble, New South Wales, Australia.

W. JEAN DODDS, D.V.M., Associate Research Scientist, Division of Laboratories and Research, New York State Department of Health, Albany; Associate Professor of Medicine (Adjunct), Albany Medical College, Albany, New York.

FRANCIS L. EARL, D.V.M., Facility Manager, Special Pharmacological Animal Laboratory, Division of Toxicology, Bureau of Foods, Food and Drug Administration, Washington, D.C.

GEORGE W. EBERHART, D.V.M., Formerly Associate Professor of Surgery, Kansas State University, Manhattan, Kansas; Formerly Clinical Veterinarian, University of California, San Diego, School of Medicine, La Jolla, California; Practitioner, Rheem Veterinary Medical Hospital, Moraga, California.

NATHAN JOEL EDWARDS, D.V.M., Shaker Veterinary Hospital, Latham, New York.

WILLIAM C. EDWARDS, D.V.M., M.S., Diplomate, American Board of Veterinary Toxicology, Associate Professor, Oklahoma State University College of Veterinary Medicine, Stillwater, Oklahoma.

STEPHEN J. ETTINGER, D.V.M., Diplomate, American College of Veterinary Internal Medicine, Internal Medicine and Cardiology, Berkeley Veterinary Medical Group, Berkeley; Associate Clinical Professor, School of Veterinary Medicine, University of California, Davis, California.

A. THOMAS EVANS, D.V.M., M.S., Assistant Professor, Michigan State University; Michigan State University Veterinary Clinic, East Lansing, Michigan.

S. A. EWING, D.V.M., Ph.D., Professor, College of Veterinary Medicine, University of Minnesota, St. Paul, Minnesota.

GEORGE E. EYSTER, V.M.D., M.S., Associate Professor, Michigan State University; Michigan State University Veterinary Clinic, East Lansing, Michigan.

R. FARNSWORTH, D.V.M., M.S., Associate Professor, College of Veterinary Medicine, University of Minnesota, St. Paul, Minnesota.

BRIAN R. H. FARROW, B.V.Sc., Ph.D., M.A.C.V.Sc., Associate Professor of Veterinary Medicine, University of Sydney, Sydney, Australia.

CHARLES S. FARROW, D.V.M., Assistant Professor, Department of Clinical Sciences, Western College of Veterinary Medicine, University of Saskatchewan, Saskatoon, Saskatchewan, Canada.

LLOYD C. FAULKNER, D.V.M., Ph.D., Diplomate, American College of Theriogenologists, Professor and Chairman, Department of Physiology and Biophysics, Colorado State University, College of Veterinary Medicine and Biomedical Sciences, Fort Collins, Colorado.

EDWARD C. FELDMAN, D.V.M., Staff, Internal Medicine Service, Berkeley Veterinary Medical Group, Berkeley, California.

WILLIAM ROY FENNER, B.S., D.V.M., Associate Staff Member, Department of Medicine, The Animal Medical Center, New York, New York.

DELMAR R. FINCO, D.V.M., Ph.D., Diplomate, American College of Veterinary Internal Medicine, Professor, University of Georgia, College of Veterinary Medicine, Athens; University of Georgia Veterinary Medical Teaching Hospital, Athens, Georgia.

CRAIG A. FISCHER, D.V.M., Diplomate, American College of Veterinary Ophthalmologists, St. Petersburg, Florida.

MURRAY ELWOOD FOWLER, D.V.M., Diplomate, American Board of Veterinary Toxicology and American College of Veterinary Internal Medicine, Professor of Medicine, University of California; Chief of Service, Zoological Medicine, Veterinary Medical Teaching Hospital, Davis, California.

G. FREDERICK FREGIN, V.M.D., Assistant Professor of Medicine, School of Veterinary Medicine, University of Pennsylvania; Head, Large Animal Cardiology, New Bolton Center, Kennett Square, Pennsylvania.

J. K. FRENKEL, M.D., Ph.D., Professor of Pathology, University of Kansas School of Medicine, Kansas City, Kansas.

FREDRIC L. FRYE, D.V.M., Clinical Professor of Veterinary Medicine, University of California, Davis; Donner Laboratory, University of California, Berkeley; Consultant to United States Public Health Service Hospital, San Francisco, California.

ALLAN FURR, B.S., D.V.M., M.S., Diplomate, American Board of Veterinary Toxicology, Assistant Professor, Iowa State University; Veterinary Toxicologist, Veterinary Diagnostic Laboratory, Ames, Iowa.

PAUL C. GAMBARDELLA, V.M.D., M.S., Staff Surgeon, Angell Memorial Animal Hospital, Boston, Massachusetts.

JACK MICHAEL GASKIN, D.V.M., Ph.D., Assistant Professor, Veterinary Microbiology, College of Veterinary Medicine, University of Florida, Gainesville, Florida.

KIRK N. GELATT, V.M.D., Diplomate, American College of Veterinary Ophthalmologists, Professor of Comparative Ophthalmology, College of Veterinary Medicine, University of Florida, Gainesville, Florida.

EDWARD L. GILLETTE, D.V.M., Ph.D., Diplomate, American College of Veterinary Radiology, Professor, Department of Radiology and Radiation Biology, Colorado State University, Fort Collins, Colorado.

T. GOPAL, B.V.Sc., M.S., Research Assistant in Veterinary Pathology, College of Veterinary Medicine, Kansas State University, Manhattan, Kansas.

IRA MALCOM GARY GOURLEY, D.V.M., Ph.D., Diplomate, American College of Veterinary Surgeons, Professor of Veterinary Surgery, School of Veterinary Medicine, University of California; Veterinary Medical Teaching Hospital, Davis, California.

RICHARD W. GREENE, D.V.M., Diplomate, American College of Veterinary Surgeons; Staff, Department of Surgery, The Animal Medical Center, New York, New York.

IAN RONALD GRIFFITHS, B.V.M.S., Ph.D., F.R.C.V.S., Senior Lecturer in Veterinary Surgery, University of Glasgow Veterinary School; Senior Lecturer in Veterinary Neurology, University Veterinary Hospital, Bearsden, Glasgow, Scotland.

D. P. GUSTAFSON, D.V.M., Ph.D., Diplomate, American College of Veterinary Microbiologists, Professor of Virology, School of Veterinary Medicine, Purdue University, West Lafayette, Indiana.

ROBERT M. GWIN, D.V.M., N.I.H. Fellow in Comparative Ophthalmology, College of Veterinary Medicine, University of Florida, Gainesville, Florida.

ALLEN W. HAHN, D.V.M., Ph.D., Diplomate, American College of Veterinary Internal Medicine, Professor of Veterinary Medicine and Surgery and Investigator, John M. Dalton Research Center, University of Missouri; Staff Cardiologist, Veterinary Teaching Hospital, College of Veterinary Medicine, University of Missouri, Columbia, Missouri.

MARC A. HALL, D.V.M., Small Animal Hospital, Ocoee, Florida.

RICHARD E. W. HALLIWELL, M.A., Ph.D., Vet. M.B., M.R.C.V.S., Diplomate, American College of Veterinary Internal Medicine, Assistant Professor of Dermatology, School of Veterinary Medicine, University of Pennsylvania, Philadelphia, Pennsylvania.

ROBERT L. HAMLIN, D.V.M., Ph.D., Diplomate, American College of Veterinary Internal Medicine, Professor, Ohio State University, College of Veterinary Medicine; Senior Attending Clinician, Veterinary Hospital, Columbus, Ohio.

ROBERT M. HARDY, D.V.M., M.S., Assistant Professor and Head, Division of Small Animal Medicine, Department of Small Animal Clinical Sciences, College of Veterinary Medicine, University of Minnesota, St. Paul, Minnesota.

NEIL K. HARPSTER, V.M.D., Director of Cardiology, Angell Memorial Animal Hospital, Boston, Massachusetts.

JAMES MICHAEL HARRIS, D.V.M., Montclair Veterinary Hospital, Oakland; Medical Director, International Bird Rescue-Research Center, Berkeley, California.

WILLIAM F. HARRIS, D.V.M., Veterinary Practice, Puyallup, Washington.

BENJAMIN L. HART, D.V.M., Ph.D., Professor, School of Veterinary Medicine, University of California, Davis; Behavior Specialist, Veterinary Medical Teaching Hospital, Davis, California.

COLIN E. HARVEY, B.V.Sc., M.R.C.V.S., Diplomate, American College of Veterinary Surgeons, Associate Professor of Surgery and Chief, Section of Small Animal Surgery, School of Veterinary Medicine, University of Pennsylvania, Philadelphia, Pennsylvania.

H. JAY HARVEY, D.V.M., Associate Staff, The Animal Medical Center; Department of Surgery and The Donaldson-Atwood Cancer Clinic of The Animal Medical Center, New York, New York.

JACK E. HATHAWAY, D.V.M., M.S., Manager of Veterinary Services, Professional Marketing Services Department, Ralston Purina Company, Checkerboard Square, St. Louis, Missouri.

PAUL W. HESS, D.V.M., Former Head, Cancer Therapy Unit, Henry Bergh Memorial Hospital; Former Research Associate, Memorial Sloan-Kettering Cancer Clinic, New York, New York.

RONALD W. HILWIG, D.V.M., M.Sc., Ph.D., Associate Professor of Veterinary Science, College of Agriculture, University of Arizona, Tucson, Arizona.

CHARLES H. HOBBS, D.V.M., Diplomate, American Board of Veterinary Toxicology, Radiation Biologist (Toxicologist), U.S. Energy Research and Development Administration, Washington, D.C. (on leave of absence from Inhalation Toxicology Research Institute, Lovelace Foundation for Medical Education and Research, Albuquerque, New Mexico).

RICHARD E. HOFFER, D.V.M., M.S., Diplomate, American College of Veterinary Surgeons, Associate Professor, Small Animal Surgery, New York State College of Veterinary Medicine, Cornell University; Small Animal Clinic, Cornell University, Ithaca, New York.

JEAN HOLZWORTH, D.V.M., Diplomate, American College of Veterinary Internal Medicine, Clinical Staff, Angell Memorial Animal Hospital, Boston, Massachusetts.

WILLIAM E. HORNBUCKLE, D.V.M., Staff Clinician, Angell Memorial Animal Hospital, Boston, Massachusetts.

LANCE N. HORWITZ, V.M.D., Associate in Dermatology, School of Veterinary Medicine, Small Animal Hospital, University of Pennsylvania, Philadelphia, Pennsylvania.

KATHERINE ALBRO HOUPT, V.M.D., Ph.D., Assistant Professor of Physiology and Behavioral Consultant, Veterinary Hospital, New York State College of Veterinary Medicine, Cornell University, Ithaca, New York.

ARTHUR I. HURVITZ, D.V.M., Ph.D., Diplomate, American College of Veterinary Pathologists, Chairman, Department of Pathology and Director of Research, The Animal Medical Center, New York, New York; Adjunct Assistant Professor of Pathology (part time), Columbia University, New York, New York.

DAVID L. HUXSOLL, D.V.M., Ph.D., Commanding Officer, U.S. Army Medical Research Unit, Kuala Lumpur, Malaysia.

PETER J. IHRKE, V.M.D., Associate in Dermatology, School of Veterinary Medicine, Small Animal Hospital, University of Pennsylvania, Philadelphia, Pennsylvania.

KARIM JERAJ, B.V.Sc., Resident in Internal Medicine, Department of Small Animal Clinical Sciences, College of Veterinary Medicine, University of Minnesota, St. Paul, Minnesota.

CARL R. JESSEN, D.V.M., Ph.D., Associate Professor and Head, Division of Radiology, Department of Small Animal Clinical Sciences, College of Veterinary Medicine, University of Minnesota, St. Paul, Minnesota.

GERALD JOHNSON, D.V.M., Diplomate, American College of Veterinary Internal Medicine; Staff, Department of Medicine, Animal Medical Center, New York, New York.

ROGER K. JOHNSON, D.V.M., Diplomate, American College of Veterinary Internal Medicine, Walnut Creek, California.

DUDLEY E. JOHNSTON, B.V.Sc., M.V.Sc., A.M., Diplomate, American College of Veterinary Surgeons, Professor of Surgery, School of Veterinary Medicine, Small Animal Clinic, School of Veterinary Medicine, University of Pennsylvania, Philadelphia, Pennsylvania.

GARY R. JOHNSTON, D.V.M., Resident in Radiology, Department of Small Animal Clinical Sciences, College of Veterinary Medicine, University of Minnesota, St. Paul, Minnesota.

SHIRLEY D. JOHNSTON, D.V.M., Resident, Theriogenology, Department of Large Animal Clinical Sciences, College of Veterinary Medicine, University of Minnesota, St. Paul, Minnesota.

JACOB A. JOLES, Research Student, Small Animal Clinic, State University of Utrecht, The Netherlands.

DONALD E. KAHN, D.V.M., Head, Urology Research Department, Biological Research Division, Pitman-Moore, Inc., Washington Crossing, New Jersey.

WILLIAM JAMES KAY, B.S., D.V.M., Diplomate, American College of Veterinary Internal Medicine, Chief-of-Staff, The Animal Medical Center; Adjunct Associate Professor of Neurology, New York University Medical Center, New York, New York.

ANATOLE KERN, D.V.M., Instructor, Department of Small Animal Medicine, College of Veterinary Medicine, University of Georgia, Athens, Georgia.

ROBERT W. KIRK, B.S., D.V.M., Diplomate, American College of Veterinary Internal Medicine, Professor and Chairman, Department of Small Animal Medicine and Surgery; Director, Small Animal Clinic, New York State College of Veterinary Medicine, Cornell University, Ithaca, New York.

JEFFREY S. KLAUSNER, D.V.M., Resident in Internal Medicine, Department of Small Animal Clinical Sciences, College of Veterinary Medicine, University of Minnesota, St. Paul, Minnesota.

LAWRENCE J. KLEINE, D.V.M., M.S., Diplomate, American College of Veterinary Radiology, Director of Radiology, Angell Memorial Animal Hospital, Boston, Massachusetts.

KENNETH W. KNAUER, D.V.M., M.S., Associate Professor of Veterinary Medicine and Surgery, College of Veterinary Medicine, Texas A & M University, College Station, Texas.

GARY J. KOCIBA, D.V.M., Diplomate, American College of Veterinary Pathologists, Associate Professor, Department of Veterinary Clinical Sciences, Ohio State University; Clinical Pathologist, Ohio State University Veterinary Teaching Hospital, Columbus, Ohio.

RONALD J. KOLATA, D.V.M., Associate in Surgery, Department of Clinical Studies, University of Pennsylvania School of Veterinary Medicine; Head, Trauma Emergency Service, University of Pennsylvania Veterinary Hospital, Philadelphia, Pennsylvania.

D. J. KRAHWINKEL, JR., D.V.M., M.S., Associate Professor, College of Veterinary Medicine, University of Tennessee; Director of Surgical Services, Department of Urban Practice, Veterinary Teaching Hospital, University of Tennessee, Knoxville, Tennessee.

LENNART KROOK, D.V.M., Ph.D., Professor of Pathology, New York State College of Veterinary Medicine, Cornell University, Ithaca, New York.

JEFFREY A. LaCROIX, D.V.M., Ithaca, New York.

THEODORE J. LAFEBER, D.V.M., Niles Animal Hospital, Niles, Illinois.

ARTHUR L. LAGE, D.V.M., Director of Medicine, South Shore Veterinary Associates, South Weymouth, Massachusetts; Clinical Veterinarian, Harvard University, Boston, Massachusetts.

ALEXANDER de LAHUNTA, D.V.M., Ph.D., Diplomate, American College of Veterinary Internal Medicine, Professor of Veterinary Anatomy and Director of Veterinary Medical Teaching Hospital, New York State College of Veterinary Medicine, Cornell University, Ithaca, New York.

J. GEOFFREY LANE, B. Vet. Med., F.R.C.V.S., Lecturer in Veterinary Surgery, University of Bristol; E.N.T. and Oral Surgeon, University of Bristol Veterinary Hospital, Bristol, England.

ROLF E. LARSEN, D.V.M., Veterinary Medical Associate, College of Veterinary Medicine, University of Minnesota, St. Paul, Minnesota.

V. L. LARSON, D.V.M., Ph.D., Professor, College of Veterinary Medicine, University of Minnesota, St. Paul, Minnesota.

J. D. LAVACH, D.V.M., M.S., Resident in Ophthalmology, College of Veterinary Medicine and Biomedical Sciences, Colorado State University, Fort Collins, Colorado.

IRWIN LEAV, D.V.M., Diplomate, American College of Veterinary Pathologists, Assistant Professor of Pathology, Tufts University School of Medicine; Angell Memorial Animal Hospital, Boston, Massachusetts.

DONALD H. LEIN, D.V.M., Ph.D., Diplomate, American College of Veterinary Pathologists, Associate Professor of Veterinary Medicine, New York State College of Veterinary Medicine, Cornell University; Theriogenologist, New York State College of Veterinary Medicine Teaching Hospitals, Ithaca, New York.

GEORGE E. LEWIS, JR., D.V.M., College of Veterinary Medicine, University of Illinois, Urbana, Illinois.

HUGH BILSON LEWIS, B.V.M.S., M.R.C.V.S., Diplomate, American College of Veterinary Pathologists, Associate Professor of Clinical Pathology, School of Veterinary Medicine, Purdue University, West Lafayette, Indiana.

ROBERT M. LEWIS, D.V.M., Diplomate, American College of Veterinary Pathologists, Professor and Chairman, Department of Pathology, New York State College of Veterinary Medicine, Cornell University, Ithaca, New York.

MICHAEL D. LORENZ, D.V.M., Diplomate, American College of Veterinary Internal Medicine, Associate Professor, College of Veterinary Medicine, University of Georgia, Athens, Georgia.

DONALD G. LOW, D.V.M., Ph.D., Diplomate, American College of Veterinary Internal Medicine, Professor of Veterinary Medicine, University of California, Davis; Director, Veterinary Medical Teaching Hospital, University of California, Davis, California.

ALEID A. M. E. LUBBERINK, D.V.M., Small Animal Clinic, State University of Utrecht, Utrecht, The Netherlands.

DOUGLAS M. MacCOY, B.S., D.V.M., Assistant Professor, Small Animal Surgery, New York State College of Veterinary Medicine, Cornell University, Ithaca, New York.

E. GREGORY MacEWEN, V.M.D., Chairman, Department of Medicine, and Head, Donaldson-Atwood Cancer Clinic, The Animal Medical Center; Research Associate, Memorial Sloan-Kettering Cancer Center, New York, New York.

ALAN D. MacMILLAN, D.V.M., Ph.D., Diplomate, American College of Veterinary Ophthalmologists, Assistant Professor, Department of Surgery, School of Veterinary Medicine, University of California, Davis, California.

LEONARD C. MARCUS, V.M.D., M.D., Diplomate, American College of Veterinary Pathologists, Assistant Clinical Professor of Pediatrics and of Pathology (joint appointment), Tufts University School of Medicine, New England Medical Center; Assistant Director of Health Services, State Laboratory Institute, Massachusetts Department of Public Health; Affiliate, Angell Memorial Animal Hospital, Boston, Massachusetts.

SHARRON L. MARTIN, D.V.M., M.Sc., Professor of Veterinary Clinical Sciences, Ohio State University; Attending Clinician, Ohio State University Veterinary Teaching Hospital, Columbus, Ohio.

DANIEL MATTHEEUWS, D.V.M., Professor, Department of Small Animal Medicine and Surgery, Faculty of Veterinary Medicine, State University of Ghent, Director of the Small Animal Clinic, Ghent, Belgium.

LESLIE E. McDONALD, D.V.M., Ph.D., Professor of Veterinary Medicine, University of Georgia, Athens, Georgia.

TOM MEHLHOFF, D.V.M., Resident in Clinical Pathology, Department of Veterinary Pathobiology, College of Veterinary Medicine, University of Minnesota, St. Paul, Minnesota.

K. F. MEYER, M.D., Deceased.

ROBERT M. MILLER, B.S. (Ag.), D.V.M., Staff Member, Conejo Valley Veterinary Clinic, Thousand Oaks, California.

MARK L. MORRIS, JR., D.V.M., Ph.D., Mark Morris Associates, Topeka, Kansas.

JACOB E. MOSIER, D.V.M., M.S., Diplomate, American College of Veterinary Internal Medicine, Professor of Veterinary Medicine, College of Veterinary Medicine, Kansas State University; Director, Dykstra Veterinary Hospital, Kansas State University, Manhattan, Kansas.

WILLIAM W. MUIR, D.V.M., Ph.D., Assistant Professor, Ohio State University; Head, Section of Anesthesiology, Ohio State University, Veterinary Teaching Hospital, Columbus, Ohio.

GEORGE H. MULLER, D.V.M., Diplomate, American College of Veterinary Internal Medicine, Clinical Professor of Dermatology, Stanford University Medical School, Stanford, California; Veterinary Dermatologist, Muller Veterinary Hospital, Walnut Creek, California.

JOHN ARTHUR MULNIX, D.V.M., M.S., Associate Professor, College of Veterinary Medicine and Biomedical Sciences, Colorado State University, Fort Collins, Colorado.

JOAN A. O'BRIEN, V.M.D., Diplomate, American College of Veterinary Internal Medicine, Associate Professor of Medicine, University of Pennsylvania School of Veterinary Medicine; Associate Professor and Chief, Section of Medicine, Small Animal Hospital, University of Pennsylvania School of Veterinary Medicine, Philadelphia, Pennsylvania.

FREDERICK W. OEHME, D.V.M., Ph.D., Diplomate, American Board of Veterinary Toxicology, Professor of Toxicology, Medicine and Physiology, Kansas State University, College of Veterinary Medicine; Clinical Toxicologist, Dykstra Veterinary Hospital, Kansas State University, Manhattan, Kansas.

PHILLIP N. OGBURN, D.V.M., Ph.D., Assistant Professor of Cardiology, University of Minnesota College of Veterinary Medicine; Small Animal Hospital, St. Paul, Minnesota.

PATRICIA O'HANDLEY, V.M.D., Assistant Professor, Department of Small Animal Surgery and Medicine, Michigan State University, East Lansing, Michigan.

JOHN E. OLIVER, JR., D.V.M., M.S., Ph.D., Diplomate, American College of Veterinary Internal Medicine, Professor and Head, Department of Small Animal Medicine, College of Veterinary Medicine, University of Georgia, Athens, Georgia.

PATRICIA SCHULTZ OLSON, D.V.M., M.S., Graduate Student, University of Minnesota, St. Paul, Minnesota.

STEN-ERIK OLSSON, V.M.D., M.D., Professor of Clinical Radiology, The Royal Veterinary College, Clinical Center, S-750 07 Uppsala 7, Sweden.

CARL A. OSBORNE, D.V.M., Ph.D., Diplomate, American College of Veterinary Internal Medicine; Professor and Chairman, Department of Small Animal Clinical Sciences, College of Veterinary Medicine, University of Minnesota, St. Paul; Professor, Department of Pediatrics, College of Medicine, University of Minnesota, Minneapolis, Minnesota.

GARY D. OSWEILER, D.V.M., M.S., Ph.D., Diplomate, American Board of Veterinary Toxicology, Associate Professor, Department of Veterinary Anatomy-Physiology, College of Veterinary Medicine, University of Missouri, Columbia, Missouri.

NICHOLAS E. PALUMBO, D.V.M., Professor, Division of Comparative Medicine, School of Medicine, University of Hawaii, Honolulu; Clinician, Lanai Veterinary Clinic, Pigeon City, Lanai, Hawaii.

HAROLD R. PARKER, D.V.M., Ph.D., Associate Professor of Veterinary Surgery, School of Veterinary Medicine, University of California; Veterinary Medical Teaching Hospital, University of California, Davis, California.

JOHN L. PARKS, D.V.M., Associate Staff Surgeon, The Animal Medical Center, New York, New York.

CHARLES J. PARSHALL, JR., D.V.M., Diplomate, American College of Veterinary Ophthalmologists; Veterinary Ophthalmology Clinic, Akron, Ohio.

AMIYA K. PATNAIK, D.V.M., Staff Pathologist, Department of Pathology, The Animal Medical Center, New York, New York.

DONALD F. PATTERSON, D.V.M., D.Sc., F.A.C.C., Diplomate, American College of Veterinary Internal Medicine, Chief, Section of Medical Genetics; Charlotte Newton Sheppard Professor of Medicine, School of Veterinary Medicine; Professor of Human Genetics, School of Medicine, University of Pennsylvania, Philadelphia, Pennsylvania.

ROBERT L. PEIFFER, JR., D.V.M., Diplomate, American College of Veterinary Ophthalmology, N.I.H. Fellow in Comparative Ophthalmology, College of Veterinary Medicine, University of Florida, Gainesville, Florida.

SAM F. PERRI, B.A., Research Associate, Comparative Medicine, John A. Burns School of Medicine, University of Hawaii, Honolulu, Hawaii.

DONALD L. PIERMATTEI, D.V.M., Ph.D., Diplomate, American College of Veterinary Surgeons, Surgical Practice, Golden, Colorado; Affiliate Professor of Surgery, Department of Clinical Sciences, Colorado State University, Fort Collins, Colorado.

R. CHARLES POVEY, B.V.Sc., Ph.D., M.R.C.V.S., Associate Professor, Department of Clinical Studies, Ontario Veterinary College; Small Animal Clinic, Ontario Veterinary College, University of Guelph, Guelph, Ontario, Canada.

K. W. PRASSE, D.V.M., Ph.D., Diplomate, American College of Veterinary Pathologists, Associate Professor of Veterinary Pathology, College of Veterinary Medicine, University of Georgia, Athens, Georgia.

ROBERT LEE PYLE, V.M.D., M.S., Diplomate, American College of Veterinary Internal Medicine, Associate Professor of Medicine, Colorado State University, Fort Collins, Colorado.

MALCOLM I. RAFF, Ph.D., Director of the Native Bird Facility of the Berkeley-East Bay Humane Society, Berkeley, California.

LLOYD M. REEDY, D.V.M., Diplomate, American College of Veterinary Internal Medicine, Animal Dermatology Clinic, Dallas, Texas.

JOHN S. REIF, D.V.M., M.Sc. (Med.), Associate Professor of Epidemiology and Medicine, School of Veterinary Medicine, University of Pennsylvania, Philadelphia, Pennsylvania.

RON C. RIIS, D.V.M., M.S., Diplomate, American College of Veterinary Ophthalmologists, Assistant Professor of Comparative Ophthalmology, New York State College of Veterinary Medicine, Cornell University, Ithaca, New York.

AD RIJNBERK, D.V.M., Ph.D., Professor, Small Animal Clinic, State University of Utrecht, Utrecht, The Netherlands.

N. EDWARD ROBINSON, B. Vet. Med., Ph.D., M.R.C.V.S., Associate Professor, Department of Physiology, Michigan State University, East Lansing, Michigan.

DONALD L. ROSS, D.V.M., M.S., Houston Veterinary Dental Clinic, Houston, Texas.

MARVIN L. SAMUELSON, D.V.M., Assistant Professor, Kansas State University; Small Animal Clinician, Dykstra Veterinary Hospital, Kansas State University, Manhattan, Kansas.

WILLIAM D. SCHALL, D.V.M., Associate Professor of Internal Medicine, Michigan State University, College of Veterinary Medicine, Small Animal Clinic, East Lansing, Michigan.

RONALD D. SCHECHTER, V.M.D., North Park Veterinary Hospital, San Diego, California.

GRETCHEN MARIE SCHMIDT, D.V.M., Diplomate, American College of Veterinary Ophthalmologists, Assistant Professor, Michigan State University Veterinary Clinic, Department of Small Animal Surgery and Medicine, East Lansing, Michigan.

STEPHEN M. SCHUCHMAN, D.V.M., Boulevard Pet Hospital, Castro Valley, California.

RONALD DAVID SCHULTZ, B.S., M.S., Ph.D., Assistant Professor, James A. Baker Institute for Animal Health, Cornell University, Ithaca, New York.

ROBERT M. SCHWARTZMAN, V.M.D., M.P.H., Ph.D., Diplomate, American College of Veterinary Internal Medicine, Professor of Dermatology, School of Veterinary Medicine, University of Pennsylvania, Philadelphia, Pennsylvania.

DANNY W. SCOTT, D.V.M., Assistant Professor of Comparative Dermatology, New York State College of Veterinary Medicine, Cornell University, Ithaca, New York.

FREDRIC W. SCOTT, D.V.M., Ph.D., Diplomate, American College of Veterinary Microbiologists, Director, Cornell Feline Research Laboratory; Associate Professor of Veterinary Microbiology, New York State College of Veterinary Medicine, Cornell University, Ithaca, New York.

RICHARD C. SCOTT, D.V.M., Diplomate, American College of Veterinary Internal Medicine; Staff, Department of Medicine, The Animal Medical Center, New York, New York.

STEPHEN W. J. SEAGER, M.V.B., M.R.C.V.S., M.A., Associate Professor, Department of Veterinary Physiology and Pharmacology, College of Veterinary Medicine, Texas A & M University, College Station; Associate Professor, Department of Cell Biology, and Associate Director, Institute of Comparative Medicine, Baylor College of Medicine, Texas Medical Center, Houston, Texas.

G. A. SEVERIN, D.V.M., M.S., Diplomate, American College of Veterinary Internal Medicine, and American College of Veterinary Ophthalmologists, Professor, Department of Clinical Sciences, College of Veterinary Medicine and Biomedical Sciences, Colorado State University, Fort Collins, Colorado.

SAM SILVERMAN, D.V.M., Diplomate, American College of Veterinary Radiology, James Picker Fellow in Academic Radiology, Department of Radiological Science, University of California, Davis, California.

HARRY E. SMALLEY, D.V.M., M.S., Diplomate, American Board of Veterinary Toxicology, College Station, Texas.

DAVID C. SMITH, B.A., Director of Research, International Bird Rescue–Research Center, Berkeley, California.

JEFFREY S. SMITH, B.V.Sc., M.R.C.V.S., Resident, Comparative Ophthalmology, New York State College of Veterinary Medicine, Cornell University, Ithaca, New York.

FRED K. SOIFER, D.V.M., Bellaire Boulevard Animal Clinic, Houston, Texas.

LAWRENCE R. SOMA, V.M.D., Diplomate, American College of Veterinary Anesthesiologists, Professor of Anesthesia and Chairman, Department of Clinical Studies, School of Veterinary Medicine, University of Pennsylvania, Philadelphia, Pennsylvania.

ANTHONY A. STANNARD, D.V.M., Ph.D., Diplomate, American College of Veterinary Internal Medicine, Associate Professor, School of Veterinary Medicine, University of California, Davis, California.

E. L. STEPHEN, D.V.M., Aerobiologic Division, U.S. Army Medical Research Institute of Infectious Diseases, Frederick, Maryland.

JERRY B. STEVENS, D.V.M., Ph.D., Professor, Department of Veterinary Pathobiology, College of Veterinary Medicine, University of Minnesota, St. Paul, Minnesota.

C. M. STOWE, V.M.D., Ph.D., Professor, College of Veterinary Medicine, University of Minnesota, St. Paul, Minnesota.

PETER F. SUTER, D.M.V., Diplomate, American College of Veterinary Radiology, Professor of Veterinary Radiology, School of Veterinary Medicine, University of California, Davis; Chief of Small Animal Clinics, Veterinary Medical Teaching Hospital, Davis, California.

W. THEODORE SWEENY, B.Sc., D.V.M., Hazleton Research, Raphine, Virginia.

LARRY N. SWENBERG, D.V.M., Cincinnati, Ohio.

GORDON H. THEILEN, D.V.M., Professor of Surgery, University of California, Davis; Head of Clinical Oncology, Veterinary Medicine Teaching Hospital, University of California, Davis, California.

PETER THERAN, V.M.D., Diplomate, American College of Veterinary Internal Medicine, Adjunct Associate Professor, University of Pennsylvania School of Veterinary Medicine, Philadelphia, Pennsylvania; Assistant Chief of Staff, Angell Memorial Animal Hospital, Boston, Massachusetts.

WILLIAM P. THOMAS, D.V.M., Diplomate, American College of Veterinary Internal Medicine, Instructor in Cardiology, School of Veterinary Medicine, University of Pennsylvania, Philadelphia, Pennsylvania.

FREDERICK N. THOMPSON, D.V.M., Ph.D., Assistant Professor, College of Veterinary Medicine, University of Georgia, Athens, Georgia.

JERRY A. THORNHILL, D.V.M., Berwyn Veterinary Medical Center, Berwyn, Illinois.

LAWRENCE P. TILLEY, D.V.M., Diplomate, American College of Veterinary Internal Medicine; Staff Cardiologist, The Animal Medical Center; Adjunct Assistant Professor, College of Physicians and Surgeons, Columbia University, New York, New York.

JOHN F. TIMONEY, JR., B.Sc., M.V.B., M.S., Ph.D., M.R.C.V.S., Assistant Professor, Microbiology, New York State College of Veterinary Medicine, Cornell University, Ithaca, New York.

ERIC J. TROTTER, D.V.M., M.S., Diplomate, American College of Veterinary Surgeons, Assistant Professor of Small Animal Surgery, and Chief of Surgery, Veterinary Teaching Hospitals, New York State College of Veterinary Medicine, Cornell University, Ithaca, New York.

GARY A. VAN GELDER, D.V.M., M.S., Ph.D., Diplomate, American Board of Veterinary Toxicology, Professor of Veterinary Toxicology, College of Veterinary Medicine, University of Missouri, Columbia, Missouri.

JERRY S. WALKER, D.V.M., Research Scientist, U.S. Department of Agriculture, Plum Island Animal Disease Center, Greenport, New York.

JOEL D. WALLACH, B.S., D.V.M., Postdoctoral Fellow, Veterinary Research Office, Palmer Chemical and Equipment Co., Douglasville, Georgia.

GRAHAME S. WALTON, B.V.Sc., M.R.C.V.S., Lecturer, Department of Veterinary Preventive Medicine, University of Liverpool Faculty of Veterinary Science, Liverpool, England.

A. D. J. WATSON, B.V. Sc., M.R.C.V.S., Ph.D., Lecturer in Veterinary Medicine, Department of Veterinary Clinical Studies, University of Sydney, New South Wales, Australia.

R. E. WERDIN, D.V.M., Ph.D., Associate Professor, College of Veterinary Medicine, University of Minnesota, St. Paul, Minnesota.

ERIC BRIAN WHEELDON, B.V.M.S., Ph.D., M.R.C.V.S., Research Fellow, University of Glasgow Veterinary School, Glasgow, Scotland.

ROBERT JOHN WILKINS, B.V.Sc., Dip. V.P., Staff Clinical Pathologist, The Animal Medical Center, New York, New York.

GEORGE T. WILKINSON, M.V.Sc., M.R.C.V.S., M.A.C.V.Sc., Senior Lecturer in Veterinary Medicine, Department of Veterinary Medicine, University of Queensland Veterinary School; Queensland University Small Animal Clinic and Hospital, St. Lucia, Brisbane, Australia.

JEFFREY F. WILLIAMS, B.V.Sc., Ph.D., M.R.C.V.S., Associate Professor, Department of Microbiology and Public Health, Michigan State University, East Lansing, Michigan.

JAMES W. WILSON, D.V.M., M.S., Department of Orthopedic Surgery, University of Arkansas Medical Center, Little Rock, Arkansas.

WILLIAM GERALD WINKLER, D.V.M., M.S., Chief Viral Zoonoses Section, Center for Disease Control, U.S. Public Health Service, Atlanta, Georgia.

GARY L. WOOD, D.V.M., Clinician, Animal Heart Clinic, Portland, Oregon.

SHARON G. YASKULSKI, D.V.M., Resident in Dermatology, Veterinary Medical Teaching Hospital, University of California, Davis, California.

JAMES F. ZIMMER, D.V.M., Postdoctoral Fellow in Comparative Gastroenterology, New York State College of Veterinary Medicine, Cornell University, Ithaca, New York.

BERNARD C. ZOOK, D.V.M., Diplomate, American College of Veterinary Pathologists, Associate Professor of Pathology, George Washington University School of Medicine and Health Sciences, Washington, D.C.; Research Associate, Smithsonian Institution, Washington, D.C.

# PREFACE

As the earlier editions, this sixth issue of Current Veterinary Therapy is a genuine cooperative effort of many people in our profession. The sincere and dedicated interest of each of these people is combined to present here the most advanced treatment principles now in use. The methods detailed are proven by the contributors and approved by the editors. All sections have been thoroughly revised. However, new consulting editors have organized the respiratory, dermatologic, endocrine, genitourinary and infectious disease sections, therefore new contributors and new approaches are especially prominent in those areas. The articles in the section on dietary therapy that appeared in the last edition have been dispersed throughout the text, so that nutrition is discussed along with appropriate disease entities.

The book contains new emphasis on immunologic disorders. Articles on radiographic interpretation are now included, and, in keeping with the times, the dosage and numerical data have been converted to the metric system.

The number of contributors from other countries continues to increase, and we welcome this exchange of knowledge as essential to worldwide continuing education of veterinarians.

We appreciate the profession's continued interest in Current Veterinary Therapy—it supports our belief that this is a worthwhile project. As always, we welcome constructive criticism and new suggestions for the next edition.

And last, but not least, to the W. B. Saunders Company's most cooperative staff—a hearty thank-you for making our message clear.

*Ithaca, N.Y.*                                                    ROBERT W. KIRK

# CONTENTS

SECTION

# 1

## SPECIAL THERAPY

Robert W. Kirk
*Consulting Editor*

# SECTION
# 2
# CHEMICAL AND PHYSICAL DISORDERS
Frederick W. Oehme
*Consulting Editor*

SECTION

# 3

## RESPIRATORY DISEASES

N. Edward Robinson
*Consulting Editor*

SECTION

# 4

# CARDIOVASCULAR DISEASES

Stephen J. Ettinger
*Consulting Editor*

SECTION

# 5

# HEMOLYMPHATIC DISORDERS
# AND ONCOLOGY

Jack E. Hathaway
*Consulting Editor*

SECTION

# 6

## DERMATOLOGIC DISEASES

Richard E. W. Halliwell
*Consulting Editor*

SECTION
# 7

## DISEASES OF THE EYE
Stephen I. Bistner
*Consulting Editor*

SECTION

# 8

# DISEASES OF CAGED BIRDS AND EXOTIC PETS

Fredric L. Frye
*Consulting Editor*

SECTION

# 9

## NEUROMUSCULAR DISORDERS

Alexander de Lahunta
*Consulting Editor*

SECTION

# 10

## DISEASES OF THE GASTROINTESTINAL SYSTEM

Peter Theran
*Consulting Editor*

SECTION

# 11

# METABOLIC DISORDERS
Ad Rijnberk
*Consulting Editor*

SECTION
# 12
## GENITOURINARY DISORDERS
Carl A. Osborne
*Consulting Editor*

### THE KIDNEYS

## UPPER AND LOWER URINARY TRACT

## GENITAL SYSTEM

SECTION

# 13

## INFECTIOUS DISEASES

Fredric W. Scott
*Consulting Editor*

# APPENDICES
Robert W. Kirk
*Consulting Editor*

# NOTICE

Extraordinary efforts have been made by the authors, the editors and the publisher of this book to insure that dosage recommendations are precise and in agreement with standards officially accepted at the time of publication.

It does happen, however, that dosage schedules are changed from time to time in the light of accumulating clinical experience and continuing laboratory studies. This is most likely to occur in the case of recently introduced products.

It is urged, therefore, that you check the manufacturer's recommendations for dosage, especially if the drug to be administered or prescribed is one that you use only infrequently or have not used for some time.

In addition, some drugs mentioned have been used by the authors as experimental drugs. Others have been used after official clearance for use in one species but not in others described here. This is particularly true for rare and exotic species. In these cases the authors have reported on their own considerable experience, but readers are urged to view the recommendations with discretion and precaution.

THE EDITORS

# Section

# 1

# SPECIAL THERAPY

ROBERT W. KIRK, D.V.M.
*Consulting Editor*

# FLUID THERAPY

DELMAR R. FINCO, D.V.M.
*Athens, Georgia*

Fluid therapy is a routine procedure in small animal practice. Administration of parenteral fluids has undoubtedly saved the lives of countless patients, and its value is apparent. However, perspective should be retained regarding the role of fluid therapy in the management of the patient. The clinician should constantly remind himself that fluid therapy is a form of symptomatic or supportive therapy. Once life-saving supportive procedures have been initiated, a more significant aspect of care of the patient involves establishing an etiologic diagnosis and reversing the underlying cause of disease.

Administration of parenteral fluids frequently is performed when it is unnecessary. Except in instances where rapid restoration of circulatory volume is required (shock, severe dehydration), rapid systemic distribution of a material is desired, or oral ingestion of material is contraindicated (gastrointestinal disease, impending surgery), fluids, electrolyte and nutrients should be administered *per os* by force feeding, gavage or a pharyngostomy tube. The oral route of therapy has the advantages of ease of administration, economy and lack of adverse reactions to material administered. In addition, it represents the only method of providing adequate nutrients to the patient, unless prolonged intravenous infusion of hypertonic solutions is employed.

In an effort to provide an overall view of fluid therapy in this discussion, many items of significance in therapy have not been included, and generalizations have been made, to which exceptions may exist. Supplemental readings should be consulted for more detailed discussions of fluid therapy.

## EVALUATION OF THE PATIENT

When the oral route of fluid therapy is contraindicated and the decision is made to utilize parenteral routes of therapy, the clinician should evaluate the patient as thoroughly as possible in order to provide therapy that is most beneficial. Normal homeostatic mechanisms provide a degree of latitude regarding parenteral fluid therapy, inasmuch as moderate excesses of some components may be excreted by the kidney. However, if inadequate quantities of required materials are administered, the patient will suffer from a deficit in the presence of normal homeostatic mechanisms. In instances of renal dysfunction, less latitude exists for inappropriate therapy.

Three tools are utilized to evaluate the patient for therapy: history, physical examination and clinical laboratory aids. In evaluating the patient, it is desirable to make quantitative estimates of deficits or excesses so that specific quantities of material can be delivered to the patient. When quantitative data cannot be obtained, the clinician should acquire information concerning the direction of imbalance so that qualitative therapy can be initiated.

It is helpful to consider specific aspects of the therapy separately prior to synthesis of the information into an overall plan. The specific aspects of therapy that should be considered include water balance, electrolyte deficits or excesses, acid-base balance and nutritional deficits. In addition, the functional status of the kidneys should be considered, since they are significant in homeostasis.

### WATER IMBALANCE

History provides qualitative information concerning water deficit or excess but does not give quantitative information. In contrast, quantitative estimates of water deficit can be obtained by physical examination. In general, loss of water equal to 5 per cent of body weight is the minimum amount detectable by physical examination, and loss of water greater than 15 per cent of body weight is accompanied by death due to hypovolemia. The following guidelines are useful when utilizing physical examination to assess the state of hydration.

When the dog or cat is approximately 5 per cent dehydrated, the skin has a slightly doughy, inelastic consistency. This will be

3

the only clinical sign apparent at this stage of dehydration. When evaluating the state of hydration, it is advisable to avoid examination of the skin covering the cervical area, since it is present in such a quantity that it does not immediately return to a normal position even in the normal patient. With 7 per cent dehydration, skin changes are definite. Because of its inelastic nature, the skin assumes the position to which it is pulled. At this stage of dehydration, the globe of the eye is slightly depressed in the skull. When dehydration is 10 to 12 per cent of body weight, the preceding signs are more severe. Shock may be present in debilitated animals and involuntary muscle twitching may be present. Dryness of the oral mucosa may be present. At 12 to 15 per cent dehydration, shock is marked and death is imminent.

Accurate determination of body weight may also be used to estimate alterations in body content of water. If caloric intake is adequate, alterations in body weight are due solely to changes in water content. If anorexia is present and calories are not administered, weight loss of 0.1 to 0.3 kg./day/1000 calories of daily requirement can be anticipated because of tissue catabolism. Additional weight loss should be attributed to water loss.

Clinical laboratory aids that are helpful in assessing the degree of dehydration include packed cell volume (PCV) and total plasma solids (TS) determinations. Since values for PCV and TS depend upon the ratio of solids (cells, protein) to water, it is apparent that the value obtained may reflect variation in either component. For example, a PCV in an anemic patient may be in the normal range if the patient is dehydrated, because of proportionate decrease in both solids and water. To decrease the probability of errors in interpretation, the clinician should perform both the PCV and the TS to aid in assessing the state of hydration. The chance of abnormalities in both the cell mass and total protein mass is far less than the chance of alteration in but one of the two. Values obtained from PCV and TS are used to confirm or adjust clinical estimates of dehydration rather than for specific calculations of per cent dehydration. Once therapy has been instituted, TS and PCV may be valuable in reassessing the state of hydration of the patient.

## ELECTROLYTE DEFICITS AND EXCESSES

Quantitative data concerning electrolyte deficits and excesses are difficult to obtain except in instances when serum concentration is the critical factor. For this reason, the clinician frequently must plan therapy on the basis of qualitative data. History provides good qualitative data, since electrolyte deviations have been documented for common abnormalities such as vomiting, diarrhea, renal failure and anorexia, as well as for some specific diseases.

Usually very little qualitative or quantitative information concerning electrolyte deviation can be obtained from physical examination. Exceptions are severe hypokalemia, which is characterized by severe muscle weakness, and hypocalcemia, which is characterized by neuromuscular irritation.

Laboratory determination of serum concentration of electrolytes provides valuable information when concentration of the electrolyte is critical, but may give no information when data concerning body content of the electrolyte are desired. For example, congestive heart failure may be associated with sodium retention, but serum concentration of sodium is normal because of concomitant water retention. In all instances in which serum concentration of an electrolyte is interpreted, the state of hydration of the patient should be considered. Another limitation of determinations of extracellular serum concentration of an electrolyte is that the value obtained may not accurately reflect changes in the intracellular content of ions. This limitation is particularly significant in the case of potassium because of its high intracellular and low extracellular concentration.

In summary, the information obtained from the history provides information which indicates the potential direction of electrolyte deviations. Physical examination gives information in only exceptional cases, and serum electrolyte concentration requires interpretation based on restrictions regarding state of hydration of the patient.

## ACID-BASE BALANCE

Qualitative information concerning acid-base deviations can be obtained from the history inasmuch as deviations that occur in association with common clinical signs are known. Physical examination is a poor method of evaluating acid-base status, because a poor correlation is found between clinical signs and quantitative laboratory determinations of acid-base status. Evaluation of acid-base status by physical examination is limited to suspecting respiratory acidosis or alkalosis on the basis of dyspnea or polypnea, or suspecting compensation for metabolic acidosis because of polypnea. Unfortunately, clinical evidence of dyspnea or polypnea is frequently not associated with acid-base deviations, nor is their absence a reliable indication of the absence of acid-base alterations.

Laboratory evaluation of acid-base status may vary from simple procedures such as determination of urine pH to determination of blood pH and blood gases with sophisticated equipment. A commercial kit* is available for estimation of plasma bicarbonate content. It is inexpensive and accurate if attention is paid to procedural detail. Although an electrical mixer is recommended by the manufacturer, vigorous hand shaking gives accurate results. With this kit, bicarbonate determinations can be made in any veterinary practice.

Urine pH may indicate efforts by the kidneys to secrete acid. A urine pH below 5.0 suggests a larger excretion of acid, and may be observed in patients with acidosis. A urine pH above 8.0 suggests a decreased acid excretion, and may be observed in patients with alkalosis. Urinary tract infection and diet may affect urine pH, and these factors should be considered in evaluating the data. Urine pH cannot be used to evaluate acid-base balance in the vomiting dog, because of the paradox of alkalosis and aciduria.

Whereas urine pH may give qualitative data concerning acid-base balance, determination of blood pH and $pCO_2$ or bicarbonate gives quantitative data. Determination of bicarbonate concentration alone provides data that can be useful in quantitative therapy, but the clinician must be sure that he is treating metabolic acidosis rather than compensated respiratory alkalosis.

*Harleco $CO_2$ Apparatus Set. Harleco Division, American Hospital Supply Corporation, Philadelphia, Pennsylvania, 19143.

## NUTRITION

Patients that require parenteral fluid therapy are frequently in a state of nutritional deficiency, but the specific number of calories or grams of protein that must be replaced is not readily detectable from history, physical examination or clinical laboratory procedures. Although existing nutritional deficiencies may be difficult to evaluate, data are available to guide in providing maintenance requirements for calories (Fig. 1).

## RENAL FUNCTION

A normal blood urea nitrogen (BUN) and the ability to concentrate urine provide evidence of adequate homeostatic functions with regard to water, electrolytes and acid-base balance, except in instances of rare renal diseases with unique patterns of dysfunction. In the dehydrated patient, it is common to detect a mild azotemia due to poor perfusion of the kidneys with blood. Azotemia secondary to dehydration is accompanied by production of urine with high specific gravity, and the BUN returns to normal within 72 hours if the patient is adequately hydrated.

Once the status of the patient has been evaluated with regard to water, electrolytes, acid-base balance, nutrition and renal function, the information is integrated into an overall plan of therapy, with the quantity and type of fluids administered being chosen on the basis of the estimates made.

## PHASES OF THERAPY

After evaluation of the patient as previously described, deficits or excesses that exist at the time of initial examination are treated. This therapy is referred to as the phase of repair of deficits or excesses.

Consideration must also be given to maintenance therapy if normal food and water intake is not immediately resumed. Figure 1 provides information regarding daily requirements for calories, water and electrolytes in the hospitalized dog and cat. Data in Figure 1 are used to estimate maintenance requirements, and fluids are administered to supply these requirements until oral alimentation resumes.

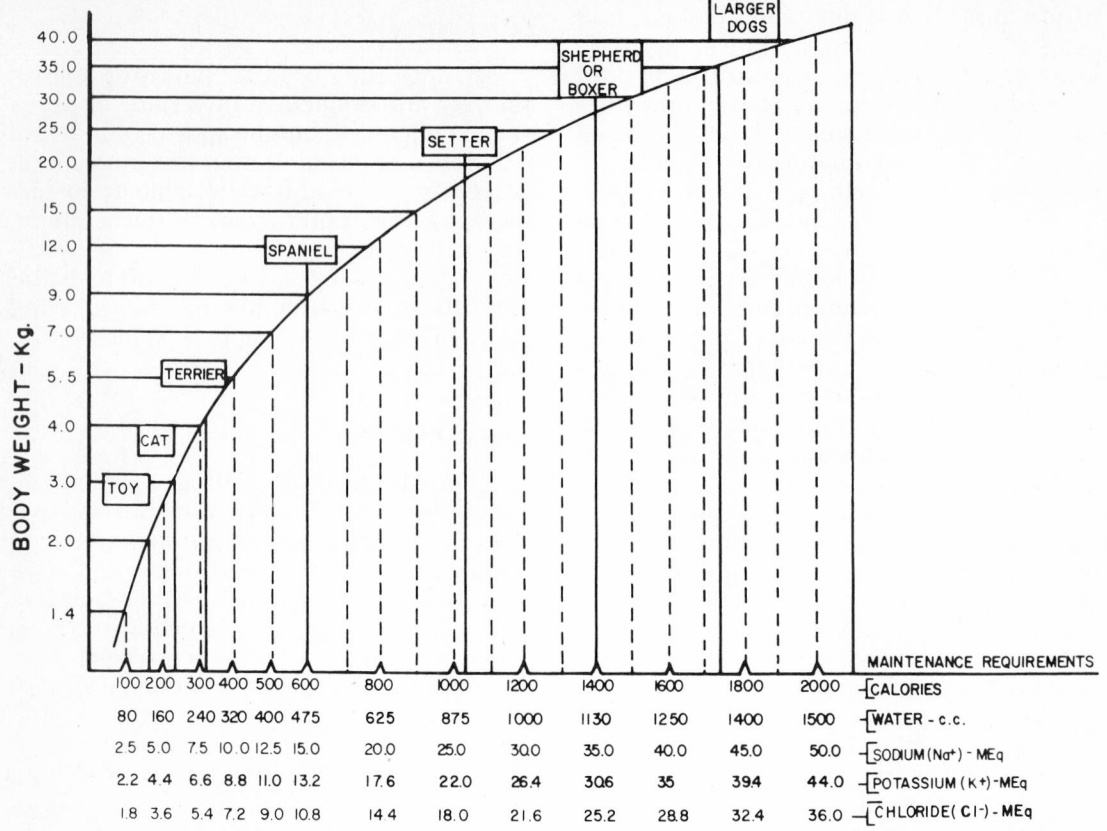

**Figure 1.** Maintenance requirements of calories, water and electrolytes of caged dogs and cats. (Modified from Harrison, J. B., Sussman, H. H., and Pickering, D. E.: Fluid and electrolyte therapy in small animals. J. Am. Vet. Med. Assn., 37:637–645, 1960.)

If the patient continues to lose body fluids in excess of normal by vomiting, diarrhea or other abnormal means, additional fluids must be administered to replace these losses. This phase of therapy is called contemporary loss therapy. The quantity of loss is estimated by visual inspection, and the composition of the abnormal loss dictates the choice of fluid for therapy.

In instances other than shock, deficit repair is completed by giving increments of fluid over the initial 24 hours, so that subsequently only maintenance and contemporary loss therapy are required. The patient is closely evaluated during and at the conclusion of deficit therapy, and adjustments in therapy are made if estimates appear erroneous.

## SPECIFIC THERAPEUTIC GOALS

### NUTRITIONAL THERAPY–CALORIES

Glucose and fructose provide approximately 4 cal. and ethanol provides about 5.6 cal/gm. These substances are most fre-

quently utilized for caloric therapy in the United States, since high caloric density parenteral lipid preparations are not available.

Although it is possible to fulfill caloric requirements with these solutions, constant infusion for over 15 hours per day is required if spillover of sugars in the urine is to be avoided. If 5 per cent dextrose is used, over 6 liters must be administered each 24 hours to fulfill maintenance requirements for a 22-kg. dog. From these figures, it should be apparent that the quantities of 5 per cent dextrose commonly administered provide but a small percentage of the caloric requirements of the dog and cat. Hypertonic solutions of dextrose (20 to 25 per cent) have been administered by slow intravenous drip via a jugular catheter in order to provide adequate calories. Although the quantity of fluid that must be administered is decreased, prolonged periods of infusion are still required.

The necessity for long-term intravenous therapy with sugars in order to fulfill caloric requirements emphasizes the desirability of providing calories *per os* whenever feasible. If parenteral therapy is the only alternative, the number of calories provided should be compared with the caloric requirements in order to retain a realistic perspective of the efficacy of the therapy provided.

## NUTRITIONAL THERAPY—AMINO ACIDS

Emaciated patients are in a negative state of nitrogen balance, and therapy with amino acids is frequently indicated. However, studies indicate that it is futile to attempt to induce positive nitrogen balance unless maintenance requirements of calories are provided. Trials in man have indicated that commercial amino acid solutions that contain 5 or 10 per cent dextrose are inadequate to promote positive nitrogen balances, because of inadequate caloric content in proportion to amino acid content.

An additional factor to consider is the low amino acid content of parenteral solutions sold by some manufacturers of veterinary products. Fortified casein or fibrin hydrolysates (Amigen®, Aminosol®) of 5 or 10 per cent concentration are adequate, since daily amino acid requirements may be fulfilled for an average-sized dog by administration of about 400 ml. of the 5 per cent solution. Some veterinary products (Ambex®, Amoplex®) contain less than 300 mg./liter of amino acids, and about 50 liters of these solutions would be required to fulfill amino acid requirements.

## PARENTERAL HYPERALIMENTATION

The term parenteral hyperalimentation has been coined to describe the technique used to induce weight gain and a positive nitrogen balance solely by long-term parenteral administration of solutions. This technique has received considerable attention in human medicine, because of reports of dramatic results obtained in cachectic patients who failed to respond to more conventional forms of fluid therapy. The procedure is indicated in those patients who are unable to eat or in whom a malfunctioning gastrointestinal tract prevents adequate absorption of nutrients. It has been used in many cases, including pediatric patients with a variety of gastrointestinal diseases, malabsorption diseases, acute renal failure,

intestinal fistulas and postoperative patients in whom oral alimentation cannot be used.

The procedure conducted in man uses 50 per cent glucose as the sole source of calories, and hydrolyzed protein as a source of amino acids. Proportionately, more amino acids are administered to pediatric patients than to adults to provide for more protein synthesis for growth. Vitamins, electrolytes and trace minerals are also administered. All components except the vitamins and trace minerals are mixed together and administered simultaneously. A concentrated solution of glucose is used in order to provide adequate calories in a smaller quantity of fluid. Because glucose at a concentration greater than 10 per cent may cause thrombophlebitis, the solution must be injected through catheters placed in large veins so that mixing of the solution with large quantities of blood may occur. To prevent hyperglycemia and hyperosmolality, the solution must be injected slowly at a constant rate 24 hours per day. Solutions are frequently administered, using a constant infusion pump, to insure accurate and constant administration. Sepsis may occur because of contamination of catheters during or after catheterization. Special laminar flow mixing hoods and bacterial filters in the fluid lines are used in an attempt to avoid sepsis. The patient is closely monitored for evidence of septicemia. Infection with bacteria and with *Candida sp.* have been reported in man.

Techniques used for parenteral hyperalimentation were applied to experimental dogs prior to their use in man. In 1949, adult dogs were infused with 50 per cent glucose and amino acid or protein preparations for up to 141 days with only electrolytes, water and vitamins given orally. Fluids were administered through catheters placed in the precava via the jugular vein. In some instances, swelling and edema of the neck and fever were noted, suggesting sepsis. Autopsy of some dogs revealed pleural effusion and thickening of the wall of the precava. Complete intravenous alimentation in adult dogs has been accomplished for 10 weeks, using fats as the predominant source of calories, and casein hydrolysate as the source of amino acids. In this experiment, dogs were given 2.25 gm. of glucose, 2.25 gm. of casein hydrolysate, 6.0 gm. of fat (soybean oil meal emulsion) and 4.7 gm. of water/kg. of body weight per day. This supplied 78 cal./kg./day.

In another study, pups were fed solely by the intravenous route from the 12th to 42nd weeks of life. They grew and developed at the same rate as littermates that were fed orally. Glucose was used as the parenteral source of calories in this study.

At the University of Georgia, these techniques have been adapted for use on clinical patients for periods up to one week. Ten per cent amino acid hydrolysate is commercially available with 500 ml. in a 1-liter bottle. Five hundred ml. of 50 per cent dextrose is aseptically transferred to the amino acid hydrolysate, giving a solution with 1 calorie per ml. for energy. Daily caloric needs are estimated from Figure 1; the number of milliliters required by the patient daily is equal to the number of calories required. The total daily requirements are administered at a constant rate over 16 hours of the day. A pediatric drop infusion set* is used to control flow rate. Only jugular veins are used for administration of the fluid to insure mixing of the hypertonic solution with large quantities of blood. Strict attention is given to all aspects of the procedure in order to avoid sepsis. Body temperature is determined twice daily, and a WBC count is performed if pyrexia occurs. The jugular catheter is removed and antibiotic therapy is initiated if leukocytosis and persistent pyrexia occur. State of hydration is monitored and additional isotonic fluids are given by subcutaneous injection if needed.

## POTASSIUM THERAPY

Most fluids used for parenteral therapy have a composition similar to that of extracellular water. Abnormalities that lead to dehydration may be associated with a loss of large quantities of potassium from the body. Frequently, the loss of potassium is equal to the loss of sodium. The rationale underlying a decision not to administer parenteral fluids that replace the potassium deficit is based on the following:

1. The knowledge that a degree of potassium deficit can exist in the patient without obvious deleterious effects.

2. The assumption that fluid therapy will be necessary for only a short interval of time (a few days), and deficits will be replaced by voluntary oral alimentation.

3. The knowledge that administration of potassium by the parenteral route must be conducted at a slow rate and with close surveillance of the patient to avoid hyperkalemia and cardiotoxicity.

If prolonged fluid therapy or a large loss of potassium occurs, therapy with potassium is indicated. The following generalizations may aid in establishing when therapy with potassium should be initiated.

1. The physical condition of the patient: If signs of hypokalemia develop, therapy is indicated.

2. Serum potassium concentration: Values below 2.5 mEq./liter in the patient that is normally hydrated are an indication for potassium therapy.

3. Prolonged support solely with parenteral fluids: If therapy exceeds five days in duration, and potassium *per os* is not provided, parenteral potassium therapy may be indicated.

4. Documentation of severe potassium loss.

Whenever feasible, oral administration of potassium should be used, since the risk of inducing hyperkalemia is minimized. Liquids and tablets containing potassium (Kaon®) are commercially available. When the oral route is available for potassium preparations, it is usually available for gavage. When gavage is performed with commercial foods, addition of potassium is unnecessary, since the potassium content of the food is adequate. If high calorie-low electrolyte concentrates are used for gavage, potassium can be added to these products.

Parenteral administration should be used in instances in which oral administration of potassium is not possible. To avoid hyperkalemia, it is recommended that potassium be administered intravenously at a rate not to exceed 0.5 mEq./kg. of body weight per hour. The subcutaneous route may also be used. Solutions containing 35 mEq./liter of potassium have been administered subcutaneously without signs of local irritation or systemic toxicity.

The quantity of potassium required in instances of deficit cannot be readily established even if plasma concentration is known, since plasma potassium concentration may not be directly related to the magnitude of the intracellular deficit. It is recommended that fluids containing 35 mEq./liter of potassium be used to fulfill deficit and maintenance requirements. The patient

---

*Baxter Laboratories, No. 2COO2, Morton Grove, Illinois.

should be reevaluated at intervals for evidence of response, and dosage adjusted accordingly.

## THERAPY OF ACID-BASE ABNORMALITIES

Most abnormalities in hydrogen ion balance result in acidosis. Severe diarrhea, uremia and diabetes mellitus are common examples of abnormalities in which metabolic acidosis may occur. Although less common, alkalosis may be encountered in the dog and cat. Profuse vomiting is the most common cause.

When metabolic acidosis is suspected or known to be present, a commitment must be made concerning the quantity of alkali to administer to the patient. Knowledge that the primary disease is associated with metabolic acidosis, and assessment of the severity of the primary disease may be used on the assumption that a parallel exists between the severity of the disease and the severity of the acidosis. Table 1 provides guidelines for therapy based on this assumption. Although the validity of this assumption is questionable, it is probable that far more patients will be helped than harmed by the use of this formula.

Urine pH can be used to evaluate efficacy of therapy. If inadequate quantities of alkali are given to the patient with metabolic acidosis, urine pH will remain acid. If excessive amounts of alkali are provided, urine pH will become alkaline.

If it is known that metabolic acidosis exists and if plasma bicarbonate concentration is known, the total bicarbonate deficit can be estimated from the following formula:

Total deficit (mEq.) = body weight (kg.) $\times$ 0.6 $\times$ (25 − plasma bicarbonate [mEq./liter]).

For example, a 10-kg. dog with plasma bicarbonate concentration of 14 mEq./liter would require 66 mEq. of bicarbonate according to the following calculations:

$$10 \times 0.6 \times (25 - 14) = 66 \text{ mEq.}$$

A decrease in plasma bicarbonate concentration may occur as a compensatory mechanism for respiratory alkalosis. In respiratory alkalosis, therapy with alkali is contraindicated. For this reason, it is important that the clinician differentiate between a

*Table 1. Estimation of Bicarbonate Deficit in Patients with Metabolic Acidosis*

| SEVERITY OF SIGNS | ESTIMATED BICARBONATE DEFICIT (mEq./liter) | BICARBONATE REQUIRED TO ALLEVIATE THE DEFICIT (mEq./kg.) |
|---|---|---|
| Mild | 5 | 3 |
| Moderate | 10 | 6 |
| Severe | 15 | 9 |

respiratory and a metabolic disorder prior to therapy. This may be done by accumulating information regarding the disease or determination of blood pH, in addition to plasma bicarbonate concentration.

Solutions that may be used for therapy of acidosis include bicarbonate, acetate and lactate. Milliequivalents of each are equal in alkalinizing potency, but the latter two must be metabolized for this activity. Contrary to popular belief, sodium lactate administration does not accentuate the acidosis associated with shock or diabetes mellitus, but it may be less effective in reversing acidosis if metabolism of lactate is impaired.

Therapy for metabolic acidosis should be administered in increments over a 24- to 48-hour period in order to avoid complications associated with rapid changes in blood pH. Administering the agent in increments also provides the clinician with the opportunity to evaluate the response to therapy and to alter dosage if the original estimate was inaccurate.

Although commercial acidifying solutions containing ammonium chloride are available for treatment of metabolic alkalosis, such solutions should be used with caution in order to avoid inducing acidosis. The alkalosis of vomiting can be adequately treated with Ringer's solution, and so more potent acidifying solutions are unnecessary.

## TRENDS OF IMBALANCES IN COMMON ABNORMALITIES

Each patient must be considered on an individual basis when planning fluid therapy. The presence or degree of fluid, electrolyte and acid-base alterations is dependent on a multiplicity of factors includ-

*Table 2. Water, Electrolyte and Acid-Base Alterations in Common Abnormalities of the Dog and Cat* *

| SIGN OR DISEASE | WATER BALANCE | ELECTROLYTE BALANCE | ACID-BASE BALANCE |
|---|---|---|---|
| Vomiting | Negative—intake lost, gastric secretions lost | Loss of large quantities of sodium and chloride in vomit; loss of potassium in vomit and in urine | Tendency toward alkalosis; serum bicarbonate and blood $pCO_2$ may be increased |
| Diarrhea | Negative—loss in feces | Loss of large quantities of sodium, potassium and chloride in feces | Tendency toward acidosis due to loss of bicarbonate in feces |
| Polyuria and renal failure | Negative balance in instances of polyuria without concomitant intake | Loss of sodium, potassium and chloride in urine; serum potassium concentration usually normal | Tendency toward acidosis due to impaired ability of kidneys to excrete hydrogen ions; serum bicarbonate concentration decreased |
| Anuria and renal failure | Small negative balance may be present but positive balance may be iatrogenically induced | Electrolyte balance variable; serum potassium concentration usually increased | Same as polyuria, renal failure |
| Anorexia | Negative due to lack of intake | Negative balance of all ions, but serum concentration may be increased because of proportionately more water loss | Tendency toward mild acidosis due to tissue catabolism |
| Congestive heart failure | Positive associated with sodium retention | Positive sodium, chloride balance but normal serum concentration; potassium balance equivocal | No alteration unless complicated by other factors |
| Diabetes mellitus | Negative—polyuria, sometimes vomiting, lack of intake | Normokalemia to slight hyperkalemia, but potential for hypokalemia with insulin therapy; probably negative sodium, chloride balance | Tendency toward acidosis; may be severe |

*Presence of abnormalities is dependent on duration and severity of signs or disease; evaluation of the individual patient should be conducted.

ing type of abnormality, duration and severity of the abnormality, body size of the pet, presence or absence of oral alimentation and state of renal function. Table 2 summarizes the trends in common abnormalities in the dog and cat.

## INTEGRATION OF DATA INTO A PLAN OF THERAPY

### SHORT-TERM VS. LONG-TERM THERAPY

If it is anticipated that therapy will be of only a few days' duration because of correction of the underlying problem, it is preferable to direct attention toward rehydrating the patient with fluids with a composition similar to that of extracellular water. Lactated Ringer's solution is satisfactory for use in such circumstances in all conditions in which acidosis is likely. Additional alkalinizing solutions may be required if acidosis is severe. Ringer's solution is indicated in instances of vomiting. If sodium excess is present but water is needed, 5 per cent dextrose may be used as an isotonic vehicle for administration of water. With acute imbalances in which short-term therapy is anticipated, caloric requirements are ignored because of the difficulty in supplying adequate calories by the parenteral route. It is anticipated that the patient will replace the caloric deficit once oral alimentation is resumed. If parenteral therapy is prolonged, calories should be provided.

Potassium loss frequently exceeds the quantity present in parenteral fluids with extracellular fluid composition. If short-term therapy is anticipated, negative potassium balance is ignored on the assumption that deficits will be replaced once oral alimentation is resumed. If therapy is more prolonged, potassium should be provided as previously indicated.

### STEPS IN PLANNING THERAPY

In order to arrive at a logical plan of therapy, the following general steps may be utilized.

### DEFICIT THERAPY

1. Estimate water deficit (body weight × per cent dehydration). Use PCV and TS to evaluate the clinical estimate. The quantity of fluid to be given has now been established.

2. Consider electrolyte deviations and the duration of therapy. For short-term losses, choose fluids with extracellular composition (lactated Ringer's solution or Ringer's solution) or choose 5 per cent dextrose in water, if water without electrolyte is required by the patient. For long-term losses, these solutions should be supplemented with potassium.

3. Consider acid-base deviations. If metabolic acidosis is present, use lactated Ringer's solution for therapy. Addition base may be required if acidosis is severe. If metabolic alkalosis is present, use Ringer's solution for therapy.

4. Nutrition. Whenever feasible, use oral alimentation. When impossible, ignore short-term losses. With long-term losses, consider caloric maintenance therapy.

### MAINTENANCE THERAPY

1. Water and electrolytes for maintenance therapy may be administered using commercial maintenance solutions. However, these solutions are hypotonic and must be given intravenously. As an alternative, 1 part of lactated Ringer's or Ringer's solution and 2 parts of 5 per cent dextrose may be used, although this regimen will be slightly deficient in potassium.

2. Caloric therapy is ignored if therapy is anticipated for less than five days. If prolonged therapy is required, constant infusion of hypertonic dextrose via indwelling jugular catheters represents the most feasible method of parenteral caloric therapy.

### CONTEMPORARY LOSS THERAPY

Contemporary loss therapy is determined by estimating the quantity of abnormal loss (vomit, diarrhea, polyuria) and administering a quantity of fluid equal to the loss. Knowing the approximate composition of the loss, the clinician can use Ringer's or lactated Ringer's solution. Supplementation with potassium or alkalinizing solution may be indicated to more closely approximate the composition of the fluid lost.

### SUPPLEMENTAL READING

Bland, J. H.: Clinical Metabolism of Body Water and Electrolytes. Philadelphia, W. B. Saunders Co., 1963.
Creno, R. J., Farrand, J., and Koch, B.: An evaluation of

the Harleco Total Carbon Dioxide Apparatus. Am. J. Med. Tech., *40*:50–54, 1974.

Hammon, P. B.: Drugs altering the fluid balance. In Jones, L. M. (ed.): Veterinary Pharmacology and Therapeutics. Ames, Iowa, Iowa State University Press, 1965.

Harrison, J. B., Sussman, H. H., and Pickering, D. E.: Fluid and electrolyte therapy in small animals. J. Am. Vet. Med. Assn., *137*:637–645, 1960.

Numerous authors: Fluid therapy in small animal practice. J. Am. Animal Hosp. Assn., *Vol. 8*:, 1972.

Pickering, D. E., and Fisher, D. A.: Fluid and Electrolyte Therapy. Portland, Medical Research Foundation of Oregon, 1959.

Tasker, J. B.: Fluid therapy. In Kirk, R. W. (ed.): Current Veterinary Therapy IV. Philadelphia, W. B. Saunders Co., 1971.

# AEROSOL THERAPY

GARY R. BOLTON, D.V.M.
*Ithaca, N.Y.*

Inhalation therapy as a method of treating respiratory diseases of animals has been largely overlooked. In the past, its effectiveness has been controversial. Even in human medicine, where much research and clinical trials have been done, there is confusion regarding its use. It has alternately been enthusiastically hailed or condemned. The specific aims of aerosol therapy are given in Table 1, and its therapeutic indications are given in Table 2.

Provision for humidification of the respiratory mucous membranes is probably the most useful application of inhalation therapy. Drying of the respiratory mucosa causes irritation. Irritation or infection of the respiratory mucosa causes swelling, bronchial gland hypertrophy, goblet cell proliferation and loss of ciliary epithelium. These changes result in impaired drainage of secretions. The nature of the secretions causes difficulty in the treatment of bron-

**Table 2.  Therapeutic Indications for Aerosol Therapy**

*Acute respiratory diseases*
  Tracheobronchitis
  Pneumonia
  Upper respiratory diseases of cats
  Bronchiolitis
  Postoperative atelectasis and pneumonia

*Chronic respiratory diseases*
  Chronic bronchitis
  Bronchopneumonia
  Collapsed trachea (with secondary tracheobronchitis)
  Emphysema
  Bronchiectasis

*Tracheostomy care*

chopulmonary disease. They may be insufficient, as in the case of acute tracheobronchitis, or they may be excessive, thick and tenacious, or inspissated, as in the case of chronic bronchitis or mucopurulent bronchopneumonia. Addition of aerosolized water thins secretions, maintains the integrity of the mucociliary pathway, and promotes efficient bronchial drainage. An additional benefit is that of soothing the irritated respiratory epithelium and relieving discomfort.

Drugs may be added to the aerosol solution. The aerosolization of drugs has caused most of the controversy regarding the use of inhalation therapy. Drugs which have been aerosolized are antibiotics, bronchodilators, detergents, bland solutions, mucolytics, steroids, enzymes and anti-foaming agents (Table 3). Drug dosages are empirical, but they probably can be transposed from the

**Table 1.  Aims of Aerosol Therapy**

1.  Humidification of respiratory mucous membranes.

2.  Deposition of minuscule amounts of potent drugs in smaller airways to obtain optimal topical therapeutic effect with minimal systemic side effects. Example: bronchodilators.

3.  Deposition of moderate amounts of relatively potent agents, or agents that are only effective topically. Examples: antibiotics, mucolytics.

4.  Deposition of relatively large amounts of bland substances which promote bronchial drainage with minimal mucosal irritation. Examples: saline, propylene glycol, detergents, glycerin.

human literature (Miller, 1970, 1973), and some are given in the veterinary literature (Mulnix, 1971).

Bemis (1976) has used antibiotics by nebulization to reduce markedly the bacterial flora of tracheal cultures. This treatment has been effective against *Bordetella bronchiseptica* in infectious bronchitis of dogs and was accompanied by clinical improvement. Treatment consisted of nebulization twice daily for three days. A diluent of 2.5 ml. of saline was used for each treatment with any *one* of the following drugs, each of which was effective in the indicated dosage per treatment: polymyxin B, 300,000 units; kanamycin, 250 mg.; gentamicin, 50 mg.

Aerosolized antibiotics ideally should be topically effective and poorly absorbed by the respiratory mucosa to minimize their systemic effects (Table 3). The antibiotics which are well absorbed by aerosol (Table 2) probably exert their effect by attaining systemic blood levels, in which case they are more effective systemically. Antibiotic aerosols are irritating and cause bronchial swelling and constriction. For this reason, they are always used in conjunction with bronchodilators. Adequate bronchial drainage is essential for effective antibiotic therapy. Antibiotic aerosol therapy for pulmonary infections is used only when the infection has been resistant to systemic therapy, or when the antibiotic's toxic effects must minimized by using it topically.

Bronchodilators have three primary effects: (1) bronchodilator action, (2) pneumodilator (alveolar) action and (3) decongestant action. Since almost all other aerosol agents cause some irritation, with edema and bronchial constriction, the bronchodilators should be a part of all aerosol drug therapy.

Detergents, mucolytics and enzymes are used when secretions are thick, tenacious and inspissated. They are irritating and are used in combination with the bronchodilators.

Bland solutions are used in large-volume, high-density mists. They are effective in mobilizing thick tenacious secretions, and are also used in conjunction with bronchodilators.

Steroid therapy has not been conclusively shown to be effective by the aerosol route. In general, steroids are rapidly absorbed, and systemic use may be preferable.

The anti-foaming agents have been used

*Table 3.  Aerosol Drugs*

1. Antibiotics
   A. Poorly absorbed from respiratory mucosa; have good application to aerosol therapy.
      (1) Bacitracin
      (2) Neomycin
      (3) Kanamycin
      (4) Vancomycin
      (5) Gentamicin
      (6) Amphotericin B
      (7) Nystatin
      (8) Polymyxin B
   B. Well absorbed from respiratory mucosa; probably not indicated for aerosol therapy.
      (1) Penicillin
      (2) Streptomycin
      (3) Chloramphenicol
      (4) Colistimethate
      (5) Carbenecillin
      (6) Tetracycline

2. Bronchodilators
   A. Isoproterenol
   B. Phenylephrine (decongestant)*
   C. Epinephrine
   D. Xanthines (theophylline, aminophylline)

3. Detergents
   A. "Alevaire"
   B. "Tergemist"

4. Bland solutions
   A. Propylene glycol (10 to 20 per cent solution)
   B. Saline
   C. Glycerin
   D. Detergents

5. Mucolytics
   A. Acetylcysteine, "Mucomyst"

6. Steroids
   A. Dexamethasone
   B. Prednisolone

7. Enzymes
   A. Pancreatic dornase

8. Anti-foaming agents
   A. Ethyl alcohol
   B. Octyl alcohol

*Not a bronchodilator; decreases airway resistance by its decongestant effect. Phenylephrine also prolongs the action of isoproterenol and epinephrine.

in man in fulminant pulmonary edema to reduce the stable foam that fills the airways and reduces tidal flow.

Oxygen therapy is also combined with aerosol therapy. Oxygen-air mixtures are used. The use of 100 per cent oxygen is avoided, since oxygen trapped in alveoli by mucous plugs is rapidly absorbed and leads to atelectasis.

## PRINCIPLES OF AEROSOL SCIENCE

There are many variables that affect the deposition and distribution of aerosols. Particle size, particle stability, physical characteristics of the respiratory system and retention time are some of the variables.

Particle size and stability affect the distribution of the aerosol. Depending on the equipment used, aerosol particles vary from 0.5 to 40 microns in size. The large particles (>5 to 10 microns) are deposited in the upper airways. Only the smaller particles (0.5 to 5 microns) will reach the lower airways and be deposited there, and only the ultrasonic nebulizers produce particles that small. Particle stability is affected by the type of solution used. Concentrated solutions or hygroscopic solutions such as propylene glycol tend to take up water from the environment, increase in size and deposit in the upper airways. Dilute solutions tend to evaporate and become smaller, reducing the amount of mist delivered to the patient, but reaching deeper into the airway. Cool-mist aerosols evaporate upon warming and decrease in particle size, while warm-mist aerosols coalesce upon cooling, and increase in particle size.

The physical characteristics of the respiratory system affect aerosol delivery. Where the air goes, the aerosol goes. If large amounts of secretion block air flow, delivery of the aerosol will be impeded. Contours of the anatomy which deflect the flow of the aerosol cause premature deposition of particles. This is particularly true in animals who normally breathe primarily through their nose. This makes it more difficult to get particles into the lower respiratory tract.

Retention time of the aerosol can be increased by depositing small particles low in the airways, or by using special breathing exercises. Since an animal will not exhale, then inhale and hold it, veterinarians must count on particle distribution.

When heated aerosol mists are used, overheating of the animal must be avoided to prevent heat prostration, since the patient usually is placed in a small sealed area while being treated. The use of unheated-mist nebulizers avoids this problem.

## EQUIPMENT AND PROCEDURES

Equipment available for use includes steam vaporizers, cool-mist vaporizers, jet nebulizers and ultrasonic nebulizers. The nebulizers can be heated or not heated, and can be used with intermittent positive pressure ventilation. Steam vaporizers and heated nebulizers have the problem of possibly overheating the animal. Cool-mist vaporizers generally do not produce enough mist to be effective. The ultrasonic nebulizer produces large amounts of mist of small particle size, and are so effective in hydrating the animal that overhydration is a possibility. When using an ultrasonic nebulizer, low flow rates are used, and the animal is weighed to assess the amount of hydration achieved. Some nebulizers available are manufactured by Ohio, DeVilbiss and Croupette. Sterilization of equipment is important. Nebulizers must be cleaned daily. One per cent acetic acid should be nebulized for 10 to 15 minutes each day, followed by water as a cleansing procedure.

Several methods are used for aerosol therapy in small animals. Sophisticated equipment is not essential. There are two methods which can be employed for home use. The easiest method is the use of the bathroom shower. The animal is placed in the bathroom with the door closed and the hot shower running. Care is taken to avoid chilling after each treatment. This method provides adequate humidification, but drugs cannot be given this way, and the animal must be checked periodically for overheating. Steam vaporizers can also be used at home by placing the animal and the vaporizer in a small closed room. Humidification of the upper airway is adequate and drugs can be added to the solution, but the effectiveness of drug therapy is questionable with this method. Overheating is also a possibility, and one must be concerned lest the animal chew the electric cord or tip over the vaporizer.

Animals who require intensive therapy should be hospitalized for treatment. For humidification, nebulization of water into a sealed cage is adequate. Provision for cooling must be available if the mist is heated. When drugs are aerosolized, the best method employs a face mask attached to the nebulizer. This way, a known amount of drug can be given. This method requires training the animal and that can be a problem. Animals that have temporary or indwelling tracheal cannulas can be nebulized using intermittent positive pressure ventilation. This is a very efficient method, but is not practical for routine treatment.

Inhalation therapy may be continuous if the condition is severe, or given intermittently two to six times daily for 15 minutes each time. When the ultrasonic nebulizer is used for continuous administration, the animal should be weighed periodically to avoid overhydration.

Adjunctive physical therapy can increase the benefits of inhalation therapy. Mild exercise or thoracic percussion following nebulization encourages the dislodging of secretions and promotes bronchial drainage. Postural bronchial drainage may be helpful. This involves placing the animal in various positions to take advantage of gravity-flow of secretions.

## CONCLUSIONS

The use of aerosol therapy in animals has excellent therapeutic potential. Results are encouraging, but much must be learned. More clinical studies are needed in the areas of administration methods and drug dosages or concentrations. The information available needs to be organized, and a logical basis for achieving therapeutic objectives must be established.

### SUPPLEMENTAL READING

Bemis, D.: Personal communication, 1976.
Miller, W. F.: Antibiotic Aerosols. *In* Kagan, B. M. (ed.): Antimicrobial Therapy. Philadelphia, W. B. Saunders Co., 1970.
Miller, W. F.: Aerosol therapy in acute and chronic respiratory disease. Arch. Intern. Med., *131*:148–155, 1973.
Mulnix, J. A.: Aerosol Therapy. *In* Kirk, R. W. (ed.): Current Veterinary Therapy IV. Philadelphia, W. B. Saunders Co., 1971.
Ruf, J. W.: Kennel cough: aerosol detergent therapy. Mod. Vet. Pract., *39*:133, 1958.

# ANTIMICROBIAL THERAPY

A. D. J. WATSON, B.V.Sc.
*Sydney, Australia*

The availability of numerous effective and inexpensive antimicrobial drugs has been of considerable value to veterinarians engaged in small animal practice. Unfortunately, it has also led to the widespread use of these agents in many unwarranted situations. The aim of treatment with antimicrobial agents is to kill or inhibit the growth of pathogenic microbes in infected animals. The use of these drugs in other situations is contraindicated because it unnecessarily exposes the patient to possible toxic reactions and increases costs to the client. In addition, it may tend to increase the prevalence of resistant organisms.

## THERAPEUTIC USE

Systemic antimicrobial therapy should be considered only when there is firm evidence of an infection of a *nontrivial* nature in the patient. Antimicrobial agents should never be used as antipyretics, placebos or substitutes for diagnosis: such "therapy" is usually ineffective and may further delay more specific diagnosis and curative treatment.

## CHEMOPROPHYLAXIS

Prophylactic administration of antimicrobial drugs may sometimes be considered for patients in which normal defense mechanisms have been severely compromised either by preexisting disease (severe malnutrition or metabolic disorders, specific immunodeficiency states, viral infections, functional urinary tract abnormalities) or as a result of therapy with corticosteroids, antimetabolites or cytotoxic agents. However, the use of antimicrobial drugs prophylactically in these situations should be considered carefully. In some instances it could be deleterious to the patient, as resistant pathogens selected by the drugs might multiply unchecked, resulting in potentially fatal infections. It may be better to avoid routine chemoprophylaxis in immunoparetic individuals, but to watch carefully for development of infection and to treat promptly if it occurs.

Whether routine prophylaxis with systemic antimicrobial agents can be justified in small animals undergoing surgery is questionable. It is probably unwarranted in simple operations involving little risk of sepsis but may be advisable for patients with lowered resistance to infection, extensive tissue trauma or gross soiling of the wound. Studies in humans have indicated that bacteria implanted in wounds at surgery can be effectively destroyed by maintaining adequate systemic levels of a bactericidal drug for the duration of surgery and for a few hours after it (Garrod *et al.*, 1973). A suitable regimen for this purpose would require administration of the chosen drug intravenously at anesthetic induction, or intramuscularly one hour beforehand, and repeat administration by the same route at 3-hourly intervals during surgery (Aronson, 1975). A short course of this type would minimize any selective effect of antimicrobial therapy on the patient's normal flora. However, it would not prevent wound infections acquired from a contaminated postoperative environment: the need for additional treatment to prevent these should be assessed in each case.

## SELECTION OF DRUGS LIKELY TO BE EFFECTIVE AGAINST THE PATHOGEN

The major requirement in selecting an antimicrobial drug is that the offending organism be susceptible to its action. A rational choice presupposes recognition of the organ or system involved and identification of the etiologic agent. Determination of susceptibility of the pathogen to antimicrobial drugs *in vitro* is an optional, further step in the process.

The selection procedure requires both clinical judgment and thought. Some clinicians seek to avoid both by using broad-spectrum antimicrobial agents routinely, in the belief that these will have some activity against most pathogens. This approach is unsatisfactory because width of spectrum does not correlate with efficacy: for example, the broad-spectrum agents chloramphenicol and tetracycline are generally less active than penicillin G against gram-positive organisms. Furthermore, broad-spectrum agents may be more likely to upset the patient's normal flora. *Habitual use of a drug merely because of the width of its spectrum implies a low standard of diagnosis on the part of the clinician.*

### DIAGNOSIS

The first prerequisite for drug selection is a clinical diagnosis based on an understanding of the nature of the disease process. This may or may not imply that the cause is a particular microorganism.

Identification of the causal organism is important because chemotherapy, to be effective, must be aimed against the pathogen rather than against the disease. Sometimes the clinical picture is sufficiently characteristic to incriminate a particular microorganism as the cause: for example, a clinical diagnosis of tetanus immediately implies *Clostridium tetani* infection. However, in many syndromes the etiologic diagnosis is more difficult to establish because the cause may be any of a number of different organisms, as in bacterial pneumonia or cystitis. When confronted by infections with specific organ or tissue involvement, knowledge of the pathogens most commonly causing infections in those sites can be most helpful (Table 1).

In some instances, further information on the nature of the causal organism can be obtained by examining gram-stained smears of exudates, body fluids or infected tissues. More precise identification may be possible if laboratory facilities permit culture of infected material *in vitro*. In either case, it is important to obtain samples before the initiation of chemotherapy, or after treatment has been withdrawn for three to five days.

Once the pathogen is identified, the drugs likely to be effective in treatment can be determined by consideration of the usual pattern of susceptibility of the organism to antimicrobial agents (Table 2). This information is most useful for microorganisms with a relatively reliable and predictable pattern of susceptibility, such as *Streptococcus* spp. and *Clostridium* spp. However, pathogens which show considerable strain variation in susceptibility to antimicrobial agents should ideally be tested for susceptibility *in vitro* to aid selection of drugs suitable for therapy.

### SUSCEPTIBILITY TESTS

Laboratory tests for antimicrobial susceptibility are indicated when the pathogen is of a type which is often resistant to antimicrobial drugs (e.g., *Staphylococcus aureus*, *Escherichia coli*, *Pseudomonas aeruginosa*,

*Table 1.  Possible Etiologic Agents in Typical Clinical Infections*

| DIAGNOSIS | COMMONLY ISOLATED ORGANISMS |
|---|---|
| Stomatitis | *Streptococcus\*, Staphylococcus\*, Proteus, Pseudomonas, Escherichia coli, Fusobacterium fusiforme, Candida albicans* |
| Tonsillitis, pharyngitis | *Streptococcus\*, Staphylococcus* |
| Bronchitis, pneumonia | *Bordetella bronchiseptica\*, Pseudomonas aeruginosa, Klebsiella, Staphylococcus aureus, Streptococcus pyogenes,* viruses |
| Pyothorax | *Pasteurella multocida\*, Escherichia coli\*, Streptococcus, Staphylococcus, Nocardia,* viruses |
| Pyodermas | *Staphylococcus aureus, Streptococcus\*, Proteus\*, Pseudomonas, Corynebacterium, Escherichia coli\*, Enterobacter aerogenes* |
| Vulvitis, vaginitis | *Proteus mirabilis\*, Escherichia coli\*, Streptococcus* |
| Metritis—chronic | *Streptococcus\*, Brucella canis, Escherichia coli, Haemophilus* |
| —acute | *Streptococcus\*, Proteus mirabilis, Escherichia coli* |
| Pyometra | *Escherichia coli\*, Streptococcus* |
| Balanoposthitis | *Escherichia coli\*, Klebsiella, Enterobacter, Proteus, Pseudomonas, Staphylococcus* |
| Cystitis | *Escherichia coli\*, Proteus mirabilis\*, Pseudomonas\*, Streptococcus, Staphylococcus* |
| Prostatitis | *Escherichia coli\*, Proteus, Pseudomonas, Streptococcus, Staphylococcus* |
| Infectious enteritis | *Salmonella\*, Escherichia coli\*, Pseudomonas (?Streptococcus, Proteus), Giardia,* coccidia, distemper virus |
| Superficial ocular infections | *Staphylococcus, Streptococcus* |
| Osteomyelitis | *Staphylococcus aureus\*, Escherichia coli\*, Streptococcus, Proteus* |
| Wound infections | *Staphylococcus\*,* coliforms\*, *Clostridium* |
| Bacterial endocarditis | *Streptococcus\*, Escherichia coli, Pseudomonas, Staphylococcus* |
| Puppy septicemias | *Streptococcus\*, Escherichia coli\*, Proteus mirabilis, Pseudomonas aeruginosa, Staphylococcus,* viruses |
| Otitis media | *Staphylococcus\*, Streptococcus\*, Pityrosporum, Pseudomonas, Escherichia coli, Proteus mirabilis* |
| Otitis externa | *Staphylococcus aureus\*, Streptococcus\*, Pityrosporum\*;* secondary: *Proteus mirabilis, Pseudomonas\*, Corynebacterium, Bacillus subtilis, Candida albicans* |
| Burns | *Pseudomonas\*, Proteus, Escherichia coli, Staphylococcus* |

Modified from Aronson and Kirk, 1975.
\*Most commonly isolated.

*Proteus* spp.). They are also advisable when the utmost antimicrobial efficacy is required, as in life-threatening infections or immunoparetic individuals.

Samples for culture should be collected prior to commencement of therapy, and the susceptibility test should be performed using a pure culture growth of the pathogen isolated from the primary specimen. The disc diffusion method (described by Kirk and Bistner, 1975) is regarded as satisfactory for routine clinical use. In critical situations antimicrobial therapy may be instituted on a "best guess" basis (Tables 1 and 2) pending the results of laboratory tests.

Although *in-vitro* susceptibility tests provide a useful guide to the selection of antimicrobial drugs, they are not infallible.

**Table 2.**   *Use of Antimicrobial Agents for Treatment of Infections*

| ORGANISM | DISEASE | DRUGS OF CHOICE | ALTERNATIVE DRUGS |
|---|---|---|---|
| *Actinomyces* | Actinomycosis | Penicillin G* | Tetracyclines |
| *Bacillus anthracis* | Anthrax | Penicillin G | Erythromycin, tetracyclines |
| *Blastomyces, Candida, Coccidioides, Histoplasma, Cryptococcus, Mucor, Aspergillus* | Pneumonia, skin and soft tissue lesions, bone lesions, disseminated disease | Amphotericin B | 2 hydroxystilbamide† (*Blastomyces*), flucytosine† (*Candida, Cryptococcus*) |
| *Bordetella bronchiseptica* | Respiratory infections | Tetracyclines | Chloramphenicol |
| *Brucella canis* | Abortions | Tetracyclines with streptomycin | —— |
| *Chlamydia psittaci* | Respiratory infections, conjunctivitis | Tetracyclines | Chloramphenicol |
| *Clostridium tetani* | Tetanus | Penicillin G* | Erythromycin |
| Clostridia, other | Gas gangrene | Penicillin G* | Tetracyclines |
| Coccidia | Coccidiosis | Sulfonamides | Nitrofurazone |
| *Escherichia coli* | Urinary tract infections | Nitrofurantoin, sulfonamides, ampicillin | Cephalosporins, chloramphenicol, tetracyclines |
|  | Other infections | Ampicillin, chloramphenicol tetracyclines | Aminoglycosides, polymyxins |
| *Fusobacterium* | Ulcerative stomatitis | Penicillin G | Tetracyclines, metronidazole |
| *Giardia* | Enteritis | Metronidazole | Quinacrine, glycobiarsol |
| *Haemobartonella* | Infectious anemia | Tetracyclines‡ | Chloramphenicol‡ |
| *Klebsiella, Enterobacter* | Respiratory, urinary tract infections | Kanamycin, gentamicin | Cephalosporins, chloramphenicol |
| *Leptospira* | Leptospirosis | Penicillin G with streptomycin | Tetracyclines |
| *Microsporum, Trichophyton, Epidermophyton* | Skin, hair and nail bed infections | Griseofulvin | —— |
| *Mycobacterium* | Tuberculosis | Isoniazid with streptomycin or *p*-aminosalicylic acid | —— |
| *Mycoplasma* | Respiratory infection(?), conjunctivitis | Tetracyclines | Chloramphenicol, macrolides |
| *Neorickettsia* | Salmon disease | Tetracyclines | Chloramphenicol |
| *Nocardia* | Nocardiosis | Sulfonamides* | Chloramphenicol, tetracyclines |
| *Pasteurella multocida* | Abscesses, respiratory infections | Penicillin G* | Tetracyclines, ampicillin |
| *Pentatrichomonas* | Trichomonal enteritis | Metronidazole | Glycobiarsol |

Modified from Aronson and Kirk 1975.                               *Continued on next page*
*Large dosage.
†Used to treat these infections in man; efficacy in dogs and cats uncertain.
‡Efficacy questionable.
§Urinary tract infections only.

*Table 2.* Use of Antimicrobial Agents for Treatment of Infections (Continued)

| ORGANISM | DISEASE | DRUGS OF CHOICE | ALTERNATIVE DRUGS |
|---|---|---|---|
| *Pityrosporum* | Skin and ear infections | 2% "tame" iodine or 25% glyceryl triacetate topically | —— |
| *Proteus mirabilis* | Urinary tract and soft tissue infections | Ampicillin, chloramphenicol, nitrofurantoin§ | Cephalosporins, aminoglycosides |
| *Pseudomonas aeruginosa* | Urinary tract and soft tissue infections, burns | Polymyxins, gentamicin | Carbenicillin, chloramphenicol |
| *Salmonella* | Gastroenteritis | Chloramphenicol | Ampicillin, nitrofurans |
| *Staphylococcus aureus* | Pyoderma, endocarditis, osteomyelitis, soft tissue infections | Penicillin G sensitive: penicillin G<br><br>Penicillin G resistant: cloxacillin, macrolides | Ampicillin, macrolides, lincomycin<br><br>Cephalosporins, chloramphenicol, lincomycin |
| *Streptococcus* | Urinary tract infections, otitis, soft tissue infections, upper respiratory infections | Penicillin G | Ampicillin, cephalosporins, erythromycin |
| *Toxoplasma* | Toxoplasmosis | Pyrimethamine with sulfonamide | —— |

§Urinary tract infections only.

Discrepancies can occur between laboratory results and treatment response because conditions *in vivo* and *in vitro* are not identical. However, as a general rule, an organism which is resistant to a particular drug *in vitro* is unlikely to be susceptible to treatment with the drug, but if the organism is susceptible *in vitro,* therapy with the drug *may* be effective.

## OTHER FACTORS INFLUENCING FINAL SELECTION OF DRUG

Whether "best guess" methods or laboratory procedures are used, the clinician is often left with a choice between several compounds likely to be active against the pathogen. In making the final selection, consideration should be given to a number of other factors involving the patient and the properties of the various drugs (Table 3).

### BACTERICIDAL VERSUS BACTERIOSTATIC ACTIVITY

Antibacterial agents can be broadly divided into two groups on the basis of their activity against bacteria *in vitro*. Some drugs have a killing (bactericidal) action at or near the minimal inhibitory concentration, while others simply inhibit bacterial growth (bacteriostatic). Agents which are generally bactericidal are penicillins, cephalosporins, aminoglycosides and polymyxins. Agents essentially bacteriostatic in activity are tetracyclines, chloramphenicol, macrolides, lincomycin, sulfonamides and nitrofurans.

While the distinction between the two groups is not absolute, it may have important implications in the treatment of infections. When bacteriostatic agents are used, the normal antimicrobial defense mechanisms of the animal must participate actively in order to cure the infection, otherwise relapse would follow cessation of treatment. Consequently, bactericidal agents are more likely to give a favorable response in individuals with impaired defense mechanisms, particularly in those with life-threatening infections. Bactericidal drugs are also preferred if concurrent corticosteroid therapy is thought necessary in an animal with a systemic infection, and

## Table 3. *Properties of Some Antimicrobial Drugs*

| | |
|---|---|
| I. PENICILLINS | Bactericidal drugs, toxic effects rare. Excretion mainly renal, hindered by probenecid orally (occasionally useful when treating systemic infections with expensive penicillins). |
| Penicillin G (benzylpenicillin) | Active mainly against gram-positive organisms, also against some gram-negative species at higher concentrations (e.g., in urine). Drug of choice against most gram-positive pathogens, except strains of *Staphylococcus aureus* producing penicillinase. Available in 3 parenteral forms—Na or K salt (short-acting), procaine salt (duration about 24 hours at usual doses) and benzathine or benethamine salt (low blood levels for at least 5 days after single injection, may be inadequate for less susceptible microbes). |
| A. *Acid-resistant*<br>Penicillin V (phenoxymethylpenicillin), phenethicillin | Similar activity to penicillin G against gram-positive organisms, but preferred for oral dosage because of greater resistance to gastric acid. |
| B. *Staphylococcal penicillinase–resistant*<br>Cloxacillin, oxacillin, nafcillin, methicillin | Generally less active than penicillin G, indicated only for infections caused by penicillinase-producing strains of *S. aureus*. Methicillin must be given parenterally, the others orally or parenterally. |
| C. *Broad-spectrum*<br>Ampicillin | Compared with penicillin G, ampicillin is slightly less active against gram-positive bacteria but more active against gram-negative bacilli. Given orally or parenterally. |
| Hetacillin | Similar properties, hydrolyzed to ampicillin *in vivo*, given orally. |
| Amoxycillin | Similar spectrum to ampicillin but with some pharmacologic advantages; veterinary value not yet clear. |
| Carbenicillin | Expensive, parenteral use only, may be useful for systemic or urinary tract infections caused by *Pseudomonas aeruginosa*, *Proteus* spp. |
| II. CEPHALOSPORINS | Bactericidal, active against many gram-positive and gram-negative bacteria. Role in veterinary therapy not completely established. In people, used against penicillin-resistant staphylococci, gram-negative bacteria (mainly in urinary tract), and as substitutes for penicillin in penicillin-sensitive patients. |
| Cephaloridine | Administered intramuscularly. High doses nephrotoxic in some species but apparently not a problem in dogs or cats. |
| Cephalexin | Administered orally, well absorbed. |
| III. AMINOGLYCOSIDES | Bactericidal, active against gram-negative bacteria, mycobacteria, some staphylococci. Absorption from gut minimal—administered parenterally for systemic or urinary tract infections (antibacterial activity enhanced in alkaline urine), orally for gut antisepsis. Excretion mainly renal. Toxic effects: damage to eighth cranial nerve (deafness, vestibular disturbance); renal damage; neuromuscular blockade (rare). |
| Streptomycin, dihydrostreptomycin | Identical activity; dihydrostreptomycin used in most veterinary preparations, but no longer recommended for people because it causes deafness more frequently than streptomycin. Bacterial strains resistant to these two emerge rapidly during treatment. |
| Neomycin | Similar activity but more toxic than streptomycin. Used systemically for short courses, only if renal function normal. Prolonged high oral dosage of neomycin (or kanamycin) may cause diarrhea, malabsorption (reversible). |
| Framycetin | Closely related to neomycin, similar properties. |
| Kanamycin | Safer systemically than neomycin, but more expensive. |
| Gentamicin | More active than other aminoglycosides against many microbes, expensive—practicable only for gram-negative pathogens resistant to other aminoglycosides, polymyxins. |
| IV. TETRACYCLINES | Bacteriostatic, active against many gram-positive and gram-negative bacteria, also mycoplasmas, rickettsias and chlamydia. Administration: oral route usually preferred, but absorption is incomplete and hindered by food or metallic salts. Intramuscular injection often painful, some intravenous formulations available. Widely distributed in body, deposited in grow- |

*Continued on next page*

Tetracycline, oxytetracycline,
  chlortetracycline, demethylchlor-
  tetracycline
(*Also* rolitetracycline, methacycline,
minocycline)

ing bone and teeth (but not necessarily active there). Excretion: mainly urine, also bile. Toxicity: gastrointestinal disturbances, necrosis at injection sites, hyperthermia, discolored teeth (if given to neonates or during gestation). Use in renal failure contraindicated because of their antianabolic effect and delayed excretion (except doxycycline).

Most commonly used tetracyclines in veterinary practice—cheaper than many of the newer derivatives (rolitetracycline, methacycline, minocycline) which offer few advantages.

Doxycycline

Low dosage form, once daily administration, may be safe in patients with renal failure.

## V. MACROLIDES

Bacteriostatic, active mainly against gram-positive cocci and clostridia, some effect against mycoplasmas, rickettsias and chlamydia.

Erythromycin

Usually second choice to penicillin G or V, which are cheaper. Generally administered orally, occasionally intramuscularly (causes pain) or intravenously. Excreted in urine and bile. Side-effects uncommon in animals, in people sometimes gastrointestinal upsets or hepatopathy with the estolate ester.

Tylosin
(*Rarely used:* oleandomycin,
  triacetyloleandomycin,
  spiramycin)

Similar indications to erythromycin. Other macrolides rarely used.

## VI. POLYMYXINS

Bactericidal, active against gram-negative bacilli, including *Pseudomonas aeruginosa* but not *Proteus* spp. Not absorbed from gut. Administered parenterally for systemic or urinary tract infections as *polymyxin B* sulfate, or methanesulfonate derivative of *colistin (polymyxin E)*. Excreted mainly in urine. Toxicity: renal damage, neurotoxicity (drowsiness, ataxia, possibly neuromuscular blockade). Gentamicin is less toxic and has tended to supplant polymyxins but polymyxins may be preferred on the basis of cost.

Polymyxin B
Colistin

## VII. MISCELLANEOUS ANTIBIOTICS
Chloramphenicol

Bacteriostatic, active against many gram-positive and gram-negative bacteria, as well as mycoplasmas, rickettsias and chlamydia. Oral administration: satisfactory for routine therapy, well absorbed. Given as tablets, capsules (absorption unimpeded by food) or suspensions of palmitate ester (provides similar blood levels to capsules at equivalent dosage). Parenteral administration: solutions in nonaqueous solvents, solutions of succinate ester, or aqueous suspensions (poorly absorbed). Excretion: 5–10% eliminated in urine as active antibiotic, the rest metabolized by liver. Toxicity: depression, decreased food intake and reversible bone marrow suppression may occur at therapeutic dose rates in cats and at higher dosages in dogs. The fatal marrow aplasia seen after use in some people has not been reported in domestic animals.

Lincomycin

Bacteriostatic, active mainly against gram-positive bacteria and some mycoplasmas. Indications and usefulness similar to erythromycin, which is cheaper. For staphylococcal infections, combined use with another antistaphylococcal agent advised because lincomycin resistance emerges readily. Excreted mainly in urine. Toxicity uncommon in animals, diarrhea in people.

Clindamycin (clinimycin)

A derivative of lincomycin, more active, some pharmacologic advantages, may eventually replace lincomycin. May be especially useful in infections due to *Actinomyces* spp.

Amphotericin B

Fungicidal, active against many fungi causing deep mycotic infections. Administration: intravenous or intraperitoneal route, prolonged course. Very toxic, low margin of safety, causes renal damage, vomiting, abdominal pain. Indications: blastomycosis, coccidioidomycosis, histoplasmosis, disseminated candidiasis, cryptococcosis, sporotrichosis, mucormycosis, aspergillosis.

*Continued on next page*

| | |
|---|---|
| Nystatin | Fungicidal, similar spectrum of activity to amphotericin B. Too toxic for parenteral use, not absorbed from the gut. Indications: topically or by mouth for superficial or intestinal candidiasis. Routine prophylactic use during tetracycline therapy (intended to prevent *Candida albicans* overgrowth) probably unwarranted. |
| Griseofulvin | Fungistatic. Indicated for dermatophyte infections of hair, skin, nails. Administered orally, absorption promoted by high fat diet. Teratogenic, avoid in pregnancy. Not effective topically. |
| VIII. SULFONAMIDES | Bacteriostatic, active against many gram-positive and gram-negative bacteria, some chlamydia and some protozoa. Generally less active than antibiotics but relatively inexpensive. Administration: usually oral, some parenteral forms available. Excretion: mainly renal. Toxicity: a variety of effects recognized, generally uncommon with correct dosage; crystalluria and renal damage avoided with highly soluble sulfonamides, alkaline urine (increases solubility), high urine flow rate. Several types available: |
| Sulfamethizole, sulfisoxazole (sulfafurazole) | *Short-acting*: rapidly absorbed and excreted, highly soluble, commonly used for urinary tract infections. |
| Sulfadiazine, sulfamethazine, sulfamerazine, triple sulfonamide mixtures | *Intermediate*: rapidly absorbed but more slowly excreted, used for systemic or urinary tract infections. |
| Sulfadimethoxine, sulfamethoxypyridazine | *Long-acting*: very slow excretion, used for systemic infections if once daily dosage advantageous. |
| Phthalylsulfathiazole | *Poorly Absorbed*: used for topical effect in bowel. |
| IX. SULFONAMIDE POTENTIATORS | The action of sulfonamides against many microbes is potentiated by combined therapy with other drugs acting on the same metabolic sequence as sulfonamides. Combinations of *trimethoprim* and sulfonamide regularly show synergistic action against many bacteria *in vitro*—often producing a bactericidal effect where each drug alone was bacteriostatic. Clinical trials have generally confirmed the potentiation, but synergy should not be expected universally during therapy because the conditions required for it to occur may not always be present *in vivo*. Veterinary preparations currently available contain trimethoprim and sulfonamide (usually sulfadiazine) in 1:5 ratio. Indications: as for broad-spectrum antibiotics. Toxicity: possibility of folate deficiency. |
| Trimethoprim | |
| Pyrimethamine | Potentiates the action of sulfonamides against protozoa, may be used with sulfonamides for toxoplasmosis, coccidiosis. Toxicity: folate deficiency. |

they are generally more effective for treating abscesses. However, there is probably little to choose between bactericidal and bacteriostatic agents for treating mild infections in otherwise healthy individuals.

**POTENTIAL TOXICITY**

The incidence of adverse reactions observed in small animals treated correctly with antimicrobial drugs is generally low. Nevertheless, most antimicrobial agents are potentially toxic and this factor must be considered when choosing between several drugs likely to be effective in a given situation.

Of the various systemic antimicrobial agents used in small animals, only the aminoglycosides, polymyxins and amphotericin B have a reputation for toxicity at therapeutic dose rates. However, the presence of disease states other than the infectious process itself may increase the risks of toxicity with many drugs. Kidney and liver diseases are particularly important in this regard, since most antimicrobial agents are excreted or metabolized by these organs. In renal or hepatic insufficiency, impaired drug elimination could lead to accumulation of toxic levels even with normal dosage. Furthermore, some antimicrobial agents are potentially nephrotoxic or hepatotoxic. For these reasons, it is preferable in patients with renal disease to avoid treatment with aminoglycosides, polymyxins, tetracyclines, cephaloridine, sulfonamides, nitrofurantoin or nalidixic acid. Likewise, caution is advised when using chloramphenicol, tetracyclines or erythromycin in animals with hepatic dysfunction.

## COST

When a number of equally effective and safe drugs are available, the one which is least expensive is obviously preferred. In addition, economic considerations will sometimes necessitate selection of an agent which is less effective but cheaper than the most active drug. High cost frequently precludes systemic therapy with polymyxins, gentamicin or carbenicillin.

## ADDITIONAL CONSIDERATIONS IN PLANNING THERAPY

### DOSE RATE AND FREQUENCY

Dose rates and treatment intervals for various antimicrobial agents are given in Table 4. Some flexibility in treatment schedules is warranted, since the optimal regimen will depend on factors which vary from infection to infection, such as the susceptibility of the organism, the extent of drug penetration into infected tissues and the activity of the host's defense mechanisms. The regimen selected must be appropriate for both the patient and the infection and should be modified if necessary in the light of the response to treatment. Dosages lower than those suggested may be satisfactory when treating urinary tract infections with drugs which are greatly concentrated in urine, but higher or more frequent dosage may be necessary to obtain adequate diffusion of the agent into deep-seated lesions or relatively avascular tissues.

### ROUTE OF ADMINISTRATION

The route chosen for administration depends on the particular drug selected, the site of infection and the state of the patient.

Oral dosage is satisfactory for mild to moderate infections and is generally convenient for outpatient treatment but may be impractical for animals which are fractious or vomiting. Further, oral administration will not produce adequate systemic concentrations of agents which are either destroyed by gastric secretions (penicillin G, carbenicillin) or poorly absorbed from the gut (aminoglycosides, polymyxins, nystatin). Drugs which are not absorbed may be useful, however, for treating localized gastrointestinal infections.

A further consideration with oral administration is that absorption of some drugs from the intestinal tract can be impaired by a variety of foods and chemicals. For example, the absorption of tetracyclines is hindered by food, milk and salts of calcium, magnesium, iron and aluminum; absorption of lincomycin is impaired by preparations of kaolin and pectin; and absorption of ampicillin is retarded by food. Consequently, it is usually advised that oral antimicrobial agents be given at least one hour before or two hours after feeding and that simultaneous oral administration of other drugs be avoided.

Parenteral therapy is generally less convenient but is advisable for severe systemic infections, where the effect of variation in intestinal drug absorption may be critical. Intravenous administration is particularly indicated in life-threatening infections and when high blood concentrations are required to overcome barriers to the penetration of antimicrobial agents. It is also useful for formulations which cause pain when injected by other routes (chloramphenicol succinate solutions). For routine parenteral therapy, most veterinarians inject antimicrobial agents intramuscularly rather than subcutaneously, although the resulting blood concentrations are often quite similar. In addition, subcutaneous administration of nonirritant preparations is generally easier in small animals and causes less pain than intramuscular injection.

### DURATION OF THERAPY

The ideal duration of antimicrobial treatment for the majority of infections is not known. However, a good general rule is to treat for a minimum of three days, and to continue for two or three days after the temperature has returned to normal and other signs of infection have subsided. Treatment for a week or less is adequate for many canine and feline infections, but more prolonged therapy may sometimes be necessary, as in bacterial urinary tract infections (minimum 3 weeks, extending up to 6 to 8 weeks), endocarditis (4 to 6 weeks), polyarthritis (3 to 4 weeks) and pneumonia (2 to 4 weeks) (Thornton, 1975).

### USE OF ANTIMICROBIAL AGENTS IN COMBINATION

Although it is generally recognized that the majority of bacterial infections can be treated successfully with a single drug, the

**Table 4.** *Conventional Regimens for Some Antimicrobial Drugs in Dogs and Cats*

| DRUG | DOSAGE | ROUTE | REPEAT DOSE |
|---|---|---|---|
| Amphotericin B | 0.25 to 0.5 mg./kg. | IV, IP | see below* |
| Ampicillin | 10 to 20 mg./kg. | PO | 8 hours |
| | 5 to 10 mg./kg. | IV,IM,SC | 8 hours |
| Cephalexin | 30 mg./kg. | PO | 12 hours |
| Cephaloridine | 10 mg./kg. | IM,SC | 8 to 12 hours |
| Chloramphenicol | 20 to 40 mg./kg. | PO | 8 hours |
| | 20 mg./kg. | IV,IM,SC | 8 hours |
| Chlortetracycline | 20 mg./kg. | PO | 8 hours |
| Cloxacillin | 10 mg./kg. | PO,IV,IM | 6 hours |
| Colistin | 1 mg./kg. | IM | 6 hours |
| Dihydrostreptomycin | 20 mg./kg. | PO | 6 hours (not absorbed) |
| | 10 mg./kg. | IM,SC | 8 to 12 hours |
| Erythromycin | 10 mg./kg. | PO | 8 hours |
| Framycetin | 20 mg./kg. | PO | 6 hours (not absorbed) |
| Gentamicin | 4 mg./kg. | IM,SC | 12 hours first day, then 24 hours |
| Griseofulvin | 20 mg./kg. | PO | 24 hours, with fat |
| | 140 mg./kg. | PO | 1 week, with fat |
| Hetacillin | 10 to 20 mg./kg. | PO | 8 to 12 hours |
| Kanamycin | 10 mg./kg. | PO | 6 hours (not absorbed) |
| | 7 mg./kg. | IM,SC | 12 hours |
| Lincomycin | 15 mg./kg. | PO | 8 hours |
| | 10 mg./kg. | IV,IM | 12 hours |
| Methicillin | 20 mg./kg. | IV,IM | 6 hours |
| Metronidazole | 60 mg./kg. | PO | 24 hours |
| Nafcillin | 10 mg./kg. | PO,IM | 6 hours |
| Neomycin | 20 mg./kg. | PO | 6 hours (not absorbed) |
| | 10 mg./kg. | IM,SC | 12 hours |
| Nitrofurantoin | 4 mg./kg. | PO | 8 hours |
| | 3 mg./kg. | IM | 12 hours |
| Nystatin | 100,000 U | PO | 6 hours (not absorbed) |
| Oxacillin | 10 mg./kg. | PO,IV,IM | 6 hours |
| Oxytetracycline | 20 mg./kg. | PO | 8 hours |
| | 7 mg./kg. | IV,IM | 12 hours |
| Penicillin G,Na or K | 40,000 U/kg. | PO | 6 hours (not with food) |
| | 20,000 U/kg. | IV,IM,SC | 4 hours |
| Penicillin G, benethamine | 40,000 U/kg. | IM | 5 days |
| Penicillin G, procaine | 20,000 U/kg. | IM,SC | 24 hours |
| Penicillin V | 10 mg./kg. | PO | 8 hours |
| Phenethicillin | 10 mg./kg. | PO | 8 hours |
| Phthalylsulfathiazole | 50 mg./kg. | PO | 6 hours (not absorbed) |
| Polymyxin B | 2 mg (20,000 U)/kg. | IM | 12 hours |
| Pyrimethamine | 1 mg./kg. | PO | 24 hours for 3 days, then |
| | 0.5 mg./kg. | PO | 24 hours |
| Streptomycin | 20 mg./kg. | PO | 6 hours (not absorbed) |
| | 10 mg./kg. | IM,SC | 8 to 12 hours |
| Sulfadiazine, sulfamerazine, sulfamethazine | 50 mg./kg. | PO,IV | 12 hours |
| Sulfadimethoxine | 25 mg./kg. | PO,IV,IM | 24 hours |
| Sulfamethizole, sulfisoxazole | 50 mg./kg. | PO | 8 hours |
| Sulfamethoxypyridazine | 50 mg./kg. | PO,IV,IM,SC | 24 hours |
| Tetracycline | 20 mg./kg. | PO | 8 hours |
| | 7 mg./kg. | IV,IM | 12 hours |
| Trimethoprim plus sulfadiazine | 15 mg.(combined)/kg. | PO | 12 hours |
| Trimethoprim plus sulfadoxine | 15 mg.(combined)/kg. | IV,IM | 24 hours |
| Tylosin | 10 mg./kg. | PO | 8 hours |
| | 5 mg./kg. | IV,IM | 12 hours |

*Amphotericin B must be diluted to 0.1 mg./ml. with 5% dextrose and water. It can be given IV 2 to 3 times weekly by slow drip (at least 2 hours). The same solution can be given intraperitoneally by slow drip (at least 30 minutes) every second day. Total accumulated dose suggested by either route is 10 to 25 mg./kg., given over a period of 2 to 3 months until clinical remission, or at least 6 weeks. It is very toxic; stop treatment if vomiting, proteinuria or an increase in BUN develops. Toxicity may preclude its use in cats (Aronson and Kirk, 1975).

tendency to use a combination of antimicrobial agents remains widespread. Jawetz (1975) has attributed this to the "vague feeling" held by most veterinarians and physicians "that if one antimicrobial drug is good, two should be better, and three should cure almost everybody of everything."

There are few clinical situations in which systemic therapy with two or more antimicrobial agents simultaneously *might* be beneficial. The indications suggested by Jawetz (1975) are as follows: to treat life-threatening infections (pending identification of the pathogen), to delay emergence of drug-resistant mutants (especially for prolonged therapy with susceptible drugs such as streptomycin), to utilize drug synergy (a rare and unpredictable phenomenon), to treat mixed systemic infections (uncommon) or to enable reduced dosage of a toxic drug.

The use of mixtures of procaine penicillin G and dihydrostreptomycin for routine antimicrobial therapy is unwarranted because it is not covered by any of these indications. Furthermore, formulations containing these two drugs in a fixed ratio are unsatisfactory, because the pharmacologic properties of the constituents do not permit safe, effective therapy with both drugs simultaneously when given in this form (Aronson and Kirk, 1975).

On the rare occasion when combined an-timicrobial therapy is indicated, the drugs should ideally be administered as individual preparations with dose rates and treatment frequencies appropriate to each drug.

## OTHER TREATMENT

In many infections, the administration of antimicrobial agents will not cure the condition without additional specific or supportive therapy. Abscesses, obstructed drainage routes and foreign bodies (calculi, sequestrations, prostheses, suture materials) frequently hinder the response to antimicrobial drugs and necessitate surgical intervention. In urinary tract infections, the efficacy of treatment can often be increased by modification of the urine pH to the optimum for the drug administered (Table 5). When necessary, the pH of urine can be raised by giving sodium bicarbonate orally, or lowered by oral administration of d,1-methionine or ascorbic acid. In some infections, supportive treatment can be of greater immediate significance than antimicrobial drug therapy: in leptospirosis, for example, correction of fluid and electrolyte imbalances associated with renal failure may be more important than eradication of the causative organism.

Although hyperthermia is common in in-

*Table 5.* *pH for Most Effective Antibacterial Activity*

| ANTIMICROBIAL DRUG | pH | 5.5 | 6.0 | 6.5 | 7.0 | 7.5 | 8.0 |
|---|---|---|---|---|---|---|---|
| Cephalothin* | | | + | + | + | + | + |
| Chloramphenicol* | | | | | | + | + |
| Colistin | | | | | | + | + |
| Erythromycin† | | | | | | | + |
| Gentamicin† | | | | | | + | + |
| Kanamycin† | | | | | | + | + |
| Lincomycin | | | | | | + | |
| Methenamine mandelate† | | + | | | | | |
| Neomycin† | | | | | | + | + |
| Nitrofurantoin† | | + | + | | | | |
| Novobiocin | | + | + | | | | |
| Oxacillin | | | + | | | | |
| Penicillin G | | + | + | + | | | |
| Polymyxin B* | | | | | | | + |
| Streptomycin† | | | | | | + | + |
| Sulfonamides‡ | | | + | + | + | + | + |
| Tetracycline* | | | + | + | + | | |
| Oxytetracycline* | | + | + | + | | | |
| Chlortetracycline† | | + | + | | | | |

Modified from Aronson and Kirk (1975).
+ Indicates optimum pH.
* The pH is not important—effectiveness of the drug is not highly dependent on pH.
† The pH is very important—effectiveness of the drug is highly dependent on pH.
‡ The pH is not important except as it affects solubility.

fections, treatment with antipyretic drugs is usually unnecessary and may obscure the natural course of the disease or the effect of the antimicrobial treatment. Likewise, corticosteroid therapy is rarely indicated and may cause positive harm by suppressing the host's defense mechanisms and masking signs of infection. Drug preparations containing mixtures of antibiotic(s) and corticosteroid(s) are particularly irrational and should rarely, if ever, be used systemically.

## SUPPLEMENTAL READING

Aronson, A. L.: The use, misuse, and abuse of antibacterial agents. Mod. Vet. Pract., 56:383–389, 1975.

Aronson, A. L., and Kirk, R. W.: Antimicrobial drugs. In Ettinger, S. J. (ed.): Textbook of Veterinary Internal Medicine. Philadelphia, W. B. Saunders Co., 1975.

Garrod, L. P., Lambert, H. P., and O'Grady, F.: Antibiotic and Chemotherapy. 4th ed. Edinburgh, Churchill-Livingstone, 1973.

Jawetz, E.: Actions of antimicrobial drugs in combination. Vet. Clin. N. Am., 5:35–50, 1975.

Kirk, R. W., and Bistner, S. I.: Antimicrobial sensitivity testing. In: Handbook of Veterinary Procedures and Emergency Treatment. 2nd ed. Philadelphia, W. B. Saunders Co., 1975.

Thornton, G. W.: Antimicrobial therapy in the dog and cat. Vet. Clin. N. Am., 5:133–141, 1975.

Weinstein, L.: Chemotherapy of microbial diseases. In Goodman, L. S., and Gilman, A. (eds.): The Pharmacological Basis of Therapeutics. 5th ed. New York, Macmillan Co., 1975.

Yeary, R. A.: Systemic toxic effects of chemotherapeutic agents in domestic animals. Vet. Clin. N. Am., 5:51–69, 1975.

# SHOCK: PATHO-PHYSIOLOGY AND MANAGEMENT

COLIN F. BURROWS, M.R.C.V.S.,
RONALD J. KOLATA, D.V.M.
and LAWRENCE R. SOMA, V.M.D.

*Philadelphia, Pennsylvania*

## INTRODUCTION

Shock is a clinical state, the central feature of which is ineffective tissue blood flow and cellular hypoxia. The course and outcome of shock depend on a number of factors, including its etiology, the time from onset to recognition and treatment and any underlying disease process. An animal in shock demonstrates progressive dysfunction of many organs at the macro-, micro- and biochemical level.

Many individual organs and metabolites have been studied in the hope that a specific organ or substance could be incriminated as the major contributor to the progressive nature of shock. In many instances a "target organ" has been identified which, in a particular shock type, supposedly contributes more than any other to the eventual demise of the patient. While this may be true in the experimental model, it is seldom true in the clinical situation.

The use of a variety of experimental animals in attempts to define general concepts can be misleading. It might be concluded, for example, that a standardized form of hemorrhagic shock would have similar physiological and pathological manifestations in a diverse number of species. However, the effects of hemorrhagic hypotension can be very different in different species. The extrapolation of information from controlled experiments to clinical situations can lead to false assumptions.

One of the more difficult aspects of the clinical management of shock is the evaluation of therapy, especially when assessment is limited to clinically applicable methods. It is difficult to establish what phase of shock a patient is in when presented. This is different from the experimental model, in which the insult can be graded and procedures standardized. In most models the refractory or reversible phase of shock is defined by rather clear-cut physiological or biochemical changes. In clinical situations in which insults may be multiple and the time from onset to presentation is variable, it takes a period of evaluation and therapy to establish the phase of shock.

As a prelude to discussion of therapy, some basic concepts of shock pathophysiology will be presented. These will enable the reader to approach shock therapy with an understanding of the underlying physiological changes.

## DEFINITION OF SYNDROME

An unavoidable task in a discussion of shock is an attempt to provide a working definition of the syndrome, preferably on an etiological and physiological basis. The word shock has been used for at least a century to describe a condition that can be initiated by a number of insults. Despite many causes (Table 1), the clinical syndrome encompasses a multitude of commonly recognizable signs. This does not mean that sepsis and hemorrhage produce identical physiological changes, but if severe enough, they can disrupt body mechanisms to such a degree that the signs of shock are evident.

Irrespective of the initial insult, shock is a condition in which tissue perfusion is inadequate. It can, for example, be created by a reduction in cardiac output, such as in hemorrhagic shock or by the intense vasoconstriction that occurs during the early phase of septic shock. Inadequate perfusion results in tissue ischemia and disruption of cellular function at all levels. The ischemia is initially confined to the nonvital vascular beds as part of an overall cardiovascular compensation. This compensation is an attempt to maintain adequate perfusion of the two circulatory beds immediately essential to life, the cerebral and coronary circulations. Reduced perfusion of the splanchnic, cutaneous and muscle beds can be sustained for a longer period of time. This

**Table 1.** *Causes of Shock*

Hemorrhage
Fluid loss
Trauma
Sepsis
Toxins
Adrenal insufficiency
Cardiac failure
Anaphylaxis

period has been defined in experimental models and is considered the breaking point between reversible and irreversible shock.

The many factors contributing to the deterioration of the animal are self-propagating. The term "refractory phase" can be used to define the period in which therapy may be sustaining physiological mechanisms but is not capable of reversing the damage that has occurred. The "irreversible phase" is the state in which no present therapy produces recovery; it is derived primarily from experimental models where it is more easily defined.

## DYNAMICS OF SHOCK

The initiating mechanisms result in a common pathway of circulatory changes (Fig. 1). Body functions are organized to compensate for these changes. A reflex compensation to hypotension occurs through both neurogenic and hormonal mechanisms. In shock produced either by acute blood loss or by a slower fluid loss due to severe diarrhea, there are reflex mechanisms attempting to adjust the discrepancy between the available vascular volume and the vascular tree. Following a reduction in effective blood volume a sympathetically mediated tachycardia occurs in an attempt to maintain cardiac output, together with a reduced perfusion of specific organ beds. This latter change results in a redistribution of the available blood volume to those organs essential for immediate survival, namely the coronary, cerebral, adrenal and arterial hepatic circulation. This is achieved by a reduced perfusion of the cutaneous, renal, splenic, muscular, portal hepatic and mesenteric beds. This massive sympathetic response is beneficial in the early stages of shock but becomes deleterious if sustained.

## METABOLISM IN SHOCK

Inadequate tissue perfusion results in a decreased supply of oxygen and energy substrates to the cell, with subsequent impairment of energy production. Forced to function anaerobically, the glycolytic cycle produces excess lactic acid, with intracellular acidosis and extracellular acidemia. The intracellular acidosis has

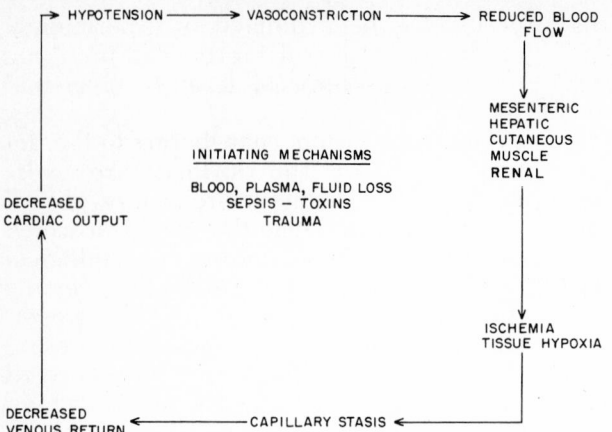

**Figure 1.** Schematic representation of overall cardiovascular changes associated with the shock state.

been implicated in the disruption of lysosomes and the release of lysosomal hydrolysates. These in turn release vasoactive peptides such as bradykinin. Myocardial depressant factor is released from the pancreas, and there is an increased escape of bacteria and their toxic products from the gut. The already impaired integrity of the capillary endothelium is decreased with a subsequent pooling of fluid in the tissues and a reduction in blood volume (Figs. 2 and 3).

Anaerobic glycolysis also results in a reduction in the amount of ATP available for energy dependent cellular functions. The cell membrane leaks potassium extracellularly and sodium intracellularly, resulting in hyperkalemia and edema of the cell and cell organelles. These changes further reduce energy production and another vicious cycle is begun. If these derangements are prolonged, irreversible cellular damage occurs, leading ultimately to vital organ dysfunction and death of the animal.

## REGIONAL BLOOD FLOW

Changes in regional blood flow are an important consideration in the pathophysiology of shock, and much work has been done to determine the changes occurring in the various vascular beds. Among the most important are the cerebral, coronary and splanchnic circulations.

### CEREBRAL CIRCULATION

Measurements of cerebral blood flow in shock show a selective preservation of the cerebral circulation compared to other or-

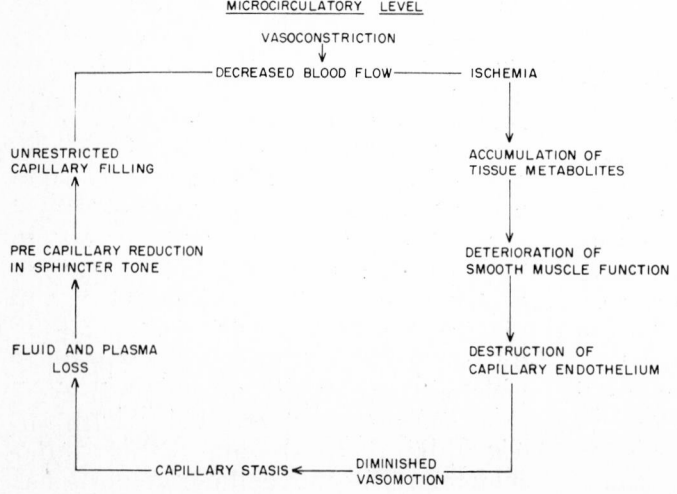

**Figure 2.** Schematic representation of alterations occurring at the microcirculatory level.

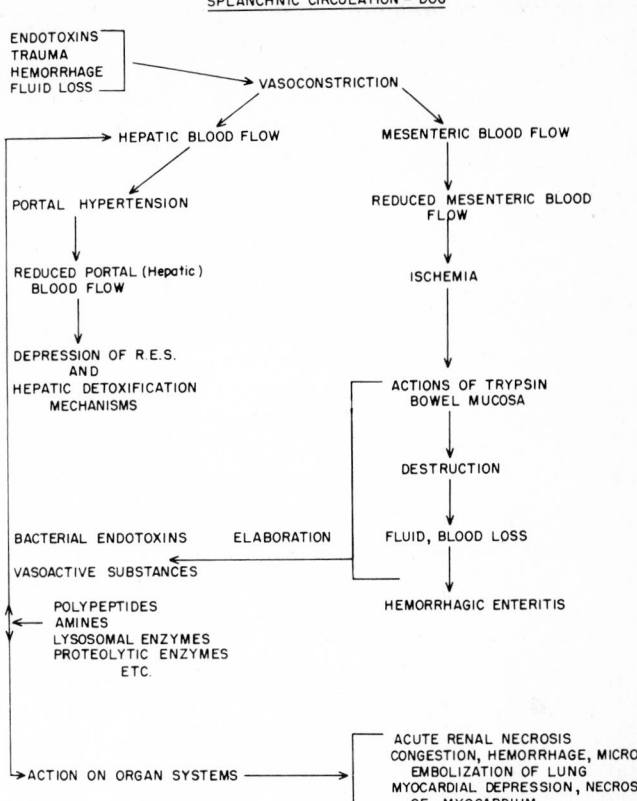

SPLANCHNIC CIRCULATION – DOG

**Figure 3.** Schematic representation of the cycle of changes in the splanchnic circulation of the dog in the refractory or irreversible stage of shock, and their effect on other organ systems.

gans. In the experimental dog, a reduction of blood pressure to a mean of between 45 and 50 mm. Hg produces transitory excitement followed by unconsciousness. Despite a reduced perfusion pressure, permanent ischemic brain damage occurs only when mean systemic blood pressure remains below this level for an extended period of time. Following volume expansion, the dog will regain consciousness and show a normal degree of alertness.

Ischemic brain damage is produced if the blood pressure is maintained at 30 to 35 mm. Hg for more than two hours. Dogs exposed to this degree of hypotension survive for at least 24 hours following volume replacement but irreversible neuronal injury and microvascular changes occur. Despite compensating mechanisms to sustain cerebral flow, it is reduced at these pressures. The relative importance of this reduction compared to the reduction in other organs is not clear, since the contribution of reduced central nervous system perfusion to the failure of other organ systems is difficult to determine.

## CORONARY CIRCULATION AND MYOCARDIAL FUNCTION

The coronary circulation, like the cerebral circulation, is preferentially preserved in shock. An important aspect of this compensatory reaction to hypotension is the elevated ratio of flow to cardiac output.

In induced hemorrhagic shock in conscious experimental animals there is little change in coronary flow following a 34 per cent reduction in cardiac output, although heart rate is increased by 90 per cent over control levels. However, following additional hemorrhage to a total of approximately 50 per cent of blood volume, coronary flow decreases to approximately half of control values. Changes in coronary flow are minimal when the mean systemic pressure is maintained above 70 mm. Hg, but as pressure falls, coronary flow begins to parallel the reduction in cardiac output. The response of the coronary circulation to stressful conditions (tilting, anesthesia, etc.) superimposed on the hypotensive period is important; despite the maintenance of flow to the coronary bed during hemorrhagic shock, its response to further stress is minimal. Therefore, movement of the animal, administration of depressants and induction of anesthesia can produce substantial changes in coronary flow and cardiovascular function.

The contribution of the reduction in myocardial function to the eventual deterioration of the cardiovascular system and the total patient is not clear. Some feel that the final common pathway to death is primarily myocardial dysfunction, while others feel that the deterioration of the peripheral microcirculation is the major change.

Many factors that contribute to the progressive reduction in cardiovascular function are not necessarily due to damaged heart muscle. These include depression due to reduced perfusion, reduction in venous return, reduction in coronary oxygen tension, acidosis and substances released from hypoperfused tissues. A biologically active dialyzable low molecular weight substance, labeled myocardial depressant factor (MDF), has been isolated from animals in shock. This substance depresses myocardial contractility in both isolated cat papillary muscle and the intact animal. MDF production is not limited to hemorrhagic shock but can be found following splanchnic ischemia, pancreatitis and injection of endotoxins.

The reduction in cardiovascular function and increase in heart rate and peripheral resistance are changes which can be reversed following the replenishment of circulating blood volume. Studies of ventricular function following volume replacement show some depression compared to control but indicate that the heart is capable of responding to an increased fluid load. Cardiac output and stroke work can be improved by massive infusion of fluids and blood over a short period of time, even during the irreversible stages of shock. Myocardial stores of adenosine triphosphate, creatinine phosphate and glucose are not depleted, indicating that metabolic energy synthesis and storage is not significantly altered. Myocardial function in fact is sustained for as long as venous return is adequate. Diminished venous return due to vascular fluid leakage seems to be the crucial factor in the final deterioration of cardiovascular function and tissue perfusion.

## MESENTERIC CIRCULATION AND INTESTINAL HEMORRHAGE IN THE DOG

Following volume replacement in severe hemorrhagic, traumatic or septic shock in the dog, a common finding is intestinal necrosis and hemorrhage. This lesion has prompted a great deal of attention to the role of the mesenteric circulation in the refractory phase of shock. Some have referred to this organ as the "shock organ" or "target organ" in the dog, but it may have been a source of erroneous assumption insofar as the pathophysiology of shock in other species, especially man, is concerned.

Splanchnic blood volume represents approximately 20 per cent of the dog's total blood volume and is a potential source of blood for temporary redistribution. Besides the mesenteric circulation, the splanchnic circulation includes the spleen, a very labile organ, and the liver, a vital organ because of its many metabolic and detoxification functions. Flow to all these organs is reduced during shock, but the marked reduction in mesenteric flow results in intestinal ischemia during hypotensive and septic shock. One explanation for this might be the anatomic difference in the distribution of arterial plexuses in the subepithelial area of the villi in the dog as compared to other species.

If the experimental animal is sacrificed during the early phases of hemorrhagic shock prior to reinfusion of fluid, the gastrointestinal tract is found to be reduced in volume and grossly pale and the vessels are smaller than normal. Microscopically the submucosal structures are intact, but changes are noted in the mucosal architecture with some sloughing of the tips of the villi. The microvasculature is devoid of erythrocytes, reflecting the reduced perfusion. However, following the reestablishment of blood volume, the gastrointestinal tract becomes congested, and varying degrees of hemorrhagic enteritis are noted. Blood and fluids are lost into the gut lumen. This stage of shock can be termed the "irreversible" or "refractory" phase, in that replacement in many cases cannot sustain losses, and any response to transfusion and fluid replacement is only temporary. Furthermore, accumulated metabolites washed into the systemic circulation have many profound and deleterious effects on the animal (Fig. 3).

It has been demonstrated that this characteristic hemorrhagic enteritis can be eliminated by the removal of the pancreatic secretions trypsin and chymotrypsin. This has been accomplished surgically in experimental dogs by ligating the pancreatic ducts 8 to 10 days prior to the shock period, or by direct injection of a trypsin inhibitor (Aprotinin, Trasylol®) (Delbay) into the gut prior to the shock state. This is not related to the quantity or type of enzymes in the gut lumen but to ischemic damage and autodigestion of the mucosal barrier, which allows leakage of blood and fluids following reestablishment of intestinal blood flow. Dogs given commercial pancreatic extract subsequent to pancreatic duct ligation show similar changes in the gut following hemorrhagic shock.

## PULMONARY FUNCTION

Three overlapping categories of pulmonary involvement related to trauma and shock can be distinguished in the dog. Obviously in many clinical cases the categorization may not be absolute, and there is inherent danger in attempting such distinction. However, categorization permits discussion of the disparate pathophysiological mechanisms involved. The three categories of pulmonary involvement are (1) progressive pulmonary insufficiency, (2) nonpenetrating blunt pulmonary trauma and (3) pulmonary damage related to refractory or irreversible shock.

### PROGRESSIVE PULMONARY INSUFFICIENCY (PPI)

The effect of cardiovascular shock on pulmonary function has been the subject of extensive clinical and experimental investigations in various species. A major area of consideration has been post-traumatic pulmonary failure or progressive pulmonary insufficiency, a condition first described during the late 1960's. Since then it has become a prominent syndrome, owing primarily to more effective initial shock therapy. Following severe trauma, hemorrhage, sepsis, burns or major operations, more patients are surviving the initial insult but a certain

percentage progress to pulmonary insufficiency and may die of hypoxia. Cases have also been seen in veterinary medicine, owing to the marked improvement in shock therapy and intensive patient care.

Progressive pulmonary insufficiency is a consequence of severe shock and follows successful resuscitation. The time period may be from a few hours to five days after injury. The cases observed in this clinic showed evidence of pulmonary failure within 48 hours. There is considerably more clinical experience in man, and the syndrome is characterized as having four somewhat separable phases.

*Phase one* is the injury and resuscitation period, which includes the low flow aspects of the shock state; transfusion of large volumes of fluid, blood or plasma; and the reestablishment of circulatory homeostasis. It may also include surgery, anesthetic agents, depressants and various other drugs (Table 2). The recovery from the initial insult may proceed uneventfully. Favorable to complete recovery is maintenance of circulating homeostasis without fluid and drug support, reestablishment of near normal acid-base balance and urinary output and maintenance of adequate arterial oxygen tension without oxygen therapy and support of ventilation.

*Phase two* is associated with continued cardiovascular stability and a deterioration in the respiratory status. The initial indication of a respiratory problem is continuous hyperventilation and borderline arterial oxygen tensions. When 100 per cent oxygen is administered, an increase in oxygen tension occurs but not to levels appropriate to the inspired gas mixture. A respiratory al-

*Table 2.  Causative Factors Progressive in Pulmonary Insufficiency*

1. Ischemic pulmonary injury
2. Pulmonary infection
3. Sepsis
4. Aspiration
5. Fluid overload
6. Microemboli
   a. Fat emboli
   b. Multiple transfusions
   c. Intravascular coagulation
   d. Tissue trauma
7. Oxygen toxicity
8. Microatelectasis
9. Cerebral trauma

kalemia exists because of the continuous hyperventilation.

*Phase three* is a progression of respiratory difficulty and includes an increase in tidal volume, hypocarbia and hypoxemia. Rales become detectable, and radiographic signs of diffuse interstitial alveolar involvement are seen. There is a continuous fall in arterial oxygen tension despite 100 per cent oxygen therapy and controlled ventilation.

*Phase four* is terminal hypoxia and hypercarbia with complete pulmonary failure and cardiac arrest. The cause of progressive pulmonary insufficiency is not clearly defined, and many factors have been implicated (Table 2). The most consistent factors appear to be overhydration, microemboli and sepsis. Careful control of the factors favoring the development of PPI is important, since it is extremely difficult to treat when established. Fluid therapy should be monitored to avoid overhydration, and diuretics should be given if rales develop. Filtration of stored blood through a micropore filter during transfusion eliminates exogenous microemboli. Respiratory care in the form of frequent positional changes, coupage and periodic induction of coughing is helpful in preventing retention of secretions, hypostatic congestion and atelectasis.

## NONPENETRATING BLUNT PULMONARY TRAUMA

Injuries of the thorax and upper abdomen caused by automobile accidents or other impact or crushing trauma are commonly seen in small animals. In injuries causing pneumothorax, hemothorax or diaphragmatic hernia, the degree of respiratory distress is related to the extent of lung collapse. The dog may have incurred other injuries that will influence the prognosis, but the latter is generally good subsequent to removal of air or blood and reexpansion of the lung; these injuries seldom involve the lung directly.

Pulmonary contusion results from direct blunt trauma transmitted to the underlying lung, producing rapid compression and reexpansion. This disruption of the pulmonary parenchyma produces tearing of alveoli and small pulmonary capillaries, with interstitial and intra-alveolar hemorrhage. A major vessel tear produces a hematoma. Signs of pulmonary contusion are tachypnea, rales and hemoptysis. The radiographic appearance is one of parenchymal consolidation in a pattern inconsistent with pulmonary edema, pneumonia or aspiration. The prognosis can be good, depending upon the extent of lung involvement. The injury may be so mild that the diagnosis is based solely on radiographic examination. Hemorrhage into an airway with rales and hemoptysis has a very poor prognosis.

Trauma in both the chest and upper abdomen may cause hepatic damage and hemorrhage. Often, the abdominal hemorrhage becomes the prime concern, and the pulmonary involvement becomes obvious only during the resuscitative or operative period. The sequence of events is (1) severe trauma to chest and upper abdomen, (2) hepatic damage, (3) general anesthesia and surgical manipulation of the liver and (4) respiratory failure and death. At necropsy the lungs are not collapsed, are heavy and congested and show interstitial and intraalveolar hemorrhage.

Surgical manipulation of the liver seems to be instrumental in pulmonary involvement and has been observed in man, in this hospital, and in the experimental dog. During surgical repair, emboli of liver tissue, bile salts and toxic or vasoactive substances are released into the vena cava and pass to the lung, resulting in pulmonary insufficiency.

## PULMONARY DAMAGE RELATED TO REFRACTORY SHOCK

Abundant literature exists in reference to pulmonary damage secondary to hemorrhagic, septic, and traumatic shock and shock produced by regional ischemia. The pulmonary pathology includes atelectasis, congestion, alveolar and parenchymal edema and hemorrhage. The pathologic changes are related to the severity and length of the shock state. Contrary to progressive pulmonary insufficiency, the pulmonary lesions are contributory to but are not the primary cause of death. The pathologic changes are part of the overall generalized effect of the shock state on body systems. The two mechanisms which may be involved in the pulmonary pathologic changes in dogs in shock are (1) release and absorption of toxins, vasoactive substances and metabolites from ischemic and damaged tissue (Fig. 3) and (2) infusion of stored blood that contains particulate debris and platelet microaggregations.

In the dog, experimental pulmonary lesions can be prevented by blockage of the actions of trypsin on the gastrointestinal tract. In the clinical situation, pulmonary lesions can be minimized by quickly reestablishing normal blood flow to damaged and ischemic tissues.

The filtration of blood through fiberglass filters (Pall) prevents pulmonary damage during shock. This is through the removal of the microaggregates that would otherwise be filtered by the lung.

## RENAL FUNCTION

Acute failure of renal function in shock is fortunately an uncommon occurrence. It is seen mainly in the older animal with a reduced nephron population; when severe tissue damage has occurred, resulting in the presence of circulating myoglobin and hemoglobin; or in dogs with a combination of hypovolemia and endotoxemia such as can occur in pyometra. The exact pathogenesis of shock-induced renal failure is unclear, but it is generally agreed that prolonged hypotension and poor renal perfusion are the principal factors. Associated with this is the activity of vasoactive hormones such as renin-angiotensin and the catecholamines. Renal vasoconstriction is typically patchy and confined to the cortex and may persist even after the return of systemic blood pressure to normal. If vasoconstriction persists for more than 12 to 24 hours, renal tubular damage occurs.

The changes brought about by prolonged vasoconstriction are manifested clinically by oliguria, isosthenuria, glycosuria and the presence of renal tubular cells in the urinary sediment. Confirmation can be made from the clinical signs of increasing depression, the onset of vomition and signs compatible with metabolic acidosis. Laboratory confirmation is made by increases in serum creatinine, serum potassium and blood urea nitrogen.

In most cases, the changes produced by prolonged hypotension are reversible, and it is uncommon for oliguric renal failure to occur in the shocked animal if adequate volume replenishment is initiated early.

## CLINICAL SIGNS AND INITIAL EVALUATION

The initial evaluation of the animal in shock requires only a few moments and yet is of vital importance in estimating the severity of the shock state and in formulating immediate resuscitative procedures. A rapid physical examination is made almost subconsciously by the experienced clinician, who will examine such factors as the color and refill time of the mucous membranes, state of hydration, character and rate of the pulse, rate and rhythm of the heart and respiration and mental state of the patient. The more abnormal these are, the more severe the state of shock.

The classic signs of shock are related primarily to the integrity and function of the cardiovascular system (Table 3). Tachycardia is often present, reflecting the response of the system to a decreased blood volume. Hypotension is evidenced by a narrowing of the pulse pressure and absence of a pulse in small peripheral arteries such as the labial or dorsal pedal. The mucous membranes may be pale or muddy and usually have a slow refill time. If refill time is longer than 2 seconds, peripheral perfusion is inadequate. Mucous membrane color is of limited use in evaluating the state of shock. Evidence of peripheral and cutaneous vasoconstriction can be detected by palpation of cold extremities. Body temperature varies widely and is consequently of limited use in evaluation. Hyperventilation, which is present in even the mildest shock case, results from acidemia, pain, fear, excitement, hypotension and hypoxia. The character, rate, rhythm and sounds of respiration are important in estimating the extent of pulmonary involvement. Cerebral hypoxia is manifested by a depressed sensorium and in severe cases by dilated pupils. Inadequate muscle perfusion is reflected by generalized weakness.

***Table 3.*** *Signs of Shock*

---

1. Tachycardia
2. Hypotension
   a. Reduced pulse pressure
   b. Poor capillary refill
   c. Muscle weakness
3. Depressed sensorium
4. Hyperventilation
5. Decreased urinary output

---

The severity of the shock state can only be estimated by considering and evaluating all the above parameters. After initial evaluation and resuscitation, a more detailed examination must be made. This includes an accurate history and a thorough examination to facilitate decisions regarding specific therapy or further diagnostic procedures.

## TREATMENT OF SHOCK

Many factors determine the treatment of shock, and each patient requires management on an individual basis. Because of the rapid changes in body functions, management necessitates continuous monitoring and intensive patient care. Therapy may have to be altered repeatedly, since shock is never a self-limiting disease in which therapy can be prescribed and administered on a timed basis until a cure is achieved. The etiology will obviously determine definitive therapy, but there are a number of specific treatments which are carried out as part of the initial therapy of any type of shock.

### PRIORITIES OF SHOCK MANAGEMENT

The essential steps in the initial management of the shocked patient are
1. Insure adequate ventilation and oxygenation.
2. Arrest hemorrhage if present.
3. Initiate volume replacement.
After these initial procedures have been carried out, reevaluation will be necessary to identify the requirements for further therapy. This may include one or more of the following steps:
1. Regulation of acid-base disturbances.
2. Glucocorticosteroids.
3. Antibiotics.
4. Mannitol.
5. Vasoactive drugs.
6. Oxygen.

### SPECIFIC THERAPY

#### AIRWAY

Deficient ventilation is a serious factor contributing to the unfavorable course of shock and may be caused by many factors, e.g., airway obstruction, pulmonary trauma, splinting of respiratory muscles and central nervous system depression. Animals with thoracic trauma may have pulmonary parenchymal hemorrhage, pneumothorax, hemothorax or ruptured diaphragm. All can contribute to hypoxia and respiratory acidosis, exacerbating the concomitant metabolic acidosis.

If, on presentation, the patient shows signs of respiratory distress, the first and most important step is to insure an adequate airway. Endotracheal intubation is the most rapid method; a cuffed tube is essential to prevent aspiration and enables the use of assisted or controlled ventilation if required. Suction should be employed to clear the tracheobronchial tree of excessive mucus, blood or foreign material. If the patient has been successfully intubated, resistance to the tube can be overcome by taping the mouth shut and using a tape roll as a bite block. If ventilation is inadequate, it should be assisted with the use of a self-inflating bag or mechanical ventilator. In many cases, the addition of oxygen to the spontaneously breathing animal may be sufficient to abolish hypoxia. If the animal is conscious and ventilating, oxygen can be administered by intratracheal catheter or mask. Respiratory distress may also be due to pleural rupture or pulmonary contusion, but in these cases, oxygen administration alone will not completely reverse the dyspnea. Since auscultation, percussion and thoracocentesis are sufficient to diagnose pneumothorax, corrective measures should be initiated immediately without confirmatory radiographic examination. Treatment of pneumohemothorax is straightforward. The chest is clipped and prepared with alcohol and iodine. A 16-gauge plastic catheter is inserted bilaterally at midlevel through the 7th or 8th interspace into the thoracic cavity, and air or blood is aspirated. This therapy usually suffices, but chest tube drainage can be established later if air or blood loss is excessive.

#### CONTROL OF HEMORRHAGE

Any obvious hemorrhage should be controlled by direct pressure, bandaging or ligation. Internal hemorrhage may warrant immediate surgical intervention following a period of intensive fluid replacement.

## VOLUME REPLACEMENT

The reestablishment of adequate tissue perfusion is the key to the successful treatment of any form of shock. In most types, this is achieved by the administration of crystalloids, blood or plasma. In cardiogenic and some cases of septic shock, however, rapid fluid replenishment, while important, is not always a major initial consideration.

**Crystalloids.** Lactated Ringer's solution has been commonly used for resuscitation, but several better balanced multielectrolyte solutions are now available. Besides some changes in ionic concentration and a higher osmolarity, the most important change in these fluids is the substitution of gluconate or acetate for lactate. These solutions are recommended in large volumes for initial resuscitation.

Adequate tissue oxygenation results from a combination of perfusion and hemoglobin oxygen saturation. There is, therefore, a limit to the amount of crystalloid that can be infused without hemodilution and a reduction in oxygen delivery, which occurs at hematocrits below 25 per cent. At hematocrits above 50 per cent, blood viscosity is increased, with a subsequent decrease in tissue perfusion; oxygen delivery is reduced despite high hemoglobin levels. While a balanced salt solution is adequate for replacement in most shocked animals, some diseases require definitive ion replacement. A guide to these is given in Table 4.

### Replacement Therapy

ASSESSMENT OF VOLUME REQUIREMENT. Clinical estimations of fluid and blood loss are inaccurate and generally low. Many techniques and sample calculations for estimating fluid deficit have been quoted in the veterinary literature. However, at best these give a very rough assessment and invariably underestimate fluid requirements. This is because they use the normal animal as the basis for their assumptions. It is advisable to ignore such calculations and adopt an open-minded approach to the question of replacement volume in shock. Obviously, a rough volume will have been assessed from such factors as the size of the patient and nature and severity of the shock state and such criteria as skin turgor and initial hematocrit (Hct), but the exact

*Table 4. Guide to Fluid and Electrolyte Therapy in Common Shock States*

1. *Hypovolemic and Hemorrhagic Shock:*
   Give balanced electrolyte solution in mild shock and whole blood or packed cells if the hematocrit falls below 25%. Give plasma if total solids fall below 4 gm./100 ml. If the patient is azotemic, give a potassium-free solution until diuresis occurs or the serum potassium concentration is ascertained.
2. *Severe Diarrhea:*
   Give a balanced electrolyte solution. Sodium bicarbonate if acidotic, and potassium chloride supplementation after diuresis occurs.
3. *Severe Vomiting:*
   Give normal saline. Add KC1 after diuresis up to a maximum of 40 mEq./l. for maintenance.
4. *Renal Failure:*
   Avoid potassium-containing solutions. Give NaCl or ½ strength dextrose and saline until serum potassium concentration is ascertained or diuresis occurs. Animals with chronic renal failure are potassium-depleted. Avoid potassium-containing fluids until shock is controlled and the serum potassium concentration is ascertained. Potassium supplementation may be required.
5. *Ketoacidotic Diabetics:*
   Give normal saline. Add KC1 when diuresis occurs. Large quantities of supplemental potassium will be required, because diabetics are potassium-depleted and insulin lowers serum potassium concentrations.
6. *Pancreatitis and Peritonitis:*
   Balanced electrolyte solution. Supplemental potassium will be required. Give plasma if total solids fall below 4 gm./100 ml.

volume can only be assessed according to the response of the patient as fluids are infused. The technique is in effect a titration of fluid volume against the various monitoring techniques to be described later. Thus, in traumatic shock, a return of heart rate, capillary refill and urine output toward normal might be considered the end point, while in the severely dehydrated patient a return of Hct, total solids (TS), vital signs and urine output toward normal would indicate adequate volume replacement.

ROUTE OF ADMINISTRATION. In the severely depleted patient, fluids should be given as rapidly as possible. This is best achieved with a short (over-the-needle) 16- or 18-gauge catheter in a peripheral vein. In large dogs, two such catheters should be inserted. If central venous pressure is to be measured, a central venous catheter should be inserted when convenient. In most animals, a 17-gauge through-the-needle catheter (e.g., Intracath®) can be used, but in obese dogs and in some cats, direct visual insertion of the catheter into the jugular vein by cutdown catheterization is indicated.

As the monitored parameters begin to return to normal, the rate of administration can be slowed accordingly.

**Maintenance Therapy and Replacement of Ongoing Losses.** Following the return of blood volume to normal, the patient should continue to receive fluids but at a slower rate. Most shock patients continue to lose body fluids at a faster than normal rate because of increased capillary permeability together with increased renal and respiratory losses. Although ADH secretion is increased as a result of hypotension, the kidneys are unable to produce maximally concentrated urine because of changes in renal blood flow which result in reduced medullary osmolarity. The increased respiratory rate of shocked animals results in additional respiratory water loss.

Maintenance volumes of up to 80 ml./kg./24 hours (double the normal value) are usually indicated to replace these losses. Fluids should be given at this rate for 1 to 3 days and reduced as the patient returns to homeostasis. In those animals with diseases associated with an excessive ongoing fluid loss such as peritonitis or diarrhea, additional volume replacement is indicated.

Hypokalemia is a common finding in the postshock state, particularly if adequate volume replacement has been given. While not too important in mild shock, hypokalemia can markedly increase morbidity and recovery time in severely shocked animals. Commercially available fluids contain insufficient potassium to correct this deficit, and for this reason, if the animal is not eating, extra potassium chloride should be added to the maintenance fluids. Provided that the animal is producing urine, 20 mEq. of KCl should be added to every 500 ml. of fluid. This is a safe amount and prevents hypokalemia in all but the most severely affected animal.

**Blood.** Whole blood or packed cells are indicated in severe hemorrhagic and traumatic shock. The need for blood cannot be determined from the initial hematocrit, and the decision to transfuse is usually a matter of clinical judgment. Animals with hemorrhage of up to 30 per cent of blood volume (a category in which most hemorrhagic shock patients fall) do not generally require trans-fusion, crystalloid replacement alone being adequate. Blood transfusion after initial replacement therapy should be considered if hemorrhage is severe. Blood should be stored in citrate-phosphate-dextrose (CPD), be from an A-negative donor or be cross-matched before administration.

The platelet aggregations, fibrin particles and other microparticles which accumulate in stored blood have a deleterious effect upon the pulmonary circulation, especially in animals with preexisting pulmonary damage. To obviate this potentially dangerous phenomenon, blood should be either fresh, transfused into an artery or filtered through commercially available microfilters, which are much finer than the filters on blood administration sets.

**Plasma.** Plasma is essential to maintain oncotic pressure in shock involving severe protein loss such as occurs in peritonitis and large volume hemorrhage. It should be given in sufficient quantity to return plasma protein levels toward normal.

**Colloids.** Therapy with high molecular weight solutions (dextran) has been advocated but is now out of favor in the therapy of most types of shock. Dextrans exert an osmotic effect and rapidly expand the circulating blood volume at the expense of the extracellular fluid; they should therefore be administered together with a balanced salt solution. They are indicated to maintain serum oncotic pressure when plasma is unavailable.

## FURTHER THERAPY

### REGULATION OF ACID-BASE DISTURBANCES

Most shock states are associated with a metabolic acidosis, the degree of acidemia being related to the extent and duration of tissue hypoperfusion. If capable, the shocked animal hyperventilates, often to the extent of being alkalotic on presentation, especially those in traumatic or hemorrhagic shock. The increased ventilation is a response to hypotension, excitement and the developing metabolic acidosis. The ventilatory response, however, is never sufficient to counter fully the metabolic acidosis that develops during severe hypoperfusion states.

Acidosis will be exacerbated in the comatose, anesthetized (spontaneously breathing) patient or in those with severe thoracic trauma. Massive blood transfusions also contribute to the metabolic acidosis.

Recovery from this acid-base disturbance can proceed rapidly following the restoration of tissue perfusion and cardiovascular function. Carbon dioxide will be eliminated by the respiratory system, and the liver rapidly metabolizes lactate and any transfused citrate.

Adjustment of acid-base status is best done after the measurement of arterial pH and $PCO_2$ and the circulation of bicarbonate concentrations and base deficit. The amount necessary to adjust pH to near normal levels is estimated from measured values, and a calculated amount of sodium bicarbonate is given intravenously.* Since blood gas and pH analyses are not often available to the practitioner, sodium bicarbonate solution should be administered at a dosage of 1 to 4 mEq./kg. according to requirements. Half the amount should be given slowly intravenously and the remainder added to the intravenous fluid and given over the next 4 to 6 hours. A mild degree of acidosis is not deleterious or in need of correction. The majority of shocked animals seen in clinical practice do not require bicarbonate therapy.

## GLUCOCORTICOSTEROIDS

Examination of data relating to the use of glucocorticosteroids in shock shows that these drugs have many desirable effects. They help preserve the integrity of cell and cell organelle membranes, favorably alter cellular metabolism, improve oxygen transport, alter microvascular hemodynamics and decrease anaphylotoxin production in septic shock.

Despite recognition of these effects, controversy still exists over the efficacy of glucocorticosteroids in every shock state. This controversy results from the large number of different shock models and experimental protocols and the paucity of objective clinical data confirming their value. While definitive information describing the role of glucocorticosteroids in the treatment of all shock states is still unavailable, these drugs have been shown to be of some value

in the treatment of septic and cardiogenic shock. Their use in other shock states, however, is not contraindicated.

Massive (pharmacologic) doses of the aqueous soluble salts of these drugs must be given very early in the course of treatment to be of maximal benefit.

It has been shown experimentally that if nonpharmacologic doses are used, few of the biochemical defects caused by shock will be reversed or eliminated, and survival of the test animals will be similar to that of the untreated animals. Pharmacologic doses are hydrocortisone, 150 to 300 mg./kg.; prednisolone, 15 to 30 mg./kg.; and dexamethasone, 4 to 8 mg./kg. These doses are not harmful if given for short periods (24 to 48 hours) and can be withdrawn without tapering. These drugs are available for intravenous administration as the water-soluble sodium succinate and phosphate salts. Dexamethasone is also available in a polyethylene glycol suspension (Azium®). Aqueous solutions are expensive but are necessary to achieve rapidly the necessary high tissue concentrations. Because of the economic constraints of veterinary practice, the slower acting and less expensive dexamethasone suspension (Azium), though less than ideal, can be given concurrently with a loading dose of the aqueous salt. The suspension should be given every 4 hours for as long as is necessary.

While use of glucocorticosteroids may be a valuable adjunct in the treatment of shock, it is important to recognize that they are no substitute for specific shock therapy.

## ANTIBIOTICS

The precise role of bacteria and their products in the genesis of clinical shock from causes other than sepsis remains to be elucidated. Broad-spectrum antibiotic therapy is recommended for purely prophylactic reasons, however, following extensive tissue damage and operative procedures. Septic shock cannot be effectively treated until infection is controlled, and in such cases broad-spectrum bactericidal antibiotics such as gentamicin, cephalosporin or ampicillin should be given intravenously in high doses. Specific antibiotic therapy is indicated after the offending organism has been identified and its sensitivity determined.

---

*The bicarbonate requirement is calculated from the following equation: bicarbonate deficit (mEq./liter) = base deficit (mEq./liter) $\times$ 0.3 $\times$ body weight in kg.

## MANNITOL

Renal blood flow ceases when the blood pressure falls below 50 to 60 mm. Hg. The functional result of this is oliguria or anuria. The canine and feline kidney is able to survive several hours of markedly reduced blood flow, and in most animals the defect is only temporary, urine output being restored with the reestablishment of normal blood pressure and renal perfusion. To establish urine output, mannitol should be given only after circulatory stability is achieved and when there is no evidence of lower urinary tract injury. The effect of mannitol is fourfold: (1) it increases circulating blood volume by an osmotic effect, (2) it retains water within the proximal nephrons, (3) it has a direct effect in increasing renal blood flow and (4) it reduces renal cellular edema. Mannitol, which is available as a 25 per cent solution, should be diluted with an equal volume of normal saline and given intravenously (0.5 to 2.0 gm./kg.). Dosage should not exceed 2 gm./kg. in a 24-hour period. If diuresis is not evident within an hour, furosemide should be given intravenously at a dose of 2 mg./kg.; if not effective, the dose should be doubled.

## VASOACTIVE DRUGS

The use of vasopressors has declined as a more rational approach to shock therapy has developed. These drugs should never be used in the initial therapy of hypovolemic or septic shock and should be reserved for extreme situations in which cardiovascular collapse is imminent.

The use of vasodilators such as chlorpromazine or isoproterenol has been suggested for some types of shock; their use is based on the assumption that restoration of blood flow through the tissues rather than the artificial maintenance of arterial pressure is the therapeutic aim. The use of these agents is indicated only after adequate fluid replacement, since they exacerbate hypotension and cardiovascular collapse in the hypovolemic patient. They are indicated in septic shock, especially in the later phases, and have no role in initial shock therapy.

Isoproterenol is a beta stimulator that can be used as a continuous IV drip (Table 5) in septic, traumatic and hypovolemic shock. It increases myocardial contractility and is a vasodilator. Since both these actions result

*Table 5.   Vasoactive Drugs*

| Vasopressors | Dose |
|---|---|
| 1. Methoxamine HCl | 0.2 mg./kg. IV or IM |
| 2. Ephedrine HCl | 10–20 mg. IV or IM |
| 3. Levarterenol bitartrate | (0.2% solution) 1–2 ml. diluted in 100 ml. IV slowly |
| Vasodilators | |
| 1. Isoproterenol HCl* | (0.02% solution) 0.05–0.10 ml. diluted in 100 ml. IV slowly |
| 2. Chlorpromazine HCl | 0.5–1 mg./kg. slowly IV |

*Isoproterenol lowers peripheral vascular resistance and diastolic pressure falls, but the positive inotropic and chronotropic actions of the drug maintain or raise the systolic pressure, although mean pressure is reduced.

in increased tissue perfusion, isoproterenol is a useful drug in refractory shock. It can induce arrhythmias and thus the heart rate and rhythm must be monitored closely. The rate of administration should be adjusted so that, depending on the size of the patient, the heart rate does not rise above 160 to 200 beats/min.

## OXYGEN THERAPY

Oxygen is indicated whenever a reduced arterial oxygen tension has been measured or is suspected. Hypoxemia is manifested by tachypnea in the face of adequate blood volume, the presence of ventricular arrhythmias, restlessness and occasionally cyanosis. These clinical signs must be used in lieu of blood gas measurements, since the necessary equipment is too expensive and complex for most veterinary practices. However, a blood oxygen analyzer that is simple to operate is available commercially. This machine can be used to diagnose hypoxia and to monitor subsequent therapy. An increase in the inspired oxygen concentration from 20 to 30 or 40 per cent provides adequate tissue oxygenation in most cases of hypoxia. However, in some animals 100 per cent oxygen with controlled ventilation may be necessary. Oxygen therapy in the conscious animal must be a compromise between the patient's requirements and the amount of restraint it will tolerate. There are several techniques of oxygen administration.

**Intratracheal Catheters.**   This technique is extremely well tolerated by most animals and is the most efficacious and economic method for long-term administration. After appropriate skin preparation and infiltration of a local anesthetic, a 14- or 16-gauge, 6- to 8-inch plastic catheter is inserted percutaneously into the trachea in the ventral midline of the neck in the midcervical region. The catheter is attached to an oxygen delivery tube and taped to the neck. For long-term administration (> 4 hours), oxygen must be humidified in order to prevent ciliary damage and dehydration through drying of the respiratory mucous membranes. This is best achieved by passing the oxygen through a commercially available humidification unit. Depending on size and respiratory rate, flow rates of 0.5 to 3.0 liters/min. are adequate.

**Nasal Catheters.** This technique is effective for short-term administration in the depressed patient. A soft 5 to 8 Fr. rubber catheter is coated with local anesthetic cream and passed up the nose, so that the tip comes to lie in the nasopharynx. The catheter is then taped in place. Before insertion, the catheter should be measured against the patient and marked to insure accurate placement in the nasopharynx. Flow rates of 2 to 4 liters/min. are generally adequate. This technique should not be used for more than 4 hours without humidified oxygen.

**Masks.** Masks are useful in emergency situations when intubation is difficult or impractical. They require high flow rates to prevent carbon dioxide accumulation and have the disadvantage that many patients resent them, struggle and negate the benefits of additional oxygen.

**Oxygen Compartments.** Mobile oxygen compartments consisting of a sealed cage, air conditioner, $CO_2$ absorber, humidifier, thermostat and oxygen analyzer are now commercially available. These units enable the temperature, humidity and oxygen concentration within the sealed cage to be accurately regulated.

Sealed oxygen cages have no humidity or temperature control but are much cheaper. Oxygen concentrations are related to flow, size of cage and frequency of opening. Overheating of the patient is common in these units.

A pediatric incubator is useful for oxygen supplementation in the small dog, cat or exotic animal. These units have a more effective temperature and humidity control but suffer many of the same disadvantages as oxygen cages.

Oxygen concentrations above 40 per cent are rarely achieved in any of these units; while this concentration is adequate for most patients, oxygenation ultimately depends upon the ventilatory capacity of the patient. If ventilation is inadequate, controlled ventilation should be considered.

## GENERAL PRECAUTIONS IN SHOCK THERAPY

1. *Never permit unnecessary movement of the patient.* Rapid changes in position, such as lifting, rotation or rapid movement on a cart, are contraindicated. Shocked animals' compensatory reflex mechanisms for both cardiovascular and respiratory adjustment are minimal; positional changes which are of no consequence in the normal animal can be disastrous in the shock state.

2. *Never delay therapy.* Always insure an adequate airway and administer intravenous fluids. If surgery is needed, it should be limited to procedures essential for correction of the initiating factors. Additional diagnostic procedures such as radiographic examination should only follow initial resuscitative procedures.

3. *Delay analgesic administrations.* Analgesics and sedatives should not be given until the condition of the animal has been carefully assessed and volume replacement initiated. All narcotics, tranquilizers and barbiturates depress cardiovascular and respiratory function. Restlessness and delirium may be due to hypoxia, not discomfort or pain, indicating the need for oxygen, not depressants.

4. *Never subject the animal to deep planes of anesthesia.* All the currently used inhalation anesthetics depress the sympathetic nervous and cardiovascular systems. As with the administration of other depressants, anesthesia must be administered carefully and only in concentrations that will produce the minimal necessary plane. *No* situation requires immediate surgical treatment before an airway is established, external hemorrhage controlled and volume replacement commenced.

### EPILOG TO THERAPY

It is not enough to give the shocked patient intravenous fluids, place it in a cage and leave observation and care to a less skilled person. Proper care demands intensive therapeutic and nursing support. After initial resuscitation and therapy, continuous attention to the patient's comfort, warmth, nutrition, oxygenation and hydration often make the difference between life and death. The therapy of shock may last from a few hours to several days. Close observation and therapy must not cease until the patient is stable. Stability is evidenced by the maintenance of cardiovascular function without fluid or drug support, a return of normal urine output, maintenance of adequate oxygenation at normal ventilatory rates and improvement of acid-base balance.

### SUMMARY OF SHOCK THERAPY

1. Insure adequate airway and ventilation.
2. Control serious external hemorrhage.
3. Place large-bore catheter in a peripheral vein. Obtain a blood sample for basic biochemical data, Hct, TS and crossmatching.
4. Begin volume replacement at a rate commensurate with degree of hypotension.
5. Conduct rapid physical examination. Decide on further diagnostic and therapeutic procedures.
6. Insert catheters to monitor CVP and urine output.
7. Determine response to initial therapy; record all parameters monitored and treatment given.
8. Begin appropriate adjunctive therapy:
   a. Acid-base correction
   b. Antibiotics
   c. Steroids
9. Give blood or plasma, if indicated.
10. Reassess animal's condition after therapy and reevaluate diagnosis as necessary.

## MONITORING TECHNIQUES

Monitoring, derived from the Latin *monere*—to warn, is the observation, measurement and recording of clinical and physiological variables. Shocked patients present a complex of constantly changing physiological functions, and it is essential for the clinician to be continually aware of these, so that therapy can be changed in response to the patient's changing needs. For these reasons, monitoring must be considered an integral part of shock therapy.

Monitoring can conveniently be divided into two types: clinical, which requires skilled staff but very little equipment, and physiological, which requires more equipment but which reveals correspondingly more information on specific organ function.

### CLINICAL MONITORING

**Temperature.** The temperature of the shocked patient can vary widely. Temperature is best monitored with a continuously recording electronic thermometer and thermistor probe, since this avoids repeatedly disturbing the patient. If the temperature falls below 100° F., the patient should be warmed, using a heating pad, blanket or lamp. Replacement fluids are best prewarmed to 37° C., since cold fluids further reduce body temperature, especially when given in large volumes.

Subjective evaluation of the temperature of the extremities of patients in shock is a time-honored means of assessing peripheral circulation. Skin temperature correlates well with cardiac output and peripheral blood flow and can be used as a means of prognosis during treatment. This technique is valuable in veterinary practice because it is rapidly performed, is noninvasive and does not require highly skilled personnel or expensive equipment.

The maximal value of this technique is achieved if frequent measurements are made and recorded during resuscitation. Temperature can be taken either with an electronic thermometer and thermistor probe or with a mercury thermometer, having a range of 70 to 110° F. (15 to 45° C.). Measurements are most conveniently made between the toe pads. The temperature of the skin between the pads is usually 1 to 5° less than that of the rectum and approximately 27 to 30° F. (14 to 16° C.) greater than normal room temperature (66 to 74° F.). In shock the skin/rectal temperature difference is greater than 5°. As the animal responds favorably to treatment, peripheral circulation is improved and the temperature differential returns toward normal. These measurements provide accurate prognostic information regarding the effectiveness of therapy.

**Pulse.** The return of pulse rate rhythm and character toward normal as therapy progresses in the shocked patient is a good prognostic sign. After homeostasis is achieved, changes in the pulse can be the first sign of infection, hypoxia or ongoing fluid loss. For these reasons it is important that the pulse be checked and findings recorded frequently throughout therapy. Because of the redistribution of blood flow in shock, it is advisable to check the pulse in more than one site. For example, while a pulse may still be detected in the femoral artery, its absence in a peripheral artery is indicative of serious hypovolemia or intense vasoconstriction.

**Respiration.** Changes in rate, rhythm and character should be noted carefully. A gradual increase in rate may be the first sign of hypoxia or of the development of pulmonary diseases such as shock lung, pulmonary edema, aspiration pneumonia or secondary pneumonia. Regular auscultation of all lung fields is important. Fluid rales or an increased harshness in the respiratory sounds can be the first sign of overhydration, incipient pulmonary disease or a failing myocardium. Most shocked patients will show an initial increase in the rate and depth of ventilation unless they are depressed or injured to such an extent that they cannot respond. A return of rate and tidal volume toward normal is a favorable prognostic sign.

**Palpation.** Palpation tends to be neglected as a monitoring technique in the critical patient. Palpation can be used as a rough assessment of the temperature of the extremities. In the hypovolemic animal the extremities are cool, indicating lowered peripheral perfusion; rewarming is an indication of an improved circulation, a favorable response to therapy and increased heat loss to the environment. Careful palpation of the extremities is also useful in detecting edema. Asymmetrical temperature differences may indicate inflammation or locally impaired circulation.

**Capillary Refill.** Capillary refill is an indication of peripheral perfusion. A refill time of more than 2 seconds is abnormal, indicating hypotension, hypovolemia or peripheral vasoconstriction. Injected membranes indicate sepsis or polycythemia, while pale membranes indicate anemia or poor tissue perfusion. Membrane color is a poor indicator of tissue perfusion and oxygenation. Cyanosis is usually a very late indicator of hypoxemia.

## PHYSIOLOGICAL MONITORING

**Hematocrit and Total Solids.** The serial measurement of these parameters is one of the simplest and most effective shock monitoring techniques. Although individually these parameters provide little definitive information about the circulating blood volume, when used conjointly they provide some of the information necessary to manipulate volume replacement efficiently. The hematocrit (normal 35 to 48 per cent) is important in determining changing red cell plasma ratios, and the total solids (normal 5.5 to 8.0 gm./100 ml.) are rough indicators of plasma protein concentration.

Serial measurements are indicated in all shock patients but are of less use in hemorrhagic shock than in other types of shock. If the animal has suffered water loss, both the hematocrit (Hct) and the total solids (TS) will be increased. In cases of plasma loss through exudation such as in peritonitis or thermal burns, the Hct is increased while the TS may be normal or low. In hypovolemia with anemia, the Hct may be misleadingly normal while the TS is usually increased. The Hct and TS are not markedly changed in early hemorrhagic shock; these values fall only as fluid compartment shifts compensate for loss of blood volume or as crystalloid replacement therapy progresses. The initial Hcts cannot therefore be used to assess the extent of hemorrhage. Following therapy, the TS returns to normal more rapidly than does the Hct, and a steady or increasing TS therefore provides an early indication that transcapillary loss may have ceased.

The difference in Hct between a peripherally and a centrally drawn blood sample can be of prognostic value in assessing the response to therapy. Normally the central Hct is about 3 per cent less than the peripheral. Differences in excess of this indicate peripheral hypoperfusion. If the differential continuously increases, the prognosis is grave. Most often this can be deduced from other signs, but, on the other hand, a narrowing may be among the first indications of an improved peripheral circulation.

During volume replacement, serial Hct and TS determinations will indicate whether the most appropriate replacement fluid is blood, plasma or a balanced salt solution. The Hct and TS should be maintained within the normal range, if possible, but a decrease in Hct to 25 per cent can be tolerated without a significant decrease in tissue oxygen delivery in animals with normal pulmonary function. Pulmonary edema is not usually a threat until the TS falls below 4 gm./100 ml. Conversely, the Hct should not be permitted to rise above 50 per cent, since tissue perfusion is decreased and cardiac work is increased because of the increased blood viscosity.

**Electrocardiogram.** Ideally, an electrocardiogram should be taken for all shocked animals at or soon after admission to act as a baseline with which to compare later changes. Depending on the cause of shock, animals can demonstrate a wide range of electrocardiographic abnormalities. Most result from electrolyte imbalances, hypoxia or cardiac contusion. Tachycardia can result from pain, fever, anoxia or hypovolemia. Premature ventricular contractions (PVCs) are seen in hypoxia and cardiac contusion. Oxygen therapy may eliminate arrhythmias caused by hypoxia. If abnormalities are detected, a complete diagnostic electrocardiogram should be taken, but for monitoring, lead II is sufficient.

**Central Venous Pressure.** The measurement of central venous pressure (CVP) has become an invaluable aid in estimating the fluid requirements of the shocked patient. It is measured from the anterior vena cava and depends on the volume of blood returning to the heart (the effective blood volume) and the efficiency of the cardiac pump. An alteration in either of these factors will tend to change the CVP. A low CVP implies a deficit in the circulating blood volume (note that it only *implies* a deficit, it does not indicate one) and a high CVP implies a failing myocardium or fluid overload. CVP measurement should always be used in the severely shocked patient or when a patient fails to respond to what is believed to be adequate volume replacement. The CVP is particularly helpful in the older animal or when cardiac failure complicates the clinical picture.

The CVP is measured using a catheter inserted via the external jugular vein into the anterior vena cava. The strictest aseptic precautions should be used whenever a catheter is introduced. Failure to do so has resulted in a large number of cases of fatal bacteremia from infected catheters. Several varieties of plastic catheters and cannulae

for recording CVP are produced commercially. The shortest catheter that will reach the anterior vena cava should be used, because the sensitivity of CVP recording and the rate at which intravenous fluids can be given through the catheter are a function of its length and diameter. In addition, myocardial injury due to the introduction of too long a catheter has been reported. A saline manometer is the simplest and cheapest method of recording central venous pressure. Its two main disadvantages are that it does not permit a permanent continuous record to be made and that a rise in pressure fills the catheter with blood, which is liable to clot. After insertion, the intravenous catheter is connected via a three-way stopcock to the manometer, and the third limb of the stopcock is connected to an infusion set from which the system can be primed and infusions can be given when a recording is not being taken. A fluctuation of 2 to 5 mm. in the saline level with each respiration indicates that the catheter tip is correctly sited and that an accurate reading is being taken.

The actual level of CVP recorded varies widely from individual to individual and also depends on the level at which the zero of the manometer is set. The most satisfactory zero level is the center of the sternum with the dog or cat lying on its side. With this as zero, the CVP of the dog or cat normally varies between 0 and 5 cm. of water. Values consistently above 8 to 10 cm. usually indicate an expanded blood volume, and if this value is obtained, fluid administration should be slowed or stopped. Values above 15 cm. water indicate right heart failure. A rising CVP in the face of falling blood pressure, reduced palpable pulse pressure, increased capillary refill time and rales indicates myocardial failure, overhydration or cardiac tamponade.

Several factors should be borne in mind when evaluating CVP:

1. Use trends rather than single values.
2. Measure at the same level with the patient in the same position.
3. Changes of less than 3 cm. water between readings, unless consistent, are not significant and can be due to positional changes.
4. The CVP fluctuates markedly in sequence with respiration when controlled ventilation is used.
5. Vasoactive drugs can cause a veno-

constriction that can result in a large incremental rise in CVP.

6. Mechanical occlusion of the catheter by clots or kinks can cause a false elevation of CVP. If the column of fluid does not fluctuate freely with respiration during measurement, mechanical flaws should be suspected.

7. When not in use, the catheter should be flushed with heparinized saline (2000 IU/liter every 6 hours) to prevent clot formation.

CVP monitoring is more a guide to overhydration than an indication of adequate fluid administration.

**Urine Output.** The rate of urine production is proportional to the GFR and is therefore a measure of renal perfusion and, indirectly, of arterial blood pressure. GFR is maintained at a constant level over a wide range of blood pressures but ceases when arterial pressure falls below 60 mm. Hg. Reduced urine output is therefore an indicator of reduced organ perfusion and hypotension; likewise a return of urine output in a previously anuric animal is a good prognostic sign.

Urine output is best monitored with an indwelling urinary catheter. It is far better to possess accurate knowledge of the rate of urine formation than to adopt a wait-and-see attitude or attempt to ascertain whether the animal is forming urine by palpating the bladder or compressing the abdomen. By the time oliguria has been confirmed using these latter techniques, it may well be too late to reestablish renal function pharmacologically.

In the male dog, catheter placement is simple. A soft rubber urinary catheter is inserted and secured by means of a piece of tape attached to the end of the catheter. The tape is then sutured to the prepuce. A pediatric 8 French Foley catheter is suitable for most female dogs. A length of stainless steel wire placed in the catheter lumen adds stability to facilitate insertion. After catheter placement, the bladder should be emptied of all urine and monitoring should be started. For continuous measurement, the catheter is attached to a fluid delivery tube and an empty intravenous fluid bottle, which acts as a graduated collection reservoir. For intermittent measurement (in the more active patient), the catheter can be occluded with a plastic plug (needle cover

or venoset cover) and emptied hourly with a syringe and three-way stopcock.

The normal cat or dog should produce 0.5 to 1.0 ml. of urine/kg. body weight/hour. If this volume is not produced after fluid volume expansion has been achieved and blood pressure has returned to normal, a test dose of a diuretic such as mannitol or furosemide should be considered, provided that the bladder is not ruptured.

Sterile technique is vital in urinary catheter placement. In order to minimize the chance of infection, the catheter should be removed as soon as the patient is stable, i.e., when urine production has been normal for several hours or when the patient is able to urinate without soiling itself.

**Blood Pressure.** Blood pressure monitoring by either direct or indirect means is a feasible and clinically useful technique. Direct monitoring requires arterial catheterization, but the measurements are accurate and the catheter can also be used to obtain arterial blood samples. An 8-inch 16- to 19-gauge catheter is placed either percutaneously or by cutdown into the femoral artery. An injection cap is applied to the catheter and both are then taped to the animal's leg. An 18-gauge needle attached by a short length of tubing to a sphygmomanometer is inserted through the injection cap, permitting measurements to be made as necessary. When not in use, the catheter should be flushed with heparinized saline solution every 4 hours to prevent occlusion.

Indirect measurements of blood pressure can be made from the dorsal pedal artery using an Arteriosonde® sphygmomanometer. This device is not highly accurate but provides clinically useful information. The pressure obtained depends to some extent on the method of measurement, but the range 90 to 140 mm. Hg is considered normal in the dog and cat. As with CVP measurement, however, it is not the specific value that is important but the return to normal as therapy progresses.

Blood pressure can also be estimated by palpation. Although the values obtained are only approximations, the technique is clinically useful. If the femoral pulse is absent or very difficult to detect, blood pressure is 50 mm. Hg or less. If the femoral pulse is detectable but weak and the dorsal pedal pulse is absent or barely detectable, the blood pressure is between 50 and 70 mm. Hg.

**Blood Chemistries.** Except in simple hemorrhagic shock, blood chemical changes should be monitored. A knowledge of the specific disturbance associated with individual diseases is obviously essential, but some disturbances are common to many diseases and should be monitored routinely. Included in the parameters which might be monitored at least once daily are electrolytes ($Na^+$, $K^+$, $Cl^-$); enzymes (SGPT, SAP); and creatinine and/or BUN. Commercial "profiles," which are often cheaper than the cost of individual tests, provide a good method of monitoring these biochemical changes.

## CONCLUSION

Although physiologic monitoring is a valuable adjunct to patient care, it cannot replace close patient observation by trained personnel. Every shocked patient needs continuous monitoring until it is stable, but the extent and type must be adapted to the patient's requirements. No matter what parameters are monitored, it is mandatory that they be recorded and form a part of the patient's hospital records. It is of vital importance to keep a record of all signs, monitored parameters, laboratory studies and therapy. One person cannot remember all the facts pertinent to a case. If an adequate record is kept, trends can be noted and appropriate therapeutic measures taken. Many expensive and complex monitoring devices are available, but, as with all sophisticated equipment, they are no substitute for clinical acumen and careful patient observation.

*List of Equipment Described in Text:*
Ambubag: Airshields Inc., Hatboro, PA.
Arteriosonde Sphygmomanometer: Hoffmann La-Roche, Inc., Cranbury, NJ.
Azium (dexamethasone): Schering Pharmaceuticals, Bloomfield, NJ
Chest Trocar and Cannula: Sherwood Medical Industries, Ltd., St. Louis, MO.
Continuous Recording Thermometer: Yellow Springs Corp., A.H. Thomas, Philadelphia, PA.
Cutdown Catheter: Becton-Dickinson, Rutherford, NJ.
CVP Manometer Set: Bard-Parker (division of Becton-Dickinson), Rutherford, NJ.
Foley Catheter: (8 Fr. Pediatric) Bard-Parker (division of Becton-Dickinson), Rutherford, NJ.
Goldberg Refractometer: American Optical Company, Buffalo, NY.
Injection Cap: Becton-Dickinson, Rutherford, NJ.
Intensive Care Oxygen Therapy Unit: Kirschner Scientific, Seattle, WA.
Intracath (through-the-needle catheter): Deseret Pharmaceutical Company, Sandy, UT.
Jet Humidifier: #217-6003-800 (oxygen humidification unit), Ohio Medical Products, Madison, WI.
Longdwell Catheter (over-the-needle catheter): Becton-Dickinson, Rutherford, NJ.
Oxygen Analyzer: Biomarine Industries, Malvern, PA.
Pall Filter: Pall Corporation, Glen Cove, Long Island, NY.
Rubber Urinary Catheter: Sherwood Medical Industries, Ltd., St. Louis, MO.
Sphygmomanometer: 9068D Medisco Inc., Broadway, New York, NY.
Squeeze Bag and Non-rebreathing Valve: North American Drager, Telford, PA.
Temperature Pads: Gaymar Ind., Buffalo, NY.

---

# CAUSES AND TREATMENT OF NEONATAL DEATHS

J. E. MOSIER, D.V.M.
*Manhattan, Kansas*

The adage "an ounce of prevention is worth a pound of cure" is especially applicable to the problem of neonatal death. Prevention is best approached by acquiring an understanding of the contributing factors and causes of neonatal disease. Admittedly, there are many facets which are either unknown or poorly understood. Current theses may be proved completely erroneous as new information is compiled and integrated with existing information. Nevertheless, recommendations designed to prevent death in the newborn must be based on and supported by existing knowledge.

For purposes of this discussion, the term "neonate" will apply to puppies from birth to three weeks of age. Problems encountered more commonly in puppies after three weeks of age will not be discussed.

Available statistics indicate a neonatal loss of approximately 23 per cent in the first three weeks of life under average kennel conditions. More carefully planned and operated kennels report a loss of approximately 10 per cent. Analysis of the difference between the two figures suggests that selection of breeding stock, nutrition, housing, sanitation and kennel management are critical factors.

## SELECTION OF BREEDING STOCK

Breeding stock should be assessed from the standpoint of reproductive capability. In the absence of specific information concerning a particular individual, the reproductive history of both the dam and sire may prove beneficial. Constant inbreeding will affect the reproductive potential and the vigor of the offspring unless breeding stock are selected with these points in mind. Age of the breeding stock may influence the death rate. The very young bitch is subject to prolonged nesting, whereas the old bitch is more likely to exhibit prolonged parturition. Practical experience suggests that the prime reproductive period ranges from two to six years. Exceptions to this rule are frequent; however, in assessing neonatal loss, the age of the dam as a contributing factor may be very real.

## NUTRITION

Malnutrition must be considered as the primary cause of puppy mortality. Malnutrition may occur in the bitch as a result of inadequate intake, food of low digestibility, deficiency of certain ingredients, unbalanced diet and inability of the bitch to absorb certain nutrients. Malnutrition in the neonate is most likely to result from ineffectual nursing but may be due to inadequate intake, abnormal quality of the milk, oversupplementation and inability to digest the milk.

Examination of the blood from the bitch for the values of hemoglobin and total protein may reflect the adequacy of diet or health of the individual. Values below 10 and 5 gm./100 ml., respectively, permit the prediction of above average puppy mortality. To the experienced clinician, the appearance of the hair coat activity and general condition of the bitch will reflect the state of nutrition.

Good quality balanced dog food is generally quite adequate for reproduction. Supplemental protein may be necessary in toy breeds, in parasitized bitches and in those females which are less than optimally nourished at time of breeding. Puppy vigor correlates well with intake of animal protein. The addition of 0.25 to 1 oz. of raw liver three times weekly to the bitches' diet may be highly beneficial.

Failure of the neonate to gain weight is frequently indicative of malnutrition. Strong vigorous puppies show weight gain within 24 hours of birth and should continue to gain daily throughout the neonatal period. A rule of thumb is the doubling of weight by the 10th day. A more precise guide is to anticipate the gain of 2.2 gm./day for each kilogram of anticipated adult weight. Puppies which do not gain as anticipated or which appear small should have supplemental feeding with simulated bitch's milk starting at 12 hours of age.

Puppies which succumb during the neonatal period and which have been subjected to prenatal malnutrition will have liver:brain ratios of less than 1.5:1 and a relative absence of perirenal fat. While genetics may contribute to abnormal liver:brain ratios, the most common factor would seem to be inadequate nutrition. Puppies born alive of malnourished, diseased or physiologically abnormal bitches are depleted at birth. The characteristic vigor and muscle tone of the healthy pup is absent. Such puppies should be placed in an environmental temperature of 85° to 90° F. and given small quantities of simulated bitch's milk at two-hour intervals during the first 48 hours. The milk may be enriched with glucose and liver juice. If untreated, the puppies are usually ineffectual nursers, rapidly become hypoglycemic and may die 6 to 36 hours after birth.

Puppy deaths occurring within the first 24 hours of birth may reflect physiologic immaturity. Incomplete development of the terminal air space, weak chest muscles, hypoglycemia, hypoprothrombinemia and periodic respiration are suggestive. Necropsy of the puppies may reveal nonfunctioning areas of lung tissue. This finding suggests either immaturity or aspiration of amniotic fluid. Abnormal liver:brain ratio is a common finding.

### HYPOXIA

The intensity of the initial gasp of air may be critical. The alveolar spaces are only potential until the puppy begins the act of breathing with the first inspiration. Secretions within the alveolus produce a cohesive action which must be overcome by the inspiratory force. In the human infant it is estimated that a force equal to that exerted by a column of water 15 to 23 mm. high is needed to expand the lung alveoli fully. Lesser force will result in a more gradual expansion and sometimes marginal respiration during the first 72 hours of life.

Pressure on the umbilical vessels caused by a large pup in a small birth canal with delayed delivery or premature separation of the placenta may initiate an inspiratory act.

When the puppy is still in the birth canal and especially if the presentation is breech, inhalation of placental fluids will occur, thus resulting in embarrassment to the respiratory function during the first few days of life. Aspiration of pharyngeal fluid, swinging the puppy in a manner designed to remove fluid from the bronchial tree or enrichment of inspired air with oxygen will enhance survival.

Restraining the puppy at a 45 degree angle with the head lower than the rear quarters for a period of 30 to 60 minutes may be helpful. This is best accomplished by gently taping the puppy to a board and then placing the puppy in an incubator with the board at the proper angle. Resentment of restraint will cause the puppy to cry. The resulting inspiratory pressure will serve to expand nonfunctional alveoli, and the position is conducive to postural drainage.

It is important to note that the hypoxic puppy will be an ineffectual nurser. Adequate airway, expanded alveoli and effective respiration are essential to puppy vigor. Immaturity and pulmonary abnormalities such as hyaline membrane disease should be considered when hypoxia exists.

### HYPOTHERMIA

During the first three weeks of life, puppies are particularly subject to environmental temperature changes. The thermoregulatory system of the newborn lacks the capability of preventing a serious drop in rectal temperature. Given an inadequate intake of nutrients, abnormal physical condition or maternal neglect, the puppy's body temperature will fall. Cold skin temperature may result in bitch culling. The puppy becomes separated from and is ignored by the bitch. Rectal temperatures below 94° F. are accompanied by ineffectual nursing. Affected puppies cry in a plaintive manner and if untreated will die in a matter of hours.

Treatment consists of warming the puppy slowly. The radiant heat of the human body can be utilized by placing the puppy in an inside coat pocket. Other methods include the use of an incubator with rheostat control, heat lamps, heating pads or warm water. Care should be taken to warm the puppy slowly. Too rapid warming increases the oxygen needs for the peripheral tissue while the slow respiratory and cardiac rates preclude adequate tissue oxygenation.

The warming process should require 1 to 3 hours, depending on the degree of chilling. The oral administration of 5 to 10 per cent glucose can be utilized to prevent dehydration and hypoglycemia during the warming process. A subcutaneous injection of equal parts 5 per cent glucose and lactated Ringer's solution at the rate of 1 cc. per 30 grams of body weight, along with 0.01 to 0.10 mg. Mephyton® has proved beneficial. It is best given as the rectal temperature approaches 94° F. on its return to normal levels.

Puppies which have been rejected by the bitch because of cold skin temperature will be accepted by the bitch once the skin temperature is within normal range for young puppies.

### HEMORRHAGIC DISEASE

Puppies dying 24 to 96 hours following birth, with signs of lethargy, weakness and rapid decline in condition, should be examined for hemorrhage. Hemorrhagic lesions may occur on lips or tongue, in the subcutaneous or pulmonary tissue, and intraperitoneally.

Recognition that all newborn puppies are borderline hypoprothrombinemic will support a decision to administer vitamin $K_1$ to the remaining puppies and to prescribe vitamin K to other bitches in the kennel during the last 30 days of gestation.

Intraperitoneal hemorrhage within the first 24 hours may indicate that the bitch has severed the umbilical cord too close to the body and subsequent retraction of the umbilical vessel into the peritoneal cavity has resulted in fatal hemorrhage. Differential diagnosis includes the finding of the stump of blood vessel and clotted blood.

Petechial hemorrhage in the tissue may result from toxemia, bacteremia or hypoxia. Puppies dying of cardiopulmonary failure will have petechial or ecchymotic hemorrhage, especially of the lungs. Ecchymotic hemorrhage of the kidneys, liver and sometimes of the lungs is characteristic of puppy viremia. Pulmonary hemorrhage is a common finding where chilled puppies are warmed too rapidly. Pericardial hemorrhage occurs when puppies are subjected to extremely high temperature ranges, 39.5° to 40° C. (103° to 104° F.). Because of the variety of causes, the significance of hemorrhage in the neonate will be dependent on thorough history, complete examination and laboratory findings.

## "TOXIC MILK" SYNDROME

A crying, bloated puppy, age four days to two weeks, should be examined for a red edematous rectum. These signs, associated with an apparently healthy bitch, are suggestive of uterine subinvolution and the "toxic milk" syndrome. Differential diagnosis between this condition and sick puppies associated with metritis in the bitch is dependent on the presence or absence of illness in the bitch. Affected puppies should be separated from the mother, placed in an environmental temperature of 85° to 90° F. and given 5 per cent glucose orally until the bloating has receded. When bloat is no longer present, simulated bitch's milk is given at regular intervals for the remainder of a 24-hour period. Abdominal palpation of the bitch may reveal an enlarged uterus or uterine segment. Intrauterine instillation of a furacin/estrogen combination is followed by two days of therapy with ergotamine and four days of systemic antibiotic treatment.

The puppies can be returned to the bitch on the day following institution of therapy.

The routine administration of oxytocin or ergotamine and penicillin following whelping has proved generally effective in preventing subinvolution in the bitch and an associated "toxic milk" syndrome in the neonate.

## PUPPY VIREMIA

Puppy viremia, as described by Carmichael (1970), is due to a herpesvirus that is said to replicate optimally at a temperature of 95° to 96° F. Since the rectal temperature of the neonatal puppy does not reach the 101° F. characteristic of the adult until the third to fourth week, it is reasonable to assume that the critical period for puppy viremia may be related to the low rectal temperature of the neonate. Puppies reaching 21 days of age are not likely to develop the disease. Puppy viremia is characterized by sudden illness, constant crying and pain, followed by death 12 to 18 hours after the onset of clinical signs. Necropsy lesions include characteristic hemorrhage in the kidney, pulmonary congestion, hemorrhage of the liver and sometimes an accumulation of clear fluid in the pleural cavity. Puppies are usually affected between the ages of 8 and 20 days. Treatment consists of placing the affected litter in an environmental temperature of 100° F. for a minimum of three hours. During this period, close supervision is essential. Water should be given orally at 15-minute intervals to avoid dehydration. After the three-hour period, puppies are placed in an environmental temperature of 95° F. for the remainder of the 24-hour treatment. Any puppy which is showing signs (i.e., crying) has, in our experience, already suffered hemorrhage; should it survive, it will become a prime candidate for chronic kidney disease during the first year of life. As a consequence, our current recommendation is to treat only those who have not started the constant crying.

## PUPPY SEPTICEMIA

Puppy septicemia may occur at any time between the ages of 1 and 40 days. Very young puppies become hypothermic, hypoglycemic and dehydrated. Death usually occurs 12 hours after onset of the illness. Older puppies have abdominal distention and rapid respirations, cry intermittently and die after 18 hours. One puppy affected is soon followed by a second puppy in a matter of a few hours and so on until most, if not all, of the litter is affected. Necropsy lesions may include gas-distended intestines and congestion of the body organs. The typical syndrome includes normal gestation and parturition, normal energetic breast feeding, and puppies which become prostrate and die 24 to 48 hours after birth. Frequently, the total litter is dead by the sixth day.

A positive diagnosis is based on culture of the heart blood within one hour of death. Organisms which have been incriminated include: *E. coli, Pseudomonas, Streptococcus, Staphylococcus* and *Klebsiella.* Streptococcal infections have been particularly prominent in kennel situations. Septicemia is frequently associated with inadequate ventilation, high humidity and bacterial contamination.

Treatment consists of separating the puppies from the bitch and placing them in an environmental temperature of 85° to 90° F. Lactated Ringer's solution is given subcutaneously, and elixir of Benadryl and chloramphenicol, orally. If bloating is extreme, trocarization with a 22-gauge needle is indicated to provide essential relief. Polymyxin and streptomycin, instead of chloramphenicol, have been used in selected cases.

Prevention of puppy septicemia is dependent on sanitation, environmental humidity control and adequate ventilation as well as control of infection in the bitch. Failure to ingest colostrum due to ineffectual nursing may predispose puppies to septicemia. Administration of bacterins to the bitch during the gestation period has been useful in problem kennels.

Metritis or mastitis in the bitch may result in the puppies developing septicemia or toxemia. Toxins of *Staphylococci* and *Streptococci* reportedly cause a disappearance of cerebral cortical activity, protracted collapse, slowing of the heart and respirations and hypothermia. Enterotoxins induce mitochondrial degeneration, inhibit mitosis and decrease the rate of epithelial replacement in the intestines. Bacteria in the digestive tract have a predilection for the immature cells emerging from the intestinal crypts. In addition, they inhibit antibody absorption.

## PRINCIPLES OF THERAPY

Prevention of individual neonatal mortality is based on an understanding of the physiology of the newborn. Clinicians working with the young puppy recognize that the pressor reflex does not develop until the fourth day, the carotid sinus and carotid center do not respond to a fall in blood pressure until the fourth week, and the shivering reflex develops about the sixth day. Other factors such as a mean arterial blood pressure averaging 81 mm. Hg for the first 20 days, a glomerular filtration rate 21 to 25 per cent of that of an adult at birth, a tubular secretion rate which at two weeks of age is 12 to 18 per cent of the rate at eight weeks of age, and a water requirement of 130 to 200 ml./kg./day contribute to the similarity of signs noted in sick puppies with illnesses from a variety of causes.

During the neonatal period, most illnesses are characterized by dehydration, hypoglycemia and hypothermia. Sick puppies will cry and may develop diarrhea. The management of sick neonatal puppies demands attention to a variety of therapeutic modalities.

An environmental temperature of 85° to 90° F. and a relative humidity of 55 to 65 per cent are essential when puppies are separated from their mother. Hydration should be maintained by subcutaneous and oral fluids at the rate of 130 to 200 ml./kg. of body weight/day. Hypoglycemia is combatted by giving 5 to 10 per cent glucose orally at frequent intervals. One-tenth to 0.01 mg. vitamin $K_1$ will prevent serious hypoprothrombinemia. Thirty to forty per cent oxygen in the inspired air is indicated in the chilled puppy as procedures for slow warming are instituted. Feeding of milk formula is to be avoided in any puppy with a rectal temperature below 94° F. Chilled puppies should receive only 5 to 10 percent glucose by mouth until the body temperature returns to 94° F. or above. Thereafter, the caloric intake should be carefully calculated. One hundred and thirty calories per kilogram of body weight for the first week, 150 cal./kg. of body weight for the second week and 180 to 200 cal./kg. of body weight for the third and fourth weeks in four divided feedings will be adequate for strong, vigorous puppies. Excess caloric intake from overfeeding will result in a diarrhea in puppies. Dilution of the formula by the addition of 30 per cent more water and the use of an antacid such as 1 to 3 cc. of milk of magnesia repeated twice at 3-hour intervals will be beneficial where overfeeding has resulted in diarrhea. Deficient caloric intake will result in failure of growth and, if markedly deficient, hypoglycemia.

Finally, one must acknowledge the potential of infection such as distemper, canine hepatitis, leptospirosis, brucellosis and overwhelming parasitism as a cause of neonatal mortality. The diagnosis of such diseases is dependent on accurate histories, careful examination of the bitch, necropsy findings and laboratory confirmation. Signs induced by the infections may not resemble the signs noted in the more mature puppy.

**SUPPLEMENTAL READING**

Carmichael, L. E.: Herpesvirus canis: aspects of pathogenesis and immune response. J. Am. Vet. Med. Assn., *12*:1714–1721, 1970.

# PERITONITIS

DOUGLAS M. MacCOY, D.V.M.
*Ithaca, New York*

Peritonitis is an inflammatory response of the peritoneum. It is a primary disease only in the cat (feline infectious peritonitis). In all other domestic animals, peritonitis is secondary to a primary disease. Peritonitis may be the major sign of a primary disease, as with bowel perforation, or may completely obscure the signs of a primary disease, as with acute necrotizing pancreatitis.

Peritonitis is recognized in two forms, localized and diffuse. The primary cause of a localized peritonitis is often identical with that of a diffuse peritonitis. In the localized form, the body defense mechanisms are successful in walling off the insult. However, localized peritonitis may develop into diffuse peritonitis. Localized peritonitis is less lethal, and its signs and systemic effects less pronounced than the diffuse form.

Diffuse peritonitis affects a membrane capable of rapid fluid and chemical exchange, which has a surface area equal to that of the patient's skin. As a result diffuse peritonitis has profound effects on virtually all body systems and is fatal if not recognized early and treated vigorously.

## ETIOLOGY

There are three broad etiologic classifications of peritonitis (chemical, bacterial and combined). In chemical peritonitis, the initial reaction is strictly caused by chemical irritation. Trauma or surgical procedures may cause leakage of bile, pancreatic enzymes, hydrochloric acid or urine. Bacterial counts are low in the acute phase, although significant bacterial invasion is inevitable if the reaction is sustained. Bacterial peritonitis results from rupture of the gastrointestinal tract distal to the duodenum, penetration of the abdominal wall or extension of infection from the urogenital system. Combined chemical and bacterial peritonitis is seen most commonly when trauma has resulted in simultaneous injury to many abdominal organs. This form also occurs with severe or long-standing chemical peritonitis, in which increased intestinal wall permeability due to inflammation and ileus allows large numbers of bacteria to enter the peritoneal space.

## PATHOGENESIS

The pathogenesis of peritonitis is complicated because of the simultaneous interaction of a large number of body systems. Following the initial response to the irritative stimulus—no matter what it is—there is immediate local vasodilatation. Damage to capillary walls increases their permeability. Plasma accumulates, with fibrin formation, local adhesions and ileus. Chemotactic invasion by neutrophils and macrophages begins, followed later by lymphocytes. At this stage, body defenses may succeed in localizing the irritant, removing the irritant material and organizing fibrin adhesions.

If localization fails, there is continued accumulation and dissemination of irritant materials. Diffuse vasodilation is followed by a massive shift of fluids and protein to the peritoneal space. Peripheral vasoconstriction and increased cardiac output occur to prevent hypotension from this loss of circulatory volume. The viscera are coated with fibrin. There is a massive shift of neutrophils to the affected areas. Fibrin adhesions, aided by ileus, may succeed in localizing the irritants at this point, and eventually resolving the peritonitis.

If the body defenses are unable to contain the reactions, continued fluid shifts, visceral pooling and accumulation of toxic metabolites result in uncompensated hypovolemia, with cardiovascular collapse and death.

Few animals (0 to 32 per cent) survive the effects of a diffuse peritonitis without supportive therapy. Three components are needed for this high mortality: a diffuse inflammatory response, live bacteria and the presence of materials which enhance bacterial virulence. The mixed bacterial flora found in a diffuse peritonitis exerts a synergistic effect on bacterial virulence. Proteins, such as hemoglobin, found in peritoneal exudates also enhance bacterial virulence. A 4 gm./100 ml. hemoglobin solution, a level commonly reached by peritoneal exudates, may cause an otherwise innocuous bacterium to become extremely lethal.

## PATHOPHYSIOLOGY

Diffuse peritonitis affects virtually all body systems. However, the cardiopulmonary system and hydrogen ion concentration control systems are the most profoundly affected.

The pathophysiology of all forms of peritonitis is essentially the same. As soon as a negative fluid balance exists, cardiac output must be increased to maintain adequate tissue perfusion. Peripheral and renal blood flow decrease in response to vasopressors. As the irritant material spreads, capillary walls lose integrity and interstitial and splanchnic fluid pooling occurs. Damaged tissues release additional catecholamines which cause local venous spasm and intensify visceral pooling. Cardiac output more than doubles in response to this hypovolemia. This increased cardiac output persists for the first week in spite of therapy, demanding increased energy and

respiratory support. As peritoneal inflammation continues, further capillary wall degeneration occurs, allowing a massive fluid, plasma protein and hemoglobin shift to the peritoneal space. Serum calcium levels are dependent on exchange with protein-bound calcium, so the protein shift results in a hypocalcemia.

Hemoconcentration with increased viscosity increases cardiac workload. Ileus, secondary to the inflammatory reaction, allows further intraluminal fluid pooling.

Maintenance of cardiac output has required further peripheral vasoconstriction and shunting, so renal, deep muscle and visceral perfusion have been reduced. Potassium accumulates due to both (1) the reduced glomerular filtration rate and (2) its increased release from damaged tissues. Local anaerobic glycolysis has begun in response to lowered tissue oxygen tension, resulting in accumulation of lactic acid and other acid metabolites. This combined with bacterial acid metabolites overwhelms the blood buffers, producing acidosis. Respirations are stimulated to reduce blood $CO_2$ concentrations and correct the metabolic acidosis. The muscular activity of respiration requires further energy and cardiac output and produces more acid metabolites. If there is severe abdominal pain, abdominal guarding may compromise respiration, aggravating the existing acidosis. Pyrexia compounds the problem by raising the metabolic rate and increasing energy requirements.

As cardiac output falls and oxygen tension decreases, the sodium pump fails, with release of cellular potassium aggravating the hyperkalemia of renal shutdown. Acidosis, hyperkalemia, hypocalcemia and toxin accumulation further decrease cardiac output in a vicious cycle that ends in cardiovascular collapse and death.

## DIAGNOSIS

Physical signs of peritonitis usually fall into two classes, either vague signs of abdominal distress (vomiting, anorexia, pyrexia, ileus) or an acute abdomen (splinting, pyrexia, ileus, abdominal fluid, and shock). The presence of abdominal pain on palpation is variable and much more likely to be present with localized than with diffuse peritonitis. Abdominal palpation may also reveal the primary disease.

Laboratory tests are not diagnostic. In localized peritonitis, slight hemoconcentration and leukocytosis with neutrophilia may be noted. In generalized peritonitis, there is usually hemoconcentration, hypoproteinemia and neutropenia in later stages. Radiography may demonstrate the presence of abdominal fluid or the radiographic pattern of a primary disease. Abdominocentesis, or preferably peritoneal lavage, may reveal the presence of an exudate, urine, intestinal contents or bile. Final diagnosis often may be made only at laparotomy. Surgical exploration should not be delayed. With adequate supportive therapy, mortality from a negative celiotomy is less than 5 per cent. If celiotomy provides the diagnosis of peritonitis, the first step in therapy has been taken.

## MEDICAL MANAGEMENT

Practically all cases of shock due to peritonitis are reversible if the offending lesion is identified and corrected promptly. Continued sepsis invariably results in patient deterioration and death.

Oxygen therapy counteracts the lowered tissue oxygen tension present from respiratory depression and lowered cardiac output. Fluids and electrolytes are given at the maximum safe rate, as determined by monitoring central venous pressure (CVP). CVP should not be raised above 10 cm. of water. Urine output must be monitored. During the first 15 to 20 minutes of fluid administration urine flow should begin and reach a rate of 2 to 6 cc./kg./hr. Persistent oliguria indicates renal shutdown, which may result in overhydration of the patient if uncorrected. To enhance renal blood flow and glomerular filtration rate, 10 gm. per 100 ml. dextrose solution may be administered intravenously at 60 ml./kg. as rapidly as CVP allows. If diuresis does not occur after the first third of the dose of dextrose, furosemide should be given intravenously at 2 mg./kg. If anuria or oliguria (less than 1 to 4 cc./kg./hr.) persists, fluid administration must be guided by CVP. Once the fluid deficit is corrected, and diuresis initiated, urine flow is maintained by continued fluid administration. The most significant complication of diuresis is potassium depletion. Serial serum potassium determinations should be done to avoid this possibility.

Early in the disease electrolyte losses are balanced, therefore lactated Ringer's solution is an ideal replacement. If the animal is extremely depressed, or if the electrocardiograph indicates hyperkalemia 2.5 gm. per 100 ml. dextrose solution in saline should be used instead of lactated Ringer's solution until serum potassium levels are known. If oliguria persists, serum chloride should be monitored to avoid iatrogenic hyperchloremia which increases acidosis. If there is no response to fluid replacement, colloid therapy or administration of fresh whole blood is indicated.

Acidosis may be evaluated clinically for initial therapy. Low, moderate or severe acidosis is treated with 3, 6 or 9 mEq. of sodium bicarbonate per kg., respectively. One-half the dose may be given slowly intravenously; the rest is mixed with the intravenous fluids. Laboratory evaluation of acid-base balance should be done as soon as feasible to permit more accurate treatment and evaluation of initial therapy. In severe acidosis with protein loss and accumulation of necrotic debris, significant sequestration of calcium can occur. Sodium bicarbonate therapy will also temporarily reduce serum calcium. Therefore serum calcium levels should be determined and corrected as needed before giving large amounts of sodium bicarbonate. The usual calcium dose is 10 to 30 ml. of a 10 gm./100ml. calcium gluconate solution administered by slow intravenous injection with monitoring of cardiac rhythm. This procedure will prevent myocardial failure from iatrogenic hypocalcemia.

In severe hypoproteinemia, hypo-osmolar plasma will complicate fluid therapy. This should be corrected by the administration of plasma, canine albumin or colloids.

Intravenous broad-spectrum antibiotics are started with initial fluids. This treatment alone raises the survival rate to over 50 per cent. Intravenous administration of sodium penicillin at 120,000 IU/kg. q4h or sodium ampicillin at 6 mg./kg. q6h provides good coverage. Kanamycin, cephaloridine or procaine penicillin G with dihydrostreptomycin may be used intramuscularly. However, reduced peripheral blood flow may compromise their absorption and distribution.

Analgesics do not seem as important in animals as in man. When they are necessary, nondepressant agents with minimal hypotensive effects (such as pentazocine lactate* at 3 to 4 mg./kg.) are preferable to depressant agents such as meperidine hydrochloride.†

Corticosteroids are important in shock therapy. Hydrocortisone sodium succinate‡ at 22 mg./kg. by intravenous bolus or dexamethazone alcohol§ at 4 to 10 mg./kg. given slowly intravenously is effective in improving peripheral circulation, increasing cardiac output, stabilizing lysosomal membranes, reestablishing capillary integrity and providing a protective action against endotoxins.

## SURGICAL MANAGEMENT

Experiments in dogs with induced peritonitis indicate surgical peritoneal lavage alone was equal to treatment with antibiotics alone; 40 to 60 per cent recovered in each group. When antibiotic treatment and surgical lavage were combined, the survival rate increased to 80 per cent. If treatment is extended with intermittent postoperative peritoneal lavage, the figure rises to 85 per cent.

There is little point in delaying surgical intervention except to stabilize the patient. In some instances, when the patient is in severe distress from continued peritoneal soilage, presurgical stabilization is impossible. In these circumstances mortality rates are much higher. Occurrence of intraoperative shock is rare and is an indication of inadequate preoperative preparation and intraoperative support.

Long, complicated procedures should not be attempted. The surgeon should utilize familiar simple repair techniques in correcting the primary disease. Adhesions are separated as gently as possible to allow complete cleansing of the abdomen. After the primary disease is corrected, peritoneal lavage is used to remove debris, blood and chemical irritants. Warm physiologic saline is used to fill the abdomen while the viscera are gently manipulated. The solution is then removed by suction. The process is repeated until the lavage fluid is clear. A final

lavage is done with a solution of 10 cc. of Betadine Whirlpool Concentrate® (Purdue-Frederick Company, Yonkers, N.Y. 10701) (*not soap*) mixed in one liter of saline or lactated Ringer's solution. Povidine iodine has a wider spectrum of antimicrobial activity than any single antibiotic, is less irritating than most antibiotics, does not significantly alter the pH or osmolality of the saline or Ringer's solution, and has a wide margin of safety. After the lavage, instruments, drapes and gloves are changed.

Before closure, a drain made from fenestrated Silastic® tubing* of appropriate size is placed at the site of the primary lesion and brought through the ventrolateral abdominal wall. It should traverse a short subcutaneous tunnel and emerge from the skin away from the celiotomy incision. This drain is fixed to the skin with a surrounding horizontal mattress suture of nonabsorbable material. A four-layer abdominal closure is performed with a continuous suture of absorbable material for peritoneal closure, simple interrupted sutures of monofilament stainless steel for linea alba closure, simple interrupted sutures of absorbable material for subcutaneous tissues and simple interrupted sutures of nonabsorbable material for skin closure.

## POSTOPERATIVE CARE

Postsurgically, broad-spectrum antibiotics are given until the abdominal drain is removed. It is wise to culture the interior tip of the drain after removal and modify antibacterial therapy as indicated by sensitivity tests. Antibiotics are continued for a minimum of five days following drain removal.

Intermittent peritoneal lavage is performed two to three times daily using 20 cc./kg. of body weight of the same Betadine®-saline solution used for intraoperative lavage. The exterior of the drain is cleaned with antiseptic, and the warmed solution is allowed to run through the drain by gravity flow. If the animal experiences discomfort or dyspnea, the flow is discontinued. When the abdomen has been filled, the drain is clamped and the solution is left in place for 10 to 20 minutes. If possible, the

---

*Talwin®, Winthrop Laboratories, Division of Sterling Drug Inc., New York, N.Y. 10016.

†Demerol®, Winthrop Laboratories, Division of Sterling Drug Inc., New York, N.Y. 10016.

‡Solu-Cortef®, Winthrop Laboratories, Division of Sterling Drug Inc., New York, N.Y. 10016.

§Azium®, Dept. of Veterinary Medicine, Pfizer Inc., New York, N.Y. 10017.

*Silastic®, Dow-Corning Corporation, Medical Products Divison, Midland, Michigan 48640.

animal may be walked during this time to aid in distribution of the lavage solution. The clamp is then removed until the next lavage, allowing free drainage of the lavage solution and any exudate. Some of the lavage solution will be absorbed, so that returned volume rarely equals infused volume. During the period of intermittent lavage the animal should be maintained on an elevated, open mesh rack to prevent soiling of the drain and patient. An Elizabethan collar is advisable to prevent patient removal of or damage of the drain.

Lavage is continued until the signs of peritonitis have resolved and the lavage fluid has remained clear on two successive lavages. Drains have been left in up to 14 days with no significant complications. Superficial minor skin infections may occur around the drain but quickly resolve upon its removal. When the drain is removed, the skin wound is closed with a single suture.

There is some evidence to indicate that lavage delays healing. In cases of intestinal resection or hollow viscus closure, fibrin accumulation and omental adhesion at the surgical site are prevented. Therefore repairs must maintain their own integrity without relying on fibrin or omental sealing. Double-layer closure with nonabsorbable suture material for the second layer is proper technique when postoperative lavage is to be used. If failure does occur, it is readily identified by the change in tube drainage.

Serum electrolytes must be monitored during the period of lavage. Electrolyte exchange occurs readily, with hypokalemia as the most important complication. Hypoproteinemia resulting from peritoneal exudation and/or anorexia must also be corrected.

Oral caloric support should begin as soon as possible because it is impractical to meet an animal's needs by intravenous materials. Until that time, 50 gm./100 ml. dextrose solution may be used to decrease the negative energy balance. This solution is extremely hypertonic and must be given very slowly to prevent severe osmotic diuresis, fatal expansion of circulating fluid volume, excessive erythrocyte destruction and severe phlebitis. Parenteral vitamin support, especially of water-soluble vitamins, is also necessary during this period. Parenteral fluid maintenance at 40 to 60 ml./kg. per day should be continued until the animal reliably maintains hydration by oral intake.

## COMPLICATIONS

There are several complications of peritonitis, all of which are life-threatening and therefore demand immediate vigorous therapy. Hyperthermia in excess of 105° F. may occur before, during or after surgery. It results in rapid tissue destruction, especially of nervous tissue, plus severe cardiopulmonary stress. Treatment is whole body immersion in ice cold water, vigorous shock therapy and chemical vasodilation with chlorpromazine hydrochloride at 0.05 mg./kg. to a maximum dose of 25 mg./patient given intravenously to facilitate radiant heat loss. The ice water immersion is discontinued when rectal temperature reaches 103° F. In some cases, the thermoregulatory mechanism appears to be disturbed and body temperature varies widely.

Disseminated intravascular coagulation (DIC) may occur with any severe debilitating disease and is a very common sequela to hyperthermia. Treatment is by heparinization at 50 to 100 IU (1 to 2 mg.) of sodium heparin per kg. q4-8h until clotting factors are seen in peripheral blood. Also give shock doses of steroids and platelet transfusions and correct the primary disease.

Acute pancreatitis may occur following peritoneal insult, hyperthermia or DIC. Treatment of this disorder is well described in the article on "Acute Pancreatitis."

Bacterial endocarditis, polyarthritis and multifocal abscesses may be seen subsequent to the bacteremia associated with peritonitis.

Finally, dehiscence of surgical repairs may occur with recontamination of the abdomen. Treatment is reoperation and correction of the failure.

### SUPPLEMENTAL READING

Artz, C. P., et al.: Further studies concerning the pathogenesis and treatment of peritonitis. Ann. Surg., *155* (5):756, 1962.
Barnett, W. O., and Hardy, J. D.: Shock in peritonitis—mechanisms and management. Surg. Clin. N. Am., *42*:1101, 1962.
Burnett, W. E., et al.: The treatment of peritonitis using peritoneal lavage. Ann. Surg., *145*(5):675, 1957.
Clowes, G. H. A., Jr., et al.: Circulatory and metabolic

alterations associated with survival or death in peritonitis. Ann. Surg., *163*:866, 1966.

Filler, R. M., et. al.: Lethal factors in experimental peritonitis. Surgery, *60*(3):671, 1966.

Hoffer, R. E., et al.: Treatment of acute peritonitis in dogs by intermittent peritoneal lavage. J.A.A.H.A., *6*(3):182, 1970.

Lavigne, J. E., et al.: The treatment of experimental peritonitis with intraperitoneal Betadine solution. J. Surg. Res., *16*:307, 1974.

Parks, J., et al.: Peritoneal lavage for peritonitis and pancreatitis in twenty-two dogs. J.A.A.H.A., *9*:442, 1973.

Rosato, E. F., et al.: Peritoneal lavage treatment in experimental peritonitis. Ann. Surg., *175*(3):384, 1972.

# VETERINARY MANAGEMENT TECHNIQUES IN CANINE BREEDING COLONIES

W. THEODORE SWEENY, D.V.M.
*Lexington, Virginia*

There are three classes of dog breeders: the owner of one animal who desires one or two litters for personal satisfaction, the professional breeder of quality registered stock and the large commercial breeder of thousands of animals (usually beagles) for use by the research community. In addition there are organizations that "condition" dogs to varying degrees; since these people are not true breeders, they will not be considered here. Dogs bred by the "backyard breeder" are not within the scope of this topic and must be treated on a one-on-one patient-doctor basis. The methods to be discussed here apply to the professional breeder of registered dogs (which includes individuals who breed for resale to the franchised pet shop trade).

Preventive medicine is the key to a successful program. The veterinarian must make every attempt to gain total authority over all health programs. Once this is accomplished, you have achieved the ultimate practice situation. You can establish all programs and supervise the activities of technicians in implementation of these programs. Once your system is established, it is necessary to assume the role of administrator. A program is only as good as the people who carry it through, and all activities must be monitored and good records must be maintained.

## ENVIRONMENTAL CONSIDERATIONS

Each kennel or colony has environmental factors peculiar to its particular circumstances but some general principles deserve mention. Proper air circulation is the most important single environmental factor in disease control, especially respiratory disease. If the facility houses the dogs inside, air changes should include a high percentage of outside air, since recirculation of inside air merely spreads any contaminants that may be present. Suspended cages are mandatory for control of internal parasites. Systems for feeding, watering and waste disposal vary widely; as long as basic sanitary measures are practiced, there should not be a problem.

## VACCINATIONS

Vaccination programs are probably the best example of preventive medicine. There is absolutely no excuse for any morbidity or mortality from canine distemper, infectious canine hepatitis, leptospirosis or canine parainfluenza in a breeding colony. Experience shows that approximately 90 per cent of pups carry significant levels of maternal antibody at 8 weeks of age and 90 per cent do not carry significant levels by 9 weeks of age. This will vary from colony to colony depending upon the vaccination program in the bitches, vaccines used, etc., so the status in the colony in question should be evaluated before a particular vaccination regimen is established. Distemper and hepatitis for the first vaccination followed in one month by distemper-hepatitis-leptospirosis-parainfluenza and one month later by distemper-hepatitis-leptospirosis-parainfluenza again is recommended. Bitches and studs should receive boosters yearly. It is not necessary to vaccinate routinely for rabies in a closed colony housed indoors; if you are dealing with an outdoor facility, however, it is wise to vaccinate for rabies.

## NUTRITION

Any reliable dog food manufacturer provides a well-balanced product. The use of pet "concoctions" is discouraged because the nutritionists who formulate commercial dog food are more knowledgeable in this area than veterinarians. Bitches and studs are fed once a day or *ad libitum*. Pups are creep-fed a gruel meal at 4 weeks of age while they are still with the bitch. The bitch can be tied in the corner of the cage at meal time to prevent interference with the puppies. Weaning should be done according to litter size, but the average age is 6 weeks. Feeding can be scheduled for three times a day until 3 months of age, two times a day from 3 to 8 months of age and then once a day. Feeding can also be *ad libitum*.

## PARASITES

### INTERNAL PARASITES

Preventive medicine, again, cannot be overemphasized. The most important single factor in internal parasite control is the use of elevated cages with wire bottoms which allow the feces to pass through. This, to a great extent, breaks the life cycle of ascarids, whipworms and hookworms. In addition, I administer anthelmintics effective in elimination of the above three parasites at 30, 40 and 50 days of age. This applies to all pups and is done regardless of whether or not the results are positive on fecal flotation. Monthly microscopic examinations are conducted from this point until the animals are sold, and treatment is initiated on the basis of the microscopic findings. If this regimen (including the caging) is followed, ascarids, hookworms and whipworms are a very rare finding in pups over 2 months of age. Bitches are treated along with the pups (when the pups are 30, 40 and 50 days of age) and again if their offspring show positive infestation at later dates. Fecal flotations are conducted on bitches and studs routinely every month, and treatment is instituted on an individual basis for any animal with positive findings. Monthly microscopic examinations of bitches' feces may be negative (sometimes for years) and yet their puppies will often harbor ascarids. This would lend credence to those who feel that high levels of progesterone during pregnancy stimulate larval migration.

Tapeworms should not be a problem in a closed colony. There should be routine preventive dipping programs that virtually eliminate fleas, and although rodents seem to resist elimination, they can be controlled.

Coccidiosis, because it seems to be precipitated by stress, is an enigma. The stress of travel often causes puppies to die during or immediately following shipping. When it is diagnosed, treat with sulfonamides. Because of the nature of the organism, one can never be confident that this therapy is truly successful.

Strongyloides is another enigmatic organism mainly because of the difficulty encountered in routine diagnosis. If this organism is found, thiabendazole seems to be the treatment of choice.

### EXTERNAL PARASITES

Demodectic mange and ear mites are the primary external parasite problems. Fleas and ticks are not a problem but their prevention should be part of your program. Monthly, every dog over 3 months of age is dipped in a Ronnel® solution, and mineral oil is instilled in their ears. These procedures are conducted alternately every two weeks. Although this is probably a more drastic program than necessary, it will eliminate ear mites and seems to control demodectic mange. Demodex is insidious and can become a problem of major proportion. Until this parasite is more completely understood, control rather than treatment is in order.

## DISEASES
## OF THE INFANT

Accurate mortality records are necessary if the veterinarian expects to formulate effective preventive and therapeutic regimens. Every pup that dies (including those dead at birth) should be examined and the findings entered in a permanent necropsy book. The necropsy book should include the following entries: the parents, sex of the deceased pup, date of death, age at death, whether or not the pup was dead at birth, and, of course, your diagnosis. Monthly and annual totals of pups dead at birth and of those that were born alive and died later as well as the number of deaths by etiologic category should be calculated. In my experience, a program is acceptable if mortality (including those dead at birth) can be kept at 25 per cent or less. By maintaining good records and acting on the problem areas discerned from these records, the mortality can be decreased even further.

### HERPES VIRUS

This acute fulminating syndrome fits the description formerly called "fading puppy syndrome." The petechial and ecchymotic hemorrhages seen throughout but especially in the capsule of the kidney at necropsy are almost pathognomonic. The puppies rarely live more than ten days. The entire litter usually succumbs, and treatment is discouraging. Treatment with serum from bitches known to be positive has had limited success. This disease is almost always seen in bitches whelping their first litter in the colony; evidently the virus is perpetuated in a colony which stimulates continual self-immunization and protection. This is significant in that a bitch that loses a litter because of this virus should not be eliminated from the colony.

### TOXEMIAS AND SEPTICEMIAS

The most common toxemia occurs when the bitch has mastitis. The syndrome is acute and fulminating, so the pups must be removed from the bitch and either nursed by hand or placed on another bitch. Treatment is discouraging. Streptococcal septicemias are occasionally seen in older puppies. The head swells, the eyes are often closed because of the swelling, pharyngeal lymph nodes are swollen and there is usually anorexia and depression. Treatment with ampicillin is quite rewarding. Pups will often show similar symptoms from localized lesions that result from fighting, and treatment for such lesions is the same. Septicemias from a wide variety of bacteria occur, and a definitive diagnosis is difficult or impossible; symptomatic treatment is the only practical approach.

### PUSTULAR DERMATITIS

This syndrome is quite common in pups. It is usually seen before weaning and may affect the entire litter. It is caused by a staphylococcus and is characterized by pustules anywhere on the body, but usually on the head, and a rough, scaly hair coat. The affected area should be clipped and furacin ointment should be applied. Recovery is rapid and uneventful.

### RESPIRATORY DISEASES

This is the most critical area for the kennel or colony veterinarian. Environmental control is the key to respiratory disease control because drafts, chilling, high humidity, etc., are predisposing factors. The very young pup (under 3 weeks) is less prone (probably because of mechanical and systemic protection by the bitch) than the pup between 4 and 12 weeks of age. Organisms such as *Bordetella bronchiseptica* and the parainfluenza virus are primarily a nuisance in older dogs where they cause the "kennel cough" syndrome but very low mortality. These same organisms in synergism with secondary invaders can cause high mortality in the 4- to 12-week-old pup. Parainfluenza can be controlled by vaccination but Bordetella cannot. Once you make certain that everything possible has been accomplished to control the environment, the treatment program is like that for any other pneumonia. The important point here is to initiate treatment early; once the lungs become consolidated, recovery is rare. Nebulization is recommended for pups with congestive pneumonia. If an especially virulent organism is involved, culture and sensitivity tests can be of value; however, you can never be certain of the possible role of viruses. Fogging with a product such as Nolvasan® has merit, but care must be taken since excessive fogging can cause irritation of the mucous membranes of the eyes and nose as well as get the pups wet, which can lead to chilling.

## MISCELLANEOUS AFFLICTIONS

Both nutritional and infectious diarrhea occur and are handled according to the cause. Prolapse of the rectum is not uncommon. Amputation is preferred over the use of purse-string sutures for prolapsed rectum because there is less recurrence.

# DISEASES OF THE ADULT

This discussion will include only those diseases of particular importance to a breeder.

## BRUCELLA CANIS

This disease was virtually unknown 12 years ago; today, it is the breeder's number one enemy. An entire chapter on *Brucella canis* appears later in this text, so this discussion will be limited to the salient points. This is an insidious disease, and with the exception of abortion, the symptoms are not dramatic. Treatment is possible but does not eliminate the carrier state and should be instituted only under exceptional circumstances. The owner should be advised in depth concerning the potential risk to the remainder of the colony and to humans. A control program consisting of periodic testing with subsequent elimination of reactors is the only way in which Brucella can be permanently eliminated. The following is the recommended testing program using the tube agglutination test with the antigen standardized by the U.S.D.A. (There is also a slide agglutination test available which is useful for screening and much less involved than the tube agglutination test.)

1. Test all breeding animals monthly until there are no reactors.

2. Eliminate all animals known to be positive and place all animals that have had any direct contact in isolation quarters with a separate caretaker; this includes puppies.

3. Thoroughly disinfect cages and ancillary articles of infected dogs with steam.

4. Once the entire population is negative, test every three months for a year, then every six months for a year, and yearly thereafter.

5. If positive animals are found at any time, resume monthly testing.

6. If new dogs are introduced, insist that they be accompanied by a recent negative test. Keep these dogs in isolation until three additional negative tests have been conducted at monthly intervals.

## MASTITIS

Mastitis can be fatal to the bitch but usually is not. The main concern is the puppies. The bitch should be treated with broad-spectrum antibiotics, and the pups should be removed. The significant point to remember is that the disease will usually recur on subsequent lactations. The fact that the bitch contracted mastitis should be noted on her record; if she manifests the condition a second time, she should be eliminated as a breeder.

## ECLAMPSIA AND PSEUDOCYESIS

These two conditions are mentioned because they are reproductive syndromes and, as such, are important in a colony situation. Incidence in a colony bitch is extremely low and therefore should not be a factor in health programs. A definitive reason for the near absence of these conditions cannot be offered here, but the presence of a standardized regimen (especially diet) seems to be a plausible explanation.

# REPRODUCTIVE CONSIDERATIONS

## HEAT DETECTION

Bitches should be examined for estrus three times a week. Occasionally, an animal will exhibit what may be called a "false heat"; there will be a slight hemorrhagic discharge but no accompanying swelling. In a day or two there are no signs of estrus. These dogs will usually have a normal heat period two or three weeks after the false heat. Most bitches do not come in season every six months but they do have their own consistent cycle.

If vaginal prolapse develops, it almost always occurs while a bitch is in heat. It is usually limited to the ventral vagina and in most cases will recede spontaneously when estrus is completed. Natural mating is often successful and should be attempted before resorting to artificial insemination in these cases. This condition usually recurs during successive heat periods.

## MATING

Bitches can be bred on their first heat unless they are extremely small or unless they come in season at an unusually early age. If a bitch is small, she probably should not have been picked as a breeder in the first place. Breeding should begin when the vaginal discharge changes to a straw color rather than on a specific day after the female comes in heat, and can be repeated every other day until the bitch refuses the stud. Breeding on the basis of vaginal cytology is neither practical nor necessary in a colony situation. Artificial insemination is used when necessary, such as when the animal refuses natural insemination or when anatomical factors prevent it.

Studs should not mate with more than one bitch per week. Antibiotics should be instilled in the prepuce after each mating to aid in prevention of disease transfer to other bitches. Mastitis syringes are convenient for this. Monthly microscopic examinations on semen should be conducted as a preventive measure. This procedure can be misleading, since too often a sample will have very poor characteristics and yet the stud continues to produce normal viable litters. Therefore it is not wise to eliminate a stud solely on the basis of semen evaluation; in addition, he should be test bred to at least two bitches.

## PREGNANCY DIAGNOSIS

The value of pregnancy diagnosis lies not in detection of those bitches who are pregnant but of those who are not. It is not enough simply to be aware that a certain percentage of your brood stock did not deliver offspring in a given month or year; you must know why they did not whelp. What might be considered a misconception could have been an animal that conceived and subsequently resorbed or even aborted. Every instance in which a mating does not terminate in whelping should be delineated as either a misconception, a resorption or an abortion, and every attempt should be made to determine the cause: Was the stud sterile? Was the cause mechanical? Was it *Brucella canis?*

The ideal time to palpate is 21 to 25 days after breeding, at which time implantation is complete and the bitch is thin enough that mechanical manipulation of the abdominal viscera can be accomplished without undue difficulty. As is the case with cattle and horses, proficiency is obtained only through practice.

## WHELPING

All assignments relative to whelping and postparturient care of the bitch and pups should be delineated on a preprinted card attached to the cage. The caretaker is instructed to initial the card after each task is completed. This assures the veterinarian that the duties have been properly completed and provides a simple way of checking as you make your rounds. At least a week before the bitch is due to whelp, she is moved to the whelping room and dipped (to control mange), the toenails are clipped (to prevent mechanical damage to the pups) and the ears are cleaned and examined for ear mites.

At parturition either a disposable cardboard whelping box or paper can be utilized. Do not use wooden whelping boxes because they cannot be disinfected properly. Forceps need not be used routinely for delivery, since forceps may be more likely to damage pups than delivery by manual manipulation. If uterine inertia is evident, posterior pituitary extract can be used twice at 20-minute intervals. If this is not successful, manual removal should be attempted. Cesarean section should be performed only as a last resort. When parturition is complete, palpate to be certain all pups have been delivered. Administration of an ergot preparation at this time prevents hemorrhage in addition to contracting the uterus.

Puppies should be examined for congenital anomalies and lacerations immediately after birth. The umbilical cords should be examined closely and iodine should be applied. Oxygen may be administered to pups in respiratory distress at birth. Heat lamps are essential if the temperature is below 70° F.; however, care must be exercised in placement of the lamps to avoid overheating the bitch. Orphan pups can be placed on a foster mother, if available, or fed one of the artificial diets.

# INDEX OF DIETETIC MANAGEMENT

M. L. MORRIS, JR., D.V.M.
*Topeka, Kansas*

## INTRODUCTION

The dietetic management of disease is an extremely useful tool for the veterinary clinician. The Index of Dietetic Management is a list of clinical conditions in which dietetic management can be beneficial in treating dogs and cats. The specific diseases, syndromes or clinical signs discussed have both nutritional and non-nutritional etiologies. Too often clinicians believe that dietetic management applies exclusively to diseases caused by diet. However, this is not the case, as many conditions with a cause unrelated to diet can be managed successfully with supportive dietary adjustment.

The information about each condition is organized into (1) a brief discussion of the condition; (2) a statement of the dietary objective(s); (3) management to accomplish the dietary objective(s); (4) special considerations; and (5) the recommended diet(s).

When implementing a system of dietetic management into a veterinary practice, it is important to discuss the following with clients:

—The reason why you are changing the pet's diet.

—The objectives to be accomplished by changing the diet.

—The degree of importance that the dietary program has in the disease or condition present.

—The reason why the program should be followed faithfully.

—The period of time the animal will need to be fed the special diet.

## ANEMIAS

A shortage of specific nutrients can become the limiting factor in erythrocyte replacement. When required, the dog's red blood cell manufacture can occur at six times the normal rate. Cats suffer from anemia more often and more severely than dogs. Anemias of nutritional origin generally respond well to dietetic therapy.

### OBJECTIVE

To supply adequate amounts of nutrients needed to support erythropoiesis.

### MANAGEMENT

1. Increase the protein level of the diet by adding 1 part, by weight, of muscle meat, liver, kidney, cottage cheese or eggs to each 3 parts of customary food. This dietary alteration is not required if the patient is consuming a high-protein diet.

2. Increase the level of B-complex vitamins. Supply at least 24 $\mu$g. folic acid, 1.0 mg. niacin, 120 $\mu$g. pyridoxine and 3.6 $\mu$g. vitamin $B_{12}$ per kilogram of body weight daily. When a response is observed, feed a diet nutritionally adequate for growth.

3. Increase the iron, cobalt and copper intake with metallic salts by administering a sufficient quantity of a trace mineral supplement to supply at least 7.0 mg. iron, 1.0 mg. copper and 0.30 mg. cobalt/kg. body weight daily.

### SPECIAL CONSIDERATIONS

1. If an intestinal block limits utilization of iron from the diet, administer 10 mg. iron/kg. body weight weekly, parenterally, in divided doses.

2. In copper deficiency, provide 2 mg/kg. body weight daily of copper in the diet with metallic salt.

3. In cobalt deficiency, provide 0.5 mg./kg. body weight daily of cobalt in the diet with metallic salt or equivalent $B_{12}$ activity.

4. In B-complex deficiency, provide a therapeutic B-complex preparation supplying 24 $\mu$g. folic acid, 1.0 mg. niacin and 120 $\mu$g. pyridoxine/kg. body weight daily.

5. Iron deficiency in kittens can be corrected by administering peroral ferrous sulfate in doses of from 0.03 gm. to 0.06 gm. per animal, depending on size.

## RECOMMENDED DIET

A high-quality protein diet with an increased level of vitamins and trace minerals should be given. A diet specifically designed to meet the increased requirements of growth is useful in managing anemias of nutritional origin. In severe cases of anemia, ½ oz. of fresh liver should be added to each pound of food.

## ANOREXIA

While the cause of anorexia may be psychological, traumatic or disease-produced, the result is invariably the same. The animal's body is deprived of the nutrients needed for its metabolic machinery to repair, replace and recover. The cause of anorexia may be due to factors other than organic disease, such as oral trauma, muscular paralysis, physical obstruction, etc. Thus, it is essential to determine the cause of anorexia. If oral alimentation is not contraindicated, it is important to provide nourishment for the patient. This is accomplished by artificial alimentation to supply nutrients important for convalescence and healing.

## OBJECTIVE

To provide a balanced and adequate nutrient source, by means of intragastric intubation, in the minimum volume practical.

## MANAGEMENT

1. Administer daily 60 to 80 Calories/kg. body weight derived primarily from fat and carbohydrate. (One t. corn syrup equals about 20 calories; 1 t. corn oil equals about 40 calories.)
2. Administer daily at least 2.0 gm. protein/kg. body weight of a biologic value of 80 or greater by using eggs or milk protein. (One egg contains 6 gm. protein; 1/6 cup cottage cheese contains about 5 gm. protein).
3. Administer vitamins at growth levels.

## CONSIDERATIONS

If large quantities of fluids and/or electrolytes are being lost, replace by oral alimentation if possible. If the animal is vomiting, fluid loss should be replaced parenterally.

## RECOMMENDED DIET

Mix in a blender:
    20 oz. water
      8 oz. Prescription Diet® i/d®
      2 oz. vegetable oil
Contains 30 Cal. and 25 ml. water/oz. Administer 2 to 3 oz./kg. body weight daily. Supply additional water to replace abnormal losses.

If the patient (dog or cat) has been anorectic for more than two days, divide initial daily dose into 2 or 3 feedings. After one or two days of divided feedings, the entire daily dose can be administered at one time. Usually by the second day voluntary eating has begun and intragastric intubation can be discontinued.

## CONGESTIVE HEART FAILURE

The kidney as well as the heart is involved in congestive heart failure. Sodium retention by the kidney, triggered by a hormonal reaction caused by the heart failing to maintain satisfactory output, is responsible for the congestion, edema and ascites seen clinically. Relief of sodium accumulation by using dietetic therapy is an important part of clinical management of congestive heart disease. The degree of sodium restriction required depends upon the severity of congestion. The more severe the congestion, the less sodium intake allowed.

## OBJECTIVE

To meet the animal's nutritive requirements with a diet that restricts sodium intake.

## MANAGEMENT

1. Estimate the sodium intake by obtaining a diet history. Restrict sodium intake in accordance with the severity of congestion. The table below provides the approximate average sodium content of various types of foods.

| TYPE OF FOOD | AV. MG. SODIUM/ 100 GM. DRY DIET |
|---|---|
| Canned (av. of 8) | 884 |
| Soft Moist (av. of 4) | 716 |
| Dry (av. of 4) | 442 (mild sodium restriction) |
| Prescription Diet® k/d® | 248 (moderate sodium restriction) |
| Prescription Diet® h/d® | 32 (strict sodium restriction) |

A diet containing 7 mg. sodium/100 gm. dry diet will meet the sodium requirement of the normal adult dog.

Dogs with severe congestion require strict sodium restriction. Those with mild or moderate congestion can be fed diets with higher sodium levels.

2. During active diuresis increase B-complex vitamins to levels comparable to 1 gm. brewers' yeast/2 kg. body weight daily, or the equivalent with a B-complex vitamin preparation. Those preparations containing sodium salts of the vitamins should be avoided. Brewers' yeast contains about 1.25 mg. sodium/gm. This quantity should be figured into the total sodium intake.

3. Feed an acid-ash diet. The metabolic acids combine with sodium and enhance diuresis.

4. Supply drinking water *ad lib*. If sodium content of tap water exceeds 150 ppm., provide distilled water during diuresis or until congestion is relieved.

5. Instruct owner to avoid use of softened water for dogs with congestive heart failure. Most homes with water softeners have a source of nonsoftened water.

## CONSIDERATIONS

1. If renal failure is also present, avoid use of sodium salts. Give priority to the more severe condition.

2. Obesity, which may accompany congestive heart disease, increases its severity. Reduce total food intake. Most reducing diets are contraindicated because of their sodium content.

3. Edema and ascites, often mistaken for obesity, may conceal emaciation. Following diuresis, if emaciation becomes evident, add 2 T. corn oil plus 1 oz. muscle meat to each pound of food fed.

4. For animals with fixed eating habits, add *small* quantities of low-sodium foods

**Table 1.**  *Table Foods Allowed and Omitted for Patients on a Low-Sodium Diet*

| LOW-SODIUM FOODS | FOODS TO AVOID |
|---|---|
| Beef | All processed meats, cheeses, breads, cereals |
| Domestic rabbit | |
| Chicken | Carrots |
| Horsemeat | Heart |
| Lamb | Kidney |
| Fresh-water fish | Liver |
| Egg yolks | Salted fats (butter, margarine) |
| Oatmeal | |
| Corn | Salted snacks and nuts |
| Rice | Whole egg |
| Farina | |

relished by the individual to tempt him to eat the prescribed diet (see Table 1).

## RECOMMENDED DIET

Dogs with mild or moderate degrees of congestive heart failure can be maintained on diets containing a higher level of sodium. The proper diet to use depends upon what diet the dog was eating when congestion developed. Change to a diet with lower sodium content (see above).

Since many cases of congestive heart failure are not diagnosed until they are advanced, a diet producing strict sodium restriction is well suited for the majority of cases. To accomplish this degree of sodium restriction, the diet must contain less than 60 mg. sodium/100 gm. dry diet. This can be accomplished by use of a dietary food, such as Prescription Diet® h/d®, or a homemade low-sodium diet.

### LOW-SODIUM DIET

¼ lb. lean ground beef
1 cup cooked rice
1 cup dietary pack canned corn (low-sodium), drained solids
1 T. corn oil
2 t. dicalcium phosphate

A balanced vitamin-mineral supplement in a quantity sufficient to provide the daily requirement for each vitamin and trace mineral. Avoid those that contain salt or sodium salts. Braise the meat, retaining fat. Add the remaining ingredients and mix. Yield: 1 lb.

### ANALYSIS

| | |
|---|---|
| Protein | 8.0% |
| Fat | 5.6% |
| Carbohydrate | 16.0% |
| Sodium* | 0.01% |
| Calories | 700 Cal./lb. |

*50 mg. sodium/100 gm. dry diet

## FEEDING GUIDE

Feed sufficient amount to maintain normal body weight.

| BODY WEIGHT | APPROXIMATE DAILY FEEDING |
|---|---|
| 5 lb. | ⅓ lb. |
| 10 lb. | ½ lb. |
| 20 lb. | 1 lb. |
| 40 lb. | 1¾ lb. |
| 60 lb. | 2⅓ lb. |
| 80 lb. | 2¾ lb. |
| 100 lb. | 3½ lb. |

Instruct the owner to feed only the low-sodium diet. All snacks, tidbits and treats, especially table food, must be eliminated.

## COPROPHAGY

Although frequently encountered, the actual causes of coprophagy are not well established. It may be due to such factors as boredom, nutrient deficiency or an insufficiency of the digestive enzymes amylase, lipase or protease. Dogs may eat their own or another animal's feces, which contain unabsorbed digestive enzymes, to replace deficient digestive enzymes.

### OBJECTIVE

To (1) provide a balanced diet adequate in all nutrients and (2) supply a dietary source of digestive enzymes.

### MANAGEMENT

1. Feed a good-quality diet, nutritionally adequate for the particular stage of the life cycle.
2. Instruct the client to sprinkle commercial meat tenderizer, such as Adolph's®, on the dog's food in the same manner as salting one's own food. Unseasoned meat tenderizer should be used for dogs with known gastrointestinal disorders, as ingredients used in the seasoned type may irritate the dog's gastrointestinal tract.

## DIABETES MELLITUS

For dogs afflicted with diabetes mellitus, it is essential that the quantity and quality of the diet be uniform from day to day so that the insulin dosage can be standardized. Ideally, the diet, exercise, environmental temperature and insulin dosage should be standardized so that body weight and blood glucose level are maintained nearly constant.

### OBJECTIVE

To maintain a constant balance between caloric intake and insulin dosage.

### MANAGEMENT

1. Feed the same quantity of a diet uniform in ingredients, both in quality and quantity, so that a consistent insulin dosage can be established.
2. Reduction of carbohydrates in the diet *may* allow reduction in insulin dosage.

### RECOMMENDED DIET

A high-protein, high-fat diet designed for puppy growth can be used for most dogs. For dogs with reduced renal function, a uniform low-protein diet, such as Prescription Diet® k/d®, may be necessary.

## DIARRHEA

Diarrhea is a major clinical sign of intestinal disorders. It can result from a variety of causes. Acute diarrhea, as a consequence of hypermotility, may be self-limiting or can be controlled by immediately applying proper medical and dietetic management. Chronic diarrhea, as the result of digestive disorders and/or malabsorption syndromes, requires an accurate determination of the cause. The diet must be recognized not only as an important part of the therapeutic regime, but also as a possible etiologic agent.

### OBJECTIVE

To provide foods which are easily digested to allow healing of the affected portion of the gastrointestinal tract.

### MANAGEMENT

1. Reduce crude fiber in the diet below 1.5 per cent on a dry weight basis. (The percentage on a dry weight basis is calculated by dividing the percentage of the nutrient in the total product by the percentage of dry matter.)

2. Feed a moderate amount of highly digestible protein from cottage cheese or eggs, at the rate of 4 gm./kg. body weight daily. Large quantities of muscle meats, meat by-products and coarse cereals are contraindicated.

3. Fat in excess of 12 per cent of the diet on a dry weight basis should be avoided.

4. Provide easily digested carbohydrates, with a low fiber content, from foods such as corn syrup, cornstarch, rice, farina and dextrose.

5. Foods containing more than 10 per cent sucrose or lactose should be avoided.

6. If individual foods, such as cottage cheese or eggs, constitute the majority of the diet, a source of potassium should be added to replace that lost in the feces.

## CONSIDERATION

In cases of severe chronic diarrhea or when vomiting occurs, parenteral fluid therapy should be instituted to replace lost fluids and electrolytes.

## RECOMMENDED DIET

Most diseases of the gastrointestinal tract demand a soft, bland, nonstimulating, low-fiber diet that is easily digested. This diet is available commercially as Prescription Diet® i/d®, or a homemade soft bland diet can be fed.

### SOFT BLAND DIET

½ cup farina (Cream of Wheat®) cooked to make 2 cups
1½ cups creamed cottage cheese
1 large egg, hard-cooked
2 T. brewers' yeast
3 T. sugar
1 T. corn oil
1 T. potassium chloride
2 t. dicalcium phosphate

A balanced vitamin-mineral supplement in a quantity sufficient to provide the daily requirement for each vitamin and trace mineral. Cook farina according to package directions. Cool. Add remaining ingredients to farina and mix well. Yield: 2 lb.

| ANALYSIS | |
|---|---|
| Protein | 7.0% |
| Fat | 2.7% |
| Carbohydrate | 9.6% |
| Moisture | 77.5% |
| Calories | 440 Cal./lb. |

## FEEDING GUIDE

Feed sufficient amount to maintain normal body weight.

| BODY WEIGHT | APPROXIMATE DAILY FEEDING |
|---|---|
| 5 lb. | ⅔ lb. |
| 10 lb. | 1 lb. |
| 20 lb. | 1⅔ lb. |
| 40 lb. | 2¾ lb. |
| 60 lb. | 3¾ lb. |
| 80 lb. | 4¾ lb. |
| 100 lb. | 5½ lb. |

## FEVER

Fever increases metabolic rate and caloric need. If accompanied by complete anorexia the necessity of managing this increased need is greater.

## OBJECTIVE

To supply sufficient calories to meet increased metabolic needs attendant with an elevation in body temperature.

## MANAGEMENT

Increase the dog's caloric intake by 6 Calories/kg. body weight daily for each degree of fever (°F.). This can be accomplished by adding corn oil to the diet (1 t. corn oil contains about 40 Calories).

## CONSIDERATION

In prolonged fever with proteinuria, feed a diet designed for growth or add ⅓ cup cottage cheese or 2 hard-cooked eggs to each pound of maintenance diet.

## RECOMMENDED DIET

A high-protein diet with readily available energy sources. If food intake is reduced, feed as described under "Anorexia," page 60.

## FLATULENCE

Flatulence is due primarily to gas formation from bacterial fermentation and putrefaction of ingested food or excess swallowing of air. The condition can be acute or chronic, although acute flatulence is seen only occasionally in dogs and cats. The influence of foods on gas formation in dogs is highly variable. A diet or foodstuff which results in flatulence in one dog may have little effect in another.

## OBJECTIVE

To avoid feeding foods which encourage fermentation, putrefaction and gas formation, or in a manner that encourages aerophagia.

## MANAGEMENT

1. Avoid feeding foods high in soybean products, potatoes, root vegetables, beans, cabbage, cauliflower, onions, etc.
2. Avoid feeding large quantities of milk as it may cause digestive upsets, allowing increase in putrefactive bacteria.
3. Avoid high-protein diets composed of meat or fish by-products.
4. Feed two or three small meals daily.

## RECOMMENDED DIET

Diet depends upon the cause. A soft bland diet (see "Diarrhea," p. 62) in frequent, small amounts may be helpful. Otherwise, feed commercial foods that do not contain the aforementioned gas-producing foods. A dietary food with a restricted amount of protein may prove helpful in some cases.

## FOOD-INDUCED ALLERGY

Accurate diagnosis is as important as management. Provocative exposure is the most accurate method of diagnosing food-induced allergy. Once the diagnosis is confirmed, the veterinarian should work toward identifying foods which are nonallergenic to the patient, rather than determining those which produce a reaction. When a sufficient number of foods that do not produce an allergic response have been discovered, a diet should be recommended that fulfills the animal's nutritional requirements.

## OBJECTIVE

To eliminate from the diet foods that produce an allergic response.

## MANAGEMENT

Conduct elimination trials using a diet composed of foods not commonly found in the patient's diet or those which have a low probability of producing an allergic response. Maintain the patient on the hypoallergenic diet and distilled water. Expose the patient to foods, one at a time, beginning with tap water, to discover offending foods. The real aim of provocative exposure is to determine foods the patient *can* eat, from which a diet can be compounded.

## CONSIDERATION

When a homemade diet composed of a restricted number of ingredients is used for management, the vitamins and minerals, especially calcium and phosphorus, must be balanced to meet the requirements of the dog. For short-term diagnostic trials this is not critical.

## RECOMMENDED DIET

A hypoallergenic diet containing ingredients not commonly fed should be prescribed. This diet is available commercially as Prescription Diet® d/d®, or a homemade hypoallergenic diet can be fed.

HYPOALLERGENIC DIET
4 oz. cooked lamb*
1 cup cooked rice
1 t. corn oil
1½ t. dicalcium phosphate

*Do not season during cooking. Discard excess fat. Balanced vitamin-mineral supplement in a quantity sufficient to provide the daily requirements for each vitamin and trace mineral. Combine all ingredients and mix well. Yield: ¾ lb.

| ANALYSIS | |
|---|---|
| Protein | 10.0% |
| Fat | 8.0% |
| Carbohydrate | 15.3% |
| Moisture | 65.0% |
| Calories | 800 Cal./lb. |

## FEEDING GUIDE

Feed sufficient amount to maintain normal body weight.

| BODY WEIGHT | APPROXIMATE DAILY FEEDING |
|---|---|
| 5 lb. | ⅓ lb. |
| 10 lb. | ½ lb. |
| 20 lb. | 1 lb. |
| 40 lb. | 1½ lb. |
| 60 lb. | 2 lb. |
| 80 lb. | 2½ lb. |
| 100 lb. | 3 lb. |

## FRACTURES

Intensive mineral therapy is not needed for fracture healing, since the mineral for calcification of the callus comes from the surrounding bone, not from circulating blood. Thus, a balanced diet, such as that recommended for puppy growth, contains adequate minerals for healing fractures.

### OBJECTIVE

To supply the nutritive requirements necessary for normal growth and calcification of bone.

### MANAGEMENT

Supply a diet known to be adequate for bone growth.

### CONSIDERATIONS

1. In cases where the diet is suspected as being marginal in animal protein, muscle meat, cottage cheese or eggs should be added to make up not more than 25 per cent of the diet.

2. If the diet contains more than 25 per cent animal tissue (meat or meat by-products), be certain the calcium:phosphorus ratio exceeds 1:1. Many homemade diets or commercial foods heavily supplemented with meat have a calcium:phosphorus ratio less than 1:1.

### RECOMMENDED DIET

A well-balanced diet with proper levels of minerals is the diet of choice. A wide variety of good-quality products designed for puppy growth are available and satisfactory.

## HEPATIC DISEASE

As the largest organ in the body, the liver performs the greatest number of body functions vital to life. Thus, a dog afflicted with severe liver disease is likely to suffer from a number of intrinsic disorders involving metabolism. Fortunately, the liver has a remarkable healing ability if it is rested. Proper dietetic management can reduce the stress placed on the liver by lowering the demand for its functions. The length of time dietetic management is required depends on the specific cause. For acute conditions three or four weeks may be adequate, while chronic liver disease demands long-term management.

### OBJECTIVE

To (1) reduce the need for liver functions, such as gluconeogenesis, fat conversion, deamination and transamination of amino acids, uric acid conversion and bile secretion; and (2) restore liver glycogen.

### MANAGEMENT

1. Provide readily available energy using carbohydrate sources, such as starch, rice, dextrose or corn syrup. Avoid higher-fiber cereal by-products as used in many dry dog foods.

2. Feed easily digested protein with a biologic value of 75 or above at rates of 3.0 to 4.0 gm./kg. body weight daily. Egg or milk protein is recommended; avoid lower-quality protein sources such as meat or poultry by-products and meat or fish meals.

3. Restrict uric acid precursors (nucleic acid–containing foods) to reduce the need for uric acid conversion. Such foods include fish meal, shellfish and glandular foods such as spleen, thymus, liver, kidney and other meat by-products.

4. Avoid feeding a diet that contains more than 12 per cent fat on a dry weight basis.

### CONSIDERATIONS

1. In methionine or choline deficiencies, or when low-protein diets (below 15 per cent) are fed, give one capsule of Caniheptin®/10 kg. body weight daily for 3 days.

2. In chronic conditions with ascites, sodium should be restricted to at least 60 mg./100 gm. dry diet.

### RECOMMENDED DIET

A soft bland diet consisting of an egg–cottage cheese–rice combination is easily digested and efficiently metabolized by the dog with liver disease. This diet is available commercially as Prescription Diet® i/d® or the homemade soft bland diet can be fed. (See "Diarrhea," p. 62.)

## NUTRITIONAL SECONDARY HYPERPARATHYROIDISM

Frequently referred to as the all-meat syndrome, this disease is caused by the prolonged consumption of a diet low in calcium or with a severely inverse calcium to phosphorus ratio. It is seen most often in animals consuming exclusive meat diets or diets composed primarily of animal tissues.

### OBJECTIVE

To provide a balanced diet, especially in respect to the calcium:phosphorus ratio, and total amounts of those minerals.

### MANAGEMENT

Provide calcium and phosphorus in readily available forms, at the rate of at least 480 mg. calcium and 400 mg. phosphorus/kg. body weight daily, for dogs. For cats, half this amount is adequate.

### CONSIDERATIONS

Do not administer excessive amounts of vitamins and minerals during treatment. Hypervitaminosis D or trace mineral deficiencies may result.

### RECOMMENDED DIET

A balanced diet designed for growth should be fed.

## FUNCTIONAL HYPOGLYCEMIA

Hypoglycemia is a metabolic disorder of carbohydrate metabolism characterized by low serum glucose levels. To manage dogs with hypoglycemia successfully, it is necessary to provide a continuous supply of nutrients that are metabolized to form glucose. Wide fluctuations in the blood glucose level is thus avoided.

### OBJECTIVE

To supply, frequently, precursors of blood glucose which are slowly converted by the body to blood sugar.

### MANAGEMENT

1. Increase the frequency of daily feedings to at least four.
2. Supply calories in the form of protein, fat and complex carbohydrates. Avoid simple sugars, such as sucrose. Complex carbohydrates, such as the starches found in cereals, are digested more slowly than simple sugars.

### CONSIDERATIONS

1. During an acute attack, feed sugar, preferably glucose, at a rate of 2 T./10 kg. body weight. Use table sugar (sucrose) in an emergency, at the same rate.
2. Feed additional food to working dogs during periods of exercise. Include a light, high-protein meal prior to exercise and 100- to 150-calorie, high-carbohydrate snacks every 4 hours during exercise.

### RECOMMENDED DIET

A high-quality protein diet containing complex carbohydrate sources should be given. Avoid soft moist pet foods containing sucrose.

## HYPOTHYROIDISM

As with most endocrine disturbances, replacement therapy is necessary for the lifetime of the patient. A high-quality diet with a consistent formulation is essential in managing and evaluating the patient's condition and response to therapy.

### OBJECTIVE

To feed a balanced diet uniform in composition and quality to enable evaluation of replacement therapy.

### MANAGEMENT

Feed a good-quality, balanced diet produced from a fixed formula. Many dietary foods meet this criterion. Select the one which meets the needs of the patient. Many commercial pet foods are produced from open formulas; thus, their composition varies, making it difficult to evaluate medical therapy.

## OBESITY

Obesity has become the most common diet-induced condition seen in dogs. Cats rarely become obese. Obesity is the result of an excessive caloric intake in relation to energy expenditure. To produce weight loss in the dog, it is necessary to reduce caloric intake below expenditure. This is accomplished by decreasing food intake or feeding a special reducing diet. Merely reducing the amount of the dog's regular diet may create deficiencies of nutrients needed for burning excess body fat. Also, the dog will become ravenously hungry and seek other sources of food. Without an actual change in diet, most reducing programs fail. Accomplish *caloric* reduction by replacing most of the fat and digestible carbohydrates with indigestible carbohydrates and fiber. The dog eats the accustomed amount of food, but receives fewer digestible calories.

### OBJECTIVE

To reduce the caloric intake of the obese animal and regulate the caloric intake of the obesity-prone animal.

### MANAGEMENT

To accomplish a successful weight-reduction program:

1. Establish rapport with the owner. Explain obesity and its dangers.

2. Conduct a complete physical examination to eliminate conditions that mimic or complicate obesity.

3. Obtain an accurate diet history. Attempt to maintain time and frequency of feeding, changing only the amount fed and the diet. Type of diet (prepared or homemade) should remain constant.

4. Establish and tell the owner the dog's optimal weight. This establishes the goal of the program.

5. Estimate the time required to reach optimal weight. Dogs up to 10 kg. optimal weight lose 0.5 kg./week; from 10 to 20 kg., lose 1.0 kg./week; and above 20 kg., lose 1.5 kg./week. The majority of obese dogs will reach optimal weight in 8 to 10 weeks when fed at 60 per cent of the caloric requirements to maintain *optimal* weight.

6. Encourage the owner to weigh the dog weekly, keep a written record, and get the family involved in increasing the dog's exercise.

7. Provide the necessary diet information, including diet and amount to feed, based on optimal weight, not obese weight.

8. Recommend the proper diet to maintain weight when optimal weight is attained. The reducing diet can be continued in quantity sufficient to maintain optimal weight.

### RECOMMENDED DIET

A reducing diet should contain not more than 350 digestible calories per lb. of canned food and supply at least 4.0 gm. protein/kg. body weight daily. This can be accomplished by restricting fat and replacing digestible carbohydrates with indigestible fiber (cellulose flour) or vegetables. Such a diet is available commercially as Prescription Diet® r/d®, or a homemade reducing diet can be fed.

#### REDUCING DIET

¼ lb. lean ground beef
½ cup cottage cheese, *uncreamed*
2 cups carrots, canned solids
2 cups green beans, canned solids
1½ t. dicalcium phosphate

Balanced vitamin-mineral supplement in a quantity sufficient to provide the daily requirements for each vitamin and trace mineral. Cook beef, drain fat and cool. Add remaining ingredients. Yield: 1¾ lb.

#### ANALYSIS

| | |
|---|---|
| Protein | 7.0% |
| Fat | 1.7% |
| Carbohydrate | 5.0% |
| Moisture | 85.0% |
| Calories | 300 Cal./lb. |

### FEEDING GUIDE

| OPTIMAL BODY WEIGHT | APPROXIMATE DAILY FEEDING |
|---|---|
| 5 lb. | ⅓ lb. |
| 10 lb. | ⅔ lb. |
| 20 lb. | 1 lb. |
| 40 lb. | 1¾ lb. |
| 60 lb. | 2½ lb. |
| 80 lb. | 2¾ lb. |
| 100 lb. | 3¼ lb. |

## ORPHANED PUPS AND KITTENS

When it becomes necessary to hand-rear orphaned pups and kittens, the first priority is a milk replacement to supply adequate nutrition. Control of environmental factors such as maintenance of temperature at 80 to 90° F., humidity at 40 to 50 per cent and the elimination of disturbances is also important.

### OBJECTIVE

To replace the milk that would normally be provided by the lactating female. This requires supplying a balanced nutrient source capable of supporting growth.

### MANAGEMENT

1. Provide energy from fats and carbohydrates at the following schedule:

1st week......120 Cal./kg. body weight daily
2nd week ....140 Cal./kg. body weight daily
3rd week.....160 Cal./kg. body weight daily
4th week
  to weaning 180 Cal./kg. body weight daily

2. Provide protein of a biologic value of 90 or greater from milk and egg protein at the rate of at least 5.4 gm./kg. body weight until weaning.
3. Provide minerals balanced at growth levels, paying particular attention to a calcium:phosphorus ratio of 1.0:0.9.
4. Provide adequate amounts of vitamins to support growth without oversupplementation.
5. Slight underfeeding is preferable to overfeeding. Divide the daily food allowance into 4 to 6 feedings.
6. All materials used should be clean and sterilized and the formula warmed to body temperature before feeding.
7. To substitute for the female's licking activity, the anal region of the young should be wiped at each feeding to stimulate elimination until they are able to do it by themselves.
8. Weigh the young daily to insure that weight gain is achieved.

### RECOMMENDED DIET

Commercial milk replacements, such as Esbilac® and KMR®, provide adequate nourishment for orphaned pups and kittens. These products also can be used to supplement the efforts of a dam with inadequate milk supply. Replacement milk can be administered by a doll bottle and nipple, a premature baby bottle, or an intragastric stomach tube. Begin weaning to solid food at 3 weeks of age or as soon as possible. Mix milk replacement with soft bland diet (see "Diarrhea," p. 62) as first food. Convert to a growth diet at 5 or 6 weeks of age.

## PANCREATIC INSUFFICIENCY

Regardless of the specific cause, pancreatic insufficiency invariably leads to maldigestion of protein, fat and some starch. It is essential in cases of pancreatic insufficiency to replace the normal pancreatic secretion and provide a uniform, consistent diet to evaluate drug or enzyme replacement therapy accurately.

### OBJECTIVE

To reduce the intake of foods which require extensive digestion by pancreatic enzymes.

### MANAGEMENT

1. Feed an easily digested low-fat and low-fiber diet.
2. Supply carbohydrates such as glucose, sucrose, cornstarch or rice.
3. Reduce fat to a level not to exceed 12 per cent on a dry weight basis.
4. Feed bland proteins from milk or eggs at restricted levels to avoid excessive intestinal putrefaction.
5. Administer vitamin A at 400 I.U./kg. body weight daily and vitamin D at 30 I.U./kg. body weight daily, orally.
6. Add Viokase® or Catazym® to food. Incubate for 20 minutes prior to feeding.

### RECOMMENDED DIET

A soft bland diet with restricted fat is ideal for nourishing patients with pancreatic insufficiency. The homemade soft bland diet (see page 63) or Prescription Diet® i/d® can be fed.

## PANSTEATITIS

Pansteatitis, or "yellow fat disease," is a nutritional disease caused by a diet containing excessive unstabilized, unsaturated fatty acids. The disease is most common in cats consuming diets composed mainly of unstabilized red tuna fish. Enough vitamin E is now added to most commercial rations to adequately stabilize the fatty acids and prevent the disease.

## OBJECTIVE

To restrict the feeding of foods with a high content of unsaturated fatty acids.

## MANAGEMENT

Eliminate the feeding of foods containing high levels of unstabilized, unsaturated fats. Feed only commercial rations which have vitamin E added.

## PUERPERAL TETANY

More commonly known as eclampsia, puerperal tetany usually occurs from one to three weeks post partum but can occur later. The main problem is a low plasma calcium level. This may result from the failure of the calcium homeostatic mechanism to compensate for the increased loss in the milk, but the exact mechanism is unknown.

## OBJECTIVE

To provide a diet which maintains a normal plasma calcium level in the lactating female.

## MANAGEMENT

Feed a diet which contains at least 1.4 per cent calcium on a dry weight basis, with a calcium:phosphorus ratio of at least 1.2:1.

## CONSIDERATIONS

1. Vitamin D therapy may be instituted during the last week of gestation. Doses of 10,000 to 25,000 I.U. daily can be tolerated. Massive doses should be avoided.

2. It may be necessary to remove the young from the female and terminate lactation to maintain a normal blood calcium level. If the young are not ready for weaning, they should be hand-reared and fed a milk replacement (see "Orphaned Pups and Kittens," p. 68). Withdrawal from the bitch for a 24-hour period is sometimes helpful.

## RECOMMENDED DIET

Any balanced diet that has been shown to be nutritionally adequate for reproduction and contains at least 1.4 per cent calcium on a dry weight basis should be given. Diet modification may not modify the natural pathogenesis.

## RENAL FAILURE

Both dogs and cats may suffer from various types of kidney disease producing renal failure. Diseased kidneys are not able to rid the body of the waste products of protein metabolism. Regardless of the specific cause of renal failure, the dietetic management is the same, i.e., restriction of protein intake. The degree of restriction required depends upon the severity of renal failure in the individual case.

## OBJECTIVE

To reduce the nitrogenous wastes and maintain energy and nutrient intake by feeding restricted quantities of protein of high biologic value, thereby reducing the need for renal function.

## MANAGEMENT

1. Reduce protein excess in accordance with the severity of renal failure. Estimate the protein intake by obtaining a diet history.

Most diets composed of human table foods are high in protein and produce large excesses. The following table provides the average protein in excess of requirement and the percentage of protein excess for a 15-kg. dog eating the various types of commercial foods at a rate sufficient to meet its daily energy needs.

| | PROTEIN EXCESS | |
| | | % Protein |
| TYPE OF FOOD | gm./day | Requirement |
| --- | --- | --- |
| Canned all meat* | 92 | 450 |
| Canned ration* | 80 | 400 |
| Soft Moist* | 55 | 275 |
| Dry* | 49 | 250 |
| Dietary† | 20 | 100 |

*Av. of 3 leading brands.
†Prescription Diet® k/d® (canned).

For most dogs, moderate protein restriction is sufficient initially. This can be accomplished by feeding a food that contains not more than 20 per cent protein calories and supplies not more than 3.0 gm. protein/kg. body weight daily.

As renal function declines, the quantity of excess protein must be reduced. In severe renal failure, strict protein restriction (1.2 gm. protein/kg. body weight daily) must be instituted to prevent uremia. As protein intake is reduced, biologic value must approach 100.

2. For cats, feed not more than 4.0 gm. protein/kg. body weight daily. Protein calories should not exceed 25 per cent of the diet.

3. Feed a diet that contains not more than 0.5 per cent phosphorus.

4. Feed a diet containing at least 0.2 per cent sodium on a dry weight basis.

5. Provide water *ad lib*.

## CONSIDERATIONS

1. During acute renal shutdown, feed a protein-free diet. Meet the animal's caloric needs with simple sugars (glucose or cornstarch), fats and oils.

2. During severe renal proteinuria (4+), add 1 egg or ⅓ cup cottage cheese for every 4 oz. of restricted protein diet fed, or feed a diet designed to meet the protein requirements of growth.

3. During initial stages of renal failure with polydipsia, polyuria and uremia, give a B-complex vitamin preparation. Brewers' yeast is contraindicated because of its protein content.

4. During uremia, administer additional sodium as sodium chloride or bicarbonate. Once the animal is compensated, these may be discontinued.

## RECOMMENDED DIET

A restricted protein diet which meets the nutritional needs of the patient but restricts excesses should be given. This diet is available commercially as Prescription Diet® k/d®, or a homemade restricted protein diet can be fed to dogs. Cats with renal failure can be fed Feline k/d®. Since cats are usually fed high-protein diets, homemade restricted protein diets for cats have not proved very satisfactory owing to their low palatability and the tendency of the owner to add protein foods to overcome this problem.

If strict protein restriction is required, add nonprotein calories to the dietary food. Start by adding 3 T. of sugar or 1 T. of vegetable oil/lb. of food. Increase as required to prevent buildup of nonprotein nitrogen blood constituents. If the homemade diet is being fed, reduce the ground beef.

RESTRICTED PROTEIN DIET
¼ lb. ground beef (regular)*
1 large egg, hard-cooked
2 cups cooked rice
1 t. calcium carbonate
3 slices white bread, crumbled

*Do not use lean ground round or chuck.

A balanced vitamin-mineral supplement in a quantity sufficient to provide the daily requirement for each vitamin and trace mineral. Braise the meat, retaining fat. Combine all ingredients and mix well. This mixture is somewhat dry and the palatability can be improved by adding a little water (not milk). Yield: 1¼ lb.

ANALYSIS

| | |
|---|---|
| Protein | 6.4% |
| Fat | 5.0% |
| Carbohydrate | 21.0% |
| Calories* | 740 Cal./lb. |

*This diet supplies 17 per cent protein calories, 30 per cent fat calories and 53 per cent carbohydrate calories.

## FEEDING GUIDE

Feed sufficient amount to maintain normal body weight.

| BODY WEIGHT | APPROXIMATE DAILY FEEDING |
|---|---|
| 5 lb. | ¼ lb. |
| 10 lb. | ½ lb. |
| 20 lb. | 1 lb. |
| 40 lb. | 1½ lb. |
| 60 lb. | 2 lb. |
| 80 lb. | 2½ lb. |
| 100 lb. | 3 lb. |

## SKELETAL DISEASES

The differential diagnosis of skeletal diseases of nutritional origin under clinical conditions is difficult, at best. One continuing diagnosis that always can be made is that the animal is consuming an unbalanced diet. The obvious method of therapy is to change the diet to one of known adequacy rather than to attempt the supplementation of a deficient ration, particularly if the deficiency is unknown.

## OBJECTIVE AND MANAGEMENT

To provide a balanced diet, nutritionally adequate for the particular stage of the life cycle.

### CONSIDERATIONS

1. During the rare instance when vitamin D is deficient, administer in the diet at the rate of 30 I.U./kg. body weight daily, which is equivalent to 0.5 ml. of cod liver oil/kg. body weight daily.
2. Do not administer excessive amounts of vitamins and minerals during treatment. If the diagnosis is correct, healing will take place rapidly on a nutritionally balanced growth diet. If the diagnosis is incorrect, neither the diet nor supplements will correct the condition. This approach eliminates the chance of producing hypervitaminosis or trace mineral deficiencies.

### RECOMMENDED DIET

A balanced diet which has been shown to be adequate for growth.

## SOFT TISSUE WOUNDS

Soft tissue wounds place heavy stress on the body. Recovery can be delayed unless those nutrients essential to tissue repair are adequately supplied. As a major component of tissue, protein becomes vitally important in repair and replacement. Carbohydrates and fats are important as well because they supply energy and, thus, spare protein.

### OBJECTIVE

To provide a diet adequate in those items essential to tissue repair, primarily protein and energy.

### MANAGEMENT

If the previously fed diet has been marginal in animal protein, add meat, cottage cheese or egg to constitute 25 per cent of the diet by weight.

### RECOMMENDED DIET

A high-protein, high-energy diet which meets the nutrient requirements for growth can be fed to patients with soft-tissue wounds.

## STARVATION

When an animal receives an inadequate amount of any nutrient, inanition results. It is usually the result of some physical or environmental stress rather than a pathologic one. This condition occurs when an animal (1) is not provided with enough food, (2) purposefully does not consume food, or (3) is physically unable to consume enough food. The condition may be overcome by increasing either the quantity or the nutrient density of the diet consumed. The following are some of the conditions which may be encountered and the management principles which apply to them.

1. *Growth.* Double the maintenance nutrient intake. Feed *ad lib.*
2. *Lactation.* Increase the maintenance food intake gradually to about 3 or 3½ times, during the 4th and 5th weeks. Feed *ad lib.* To maintain body weight it may be necessary to increase caloric density of food. This can be accomplished by adding 1 T. of fat/ lb. of canned food, or 3 T./lb. of dry food.
3. *Parasitism.* Increase food intake according to parasite load and anemia. Feed *ad lib* and treat.
4. *Poor palatability or fixed eating habits.* Modify the diet so that the animal will accept minimum daily requirements.
5. *Physical and psychological stress.* An animal experiencing temporary stress which increases the energy requirement should be provided with additional energy by adding fat, such as corn oil, at the rate of 3 T./lb. of dry food daily. Animals under continuous stress should be fed a high-energy concentrated ration, such as Science Diet® Maximum Stress Diet, or a homemade diet supplying at least 4,000 Cal./kg.
6. *Abandonment.* Begin feeding at about half the normal intake level and progress to full feeding gradually over a three-day period.

## SURGERY (GASTROINTESTINAL)

The condition of the animal prior to surgery and the segment of the gastrointestinal tract to be invaded are the major considerations when formulating a nutritional program for patients undergoing gastrointestinal surgery. General presurgical considerations include correct body weight, positive nitrogen balance and adequate carbohydrate and vitamin stores.

Postsurgical patients have a priority need for fluids, electrolytes, calories and protein, in that order.

## OBJECTIVE

To provide adequate high-quality protein and energy necessary for tissue repair and regeneration.

## MANAGEMENT

### Esophagus

1. Withhold oral alimentation for 1 to 4 days, postsurgically.
2. Administer fluid therapy if needed.
3. Restore normal alimentation, beginning with liquids, such as salted meat broth or Hospital Diet® Starter. After 48 to 96 hours, gradually incorporate small amounts of a soft bland diet with the liquids so that the animal is eating a normal diet within 10 to 14 days.

### Stomach

1. Avoid bulky foods. Feed liquid prepared diets, such as Esbilac® or Starter.
2. Change gradually to a soft bland diet (see page 63).
3. Add dilute HCl to the water at the rate of 15 drops/pint.

### Intestine

1. Nothing should be given when ileus is encountered following enterotomy (24 to 96 hours).
2. Oral alimentation should be started with the return of intestinal peristalisis. Offer small quantities of a soft bland diet and fluid frequently (4 to 6 times daily).

### Gastric Dilatation

1. Avoid feeding and watering following strenuous exercise. Introduce food and water gradually.
2. Feed a soft bland, low-fat diet in three or four meals daily. Do not allow the patient to gorge on either food or water.
3. Clean, fresh water should be available at all times and strenuous exercise should be avoided immediately following eating.

## URINARY OBSTRUCTION (UROLITHIASIS), FELINE

The mechanism that disposes an animal to urolithiasis is unknown. Infectious agents, phosphorus and magnesium have been implicated. Efforts at reducing the severity or preventing the recurrence of urolithiasis may be supplemented by dietetic measures. Since the minerals necessary to produce a urolith must be present in the urine if the stone is to be formed, dietary management is aimed at reducing the concentration of urinary minerals and maintaining a pH unfavorable to the formation of the particular urolith.

## OBJECTIVE

To feed a diet which maintains an acid pH and results in reduction of the urinary concentrations of minerals, especially magnesium and phosphorus.

## MANAGEMENT

1. Restrict the ash in the diet to not more than 5 per cent on a dry weight basis.
2. Restrict the diet to rations containing less than 0.15 per cent magnesium and 0.6 per cent phosphorus, on a dry weight basis.
3. Increase B-complex vitamins to provide an amount comparable to 0.25 gm. brewers' yeast/kg. body weight daily.
4. Increase water intake by administering salt at the rate of 500 mg./kg. body weight daily, or approximately 5 gm. salt (1 t.)/lb. canned food. Insure access to fresh water.

## CONSIDERATIONS

In vitamin A deficiency, administer it at the rate of 400 I.U./kg. body weight daily.

## RECOMMENDED DIET

Feed a low-ash dietary food such as Feline c/d®.

## VITAMIN-RELATED DISEASES

Vitamins have received more attention than they deserve in relation to their value in the treatment of disease. They should be used only when a specific vitamin deficiency exists, never as a cure-all for undiagnosed nutritional and metabolic disorders.

The following is a list of vitamin-related diseases which may occur in cats and dogs.

**Vitamin A:**   Cats are unable to utilize the

precursor b-carotene. Thus, preformed vitamin A must be supplied in their diet. With the exception of liver, many commonly fed foods are poor sources of preformed vitamin A. For this reason, acute and chronic vitamin A deficiency may occur in cats. However, hypervitaminosis A can occur in cats consuming an exclusive liver diet.

As for dogs, hypervitaminosis A from oversupplementation is seen more frequently than deficiency.

**Vitamin D.** Rickets can occur as a result of an imbalanced calcium:phosphorus ratio and inadequate vitamin D intake in young growing animals housed indoors. In adults, the result is osteomalacia. More danger actually exists from excesses of vitamin D rather than deficiencies. Hypervitaminosis D produces renal and vascular calcification.

**Vitamin E.** See "Pansteatitis," p. 68.

**Vitamin B-complex.** Because they are water-soluble, the B-complex vitamins are rarely toxic. Deficiencies are likely to occur when the animal is losing large quantities of fluids, such as in vomiting and diarrhea, or when food intake is reduced for any reason. When B-complex deficiencies are present, these vitamins should always be given as the complex in preparations containing at least five times the minimum daily requirement of each vitamin.

# A CATALOG OF GENETIC DISORDERS OF THE DOG

DONALD F. PATTERSON, D.V.M.
*Philadelphia, Pennsylvania*

With the increasing sophistication of diagnostic procedures and the declining importance of infectious, parasitic and nutritional diseases has come a growing awareness that a significant proportion of disease conditions in the dog has a genetic cause. While individual genetic diseases may be rare in the general population, they often occur with a high frequency within individual kennels or even in entire breeds. For those concerned, the economic and emotional impact may be great. The ability of the veterinarian to deal effectively with such problems depends upon a general knowledge of genetics and specific information regarding the diagnostic and genetic features of the disease in question. The latter information tends to be widely scattered and not readily available to the veterinarian. As a partial solution to this problem, the author has compiled this catalog, listing disorders with a major genetic component mainly according to the organ system primarily involved. The breeds known to be affected are given, along with the mode of inheritance when known.* The reader is directed to selected references for further details. No attempt has been made to include all references on a given condition.

It will be recognized that in many of the disorders listed there is ample evidence of a genetic cause but the lack of definitive genetic studies precludes the listing of the mode of inheritance. Family studies and breeding experiments will be needed to clarify these questions, and it is hoped that practicing veterinarians who have the opportunity to see these and as yet unidentified genetic disorders will be stimulated to undertake such observations.

---

*Throughout the catalog, modes of inheritance will be designated according to the following key: R, autosomal recessive; D, autosomal dominant; ID, incomplete dominant; XR, X-linked recessive; XD, X-linked dominant; P, polygenic; and ?, unknown or in question.

*Table 1.*   *The Blood*

| CONDITION | BREED(S) | MODE | SELECTED REFERENCES |
|---|---|---|---|
| Afibrinogenemia | St. Bernard | D | Kammermann et al. (1971) |
| Blood group incompatibility (mainly A system) | All breeds | D* | Dewit et al. (1969)<br>Swisher et al. (1962)<br>Young et al. (1951) |
| Chondrodysplasia-anemia syndrome | Alaskan malamute | R | Fletch et al. (1975) |
| Cyclic neutropenia (gray collie syndrome) | Collie | R | Ford (1969)<br>Lund et al. (1967, 1970a, 1970b)<br>Cheville (1968)<br>Cheville et al. (1970)<br>Dale et al. (1971) |
| Factor VII deficiency | Beagle<br>Alaskan malamute | R | Rowsell (1963)<br>Dodds (1974a) |
| Hemophilia A (factor VIII deficiency) | Irish setter | XR | Hutt et al. (1948)<br>Field et al. (1946)<br>Graham et al. (1949) |
|  | German shepherd, collie | XR | Rowsell (1963) |
|  | Labrador retriever | XR | Archer and Bowden (1959) |
|  | Beagle | XR | Brock et al. (1963) |
|  | Shetland sheepdog | XR | Wurzel and Lawrence (1961) |
|  | Greyhound | XR | Sharp and Dike (1963) |
|  | Weimaraner | XR | Kaneko et al. (1967) |
|  | Chihuahua | XR | Kaneko et al. (1967) |
|  | Antarctic sledge dog | XR | Bellars (1969) |
|  | Vizsla | XR | Buckner et al. (1967) |
| Hemophilia B (Christmas disease, factor IX deficiency) | Cairn terrier | XR | Rowsell et al. (1960) |
| Factor X deficiency | Cocker spaniel | ID | Dodds (1973) |
| Factor XI deficiency | Springer spaniel | ID | Dodds and Kull (1971) |
| Hyperlipoproteinemia | Miniature schnauzer | ? | Rogers et al. (1975) |
| Nonspherocytic hemolytic anemia (pyruvate kinase deficiency) | Basenji | R | Tasker et al. (1969)<br>Ewing (1969)<br>Searcy et al. (1971)<br>Standerfer et al. (1974) |
|  | Beagle | ? | Prasse et al. (1975) |
| Platelet function defects | Otterhound, basset<br>Foxhound, Scottish terrier | ID | Dodds (1967)<br>Dodds (1974a) |
| Von Willebrand's disease | German shepherd, miniature schnauzer, Golden retriever, Scottish terrier, Doberman pinscher | ID | Dodds (1974b, 1975) |

*Genes determining blood group substances are inherited as dominants in that one dose of the gene resulting in the presence of the antigen is sufficient to give a detectable reaction. For example A+ blood transfused into an A− dog elicits anti-A antibodies whether the donor is homozygous or heterozygous for the A+ allele. Natural isoantibodies against the blood group antigens are absent or weak in dogs. Hemolytic disease of newborn pups and transfusion reactions usually depend on prior immunization of A− individuals with A+ blood by transfusion.

## SELECTED REFERENCES:

### The Blood

Archer, R. K., and Bowden, R. S. T.: A case of true hemophilia in a Labrador dog. Vet. Rec., 71:560–561, 1959.

Bellars, A. R. M.: Hereditary disease in British antarctic sledge dogs. Vet. Rec., 85:600–607, 1969.

Brock, W. E., et al.: Canine hemophilia. Arch. Path., 76:464–469, 1963.

Buckner, R. G., et al.: Hemophilia in the Vizsla. J. Small Animal Pract., 8:511–519, 1967.

Cheville, N. F.: The gray collie syndrome. J. Am. Vet. Med. Assn., 152:620–630, 1968.

Cheville, N. F., Cutlip, R. C., and Moon, H. W.: Microscopic pathology of the gray collie syndrome. Path. Vet., 7:225–245, 1970.

Dale, D. C., et al.: Cyclic urinary leukopoietic activity in gray collie dogs. Science, 173:152–153, 1971.

Dewit, C. D., et al.: The practical importance of blood groups in dogs. J. Small Animal Pract., 8:285–289, 1969.

Dodds, W. J.: Familial canine thrombocytopathy. Thromb. Diath. Haemorrh. (Suppl. 26):241–248, 1967.

Dodds, W. J.: Canine factor X (Stuart-Prower factor) deficiency. J. Lab. Clin. Med., 52:560–566, 1973.

Dodds, W. J.: Hereditary and acquired hemorrhagic disorders in animals. In Spaet, T. H. (ed.): Progress in Hemostasis and Thrombosis, Vol. II. New York, Grune and Stratton, 1974a, pp. 215–247.

Dodds, W. J.: Blood coagulation, hemostasis and thrombosis. In Melby, E. C., and Altman, N. H. (eds.): Handbook of Laboratory Animal Science, Vol. II. Cleveland, CRC Press, 1974b.

Dodds, W. J.: Bleeding disorders. In Ettinger, S. J.: Textbook of Veterinary Internal Medicine, Vol. II. Philadelphia, W. B. Saunders Co., 1975.

Dodds, W. J., and Kaneko, J. J.: Hemostasis and blood coagulation. In Kaneko, J. J., and Cornelius, C. E.: Clinical Biochemistry of Domestic Animals. New York, Academic Press, 1971.

Dodds, W. J., and Kull, J. E.: Canine factor XI (plasma thromboplastin antecedent) deficiency. J. Lab. Clin. Med., 78:746–752, 1971.

Ewing, G. O.: Familial nonspherocytic hemolytic anemia of basenji dogs. J. Am. Vet. Med. Assn., 154:503–507, 1969.

Field, R. A., Rickard, C. G., and Hutt, S. B.: Hemophilia in a family of dogs. Cornell Vet., 36:285–300, 1946.

Fletch, S. M., Pinkerton, P. H., Brueckner, P. J.: The Alaskan malamute chondrodysplasia (dwarfism-anemia) syndrome. J.A.A.H.A. (review), 11:353–361, 1975.

Ford, L.: Hereditary aspects of human and canine cyclic neutropenia. J. Hered., 60:293–299, 1969.

Graham, J. B., et al.: Canine hemophilia, observations on the course, the clotting anomaly and the effects of blood transfusion. J. Exper. Med., 29:98–111, 1949.

Hutt, F. B., Rickard, C. G., and Field, R. A.: Sex-linked hemophilia in dogs. J. Hered., 39:2–9, 1948.

Kammermann, B., Gmur, J., and Stünzi, H.: Afibrinogenämie beim Hund. Zentralbl. Vet. Med., 18A:192–205, 1971.

Kaneko, J. J., Cordy, D. R., and Carlson, G.: Canine hemophilia resembling classic hemophilia A. J. Am. Vet. Med. Assn., 150:15–21, 1967.

Lund, J. E., Gorham, J. R., and Padgett, G. A.: Canine cyclic neutropenia: diagnosis and treatment. Vet. Med. Rev., 1:33–42, 1970a.

Lund, J. E., Padgett, G. A., and Gorham, J. R.: Additional evidence on the inheritance of cyclic neutropenia in the dog. J. Hered., 61:47–49, 1970b.

Lund, J. E., Padgett, G. A., and Ott, R. L.: Cyclic neutropenia in grey collie dogs. Blood, 29:452–461, 1967.

Prasse, K. W., Crouser, D., Beutler, E., Walker, M., and Schall, W. D.: Pyruvate kinase deficiency anemia with terminal myelofibrosis and osteosclerosis in a beagle. J. Am. Vet. Med. Assn., 166:1170–1175, 1975.

Rogers, W. A., Donovan, E. F., and Kociba, G. J.: Idiopathic hyperlipoproteinemia in dogs. J. Am. Vet. Med. Assn., 166:1087–1100, 1975.

Rowsell, H. C.: Hemorrhagic disorders in dogs: their recognition, treatment and importance. "The newer knowledge about dogs." 12th Gaines Veterinary Symposium, East Lansing, Michigan, January 23, 1963.

Rowsell, H. C., et al.: A disorder resembling hemophilia B (Christmas disease) in dogs. J. Am. Vet. Med. Assn., 137:247–250, 1960.

Searcy, G. P., Miller, D. R., and Tasker, J. B.: Congenital hemolytic anemia in the basenji dog due to erythrocyte pyruvate kinase deficiency. Canad. J. Comp. Med., 35:67–70, 1971.

Sharp, A. A., and Dike, G. W. R.: Hemophilia in the dog: treatment with heterologous antihaemophilic globulin. Thromb. Diathes. Haemorrhagica, 10:494–501, 1963.

Standerfer, R. J., Templeton, J. W., and Black, J. A.: Anomalous pyruvate kinase deficiency in the basenji dog. Am. J. Vet. Res., 35:1541–1543, 1974.

Swisher, S. N., Young, L. E., and Trabold, N.: *In vitro* and *in vivo* studies of the behavior of canine erythrocyte-isoantibody systems. Ann. New York Acad. Sci., 97:15–25, 1962.

Tasker, J. B., et al.: Familial anemia in the basenji dog. J. Am. Vet. Med. Assn., 154:158–165, 1969.

Wurzel, H. A., and Lawrence, W. C.: Canine hemophilia. Thromb. Diathes. Haemorrhagica, 6:98–103, 1961.

Young, L. E., et al.: Hemolytic disease in newborn dogs. Blood, 6:291, 1951.


## SELECTED REFERENCES:

### Bones and Joints

Amlöf, J.: On achondroplasia in the dog. Zentralbl. Vet. Med., 8:43–56, 1961.

Bardens, J. W.: Congenital malformation of the foramen magnum in dogs. S. West. Vet., 18:295–298, 1965.

Bradley, I. W.: Non-union of the anconeal process in the dog. Aust. Vet. J., 43:215–216, 1967.

Burns, M., and Fraser, M. N.: Genetics of the Dog: The Basis of Successful Breeding. Philadelphia, J. B. Lippincott Co., 1966.

Calkins, E., Kahn, D., and Diner, W. C.: Idiopathic familial osteoporosis in dogs: "osteogenesis imperfecta." Ann. New York Acad. Sci., 64:410–423, 1956.

Carlson, W. D., and Severin, G. A.: Elbow dysplasia in the dog. J. Am. Vet. Med. Assn., 138:295–297, 1961.

Carrig, C. B., and Seawright, A. A.: A familial canine polyostotic fibrous dysplasia with subperiosteal cortical defects. J. Small Animal Pract., 10:397–405, 1969.

Cawley, A. J., and Archibald, J.: Ununited anconeal processes of the dog. J. Am. Vet. Med. Assn., 136:454–458, 1959.

Chester, D. K.: Multiple cartilaginous exostoses in two generations of dogs. J. Am. Vet. Med. Assn., *159*:895–897, 1971.

Corley, E. A., and Carlson, W. D.: Radiographic, Genetic, and Pathologic Aspects of Elbow Dysplasia. Proceedings of the American Veterinary Medical Association, 102nd Annual Meeting, 1965.

Curtis, R. L., English, D., and Kim, Y. J.: Spina bifida in a "stub" dog stock, selectively bred for short tails. Anat. Rec., *148*:365, 1964.

deBoom, H. P. A.: Anomalous animals. S. Afr. J. Sci., *61*:159–171, 1965.

Fletch, S. M., and Pinkerton, P. H.: Animal model: inherited hemolytic anemia with stomatocytosis in the Alaskan malamute dog. Am. J. Path., *71*:477–480, 1973.

Fletch, S. M., et al.: Clinical and pathologic features of chondrodysplasia in the Alaskan malamute. J. Am. Vet. Med. Assn., *162*:357–361, 1973.

Fletch, S. M., Pinkerton, P. H., and Brueckner, P. J.: The Alaskan malamute chondrodysplasia (dwarfism-anemia) syndrome. J.A.A.H.A. (review), *11*:353–361, 1975.

Fox, M. W.: Abnormalities of the canine skull. Canad. J. Comp. Med. Vet. Sci., *9*:219–222, 1963.

Fox, M. W.: The otocephalic syndrome in the dog. Cornell Vet., *54*:250–259, 1964.

Gardner, D. L.: Familial canine chondrodystrophia foetalis (achondroplasia). J. Path. Bact., *77*:243–247, 1959.

Geary, J. C., Oliver, J. E., and Hoerlein, B. F.: Atlanto-axial subluxation in the canine. J. Small Animal Pract., *8*:577–582, 1967.

Gee, B. R., and Doige, C. E.: Multiple cartilaginous exostoses in a litter of dogs. J. Am. Vet. Med. Assn., *156*:53–59, 1970.

Green, E. L.: Mutant stocks of cats and dogs offered for research. J. Hered., *48*:56–57, 1957.

Grüneberg, H., and Lea, A. J.: An inherited jaw anomaly in long-haired dachshunds. J. Genet., *39*:285–296, 1940.

Hansen, H. J.: A pathologic-anatomical study on disc degeneration in the dog. Acta Orthopaed. Scand., *11*:117, 1952.

Hansen, H. J.: The body constitution of dogs and its importance for the occurrence of disease. Nord. Vet. Med., *16*:977–987, 1964.

Hansen, H. J.: Historical evidence of an unusual deformity in dogs ("short-spine dog"). J. Small Animal Pract., *9*:103–108, 1968.

Henricson, B., and Olsson, S. E.: Hereditary acetabular dysplasia in German shepherd dogs. J. Am. Vet. Med. Assn., *135*:207–210, 1959.

Henricson, B., Norberg, I., and Olsson, S. E.: Huftgelenksdysplasie beim Hund. Nord. Vet. Med., *17*:118–131, 1965.

Henricson, B., Norberg, I., and Olsson, S. E.: On the etiology and pathogenesis of hip dysplasia: a comparative review. J. Small Animal Pract., *7*:673–688, 1966.

Hime, J. M.: An unusual spinal condition in foxhounds. Vet. Rec., *75*:644, 1963.

Hime, J. M., and Drake, J. C.: Osteochrondrosis of the spine in the foxhound. Vet. Rec., *77*:445–449, 1965.

Hodgman, S. F. J.: Abnormalities and defects in pedigree dogs. I. An investigation into the existence of abnormalities in pedigree dogs in the British Isles. J. Small Animal Pract., *4*:447–456, 1963.

Hutt, F. B.: Genetic selection to reduce the incidence of hip dysplasia in dogs. J. Am. Vet. Med. Assn., *151*:1041–1048, 1967.

Hutt, F. B.: Genetic defects of bones and joints in domestic animals. Cornell Vet., *58*:104–113, 1968.

Jubb, K. V. F., and Kennedy, P. C.: Pathology of Domestic Animals. New York, Academic Press, 1964.

Keeler, C. E., and Trimble, H. C.: The inheritance of dew claws in the dog. J. Hered., *29*:145–148, 1938.

Knight, G. C.: Abnormalities and defects in pedigree dogs. III. Tibiofemoral joint deformity and patella luxation. J. Small Animal Pract., *4*:463–464, 1963.

Kodituwakku, G. E.: Luxation of the patella in the dog. Vet. Med., *74*:1499–1508, 1962.

Ladrat, J., Blin, J. C., and Lauvergne, J. J.: Ectomélie bithoracique Héréditaire chez le chien. Ann. Génét. Sél. Anim., *1*:119–130, 1969.

Lee, R., and Fry, P. D.: Some observations on the occurrence of Legg-Calvé-Perthes disease (coxaplana) in the dog, and an evaluation of excision arthroplasty as a method of treatment. J. Small Animal Pract., *10*:309–317, 1969.

Lettow, E., and Dammrich K.: Beitrag zur Klinit und Pathologie der Osteogenesis Imperfecta bei Junghunden. Zentralbl. Vet. Med., *7*:936–966, 1960.

Lodge, D.: Two cases of epiphyseal dysplasia. Vet. Rec., *79*:136–138, 1966.

Loeffler, K.: Glenkanomalien als Problem in der Hundezucht. Dtsch. Tieraerztl. Wochenschr., *71*:291–297, 1964.

Loeffler, K., and Meyer, H.: Erbliche Patellarluxation bei Toy-Spaniels. Dtsch. Tieraerztl. Wochenschr., *68*:619–622, 1961.

Moltzen-Nielsen, H.: Calvé-Perthes Krankheit, Malum Deformans Juvenilis Coxae bei Hunden. Arch. Wiss. Prakt. Tierheilk, *72*:91, 1937.

Palmer, A. C., and Wallace, M. S.: Deformation of cervical vertebrae in Basset hounds. Vet. Rec., *80*:430–433, 1967.

Parker, A. J., and Park, R. D.: Atlanto-axial subluxation in small breeds of dogs. Diagnosis and pathogenesis. Vet. Med./Small Animal Clin., *68*:1133–1137, 1973.

Phillips, J. M.: "Pig jaw" in cocker spaniels. Retrognathia of the mandible in the cocker spaniel and its relationship to other deformities of the jaw. J. Hered., *36*:177–181, 1945.

Pick, J. R., et al.: Subluxation of the carpus in dogs. An X chromosomal defect closely linked with the locus for hemophilia A. Lab. Invest., *17*:243–248, 1967.

Priester, W. A.: Sex, size and breed as risk factors in canine patella dislocation. J. Am. Vet. Med. Assn., *160*:740–742, 1972.

Pullig, T.: Inheritance of a skull defect in cocker spaniels. J. Hered., *44*:97–99, 1952.

Pullig, T.: Anury in cocker spaniels. J. Hered., *44*:105–107, 1953.

Pullig, T.: Brachyury in cocker spaniels. J. Hered., *48*:75–76, 1957.

Rasmussen, P. G.: Multiple epiphyseal dysplasia in a litter of beagle puppies. J. Small Animal Pract., *12*:91–96, 1971.

Rasmussen, P. G.: Multiple epiphyseal dysplasia in beagle puppies. Acta Radiol. (Suppl. 319):251–254, 1972.

Riser, W. H.: An analysis of the current status of hip dysplasia in the dog. J. Am. Vet. Med. Assn., *144*:709–721, 1964.

Riser, W. H., and Shirer, J. F.: Correlation between canine hip dysplasia and pelvic muscle mass: a study of 95 dogs. Am. J. Vet. Res., *28*:769–777, 1967.

Riser, W. H., Parkes, L. J., and Shirer J. F.: Canine craniomandibular osteopathy. J. Am. Rad. Soc., *VIII*:23–31, 1967.

Riser, W. H., et al.: Influence of early rapid growth and

### Table 2.   *Bones and Joints\**

| CONDITION | BREED(S) | MODE | SELECTED REFERENCES |
|---|---|---|---|
| Achrondroplasia, limbs | Dachshund, basset | ID | Stockhard (1941) |
| Anury (tail-less) | Cocker spaniel | R? | Pullig (1953) |
| Brachydactyly | | R? | Green (1957) |
| Brachyury (short tail) | Cocker spaniel, beagle, English bulldog | R? | Pullig (1957), Curtis et al. (1964) |
| Carpal subluxation | Irish setter | XR | Pick et al. (1967) |
| Cartilaginous exostoses | Mixed | ? | Gee and Doige (1970), Chester (1971) |
| Cervical vertebral deformity (spondylolisthesis) | Basset, Great Dane | ? | Palmer and Wallace (1967), Wright et al. (1973), Selcer and Oliver (1975) |
| Craniomandibular osteopathy | West Highland white, Scottish terrier, Cairn terrier, Labrador retriever | ? | Jubb and Kennedy (1964), Riser et al. (1967) |
| Cranioschisis (skull fissures) | Cocker spaniel | R? | Pullig (1952) |
| Dwarfism (chondrodysplasia with anemia) | Alaskan malamutes | R | Smart and Fletch (1971), Subden et al. (1972), Fletch et al. (1973), Fletch and Pinkerton (1973), Fletch et al. (1975) |
| Ectromelia | —— | R | Ladrat et al. (1969) |
| Epiphyseal dysplasia | Beagle | R? | Rasmussen (1971, 1972) |
| Epiphyseal dysplasia (pseudoachondroplastic) | Miniature poodle | R | Gardner (1959), Amlöf (1961), Lodge (1966) |
| Foramen magnum enlargement | | ? | Bardens (1965) |
| Hip dysplasia | Most breeds, notably German shepherds | P | Schales (1957, 1959), Riser (1964), Riser et al. (1964, 1967), Henricson et al. (1965, 1966), Henricson and Olsson (1959), Hutt (1967) |
| Intervertebral disc degeneration | Chondrodystrophoid breeds: cocker spaniel, dachshund, Pekingese, beagle | ? | Hansen (1952, 1964), Vaughan (1958) |
| Legg-Calvé-Perthes disease | Small breeds | ? | Moltzen-Nielsen (1937), Wamberg (1961), Lee and Fry (1969) |

*Skeletal conformation, generally. Aside from crossing strongly contrasting breeds, little definitive analysis of the genetic basis for skeletal variation has been attempted. The most extensive studies are those of Stockard (1941), who performed standard mendelian crosses, including $F_2$ and back-crosses, between different breeds. In these studies, there was a tendency for the $F_1$ to be intermediate between the parental types, and a single back-cross of the $F_1$ to either parental breed produced pups which closely resembled that breed.

While single gene defects, in some instances, can have marked effects on the form of the skeleton (as in achrondroplasia), reports that minor variations in skeletal conformation are determined by single genes should be viewed with skepticism. Variations from the ideal type in purebred dogs are more likely to represent the influence of polygenic inheritance, "abnormal" individuals merely representing the extremes of variation possible under a polygenic system of determinants.

From a practical point of view, selection for body conformation, as important to the dog breeder, may be regarded as a problem of selecting for polygenic traits. A further discussion of this may be found in the book by Burns and Fraser (1966).

*Continued on next page*

### Table 2.    Bones and Joints (Continued)

| CONDITION | BREED(S) | MODE | SELECTED REFERENCES |
|---|---|---|---|
| Ondontoid process dysplasia | Miniature poodle, Pomeranian, Yorkshire terrier | ? | Geary et al. (1967), Parker and Park (1973) |
| Osteogenesis imperfecta | Bedlington terrier, elkhound, poodle | ? | Jubb and Kennedy (1964), Calkins et al. (1956), Lettow and Dammrich (1960) |
| Otocephaly (partial agnathia, hydrocephaly, parietal fontanelle defects) | Beagle | P? | Fox (1963, 1964) |
| Over- and undershot jaw | Cocker spaniel, long-haired dachshund | ? | Phillips (1945), Grüneberg and Lea (1940), Ritter (1933), Stockard (1941) |
| Patellar luxation | Toy breeds | ? | Hodgman (1963), Kodituwakku (1962), Loeffler and Meyer (1961), Knight (1963), Hutt (1968), Priester (1972) |
| Polydactyly (rear dew claws) | Many breeds | D? | Keeler and Trimble (1938), Whitney (1947) |
| Polyostotic fibrous dysplasia | Doberman | ? | Carrig and Seawright (1969) |
| Short skull | Bulldogs, Pekingese, Brussels griffin, other breeds | ? | Stockard (1941) |
| Short spine | Shiba-Inu (Japan), greyhound | R | deBoom (1965), Hansen (1968), Suu (1956, 1957) |
| Spina bifida | English bulldogs | ? | Curtis et al. (1964) |
| Spondylosis deformans | Boxer | ? | Zimmer and Stähli (1960) |
| Ununited anconeal process | German shepherd, cocker spaniel, Labrador retriever | P? | Cawley and Archibald (1959), Vaughan (1962), Loeffler (1964), Bradley (1967), Carlson and Severin (1961), Corley and Carlson (1965) |
| Vertebral osteochondrosis | Foxhounds | ? | Hime (1963, Hime and Drake (1965) |

weight gain on hip dysplasia in the German shepherd dog. J. Am. Vet. Med. Assn., *145*:661–668, 1964.

Ritter, R.: Konnen Anomalien des Gebisses Gezuchtet Werden? Dtsch. Zahn Mund. Kieferheilk., *4*:235–257, 1933.

Schales, O.: Heredity patterns in dysplasia of the hip. N. Am. Vet., *38*:152–155, 1957.

Schales, O.: Congenital hip dysplasia in dogs. Vet. Med., *54*:143–148, 1959.

Selcer, R. R., and Oliver, J. E., Jr.: Cervical spondylopathy—wobbler syndrome in dogs. J.A.A.H.A., *11*:175–179, 1975.

Smart, M. E., and Fletch, S.: A hereditary skeletal growth defect in purebred Alaskan malamutes. (Letter to the Editor.) Canad. Vet. J., *12*:31–32, 1971.

Stockard, C. R.: The Genetic and Endocrinic Basis for Differences in Form and Behavior as Elucidated by Studies of Contrasted Pure-line Dog Breeds and Hybrids. American Anatomical Memoirs. Philadelphia, Wistar Institute of Anatomy and Biology, 1941.

Subden, R. E., et al.: Genetics of the Alaskan malamute chondrodysplasia syndrome. J. Hered., *63*:149–152, 1972.

Suu, S.: Studies on the short-spine dogs. I. Their origin and occurrence. Res. Bull. Fac. Agric. Gifu. Univ., *7*:127–134, 1956.

Suu, S., and Ueshima, T.j; Studies on the short-spine dogs. II. Somatological observation. Res. Bull. Fac. Agric. Gifu. Univ., *8*:112–128, 1957.

Vaughan, L. C.: Studies on intervertebral disc protrusion in the dog. I. Aetiology and Pathogenesis. Brit. Vet. J., *114*:105–112, 1958.

Vaughan, L. C.: Congenital detachment of the processus anconeus in the dog. Vet. Rec., *74*:309–311, 1962.

Wamberg, K.: Huftgelenksleiden des Hundes. Mh. Vet. Med., *16*:884–891, 1961.

Whitney, L. F.: How to Breed Dogs. New York, Orange Judd Publishing Co., Inc., 1947.

Wright, F., Rest, J. R., and Palmer, A. C.: Ataxia of the Great Dane caused by stenosis of the vertebral canal: comparison with similar conditions in the Basset Hound, Doberman Pinscher, Ridgeback and the thoroughbred horse. Vet. Rec., *92*:1–6, 1973.

Zimmer, E. A., and Stähli, W.: Erbbedingte Versteifung der Wirbelsaule in einer Familie deutsche Boxer. Schweiz. Arch. Tierheilk., *102*:254–264, 1960.

## SELECTED REFERENCES:
### Cardiovascular and Lymphatic Systems

James, T. N., and Drake, E. H.: Sudden death in Doberman pinschers. Henry Ford Hosp. Med. Bull., *13*:183–190, 1965.

James, T. N., and Drake, E. H.: Sudden death in Doberman pinschers. Ann. Intern. Med., *68*:821–829, 1968.

Ladds, P. W., Dennis, S. M., and Leipold, H. W.: Lethal congenital edema in bulldog pups. J. Am. Vet. Med. Assn., *159*:81–86, 1971.

Lüginbuhl, H., et al.: Congenital hereditary lymphoedema in the dog. Part II. Pathological studies. J. Med. Genet., *4*:153–165, 1967.

Moore, E. N., Boineau, J. P., and Patterson, D. F.: Incomplete right bundle branch block. An electrocardiographic enigma and possible misnomer. Circulation, *44*:678–687, 1971.

Mulvihill, J. J.: Comments on the epidemiology of congenital heart disease in dogs. Birth Defects: Original Article Series, Vol. XV, Cardiovascular System. National Foundation, pp. 175–177, 1972.

Naylor, R. J.: Regurgitation in pups. I. Persistent aortic arches. J. Am. Vet. Med. Assn., *130*:283–284, 1957.

Patterson, D. F.: Epidemiologic and genetic studies of congenital heart disease in the dog. Circ. Res., *23*:171–202, 1968.

Patterson, D. F., and Pyle, R. L.: Genetic aspects of congenital heart disease in the dog. "The newer knowledge about dogs." 21st Annual Gaines Veterinary Symposium, Ames, Iowa, 1971.

Patterson, D. F., Pyle, R. L., and Buchanan, J. W.: Hereditary cardiovascular malformations of the dog. Birth Defects: Original Article Series, Vol. XV, Cardiovascular System. National Foundation, pp. 100–174, 1972.

Patterson, D. F., et al.: Congenital hereditary lymphoedema in the dog. Part I. Clinical and genetic studies. J. Med. Genet., *4*:145–152, 1967.

Patterson, D. F., et al.: Hereditary patent ductus arteriosus and its sequelae in the dog. Circ. Res., *39*:1–13, 1971.

Patterson, D. F., et al.: Hereditary defects of the conotruncal septum in keeshond dogs. Pathologic and genetic studies. Am. J. Cardiol., *34*:187–205, 1974.

## Table 3. *Cardiovascular and Lymphatic Systems*

| CONDITION | BREED(S) | MODE | SELECTED REFERENCES |
|---|---|---|---|
| Patent ductus arteriosus | Poodle, (collie, Pomeranian, cocker spaniel) | P | Patterson (1968), Patterson et al. (1971), Patterson and Pyle (1971), Patterson et al. (1971, 1972), Mulvihill (1971) |
| Subaortic stenosis | Newfoundland, (boxer, German shepherd) | P | Patterson (1968), Patterson and Pyle (1971), Patterson et al. (1971, 1972), Mulvihill (1971) |
| Conotruncal septum defects, including tetralogy of Fallot | Keeshond | P | Patterson et al. (1974) |
| Valvular pulmonic stenosis | Beagle, (English bulldog, fox terrier, Chihuahua) | P | Patterson (1968), Patterson and Pyle (1971), Patterson et al. (1972) |
| Persistent right aortic arch | German shepherd (Irish setter) | P | Naylor (1957), Patterson (1968), Patterson and Pyle (1971), Mulvihill (1971), Patterson et al. (1972) |
| Atrial septal defect and other cardiac defects | Boxer | ? | Pyle and Patterson (1972) |
| Congenital lymphedema | Labrador-poodle cross | D | Patterson et al. (1967), Luginbuhl et al. (1967) |
| Congenital anasarca | English bulldog | ? | Ladds et al. (1971) |
| Incomplete right bundle branch block (focal right ventricular hypertrophy) | Beagle | ? | Moore et al. (1971) |
| His bundle degeneration (suspected cause of sudden death) | Doberman | ? | James and Drake (1965, 1968) |

Parentheses indicate breeds in which definitive genetic studies have not been made but in which epidemiologic evidence suggests a genetic cause.

## Table 4.   *Chromosomal Abnormalities*

| ABNORMALITY | BREED AND PHENOTYPE | SELECTED REFERENCES |
|---|---|---|
| Semibalanced autosomal translocation | Mongrel, male, cleft lip and maxilla, congenital heart disease, 77 chromosomes including large submetacentric translocation chromosome | Shive et al. (1965), Patterson et al. (1966) |
| Semibalanced autosomal translocation | Miniature poodle, female, chondrodysplastic dwarfism, 77 chromosomes including a large subtelocentric translocation chromosome | Hare et al. (1967) |
| Extra minute chromosome | Male cocker spaniel, congenital heart disease, 79 chromosomes including extra minute chromosome | Shive et al. (1965), Patterson et al. (1966) |
| XXY | German short-haired pointer, male, with testicular hypoplasia and congenital heart disease; XXY sex chromosome constitution | Clough et al. (1970) |

For a general discussion of cytogenetics in the dog and cat, see Hare et al. (1966). Studies of the karyotype of various breeds, including the Malayan telomian dog, have not shown any apparent differences between breeds (Borgaonkar et al., 1968). Giemsa banding studies by Selden et al. (1975) have recently further defined the canine karyotype.

Pyle, R. L., and Patterson, D. F.: Multiple cardiovascular malformations in a family of boxer dogs. J. Am. Vet. Med. Assn., *160*:965–976, 1972.

**SELECTED REFERENCES:**

**Chromosomal Abnormalities**

Borgaonkar, D. S., et al.: Chromosome study of four breeds of dogs. J. Hered., *59*:157–160, 1968.
Clough, E., et al.: An XXY sex-chromosome constitution in a dog with testicular hypoplasia and congenital heart disease. Cytogenetics, *9*:71–77, 1970.
Hare, W. C. D., et al.: Cytogenetics in the dog and cat. J. Small Animal. Pract., *7*:575–592, 1966.
Hare, W. C. D., et al.: Bone chondroplasia and a chromosomal anomaly in the same dog. Am. J. Vet. Res., *28*:583–587, 1967.
Patterson, D. F., et al.: Congenital malformations of the cardiovascular system associated with chromosomal abnormalities: a report of the clinical, pathologic, and cytogenetic findings in 2 dogs. Zentralbl. Vet. Med., *13*:669–686, 1966.
Selden, J. R., et al.: The Giemsa banding pattern of the canine karyotype. Cytogenet. Cell Genet., *15*:380–387, 1975.
Shive, R. J., Hare, W. C. D., and Patterson, D. F.: Chromosome studies in dogs with congenital cardiac defects. Cytogenetics, *4*:340–348, 1965.

**SELECTED REFERENCES**

**Digestive System**

Aitchison, J.: Incisor dentition in short muzzled dogs. Vet. Rec., *76*:165–169, 1964.
Burstone, M. S., Bond, E., and Litt, R.: Familial gingi-

## Table 5.   *Digestive System*

| CONDITION | BREED(S) | MODE | SELECTED REFERENCES |
|---|---|---|---|
| Cleft lip and palate | Staffordshire terrier, dachshund, cocker spaniel<br>English bulldog<br>Beagle<br>Shih-Tzu | P? | Jurkiewicz (1965), Jurkiewicz and Bryant (1968)<br>Gardner (1954), Pearce (1969)<br>Horowitz and Chase (1970)<br>Cooper and Mattern (1970) |
| Dentition abnormal | Boxer, English bulldog | ? | Aitchison (1964) |
| Esophageal achalasia | Wire-haired fox terrier<br>Greyhound<br>German shepherd | ? | Osborne et al. (1967)<br>Spy (1963)<br>Earlam et al. (1967) |
| Gingival hyperplasia | Boxer | ? | Burstone et al. (1952) |
| Glossopharyngeal defect (bird tongue) | Not given | R | Hutt and deLahunta (1971) |
| Hepatitis (copper storage) | Bedlington terrier | R? | Hardy et al. (1975) |

## *Table 6.* *The Ear*

| CONDITION | BREED(S) | MODE | SELECTED REFERENCES |
|---|---|---|---|
| Deafness (cochlear degeneration) | Dalmation | ? | Hudson and Ruben (1962), Anderson et al. (1968) |
| | Collie | ? | Lurie (1948) |
| | Foxhound | ? | Adams (1956) |
| | White dogs of various breeds | ? | Young (1955) |

These represent instances of hereditary deafness other than that produced by the merle gene. As in other animals, deafness often is associated with depigmentation. In none of the above reports was the mode of inheritance well defined. Deaf dogs are usually born of normal parents. The studies of Anderson et al. (1968) in Dalmatians are the most extensive. They yielded results which are not consistent with any simple genetic hypothesis. Although the anatomic defect in all of the above examples appears to be an abnormal development or early degeneration of the cochlea, the defect occurs in varying degrees, and may involve one or both sides. This wide range of variation in the phenotype, plus a lack of accurate means of determining minor degrees of hearing loss in the dog, make genetic analysis difficult.

val hypertrophy in the dog (boxer breed). Arch. Path., *54*:208–212, 1952.

Cooper, H. K., Jr., and Mattern, G. W.: Genetic studies of cleft lip and palate in dogs (a preliminary report). Carnivore Genetics Newsletter No. 9:204–209, 1970.

Earlam, R. J., Zollman, P. E., and Ellis, F. H., Jr.: Congenital oesophageal achalasia in the dog. Thorax, 22:466–472, 1967.

Gardner, J. E., Jr.: Report of a survey on cleft palates in the English bulldog. Bulletin of the Bulldog Club of New Jersey, September, 1954.

Hardy, R. M., Stevens, J. B., and Stowe, C. M.: Chronic progressive hepatitis in Bedlington terriers associated with elevated liver copper concentrations. Minn. Vet., *15*:13–24, 1975.

Horowitz, S. L., and Chase, H. B.: A microform of cleft palate in dogs. J. Dent. Res., *49*:892, 1970.

Hutt, F. B., and deLahunta, A.: A lethal glossopharyngeal defect in the dog. J. Hered., *62*:291–293, 1971.

Jurkiewicz, M. J.: A genetic study of cleft lip and palate in dogs, S. Forum, *16*:472–473, 1965.

Jurkiewicz, M. J., and Bryant, D. L.: Cleft lip and palate in dogs: a progress report. Cleft Palate J., *5*:30–36, 1968.

Osborne, C. A., Clifford, D. H., and Jessen, C.: Hereditary esophageal achalasia in dogs. J. Am. Vet. Med. Assn., *151*:572–581, 1967.

Pearce, R. G.: Anomalies of the English bulldog. Southwest Vet. J., *22*:218–220, 1969.

Spy, G. M.: Megaesophagus in greyhounds. Vet. Rec., *75*:853, 1963.

### SELECTED REFERENCES:

#### The Ear

Adams, E. W.: Hereditary deafness in a family of foxhounds. J. Am. Vet. Med. Assn., *128*:302, 1956.

Anderson, R., et al.: Genetic hearing impairment in the Dalmation dog. Acta Otolaryngologica (Suppl. 232), 1968.

Hudson, W. R., and Ruben, R. J.: Hereditary deafness in Dalmations. Arch. Otolaryngol., *75*:213, 1962.

Lurie, M. H.: The membranous labyrinth in the congenitally deaf collie and Dalmation dog. Laryngoscope, *58*:279, 1948.

Young, G. B.: Inherited defects in dogs. Vet. Rec., *67*:15–19, 1955.

### SELECTED REFERENCES:

#### Endocrine and Metabolic Disorders

Bardens, J. W.: Glycogen storage disease in puppies. Vet. Med. Small Animal Clin., *61*:1174–1176, 1966.

## *Table 7.* *Endocrine and Metabolic Disorders*

| CONDITION | BREED(S) | MODE | SELECTED REFERENCES |
|---|---|---|---|
| Copper storage | Bedlington terrier | R? | Hardy et al. (1975) |
| Cystinuria | (See Table 13, Urinary System.) | | |
| Diabetes mellitus* | Dachshund | ? | Wilkinson (1960) |
| | Miniature poodle | ? | Gershwin (1975) |
| Goiter | Fox terrier | ? | Brouwers (1950) |
| High uric acid excretion | (See Table 13, Urinary System.) | | |
| Glycogen storage disease | "Toy breeds,"† Lapland dog | ? | Bardens et al. (1961), Bardens (1966), Mostafa (1970) |

*The large number of cases of diabetes mellitus in dachshunds in one study suggested a genetic influence. However, the population base was poorly defined (actual prevalence rates in dachshunds unknown) and no direct genetic studies have been made.

†Poorly defined syndrome supposedly characterized by hypoglycemia in pups 6 to 12 weeks old. There is reputed to be glycogen infiltration of liver, kidney and myocardium in some cases.

Bardens, J. W., Bardens, G., and Bardens, B.: A Von Gierke-like syndrome. Allied Vet., 32:4–7, 1961.

Brouwers, J.: Goitre et heredite chez le chien. Ann. Med. Vet., 94:173–174, 1950.

Gershwin, L. J.: Familial canine diabetes mellitus. J. Am. Vet. Med. Assn., 167:479–480, 1975.

Hardy, R. M., Stevens, J. B., and Stowe, C. M.: Chronic progressive hepatitis in Bedlington terriers associated with elevated liver copper concentrations. Minn. Vet., 15:13–24, 1975.

Mostafa, I. E.: A case of glycogenic cardiomegaly in a dog. Acta Vet. Scand., 11:197–208, 1970.

Wilkinson, J. S.: Spontaneous diabetes mellitus. Vet. Rec., 72:548–558, 1960.

## SELECTED REFERENCES:

### The Eye

Aguirre, G. D.: Hereditary retinal disease in small animals. Vet. Clin. N. Am., 3:515–528, 1973.

Aguirre, G. D., and Rubin, L. F.: Progressive retinal atrophy (rod dysplasia) in the Norwegian elkhound. J. Am. Vet. Med. Assn., 158:208–218, 1971.

Andersen, A. C., and Shultz, F. T.: Inherited (congenital) cataract in the dog. Am. J. Path., 34:965–975, 1958.

Ashton, N., Barnett, K. C., and Sachs, D. D.: Retinal dysplasia in the Sealyham terrier. J. Path. Bact., 96:269–272, 1968.

Barnett, K. C.: Canine retinopathies. II. The miniature and toy poodle. J. Small Animal Pract., 6:93–109, 1965.

Barnett, K. C.: Primary retinal dystrophies in the dog. J. Am. Vet. Med. Assn., 154:804–808, 1969.

Barnett, K. C.: Types of cataract in the dog. J.A.A.H.A., 8:2–9, 1972.

Barnett, K. C., and Knight, G. C.: Persistent pupillary membrane in the basenji. Vet. Rec., 85:242, 1969.

Barnett, K. C., et al.: Hereditary retinal dysplasia in Labrador retrievers in England and Sweden. J. Small Animal Pract., 10:753–759, 1970.

Bedford, P. G. C.: The aetiology of primary glaucoma in the dog. J. Small Animal Pract., 16:217–239, 1975.

Black, L.: Progressive retinal atrophy. A review of the genetics and an appraisal of the eradication scheme. J. Small Animal Pract., 13:295–314, 1972.

Burns, M., and Fraser, M. N.: The Genetics of the Dog: The Basis of Successful Breeding. Philadelphia, J. B. Lippincott and Co., 1966.

Cogan, D. G., and Kuwabara, T.: Photoreceptive abiotrophy of the retina in the elkhound. Path., Vet., 2:101–128, 1965.

Donovan, E. F., and Wyman, M.: Ocular fundus anomaly in the collie. Proceedings of the 102nd Annual Meeting. J. Am. Vet. Med. Assn., 147:1465–1469, 1965.

Donovan, R. H., and Macpherson, A. M.: The inheritance of chorioretinal change and staphyloma in the collie. Carnivore Genetics Newsletter, 5:85–89, 1968.

Formston, C.: Observations on subluxation and luxation of the crystalline lens in the dog. J. Comp. Path., 55:168–184, 1945.

Gelatt, K. N., and McGill, L. D.: Clinical characteristics of microphthalmia with colobomas of the Australian shepherd dog. J. Am. Vet. Med. Assn., 167:393–396, 1973.

Heywood, R.: Juvenile cataracts in the beagle dog. J. Small Animal Pract., 12:171–177, 1971.

Hodgman, S. F. J.: Abnormalities and defects in pedigree dogs. I. An investigation into the existence of abnormalities in pedigree dogs in the British Isles. J. Small Animal Pract., 4:447–456, 1963.

Hodgman, S. F. J., et al.: Progressive retinal atrophy in dogs. I. The disease in Irish setters (red). Vet. Rec., 61:185–189, 1949.

Host, P., and Sreison, S.: Hereditary cataract in the dog. Norsk, Vet. Tidsskv., 48:244–270, 1936.

Keep, J. M.: Clinical aspects of progressive retinal atrophy in the cardigan Welsh corgi. Aust. Vet. J., 48:197–199, 1972.

Kittel, H.: Uber Dermoide der Kornea am Spaltbildungen der Lider am Ange von Bernhardinerhunden. Dtsch. Tierearztl. Wochenschr., 52:793–797, 1931.

Koch, S. A.: Cataracts in interrelated old English sheepdogs. J. Am. Vet. Med. Assn., 160:299–301, 1972.

Lawson, D. D.: Luxation of the crystalline lens in the dog. J. Small Animal Pract., 10:461–463, 1969.

Lovekin, L. G.: Primary glaucoma in dogs. J. Am. Vet. Med. Assn., 145:1081–1091, 1964.

Lovekin, L. G., and Bellhorn, R. W.: Clinicopathologic changes in primary glaucoma in the cocker spaniel. Am. J. Vet. Res., 29:375–385, 1968.

Magnusson, H.: About retinitis pigmentosa and consanguinity in dogs. Arch. Verhg. Ophthal., 2:147–163, 1911.

Magrane, W. G.: Congenital anomaly of the optic disc in collies. N. Am. Vet., 34:646, 1953.

Martin, C. L., and Leach, R.: Everted membrana nictitans in German shorthaired pointers. J. Am. Vet. Med. Assn., 157:1229–1232, 1970.

Martin, C. L., and Wyman, M.: Glaucoma in the Basset hound. J. Am. Vet. Med. Assn., 153:1320–1327, 1968.

Parry, H. B.: Degenerations of the dog retina. II. General progressive atrophy of hereditary aetiology. Brit. J. Ophthalmol., 37:487–502, 1953.

Parry, H. B.: Degenerations of the dog retina. VI. Central progressive atrophy with pigment epithelial dystrophy. Brit. J. Ophthalmol., 38:653–668, 1954.

Roberts, S. R.: Superficial indolent ulcer of the cornea in boxer dogs. J. Small Animal Pract., 6:111–115, 1965.

Roberts, S. R.: Three inherited ocular defects in the dog. Mod. Vet. Pract., 48:30–34, 1967.

Roberts, S. R., and Helper, L. C.: Cataracts in Afghan hounds. J. Am. Vet. Med. Assn., 160:427–432, 1972.

Rubin, L. F.: Hereditary retinal detachment in Bedlington terriers. A preliminary report. Small Animal Clin., 3:387–389, 1963.

Rubin, L. F.: Heredity of retinal dysplasia in Bedlington terriers. J. Am. Vet. Med. Assn., 152:260–262, 1968.

Rubin, L. F.: Cataract in golden retrievers. J. Am. Vet. Med. Assn., 165:457–458, 1974.

Rubin, L. F., and Flowers, R. D.: Inherited cataract in a family of standard poodles. J. Am. Vet. Med. Assn., 161:207–208, 1972.

Rubin, L. F., Bourns, T. K. R., and Lord, L. H.: Hemeralopia in dogs: heredity of hemeralopia in Alaskan malamutes. Am. J. Vet. Res., 28:355–357, 1967.

Rubin, L. F., Koch, S. A., and Huber, R. J.: Hereditary cataracts in miniature schnauzers. J. Am. Vet. Med. Assn., 154:1456–1458, 1969.

Saunders, L. Z.: Congenital optic nerve hypoplasia in collie dogs. Cornell Vet., 42:67–80, 1952.

Sorsby, A., and Davey, J. B.: Ocular associations of dappling (or merling) in the coat colour of dogs. I.

*Table 8.  The Eye*

| CONDITION | BREED(S) | MODE | SELECTED REFERENCES |
|---|---|---|---|
| Cataract | Boston and Staffordshire terrier | R? | Barnett (1972) |
| | Afghan hound | R? | Roberts and Helper (1972) |
| | Pointer | D? | Host and Sreison (1936) |
| | Beagle | D? | Andersen and Shultz (1958), Heywood (1971) |
| | German shepherd | D | von Hippel (1930) |
| | Golden and Labrador retriever | D | Barnett (1972), Rubin (1974) |
| | Old English sheepdog | R? | Koch (1972) |
| | Miniature schnauzer | R? | Rubin et al. (1969) |
| | Standard poodle | R? | Rubin and Flowers (1972) |
| Collie eye anomaly (chorioretinal dysplasia, posterior scleral ectasia) | Collie (all color varieties) | R* | Donovan and Wyman (1965), Yakely et al. (1968) (See also Symposium on Collie Eye Anomaly. J. Am. Vet. Med. Assn., 155:859–878, 1969) |
| | Shetland sheepdog | ? | Aguirre (1973) |
| Conjunctival dermoid cyst | German shepherd | ? | Szczudlowska (1967) |
| Corneal cyst | St. Bernard | ? | Kittel (1931) |
| Corneal ulceration | Boxer | ? | Roberts (1965) |
| Entropion | Various breeds | ? | Burns and Fraser (1966), Hodgman (1963) |
| Everted membrana nictitans | German short-haired pointer | ? | Martin and Leach (1970) |
| Glaucoma | Basset hound Wire-haired fox terrier, cocker spaniel | ? | Martin and Wyman (1968) Lovekin (1964), Lovekin and Bellhorn (1968), Formston (1945) |
| | English cocker spaniel | ? | Bedford (1975) |
| Hemeralopia (day blindness) | Alaskan malamute | R | Rubin et al. (1967) |
| Heterochromia iridis ("walleye") | Collie, Shetland sheepdog, dachshund, Great Dane, Australian shepherd, other breeds with merle gene | ID† | Sorsby and Davey (1954), Gelatt and McGill (1973) |
| Lens luxation | Sealyham terrier | ? | Lawson (1969) |
| | Fox terrier | ? | Formston (1945) |
| Optic nerve hypoplasia | Collie | ? | Saunders (1952), Magrane (1953) |
| Persistent pupillary membrane | Basenji | D? | Roberts (1967), Barnett and Knight (1969) |
| Progressive retinal atrophy‡ (generalized) | Irish setter, Gordon setter | R | Magnusson (1911), Hodgman et al. (1949), Parry (1953) |
| | Miniature and toy poodle, English cocker spaniel | R | Barnett )1965) |
| | Norwegian elkhound | R | Cogan and Kuwabara (1965), Aguirre and Rubin (1971) |
| | Cardigan Welsh corgi | ? | Barnett (1969), Keep (1972) |

*Continued on next page*

*It is reasonable to believe that the varied stigmata are the result of a pleiotropic single gene with variable expressivity, depending on the genetic background. It has been postulated, however, that staphyloma is inherited as a single autosomal dominant which is expressed only in the presence of recessively inherited chorioretinal change (Donovan and Macpherson, 1968).

†Merled or dappled dogs are heterozygous for M, an incompletely dominant gene with pleiotropic effects. In heterozygotes (Mm), there is often heterochromia of the iris, or both irises may be blue. Homozygotes (MM) frequently have severe eye anomalies, including microphthalmia and colobomas of the iris and choroid, and are often blind and deaf.

‡There is no evidence that PRA in different breeds results from the same gene mutation. See Black (1972) for a more complete review of the literature.

*Table 8.   The Eye (Continued)*

| CONDITION | BREED(S) | MODE | SELECTED REFERENCES |
|---|---|---|---|
| Progressive retinal atrophy (central) | Labrador retriever | ? | Parry (1954) |
| | Border collie | ? | Barnett (1969) |
| | Golden retriever | ? | |
| | English springer spaniel | ? | |
| Retinal dysplasia (congenital retinal detachment) | Sealyham terrier | R? | Ashton et al. (1968) |
| | Bedlington terrier | R | Rubin (1963, 1968) |
| | Australian shepherd | ? | Gelatt and McGill (1973) |
| | Labrador retriever | R | Barnett et al. (1970) |

Clinical and genetical data. J. Genet., *52*:425–440, 1954.

Szczudlowska, M.: Dermoid cyst of the eye in relation to heredity and overfeeding. Med. Vet., *23*:567–569, 1967.

von Hippel, E.: Embryologische Untersuchungen über Verebung angeborener Kataract, über Schichter des Hundes sowie über eine besondere Form von Kapelkarakt. Graefes Arch., *124*:300–324, 1930.

Yakely, W. L., et al.: Genetic transmission of an ocular fundus anomaly in collies. J. Am. Vet. Med. Assn., *152*:457–461, 1968.


SELECTED REFERENCES:

Neuromuscular System

Bernheimer, H., and Karbe, E.: Morphologische und neurochemische Untersuchungen von 2 Formen der amaurotischen Idiotie des Hundes: Nachweis einer $G_{m2}$-Gangliosidose. Acta Neuropathologia (Berlin), *16*:243–261, 1970.

Bielfelt, S. W., Redman, H. C., and McClellan, P. O.: Size and sex-related differences in rates of epileptiform seizures in a purebred beagle colony. Am. J. Vet. Res., *32*:2039–2048, 1971.

Björck, G., Dyrendahl, S., and Olsson, S. E.: Hereditary ataxia in smooth-haired fox terriers. Vet. Rec., *69*:871–876, 1957.

Burns, M., and Fraser, M. N.: Genetics of the Dog. The Basis of Successful Breeding. Philadelphia, J. B. Lippincott Co., 1966.

Cordy, D. R., and Snelbaker, H. A.: Cerebellar hypoplasia and degeneration in a family of airedale dogs. J. Neuropath. Exp. Neurol., *11*:324–328, 1952.

Croft, P. G., and Stockman, M. H. R.: Inherited defects in dogs. Vet. Rec., *76*:260–261, 1964.

Douglas, S. W., and Palmer, A. C.: Idiopathic demyelination of brain-stem and spinal cord in a miniature poodle puppy. J. Path. Bact., *82*:67–71, 1961.

Dykman, R. A., Murphree, O. D., and Peters, J. E.: Like begets like: behavioral tests, classical autonomic and motor conditioning and operant conditioning in two strains of pointer dogs. Ann. New York Acad. Sci., *159*:976–1007, 1969.

Eberhart, G. W.: Epilepsy in the dog. Gaines Vet. Symp., *18*:20, 1959.

Fankhauser, R., Luginbühl, H., and Hartley, W.: Leukodystrophie vom typus Krabbe beim Hund. Schweiz. Arch. Tierheilk., *105*:198–207, 1963.

Fletcher, T., Kurtz, H., and Low, D.: Globoid cell leukodystrophy (Krabbe type) in the dog. J. Am. Vet. Med. Assn., *149*:165–172, 1966.

Freak, M. J.: The whelping bitch. Vet. Rec., *60*:295–301, 306, 1948.

Gambetti, L. A., Kelly, A. M., and Steinberg, S. A.: Biochemical studies in a canine gangliosidosis. J. Neuropath. Exper. Neurol., 29:137, 1970.

Hagen, L. O.: Lipid dystrophic changes in the central nervous system in dogs. Acta Path. Microbiol. Scand., *33*:22–35, 1953.

Hartley, W. J.: Ataxia in Jack Russell terriers. Acta Neuropathologica (Berlin), 26:71–74, 1973.

Hegreberg, G. A., and Padgett, G. A.: Inherited progressive epilepsy of the dog with comparisons to Lafora's disease of man. Fed. Proc., 35:1202–1205, 1976.

Hodgman, S. F. J.: Abnormalities and defects in pedigree dogs. I. An investigation into the existence of abnormalities in pedigree dogs in the British Isles. J. Small Animal Pract., 6:447–456, 1963.

Johnson, G. R., Oliver, J. E., and Selcer, R.: Globoid leukodystrophy in a Beagle. J. Am. Vet. Med. Assn., *167*:380–384, 1975.

Karbe, E., and Schiefer, B.: Familial amaurotic idiocy in male German shorthair pointers. Path. Vet., *4*:223–232, 1967.

Kollarits, J.: Permanent trembling in some dog breeds as hereditary degeneration (in German). Schweiz. Med. Wochenschr., *54*:431–432, 1924.

Koppang, N.: Lipodystrophia cerebri hos engelskette. Beretn. Nord. Vet. Med., *2*:862–867, 1963.

Koppang, N.: Familiare Glykosphingolipoidose des Hundes Juvenile Amaurotische Idiotie. Ergebn. Allg. Path. Anat., *47*:1–43, 1966.

Koppang, N.: Neuronal ceroid-lipofuscinosis in English setters. J. Small Animal Pract., *10*:639–644, 1970.

Krushinskii, L. V.: Animal Behavior: Its Normal and Abnormal Development. New York Consultants Bureau, 1962.

Lane, J. G., and Holmes, R. J.: Fly catching: Hallucinatory behavior by Cavalier King Charles Spaniels. Grunsell, C. S. G., and Hill, F. W. G. (eds.): Vet Annual. Bristol, England, J. Wright and Sons, Ltd., 1972.

Lawler, D. C.: Epilepsy in dogs. New Zealand Vet. J., *19*:53, 1971.

McGrath, J. T.: Neurologic Examination of the Dog with Clinicopathologic Observations. 2nd ed. Philadelphia, Lea and Febiger, 1960.

McGrath, J. T.: Spinal dysraphism in the dog. Path. Vet., 2(Suppl.):1–36, 1965.

McGrath, J. T., Kelly, A. M., and Steinberg, S. A.: Cerebral lipidosis in the dog. J. Neuropath. Exper. Neurol., 27:141, 1968 (Abstr.).

Meyers, K. M., Padgett, G. A., and Dickson, W. M.: The genetic basis of a kinetic disorder of Scottish terrier dogs. J. Hered., *61*:189–192, 1970.

Patel, V., Koppang, N., Patel, B., and Zeman, W.: p-Phenylenediamine-mediated peroxidase deficiency in English Setters with neuronal seroid lipofuscinosis. Lab. Invest., 30:366–368, 1974.

Sanda, A., and Krizenecky, J.: Genetic basis of necrosis of digits in shortcoated setters. Vet. Bull., 36:2764, 1960.

Sanda, A., and Pivnik, L.: Necrosis of the toes in Pointers. Vet. Bull., 34:2283, 1964.

Scott, J. P., and Fuller, J. L.: Genetics and the Social Behavior of the Dog. Chicago and London, University of Chicago Press, 1965.

Steinberg, S. A.: Clinicopathologic conference. J. Am. Vet. Med. Assn., 143:404–410, 1963.

### Table 9. Neuromuscular System

| CONDITION | BREED(S) | MODE | SELECTED REFERENCES |
|---|---|---|---|
| Ataxia | Fox terrier (Sweden) | R? | Björck et al. (1957) |
|  | Jack Russell terriers | R? | Hartley (1973) |
| Behavioral abnormalities* | Several breeds, including poodle, cocker spaniel, German shepherd | P? | Stockard (1941), Thorne (1944), Freak (1948), Krushinskii (1962), Hodgman (1963), Burns and Fraser (1966), Thompson and Melzack (1956), Dykman et al. (1969), Lane and Holmes (1972) |
| Cerebellar hypoplasia | Airedale | ? | Cordy and Snelbaker (1952) |
| Cerebrospinal demyelination | Miniature poodle | ? | McGrath (1960), Douglas and Palmer (1961), Steinberg (1963) |
| Epilepsy | Keeshond, poodle | R? | Croft and Stockman (1964), Eberhart (1959) |
|  | Beagle | ? | Bielfelt et al. (1971) |
|  | Tervueren shepherd (Netherlands) | | Van der Velden (1968) |
|  | German shepherd | ? | Lawler (1971) Hegreberg and Padgett (1976) |
| Familial amaurotic idiocy† (GM$_2$ gangliosidosis) | German short-haired pointer | R? | Karbe and Schiefer (1967), McGrath et al. (1968), Bernheimer and Karbe (1970), Gambetti et al. (1970) |
| Globoid leukodystrophy | Cairn terriers, West Highland white terriers | R | Fankhauser et al. (1963) Fletcher et al. (1966) Suzuki et al. (1970, 1974) |
|  | Beagle | | Johnson et al. (1975) |
| Hydrocephalus | English bulldog | ? | Stockard (1941) |
|  | Cocker spaniel | | Scott and Fuller (1965) |
| Muscular dystrophy | Irish terrier | XR? | Wentink et al. (1972) |
| Neuronal ceroidlipofuscinosis | English setters | R | Hagen (1953), Koppang (1963, 1966, 1970), Patel et al. (1974) |
| Neuropathic necrosis, digits | Pointers | R? | Sanda and Pivnik (1964, 1966) |
| Scottie cramp | Scottish terriers | R | Meyers et al. (1970) |
| Syringomyelia | Weimaraner | ? | McGrath (1965) |
| Trembling | Airedale | ? | Kollarits (1924) |

*Reported by Karbe and Schiefer (1967) to be X-linked, but evidence is insufficient. Probably autosomal recessive, based on data from McGrath et al. (1968).

†Interbreed differences in behavior. The extensive studies by Scott and Fuller (1965) on the genetic basis of interbreed differences in behavioral characteristics leave little doubt that behavior is, to a large degree, genetically determined. Genetic analysis showed, however, that the differences in such traits as aggressiveness, trailing ability, vocalization and ability to learn certain tasks are usually not determined by single genes. There is no evidence to support a conclusion that certain behavioral characteristics are "linked" or in some other way causally related to body type. The fact that breeds of a certain body type have a certain form of behavior appears more likely to be the result of the simultaneous artificial selection for two independent hereditary characteristics.

Stockard, C.: An hereditary lethal for localized motor and preganglionic neurones with a resulting paralysis in the dog. Am. J. Anat., 59:1–53, 1936.

Stockard, C. R.: The Genetic and Endocrinic Basis for Differences in Form and Behavior as Elucidated by Studies of Contrasted Pure-Line Dog Breeds and Hybrids. American Anatomical Memoirs. Philadelphia, Wistar Institute of Anatomy and Biology, 1941.

Suzuki, Y., et al.: Studies in globoid leukodystrophy: enzymatic and lipid findings in the canine form. Exper. Neurol., 29:65–75, 1970.

Suzuki, Y., Miyatake, T., Fletcher, J. F., and Suzuki, K.: Glycosphingolipid B galactosidases. J. Biol. Chem., 249:2109–2112, 1974.

Thompson, W. R., and Melzack, R.: Early environment. Sci. Am., 194:38–42, 1956.

Thorne, F. C.: the inheritance of shyness in dogs. J. Gen. Psychol., 65:275–279, 1944.

Van der Velden, N. A.: "Fits" in tervueren shepherd dogs: a presumed hereditary trait. J. Small Animal Pract. 9:63–70, 1968.

Wentink, G. H., et al.: Myopathy with a possible recessive X-linked inheritance in a litter of Irish terriers. Vet. Path. 9:328–349, 1972.

## SELECTED REFERENCES:

### Other Structural Malformations

Fox, M. W.: Inherited inguinal hernia and midline defects in the dog. J. Am. Vet. Med. Assn., 143:602–604, 1963.

Hodgman, S. F.: An investigation into the existence of abnormalities in pedigree dogs in the British Isles. J. Small Animal Pract., 6:447–456, 1963.

Koch, W.: New pathological hereditary characters in the dog. Z. Iwdukt. Abstamm. Vererb. L., 70:503–506, 1935.

Leonard, H. C.: Collapse of the larynx and adjacent structures in the dog. J. Am. Vet. Med. Assn., 137:360–364, 1960.

Leonard, H. C.: Surgical correction of collapsed trachea in dogs. J. Am. Vet. Med. Assn., 158:598–600, 1971.

Pendergrass, T. W., and Hayes, H. M., Jr.: Cryptorchism and related defects in dogs: Epidemiologic comparisons with man. Teratology, 12:51–56, 1975.

Phillips, J. M., and Felton, T. M.: Hereditary umbilical hernia. J. Hered., 30:433–435, 1939.

Suter, P. F., Colgrove, D. J., and Ewing, G. O.: Congenital hypoplasia of the canine trachea. J.A.A.H.A., 8:120–127, 1972.

Willis, M. B.: Abnormalities in pedigree dogs. V. Cryptorchidism. J. Small Animal Pract., 4:469–474, 1963.

## SELECTED REFERENCES:

### The Skin

Burgisser, H., and Hinterman, J.: Kystes dermoides de la tête chez le boxer. Schweiz. Arch. Tierheilk., 103:309–312, 1961.

Editorial. The hairless dog. J. Hered., 8:519–520, 1917.

Gaspar, J.: Analyse der erbfaktoren des schadels bei einer Paarung von Ceylon-Nackthund X Dackel. Jena Z. Naturw., 65:245–274, 1930.

Hegreberg, G. A., et al.: Cutaneous asthenia in dogs. Newer knowledge about dogs. 16th Gaines Vet. Symp.:3–5, 1966.

Hegreberg, G. A., et al.: A connective tissue disease of dogs and mink resembling the Ehlers-Danlos syndrome of man. II. Mode of inheritance. J. Hered., 60:249–254, 1969.

Hegreberg, G. A., Padgett, G. A., and Henson, J. B.: Connective tissue disease of dogs and mink resembling Ehlers-Danlos syndrome of man. III. Histopathological changes of the skin. Arch. Path., 90:159–166, 1970a.

Hegreberg, G. A., Padgett, G. A., Ott, R. L., and Henson, J. B.: A heritable connective disease of dogs and mink resembling Ehler-Danlos syndrome of man. I. Skin tensile strength properties. J. Invest. Derm., 54:377–380, 1970b.

Hofmeyer, C. F. B.: Dermoid sinus in the ridgeback dog. J. Small Animal Pract., 4:5–8, 1963.

Hutt, F. B.: Inherited lethal characters in domestic animals. Cornell Vet., 24:1–25, 1934.

Kohn, F. G.: Beitrag zur Kenntnis der Haut des Nackthundes. Zool. Jb. Anat., 31:427–438, 1911.

Mann, G. E., and Stratton, J.: Dermoid sinus in the Rhodesian ridgeback. J. Small Animal Pract., 7:631–642, 1966.

Schwartzman, R. M., Rockey, J. H., and Halliwell, R. E.: Canine reaginic antibody: characterization of the spontaneous anti-ragweed and induced anti-dinitrophenyl reaginic antibodies of the atopic dog. Clin. Exper. Immunol., 9:549–569, 1971.

Selmanowitz, V. J., Kramer, K. M., and Orentreich, N.:

## Table 10.  *Other Structural Malformations*

| CONDITION | BREED(S) | MODE | SELECTED REFERENCES |
|---|---|---|---|
| Cryptorchidism | Most breeds | R? | Willis (1963) Pendergrass and Hayes (1975) |
| Elongated soft palate | Brachycephalic breeds | ? | Hodgman (1963) |
| Inguinal and midline hernias | Collies, cocker spaniels, bull terriers, basenjis | ? | Phillips and Felton (1939), Fox (1963) |
| Laryngeal malformations | Skye terrier | ? | Koch (1935), Leonard (1960) |
| Tracheal collapse | Toy breeds, especially toy poodle, Pomeranian | ? | Leonard (1960, 1971) |
| Tracheal hypoplasia | English bulldog | ? | Suter et al. (1972) |

### Table 11. *The Skin*

| CONDITION | BREED(S) | MODE | SELECTED REFERENCES |
|---|---|---|---|
| Atopic dermatitis | Beagle, Dalmatian, Scottish terrier, wire-haired fox terrier | ? | Schwartzman et al. (1971) |
| Black hair follicular dysplasia | Mongrel | ? | Selmanowitz et al. (1972) |
| Cutaneous asthenia (hyperelasticity, fragility) | Springer spaniel | D | Hegreberg et al. (1966, 1969, 1970a, 1970b) |
| Dermoid sinus | Rhodesian ridgeback | ? | Hofmeyer (1963), Mann and Stratton (1966) |
|  | Boxer | ? | Burgisser and Hinterman (1961) |
| Ectodermal dysplasia | Miniature poodle | ? | Selmanowitz et al. (1970) |
| Hairlessness | Mexican hairless, other hairless breeds | D* | Editorial (1917), Gaspar (1930), Hutt (1934), Kohn (1911), Thomsett (1961), Zulueta (1945) |

*The Mexican hairless and other hairless breeds are reported to be heterozygous for a dominant gene for hairlessness. Reportedly, in the homozygous state, the gene is lethal, producing complete occlusion of the lower esophagus. Recessive forms of hairlessness probably occur occasionally in other breeds.

Congenital ectodermal defect in miniature poodles. J. Hered., *61*:196–199, 1970.

Selmanowitz, V. J., Kramer, K. M., and Orentreich, N.: Canine hereditary black hair follicular dysplasia. J. Hered., *63*:43–44, 1972.

Thomsett, L. R.: Congenital hypotrichia in the dog. Vet. Rec., *73*:915–917, 1961.

Zulueta, A. de: The hairless dogs of Madrid. Proc. VIII Int. Cong. Genet.:687–688, 1945.

**SELECTED REFERENCES:**

**Susceptibility to Disease**

Baker, J. A., et al.: Breed response to distemper vaccination. Proc. Animal Care Panel, *12*:157–162, 1962.

Bierwaltes, W. H., and Nishiyama, R. H.: Dog thyroiditis: occurrence and similarity to Hashimoto's struma. Endocrinology, *83*:501–508, 1968.

### Table 12. *Susceptibility to Disease*

| CONDITION | BREED(S) | SELECTED REFERENCES |
|---|---|---|
| Colibacillosis | Basenji | Fox (1965) |
| Distemper | Beagle, bloodhound, pointers | Whitney (1948), Baker et al. (1962) |
| Eosinophilic panostitis | Beagle, bloodhound, pointers | Cotter et al. (1968) |
| Lupus erythematosus | German shepherd | Lewis and Schwartz (1971) |
| Neonatal death, generally* | Purebred vs. mixed | Scott and Fuller (1965) |
| Neoplasms† |  |  |
|   Melanoma | Breeds with red or black coat color | Cotchin (1955), Brodey (1970) |
|   Osteosarcoma | Giant breeds | Owen (1962), Tjalma (1966), Brodey (1970) |
|   Pituitary tumors | Boston terrier | Luginbuhl (1963) |
|   Hair follicle tumors | Kerry blue terrier | Brodey (1970) |
|   Mast cell tumors | Boxer, Boston terrier | Peters (1969) |
|   Skin neoplasms, generally | Cocker spaniel | Brodey (1970) |
|   Aortic and carotid body tumors | Boxer, Boston terrier | Brodey (1970) |
| Thyroiditis | Beagle | Bierwaltes and Nishiyama (1968) |

*The much higher neonatal death rate in the offspring of purebred dogs than in the offspring of crosses between breeds suggests that deleterious recessive genes in the homozygous state are involved.

†As in other species, the high incidence of certain neoplasms in certain strains or breeds may be the result of vertical transmission of oncogenic viruses. Their expression, however, probably depends upon the genotype of the host.

### Table 13.   *Urinary System*

| CONDITION | BREED(S) | MODE | SELECTED REFERENCES |
|---|---|---|---|
| Cystine stones (cystinuria) | Dachshund, Irish terrier, poodle, Welsh corgi, Labrador retriever, Great Dane, German shepherd, Cairn terrier, Scottish terrier | XR? | Brand and Cahill (1936), Brand et al. (1940), Holtzapple et al. (1969), Bovee and Segal (1971), Tsan et al. (1972) |
| Renal aplasia (unilateral) | Beagle | R? | Fox (1964), Vymetral (1965) |
| Renal cortical hypoplasia | Cocker spaniel, dachshund, Doberman pinscher, Norwegian elkhound, malamute | R? | Murti (1965), Krook (1957), Persson et al. (1961), Kaufman et al. (1969), Finco et al. (1970) |
| Renal tubular dysfunction | Basenji | ? | Easly and Breitschwerdt (1976) |
| Uric acid stones (high uric acid excretion) | Dalmation | R | Trimble and Keeler (1938), Keeler (1940), Harvey, and Christensen (1964), Ts'Ai-Fan Yu et al. (1971) |

Brodey, R. S.: Canine and feline neoplasia. *In* Advances in Veterinary Science. Vol. 14. New York, Academic Press, 1970.

Cotchin, E.: Melanotic tumours of dogs. J. Comp. Path., 2:115–129, 1955.

Cotter, S. M., Griffiths, R. C., and Leav, I.: Enostosis in young dogs. J. Am. Vet. Med. Assn. 153:401–410, 1968.

Fox, M. W., Hoag, W. G., and Strout, J.: The epidemiology, pathogenicity, and breed susceptibility of endemic coliform enteritis in the dog. J. Lab. Animal Care, 15:194–200, 1965.

Lewis, R. M., and Schwartz, R. S.: Canine systemic lupus erythematosus. Genetic analysis of an established breeding colony. J. Exp. Med., 134:417–438, 1971.

Luginbuhl, H.: Comparative aspects of tumors of the nervous system. Ann. New York Acad. Sci., 108:702–721, 1963.

Owen, L. N.: The differential diagnosis of bone tumors in the dog. Vet. Rec., 74:439–446, 1962.

Peters, J. A.: Canine mastocytoma: excess risk related to ancestry. J. Nat. Cancer Ins., 42:435–443, 1969.

Scott, J. P., and Fuller, J. L.: Genetics and the Social Behavior of the Dog. Chicago, University of Chicago Press, 1965.

Tjalma, R. A.: Canine bone sarcoma: Estimation of relative risk as a function of body size. J. Nat. Cancer Inst., 36:1137–1150, 1966.

Whitney, L. F.: How to Breed Dogs. New York, Orange Judd Publishing Co., 1948.

## SELECTED REFERENCES:

### Urinary System

Bovee, K. C., and Segal, S.: Canine cystinuria and cystine calculi. The newer knowledge about dogs. Proceedings of the 21st Gaines Veterinary Symposium. 1971.

Brand, E., and Cahill, G. F.: Canine cystinuria, III. J. Biol. Chem., 15:114, 1936.

Brand, E., Cahill, G. F., and Kassell, B.: Canine cystinuria. V. Family history of two cystinuric dogs and cystine determinations in dog urine. J. Biol. Chem., 133:431–436, 1940.

Easley, J. R., and Breitschwerdt, E. B.: Glucosuria associated with renal tubular dysfunction in three basenji dogs. J. Am. Vet. Med. Assn., 168:938–943, 1976.

Finco, D. R., et al.: Familial renal disease in Norwegian elkhound dogs. J. Am. Vet. Med. Assn., 156:747–760, 1970.

Fox, M. W.: Inherited polycystic mononephrosis in the dog. J. Hered., 55:29–30, 1964.

Harvey, A. M., and Christensen, H. N.: Uric acid transport system: apparent absence in erythrocytes of the Dalmatian coach hound. Science, 145:826–827, 1964.

Holtzapple, P. G., et al.: Amino acid uptake by kidney and jejunal tissue from dogs with cystine stones. Science, 166:1525–1527, 1969.

Kaufman, C. F., Soirez, R. F., and Tasker, J. P.: Renal cortical hypoplasia with secondary hyperparathyroidism in the dog. J. Am. Vet. Med. Assn., 155:1679–1685, 1969.

Keeler, C. F.: The inheritance of predisposition to renal calculi in the Dalmatian. J. Am. Vet. Med. Assn., 96:507–510, 1940.

Krook, L.: The pathology of renal cortical hypoplasia in the dog. Nord. Vet. Med., 9:161–176, 1957.

Murti, G. S.: Agenesis and dysgenesis of the canine kidneys. J. Am. Vet. Med. Assn., 146:1120–1124, 1965.

Persson, F., Persson, S., and Asheim, A.: Renal cortical hypoplasia in dogs. A clinical study on uraemia and secondary hypoparathyroidism. Acta Vet. Scand., 2:68–84, 1961.

Trimble, H. D., and Keeler, C. E.: The inheritance of high uric acid excretion in dogs. J. Hered., 29:280–289, 1938.

Ts' Ai-Fan Yu, et al.: Low uricase activity in Dalmatian dogs simulated in mongrels given uronic acid. Am. J. Physiol., 220:973–979, 1971.

Tsan, M., et al.: Canine cystinuria: Its urinary amino acid pattern and genetic analysis. Am. J. Vet. Res., 33:2455–2461, 1972.

Vymetral, F.: Renal aplasia in beagles. Vet. Rec., 77:1344–1345, 1965.

# Section

# 2

# CHEMICAL AND PHYSICAL DISORDERS

FREDERICK W. OEHME, D.V.M.
*Consulting Editor*

# EMERGENCY AND GENERAL TREATMENT OF POISONINGS*

E. MURL BAILEY, D.V.M.
*College Station, Texas*

Many acutely ill animals are diagnosed as poisoned when no other diagnosis can be readily ascertained. For this reason, the treatment and management of acutely ill animals should be directed toward preserving the life of the animal, regardless of the etiology(ies).

The veterinary clinician should direct his efforts toward treating the signs exhibited by the affected animal unless the correct diagnosis is obvious. Preexisting conditions and the diagnosis should be determined following stabilization of the patient.

Special goals of therapy in cases of intoxications are

(1) Emergency intervention and prevention of further exposure.

(2) Delaying further absorption.

(3) Application of specific antidotes.

(4) Hastening elimination of the absorbed toxicant.

(5) Supportive therapy.

## PRELIMINARY INSTRUCTIONS TO CLIENTS

Veterinarians are frequently contacted by telephone concerning an intoxicated animal. The preliminary instructions given at this time can be important to the success of subsequent therapeutic measures.

The client should be instructed to protect the animal as well as the people in contact with the affected animal. This may include keeping the animal warm and avoiding any other stress phenomena. Onlookers should be warned about the condition of the animal, and it may be desirable to place a muzzle on the animal.

If the animal's exposure was topical, the client should be instructed to cleanse the animal's skin or eye with copious amounts of water. The client should also be instructed to be careful to avoid exposure to the toxicant and should use some type of protective clothing if available.

In many instances, the client will be concerned about inducing emesis in the animal. The clinician should cite the contraindications to emesis, i.e., CNS depression; ingestion of petroleum distillates, acids or alkalis. Emetic preparations and techniques easily available to the lay individual, such as syrup of ipecac, hydrogen peroxide, table salt and sticking the finger in the back of the animal's mouth, are generally ineffective and sometimes dangerous.

If the client is very insistent about administering medication, he should be advised to allow the animal to drink as much water as it wants. This will act as a diluent. In most cases, one may also advise the administration of milk or egg whites. The client should be cautioned not to administer anything by mouth if the animal is convulsing, depressed or unconscious.

It is imperative that the client not waste time. The animal should be brought to the veterinarian as soon as possible (or the veterinarian should be summoned). The owner should be instructed to bring vomitus and/or suspected materials or their containers with the animal. In many instances valuable time can be saved by applying the proper therapeutic measures if the suspected intoxicant is known. This suspected material may also be valuable from a medicolegal aspect. The client should be advised to bring the specimens in clean plastic containers or glass jars and should be cautioned not to contaminate the material.

## EMERGENCY INTERVENTION

The most important aspect of emergency treatment of intoxications is to insure adequate physiologic function. All the an-

*Supported in part by Texas Agricultural Experiment Station, Project No. 01981.

tidotal procedures available to the clinician will be to no avail if the animal has lost one or all of the vital functions. This may include establishment of a patent airway, artificial respiration, cardiac massage (external or internal) and perhaps the application of defibrillation techniques. Following stabilization of the vital signs, the emergency clinician may proceed with subsequent therapeutic measures.

## DELAYING ABSORPTION

Preventing the animal from absorbing additional intoxicant is a major factor in treating cases of intoxication. In many instances intoxication may be prevented in this manner if the animal was actually observed ingesting or being in contact with suspected material. Removal of the animal from the affected environment is a necessary first step to prevent further absorption. Hopefully, bringing the animal to the veterinary clinic or hospital will suit this purpose. It also may entail washing the animal's skin to remove the noxious agent. If an external toxicant is involved, caution must be exercised to avoid contamination of all persons handling the case. In addition, the judicious use of emetics, gastric lavage techniques, adsorbents and cathartics will further aid in the prevention of further absorption of toxic materials that are ingested.

### INDUCTION OF EMESIS

Emesis may be considered as a method of emptying the stomach of toxic materials. Some commonly available agents are not too reliable, and emesis may be of little value after 1 to 2 hours following exposure to a toxicant.

Syrup of ipecac is considered a general emetic. Its mechanism is gastric irritation rather than central stimulation. The dose of ipecac for small animals is 1 to 2 ml./kg., but it is only about 50 per cent effective. This agent should never be used when activated charcoal is part of the therapeutic regimen, since it markedly reduces the effectiveness of the charcoal.

Other agents such as copper sulfate, table salt or hydrogen peroxide have been advocated as locally acting emetics. However, the effectiveness of these agents is questionable.

Apomorphine is the most effective and most reliable emetic available. The effective dose in most small animals is 0.04 mg./kg. IV or 0.08 mg./kg. IM or SC. Apomorphine may cause respiratory depression, and protracted emesis may develop following its use. These signs may be effectively controlled with appropriate narcotic antagonists injected IV (naloxone, Narcan®: 0.04 mg./kg.; levallorphan, Lorfan®, 0.02 mg./kg.; or nalorphine, Nalline®; 0.1 mg./kg.). In addition to the general contraindications of emetics, apomorphine may be further contraindicated in cases where additional CNS depression must be avoided.

The contraindications for induction of emesis are unconscious or severely depressed animals, intoxication by petroleum distillates, tranquilizers or other antiemetics. If the time interval following exposure to the toxicant is greater than 1 to 2 hours, most of the toxicant will have passed to the duodenum. Intoxication with acids or alkalis may be diagnosed when corrosive changes are present in and around the mouth, forepaws and other areas on the cranial portions of the body. If emesis were induced, caustic agents would cause additional damage to the esophagus and oral cavity. In addition, these agents generally weaken the gastric wall, which could easily be ruptured during forceful emesis.

Activated charcoal may increase the efficacy of emesis. If charcoal is to be utilized, the clinician should first induce emesis with apomorphine, administer the charcoal, and reinduce emesis with a subsequent IV dose of apomorphine.

Any vomitus should be saved for analysis, especially if there are any medicolegal considerations. The clinician should consider any intoxication as grounds for a possible court case and should conduct treatment accordingly.

### GASTRIC LAVAGE

Gastric lavage is an emergency procedure which has at times been maligned as being relatively inefficient. Changes in technique (e.g., using a larger tube, more volume and more frequent lavages) have made this a very reliable procedure when undertaken within 2 hours of exposure to an ingested toxicant.

The animal should be unconscious or under light anesthesia. A cuffed endotracheal tube should be placed within the trachea. The distal end of the tube should protrude 2 inches beyond the teeth. This will increase the animal's dead space but is required to prevent any inhalation of lavage fluid. The head and thorax should be lowered slightly but not enough to compromise respiration due to the weight of the abdominal viscera. Pre-measure the stomach tube from the tip of the animal's nose to the xiphoid cartilage. In all cases, use as large a stomach tube as possible. A good rule is to use the same size stomach tube as cuffed endotracheal tube (1 mm. = 3 French). The volume of water or lavage solution to be used for each washing is 5 to 10 ml./kg. of body weight. Following the infusion of the solution, the fluid should be aspirated from the stomach via the stomach tube with either a large aspirator bulb or a 50-ml. syringe. The infusion and aspiration cycle of the lavage solution should be repeated 10 to 15 times. Activated charcoal in the solution will enhance the effectiveness of this procedure.

Some precautions to be taken with this technique are (1) use low pressure to prevent the forcing of the toxicant into the duodenum, (2) reduce the infused volume in obviously weakened stomachs and (3) make sure not to force the stomach tube through either the esophagus or the stomach wall.

## Adsorbents

Activated charcoal is probably the best adsorbing agent available to the practitioner. Although it does not detoxify toxicants, it will effectively prevent absorption of a toxicant if properly utilized. Activated charcoal can be effectively utilized with emetic and gastric lavage techniques.

The proper type of activated charcoal for treatment in toxications is of vegetable, not mineral or animal, origin. There are several commercial types of activated charcoal available: Norit® (American Norit), Nuchar C® (West Virginia Pulp and Paper) and Darco G-60® (Atlas Chemical). Compressed activated charcoal tablets are also available. These tablets are easier to handle than the powdered charcoal but are apparently not as effective.

A bathtub or some other easily cleaned area is the best place to administer the activated charcoal to small animals. The proper technique for utilizing activated charcoal is as follows: (1) Make a slurry of the charcoal using water. The proper dose is 2 to 8 gm./kg. body weight in a concentration of 1 gm. charcoal/3 to 5 ml. water. (2) Administer the charcoal by a stomach tube using either a funnel or a large syringe. (3) Thirty minutes following administration of the charcoal, a cathartic of sodium sulfate should be administered. This technique may be modified if the charcoal is used in conjunction with emetic or lavage techniques. However, with either technique, some charcoal should remain in the stomach and should be followed by a cathartic to prevent desorption of the toxicant.

Activated charcoal is highly adsorptive for many toxicants, including mercuric chloride, strychnine, other alkaloids including morphine and atropine, barbiturates and ethylene glycol. It is ineffective against cyanide.

Syrup of ipecac will negate some of the adsorptive characteristics of the activated charcoal. The "universal antidote," consisting of 2 parts activated charcoal, 1 part MgO and 1 part tannic acid, is very inefficient, since the MgO and tannic acid decrease the adsorptive capability of the charcoal. Burned or charred toast as described in some emergency texts is highly ineffective as an adsorbing agent.

## Cathartics

Sodium sulfate is a more efficient agent for evacuation of the bowel than magnesium sulfate and is the preferable agent to use, especially with activated charcoal. There is also some danger of CNS depression due to the magnesium ion. However, either agent may be used in an emergency. The oral dose of sodium sulfate is 1 gm./kg.

Mineral oil or vegetable oils are of value if lipid-soluble toxicants are involved. Mineral oil (liquid petrolatum) is inert and unlikely to be absorbed. Vegetable oil, however, is more likely to be absorbed and therefore may be contraindicated. Regardless of the type of oil utilized, it should be followed by a saline cathartic in 30 to 40 minutes.

A colonic lavage or high enema may be of value to hasten the elimination of toxicants from the gastrointestinal tract. Warm water with castile soap makes an excellent enema solution. Hexachlorophene soaps should be

***Table 1.*** *Locally Acting Antidotes Against Unabsorbed Poisons and Principles of Treatment\**

| POISON | ANTIDOTE AND DOSE OR CONCENTRATION |
|---|---|
| Acids, corrosive | Weak alkali—Magnesium oxide solution (1:25 warm water) internally. *Never give sodium bicarbonate!* Milk of Magnesia—1 to 15 ml. Flush externally with water. Apply paste of sodium bicarbonate. |
| Alkali, caustic | Weak acid—Vinegar (diluted 1:4), 1%. Acetic acid or lemon juice given orally. Diluted albumin (4 to 6 egg whites to 1 qt. tepid water) followed by an emetic and then by a cathartic, because some compounds are soluble in excess albumin. Local—flush with copious amounts of water and apply vinegar. |
| Alkaloids | Potassium permanganate (1:5000 to 1:10,000) for lavage and/or oral administration. Tannic acid or strong tea (200 to 500 mg. in 30 to 60 ml. of water) except in cases of poisoning by cocaine, nicotine, physostigmine, atropine and morphine. Emetic or purgative should be used for prompt removal of tannates. |
| Arsenic | Sodium thiosulfate—10% solution given orally (0.5 to 3.0 gm. for small animals). Protein—evaporated milk, egg whites, etc. Tannic acid or strong tea. |
| Barium salts | Sodium sulfate and magnesium sulfate (20% solution given orally). Dosage: 2 to 25 gm. |
| Bismuth salts | Acacia or gum arabic as mucilage. |
| Carbon tetrachloride | Empty stomach; give high protein and carbohydrate diet; maintain fluid and electrolyte balance. Hemodialysis is indicated in anuria. Epinephrine is contraindicated (ventricular fibrillation!). |
| Copper | Albumin (as for Alkali above). Sodium ferrocyanide in water (0.3 to 3.5 gm. for small animals). Magnesium oxide (as for Acids above). |
| Detergents, anionic (Na, K, $NH^+_4$—salts) | Milk or water followed by demulcent (oils, acacia, gelatin, starch, egg white, etc.). |
| Detergents, cationic (chlorides, iodides, etc.) | Soap (castile, etc.) dissolved in 4 times its bulk of hot water. Albumin (as for Alkali above). |
| Fluoride | Calcium (milk, lime water or powdered chalk mixed with water) given orally. |
| Formaldehyde | Ammonia water (0.2% orally) or ammonium acetate (1% for lavage). Starch—1 part to 15 parts hot water added gradually. Gelatin soaked in water for ½ hour. Albumin (as for Alkali above). Sodium thiosulfate (as for Arsenic above). |
| Iron | Sodium bicarbonate—1% for lavage. |
| Lead | Sodium or magnesium sulfate given orally. Sodium ferrocyanide (as for Copper above). Tannic acid (as for Alkaloids above). Albumin (as for Alkali above). |
| Mercury | Protein—Milk, egg whites (as for Alkali above). Magnesium oxide (as for Acids above). Sodium formaldehyde sulfoxylate—5% solution for lavage. Starch (as for Formaldehyde above). Activated charcoal—5 to 50 gm. |
| Oxalic acid | Calcium—Calcium hydroxide as 0.15% solution. Other alkalis are contraindicated because their salts are more soluble. Chalk or other calcium salts. Magnesium sulfate as cathartic. Maintain diuresis to prevent calcium oxalate deposition in kidney. |
| Petroleum distillates (aliphatic hydrocarbons) | Olive oil, other vegetable oils or mineral oil given orally. After ½ hour, sodium sulfate as cathartic. Both emesis and lavage are contraindicated. |
| Phenol and cresols | Soap-and-water or alcohol lavage of skin. Sodium bicarbonate (0.5%) dressings. Activated charcoal and/or mineral oil given orally. |

\*Modified from Szabuniewicz et al. (1971).

*Continued on next page*

**Table 1.** *Locally Acting Antidotes Against Unabsorbed Poisons and Principles of Treatment (Continued)*

| POISON | ANTIDOTE AND DOSE OR CONCENTRATION |
|---|---|
| Phosphorus | Copper sulfate (0.2 to 0.4% solution) or potassium permanganate (1:5000 solution) for lavage. |
| | Turpentine (preferably old oxidized) in gelatin capsules or floated on hot water. Give 2 ml. 4 times at 15-minute intervals. |
| | Activated charcoal. |
| | Do not give vegetable oil cathartic. Remove all fat from diet. |
| Silver nitrate | Normal saline for lavage. |
| | Albumin (as for Alkali above). |
| Unknown | Activated charcoal (replaces universal antidote). For small animals—5 to 50 gm. in gelatin capsules or, via stomach pump, as a slurry in water. Follow by emetic or cathartic and repeat dosage. |

avoided. There are several commercial enema preparations available which act as osmotic agents.

## LOCALLY ACTING ANTIDOTES

There are numerous locally acting antidotes and therapeutic regimens reported for preventing the absorption of toxicants. The nonspecific antidotal procedures for some of the more common toxicants are described in Table 1.

## SPECIFIC ANTIDOTES

There are a few specific antidotal agents available for some of the more common animal toxicants. A list of these specific antidotal procedures is presented in Table 2.

Caution should be exercised with the use of some of the more specific antidotes, since many of these agents are themselves toxic. In certain chronic metallic intoxications such as lead poisoning, the use of chelating agents has precipitated the acute metallic intoxication. Consequently, the dosage of chelating agents should be reduced in some chronic metal intoxications.

## ELIMINATION OF ABSORBED TOXICANTS

Absorbed toxicants are generally excreted via the kidneys. Some toxicants may be excreted by other routes (bile-feces, lung, other body secretions). Renal excretion can be manipulated in many instances. Urinary excretion of toxicants may be enhanced by the use of diuretics or altering the pH of the urine.

The use of diuretics to enhance urinary excretion of toxicants requires adequate renal function and hydration of the affected animal. Once these requisites are established, diuretics are indicated. Monitoring of urinary output is essential in these animals, and a minimum urinary flow of 0.1 ml./kg./min. is necessary. The diuretics of choice are mannitol and furosemide (Lasix®). Both of these agents are very potent diuretics. The dosage for mannitol is 2 gm./kg./hr. and for furosemide is 4 mg./kg.

Alteration of urinary pH to expedite the excretion of toxicants and foreign chemicals is a classic pharmacologic technique. The technique relies on the physiochemical phenomenon that ionized compounds do not readily traverse cell membranes and hence are not reabsorbed by the renal tubules. Consequently, acid compounds such as acetylsalicylic acid (aspirin) and some barbiturates remain ionized in alkaline urine, and alkaline compounds such as amphetamines remain ionized in acidic urine. As a result, urinary excretion of many toxic compounds may be enhanced by modifying the urine pH. Urinary acidifying agents include ammonium chloride (200 mg./kg./day in divided doses) and ethylenediamine dihydrochloride (Chlorethamine®, 1 to 2 tablets 3 times a day for the average sized dog.) Sodium bicarbonate may be used as an alkalinizing agent.

Peritoneal dialysis is indicated when an intoxicated animal exhibits oliguria or anuria. It is a rather time-consuming but effective technique in many conditions. The procedure requires the use of two separate solutions, and the solutions must be ex-

### Table 2. *Systemic Antidotes and Dosages**

| TOXIC AGENT | SYSTEMIC ANTIDOTES | DOSAGE AND METHOD FOR TREATMENT |
|---|---|---|
| Amphetamines | Chlorpromazine | 1 mg./kg. IM, IP, IV; administer only half dose if barbiturates have been given; blocks excitation. |
| Arsenic, mercury and other heavy metals except silver, selenium and thallium | Dimercaprol (BAL) | 10% solution in oil; give small animals 2.5 to 5.0 mg./kg. IM every 4 hours for 2 days, three times a day for the next 10 days or until recovery. NOTE: In severe acute poisoning 5 mg./kg. dosage should be given only first day. |
| | N-Acetyl-D.L.-penicillamine (only for mercury poisoning) | Developed for chronic mercury poisoning, now seems most promising drug; no reports on dosage in animals. Dosage for man is 250 mg. orally, every 6 hours for 10 days (3 to 4 mg./kg.) |
| Atropine— | | |
|   Belladonna alkaloids | Physostigmine salicylate | 0.01 to 0.6 mg./kg. |
|   Barbiturates | Pentylenetetrazol | 10% solution; give small animals 10 to 20 mg./kg. IV or IM, repeated at 15 to 30 minute intervals as needed. |
| | Doxapram | 2% solution; give small animals 3 to 5 mg./kg. IV only, repeated as necessary. |
| | Bemegride | 3% solution; give small animals 5 to 10 mg./kg. IV only, by slow infusion or in intermittent doses. |

NOTE: All of the above are reliable only when depression is mild; in deeper levels of depression, artificial respiration (and oxygen) is preferable.

| | | |
|---|---|---|
| Bromides | Chlorides (sodium or ammonium salts) | 0.5 to 1.0 gm. daily for several days; hastens excretion. |
| Carbon monoxide | Oxygen | Pure oxygen at normal or high pressure, or oxygen with 5% carbon dioxide; artificial respiration; blood transfusion. |
| Cholinergic agents | Atropine sulfate | 0.02 to 0.04 mg./kg. as needed. |
| Cholinesterase inhibitors | Atropine sulfate | Dosage is 0.2 mg./kg., repeated as needed for atropinization. Treat cyanosis (if present) first. Blocks only muscarinic effects. Atropine in oil may be injected for prolonged effect during the night. *Avoid atropine intoxication!* |
| Cholinergic agents and cholinesterase inhibitors (organophosphates, some carbamates; but not carbaryl, dimethan or carbam piloxime, etc.) | Pralidoxime chloride (2-PAM) | 2% solution; give 20 to 50 mg./kg. IM or by slow IV injection (maximum dose is 500 mg./min.), repeat as needed. 2-PAM alleviates nicotinic effect and regenerates cholinesterase. Morphine, succinylcholine and phenothiazine tranquilizers are contraindicated. |
| Copper | D-Penicillamine | Dose for animals not established. Dose for man is 1 to 4 gm. daily in divided doses (250-mg. tablets). |
| Coumarin-derivative anticoagulants | Vitamin K₁ | 5% stable emulsion. Give 5 mg./kg. IM for 3 days. |
| | Whole blood or plasma | Blood transfusion, 25 ml./kg. |
| Curare (tubocurarine) | Neostigmine methylsulfate | Solution: 1:500 or 1:2000 (1 ml.= 2 mg. or 0.5 mg.). Dose is 0.05 mg./5 kg. SC. Follow with IV injection of a 1% solution of atropine (0.04 mg./kg.). |

---

*Modified from Szabuniewicz et al. (1971).

*Continued on next page*

**Table 2.** *Systemic Antidotes and Dosages\* (Continued)*

| TOXIC AGENT | SYSTEMIC ANTIDOTES | DOSAGE AND METHOD FOR TREATMENT |
|---|---|---|
| Cyanide | Edrophonium chloride Artificial respiration | 1% solution; give 0.05 to 1.0 mg./kg.IV. |
| | Methemoglobin (sodium nitrite is used to form methemoglobin) | 1% solution of sodium nitrite, dosage is 16 mg./kg. IV. Follow with: |
| | Sodium thiosulfate | 20% solution at dosage of 30 to 40 mg./kg. IV. If treatment is repeated, use only sodium thiosulfate. NOTE: Both of the above may be given simultaneously as follows: 0.5 ml./kg. of combination consisting of 10 gm. sodium nitrite, 15 gm. sodium thiosulfate and distilled water q.s. 250 ml. Dosage may be repeated once. If further treatment is required, give only 20% solution of sodium thiosulfate at level of 1 ml./kg. |
| Digitalis glycosides, oleander and Bufo toads | Potassium chloride | Dog: 0.5 to 2.0 mg. orally in divided doses, or in serious cases, as di- drip (ECG control is essential). |
| | Diphenylhydantoin sodium | 25 mg./min. IV until control is is established. |
| | Propranolol (beta blocker) | 0.5 to 1.0 mg./kg. IV or IM as needed to control cardiac arrhythmias. |
| | Atropine sulfate | 0.02 to 0.04 mg./kg. as needed for cholinergic control. |
| Fluoride | Calcium borogluconate | 3 to 10 ml. of 5 to 10% solution. |
| Fluoroacetate (compound 1080) | Glyceryl monoacetin | 0.1 to 0.5 mg./kg. IM hourly for several hours (total 2 to 4 mg./kg.); or diluted (0.5 to 1.0%) IV (danger of hemolysis). Monoacetin is available only from chemical supply houses. |
| | Acetamide | Animal may be protected if acetamide is given prior to or simultaneously with 1080 (experimental). |
| | Phenobarbital or pentobarbital | May protect against lethal dose (experimental). |
| Hallucinogens (LSD, phencyclidine-PCP) | Phenothiazine tranquilizers or pentobarbital | Follow with symptomatic treatment. |
| Heparin | Protamine sulfate | 1% solution; give 1.0 to 1.5 mg. to antagonize each 1 mg. of heparin; slow IV injection. Reduce dose as time increases between heparin injection and start of treatment. (After 30 minutes, give only 0.5 mg.) |
| | Hexadimethrine | 1 mg. for each 1 mg. heparin, by slow IV injection. Hexadimethrine is a synthetic product and causes fewer side effects than protamine. |
| Iron salts | Desferrioxamine (deferoxamine) | Dose for animals not yet established. Dose for man is 5 gm. of 5% solution given orally, then 20 mg./kg. IM every 4 hours. In case of shock, dose is 40 mg./kg. by IV drip over 4-hour period; may be repeated in 6 hours, then 20 mg./kg. by drip every 12 hours. |

\*Modified from Szabuniewicz et al. (1971).

*Continued on next page*

*Table 2.   Systemic Antidotes and Dosages\* (Continued)*

| TOXIC AGENT | SYSTEMIC ANTIDOTES | DOSAGE AND METHOD FOR TREATMENT |
|---|---|---|
| Lead | Calcium disodium edetate (EDTA), EDTA and BAL | Dosage: Maximum safe dose is 75 mg./kg./24 hours (only for severe case). EDTA is available in 20% solution; for IV drip, dilute in 5% glucose to 0.5%; for IM, add procaine to 20% solution to give 0.5% concentration of procaine. BAL is given as 10% solution in oil. Treatment: (1) In severe case (CNS involvement of >100 mg. Pb/100 gm. whole blood) give 4 mg./kg. BAL only as initial dose; follow after 4 hours, and every 4 hours for 3 or 4 days, with BAL and EDTA at separate IM sites; skip 2 or 3 days and then treat again for 3 to 4 days. (2) In subacute case or <100 mg. Pb/100 gm. whole blood, give only 50 mg. EDTA/kg./24 hours for 3 to 5 days. |
| Methanol and ethylene glycol | Ethanol | Give IV, 1.1 gm./kg. of 25% solution, then give 0.5 gm./kg. every 4 hours for 4 days. To prevent or correct acidosis, use sodium bicarbonate IV. Sodium bicarbonate: 0.4 gm./kg. Activated charcoal: 5 gm./kg. orally if soon after ingestion. |
| Methemoglobinemia-producing agents (nitrites, chlorates, etc.) | Methylene blue | 1% solution (maximum concentration), give by *slow* IV injection, 8.8 mg./kg.; repeat if necessary. To prevent fall in blood pressure in cases of nitrite poisoning, use a sympathomimetic drug (ephedrine, epinephrine, etc.). |
| Morphine and related drugs | Nalorphine hydrochloride | Give IV, 1.0 to 2.5 ml. of solution containing 5 mg. nalorphine per ml. Do not repeat if respiration is not satisfactory. |
|  | Levallorphan tartrate | Give IV, 0.1 to 0.5 ml. of solution containing 1 mg./ml. NOTE: Use either of the above antidotes only in acute poisoning. Artificial respiration may be indicated. Activated charcoal is also indicated. |
| Oxalates | Calcium | Treatment: 23% solution of calcium gluconate IV. Give 3 to 20 ml. (to control hypocalcemia). |
| Phenothiazine derivatives | Methylamphetamine | 0.1 to 0.2 mg./kg. IV; also transfusion. |
|  | Diphenhydramine HCl | For CNS depression 2 to 5 mg./kg. IV for extrapyramidal signs. |
| Phytotoxins and botulin | Antitoxins | As indicated for specific antitoxins. Examples of phytotoxins: ricin, abrin, robin, crotin. |
| Red squill | Atropine sulfate, propranolol | As for digitalis glycosides poisoning, above. |
| Strontium | Calcium salts | Usual dose of calcium borogluconate. |
|  | Ammonium chloride | 0.2 to 0.5 gm. orally 3 or 4 times daily. |

\*Modified from Szabuniewicz et al. (1971).

*Continued on next page*

**Table 2.** *Systemic Antidotes and Dosages\* (Continued)*

| TOXIC AGENT | SYSTEMIC ANTIDOTES | DOSAGE AND METHOD FOR TREATMENT |
|---|---|---|
| Strychnine and brucine | Pentobarbital | Give IP or IV to effect; higher dose is usually required than that required for anesthesia. Place animal in warm, quiet room. |
| | Amobarbital | Give by slow IV injection to effect. Duration of sedation is usually 4 to 6 hours. |
| | Methocarbamol | 10% solution; average first dose is 149 mg./kg. IV (range: 40 to 300 mg.) repeat half dose as needed. |
| | Glyceryl guaiacolate | 110 mg./kg. IV, 5% solution. Repeat as necessary. |
| Thallium | Diphenylthiocarbazone | Dog: 70 mg./kg. orally, 3 times a day for 6 days. Hastens elimination, but is partially toxic. |
| | Prussian blue | 0.2 gm./kg. in 3 divided doses daily. |
| | Potassium chloride | Give simultaneously with thiocarbazone or Prussian blue, 2 to 6 gm. orally daily in divided doses. |

\*Modified from Szabuniewicz et al. (1971).

changed every 30 to 60 minutes. Two dialyzing solutions which may be used are 5 per cent dextrose in 0.45 per cent NaCl with 15 mEq./l. of potassium as potassium chloride and 5 per cent dextrose in water with 44.6 mEq. of bicarbonate and 15 mEq. of potassium added. Other dialyzing solutions may be utilized.

The process of peritoneal dialysis involves the infusion of 10 to 20 ml./kg. of the one dialyzing solution into the peritoneal cavity, waiting the prescribed length of time, withdrawing the first dialyzing solution and infusing the second solution. The infusion and withdrawal cycles with alternating solutions should be maintained for 12 to 24 hours or until normal renal function is restored. The pH of the dialyzing solutions may be altered to maintain the ionized state of the offending compound.

## SUPPORTIVE MEASURES

Supportive measures are very important in intoxications. These measures include control of body temperature, maintenance of respiratory and cardiovascular function, control of acid-base imbalances, alleviation of pain and control of central nervous system disorders.

### BODY TEMPERATURE CONTROL

Hypothermia may be controlled with the use of blankets and by keeping the animal in a warm, draft-free cage. Infrared lamps or heating pads should be used with caution and under constant observation. A pad with circulating warm water may be of greater value and less dangerous than lamps or conventional heating pads. This type of pad is convenient for both emergency and surgical use (Aquamatic K Pad®, American Hospital Supply).

Hyperthermia is controlled through the use of ice bags, cold water baths, cold water enemas or cold peritoneal dialysis solution. Regardless of the type of temperature control required, it is vitally important that the animal's body temperature be constantly monitored to insure that overcorrection does not occur.

### RESPIRATORY SUPPORT MEASURES

Adequate respiratory support requires the presence of an adequate, patent airway, which may be obtained with either a cuffed endotracheal tube in an unconscious animal or a tracheostomy performed under local anesthesia. An emergency tracheostomy tube may be made from a cuffed endotracheal tube which has been shortened to reduce the dead space.

A respirator such as a Bird Respirator® or Ohio® ventilator is of greater value in cases of respiratory depression; however, an anesthetic machine may be utilized with manual compression of the bag. A mixture of 50 per cent oxygen and 50 per cent room air is generally adequate unless there is a thickened respiratory membrane, in which case 100 per cent oxygen is necessary.

The use of analeptic drugs in cases of severe respiratory depression or apnea is questionable owing to the short duration of their effects and to other undesirable side effects. Positive pressure ventilatory support is of greater value.

## CARDIOVASCULAR SUPPORT

Cardiovascular support requires the presence of an adequate circulating volume, adequate cardiac function, adequate tissue perfusion and adequate acid-base balance. Volume and cardiac activity are of immediate concern; perfusion and acid-balance, although of no lesser concern, are not of immediate concern.

In the presence of hypovolemia due to loss of both cells and volume, whole blood is the necessary agent. A good rule is to give a sufficient quantity of whole blood to raise the packed cell volume to 75 per cent of the animal's estimated normal level.

Hypovolemia due to fluid loss alone can be treated with the administration of lactated Ringer's solution or plasma expanders. Central venous pressures should be monitored in these cases to prevent overloading the heart with too much volume, too rapidly.

Tissue perfusion should also be monitored periodically to determine the adequacy of the replacement therapy. In some cases it may be necessary to administer massive doses of corticosteroids intravenously to restore adequate tissue perfusion (dexamethasone, Azium®, 2 to 10 mg./kg.).

Cardiac activity can be aided by the application of closed-chest cardiac massage for immediate requirements, but the administration of pharmaceutical agents which can stimulate ionotropic and chronotropic activity must also be undertaken in most instances. One of these agents is calcium gluconate infused very slowly IV. This agent is also reported to be a good nonspecific measure in many toxicities. Other agents include glucagon, 25 to 50 $\mu$g./kg. IV, and digoxin, 0.2 to 0.6 mg./kg. IV. Care must be taken to avoid overdose with cardioactive agents, since they are highly toxic to the myocardium.

## ACID-BASE IMBALANCE

Control of acid-base balance problems is primarily a matter of physiologically maintaining an animal in a homeostatic condition. The most common acid-base disturbance seen in animals is acidosis, mainly of metabolic origin. However, acidosis or alkalosis may occur in cases of intoxication.

In correcting acidosis, not of respiratory origin, sodium bicarbonate, administered IV at a dosage rate of 2 to 4 mEq./kg. every 15 minutes, is the drug of choice. Other alkalinizing solutions including 1/6 molar sodium lactate, 16 to 32 ml./kg.; lactated Ringer's solution, 120 ml./kg.; or THAM buffer, 300 mg./kg. Bicarbonate is generally the easiest to administer with respect to volume and requires no metabolic conversion. Caution must be exercised with all alkalinizing agents against the induction of alkalosis.

Alkalosis, unless drug-induced, does not generally occur in animals. However, if alkalosis is present, the IV administration of 0.9 per cent NaCl (physiological saline), 10 ml./kg., is usually sufficient for initial therapy. This should be followed by the oral administration of ammonium chloride, 200 mg./kg./day in divided doses. As in the case of acidosis, the clinician should be cautioned about the overtreatment of the alkalotic patient.

## PAIN

Another important supportive measure in cases of intoxication is the control of pain. A minimal dose of morphine (dogs, 1 to 2 mg./kg.; cats, 0.1 to 0.2 mg./kg.) or meperidine (Demerol®) (dogs, 5 to 10 mg./kg.; cats, 1 to 2 mg./kg.) is indicated in animals showing pain as a result of intoxications.

## CENTRAL NERVOUS SYSTEM DISORDERS

Management of central nervous system disorders, in cases of intoxication, is simple in appearance but complex in actuality. The type of therapy will depend upon the presence of depression or hyperactivity. Either disorder can easily be turned into the opposite problem by overzealous therapeutic measures.

**CNS Depression.** CNS depression can also be considered respiratory depression, since the management of the two conditions is very similar. Although the IV administration of analeptic agents such as doxapram (Dopram®), 3 to 5 mg./kg.; bemegride (Mikedimide®), 10 to 20 mg./kg.; or pentylenetetrazol (Metrazol®), 6 to 10 mg./kg. is reported to be efficacious in these conditions, their actions are short-lived, and CNS depression can return if the animals are not monitored continuously. Another disadvantage is that analeptics can also induce convulsions. Artificial respiration or respiratory support is of greater value in animals exhibiting CNS depression and may be the treatment of choice for most CNS depression syndromes.

**CNS Hyperactivity.** Cases of CNS hyperactivity including convulsions can be managed by the administration of CNS depressants or tranquilizers. Pentobarbital sodium is generally the agent of choice for convulsions and hyperactivity. Care must be taken, since in many cases a respiratory depressing dose may be required to alleviate the signs. In these cases, respiratory support is mandatory. Inhalant anesthetics have been reported as excellent for long-term management of CNS hyperactivity, but this removes the inhaler from surgery-room use for extended periods. Central-acting skeletal muscle relaxants and minor tranquilizers have been reported for use with convulsant intoxicants. Some of these include methocarbamol (Robaxin®), 110 mg./kg. IV; glyceryl guaiacolate (Gecolate®), 110 mg./kg. IV; and diazepam (Valium®), 0.5 to 1.5 mg./kg. IV or IM. In other cases of CNS stimulation due to amphetamines and some hallucinogens such as LSD and phencyclidine, phenothiazine tranquilizers have produced adequate control. Regardless of the regimen of therapy for CNS hyperactivity, the animals should be placed in a quiet, dark room to prevent additional stimulation due to auditory or visual stimuli.

## POISON CONTROL CENTERS AND DIAGNOSTIC LABORATORIES

Poison Control Centers or Animal Diagnostic Laboratories can be of great value to the clinician in cases of suspected intoxications, especially when labels or containers are presented with the acutely ill animal. When the suspected compound and the signs exhibited by the animal do not concur, the signs should be treated and the label should be disregarded.

The diagnosis should be confirmed by chemical analysis, even though this may occur after the fact. An accurate diagnosis, as well as detailed records, may help the veterinarian faced with subsequent cases from the same intoxicant. Detailed records will also be invaluable considerations in any medicolegal proceedings.

(See also "Poison Control Centers," below.)

### SUPPLEMENTAL READING

Aronson, A. L.: Chemical poisonings in small animal practice. Vet. Clin. N. Am., 2(2):379–395, 1972.
Szabuniewicz, M., Bailey, E. M., and Wiersig, D. O.: Treatment of some common poisonings in animals. V.M.S.A.C., 66:1197–1205, 1971.
Thienes, C. H., and Haley, T. J.: Clinical Toxicology. Philadelphia, Lea & Febiger, 1972.

# POISON CONTROL CENTERS

FREDERICK W. OEHME, D.V.M.
*Manhattan, Kansas*

Fortunately for the practitioner faced with an unknown or confusing poisoning, or for the veterinarian treating a patient that consumed a quantity of an unfamiliar compound, there are centers of toxicity information available. A large number of government-sponsored Poison Control Centers are located in selected human hospitals throughout the United States and Canada:

In New York City:
  Poison Information Center
  New York City Department
    of Health
  Bureau of Laboratories
  455 First Avenue
  New York City 10016
  Telephone: 212-340-4495

In Chicago, three centers are
available:
  The Chicago Master Center
  Rush-Presbyterian-St. Luke's
    Medical Center
  1753 West Congress Parkway
  Chicago 60612
  Telephone: 312-942-5969

Poison Control Center
St. Mary of Nazareth Hospital
  Center
1120 North Leavitt Street
Chicago 60622
Telephone: 312-292-5391

Poison Control Center
South Chicago Community
  Hospital
2320 East 93rd Street
Chicago 60617
Telephone: 312-978-2000,
  ext. 264, 265 or 297

In Fort Worth, Texas:
  Poison Control Center

W. I. Cook Children's Hospital
1212 West Lancaster Avenue
Fort Worth 76102
Telephone: 817-336-5521, ext.
  17, or at night 336-5527

In Los Angeles, California:
  Poison Control Center
  The Thomas J. Fleming
    Memorial Center Children's
    Hospital of Los Angeles
  Post Office Box 54700
  4650 Sunset Boulevard
  Los Angeles 90054
  Telephone: 213-664-2121

The National Clearing House for Poison Control Centers publishes a detailed listing of the currently staffed Poison Control Centers in their Bulletin. This bulletin is available through the United States Department of Health, Education, and Welfare, Food and Drug Administration, Bureau of Foods, 5401 Westbard Avenue, Bethesda, MD 20016. From this listing practitioners may locate the center nearest to them that can afford them rapid emergency information.

Although the quality of reference materials and the service provided varies somewhat from hospital to hospital, these centers are usually supplied with the latest information available on toxic ingredients in vari-

ous medicines, herbicides, pesticides and other registered commercial (and some noncommercial) products. In the absence of a detailed listing of Poison Control Centers, practitioners should contact their local hospital to determine the telephone number of the nearest Poison Control Center. They then should make initial contact to determine the most efficient procedure for securing information on toxic materials in emergencies.

The rapid determination of toxic ingredients, expected signs or lesions and the recommended treatment may then be no more than a telephone away.

---

# USE OF LABORATORIES FOR THE CHEMICAL ANALYSIS OF TISSUES

WILLIAM B. BUCK, D.V.M.
*Ames, Iowa*

An accurate diagnosis is the single most important factor in dealing with animal toxicoses. Once the cause of a problem is known, specific treatment and prevention can be initiated. Prior to that time, however,

the veterinarian is limited to supportive and symptomatic therapeutic measures. The toxicologic diagnosis is based upon a knowledge of pertinent criteria in the case, qualified laboratory evaluation of proper specimens, and intelligent interpretation of laboratory results in light of the circumstances associated with the problem.

When the practicing veterinarian desires to consult with a diagnostic laboratory or another colleague in an effort to establish a diagnosis, certain fundamental information should be given: veterinarian's name and address; owner's name and address; and species, breed, sex, age and weight of animal. Certain specific factors should be included: (1) type of area in which the animal lives, whether city or farm; (2) whether it roamed at will or was tied or maintained in the house; (3) the distance to the nearest dump, grain elevator or other source of poison; (4) history of rodenticide or other pesticide use on the home premises; and (5) history of treatment for parasites and immunizations within the past two or three weeks.

## CHEMICAL ANALYSES

Chemical evidence is often an indispensable aid in diagnosing toxicologic problems. Used properly and in the right perspective, chemical analyses provide the single most important diagnostic criterion. There are limitations, however, to the value of chemical analyses. Rarely should chemical results be used alone in making a diagnosis. Positive chemical data plus history, clinical signs and postmortem findings may provide evidence to arrive at an accurate diagnosis. One should never request a chemistry laboratory to simply "analyze for poisons" because an animal died of unknown causes. There are thousands of toxic chemicals and plants, and analyses for all of them would be impossible not only because of the limited amount of sample available but also because the cost would be prohibitive. Also, there are many toxic plants and even some chemical agents for which no chemical analytical procedures are available.

Although there are some toxicologic tests suitable for the veterinary hospital or clinical laboratory, many procedures for toxicologic analyses are complicated, time consuming and require expensive equipment. Unfortunately, many of the screening qualitative tests for toxicants are not worth the time it takes to perform them. An example is the Reinsch test for arsenic and mercury. When performed by an inexperienced individual, this test is worse than no test at all.

Several metals such as arsenic, mercury and antimony will give a positive reaction to this test. Also, sulfur and other elements found in biologic specimens will give false positives with the Reinsch test. Thus, unless a laboratory is adequately staffed and equipped for analytical chemistry procedures, little significance can be placed on toxicologic screening tests. False-positive or false-negative results can be disastrous, especially when one considers that a majority of toxicoses involve potential litigations. One can find himself in an embarrassing position when he is unable to rely upon his analytical procedures in making a toxicologic diagnosis. Perhaps a certain amount of screening and preliminary tests can be performed by a veterinary clinic for the sole purpose of aiding in treatment rationale, but the clinic should rely upon subsequent chemical confirmation by a qualified toxicology laboratory.

The minimum equipment necessary for an analytic chemistry-toxicology laboratory includes an atomic absorption spectrophotometer, a colorimeter or ultraviolet spectrophotometer, and a gas-liquid chromatograph or thin-layer chromatographic equipment. Facilities for ashing or digesting specimens, such as a perchloric acid hood and a muffle furnace, should be available, as well as analytical balances, specialized glassware and other routine analytic chemistry laboratory equipment. The cost of equipping such a laboratory would be prohibitive to all except a large group practice or hospital.

## SUBMITTING SPECIMENS FOR LABORATORY EVALUATION

When submitting specimens to a diagnostic laboratory, certain considerations should be made. The importance of supplying a complete account of history, signs and lesions with specimens submitted for laboratory evaluation cannot be overemphasized. Such information will enable the toxicologist to select toxicants intelligently for which to make analyses. This is especially important when a test for the toxicant originally suspected proves negative. A chemist still has the opportunity to test for other poisons if adequate specimens have been submitted.

The choice of specimen is important in making a chemical analysis. Specimens should be taken free of chemical contamination and debris and should not be washed because of the possibility of removing residues of the toxic agent or of contaminating the specimen with the water. Keep in mind that one is often dealing with trace amounts of a particular chemical, and even the slightest contamination may produce erroneous results. Tissue specimens should be frozen and packaged to arrive at the laboratory while still frozen. Serum and blood should not be frozen but kept refrigerated. Always package specimens of various organs separately. Use clean glass or plastic containers that can be tightly sealed. Always label each specimen with the owner's name, animal name or number, and tissue or specimen in the container. Never add preservatives such as formalin to specimens unless there is a specific reason for doing so and such information is included along with the specimen. Always send more material than you think is necessary. It is easier to throw away excess specimen than to obtain more specimen after the carcass has been discarded.

Serum cations and enzymes may be very helpful in the diagnosis of certain toxic and metabolic conditions. To obtain meaningful results, several general rules for collection and preservation of serum should be followed. Always collect blood with clean equipment and transfer it to clean vials or tubes. Avoid excessive aspiration pressure, splashing or time lag during collection to minimize hemolysis. Make every effort to avoid trauma to the unclotted or clotted sample. Allow sufficient time for the blood to clot and begin to retract, usually about one hour. Always try to remove serum from the clot within two hours. This may be done by carefully pouring off serum from the retracted clot or by centrifugation. After the serum is separated from the clot, it can be frozen and transported with ice.

Specimens that should be submitted from a live animal include: 5 ml. of serum with clot removed; 10 ml. of whole blood; 50 ml. of urine; and 200 gm. of bait, vomitus or other such materials.

Specimens that should be submitted from a dead animal include: 5 and 10 ml. of serum and whole blood, respectively, if available; 50 ml. of urine; and 100 gm. each of liver, kidney, spleen and body fat. The entire brain should be submitted. Many disorders resembling poisons can be differentiated by brain lesions. If an infectious or inflammatory process is suspected, separate the brain longitudinally, fix half in 10 per cent buffered formalin, and freeze the other half. Up to 500 gm. of stomach contents should be included.

Plastic bags, newspaper, canned ice and cardboard are good materials to use for transporting specimens to a laboratory for examination. Liquids such as blood, urine, stomach contents and water should be shipped in a glass or heavy plastic container that can be sealed. Wrap each labeled specimen well in newspaper and package for mailing unless they can be delivered in person which, of course, is the most desirable. Always wrap the specimens individually for mailing so that the contents cannot leak and contaminate other mail or other specimens.

If one is in doubt about proper tissues for analysis or the availability of confirmatory tests, much time, effort and confusion can be avoided by placing a telephone call to the laboratory.

## SPECIMENS FOR DIAGNOSIS OF SPECIFIC TOXICANTS

The procedures for sending in specimens as outlined under the heading, "Submitting Specimens for Laboratory Evaluation," are suitable for the detection of most toxicants. There are instances, however, where special considerations regarding chemical analysis and pathologic evaluation are required. Some specific examples for specific toxicants are given in Table 1.

## INTERPRETATION OF LABORATORY RESULTS

Interpretation of the significance of chemical data should be done carefully, taking into consideration other evidence presented with the case. Positive chemical findings are not always evidence of intoxication, nor do negative findings always indicate that a toxicosis did not occur. For example, finding chlorinated hydrocarbon insecticides in the fatty tissues of an animal only indicates that the animal was exposed to the pesticide, not that the insecticide produced a toxicosis. On the other hand, failure to find certain organophosphorous insecticides in the body tissues would not guarantee that the animal had not been poisoned by such a chemical. In the case of most chlorinated hydrocarbon insecticides, the animal may store a considerable amount of the chemical in its tissues without appar-

*Table 1.* *Specimens Required for Specific Tests*

| POISON OR ANALYSIS REQUESTED | SPECIMEN REQUIRED | AMOUNT OF SPECIMEN DESIRED | COMMENTS |
|---|---|---|---|
| Ammonia° | Whole blood or serum<br>Stomach contents<br>(composite)<br>Urine | 5 ml.<br><br>100 gm.<br>5 ml. | Frozen (1–2 drops of saturated $HgCl_2$ may be used instead of freezing rumen contents) |
| ANTU | Stomach and intestine<br>contents<br>Liver | <br>200 gm.<br>200 gm. | Can be detected only within 12–24 hours after ingestion |
| Arsenic | Liver<br>Kidney<br>Feed<br>Stomach contents<br>Urine | 50 gm.<br>50 gm.<br>100 gm.<br>100 gm.<br>50 ml. | |
| Calcium | Serum<br>Feed | 2 ml.<br>25 gm. | Serum must *not* be hemolyzed; separate clot before transit |
| Carbon monoxide | Whole blood | 15 ml. | |
| Chloride | See Sodium | | |
| Chlorinated hydrocarbon insecticides | Brain<br>Body fat<br>Stomach contents<br>Liver<br>Kidney<br>Whole blood | ½ cerebrum<br>100 gm.<br>100 gm.<br>50 gm.<br>50 gm.<br>10 ml. | Must not be contaminated with hairs or stomach contents; preferable to use chemically clean glass jars; avoid plastic containers |
| Copper | Kidney<br>Liver<br>Whole blood<br>Feces | 50 gm.<br>50 gm.<br>10 ml.<br>100 gm. | |
| Cyanide | Whole blood<br>Liver<br>Forage, silage<br>Other materials | 10 ml.<br>50 gm.<br>100 gm.<br>100 gm. | Freeze specimen promptly in air-tight container |
| Ethylene glycol | Serum<br>Kidney (in formalin)<br>Urine | 10 ml.<br>Whole organ<br>10 ml. | One kidney, both in small animals |
| Fluoroacetate | Stomach contents<br>Kidney<br>Urine<br>Liver<br>Other materials | All available<br>One whole<br>50 gm.<br>50 gm.<br>100 gm. | Frozen |
| Nitrates | Water<br>Forage, silage<br>Whole blood<br>(methemoglobin)<br>Other materials | 50 ml.<br>100 gm.<br><br>10 ml.<br>100 gm. | |
| Organophosphorous insecticides | Brain<br>Body fat<br>Stomach contents<br>(composite)<br>Blood (heparinized)<br>Urine<br>Feed | 50 gm. (cerebrum)<br>50 gm.<br><br>50 gm.<br>10 ml.<br>50 ml.<br>100 gm. | |
| Oxalates | Fresh forage<br>Kidney (in formalin) | 6–8 plants<br>Whole organ | Do *not* chop plants; freeze promptly<br>One kidney, both in small animals (qualitative test only) |
| Phenols | Stomach contents<br>Other materials | 500 gm.<br>200 gm. | Pack in air-tight container |
| Phenothiazines | Feed or other materials | 50 gm. | |

°A total of 5 ml. of nonhemolyzed serum is sufficient to conduct several clinical tests.

*Continued on next page*

*Table 1.    Specimens Required for Specific Tests (Continued)*

| POISON OR ANALYSIS REQUESTED | SPECIMEN REQUIRED | AMOUNT OF SPECIMEN DESIRED | COMMENTS |
|---|---|---|---|
| Phosphates | Serum | 5 ml. | |
| | Bone | 25 gm. | |
| | Other materials | 100 gm. | |
| Thallium | Urine | 10 ml. | |
| | Kidney | 50 gm. | |
| | Liver | 50 gm. | |
| Urea | Feed | 100 gm. | |
| | Other materials | 500 gm. | |
| | See also Ammonia | | |
| Warfarin | Liver | 100 gm. | |
| | Feed | 100 gm. | |
| | Other materials | 100 gm. | |
| Zinc | Liver | 50 gm. | |
| | Kidney | 50 gm. | |
| | Other materials | 100 gm. | |

ent harmful effects. With organophosphorous compounds, the body may metabolize them so rapidly that they are not detectable by chemical analysis.

## LABORATORIES OFFERING TOXICOLOGY-CHEMICAL ANALYTIC SERVICE

In April, 1976, the Veterinary Services Diagnostic Laboratory, Animal and Plant Inspection Services, USDA, Ames, Iowa, made a survey of public and private veterinary diagnostic laboratories in the United States. The following is a list of those laboratories reporting capabilities for general toxicology-chemical analyses. For a more complete listing, refer to the Directory of Animal Disease Diagnostic Laboratories, 1975, U.S. Government Printing Office, Washington, D. C.

*Alaska*

Alaska State-Federal
Laboratory
P.O. Box 720
Palmer, Alaska 99645
907-745-3236

*Arizona*

Arizona State Department of
Health
1716 West Adams Street
Phoenix, Arizona 85007
602-765-4552

Department of Veterinary
Science
University of Arizona
Tucson, Arizona 85721
602-884-2355

*Arkansas*

Arkansas Livestock and
Poultry Commission
Diagnostic Laboratory
2915 South Pine
Little Rock, Arkansas 72204
501-371-1321

*California*

County of Los Angeles
Department of Health
Services Division
12824 Horton Avenue
Downey, California 90242
213-923-0641

Wildlife Investigations
Laboratory
987 Jedsmith Drive
Sacramento, California 95819
916-465-0157

*Colorado*

Colorado State University
Diagnostic Laboratory
Fort Collins, Colorado 80521
303-491-6128

*Connecticut*

Department of Pathobiology
Box U-89
University of Connecticut
Storrs, Connecticut 06268
203-486-4000

*Delaware*

Eastern Shore Laboratories,
Inc.
P.O. Box 657
Laurel, Delaware 19956
301-749-2284

*Florida*

Kissimee Animal Disease
Diagnostic Laboratory
P.O. Box 460
Kissimee, Florida 32741
305-847-3185

**Georgia**

Diagnostic and
Investigational
Laboratories
Route 2 Brighton Road
Tifton, Georgia 31794
912-386-3340

Diagnostic Assistance
Laboratory
College of Veterinary
Medicine
University of Georgia
Athens, Georgia 30601
404-542-5568

**Hawaii**

Department of Agriculture
Veterinary Laboratory
Branch
1428 South King Street
Honolulu, Hawaii 96814
808-941-3071 (ext. 158)

**Idaho**

Livestock Disease Control
Laboratory
P.O. Box 7249
Boise, Idaho 83707
208-554-3111

**Illinois**

Laboratories of Veterinary
Diagnostic Medicine
University of Illinois
Urbana, Illinois 61801
217-957-1620

Regional Diagnostic
Laboratory
235 North Walnut Street
Centralia, Illinois 62801
618-532-6701

**Indiana**

Animal Disease Diagnostic
Laboratory
School of Veterinary
Medicine
Purdue University
West Lafayette, Indiana
47907
317-749-2496

**Iowa**

Veterinary Diagnostic
Laboratory
College of Veterinary
Medicine
Iowa State University
Ames, Iowa 50010
515-294-1950

**Kansas**

Comparative Toxicology
Laboratory
College of Veterinary
Medicine
Kansas State University
Manhattan, Kansas 66506
913-532-5679

**Kentucky**

Central Kentucky Animal
Disease Diagnostic
Laboratory
Rural Route 6 Newton Pike
Lexington, Kentucky
40505
606-253-0571

Kentucky Department of
Agriculture Animal
Diagnostic Laboratory
North Drive
Hopkinsville, Kentucky
44240
505-886-3959

**Louisiana**

Northwest Louisiana
Livestock Diagnostic and
Research Laboratory
P.O. Box 4297
N.S.U.
Natchitoches, Louisiana
71457
318-352-6272

**Maine**

Maine Poultry Consultants
Box 262
Waterville, Maine 04901
207-873-3405

**Massachusetts**

Large Animal Diagnostic
Laboratory
Paige Laboratory
University of Massachusetts
Amherst, Massachusetts
01002
413-545-2427

**Michigan**

Michigan Department of
Agriculture Laboratory
Division
1615 South Harrison Road
East Lansing, Michigan
48823
517-253-6410

Veterinary Diagnostic
Laboratory
Michigan State University
East Lansing, Michigan
48823
517-373-1683

**Minnesota**

Veterinary Diagnostic
Laboratories
College of Veterinary
Medicine
University of Minnesota
St. Paul, Minnesota 55101
612-373-0774

**Mississippi**

Mississippi Veterinary
Diagnostic Laboratory
P.O. Box 4356
Jackson, Mississippi
601-354-6091

**Missouri**

Bureau of Laboratory
Services
Missouri Division of Health
Broadway State Building
Jefferson City, Missouri
65101
314-751-3334

Fish-Pesticide Research
Laboratory
Bureau of Sport Fisheries
and Wildlife
Columbia, Missouri 65201
314-442-2271 (ext. 3101)

Ralston Purina Veterinary
Laboratories
Checkerboard Square
St. Louis, Missouri 63188
314-982-2611

Veterinary Medical
Diagnostic Laboratory
School of Veterinary
Medicine
University of Missouri
Columbia, Missouri 65201
314-882-6811

*Montana*

State of Montana Animal
Health Division
Diagnostic Laboratory
P.O. Box 997
Bozeman, Montana 59715
406-586-5952

*Nebraska*

Harris Laboratories, Inc.
P.O. Box 80837
Lincoln, Nebraska 68502
402-432-2811

Veterinary Science
Laboratory
University of Nebraska
North Platte, Nebraska 69101
308-532-3611

*North Carolina*

Rollins Animal Disease
Diagnostic Laboratory
P.O. Box 12223 Cameron
Village Station
Raleigh, North Carolina
27606
919-829-3986

*North Dakota*

North Dakota State
University Veterinary
Diagnostic Laboratory
Fargo, North Dakota 58102
701-237-7511

*Ohio*

Ohio Department of
Agriculture Animal
Disease Diagnostic
Laboratory
Reynoldsburg, Ohio 43068
614-866-6362

*Pennsylvania*

Pennsylvania Department of
Agriculture
Bureau of Animal Industry
Laboratory
Summerdale, Pennsylvania
17093
717-637-8808

*South Dakota*

Animal Disease Research
and Diagnostic Laboratory
South Dakota State
University
Brookings, South Dakota
57006
605-688-5171

*Tennessee*

C. E. Kord Animal Disease
Laboratory
P.O. Box 40627 Mel. Station
Nashville, Tennessee 37204
615-853-1559

*Texas*

Texas Veterinary Medical
Diagnostic Laboratory
Drawer 3040
College Station, Texas 77840
713-845-3414

*Utah*

Intermountain Laboratories,
Inc.
870E 7200 South
Midvale, Utah 84047
801-561-2244

State Chemists Office and
State-Federal Cooperative
Laboratory
412 Capitol Building
Salt Lake City, Utah 84114
801-533-5421

Utah State University
Veterinary Diagnostic
Laboratory
Logan, Utah 84321
801-586-7011 (ext. 7584)

*Virginia*

Department of Veterinary
Science
Virginia Polytechnic and
State University
Blacksburg, Virginia 24061
703-951-6376

Division of Animal Health
and Dairies Research
Laboratory
116 Reservoir Street
Harrisonburg, Virginia 22801
703-434-3897

Division of Animal Health
and Dairies Regulatory
Laboratory
Box 4191
Lynchburg, Virginia 24502
804-846-8860

Division of Animal Health
and Dairies Regulatory
Laboratory
234 West Shirley Avenue
Warrenton, Virginia 22186
703-347-3131

*Washington*

Western Fish Disease
Laboratory
Building 204—Sand Point
Naval Support Activity
Seattle, Washington 98115
206-392-3500

*West Virginia*

State Federal Cooperative
Animal Health Laboratory
Room B-86 Capitol Building
Charleston, West Virginia
25305
304-885-2231

*Wisconsin*

Central Animal Health
  Laboratory
6101 Mineral Point Road
Madison, Wisconsin 53705
608-366-2465

Consultant Services in
  Veterinary Pathology
130 Warren Street
Beaver Dam, Wisconsin
  53916
414-887-1371

*Wyoming*

Wyoming State Veterinary
  Laboratory
Box 950
Laramie, Wyoming 82070
307-742-6638

### SUPPLEMENTAL READING

Buck, W. B.: Laboratory toxicologic tests and their interpretation. J. Am. Vet. Med. Assn., *155*:1928–1941, 1969.

Buck, W. B., Osweiler, G. D., and Van Gelder, G. A.: Clinical and Diagnostic Veterinary Toxicology. Dubuque, Iowa, Kendall-Hunt Publishing Co., 1973.
Radeleff, R. D.: Veterinary Toxicology. 2nd ed. Philadelphia, Lea & Febiger, 1970, pp. 25–28.

# COMMON POISONINGS IN SMALL ANIMAL PRACTICE

GARY D. OSWEILER, D.V.M.
*Columbia, Missouri*

Small animal poisoning is often associated with acute or peracute onset of severe clinical signs which progress rapidly to death or recovery. Many times an animal's owner is not aware of access to foreign materials which could be toxic. In other instances, the client is firmly convinced that malicious poisoning has occurred. Dogs and cats previously in apparent good health may be found dead, and this situation frequently gives rise to suspicions of poisoning in the minds of client and veterinarian alike. There is also some tendency to consider as poisoning those disease states which can't be explained by other means. Perhaps the most common toxicologic diagnosis made is "poisoning" due to undetermined etiology.

The actual confirmed incidents of intoxication by specific materials constitute a very small portion of small animal medicine diagnoses. The topics covered in this section on chemical and physical disorders constitute the "common" specific poisonings, i.e., those intoxications most often diagnosed clinically and/or confirmed chemically. The purposes of this chapter are (1) to review some of the limitations which prevent better diagnosis of poisoning and (2) to classify the sources and situations

from which poisonings commonly arise with some perspective on their importance.

To complete the goals of establishing a tentative clinical diagnosis, determining the source and educating the client in avoidance of further problems, one must rely primarily upon clinical assessment of the patient and upon careful and thorough questioning of the client regarding possible or probable sources of toxicants. The history and clinical exam are inseparable in toxicology and must be evaluated in light of one another. As with all diagnostic medicine, several tentative diagnoses may come to mind in poisoning cases. These must then be systematically eliminated or confirmed using all possible or available factors as aids in the process.

All pertinent facts and statements should be recorded in writing. This will serve later to review the facts and point out any inconsistencies or trends in the history. It may aid in invalidating indications of poisoning. Conversely, in the occasional malicious or negligent poisoning the written details are invaluable corroboration of the diagnostic procedure.

Animal and environmental factors that may modify responses to various poisons should be carefully noted. Was the animal young? Old? Chronically ill? Recently medicated? Changed in location? As Clarke and Clarke (1967) state with particular emphasis, almost any food or drug can be toxic if administered in too high a dosage, too frequently, too rapidly or to a highly susceptible animal. Thus, a poison source is a hazard only when the conditions of exposure exceed the tolerance of the animal for that material.

A knowledge of the circumstances associated with poisoning is very useful and may provide a key for making a proper diagnosis. Most of the history may have no bearing on intoxication but important points may be gleaned from it. The presence of poisons such as rodenticides, insecticides, drugs, paints, fertilizers, petroleum products and other chemicals on the premises, or a history of their use or availability for animal exposure should be ascertained. One should be prepared to estimate the amount or degree of possible exposure to these chemicals. The food and water supply should be checked carefully for the presence of toxic plants, molds, algae, fungi or other toxicants. Other important facts that should be obtained include the course of events in hours or days as well as the breed, sex, feeding program, history of past illnesses and immunization record of the animal.

Circumstantial evidence has greater value if one can determine that animals have consumed or were definitely exposed to a particular toxic agent. One should guard against diagnosing lead poisoning simply because lead paint is found on the premises, or plant poisoning(s) unless there is evidence that the suspected plant was consumed in sufficient quantity to produce toxicosis. Circumstantial evidence should be viewed as just one factor; other types of evidence must be present to reach an accurate diagnosis which could be used as input to determine which are the "common" confirmed poisonings. The veterinarian must decide, on the merits of each case, how much effort goes into reviewing the factors in a potential poisoning. When surveys or summaries are made concerning frequency of poisoning (or other diseases) one should always question the degree of surety with which diagnoses were made.

In addition to lack of circumstantial or clinical evidence (the clinician's part), lack of chemical or analytical data may be a problem. For some toxicants, such as plant toxins or animal venoms, diagnostic chemical analyses are not available or are not practical. In other cases, the cost of analyzing for many poisons is prohibitive.

Thus, our view of what is a common poison is limited by the effort expended in gathering accurate and detailed history, the thoroughness of the clinical and clinicopathological exam and the availability of confirmatory chemical analyses.

## CLASSIFICATION OF POISONS

Toxic materials may be classified in many ways. In many cases it is useful to group them according to where they occur or why they are used. Thus, insecticides would be potential toxicants if the owner had just sprayed extensively for roaches, and plant poisoning is more likely if the season is spring and flowers, shrubs and vines are abundant around the home.

Toxins may be grouped according to the following general headings:

A. Natural Hazards
   1. Plants, seeds
   2. Fungi, algae
   3. Mycotoxins
   4. Zootoxins (snakes, toads, insects, etc.)
   5. Poisonous minerals in food or water
B. Man-made Hazards
   1. Industrial contamination
   2. Pesticides and economic poisons
   3. Domestic materials
   4. Drugs
   5. Food and water

### NATURAL TOXINS

Toxic plants and seeds are found in many homes and places of business. While the dog and cat are not foragers, both species have been known to consume various plants or portions thereof (e.g., grass-eating dogs and catnip-loving cats). Poisoning by oleander, dumb cane, castor bean, chokecherry, jimsonweed, morning-glory and mushrooms has been recorded as occurring in small animals.

Fungi, mycotoxins and blue-green algae have caused poisoning in pets. Most notable of the fungi are the *Amanita* spp. *A. phalloides* produces a fatal gastroenteric and hepatotoxic reaction, while *A. muscaria* causes signs which mimic cholinergic drugs and which are alleviated by atropine. Mycotoxins of *Aspergillus flavus* (aflatoxin) and *Penicillium* sp. are toxic to dogs, and outbreaks of aflatoxicosis from contaminated dog food have been observed. Most effects of the aflatoxins are recorded in dogs and are exerted on the liver, kidney and blood-vascular system. Diagnosis of mycotoxicosis is difficult, since effects may be delayed, and a source of toxin may no longer be available. Algal blooms in late summer are associated with gastroenteritis, hepatotoxicity and "fast-death" in many species including dogs.

Certain toxic animals, insects and snakes are a hazard to pets in some locations of North America. Most problems are reported from the southern and southwestern United States. Snake bites (rattlesnake, copperhead and coral snake) and toad poisoning from *Bufo* spp. are the most frequently reported problems. Animal venoms and toxins characteristically affect the nervous system, cause tissue necrosis, induce hemorrhage or hemolysis or induce an allergic response.

Mineral poisoning in food or water is rare in small animals. Arsenical contamination of grain or availability of rodent baits containing toxins such as phosphorus, arsenic, inorganic fluorides or barium may occasionally occur. Cured meat or the water from cooked cured meats may be high in nitrites and result in methemoglobinemia. Since pets generally consume from the same water supply as man, acute waterborne poisoning is relatively rare.

## MAN-MADE SOURCES OF POISONS FOR PET ANIMALS

The sources of potential poisons are legion and are exceeded only by the toxicants themselves. Some 2,000 chemicals and drugs are considered dangerously toxic, and new chemicals with potential toxicity are being introduced at the rate of 1,500 or more each year.

In order to consider even the broadest possibilities, one must be equipped with at least some ready reference works which give detailed information about the more common poisoning problems. In addition, it is helpful to know the areas and uses where the more toxic chemicals, plants and ven-

oms are found. Furthermore, the general clinical effects associated with toxic substances should be kept as a cross reference.

## INDUSTRIAL CONTAMINATION

The gases, vapors, dusts and water pollutants which plague man are available to the companion animals which share his environment. Carbon monoxide, oxides of nitrogen and sulfur and various pneumoconioses should be considered when evaluating respiratory problems in small animals. Water pollutants such as nitrates have been associated experimentally with hydrocephalus in young dogs. However, little work has been done specifically relating pollutants to disease problems in the small animal population.

## PESTICIDES AND ECONOMIC POISONS

These materials, especially the rodenticides and insecticides, appear most often as accidental and malicious poisons in small animals. This comes from the fact that they are designed to be toxic to similar biologic mechanisms and that they are used largely by laymen in areas frequented by pets. Proper use and storage of such products would eliminate most of these problems.

The important economic poisons in small animal toxicology are discussed in individual chapters in this section.

## DOMESTIC MATERIALS

A great number of products used in homes or businesses contain toxic materials. Many of these are listed in the article on "Common Potential Sources of Small Animal Poisoning." These materials are usually packaged and should not be available to pets if properly used and stored. Since most pets (perhaps primates excepted) do not remove caps or lids, and since they can be effectively locked away from these materials when in use, there is little excuse other than negligence for poisoning by these products. Many of these chemicals are volatile or corrosive, and often they are able to penetrate intact skin.

Clarke (1975) reports that overheated frying pans coated with nonstick materials emit a vapor toxic to birds. The fluorinated propellants (freons) may cause acute respiratory and cardiovascular abnormalities with fatal consequences in pets.

Cats are peculiarly susceptible to many domestic products, and a good review of this subject has recently been written (Atkins and Johnson, 1975).

## DRUGS

Pets occasionally gain access to drugs of abuse through living with an owner who is inclined to their use. Most common is the consumption of marijuana cigarettes generally with resultant nonfatal hallucination for one or two days.

Many therapeutic agents can give rise to adverse reactions when used in veterinary medicine. Adverse drug reactions reported through the Food and Drug Administration for the first quarter of fiscal year 1976 included the following:

| ANIMAL | DRUG | NUMBER INVOLVED |
|---|---|---|
| Canine | Caparsolate | 2 |
| | Cythioate | 1 |
| | Dichlorvos | 2 |
| | Diethylcarbamazine | 27 |
| | Disophenol | 1 |
| | Phthalofyne | 1 |
| | Fentanyl and Droperidol | 3 |
| | Halothane | 1 |
| | Methoxyflurane | 6 |
| | Xylazine | 1 |
| Feline | Ketamine | 12 |
| | Xylazine | 1 |

Robens (1972) reviewed animal drug toxicities with results as follows:

Generally, the side effects and therapeutic incompatibilities of drugs are known prior to their release. Individuals prescribing or using therapeutic agents should be familiar with the side effects, adverse reactions and contraindications of all such drugs. A discussion of drug-induced and adverse reactions will be found in a separate chapter within this section.

## FOOD AND WATER

Food poisoning or garbage intoxication is more frequently diagnosed than any other intoxication. Mold toxins, bacterial exotoxins, bacterial endotoxins and toxic products from putrefaction may be involved separately or in concert with one another. Much more work is needed in studying the physiologic response of small animals to contaminated or tainted foods. This subject is treated more fully elsewhere in this section.

## FREQUENCY OF SMALL ANIMAL POISONING

From the foregoing plethora of potential poisons, the clinician must judge which are most likely. In addition, those toxins most probably encountered should be well understood and dealt with as specifically and thoroughly as possible. To this end, it is sometimes helpful to know what one's colleagues have encountered as problems.

In 1969 a survey was conducted of the American Animal Hospital Association

| DRUG | ABNORMAL RESPONSE |
|---|---|
| Corticosteroids | Muscle weakness in dogs; premature parturition. |
| Estrogens | Alopecia; ovarian tumors at high dose; endometrial hyperplasia; aplastic anemia; infertility in mice, mink and guinea pig. |
| Progesterone | Endometrial hyperplasia; masculinization of female fetus (dogs). |
| Tetracyclines | Vomition (when given large doses IV); chelation with calcium phosphate; colors developing bone and teeth yellow; metabolites may be nephrotoxic. |
| Streptomycin | Vestibular nerve toxicity in cats. |
| Dihydrostreptomycin | Auditory nerve toxicity in cats. |
| Chloramphenicol | Prolongs pentobarbital anesthesia; hematopoietic depression (cat and dog). |
| Gentamycin | Vestibular nerve toxicity and nephrotoxicity in cats. |
| Nitrofurans | Systemic administration may produce vomiting, diarrhea, peripheral neuritis, ocular dysfunction. |
| Disophenol | Therapeutic dose is 6 to 10 mg./kg. while more than 15 mg./kg. is toxic; causes cardiac insufficiency, dyspnea, vomition and hyperthermia. Lesions are pulmonary congestion, cardiac fatty change. |
| Tolbutamide | Hepatotoxic to dogs at 30 mg./kg./day. |
| Neomycin | Nephrotoxic to cats; transient neuromuscular block. |
| Diuretics (ethacrynic acid and furosemide) | Inner ear degeneration—both temporary and permanent. |

membership and of veterinary college teaching hospitals. Those results are presented in Table 1. One must remember that such surveys are only as good as the input data. In many cases, the diagnoses were not confirmed by chemical analyses nor was a source determined. However, the information does reflect the diagnoses which appeared clinically to be caused by specific compounds.

The data presented in Table 1 are a composite of both canine and feline poisoning. By far, the greatest number of diagnosed toxicoses occur in dogs. The peculiar sensitivity of cats to phenolics and chlorinated aryl hydrocarbons, however, results in more frequent poisoning of cats by such compounds with ring structures, which they are unable to metabolize.

The author has recently rechecked with selected practices and institutions. In general, the same diagnoses are being made.

However, certain differences appear to be developing. Some of these are as follows:

1. Poisoning by ANTU rodenticide is diagnosed only rarely and is usually based on the lesion rather than determination of the source. Organophosphate insecticides and the herbicide paraquat may cause similar pulmonary lesions.
2. Thallium poisoning is almost never reported. The few cases that are found have been from metropolitan areas of Chicago and the eastern seaboard. Thallium is no longer available as a pest control agent.
3. Sodium fluoroacetate (Compound 1080) poisoning is reported with increasing frequency among the rodenticides—especially in the Midwest. It is most often associated with commercial or governmental pest control. Compound 1080 is one of the few agents toxic enough to cause secondary intoxication in *Canidae* which consume poisoned animal pests. Part of the increased incidence is probably due to greater awareness of the ef-

**Table 1.** *Reported Clinical Diagnoses of Small Animal Toxicoses in the United States*

| | NORTHEAST | SOUTHEAST | SOUTHWEST | WEST | MIDWEST | NATIONAL TOTAL |
|---|---|---|---|---|---|---|
| **Rodenticides** | | | | | | |
| ANTU | 2 | 5 | 1 | 7 | 6 | 21 |
| Thallium | 45 | 19 | 8 | 3 | 49 | 124 |
| Warfarin | 60 | 27 | 35 | 39 | 118 | 279 |
| Strychnine | 78 | 60 | 57 | 66 | 154 | 415 |
| Compound 1080 | | | | | | |
| Zinc phosphide | 3 | 1 | | | 2 | 6 |
| | | | | | | |
| **Pesticides** | | | | | | |
| Arsenic | 11 | 21 | 12 | 43 | 58 | 145 |
| Chlorinated hydrocarbons | 19 | 38 | 28 | 21 | 66 | 172 |
| Organophosphates | 48 | 69 | 33 | 20 | 99 | 269 |
| Metaldehyde | | 2 | | 117 | | 119 |
| | | | | | | |
| **Glycols** | | | | | | |
| Antifreeze | 6 | 2 | 4 | | 20 | 32 |
| | | | | | | |
| **Heavy Metals** | | | | | | |
| Lead | 17 | 3 | 1 | 3 | 43 | 67 |
| Mercury | | | | | 2 | 2 |
| | | | | | | |
| **Miscellaneous** | | | | | | |
| Acid | | 3 | 3 | 3 | 12 | 21 |
| Alkali | 3 | 2 | 1 | 3 | 12 | 21 |
| Phenols | | | 2 | 1 | 13 | 16 |
| Quaternary ammonia | 2 | | | | | 2 |
| Food intoxication | 118 | 111 | 85 | 219 | 394 | 927 |
| Phosphorus | | | 1 | | 2 | 3 |
| Toxic plants | 5 | | 5 | 5 | 10 | 25 |
| Fungi | 122 | 15 | | 11 | | 148 |
| Snakes | 16 | 85 | 58 | 46 | 9 | 214 |
| Toads | 4 | 35 | 53 | 3 | 5 | 100 |
| **Totals** | 559 | 498 | 387 | 610 | 1074 | 3128 |

fects of 1080 and to greatly improved detection methods for the toxin.

4. Organophosphate and carbamate toxicoses continue to result in almost the entire number of reported insecticide poisonings. Most chlorinated hydrocarbon insecticides have been severely curtailed for both home and agricultural use. Although some chlordane and lindane products may be found on retail shelves, the registration of chlordane may soon be deleted. Young animals are more susceptible than adults to poisoning by chlorinated hydrocarbon insecticides. As a species the cat is more susceptible to at least some of the chlorinated hydrocarbons. The dog, however, is peculiarly sensitive to toxaphene, and this chemical is one of the few chlorinated hydrocarbons still approved and in widespread use.

5. An insecticide-related problem, flea-collar dermatitis, continues to be a problem, especially for dogs. Keeping the collar dry, properly sized and loosely fitted prevents the majority of problems.

6. Antifreeze (ethylene glycol) poisoning is a persistent and perennial problem and increasingly is recognized in cats as well as in dogs. Ethylene glycol is a season-related toxicant, with an increased incidence being seen in fall and early winter.

7. Strychnine poisoning continues to be a leading cause of chemical poisoning in dogs and is commonly implicated in malicious poisoning. It is readily recognized clinically and chemically and is of high toxicity to dogs.

8. Many of the animals seen with anticoagulant poisoning are treated and saved. Large amounts of the commonly used 0.025% baits must be consumed for exposure to result in fatality.

9. In the author's opinion, more poisoning from the rodenticide zinc phosphide may occur than is reported. The clinical signs of zinc phosphide toxicosis are variable, and death may be acute after a latent period. Furthermore, there is no good chemical test in routine use for zinc phosphide.

10. Metaldehyde poisoning from commercial snail baits occurs in warm, damp climates and is associated with the method of snail or slug baiting. If small piles are carelessly left accessible in the garden, dogs in particular may consume the bait.

11. Lead poisoning, in addition to the encephalitic form, may go unrecognized as a syndrome of anorexia, weakness, mild colic and occasional vomiting. These signs often occur prior to neurologic involvement.

12. The herbicide 2,4-D, commonly used for lawn weed control, is relatively more toxic to the dog than to other species. However, based on toxicity data and applicable rates to lawns, direct contact with treated lawns is not likely to cause poisoning. However, improperly disposed spray mixtures or pools of diluted spray could be a hazard to dogs.

13. Poisonous toads and venomous animals are mainly geographic problems of the southern states. They are discussed in separate chapters of this section.

14. Actual poisoning by plants is in the author's opinion rare in small animals. The most frequent response to ingested plants is nausea, vomition, and salivation. While certain seeds, bulbs and leaves are highly toxic, only the occasional young inquisitive animal, or those pets with depraved appetites or insufficient food are likely to consume plants.

Aside from the few generalizations made here, there is no definitive evidence of any one overwhelming toxicology problem. Certainly, clinical toxicoses of small animals pose a formidable diagnostic challenge. They must be dealt with clinically but can only be defined by a well-organized, coordinated gathering of evidence made in light of the potential hazards available and confirmed by chemical and clinical corroboration. The final step is to educate the client to avoid such hazards or to keep and use hazardous materials in their proper place.

## SUPPLEMENTAL READING

Arena, J. M.: Poisoning. Toxicology, Symptoms, Treatments. 3rd ed. Springfield, Illinois, Charles C Thomas, 1974.

Atkins, C. E., and Johnson, R. K.: Clinical toxicities of cats. Vet. Clin. N. Am., 5:623–652, 1975.

Buck, W. B., Osweiler, G. D., and Van Gelder, G. A.: Clinical and Diagnostic Veterinary Toxicology. Dubuque, Iowa, Kendall-Hunt Publishing Co., 1973.

Bureau of Veterinary Medicine. Memo: Summary of Adverse Reactions to Animal Drugs. Bureau Vet. Med. Memo No. 20, Rockville, Maryland, August, 1975.

Catcott, E. J. (ed.): Canine Medicine. Wheaton, Illinois, American Veterinary Publications, 1968.

Clarke, E. G. C.: Pets and poisons. J. Small Animal Pract., *16*:375–380, 1975.

Clarke, E. G. C., and Clarke, M. L.: Garner's Veterinary Toxicology. 3rd ed. Baltimore, The Williams & Wilkins Co., 1967.

Diechman, W. B., and Gerarde, H. W.: Toxicology of Drugs and Chemicals. 4th ed. New York, Academic Press, 1969.

Gleason, M. N., Gosselin, R. E., and Hodge, H. C.: Clinical Toxicology of Commercial Products. Baltimore, The Williams & Wilkins Co., 1971.

Kirk, R. W. (ed.): Current Veterinary Therapy V. Philadelphia, W. B. Saunders Co., 1974.

Kirk, R. W., and Bistner, S. I.: Handbook of Veterinary Procedures and Emergency Treatment. 2nd ed. Philadelphia, W. B. Saunders Co., 1975.

Malone, J. C.: Diagnosis and treatment of poisoning in dogs and cats. Vet. Rec., *84*:161–166, 1969.

Osweiler, G. D.: Incidence and diagnostic considerations of major small animal toxicoses. J. Am. Vet. Med. Assn., *155*:2011–2015, 1969.

Radeleff, R. D.: Veterinary Toxicology. 2nd ed. Philadelphia, Lea & Febiger, 1970.

Robens, J. F.: Animal drug toxicities. Veterinary Toxicology Training and Review Workshop. Ames, Iowa, February 21–26, 1972.

Szabuniewicz, M.: Treatment of some common animal poisonings. Vet. Med./Small Animal Clin., December, 1971, pp. 1197–1205.

# STRYCHNINE POISONING

GARY D. OSWEILER
*Columbia, Missouri*

## SOURCE

Strychnine is an indole alkaloid. The commercial sources of strychnine are primarily from Southeast Asia, being derived from seeds of the plants *Strychnos nux-vomica* and *Strychnos ignatii*. It was first used in medicine in about 1540 and has been used in Europe as an animal poison since the sixteenth century.

Present-day usage of strychnine is primarily as a ruminatoric (tartar emetic), stimulant and pesticide. However, there is no modern rational basis for the use of strychnine in therapy. Its principal pesticidal applications are for rat, gopher, mole and coyote control. Many commercial forms are pelleted and are dyed either bright green or red. Strychnine is available to the public through many retail outlets. It is one of the most commonly recognized causes of accidental and malicious poisoning in the dog.

Brucine is a structurally close relative of strychnine and has physiologic effects similar to strychnine (although less potent). The morphine alkaloids thebaine, morphine and codeine are structurally similar to strychnine in many respects but have obvious depressant activity rather than the excitatory properties of strychnine.

## TOXICITY

Strychnine is a highly toxic compound to most domestic animals. The approximate oral lethal toxicity to various animals is as follows:

| | |
|---|---|
| bovine | 0.5 mg./kg. |
| equine | 0.5 mg./kg. |
| porcine | 0.5-1.0 mg./kg. |
| canine | 0.75 mg./kg. |
| feline | 2.0 mg./kg. |
| fowl | 5.0 mg./kg. |
| rat | 3.0 mg./kg. |

Parenteral strychnine is 2 to 10 times more toxic than oral strychnine.

## MECHANISM OF ACTION

The physiologic effect of strychnine is to allow uncontrolled and relatively diffuse spinal reflex activity to proceed basically unchecked. All striated muscle groups are affected, but the relatively more powerful extensors predominate to produce symmetrical and generalized rigidity and tonic seizures. Gross or microscopic changes in the neurons, axons or myelin sheath have not been observed.

Strychnine appears to affect the central nervous system directly by selectively antagonizing certain types of spinal inhibition. It interferes with postsynaptic inhibition in the spinal cord and medulla. Thus, the moderating and controlling effects in the reflex are eliminated. Examples of postsynaptic inhibition are the inhibitory influences between motoneurons of antagonistic muscle groups and the recurrent spinal inhibition mediated by Renshaw cells.

The amino acid glycine is an accepted inhibitory transmitter in the spinal cord and medulla. Strychnine reversibly and selectively antagonizes glycine in the spinal cord and medulla, possibly by a competitive type of antagonism. Postsynaptic membrane permeability is changed, and the net effect is that strychnine reduces the inhibitory postsynaptic potential normally controlled by glycine.

## CLINICAL SIGNS

Clinical signs of strychnine poisoning appear within 10 minutes to 2 hours after ingestion of the poison. Early signs are apprehension, nervousness, tenseness, and stiffness. Palpation in early stages reveals tense abdomen and rigid cervical musculature. Violent tetanic seizures may appear spontaneously or be initiated by stimuli such as touch, sound or a sudden bright light. There is extreme and overpowering extensor rigidity causing the animal to assume a "sawhorse" stance. The strength of the tetanic spasm may throw the animal off its feet. The legs and body are stiff, the neck is arched, ears are erect and the lips are pulled back from the teeth. Breathing may cease momentarily. Duration of a tetanic convulsion may vary from a few seconds to a minute or more. Intermittent periods of relaxation are observed but become less frequent as the clinical course progresses. During convulsions the pupils are dilated, and cyanotic mucous membranes are evidence of anoxia. Convulsive seizures become more frequent and death eventually occurs from exhaustion or anoxia during a tetanic seizure. The entire syndrome, if untreated, is often less than 1 to 2 hours.

## PHYSIOPATHOLOGY

Rigor mortis occurs rapidly after death from strychnine poisoning. Relaxation of body musculature also follows in more rapid than normal succession. No gross or microscopic lesions characteristic of strychnine poisoning can be consistently detected. Cyanosis, petechial or ecchymotic hemorrhages and traumatic lesions are evidence of a violent and hypoxic state. Characteristically, the stomach of strychnine-poisoned animals is filled with food or bait which has not been completely digested.

Absorbed strychnine is transported in the blood by both plasma and erythrocytes but is rapidly passed from blood to tissue. It does not appear to concentrate in nervous tissue.

Excretion is accomplished in urine and via secretion into the stomach. The ionization of strychnine, a basic drug, is influenced by pH. Thus ion-trapping of strychnine occurs in the acid conditions of the stomach, and urinary excretion may be enhanced by acidification of the urine.

## DIAGNOSIS

Tentative diagnosis is usually based on history of ingestion, characteristic clinical signs and lack of lesions. Similar clinical signs may be caused by chlorinated hydrocarbons, zinc phosphide, metaldehyde, lead, hypocalcemia and acute hepatic necrosis.

Samples for analysis should include stomach contents, liver, kidney, urine and central nervous system. In addition, baits or vomitus should be kept for analysis. Most chemical confirmations of strychnine poisoning are from stomach contents or liver. In many cases, animals die so rapidly that urinary excretion has been insignificant.

In some field cases suspected to be strychnine poisoning, pentobarbital is administered to control the convulsions. Since pentobarbital is metabolized in the liver and has amine properties like alkaloids, it may react with iodoplatinate to give a spot on thin-layer chromatography (TLC) which might be confused with strychnine. Cases where pentobarbital might occur and give false positives are those which give negative results for stomach contents but positive results for the liver.

Biologic verification of strychnine poisoning may be accomplished by the following procedure:

1. Extract stomach contents or urine mixing with equal volume of acid.

2. Centrifuge or filter the acid extract.

3. Neutralize the supernate with ammonium hydroxide to a range of pH 7.0 to 8.0.

4. Inject 0.5 ml. in the dorsal sac of a frog or intraperitoneally in a mouse.

5. Typical strychnine convulsive seizures usually occur within 2 to 4 minutes.

## TREATMENT

Of prime concern in strychnine poisoning is the maintenance of relaxation and prevention of asphyxia. In emergency situations, pentobarbital in doses just sufficient to maintain relaxation is acceptable. However, more prolonged maintenance of relaxation may be accomplished by inhalation anesthesia or by administration of methocarbamol (150 mg./kg.) and continued maintenance as needed. Because respiratory paralysis and repeated hypoxia of the CNS may occur in strychnine poisoning, facilities for artificial ventilation and administration of oxygen should be readily available.

Other successful therapeutic regimens for strychnine toxicosis have included use of diazepam or glyceryl guaiacolate ether, both of which have central muscle relaxant properties. Glyceryl guaiacolate has been employed at 110 mg./kg. intravenously with repeated maintenance doses as needed. In man, 10 mg. of diazepam has been utilized intravenously and repeated as needed. The animal dosage for diazepam is 2.5 to 20 mg. intravenously or orally.

The advantage of combination therapy is primarily the reduction of exposure to high levels of barbiturates for prolonged periods.

Early induction of vomiting with apomorphine is recommended, provided the animal is not in a hyperesthetic or convulsive state. Rapid recovery from strychnine toxicosis may be enhanced by prompt application of the enterogastric lavage technique described by Frye (1974).

If anesthesia must be maintained, gastric lavage can be employed using 1 to 2 per cent tannic acid or 1:2,000 potassium permanganate. Following this, activated charcoal and sodium sulfate may be left in the stomach to aid adsorption and more rapid elimination of the alkaloid.

Forced diuresis with 5 per cent mannitol in 0.9 per cent sodium chloride administered at the rate of 7 ml./kg./hour and acidification of the urine with 150 mg./kg. body weight of ammonium chloride orally will enhance excretion of strychnine. This must be subsequent to establishment of adequate urine flow.

Toxic doses of strychnine will be depleted from the body within 24 to 48 hours. One must expect to continue maintenance relaxation and sedation for 12 to 48 hours. It should be emphasized that the sedation time can be considerably shortened if prompt and aggressive action is taken to clear the gastrointestinal tract, inactivate unabsorbed strychnine and hasten elimination of alkaloid via diuresis and ion-trapping.

When prompt and thorough action is taken, recovery of a high proportion of strychnine poisoning cases can be expected.

## SUPPLEMENTAL READING

Bailey, E. M., and Szabuniewicz, M.: The use of glyceryl guaiacolate ether in the treatment of strychnine poisoning in the dog. Vet. Med./Small Animal Clin., 70:170–174, 1975.

Clarke, E. G. C., and Clarke, M. L.: Garner's Veterinary Toxicology. 3rd ed. Baltimore, The Williams & Wilkins Co., 1967.

Curtis, D. R., and Johnston, G. A. R.: Convulsant alkaloids. In Simpson, L. L., and Curtis, D. R. (eds.): Neuropoisons, Vol. New York, Plenum Press, 1974.

Franz, D.: Central nervous system stimulants. In Goodman, L. S., and Gilman, A. (eds.): The Pharmacologic Basis of Therapeutics. 5th ed. New York, Macmillan Co., 1975.

Frye, F. L.: Enterogastric lavage in small animal practice. Vet. Med./Small Animal Clin., 69:835–836, 1974.

McConnell, E. E., van Rensburg, I. B. S., and Minne, J. A.: A rapid test for the diagnosis of strychnine poisoning. J. S. Afr. Vet. Med. Assn., 42(1):81–84, 1971.

MacKinnon, J., Waite, P. R., and Hilbery, A. D. R.: Accidental poisoning in animals. Vet. Rec., May 5, 92:489, 1973.

Maron, B. J., Krupp, J. R., and Tune, B.: Strychnine poisoning successfully treated with diazepam. J. Ped., April, 78:697–699, 1971.

Osweiler, G. D.: Strychnine poisoning. In Kirk, R. W.: Current Veterinary Therapy V. Philadelphia, W. B. Saunders Co., 1973.

Radeleff, R. D.: Veterinary Toxicology. Philadelphia, Lea & Febiger, 1964.

# ANTU POISONING

WILLIAM F. HARRIS, D.V.M.
*Puyallup, Washington*

In the dog and cat, ANTU produces a marked hemorrhagic congestion of the heart, lungs, stomach, intestine, kidneys and liver, with effusion of dramatic quantities of clear fluid into the thoracic and pericardial cavities. Most symptomatic cases proceed to a postmortem diagnosis as therapy is of little value.

ANTU (1[1-naphthyl]-2-thiourea) ($C_{10}H_7NHCSNH_2$) is an effective rodenticide against the Norway rat (*Rattus norvegicus*). It is a bitter-tasting but odorless white crystalline powder which is practically insoluble in water. It has a molecular weight of 202.28. It will kill adult rats at 3 to 6 mg./kg. body weight. It is commonly used as a 1 per cent concentration in bait. The use of ANTU has been prohibited in several states and restricted in others, so that poisoning of pet animals is relatively uncommon. The lethal dose for the dog is in the range of 10 to 40 mg./kg. body weight. For the cat, the lethal dose is 75 to 100 mg./kg. body weight. Young dogs in good condition have a much higher tolerance than do older dogs. If the stomach is full of food when the drug is ingested, the probability of lethal results is increased. This is due to the protective effect afforded by the food against the irritant effect ANTU has on the gastric mucosa. The longer the material is retained in the stomach, the greater the probability of lethal consequences. Some animals will vomit soon after ingestion of the toxic agent and may survive an otherwise lethal dose.

The signs, lesions, postmortem observations and histopathologic findings associated with ANTU toxicity are typified by an experimental poisoning: A 22-kg. entire female basset hound in good health and just past estrum was given 550 mg. of the undiluted chemical (25 mg./kg. body weight) in a moderate feeding of dog food 1½ hours after a regular feeding. No remarkable changes were noted for 6 to 7 hours except for an increasing restlessness. At 7 hours, the mucosa and conjunctivae began to assume a cherry-red congestion with some mucopurulent ocular discharge. There was an increase in respiratory rate and depth. The heart rate had increased and the character of the pulse was weak and thready. At 9 hours, vomiting was noted which recurred at infrequent intervals until death occurred at 14 hours post ingestion. As the signs became more pronounced, the restlessness gave way to lethargy. The dog assumed a sitting position with its forelegs extended and placed wide apart. The muzzle was extended and the eyelids drooped, with the nictitating membrane covering most of the cornea. The extremities were cold. There was a rapid progression of the critical signs until death occurred quietly and without struggle.

The predominant gross lesion on postmortem examination was hyperemia and congestion involving the gastric and upper intestinal mucosa and the lungs. The pericardium and the thorax contained close to a liter of clear straw-colored fluid free of fibrin.

Sections through organ and tissue specimens showed a diffuse and severe hemorrhagic congestion of all organs, with particularly striking changes in the heart, lungs, kidneys, submucosal layers of the stomach and mucosal layers of the intestine.

The lungs had a striking pulmonary edema with congestion of all segments of the vascular tree. The alveolar spaces were uniformly filled with proteinaceous edema fluid. Sections through the heart showed rather markedly degenerative changes which undoubtedly would have progressed to frank necrosis had the animal survived for a sufficient period of time. An additional characteristic of these changes was lack of inflammatory exudate. The gastric mucosa in particular was remarkably well preserved and showed little change other than the congestion seen in the submucosal layers. No toxic changes were evident in either the liver or kidney sections, which showed only the severe congestion described.

This description of a basset hound experimentally poisoned with ANTU is, in every respect, typical of approximately 30 dogs encountered as field cases. There were no survivors. Therapy is of little value unless the chemical can be removed from the stomach within a short time. In most cases the thoracic lesions are well advanced before the dog's condition becomes a cause for concern to its owner. By the time the affected animal reaches the veterinary hospital, the pathologic changes are usually irreversible.

In the dog, apomorphine hydrochloride (0.04 IV or 0.08 mg./kg. IM or SC), if promptly administered, might prove helpful in evacuating the stomach, along with gastric lavage. Apomorphine is a respiratory sedative and contraindicated after the onset of signs. Atropine sulfate may be helpful in early stages or in mild cases of toxicity. Venoclysis is contraindicated because it adds to the supply of available fluids to produce edema and effusion into body spaces and thereby contributes to respiratory embarrassment.

The diagnosis is based on history and the characteristic clinical signs, postmortem findings and histopathologic changes. Attempted identification of ANTU in the tissues by chemical tests is not a dependable diagnostic criterion because the chemical is usually gone from the tissues before the postmortem examination occurs.

SUPPLEMENTAL READING

Garner, R.: Garner's Veterinary Toxicology. 3rd ed. Baltimore, The Williams & Wilkins Co., 1967, p. 264.
Radeleff, R. D.: Veterinary Toxicology. 2nd ed. Philadelphia, Lea & Febiger, 1969, p. 189.

---

# SODIUM FLUORO-ACETATE (COMPOUND 1080) POISONING

WILLIAM C. EDWARDS
*Stillwater, Oklahoma*

Sodium fluoroacetate, or compound 1080, and related compounds such as fluoroacetamide and fluoroacetic acid are generally colorless, odorless and tasteless. These highly toxic compounds have been investigated by the governments of some countries for their potential as chemical warfare agents. In the United States the use of sodium fluoroacetate is now limited by law to licensed pest-control operations. These compounds are usually mixed with a black dye and are used with bread, bran, cereals or other baits. Fluoroacetate has been a popular rodenticide and insecticide for use around sewers, ship holds, grain storage elevators and mills.

There has been considerable concern about the use of fluoroacetate in areas where biological chain reactions may occur. Such instances have occurred where pet animals have been poisoned by eating the flesh of rodents or birds killed by compound 1080.

Fluoroacetate is an extremely toxic compound. Dogs are quite susceptible, and the lethal dose may be as little as 0.05 mg./kg. Rats and mice are more resistant than dogs and cats and the lethal dose ranges from 5.0 to 8.0 mg./kg.

Paradoxically, fluoroacetate would not be particularly toxic if it were not for its biotransformation to fluorocitric acid by the host. This phenomenon is referred to as lethal synthesis." Fluoroacetate replaces cellular acetyl coenzyme A, which combines with oxaloacetic acid in the citric acid (Krebs) cycle to form fluorocitric acid. Fluorocitric acid then inhibits the enzyme aconitase in the citric acid cycle. There is a build-up of citric acid and interference with cellular respiration which results in central nervous and cardiovascular disturbances.

The time required for lethal synthesis accounts for the ½- to 2-hour latent period from the time of exposure until clinical signs appear.

## CLINICAL SIGNS

Fluoroacetate may be absorbed from the gastrointestinal tract, respiratory tract or abraded skin. The most common route of exposure in domestic animals is ingestion. Within the ½- to 2-hour latent period vomiting usually occurs. There is often a prodromal period of short duration in which the animal shows apprehension, panting and nervousness. When signs commence, the onset is acute and the course rapid.

There are marked species differences in symptomatology. Man, monkeys, horses and rabbits exhibit cardiac arrhythmias, cardiovascular collapse and ventricular fibrillation while CNS signs may be incidental. Dogs usually show intermittent central nervous excitation and depression and may die in convulsions or of subsequent respiratory paralysis. Cats may show both the cardiovascular and central nervous signs but the cardiac arrhythmias usually predominate.

The clinical signs of fluoroacetate poisoning in the dog include initial vomition, urination and repeated defecation, often with tenesmus. During the initial period, restlessness, hyperirritability and aimless wandering or running fits may be observed. There may be periods when the dog will collapse from exhaustion following a running fit or tonic-clonic seizures with paddling. During these periods of collapse the dog is not responsive to external stimulation which aids in the differential diagnosis to exclude strychnine as the cause of poisoning.

Convulsions eventually become weaker and more frequent and death usually occurs from exhaustion and respiratory failure within 2 to 12 hours after onset of signs. Animals which die from fluoroacetate poisoning develop rigor mortis very rapidly, with the limbs usually rigidly extended.

## DIAGNOSIS

The diagnosis of fluoroacetate poisoning is usually made on the basis of circumstantial evidence and clinical signs. Chemical analysis of tissues for fluoroacetate or fluorocitrate is very difficult, but vomitus can be submitted to a forensic toxicology laboratory when available.

There are no pathognomonic lesions associated with fluoroacetate poisoning. There is generalized cyanosis of the mucous membranes, and the liver and kidney usually show marked congestion. The heart is usually flaccid and may show subepicardial hemorrhages.

Affected animals will have hyperglycemia and this may be of diagnostic importance. Elevated citrate levels in kidney tissue may also aid in the confirmation of the clinical diagnosis. The differential diagnosis must include strychnine, chlorinated hydrocarbons, plant alkaloids, organophosphate pesticides, garbage intoxication, epilepsy, eclampsia and lead poisoning.

Strychnine-poisoned dogs usually do not vomit nor is there the extreme running and yelping associated with fluoroacetate poisoning. Strychnine-poisoned dogs also respond with convulsive seizures to external stimulation, whereas fluoroacetate convulsions cannot be induced by noise or touch. Chlorinated hydrocarbon poisoning is manifested by intermittent epileptiform convulsions, muscle fasciculation and champing fits. The body temperature may be markedly elevated with chlorinated hydrocarbon poisoning and eclampsia.

Garbage poisoning in dogs may cause muscle weakness, vomiting and diarrhea but seldom causes the severe convulsions and running fits or paddling seen with compound 1080. The clinician should recall that fluoroacetate poisoning is an acute syndrome with death ensuing in 2 to 12 hours, whereas lead poisoning, true epilepsy and chlorinated hydrocarbon poisoning are usually more chronic in nature.

Whenever fluoroacetate poisoning is diagnosed the local authorities and poison information centers should be notified because of the potential for biological chain reactions and possible human exposure. Other animals in the household should be protected by finding the fluoroacetate source and cleaning up any vomitus.

## TREATMENT

There is no specific antidote for fluoroacetate poisoning. Emergency measures to control the violent convulsions, acidosis and cyanosis should be of the first priority. A basal anesthetic such as an ultra–short-acting barbiturate and gas anesthesia may be used to control the convulsions. Glyceryl monoacetate (monoacetin) has been recommended to block the acetate-to-citrate lethal synthesis, and intravenous calcium gluconate may be of value as an additional means of controlling convulsions and combating possible hypocalcemia.

### Outline of Treatment for the Veterinarian

1. Immediately after exposure, induce vomiting or perform gastric lavage.

2. Administer glyceryl monoacetate (monoacetin) intramuscularly, if available at the rate of 0.125 gm./kg. If glyceryl monoacetate is unavailable, administer 50 per cent ethyl alcohol and 5 per cent acetic acid orally at the rate of 2 ml./kg. of each.

3. Control convulsions with short-acting barbiturate or gas anesthesia.

4. Provide oxygen therapy and artificial resuscitation as required.

5. Monitor cardiac status with ECG if possible.

### SUPPLEMENTAL READING

Buck, W. B., Osweiler, G. O., and Van Gelder, G. A. Clinical and Diagnostic Veterinary Toxicology. Dubuque, Iowa, Kendall-Hunt Publishing Co., 1973

Gleason, M. N., Gosselin, R. E., Hodge, H. C., and Smith, R. P.: Clinical Toxicology of Commercial Products. Baltimore, The Williams & Wilkins Co. 1969.

# WARFARIN AND OTHER ANTI-COAGULANT POISONINGS

WILLIAM B. BUCK, D.V.M.
*Ames, Iowa*

The anticoagulant rodenticides are structurally related to coumarin. All have the basic coumarin or indandione nucleus.

4-Hydroxycoumarin          Indane-1,3-dione

Three common rodenticides used extensively by professional exterminators and the layman are:

*Warfarin,* 3 (alpha-phenyl-beta-acetylethyl)-4-hydroxycoumarin (D-Con)

*Pindone,* 2-pivalyl-1,3-indandione (Pival)

*Diphacinone,* 2-diphenylacetyl-1,3-indandione (Diphacin)

Various other products are available. They vary in their side chains, solubility and toxicity but contain the same basic nucleus. Many anticoagulant rodenticides incorporate sulfaquinoxaline in the bait to enhance the toxicity.

## TOXICITY

The anticoagulant rodenticides are a potential hazard to all mammals and birds. Dogs and cats appear to be most frequently affected, and swine are occasionally poisoned by warfarin. The toxicity of these compounds varies widely from one to another. Susceptibility also varies among species. Massive single exposure or repeated low dosages may cause poisoning. Table 1 gives some values for warfarin toxicity in various species.

The toxicity of the indandione products varies among compounds, but toxicity generally ranges from 50 to 100 mg./kg. single dose in dogs.

Several factors may influence the toxicity of coumarin and indandione compounds. Vitamin K deficiency resulting from high dietary fat intake or prolonged oral antibiotic therapy may increase the susceptibility of animals to warfarin. Likewise, liver disease makes animals more sensitive to a loss of prothrombin production. Concomitant administration of adrenocorticosteroids may increase the susceptibility of animals to competitive displacement from the plasma binding sites. The half-life of plasma warfarin is markedly reduced by barbiturates (amobarbital, secobarbital) and meprobamate.

## MECHANISM OF ACTION

The anticoagulant rodenticides interfere with the normal synthesis of clotting factors by the liver. Their major effect is due to inhibition of prothrombin synthesis as a result of interference with the action of vitamin K. The coumarins do not destroy prothrombin, although they may interfere with the con-

**Table 1.** *Values for Warfarin Toxicity*

| SPECIES | SINGLE DOSE | REPEATED DOSES |
|---|---|---|
| Rats | 50 to 100 mg./kg. | 1 mg./kg. for 5 days |
| Dogs | 50 mg./kg. | 5 mg./kg. for 5 to 15 days |
| Cats | 5 to 50 mg./kg. | 1 mg./kg. for 5 days |
| Swine | 3 mg./kg. | 0.05 mg./kg. for 7 days |
| Ruminants | | 200 mg./kg. for 12 days |
| Poultry | 50 per cent of body weight of feed containing 0.1 mg./kg. | |

121

version of prothrombin to thrombin. There is also a definite depression of factors VII, IX and X in the serum of warfarin-poisoned animals. Platelet adhesiveness may be slightly decreased, but platelet counts are not depressed.

There does not appear to be any direct hepatotoxic action from warfarin. Hypoxia and anemia, as a result of hemorrhage, may cause liver necrosis as a sequel to the basic lesion.

## CLINICAL AND PATHOLOGIC SIGNS

The clinical signs of coumarin or indandione poisoning reflect some manifestations of hemorrhage. Onset may be acute, and occasionally animals are found dead with no previous signs of illness. This is especially true when hemorrhage in the cerebral vasculature, pericardial sac, mediastinum or thorax occurs. In subacute cases, animals are anemic and weak; and pale mucous membranes, dyspnea, hematemesis, epistaxis and bloody feces are common signs. Scleral, conjunctival and intraocular hemorrhage may be seen. With severe blood loss, weakness and staggering or ataxia are observed. Blood loss and pulmonary hemorrhage are reflected in dyspnea with moist rales and blood-tinged froth around the nose or mouth. Cardiac rate is irregular and heartbeat is weak. Extensive external hematomata may occur, especially in areas of trauma. Swollen, tender joints are commonly seen. If hemorrhage involves the brain, spinal cord or subdural space, CNS signs will be manifest as paresis, ataxia, convulsions or acute death. When the course of poisoning is prolonged, autolysis of impounded blood can cause icterus.

## DIAGNOSIS

Warfarin poisoning should be differentiated from other hemorrhagic disorders. Some of these are aflatoxicosis, thrombocytopenia, radiation injury, infectious canine hepatitis and vitamin K deficiency (especially in poultry and swine). Clinical pathology utilizing clotting time, prothrombin time, hematocrit, differential leukocyte count and clot retraction may be employed if doubt exists. Plasma warfarin levels from live animals or liver warfarin levels in necropsy specimens can aid in confirming the diagnosis.

## TREATMENT

Warfarin-poisoned animals should be handled to minimize trauma. Sedation or light anesthesia can aid in gentle manipulation. If respiratory difficulty or severe anemia is encountered, oxygen therapy may prolong life until treatment can be continued. In acute cases, fresh or stored whole blood should be administered to supply prothrombin and factors VII, IX and X. Give 20 ml./kg. intravenously. Half the dose should be given rapidly and the remainder at about 20 drops/minute. If blood loss has been minimal, plasma can be used instead of whole blood, since it contains the clotting factors. If dyspnea continues to be a problem, a thoracic radiograph is indicated. Thoracentesis to remove excess blood may save an animal's life and make further therapy possible.

Vitamin K ($K_1$) should be administered intravenously (15 to 75 mg.) as a 5 per cent suspension in 5 per cent dextrose. Keep fluids to a minimum. Poisoned animals need blood more than extracellular fluid. Vitamin $K_1$ begins to reverse the hypoprothrombinemia in about 30 minutes, but several hours are required for full clinical response.

Animals should be kept warm and free of physical trauma for at least 24 hours. Convalescent animals may be given oral vitamin K (menadione) for four to six days to allow for complete degradation of the circulating warfarin.

### SUPPLEMENTAL READING

Buck, W. B., Osweiler, G. D., and Van Gelder, G. A. Clinical and Diagnostic Veterinary Toxicology Dubuque, Iowa, Kendall-Hunt Publishing Co., 1973.
Lawson, J., and Doncaster, R. A.: A treatment for warfarin poisoning in the dog. Vet. Rec., 77:1183, 1965.
Nagashim, R., O'Reilly, R. A., and Levy, G.: Kinetics of pharmacologic effects in man: anticoagulant action of warfarin. Clin. Pharmacol. Therap., 10:22, 1969.

# METALDEHYDE POISONING

MARVIN L. SAMUELSON, D.V.M.
*Manhattan, Kansas*

Metaldehyde is frequently found as an ingredient in snail and slug poisons. Consequently intoxication in dogs occurs mostly in those areas where and during seasons when these pests are prevalent.

Metaldehyde is commonly used in meal form and spread as bait. Liquid and pellet forms are also used. Dogs are frequently presented on weekends and in early evening hours. This may coincide with the increase in yard care including application of this pesticide which goes on at these times.

Dogs seem to be attracted to some preparations. Efforts by manufacturers and government agencies to make the preparations less attractive to dogs should reduce the incidence. Additional help may come by educating users to spread the substance and keep dogs away until the material is worked into the ground cover.

Metaldehyde is a polymer of acetaldehyde, insoluble in water and somewhat slowly absorbed from the digestive tract. It is metabolized primarily by the liver.

Metaldehyde is sometimes found in combination with arsenicals and organophosphates. These agents present separate problems and should be treated accordingly.

The $LD_{50}$ of metaldehyde for the dog as reported in the literature is quite variable, 60 to 500 mg./kg. Dogs have survived 750 mg./kg. Morbidity and mortality may be dependent on the condition of the digestive tract and other health factors. Obese dogs and those with liver disease seem much more vulnerable.

## CLINICAL SIGNS

Signs of incoordination, muscle tremors, anxiety, hyperesthesia and salivation are common in the early stages. As the tremors increase, the dog falls over and the limbs are extended. The tremors differ from those of strychnine as they are continuous and are not influenced by external stimuli. Marked hyperthermia and severe acidosis may follow.

## TREATMENT

The aims of clinical care are to evacuate the digestive tract, control tremors, prevent aspiration, combat acidosis and support liver function.

Apomorphine, 40 $\mu$g./kg. IV is indicated if the dog is still standing. After vomition and depending on the intensity of tremors, sedation is useful. Diazepam, 2 to 5 mg./kg. IV (Valium), or triflupromazine, 0.2 to 2.0 mg./kg. IV (Vetame), is usually adequate. Muscle relaxants may be helpful, especially when used with barbiturates.

In cases where the patient is prostrate and the tremors are intense, sedation is indicated prior to evacuation of the stomach. This stage is critical and there is danger of aspiration if vomition occurs. Aspiration is a major cause of death.

Barbiturates alone or in combination with muscle relaxants may be used to sedate the patient just to the point of controlling tremors and the placement of an endotracheal tube. Metaldehyde seems to produce some alternation of excitement and depression. This feature necessitates the use of minimal doses of depressants. The barbiturate should be used in minimal doses to effect control and should be maintained by intravenous drip via catheter. Avoid deep anesthesia. The metaldehyde patient may be controlled with less than one fourth the usual dose of barbiturate and maintained by very low doses via intravenous drip. The patient should be suspended with the head lower on the table while gastric lavage is accomplished.

Lactated Ringer's solution aids in combating acidosis and dehydration and serves as a vehicle for the depressants. A severe case may require continuous care for 24 hours or more. Lipotrophic agents may aid in aftercare.

The prognosis is always guarded, though most patients recover. Losses occur mostly from aspiration, acidosis and liver failure.

# THALLIUM INTOXICATION

CARL E. ARONSON, Ph.D.
*Philadelphia, Pennsylvania*

Thallium is an element classified among the heavy metals. Its most common salts, thallous acetate ($TlC_2H_3O_2$) and thallous sulfate ($Tl_2SO_4$), are whitish crystalline substances that are odorless, tasteless and very water-soluble.

In the past, thallium salts were employed in the treatment of a wide variety of human illnesses including venereal diseases, gout, dysentery and ringworm. In addition, thallium was used as the active ingredient in certain depilatory preparations. Until recently, thallium was also employed as a fungicide, pesticide and rodenticide. Thallium-containing rodenticides were often sold in the form of corn saturated with thallous sulfate, and accidental ingestion of these products by domestic animals resulted in numerous deaths. The general distribution of such rodenticides, however, was banned in 1965 by the U. S. Department of Agriculture and their manufacture was halted in 1972.

Strict enforcement and a program of surveillance by the U. S. Environmental Protection Agency has markedly reduced the number of documented cases of thallium intoxication treated by veterinarians, but it remains a problem in some urban areas. In Philadelphia, for example, several dogs were diagnosed and treated for thallium poisoning during 1975 at the Small Animal Hospital of the University of Pennsylvania's School of Veterinary Medicine.

The $LD_{50}$ for most species is approximately 10 to 15 mg./kg., and a 20 to 25 mg./kg. dose is almost always fatal. Thallium is rapidly absorbed from the gastrointestinal tract, the primary route of entry into the body in most cases of accidental poisoning. Absorption does occur through the skin, but exposure to toxic levels via this route is uncommon in animals. Distribution of thallium throughout various tissues of the body occurs fairly evenly with the highest concentration being found in the kidney approximately 24 hours after oral ingestion.

Peak blood levels occur 2 to 4 hours following ingestion.

While the presence of thallium may be detected in the urine of affected animals within several hours after exposure, its pattern of excretion via the urine and feces indicates that it is cleared from the body very slowly (approximately 4 per cent during the first day, 37 per cent in 7 days and 60 per cent after 28 days). Because of thallium's slow rate of clearance, repeated ingestion of small quantities may lead to its accumulation and levels sufficient to produce clinical signs of toxicity.

Like other heavy metals, thallium presumably causes its toxic effects by interacting with structural and enzymatic protein at both cellular and subcellular levels. There are strong indications that it interferes with the actions of mitochondrial enzymes, thereby inhibiting metabolic pathways associated with the process of oxidative phosphorylation. There is also evidence that thallium exchanges for potassium in excitable tissues such as muscle and nerve.

## CLINICAL SIGNS

Because of its relatively widespread tissue distribution, thallium attacks most body systems with varying degrees of severity. Consequently, it produces a wide variety of clinical signs the nature of which are dose- and time-related.

The importance of obtaining a complete history cannot be overstressed, since many of the initial signs produced by thallium are relatively nonspecific and may make an accurate early diagnosis difficult. Owners are often extremely hesitant to admit that their pets have been allowed to run unattended or that rodenticides have been used on or in the vicinity of their property. It is imperative that thallium be identified as the causative agent as promptly as possible whenever it is even remotely suspected. Failure to recognize the problem and institute proper treatment will greatly limit the animal's chances for recovery.

## Acute and Subacute Toxicity

GASTROINTESTINAL SYSTEM. Most animals poisoned with thallium present signs of gastrointestinal disturbance ranging from mild upset to severe hemorrhagic gastroenteritis. They frequently vomit and often have diarrhea, their stools being black and tarry. Since they appear weak and act depressed, it is not usual for such animals to be partially or totally anorexic. There may also be evidence of abdominal pain. Oral and visible mucous membranes begin to take on a characteristic "brick red" appearance as early as two to four days after exposure and ulceration of these tissues may occur. Lingual lesions have been reported in cats.

RESPIRATORY SYSTEM. Early in the course of the disease, one should be alert for signs of labored breathing and/or dyspnea. Thallium causes eventual destruction of cilia in the respiratory tract which may lead to complications, including pneumonia. Polypnea, cough and nasal discharge are not uncommon.

NERVOUS SYSTEM. Neurologic disturbances ranging from mild to severe occur in many animals. They include convulsions, hyperexcitability, tetany, ataxia or paresis. As the illness progresses the patient may become comatose.

RENAL SYSTEM. Thallium-induced renal damage may result in the appearance of casts in the urine, proteinuria and an elevation in BUN.

MISCELLANEOUS. Skin lesions generally appear in those thallium-poisoned animals which live 4 to 5 days after exposure. Initially, a mild to moderate erythema develops about the ears and nose, and it subsequently spreads to include the axilla and inguinal regions. At this stage interdigital areas may just appear erythematous, but as the disease progresses, inflammation and swelling may develop to the point where standing and walking become extremely difficult and painful. Foot pads frequently take on a "hard pad"–like appearance. Lesions tend to be most pronounced in frictional areas subjected to constant abrasion during normal body movement. Some areas become necrotic and slough plaquelike pieces of superficial epithelium while others are pustular in character. The latter frequently ooze, the result being open, raw lesions which eventually form scabs.

Spontaneous loss of hair begins at about the seventh day and usually occurs first in those areas subject to abrasion. At this stage, hair can easily be plucked from the skin with little or no apparent discomfort to the patient. If the animal lives long enough (7 to 10 days) large patches of hair will begin to be lost spontaneously over much of the body. In those animals which recover, hair loss is temporary but repeated exposure to thallium may cause permanent damage to hair follicles.

About the same time that the oral mucosa of most animals develops a characteristic "brick red" appearance (2 to 4 days), changes also occur in the eye. Conjunctivitis and scleral injection develop, and a mucopurulent discharge which resembles that seen in distemper may be present.

## Chronic Toxicity

In cases of chronic toxicity, some of the clinical signs commonly observed are generally considerably less dramatic than those associated with episodes of acute and subacute intoxication. Gastrointestinal and neurologic signs may be minimal in such animals, but alopecia is generally quite pronounced. Animals suffering from chronic exposure to thallium succumb most often as a result of secondary complications such as pneumonia.

### LABORATORY FINDINGS

Hemotologic changes reported in thallium-poisoned dogs include eosinopenia, neutrophilia, immature leukocytosis and lymphopenia, while urine from such animals may show an increase in specific gravity accompanied with proteinuria and possibly bilirubinuria. Glycosuria may also occur. Prerenal uremia usually leads to an elevation of BUN, but such elevation may also be associated with nephrotoxicity. Examination of sediment in the urine may reveal the presence of casts, red blood cells, large numbers of white blood cells and epithelial cells.

The presence of any thallium in the urine, no matter how small the amount, should be considered highly significant.

## PATHOLOGIC FINDINGS

The lesions found in thallium-poisoned animals are not generally considered pathognomonic but appear to vary as a function of the amount of thallium ingested and the time course of the illness.

GROSS LESIONS. In acute cases, severe gastroenteritis and inflammation of the respiratory mucosa are often observed. A number of animals show evidence of cardiac hypertrophy, epicardial and endocardial hemorrhages, necrosis and degeneration of cardiac muscle. In some cases, fatty degeneration and necrosis of the liver may also be seen. Hemorrhages and congestion of the spleen, kidneys and lungs have been reported. Cutaneous erythema, pustular lesions and alopecia may occur, but in chronic cases, cracking of the skin and severe alopecia may be the only lesions evident.

MICROSCOPIC LESIONS. Thallium produces varying degrees of necrosis in several tissues including the heart, kidneys, brain, liver and skeletal muscle. Testicular degeneration has also been reported. Skin changes are extensive and hyperkeratosis, parakeratosis, hyperemia and a degree of hyalinization may be observed.

Within the central nervous system, the brain may show evidence of nerve body degeneration and demyelination while perivascular cuffing may occur in the basal ganglia, pons and temporal cortex.

## DIAGNOSIS

If an animal's history and clinical signs remotely suggest the possibility of thallium intoxication, a urine sample should be obtained, by catheter if necessary, and examined for the presence of thallium. The Gabriel-Dubin method is quick, simple and very sensitive. Since it requires no expensive equipment, it can readily be accomplished as an office procedure. While the test does not generally produce false positives, it may give false negatives if proper attention is not given to the preparation and storage of certain reagents as indicated below.

### Reagents

1. *Bromine Solution:* Saturate distilled water with free bromine until free bromine can be seen in the bottom of the glass-stoppered amber bottle in which this solution is to be kept. Allow the solution to stand at least 12 hours, preferably overnight, before use. The test will *not* work properly and false negatives will result unless this solution is kept saturated, hence the reason for the presence of an excess of free bromine. This reagent should be examined carefully before being used. WARNING! Do not allow this solution to come in contact with skin because bromine is very corrosive. Use a solution of sodium thiosulfate to neutralize the bromine in the event of a spill or contact with skin.

2. *Sulfosalicylic Acid:* 10% solution (W/V). (Dissolve 10 grams in a total volume of 100 ml. of distilled water.)

3. *Concentrated HCl*

4. *Rodamine B:* 0.05% solution (W/V) in concentrated HCl. (Dissolve 0.05 grams of Rodamine B in a total volume of 100 ml. of concentrated HCl.)

5. *Benzene:* (WARNING! Benzene is toxic. It should be used with "adequate ventilation" in a fume hood if available. Avoid contact with skin!)

6. *Thallium Standard:* 0.1% solution (W/V). (Dissolve 0.1 gram of thallous sulfate or acetate in a total volume of 100 ml. of distilled water.)

### Procedure

1. Prepare three tubes and label them "blank," "standard" and "unknown."

2. Add approximately 4 drops of water to the "blank," 4 drops of standard thallium to the "standard" and 4 drops of the urine in question to the "unknown" tube.

3. Add bromine water, drop by drop, to each tube until a yellow color remains.

4. Add sulfosalicylic acid, drop by drop, to each tube until the bromine color just disappears.

5. Add one drop of concentrated HCl to each tube.

6. Add 1 to 2 drops of Rodamine B to each tube.

7. Add approximately 0.5 ml. benzene, mix carefully and allow layers to separate.

8. A *positive* test is indicated by the presence of a reddish to purple color in the *upper benzene layer*. The color in the lower aqueous layer is of no importance.

9. When a faint positive is suspected, carefully remove an aliquot of the benzene layer (ONLY!) from the sample in question and transfer it to a clean tube. Holding it against a plain white background, compare it with benzene layers removed from the blank and standard in the same manner.

10. When viewed in the dark under ultraviolet light, the *benzene layer* of a *positive* test will emit a yellow-green fluorescence while no fluorescence will be seen if the test is negative.

DIFFERENTIAL DIAGNOSIS. Especially in its early stages, thallium intoxication may easily be confused with several other illnesses. In young dogs, for example, the mucopurulent discharge from the eyes may closely resemble that which occurs in canine distemper. It must also be differentiated from signs produced by the severe infestations that may occur in canine heartworm disease. Other types of heavy metal intoxication, skin conditions of similar appearance, hepatitis and nonspecific gastrointestinal upsets caused by a variety of other factors must also be taken into consideration when establishing a diagnosis.

While restrictions on the sale, manufacture and use of thallium-containing products have caused a decrease in the number of animals poisoned with thallium, they have also been responsible for a tendency on the part of some veterinarians to overlook and/or discount thallium because they no longer recognize or consider it to be a problem.

# TREATMENT

Every effort should be made to remove thallium from the gastrointestinal tract immediately after ingestion to minimize its rapid absorption. Stomach lavage or emetics such as apomorphine or equal parts of mustard and table salt may be administered and a Fleet enema may also be indicated. If, however, several hours have elapsed between ingestion and treatment, it is questionable whether these procedures will actually benefit the patient, since toxic quantities will most likely already have been absorbed and circulated throughout the body.

While several chelating agents have been employed, with varying degrees of success, to detoxify thallium and promote its excretion, diphenylthiocarbazone (dithizone) has proved most beneficial. In dogs, diphenylthiocarbazone (50 to 70 mg./kg.) may be administered orally 3 times per day for a period of up to five days. The patient should be closely watched, however, because diphenylthiocarbazone has been reported to cause cataracts and blindness in dogs. In chronic poisoning a lower dosage level than that indicated above should be used. Its use in cats at the same levels employed in dogs is not currently recommended, since adverse effects, including depression and jaundice, have been reported.

Prussian blue (ferric-cyanoferrate) (100 mg./kg.) may be administered orally 3 times per day. This agent is considered by some to be more effective than diphenylthiocarbazone after an initial 24 hours of treatment with diphenylthiocarbazone. Prussian blue interferes with the enterohepatic circulation of thallium and increases its fecal excretion.

Oral administration of potassium chloride (2 to 6 grams per day) in divided doses has been shown to be of value, since it aids in the maintenance of plasma potassium levels as chelated thallium is displaced from cells and replaced by potassium. The irritant effect of this salt on the gastrointestinal tract, however, may cause vomiting. Furthermore, it should not be used unless there is ample evidence that the patient's renal function is adequate. Potassium chloride administration should be discontinued once the animal shows signs of clinical improvement and minimal evidence of weakness. Hyperkalemic animals are prone to develop cardiac arrhythmias which may prove fatal.

Treatment of thallium-poisoned animals with the calcium chelate of disodium ethylenediaminotetraacetic acid (CaEDTA), dimercaprol (BAL) or penicillamine (Cuprimine® [Merck]) is not recommended, even though these drugs are highly effective in combating certain other types of heavy metal intoxication. The use of NaI and sodium thiosulfate is of questionable value and no longer advised.

# ANCILLARY TREATMENT

Good nursing care and supportive measures are essential in the treatment of thallium intoxication. The acidosis which sometimes develops may be treated with sodium bicarbonate (0.3 to 3.0 grams per day) and parenteral electrolyte replacement therapy may be required to combat and/or prevent dehydration.

Barbiturates and related drugs may be used to control convulsions and other disturbances of the central nervous system.

Animals should be fed soft, palatable foods which are easy to digest and nutritious. These include cooked cereals, boiled meats such as ground beef, boiled eggs, baby foods and prescription diets intended for dogs suffering from intestinal diseases. Force feeding and/or use of a pharyngostomy tube may be required. Administration of emollients and anticholinergic drugs to protect injured intestinal mucosa and reduce hypermotility may prove beneficial. Parenteral administration of therapeutic levels of vitamin B complex on a daily basis is also recommended.

Antibiotic therapy is often necessary to combat a variety of secondary infections, including those of the skin, eyes and respiratory tract. If glucocorticoids are given, they should be administered with caution depending on the animal's renal status.

## PROGNOSIS AND COURSE

The degree of intoxication and the promptness with which proper treatment is initiated are the two most important factors which govern the prognosis in thallium-poisoned animals.

Animals suffering from mild intoxication which receive prompt treatment stand a fair to good chance for recovery. However, as both the dose of thallium ingested and the time between exposure and treatment increase, the animal's chances for survival greatly diminish.

## SUPPLEMENTAL READING

Buck, W. B., Osweiler, G. D., and Van Gelder, G. A.: Clinical and Diagnostic Veterinary Toxicology. Dubuque, Iowa, Kendall-Hunt Publishing Co., 1973.

Budinger, J. M.: Diphenylthiocarbazone blindness in dogs. Arch. Path., 71:304, 1961.

Casarett, L. J., and Doull, J. (eds.): Toxicology—The Basic Science of Poisons. New York, Macmillan Co., 1975.

Clarke, E. G. C., and Clarke, J. L.: Garner's Veterinary Toxicology. 3rd ed. Baltimore, The Williams & Wilkins Co., 1967.

Doak, R. L., et al.: Thallium intoxication: a specific antidote, supportive therapy and clinical evaluation. Vet. Med./Small Animal Clin., 60:1227, 1965.

Gabriel, K. L., and Dubin, S.: A method for the detection of thallium in canine urine. J. Am. Vet. Med. Assn., 143:772, 1963.

Heylauf, H.: Ferric-cyanoferrate: an effective antidote in thallium poisoning. Europ. J. Pharmacol., 6:340–344, 1969.

Lee, A. G.: The Chemistry of Thallium. New York, Elsevier Publishing Company, 1971.

Mather, G. W., and Low, D. G.: Thallium intoxication in dogs. J. Am. Vet. Med. Assn., 137:544, 1960.

Radeleff, R. D.: Veterinary Toxicology. Philadelphia, Lea & Febiger, 1964.

Schwartzman, R. M., and Kirschbaum, J. O.: Cutaneous histopathology of thallium poisoning. Small Animal Clinician, 2:30, 1962.

Skelley, J. F., and Gabriel, K. L.: Thallium intoxication in the dog. Ann. N.Y. Acad. Sci., 111:612, 1964.

Wilson, J. R.: Thallotoxicosis. J. Am. Vet. Med. Assn., 139:1116, 1961.

Zook, B. C., Holzworth, J., and Thornton, G. W.: Thallium poisoning in cats. J. Am. Vet. Med. Assn., 153:285, 1968.

# LEAD POISONING

BERNARD C. ZOOK, D.V.M.
*Washington, D.C.,*

*and* JAMES L. CARPENTER, D.V.M.
*Boston, Massachusetts*

Lead poisoning is one of the most common toxicologic disorders in dogs. About one of every 25 dogs under six months of age, hospitalized at the Angell Memorial Animal Hospital in Boston, has been poisoned by lead. The incidence of subclinical lead intoxication is also apparently very high, especially in dogs living in slum areas or found in city pounds. It is suspected that stress may precipitate clinical signs in these dogs, and some evidence suggests that subclinical plumbism predisposes to infectious diseases.

Lead poisoning may occur at any age, but most affected dogs are between two and eight months of age. Teething and the bizarre appetites of young dogs result in the gnawing on and ingestion of strange substances, and man has unwittingly provided abundant sources of lead within easy access.

Lead poisoning occurs more frequently in summer and fall, possibly because of the influence of vitamin D on the intestinal absorption of lead. Good weather may also allow access to more sources of lead.

## SOURCES OF LEAD

The sources of lead are varied and numerous, the most common being lead-containing paint. Interiors of dwellings painted before 1940 often contain layers of lead-based paint. Leaded paints are sometimes mistakenly used indoors and thus may be accessible to dogs in new as well as old dwellings. Exteriors of buildings (including dog houses) are frequently covered with leaded paint, as are fences and painting materials. Soil and vegetation may be contaminated with lead as a result of the weathering of lead pigments from painted structures.

Other sources of lead include linoleum; batteries; plumbing materials; putty; lead foil; solder; golf balls; certain roof coverings, lubricants and rug pads; acid (soft) drinking water from lead pipes or in improperly glazed ceramic water bowls; and lead weights or objects such as fishing sinkers, drapery weights and toys. Soil along streets and roadways may contain small amounts of lead from automobile exhaust fumes. Soil contaminated with lead from paint or auto exhausts is not a likely source of poisoning, but may contribute somewhat to the total body burden of lead. Some pet foods have been found to contain up to 7 ppm lead. Dog food is unlikely to be a sole source of lead poisoning, but it certainly contributes to a dog's overall lead burden.

The history may or may not suggest exposure to lead. Recent remodeling of dwellings, especially old dilapidated houses, including removal of old paint, plaster or linoleum, or application of new lead-based paints, is a common history. In many instances, it is impossible to determine which of many possible sources of lead has poisoned a particular dog.

## DOSE, ABSORPTION AND EXCRETION OF LEAD

Diets containing 100 ppm lead, and doses as low as 0.3 mg./kg./day, have been found to be toxic to immature dogs after several months' ingestion. Young dogs retain about 36 per cent of their dietary lead, whereas adults retain only about 10 per cent. Lead is eliminated very slowly and largely in the feces; only about 1 per cent of lead excreted is found in the urine.

## CLINICAL SIGNS

Clinical signs of lead poisoning in dogs are referable to the gastrointestinal and nervous systems. Usually both systems are clinically involved, but sometimes only one is. A period of gastrointestinal disturbances may be followed by a quiescent stage, after which convulsions, champing fits or other signs of serious nervous derangement predominate. Such histories and clinical signs in young dogs have led to erroneous diagnoses of canine distemper.

Gastrointestinal signs occur in about 90 per cent of dogs. Colic, often a pronounced sign, is manifested by whining, restlessness, abnormal positions, tensing of abdominal muscles and crying when the abdomen is palpated. Colic is apparently the result of smooth muscle spasms induced by lead. Intermittent vomiting and partial anorexia are frequent. Burtonian (lead) lines in the gums are rarely, if ever, found in dogs.

Neurologic changes caused by lead may be responsible for a variety of clinical disorders. Hysteria, characterized by sudden excitement or apparent fear and the dog's running wildly about while barking continuously, is a typical manifestation. Our experience indicates that 90 to 95 per cent of dogs with hysteria have lead poisoning. Grand mal seizures are also common and may be accompanied by frothing and champing of the jaws. Fever is generally absent; however, body temperature is often elevated during and briefly following nervous seizures. Heat stroke and lead poisoning may occur together, perhaps by one disease bringing about clinical signs of the other.

Other signs of brain or nerve injury, in approximate order of frequency, are nervousness, whining, behavioral changes (i.e., aggressiveness, hiding, failing to respond to commands), retraction of the eyeball with resultant protrusion of the nictitating membrane, myoclonus, photophobia, miosis, incoordination, paresis, stupor, esophageal paralysis and amaurosis.

Differential diagnoses, based on history and clinical signs, include poisoning by other sources, intestinal parasitism, intussusception, acute pancreatitis, heat stroke, infectious canine hepatitis, encephalitis, rabies and, above all, canine distemper. It may be difficult or impossible to distinguish these diseases by history and physical examination alone.

## RADIOGRAPHIC FINDINGS

Radiographic findings can at times be helpful in diagnosis. Ingested substances that contain lead are quite radiopaque and readily visible on abdominal radiograms. At the time clinical signs develop, however, lead may no longer be detected in the gastrointestinal tract. Furthermore, gravel or chips of bone may be radiographically indistinguishable from lead-containing substances. Examination of feces for chips of paint or bone may suggest the nature of substances in the gastrointestinal tract that were visualized by radiography.

The metaphyses of long bones may develop lead lines in immature dogs with poisoning of over 10 days' duration. These radiopaque bands occur in many bones, including ribs, but are best seen just proximal to the open epiphyses of the distal radius, ulna and metacarpal bones. This change is the result of the incorporation of lead into sites of active bone formation, causing a dense zone of mineralized cartilage and bone in the metaphysis called metaphyseal sclerosis. Similar radiographic changes are reported in phosphorus and vitamin D intoxication.

## LABORATORY FINDINGS

The hematologic findings in dogs with lead poisoning are so consistent and characteristic that they are almost pathognomonic. A well stained direct smear of the peripheral blood provides an excellent screening test. Typical blood changes precede clinical signs except in rare, very acute poisonings, and they are found in all stages of the disease.

Corrected white blood cell counts are often elevated because of a neutrophilic leukocytosis. A shift to the left is common. The hematocrit is usually normal, but mild to moderate hypochromic anemia develops in chronic poisoning. Of prime importance is the finding of large numbers of nucleated red blood cells in the peripheral blood smear (Fig. 1). Nucleated red blood cells are found in the blood of nearly all lead-poisoned dogs. The number may vary from one to more than 300/100 white blood cells, but 10 to 40/100 white blood cells is com-

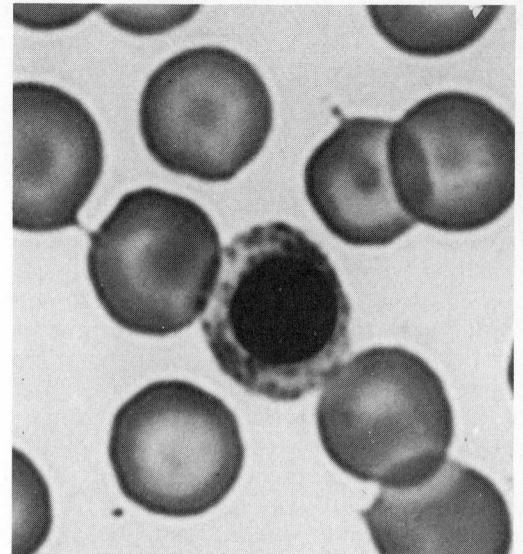

**Figure 1.** Nucleated erythrocyte with basophilic stippling in dog with lead poisoning. Wright-Giemsa stain.

mon. Basophilic stippling of red blood cells is another almost constant feature of the disease. Stippled red blood cells contain clusters of very fine blue dots or larger (0.5 to 1.0$\mu$m.) blue-black granules. Stippled cells are best found in unfixed direct smears stained with neutral Wright-Giemsa stain. Polychromatophilia, anisocytosis, poikilocytosis and target cells are also numerous.

Moderate numbers of nucleated red blood cells and a few stippled red blood cells may be found in some dogs with marked and prolonged anemias, e.g., autoimmune hemolytic anemia. Older dogs that have visceral hemangiosarcomas are usually anemic and have numerous nucleated red blood cells, but rare or no stippled red blood cells. To our knowledge, no other diseases of dogs are associated with many nucleated and stippled red blood cells.

The finding of numerous nucleated, stippled and other immature red blood cells in the absence of severe anemia is characteristic. Blood may be taken for lead analysis to confirm the diagnosis, but treatment for lead poisoning should be started immediately.

Results of other laboratory tests, such as blood urea nitrogen, creatinine, transaminase, amylase, blood glucose, sedimentation rate and Coombs' test, are normal. Bone marrow examination discloses an increase of erythroid elements. Elevated reticulocyte counts and the finding of many immature red blood cells in peripheral blood smears indicate early release of erythroid cells from the hyperplastic bone marrow. The urine usually contains granular casts; often mild proteinuria and sometimes glycosuria are found. The cerebrospinal fluid may have a normal pressure, protein and cell content.

## DIAGNOSIS

The finding of many nucleated and stippled erythrocytes in a dog that is not markedly anemic is, as mentioned above, essentially diagnostic. Lead poisoning can be confirmed by finding excess lead in the blood. Many diagnostic laboratories perform analysis for lead in blood; however, the results from some laboratories are not always reliable. Most methods require 10 ml. of whole, oxalated or heparinized blood in a clean, lead-free vial. Versenate (EDTA) anticoagulant interferes with some methods. The finding of 60 $\mu$g. or more of lead/100 ml. of blood (0.6 ppm) is virtually diagnostic of lead poisoning in dogs. Blood lead values of 40 to 50 $\mu$g./100 ml. (0.4 to 0.5 ppm) are abnormally high and indicate lead poisoning if associated with typical signs and hematologic findings.

Samples of liver obtained post mortem and analyzed for lead provide the best single diagnostic test for lead poisoning. The upper limit of normal is 3.5 ppm (wet weight); 5 ppm or more is virtually diagnostic. Samples of hair, feces or single specimens of urine for lead analysis are not recommended. Urine specimens taken just before and 24 hours after starting chelation therapy (calcium disodium edetate [CaEDTA] at the dosage administered for regular treatment) disclose a tenfold to sixty-fold increase in urine lead output in dogs with lead poisoning. Although this test is reliable, it is difficult to obtain the specimens and is expensive and time-consuming.

## TREATMENT

Untreated, lead intoxication is often fatal, but fortunately effective therapy is available.

The purposes of therapy in lead poisoning are to remove lead, if present, from the gastrointestinal tract so that further absorption is prevented, to remove lead from the blood and body tissues rapidly, and to alleviate marked neurologic signs in individual cases that require it.

Lead should be removed from the gastrointestinal tract prior to chelation therapy, as chelating agents may enhance the absorption of lead from the intestines. Lead-containing substances are most often found in the large intestine. Enemas, such as Fleet enema, effectively remove these materials. Emetics can remove lead-containing substances from the stomach. Surgery may be required to remove lead objects too large (as determined by radiography) for safe passage by other methods.

Lead that has been absorbed into the body is effectively removed by one of several chelating agents. These agents combine with lead (and other substances such as calcium), forming a nontoxic complex that is rapidly removed from the blood by the kidneys. The chelating agent of choice is CaEDTA, which has been shown to be effective in treating lead poisoning in a wide variety of animals. The CaEDTA must be administered as the calcium chelate in order to prevent hypocalcemia. Renal damage has occurred in man due to excessive CaEDTA; however, we have found no evidence of any side effects in dogs. Nonetheless, the daily dose should not exceed 2 gm., and therapy should not be continued for more than five consecutive days.

CaEDTA is given at the rate of 100 mg./kg. of body weight daily for five days. The daily dose is divided into four equal portions and administered subcutaneously after dilution to a concentration of about 10 mg. CaEDTA/ml. of 5 per cent dextrose solution. Higher concentrations of CaEDTA can cause painful reactions at injection sites.

CaEDTA given at recommended doses and properly divided four times daily is extremely effective; the results are often dramatic. In most cases, vast clinical improvement occurs within 48 hours—often sooner. Dogs that respond slowly or have a pretreatment blood level of lead of more than 100 $\mu$g./100 ml. (1.0 ppm) should be given a second five-day treatment five days after completion of the first series. This second treatment prevents recurrence of clinical signs, provided the dog is not allowed to consume more lead after discharge from the hospital.

A combination of British anti-lewisite

(BAL) and CaEDTA has been used with success in children poisoned by lead. Although it may be just as effective in dogs, it is difficult to imagine much improvement over CaEDTA alone, in which the dosage and course of treatment are well established.

Penicillamine (Cuprimine® [Merck]), oral chelating agent of proven value in treating lead-poisoned children, offers promise for dogs. Penicillamine, given orally, has a distinct advantage over CaEDTA, which must be repeatedly injected subcutaneously, requiring at least five days of hospitalization. Clinical trials to date indicate that penicillamine is effective in promoting urinary excretion of lead and alleviating clinical signs, although it is somewhat less effective than CaEDTA.

Penicillamine, given in a dose of 100 mg./kg. body weight daily, has some undesirable effects, such as vomiting, listlessness and partial anorexia. At present, penicillamine can be recommended for dogs that are not seriously ill or do not have marked neurologic disorders or persistent vomiting. If an owner refuses to hospitalize his dog, penicillamine can be prescribed; however, the owner should be warned that the side effects may occur and that any lead ingested while on treatment is apt to be absorbed more completely than without treatment.

It seems that penicillamine might also be beneficial in combination with CaEDTA. It may be that CaEDTA needs to be given for only a few days, followed by penicillamine. This regimen should assure adequate hydration, promote renal function and help reduce the care and cost of treatment. Penicillamine might also be useful in treating dogs that recovered slowly from a five-day course of CaEDTA or had an initial blood lead level of more than 100 $\mu$g./100 ml. (1.0 ppm) and therefore should be treated again.

[*Editor's Note:* Recently, Center and Aronson have reported adverse reactions with the use of CaEDTA in dogs suspected of lead poisoning. The initial signs are depression, anorexia, vomiting and diarrhea. The drug depresses turnover of DNA, and its early effect is to reduce the normal rapid regrowth of epithelial cells of the villi of the small intestine. These toxic effects may be lessened by administering the drug on alternate days only. The drug should be withdrawn at the first appearance of any of the above signs, and good nursing care should be instituted. Oral zinc supplementation may aid in reversing toxic manifestations.]

## ANCILLARY TREATMENT

Nonspecific therapy in canine lead poisoning is directed primarily against severe neurologic signs. Chelating agents apparently do not cross the blood-brain barrier. Administration of barbiturates or tranquilizers may be necessary to control seizures or allay severe nervousness or aggression. These drugs are seldom necessary after 48 hours of chelation therapy. Dexamethazone or mannitol may be used in an effort to relieve cerebral edema. Permanent mental deficiencies and recurrent seizures are common sequelae of lead poisoning in children. Thus, it seems appropriate to treat lead encephalopathy in dogs as well, because these drugs not only appear to speed clinical recovery, but also may prevent permanent brain damage. Other symptomatic or supportive treatment is seldom required.

## PROGNOSIS

Prognoses in untreated cases of lead poisoning are unfavorable; fatal termination may be expected. Although clinical signs have been known to disappear after cage rest or anticonvulsant therapy, they usually return. Prognoses in cases treated promptly and adequately depend upon the degree and duration of neurologic involvement and, to a lesser extent, upon the amount of lead found in the blood. Continuous or uncontrolled convulsions warrant an unfavorable prognosis. Dogs with 100 $\mu$g. or more of lead/100 ml. of blood tend to recover slowly, and signs may recur if a second course of therapy is not given. If there are no neurologic signs, or if they are mild or readily controlled by ancillary treatment, the prognosis is favorable. If the recommended course of treatment is zealously implemented, recovery should be rapid and complete in about 95 per cent of cases.

## PROPHYLAXIS

Prevention of further exposure to lead is, needless to say, an important part of the general treatment. The owner should be made aware of the nearly countless possible sources of lead (some of which are hazards to children as well as to dogs, especially lead paints). Many people are apparently unaware of the danger of lead-containing paint, or erroneously believe that modern paints do not contain lead. Pet owners should be instructed to recognize and remove sources of lead or confine dogs to safe surroundings.

## PATHOLOGIC FINDINGS

Gross necropsic findings are generally not remarkable; however, careful examination may reveal chips of paint or other lead-containing substances in the gastrointestinal tract. White bands are sometimes found in transversely sectioned metaphyses of immature dogs. Microscopic study may disclose acid-fast intranuclear inclusion bodies in renal proximal tubular cells, and less often in hepatocytes. These inclusions are essentially pathognomonic of lead poisoning, but are not found in all cases. Lesions in the brain include degenerative changes in small vessels, hemorrhages, laminar necrosis, and proliferation of capillaries and gliosis in chronic encephalopathies.

## LEAD POISONING IN OTHER PETS

Monkeys dwelling in cages painted with leaded paint are commonly poisoned by lead. It is suspected that the curious nature and indiscriminate eating habits of young Old World primates make them highly susceptible to lead ingestion. Convulsions, with or without blindness, are often the first manifestations. Blood changes may be absent or minimal; basophilic stippling may or may not be present. Radiographic lead lines may be seen in the bones of growing primates. Blood lead values over 80 $\mu$g./100 ml. (0.8 ppm) should be considered strong evidence of lead poisoning, although higher levels have been observed in asymptomatic monkeys.

Cats are rarely poisoned by lead; only four cases have been reported. Only two cases were found after diligent search among this hospital's admissions. Cats, unlike dogs and Old World monkeys, are very selective eaters and seldom gnaw on or ingest nonfood substances; they are thus not subject to most sources of lead. Because of their fastidious fur-cleaning habits, however, they may ingest lead-containing dusts or other substances that contaminate their coat. The two cases observed had neurologic signs and hematologic changes similar to those in dogs.

Parrots may pick at and ingest peeling paint or, if the bars of their cages are painted, they may ingest the paint while clambering about or trimming their beaks. At least two pet parrots and numerous zoo parrots are known to have died of lead poisoning. No hematologic changes were seen in the parrots studied. Any curious pet with indiscriminate eating habits and exposure to lead is a likely candidate for lead intoxication.

Treatment of three monkeys and two cats with CaEDTA has proven successful. Dosages and methods of administration were the same as for dogs.

### SUPPLEMENTAL READING

Center, S. A., and Aronson, A. L.: Calcium EDTA toxicity in a dog. J. Am. Vet. Med. Assn., in preparation, 1977.

Zook, B. C.: The pathologic anatomy of lead poisoning. Vet. Pathol., 9:310–327, 1972.

Zook, B. C., Carpenter, J. L., and Leeds, E. B.: Lead poisoning in dogs. J. Am. Vet. Med. Assn., 155:1329–1342, 1969.

Zook, B. C., Carpenter, J. L., and Roberts, R. M.: Lead poisoning in dogs: occurrence, source, clinical pathology and electroencephalography. Am. J. Vet. Res., 33:891–902, 1972.

Zook, B. C., et al.: Lead poisoning in dogs: analysis of blood, urine, hair, and liver for lead. Am. J. Vet. Res., 33:903–909, 1972.

# ARSENIC POISONING

ALLAN FURR, D.V.M.
*Ames, Iowa*

The increasing restrictions on the use of inorganic arsenicals in pesticide formulations have resulted in a noticeable decrease in the incidence of confirmed arsenic toxicoses in pet animals. There are, however, occasional episodes of poisoning in animals that have been accidentally exposed to improperly handled supplies of arsenicals that are no longer permitted and to improperly used approved compounds, such as ant poisons, herbicides and insecticides.

The route of exposure is usually by ingestion, thus the veterinarian is concerned with treating either an acute or a peracute condition. The arsenic compounds are considered to be highly toxic with a rapid onset of clinical signs. Often, the affected animal is found dead with no clinical signs having been observed.

The toxicity and rapidity of onset are variable, depending upon the age and the species of animal. The chemical form and solubility of the toxicant also play a role in the course of the clinical syndrome. Inorganic arsenicals inhibit the sulfhydryl enzyme systems which are essential for normal cellular respiration and for metabolism of fats and carbohydrates.

The onset of clinical signs is usually rapid, from 30 minutes to several hours, after ingestion. The initial signs are restlessness, nausea and repeated vomition. There is severe abdominal pain; the animal becomes weak and develops a watery diarrhea that may contain flecks of blood and mucosal tags. The pulse becomes feeble and fast. The respiratory rate generally increases while the temperature may be below normal, normal or above normal, depending on the physical stress of the animal. The animal becomes severely depressed and regresses into shock due to dehydration as a result of vomition and diarrhea. In addition, there is a transudation of fluids due to the disruption of the integrity of the capillaries and extensive hemorrhaging, especially of the alimentary tract. Collapse and death can rapidly occur after the onset of clinical signs.

Therapeutic measures are intended to either remove or inactivate the unabsorbed material in the intestine, protect the alimentary tract, reverse the toxic syndrome and restore the homeostatic equilibrium of the animal.

The animal that is not showing clinical signs but is suspected to have ingested an arsenic compound is given a gastric lavage with warm water followed by apomorphine (SC) to induce vomition. Following evacuation of the alimentary tract, the animal can be given a preventive IM injection of BAL (Dimercaprol) at 5 mg./kg. of body weight, repeated in 3 to 4 hours at 2 mg./kg. if indicated. Also recommended is the administration of sodium thiosulfate (10 per cent solution) at up to one gram per day divided into four doses. The addition of ascorbic acid at up to one gram a day has been found to be beneficial. Sodium thiosulfate and ascorbic acid have a wide margin of safety, whereas BAL is relatively toxic.

The animal that has already developed advanced clinical signs and has already evacuated the alimentary tract is treated heroically, with a grave prognosis being rendered. BAL is not very effective in advanced cases but is still used. Sodium thiosulfate and ascorbic acid should be administered and repeated at 6-hour intervals. Whole blood at 10 ml./kg. or plasma extenders should be given IV to restore the blood volume. If neither blood nor plasma extenders are available, the animal should be rehydrated with lactated Ringer's solution. Supportive therapy with fluids, B-complex vitamins and amino acids should be continued as indicated throughout the course of the syndrome. Antibiotics should be used to prevent invasion by opportunistic bacteria. The animal should be kept warm and comfortable in a draft-free area.

When the animal has recovered sufficiently, small amounts of high-quality protein food should be given with a limited amount of water until the alimentary tract will tolerate a normal diet.

Samples of urine, vomitus and the suspected toxicant should be chemically analyzed for the presence and quantity of arsenic to provide a confirmatory diagnosis.

### SUPPLEMENTAL READING

Buck, W. B., Osweiler, G. D., and Van Gelder, G. A. : Clinical and Diagnostic Toxicology. Dubuque, Iowa, Kendall-Hunt Publishing Co., 1973.

Goodman, L. S., and Gilman, A.: The Pharmacological Basis of Therapeutics. 4th ed. The Macmillan Co., 1970.

Kirk, R. W. (ed.): Current Veterinary Therapy V. Philadelphia, W. B. Saunders Co., 1974.

Radeleff, R. D.: Veterinary Toxicology. 2nd ed. Philadelphia, Lea & Febiger, 1970.

Rossoff, I.: Handbook of Veterinary Drugs. New York, Springer Publishing Co., 1974.

---

# ANTIFREEZE (ETHYLENE GLYCOL) POISONING

FREDERICK W. OEHME, D.V.M.
*Manhattan, Kansas*

Antifreeze toxicity is a common poisoning in small domestic animals. The major toxic component is ethylene glycol, which comprises 95 per cent or more of most commercial antifreeze preparations. Dogs and cats have frequently consumed radiator drainage containing antifreeze, probably due to its sweet taste. The incidence of antifreeze poisoning increases significantly in the fall of the year, when radiators are being drained and new antifreeze is being incorporated into automobile and other machinery-cooling systems. The toxic dose that has been reported in dogs varies from 4.2 to 6.6 ml. of ethylene glycol/kg. of body weight. Interestingly, the fatal dose of ethylene glycol in cats has been given as only 1.5 ml./kg.

## CLINICAL SYNDROMES

The clinical diagnosis and treatment of ethylene glycol poisoning are difficult since animals progress through varying stages of signs, and the clinician may be presented with the patient at any phase of the syndrome. The basis of ethylene glycol toxicity is twofold: (1) acute toxicity and acidosis due to rapid absorption of a large dose from the digestive tract; or if the amount of ethylene glycol absorbed is small and time permits, (2) the metabolism of ethylene glycol through a series of metabolites to oxalic acid which then combines with calcium to form a calcium oxalate complex that is deposited in the renal tubules, causing tubular epithelial damage, renal failure and death due to uremia. Thus the clinician may be presented with dogs or cats in the acute acidotic phase or with the animal in the more chronic uremic syndrome resulting from renal failure.

**Acute Ethylene Glycol Poisoning.** Absorbed ethylene glycol doses in excess of approximately 6 ml./kg. of body weight characteristically produce an acute depression and death within 12 to 36 hours after ingestion. If observed, initial clinical signs of apprehension, moderate depression and mild ataxia are seen 30 to 60 minutes after ethylene glycol ingestion. Vomiting frequently occurs and progressive depression, incoordination and ataxia are followed by paresis and coma. Coma usually occurs 6 to 12 hours after ingestion and progresses to death. Although convulsions are not common, some patients may display involuntary forced muscular activity ("paddling") in the terminal phases of poisoning.

Postmortem examination predominantly reveals various degrees of digestive tract hyperemia. In addition, acute congestion of body tissues and swelling of the kidneys may be observed, but the latter is more common with animals surviving longer periods of time. Examination of urine sediments will show increasing numbers of oxalate crystals beginning approximately six hours after ingestion. Such crystals in the urinary sediment or those observed in kidney impression smears or upon histopathologic examination of kidney tissue are useful diagnostic aids. However, the clinician should realize that small numbers of oxalate crystals may be observed in the urinary sediment of normal dogs.

**Chronic Ethylene Glycol Poisoning and Uremia.** Dogs and cats surviving more than 24 hours exhibit increasing levels of blood urea nitrogen. The clinical signs described for the acute syndrome are present but in milder degrees. Vomiting and progressive depression with ataxia and eventual paresis may occur 3 to 10 days following ingestion of ethylene glycol. Such animals have ingested smaller amounts of ethylene glycol or may have vomited significant portions of the compound prior to absorption from the stomach. Increasing thirst is initially apparent, but renal failure results in small amounts of dark-colored urine being voided and eventual anuria. Blood urea nitrogen levels are often in excess of 200 mg./100 ml. when coma develops. Muscle fasciculations, paddling of the limbs in slow running movements, occasional periods of diffuse and general muscle contractions, and neuromuscular manifestations of uremia may be seen. The terminal uremia leads to death.

Postmortem examination of these animals reveals cachexia, dehydration, oral ulcerations and a hemorrhagic gastritis. The kidneys may be swollen. Impression smears of the kidneys reveal abundant numbers of oxalate crystals; these are readily observed primarily in the proximal tubules when histopathologic examination utilizing polarized light is performed. In addition to the presence of oxalate crystals, cystic tubules, congestion, proteinaceous casts and varying degrees of tubular epithelial damage are observed.

## DIAGNOSIS

The clinical signs of ethylene glycol poisoning are predominantly vomiting, progressive depression and coma with or without neuromuscular activity. These are extremely difficult to differentiate from other causes of similar signs during the acute syndrome, but the presence of numerous oxalate crystals in urinary sediment may be

of value. Other intoxications, acute metabolic acidoses and neuromuscular injuries and diseases must also be differentiated from ethylene glycol poisoning. Animals with rising blood urea nitrogen levels and the presence of abundant oxalate crystals in urinary sediment should be suspected of having ethylene glycol poisoning.

Commercial laboratories are capable of determining ethylene glycol or oxalate levels in whole blood samples. Practitioners with such facilities available may utilize them for diagnostic benefit. On histopathologic examination of kidney sections, the observation of abundant calcium oxalate crystals in the tubular lumen under polarizing light is characteristic.

## TREATMENT

Successful therapy of antifreeze poisoning is based upon a favorable combination of several factors: (1) limited ingestion and absorption of ethylene glycol; (2) rapid diagnosis and initiation of treatment following poisoning; and (3) faithful application of a systematic therapeutic regimen of ethanol and sodium bicarbonate.

Animals receiving unusually large dosages of ethylene glycol (in excess of 10 ml./kg. of body weight in dogs; in excess of 8 ml./kg. of body weight in cats) are incapable of responding to any therapy. The rapid absorption and metabolic conversion of the ethylene glycol to a series of acids results in an acute acidosis and prompt death. Animals ingesting such large quantities of ethylene glycol are rarely seen except in a comatose condition, at which time diagnosis is extremely difficult and biologic response to antidotal therapy improbable.

Animals receiving lethal amounts of ethylene glycol respond to therapy in direct relation to the promptness with which therapy is instituted. In general, dogs will recover from twice the lethal dose of ethylene glycol if treatment is instituted within 12 hours following ingestion. Cats respond to therapy for three times the lethal dose of ethylene glycol if therapy is instituted at least eight hours following ingestion. This observation is logical when one realizes that the ethylene glycol, in itself, is relatively nontoxic; it is the metabolites that induce the toxicosis. Hence, the longer the period of time allowed for metabolism to occur before therapy is instituted, the less the chance of successful treatment and recovery.

Successful therapy of ethylene glycol poisoning in dogs and cats depends upon the repeated systemic administration of solutions of 20 per cent ethanol and 5 per cent sodium bicarbonate. In dogs, the optimal dosage levels are 5.5 ml. of 20 per cent ethanol/kg. of body weight given intravenously and 8 ml. of 5 per cent sodium bicarbonate/kg. of body weight given intraperitoneally. This treatment level must be repeated every four hours for a total of five treatments, and then every six hours for four additional treatments. In cats, lower enzyme levels require that the dosage be altered. Five milliliters of 20 per cent ethanol and 6 ml. of 5 per cent sodium bicarbonate are given per kilogram of body weight, both intraperitoneally. This is administered every six hours for a total of five treatments, and then given four more times at eight-hour intervals.

The treatment rationale is based upon ethanol blocking the enzymes responsible for metabolizing the ethylene glycol to the more toxic end-products. Hence only limited oxalic acid is produced and reduced calcium oxalate formation and renal deposition of crystals occur. The administration of sodium bicarbonate prevents and reverses the acidosis, favors increased excretion of the unmetabolized ethylene glycol and reduces calcium oxalate formation by altering urinary pH. Renal excretion of unchanged ethylene glycol is further enhanced by the volume of fluids being administered and the availability of frequent small amounts of drinking water to animals undergoing therapy.

Even though the amount of ethylene glycol ingested by spontaneously poisoned animals is often impossible to determine, clinical evaluation and prognosis is possible approximately 12 to 16 hours into the therapeutic regimen. Animals regaining consciousness, drinking water and perhaps walking with difficulty after the third or fourth treatments may reasonably be estimated to have absorbed limited amounts of ethylene glycol. The prognosis for recovery with completion of the entire treatment schedule is fair to good. Animals undergoing therapy that do not regain consciousness between treatments have a poor potential for recovery. Likewise, dogs presented in coma with suspected ethylene glycol ingestion must be given poor prognoses. Such animals are frequently in a terminal state of either acute intoxication or in the more chronic renal syndrome with uremia. Such animals will not respond to ethanol-bicarbonate therapy.

While not readily available under most clinical circumstances, the application of hemodialysis and fluid therapy would be useful in comatose ethylene glycol-poisoned animals. Peritoneal dialysis is a practical compromise for hemodialysis, but does not provide the effective cleansing of biological fluids achieved by the latter. Until the present experimental resins and other techniques are further developed for practical "cage-side" use in dialyzing whole blood of foreign compounds, the prompt and conscientious application of ethanol and sodium bicarbonate remains the most effective treatment for antifreeze (ethylene glycol) poisoning in dogs and cats.

### SUPPLEMENTAL READING

Beckett, S. D., and Shields, R. P.: Treatment of acute ethylene glycol (antifreeze) toxicosis in the dog. J. Am. Vet. Med. Assn., *158*:472–476, 1971.

Kersting, E. J., and Nielsen, S. W.: Ethylene glycol poisoning in small animals. J. Am. Vet. Med. Assn., *146*:113–118, 1965.

Kersting, E. J., and Nielsen, S. W.: Experimental ethylene glycol poisoning the the dog. Am. J. Vet. Res., *27*:574–582, 1966.

Nunamaker, D. M., Medway, W., and Berg, P.: Treatment of ethylene glycol poisoning in the dog. J. Am. Vet. Med. Assn., *159*:310–314, 1971.

Penumarthy, L., and Oehme, F. W.: Treatment of ethylene glycol toxicosis in cats. Am. J. Vet. Res., *36*:209–212, 1975.

Sanyer, J. L., Oehme, F. W., and McGavin, M. D.: Systematic treatment of ethylene glycol toxicosis in dogs. Am. J. Vet. Res., *34*:527–534, 1973.

# ORGANO-PHOSPHATE AND CARBAMATE INSECTICIDE POISONING

HARRY E. SMALLEY, D.V.M.
*College Station, Texas*

Recent restrictions on the use of chlorinated hydrocarbon insecticides have emphasized the role that other, less persistent insecticidal compounds must play in the control of insects on domestic animals. Even though some of the alternate insecticides—such as the organophosphate (O-P) and carbamate insecticides—may be much more toxic than the bulk of the chlorinated hydrocarbon insecticides, their lack of persistence in the environment and general lack of residual action in the animal make the O-P and carbamate insecticides more ecologically acceptable.

Although there are some important differences between the O-P and carbamate insecticides, which will be briefly discussed later, the two classes of chemicals are usually discussed together because their primary mode of action is similar. This common action is inhibition of the enzyme acetylcholinesterase. Acetylcholinesterase is an enzyme common to insects and mammals which functions to remove toxic amounts of acetylcholine at nerve synapses and endings; acetylcholine mediates the nerve impulse at neuromuscular junctions and parasympathetic nerve endings. An excess of acetylcholine causes a toxic condition leading to death because of failure of respiration. The nerves most directly affected by an excess of acetylcholine are preganglionic fibers to autonomic ganglia; postganglionic, cholinergic fibers to smooth and cardiac muscle and to secretory cells; and motor nerves to striated muscle. Any abnormal accumulation of acetylcholine elicits specific reactions: a small amount in excess produces abnormal increase in function; a large amount in excess rapidly pro-

duces a decrease in function—to wit, paralysis. Because of the type of nervous stimulation and paralysis, these insecticides are considered to be muscarinic as well as nicotinic in action. The first O-P insecticide was developed in Germany as a substitute for nicotine—tetraethyl pyrophosphate (TEPP)—which was in short supply during World War II. TEPP is considered to be one of the most toxic of the organophosphates, and other extremely toxic compounds were developed as potential chemical warfare agents—sarin, tabun and schradan. These are considered "nerve gases" and are not used as insecticides. Efforts to find more stable compounds led Schrader, in 1944, to synthesize parathion, which, because of its broad range of insecticidal activity and stability, has become one of the most widely used insecticides.

Academically, parathion is not considered toxic. Biotransformation of parathion to its oxygen analog—paroxon—is accomplished in the body by enzyme action; paroxon is extremely toxic. Regardless of the subtle distinction, the "cause-effect" relationship has led to common acceptance of the extreme toxicity of parathion in both insects and mammals.

Although there may be localized effects depending on the type of exposure, systemic effects rapidly become preeminent. Any type of exposure can lead to poisoning—inhalation, dermal, oral, parenteral, ocular, etc.—and, depending on the dose, can cause poisoning. Reaction time, i.e., the time between exposure and reaction, is again dependent on the dose; it may be 2 to 3 minutes with large, overpowering doses, or may be several hours with smaller

138

doses. Minor reactions, generally localized, are seldom seen clinically and have few effects; minor exposure to an aerosol may be noticed only as a slight increase in salivation, or perhaps miosis. Most clinical cases have progressed to the point where the reaction is so obvious that the owner becomes greatly concerned, and the effects have proceeded to the point of a physiologic and toxicologic crisis. Again, the duration of O-P poisoning depends on the dose received, but since the clinician has no idea of the amount of exposure, he must proceed with examination and treatment on an emergency basis.

As you would expect, signs of poisoning reflect the biochemical lesions seen in the nervous system. There are muscular tremors or fasciculations, varying from slight to extreme, which generally progress from the posterior to the anterior of the body. There is, typically, profuse salivation, which, with involuntary champing, causes the mouth to foam and leads laymen to an unwarranted diagnosis. Lacrimation, or tearing, is obvious as is the relaxation of sphincter muscles, causing involuntary urination and defecation. Respiratory signs are alarming and will proceed to paralysis unless treated. Further clinical examination is unnecessary but would reveal a blanching of mucous membranes, tachycardia, elevated blood pressure and hyperglycemia. More often, a quick, searching question to the owner elicits the most probable cause which, with the gross observations, serves to establish a tentative diagnosis, or at least a basis on which to start treatment.

In the laboratory, measurement of the degree of acetylcholinesterase inhibition serves to establish the exposure of the animal to a cholinesterase-inhibiting compound. Tests are based on the kinetics of the reaction in the blood and may serve as corroboration of the clinical diagnosis and may prove to be important in forensic or legal procedures.

A number of the O-P insecticides cause a further sign of poisoning—a paralysis of one, or occasionally both, of the hind limbs. The classic example is Tri-ortho-cresyl-phosphate (TOCP), a chemical often used as an additive to oils which may be under extremes of heat and pressure, such as around oil rigs. Other tri-aryl-phosphates may cause the same condition, which was first described in man during the Prohibition era.

Jamaica ginger, a potent drink, was frequently used with certain additives, leading to a condition in man called "Jake-leg" or "ginger-leg." The cause in both man and animals was found to be similar, the symptoms were similar and the lesion—a progressive demyelination of peripheral nerves—was similar. Another similarity, and even more interesting, is that the action is delayed, i.e., paralysis may not become severe for several days to weeks following exposure. This sign of poisoning is of academic interest because the cholinesterase-inhibitory action is paramount.

There is some evidence of teratogenic action of some of these insecticides but, again, this is not of great importance to the clinician facing a crisis.

## TREATMENT

The veterinarian who is confronted with a shivering, slobbering, defecating, urinating animal in obvious respiratory distress—with an extremely concerned owner—must depend on his own experience and knowledge and proceed with treatment.

Very soon after the elucidation of action of the O-P compounds, the antagonistic action of atropine was deduced pharmacologically. Atropine is, however, specific only in counteracting some of the more important effects of acetylcholine excess, and specific antidotes were developed later.

The first consideration in any emergency is maintenance of the life processes. Thus, if the animal's respiratory distress has progressed to the point of cessation, artificial respiration must be given. If the patient is in convulsions, they can be relieved with ether administration or trimethadione. Do not administer succinylcholine, morphine or any of the phenothiazine derivative tranquilizers.

Once the patient is somewhat stabilized as to respiration or convulsions, intravenous administration of an aqueous solution of atropine sulfate should be given. Depending on the size of the animal, one fourth of the total calculated dose should be given intravenously and the remaining three fourths should be given intramuscularly or subcutaneously. The total dose should not exceed 2 mg. The response of the patient is almost magical, occurring within a very few minutes, and is very impressive to the owner. Care must be taken, however, to observe the patient closely for several days—at least 48 hours—because the dose of O-P may be of such magnitude that it overwhelms the action of atropine in time, and the erstwhile recovered patient may die that night. This aspect of O-P poisoning is often neglected and is of such importance that we may very easily say that atropine should be given "to effect." The evils of atropinization (excessive administration of atropine) can easily be seen by the "dry mouth" effect, but this is certainly less evil than O-P poisoning.

Once the patient is stabilized, any apparent source of poisoning should be removed, e.g., washing the animal if exposure was by spraying or dipping, gastric lavage in cases of ingestion.

Specific O-P poisoning can be alleviated as well by 2-PAM (pyridoxine-2-aldoxime, Protopam Chloride®). Protopam will specifically reverse the inhibition of cholinesterase at 10 to 100 mg./kg. of body weight. *2-PAM is contraindicated in poisonings by carbamate insecticides.*

The specific insecticide suspected of poisoning should be determined from the owner. Atropine alone is the specific antidote for carbamate poisoning and is a general or symptomatic antidote for O-P poisoning. In general, the inhibition seen in carbamate toxicities is temporary and of a transient nature, but the magnitude of the dose may be so overwhelming that corrective action should be taken early. Additionally, it has been shown that forced diuresis is of value in rapid excretion of some carbamate compounds.

Activated charcoal, given as an oral slurry, has had some beneficial effects in adsorbing ingested poisons.

Although the toxicant action of both O-P insecticides and carbamate insecticides is the same (which is why I have not distinguished them here), there are important differences, foremost of which is that the cholinesterase-inhibiting action of the carbamate insecticides is reversible. The use of 2-PAM or Protopam in carbamate poisonings will exacerbate the symptoms instead of alleviating them.

The relative acute toxicities of most toxicants are determined in the laboratory using a single oral dose in the rat and are recorded as $LD_{50}$. Naturally there are exceptions to these toxicities depending on sex (males are more susceptible); age (usually the young are more susceptible, but not always); state

of nutrition; state of pregnancy; species (dog is more susceptible to diazinon); etc. Very seldom does the clinician see cases of chronic poisoning, and his/her on-the-spot estimate of the situation is much more pertinent to the case at hand than many of the exceptions noted in the literature. The common names of various O-P insecticides are given in Table 1, along with the trade names most often seen or used; by referral to this list, the practitioner may identify the insecticide cited by the patient's owner as being most suspect. The $LD_{50}$ (acute oral in

**Table 1.** *Organophosphate Insecticides with Acute Oral $LD_{50}$ Values in Rats*

| INSECTICIDE | ORAL $LD_{50}$ (mg./kg.) |
|---|---|
| Phorate | 1 |
| Thimet® | |
| TEPP | 1.1 |
| Tetron® | |
| Nifos T® | |
| Vapotone® | |
| Demeton | 2 |
| Systox® | |
| Fensulfothion | 2 |
| Dasanit® | 2 |
| Mevinphos | 3 |
| Phosdrin® | |
| Parathion | 3 |
| Thiophos® | |
| Carbophenothion | 6 |
| Trithion® | |
| Disulfoton | 6.8 |
| Di-Syston® | |
| EPN | 7 |
| Dyfonate® | 8 |
| Azinphosmethyl | 13 |
| Guthion® | |
| Gusathion® | |
| Coumaphos | 13 |
| Co-Ral® | |
| Asuntol® | |
| Muscatox® | |
| Ethion | 13 |
| Niollate® | |
| Methyl parathion | 14 |
| Chlorfenvinphos | 15 |
| Supona® | |
| Birlane® | |
| Phosphamidon | 15 |
| Dimecron® | |
| Dioxathion | 19 |
| Delnav® | |
| Azodrin® | 21 |
| Bidrin | 22 |
| Dichlorvos | 25 |
| DDVP | |
| Vapona | |
| Famphur | 35 |
| Famophos | |
| Warbex® | |

*Continued on next page*

**Table 1.** *Organophosphate Insecticides with Acute Oral LD$_{50}$ Values in Rats (Continued)*

| INSECTICIDE | ORAL LD$_{50}$ (mg./kg.) |
|---|---|
| MOCAR® | 61 |
| Diazinon | 66 |
| Dursban® | 97 |
| Dowco 179® | |
| Methyl Trithion® | 98 |
| Ciodrin® | 125 |
| Imidan® | 147 |
| Prolate® | |
| Phosmet | |
| Dimethoate | 155 |
| Cygon® | |
| Fenthion | 178 |
| Baytex® | |
| Dichlofenthion | 270 |
| VC-13® | |
| Naled | 430 |
| Dibrom® | |
| Trichlorfon | 450 |
| Dipterex® | |
| Dylex® | |
| Neguvon® | |
| Ruelene® | 660 |
| Chlorothion | 880 |
| Malathion | 885 |
| Cythion® | |
| Ronnel | 906 |
| Korlan® | |
| Trolene® | |
| Nankor® | |
| Viozene® | |
| Fenchlorphos® | |
| Abate® | 1000 |
| Bithion® | |
| Rabon® | 4000 |
| Gardona® | |

rats) is given for comparative purposes. Table 2 gives the same information for the carbamate insecticides.

## SUPPLEMENTAL READING

Buck, W. D., Osweiler, G. D., and Van Gelder, G. A.: Clinical and Diagnostic Veterinary Toxicology. Dubuque, Iowa, Kendall-Hunt Publishing Co., 1973.

Casarett, L. J., and Doull, J.: Toxicology—The Basic Science of Poisons. The Macmillan Co., New York, 1975.

Kay, K.: Toxicology of pesticides: Recent advances. Env. Res. 6:202–243, 1973.

Matsumura, F.: Toxicology of Insecticides. New York, Plenum Press, 1975.

**Table 2.** *Carbamate Insecticides with Acute Oral LD$_{50}$ Values in Rats*

| INSECTICIDE | LD$_{50}$ (mg./kg.) |
|---|---|
| Aldicarb | 0.8 |
| Temik® | |
| Carbofuran | 5 |
| Furadan® | |
| Zectran | 37 |
| Aminocarb | 50 |
| Matacil® | |
| Propoxur | 83 |
| Baygon® | |
| Undan® | |
| Blattanex® | |
| Bux® | 87 |
| Methiocarb | 100 |
| Mesurol® | |
| Mobam | 150 |
| Landrin | 178 |
| Carbaryl | 300 |
| Sevin® | |

# CHLORINATED HYDROCARBON INSECTICIDE TOXICOSIS

GARY A. VAN GELDER, D.V.M.
*Columbia, Missouri*

Chlorinated hydrocarbon insecticide toxicosis in companion animals primarily results from bathing or dipping the animal in excessive concentrations of the compound. In a 1969 survey of 3452 toxicoses in small animals, approximately 5 per cent involved chlorinated hydrocarbon insecticides. With the increasing emphasis on the use of organophosphate and carbamate insecticides, the incidence of chlorinated hydrocarbon toxicosis will probably decrease. The syndrome involves hyperexcitability, hyperesthesia, tonic-clonic convulsive seizures and often periods of depression. A good history and occasionally laboratory tests are needed to differentiate this toxicosis from infectious encephalopathies and other toxicoses, such as those caused by lead, strychnine, compound 1080 or bacterial toxins. The more frequently encountered chlorinated hydrocarbon insecticides in companion animals include methoxychlor, toxaphene, lindane and chlordane. The compounds are absorbed through the intact skin.

## Clinical signs

The toxicosis begins with a period of hyperexcitability during which there may be exaggerated responses to stimulation by sound, light and touch. Some animals may seem apprehensive. Spontaneous muscle twitching will follow the initial period of hyperexcitability. The spontaneous tremors and fasciculations usually begin in the facial region and progress caudally to involve all the skeletal muscles. This may progress into a tonic-clonic convulsive seizure. The head will be drawn back, accompanied by champing of the jaws and retractions of the lips. The convulsion may start with the animal standing, followed by collapse into lateral recumbency. Rapid paddling of both the front and rear limbs will occur. During the seizure, there may be considerable foam about the mouth, which should not be confused with the excessive salivation seen in organophosphate insecticide poisoning. The animal will experience varying degrees of respiratory paralysis during a seizure. Body temperature may be elevated especially following a seizure.

Seizures will terminate as rapidly as they begin. Depending on the duration and severity, the animal may be inactive and depressed for a few minutes or hours, followed by apparent recovery. A series of seizures may occur. Seizures can be initiated by suddenly presented sensory stimulation such as turning on a light or a sudden loud noise. Handling the animal to restrain it or to give medication may also precipitate another seizure. The animal is less prone to another seizure during the period immediately after the termination of a seizure.

It is not possible accurately to predict the outcome based on the occurrence of clinical signs. Occasional animals will die during seizures. Others will go through several episodes, be very depressed for hours afterward and recover completely over a period of several days.

## Aims of treatment

The treatment is essentially nonspecific, since there is no specific antidote for the chlorinated hydrocarbon insecticides.
1. Sedate the animal to control the convulsive seizures.
2. Remove the source of exposure.
3. Keep the animal in a quiet, darkened area.
4. Provide fluids in protracted cases.

## Treatment

The animal should first be lightly anesthetized with a barbiturate to control convulsive seizures. In cases of dermal exposure, the animal should be bathed immediately with warm, soapy water.

Oral exposures present a more difficult problem. If initiated in the early stage, a saline gastrointestinal lavage will greatly reduce exposure. Maximal benefit can be expected during the first 2 hours following exposure. Emetics should be used with caution, especially in animals showing clinical signs, since the administration of the emetic may initiate a seizure resulting in aspiration of vomitus.

The administration of activated charcoal will limit absorption from the gastrointestinal tract.

## Ancillary treatment

In protracted cases, intravenous fluids plus glucose should be given. The chlorinated hydrocarbon insecticides affect the liver and are primarily eliminated in the urine. Therefore, the maintenance of renal function and provision of adequate energy is important.

## Contraindications

Oily cathartics should never be used, since this will increase absorption of chlorinated hydrocarbon insecticides from the gastrointestinal tract. The use of barbiturate anesthetics, as opposed to other anesthetic agents, is strongly encouraged. Based on limited experimental work by the author, there is some evidence to suggest that phencyclidine derivative drugs (e.g., Sernylan) should not be used to sedate chlorinated hydrocarbon-poisoned animals, since these drugs may potentiate the neurologic effects.

## CONVALESCENCE

If the source of exposure is removed, recovery should be uncomplicated. If the source of exposure is unknown, it is good practice to change feed, water and bedding, especially if the poisoning occurred shortly after a new source was introduced. The animal should not be allowed to roam freely until an extensive search of the habitat has been made to insure that any potential source of exposure has been removed.

## SPECIAL DIAGNOSTIC CONSIDERATIONS

In cases where the source of exposure is unknown or where malicious poisoning is suspected, samples of the vomitus or feces should be collected and saved for chemical analysis. Whole blood samples (10 ml.) from live animals can also be subjected to chemical analysis to identify the compound involved. In cases involving death, 200-gm. tissue samples of brain, liver, fat and kidney should be collected at necropsy for later chemical analysis. Some toxicologists prefer residue analysis of brain tissue, since clinical signs correlate better with brain insecticide levels than with levels in other tissues. There are no specific lesions observable at necropsy.

It is not always necessary to identify the insecticide involved. But occasional cases involving a number of animals may necessitate identifying the specific insecticide present in order to determine the source.

### SUPPLEMENTAL READING

Buck, W., Osweiler, G. D., and Van Gelder, G. A.: Clinical and Diagnostic Veterinary Toxicology. Dubuque, Iowa, Kendall-Hunt Publishing Co., 1976.

Clarke, E. G. C., and Clarke, M. L.: Garner's Veterinary Toxicology. Baltimore, The Williams & Wilkins Co., 1967.

Radeleff, R. D.: Veterinary Toxicology. 2nd ed. Philadelphia, Lea & Febiger, 1970.

# HERBICIDE AND FUNGICIDE POISONING*

E. MURL BAILEY, D.V.M.
College Station, Texas

Herbicides and fungicides have been used in American agriculture for over 20 years. Subsequently, their use in and around homes has increased the hazard for intoxication of dogs and cats. Relatively little has been published on the toxicity of herbicides and fungicides in small animals. To date, intoxications in small animals caused by these agents have not been recognized as important.

The occurrence of intoxications caused by herbicides and fungicides is rare, even with the application of the agents to plants and especially in animals which do not rely upon plants as foodstuffs. With improper storage of these toxic agents, there is a hazard of poisoning in cats and dogs because of the inquisitive nature of these animals. The reported distastefulness of most chemicals even further reduces the amount ingested. The clinical signs generally associated with experimental intoxications due to these agents in dogs and cats are nonspecific gastroenteritis disturbances, listlessness and depression. Staggering and other neuromuscular signs may be present.

The treatment of intoxicated animals is, for the most part, symptomatic. Arsenicals, mercurials and sodium chlorate have specific treatments if the condition is diagnosed soon enough.

*Supported in part by Texas Agricultural Experiment Station, Project No. 01981.

### Table 1.  Some Common Herbicides

| CHEMICAL GROUP | COMMON NAMES |
| --- | --- |
| Chlorophenoxy compounds | 2,4-D, 2,4,5-T |
| Chlorinated aliphatic acids | Erbon, Trichloroacetic acid |
| Amide compounds | Bensulide, Chlorthiamid |
| Carbamate | Chlorpropham |
| Thiocarbamate | Pebulate, Vernolate |
| Phenyl urea | Norea, Chloroxuron, Linuron |
| Arsenicals, inorganic | $K_3As_3O_3$ |
| Arsenicals, organic | Monosodium metha-nearsonate (MSMA) (DSMA) |
| Substituted dinitroanaline compounds | Trifluran, Benefin |
| Dipyridyl compounds | Paraquat, Diquat |
| Phthalmic acid compounds | Naptalam, Dinoseb |
| Sodium chlorate | Sodium chlorate |
| Triazines | Atrazine, Prometone |
| Dinitrophenols | Dinitro-o-cresol |

Tables 1 and 2 are listings of some of the more commonly used herbicides and fungicides.

### SIGNS OF INTOXICATION

Clinical signs associated with herbicide intoxications in small animals are nonspecific. These signs include anorexia, muscular weakness, myotonia, vomiting, diarrhea and death. There may be a contact dermatitis associated with agents such as trichloroacetic acid and paraquat. In addition, paraquat poisoning may induce cyanosis and convulsions. Sodium chlorate, a methemoglobin former, may produce cyanosis, respiratory distress and chocolate-brown–colored blood.

Clinical signs observed with fungicide poisoning may be similar to those observed in herbicide intoxication. In addition, there may be greater involvement of the central nervous system, including ataxia, tremors, collapse, depression and rapid respiration.

### Table 2.  Some Common Fungicides

| CHEMICAL GROUP | COMMON NAMES |
| --- | --- |
| Chlorophenols | Pentachlorophenol |
| Organomercurials | Ceresan-M |
| Organotin | Triethyltin |
| Chloroneb | Demosan |
| Organozinc | Zineb |
| Organosulfur | Captan |
| Volatile fumigant | Methylbromide |

Lesions observed in animals poisoned by herbicides or fungicides are mainly located in the gastrointestinal tract. Severe gastroenteritis with ulcerations may be found. In addition, congestion of the cerebral vessels may occur.

### AIMS OF TREATMENT

Treatment of herbicide or fungicide intoxications, with the exception of sodium chlorate, arsenicals or mercurials, is primarily symptomatic. Consequently, the treatment of acute intoxications caused by these toxic agents, as with all poisons, is directed toward the following:

1. Emergency intervention.
2. Application of mechanical or chemical antidote.
3. Hastening elimination of absorbed intoxicants.
4. Symptomatic or supportive therapy.
5. Elimination of the source of the toxic material. For more information, refer to the article on "Emergency and General Treatment of Poisonings."

### TREATMENT

**Nonspecific Treatment.** Treatment of most poisonings caused by herbicides or fungicides is symptomatic and supportive in nature because of the lack of specific antidotes. The recommendations in the introductory chapter on treatment of poisonings should be followed in treating animals poisoned by these agents.

**Specific Antidotes.** Early emergency measures for arsenic poisoning include oral administration of evaporated milk or egg white, followed in 5 to 10 minutes by an emetic such as apomorphine, 3 to 6 mg. administered subcutaneously. The owner of the animal can be instructed to perform the oral administration and subsequently could administer ipecac or powdered mustard to induce vomiting.

Following admission to the clinic or after observing advanced signs of arsenical intoxication, dimercaprol (BAL) should be administered at the rate of 6 mg./kg. body weight three times a day until the animal recovers. Other supportive measures should be instituted such as administration of digestive tract protectives and parenteral solutions to repair the fluid loss and acidosis. The clinician is directed to the article on

"Arsenic Poisoning" for further information.

Animals poisoned by sodium chlorate, a methemoglobin former, should be given methylene blue (1 per cent solution), 1 ml./kg. body weight. The methylene blue must be given slowly, and the animal must be closely observed because methylene blue in an overdose is also a methemoglobin former. Because sodium chlorate is not rapidly biotransformed, a poisoned animal may have to be re-treated for one to two days to insure proper recovery. Following institution of therapy for the methemoglobinemia, protectives and demulcents, such as evaporated milk or egg white, should be given orally followed by a purgative such as milk of magnesia. Other supportive measures such as fluid and electrolyte therapy should also be instituted.

In poisonings caused by organic mercurial fungicides, signs may not become apparent until permanent nerve damage has occurred. BAL, as used for arsenical poisonings, may be of value along with other supportive measures.

## PREVENTION AND PROPHYLAXIS

Proper storage of lawn, garden and agricultural chemicals is the best preventive measure against herbicide or fungicide intoxication in pet animals. This precaution will help to keep poisonings caused by these agents to a minimum.

## SUPPLEMENTAL READING

Dalgaard-Mikkelsen, S. V., and Poulsen, E.: Toxicology of herbicides. Pharmacol. Rev., *14*:225–250, 1962.

Palmer, J. S.: Toxicity of 45 organic herbicides to cattle, sheep, and chickens. U.S. Dept. of Agriculture Production Research Report, No. *137*:41, 1971.

Radeleff, R. D.: Veterinary Toxicology. 2nd ed. Philadelphia, Lea & Febiger, 1970.

# POISONINGS FROM PHENOLIC CHEMICALS

FREDERICK W. OEHME, D.V.M.
*Manhattan, Kansas*

Phenol (carbolic acid) is an extremely poisonous compound and has in the past been used in various disinfectant preparations. Derivatives of phenol were prepared to reduce the toxicity but retain the germicidal properties of this group; hence phenol is no longer used in most commercially available disinfectants but is replaced with one or more related phenolic compound(s). By adding chlorine and other radicals to the benzene ring of phenol, chemists have developed materials commercially useful as wood preservatives, fungicides or herbicides, antiseptics and photographic developers. Such chemicals are frequently found around homes and commercial establishments, and animals may be exposed via accidental application (such as falling in a barrel of wood preservative) or by direct application to the animal by the uninformed owner. In the latter case, animals may be housed in freshly preserved wooden structures, or overzealous owners may directly apply large quantities of disinfectants or antiseptics to the pet and to its immediate surroundings.

While most animals are capable of physiologically and biochemically handling, detoxifying and excreting reasonable quantities of phenolic chemicals, the absorption of large amounts of these materials is potentially toxic to any species. Animals of the feline species, however, have an inherent deficiency in the enzymes necessary to metabolize and excrete phenolic chemicals and, compared to dogs, are capable of handling approximately one-third the quantity of phenolic compounds. In addition, the metabolizing enzymes necessary for detoxification of phenolics usually develop maximum capability only several weeks following birth. Hence, the application of phenolic compounds to very young animals presents additional problems in their detoxification and excretion. At the present time, phenolic chemicals seem most hazardous to biochemically immature individuals of the feline species.

The possibility of chronic low-level exposure to phenolic compounds was recently studied in immature and adult dogs and cats. Animals were given 25 every-other-day doses of the calculated amount of a phenolic disinfectant contained in a 4-second burst of aerosol spray from a proprietary product. Although biologic accumulation of the phenolic chemical occurred, no animals exhibited any adverse clinical effects or showed any pathologic changes during or after the 25-dose exposure. This suggests that under routine use, exposure to moderate amounts of phenolic-containing disinfectants should be nontoxic, even to immature dogs or cats.

However, the possibility of overly conscientious owners exposing animals to excessive chemical concentrations, or for enzyme deficiencies to occur in highly inbred species or individual animals, still presents the potential for development of toxicity in isolated and unusual circumstances. Thus the practitioner must be aware of the development of toxicity not only from overt large-scale exposure due to accidental ingestion or application, but also from the well-intentioned overuse of phenolic compounds or in the individual animal that is biochemically hyperreactive to phenols.

## CLINICAL SYNDROME

Since phenol is seldom available to domestic animals, most intoxications result from the phenolic derivatives previously mentioned. These are all rapidly absorbed either through the intact skin or from the digestive tract. Early signs include incoordination, mild muscular fasciculations, depression leading to coma, and deepening coma with terminal respiratory failure. Dogs tend to exhibit more severe muscular involvement, although frank convulsions are usually not seen. Prolonged coma is common in the cat. If amounts of phenolics are absorbed slowly, such as from skin application, increased red cell fragility and intravascular hemolysis occur. A progressive icterus is then observed prior to death. The application of concentrated solutions of phenolic chemicals may be corrosive to applied surfaces, to the digestive tract and to mucous membranes.

The clinical course of phenolic chemical poisoning is largely determined by the amount and type of phenol-chemical absorbed. Larger concentrations result in acute toxicity, initial signs one-half hour following application, and death within 12 to 24 hours. Other individuals receiving smaller amounts may become depressed for several hours, vomit occasionally and then progress into neurologic and respiratory depression, with death occurring after several days. Cats and other members of the feline species more characteristically develop the acute syndrome, with death occurring 24 to 36 hours following exposure. This more severe response is largely due to the inherent inability of cats to detoxify and excrete the phenolic compounds, resulting in rapidly rising blood levels and tissue accumulation of the toxic chemical.

Necropsy lesions are not spectacular, but are consistent with the expected effects of the protein-precipitating phenolic chemicals. Surface tissues may be irritated and show coagulation necrosis. Congestion of internal organs may be seen, and generalized icterus, reflecting intravascular hemolysis, may be present. Occasionally the skin surface or digestive tract contents may have a characteristic odor of the phenolic-containing material. Microscopic lesions are limited to coagulation necrosis of contacting epithelial cells, early hepatocyte degeneration, and nonspecific glomerular and tubular nephrotoxic alterations.

## DIAGNOSIS

History and evidence of contact with phenolic-containing materials are invaluable for the early diagnosis of poisoning due to phenolic chemicals. The clinical signs are not sufficiently specific to allow diagnosis on that basis alone. However, the presence of icterus in an animal with progressively deepening coma and mild muscular fasciculations should suggest the possibility of phenolic intoxication.

A rapidly performed presumptive screening test for phenolic compounds may be utilized on urine from animals suspected of suffering from phenolic poisoning. Two simple tests are available, and the combination of both giving positive reactions is presumptive evidence of poisoning. In the first procedure, 1 ml. of a 20 per cent aqueous solution of ferric chloride is added to 10 ml. of urine. A resulting purple color is positive. In the second test, 10 ml. of suspected urine is boiled with 1 to 2 ml. of Millon's reagent. Millon's reagent is made by dissolving 10 gm. of mercury in 20 ml. of nitric acid, diluting with an equal amount of distilled water, allowing the mixture to stand for two hours and then decanting the excess water. A positive reaction with urine results in a red color.

## TREATMENT

A specific treatment for phenolic intoxication is not available. Exposed animals should be rid of any unabsorbed chemical by washing with abundant soap or by inducing vomiting. Oral administration of activated charcoal is effective in binding unabsorbed phenolic chemicals present in the digestive tract contents. Supportive therapy, including the maintenance of normal body temperature and respiration and the administration of fluids, should be included in therapy. The administration of glucose may have some benefit in reducing liver damage and maintaining renal function. Despite the hypothesized action of phenol in causing the accumulation of acetylcholine at nerve-muscle junctions, the administration of atropine to poisoned individuals has not been found to be of any prophylactic or therapeutic benefit. Recovery from phenolic poisoning is largely determined by the total absorbed dose and the animal's ability to detoxify and excrete the toxic chemical.

### SUPPLEMENTAL READING

Oehme, F. W.: New information on the toxicity of phenolic compounds in small animals. Proceedings of the 21st Gaines Veterinary Symposium, Iowa State University, Ames, Iowa. October 20, 1971, p. 8–15.
Rachofsky, M. A., and Oehme, F. W.: Comparative and age-related pharmacodynamics for single and multiple doses of o-phenylphenol. Toxicol. Appl. Pharmacol., 37:93, 1976.

# COMMON POTENTIAL SOURCES OF SMALL ANIMAL POISONINGS

GARY D. OSWEILER, D.V.M.
*Columbia, Missouri*

When a potential intoxication is presented, the first concern is usually the accurate assessment of the clinical status of the animal and the prompt incorporation of procedures to support life and control clinical signs. Immediately thereafter, or concurrent with emergency management, a tentative diagnosis should be made.

Part of the input to determine that diagnosis is a review of potential toxicants to which an animal may have been exposed. Appropriate questioning of the client may aid in establishing potential sources. From among the thousands of potentially toxic chemicals in the world, one usually attempts to consider those which are (1) in the animal's environment, (2) toxic enough to constitute a hazard if exposure occurs, (3) available to the animal and (4) generally capable of causing the signs being manifested.

From the article "Common Poisonings in Small Animal Practice," it may be seen that the number of intoxications diagnosed is rather small and concerns mainly natural toxins and economic poisons. Those toxins

### Table 1.   *Sources of Poisonous Plants*

| LOCATION | EXAMPLES |
|---|---|
| House Plants | Daffodil, oleander, poinsettia, dumb cane, mistletoe, philodendron |
| Flower Garden | Delphinium, monkshood, foxglove, iris, lily-of-the-valley |
| Vegetable Garden | Rhubarb, spinach, tomato vine, sunburned potatoes |
| Ornamentals | Oleander, castor bean, daphne, golden chain, rhododendron, lantana |
| Trees and Shrubs | Cherries, peach, oak, elderberry, black locust |
| Woodland Plants | Jack-in-the-pulpit, moonseed, May apple, Dutchman's-breeches |
| Swamp Plants | Water hemlock, mushrooms |
| Field Plants | Buttercup, nightshade, poison hemlock, jimsonweed, pigweed |
| Range Plants | Locoweed, lupine, halogeton |
| Grain Contaminants | Crotalaria, corn cockle, ergot |
| Cultural Changes | Nitrate, cyanide, herbicides, insecticides |

in the animal's environment generally include products in and around the home, those involved in pest control and those which are available in the natural or altered environment. Key questions should be directed to the client to establish what products, plants or animals are kept or available in or near the home. Recent use of such materials, where they are stored and recollection of spillage should be reviewed with the client. The species, age, eating habits and freedom of the affected animal should be known. For example, it is important to remember that the dog that roams the neighborhood nightly is exposed to "common sources" different from those of the constantly housed animal.

Each geographic area of North America has its own peculiar common sources, as detailed in the article on common poisonings (cited above). Indigenous plants, venomous reptiles, snail baits, rust inhibitors and anti-

### Table 2.   *Some Toxins of Zoologic Origin*

| ORGANISMS | LOCATIONS | GENERAL PROBLEMS ENCOUNTERED |
|---|---|---|
| *Snakes* | | |
| Pit vipers | Terrestrial; Eastern U.S.A. | Necrosis, inflammation, |
| Rattlesnake | through South Central, | anaphylaxis |
| Copperhead | Midwest and Southwest | |
| Water moccasin | | |
| Coral snake | Southeast U.S.A., mainly Florida | Neuroparalytic, loss of sensation |
| *Lizards* | | |
| Gila monster | Terrestrial; primarily | Inflammation, vomition, shock |
| Mexican beaded lizard | Southwest U.S.A. | |
| *Toads* | | |
| *Bufo* sp. | Terrestrial-aquatic; Southern and | Parotid glands exude a cardio- |
| | Southwestern U.S.A. | toxic and cholinergic toxin |
| *Spiders* | | |
| Black widow | Terrestrial | Neuromuscular; |
| Brown recluse | | wound heals with difficulty; |
| Tarantula | | infection from the bite |
| *Insects* | | |
| Fire ant | Terrestrial; Southern and | Painful, necrotizing bite; |
| Wasps | Southwestern U.S.A. | inflammation and anaphylaxis |
| Bees | | |
| *Invertebrates* | | |
| Jellyfish | Aquatic-marine | Pain, swelling, cramps, nausea, |
| Coral | | CNS derangement |
| Sea anemone | | |
| Sea urchin | | Burning sensation, inflammation, paralysis |
| *Vertebrates* | | |
| Fish | Aquatic-marine | Sharp pain, inflammation |
| Stingray | | |
| Catfish | | |
| Scorpion fish | | |

freeze solutions are but a few examples of toxicants which may be more prevalent in particular geographic areas.

This section, Chemical and Physical Disorders, covers in some detail the common sources generally associated with commonly diagnosed intoxications. However, Tables 1, 2 and 3 are presented here to offer a broad review of the scope of commonly available substances which may occasionally be toxic. These tables should be used to suggest specific potentially toxic

*Table 3.  Some Chemical Products Hazardous to Pets*

### ARTS AND CRAFTS SUPPLIES

*Antiquing Agents*
  Methyl ethyl ketone
  Turpentine
*Oil Paints and Tempera Paints*
  Pigment salts of lead, arsenic, copper and cadmium
*Pencils, Indelible*
  Crystal violet

### PHOTOGRAPHIC SUPPLIES

*Developers*
  Borates
  Bromides
  Iodides
  Thiocyanates
*Fixatives*
  Sodium thiosulfate
*Hardeners*
  Aluminum chloride
  Formaldehyde

### AUTOMOTIVE AND MACHINERY PRODUCTS

*Antifreeze, Fuel System De-icer*
  Ethylene glycol
  Isopropyl alcohol
  Methanol
  Rust inhibitors
    a. Borates
    b. Chromates
    c. Zinc chloride
*Brake Fluids*
  Butyl ethers of ethylene glycol and related glycols
  Ethyl ethers of ethylene glycol and related glycols
  Methyl ethers of ethylene glycol and related glycols
*Carburetor Cleaners*
  Cresol
  Ethylene dichloride
*Corrosion Inhibitors*
  Borates
  Sodium chromate
  Sodium nitrate
*Engine and Motor Cleaners*
  Cresol
  Ethylene dichloride
  Methylene chloride
*Frost Removers*
  Ethylene glycol
  Isopropyl alcohol
*Lubricants*
  Barium compounds
  Isopropyl alcohol
  Kerosene
  Lead compounds
  Stoddard solvent
*Motor Fuel*
  Gasoline
  Kerosene
  Tetraethyl lead

*Radiator Cleaners*
  Boric acid
  Oxalic acid
  Sodium chromate
*Shock Absorber Fluids*
  Petroleum ether
*Tire Repair*
  Benzene
*Windshield Washer*
  Ethylene glycol
  Isopropyl alcohol
  Methyl alcohol

### CLEANERS, DISINFECTANTS, SANITIZERS

*Cleaners, Bleaches, Polishes*
  Ammonium hydroxide
  Benzene
  Carbon tetrachloride
  Hydrochloric acid
  Methyl alcohol
  Naphtha
  Nitrobenzene
  Oxalic acid
  Phosphoric acid
  Sodium fluoride
  Sodium or potassium hydroxide
  Sodium hypochlorite
  Sodium perborate
  Sulfuric acid
  Trichloroethane
  Turpentine
*Disinfectants, Sanitizers*
  Acids
  Alkalis
  Hypochlorites
  Iodophors
  Paradichlorobenzene
  Phenol, Cresols
  Phenyl mercuric acetate
  Pine oil
  Quaternary ammonium

### HEALTH AND BEAUTY AIDS

*Athlete's Foot*
  Caprylic acid
  Copper
  Propionic acid
  Sodium
  Undecylenic acid
  Zinc salts
*Bath Preparations*
  Bath oils
  Perfume
  Sodium lauryl sulfate
  Trisodium phosphate

*Continued on next page*

*Table 3.*   *Some Chemical Products Hazardous to Pets (Continued)*

**Corn Removers**
Phenoxyacetic acid
Salicylic acid
**Deodorants and Antiperspirants**
Alcohol
Aluminum chloride
**Diet Pills**
Amphetamines
Diuretics
Thyroid hormone
**Eye Make-up**
Boric acid
Peach kernel oil, q.s.
**Hair Preparations**
Cadmium chloride
Cupric chloride
Dyes, tints
Ferric chloride
Lead acetate
Permanent wave lotions
Pyrogallol
Silver nitrate
Thioglycolic acid
**Headache**
Aspirin
Phenacetin
**Laxatives**
IRRITANT OR STIMULANT LAXATIVES
Aloes
Aloin
Cascara sagrada
**Liniments**
Camphor
Chloroform
Oil of wintergreen (methyl salicylate)
Pine oil
Turpentine
**Nailetics**
Acetone
Alcohol
Benzene
Ethyl acetate
Nail enamel
Nail polish
Nail polish remover
Toluene
Tricresyl phosphate
**Ointments**
Benzoic acid
Borates
Caprylic acid
Menthol
Mercury compounds
Oil of wintergreen (methyl salicylate)
Phenols
Salicylic acid
**Perfumes, Toilet Waters and Colognes**
Alcohol
Essential oils
Floral oils
Perfume essence
**Shampoos**
Sodium lauryl sulfate
Triethanolamine dodecyl sulfate
**Shaving Lotions**
Alcohol
Boric acid

**Somnolents (Sleeping Pills)**
Barbiturates
Bromides
**Stimulants**
Amphetamine
Caffeine
**Suntan Lotions**
Alcohol
Tannic acid and derivatives

PAINTS AND RELATED PRODUCTS
**Caulking Compounds**
Barium
Chlorinated biphenyl
Chromium
Lead
Mineral spirits
Petroleum distillate
Xylene
**Driers**
Cobalt compounds
Iron compounds
Manganese compounds
Vanadium compounds
Zinc compounds
**Lacquer Thinners**
Aliphatic hydrocarbons
Butyl acetate
Butyl alcohol
Toluene
**Paint**
Arsenic oxide
Coal tar
Cuprous oxide
Lead chromate
Petroleum ether
Pine oil
Red lead oxide
Zinc chromate
**Paint Brush Cleaners**
Benzene
Kerosene
Naphthas
**Paint and Varnish Cleaners**
Ethylene dichloride
Kerosene
Naphthalene
Trisodium phosphate
**Paint and Varnish Removers**
FLAMMABLE
Benzene
Cresols
Phenols
Toluene
NONFLAMMABLE
Methylene chloride
Toluene
**Preservatives**
BRUSH
Kerosene
Turpentine
CANVAS
2-Chlorophenylphenol
Pentachlorophenol

*Continued on next page*

*Table 3.   Some Chemical Products Hazardous to Pets (Continued)*

FLOOR
   Magnesium fluorosilicate
WOOD
   Copper naphthenate
   Copper oleate
   Mineral spirits
   Pentachlorophenol
   Zinc naphthenate

### PEST CONTROL

*Birds*
   Endrin
   Toluidine
*Fungicides*
   Captan
   Copper compounds
   Maneb
   Mercurials
   Pentachlorophenol
   Thiram
   Zineb
*Insects and Spiders*
   Baygon
   Carbaryl
   Chlordane
   Diazinon
   Dichlorvos
   Kelthane
   Mirex
   Paradichlorobenzene
   Pyrethrins
   Rotenone
   Toxaphene
*Lawn and Garden Weeds*
   Arsenic
   Chlordane
   Dacthal
   Pentachlorophenol
   Trifluralin
   2,4-D
*Rats, Mice, Gophers, Moles*
   Arsenic
   Barium carbonate
   Dicoumarol
   Phosphorus
   Sodium fluoroacetate

   Strychnine
   Thallium (rare)
   Warfarin
   Zinc phosphide
*Snails, Slugs*
   Metaldehyde

### SAFETY PRODUCTS

*Fire Extinguishers*
   LIQUID FIRE EXTINGUISHERS
      Carbon tetrachloride
   MISCELLANEOUS FIRE EXTINGUISHERS
      Methylbromide
   POWDER EXTINGUISHERS
      Borax compounds
*Nonskid Products*
   Stoddard solvent
   Methyl ethyl ketone

### SOLVENTS

*Alcohols*
*Chlorinated Solvents*
   Carbon tetrachloride
   Methylene chloride
   Orthodichlorobenzene
   Trichloroethylene
*Esters*
   Amyl acetate
   Ethyl acetate
   Isopropyl acetate
   Methyl acetate
*Hydrocarbons*
   Aromatics, chiefly benzene, toluene and xylene
   Naphthenes
*Ketones*
   Acetone
   Methyl ethyl ketone
*Other Common Solvents*
   Aniline
   Carbon disulphide
   Cresylic acid
   Kerosene
   Mineral spirits
   Phenols
   Turpentine

agents found in many homes and businesses. Table 4 enumerates some data valuable in establishing exposure to various sources.

When access or potential exposure to the materials listed is established, additional details may be found in this section or in the references listed at the end of this article.

Knowledge of sources and the pattern of exposure which occurred (e.g., accidental, malicious) can serve as a focus for education of the client in safe use of toxic materials to prevent further danger to either animals or man.

### SUPPLEMENTAL READING

Arena, J. M.: Poisoning. Toxicology, Symptoms, Treatments. 3rd ed. Springfield, Illinois, Charles C Thomas, 1974.

Atkins, C. E., and Johnson, R. K.: Clinical toxicities of cats. Vet. Clin. N. Am., 5:623–652, 1975.

Buck, W. B., Osweiler, G. D., and Van Gelder, G. A.: Clinical and Diagnostic Veterinary Toxicology. Dubuque, Iowa, Kendall-Hunt Publishing Co., 1973.

Bureau of Veterinary Medicine. Memo: Summary of Adverse Reactions to Animal Drugs. BVMM-20, Rockville, Maryland, August, 1975.

Catcott, E. J. (ed.): Canine Medicine. Wheaton, Illinois, American Veterinary Publications, 1968.

Clarke, E. G. C.: Pets and poisons. J. Small Anim. Pract., 16:375–380, 1975.

*Table 4.  Small Animal Toxicology History*

Date: _____  Case: _____  Owner: _____
D.V.M.: _____  Name: _____  Address: _____
Address: _____  Species: _____  _____
_____  Breed: _____
_____  Weight: _____  Phone: _____
Phone: _____  Age: _____ Sex: _____  Delivered by: _____

Illnesses within the past 6 months  _____
Vaccinations within the past year    _____ rabies         _____leptospirosis
                                     _____distemper   _____hepatitis      _____other
Medications, sprays, dips, wormers, etc., given within the past month (type and date)  _____
When was this animal last seen by a veterinarian?  _____

How long was this animal sick?_____days _____months _____hours
If found dead, how long since last seen alive and healthy? _____days _____hours

History of confinement:      _____roamed occasionally (supervised)      _____roamed at will
                             _____roamed occasionally (unsupervised)  _____always housed
                             _____always penned or tied               _____other
Animal lived near or on (check more than one if applicable):
_____industrial buildings      _____garbage dump      _____small town      _____city
_____commercial buildings      _____railroad          _____suburb          _____other
_____automotive garage         _____grain elevator    _____farm

Has the patient always lived in this locality?  _____yes _____no
If no, please explain: _____
Have there been any changes in food, water or location in recent days? _____yes _____no
If yes, please explain:  _____
What is the patient normally fed? _____
When was this animal last fed? _____

What types of mouse or rat poisons, insecticides, weed killers, etc., are used on or near your property? _____
_____

Have other animals in your home or neighborhood had similar problems? _____
_____

Clinical signs:
                          _____convulsions   _____depression   _____weakness
_____difficult urination  _____blindness      _____stiffness     _____diarrhea
_____difficult breathing  _____salivation     _____bleeding      _____thirst
_____vocalization         _____excitement     _____vomiting      _____other

Tentative diagnoses:




Use back of sheet for additional history and comments.

Clarke, E. G. C., and Clarke, M. L.: Garner's Veterinary Toxicology. 3rd ed. Baltimore, The Williams & Wilkins Co., 1967.

Diechman, W. B., and Gerarde, H. W.: Toxicology of Drugs and Chemicals. 4th ed. New York, Academic Press, 1969.

Gleason, M. N., Gosselin, R. E., and Hodge, H. C.: Clinical Toxicology of Commercial Products. Baltimore, The Williams & Wilkins Co., 1971.

Kirk, R. W. (ed.): Current Veterinary Therapy V. Philadelphia, W. B. Saunders Co., 1974.

Kirk, R. W., and Bistner, S. I.: Handbook of Veterinary Procedures and Emergency Treatment. 2nd ed. Philadelphia, W. B. Saunders Co., 1975.

Malone, J. C.: Diagnosis and treatment of poisoning in dogs and cats. Vet. Rec., 84:161–166, 1969.

Osweiler, G. D.: Incidence and diagnostic considerations of major small animal toxicoses. J. Am. Vet. Med. Assn. 155:2011–2015, 1969.

Radeleff, R. D.: Veterinary Toxicology. 2nd ed. Philadelphia, Lea & Febiger, 1970.

Robens, J. F.: Animal drug toxicities. Veterinary Toxicology Training and Review Workshop. Ames, Iowa, February 21–26, 1972.

Szabuniewicz, M.: Treatment of some common animal poisonings. Vet. Med./Small Animal Clin., December, 1971, pp. 1197–1205.

# ADVERSE DRUG REACTIONS

C. M. STOWE, V.M.D.,
R. FARNSWORTH, D.V.M.,
R. HARDY, D.V.M.,
J. KLAUSNER, D.V.M.,
V. L. LARSON, D.V.M.,
*and* R. E. WERDIN, D.V.M.*
St. Paul, Minnesota

Clinical drug experience is an area that relates clinical sciences to toxicology and pharmacology. It has developed exponentially during the past 15 years and is now formally recognized and supported at various veterinary colleges by the FDA. Practicing veterinarians also contribute significantly by voluntarily reporting adverse reactions.

It is difficult at times to differentiate terms such as "side effects," "toxic reactions," "adverse experience" and "adverse reaction." Generally, "adverse experience" and "adverse reaction" refer to an unexpected response (not *necessarily* overtly deleterious) to a drug used for therapeutic or diagnostic purposes. More specifically, the FDA defines an adverse reaction as (1) any unexpected change in a bio- or clinico-chemical value, (2) any functional or behavioral change of an organ or organ system, (3) any structural change and (4) any ineffective drug response (assuming rational use).

An ever-present hazard in judging an adverse reaction is the *post hoc, ergo propter hoc* fallacy—"after this, therefore on account of this." To incriminate a drug for an unexpected or untoward effect or for failing to do what was expected may not be fair. Furthermore, the problem is compounded when two or more drugs are used. Trying to unravel such complex situations and arrive at logical judgments concerning a drug's complicity is extremely difficult. For these reasons, it is advisable for judgments to be made by a group of clinicians rather than by one.

Another problem derives from the fact that drugs are often used "ex label," i.e., for therapeutic objectives other than those on the label or insert, but these drugs may, nevertheless, be therapeutically sound. On the other hand, drugs may sometimes be used for invalid reasons, or even in contradiction to label warnings. Adverse reactions occurring under such circumstances should nevertheless be reported (anonymously, if preferred) as an adverse clinical experience. The point is that everyone learns from these mistakes.

The pharmaceutical industry may feel that reporting of adverse reactions poses a threat at times. This is not true, because a broadly scoped program of clinical drug experience will uncover problem areas and encourage development of drugs having greater benefit:risk ratios. No drug is devoid of adverse effects at some time.

The following table presents adverse reactions which have occurred with various drugs *as they have been used*; no attempt has been made to judge whether such usage was valid. What may appear to be invalid to an observer at a different time and place may have seemed eminently logical to the veterinarian "on the firing line." This is consistent with the professional principle that a veterinarian may use whatever drug(s) he deems desirable, with the understanding that serious misjudgments might leave him vulnerable to allegations of misuse.

*The authors wish to express their earnest appreciation to the practicing veterinarians in Minnesota and elsewhere who have so generously informed them of adverse and toxic reactions which they have encountered in their practices.

## Veterinary Adverse Drug Reactions—30-Month Summary in Small Animals

### I. CENTRAL NERVOUS SYSTEM DEPRESSANTS

| Drug(s) | Species* | Nature of Adverse Reactions | Treatment | Outcome | Comments |
|---|---|---|---|---|---|
| Acepromazine® | D(3) | "Extrapyramidal reactions." | None | One recovery in 5-10 min.; two fatal. | Extensor rigidity, opisthotonos, dyspnea, collapse, cardiac irregularity. |
| " | D(4) | Prolonged depression (½-1½ days). | None | Recovery. | |
| " | D(2) | Lack of sedation; aggressiveness. | Anesthesia | Satisfactory recovery. | |
| Promazine | D(6) | "Extrapyramidal reactions." | None | Recovery. | Similar to above. Frequency probably related to IV dose and rate of injection. |
| Piperacetazine | D | Alternate depression and restlessness. | None | Recovery. | |
| Innovar® | D(10) | Excitement, agitation, vocal activity, extensor rigidity, hyperthermia (1), prolonged depression (2) for 1-2 weeks, hallucinations (1). | Levallorphan | Prompt reversal of signs. Gradual recovery. | |
| Rompun® (xylazine) | D(5) | Cardiac irregularity, A-V disassociation, systolic murmurs. | None | Recovery in 1-2 hours. | Hyperglycemia common with xylazine. |
| " | D(4) | Muscle tremors, clonic spasms, convulsive seizures. | None | Recovery in 1-2 hours. | |
| " | D(3) | Ineffective for capture of wild dogs. | | Recovery. | Nicotine resorted to. |
| " | D(1) | Urticaria, hives. | Antihistamine | | |
| " | D(2) | Profound depression, respiratory failure. | Fluids, $O_2$ | Two dogs died. | |
| Rompun® (xylazine) plus Surital® | C | Vomiting, prolonged recovery (18 hours). | None | Recovery. | Use combination cautiously. |
| Rompun® plus ketamine | C | Respiratory arrest. | $O_2$ | Recovery. | Hyperglycemia also occurs. |
| Ketamine | C(3) | Prolonged depression, coma, death. | $O_2$, fluids | Death. | |
| " | C(2) | Prolonged depression, recovery in 1-3 days. | $O_2$, fluids | Recovery. | |
| " | C | Tonic-clonic convulsions. | Diazepam (IV) | Convulsions controlled. | |
| " | LC | Excitement, convulsions, inadequate analgesia. | Promazine | One died (ocelot). | Tiger, jaguar, ocelot. |

| Drug | (See comments) | Respiratory failure, death. | None | Death. | Canadian goose. |
|---|---|---|---|---|---|
| Ketamine, Acepromazine®, halothane | (See comments) | Respiratory failure, death. | None | Death. | Canadian goose. |
| Valium® (diazepam) | D(2) | 15 mg. ineffective in controlling strychnine convulsions. | Pentobarb (IV) | Recovery. | Essential to monitor dogs for 36-72 hours. |
| " | D(2) | Controlled zinc phosphide convulsions for only 3-5 min. | Pentobarb (IV) | Eventual death. | No known antidote to $Zn_3P_2$. |
| Dilantin® (3 months to 2 years) | D(2) | Pancytopenia, thrombocytopenia. | Ceased drug | Gradual recovery. | Other antiepileptics used. |
| Primidone® | D | Poor control of seizures. | Dilantin | Successful control. | |
| " | D | Macrocytic anemia. | Ceased drug | Dyscrasia disappeared. | |
| Glyceryl guaiacol ether (5% IV) | D(2) | Relief from strychnine convulsions of brief (10-15 min.) duration. | Pentobarb (IV) | Recovery. | |
| Metofane® (plus xylazine) | C | Prolonged recovery (3-4 days). | Fluids | Eventual recovery. | Caution. Metofane® may be metabolized to $F^-$ and oxalate. |
| Aspirin | D | Anorexia, "nervousness," ataxia. | None | Recovery in 1-2 days. | |
| Repose® (Pentobarbital) | D | Sudden extensor rigidity, opisthotonos prior to apnea. | None | Euthanasia. | |
| Pentobarbital | D | Excited and barked before respiratory failure. | None | Euthanasia. | Uncommon with proper administration. |
| Althesin® (CT1341) | K | Inadequate anesthesia. | Injected additional drug | Satisfactory brief anesthesia. | |
| " | C(12) | Rubbing nose. | None | Recovery in 1 hour. | Common response to Althesin®. |
| " | R | Prolonged anesthesia, apnea, death (3). | None | Death. | Owl, 2 hawks. |
| Fentanyl | C | Excitement, mania. | None | Gradual recovery. | Classic opiate excitement. |
| " | C | Ineffective; no response, no analgesia. | — | | |
| Halothane | C | Apnea, cardiac arrest. | Epinephrine (IC) | Cat recovered. | Epinephrine sometimes ineffective. |
| Thiamylal (Surital®) | D(3) | Prolonged recovery; saline and glucose deeper barbiturate anesthesia. | Saline-dextrose | Deeper depression. | Well-known phenomenon with barbiturates. |

* D=dog, C=cat, P=puppy, K=kitten, LC=large feral cats, R=raptors, SM=squirrel monkey. Number in ( ) is number of animals involved.

*Continued on next page*

## Veterinary Adverse Drug Reactions—30-Month Summary in Small Animals (Continued)

### I. CENTRAL NERVOUS SYSTEM DEPRESSANTS

| Drug(s) | Species* | Nature of Adverse Reactions | Treatment | Outcome | Comments |
|---|---|---|---|---|---|
| Surital® and Metofane® | D | Sudden pulmonary edema. | Atropine and oxygen | Dog died. | Unexplained adverse response. |
| " | C | Slow recovery. Died overnight. | | No lesions. | Possible $F^-$ toxicity. |
| Meperidine, phenobarbital, Valium® | D | Anal gland irritation and pain. Treated by physician. Deep depression, respiratory failure, death. | $O_2$, fluids | Dog died. | Additive depression by 3 depressant drugs. |
| Catnip (*Nepeta cataria*) | C(2) | Prolonged CNS depression (4-7 days). | Fluids | | Probably overdose from catnip toys. |

### II. ANTIBACTERIAL AGENTS

| Drug(s) | Species* | Nature of Adverse Reactions | Treatment | Outcome | Comments |
|---|---|---|---|---|---|
| Amphotericin B | D(2) | Muscle trembling, mild convulsions. | None | Continued treatment q-48 hrs. | Toxic drug. Essential to monitor BUN. |
| " | D(1) | Elevated BUN (40-50). | None | Continued with BUN monitoring. | |
| " | D(1) | Drug fever. | None | | |
| Chloramphenicol | C | Ataxia, nystagmus, posterior hemiparalysis. | Ceased drug | Gradual recovery. | |
| Chloramphenicol with fibrinolysin | D | Ineffective response. | Other antibiotics | Dog died. | |
| Cyclophosphamide | D | Severe hemorrhagic cystitis. | 2% $AgNO_3$ in bladder | Euthanasia. | |
| Gentamicin | K | Ataxia, incoordination after 4-6 days. | Ceased drug | Recovery. | Well-known effect of aminoglycosides. |
| Lincomycin, novobiocin | SM | Acute anaphylactoid reaction. | None | Monkey died. | |
| Nitrofurans: Furacin® | D(2) | Ataxia, convulsions. | Ceased drug | One died. | Common reaction in calves and pigs. |
| Furazolidone | P(6) | Muscle trembling, excitement, convulsions. | Ceased drug | Recovery in 5 out of 6 | Common adverse effect in calves and pigs |

| Drug | Animal* | Signs | Treatment | Result | Comments |
|---|---|---|---|---|---|
| Nystatin | D | Ineffective in Moraxella sinusitis. | Neomycin, streptothricin | Recovery. | Ineffective drug response. |
| **Penicillins:** Na Salt (IV) | D | Ataxia, muscle tremors, grand mal–type seizures. | Ceased drug; phenobarb and diazepam (IV) | Recovery. | Probably CNS toxicity due to high CNS levels. |
| Procaine | D | Sudden collapse, defecation, urination. | None | Recovery in 1-2 hours. | Probable acute anaphylactoid reaction. |
| Ampicillin | D | Swelling of eyelids, jowls; rubbing of ears. | Ceased drug | Signs regressed in 1-2 days. | Hypersensitivity common with penicillins. |
| " | K | Ataxia. | Ceased drug | Recovery. | |
| Penicillin-streptomycin | C | Vomited following IM treatments. Also vomited with tetracycline and novobiocin. | None | Recovery. | |
| **Sulfonamides:** Methoxy-pyridazine | C(2) | Alopecia. | Ceased drug | Gradual return of hair. | |
| Quinoxaline | P(15) | Spontaneous hemorrhagic syndrome, multiple hemorrhages through body. Prothrombin times over 10-15 min. | Ceased drug, emulsified vitamin K (IV) | 15 out of 104 died. | Sulfaquinoxaline a poor choice; menadione unreliable; emulsified vitamin K rapidly reverses the prothrombin time. |
| **Tetracyclines:** Oxy-TC | D(2) | Anorexia, constipation, flatus, tenesmus, drug fever. | Ceased drug | Recovery in 1-3 days. | Alteration of gut flora. Also seen in large animals. |
| Oxy-TC–novobiocin | D | Anorexia, drug fever to 104° F. | Reduced dosage | Recovery. | |
| TC | C(2) | Ineffective response. | Changed to Tylosin® | | Tetracyclines supposedly effective against *Hemobartonella*. |
| " | C | Drug fever (103-104° F.) after 2 days of therapy. | Ceased drug | Fever regressed. | Drug fever reported fairly commonly. |
| Tylosin | C | Ineffective drug response. | Penicillin | Recovery. | Organism not identified. |

\* D=dog, C=cat, P=puppy, K=kitten, LC=large feral cats, R=raptors, SM=squirrel monkey. Number in ( ) is number of animals involved.

*Continued on next page*

*Veterinary Adverse Drug Reactions—30-Month Summary in Small Animals (Continued)*

### III. ANTIPARASITIC DRUGS

| Drug(s) | Species* | Nature of Adverse Reactions | Treatment | Outcome | Comments |
|---|---|---|---|---|---|
| Caparsolate® (thiacetarsamide) | D(20) | Elevated serum transaminase (SGPT); no concurrent clinical signs. | None | Recovery, effective. | Very common reaction. Caution in preexisting liver damage. |
| " | D(2) | Anorexia, icterus, depression lasting 2 weeks. | Fluids, vitamins | Recovery after several weeks. | Potentially hazardous drug to liver and kidney. |
| " | D(4) | Glycosuria, proteinuria (4+). | Fluids, vitamins | Gradual recovery. | " " |
| Dinitrophenol (DNP) | P(5) | Hyperthermia, polyuria, polydipsia. | None | Five died. | Owner administered. Narrow safety margin. |
| " | D(4) | " | Cold water | Two died. | " |
| Levamisole | D(3) | Salivation, mydriasis, diarrhea, tremors, collapse, death (1). | Ceased drug; Acepromazine® or barbiturates | One died. | Doses of 2 to 2.5 mg./kg. apparent narrow margin; similar toxicity in large animals. |
| Quinacrine (Atabrine®) | D | Depression, vomiting, anorexia. | Divided doses | Regimen completed. | Quinacrine often a problem in dogs. |
| " | D | Weakness, trembling after 7th dose. | Gave with meals | " | |
| " | D | Marked ataxia. | Ceased drug | | |
| " | P | Hypersensitive to sound. Tilting of head, circling, reverse walking, chorea, partial blindness, anuria. | Fluids, furosemide | Gradual recovery. | Severe CNS effects; renal function essential. |
| Arecoline-tetrachlorethylene | D(2) | Ataxia, depression lasting 1-2 days. | Fluids, B vitamins | Recovery. | OTC† remedy, home use. |
| Organophosphates: Ruelene® | D | Miosis, salivation, muscle tremors, convulsions, death. | Atropine (IV and SQ) | Dog died | Classic organophosphate signs |
| Dermaton® | D | Red, swollen, pruritic areas on skin. | Washed skin | Recovery. | Topical recovery. |
| Malathion | D | Miosis, head tilting and pressing, circling, death. | Atropine, Kao-pectate | Dog died. | |
| Piperazine | D | Abdominal pain, shock, >CVP. | Sparine (IV) | Nutmeg liver. <CVP. Fresh hepatic hemorrhage; portal vessels hemorrhagic. Death. | Unexplained death. |
| Thenium closylate | P(3) | Sudden, shocklike syndrome; coma, death 2-8 hours later. | Fluids (IV), antibiotics, steroids | Three pups died. | |

IV. MISCELLANEOUS DRUGS

| Drug(s) | Species* | Nature of Adverse Reactions | Treatment | Outcome | Comments |
|---|---|---|---|---|---|
| Nicotine | D(3) | Tremors, dyspnea, excitement, paralysis, apnea, death. | None | Three died (wild dogs). | Dose of nicotine for capture is difficult to judge. |
| Quinidine | D(2) | Nausea and vomiting. | Reduced dose; Lidocaine | Controlled vomiting and ventricular tachycardia. | Difficult to adjust dosage of cardiac glycosides. |
| Digoxin | D | Developed ascites on maintenance doses of digoxin for a year. Sudden death. | None | Dog (6 lb.) died. | Reduce dosage at each administration. |
| d-Penicilla-mine (Cupri-mine®) | D | Vomiting, within 1-3 hours after administration. | Ceased drug | — | " " |
| " | C | Vomiting 2-3 hours after administration. | Continued therapy | Signs of Pb poisoning regressed. | |
| Cream of tartar (NaK tartrate) | D | Anorexia, depression, death. (Used for coprophagia.) | None | Died. Necrosis of renal tubules and Henle loops. | Tartrates exert well-known toxic effects on kidney. |
| Dexamethasone (with peni-cillin and streptomycin) | D | Dog with pulmonary blastomycosis. *Marked* worsening of disease. | Amphotericin B | Recovery in 3-4 weeks. | Steroids must be avoided in systemic mycoses. |
| Dexamethasone | D(2) | Polyuria, polydipsia. | Ceased drug | — | Common adverse reaction to steroids. |
| Atropine | D(2) | Organophosphate poisoning. Atropine-controlled salivation, miosis, bronchospasm. Dog died. | None | Dog died. | Atropine not always successful (nor is 2-PAM). |
| Ruelene® | D | Miosis, salivation, muscle tremors, convulsions, death. | Atropine (IV and SQ) | Dog died. | Classic organ-phosphate signs. |
| Ovaban® (megestrol acetate) | D(2) | Depressed, voracious appetite, gain in weight, polyuria, polydipsia. | Reduced dose, continued therapy | — | |
| Fluorescein (IV) | D | Acute anaphylactoid shock, collapse, hemorrhagic diarrhea. | Fluids, HCO₃, steroids | Recovery. | |
| ACD blood collection (given IV) | D(3) | Immediate tremors, convulsions. (Overdose of ACD in relation to blood volume injection.) | Ceased administration | Recovery. | Inadequate blood withdrawn from donor. |

* D=dog, C=cat, P=puppy, K=kitten, LC=large feral cats, R=raptors, SM=squirrel monkey. Number in ( ) is number of animals involved.

† Over-the-counter remedy.

In our experience in treating small animals over a 30-month period, CNS depressants and anesthetics were most often involved in adverse reactions. In this connection, the anesthetic mortality rate was 1.48/1000 hours, with halothane, methoxyflurane, thiobarbiturates, ketamine, xylazine and nitrous oxide being used and implicated in that decreasing order. Methoxyflurane is of interest because potentially it is metabolized to fluoride ions, which are nephrotoxic. Anesthetic morbidity in experimental animals and man seems to correlate with the depth and duration of anesthesia and with rising levels of serum fluoride.

In a broader sense, adverse reactions involving the nervous system are perhaps not surprising in view of this system's complexity. However, adverse manifestations exhibited by one organ system could well be the result of impaired hepatic metabolism or renal excretion. An increased frequency of adverse drug reactions in man is associated with renal dysfunction.

With respect to the liver, the frequency of adverse reactions increases as its function becomes more impaired, particularly when barbiturates, tranquilizers and other drugs which undergo hepatic biotransformation are used. With this in mind, and in view of the public's general awareness of drug toxicity, a practitioner might want to consider evaluation of serum transaminase, BUN, CPK and urine analysis, CBC or other parameters when potentially troublesome drugs are employed. By doing so, the vet-

erinarian might be in a better position to predict and forestall serious adverse reactions.

Other factors which seem to be involved in adverse reactions are the presence of infectious diseases, possibly because drug distribution and metabolism may be significantly altered in the presence of infection. Another important factor is a history of prior drug reactions, i.e., animals with a history of adverse reactions are more likely to experience adverse reactions to the same or other drugs in the future. This fact underscores the importance of obtaining a careful and detailed history.

When two or more drugs are employed simultaneously, the likelihood of adverse reactions is sharply increased. Extensive experience in human medicine demonstrates this quite clearly, and while it *seems* to be true in veterinary medicine, our experience is not sufficiently extensive at present to draw a firm conclusion, despite its intuitive appeal.

## SUPPLEMENTAL READING

Ballin, J. C.: The ADR numbers game revisited (Editorial). J.A.M.A., 234:1257, 1975.

Gralla, E. J.: Adverse drug reactions. Vet. Clin. N. Am., 5:699, 1975.

Gralla, E. J.: Drug interaction. Vet. Clin. N. Am., 5:717, 1975.

Harvey, T.: Drug induced reactions. In Kirk, R. W.: Current Veterinary Therapy V. Philadelphia, W. B. Saunders Co., 1974.

Karch, F. E., and Lasagna, L.: Adverse drug reactions. J.A.M.A., 234:1236, 1975.

---

# TERATOGENESIS

F. L. EARL, D.V.M.
*Washington, D.C.*

The discovery that the family pet has produced an abnormal offspring may be shocking to some owners while to others it may be a curiosity which needs only an explanation. Most clients today are too sophisticated to attribute its cause to some old wives' tales from which the word "terata," meaning monster, was derived. When a birth defect occurs in an offspring, the natural tendency is to attribute such a condition to heredity; miniaturization of breeds has resulted in a number of abnormalities such

as cardiac defects, hip dysplasia, malocclusion of the teeth, eye defects and aggressiveness. However, exposure to certain teratogenic drugs or other chemical agents during the crucial period of uterine development may also result in teratism. Infective viruses and physical injury to the pregnant mother should not be overlooked as potential causes of malformed offspring. Conceivably, excesses or deficiencies of certain nutritional factors can cause embryonic abnormalities but such etiologic causes are more in the experimental realm than in practice.

Embryologists postulate that biochemical inducers are responsible for the induction of an organ system. Once induced, complete development of the system is assured. In theory, inhibition of the inducer prevents the development of the system, but in practice this explanation of embryonic development does not account for all birth defects.

Teratogenesis is not as predictable in larger laboratory animals (dogs, cats, pigs, etc.) as in smaller laboratory animals (e.g., rodents). The feeding of experimental compounds to dogs after coitus but before implantation (18 days) may not affect the fetus unless the formation and attachment of the placenta are inhibited. This inhibition may result in resorption of the zygotes and a nonpregnant or pseudo-pregnant female. However, if formation of the placenta does occur, the compound may be embryotoxic rather than teratogenic.

Intrauterine deaths are usually not examined to determine the cause of death; therefore little information is available on the nature of such deaths. Experimentally, various chemicals have caused necrosis of the placenta at the maternal attachment, resulting in a narrowed placental band and a dwarf fetus, dead or dying shortly after birth. Resorption of the dead fetus occurs rapidly (within 2 weeks or less), and the only evidence that a fetus ever existed will be the small maternal band found at necropsy. A 5 per cent resorption rate of implanted fetuses is normal in dogs.

Subsequent pregnancies are not affected even if all pups are resorbed. Endometrial dysfunction is believed to be the cause of these intrauterine deaths. However, competition for uterine space and recessive genetic factors should not be overlooked as possible causes of stillbirth or dead fetuses. Inbreeding may result in high neonatal mortality while crossbreeding results in "hybrid vigor." A recessive gene may cause such an effect in homozygous offspring, whereas the heterozygote perpetuates the lethal factor; for example, examination of some dead fetuses showed anomalies like cleft palate/harelip, patent foramen ovale or ductus arteriosus, patent fontanelle, imperforate anus, hydrocephalus, atelectasis and other inherited glycolytic enzyme deficiencies or hemoglobinopathies. Familial amaurotic idiocy, hemophilia A and B, sub-

luxation of the carpus and cystinuria are considered to be transmitted on the X-chromosome of dogs.

Malformation of the mouth involving the teeth usually occurs mostly in toy breeds (Maltese, papillon, Pekingese, Pomeranian, etc.). In some breeds that have a very short face, the teeth are crowded, producing an abnormality.

Spontaneous malformations do occur in the form of dipygus tripus (two right rear limbs), spina bifida, cranioschisis and exophthalmos. Some of these conditions have been reported to occur following a bad fall on or about the 14th day of pregnancy, with a resulting 2-day coma during the presomite stage of development.

Functional disorders may result from developmental causes. Pylorospasm may not be detected until the dog is 4 to 6 weeks of age. Paraplegia has resulted from the progressive degeneration of the motor neurons of the lumbar portion of the spinal cord; atrophy of certain muscles in the rear limbs caused the paraplegia. Myasthenia gravis pseudoparalytica has been observed in dogs; it is a matter of conjecture whether it has been inherited or acquired.

Anomalies of the central nervous system can result in impaired sight, awkward and clumsy gait and fits. Usually an increased irritability of the skin and foot pads is associated with the onset of fits because the skin and the nervous system have the same embryologic origin.

Renal agenesis of one kidney usually affects males more than females and involves the left kidney more than the right. This condition is known to occur in approximately 0.2 per cent of necropsies. The functional kidney undergoes hypertrophy to compensate for the absence of the other kidney. Although cryptorchidism and perineal hypospadias may be associated with renal agenesis, urinary difficulties have been reported from renal agenesis only. This condition does not appear to be caused by an inherited defect but rather by a developmental deviation associated with metanephros independent of the developing metanephric tubules of the mesonephros in individual dogs.

Reports of teratogenic abnormalities attributable to accidental ingestion of foreign substances (teratogen) or injection of drugs are rare, probably because animals must be exposed to teratogens at a time when the embryo is susceptible. The embryo undergoes at least three critical stages of development. These stages can roughly be divided into (1) the stage before germ layer formation, (2) the embryonic stage and (3) the fetal stage.

The specific mechanisms of many teratogenic events are not clearly understood. One hypothesis is that the teratogen is nonspecific and the malformation which has occurred is dependent upon the organogenetic event in progress at the time of the insult. Thus many different malformations could result from a single teratogenic stimulus given at different critical periods of embryogenesis. An alternate hypothesis is that certain teratogens are site-specific; they induce malformations only in certain developing organ systems. Heavy metals, for example, are site-specific teratogens because they enter into a variety of rather specific enzymatic reactions.

The most critical time is the period of the germ layer formation and implantation of the embryo (postcoitus, day 17 to 18 in dogs and 13 to 14 in cats). A striking teratogenic effect can occur within hours during this critical period. This was readily demonstrated with such compounds as thalidomide. When the zygote is free-floating in the uterus before implantation, direct teratogenic effects upon the embryo are not thought to be possible. If the concentration of the teratogen is great enough, placentation is prevented and embryonic deaths occur.

Present laws do much to prevent the careless handling of prescribed drugs. However, a practitioner should not overlook the possibility of teratogenic insults produced by carelessness on the part of the owner in leaving drugs or pesticides accessible to curious pets. Theoretically, it might be possible for a pet to be exposed to enough high-potency vitamin A capsules (125,000 I.U./kg.) or substances such as mescaline (peyote) to cause teratogenesis. The minimal teratogenic dose of vitamin A is not known. Mescaline causes malformation of the brain, spinal cord, liver and other viscera in hamsters, and these potential effects might occur in other pets if mescaline were accessible to them.

The possibility that teratogenesis would result from an acute dose of a teratogen after organogenesis has occurred (after 30 to 35 days) is rather remote. After this period, the fetus is completely formed and merely grows until parturition. However, tissues undergoing growth and/or maturation, such as the cerebellum and some cardiovascular and urogenital structures, can become deformed; these deformities later manifest themselves as learning and reproductive difficulties when the offspring begin to mature. Occasionally, anasarcous pups are seen.

The amount of the teratogen ingested does not appear to be as important as the time it was consumed. Apparently, there is a critical period at the time of implantation when a low blood level of the teratogen will cause teratogenic effects. Higher doses or doses given before or after implantation do not have the same effect. There are, of course, exceptions to these potential teratogenic agents.

The veterinary practitioner should establish a policy of not administering drugs, biologics or injectables to pregnant bitches or queens, especially during the first half of pregnancy. Injectables should not be given even in late pregnancy. Subcutaneous injections of testosterone propionate into the dam between days 35 and 42 of the pregnancy are believed to have caused ovarian hermaphroditism in two pups, manifested by hypoplastic penis and undescended testicles. A third pup had an enlarged clitoris in which a bony corpus was noted clinically as well as by x-ray technique. The injection of 25 mg. of progesterone intramuscularly, followed by norethindrone orally at 2.5 mg./day, resulted in masculinization of the external genitalia of the female pups of a pregnant boxer. These compounds were administered during the period of gestation when the external genitalia were being formed, causing a more extensive fusion of the labia than normal. Corticosteroids should not be administered to pregnant females. Deformed forelegs, phocomelia and ankylosed forelegs have been observed in a litter of cocker spaniel pups in which the dam was treated with dexamethasone during the latter half of gestation. There are indications that corticosteroids may be the cause of an increase in the number of anasarcous pups in the brachycephalic breeds.

Griseofulvin is believed to have produced cleft palates in 6 of 7 pups born after the daily administration of 750 mg. to a golden retriever bitch 4 weeks preceding and throughout pregnancy. The bitch had no history of abnormal litters from previous or subsequent matings. Experimentally, the daily administration of 35 mg. griseofulvin per kg. to beagle bitches for as little as one week to as long as the entire period of gestation resulted in resorptions and small, weak, short-haired pups with multiple subcutaneous hemorrhages of the head, extremities and abdomen. A cleft palate was observed in 1 of 3 kittens from a queen administered a similar dose throughout pregnancy. Teratogenic effects in the offspring of cats given griseofulvin clinically during pregnancy included shortened tails, shortened hind limbs, absence of phalanges and fused phalanges of the posterior limbs.

The possibility of nutritionally induced teratogenesis is remote. A nutritional deficiency producing a clinical case of teratogenesis would be almost impossible except under laboratory conditions. The same would be true of an environmental contaminant. Exposure to 0.1 mg./kg. methyl mercury chloride (MeHgCl) before and during gestation for 129 days produced abnormal development in 1 of 10 litters, including omphalocele, cleft palate, patent fontanelles, superfluous phalanges and enlarged kidneys. Pregnant cats given MeHgCl at 0.25 mg./kg. daily had an increased incidence of abortions and fetal abnormalities. In surviving fetuses, histopathology revealed a reduced neuronal population in the external granular layer of the cerebellum. A kitten from a queen treated with bis-ethyl mercuric sulfide displayed an unsteady gait and a disturbance of posture fixation two weeks after birth; the kitten died 3 months later. Granular atrophy of the cerebellum was present in both the mother and the affected kitten. Cats and dogs should not be fed the meat of animals accidentally exposed to alkyl mercury or fish containing high levels of mercury residues because it may produce not only teratogenic effects in the offspring but also blindness in the dam. It is highly improbable that environmental lead contamination could cause a teratogenic problem in pets, since few effects have been observed from experimental tests on larger laboratory animals (dogs, swine, sheep, goats and cattle) fed extremely high doses of lead salts.

Many pesticides have been shown experimentally to be teratogenic. Carbaryl, a reversible cholinesterase inhibitor, administered in the diet to pregnant bitches at levels as low as 6.25 mg./kg. throughout pregnancy caused teratism in 11.6 per cent of 186 pups. Fetal abnormalities include abdominal-thoracic fissures with varying degrees of intestinal agenesis and displacement, brachygnathia, ecaudate pups, failure of skeletal formation and superfluous phalanges. Uterine atony causing dystocia was also frequent. Other pesticides found to be teratogenic were Diazinon®, captan and lindane. Drugs shown to produce experimental teratogenesis in dogs are aminopterin, hydroxyurea, hydroxyzine (Atarax®) and thalidomide. Administration of thalidomide to dogs did not produce the phocomelia seen in man. In fact, dogs were not a good model for thalidomide, as teratogenic effects were difficult to demonstrate. The teratogenic effects of thalidomide on the offsprings of cats are primarily cardiovascular defects.

Viruses (German measles, mumps, etc.) and protozoa (toxoplasmosis) have been shown to cause congenital defects in man. Similarly, feline panleukemia virus has an affinity for dividing cells, making the cerebellum especially vulnerable to *in-utero* infections prior to birth and in early neonatal life. Degeneration and hypoplasia of the cerebellum and other visceral abnormalities have been observed. Ataxia has been seen in kittens from affected cats. Although congenital infections of toxoplasmosis occur in dogs and cats, developmental defects attributable to *in-utero* infection have not been reported.

Improper neonatal husbandry may produce a condition called "swimmer" pup. This condition is noted in 1 to 2 days after birth and becomes progressively worse. Such a pup has a broad, flat chest and is unable to get its feet under it. This broad, flat chest might be interpreted as a congenital abnormality. These pups are usually seen in litters of only 1 to 2 pups. The dams are prolific milk producers and have been housed in whelping boxes with slick floors. This abnormality results from inactivity and overeating, i.e., not enough exercise from crawling over littermates and no incentive to move, combined with easy access to large amounts of milk. Large litters afford competition among the pups, which corrects all these factors by decreasing milk consumption and forcing competitive exercise by crawling over one another. The slick floors could be corrected by covering them with a rug or hardware cloth.

When an abnormal fetus or offspring is

presented to the practitioner, a careful history should be obtained from the owner. It should be determined whether the dam has been exposed to any drugs, biologics or infections or has undergone any unusual changes during pregnancy. The breeding history of the sire and dam should be obtained, if possible, for three generations to determine if there were previous teratogenic defects. The obvious causes should not be overlooked before more obscure reasons are investigated.

Clients with dogs or cats used for breeding should be advised that dams should not be given any drugs or biologics during pregnancy. A history of unusual happenings should be maintained during pregnancy and should be carefully reviewed if fetal abnormalities are found at birth. Such defects should not be corrected by cosmetic surgery on a breeding animal unless it can be determined that the defect is not of genetic origin. If there is any question as to the origin of the defect, the animal should be neutered before sexual maturity.

## SUPPLEMENTAL READING

Earl, F. L.: Developmental abnormalities in the dog. In Benirschke, K. et al. (eds.): Pathology of Laboratory Animals. New York, Springer–Verlag, in press.

Earl, F., Miller, E., and Van Loon, E. J.: Teratogenic research in beagle dogs and miniature swine. In Spiegel, A. (ed.): The Laboratory Animal in Drug Testing. Stuttgart, Gustav Fischer Verlag, 5th Symposium of the International Committee on Lab. Animals (ICLA), Hanover, Germany, 1973, pp. 233–248.

Earl, F., Miller, E., and Van Loon, E. J.: Reproductive, teratogenic and neonatal effects of some pesticides and related compounds in beagle dogs and miniature swine. In Deichmann, W. B. (ed.): Pesticides and the Environment: A Continuing Controversy. Vol. 2. New York City, International Medical Book Corp., 1973, pp. 253–266.

Earl, F. L., and Vish, T. J.: Teratogenicity of heavy metals. In Oehme, F. W. (ed.): Toxicity of Heavy Metals in the Environment. New York, Marcel Dekker, in press.

Fox, M. W.: Diseases of possible hereditary origin in the dog: A bibliographic review. J. Hered. 56:169–176, 1965.

Kalter, H. : Teratology of the Central Nervous System. Chicago, University of Chicago Press, 1968.

Robens, J. F.: Teratogenesis. In Kirk, R. W. (ed.): Current Veterinary Therapy V. Philadelphia, W. B. Saunders Co., 1974.

---

# CARCINOGENESIS

T. GOPAL, M.V.Sc.
*Manhattan, Kansas*

The normal behavior of a cell in the biologic system can be changed into neoplasia by the influence of various factors. Such a transformed cell is capable of further multiplication without any restraint on its growth and hence is designated as *cancerous*. The initiation process, *carcinogenesis*, comprises a complex of sequential events within the cell that eventually lead to *cancer*. Agents or factors responsible for initiating cancer are termed *carcinogens*. The study of carcinogens and carcinogenesis broadly includes the study of cancer and its pathogenesis.

## INCIDENCE

Despite the fact that cancer can be induced by various etiologic agents, as evidenced by controlled experimentation in animals and circumstantial evidence in humans, the question remains unanswered as to the specific cause of some naturally and spontaneously occurring neoplasms in animals. The incidence of cancer in animals is mostly recognized by clinical signs, and many times it is encountered as an incidental finding during necropsy. The effect is seen, but not the cause.

## MODIFYING FACTORS

The commonly observed spontaneously occurring neoplasms in animals suggest that genetic composition of the host is the most important intrinsic factor determining individual susceptibility and resistance. The genetic component can be modified by various endogenous factors, such as heredity, age, sex, species and breed. Other individual physiologic variations of hormonal, metabolic and biochemical activities, which upset the normal homeostatic restraint on cell growth, also contribute to the initiation of carcinogenesis.

Animal neoplasms probably result from favorable host genetic composition acted upon by one or more interacting exogenous factors, such as various physical, chemical or biologic agents, in combination. The information on the incidence of animal cancer suggests that many etiologic agents associated with human cancer may also be responsible for animal cancer. This is probably true, since domestic animals often share the same environment as man.

## SOURCES

Most of the environmental carcinogens are found naturally, but some of them find their way into the environment intentionally or accidentally. The increasing incidence of human cancer and the experimental induction of cancer using newly synthesized chemicals support the fact that man-made environmental carcinogens will result in a continued distinct hazard to human and animal health.

The effect of slow-growing viruses in the environment combined with low-grade exposure to various chemical pollutants has increased the risk of cancer. The possibility that many dormant viruses are capable of triggering carcinogenesis has been suspected for many years, and the evidence accumulated by recent studies supports this concept.

## ETIOLOGIC AGENTS

**Physical Agents.** Many of the physical agents carcinogenic in man are also carcinogenic in animals. Ultraviolet rays and ionizing radiation are major initiators of malignancy in experimental animals. Radioactive fallout from nuclear reactions has the potential for carcinogenic effects in animals.

Experimental studies in different species of animals with various radioactive substances have confirmed the carcinogenic effects of ionizing radiation. Whole-body radiation in dogs has produced cancer of the thyroid and has caused leukemias. Inhalation and ingestion of radioactive compounds have resulted in cancer.

Chronic irritation, as in some horn cancers in East Indian cattle, and the presence of certain parasites, like *Spirocerca lupi* in dogs and *Gasterophilus* spp. in horses, have been incriminated as initiators of cancer.

**Chemical Agents.** Owing to the increased use of synthetic chemicals in agriculture, medicine and industry, chemical carcinogens have received considerable attention. The frequency with which these substances appear and their potential properties of carcinogenic activity in man and animals have gained much importance. Some of them are intentionally included in foods as additives and preservatives, and others are included as drugs for therapy and increased food production. Others unintentionally find their way into the environment as synthetic fertilizers, insecticides, growth promoters and industrial and automobile effluents.

Some of the known animal carcinogens are 2-naphthalamine, benzidine, 4-aminobiphenyl, 2-acetylaminofluorene, N-methyl-4-aminoazobenzene, dimethylnitrosamine, diethylstilbestrol and polycyclic aromatic hydrocarbons. Among the naturally occurring carcinogens are aflatoxins, cycasins and pyrrolizidine alkaloids.

The mechanism of chemical carcinogenesis varies with the chemical and its biologic behavior in a given species of animal. There is wide individual variation. Many theories have been suggested concerning the actual mechanism. In general, a common mechanism is suggested in which the chemical carcinogen acts by altering or destroying the preexisting genetic information in the normal host cell. In a simple way, a chemical carcinogen behaves by "hitting and running," leaving behind an altered cell. This is probably true for many chemicals, since they are often not present in the system during the actual growth of the cancer.

This suggests that the initial reaction between carcinogen and target cell may be of short duration and is most likely irreversible. In other instances, the chemical undergoes activation by various enzymatic systems to an ultimate carcinogen which is highly reactive with cellular components, particularly those involved with genetic control of cell growth, i.e., DNA, RNA and proteins.

Virtually all chemical carcinogens interact with DNA to produce alkylation, acylation and depurination reactions. Recent evidence suggests that DNA is the genetic material that plays a key role in maintaining the functional integrity of the cell; after DNA's interaction with a chemical carcinogen, faulty information will be transferred during DNA replication. If the interaction occurs when DNA is replicating, the effect is immediate and permanent. However, if the carcinogen interacts with other macromolecular components of the cell, like RNA or other proteins, the change has to be incorporated into DNA at a later stage. This will lead to slow carcinogenesis. Whether interaction with the genetic component of the cell produces spontaneous transformation or a slow transformation, the ultimate effect is the same. In immediate transformation the affected cell produces cancerous cells directly; the slow transformation process is successively transmitted through several generations until a population of completely transformed cells results.

**Biologic Agents.** Biologic carcinogens include a broad group of viruses of the RNA and DNA type. Studies of virus-induced neoplasms in birds and mammals indicate that the genetic material contained in the virus results in altered genetic control of the host cell, with subsequent transfer of information to successive generations. The DNA or RNA component of the virus is incorporated in the DNA or RNA of the cell and initiates cancer. Virus-induced malignancies include avian leukosis, sarcomas and cutaneous papillomas in a wide range of animals. Leukemia and lymphosarcomas are frequently encountered in cats.

Certain parasites are associated with cancer of animals. *Spirocerca lupi*-induced sarcomas in dogs and cancer associated with *Ganglionema neoplasticum* in rats are some of the examples. The initiation of cancer by these agents has been attributed to chronic irritation rather than to chemical factors. Although the occurrence of carcinogenic metabolites has not been established, the possibility should not be overlooked.

The incidence of transmissible venereal lymphogranuloma in dogs is rare in the United States, but isolated cases are reported. The neoplastic cell is not the somatic component of the host but rather is mechanically transmitted by coitus. Under favorable conditions of susceptibility the transplanted cell gives rise to successive neoplastic generations. Since there is no involvement of the host cell material, it appears that the host is used for the *in-vivo* propagation of the neoplastic cell.

## SUPPLEMENTAL READING

Farber, E.: Mechanisms by which chemicals initiate cancer. J. Clin. Pharmacol., *15*:24–28, 1975.

Heidelberger, C.: Chemical carcinogenesis. Ann. Rev. Biochem., *44*:79–121, 1975.

Meier, H.: Epizootiology of cancer in animals. Ann. N.Y. Acad. Sci., *108*:617–1326, 1963.

Moulton, J. E.: Tumors in Domestic Animals. Berkeley, California, University of California Press, 1961.

Temin, H. M.: On the origin of the genes for neoplasia. Cancer Res., *34*:2835–2841, 1974.

Wolff, A. H., and Oehme, F. W.: Carcinogenic chemicals in food as an environmental health issue. J. Am. Vet. Med. Assn., *164*:623–629, 1974.

# BITES AND STINGS OF VENOMOUS ANIMALS

FREDRIC L. FRYE, D.V.M.
*Berkeley, California*

## INTRODUCTION

While not an everyday occurrence in most veterinary practices, the occasional case of a patient who has been envenomated by a biting or stinging animal makes this a subject of more than academic interest. Depending upon the frequency at which these cases are clinically seen, the practitioner may find it advisable to stock his pharmacy with specific and/or polyvalent antivenins and other emergency drugs so that they may be readily available if and when the need arises. If the incidence of venomous bites and stings is very low, these materials can usually be obtained from most municipal hospital emergency departments.

## SNAKE BITES

In North America, there are only four principal poisonous snakes. They are confined to two subfamilies: the *Crotalidae*, or pit vipers, encompass the rattlesnakes, the copperhead, the "cottonmouth" water moccasin and the Mexican cantil. The second subfamily, *Elapidae*, embraces those snakes of the genus *Micrurus*, the colorful coral snakes of the southern United States and Mexico. The coral snakes are related to the Old World cobras and kraits. Most of the rattlesnakes are assigned to the genus *Crotalus*, but there are also a few small rattlesnakes, such as the massasauga and pygmy rattlesnakes, which are within the genus *Sistrurus*.

Most of the pit vipers are identified by their lance- or arrow-shaped heads with rather prominent temporal width, well set-off from a narrower neck. Their skins are rough-textured owing to the presence of "keels," which are located in the center of each dermal scale along the dorsal and lateral surfaces of their bodies. Most have vertically elliptical pupils, and all have a deep pit located between their nostrils and anterior canthi. This pit is associated with an organ which is sensitive to infrared radiation detection.

The coral snakes are usually smaller than most pit vipers, with indistinct heads that are not much wider than the necks which support them, and they have smooth scales. They are also very brightly colored with bands in shades of vivid red, yellow or white, and jet black. While other snakes of the harmless kingsnake genus, *Lampropeltis*, may very closely mimic the poisonous coral snakes, an important differentiation can be made: only in the coral snake are bands of red and yellow in juxtaposition. The kingsnakes, or "false coral snakes," have these colors interposed between bands of black. Whereas the pit vipers are equipped with long, hollow and hinged fangs which are deployed when the mouth is opened widely, the coral snakes have short, grooved and fixed fangs which must be brought into functional use by the snake's making a deliberate bite and actually chewing upon the victim in order to embed the fangs and introduce the venom.

There are many other structural differences among these animals, but it should suffice to mention that when presented with

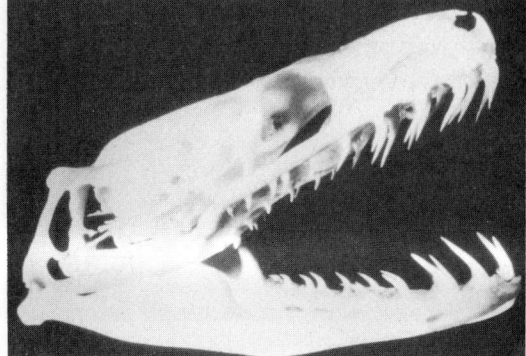

**Figure 1.** Typical dental configuration of a nonvenomous snake. This is the skull of a boa constrictor. (Courtesy of Nathan W. Cohen, Ph.D.)

an obvious, or even suspected, snakebite victim, the major emphasis will be directed toward treating the patient rather than making a finite taxonomic identification of the biting snake. Frequently, the snake has left the scene long before its victim is even noted to have been envenomated.

The bite of a nonvenomous snake usually appears as a semilunar or "U"-shaped row of tiny punctures made by the snake's teeth. There is minimal pain and induration in the area, and even these signs subside quickly. The mere swabbing of the punctures with hydrogen peroxide and an antiseptic should suffice in most cases.

The pit vipers, owing to their more open habitats. often will strike upon being disturbed; the more secretive coral snakes usually will have to be mauled or stepped upon before being induced to bite. Even then, coral snakes will have to hold fast to their victim and chew at the same time, as previously described. The fang arrange-

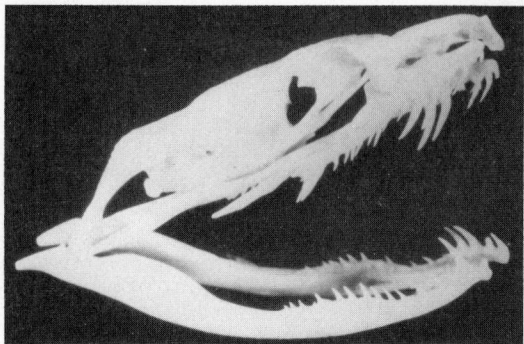

**Figure 2.** Skull of a rear-fanged snake. Note the rear fangs, which necessitate an active chewing upon a victim in order to envenomate a victim effectively. (Courtesy of Nathan W. Cohen, Ph.D.)

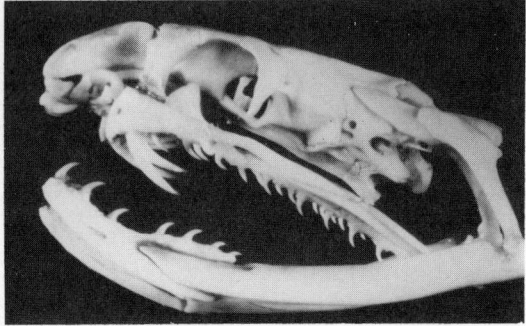

**Figure 3.** Skull of a typical Elapid snake, an Indian cobra. Note the forward location of the short fangs. (Courtesy of Nathan W. Cohen, Ph.D.)

ments of typical venomous snakes are illustrated in Figures 2 to 4. Although there are some rear-fanged snakes which conceivably could envenomate companion animals, the extreme rarity of such occurrences will eliminate them from this discussion. Their fangs are placed well back in their mouths; their venoms are more adapted to immobilizing cold-blooded prey; and a meaningful bite, producing signs of envenomation, would necessitate considerable chewing on the part of the snake with concurrent acquiescence on the part of the victim!

## PATHOGENESIS

Most snake venoms are principally proteinaceous and consist of enzymes and toxins. Some of the identified enzymes are

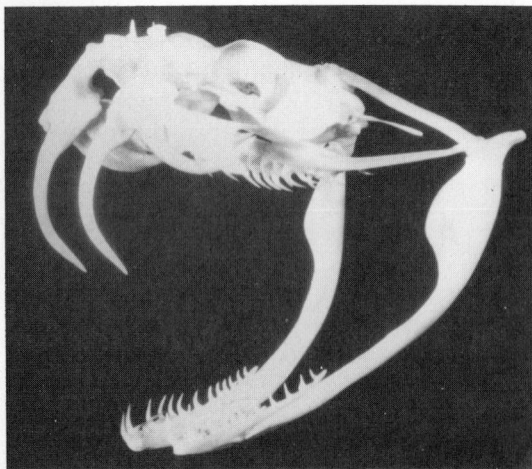

**Figure 4.** The fang placement typical to those viperine snakes such as rattlesnakes, water moccasin and the Old World vipers. (Courtesy of Nathan W. Cohen, Ph.D.)

hyaluronidase, L-amino-oxidase, various proteases, phospholipases, phosphatases and coagulases. Numerous hemolysins and neurotoxins have also been characterized by chromatography.

Most of the pit vipers possess venoms which are predominately active in producing hemolysis and tissue necrosis. Some also contain specific neurotoxins which vary with the individual species. The coral snakes, on the other hand, are adapted to employing neurotoxic venoms which are more potent on a volumetric basis than most hemotoxic venoms. The small size of the coral snake limits the actual volume of venom which can be injected during a single biting experience. These neurotoxins produce multiple neuromuscular blocks which result in a wide variety of autonomic and central nervous system signs. Cardiorespiratory failure is a frequent sequel to a severe, untreated envenomation by a venomous elapid snake.

In most cases, snake venoms are absorbed via the lymphatic system. A direct injection into a vein may prove fatal within a very brief time.

The gravity of a given snakebite depends upon many variables: the body weight, body composition (fat or lean) and general health of the patient; the presence or absence of a thick fur coat or subcutaneous fat layer which may absorb the venom or impede its absorption; and the condition of the snake itself. The species of the snake, *its* general health, the interval since its last feeding, the virulence of its venom, the length and strength of its fangs and the total volume of venom injected are also important considerations. Finally, the presence of pathogenic bacteria either within the snake's mouth or upon the skin of the victim may also affect the eventual result of the bite.

## PHYSICAL SIGNS

In the case of a bite by a pit viper, the major *immediate* signs following the injection of venom are pain, swelling, erythema and serum or lymphatic transudation from the fang punctures. As time passes, the swelling and pain extend proximally and distally from the bite. This swelling can often reach alarmingly massive proportions. Frank hemorrhage, beginning as petechiation and extending through ecchymoses to hemolytic effusions, is seen. Eventually, the tissues distal to the bite may become somewhat anesthetized. More general systemic signs of envenomation are salivation, diarrhea, hyperpnea and sometimes convulsions. As signs of shock progress, the pulse rate increases and the pulse itself becomes thready, the body temperature falls and respiratory collapse may ensue. If the victim survives the initial period following envenomation, the body temperature tends to rise as necrosis and infection proceed.

Because of the plethora of microorganisms which may be present in the mouths of snakes, serious wound-borne infections frequently accompany snakebites. These organisms find a very suitable growth medium in the warm and moist environment surrounding the bite. In such a milieu, there is no shortage of nutrients, and pathogens rapidly multiply. Clostridial bacteria are common inhabitants of reptilian oral cavities.

The bite of a coral snake, being basically a neurotoxic activity, will reflect the action of the venom upon neuromuscular function; therefore symptoms manifested will be pain, salivation, vomition, diarrhea, urinary incontinence and cardiorespiratory collapse due to the cholinesterases and related components of the venom. Some hemolytic activity may also be exhibited, but the majority of the signs will reflect the neurotoxic character of the venom.

## TREATMENT

Obviously, the presence of actual fang wounds consisting of one or two small punctures should be ascertained. Depending upon the distance between the two punctures, an estimate of the size of the snake can be made. In practice, however, the clinician will find that his or her time will be adequately consumed in merely trying to overcome the effects of the bite and will probably leave the intellectual pursuit of snake size to a more propitious moment. At least, the practitioner finding a widely spaced pair of punctures can assume that a relatively large volume of venom may have been injected and a correspondingly large amount of antivenin may be required to neutralize the venom.

Classically, the recommended treatment for poisonous snakebite has consisted of immobilization, pain relief, application of a suitable tourniquet to limit the spread of the venom, incision and removal of as much venom as possible, neutralization of absorbed venom and sound supportive therapy including antibiotic and parenteral fluid administration. Other measures will be discussed here.

Unless the bite has occurred on the head, trunk or genitalia, a flat tourniquet should be applied proximal to the site of envenomation to impede the spread of venom. This tourniquet need compress only the lymphatic flow from the area where the bite occurred; it need not stop venous and arterial circulation, since this may only aggravate the swelling. A flat latex rubber drain tube makes an excellent tourniquet for this purpose. If the operator can slip a finger beneath the tourniquet when it is in place, it is tight enough. This constriction should be left *in situ* for about 45 to 60 minutes at a time. More frequent changes may only enhance the lymphatic return centrally.

In man, the use of suction to aid in the removal of venom from a bite has become standard practice. In veterinary medicine, the furry companion animals one is most likely to see as snakebite victims pose a difficult problem: even after clipping or shaving the bite area and applying water, lubricating jelly or Vaseline®, the maintenance of sufficient suction leaves much to be desired. In some cases, when judgment deems it applicable, it should be attempted.

The bite area should be quickly prepared for incision by routine clipping of the hair or fur and scrubbing of the skin with an appropriate antiseptic. A single linear (not cruciate) incision is carried to a depth of at least 5 millimeters and should connect the two fang marks. Some authorities advise the total excision of an elliptical piece of skin and subcutaneous tissue surrounding and beneath the bite wounds. This may be necessary in some cases, but this author has never resorted to this procedure.

If the swelling progresses rapidly in spite of all ancillary treatment, additional incisions have proved useful. These are most advantageously made about 1 centimeter long and about 5 millimeters deep and should be made longitudinally to avoid severing vital soft tissue structures. These secondary incisions should be made along the front of the advancing swelling in such a manner that serum may ooze directly from them as cellulitis develops.

When deemed appropriate, a modified Robert Jones dressing may be applied to help immobilize the limb and absorb tissue fluids and venom from the incisions. Not only will such a dressing aid in absorption, but it will also reduce lymphatic flow and minimize the pain typical of such bites. Naturally, if such a dressing is employed, remember to service the tourniquet at intervals.

In the author's opinion, the use of local hypothermia is advantageous in limiting tissue necrosis and pain. Ice packs have proved quite suitable for this purpose and should be applied and changed whenever necessary. Local frostbite or freezing of the already damaged tissues must be avoided. The ice packs can be wrapped in towels to obviate this problem.

Under ideal circumstances, the patient should be treated in the hospital. Appropriate veins are catheterized, and a continuous intravenous infusion of lactated Ringer's solution is maintained. This route will insure a ready means for delivering those medications which are most satisfactorily administered intravenously.

If antivenin is available to the clinician, it should be reconstituted with its accompanying diluent (Table 1). Equal volumes are injected intramuscularly and intravenously. This antivenin should not be injected directly into the actual bites themselves. Some authorities advocate the intraarterial injection of antivenin, claiming a more rapid action in neutralizing the absorbed venom. The commercial laboratories which produce these antivenins recommend the intravenous and intramuscular routes of administration only, and this author has found these routes efficacious when treating the bites of pit vipers. The actual amount of antivenin to be used depends upon the advance or regression of swelling and any accompanying systemic signs. For many small companion pet animals, a single ampule may be sufficient. In others, several doses may be required.

Adjunctive therapy with adrenal corticosteroids also has its proponents and opponents. This author believes that they *are* indicated in severe envenomations to help reduce both local and widespread systemic effects of the venom. Additionally, since most of the antivenins are of noncanine origin, these steroids may obviate any untoward serum reactions from this heterologous source. For pain relief, meperidine

**Table 1.**   *Specific Antivenins in Treatment of Bites and Stings of Animals in North America*

| PRODUCT | MANUFACTURER | APPLICATION |
| --- | --- | --- |
| Antivenin Crotalidae, Polyvalent® (North and South American antisnakebite serum)* | Wyeth Laboratories, Marietta, Pa. | For antiserum treatment of snakebites by pit vipers, family *Crotalidae*, including *Crotalus, Agkistrodon, Sistrurus, Bothrops, Lachesis* and *Trimeresurus.* |
| Antivenin (*Latrodectus mactans* antivenin) Lyovac® | Merck, Sharp and Dohme, Philadelphia, Pa. | For antiserum treatment of black widow spider bites. Also shown to be effective in treatment of redlegged widow spider bite. |
| Suero Antialacran Myn®, S.A. (polyvalent) | Laboratorios Myn, Av. Coyoacan 1707, Mexico 12, D.F. | For antiserum treatment of scorpion stings by the following species of the genus *Centruroides*: *C. suffusus suffusus, C. noxius, C. 1. limpidus, C. 1. tecumanus, C. 1. infamatus* and *C. sculpturatus.* |

*The U.S. Department of Agriculture recently licensed the first polyvalent antivenin specifically recommended for treating dogs bitten by rattlesnakes, copperheads, water moccasins and related pit vipers. The new product is identical to the antivenin used to treat humans bitten by these snakes. It is produced by Wyeth Laboratories of Marietta, Pennsylvania, and is marketed by Fort Dodge Laboratories of Fort Dodge, Iowa.

HCl has proved to be the most effective to date. The addition of antihistamines such as diphenylhydramine HCl, Pyribenzamine® HCl, chlorpheniramine maleate, etc., also has had its supporters and detractors. In most cases treated by this writer, one of these agents has been used with what are believed to be beneficial results. The benefit of administering calcium gluconate in snakebite therapy is conjectural, but probably is, at worst, harmless; it might conceivably be useful. Lastly, a *bactericidal* injectable antibiotic or combination of antibiotics should be employed to help the patient combat infection.

If respiratory distress is evident, assistance should be initiated with the use of oxygen cages, masks or artificial respiration. If it is absolutely necessary, a small animal patient can be fully anesthetized and placed upon an assist-breathing apparatus while local and systemic therapy progresses. Obviously, this will simplify restraint and relieve pain, but it does impose another variable and additional stress upon the patient.

## VENOMOUS LIZARD BITES

There are only two poisonous lizards in the world and both are residents of North America. They are the Gila "monster" of Arizona and the Mexican beaded lizard. Both of these large, colorful lizards belong to a single genus, *Heloderma*. The Gila monster is a squat, bead-skinned animal with stout jaws and a fat tail. Its usual colors are pink-orange and black. The somewhat larger Mexican beaded lizard has a more streamlined tail configuration and presents less of a stubby appearance. Coloration consists of yellow and black random bars and whorls. Both species are rather sluggish and do not usually display a propensity to strike *per se*, but rather, if tormented, will deliberately bite and chew tenaciously. Once having clamped their powerful jaws, these lizards usually will not release their grip without some inducement in the form of a pry bar or tire iron.

Both lizards have four pairs of modified salivary glands located in the lower jaw which secrete their venom directly into the oral cavity; the stout teeth are thereby bathed in toxic salivary secretions. Grooves in the teeth provide an effective means for delivering the venom to the lizards' prey or tormentors.

There are several documented cases of human envenomation arising from the careless handling of these reptiles. A dog who would maul or mouth one of these lizards could, quite conceivably, be bitten and poisoned.

The clinical signs of venomous lizard bites are similar to those produced by the pit vipers plus some neurotoxic manifestations as well. While there are no specific antivenins made to neutralize the venoms of these two animals, the treatment is almost identical to that for snakebite. Several authors recommend local hypothermia as an adjunct to other medical management. *The one major departure from routine snakebite therapy is the contraindication for meperidine HCl (Demerol®) in controlling the pain associated with the venom from* Heloderma. *Apparently meperidine HCl is synergistic with the venom of these reptiles and only compounds the toxicity when used.* This effect has not been shown in conjunction with the treatment of other venomous reptile bites.

## SPIDER, SCORPION, CENTIPEDE AND OTHER ARTHROPOD BITES AND STINGS

While the veterinary clinician may often be presented with a patient whom he may *suspect* of having been bitten or stung by an arthropod, it is rare when the actual biting or stinging "beastie" is identified; the exceptions, of course, are bees and wasps, which the animals' owners may actually have seen. The suspicion is usually the result of the clinical signs associated with such stings or bites. These signs are intense pain, erythema, swelling, salivation, diarrhea, vomiting and general malaise. In severe envenomation, cardiorespiratory collapse may be seen.

### SPIDER BITES

The only significant spider species living in North America capable of producing clinical signs justifying medical management are (1) the black widow spider, *Latrodectus mactans*; (2) the red-legged widow spider, *Latrodectus bishopi*; (3) the brown recluse spider, *Loxosceles reclusa*; and (4) the common brown spider, *Loxosceles unicolor*.

From the standpoint of treatment, the two widow spiders produce venoms which induce signs which may last several days and are related to the neurotoxic character of their components. Specific and polyvalent antivenins are available which are somewhat cross-protective but are only rarely employed in treating companion animals.

The bites of the two brown spiders of the genus *Loxosceles*, on the other hand, produce more chronic effects. Typically, the area of the bite ulcerates, leaving a necrotic center. This indolent ulcer may not heal spontaneously for several months. Often, total excision of the chronic lesion and skin grafting may be necessary to effect a cure.

For the acutely ill patient affected with a widow spider bite, general supportive therapy consists of intravenous fluids, adrenal corticosteroids, antihistamines and meperidine HCl. Prophylactic antibiotics are also advised. There have been several reports in the medical literature indicating that calcium and magnesium ions, specifically, relieve the serious voluntary muscular spasms. These salts may be administered intravenously as calcium gluconate and magnesium sulfate, respectively, in appropriate dosages. It is of interest to speculate whether a specific muscle relaxant such as methocarbamol (Robaxin®*) would act to lessen these muscle signs. This might prove to be a rational adjunct to the treatment of the widow spider bites.

### SCORPION STINGS

While scorpions are widely distributed throughout much of North America, there are, fortunately, only a few species of potentially lethal scorpions in the United States. Most of these arachnids belong to the genus *Centruroides*. The actual incidence in veterinary medicine of known cases of scorpion stings has not been established but is apparently quite low. Many stings probably go unnoticed and therefore undiagnosed.

Because of the neurotoxic action of scorpion venoms, especially upon the autonomic nervous system, the clinical signs following envenomation by a scorpion sting are pain, muscular contractions, salivation,

*A. H. Robbins.

respiratory paralysis, bronchoconstriction, piloerection, vasoconstriction, hypertension and mydriasis.

The venom is contained within the terminal bulb, or *telson*, which is located at the end of the scorpion's tail. At its terminus, the telson bears a partially recurved sting. When the scorpion is feeding, annoyed or restrained, it elevates its tail and strikes or drives this sting into the flesh of its prey or tormentor. At the same time, voluntary muscles contained within the telson contract, expressing the venom through the hollow sting and into the soft tissues of its victim.

The clinical signs following a scorpion sting depend upon the species of the scorpion, body weight and condition of its target animal, amount and virulence of the injected venom and many of the same criteria as in snakebite.

The advised treatment is based upon combating the neurotoxic effects of the venom. Specific antivenin for the neutralization of the venom of *Centruroides* spp. is available but rarely employed in companion animals. Atropine sulfate has been shown to have a specific antagonistic effect against many of the signs relating to scorpion venom. Intravenous antihistamines, corticosteroids, meperidine HCl and lactated Ringer's solution may be indicated as each case dictates.

### CENTIPEDE BITES

While centipedes are potentially capable of producing painful bites with their powerful mouthparts, specific envenomation in the United States is virtually unknown. Symptomatic treatment consists of local wound treatment and, if necessary, analgesic medication.

### BEE, WASP AND ANT STINGS AND BITES

Bee and wasp venoms are both neurotoxic and hemolytic in their pharmacodynamic action. Multiple stings may cause systemic illness in some individuals, and a solitary sting can cause peracute anaphylactic reactions in the hypersensitive patient. In the normal individual, the usual reaction to the sting of a bee or wasp is acute pain, erythema, local induration, edema and, later, pruritus. Hypersensitive individuals, if stung by a single bee or wasp, may exhibit anaphylactoid signs, with urticaria, nausea, vomiting, diarrhea, edema of the head, laryngeal edema, dyspnea, hypotension and death.

Most ants inject formic acid when biting, and this usually produces local pain and swelling. The fire ant, *Solenopsis invicta*, is now spreading its range into the southern United States. Its bites produce surrounding vesiculation. Treatment is symptomatic.

Treatment, depending upon the severity of the signs, consists of antihistamines, local hypothermia, application of wet soaks of sodium bicarbonate and sometimes adrenal corticosteroids. In acute emergencies, subcutaneous injections of epinephrine in doses of 0.20 to 0.50 ml. of a 1:1000 aqueous solution may be given, as required, every 30 minutes. Oxygen administration may be necessary if dyspnea and cyanosis develop.

## TICK BITES AND TICK PARALYSIS

In most cases of simple tick bite, the only sign other than the attached tick is an indurated lesion at the site of the bite itself which may be pruritic for a day or two. Occasionally, a more systemic reaction is exhibited owing to the action of neurotoxins, present in the saliva of the tick, which are injected at the time the tick feeds.

In some individuals, a syndrome characterized by sudden onset of motor paresis and paralysis may develop. Diarrhea may also be present. The ticks which usually produce this syndrome are gravid females which attach themselves to the heads and necks of their hosts. Apparently, these ticks must be attached for several days before signs develop. The ticks most commonly associated with tick paralysis are *Dermacentor andersoni, D. variabilis, Amblyomma americanum* and *A. maculatum*.

Treatment consists of removing the intact ticks from the host. Signs of paralysis usually subside quickly following removal of the engorged tick(s).

Finally, shrews of the genus *Blarina* have been shown to possess toxic saliva, but convincing clinical cases of animals other than man and the shrews' prey species being bitten have not been reported. In humans, the signs of toxicity are limited to local tissue reactions and transient paresthesia. Treatment is symptomatic.

# TOAD POISONING

N. E. PALUMBO, D.V.M.
*Lanai City, Hawaii*

*and* S. PERRI, B.A.
*Honolulu, Hawaii*

There is little question that the introduction during the past four decades of the giant tropical toad, *Bufo marinus*, into the southern states, and especially into Hawaii, has paid great dividends in controlling undesirable insect pests. These toads, however, are capable of producing a potent toxin in their large, warty, paired parotid glands, which are roughly oval in shape, are situated behind the border of the tympanum and extend backward over the shoulders. Numerous pinhole openings can be seen on the surface skin of these glands from which a thick, pasty, yellow-white toxin can be manually expressed. These toads therefore represent a threat to unsuspecting people who may mistake them for frogs and consume their skin, as has been documented in Hawaii, or who may be exposed to the toad's toxin through an open wound, as has been reported in Florida. More common, of course, is the threat of this potent toxin to animals mouthing the toads.

Although we have seen feline intoxications in rare instances, the principal cause for concern has been the threat to dogs. The lethargic hopping of the awkward toad will often attract dogs at dusk when other kinds of activity are minimal. These dogs will grasp the toad in their mouths, causing compression of the toad's parotid glands and expression of the toxin. Absorption of the toxin through the buccal and gastric mucosa apparently is quite rapid, resulting in a variety of symptoms which may culminate in death. The *Bufo marinus* in Florida, possibly because of diet, climate or genetic factors, seems to produce a more potent toxin than that produced by the Hawaiian *Bufo marinus*. The death rate in Hawaii of exposed and untreated dogs is approximately 5 per cent as compared to nearly 100 per cent in Florida. In Texas, the death rate is also low.

The dog that "mouths" a toad will exhibit variable symptoms depending upon its age, concurrent disease, amount of toxin absorbed in relation to its total body weight and length of time since exposure; the signs range from slight salivation to cyanosis and convulsive seizures. Obviously many other conditions could be confused with toad poisoning, and a history of having seen the dog "mouth" a toad will be sufficient evidence in a sick animal to warrant initiation of immediate antitoad-poisoning therapy.

## COMPOSITION OF THE BUFO TOXIN COMPLEX

There are 12 species of Bufo toads distributed worldwide. The parotid gland secretions of all toads contain bufagins, bufotoxins, bufotenins and other compounds. Bufotoxins are the conjugation product of the specific bufagin with one molecule of suberyl arginine. Bufotenins are organic bases containing an indole ring in the molecule. The action or effect of bufagins is one described as digitalis-like, often resulting in ventricular fibrillation; the action of bufotoxin is similar. Bufotenins have, for the most part, an oxytocic action accompanied frequently with a marked pressor action.

Other compounds found in *Bufo marinus* toxin are epinephrine, cholesterol, ergosterol and 5-hydroxytryptamine (5-HT). The last is also known as serotonin, or "serum vasoconstrictor." The highest biologic concentration of 5-HT occurs in the skins of certain toads. The physiologic role of 5-HT in bufo intoxication in the dog is not fully appreciated at this time. 5-HT is rapidly degraded in the gastrointestinal tract but might participate in the intoxication should some of the toxin be inspired via the respiratory tract.

## PHARMACODYNAMICS OF BUFO INTOXICATION IN THE DOG

A syndrome resembling canine bufo intoxication was reproduced by giving ouabain and epinephrine intravenously in a rat study. A synergistic effect was found to exist between the glycoside and the catecholamine; sublethal doses of each given simultaneously were shown to be lethal.

When bufotoxin is given intravenously to a dog, the response is similar to that seen experimentally in the rat—rapid rise in blood pressure, cardiac arrhythmias and dyspnea. However, when the same amount of bufotoxin is given orally to the dog, the onset of signs is slower, and there is no pressor effect. Following oral administration of a lethal dose of bufotoxin to an anesthetized dog, one finds a gradual deterioration of the ECG with progressive negative ventricular deflection, which eventually results in ventricular fibrillation and death if untreated. Respiratory rate and depth increase without any appreciable increase in blood pressure.

The fact that oral intoxication in the dog is not associated with increased blood pressure (and so is markedly different from the intravenous intoxication) is due to the inactivation of catecholamines by the digestive tract and liver. Toxic intravenous or oral doses of bufotoxin in the dog result in a moderate increase in packed cell volume, hemoglobin content, icterus index and concentrations of blood glucose and serum urea nitrogen, serum potassium and serum calcium. The sedimentation rate increases. Serum sodium and chloride concentrations decrease slightly, but serum inorganic phosphorus content decreases markedly. Total protein usually decreases slightly owing to loss of albumin. The total white blood cell count decreases, principally because of neutropenia. After an initial spike in SGOT activity, which may be due to the stress and struggle associated with the intoxication, this enzyme tends to return slowly to baseline values. Neither the SGPT nor alkaline phosphatase levels change appreciably.

## TRADITIONAL THERAPY: AN ANALYSIS OF THE RATIONALE

There is a wide range of preferred treatments for this kind of intoxication. Some of the preferred regimens of therapy reported to yield good rates of cure are actually conflicting. Not only is one confused by the conflicting recommendations of veterinary clinicians who have been intimately involved in solving the problem of bufo intoxication in sick pets, but there is much additional confusion to be found in the general scientific and veterinary literature.

In the past, preferred treatments for canine toad intoxication included atropine, prednisone, antihistamines, calcium gluconate, tranquilizers and anesthesia (barbiturates).

Atropine is frequently used symptomatically to dry mucous membranes in the respiratory system and to depress salivary secretions. Its action on the heart is to block the vagal effect, thus abolishing the normal slowing reflex. For these reasons, atropine may well be used in the treatment of bufo intoxication. It should be recognized, however, that atropine is not likely to produce any essential antitoxic effect on the myocardium, and that swabbing may equally well accomplish drying of the mouth. Thus atropine is not a specific antidote to the disease as we envision it. In animals that may have inspired foamy saliva containing the toxin into the respiratory tract, the 5-HT could conceivably cause bronchoconstriction. In these cases, the effect of atropine in clearing the airway will be desirable, but a specific antagonist of 5-HT would be more efficacious.

Calcium gluconate must be given intravenously but some of its toxic side effects cause heart block and ventricular fibrillation, the usual terminal events in bufo intoxication. One of the actions ascribed to calcium is the maintenance of membrane permeability. Digitalis intoxication inhibits ATPase activity in cell membranes, affecting the $Na^+/K^+$ pump and increasing $Ca^{++}$ permeability. This effect is aggravated by giving additional $Ca^{++}$ or by further depletion of $K^+$, and is improved by decreasing $Ca^{++}$ or by adding $K^+$. Calcium and digitalis have similar effects on the myocardium, and calcium may provoke arrhythmias and even ventricular fibrillation in the digitalized subject.

Antihistamines and steroids may also provide additional benefit by reducing the effects of bufotoxin on the mucous membranes of the mouth and other organs. Again, in this instance we do not envision these drugs as having any direct or vital beneficial effect.

Pentobarbital anesthesia increases canine tolerance to bufo intoxication. In one experiment, dogs given bufotoxin and anesthetized within 5 minutes could tolerate a dose that would prove fatal to nonanesthetized dogs. The major difference in the anesthetized animal's behavior seemed to be the marked decrease in the amount of mouthing, salivation and labored respirations. Presumably this activity may increase absorption through the pharynx and mouth or perhaps even through the respiratory tract, where there could be the additional effect of serotonin and catecholamines. To a lesser extent, but possibly through the same general mechanisms of action, tranquilizers serve to protect animals soon after exposure. Thiamylal sodium, a short-acting barbiturate, is contraindicated, since its action is too brief and it may produce cardiac arrhythmias which may predispose the dog to ventricular fibrillation.

The oldest and possibly one of the best ways of handling the early intoxication is to rinse the dog's mouth promptly with water. A garden hose serves well for this purpose. Inducing vomiting is another popular method of rendering first aid.

## DISCUSSION

If propranolol HCl, a beta-adrenergic blocking agent, is given to a dog exposed to a lethal oral dose of bufotoxin prior to the onset of ventricular fibrillation, or immediately following its onset, the ECG makes a spectacular reversal to normal.

Bufo intoxication in the dog is presumed to be due to the glycoside portion of the bufotoxin complex and is possibly potentiated by endogenous catecholamines. The mechanism of action of propranolol as an antidote is suspected to be due to this drug's ability to antagonize the glycosides' stimulatory effect on sympathetic nerves, thus blocking the release of endogenous catecholamines. This action then limits the intoxication essentially to a pure glycoside intoxication, which the dog can handle more effectively.

Propranolol effectively blocks the cardiac actions of catecholamines in dosages of 0.2 mg./kg.; at the high dosage we use (5 mg./kg.) the drug still possesses its β-adrenergic blocking action but presumably is exerting a quinidine-like action in reversing the arrhythmias associated with digitalis intoxication. D-Propranolol, which as no β-blocking activity, is equally as effective as L-Propranolol (a $\beta$-adrenergic blocker) in antagonizing digitalis-induced arrhythmias. Another interesting hypothesis on the mechanism of action of propranolol as an antiarrhythmic agent is that it may act as a neurodepressant on cardiac sympathetic innervation. (See Editor's Note at end of article.)

Potassium therapy is well established as standard therapy in glycoside intoxication. The danger of causing toxic side effects from improper administration if $K^+$ is also documented. Propranolol has been shown to cause massive leakage of $K^+$ from red blood cells, which results in an alteration of the Gibbs-Donnan equilibrium across the red blood cell membrane. Propranolol therapy results in elevated serum $K^+$ levels which may also be of therapeutic value.

Elderly humans appear to be especially labile to digitalis intoxication, so if in the case of cardiac glycoside intoxication one may extrapolate from man to dog, then one may guess that old, sick dogs with preexisting heart disease would be more susceptible to bufo intoxication than would be young, healthy dogs.

## A NEW SUGGESTED THERAPEUTIC REGIMEN

On the basis of our observations and clinical experience, a new and more specific approach to the treatment of *Bufo marinus* intoxication in the dog is suggested in this order:

1. Determine whether the history is compatible with toad intoxication.

2. Give 5.0 mg. propranolol/kg. body weight intravenously and rapidly.

3. Anesthetize with pentobarbital, intubate and rinse the oral mucous membranes with water.

4. Repeat propranolol administration in 20 minutes if necessary (5.0 mg./kg.).

5. If considered appropriate, administer $K^+$ by slow intravenous drip, while monitoring with ECG (lead II).

[*Editor's Note*: The doses of propranolol described in this article were used by the authors *only* to treat early cases of toad-poisoning. Similar doses given to patients with cardiac or other diseases may produce severe and untoward reactions.]

## SUPPLEMENTAL READING

Knowles, R. P.: The poison toad and the canine. Vet. Med./Small Animal Clin., January, 1964, pp. 38–42.

Otani, A., Palumbo, N., and Read, G.: Pharmacodynamics and treatment of mammals poisoned by *Bufo marinus* toxin. Am. J. Vet. Res., *30*:1865–1872, 1969.

Palumbo, N., Perri, S., and Read, G.: Experimental induction and treatment of toad poisoning in the dog. J Am. Vet. Med. Assn., *11*:1000–1055, 1975.

Russell, R. L.: Toad poisoning. In Kirk, R. W. (ed.) Current Veterinary Therapy III. Philadelphia, W. B Saunders Co., 1966, pp. 621–622.

# GARBAGE- AND FOOD-BORNE INTOXICATIONS (ENTERO-TOXEMIAS)

GEORGE W. EBERHART, D.V.M.
*Moraga, California*

Among the disease problems most commonly encountered in the dog and cat, the digestive tract is frequently involved. Garbage- and food-borne intoxications stem from the absorption of toxins from the intestine. These toxic compounds may be preformed (as the powerful neurotoxin of botulism and the enterotoxin of staphylococcal poisoning) or may arise from toxin-producing bacteria multiplying in the bowel. When these absorbed substances overwhelm the elimination, defensive and detoxification mechanisms of the body, the signs of enterotoxemia appear. Any facto that introduces these bacteria to the gastrointestinal canal and favors their excessive growth therein, favors absorption of their toxins or interferes with the function of the detoxifying system (liver, kidneys, etc.) tends to promote the development of either an acute or a chronic enterotoxemia syndrome.

The normal bacterial flora of the dog's bowel represents five primary types, according to Sudduth (1971): *Escherichia coli, Clostridium perfringens, Lactobacillus acidophilus,* enterococcus and bacteroides. Although these organisms are fermentative or putrefactive, they ordinarily grow and produce toxins only in an alkaline medium. During their growth, however, their by-products (ammonia and amines) produce greater alkalinity which further increases their multiplication. Gas accumulates intraluminally which increases absorption of toxic products and decreases peristalsis due to distention and stretching of the gut wall. The proximal segment of small intestine is especially efficient in absorptive capacity. However, the normal physiology of the small intestine tends to inhibit bacterial growth proximal to the ileum by maintaining an acid medium, and by peristalsis, which ordinarily prevents the retrograde flow of colon contents into the ileum.

Any inflammation of the bowel wall lowers its resistance to invasion of toxins and microorganisms. Allergenic substances, including foods, pollens, yeasts and fungi, will cause an inflamed mucosa in a hypersensitive animal.

Such foodstuffs as milk, buttermilk, cottage cheese and yogurt owe their therapeutic value to the fact that they donate *Lactobacillus acidophilus* organisms to the stomach and small bowel, and provide a favorable acidic ecology for their propagation. The pharmaceutic compounds such as Bacid, Lactonoc and Lactinex should fulfill the same objective.

## ETIOLOGY

1. Ingestion of garbage, decomposed food, carrion and decaying organic substances (compost).

2. In puppies especially, overeating of highly fermentable and low digestible foods.

3. Eating foreign materials such as bones, horse and cow manure.

4. Achlorhydria—this frequently results in small bowel pH above 6 which allows putrefactive growth.

## CLINICAL SIGNS

In the peracute form of food-borne intoxications, gastritis which is signaled by vomiting usually occurs. In the dog, vomiting is a well developed reflex, and frequently serves as the cure for food poisoning if it occurs early enough. In the acute and subacute stages, the cardinal signs are vomiting, pain in the cranial part of the abdomen and malaise. These occur within two to six hours following the ingestion of the noxious material. If these signs persist and go untreated, diarrhea usually follows and is sometimes hemorrhagic in nature. Shock, characterized by mucosal pallor, tachycardia and shallow respiration, occurs when the endotoxins have invaded and overwhelmed the reticuloendothelial system, primarily the liver.

Enterotoxemia from food-borne origins in its more chronic form is typified by increased flatulence, halitosis, feces covered with mucus, decreased vigor and vitality and sometimes a soreness and stiffness suggestive of rheumatoid arthritis. Fatness and atonic skin with lusterless haircoat are not unusual, and a rancid seborrheic odor from the body is common.

Botulism is caused by neurotoxins produced by *Clostridium parabotulinum* (types A and B) or *Clostridium botulinum* (types C, D and E). Botulin neurotoxin effect on the dog resembles that of curare, and respiratory failure is the most common cause of death. The author has attended three dogs with signs of botulism in which the history supported such diagnosis. One dog, a six-year-old male Australian shepherd, was presented with complete paralysis of all the voluntary muscles except the ocular group, which allowed him to blink his eyes. The owner had fed him and a Siamese cat two chickens that apparently had died of "limberneck" (botulism). The dog was hospitalized and given p/d mixed with enough milk to liquefy it for administration through a stomach tube once daily; he was also given a low enema once daily. This shepherd recovered gradually, with return of muscle function in a three-week period.

[*Editor's Note:* Dogs as a species are quite resistant to botulinum toxin.]

## DIAGNOSIS

The diagnosis of food-borne poisons is based on the history, presenting signs and the elimination of other probable causes. In peracute and acute food poisoning, rapid development of shock correlated with the history leads one to suspect enterotoxic conditions, if no other pathophysiology is evident. Sudduth (1971) maintains that a high level of urinary indican is highly suggestive of enterotoxemia.

## TREATMENT

In the peracute stage of food-borne intoxication, it is important to evacuate the stomach if ingesta are still present. We prefer to administer apomorphine subcutaneously or into the conjunctiva for this purpose. If the abdomen seems distended excessively, an enema is given to evacuate the colon, and we usually continue the process until emesis occurs. Azimycin intramuscularly at the rate of 1 ml./7 kg. of body weight is given, as well as parenteral B complex. If clinical shock is manifested, 100 mg. of hydrocortisone sodium succinate (Solu-Cortef® [Upjohn] or Cortisate® [H. C. Burns]) is given intravenously along with 5 per cent dextrose in lactated Ringer's solution.

About one hour following stomach evacuation, we give Sulkamycin® tablets (Norden) at the rate of 1 tablet per 7 kg. of body weight, and this is continued every eight hours for three doses. Chloramphenicol (50 mg./kg. divided into three doses daily) is very effective in controlling the gastrointestinal infection as well as in helping to prevent systemic complications. This is given for four to five days. Food and water are withheld for 24 hours, and a gradual return to oral food begins with either i/d or k/d feedings three times daily. At the end of the antibiotic treatment, we commence the administration of Bacid® (Fisons) or Lactonoc® capsules (Norden) three times daily for one week. If the owner prefers not to remain on the Prescription Diet® (Hill) regimen, he is instructed to return to the original commercial diet on a gradual basis, mixing 3 parts i/d or k/d to 1 part commercial diet. Every two days, he increases his commercial food by one-fourth, so that in eight days he has reconditioned his dog's gastrointestinal tract and taste buds to the original diet (assuming the food was of good quality). In most cases, cottage cheese and cooked egg are advised to be added to most commercial dog foods.

Management of the chronic enterotoxemia patient can become involved. This writer has simplified the dietary approach by recommending an appropriate Prescription Diet, such as i/d, for maintaining a balanced diet of high biologic value. Animals suffering with urinary system disorders are usually prescribed k/d, unless they fare better on i/d diet.

For intractable cases of diarrhea, Van Kruiningen (1973) has suggested treatment with Tylan® (Lilly). This is a powder-form preparation of tylosin and vitamins usually administered to pigs. Our experience with this product has been most rewarding, and our results are in agreement with Van Kruiningen's observations. He recommends 1 teaspoonful of Tylan powder to 1 lb. of food. This is continued for three months. Should the diarrhea recur upon the discontinuance of the drug, it is possible that the dog may need it all its life.

### SUPPLEMENTAL READING

Sudduth, W. H.: Enterotoxemia. In Kirk, R. W. (ed.) Current Veterinary Therapy IV. Philadelphia, W. B Saunders Co., 1971.
Van Kruiningen. H. J.: Gastroenterology Seminar. Contra Costa County Veterinary Medical Association Walnut Creek, Calif., March 18, 1973.

# POISONING AND INJURY BY PLANTS

BILLY R. CLAY, D.V.M.
*Stillwater, Oklahoma*

Diagnoses of acute poisoning by plants are infrequently made by small animal veterinarians. This may reflect a lack of occurrence but it may also reflect the nondefinitive nature of symptoms produced by a large number of toxic plants. From a 1973 Oklahoma survey of 20 metropolitan small animal practices it was learned that 21 per cent of their cases were gastrointestinal disorders and 56 per cent of those were of undetermined etiology. With unknown etiology for more than half the gastrointestinal cases and with such a large number of ornamental and field plants as potential gastrointestinal irritants (Table 1), it is likely that some of these cases may be attributed to plants or plant parts. This is further supported by the fact that dogs and cats will, from time to time, consume varying amounts of vegetation, especially grass. In the absence of grass, however, other plants are often acceptable, some of which may be hazardous.

Aside from this "natural" foraging behavior, there are a variety of factors and circumstances which may influence animals to consume or come in contact with noxious plants. Age, boredom, feeding habits of the owner and new or altered surroundings have all been observed to reflect the conditions of poisoning or injury by plants.

## CONDITIONS OF POISONING OR INJURY

**Age.** Mature animals are less likely to become affected by noxious plants than are immature ones. Teething puppies will chew on any accessible item about the household or kennel. Some readily available yet potentially dangerous items are tobacco; nuts; onions; garden bulbs or rhizomes (daffodil, hyacinth, autumn crocus, star-of-Bethlehem, iris); pits from cherries, apricots or peaches; necklaces of precatory bean, Sophora or castor bean; morning-glory seeds; marijuana; or nutmeg. There are recent accounts in the literature of intoxications in young animals from ingestion of cigarettes, chokecherry leaves, philodendron leaves and hashish.

**Boredom.** Confinement of animals of any age may result in boredom and subsequent chewing or ingestion of noxious agents. Plants are oftentimes the most accessible items. Penned or caged pets may readily accept nearby vegetation, whereas the same animal when allowed freedom may show no interest in the plant. This was vividly demonstrated in a toxicity case involving a one-year-old German shepherd male dog referred to the Oklahoma State University College of Veterinary Medicine. The dog was allowed freedom in the owner's backyard until he built a 100-square-foot pen in one corner where the dog was subsequently confined. Included in the pen was a Japanese yew shrub, *Taxus cuspidata*, which soon attracted the dog's attention. Shortly thereafter, the owner noted that a considerable amount of bark was stripped from the base of the shrub and that the animal had vomited. During the next two hours the dog developed muscular weakness and coma and died. Shreds of bark were found in the stomach at postmortem examination.

In another instance a confined dog was poisoned following consumption of leaves from a nearby chokecherry bush, *Prunus virginiana*. The chokecherry, like other members of the genus *Prunus* (Table 1, item XI) contains hydrocyanic acid, one of few plant toxins treatable by specific antidote. Sodium nitrite (20 mg./kg.) and sodium thiosulfate (70 mg./kg.) administered intravenously in 25 milliliters of distilled water will prevent further cyanide inhibition of the cytochrome-enzyme complex and will aid in renal excretion of the toxin.

Pets confined to the house will sometimes chew or consume potted plants. Reports of dieffenbachia and philodendron consumption by cats are often received by the author. One case involving death of an iguana was traced to a *Kalanchoe blossfeldiana* plant which had been consumed entirely. No feeding trials were conducted to verify the toxicity of Kalanchoe to iguanas; therefore, the plant remains as suspect only.

Holiday seasonal introduction of plants to the home may arouse the curiosity of bored or young pets. Ingestion of poinsettia, mistletoe, English holly berries, pine tree needles and water from around Christmas trees has been reported to produce gastroenteritis in dogs and cats.

**Feeding Habits of the Owner.**  Feeding of kitchen scraps may also become a source of plant toxicants. With both meat and vegetable matter included in the feeding regimen, gluttonous animals may consume all. This may be a source of sprouted potato peels; peach, cherry or apricot pits; rhubarb leaf blades; onions; etc.

Commercial diets can also be a source of plant toxins. The mysterious hepatitis X disease of dogs was traced to toxic levels of aflatoxins in a commercial dog food. Aflatoxins are metabolites of the fungi *Aspergillus flavus* and other Aspergilli which are potent hepatoxins and carcinogens. These and other toxin-producing saprophytic fungi are common inhabitants of molded grains which, on occasion, may be added to commercial pet foods. Ergot, the parasitic fungus of cereal grains, might also appear as a contaminant. The gangrene of extremities produced from its vasoconstrictive and occlusive effects is historically characteristic. Gossypol, another plant toxin of historical significance, has been found in diets containing improperly processed cottonseed meal. The monogastric animal is most susceptible to this chronic debilitating poison, which is believed to produce heart failure through impairment of oxidation-reduction reactions. Two separate incidences of gossypol poisonings in dogs have been reported.

With increased interest in commercial pet foods as a part of the human diet, it is likely that intensified regulatory inspection of ingredients and preparations will reduce the chances for contamination in the future. However, complete exclusion is virtually impossible; therefore, the clinician should remain cognizant of these possible sources of toxins.

**New Surroundings.**  In our mobile society pets are constantly subjected to new surroundings. The curious and less selective ones may be encouraged to "forage" on unfamiliar vegetation which could lead to ill effects. Perhaps a more common malady under these circumstances, however, is mechanical injury or chemical irritation resulting from contact with the numerous plants armored with spines, barbs, awns or stinging hairs. A list of these potentially injurious plants is shown in Table 1, item XII.

Perhaps the most frequent injuries are those produced from penetration of mucous membranes by grass awns and other floral parts. Members of the genus *Stipa* are most notable among this group owing to the extensive migration of its floral parts in animal tissues following penetration. The awn and anterior floret of some species possess retrorse (posteriorly directed) barbs which prevent backward movement and easy removal from tissues. These foreign bodies have been recovered from abscesses of the mouth, nasum, orbit, post orbitum, mediastinum, pericardium, spinal canal, bursae of joints and elsewhere. Entire florets of wild barleys (*Hordeum spp.*) and bromes (*Bromus spp.*) have also been recovered from the tissues between the toes, metacarpals and metatarsals, where they produce severe lameness due to infection, fistulous tracts, swelling and pain.

Sandburs (*Cenchrus pauciflorus*), goatheads (*Tribulus terrestris*) and numerous cacti become hazards to working dogs introduced to an area where these plants are abundant. The performance of the dog will be severely impaired upon first exposure and may become permanent if the animal is not protected. The spines of sandburs are curved at the tips, which prevents easy removal. They may remain as an irritant in the digital pads or mucous membranes for extended periods but they rarely produce abscess formation.

Burdock (*Arctium lappa*), a member of the Composite family, possesses small hooks on the flower bracts (involucre), which at maturity become dislodged and caught in the hair of dogs. In the process of grooming, the dog may get the hooks embedded in the tongue and mouth, where they become the nidus for a granular stomatitis. Removal of these is best accomplished by scraping the inflamed areas with a scalpel blade held perpendicular to the tissues.

Contact with nettles (*Urtica spp.* and *Laportea spp.*) is another source of injury to pets. Hunting dogs frequently encounter these in areas where they are common. Abundant stinging hairs are present on these plants which contain varying amounts of acetylcholine, histamine, serotonin, formic acid and perhaps other active compounds. Upon contact the dog may show symptoms of salivation, pawing at the mouth, emesis, respiratory distress, slow and irregular heartbeat, muscular weakness and occasionally death. A similar syndrome is seen with some of the species of *Cnidoscolus* (nettle spurge).

## DIAGNOSIS AND TREATMENT

Diagnosis of plant poisons like many other poisons is often achieved after gastric evacuation and/or symptomatic therapy is begun. In any case it behooves the veterinarian to make every effort to identify the offending agent.

If the client has not observed consumption or contact with possible injurious plants, then the case history should be gathered in such a manner that the presence of these plants would be revealed. In collection of the history the clinician should keep in mind the factors that might contribute to toxicosis so that the client may be advised to alter his management to prevent future occurrences.

Upon recognition that a plant is the toxin source, the often difficult task of identification remains. With the aid of Table 1 perhaps the task can be made less difficult. Other references which should prove helpful include the following:

1. Harden, J. W., and Arena, J. M.: Human Poisoning from Native and Cultivated Plants. 2nd ed. Durham, North Carolina, Duke University Press, 1974.
2. Kingsbury, J. M.: Poisonous Plants of the United States and Canada. Englewood Cliffs, New Jersey, Prentice-Hall, Inc., 1964.
3. Lampe, K. F., and Fagerstrom, R.: Plant Toxicity and Dermatitis: A Manual for Physicians. Baltimore, The Williams & Wilkins Co., 1968.
4. Poison Information Centers.
5. County Extension Directors.
6. Florists.

If additional assistance is needed, fresh plant specimens or washed plant parts from vomitus or stomach washings may be submitted to diagnostic laboratories or qualified toxicologists. Plant specimens collected for identification should include representative leaves, stems and a flower, if possible. These may be placed in an airtight plastic bag where they will remain preserved for as long as seven days, providing they are kept refrigerated. If the specimen is dried, it should be shipped with well-insulated packing to prevent fragmentation in transit. All specimens should be accompanied by a description of the plant and a detailed history.

The patient that is presented with acute intoxication should always be handled as an emergency according to the basic guidelines presented in an earlier article in this book entitled, "Emergency and General Treatment of Poisonings." In summary, the veterinarian should:

1. Institute supportive therapy necessary to maintain life.
2. Establish a tentative diagnosis upon which to base rational therapy.
3. Institute antidotal procedures or remove the toxin.
4. Identify the plant or plant part and determine its source.
5. Educate the client concerning the hazards and avoidance of such occurrences in the future.

When signs of lameness, fistulous tracts, stomatitis, conjunctivitis, otitis, abscessation, suppurative pleuritis or other signs of foreign bodies exist, the veterinarian should be alerted to the possibility of penetration by plant parts. Manual or surgical removal and antibiotic therapy for secondary bacterial infections are indicated. Infections by common soil organisms of the genus *Nocardia* or *Actinomyces* are often associated with migrating plant foreign bodies.

If a diagnosis of mushroom poisoning is made, the clinician, most likely, will need special assistance for identification of the specimen. There are approximately 13,500 species of Basidiomycete mushrooms, of which only about 70 are known to be toxic. Identification of some of these presents a challenge even to the trained mycologist.

Symptoms vary considerably with different mushrooms. Most produce gastroenteritis with vomiting either immediate or delayed 6 to 12 hours. Those that produce delayed effects usually produce liver damage and jaundice. In addition to gastroenteritis, any of the symptoms of salivation, cardiac depression, tetany, transient

**Table 1.** *Potentially Dangerous Plants—Toxic Effects and Early Symptoms\**

| COMMON NAME | SCIENTIFIC NAME | TOXIN AND EARLY SYMPTOMS |
|---|---|---|
| **I. Oral, Pharyngeal and Esophageal Irritants** | | |
| Alocasia | *Alocasia spp.* | Needle-like calcium |
| Caladium | *Caladium spp.* | oxalate crystals and/or |
| Calla lily | *Zantedeschia aethiopica* | irritant sap in all |
| Dumbcane | *Dieffenbachia spp.* | parts that produce |
| Elephant's-ear | *Colocasia spp.* | *salivation* and edema |
| Green dragon, | | of oral and pharyngeal |
|   Oregon root | *Arisaema dracontium* | mucosa. |
| *Jack-in-the-pulpit,* | | |
|   Indian turnip | *Arisaema triphyllum* | |
| Malanga | *Xanthosoma spp.* | |
| Philodendron | *Philodendron spp.* | |
| Skunk cabbage | *Symplocarpus foetidus* | |
| **II. Gastric Irritants** | | |
| Amaryllis | *Amaryllis spp.* | Alkaloid, lycorine, |
| Daffodil | *Narcissus spp.* | unknown toxin in seed |
| Wisteria | *Wisteria spp.* | of wisteria; immediate |
| | | *nausea* and *emesis.* |
| **III. Intestinal Irritants** | | |
| Balsam pear | *Momordica charantia* | Saponins in fruit |
| English ivy | *Hedera helix* | or seed; *salivation,* |
| Horse chestnut, | | immediate *nausea* and |
|   buckeye | *Aesculus spp.* | *emesis, abdominal* |
| Mock orange | *Poncirus spp.* | *pain* and *diarrhea.* |
| Pongam | *Pongamia pinnata* | |
| Rain tree, | | |
|   monkey pot | *Samonia samon* | |
| Soapberry | *Sapindus saponaria* | |
| Yam bean | *Pachyrhizus erosus* | |
| Bloodberry, | | Resins in leaf or |
|   baby-pepper | *Rivina humilis* | fruit and in root of |
| Daphne, | | pokeweed and iris; |
|   spurge laurel | *Daphne spp.* | immediate *nausea* and |
| Iris, flag | *Iris spp.* | *emesis, abdominal* |
| Lords and ladies | *Arum spp.* | *pain* and *diarrhea.* |
| Pokeweed | *Phytolacca americana* | |
| American yew | *Taxus canadensis* | Foliage, bark or |
| English yew | *Taxus baccata* | seed contains taxine; |
| Japanese yew | *Taxus cuspidata* | immediate *nausea* and |
| Western yew | *Taxus breviflora* | *emesis, abdominal pain,* |
| | | *mydriasis* and *arrhythmia.* |
| Baneberry | *Actaea spp.* | Protoanemonin glycoside, |
| Clematis | *Clematis spp.* | immediate *emesis, diarrhea* |
| | | and *rash.* |
| **IV. Miscellaneous Gastrointestinal Irritants and Cathartics** | | |
| Bird-of-paradise | *Poinciana gilliesii* | Miscellaneous G.I. |
| Buckthorn | *Rhamnus spp.* | irritant compounds; |
| Candlenut | *Aleurites spp.* | all produce *immediate* |
| Christmas candle | *Pedilanthus tithymaloides* | *nausea* and *emesis* with |
| Clusia | *Clusia rosea* | *abdominal pain* and |
| Common box | *Buxus sempervirens* | *diarrhea.* Nervous or |
| English holly | *Ilex aquifolium* | renal involvement |
| Euonymus | *Euonymus spp.* | follows with some. |
| Honeysuckle | *Lonicera tatarica* | |
| Poinsettia | *Euphorbia pulcherrima* | |
| Privet | *Ligustrum spp.* | |
| Yellow allamanda | *Allamanda cathartica* | |

\*Adapted from Lampe, K. F., and Fagerstrom, R.: Plant Toxicity and Dermatitis: A Manual for Physicians. Baltimore, The William and Wilkins Co., 1968.

*Continued on next page*

*Table 1.  Potentially Dangerous Plants–Toxic Effects and Early Symptoms (Continued)*

| COMMON NAME | SCIENTIFIC NAME | TOXIN AND EARLY SYMPTOMS |
|---|---|---|
| **V. *Delayed Gastrointestinal Effects*** | | |
| Black locust | *Robinia pseudoacacia* | Toxalbumins; *delayed* |
| Castor bean | *Ricinus communis* | *emesis, abdominal pain,* |
| Coral plant | *Jatropha multifida* | *diarrhea* (followed by |
| Rosary pea, | | constipation with |
|   precatory bean | *Abrus precatorius* | Robinia), *depression* or |
| Sandbox tree, | | *coma* and *hypotension.* |
|   monkey pistol | *Hura crepitans* | |
| | | |
| Bittersweet | | |
|   nightshade | *Solanum dulcamara* | Solanine glycoalkaloid; |
| Chalice-vine | *Solandra spp.* | *delayed emesis, abdominal* |
| Ground cherry | *Physalis spp.* | *pain, diarrhea* and dry |
| Jerusalem cherry | *Solanum pseudocapsicum* | oral mucous membranes in |
| Jessamine | *Cestrum spp.* | Cestrum, cardiac activity |
| Potato | *Solanum tuberosum* | with Jerusalem cherry. |
| | | |
| Garden sorrel | *Rumex acetosa* | Oxalic acid; *delayed* |
| Rhubarb | *Rheum rhaponticum* | *emesis, abdominal pain,* |
| Virginia creeper | *Psedera quinquefolia* | *diarrhea, depression* or |
| | | *coma.* |
| | | |
| Autumn crocus | *Colchicum spp.* | Colchicine; *delayed* |
| Glory lily | *Gloriosa spp.* | *emesis, abdominal pain* and *diarrhea.* |
| | | |
| **VI. *Cardiovascular Disturbances*** | | |
| Foxglove | *Digitalis purpurea* | Digitalis; *immediate* |
| Lily-of-the-valley | *Convallaria majalis* | *nausea* and *emesis,* |
| Oleander | *Nerium spp.* | *abdominal pain, brady-* |
| Yellow oleander | *Thevetia peruviana* | *cardia* and *arrhythmias.* |
| | | |
| Aconite, monkshood | *Aconitum napellus* | Aconite; *immediate* |
| Larkspur | *Delphinium spp.* | *nausea, tremors* and |
| Western monkshood | *Aconitum columbianum* | *convulsion, bradycardia, arrhythmias* and *dyspnea.* |
| | | |
| **VII. *Nicotine-like Action*** | | |
| Cardinal flower, | | |
|   Indian tobacco | *Lobelia spp.* | Cytisine, coniine, |
| Goldenchain | *Laburnum anagyroides* | nicotine or lobeline; |
| Kentucky coffee-tree | *Gymnocladus dioica* | *salivation, immediate* |
| Mescal bean | *Sophora spp.* | *nausea* and *emesis,* |
| Poison hemlock | *Conium maculatum* | *tachycardia.* |
| Tobacco | *Nicotiana spp.* | |
| | | |
| **VIII. *Atropine Action*** | | |
| Angel's trumpet | *Datura arborea* | |
| Belladonna, deadly | | |
|   nightshade | *Atropa belladonna* | Atropine; *mydriasis* |
| Henbane | *Hyoscyamus niger* | (cat), *hyperthermia,* |
| Jessamine | *Cestrum spp.* | *tachycardia, dry* |
| Jimsonweed, | | *mouth* and *dyspnea.* |
|   thorn apple | *Datura spp.* | |
| Matrimony vine | *Lycium halimifolium* | |
| | | |
| **IX. *Convulsants*** | | |
| Chinaberry | *Melia azedarach* | Various compounds; |
| Coriaria | *Coriaria spp.* | *convulsions.* |
| Moonseed | *Menispermum canadense* | |
| Nux vomica | *Strychnos nux-vomica* | |
| Water hemlock | *Cicuta maculata* | |

*Continued on next page*

**Table 1.** *Potentially Dangerous Plants—Toxic Effects and Early Symptoms (Continued)*

| COMMON NAME | SCIENTIFIC NAME | TOXIN AND EARLY SYMPTOMS |
|---|---|---|
| **X. *Behavioral Alterants, "Hallucinogens"*** | | |
| Marijuana | *Cannabis sativa* | Tetrahydrocannabinols |
| Morning-glory | *Ipomoea spp.* | Lysergic acid |
| Periwinkle | *Vinca rosea* | monoethylamide |
| Nutmeg | *Myristica fragrans* | Myristicin |
| Peyote, mescal | *Lophophora williamsii* | Mescaline |
| | | |
| **XI. *Cyanogenetic Action*** | | |
| Apricot, almond, peach, cherry, choke-cherry, wild cherry | *Prunus spp.* | Cyanogenetic glycosides; *emesis, dyspnea, stupor,* and *coma; bright red venous blood.* |
| Hydrangea | *Hydrangea macrophylla* | |
| Japanese plum | *Eriobotrya japonica* | |
| | | |
| **XII. *Contact Irritants or Mechanical Injury*** | | |
| Nettle | *Urtica chamaedryoides* | Acetylcholine, histamine, serotonin and formic acid; *salivation, emesis, bradycardia, arrhythmia* and *dyspnea.* |
| Nettle | *Laportea canadensis* | |
| Nettle spurge | *Cnidoscolus stimulosus* | |
| Stinging nettle, bull nettle | *Urtica dioica* | |
| | | |
| Burdock | *Arctium lappa* | Awns, florets, barbs, spines, hooks; *stomatitis, conjunctivitis, abscesses, fistulous tracts, reduced performance, hemmorhage* or *lameness.* |
| Blackberry | *Rubus spp.* | |
| Cacti | Numerous genera | |
| Carolina nightshade | *Solanum carolinense* | |
| Foxtail | *Setaria spp.* | |
| Goathead | *Tribulus terrestris* | |
| Honey locust | *Gleditsia triacanthos* | |
| Needlegrass | *Stipa spp.* | |
| Sandbur | *Cenchrus pauciflorus* | |
| Tripleawn | *Aristida spp.* | |
| Wild barleys | *Hordeum spp.* | |
| Wild bromes | *Bromus spp.* | |

excitement or possibly hallucinations may be seen with toxicosis due to mushrooms. Some of the genera of toxic mushrooms that the veterinarian may encounter are *Agaricus, Boletus, Inocybe, Amanita, Conocybe, Psilocybe, Galerina, Pholiota, Clitocybe, Lactarius, Scleroderma* and *Paxillus.*

# RADIATION TOXICITY

CHARLES H. HOBBS, D.V.M.
*Washington, D.C.*

The subject of radiation toxicology is quite broad and inclusive. Ionizing radiation, to which this discussion is limited, is known to be acutely toxic, teratogenic, carcinogenic and mutagenic. It has been stated that more is known about the effects of radiation than is known about any other agent to which man and animals are exposed. Perhaps of greatest concern are the long-term effects of radiation on man and his environment from the increasing use of radiation by man. Of far more practical importance than radiation toxicity in the practice of veterinary medicine is the practice of radiation safety. All veterinarians who utilize radiation for diagnosis and therapy must be concerned with the prevention of radiation toxicity to themselves, their employees, clients and patients.

Ionizing radiation is a term applied to

radiations that give rise, either directly or indirectly, to ionizations when they interact with matter. While the precise mechanism of radiation toxicity is not known, it is considered to be related in some way to the production of ions within the cell. Ionizing radiations comprise electromagnetic radiations, such as gamma and x-rays, and particulate radiation, such as alpha particles, beta particles, electrons, neutrons and protons. X-rays originate from outside the nucleus of atoms, and gamma rays originate from unstable atomic nuclei releasing energy to gain stability. These rays have penetrating power directly related to the energy of the photon. For example, gamma or x-rays with energies of 300 KeV. would be more penetrating than those with energies of 50 KeV. Alpha ($\alpha$) and beta ($\beta$) particles result from the radioactive decay of unstable elements termed radionuclides. An alpha particle is identical to a helium nucleus, consisting of two neutrons and two protons. It results from the radioactive decay of heavy elements such as uranium, plutonium, thorium and radium. Because of their large mass, +2 charge and slow speed, alpha particles transfer their energy to atoms in a medium (i.e., biologic tissues) over a short range and thus have a high linear energy transfer (LET). For this reason alpha particles produce relatively large amounts of damage in tissues but do not penetrate far. Beta particles are electrons resulting from the conversion of a neutron to a proton in the nucleus of an atom. Iodine-131, carbon-14, strontium-90 and cerium-144 are examples of radionuclides that emit beta particles on decay. Beta particles have a greater range and penetrating power but have a lower linear energy transfer than alpha particles.

The roentgen (R) is a unit of radiation exposure related to the amount of ionization produced in air by gamma or x-rays. A roentgen equals $2.58 \times 10^{-4}$ coulombs per kilogram of air. The rad is the unit of radiation-absorbed dose and is a measurement of energy deposition in any medium by all types of ionizing radiation. One rad equals 100 ergs/g. in any medium. In the case of gamma radiation over the commonly encountered range of photon energy, the energy deposition in tissue for a dose of 1 R is about 0.96 rad. The dose equivalent, expressed as rem, is the product of the absorbed dose in rads times the unitless quantities of radiation quality and other factors,

such as the distribution of the dose within the target tissue. In practice the latter factors are generally taken as 1. The quality factor is based on the linear energy transfer of the type of radiation. The quality factor of x-rays, gamma-rays and beta particles is generally considered to be 1. A quality factor of 10 is generally accepted for alpha particles. Thus, a radiation dose of 10 rads from alpha radiation would be equivalent to a dose of 100 rems and would be expected to cause equal biologic damage to a dose of 100 rads from beta, gamma or x-irradiation.

The sources of exposure of man and animals to ionizing radiation fall into four major groups: (1) natural sources, such as cosmic and terrestrial x-irradiation, and internally deposited, naturally occurring radionuclides, such as radium and potassium-40; (2) health science applications of radiation by the healing arts; (3) nuclear reactions, such as nuclear power reactors and nuclear weapons; and (4) other sources, such as industrial x-ray machines. The degree of exposure to the latter three groups is subject to change depending on the intelligent and judicial use of radiation by man. The exposure of man to natural sources of radiation results in an average dose-rate of about 100 millirems per year to the population of the United States. This dose can vary considerably from region to region. The other major source of radiation dose to the population is the medical use of radiation. The average dose-rate to the population from this source has been estimated to be about 70 millirems per year. However, from certain diagnostic procedures the dose to an individual may be much higher. For example, the dose for a diagnostic upper gastrointestinal examination on a human patient has been reported to average 1.6 rads at midfield. A maximal midline exposure dose to dogs given a relatively extensive radiographic examination involving 11 radiographs has been reported to be about 70 millirems. The proper use of radiographic techniques, equipment and careful selection of patients to be examined could substantially reduce the dose to the population from the medical uses of radiation.

## EARLY RADIATION EFFECTS

The early effects of exposure to ionizing radiation result primarily from cell death. The radiosensitivity of cells is generally related to their turnover rate. Cells that frequently undergo mitosis are generally more radiosensitive than cells that seldom undergo mitosis.

Exposure of the whole body to penetrating radiation of various types is likely to occur only from severe accidents or nuclear warfare. Manifestations of early radiation effects occur only after relatively high doses (above about 50 rads) delivered at relatively high dose-rates (several rads/hr). These acute early effects appear to be threshold phenomena and are dose-rate dependent; their incidence and severity increase non-linearly with dose.

At whole-body doses approaching 5000 rads, death results within 48 hours of exposure apparently from neurologic and cardiovascular collapse (central nervous system syndrome). When the total-body exposure is between 1000 and 5000 rads, death generally occurs between 5 and 10 days after exposure in most species. In this case death is associated with bloody diarrhea and destruction of the gastrointestinal mucosa (gastrointestinal syndrome). Penetrating whole-body doses of from 50 to 1000 rads cause symptoms related primarily to injury of the bone marrow (hematopoietic syndrome). The dose lethal to 50 per cent of beagle dogs within 30 days ($LD_{50/30}$) is about 250 rads midline absorbed dose. At doses near the $LD_{50}$ the dogs that die generally die within 10 to 25 days after exposure. Most dogs that receive doses of less than about 150 rads can be expected to survive, and dogs exposed to less than 50 rads will show few symptoms. The $LD_{50/30-day}$ dose varies markedly from species to species. Typical $LD_{50/30-day}$ doses for various species are mice~625, rats~800 and monkeys~550 rads. The treatment for acute radiation exposure in the near lethal range is essentially the same as that for any pancytopenia.

Exposure of portions of the body to high doses at high dose-rates results in tissue death in the area irradiated. Erythema and ulceration of the skin may occur at skin doses of 500 rads or more. Doses in this range are commonly used in radiotherapeutic applications. Cataracts are another complication of local area irradiation. The germ cells of both sexes are radiosensitive. In males, acute doses of from 10 to 100 rads will cause a dose-related depression of the sperm count, which recovers slowly. In females, destruction of oocytes results in

permanent sterility due to a lack of stem cells in the adult ovary.

Radiation is also teratogenic. Radiation received by the embryo during early gestation is likely to cause developmental abnormalities, particularly microencephaly or impaired body growth. This is generally observed at doses greater than 100 rads and only when the radiation is received during early pregnancy. However, some authors have recommended therapeutic abortions for women who have received doses of 5 to 10 rads during early pregnancy. The developing fetus may also be very sensitive to the induction of neoplasms when irradiated *in utero*, even toward the end of gestation.

## LATE EFFECTS OF RADIATION EXPOSURE

Over the past few years there has been increased concern that even very low doses of radiation may produce harmful biologic effects, particularly in man. Experimental animal data have clearly established that ionizing radiation is both carcinogenic and mutagenic at relatively high doses generally delivered at high dose-rates. However, owing to uncertainties over the shape of the dose-response curve and the lack of definitive proof of a threshold (a dose below which no effect will be produced), concern exists for the effects of irradiation at doses and dose-rates that extend down to doses that may be received from the environment or from diagnostic radiography.

As a result of extensive studies by the Atomic Energy Commission (now the Energy Research and Development Administration) and other government agencies, much information is available on the effects of low doses of radiation in experimental animals. The primary experimental animal for these studies has been the mouse, but several large studies have utilized beagle dogs. It appears that ionizing radiation is potentially carcinogenic to all tissues under the proper circumstances. Typically, following exposures of the total body or a significant portion of the bone marrow to ionizing radiation, leukemia is the cancer with the shortest latent period; other malignant neoplasms appear at later times. In general the lower the total dose received, the longer the latent periods for neoplasms have been. In dogs exposed to near-lethal doses of radiation, the latent period for leukemia ha been observed to be about 2 years. Dogs exposed to relatively low doses of radiation from inhaled plutonium have developed lung tumors. At the lowest doses studied, the lung tumors appeared near the end of the dogs' life span.

Ionizing radiation produces gene mutations and chromosome aberrations. As was the case for cancers produced by radiation, radiation-induced mutations are not generally different from "spontaneous" mutations. However, most evidence indicates that any increase in the genetic mutation rate will be harmful to a population on a long-term basis. It has been estimated that the doubling dose for mutations in man is between 20 and 200 rem.

## INTERNALLY DEPOSITED RADIONUCLIDES

The toxicity of radioactive materials that gain entry into the body from inhalation, ingestion or injection depends on the temporal and spatial dimensions of the radiation dose pattern which results in the irradiated tissues. The radiation dose pattern is governed by the physical and chemical characteristics of the element which influence its distribution within the body and its retention, as well as by such factors as the physical half-life of the radionuclide and the type of radiation emissions from the material, i.e., alpha or beta particles or gamma rays.

For example, radioiodine, irrespective of the route of administration, is rapidly absorbed into the bloodstream and concentrated by the thyroid. These characteristics of radioiodine have been utilized in nuclear medicine for both therapeutic and diagnostic purposes. However, the radiation dose from the radioiodine may also result in thyroid neoplasms, particularly in young members of a population.

There are numerous other radionuclides of concern because of their use in nuclear medicine, and because of the potential for accidental exposure of man and animals by various means. Of these radionuclides, fission products ($^{90}$Sr, $^{144}$Ce and $^{91}$Y) and transuranics ($^{238}$Pu, $^{239}$Pu, $^{241}$Am and $^{244}$Cm) may be released from certain nuclear operations. While the potential for their release is very small, there is the potential for the production of deleterious biologic effects in both occupationally and environmentally

exposed populations. The toxicity of these radionuclides has been the subject of a great deal of research, much of which has utilized beagle dogs.

## RADIATION PROTECTION STANDARDS AND RADIATION SAFETY

The use of radiation in veterinary medicine should have as its objective obtaining maximal diagnostic or therapeutic results with a minimal radiation exposure to the animal patient, the radiologic personnel and the general public. It must be recognized that reduction in the dose to the animal patient will generally result in a proportional decrease in exposure of people. The subject of radiation protection in veterinary medicine has recently been the subject of a publication by the National Council on Radiation Protection and Measurements (NCRP Report No. 36). The guidelines in that report should be followed for all uses of radiation in veterinary medicine. There is no excuse for excessive exposure to radiation in the practice of veterinary medicine, and all possible measures must be taken to reduce the dose to the patient and personnel to as low as practicable levels.

The reduction in exposure from external radiation sources such as x-ray equipment can be accomplished by increasing the distance from the source, by reducing the duration of exposure and by using protective barriers between the individual and the source. All personnel involved with the use of radiation, and even persons potentially exposed to the radiation, should wear monitoring devices. These consist of film badges, ionization chambers and thermoluminescent materials that are sensitive to the type of radiation to be measured. Records of the exposure as determined by these monitoring devices must be maintained. A log which contains the date of exposure, kilovoltage, exposure time, operator and identification of the animal patient must be maintained for all types of radiation devices.

It should be recognized that pregnant and potentially pregnant women and individuals under 18 years of age must not hold animal patients during examination or treatment and that, whenever possible, restraints or anesthesia should be used so that the animal need not be held during irradiation. When it is necessary to hold the animal, all personnel should be equipped with properly maintained lead gloves and aprons and even then should not expose any part of the body to the direct radiation beam. The use of fluoroscopy should be kept to a minimum, and fluoroscopy should not be used as a substitute for radiography.

The public has become increasingly aware of the dangers of ionizing radiation. In many cases the dangers of irradiation may have been exaggerated, and the public may not be aware of the many modifying factors that can lessen the hazard. However, if one assumes a linear dose response with no threshold, any radiation dose will be associated with some harm. In this case any radiation exposure is associated with a risk versus benefit judgment of the value of the radiation dose (i.e., diagnosis) versus its harmful effect. While there is evidence to suggest that at least for some types of radiation there exists a threshold below which no adverse effect will occur, the generally conservative approach of not assuming a threshold has been used for the development of radiation protection standards in use today. It is the responsibility of all veterinarians who use radiation to keep exposures to as low as practicable levels. In addition, the costs of any legal action resulting from improper practices will more than exceed the costs of the use of proper equipment, monitoring devices and protective measures to prevent exposure of personnel.

## SUPPLEMENTAL READING

Behrens, C. F., et al. (eds.): Atomic Medicine. 5th ed. Baltimore, The Williams and Wilkins Co., 1969.
Biological Effects of Ionizing Radiation (BEIR) Advisory Committee: Report: The Effects on Populations of Exposure to Low Levels of Ionizing Radiation. National Academy of Sciences, National Research Council, Washington, D.C., 1972.
Carlson, W. D.: Radiation safety. In Carlson, W. D.: Veterinary Radiology. 2nd ed. Philadelphia, Lea & Febiger, 1967.
Fabrikant, J. I.: Radiobiology. Chicago, Year Book Medical Publishers, 1972.
Hobbs, C. H., and McClellan, R. O.: Radiation toxicity. In Casarett, L. J., and Doull, J. (eds.): Toxicology: The Basic Science of Poisons. New York, Macmillan Co., 1975.
National Council on Radiation Protection and Measurements: Radiation Protection in Veterinary Medicine. NCRP Report No. 36, National Council on Radiation Protection and Measurements, 4201 Connecticut Ave., N.W., Washington, D.C. 20008, 1970.
National Council on Radiation Protection and Measurements: Basic Radiation Protection Criteria. NCRP Report No. 39, National Council on Radiation Protection and Measurements, 4201 Connecticut Ave., N.W., Washington, D.C. 20008, 1971.
Stannard, J. N.: Toxicology of Radionuclides. Ann. Rev. Pharmacol., *13*:325–357, 1973.

# SMOKE INHALATION

C. S. FARROW, D.V.M.
*Saskatoon, Saskatchewan*

The initial signs of smoke inhalation are often deceptively subtle and, therefore, may lead to something less than intensive care as well as a falsely optimistic prognosis. This is not to say that every case of smoke inhalation bodes the worst; on the contrary, many affected patients go on to an uncomplicated recovery. However, one is advised to become aware of the pathologic substrate which underlies the comparatively complicated clinical spectrum associated with this disorder. With this knowledge, the clinician may then formulate an appropriate and effective management program in the context of a high degree of prognostic accuracy.

## PATHOPHYSIOLOGY

Of primary concern in evaluating potential damage to the respiratory system are the heat of the fire, the lack of oxygen and the amount of carbon monoxide produced by combustion. A secondary consideration is the presence of other gases, perhaps poisonous, derived from the pyrolytic process.

A hyperthermic atmosphere, even devoid of noxious fumes, can seriously damage the lung; the greater the specific heat delivered to the lung parenchyma, the more disastrous the damage becomes. Even larger numbers of calories are released when partial combustion of an inflammatory vapor is completely oxidized deep within the respiratory tree.

The implications of oxygen deprivation are obvious and need not be detailed. Suffice it to say that a shift in cellular respiratory mechanisms will occur, producing varying degrees of metabolic acidosis. Blood gas studies indicate that arterial lactate-pyruvate levels do not rise significantly at oxygen tension levels above 50 torr. Damage to the central nervous system and myocardium is directly attributable to cellular hypoxia.

Carbon monoxide is a lethal poison. Produced by incomplete combustion and having a combining power with hemoglobin that is 300 times greater than that of oxygen, this deadly gas is rapidly absorbed by the lung. The ensuing carboxyhemoglobinemia leads to asphyxia and subsequent death if hemoglobin saturation exceeds 60 per cent. Pathologic changes are absent in nonfatal cases, although transient metabolic derangement may occur.

## POTENTIAL INHALANTS

Modern households include myriad synthetics among their furnishings. It may be supposed *a priori* that since synthetics are diverse in nature they may give rise to combustion products more toxic than those given off by more traditional materials such as wood or natural textiles. Actually, plastics are carbon compounds and will give rise to carbon dioxide, carbon monoxide and, depending on chemical composition, other gases or toxic fumes. The plastics, together with rubber and textiles, are organic compounds composed of a combination of monomers referred to as macromolecules. Their uses are diverse and their household distribution is widespread. Carpets, drapes, upholstery fabrics, insulation materials, paints and numerous items of wearing apparel constitute only a brief list of macromolecular applications.

## EARLY PULMONARY CHANGES

Both smoke and heat exact a high physiologic tribute from the patient. The end result is acute respiratory failure brought about by a combination of alveolar hypoventilation and an unsatisfactory correlation between alveolar ventilation and capillary perfusion. The events which transpire during the interim include denuding of the respiratory mucosa, occlusion of pulmonary air space, massive pulmonary edema and a marked alteration in respiratory mechanics. Normal pulmonary protective mechanisms are inactivated or actually operate to the patient's detriment.

As hot smoke begins to penetrate the upper airways a combination of mechanical, chemical and thermal stimuli act upon the vagal receptors located within the sensitive mucous membranes of the throat and proximal airways. The result is cough, often intractable and paroxysmal in nature. Carbonaceous accumulations rapidly induce severe cellular pathologic changes. This damage is manifested initially in the form of intracellular edema, resulting in increased permeability and/or structural deterioration. Production of mucus increases markedly, as does the action of the ciliated epithelium. Intraluminal secretions accumulate, initially mobilized by the combined actions of the mucociliary blanket, subepithelial lymphatics and phagocytes. Reflex constriction of the bronchioles retards the influx of irritating fumes but, in so doing, presents a similar ventilatory impairment.

The positive effects of these pulmonary defense mechanisms are soon obviated as the pulmonary secretions become inspissated because of the low humidity created by the heat of the fire. This increased mucus viscosity results in slowing of the mucociliary system and eventually in obstruction of the smaller airways. Phagocytosis is compromised by a coating of coagulated transudate, making effective clearing of intrapulmonary debris difficult. Bronchiolar constriction is soon relaxed, owing to smooth muscle fatigue rapidly brought about by constant stimulation.

As the inflammatory crescendo builds, numerous vasoactive substances may be liberated, depending on the magnitude and duration of the inflammatory response. These events also contribute to abnormal liquid accumulations within the major conducting airways and, to a lesser extent, the peribronchial tissues.

## PULMONARY EDEMA

As smoke invades the inner recesses of the pulmonary exchange system, a marked alteration in both alveolar epithlelial and capillary endothelial premeability occurs.

The result is acute pulmonary edema. Measurements of proteins in edema fluid from human patients with altered permeability have shown protein concentrations approximating those of plasma. Even fibrinogen has been identified in this liquid.

These findings suggest that the leak of plasma-like liquid into the interstitium and alveolar spaces, with subsequent denaturation of protein and conversion of fibrinogen to fibrin, explains the development of hyaline membranes (acute adult respiratory distress syndrome). The breakdown of protein in local interstitial and alveolar spaces results in the possible release of protein-bound toxic substances (causing further inflammation) and increased interstitial alveolar oncotic pressures (causing further liquid accumulation).

The formation of pulmonary edema, particularly alveolar, leads to a patchy rise in surface tension and alveolar instability. The net result is a decrease in surface activity, resulting in alveolar collapse and concomitant ventilation-perfusion abnormalities.

As the edema fluid builds within the lung, the work of breathing is significantly increased. A reduction in pulmonary compliance and a commensurate elevation in resistance result in acute respiratory distress or the so-called "stiff-lung" syndrome.

Clearing of alveolar compartments of carbon particles less than 10 microns in diameter is achieved by phagocytosis. The phagocyte is incapable of digesting an inorganic particle and therefore carries the engulfed (but not digested) particle to the region of the alveolar duct. This is the level of termination of both ciliated epithelium and the lymphatic system. Disposition may then be accomplished by ciliary action that sweeps the phagocyte and its carbon passenger upward; or the cell may enter the lymphatic system and arrive in nearby lymphoid collections or hilar nodes. These entrapment mechanisms are not nearly so successful against liquids and therefore would not be anticipated to function well in the current context where the intraalveolar carbon particles are suspended in edema fluid. Clearance through the lymphatic system is retarded owing to a decrease in pulmonary ventilation as a result of the numerous obstructive phenomena previously detailed. Dependent on parenchymal air space movement for external pressure flow, the deep lymphatic contents remain static. Ciliary action is severely compromised, as described earlier. Under these adverse conditions, the alveoli are virtually incapable of being cleared of irritating carbon particles.

## BLOOD GASES

Blood gas analysis in the smoke-inhalation patient has revealed that carbon dioxide tension is seldom increased, generally ranging between 30 and 40 torr. The elevation, when present, is often associated with upper respiratory failure. The pH values are frequently between 7.45 and 7.50, an indication of classic respiratory alkalosis.

Plasma bicarbonate levels are frequently lower than normal, ranging from 17 to 24 mEq./l. This decreased arterial bicarbonate would appear to reflect renal compensation for reduced carbon dioxide tension. There may also be a variable element of bicarbonate reduction due to an interaction with the increased lactic acid levels seen. Keto acids may represent a further aggravation of metabolic acidosis and commensurate bicarbonate reduction.

The normal oxygen tension in hospitalized burn patients is constantly below textbook values. A definition of "normal" employed by one prominent burn clinician is "the lowest oxygen tension that has not been seen in association with clinical signs of respiratory difficulty." In man, this figure has generally been about 75 torr. The physiologic basis for this hypoxemia is thought to be a reduction in the volume of alveolar ventilation.

Arterial lactate-pyruvate studies aimed at uncovering tissue anoxia have shown that little, if any, tissue oxygen deficit exists when values for arterial oxygen tension are above 50 torr. In the early period after smoke inhalation, however, large-scale tissue hypoxia undoubtedly occurs owing to the combined effects of reduced cardiac output and pulmonary insufficiency. The presence of burns will contribute to anoxic events both at burn sites and, systemically, via the production of burn factor, a myocardial depressant.

## PNEUMONIA

Patients who survive the first 48 hours after significant smoke inhalation will develop bronchopneumonia almost without exception. Prophylactic antibiotics have proved to be of little benefit in preventing or lessening the severity of this infectious complication. The progressive involvement of the lungs with bronchopneumonia occurs gradually as a result of the patient's inability to clear the abundant mucus which is blocked by mucosal sloughs and mucous plugs or is not mobilized as the result of extensive loss of ciliary function. These functional blocks provide sanctuaries where bacteria can proliferate and invade previously uninvolved lung.

## POSTMORTEM FINDINGS

Pathologic changes found in man at autopsy correlate closely with the necropsy findings described in the dog. The respiratory mucosa is severely denuded and may be completely replaced by an inflammatory membrane. Pulmonary congestion is marked and is accompanied by severe edema of the pulmonary air spaces. The smaller bronchi are consistently plugged with epithelial debris and edema fluid, with resulting atelectasis distal to the plugs. As described above, if the patient survives the first 48 hours, evidence of superimposed bacterial infection is found. In the event of early death, the alveoli contain edema fluid, cellular debris and fibrin. Later demise results in the finding of polymorphs, serous exudate and debris within the alveoli, in addition to hyaline membranes and partial destruction of alveolar walls.

## MANAGEMENT

### CLINICAL STAGES

Of paramount importance in the management of the smoke-inhalation patient is the fact that the pathogenetic mechanisms previously discussed result in a highly predictable clinical course which, in man (and in experimental animals including the dog), involves three clinical stages. The first stage is one of acute respiratory distress beginning almost immediately and lasting up to 36 hours. In some instances the onset of this period may be delayed up to 18 hours. The second stage begins within the first few hours (in some instances, minutes) and involves the formation of pulmonary edema. Duration rarely exceeds two or three days. Pneumonia constitutes the final stage.

In a pulmonary burn of any significant magnitude, development of the final stage is probably initiated immediately but is clinically undiscernible until the third or fourth clinical day. Its duration depends on the severity of the burn, the specific offending organism and the use of prophylactic antibiotics (which may actually prolong the pneumonia); however, it rarely lasts less than one week.

### PHYSICAL SIGNS

Signs observed at the time of admission, in addition to the consistently predictable clinical course, may be helpful in prognosis. Signs considered unfavorable include pulmonary rales, cyanosis and blood-tinged cough products. The absence or diminution of chest sounds should not cause premature optimism, especially if they occur within the first 24 hours after earlier abnormal lung sounds have been detected. This silence may represent atelectasis rather than improvement. Radiographs will serve to resolve this dilemma.

The physiologic implications of cyanosis are obvious. One is cautioned that the cherry-red color caused by carboxyhemoglobinemia may mask cyanosis. Evaluation of the shocklike state of smoke-inhalation patient for mucous membrane color may be hazardous, since constriction of the peripheral capillary bed allows for little circulating blood. The danger of overlooking or failing to recognize hypoxia is great.

Blood-tinged cough products indicate the degree of cellular disruption in the upper airways and must be considered a dire prognostic finding. Conversely, purulent material in the sputum on the third or fourth day should be expected, since it represents an effort to clear the airways of accumulated cellular debris and mucus in addition to associated phagocytic elements.

### RADIOLOGY

Dorsoventral and lateral thoracic radiographs are recommended during the early postadmission period after initial treatment has been given. Subsequent radiographs are taken as indicated until such time as the patient is stabilized. Progress checks at two and four weeks are advised. Recrudescence may warrant additional studies.

Roentgenographic findings in the early postinhalation period will include patchy pulmonary densities throughout the lung field because of alveolar flooding resulting from the rapid-forming pulmonary edema. The stomach is frequently distended with air owing to aerophagia. This occurrence may prove a source of secondary interpretive difficulty, since the stomach presses on the diaphragm, mechanically impeding thoracic excursion and thereby relatively increasing existing pulmonary densities.

During the next 36 hours, as tissue slough begins and sepsis is initiated, atelectasis is frequently noted. Its presence is suggested by a mediastinal shift as seen in the dorsoventral or ventrodorsal projection. In the lateral view one may see a linear density pattern and occasional vascular crowding. These changes are caused by the alveoli distal to a bronchial plug undergoing absorption of contained air, with a resulting collapse of the affected area. The collapsed area itself, containing less air than surrounding tissue, appears as an area of increased density. The adjacent blood vessels are displaced toward the collapsed tissue and appear crowded together. With effective coughing, the regions of atelectasis may shift from lobe to lobe or vanish altogether. In the case of the older patient, depletion of the oxygenating capacity of a part of the lungs may be associated with compensatory emphysema in other portions. Radiographic signs of pneumonia may be present in the form of interstitial and/or alveolar patterns.

## CONSERVATIVE THERAPY VS. RESPIRATORY SUPPORT SYSTEMS

Treatment of acute respiratory failure associated with smoke inhalation must be performed in an intensive manner. Initial efforts are directed toward restoration of normal gas exchange and management of shock, if present. Treatment, in general, falls into two categories: conservative and supportive.

Conservative therapy is reserved for the conscious patient who is not felt to require a respiratory support system. Objective determination of the need for a respiratory support system is best based on arterial blood gas analysis, preferably serial. In the absence of this capability one must rely on close patient observation and clinical acumen. Elements of conservative therapy consist of oxygen enrichment of the inhaled air, humidification, steroids and diuretics. Additionally, one may wish to employ sodium bicarbonate, analgesics and/or sedatives.

Intervention with a respiratory support system depends on two major considerations: (1) Can the patient ventilate properly? and (2) If so, can a gas exchange compatible with life be maintained? Respiratory support may be required at the time of presentation (as in the case of the unconscious animal requiring immediate resuscitation) or at some later time when the lung can no longer compensate for the existing inflammatory burden. Respiratory support systems with the capability of maintaining postend-expiratory pressure within the alveoli are usually unavailable to the veterinary practitioner. Lack of existing manpower, patient logistics and attendant costs further lessen the feasibility of this procedure. Short-term efforts may be mounted using anesthesia hardware present in most practices. Emphasis, therefore, will be on conservative management techniques.

## OXYGEN THERAPY

Of primary concern in the smoke-inhalation patient is correction of the existing cellular hypoxia. This is best accomplished with an oxygen-enriched atmosphere, i.e., an oxygen cage. While the matters of oxygen concentration and length of administration require consideration, it should be understood that there are no specific contraindications to oxygen therapy. In man, it has been suggested that no patient receive greater than 40 per cent oxygen unless the oxygen tension is less than 60 torr, and that the period of administration not exceed 36 hours.

Excessive oxygen exposure has several undesirable effects on animal lungs, including diminished replication of endothelial cells, accumulation of interstitial and alveolar fluid, deposition of hyaline membranes and interference with the formation and/or function of alveolar surfactant. These changes have the effect of decreasing the uptake of oxygen, both by impeding diffusion across the alveolar-capillary barrier and by increasing the passage of venous blood through unventilated lung tissues. In actuality, one may probably use oxygen concentrations well above the maximal level considered above, since the existing pulmonary damage will most likely prevent the achievement of a correspondingly increased oxygen content. This supposition is strengthened by experimental work with rabbits which has shown that protection from oxygen poisoning which ordinarily occurs in rabbits exposed to 80 to 90 per cent oxygen can be achieved by prior instillation of diphosgene, an agent which damages the respiratory tract.

Weaning from increased oxygen levels should begin at the earliest possible opportunity and should be accomplished gradually.

## HUMIDIFICATION

Addition of humidification during oxygen enrichment of the atmosphere, as well as during the early recuperative period, is to be encouraged. Humidification decreases the viscosity of oral and pharyngeal secretions, restores moisture to bronchial mucosa and humidifies the inspired gases, thereby preventing drying of pulmonary secretions. Hazards attendant to humidification include an increased metabolic demand as a result of shivering if the ambient temperature becomes too cold. Conversely, if the ambient temperature is too hot, humidification interferes with heat loss and leads to elevated temperature, increased oxygen consumption and eventually an increased cardiac workload. Finally, if the humidity is allowed to remain excessively high for too long, a positive water balance may result owing to increased absorption, producing a commensurate overhydration and increased cardiac workload. Thus, it is suggested that humidification within an enclosed space be temperature-controlled if at all possible. If this is not possible, simple air circulation and close patient monitoring are mandatory.

## DIURETICS

Loop diuretics such as furosemide are an essential element in combating pulmonary edema in the smoke-inhalation patient. The intravenous route is preferred initially, the subcutaneous and oral forms being used only after water balance has begun to shift. The use of this therapeutic agent requires close observation of both patient hydration and urinary output. Free access to water is desirable. Dosage will vary according to the patient's body weight and the severity of existing pulmonary edema. An initial dose of 4 mg./kg. body weight is given in the more severely affected patients; dose reduction is predicated on response.

## CORTICOSTEROIDS

*Steroid therapy, oxygen and diuretics constitute the clinician's primary means of managing the smoke-inhalation patient.* The glucocorticoid hormones not only exert a suppressive effect on inflammatory reactions (regardless of the nature of the inflammatory stimulus) but function in an anti-immunologic capacity as well.

Corticosteroids inhibit the inflammatory response, in part, by their actions on the vast capillary network of the lung. The degree of anti-inflammatory activity appears to be quantitatively related to the concentration of hormonally active steroid present at the site of inflammation. Normally, capillary integrity and the response of vasoconstriction to norepinephrine are monitored by corticosteroid hormones. Moreover, glucocorticoids oppose the increase in capillary permeability characteristic of acute inflammation which is produced by factors such as histamines and kinins. The accumulation of pulmonary fluids is reduced, since the capillaries are less likely to leak proteins and fluid. Migration of macrophages and leukocytes into the inflamed area is impeded because steroids inhibit endothelial sticking of leukocytes and diapedesis through the capillary wall. Finally, formation of granulation tissue is retarded by an inhibitory action of glucocorticoids on the formation of fibroblasts and collagen.

The immunology of pulmonary injury is also favorably influenced by steroid therapy. This fact takes on added importance in the smoke-inhalation patient who, as stated previously, will always develop some degree of pneumonia. This constant feature of smoke-inhalation trauma is a complex pathophysiologic situation involving not only particular infecting bacteria but the function of neutrophils and macrophages, immunoglobulin metabolism and cell-mediated and humoral immunity. These factors explain, in part, the matter of patient debilitation or susceptibility. Once tissue injury begins, degraded proteins may be ingested by cells in an attempt to clean up the debris. However, the ingestion of such particles by cells can result in release of lysosomal enzymes which induce further injury. This processing of altered protein may result in release of newly antigenic substances (partially degraded host materials) and may perpetuate the immune inflammatory reaction. Steroids, by interfering with uptake and subsequent digestion of debris, would thereby limit the inflammatory reaction, It is not difficult to realize that these anti-immunologic, anti-inflammatory effects are not gained without a price. The inhibition by corticoids of ingestion and/or the digestion of microorganisms by macrophages may permit the insidious, often occult, onset of infection.

Intravenous prednisolone is given initially at a level of 4 mg./kg. body weight, followed by dexamethasone (4 mg./kg. body weight) every six hours for a minimum of two days. Passage of an intravenous catheter facilitates administration of the steroid. After the patient's condition stabilizes, a parenteral route is used, the dosage level being adapted to the patient's specific requirements and continued for at least two weeks.

## ANALGESICS

Morphine sulfate, given subcutaneously at a dose rate of 0.2 mg./kg. body weight, has been highly instrumental in successful management of the smoke-inhalation patient. The primary pain-relieving properties of this potent analgesic provide relief from the sense of dyspnea by abolishing pain and, possibly, by decreasing total body metabolism, thus reducing the work of breathing. Of additional benefit are the peripheral pooling of blood (a welcome feature in managing the pulmonary edema) and positive circulatory effects in the nonambulatory patient. Vomiting is not a common occurrence.

Maximal effect is reached in 60 minutes via the subcutaneous route, and effective analgesia lasts from three to six hours. The intravenous route is significantly more rapid (three to five minutes) but is attended by an equally rapid respiratory depression. The subcutaneous route permits the narcotic to be given when the patient is placed in the oxygen-rich environment. It also provides relief of tissue anoxia and release of carbon monoxide prior to the onset of alteration in the sensitivity of respiratory chemoreceptors. In addition, narcotic analgesia can be reversed with nalorphine if necessary.

## BICARBONATE

As described earlier, plasma bicarbonate levels are usually mildly reduced in the pulmonary-burn patient. The need for alkali replacement is currently uncertain. Sodium bicarbonate is advised in patients requiring respiratory support and those with a concomitant shock syndrome. Dose levels are determined most accurately by blood gas analysis. An empirical dosage of 1.0 to 2.0 mEq./kg. body weight is suggested if bicarbonate determination is unavailable.

## ANTIBIOTICS

Little or no benefit is to be expected from the prophylactic use of antibiotics in the prevention of pneumonia in the smoke-inhalation patient; to the contrary, they may actually increase the degree of severity. A more rational approach is to allow the patient's natural defenses an opportunity to combat the infection. Failing this, a transtracheal aspiration may be performed with specific antibiotic therapy predicated on cultural findings.

### SUPPLEMENTAL READING

Farrow, C. S.: Smoke inhalation in the dog: Current concepts of pathophysiology and management. Vet. Med./Small Animal Clin., 70:404–422, 1975.

Kirkpatrick, C. H., and Rosenthal, A. S.: Anti-immunologic and anti-inflammatory effects of steroid therapy. In Azarnoff, D. L. (ed.): Steroid Therapy. Philadelphia, W. B. Saunders Co., 1975.

Suter, P. F., and Ettinger, S. J.: Pulmonary edema. In Ettinger, S. J. (ed.): Veterinary Internal Medicine. Vol. 1. Philadelphia, W. B. Saunders Co., 1975.

# THERMAL INJURIES

C. S. FARROW, D.V.M.
*Davis, California*

## INTRODUCTION

Thermal injuries, excluding friction burns and abrasions, are relatively uncommon in pet animals. Comparatively little information is available on this subject in the veterinary literature. Many of these injuries occur as a direct result of owner carelessness and, therefore, may be considered preventable. Burn trauma is unique, and a basic understanding of the underlying pathophysiology is necessary in order to formulate and carry out an effective management program. This discussion will deal with the classification, etiology, pathophysiology and management of thermal injuries.

## CLASSIFICATION

Burns are classified according to the depth and extent of the injury. The depth of injury is expressed as the degree of burn. Classically, there are three categories, progressing from first degree, which is the mildest, to third degree, which is the most severe. Another classification, based on a combination of the depth and extent of involvement, can be employed to divide thermal injuries into major and minor burns.

Generally, first-degree burns are considered minor. Second- and third-degree burns involving less than 10 per cent of the body are also considered minor. Combinations of second- and third-degree burns involving more than 20 per cent of the body are considered major.

A first-degree burn is indicated by the presence of redness (often difficult to appreciate if the overlying hair coat is intact, or the skin heavily pigmented), mild swelling and pain to the touch. Management is minimal and resolution rapid. There is no disfigurement.

Second-degree burns are characterized by blistering (especially in flame and scald injuries) and a considerable amount of pain and swelling. If infection can be prevented, disfigurement will be minimal. Healing generally takes place in 2 to 4 weeks.

Third-degree burns are the most serious kinds of thermal injuries and, depending on the extent of involvement, may be life-threatening. Full-thickness skin loss occurs, including loss of hair follicles and glandular structures. The injured skin may be charred in appearance or appear as an eschar. Cutaneous sensation is absent, and the surface of the injury site will not bleed if incised. In extreme cases, the skin is totally destroyed, exposing underlying tissues. Infection and disfigurement are usual features of this burn type, with healing often being protracted.

An accurate evaluation of the extent of the burn injury is important for proper management, especially fluid therapy. A diagram is provided to facilitate this estimation (Fig. 1). The considerable variation in relative individual surface areas among different breeds, as well as the changes which take place during growth, should be appreciated and taken into consideration when this chart is used.

## ETIOLOGY

Causes of thermal injury to pet animals include (1) friction or abrasion burns, (2) chemical "burns," (3) direct heat burns, (4) flame burns, (5) scald burns, (6) electrical burns and (7) lightning burns.

*Friction or abrasion burns* occur most frequently to the dog as a result of being hurled against or dragged along the pavement following an encounter with an automobile. This type of injury may also occur to the foot pads following vigorous physical activity on a highly abrasive surface, such as asphalt. Detachment of the pad surface may occur owing to excessive shear forces created by sudden stops and abrupt turns.

Wound contamination invariably occurs in the form of hair, dirt and road debris. Although one might predict *a priori* that infection is almost a certainty, many badly con-

195

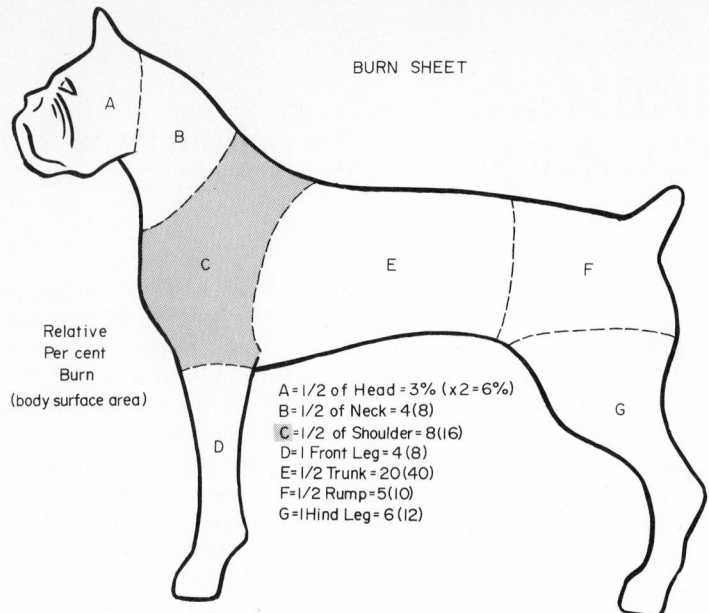

BURN SHEET

Relative
Per cent
Burn
(body surface area)

A = 1/2 of Head = 3% (x 2 = 6%)
B = 1/2 of Neck = 4(8)
C = 1/2 of Shoulder = 8(16)
D = 1 Front Leg = 4 (8)
E = 1/2 Trunk = 20(40)
F = 1/2 Rump = 5(10)
G = 1 Hind Leg = 6 (12)

**Figure 1.**

taminated wounds heal rapidly without clinical evidence of infection.

*Chemical agents* in general do not "burn" in the sense that they do not destroy tissue by hyperthermic activity, although some do act in this fashion. Rather, as a class, they comprise entities which coagulate protein by means of reduction, oxidation, salt formation, corrosion, protoplasmic poisoning, metabolic competition, inhibition, desiccation or the ischemic concomitants of vesicant activity. In addition to being classified by chemical activity, these agents may be separated on the basis of predominant chemical class: acids, alkalis and vesicants. Animal contacts often take place in storage areas, such as the garage, where such compounds are often placed in an effort to keep them out of the reach of children.

*Direct heat* injuries may result from myriad contacts, most of which are preventable. The family kitchen is a prime locale for such injuries. Cats frequently sustain severe foot pad burns when they unknowingly step on a recently heated burner. In the warmer months, dogs and cats may sustain serious tongue burns from licking barbecue grills. The extensive use of dry dog foods to which excessively hot water has been injudiciously added may result in burn injury not only to the tongue and mouth but to the esophagus and stomach as well.

*Flame burns* are becoming more common, usually as the result of home or apartment fires, and are often accompanied by smoke inhalation. (*Note:* The absence of obvious burn injury in the facial region should not serve to preclude the possibility of smoke inhalation.) The degree and extent of such injuries are usually severe. Although it is certainly a sad commentary on the times in which we live, animals doused with flammable liquids and then deliberately ignited may be presented to the veterinary clinician. The odor of gasoline should alert one to such a possibility.

*Scald burns* frequently take place in the kitchen and often are the result of the inadvertent spillage of hot water on food-seeking pets situated at or near the stove or counter surfaces. Again, this is a preventable injury.

*Electrical burns* are almost entirely limited to young puppies often confined in the home and without supervision. Lamp and appliance cords, by virtue of their ubiquitous distribution, are the prime offenders, and if bitten deeply usually cause coagulation necrosis of portions of the oral cavity. Severe neuricentric cardiopulmonary complications may result in death; however, this is the exception rather than the rule.

*Lightning burns* are rare and, unfortunately, often fatal. They are most prevalent in the midwestern part of the country. Large amounts of static electricity build up within clouds from the collision between particles of ice carried by updrafts and downdrafts.

This results in the development of a large negative charge at the bottom of the cloud, which is then discharged to earth by a lightning bolt. The current contained in such a bolt has been estimated to vary between 12,000 and 200,000 amps, and the time required for passage to earth lies between 1/100 and 1/1000 of a second.

## PATHOPHYSIOLOGY

The pathologic alterations in the skin and underlying tissues will vary depending on the intensity of the heat and duration of the exposure. Local, regional and systemic disorders combine to alter radically the biostability and defense capability of the patient.

**Early Changes.** Thermal injuries will involve variable degrees of dermal and subdermal destruction, depending on their severity. Inflammation, with its attendant vascular manifestations, serves to prime the pathologic pump and sets the stage not only for local and regional pathologic changes but for serious systemic complications as well.

Very shortly following the initial burn, the local and regional vasculature, especially capillary beds, undergoes a marked dilatation, with a subsequent increase in permeability. This later alteration is largely humorally mediated, with histamine, serotonin and possibly catecholamines playing significant roles in the development of this phenomenon. The result is severe and sustained fluid loss.

As the inflammatory fluid builds within the interstitium, a concomitant increase in pressure occurs. This change is hardest felt by the thin-walled elements of the vasculature—the veins and lymphatics. Eventually, venous and lymphatic thrombosis occurs, producing additional edema and extravasation of the formed elements of the blood and lymph. Dermal ischemia follows shortly.

Severe protein loss invariably accompanies major burn injury and results in a marked drop in oncotic pressure, which in turn aggravates edema formation at the expense of the intravascular fluid compartment. The greater the intravascular fluid loss, the more pronounced the hypovolemia and its attendant features. Cardiovascular compensation is effective to a point, beyond which the necessary vital organ perfusion is no longer adequate. The net effect is severe and profound shock! An additional manifestation of severe protein loss, which is often overlooked, is decreased transport capacity due to albumin loss. This is especially true if there are hepatic complications which interfere with replenishment.

Structural and functional changes affect both erythrocytes and leukocytes. The red blood cells, in addition to being directly hemolyzed, may be structurally altered in such a way that they either are sequestered by the spleen or suffer a premature death within the confines of the circulatory system owing to an increase in membrane fragility. The neutrophils demonstrate an as yet unexplained phenomenon in which their intracellular bactericidal ability is significantly reduced without a commensurate drop in phagocytic function. This latter alteration, in part, explains the patient's increased susceptibility to infection.

**Later Changes.** Many important postburn complications may occur in both the early and the late postburn periods. The most important of these is infection. Arising at or near the site of severest injury, infective agents not only may lobby against local healing but may be disseminated to the general circulation and produce septicemia. Death rapidly ensues. Gaining an infective foothold is not difficult considering the widespread dermal disruption and the nature of the exposed edematous tissues, rich in potential bacterial growth media. Add to this the retarded bactericidal ability of the white cell population, and the generalized reduction in immunocompetence, and it is not difficult to appreciate that practically all major burns become infected.

Other, and considerably more variable, complications include cardiopulmonary and hepatic disorders. Cardiac function may be detrimentally altered or, in some instances, fail, owing to an unidentified protein substance produced at or near the burn site and known as "burn factor." Besides possessing strong myocardial depression capability, this substance may have a widespread detrimental influence on the vasculature, including the vast capillary network of the lung.

Postburn pneumonitis often complicates a major burn and can result in the acute demise of the patient as a result of pulmonary decompensation. The alveolar macrophage, although initially hyperactive against bacterial intruders during the first 24 to 48 hours following the injury, fails to undergo increased production. Since the monocyte is currently felt to be the precursor of the alveolar macrophage, the matters of abnormal monocyte production, release, distribution and migration are currently being examined at the extrapulmonary level.

Burn-related hepatic disease usually takes the form of a nonspecific, reactive hepatitis. Decreased cardiac output, increased blood viscosity and associated splanchnic vasoconstriction all are major contributors. In cases where jaundice develops, intracellular canalicular cholestasis is indicated, apparently resulting from reduced hepatocyte secretion of conjugated bilirubin due to an oxygen-poor (and energy-dependent) Golgi system.

Lymphocytopenia, delayed allograft rejection time and increased susceptibility to infection have been offered as evidence of a decrease in patient immunocompetency.

**Changes in Acute Electrical Injuries.** Acute electrical injuries produce many of the pathophysiologic alterations described above. They also produce changes which are quite etiospecific. For example, an animal struck by lightning becomes highly charged. If the animal is grounded or in contact with a metal object, the current will pass through the body, and entry and exit burns can be identified. The degree of injury is related to (1) the amount of current, (2) the passage time and (3) local tissue resistance. If immediate grounding does not take place, arcing of the current to an adjacent object frequently occurs.

Another specific and often insidious tissue change produced by acute electrical injury is deep muscle necrosis. This injury results from the conversion of electrical to thermal energy as the current passes through the body. The extent and, in some instances, the existence of this kind of injury may be difficult to determine, since it frequently appears in so-called "core" locations with relative sparing of the associated superficial musculature. This distribution pattern of muscular injury is attributed to the greater heat retention capacity of bone and its commensurate protracted heat dissipation time.

## MANAGEMENT

The management of a pet animal which has sustained a major thermal injury has four primary objectives: (1) to save life, (2) to relieve pain, (3) to close the wound and (4) to minimize or correct deformities.

The major life-threatening problems encountered in the management of a severely burned patient are (1) shock, (2) malnutrition, (3) infection, (4) reduced immunocompetency and (5) other organ-system complications. In light of these many potential complications, it is imperative that the clinician and client alike appreciate the length to which each must go in order to effect the survival of the patient. Moreover, it should be made clear from the outset that even with heroic efforts, the animal may still succumb to its injuries.

*Minor burns* are not life-threatening and can usually be treated on an outpatient basis. The responsible owner can carry out much of the necessary treatment at home. Periodic return visits will allow the clinician to evaluate the progress of the injury and to amend home care when indicated. Prognosis, in most instances, will be favorable. An outline of specific management recommendations for the minor burn patient is provided (Table 1).

*Major burns* are potentially life-threatening, and their management should reflect this fact! If the patient requires resuscitation or is in need of respiratory support, the clinician must direct his therapeutic energies accordingly. A brief physical

**Table 1.** *Outline for Initial Management of Minor Thermal Injuries*

1. Be relatively certain the injury is in fact minor. (See text for classification of thermal injuries.)
2. Gently remove the overlying hair coat. Anesthesia may be required, especially if the injury is very painful.
3. Cleanse the injury site with cool saline or Ringer's solution. A *very mild* soap may also be used.
4. Debride devitalized tissues and blisters, if present.
5. Apply topical antimicrobial ointment. Furacin, silver sulfadiazine and Garamycin cream are all effective. Sulfamylon® and Betadine® cause considerable patient discomfort and should be avoided.
6. Apply multiple gauze pads or, preferably, burn dressings and secure with stockinette or an Ace-type bandage.
7. Advise owner to return for checkup in 24 hours, at which time the dressing is removed and the burn is inspected and rebandaged if necessary.
8. Advise capable owners about how to carry out home treatment. These instructions should include soaking of the wound in cool $H_2O$, the application of medicated ointment and the appropriate bandaging techniques.
9. The owner should return for subsequent checkups as needed.

examination should be conducted to ascertain both the extent and the depth of the injury, as well as the patient's general condition. The time of the injury should be recorded with subsequent treatment related to this point. The patient should be hospitalized, the owner should be given a provisional prognosis and aggressive therapy should be begun. An outline of initial management procedures in major thermal injuries is provided (Table 2). Following stabilization, the patient should be reexamined in order to identify any injuries that may have been overlooked during the initial examination.

*Airway and pulmonary disorders* do not correlate well with the degree and extent of thermal injury and, therefore, should be suspected if the patient has had significant smoke exposure. Specific management recommendations are provided in the article "Smoke Inhalation" presented earlier in this text.

*Fluid and electrolyte* recommendations often are provided in specific formulas.* These recommendations should be considered as general guidelines only. There is no substitute for close and frequent monitoring of the patient's vital signs, urine output, electrolytes, hemoglobin and hematocrit. Recent experience in burn shock resuscitation indicates that a combination of 5 per cent dextrose and lactated Ringer's solution, given in comparatively large volume, is the most satisfactory form of fluid therapy.

Whole blood no longer enjoys its previous position of favor; however, it will provide multiple benefits, including (1) increased oxygenating capacity, (2) intravascular toxin dilution, (3) enhanced restitution of damaged endothelial tissues and (4) partial restoration of extravasated colloids. Blood transfusions should be delayed for at least 24 hours following the burn, since existing vascular alterations will result in considerable waste. Furthermore, accumulated serum albumin, lost within the damaged tissues, will result in increased fibrosis as healing progresses. This shift in body fluid from the intravascular into the interstitial compartment usually ceases 24 to 48 hours following the burn.

Oral fluids should be withheld for at least 48 hours. This is done to prevent inhalation disorders associated with vomiting. Additionally, it will diminish the chances of a dilutional hyponatremia or water intoxication.

*Pain relief* is best accomplished with morphine sulfate or one of its derivatives; satisfactory synthetics are also available. Dose and route of administration are dependent not only on the degree of patient discomfort but on circulatory and renal status as well. Secondary pain relief can also be provided in the form of wound coverings to include ointments, dressings, skin grafts and artificial skin. Cold compresses, or cold water immersion in the case of extremital burns, will also ease patient discomfort.

*Cleansing, initial débridement and dressing.* In wounds with little or no contamination, irrigation with large amounts of saline usually suffices to cleanse the surface. At the same time, all devitalized tissue should be debrided, and any blisters, even though

---

**Table 2.** *Outline for Initial Management of Major Thermal Injuries*

1. Establish an airway and administer oxygen or assisted ventilation as needed.
2. Weigh the animal and record the weight.
3. Obtain baseline CBC, electrolytes, BUN and glucose determinations.
4. Begin fluids: one-third 5 per cent dextrose/two-thirds lactated Ringer's given IV; administer at a rate of 10-20 ml./kg./hr. in dogs, and 5-10 ml./kg./hr. in cats. Watch patient closely for signs of fluid overload.
5. Relieve pain with:
   a. Narcotic or narcotic derivative.
   b. Cool saline compresses.
   c. Extremital immersion (saline best but water acceptable).
6. Debride loose flesh and remove any foreign material.
7. Cleanse wound with cool saline—avoid hexachlorophene!
   a. If wound is comparatively clean, copious irrigations are adequate.
   b. If moderately contaminated or previously treated with a home remedy, gentle sponging of the wound with a mild soap is indicated.
8. Assess degree and extent of injury and record.
9. Apply antibiotic ointment and burn dressings.
10. Place urinary catheter and keep track of output.
11. Start burn record, beginning from time of injury.
12. Carefully evaluate patient for signs of smoke inhalation (to include thoracic radiographs).
13. Consider early graft procedure once patient has been stabilized.
14. Place patient in an isolated environment and employ sterile techniques where possible, i.e., masks, gowns, etc.
15. Formulate a detailed treatment plan with special attention paid to graft techniques and the possibility of additional organ-system complications.
16. Give the owner a status report, including a prognosis.

---

*Evan's Formula, Brooke Army Formula.

intact, should be opened and removed. This maneuver is essential if optimal results are to be obtained with topical agents.

If frank contamination is present, the wound may be gently sponged with a mild detergent soap. Since hexachlorophene is rapidly absorbed through the burned tissues in sufficient quantities to produce neurotoxic effects and convulsions, preparations containing this agent should be avoided.

Two schools of thought exist relative to the manner in which burns should be initially dressed. The open method consists of the application of topical ointments to the wound site, without an overlying dressing. This method is not practical with pet animals. The second, or so-called closed method, involves covering the burn site with a burn dressing in addition to a topical ointment and is well suited to veterinary needs. Burn pads consist of multiple layers of single-ply cheesecloth and are commercially available in sheets 18 x 36 inches in size. These may be readily cut to fit any particular wound and can be secured in place with a combination of tape and stockinette.

*Topical antibiotics* have had a statistically significant effect on the control of burn-wound sepsis and have improved the chances of survival in patients suffering burns involving up to 60 per cent of their bodies. Choice of a specific antibiotic ointment should be predicated on the following considerations: (1) antibacterial/antifungal activities, (2) absence of pain-producing qualities, (3) diffusibility, (4) potential toxicity if consumed by the patient, (5) duration of action and (6) influence on regional fluid and electrolyte loss.

Silver sulfadiazine and nitrofurazone fulfill most of these criteria. Mafenide (Sulfamylon®) is a proven product but causes considerable patient discomfort shortly following application. It also is a potent carbonic anhydrase inhibitor and can create severe alkalosis with prolonged use. Mafenide has no antifungal properties. Betadine® also causes a great deal of patient discomfort when applied to a burn site. Garamycin cream is satisfactory but very costly. Silver nitrate has been reported to cause severe fluid and electrolyte imbalances, in addition to having poor penetration qualities.

*Systemic antibiotics*, given prophylactically to the major burn patient, have no proven efficacy in preventing either cutaneous or systemic infections. On the contrary, prophylactic antibiotics may alter the flora of the burn wound, with resultant emergence of antibiotic-resistant organisms. Recent investigation involving the prophylactic treatment of human burn patients with high levels of penicillin G showed twice the number of subsequent infections in the treated group as compared with the untreated group. This study and others like it leave very serious doubt as to the advisability of giving prophylactic systemic antibiotics to burn patients.

*Wound closure* is the primary goal in burn therapy and may take multiple forms to include various kinds of grafts as well as commercially available synthetic skin. The metabolic effects associated with early burn wound closure consist of a decrease in evaporative water loss from the burn wound, a diminution of exudative protein and blood loss, marked decrease of pain and metabolic rate, improvement in nutrition and protection of the patient from external invasive infections.

*Grafts* are classified according to origin, with autografts originating from the patient, homografts coming from another of the same species and hetero- or zenografts being provided by a different species.

Autografts obviously provide the most effective physiologic wound closure, although "taking" is often delayed owing to a general and relatively prolonged reduction in healing capacity. Skin obtained from another of the same species (homograft) makes an effective *temporary* closure with rejection occurring by the 10th day. If the burn is not overly deep, the underlying bed of granulation tissue, which formed beneath the rejected graft, will provide the necessary impetus for local reepithelization. Porcine heterografts have been demonstrated to be nearly as effective as homografts for biologic dressing and are available commercially. Currently, it is recommended that such grafts be employed as temporary dressings; these should be changed every fifth day.

Grafting, as with any surgical procedure, requires a plan and a modicum of experience. If one is not familiar with such techniques, appropriate surgical texts (largely human) should be studied before grafting is attempted. It must be emphasized that grafts are a *necessary* part of the treatment of a severely burned patient, and that they must be used early in the clinical course. To delay in the hope that simple dressings will be sufficient is to invite failure and, in all likelihood, the demise of the patient. As stated earlier, total commitment is required to save the critically burned patient, and grafts are an integral part of this commitment.

*Metabolic and nutritional* derangements are commonly encountered in major thermal injuries and may be so severe as to result in the death of the patient.

Hypermetabolic phenomena exhibited by burn patients have generally been attributed to a marked increase in heat loss, a consequence of augmented evaporative water loss through the thermally damaged skin. Evaporative water loss in excess of 300 ml./hour has been documented in man, accounting for heat losses of greater than 4000 Kcal./24 hours. Recent research, however, indicates that increased evaporative water loss is not primarily responsible for the hypermetabolic state following burns. Based largely upon metabolic studies performed in thermally injured experimental animals, the current evidence appears to point to the central nervous system, particularly the hypothalamus, as the seat of difficulty.

The major manifestations of the hypermetabolic state are severe weight loss, negative nitrogen balance and retarded wound healing. The extent of the catabolic response seems to parallel the severity of the burn. Protein catabolism does not proceed uniformly in all tissues. Vital organs such as the heart and liver are maintained at the expense of muscle protein. Increased caloric demands are primarily met by the stores of body fat (÷ 80 per cent), while endogenous protein supplies only about 20 per cent of the bodily needs. It therefore becomes obvious that the condition of the patient at the time of the burn injury will be a prime prognostic consideration.

Prevention of protein depletion is accomplished by increasing the patient's daily consumption of both calories and nitrogen. In the case of major burns, the injured animal should receive approximately 3 to 5 times the normal daily requirement of nitrogen and at least 2 to 4 times the normal daily caloric requirement. This supplementation should consist of a high-caloric, high-protein diet, preferably given by mouth and continued on a gradually reduced basis for up to 3 months. Wound healing may serve as a rough indication as to when heavy supplementation may be discontinued. Protein hydrolysates should be handled only by those thoroughly familiar with their use, since they can be associated with myriad untoward effects. Glucose solutions are of benefit during the early postburn period but are totally inadequate thereafter.

*Burn-wound sepsis* is the most frequently encountered complication in any form of thermal injury. Septicemia is responsible for the greatest number of deaths in those patients who survive the initial injury.

Bacterial organisms most frequently cultured from burn wounds include *Staphylococcus* and *Pseudomonas* species. These organisms are also cultured from the blood in those patients who become septicemic. Fungal organisms, such as *Candida*, are now a major problem in human burn patients. Until evidence is offered to the contrary, one should suspect such organisms as potential secondary invaders in burned pet animals.

The prevention of burn-wound sepsis is very difficult in major burn patients. It is best accomplished by a combination of early wound closure, topical antibiotics and the maintenance of environmental isolation to the extent that this is possible. The last point is especially true while the patient is hospitalized. Whenever possible, sterile technique should be employed in handling the patient; this will add to the chances of survival.

Topical antibiotics and wound closure were discussed previously and need not be described here. As indicated earlier, prophylactic systemic antibiotics are to be discouraged. Multiple wound sites should be cultured 24 hours following the initial burn and every third day thereafter, with antibiotic therapy directed at specific bacterial populations.

Immunologic control of *Pseudomonas* infections using both vaccine and hyperimmune globulins in human burn patients has been reported. Judgment concerning these procedures awaits further veterinary experience.

*Additional complications* frequently encountered in major burn patients include acute liver disorder, anemia, pneumonia, nephrosis, seizures and a generalized reduction in immunocompetency. Most of these complications occur with sufficient frequency to be anticipated during the patient's period of hospitalization. Biochemical surveillance, in combination with a high index of suspicion, will provide for the early identification of such disorders if they should occur. Specific management methods for these body systems are covered elsewhere in this text.

In conclusion, one should be aware that many excellent human burn centers exist throughout the country, and their staffs are usually very willing to provide advice and materials when consulted.

### SUPPLEMENTAL READING

Fuller, I., and Archambeault, C.: Nursing the Burned Patient. Institute for Burn Medicine, Ann Arbor, Mich., 1973.
Muir, I., and Bardy, T.: Burns and Their Treatment. 2nd ed. London, Lloyd-Luke, Ltd., 1974.
Polk, H., and Stone, H.: Contemporary Burn Management. Boston, Little, Brown and Co., 1971.

# HEAT STROKE (HEAT STRESS, HYPERPYREXIA)

WILLIAM D. SCHALL, D.V.M.
*East Lansing, Michigan*

Heat stroke is a sporadically encountered condition characterized by hyperthermia (rectal temperature 105° to 110° F.) and often complicated by alterations in acid-base homeostasis, disseminated intravascular coagulation and cerebral edema.

Several factors either are necessary for or may contribute to the induction of heat stroke. A prerequisite is high ambient temperature that may be as low as 90° F. but is more often 100° to 115° F. Virtually all dogs in which the condition occurs are confined in some manner. In most instances, dogs are confined to an enclosure with poor ventilation, such as an automobile or transporting crate. We have encountered dogs with heat stroke that were not enclosed but were confined by a chain outdoors. In these cases, excitement and exercise associated with animal fights appear to have precipitated heat stroke. Although exercise and excitement can significantly contribute to the induction of heat stroke in confined dogs, the condition is rare in dogs that run free, regardless of air temperature and exercise. High humidity contributes to the likelihood of heat stroke because evaporation of water from the oral and nasal cavities is reduced in spite of maximal panting. Other predisposing factors are lack of available water, brachiocephalic anatomy, obesity and decreased heat tolerance associated with young and old age.

Cats apparently can tolerate higher temperatures than can dogs. Heat stroke occurs rarely in this species.

## PATHOPHYSIOLOGY

The initial compensatory response to increased ambient temperature is panting. This mechanism of dissipating body heat is efficient and involves the unidirectional flow of air into the nasal passages and out the oral cavity. This flow maximizes evaporation and heat loss because air is exposed to the greater evaporative surface area of the nasal turbinates. The process of panting, however, is not devoid of serious consequence. Significant pulmonary exchange takes place during panting and results in respiratory alkalosis. In dogs anesthetized with pentobarbital and subjected to an environment of 114° F. at 80 per cent relative humidity, respiratory alkalosis was documented 30 minutes after initiation of the experiment. Inasmuch as blood gas determinations were not done between the time the dogs were subjected to the hot environment and 30 minutes later, the precise time of onset of respiratory alkalosis is not known. The magnitude of respiratory alkalosis in our experimental hyperthermic dogs was profound. Typically, one hour after entrance into the hot environment experimental dogs had an arterial blood pH of about 7.75 and a $PCO_2$ of less than 10 torr.

The respiratory alkalosis induced in pentobarbital-anesthetized dogs subjected to high temperature, however, eventually was modified by metabolic acidosis presumably due to muscle activity associated with panting. Most dogs had an arterial blood pH less than 7.30 three to four hours after experimental hyperthermia. The combination of respiratory alkalosis and metabolic acidosis was associated with cessation of panting and with cerebral edema and was followed by death. Although the experimental hyperthermia which we induced may not be identical to naturally occurring heat stroke, it seems likely that dogs with heat stroke, when examined by the clinician, may have respiratory alkalosis or a combination of respiratory alkalosis and metabolic acidosis. The acid-base status of the individual patient can be known only if blood gas determinations are done.

Although serum electrolyte concentrations have not been done routinely on dogs with heat stroke, serum potassium concentration is known to increase in experimental canine and feline hyperthermia. The liver and jejunum have been established as two major sources of potassium released to extracellular water, but they do not account totally for the observed hyperkalemia. Although other sources of potassium release remain unknown, it has been established that striated muscle is not the source. On the contrary, intracellular striated muscle concentrations of potassium are known to increase. The highest serum potassium concentrations coincide with the severest respiratory alkalosis. The decrease in serum potassium concentration associated with experimental hyperthermia, however, is mild and may not be clinically significant. Typical serum potassium concentrations are about 5.0 mEq./l.

Hypophosphatemia occurred in our experimental hyperthermic dogs approximately at the time of peak hyperkalemia and respiratory alkalosis. Most dogs had serum inorganic phosphorus concentrations of about 2.0 mg./dl. compared to control values of 3.5 to 4.5 mg./dl. The mechanism of the hypophosphatemia is unknown.

Other alterations in serum electrolyte concentration known to be associated with experimental hyperthermia, and hence presumed to be typical of heat stroke, have been minor and probably are the result of hemoconcentration.

The degree of hemoconcentration that occurs in heat stroke may be severe. Packed cell volumes (PCV) of 75 per cent have been reported. Whether hemoconcentration is mild, moderate or severe is probably determined by environmental humidity and duration of the animal's exposure to the environment. In pentobarbital-anesthetized dogs subjected to 114° F. at 80 per cent relative humidity until rectal temperature reached 109° F., the PCV typically increased by 30 per cent and the serum osmolality increased by 10 per cent.

Disseminated intravascular coagulation (DIC) is known to occur as a result of heat stroke in man and dog. Experimental canine hyperthermia is also known to cause DIC and has been proposed as an experimental DIC model. The precise mechanism by which hyperthermia causes DIC is unknown but is characterized by progressive thrombocytopenia, increased activated clotting time, increased partial thromboplastin time and the presence of fibrin (fibrinogen) degradation products in serum. The historical observation that some dogs with heat stroke die of a shocklike syndrome accompanied by hemorrhagic diathesis hours after seemingly complete recovery from heat stroke probably reflects the occurrence of DIC.

Another complication of heat stroke is cerebral edema. Although the mechanism by which hyperthermia induces cerebral edema is unknown, this complication is commonly present in heat stroke and experimental hyperthermia. Dogs with heat stroke and cerebral edema are initially stuporous. Involuntary paddling movements and coarse tremors are often present and the dogs appear to be unaware of their surroundings. If the edema progresses, the menace reflex is lost, and the dogs lapse into a coma. The panting reflex is abolished, the respiratory rate markedly decreases and the dogs die of respiratory arrest.

## CLINICAL FINDINGS

The physical findings in dogs with heat stroke vary depending on the duration and severity of the disease. Initially, panting, tachycardia, bright red oral mucosa and hyperthermia are the only findings. As the disease progresses, dogs become stuporous. The extremities become hot to the touch and the bright red oral mucosa becomes pale, owing to either decreased circulating volume or peripheral vasoconstriction or both. At this stage, dogs may involuntarily void watery diarrhea. If the diarrhea becomes bloody or if petechiae are present, DIC may be a complication. Finally, coma and respiratory arrest follow unless spontaneous recovery or medical intervention interrupts the pathophysiologic sequence.

Laboratory findings relate to the stage and severity of the disease and are considered in detail in the discussion of pathophysiology.

## THERAPY

Our understanding of heat stroke pathophysiology remains incomplete, and the direct relevance of some experimental hyperthermia observations remains uncertain. For these reasons, some of the therapeutic recommendations are quasiscientific and based on inference.

The first objective of therapy is to lower body temperature. Experimental work supports the clinical observation that the chief determinants of survival are duration and degree of hyperthermia. An efficient method of lowering the rectal temperature is to submerge the trunk and limbs in a tub of cold or iced water. The rectal temperature should be taken at 10-minute intervals and the dog should be removed when rectal temperature reaches 103° F., because further cooling may be followed by hypothermia. Since recurrence of hyperthermia is also possible, the rectal temperature should be determined at 10-minute intervals for at least 30 minutes after the dog is removed from the tub. Cold-water enemas have been suggested as a method of cooling but have the disadvantage of interfering with temperature monitoring. Evaporative methods of cooling which are commonly used in man are ineffective in the dog because of the hair coat. During the period of cooling, friction may be applied to the extremities to promote superficial circulation. Occasionally, severe shivering may hinder cooling. The intravenous administration of a phenothiazine tranquilizer such as chlorpromazine (1.0 mg./kg. body weight) may be used to counteract shivering.

The second objective of therapy is to prevent cerebral edema. Immediately after or immediately before submersion in cold water, dexamethasone should be administered intravenously in an anti-edema dose (1.0 to 2.0 mg./kg. body weight). This dose of glucocorticoid may also be beneficial routinely to treat and prevent shock. Intravenous infusions of mannitol (2.0 gm./kg. body weight as a 20 per cent solution over a 10-minute period) may be used if the patient is stuporous or comatose or if stupor or coma develops during therapy. Mannitol should not be administered if serious blood loss complicates heat stroke. Mannitol should be administered cautiously if DIC is documented or suspected.

Intravenous fluids are indicated if hemoconcentration is documented or if peripheral circulation failure is suspected. Fluids are of potential benefit in preventing DIC and shock but must be administered with caution because of possible induction of pulmonary edema and aggravation of cerebral edema. In the absence of specific serum electrolyte determinations, individual electrolyte replacement is contraindicated; a balanced electrolyte solution such as Ringer's is the fluid of choice. There are insufficient data from naturally occurring heat stroke and experimental hyperthermia to recommend the indiscriminate administration of calcium gluconate solutions.

Unless blood gas determinations are done, decisions regarding acid-base therapy are impossible. In the absence of specific information, fluids which have little effect on acid-base balance, such as Ringer's, should be administered.

If hemorrhagic diarrhea, excessive bleeding from venipuncture sites or hemorrhage elsewhere is present, DIC may be a complication of heat stroke. Coagulation studies may help verify the presence of DIC and ideally should include one-stage prothrombin time, activated partial thromboplastin time, activated clotting time, platelet count and the detection of increased serum concentration of fibrin (fibrinogen) degradation products. If no facilities are available for these studies, the clinician should assume that DIC is present if bleeding tendencies are noted. Therapy for DIC should be initiated with the intravenous administration of heparin (50 to 150 I.U./kg. body weight). Intravenous heparin should be repeated at 4- to 6-hour intervals until the bleeding tendency is no longer noted.

Antibiotics are often administered to dogs with heat stroke based on the assumption that patients are predisposed to infection. Broad-spectrum antibiotics are recommended for this purpose.

**SUPPLEMENTAL READING**

Barry, M. E., and King, B. A.: Heatstroke. South African Med. J., *36*:455, 1962.
Malamud, N., Haymaker, W., and Custer, R. P.: Heatstroke. Milit. Surg. 99:397, 1946.
Perchick, J. S., Winkelstein, A., and Shadduck, R. K.:

Disseminated intravascular coagulation in heatstroke. J.A.M.A., *231*:480, 1975.
Shapiro, Y., Rosenthal, T., and Sohar, E.: Experimental heatstroke. Arch. Intern. Med., *131*:688, 1973.
Spurr, G. B., and Barlow, G.: Tissue electrolytes in hyperthermic dogs. J. Appl. Physiol., 28:13, 1970.

# COLD INJURY (HYPOTHERMIA, FROSTBITE, FREEZING)

ROBERT A. DIETERICH, D.V.M.
*Fairbanks, Alaska*

Hypothermia or freezing of tissues in domestic animals as a result of environmental exposure occurs more commonly in areas located in the northern latitudes but is seen occasionally in other areas as a result of accidental cooling or freezing of a pet held captive in household refrigerators or freezers. Another frequently encountered cause of hypothermia is interference with thermoregulatory centers during surgery by anesthetics or sedatives. Hypothermia will be considered separately from freezing even though both may be present in a patient at the same time. Treatment for each condition involves different principles and they should be considered different entities.

## HYPOTHERMIA

Hypothermia is defined as the condition produced by deep cooling from external cold, drugs or failure of the temperature-regulating mechanisms which results in a profound decrease in body temperature. This definition does not include normal cooling due to circadian rhythms which produce changes in body temperature of from 1° to 2° C. Mild hypothermia is characterized by body temperatures of 30° to 32° C., moderate hypothermia by temperatures of 22° to 25° C. and profound hypothermia by temperatures of 0° to 8° C. The physiologic changes of hypothermia depend on the extent and duration of exposure. The duration of hypothermia can be characterized as acute (few hours), prolonged (several hours) or chronic (days).

Survival of animals suffering from hypothermia depends on the degree of cooling to which they are subjected. Moderate hypothermia allows survival for approximately 24 hours, while body temperatures of 15° C. shorten survival time to 5 or 6 hours. Profound hypothermia narrows survival time still further to 1 or 2 hours.

### TREATMENT

Treatment of hypothermia is directed toward rewarming and maintenance of vital body functions. Rewarming may be accomplished by external (surface) means or by internal (core) methods. External rewarming results in the body surface or shell being warmed first with the aid of warm water immersion, water or electric heating blankets, hot-water bottles or simply a warm room and blankets. Oxygen and appropriate intravenous fluid therapy may also be needed, depending on the degree of hypothermia being treated.

Internal rewarming is accomplished using peritoneal dialysis. The dialysate is heated to 50° to 55° C. and is allowed to flow into the peritoneal cavity as fast as gravity permits. After flowing through the administration tubing, the dialysate fluid will reach the abdominal cavity at a temperature of approximately 45° C. Dialysis is continued until normal body temperature is reached. Methods of procedure to carry out peritoneal dialysis are described in the article on "Peritoneal Dialysis" in this text.

The advantages of internal rewarming are several. Sometimes when external rewarming is attempted there will be vasodilatation of surface vessels and a transfer of cooled blood to the body core, bringing about a further drop in internal temperature which results in rewarming shock. Normothermia can be achieved faster with peritoneal dialysis than with external rewarming methods. Cardiac output and electrocardiogram readings return to normal rapidly after rewarming by internal methods. When using either the external or the internal rewarming method, it is important to avoid overheating and resultant hyperthermia.

After a hypothermic patient is returned to normothermia, a complete examination should be carried out to determine whether another disorder led to the lowered body temperature. Renal failure, pneumonia or malnutrition can easily lower an animal's resistance to cold exposure, and the resulting hypothermia may be only a secondary symptom.

## FROSTBITE OR FREEZING

Frostbite or freezing of tissue is rare in animals that are healthy and well nourished. Well-acclimatized long-haired animals can remain exposed to temperatures of −50° C. for indefinite periods with no ill effects. It is critical that animals exposed to very low environmental temperatures be fed adequate amounts of food to enable them to produce enough body heat to maintain normothermia. In cold regions, frostbite of the tips of the ears or tails of cats is perhaps the most common cold injury seen. This usually requires no treatment unless secondary infection is encountered. A bland ointment may be applied if needed. The scrotum of male dogs will sometimes be injured by cold from repeated contact with cold surfaces or deep snow. Erythema and scaliness or even minor sloughing of surface scrotal tissue can occur and is treated with ointments and reduced cold exposure. Continued contact with snow or cold surfaces will delay healing.

The deep-freezing of tissues is seen in animals that have been physically injured or caught in various types of wildlife traps or other circulation-inhibiting situations. Recently, major advances have been made in the treatment of severe frostbite. The owner of the frostbite patient should be encouraged to bring the injured animal directly to a veterinarian and should attempt no home treatment unless an extended period of time would pass before the animal could reach a veterinary hospital. Tissue damage and tissue necrosis are increased greatly if thawing and subsequent refreezing occur (freeze-thaw-freeze-thaw syndrome). The frozen part should be kept frozen and protected to avoid trauma during transport or handling.

### TREATMENT

Frozen tissue should be thawed rapidly in warm water (38° to 44° C.) as soon as possible after it is known that refreezing can be prevented. The frozen part should not be massaged during warming. Previously thawed parts should not be subjected to rapid rewarming. The thawed part will soon become erythematous and edematous. Large blebs usually occur, and self-mutilation by the patient should be avoided. It is best to leave the injured tissue exposed rather than to use occlusive wet dressings or petrolatum gauze. Premature débridement or other surgical intervention should not be undertaken. Treatment should be confined to protection of the part from trauma and prevention of infection. Systemic antibiotics should be administered in severe cases.

Unnecessary débridement of necrotic tissue or amputation should be delayed as healing occurs. Irreversibly damaged tissues begin to demarcate in 4 to 7 days. Often, 15 to 20 days are required for the injured tissue to reach a point at which there is a clear demarcation of the tissue to be lost, and therefore removed, and the tissue which is viable. The pads of frostbitten feet should be preserved if at all possible.

Fractures, dislocations and extensive trauma of frozen tissue should not be repaired until after thawing is complete. Fracture treatment should be conservative. A high-protein, high-caloric diet with vitamin supplements is helpful, particularly in the malnourished patient that has suffered both hypothermia and frostbite.

### SUPPLEMENTAL READING

Mills, W.: Frostbite and hypothermia, current concepts. Alaska Med., Vol. 15, No. 2, March, 1973.

Petajan, J.: Prevention and treatment of frostbite. Report No. 103, Arctic Health Research Center, Fairbanks, Alaska 99701, 1969.

Popovic, V. and Popovic, P.: Hypothermia in biology and in medicine. New York, Grune and Stratton, 1974.

# Section
# 3

# RESPIRATORY DISEASES

## N. EDWARD ROBINSON
*Consulting Editor*

# RESPIRATORY FUNCTION

N. EDWARD ROBINSON, M.R.C.V.S.,
*and* PATRICIA O'HANDLEY, V.D.M.
*East Lansing, Michigan*

Cough, dyspnea and reduced exercise tolerance are common clinical signs of respiratory disease which result from a wide variety of disturbances of normal respiratory physiology. As clinicians, we must identify, localize and correct these physiologic derangements. This discussion will attempt to provide a physiologic basis for the rational diagnosis and therapy of respiratory disease.

In normal animals, pulmonary gas exchange supplies oxygen and removes carbon dioxide at a rate matched to tissue metabolism. This highly efficient process depends on control systems to regulate both ventilation and perfusion of the lungs so that gas transport mechanisms in the blood can perform optimally. For purposes of discussion, it is useful to separate respiratory function into the processes of ventilation, perfusion, gas exchange, gas transport and control. Inefficiency in one or more of these processes will result in the clinical signs of respiratory disease.

## VENTILATION

Ventilation is the process whereby gases are moved into and out of the exchange area of the lung (alveoli and respiratory bronchioles), through the conduction airways (nares, trachea, bronchi and bronchioles). Since the conducting airways do not participate in gas exchange, they are referred to as dead space. Tidal volume is the volume of each breath, whereas minute ventilation is the volume of air exhaled per minute, the product of tidal volume and frequency (number of breaths/minute).

Inspiration is an active process with the energy supplied by the inspiratory muscles (diaphragm, external intercostals, sternocephalicus, etc.). The inspiratory muscles enlarge the thorax, thereby decreasing the intrapleural pressure. This decreased pressure is necessary to overcome lung elasticity, expand the gas exchange area and generate flow through the airways. Normally exhalation is passive, but with exercise or lung disease, expiration may become an active and exhausting process involving the abdominal muscles.

**Pulmonary Elasticity.** Pulmonary elasticity is due to the elastic and collagen fibers in lung tissue and also to the surface tension forces generated by the fluid film lining the alveoli. Elastic recoil is frequently increased in lung disease by the accumulation of acute or chronic inflammatory tissue in the lung. Such a lung has reduced compliance and is "stiffer" than normal. Decreased lung compliance will increase the work of breathing. Affected animals tend to minimize the work of breathing by taking rapid, short breaths (tachypnea). A similar pattern of breathing is observed when intrathoracic masses and fluids or lesions of the thoracic cage are present. Since these abnormalities all limit lung inflation, they are classified as restrictive diseases. In addition to altering the pattern of breathing, restrictive diseases reduce the resting lung volume, i.e., functional residual capacity (FRC). Increased compliance which increases FRC is a normal consequence of canine aging and rarely a result of pulmonary disease.

The surface tension of fluid lining the alveoli is considerably less than the surface tension of water because of a phospholipid surfactant produced by Type II alveolar cells. A lack of surfactant decreases lung compliance, producing an unstable lung which tends to collapse and develop atelectasis. This situation is observed in premature newborns because surfactant is not ordinarily formed until late in gestation. A similar situation can result if the lungs are not fully inflated by means of a sigh reflex several times per hour to reactivate surfactant. Anesthetized animals and animals with thoracic or abdominal pain may fail to sigh, but atelectasis can be prevented by providing regular deep breaths to these patients.

**The Conducting Airways.** The conducting airways consist of branching tubes with approximately 22 divisions between the trachea and the alveoli. The resistance of any tube to air flow depends upon its length but more importantly upon its diameter. The length of the conducting airways changes little, but the diameter can vary greatly as a result of accumulated secretions (e.g., bronchitis); smooth muscle contraction (e.g., allergic reactions); extraluminal masses (e.g., intrathoracic neoplasms); changes in lung volume; or changes in the transmural pressure gradient across the wall of the airways (e.g., forced expiratory effort of collapsing trachea).

Airway smooth muscle constricts in response to parasympathetic stimulation, inhaled irritants, allergic reactions and local irritation generated by infection. Sympathomimetics (e.g., isoproterenol), parasympatholytics (e.g., atropine) and xanthines (e.g., aminophylline) all relax airway smooth muscle. Lung volume is also an important factor affecting airway diameter. Airways are dilated at large lung volumes and narrowed at small volumes. The narrowing of airways at low lung volumes causes the end-expiratory wheezing typical of airway obstruction.

Transmural pressure is the pressure gradient across the wall of the airway. When outside pressure exceeds inside pressure, collapse of the airway occurs. Rigid supporting tissue (cartilage) in the walls of bronchi reduces the effect of changes in transmural pressure. In the upper airway, transmural pressure tends to collapse the airway during inspiration and dilate it during expiration. Thus, upper airway lesions tend to cause inspiratory dyspnea. However, in the intrathoracic airways, transmural pressure dilates the airway during inhalation and collapses it during exhalation so that intrathoracic airway lesions cause expiratory dyspnea. (see Figure 1, in "Interpretation of Pulmonary Radiographs," at the end of this section). Compression of the intrathoracic airways is exaggerated by an active maneuver, particularly if there is obstruction of the small airways. Repeated forced expiratory efforts resulting in tracheal compression are responsible for the honking cough in cases of collapsing trachea.

Intrathoracic airway obstruction (e.g., bronchitis or bronchiolitis) limits expiratory flow rates and prolongs expiration so that each subsequent breath begins at a larger lung volume. This cycle is repeated until a new equilibrium is reached, with the airway sufficiently dilated by the larger lung volume to allow passive exhalation. By this process, the animal has increased its FRC, which is frequently visible radiographically as a hyperlucent lung field and a flattened diaphragm. Increased FRC is diagnostic of intrathoracic airway obstruction (obstructive pulmonary disease). If increased FRC will not sufficiently dilate airways to allow passive exhalation, the animal will exhale actively. Abdominal expiration is a sign of severe airway obstruction and, if prolonged, may produce a heave line.

The total cross-sectional area of the airways becomes very large as the airways bifurcate, so that the major resistance to breathing is between the upper airway and the lobar bronchi. Small airways less than 2 mm. in diameter, which have no cartilage support, contribute little to the total airway resistance. Their importance lies in their collapsibility and susceptibility to obstruction. Reductions in lung volume caused by localized masses, pleural effusions or abdominal distention will close small airways, thus trapping gas in the alveoli distal to the site of closure. Similarly, inflammation or plugging of the small airways with secretions (e.g., bronchiolitis) will also cause gas trapping. Alveoli distal to small airway obstruction can ventilate only through collateral channels provided by either the interalveolar pores (pores of Kohn) or anastomosing respiratory bronchioles. Inadequate collateral ventilation results in inefficient gas exchange, while the absence of collateral ventilation causes atelectasis. Fortunately, dogs have extensive collateral ventilation, so atelectasis develops only following obstruction of lobar bronchi.

## PERFUSION

Blood flow to the lungs is provided by the pulmonary and bronchial circulations. While pulmonary circulation is involved in gas exchange, the bronchial circulation, being part of the systemic circulation, provides nutritional blood flow to the airways. When the pulmonary circulation is reduced, the bronchial circulation hypertrophies, but it is doubtful whether it participates greatly in maintaining gas exchange.

The pulmonary circulation is a low-pressure, low-resistance circulation with resting pulmonary arterial pressures of 22 mm. Hg systolic, 8 mm. Hg diastolic and 15 mm. Hg mean. The pulmonary circulation is greatly affected by changes in lung volume as well as by changes in intrapulmonary pressures. The pulmonary capillaries, which almost surround each alveolus with a sheet of blood, are collapsible, thin-walled tubes whose perfusion is a function of pulmonary arterial, pulmonary venous and alveolar pressures. Positive pressure ventilation will reduce capillary volume by increasing alveolar pressure, while left heart failure and exercise will increase volume by elevating intravascular pressures. The increased pulmonary blood volume of left heart failure is recognized radiographically by the increased diameter of pulmonary veins. Gravitational forces also increase intravascular pressures in dependent areas of the lung, and perfusion is always greatest in these areas. Because of vascular pooling in dependent areas, recumbent animals should be frequently turned over.

Various humoral mediators and local chemical changes cause active changes in pulmonary vascular resistance. The most potent stimulus for pulmonary vascular constriction is alveolar hypoxia, which will reduce perfusion to poorly ventilated areas of lung. In extensive lung disease, generalized hypoxic pulmonary vasoconstriction will elevate pulmonary arterial pressure and may cause right heart failure (cor pulmonale). The role of the pulmonary circulation in maintaining a relatively dry lung will not be discussed in this chapter but is well described in the article "Pulmonary Vascular Disease in the Dog."

Besides its role in gas exchange, the pulmonary circulation is the site of uptake of vasoactive agents (e.g., serotonin and prostaglandins). It also acts as a blood filter, removing emboli arising in the systemic circulation.

## GAS EXCHANGE

The clinician evaluates pulmonary gas exchange by examining the mucous membranes for cyanosis and by measuring arterial oxygen or carbon dioxide tensions ($PaO_2$ and $PaCO_2$, respectively). These evaluations describe the end result of several processes occurring in gas exchange, including alveolar ventilation, gas diffusion across the alveolar-capillary membrane and the matching of ventilation and perfusion.

Inhaled air has an oxygen partial pressure ($PO_2$) of 160 torr (mm. Hg). The upper respiratory tract adds water vapor to air, so that the $PO_2$ of the humidified air at body temperature is approximately 140 to 150 torr. In the alveoli, oxygen is removed and carbon dioxide is added to the alveolar gas, so that the average alveolar oxygen tension ($PaO_2$) is 100 torr.

While minute ventilation is the total volume of air breathed per minute, alveolar ventilation is the volume of gas participating in gas exchange per minute. Since a panting dog is primarily ventilating the dead space of the upper airways, little alveolar ventilation takes place, although minute ventilation is very large. In contrast, deep sighs increase both minute and alveolar ventilation. Normally, alveolar ventilation is controlled to maintain $PaCO_2$ at 40 torr. In alveolar hyperventilation, carbon dioxide is removed faster than it is produced by the tissues, and $PaCO_2$ decreases. This occurs during excitement and in response to hypoxemia. With hypoventilation, carbon dioxide is produced faster than it is eliminated, and $PaCO_2$ increases. Alveolar hypoventilation (respiratory failure) is a sign of advanced lung disease, thoracic trauma or central nervous system depression (e.g., anesthesia or brain injury). Changing alveolar ventilation provides a rapid means of changing blood pH, with hyperventilation eliminating hydrogen ions and hypoventilation retaining hydrogen ions.

Alveolar oxygen tension and hence arterial oxygen tension also vary with alveolar ventilation; both increase in hyperventilation and decrease in hypoventilation. However, since there are many other factors which affect arterial oxygen tension, alveolar ventilation is best evaluated by measuring $PaCO_2$.

Gases pass between the alveoli and capillary blood by diffusion. Diffusion rates are affected by both the surface area of the lung available for gas exchange (the pulmonary capillary surface) and the thickness of the alveolar-capillary membrane. Loss of surface area for gas exchange (e.g., consolidation or atelectasis) or thickening of the alveolar membrane (e.g., edema) will reduce the rate of gas diffusion. Diffusion abnormalities in respiratory disease frequently cause no problems in the resting animal because pulmonary blood flow is slow enough for diffusion to be completed. When blood flow rate increases, as in exercise, blood will leave the pulmonary capillaries before diffusion can be completed, resulting in arterial hypoxemia and reduced exercise tolerance. Diffusion abnormalities tend to decrease $PaO_2$ more than they increase $PaCO_2$ because $O_2$ is much less diffusible than $CO_2$.

For optimal gas exchange, ventilation and perfusion must be matched so that the rate of oxygen transport into the alveolus equals its rate of uptake by capillary blood. Ventilation-perfusion mismatching is the commonest cause of hypoxemia in clinical respiratory disease.

Complete or partial obstructions of pulmonary arteries (e.g., by emboli, heartworms or valvular lesions) will decrease pulmonary capillary pressure and reduce perfusion to some areas of lung tissue. This results in ventilation in excess of perfusion (alveolar dead space), which necessitates increased minute ventilation and therefore increased work of breathing.

In contrast, perfusion in excess of ventilation results from airway obstruction caused by small airway disease (e.g., bronchitis or bronchiolitis) or from airway closure due to lung compression (e.g., by pleural effusions or abdominal distention). When perfusion exceeds ventilation in an area of lung, the pulmonary capillary blood has a lower oxygen content and a higher carbon dioxide content than normal. This blood, which is referred to as venous admixture, mixes with blood from the normal alveoli to form the systemic arterial blood which is distributed to the tissues. The extreme example of venous admixture is blood flow from the right to the left side of the heart through unventilated tissue (i.e., a right-to-left shunt). Right-to-left shunts can occur through congenital cardiac defects (e.g., tetralogy of Fallot) or through pulmonary areas of atelectasis or consolidation. Venous admixture lowers $PaO_2$, which cannot be corrected by hyperventilation of the remaining normal areas of lung. This occurs because hemoglobin is almost fully saturated with oxygen when $PO_2 = 100$ torr, and hyperventilation cannot add sufficient oxygen to blood to compensate for the low oxygen content in the venous admixture. In contrast, hyperventilation of the remaining healthy lung will eliminate carbon dioxide and compensate for the carbon dioxide content of the venous admixture. Typical blood gas values resulting from venous admixture are low $PaO_2$ and a normal or low $PaCO_2$.

Raising inspired oxygen tension with oxygen therapy will frequently elevate $PaO_2$ significantly when hypoxemia results from decreased ventilation to some areas of lung. However, in right-to-left shunts, oxygen therapy will usually elevate $PaO_2$ only a small amount.

In summary, hypoxemia can result from (a) decreased inspired oxygen tension, (b) alveolar hypoventilation (detectable by measuring $PaCO_2$), (c) diffusion abnormalities, (d) ventilation-perfusion mismatching and (e) right-to-left vascular shunts. Oxygen therapy will correct hypoxemia in all of these but least in the right-to-left shunt. However, oxygen therapy itself will not correct alveolar hypoventilation, so carbon dioxide must be eliminated by increasing alveolar ventilation with some form of positive pressure respiration.

## GAS TRANSPORT

The partial pressure of oxygen in arterial blood ($PaO_2$) is approximately 100 torr. Because oxygen has a low solubility, each 100 ml. of plasma carries only 0.3 ml. of oxygen when $PaO_2$ equals 100 torr. To supply oxygen to the tissues with a reasonable cardiac output, an additional oxygen transport mechanism is necessary; this is provided by hemoglobin, each gram of which can transport 1.39 ml. of oxygen. Blood normally contains approximately 15 grams of hemoglobin per 100 ml., so that it is therefore capable of transporting 21 ml. of oxygen (i.e., blood has an oxygen content of 21 volumes per cent, or per 100 ml.). The combination of oxygen with hemoglobin is reversible and depends upon blood $PO_2$. However, the relationship between $PO_2$ and oxygen content is not directly proportional and also varies with pH, temperature and the level of 2,3-diphosphoglycerate (2,3-DPG) found in the erythrocyte.

Examination of Fig. 1 will show that above $PO_2$ levels equal to 70 torr, the oxyhemoglobin dissociation curve is flat, so that raising $PO_2$ adds very little oxygen to hemoglobin, which is then saturated. This plateau allows mammals to load oxygen onto hemoglobin while living at high altitudes or in the presence of mild cardiopulmonary disease, both of which decrease $PO_2$. Furthermore, hyperventilation

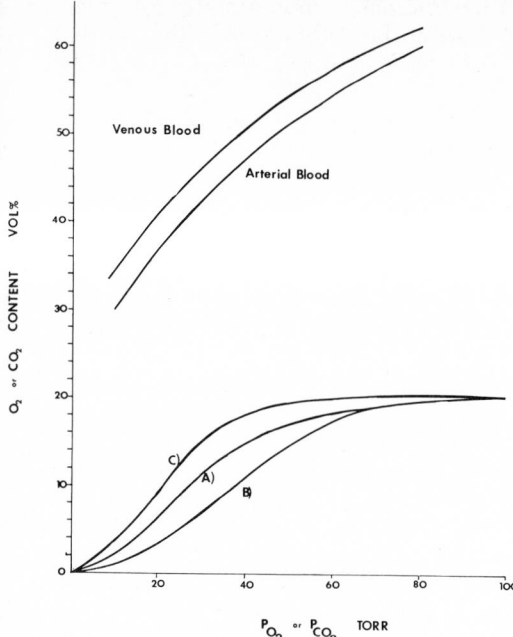

**Figure 1.** The oxyhemoglobin and carbon dioxide dissociation curves (lower and upper curves, respectively). These curves describe the relationship between partial pressure ($PO_2$, $PCO_2$) and blood gas content. Compare the plateau in the oxyhemoglobin dissociation curve above $PO_2$ = 70 torr and the lack of plateau in the carbon dioxide curves. Curve A represents blood with pH = 7.4, $PCO_2$ = 40, temperature = 39° C. and normal 2,3-DPG levels. Curve B shows the effect of decreased pH, increased $PCO_2$, increased temperature and increased 2,3-DPG. Curve C shows the effect of increased pH, decreased $PCO_2$, decreased temperature and decreased 2,3-DPG. Note that venous blood has a higher carbon dioxide content than arterial blood at a given $PCO_2$.

lowing transfusion, 24 hours are required to reestablish normal 2,3-DPG levels and thus restore the oxygen transport ability of hemoglobin.

Knowledge of the oxyhemoglobin dissociation curve should assist in diagnosis and therapy. Anemic animals are in need of hemoglobin, not increased inspired oxygen levels, which only add small amounts of oxygen to plasma. Animals with lung disease have low $PaO_2$ and need oxygen, not hemoglobin. In evaluating animals with lung disease, $PaO_2$ gives more useful information than arterial oxygen content because the latter is relatively unchanged above $PO_2$ levels of 70 torr, and only severe lung diseases decrease $PaO_2$ levels below 70 torr. Cyanosis develops when there are more than 5 grams of unsaturated hemoglobin per 100 ml. of blood. This occurs in severe cardiopulmonary disease when $PaO_2$ is less than 45 torr or because of decreased perfusion of peripheral tissues.

In contrast to oxygen, carbon dioxide is very soluble. At the normal arterial carbon dioxide tension ($PaCO_2$) of 40 torr, significant amounts of carbon dioxide are transported in solution in plasma or within erythrocytes. Most carbon dioxide combines with water to form carbonic acid, which then dissociates to bicarbonate and hydrogen ions. This reaction occurs most rapidly within erythrocytes because of the enzyme carbonic anhydrase and the presence of hemoglobin needed to buffer hydrogen ion. Carbamino compounds formed by combinations of carbon dioxide and proteins are yet another mode of carbon dioxide transport.

Carbon dioxide transport in blood requires buffers to reduce hydrogen ion activity. Because reduced hemoglobin is a better buffer than oxyhemoglobin, venous blood can carry more carbon dioxide than arterial blood, while the elimination of carbon dioxide from the lungs is assisted by oxygenation of hemoglobin. Buffers in large quantities allow blood carbon dioxide content to increase with partial pressure, whereas oxygen content is limited by the available hemoglobin (Fig. 1).

## RESPIRATORY CONTROL MECHANISMS

The inspiratory and expiratory muscles are controlled by inspiratory and expiratory neurons located in the medulla. These neu-

or oxygen therapy which increases $PO_2$ adds little oxygen to hemoglobin but does increase the amount of oxygen in solution in plasma.

Below $PO_2$ levels equal to 60 torr, the oxyhemoglobin dissociation curve is steep, indicating that oxygen content decreases rapidly as $PO_2$ decreases. This steep curve is in the range of tissue $PO_2$ and allows unloading of oxygen where it is needed. Tissue metabolism varies greatly, but only very active tissues such as heart muscle unload almost all the oxygen from hemoglobin. Increased levels of 2,3-DPG are found in chronic hypoxemia (e.g., chronic lung disease or cardiac failure) where they aid in oxygen release to the tissues. Decreased 2,3-DPG occurs in stored blood after one week, so that the ability of this blood to release oxygen to the tissues is reduced. Fol-

rons, although themselves capable of generating erratic respiration, receive input from higher brain centers, chemoreceptors and pulmonary mechanoreceptors. Respiratory centers located in the pons provide a normal respiratory rhythm. Respiration can also be modified by the cerebral cortex or the thermoregulatory center in the hypothalamus.

Chemoreceptors are located in the medulla, the carotid body and the aortic body; the latter two are referred to as peripheral chemoreceptors. The medullary chemoreceptor, which is responsible for minute-by-minute regulation of ventilation, is bathed by cerebrospinal fluid (CSF) and responds to changes in CSF pH; CSF acidosis increases alveolar ventilation, and CSF alkalosis decreases alveolar ventilation. Since carbon dioxide can diffuse across the blood-brain barrier, changes in $PaCO_2$ cause changes in CSF pH and thus alter ventilation. Similarly, metabolic acidosis and alkalosis also alter CSF pH and cause hyperventilation and hypoventilation, respectively. In chronic respiratory failure (increased $PaCO_2$), CSF pH returns to normal levels because of an increase in CSF bicarbonate. In this case, ventilation no longer depends on $PaCO_2$ but is regulated by hypoxemia. Oxygen therapy in these animals can cause apnea and death by removing the hypoxic respiratory drive.

The peripheral chemoreceptors increase ventilation in response to low $PaO_2$, high $PaCO_2$ or low pH, but their threshold to these stimuli is high. However, the peripheral chemoreceptors provide the only mechanism for detection of hypoxemia. When $PaO_2$ decreases below 60 torr, ventilation increases dramatically and overrides the medullary chemoreceptor, so that low $PaCO_2$ is a common finding with hypoxemia.

Mechanoreceptors within the lungs respond to lung inflation, lung deflation and mechanical irritation. Lung inflation stimulates stretch receptors within the airways, causing a diminished inspiratory effort. These stretch receptors probably adjust both tidal volume and frequency to minimize the work of breathing, so that tachypnea occurs in diseases with low lung compliance and slow, deep breathing occurs in airway obstructive diseases. Lung deflation produces an increased inspiratory effort. This deflation reflex may cause the regular sighs needed for reactivation of surfactant and prevention of atelectasis. Irritant receptors, found primarily in the upper trachea, are responsible for cough and, when stimulated, cause reflex bronchoconstriction in many species. The response of the irritant receptors greatly increases during and for some time after viral respiratory disease (e.g., infectious tracheobronchitis). Thus, bronchoconstriction occurs more readily in these animals when they are exposed to dust and cold air.

## SUPPLEMENTARY READING

Bates, D. V., Macklem, P. T., and Christie, R. V.: Respiratory Function in Disease. Philadelphia, W. B. Saunders Co., 1971.

Robinson, N. E., and Gillespie, J. R.: Physiology of the Respiratory System. In Ettinger, S. J. (ed.): Textbook of Veterinary Internal Medicine. Philadelphia, W. B. Saunders Co., 1975.

West, J. B.: Respiratory Physiology—The Essentials. Baltimore, The Williams & Wilkins Co., 1974.

# A DIAGNOSTIC APPROACH TO RESPIRATORY DISEASE

JOAN A. O'BRIEN, V.M.D.
*Philadelphia, Pennsylvania*

## HISTORY

Specific assessment of respiratory disease cannot be divorced from a complete history and thorough physical examination. Many disease processes can mimic and/or contribute to respiratory illness (anemia, ascites, extreme obesity). The clinician must therefore be aware of species, breed, sex and age incidence in the occurrence of respiratory disease.

The history of the animal should be obtained in an orderly fashion and should include the presenting signs, past as well as present geographic and socioeconomic environmental conditions, the health status of litter mates, an inventory of other household animals and people in the household, previous incidences of surgery or illness and the response to therapy, medications being given at present and the history of the present illness.

In detailing the history of the present illness, it is often necessary to question the client closely and repetitively to obtain a sequential picture of the disease process. The clinician must be alert for a description of signs, (e.g., vomiting, diarrhea, lameness) that can suggest a multisystem disease in which the respiratory component is the client's dominant complaint. It is also important to determine whether the onset of signs was sudden or gradual, whether the signs are intermittent or constant and whether the course of the disease seems static or progressive. The information must be obtained for each of the signs of respiratory disease described by the client.

The cardinal signs of respiratory disease are cough, dyspnea, production of abnormal secretions, noisy breathing, sneezing and change in sound production.

Coughing is perhaps the most common complaint in respiratory disease. Most owners do not realize that animals swallow most of their coughed-up secretions and will report that the cough is nonproductive. Inquiries as to whether the cough is tight and harsh or discontinuous and bubbly followed by swallowing will often differentiate the type of cough.

Noting the time when coughing occurs can be helpful. A productive cough followed by swallowing upon rising after rest is often found in chronic bronchitis. A cough which wakes the animal from sleeping is more often a sign of left congestive heart failure, while paroxysms of harsh, tight coughing of recent onset are more typical of acute viral disease. A cough which gradually becomes more productive so that secretions are coughed out of the mouth is seen in pneumonia or bronchiectasis. Laryngeal incompetence or esophageal disease may be indicated if coughing after eating or drinking is noted.

It is necessary to determine how much coughing actually occurs. Is it one or two short episodes a day or a week, or is it paroxysms lasting several minutes many times a day? Many owners do not realize that coughing is a protective mechanism against any irritation and that minor scattered episodes may simply represent reaction to pull on a choke chain or collar or reaction to inhaled irritants (dust, smoke).

Dyspnea is usually a sign of severe respiratory disease. Dyspnea in an open-mouthed cyanotic animal is obvious but evaluation may be more difficult if signs are less pronounced. An increase in the normal rate of breathing for the size of the animal is often the earliest sign of dyspnea; however, it must be distinguished from panting. This information may not be obtained unless specific inquiries are made. Subtle dyspnea may become more marked after exertion or excitement. Sudden onset of dyspnea usually suggests a more acute process (trauma, aspiration, pneumonia) but this determina-

215

tion depends, to a great extent, on the owner's observation and the patient's activity level; the prime example is in cats with empyema, where the disease process is chronic but the dyspnea appears to be of sudden onset. Dyspnea associated with noisy breathing suggests airway obstruction, whereas short, shallow, rapid breathing may indicate a restriction of lung expansion as in pleural effusion, rib fracture or pneumonia. Dyspnea must further be differentiated from the deep sighing respiration associated with metabolic acidosis.

Abnormal production of secretions may be the consequence of either upper or lower respiratory disease. Nasal discharge is a common presenting complaint reported by owners. Whether the discharge is at present, or was at one time, unilateral is important. Unilateral discharge of sudden onset may suggest a foreign body, whereas that of a more insidious onset may be indicative of a nasal tumor. The type and amount of discharge should be ascertained; serous or seromucoid discharges are common in viral infections and irritant or allergic responses, whereas purulent material suggests a chronic infection. Discharges which gradually become mixed with blood or are frankly bloody may indicate a destructive lesion such as a tumor or fungal involvement.

Abnormal secretions from the tracheobronchial tree are often swallowed. In animals with chronic bronchitis, mucoid sputum in small amounts may be expectorated after a coughing paroxysm. In some cases, swallowed secretions will be vomited after coughing and will appear as a mucoid watery material. Production of regularly noticeable amounts of purulent sputum is common in pneumonia and particularly so in bronchiectasis. Hemoptysis is usually a grave sign of respiratory disease and is most often associated with heartworm disease or lung tumors. Occasionally, it may be seen with foreign body aspiration and bronchiectasis.

Noisy breathing is a common presenting complaint of the client. Stertorous nasal breathing, more marked during sleep, may indicate a progressive nasal obstruction. The onset of or an increase in the amount of snoring is often seen in nasal and pharyngeal disease. Inspiratory wheezing or stridor is a sign of laryngeal or upper airway obstruction. The sound in tracheal col-

lapse is often described by clients as honking or rattling. It is often helpful to ask the client to describe the sound, imitate it if possible and attempt to locate it anatomically as if it were the client who were affected. Tape recordings of classic upper airway sounds that include honking, snoring and reverse sneezing may also be helpful.

Sneezing is a very common sign in nasal disease. Since it is a very effective mechanism for ridding the nasal passages of irritants, it is important that the owner be reassured that occasional minor episodes of sneezing do not indicate disease and are common, especially in toy hairy-faced breeds such as Bichons, Lhasas and Maltese terriers. Prolonged repetitive sneezing of sudden onset may indicate a nasal foreign body, while sneezing after exposure to weeds or grasses may suggest an allergy. Episodes of sneezing are very common in viral respiratory disease, especially in the cat. Sneezing associated with significant amounts of bleeding may be associated with head trauma or a destructive nasal disease. Occasionally, severe paroxysms of sneezing will result in blood-streaked mucus due to the rupture of tiny superficial blood vessels by turbulent air flow.

Laryngeal disease is often characterized by a change in voice or sound production. Since owners do not associate this sign with disease in animals, specific questions must be asked concerning change in bark, meow or purr.

## PHYSICAL EXAMINATION

The specific approach to a respiratory problem should follow only after a careful general examination. Signs of systemic involvement may include fever, emaciation, inappropriate behavior or gait, pale or inflamed mucous membranes or alterations in the skin or hair coat. The legs should be examined for signs of pain or heat suggestive of hypertrophic osteoarthropathy, and mammary tissue should be examined for possible malignancies. Funduscopic examination should be performed to determine whether viral, fungal or lymphoid infiltrations of the retina are present. The abdomen should be examined for evidence of ascites or masses that may be responsible for pulmonary metastasis or restriction of diaphragmatic movement.

The classic parameters of physical examination of the respiratory system include observation, palpation, percussion and auscultation. In practice, these examinations are often carried out jointly and continuously rather than as isolated procedures. This is certainly so in the case of observation or inspection, which is initiated upon first sight of the patient and continues throughout the examination.

Observation involves the conscious and subconscious accumulation of impressions and data that permit an assessment of the patient's status. With experience, the clinician does this automatically, but initially, one must discipline oneself to observe closely. Does the animal appear severely, moderately or only minimally ill?

The eyes should be inspected for deviation of gaze or proptosis and should be palpated for resilience. Likewise, the muzzle should be examined for swelling or fistula, and the nasal passages should be observed for normal conformation and patency of air passages. A clean glass slide held in front of the nares will help permit evaluation. In a cooperative patient, it is helpful to close the mouth, having the animal breathe on the examiner's cheek while he gently holds off one nostril at a time to estimate nasal air flow. The type of secretion should be noted. An idea of air exchange can be obtained by holding the palm of the hand in front of the nares and mouth.

The oral and pharyngeal cavity should be examined for evidence of secretions, ulceration, masses or dental disease. In a recalcitrant patient, this examination is best deferred to the very end of the physical examination or performed under anesthesia. In a cooperative patient, the dental arcade, hard and soft palate, sublingual area and pharyngeal wall can be palpated for signs of pain or changes in normal tissue. In a very few animals, the larynx may be visualized but anesthesia is usually required for this examination.

The larynx and trachea should be palpated for normal position and form. The consistency of these cartilaginous structures can vary greatly among breeds, but complete compressibility, areas of narrowing and excessive coughing after palpation are abnormal.

The bony thorax should be palpated; this is especially helpful in heavily coated animals in which the hair coat may mask emaciation, masses or abnormal rib conformation or compliance. Observations on the rate, depth and ease of respiration are often augmented by palpation during breathing. Increased tactile fremitus can be palpated in pneumonia and other diseases characterized by bronchial fluid.

The art of percussion requires practice to be effective. It is most useful in detecting extreme variation from normal (e.g., hyporesonance in pleural effusion) and in following the resolution of these processes. Unless lesions of the lung parenchyma are massive, they often cannot be detected by percussion. In all instances, percussion notes in one area should be compared with those on the opposite side of the chest. Coughing after percussion often signals an area of abnormal lung underlying the percussed area, and particular attention should be paid to that area during auscultation.

In ausculting respiratory sounds, the clinician should always use the same stethoscope, since breath sounds are transmitted differently through different stethoscopes. It is necessary to auscult the entire respiratory system, first listening for noisy breathing at the mouth and nares and then using the stethoscope to evaluate laryngeal, tracheal and bronchovesicular sounds. Obstructive upper airway noises are transmitted through the chest wall but an orderly pattern of auscultation will permit evaluation of sites of maximal intensity. In order to evaluate breath sounds, it is necessary, at least initially, for the student consciously to screen out cardiac sounds. Normal breath sounds are usually louder and somewhat harsher in very young and very small dogs and cats and are of a harsh bronchovesicular to bronchial character in a panting dog. Blowing sounds are normally heard over the trachea. In most cases, true vesicular breathing in which the expiratory component is almost silent can be heard only in a quiet, unexcited animal; thus clinicians must often evaluate whether the bronchovesicular breathing of the typical excited patient is within normal limits. It must be remembered that breath sounds may sound distant and far off in the obese, heavily coated animal.

There is no area of greater confusion than the definitions assigned to abnormal lung sounds, i.e., rales and rhonchi. There is a simple definition for each. Rales have been defined as discontinuous, bubbling, moist, short sounds which are heard most easily on inspiration as air bubbles through fluid in the lung. Rales may be fine, medium or coarse depending on the size of the airway involved, with fine rales implying fluid in small bronchioles and medium and coarse rales in proportionately larger airways. Coarse rales are often palpable through the chest wall.

Rhonchi are more musical, whistling notes produced by air moving past an obstruction in the tracheobronchial tree. They are better heard on expiration. Tumor, bronchospasm or secretions may cause further narrowing on expiration and produce rhonchi. Localized persistent rhonchi should suggest an obstruction by tumor or foreign body, while diffuse rhonchi are more typical of bronchospasm. Rhonchi can often be further classified by pitch—low-pitch, sonorous in larger bronchi and high-pitch, sibilant in smaller airways.

It is much more difficult to demonstrate abnormal auscultatory findings in the dog and cat than in a cooperative person. Deep breathing is essential to proper auscultation; therefore, every effort must be made to evaluate the patient during full respiratory efforts. Listening during panting respiration is not sufficient. Although deep breaths will follow breath-holding or exertion, they also occur with coughing. This serves the multiple purpose of allowing the type of cough to be documented, permitting breath sounds to be evaluated and demonstrating posttussive rales, if present. A cough may usually be produced by laryngeal or tracheal palpation and, in some cases, by chest percussion. The duration and type of cough produced should be noted, and the client should be questioned as to its similarity to the presenting complaint.

## SPECIAL DIAGNOSTIC PROCEDURES

### RADIOGRAPHY

Thoracic radiographs are such an essential diagnostic tool that they should not be considered a special diagnostic procedure but rather should represent an integral part of the work-up in the diagnosis of any severe, recurrent or chronic respiratory problem. (See the article on "Interpretation of Pulmonary Radiographs.")

Radiographs should include lateral and dorsoventral views of the thorax, occlusal or open-mouth films of the nasal passages, and views of the frontal sinus, so that the full extent of nasal disease can be determined. (See the articles on Rhinitis and Sinusitis in the Dog and in the Cat.)

### ENDOSCOPY

**Rhinoscopy.** Requires anesthesia. Indications: Chronic nonresponsive unilateral or bilateral nasal discharge, obstructed air flow.

Endoscopic evaluation of the nasal passages in the dog and cat is severely limited by the well-developed and convoluted turbinate pattern. It is possible, however, to visualize the rhinarium and the rostral aspects of the turbinates by using an otoscopic speculum suited to the size of the animal. The choanae and nasopharynx can be visualized by pulling the soft palate forward with tissue forceps and then using a curved, lighted, rotating laryngeal mirror* which will fit a conventional otoscopic light handle. In large breed dogs, a flexible bronchoscope, 4 mm. in diameter, can be used to examine the common meatus from the nose to the pharynx. Large areas of the nasal passages, however, can be directly visualized only through surgical exploration.

The nasal mucosa is extremely sensitive, and general anesthesia is necessary to allow examination and prevent trauma. The examiner should note the condition of mucosa, the type of secretions, any deviation of turbinates, the presence of abnormal tissue, ulcerations, bleeding sources, foreign bodies and the equality of air flow. Secretions should be gently suctioned for culture and cytologic examination.

**Laryngoscopy.** Requires anesthesia. Position: Ventral recumbency. Indications: Stridor or change in "voice."

The conventional intubating laryngoscope is adequate for visualizing the larynx. The examiner should look for deviations in normal form, color and motility. Light anesthesia is required for the accurate assessment of normal motility.

**Bronchoscopy.** Requires anesthesia. Position: Ventral recumbency. Indications: Unexplained chronic or recurrent cough or dyspnea. Therapeutic removal of obstructing secretions or foreign body (O'Brien and Roszel, 1974).

---

*Welch-Allyn laryngeal mirror.

Bronchoscopy may be performed either with standard rigid bronchoscopes* of adequate length and diameter or with the flexible fiberoptic endoscope. A flexible fiberoptic pediatric gastroduodenoscope† is an excellent, though expensive, instrument for this purpose. Its small diameter and sheath length permit its use in animals of various sizes.

Bronchoscopic examination should include the aspiration of secretions for bacteriologic and cytologic examination. The examiner should also note any evidence of ulceration, edema, infiltration, growth or change in color in the mucosa. The normal tracheobronchial tree expands with inspiration and constricts with expiration, narrowing to approximately one half its diameter with coughing. Any abnormal compliance, rigidity, immobility, fixation or deviation of the trachea, the carina or the main stem bronchi should be noted as well as type and source of secretions. Additional information may be afforded by cytologic and histologic examination of bronchial brushings or endoscopic biopsy specimens.

**Esophagoscopy.** Requires anesthesia. Position: Left lateral recumbency. Indications: Repeated episodes of aspiration pneumonia; expectorated blood of unknown origin.

The same instruments utilized in bronchoscopy are employed in esophagoscopy. Any change in mucosal characteristics and any evidence of dilation, stricture or bleeding should be noted.

**Mediastinoscopy and Thoracoscopy.** These techniques have not been developed as diagnostic procedures in animal medicine. In human medicine, they are utilized for the visualization and biopsy of either mediastinal or intrathoracic abnormalities.

## COLLECTION OF SPECIMENS FOR CYTOLOGIC EXAMINATION AND CULTURE

**Sputum.** Generally, sputum samples are not valuable sources for culture, since expectoration cannot be induced in the dog or cat. Contamination with oropharyngeal microorganisms makes the evaluation of isolates difficult. In viral outbreaks, however, culture of nasal and pharyngeal mucosa can be useful in confirming the presence of a virus. In pulmonary malignancies characterized by the production of excess secretions, sputum samples can be useful in demonstrating the presence of malignant cells.

**Bronchial Washings.** Samples of bronchial secretions may be obtained directly after instillation of sterile saline by means of a sterile aspirator inserted through a sterile bronchoscope. Self-contained prepacked sterile specimen traps* are available for collection of the aspirate. Samples may be divided into aliquots for culture and cytologic examination. Direct smears of aspirate should also be made at the time of collection. Aspirate collection under direct visualization makes possible selective and repetitive aspiration of abnormal areas but this procedure requires general anesthesia.

**Transtracheal Aspiration.** Tracheobronchial secretions may be collected by instilling aliquots of saline through an intracath.† This procedure usually requires only light sedation and infiltration with local anesthesia. After sterile preparation, a stab incision is made in the skin, the needle is passed through the cricothyroid or intertracheal membrane and the plastic intracath is carefully guided into the trachea. Nine to 10 cc. of saline is then inserted and secretions are suctioned. If the animal coughs, secretions that coat the distal end of the catheter can also be cultured if the amount of aspirated material in the syringe is marginal.

**Pleural Effusion.** (See article "Pleural Effusions.")

## CYTOLOGIC EVALUATION

*Stains:*
New methylene blue—not permanent
Wright-Giemsa—air dry; permanent
Papanicolaou or Sano trichrome—alcohol fix; permanent
Gram—permanent
Smears from nasal exudate, tracheobronchial secretions or pleural fluid may be

---

*Geo. Pilling & Sons, Fort Washington, PA 19034; ACMI, 300 Stillwater Avenue, Stamford, Connecticut 06902.
†Olympus Corp. of America, New Hyde Park, New York 11040; ACMI, 300 Stillwater Avenue, Stamford, Connecticut 06902.

*Clinical Products Specimen Trap, Chesebrough-Pond's Inc., Greenwich, Connecticut 06830.
†Deseret Pharmaceutical Co., Sandy, Utah 84070.

examined cytologically (O'Brien and Roszel, 1974; Sano, 1949).

Whenever possible, cytologic evaluation should include examination of freshly made smears as well as those of the centrifuged sediment. Smears may be useful in identifying the type of inflammation (neutrophilic or eosinophilic) and in establishing the presence of malignant cells, parasite eggs or larvae, fungal elements and bacteria. Abnormalities of bronchial epithelium, increases in goblet cells and bronchial casts can also be detected by cytologic examination. The presence of alveolar macrophages or "dust cells" indicates that a deep aspirate has been obtained from the bronchial tree. If a trichrome stain such as Papanicolaou is to be used, smears must be fixed while wet in alcohol or fixed in sprayed fixative.*

### SKIN TESTS

Skin tests for inhalant allergens can be useful in dogs in which respiratory disease

*Spray-Cyte, Clay Adams, Parsippany, New Jersey 07054.

and peripheral eosinophilia suggest an allergic component. Intradermal injections of antigen plus a histamine and saline control are read for evidence of immediate hypersensitivity within 15 to 20 minutes or Arthus reaction after 3 to 4 hours. These tests are most useful in confirming a clinical history suggestive of an allergic reaction.

Skin tests for systemic fungi and tuberculosis give rise to a delayed Type IV reaction observed after 24 to 48 hours. They may be negative in the presence of severe disease, and if positive, they may indicate only past exposure, therefore their usefulness is limited.

### SUPPLEMENTAL READING

O'Brien, J. A., and Roszel, J. F.: Bronchoscopy and bronchial cytology. In Kirk, R. W. (ed.): Current Veterinary Therapy V. Philadelphia, W. B. Saunders Co., 1974.
Sano, M. E.: Trichrome stain for tissue section, culture or smear. Am. J. Clin. Path., Vol. 19, No. 9., September, 1949.

---

# RHINITIS AND SINUSITIS IN THE DOG

J. G. LANE, F.R.C.V.S.
*Bristol, England*

## INTRODUCTION

When nasal airflow in the dog is obstructed, distress is exhibited in a number of ways, including sneezing and snorting which are reflex actions to clear the passages, while mouth-breathing provides an alternative airway. In intranasal disease, the obstruction is frequently caused by a discharge which may appear at the external nares or may evoke gagging and coughing by its presence in the nasopharynx. Veterinary attention is sought because of the distressing condition of the dog and because the nasal discharge is objectionable, particularly when bloody. Less frequently a dog may be presented exhibiting either a facial deformity or pain when the supporting bones of the nose are touched.

## CANINE NASAL DISORDERS

### ACUTE RHINITIS

In recent years a wide range of viruses have been incriminated as the primary pathogens initiating inflammation of the upper respiratory tract of dogs. Adenovirus, herpesvirus, reovirus and influenza virus have all been recovered from clinical cases of acute rhinitis, while rhinitis has always been recognized as one of the major features of generalized distemper infection. Respiratory disease caused by distemper virus may occur in the absence of alimentary and nervous signs, particularly in vaccinated dogs. Most upper respiratory tract viruses are epitheliotropic, producing focal areas of necrosis in the nasal, tracheal and bronchial mucosa. Infections are accomanied by a variable febrile response together with a rapid onset of sneezing and the production of a bilateral mucoserous discharge, except in cases of distemper where the discharge is purulent.

Some bacteria, such as *Bordetella bronchiseptica*, can act as primary pathogens of the canine upper airways, but the secondary invasion of virus-induced damage, by bacteria, Mycoplasma and fungi, plays the major role in clinical infectious rhinitis. Protective responses include mucous and serous hypersecretion, lymphoid hyperplasia, hyperemia and engorgement of the mucosa, neutrophil leukocyte infiltration and, later, mononuclear cell permeation. The degree of destruction of underlying turbinate bone depends on the dominant organism present. Necrotic epithelial elements and pus may be shed into the mucoid discharge. Ulceration of highly vascular tissue can lead to epistaxis but this is a rare sign in bacterial and Mycoplasma rhinitis.

External trauma to the nose with or without fractures of the supporting bones can disrupt the delicate turbinates, causing epistaxis. While much of this blood will be removed by sneezing and swallowing, that which remains forms an ideal substrate for bacterial growth.

Foreign materials, particularly grass seeds, awns and food particles, cause considerable nasal irritation that produces a purulent discharge and constant sneezing. Disturbances of normal deglutition may lead to food being forced into the nasal chambers. Congenital defects of the hard and soft palates, oronasal fistulae, pharyngeal paralysis, oropharyngeal neoplasia, cricopharyngeal achalasia and megaloesophagus are all conditions in which secondary rhinitis can be expected. *Linguatula serrata* has traditionally been mentioned as a cause of rhinitis, but separation of the dog from the herbivorous intermediate host as a result of improved slaughterhouse hygiene has made this condition very rare.

## CHRONIC HYPERPLASTIC RHINITIS

Prolonged irritation and stimulation of the nasal mucous membranes by uncontrolled microbial infection, intranasal foreign material, or neoplasia can cause irreversible hyperplastic changes of the epithelium, particularly of the mucous gland elements and stroma. The signs of rhinitis will persist as long as there is nasal hypersecretion.

Polyps, which are uncommon, arise when the hyperplastic reaction produces visible localized protuberances. Pedunculated polyps may appear at the external nares or extend posteriorly into the nasopharynx, causing marked dyspnea.

Irish wolfhound rhinitis is a chronic hyperplastic inflammation of the nasal cavity attributed to an upper respiratory tract virus infection with lesions also present in the trachea and bronchi. Young wolfhound puppies are affected soon after birth and those which survive show chronic signs of a bilateral purulent nasal discharge and persistent productive coughing.

## NASAL MYCOSES

A fungal infection may become established at a point in the respiratory tract where tissue damage by a primary disease, such as infection, trauma or neoplasia, has led to poor local ventilation. Thus in man, in whom primary pulmonary disease is more common than in the dog, mycotic lung lesions are correspondingly more frequent. In temperate climates the ubiquitous *Aspergillus fumigatus* is the most common fungal opportunist invader, while other mycotic agents such as *Cryptococcus neoformans* are rarely isolated from the sinuses and nasal cavities of the dog. Once infection is established, the fine trabecular structures of the turbinate bones are readily destroyed as the mycelium advances. Reproductive hyphae produced by the mycelium may form areas of white mold. Initially a unilateral purulent discharge is produced, but as destruction advances, epistaxis may occur, and the nasal septum and overlying nasal and incisive bones may be invaded in the later stages of the disease. The discharge may become bilateral and the patient may also show pain and facial distortion at the bridge of the nose. Infection may advance into the paranasal sinuses (vide infra), and breakdown of the cribriform plate has been reported.

Experiences at this center suggest that dolichocephalic breeds are most susceptible to nasal aspergillosis, and in many cases infection commences in the posterior region of the ventral maxilloturbinate before advancing anteriorly.

## SEQUESTRATION OF NASAL BONE FRAGMENTS

The maxilla, nasal, incisive and frontal bones are prone to fractures during trauma. Depression fractures can usually be managed conservatively without complication. Sometimes, however, fragments of dead bone remain in the frontal sinus or lateral wall of the nasal cavity. A typical sequestration process will follow, leading to suppuration through a superficial sinus or through the nasal airways.

## EXTENSION OF DENTAL DISEASE INTO THE NASAL CHAMBERS

Idiopathic periapical dental abscesses may arise from the maxillary carnassial teeth of the dog. On other occasions the predisposing pulpitis for a periapical abscess can be the sequel of dental caries, overt iatrogenic and traumatic dental fractures or fissure fracture. Each of the maxillary teeth of the dog is separated from the nasal chamber or maxillary recess by a layer of supporting alveolar bone. In spite of this, periapical abscesses are rarely the cause of a nasal discharge. When the roots of the carnassial tooth are involved, it is far more likely that the infection will be contained within the maxillary recess before a superficial discharging sinus develops ventral to the lower eyelid.

## INTRANASAL NEOPLASIA

Neoplasms arising from structures within the nasal chambers account for the majority of cases of dogs with persistent epistaxis, for some patients with a chronic nonhemorrhagic nasal discharge and for a small number of cases of persistent nonproductive sneezing or nasopharyngeal obstructive dyspnea. Similar signs may result from the spread of invasive tumors of adjacent organs, particularly of the oropharynx.

It is convenient to classify primary endonasal tumors as (1) carcinomas, (2) sarcomas and (3) other rare types.

The biologic behavior of primary nasal tumors is similar. Medium and medium/large breeds (20 to 40 kg.) are most susceptible, while giant and miniature types are seldom affected. Brachycephalic dogs are rarely involved, and males and females are equally represented.

The most frequent site of tumor development appears to be the ethmoturbinal region. Expansion of the soft tissue mass takes place in parallel with destruction normal structures. The tumor may occupy much of the nasal cavity on the side of origin before breaking through the medial septum or overlying nasal bone, this latter producing a facial swelling. Infrequent lines expansion are through the cribriform plate through the medial wall of the orbit (producing proptosis) or through the hard palate.

Primary endonasal tumors are only local malignant and show little tendency metastasize either to local lymph nodes to distant sites. They show a high tendency to recur following surgical removal presumably because of the difficulty of complete extirpation.

## SINUSITIS

Primary sinus diseases are rare in dogs. Those conditions which are diagnosed (and unsuccessfully treated) as primarily involving the paranasal sinuses are almost invariably extensions of disease from adjacent tissues. As suggested above, the roof of the frontal sinus may be subjected to trauma and occasionally tumors may arise from the walls of the paranasal sinuses. Infection probably reach the frontal sinuses by spread from the turbinate structures or, in the case of the maxillary recess, from a tooth root abscess. Endonasal tumors may also expand into the sinuses.

The frontal sinuses communicate with the nasal chambers through a narrow opening between the endoturbinate scrolls. Patency of this ostium is essential for the drainage normal secretions, and it readily becomes obstructed when the turbinates are diseased. A sinus mucocele then forms and is often mistakenly diagnosed as sinusitis.

## DIAGNOSIS

A routine should be adopted in the investigation of cases of nasal disease. History annotation includes the duration of symptoms, their rate of onset, any known trauma to the nose, the degree of dyspnea and the characteristics and progress of any nasal discharge. For example, a history of sudden onset of frenzied sneezing with a unilateral purulent discharge is highly suggestive an intranasal foreign body.

During the general clinical inspection the attitude and overall bodily condition of the patient are noted. Attention is paid to any nasal discharge, facial deformity or ulceration at the angles of the rhinarium. This ulceration may be excoriation resulting from persistent licking of a nasal discharge. The presence of an ocular discharge suggests interference with tear drainage through the nasolacrimal duct.

Temperature, pulse and respiratory function are assessed. In a patient with symptoms of short duration a febrile reaction suggests an acute infection. Observations of the dyspnea may help to localize the intranasal lesion. When sneezing is the dominant sign, the lesion is likely to be in the anterior area of the nasal chamber; conversely, when snorting and gagging predominate, the lesion probably lies posteriorly. A tendency to mouth-breathe suggests a severe, possibly bilateral, nasal obstruction. A simple assessment and comparison of airflow through the nasal passages can be made by holding a wisp of cotton at each nostril. Palpation of the nasal bones may reveal asymmetry or swellings as well as areas of softening or pain. At this stage a preliminary inspection of the oropharynx is made.

The patient is anesthetized for more detailed investigations. The possibility of inhalation of discharges or other fluids makes it imperative to utilize a cuffed endotracheal tube. A detailed oral examination includes inspection of the dental crowns, hard and soft palates, tonsils and oropharynx. The nasopharynx is visualized by drawing the soft palate forward before introducing an illuminated dental mirror. Anterior rhinoscopy is performed by introducing an auriscope or 5-mm. fiberscope into the nasal vestibule. Although this endoscopic procedure is usually frustrated by the presence of discharge, it is occasionally possible to see foreign bodies, fungal growths or neoplasms. Many fiberscopes have the additional facility of a biopsy channel for obtaining samples of suspicious lesions.

The following projections are used in the radiography of the nasal chambers:

1. Dorsoventral occlusal (film in mouth).
2. Tilted ventrodorsal open-mouth (Fig.
.
3. Anteroposterior (frontal sinus view) ig. 2).
4. Straight lateral.

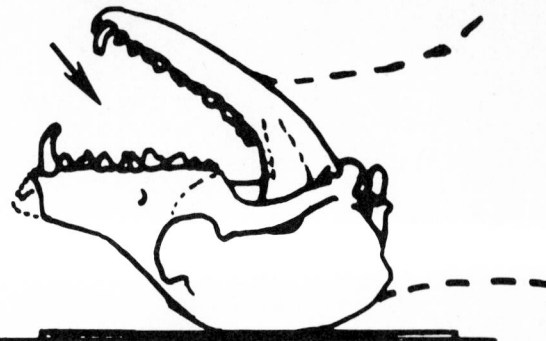

**Figure 1.** Position for the tilted ventrodorsal open-mouth projection. The beam (shown by the arrow) is angled at 20 to 30 degrees from the vertical to avoid superimposition of the mandible.

5. Lateral oblique (maxillary dental arcade view).

The open-mouth projection is necessary because the occlusal view does not permit inclusion of the frontal sinuses. As a result of the tilted beam, the open-mouth projection leads to foreshortening of the maxilloturbinates particularly, but the frontal sinuses can be visualized.

The radiologist relies on subtle contrasts of delicate trabecular bone, soft tissue and air when reading films of the nasal chambers. Optimal definition is obtained by the use of slow, double-wrapped films or cassettes with high-definition screens.

The salient radiographic features associated with endonasal disease are summarized in Table 1, together with other

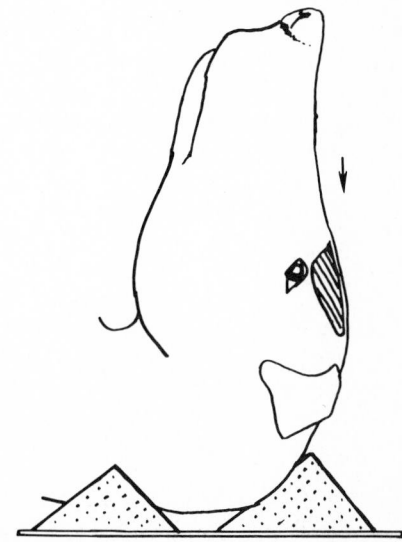

**Figure 2.** Position for the anteroposterior view skylining the frontal sinuses. Arrow shows direction of x-ray beam.

*Table 1.  Differential Diagnosis of Chronic Nasal Diseases of the Dog*

| | INTRANASAL NEOPLASIA | CHRONIC HYPERPLASTIC RHINITIS† | ASPERGILLUS FUMIGATUS INFECTION | DYSPHAGIA | POST-TRAUMATIC SEQUESTRUM | DENTAL PERIAPICAL ABSCESS | INTRANASAL PARASITISM |
|---|---|---|---|---|---|---|---|
| *Nature of Discharge* | | | | | | | |
| Purulent | * | X | X | X | X | X | X |
| Epistaxis | XX | | * | X | | | * |
| Food Material | | | | X | | | |
| Unilateral | X → | * | X → | | X | X | X |
| Bilateral | * | X | * | X | | | * |
| *Facial Deformity* | | | | | | | |
| Pain on Nasal Bone | | | | | | | |
| Obstructed Air Flow | * | * | * | | | | |
| *Radiography* | | | | | | | |
| Bone Trabecular Destruction | X | | X | | | | |
| Increased Soft Tissue Density | X | X | | | | | |
| Periapical Rarefaction | | | | | | X | |
| Sequestrum | | | | | X | | |
| Serology | | | X | | | | |
| Culture | | | X | | | | |
| Exploratory Rhinotomy | X | X | X | | | | |
| Histopathology | X | X | X | | | | X |

X = Frequent positive finding.
* = Occasional positive finding.
†This includes the Irish wolfhound rhinitis syndrome.

ndings which help one achieve a specific diagnosis. Radiographic evidence of lysis of the turbinate trabecular pattern in the absence of increased soft tissue density (Fig. ) suggests *Aspergillus fumigatus* infection. A diagnosis of nasal aspergillosis may be onfirmed by either direct smear or culture f the nasal discharge; however, these tests ay produce false negative results. Accurate diagnosis of this condition is by the gar-gel diffusion technique to confirm the resence of *Aspergillus fumigatus* antibodies in serum.

Apart from confirming a diagnosis of nasal ycosis, swabbing of the nasal discharge, icrobial culture and antibiotic sensitivity esting are not usually helpful. In most instances the organisms isolated are upper irway commensals which are acting as oportunist pathogens.

In some instances the clinician is unable ） make a definitive diagnosis without re-orting to exploratory surgery. When there reason to suspect intranasal neoplasia, hronic hyperplastic rhinitis, nasal mycosis, asal parasitism or the presence of a persis-nt foreign body in the nose, exploratory ninotomy is justified. In such cases, the nacroscopic appearance of the nasal con-nts is usually sufficient to make a diag-

nosis prior to carrying out the appropriate treatment. Excised material should be submitted for histopathologic evaluation so that an accurate diagnosis and prognosis can be made.

## TREATMENT

In acute rhinitis, therapy is directed toward elimination of the initiating factors when possible but, more frequently, toward prevention of chronic sequelae, particularly by controlling secondary bacterial invasion. Acute viral infections are treated using a broad-spectrum antibiotic cover (e.g., ampicillin, oxytetracycline or potentiated sulfonamides) for a period of 15 to 30 days, depending on the severity of the signs at the outset. The conservative management of nasal trauma must include a similar course of antibacterial medication. Posttraumatic epistaxis can usually be controlled by the application of cold compresses to the external surfaces. Only rarely is intranasal packing necessary. Fractures of the supporting bones of the nasal chambers and frontal sinuses do not usually require open reduction. Many are of the depression type and spontaneous resolution takes place with

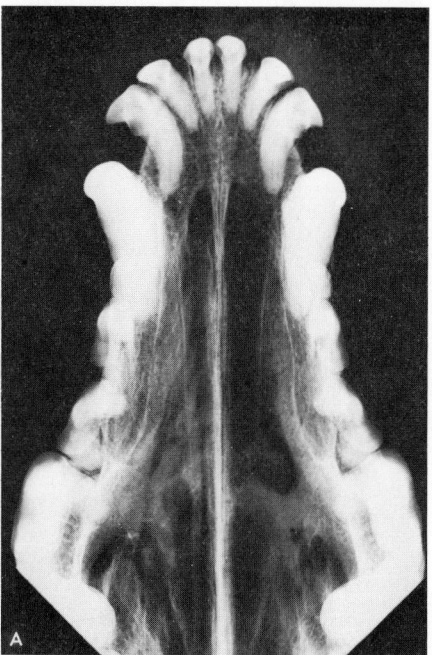

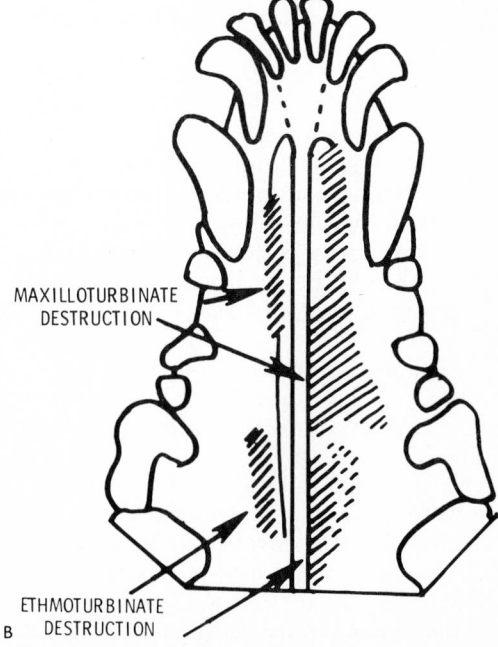

MAXILLOTURBINATE
DESTRUCTION

ETHMOTURBINATE
B   DESTRUCTION

**Figure 3.**   Radiograph (*A*) and line diagram (*B*) illustrating turbinate destruction by *A. fumigatus* infection in a order collie. (From Lane, J. G., et al.: J. Small Animal Pract., *15*:79–87, 1974. By courtesy of the Editor, Journal of nall Animal Practice.)

minimal disfigurement. When there is significant displacement and overriding of fragments, reduction followed by fixation with simple wire sutures is adequate. Severe fractures of the maxilla may require half-pin splintage.

Foreign bodies can be removed under direct vision using alligator forceps. Other, possibly hidden, foreign bodies may be dislodged from the nasal meatuses into the nasopharynx by flushing saline solution through the nostrils. This procedure is carried out under general anesthesia, and routine precautions should be taken to prevent inhalation. Gauze packing in the pharynx soaks up the irrigation fluid as well as collecting the offending matter. A short antibiotic cover is provided afterward.

Systemic or topical applications of fungistatic drugs such as amphotericin B and nystatin are usually ineffective in controlling nasal Aspergillus infection. Thiabendazole, an anthelmintic, is sometimes effective in eliminating this fungal infection. Oral administration commences at a rate of 10 mg. per kg. per day in two equal doses and is increased to 20 mg. per kg. after one week; this therapy is continued for five weeks. Thiabendazole is claimed to be nontoxic to healthy dogs at this dose rate. However, occasional patients show lassitude and intermittent vomiting toward the end of the course of treatment; a return to normal can be expected upon withdrawal of the drug.

## RHINOTOMY

Although rhinotomy is surprisingly well tolerated by dogs, it should be performed only after a full hematologic and biochemical evaluation. Whole blood transfusion is indicated for anemic dogs. If possible, rhinotomy should be postponed in dogs showing intercurrent disease such as nephritis.

The indications for exploratory rhinotomy have already been described. Rhinotomy also permits extirpation of tissues infected by fungi which have not responded to medical therapy. Total bilateral turbinectomy is necessary to eliminate extensive areas of nasal mucosa with chronic irreversible hyperplasia. Rhinotomy and curettage may be performed in those few cases of intranasal neoplasia where there is a realistic prospect of total ablation of the neoplastic tissues. However, for the majority of

confirmed canine nasal tumors, excision ca no longer be justified.

Rhinotomy is performed with the patier in ventral recumbency; anesthesia is mair tained through a cuffed endotracheal tube and the pharynx is packed with gauz sponges. A dorsal midline skin incision made from the rhinarium to a point 4 cm posterior to a line joining the supraorbita processes. The subcutis and periosteum ar elevated and reflected laterally from th midline on the affected side. The front sinus is trephined using a 6.5-mm. drill at site midway between the midline and th supraorbital process (Fig. 4); the conten are inspected, and any stagnant mucus ( pus is removed by suction. A bone flap created (Fig. 4) to permit adequate exposu of the nasal chamber and allow exploratio and curettage. The flap is fashioned with hand-saw or osteotome; it remains attache to the rhinarium anteriorly so that it can b elevated rostrally. The edges of the flap ar beveled to facilitate its replacement at th conclusion of the procedure. Diseased tu binate tissue is removed using a Volkmar spoon, and affected bone may be broke away with a rongeur; specimens are submi ted for histopathology. In those instance where neoplastic or fungal disease have e tended to the frontal sinus, the trephin hole may be enlarged using the rongeur. sinus mucocele is drained by enlarging th normal ostium with a gouge. In most cas

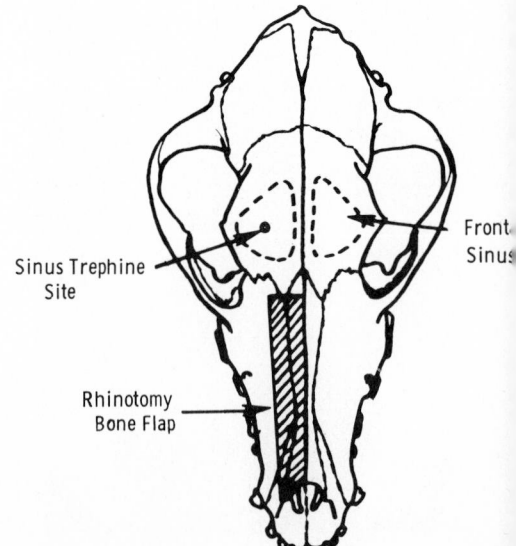

**Figure 4.** Line drawing indicating the anatom landmarks for rhinotomy in the dog.

when rhinotomy is performed, total turbinectomy is necessary on the affected side and care must be taken to extirpate all the tags of nasal mucous membrane prior to scraping clean the bony walls of the excavated nasal cavity. When bilateral exposure of the nasal chambers is required, a unilateral rhinotomy followed by ablation of the nasal septum affords an adequate exposure except in small breeds where a second rhinotomy flap may be necessary. Hemostasis is achieved by intermittent pressure-packing of the cavity; suction is used to maintain visibility. By the end of the procedure, hemorrhage has usually diminished to a slight venous ooze. In cases in which significant bleeding continues, gauze packing is left in place for 48 hours prior to withdrawal through the nostrils. For the purposes of postoperative irrigation of the sinus and nasal cavity, a polyethylene tissue-drainage tube is introduced through the sinus trephine hole and thence through the sinonasal ostium to be retained in position by skin sutures; a similar tube may be inserted into the contralateral chamber.

Closure of the rhinotomy begins by replacing the bone flap if this has not been excised. The flap is secured by the coaption of the overlying periosteal and subcuticular layers using absorbable material. The skin incision is closed with monofilament nylon. A good cosmetic result can be expected within six weeks.

Postoperative care consists of a systemic broad-spectrum antibiotic for five days and flushing with saline twice daily through the irrigation tubing. Provision of an alternative airway by tracheotomy intubation is rarely necessary, although equipment for this procedure should be available during anesthetic recovery. Postoperative subcutaneous emphysema is occasionally encountered but usually resolves spontaneously.

## PROGNOSIS

Complete excision of the diseased elements can be expected to produce remission in cases of chronic hyperplastic rhinitis and nasal aspergillosis. Long-term studies of dogs with intranasal neoplasms confirm that excision alone is followed by a very high rate of local recurrence. The occasional long-term success is achieved when the tumor arises from, and primarily involves, the maxilloturbinates, lending itself to thorough ablation. The tumor type does not seem to influence the rate of recurrence. Owners of dogs with nasal tumors should be advised that the prognosis is poor and surgery is likely to provide short-term palliation only. Studies are in progress to evaluate the possible role of radiation therapy and cryosurgery in the management of canine intranasal neoplasia.

### SUPPLEMENTAL READING

Bradley, P. A., and Harvey, C. E.: Intra-nasal tumors in the dog: an evaluation of prognosis. J. Small Animal Pract., *14*:459–467, 1973.

Denny, H. R., Gibbs, C., and Kelly, D. F.: The surgical treatment of intra-nasal tumors in the dog. Folia Vet. Latina, *V*:3, 1975.

Hoerlein, B. F.: Canine Neurology—Diagnosis and Treatment. 2nd ed. Philadelphia, W. B. Saunders Co., 1971, pp. 440–447.

Lane, J. G., Clayton-Jones, D. G., Thoday, K. L., and Thomsett, L. R.: The diagnosis and treatment of *Aspergillus fumigatus* infection of the frontal sinuses and nasal chambers of the dog. J. Small Animal Pract., *15*:79–87, 1974.

Morgan, J. P., Suter, P. F., O'Brien, T. R., and Park, R. D.: Tumors in the nasal cavity of the dog: a radiographic study. J. Am. Vet. Rad. Soc., *13*:18–26, 1972.

Wilkinson, G. T.: Some observations on the Irish wolfhound rhinitis syndrome. J. Small Animal Pract., *10*:5–8, 1969.

# RHINITIS AND SINUSITIS IN THE CAT

J. G. LANE, F.R.C.V.S.
*Bristol, England*

## INTRODUCTION

Although the presenting signs of rhinitis and sinusitis in the cat are essentially similar to those in the dog, they are usually more severe. The emphasis is on acute viral infections and their chronic consequences. Fungal and parasitic infestations and neoplasms of the nasal chambers and paranasal sinuses are uncommon in the cat. Primary sinusitis is rare, so that any efforts to carry out surgical treatment of feline frontal sinusitis without regard for the underlying rhinitis are misguided.

## FELINE NASAL DISORDERS

### ACUTE RHINITIS

Two viruses, feline viral rhinotracheitis (FVR) virus and feline calicivirus (FCV), are the primary pathogens responsible for the majority of upper respiratory tract infections in cats. These viruses have a worldwide distribution and have been isolated in approximately equal frequency from clinical cases. FVR virus usually produces severe clinical signs especially in young susceptible cats. The clinical conditions caused by FCV tend to be similar to but milder than those of FVR virus, although there is variation between strains.

Signs develop within 2 to 10 days of acquiring FVR virus infection. Paroxysms of sneezing are accompanied by the production of a clear mucoid discharge which becomes copious and mucopurulent within a few days. Simultaneously, conjunctivitis with a marked ocular discharge develops. Severe debilitation and depression with total anorexia may occur; mouth-breathing may be adopted and coughing can add to the distress. A fever in excess of 104° F. is not uncommon, and leukocytosis with a shift to the left parallels the temperature elevation; leukopenia is not observed. Occasionally with FVR virus, but more frequently with FCV infections, ulceration of the lingual and buccopharyngeal mucous membranes develops. During the early stages, natural feline cleansing activity leads to soiling of the forepaws by the oculonasal discharges. Later this washing behavior is reduced, leaving the nares encrusted, and the eyelids may be held partly closed by the tenacious exudate; contact keratitis may develop. Fatalities most often result from anorexia and dehydration and from secondary bacterial infection which may extend to produce pneumonia and pleuritis. Older and partly immune cats are less severely affected, exhibiting a mild conjunctivitis and rhinitis, yet still retaining a normal appetite.

Some FCV strains may cause an upper respiratory disease which is clinically indistinguishable from FVR virus infection. More often FCV produces a milder disease, of which oral ulceration may be the only sign.

FVR virus produces its most marked effects on the turbinate region, provoking an intense inflammatory reaction with necrosis and ulceration of the mucosa. In the growing cat, there is also a severe osteolytic response, with resorption of turbinate bone. Excessive mucus production, fibrin exudation, suppuration and the shedding of necrotic debris contribute to the oculonasal discharges. In the regenerative phase of the disease, squamous metaplasia and mucous gland hyperplasia occur; in many cats recovering from the acute phase, areas of permanently damaged nasal mucosa remain which are prone to recurrent microbial infection. FCV may produce a similar necrotizing rhinitis but there is a lesser tendency to incur secondary bacterial invasion.

Viral rhinitis is often prolonged and exacerbated by secondary infection with streptococci, staphylococci, Pasteurella or coliforms. Apart from intensifying the acute condition, bacterial invasion increases the likelihood of chronic, irreversible changes.

## CHRONIC RHINITIS AND SECONDARY SINUSITIS

Thickening of the nasal mucosa by epithelial hyperplasia and submucosal proliferation takes place during the acute phase of rhinitis. In a significant number of affected cats this response does not regress. Furthermore, areas of ulceration may not heal and thus provide foci for persistent opportunistic infection.

The role of primary nasal pathogens in the etiology of frontal sinusitis has not been established. The acute and chronic inflammatory changes which occur in the turbinate structures obstruct the normal ventilation and drainage of the sinuses through their small nasal openings. This provides a suitable environment for secondary bacterial infection, but, more important, the accumulation of secretions precipitates sinus mucocele formation. Prolonged build-up of inspissated secretions within the frontal sinuses may lead to softening of the thin overlying bone, producing a facial swelling.

Cats affected by chronic rhinitis are sometimes designated "snufflers" and exhibit intermittent bouts of sneezing and a purulent discharge which is occasionally blood-stained. The general attitude of the cat fluctuates with the nasal symptoms and the animal shows signs of not thriving. Severely affected patients become inappetent and mouth-breathe continuously.

## NASAL MYCOSES

Nasal mycoses are rare in cats. *Cryptococcus neoformans* is the most frequently encountered fungal infection, and although this may affect other organs, it shows a predilection for the upper respiratory tract. Granulomatous lesions are produced in the nasal chambers where infections may be uni- or bilateral. The presenting signs of nasal cryptococcosis are similar to those of severe chronic rhinitis. There is an intractable mucopurulent nasal discharge with persistent sneezing; extension of the lesion leads to destruction of the facial bones and the development of a swelling. There is no evidence of transmission of cryptococcosis from an infected cat to human contacts.

## INTRANASAL NEOPLASIA

Nasal tumors seldom occur in cats. Feline intranasal tumors are divided into two groups: carcinomas, which behave like canine nasal tumors, and lymphosarcomas, which often occur as a localized manifestation of a generalized condition. The signs of neoplasia are similar to those of chronic rhinitis but, as with cryptococcosis, they fail to respond to antibiotic therapy. In addition to continuous sneezing, a secondary sinus mucocele develops and eventually destruction of overlying bone takes place.

## DIAGNOSIS

The presenting signs already described justify a diagnosis of acute viral rhinitis; a marked leukocytosis adds further confirmatory evidence. Virus recovery and identification is unnecessary unless advice is to be given on the control of carrier cats in a breeding colony.

Failure of chronic rhinitis to respond to a trial parenteral broad-spectrum antibiotic alerts the clinician to consider other rarer possible diagnoses. Direct smears of the nasal discharge are taken for the identification of *Cryptococcus neoformans*. Bacterial and fungal culture and sensitivity testing will identify other pathogens. The most valuable swab material is obtained from the nasal chambers after the nares have been cleaned with an antiseptic solution. Swabs from a trephined sinus mucocele are unsatisfactory, since they do not identify the organisms which are perpetuating the underlying rhinitis. In many instances sinus swabs are sterile.

The narrow nasal vestibules limit anterior rhinoscopy, but a fungal granuloma or intranasal neoplasm is occasionally obvious at the external nares and is accessible for biopsy sampling. Posterior rhinoscopy using an illuminated dental mirror is a routine procedure in cats with nasopharyngeal dyspnea; rarely polyps are identified in this region.

In the cat, radiographic evidence contributes little toward the definitive diagnosis of intranasal diseases. The following projections are used in the radiography of the nasal chambers of the cat:

1. Dorsoventral occlusal (film in mouth).
2. Ventrodorsal (whole skull, jaws closed).
3. Straight lateral.

The occlusal view permits satisfactory exposure of the anterior areas of the nasal cavities but the frontal sinuses cannot be included. Although the anterior areas are obscured by the overlying mandible in the ventrodorsal projection, the posterior nasal chambers and frontal sinuses can be viewed (Fig. 1). The ventrodorsal open-mouth view used in the dog is not applicable to cats because the angle of beam required to eliminate the mandible leads to superimposition of the nasal chambers and the cranial vault. The skull conformation of the cat is unsuitable for skylining the frontal sinuses using an anteroposterior view.

Destruction of the turbinate trabecular pattern is expected in cases of intranasal neoplasia and fungal granuloma; this fine pattern may be seriously disrupted as a result of FVR virus osteoclasis. Breakdown of the supporting bones of the nose occurs in the later stages of neoplastic and granulomatous proliferation and, at the same time, there is increased soft tissue density within the chambers. Radiographs may be helpful in prognosis and also in determining whether there is symmetrical involvement; e.g., unilateral fluid filling of the frontal sinuses (Fig. 2) suggests that a mucocele has formed as a result of unilateral obstruction of sinus drainage.

In chronic feline nasal disease, where neoplasia or fungal granuloma is suspected, an accurate diagnosis can be reached only by biopsy sampling and histopathologic investigation of intranasal tissues. A sample can usually be obtained by introducing fine biopsy forceps through the nasal vestibule. The hemorrhage which accompanies biopsy collection is usually slight and of short duration but the procedure is best performed under general anesthesia with a cuffed endotracheal tube in position.

## TREATMENT

### ACUTE RHINITIS

There are no suitable antiviral drugs for the treatment of acute feline viral rhinitis. Management consists of special nursing and medication to eliminate secondary bacterial infection. The cat with viral rhinitis presents a risk to other hospital patients. Intensive care is required, while scrupulous hygiene is necessary to prevent cross infection. After suitable instruction, many cat owners quickly take to home-nursing of their pets, so that infected patients can be treated as outpatients. In this situation, it is irresponsible to allow infected animals to mix with other patients in the waiting area; they must be admitted directly into the treatment room. Afterward, infected surfaces and utensils are cleansed using a cationic surface-acting agent such as cetrimide (Cetavlon® [I.C.I., U.K.]*), or they are discarded.

---

*Nolvosan (Fort Dodge), available in the United States, is a similar but *not identical* product.

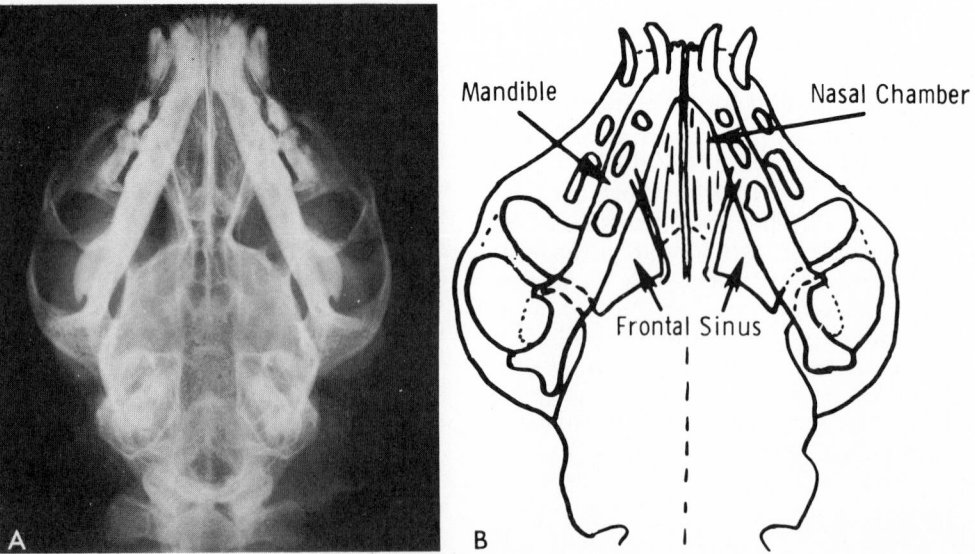

**Figure 1.** Radiograph (*A*) and line diagram (*B*) to indicate the position of the nasal chambers and frontal sinuses of the cat with the whole skull projected in the ventrodorsal position.

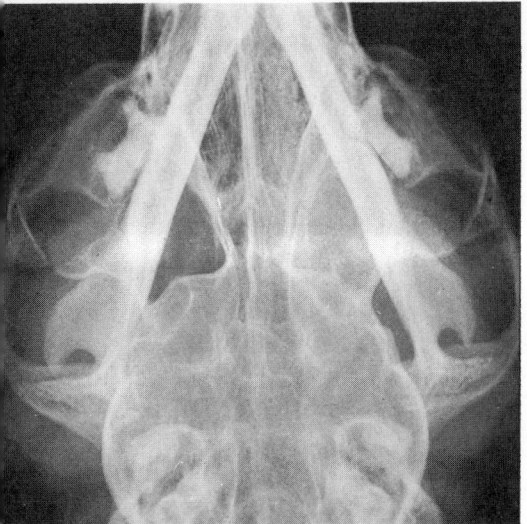

**Figure 2.** Radiograph of a cat with a persistent unilateral mucopurulent nasal discharge. There is increased density in the right nasal chamber and fluid filling of the right frontal sinus.

A dirty cat is a dejected cat; the patient with acute rhinitis must be provided with a clean, warm, well-ventilated environment and at the same time must be assisted in cleaning itself. Encrusted discharges are regularly bathed gently from around the eyes and nares; a bland ointment is then applied to these areas to prevent excoriation. Attention is paid to thorough grooming which the patient with lingual ulceration may be reluctant to carry out for itself. Cats with acute upper respiratory infections may reject their normal diet and often find strong tasting foods, such as sardines, tinned salmon or anchovies, more attractive. These aromatic foods are liquefied to make swallowing less painful as well as to increase fluid intake. If necessary, this food is reduced to a suitable consistency for feeding through a disposable syringe. Pharyngostomy intubation is indicated in cats which remain totally inappetent for longer than four days. The tube is introduced through the piriform fossa and extends into the stomach; its position is confirmed by radiography. This technique, which is not distressing to the cat, affords a convenient route for forced feeding and for the administration of medication.

Broad-spectrum antibiotic cover is provided for 14 days but may be continued for an additional 14 days in severe cases. Tablets are avoided because they are painful to swallow; for oral administration pediatric syrups are most suitable. An initial loading dose of antibiotic is provided parenterally. The following choice of antibiotics together with dose rates is suggested:

1. Ampicillin—loading dose: 7 mg./kg. subcutaneously, followed by 10 mg./kg. orally twice daily.

2. Potentiated sulfonamide—maintenance dose: 4 mg./kg. orally twice daily.

3. Oxytetracycline—loading dose: 20 mg./kg. intramuscularly, followed by 25 mg./kg. orally twice daily.

4. Tylosin (Tylan® [Lilly])—loading dose: 10 mg./kg. intramuscularly, followed by 40 mg./kg. orally three times daily.

Supportive vitamin therapy is helpful because

1. Vitamin A (1000 I.U. per day) is said to be important in assisting the regeneration of damaged mucosa.

2. Vitamin B complex preparations may stimulate the return of appetite. Vitamin $B_{12}$ ($250 \mu$g. daily) has a marked euphoric effect on depressed cats.

3. Vitamin C (up to 100 mg. daily) may shorten the recovery period.

Abdec ® drops (Parke-Davis) are suitable for oral use and, with the exception of $B_{12}$, provide the required levels of the vitamins mentioned.

Dehydration must be corrected, and fluid is best administered subcutaneously. When there is severe dehydration, the shutdown of the peripheral circulation can lead to poor absorption of fluids from this site; the intravenous route is then indicated. In the author's experience, if the cat is sufficiently depressed to lie still, the intravenous route is used, but if there is resentment and noncooperation, subcutaneous injection will be satisfactory. The objective of fluid therapy for cats with acute rhinitis is the correction of water depletion rather than of ionic imbalance. Therefore 0.18 per cent saline with 4.3 per cent dextrose is a suitable solution; concentrations of dextrose in excess of 5 per cent are irritant and are not used.

Most cats resent the restraint which is necessary for the application of nasal drops, and this method of administering decongestant inhalants is not recommended. Nebulizers and steam inhalations are preferred. Antihistaminics should be avoided, since they lead to drying up of the discharges, which then become difficult to dislodge. Corticosteroids retard the healing processes and are therefore contraindicated.

A complete reappraisal of each case of acute rhinitis should be made one week after the start of treatment. Failure to control the secondary bacterial infection may be due to the choice of the wrong antibiotic or to inadequate concentrations of antibiotic reaching the nasal chambers. Swab cultures and sensitivity tests are performed and the therapy is amended if necessary.

When rhinitis is still in the acute phase and is not responding to parenteral or oral antibiotic treatment, local administration through the frontal sinuses may be considered. Dye tests have shown that infusions made through the sinuses reach all areas of the nasal chambers. The procedure is performed under general anesthesia with a cuffed endotracheal tube. The sites of penetration of the sinuses depend on the age of the cat. In animals under 5 months of age, where the sinuses are still small, the sites lie on either side of the midline, on a line joining the lateral canthi. In adult cats, the points are more posterior, again on either side of the midline, but on a line joining the anterior borders of the supraorbital processes. Longitudinal 0.5-cm. skin incisions are made and the sinuses are entered using a 2.5-mm. intramedullary pin. Infusions are made through a closely fitting blunted needle. Using saline, the sinuses, sinus ostia and nasal chambers are flushed clear of pus and debris before the appropriate antibiotic is instilled. Indwelling tubes are not recommended for cats, and each incision is closed using a single suture of monofilament nylon before antibiotic cream is applied to the skin surface. The procedure is repeated through the original trephine holes between three and five times on alternate days.

## CHRONIC RHINITIS

There are two fundamental approaches to the treatment of this condition in which the intranasal structures are irreversibly damaged: firstly, conservative methods, whereby the recurrent opportunistic infections are tactically controlled for short periods and, secondly, a radical surgical excision of the diseased tissues.

The conservative methods are as follows:

1. Oral and parenteral antibiotic therapy based on culture and sensitivity testing of nasal swabs. The recommended choice of drugs, dose rates and duration of treatment are similar to those advised for the acute phase of rhinitis. A similar course of supportive vitamin therapy is also recommended.

2. Local infusion of antibiotics through the frontal sinuses. In the chronic phase, sinus irrigation provides temporary relief but appears to have no advantages over other conservative methods. Any temptation to vary the technique by the implantation of drainage tubes should be resisted because indwelling tubes are poorly accepted by cats and perfusion of the nasal chambers of a conscious cat is greatly resented. There can be no justification for a method which inflicts unnecessary distress without achieving permanent relief.

3. Autogenous vaccines prepared from cultures of nasal swabs will provide only temporary relief.

Radical nasal surgery is poorly tolerated by cats. Patients should be carefully selected for rhinotomy and turbinectomy when conservative treatments produce minimal improvement of the chronic rhinitis, and when repeated antibiotic therapy is unacceptable. In addition to these two groups, cats may be subjected to exploratory rhinotomy, and rarely, the excision of an intranasal tumor may be attempted. The surgical procedure for rhinotomy in the cat is similar to that in the dog, except that each nasal chamber is entered by creating a separate bone flap, the caudal limit of which is 0.5 cm. posterior to the line joining the medial canthi. Care is taken to excise all the remnants of turbinate and nasal mucous membrane, and the sinonasal ostia are enlarged to facilitate drainage. Sinus irrigation is performed postoperatively at 4-day intervals. Fluid and supportive therapy is most important pre- and postoperatively. After rhinotomy, an alternative airway is always provided by tracheotomy intubation. Pharyngostomy feeding is routinely used until normal appetite returns.

## NASAL CRYPTOCOCCOSIS

Treatment of *C. neoformans* infection may be attempted using amphotericin B. Prolonged courses of therapy may be required using intravenous infusion at a dose rate of 0.5 mg./kg., in dextrose saline, three times weekly for several months. As amphotericin B produces renal toxicity, blood urea nitrogen is monitored throughout the period of treatment; evidence of renal failure usually disappears if the drug is withdrawn promptly.

## INTRANASAL NEOPLASIA

Feline intranasal neoplasms are usually advanced when the diagnosis is confirmed, and surgical excision is rarely attempted. Furthermore, there is little justification for surgery because carcinomas show a high tendency to recur and lymphosarcomas may be part of a disseminated condition.

## PROGNOSES AND ADVICE TO OWNERS

If attention is sought and treatment is instituted at the earliest sign of infection, careful nursing combined with intensive medical therapy will lead to resolution of most cases of acute feline rhinitis. Patients which are neglected by owners or inadequately treated, and even some of those which are correctly managed, may develop chronic rhinitis.

When chronic irreversible changes have taken place within the nasal chambers of the cat, owners must be advised that there is at present no satisfactory method of treatment. Conservative medication and surgical interferences to the frontal sinuses bring only temporary amelioration. Extirpation of the diseased structures from the nasal cavities should provide a solution, but this radical procedure is often poorly tolerated by cats and fatalities may occur during the postoperative period.

A combined FVR and FCV vaccine has recently been introduced in North America. The attenuated live strains, when injected intramuscularly, are reported to produce satisfactory immunity in susceptible cats for at least six months. This vaccine may be particularly suitable for prophylaxis, e.g., before admission to a boarding cattery.

Cats which recover from upper respiratory tract viral infections may not eliminate the virus and may remain carriers. In breeding catteries and other colonies, carriers represent a reservoir for further cat-to-cat transmission. The continuous excretion of virus by the FCV carrier constantly boosts immunity within the group and keeps clinical disease at a low level. However, excretion of virus by the FVR carrier is intermittent and immunity within the colony may fluctuate. Irregular outbreaks of clinical disease can then be expected. Young kittens whose passive immunity is falling are most vulnerable where virus infections are endemic, and carriers must be identified and isolated from susceptible cats and kittens.

### SUPPLEMENTAL READING

Barrett, R. E., and Scott, D. W.: Treatment of feline cryptococcosis. J. Am. Animal Hosp. Assn., *11*:511–518, 1975.

Crandell, R. A., Rehkemper, J. A., Neimann, W. H., Gannaway, J. R., and Maurer, F. D.: Experimental feline viral rhinotracheitis. J. Am. Vet. Med. Assn., *138*:191–196, 1961.

Gaskell, R. M., and Wardley, R. C.: The carrier state of feline viral upper respiratory tract disease. Vet. Annual, Bristol, John Wright and Son, *15*:252–255, 1975.

Povey, R. C.: Feline viral respiratory disease. Vet. Rec., *84*:335–338, 1969.

Winstanley, E. W.: Trephining frontal sinuses in the treatment of rhinitis and sinusitis in the cat. Vet. Rec., *95*:289–292, 1974.

# UPPER AIRWAY OBSTRUCTION SYNDROMES IN DOGS

COLIN E. HARVEY, M.R.C.V.S.
*Philadelphia, Pennsylvania*

Many disease states can cause obstruction of the upper airway, which is manifested by noisy, snorting respiration; frequent mouth-breathing; and snoring. Poor exercise tolerance, increased respiratory effort, cyanosis and collapse are present in the more severely affected dogs. Trauma or infection can cause severe airway obstruction; however, more frequently the obstruction is a minor component of the disease; diagnostic procedures and treatment recommendations are directed at relief of the major problems. An animal with a neoplasm growing within or impinging on the airway may be presented because of airway obstruction only. Of more importance are several well-recognized clinical syndromes causing upper airway obstruction which occur in specific breeds or types of dogs, or which result from particular disease states with a narrow clinical effect. This chapter is limited to the discussion of these obstructive syndromes.

Prudent in-hospital management of any dog with airway obstructive disease must include constant observation. Excitement, stress, surgery and anesthetic recovery can all result in exacerbation of preexisting airway disease, to the point where a moderately obstructed dog can become severely or even fatally obstructed.

## AIRWAY OBSTRUCTION IN BRACHYCEPHALIC DOGS

Bulldogs, pugs, Pekingese, Boston terriers and other brachycephalic breeds usually show some degree of airway obstruction. Clinical signs are more severe when the dog is hot or during exercise and may be progressive with age. Obstructive disease is inherent in the breed conformation, resulting from the compression of the nasal cavity, pharynx, larynx and surrounding tissues into an inadequate space. Several distinct entities have been described in brachycephalic dogs: stenotic nares, overlong soft palate, eversion of the lateral ventricles, and laryngeal collapse. It is important to recognize that these conditions are listed separately because they are treatable separately; however, airway obstruction may result from a combination of these conditions, or from other factors such as edematous folds of the pharyngeal wall or roof that are often also present but not usually treated surgically. The entire nasopharyngolaryngeal airway should be examined prior to operative treatment of any part of the upper airway.

## STENOTIC NARES

Stenotic nares are common in brachycephalic dogs. The wing of the dorsal parietal nasal cartilage and the rhinarium covering it are folded medially, causing occlusion of the external nares. The principal clinical sign is complete or partial inability to breathe through the nose. This condition responds well to surgical treatment, which consists of removal of a lateral wedge of the wing of the nostril. Blood loss is minimal; hemorrhage is controlled by placement of two surgical gut sutures to appose the cut surfaces.

Surgical treatment of stenotic nares is a useful adjunct to treatment of other aspects of brachycephalic airway obstruction; however, it is very rarely indicated as the only treatment.

## OVERLONG SOFT PALATE

This condition occurs most commonly in brachycephalic dogs, although it has also been recognized in several other breeds. Noisy respiration and snoring are the most prominent clinical signs. In the normal dog the soft palate overhangs the epiglottis slightly. In dogs with overlong soft palate, the overhang is sufficient partially to occlude the glottis. The glottic obstruction is made much worse by the thickness of the palate due to inflammation and edema. Diagnosis is made by direct observation of the relationship between the soft palate and the larynx. Lateral radiographs of the neck may be helpful: in affected dogs, the nasopharyngeal airway is much reduced in size or is not seen; the soft palate shadow may appear tremendously thickened. Cooling and calming the dog and the administration of anti-inflammatory corticosteroids (prednisolone 1.0 mg./kg.) are usually effective in managing the acute case. Surgical treatment will often give permanent relief from severe obstruction, although respirations usually remain somewhat noisy. The corrective surgical procedure consists of resecting part of the soft palate. An endotracheal tube should be placed to maintain an open airway and prevent aspiration of blood. A scissor, electroscalpel or tonsil snare may be used. Very satisfactory results are obtained by cutting the palate with scissors and apposing the oral and nasal epithelial cut surfaces with fine surgical gut sutures. The tip of the epiglottis or the midpoint of the palatine tonsil may be used as a guide to the amount of soft palate to be resected: enough soft palate must be left to allow the nasopharynx to be closed during swallowing. Prednisolone (1.0 mg./kg.) is given preoperatively and on the first post-operative day to reduce surgical swelling of the palate. Soft foods are fed for one week following surgery. Resection of the soft palate is the most commonly performed surgical treatment of brachycephalic airway obstruction.

## EVERSION OF THE LARYNGEAL SACCULES

This condition occurs in some brachycephalic dogs to a degree sufficient to cause obstruction. It is thought that increased negative pressure in the laryngeal airway from increased respiratory effort causes the mucosal linings of the laryngeal saccules to become edematous and to be sucked into the glottis. The diagnosis is made at laryngoscopy by observing balls of edematous saccular tissue obscuring the true vocal cords and narrowing the glottis. Surgical correction is resection of the everted tissue with long-handled laryngeal cup forceps. Tissue forceps and scissors may be used but visualization is not as good. Hemorrhage is usually minimal. The procedure is rapid, and tracheotomy is usually not necessary, although each animal should be evaluated individually regarding the need for tracheotomy, particularly in dogs which also have some degree of laryngeal collapse.

## VOCAL CORD PARALYSIS AND LARYNGEAL COLLAPSE

Vocal cord paralysis occurs as an acquired disease in middle-aged or older large breed dogs and is occasionally seen as a congenital problem in sled dogs and Bouviers. It can also occur as a result of trauma or surgery in the neck area. Laryngeal collapse is also seen in brachycephalic dogs with severe airway obstruction. Increased negative pressure in the supraglottic area, resulting from increased respiratory effort caused by overlong soft palate or laryngeal malfunctions, causes the arytenoid cartilages and aryepiglottic folds to collapse medially and ventrally. The clinical signs associated with vocal cord paralysis and laryngeal collapse are stridulous respiration (which has been described as "roaring" in large breed dogs) and collapse on exertion. Airway obstruction may be severe enough to require immediate tracheotomy. Diagnosis is made by laryngoscopy: normal laryngeal movements are not seen under deep anesthesia even in normal dogs, so a light plane of general anesthesia is required to diagnose vocal cord paralysis by the absence of intrinsic laryngeal movement. With laryngeal collapse, the arytenoid cartilage medial surfaces are often touching and the aryepiglottic folds and arytenoid cartilage projections (corniculate and cuneiform tubercles) are soft flabby structures lying more medial than is normal. Inflammation and edema of the laryngeal mucosa are usually present. Everted laryngeal saccules are often also present.

The important factor in assessing the need for surgical correction of laryngeal collapse is the size of the glottic lumen. If this is very small relative to normal for an animal of that size, surgical treatment is necessary. If the glottis is somewhat larger, cage rest and corticosteroids followed by a cool environment and prevention of excitement may be sufficient temporarily to alleviate the condition, or soft palate resection may be sufficient to provide long-term relief for affected brachycephalic dogs.

A tracheotomy tube should be placed prior to surgical treatment of vocal cord paralysis and laryngeal collapse. The laryngeal airway (glottis) is enlarged by unilateral excision of arytenoid cartilage, aryepiglottic fold and vocal cord with long-handled laryngeal cup forceps. Scissors may be used but are less desirable, since more hemorrhage may occur. Hemorrhage is controlled by direct pressure with a gauze sponge held on the surgical site. Corticosteroids are given preoperatively (prednisolone, 1.0 mg./kg.) and for one day postoperatively. In large breed dogs, the tracheotomy tube can usually be removed a few hours after surgery. Smaller dogs, such as pugs or Boston terriers, require more time and care during the postoperative period, since their upper airway is smaller and edema is more likely to result in obstruction postoperatively. The prognosis following partial laryngectomy is good in large dogs. Because visualization during surgery is not as good and because of the increased postoperative care required, the prognosis in small dogs (Pekingese, pugs, Boston terriers) is more guarded; multiple operative procedures, each consisting of removal of a few small bites of laryngeal tissue, may be necessary to allow creation of an adequate airway while minimizing the risk of aspiration.

## TRACHEAL COLLAPSE

Tracheal collapse occurs in Chihuahuas, Pomeranians, toy poodles and other mainly nonbrachycephalic toy breed dogs. The trachea is collapsed dorsoventrally, and the dorsal membrane of the trachea is stretched and flaccid. The most marked area of collapse is usually the thoracic inlet, although often the entire length of the trachea and the major bronchi may be collapsed. The clinical signs are a low-pitched noise described as "honking," cough and signs of airway obstruction. Heart disease may coexist in older animals.

Diagnosis is based on the breed, clinical signs and palpation of a deformed, flaccid trachea. Lateral radiographs of the cervical and thoracic trachea showing severe narrowing or complete collapse are confirmatory, although false positive radiographs may result from partial obliteration of the tracheal air shadow by overlying soft tissue; fluoroscopic examination provides the most accurate clinical means of assessing the degree of normality.

As with most obstructive airway diseases, cage rest and corticosteroids (prednisolone, 0.1 mg./kg.) usually result in some clinical improvement. Low daily doses of tranquilizers (e.g., promazine, 1.0 mg/kg.) are helpful to prevent acute exacerbations. Many surgical treatments have been reported; however, adequate long-term follow-up reports are not available, and no one surgical treatment method has yet become accepted as a standard effective treatment. For these reasons, conservative medical management as above is recommended for all except the most severe recurrent cases.

### SUPPLEMENTAL READING

Amis, T. C.: Tracheal collapse in the dog. Aust. Vet. J., 50:285–289, 1974.

Bojrab,M. J.: Surgical reconstruction for collapsed tracheal rings. Proc. 40th Ann. Mtg. Am. Animal Hosp. Assn., 1973.

Harvey, C. E., and O'Brien, J. A.: Management of respiratory emergencies in small animals. Vet. Clin. N. Am., 2:243–258, 1972.

Harvey, C. E., and Venker-vanHaagan, A.: Surgical management of pharyngeal and laryngeal airway obstruction in the dog. Vet. Clin. N. Am., 5:515–535, 1975.

Knowles, R. P., and Snyder, C. C.: Chondrotomy for congenital tracheal stenosis. Proc. 34th Ann. Mtg. Am. Animal Hosp. Assn., 1967, pp. 246–249.

# CHRONIC TRACHEOBRONCHIAL DISEASE IN THE DOG AND CAT

E. B. WHEELDON, M.R.C.V.S.
*Glasgow, Scotland*

Acute viral infections are the most frequently encountered tracheobronchial diseases of the dog and cat and are a particular problem where groups of animals are housed in close concentration. Considerable research in the last 15 years has identified several different viruses and bacteria which can be isolated regularly from such cases and which can induce experimental respiratory infection. There are, however, more chronic diseases which present special problems of diagnosis and treatment. Some of these syndromes, such as "feline asthma" and bronchiectasis, are still poorly defined but others, including tuberculosis and chronic bronchitis, now have good clinical and pathologic correlation. This article is an attempt to draw attention to recent advances made in the diagnosis and treatment of chronic tracheobronchial diseases.

(Canine tracheobronchitis due to *Filaroides osleri* is dealt with elsewhere in this book.)

## CANINE CHRONIC BRONCHITIS

Recent work has revealed that a chronic bronchitis occurs in the dog which closely resembles, both clinically and pathologically, the disease of chronic bronchitis in man. The canine condition can be defined in clinical descriptive terms similar to the definition used in man: chronic bronchitis in the dog refers to the condition of subjects with chronic or recurrent excessive mucus secretion in the bronchial tree. The words chronic or recurrent may be defined as occurring on most days for at least two consecutive months in the preceding year, with the excessive mucus secretion being manifested clinically by coughing.

This is a disease of adult dogs and is found from middle age onward. Although larger breeds, such as German shepherds, can be affected, chronic bronchitis typically occurs in smaller breeds, such as poodles and terriers, and is commonly seen in obese animals. The disease has an insidious onset and a progressive course: usually by the time the dog is presented it has been coughing for several months. Coughing is often precipitated by exercise or excitement and in a proportion of cases it is productive, with gagging and expectoration. Auscultation will reveal crackling adventitious lung sounds and typically the heart has a pronounced sinus arrhythmia. This last feature is of value in the differential diagnosis of coughing due to valvular endocardosis and pulmonary edema, since in these cases there is also a gross murmur and tachycardia with a fast weak pulse. Radiographic examination discloses characteristic changes in approximately half the cases of chronic bronchitis; these changes take the form of increased bronchovascular markings extending to the periphery of the lung field resulting in parallel and annular linear opacities.

The dominant feature at postmortem examination is the excess amount of mucus present in the airways; the mucus extends throughout the tracheobronchial tree and there is often pooling at the tracheal bifurcation. Beneath the mucus, the mucosa appears roughened and opaque; microscopically, it is thickened by irregular and diffuse fibrosis, edema and mononuclear cell infiltration. Most importantly, the mucus-secreting apparatus is increased in size: tracheobronchial mucous glands proliferate and enlarge so that they completely surround the airway lumina and there is a marked increase in the number of epithelial goblet cells. In addition, there is a qualitative change in the mucus, with a shift in the production of the different types of mucosubstances.

The treatment of chronic bronchitis in the dog is still largely experimental and is based on the methods employed in human chronic bronchitis. Treatment of the condition is largely supportive, and the main aims must be to control coughing, if troublesome, and to minimize progression of the disease by preventing acute exacerbations. There is often marked alleviation of clinical signs after hospitalization and rest; this procedure can incorporate measures to control obesity if applicable. Acute exacerbations of bronchitis tend to recur and these should be treated promptly with antimicrobial drugs, care being taken to insure adequate dosage and an adequate period of treatment. Little is known of the bacteria causing exacerbations of bronchitis in the dog but *Bordetella bronchiseptica* is commonly found in these cases and this is sensitive *in vitro* to most broad-spectrum antimicrobial drugs. In man, chemotherapy is restricted to episodes where the sputum becomes purulent, indicating a definite acute exacerbation of the bronchitis. Where possible, culture of bronchial washings or swabs should be used to determine bacterial sensitivity to antimicrobial drugs. This approach will help to minimize further damage to the bronchial mucosa and reduce the deleterious changes in the airways, which result in progression of the disease.

It is generally considered that a certain amount of coughing is desirable to get rid of excess mucus, and cough suppressants are not usually prescribed unless paroxysmal coughing is causing physical exhaustion. Alternatively, the coughing may constitute a nuisance in the household, particularly if it occurs at night; in these situations, suppression of the cough by a sedative such as one of the codeine derivatives will be of importance in the overall management of the case. In recent years, mucolytics have been widely used in the treatment of the human condition; although little is known of their effects in the dog, veterinarians are now using mucolytics on an empirical basis with apparently beneficial results.

## CANINE BRONCHIECTASIS

The term bronchiectasis is used to indicate chronic dilatation of the bronchi. Although bronchiectasis undoubtedly occurs in the dog, it is an uncommon condition and is found much less frequently than, for example, chronic bronchitis. In man, the classic signs are a productive cough with purulent sputum and sometimes hemoptysis. Dogs with bronchiectasis present with a history of persistent cough which has become productive; expectoration of purulent sputum is a frequent finding. However, certain confirmation of diagnosis can only be made by bronchography; this will reveal cystic and saccular enlargements of the bronchi. Pathologic examination of affected bronchi reveals ulceration of the bronchial epithelium together with irregular destruction, fibrosis and cellular infiltration of the bronchial wall; the overall result is a weakening of the bronchial wall with distention and sacculation of the airway. The distended bronchi often contain accumulations of mucus and inflammatory cells, which form stagnant casts of material.

In the event of a clinical diagnosis being made with the aid of bronchography, treatment consists of either surgical intervention, with resection of affected segments, or medical treatment in the form of suppressive chemotherapy to control existing chronic bronchial infections and to prevent acute exacerbations. Postural drainage is an important part of treatment for the condition in man, but it is unlikely to be of value in the dog. Bronchiectasis is not usually progressive, and spread into unaffected bronchi is rare.

## TRACHEOBRONCHIAL NEOPLASIA IN THE DOG AND CAT

Primary lung tumors are rare in all the domesticated animals but they occur most frequently in the dog. The recorded incidence varies according to the population sampled, but Stünzi (1974) observed them in one per cent of the dogs submitted for postmortem examination at the Zurich Veterinary School.

Although cough is often stated to be the presenting sign in these cases, in our experience cough is frequently absent and the main presenting sign is tachypnea, which may appear to be of sudden onset and which may not be noticed by the owner. For this reason, primary lung tumors are often detected only when tachypnea is noticed in the dog being examined for other purposes. The average age of dogs suffering from lung carcinoma is approximately 11 years.

Radiography is of value in the diagnosis and differential diagnosis of pulmonary tumors; typically, the appearance is of a single mass together with a variable number of smaller peripheral metastases.

At postmortem examination, the tumors are firm, are gray-white and may have necrotic areas containing a mixture of mucus and cell debris. In addition, the regional lymph nodes often contain metastases, typically with umbilicated centers. The tumor mass may spread directly to adjacent lung lobes with involvement of the pleura. In man, primary lung tumors tend to occur in the hilar region, but in the dog the tumors tend to occur in the peripheral part of the lung. As well as differences in location of the primary tumors within the lung, there are important differences in the types of tumor. In man, the great majority of lung tumors are epidermoid and anaplastic tumors, thought to reflect the importance of irritants such as cigarette smoke in the etiology. By contrast, the great majority of lung tumors seen in the dog are adenocarcinomas; epidermoid and anaplastic carcinomas are rare.

Less is known about primary lung tumors in the cat; only a handful have been recorded in the literature. Stünzi (1974) quotes a comparable figure of 0.5 per cent in his necropsy survey. As in the dog, the most common histologic type is the adenocarcinoma and the average age of affected cats is approximately 13 years. The usual presenting signs are dyspnea together with coughing or wheezing. Again radiography is an important aid in the diagnosis of primary lung tumor in the cat.

## "BRONCHIAL ASTHMA" IN THE CAT

There have been several reports in the United States of a respiratory disease in the cat characterized by severe dyspnea and forced expirations. Coughing occurs in a proportion of cases together with cyanosis in those severely affected. Many of these cats have a systemic eosinophilia and radiographic changes characterized by increased bronchovascular markings. Eight of the 10 cases so far recorded have been in Siamese cats.

The clinical signs are relieved by epinephrine and also respond to corticosteroid therapy. Treatment consists of an initial intramuscular injection of prednisolone at a dose of 2 mg./kg. followed by oral prednisolone at the rate of 1.0 mg./kg. daily in three divided doses for five days, concluding with half this dosage for an additional five days. In the cases so far examined, the condition has tended to recur at irregular intervals.

Postmortem findings of bronchial smooth muscle hypertrophy, bronchial mucous gland hyperplasia and peribronchial infiltration by eosinophils have all been described. Despite this, the pathogenesis of this disease remains unclear and diagnosis is based largely on the response to corticosteroid therapy. It remains to be seen whether this syndrome is a form of bronchial asthma which would fulfill criteria similar to those laid down for the definition of bronchial asthma in man.

## TUBERCULOSIS IN THE DOG AND CAT

Despite the dramatic decline in the incidence of tuberculosis in man and animals, the disease has still not been eradicated. Cases of tuberculosis are still being seen in dogs and cats and these present a particular hazard to the veterinarian. Moreover, it has been demonstrated that cases of tuberculosis in the dog and cat are often the result of infection from man; thus prompt and accurate diagnosis is important from a public health aspect.

Tuberculosis may present in a variety of manifestations, including a generalized systemic disease. In the dog, the thoracic form of the disease is the most common syndrome; in the cat, in which the usual source of infection was believed to be the ingestion of contaminated milk, the abdominal form,

with involvement of the mesenteric lymph nodes, has been the usual variant described.

Pulmonary tuberculosis in the dog is characterized by dyspnea with or without tachypnea, and there is usually an accompanying cough. The history may be of progressive wasting with prolonged and fluctuating pyrexia. In the cat, the clinical signs of pulmonary tuberculosis are less well-defined but include sneezing, a wheezy cough and often a nasal discharge.

Radiographic examination will very often indicate some degree of pleural effusion and the presence of hilar lymphadenopathy —features which are both strongly suggestive of tuberculosis. However, radiography can reveal a variety of appearances, and in the more atypical cases other conditions, such as nocardiosis, should be borne in mind. Other diagnostic techniques such as throat swabs and intradermal injections of tuberculin give inconsistent results. At postmortem examination, the lungs, bronchomediastinal lymph nodes and serous membranes may all be involved. Pleural effusions are found in most of the pulmonary cases; there is a serous or serohemorrhagic effusion into the pleural cavity and pericardial sac, with firm beige or white nodules scattered over the visceral and parietal pleura. The bronchial lymph nodes are enlarged and have foci of central necrosis.

There have been several reports of the successful treatment of tuberculosis in dogs and cats with isoniazid and streptomycin; other workers have suggested inoculation with BCG to increase resistance. However, because of the possibility of transmission to man or other animals, affected animals should be euthanized.

### SUPPLEMENTAL READING

Carpenter, J. L.: Bronchial asthma in cats. In Kirk, R. W. (ed.): Current Veterinary Therapy V. Philadelphia, W. B. Saunders Co., 1974.
Snider, W. R.: Tuberculosis in canine and feline populations—review of the literature. Am. Rev. Resp. Dis., *104*:877–887, 1971.
Stünzi, H., Head., K. W., and Nielsen, S. W.: Tumours of the lung. Bull. W.H.O., *50*:9–19, 1974.
Wheeldon, E. B., Pirie, H. M., Fisher, E. W., and Lee, R.: Chronic bronchitis in the dog. Vet. Rec., *94*:466–471, 1974.

# PNEUMONIA

R. L. HAMLIN, D.V.M.
*Columbus, Ohio*

*and* DONALD KAHN, D.V.M.
*Washington Crossing, New Jersey*

## INTRODUCTION

For the purposes of this discussion, pneumonia will be defined as an inflammation of the gas exchange portions of the lung, including respiratory bronchioles and alveoli. Because the respiratory tract is a continuum extending from the nasopharynx to the alveoli, pneumonia may accompany tracheobronchitis or bronchitis. It may be observed more prevalently in brachycephalic breeds, in dogs with chronic debilitating diseases, in dogs receiving immunosuppressants or in dogs with cleft palates or left-to-right intracardiac shunts. It shows no sex or age predilection once adjusted for young dogs with congenital defects or aged dogs with debilitation.

## ETIOLOGY

Pneumonias may be classified as (a) exudative or nonexudative; (b) bronchial, lobar or interstitial; or (c) according to etiology. Causes of most pneumonias in dogs are unknown; however, when etiologies are known, they usually fall into one of the following categories:

1. *Viral*—the parainfluenza ($SV_5$); or canine adenovirus, type 2 (CAV-2).

2. *Bacterial*—usually secondary to viral infection, often *Bordetella bronchiseptica* or, more rarely, common organisms occupying the upper respiratory tract (*E. coli, Klebsiella* and *Enterobacter* spp., strep and staph spp., *Pasteurella multocida*). Neither Mycoplasma nor canine herpes virus species appear important in the pathogenesis of canine pneumonias.

3. *Systemic mycoses*—e.g., histoplasmosis, nocardiosis, or blastomycosis in regions where they are endemic (see article on "Systemic Mycotic Pneumonias").

4. *Allergic or hypersensitive reactions.*

5. *Aspiration of food or gastric contents*—particularly in dogs with megaesophagus or cleft palate, or following anesthesia.

6. *Inhalation of noxious fumes or hot gases.*

7. *Parasitic*—either the migrating stage of nonrespiratory parasites or the mature stage of lung parasites (see article on "Parasitic Diseases of the Respiratory Tract").

Although each category may be a primary cause of pneumonia, bacterial invaders may be secondary to viral or parasitic invasion or to inhalation of toxic substances.

## PATHOPHYSIOLOGY

Signs of pneumonia may result from interference with one or more functions of the lung by the etiologic agent. Exudation may result in plugging of airways or alveoli, altering ventilation or the respiratory exchange area and interfering with diffusion of gases—particularly oxygen—across the alveolar-capillary membrane. Such a "wet" lung would become stiffer than normal and require increased work of ventilation. Excessive secretions in the airways may result in active abdominal expiration, airway closure at volumes approaching or greater than functional residual capacity and ventilation-perfusion inequalities. Filling of alveoli with exudate results in right-to-left shunts. Excessive exudation may "wash out" surfactant, causing the lung to become stiffer yet and further exaggerating the ventilation-perfusion inequality and venoarterial shunting.

Nonexudative pneumonias may cause cough by irritation of airways. Pulmonary parenchyma may be replaced with fibrotic scars which decrease lung compliance, or proliferation of bronchial epithelium may increase airway resistance. Not only may pneumonias alter lung function and cause alterations in arterial blood gases and pH, but the cardiovascular system may also be affected. Pulmonary hypertension may result in right heart failure (cor pulmonale), manifested as right ventricular and atrial enlargements. Right heart dilatation may subsequently cause tricuspid regurgitation. Cough may further impede venous return and reduce cardiac output enough to cause syncope during severe paroxysms of coughing.

Large fluctuations in intrapleural pressure during coughing may impose sufficient stresses on pulmonary blood vessels that they may rupture, producing either hemoptysis or hemothorax. Weakened and stressed airways or alveoli may rupture and result in pneumothorax.

## DIAGNOSIS

Because all dogs with pneumonia do not manifest identical signs, signs of any particular pneumonia may vary according to its etiology and the response of the individual dog to the etiologic agent. Certain signs, however, are observed in a majority of dogs afflicted with pneumonia. These are tachypnea, dyspnea, cough, bronchovesicular breath sounds, fever, leukocytosis and depression with restlessness. Dogs with allergic or parasitic pneumonias may have eosinophilia—particularly in tracheal washings.

Radiographic examination is extremely important in the diagnosis of pneumonia. Increased radiodensity of the lung parenchyma may be manifested as a general hazing or ground-glass appearance to the normally dark lung fields, particularly obvious in bronchopneumonia. An interstitial pattern with linear or nodular density or with patches or puffs of increased density may indicate pulmonary mycosis. Lobar pneumonia may be manifested by well-defined regions of greatly increased density with consolidation and air bronchograms. In some cases, bronchopneumonia, like bronchitis, may not be detected radiologically.

Bronchovesicular breath sounds are expiratory sounds over the middle and diaphragmatic lobes which are louder than the normal respiratory sounds over the same regions and are usually rather harsh and high-pitched. Often these sounds are identical to the harsh, high-pitched sound heard over the trachea during a rapid exhalation of a normal dog.

Dogs with long-standing bronchopneumonia may develop fine, soft, high-pitched rales. (These may be mimicked by rolling the hair of side-burns between the thumb and first finger.) When pneumonia becomes exudative, rales may become louder, lower pitched and coarser. Rales may be present without fluid in the airways, possibly arising from opening and closing of airways. The longer the time period in which rales are heard during a single breath, the more severe the disease. Similarly, the greater the region of the thorax over which rales are heard, the more severe the disease.

Very coarse, loud, "snoring-type" sounds of extreme dyspnea are called sonorous rhonchi. These may indicate an exudative process or extreme pharyngeal or laryngeal edema. Sonorous rhonchi are heard normally in some brachycephalic breeds. Fine rales are never heard in normal dogs. If pleural effusion develops, sounds over the affected region may be soft or absent, and on percussion there is less resonance than normal over that region of the thorax. If pneumothorax develops, sounds may be soft or absent, and percussion reveals an extreme hyperresonance.

Dogs with allergic pneumonitis may manifest dyspnea and tachypnea and an "alveolar pattern" radiographically. For dogs showing such a pattern a tracheal washing should be analyzed for eosinophils.

With exudative pneumonia, dogs usually have a mucopurulent nasal discharge and may sneeze great quantities of this ropy material. A culture and sensitivity of the discharge may be useful when selecting an appropriate antibiotic.

Dogs with severely embarrassed ventilation or with large right-to-left shunts may appear cyanotic and have a reduced $PaO_2$ with normal, reduced or elevated $PaCO_2$. Most often, however, $PaCO_2$ will be normal or reduced owing to hyperventilation generated by the low $PaO_2$. Respiratory alkalosis, resulting from hyperventilation, is not uncommon in dogs with pneumonia. Only those dogs with reduced alveolar ventilation will manifest respiratory acidosis due to increased $PaCO_2$.

## DIFFERENTIAL DIAGNOSIS

Bronchitis, tracheobronchitis, tracheal stenosis or collapse, pneumothorax, bronchiectasis, left-sided congestive heart failure, thoracic tumors and lymphoma must all be considered in the differential diagnosis of a dog presented with signs of pneumonia. Many of these diseases may coexist with or predispose the dog to pneumonia.

## TREATMENT

Treatment of a dog with pneumonia is dependent upon the etiology of the pneumonia and the response made to the etiologic agent. Some young dogs with bronchopneumonia, mild fever, leukocytosis, little cough or dyspnea and adequate gaseous exchange in the lung require only a favorable environment and time for complete recovery. Other aged dogs with exudative pneumonia, copious mucopurulent nasal discharge, extreme dyspnea, hypoxemia and respiratory acidosis may require intensive antibiotic, oxygen, positive end-expiratory pressure (PEEP), bronchodilator and mucolytic therapy.

Because most bronchopneumonias are probably viral in origin, with secondary bacterial invaders, they may be treated with rest, antibiotics and oxygen therapy. The rationale for our use of antibiotics in the treatment of most pneumonias of unknown etiology is unscientific. Although we know that most pneumonias of known etiology are caused by organisms sensitive to aerosol administration of kanamycin and polymyxin once every 3 to 4 days, we still treat most pneumonias with either tetracycline or ampicillin given in high therapeutic doses. Initial treatment is for 14 days with therapy repeated for 7 to 10 consecutive days a month for the next 3 months to prevent exacerbations. This latter regimen has appeared to be effective on a clinical basis. Objective studies have shown aerosol kanamycin-polymyxin to be effective in the treatment of *B. bronchiseptica.* We prefer ampicillin and tetracycline because they are broad-spectrum, have low toxicity and do not lead to resistant strains of bacteria as easily as other antibiotics. Tetracycline should not be given to puppies because of the effect on teeth. Gentamicin and sulfonamides are also useful in the treatment of bacterial pneumonias.

With severe exudation, bronchodilators (aminophylline, Elixophylline® [Cooper]) given orally and mucolytics (acetylcysteine, Mucomyst®[Mead Johnson]) given by aerosolization are often useful. With aerosol treatment, kanamycin and polymyxin may be given every 3 to 4 days, while the Mucomyst should be given two to four times a day. Atropine and other parasympatholytics are contraindicated because they paralyze mucociliary transport, make secretions more viscous and cause mucous plugs in the airways.

Inhalation therapy with an oxygen-enriched atmosphere is often helpful with acute respiratory distress. Oxygen therapy is necessary only when $PaO_2$ is less than 60 torr. By increasing alveolar oxygen tension ($PaO_2$), the gradient driving oxygen from alveolus to capillary is increased, and better oxygenation of blood is achieved. The aim of oxygen therapy is to saturate hemoglobin, and enriching the atmosphere to 40 per cent oxygen is usually adequate. In long-standing respiratory distress, oxygen concentration should be elevated cautiously, since some of these animals have chronic hypercapnia and no longer respond to changing levels of carbon dioxide. Oxygen which removes the hypoxic drive to ventilation may result in a large increase in $PaCO_2$ with resultant carbon dioxide narcosis. Ideally, blood gases should be regularly monitored during oxygen administration to assure that increased $PaO_2$ does not reduce minute ventilation and produce hypercarbia and acidosis.

In many dogs with acute respiratory distress due to pneumonia, ventilation with high concentrations of oxygen does not effectively increase oxygenation of the blood because there are many areas of lung with reduced ventilation/perfusion ratios. A possible remedy for this ventilation/perfusion abnormality is the use of PEEP (positive end-expiratory pressure). It provides for more uniform oxygenation of alveoli by keeping airway pressure positive, thus keeping open airways that are anatomically or functionally occluded or compressed by the disease process. PEEP allows the previously unventilated exchange area to be ventilated, thus reducing ventilation/perfusion abnormalities. The disadvantages of PEEP are (1) it requires chemical restraint of the dog and intubation, (2) it requires rather elaborate equipment for administration, and (3) it may reduce cardiac output by impeding venous return. In acute respiratory distress, we have observed remarkable improvement in certain dogs treated with PEEP, but it requires extensive clinical and experimental investigation to justify its routine use in acute respiratory distress in dogs.

In allergic pneumonitis, glucocorticoids "covered" with broad-spectrum antibiotics often produce dramatic relief within 24 hours. This same regimen is useful for treating pneumonitis due to inhalation of toxic substances or hot air (e.g., dogs suffering smoke inhalation from fires). In addition, these dogs may develop severe pulmonary edema, so a potent diuretic (furosemide) is indicated. Caution must be exercised against dehydrating these dogs with too rigorous diuresis. This will reduce cardiac output and possibly cause prerenal azotemia. Because this edema results from loss of integrity of the alveolar-capillary membrane and is not cardiogenic in origin, digitalis should not be given to such dogs. In addition, dogs with respiratory distress are often more sensitive to catecholamines and digitalis, and these agents may cause lethal arrhythmias. Consequently, they should be given with extreme care, if at all.

## SUPPLEMENTAL READING

Appel, M., Pickerill, P. H., Menegus, M., Percy, D. H., Parsonson, I. M. G., and Sheffy, B. E.: Current status of canine respiratory disease. Gaines Vet. Symposium, 1970.

Creighton, S. R., and Wilkins, R. J. Bacteriologic and cytologic evaluation of animals with lower respiratory tract disease using transtracheal aspiration biopsy. J. Am. Animal Hosp. Assn., 10:227, 1974.

O'Brien, J. A., and Todd, J. D.: Bronchitis. In Kirk, W. R. (ed.): Current Veterinary Therapy IV. Philadelphia, W. B. Saunders Co., 1971.

Wilkins, R. J., and Helland, D. R.: Antibacterial sensitivities of bacteria isolated from dogs with tracheobronchitis. J. Am. Vet. Med. Assn., 161:47, 1973.

# PULMONARY VASCULAR DISEASE IN THE DOG

NEIL K. HARPSTER, V.M.D.
*Boston, Massachusetts*

Veterinary literature contains many references to cardiac dysfunction but pulmonary vascular disease has been rarely described in the dog. It is difficult to divorce cardiac function and the pulmonary circulation, since interrelationships between the two are so intimately associated. This paper examines the pulmonary circulation in cardiorespiratory disease; cardiac function will be discussed as it relates to this.

## THE LUNG CIRCULATION

The lungs are quite unique in that they have two circulatory systems in addition to a lymphatic system. These systems jointly serve in the exchange of respiratory gases.

**The Pulmonary Circulation.** The pulmonary circulation is the major circulatory system to the lungs. In contrast to the systemic circulation, the pulmonary circulation is a low pressure system capable of considerable degrees of distention. Table 1 lists the normal pressures and blood gas tensions for the pulmonary circulation of the dog. Since the pulmonary veins contain no valves, left atrial pressure may be measured indirectly by an occluding catheter placed into a small pulmonary artery (wedge pressure). Increases in pulmonary blood flow, hypoxemia, sympathetic tone and blood viscosity effect an increase in pulmonary artery pressures. Both the pulmonary arterial and wedge pressures decrease during inspiration (decrease in intrathoracic pressure) and increase during expiration (increase in intrathoracic pressure).

In addition to its function in gas exchange, the pulmonary circulation serves as a blood reservoir which regulates the venous return and thus the output of the left ventricle. This regulation is effected by various neurohumoral and hemodynamic mechanisms which can either dilate or con-

*Table 1.*  *Normal Pulmonary Values in the Dog*

| ANATOMIC SITE | PRESSURES IN MM. HG | | | PO$_2$ (MM. HG) | PCO$_2$ (MM. HG) |
| | Systolic (Range) | Diastolic (Range) | Mean (Range) | | |
|---|---|---|---|---|---|
| Right Atrium | —— | —— | 0.70† (−1.3 to +2.8) | 44 to 51 | 38 to 42 |
| Right Ventricle | 25* (16 to 35) | 0* | 11.6† (8.4 to 14.8) | 44 to 51 | 38 to 42 |
| Pulmonary Artery | 20* (15 to 25) | 10* (7 to 12) | 14.7† (8.2 to 18.2) | 44 to 51 | 38 to 42 |
| Wedge Pressure | 10* (8 to 11) | 5* (4 to 6) | 7* (6 to 8) | —— | —— |
| Femoral Artery** | —— | —— | —— | 86 to 100 | 37 to 40 |

*Data from Yarns, D. A., and Tashjian, R. J.: Cardiopulmonary values in normal and heartworm infested dogs. Am. J. Vet. Res., 28:1461, 1967.

**Blood gas values can be assumed to be equal to those in the left atrium.

†Values obtained from 10 unsedated and unanesthetized normal dogs (in cm. H$_2$0).

strict the pulmonary vascular bed. Thermal regulation is another important function of the pulmonary circulation in dogs and other mammals with limited sweat glands.

**The Bronchial Circulation.** The bronchial circulation is normally a minor contributor to the overall circulation of the lung. Single or paired bronchial arteries usually arise as branches of intercostal arteries and supply the bronchial lymph nodes, peribronchial connective tissue and bronchial mucous membranes. When the pulmonary circulation is inadequate, as in certain congenital anomalies, the bronchial circulation may expand considerably and assume a more significant role in gas exchange.

**Pulmonary Lymphatic System.** The lungs are supplied with an extensive and elaborate network of lymphatic channels located within the supporting portions of the alveolar-capillary membrane. These channels assist in removal of fluid and protein constituents which enter this membrane from the adjacent capillaries. They are functionally important in keeping the lungs dry and thus serve significantly in maintaining normal gas exchange.

## CLINICAL RECOGNITION OF PULMONARY VASCULAR DISEASE

Pulmonary vascular disease implies a process interfering with blood flow through the pulmonary circulation. This may occur as an acute process with sudden embarrassment of pulmonary blood flow or, more commonly, as a gradually progressive disease leading to pulmonary hypertension.

The dog has pulmonary hypertension when the pulmonary artery pressures exceed 25 mm. Hg systolic or 18.2 cm. of water (mean). These values can be considered to be the upper limits of normal at rest or under anesthesia. Because of the compliance of the pulmonary vascular bed, considerable and possibly irreversible changes may be present before resting pulmonary artery pressures are abnormal. Diagnosis of pulmonary hypertension is therefore facilitated by pressure recordings when vascular compliance is challenged by increased pulmonary blood flow, e.g., during exercise.

The clinical signs associated with pulmonary vascular disease will be determined in part by the underlying cause and in part by the severity of the pulmonary hypertension. These may be absent or minimal when the disease process is in its early stages. Decreased exercise tolerance may be the earliest sign. Further increases in pulmonary artery pressures result in decreased activity, exertional dyspnea, exercise-related collapsing spells and even right-sided heart failure. Clinical findings may include weight loss, mild dyspnea and/or cyanosis, abnormal lung sounds, a variety of heart murmurs and splitting of the second heart sound when pulmonary hypertension is severe. This last auscultatory abnormality is associated with late closure of the pulmonic valve. A jugular pulse, hepatomegaly and ascites will be additional findings when right-sided failure has occurred. Right-sided cardiac enlargement with or without right-sided failure resulting from impaired pulmonary function is termed cor pulmonale (pulmonary heart disease). In cor pulmonale, pulmonary artery pressures tend to be elevated at rest. Cor pulmonale can develop as the end result of gradually progressive pulmonary vascular disease or, less commonly, is due to sudden obstruction of pulmonary blood flow. In the latter case, sudden death is not uncommon.

The radiographic hallmarks of chronic cor pulmonale are right ventricular enlargement, an enlarged pulmonary artery segment (PAS) bulge and enlarged main pulmonary arties. Radiographic abnormalities tend to be absent or less characteristic in milder degrees of pulmonary hypertension, in acute cor pulmonale and when biventricular enlargement is present. On the lateral thoracic radiograph, isolated right ventricular enlargement is most typically seen as an increase in the area of cardiac-sternal contact. When right ventricular enlargement is extreme, there can be tracheal elevation and the apex of the cardiac silhouette may be lifted off the sternum. Cranial waist will be lost if the main pulmonary artery is sufficiently dilated. On the ventrodorsal thoracic radiograph, the cardiac silhouette may present a double apex when right ventricular enlargement is considerable. The distance between the right border of the cardiac silhouette and the right thoracic wall will be decreased. A PAS bulge at the 1 o'clock position may contribute to a cardiac silhouette with an inverted "D" configuration. Patchy or diffuse lung densities can assume a wide variety of distributions. These will depend upon the primary etiologic agent involved and whether or not secondary pulmonary disease processes are contributing.

Additional diagnostic procedures may be helpful and in certain instances are necessary to establish a diagnosis of pulmonary vascular disease.

**Electrocardiography.** In chronic cor pulmonale, the electrocardiogram is compatible with right ventricular hypertrophy (RVH) (Knight, 1968). Electrocardiography is less helpful in the other forms of pulmonary vascular disease which have been discussed.

**Cardiac Catheterization.** Catheterization of the right side of the heart with measurement of the main pulmonary artery pressures will occasionally be required to establish a diagnosis of chronic cor pulmonale. Abnormal elevations of pulmonary artery pressure confirm the existence of pulmonary hypertension. The inclusion of pulmonary artery angiography in the catheterization studies assists in establishing the site and extent of vascular involvement. In acute cor pulmonale, when surgical intervention is being considered, angiography is mandatory to define the site of obstruction.

Right atrial and ventricular studies should be included as part of the catheterization procedure. These permit evaluation for primary right-sided cardiac disorders as well as detection of early right-sided heart failure. When congenital heart disease or primary acquired left heart disease is felt to be contributing to the pulmonary vascular disease, left-sided cardiac catheterization studies are also indicated.

**Central Venous Pressure.** Central venous pressure (CVP), by itself, is of no assistance in differentiating between cor pulmonale and other possible causes of right-sided heart failure. When cor pulmonale is accompanied by an elevation in the CVP, the need for cardiac supportive therapy is indicated. CVP can also be used in this setting to evaluate the response to medical management.

## ETIOLOGIES OF PULMONARY VASCULAR DISEASE

Pulmonary vascular disease in the dog has many causes, both congenital and acquired (Table 2). Those causes resulting from musculoskeletal abnormalities and secondary to extracardiac hemodynamic abnormalities appear to be rare and will not be discussed here. The final result in each of the disease states described will be pulmonary hypertension, assuming sufficient chronicity and severity to effect significant pulmonary vascular changes.

**Congenital Left-to-Right Shunts.** In the presence of a pulmonary circulation with normal resistance and compliance, large congenital left-to-right intracardiac shunts tend to cause a volume overload of the left

**Table 2.** *Classification of Pulmonary Vascular Disease in the Dog*

1. Congenital Left-to-Right Shunts
   (a) Patent ductus arteriosus
   (b) Interventricular septal defects
   (c) Interatrial septal defect (with or without partial anomalous pulmonary venous drainage)
   (d) Aortopulmonary septal defect
   (e) Persistent truncus arteriosus
   (f) Persistent common atrioventricular canal
2. Pulmonary Venous Hypertension
   (a) Mitral valve insufficiency
   (b) Left ventricular failure
   (c) Cor triatriatum
3. Primary Occlusive Pulmonary Vascular Disease
   (a) Dirofilariasis
   (b) Pulmonary embolism
   (c) Pulmonary artery thrombosis
4. Diffuse Pulmonary Diseases
5. Secondary to Extracardiac Hemodynamic Abnormalities
   (a) Peripheral arteriovenous shunts
   (b) Polycythemia
6. Secondary to Musculoskeletal Abnormalities
   (a) Thoracoplasty
   (b) Pectus excavatum

ventricle and may result in left-sided heart failure at an early age. When the shunt is smaller and increased pulmonary blood flow occurs over a longer period, pulmonary hypertension and cor pulmonale may be the final results. In this setting, pulmonary hypertension results from medial and intimal changes in the pulmonary arteries secondary to chronic increased blood flow, although some feel that congenitally abnormal pulmonary vascular resistance may play a role. When the pulmonary arterial pressures become extremely elevated, right-sided heart failure or Eisenmenger's syndrome may develop. In Eisenmenger's syndrome, pulmonary hypertension is so severe that blood flow through the shunt reverses and becomes right-to-left. This syndrome must be distinguished from Eisenmenger's complex, a specific congenital cardiac anomaly in which an interventricular septal defect is accompanied by an overriding aorta.

The clinical signs associated with these complicated congenital anomalies do not differ significantly from those discussed previously. Stress- and exercise-related collapsing spells and sudden death are not uncommon. Abdominal enlargement may be the primary complaint when right heart failure is present.

The clinical findings on physical examination may be quite confusing if the congenital heart disease was previously undetected. Varying degrees of dyspnea and cyanosis may be present. Lung sounds are typically normal on auscultation. The heart murmurs normally expected with these congenital anomalies may be considerably altered or even absent. The second heart sound may be distinctly split. Cardiac arrhythmias are frequent. A jugular pulse, hepatomegaly and ascites are present when right heart failure has occurred.

A diagnosis of pulmonary hypertension secondary to congenital left-to-right intracardiac shunts may be suggested on the basis of clinical signs, physical findings and radiography, especially when congenital heart disease was previously known to be present. Biventricular enlargement is the expected finding on thoracic radiographs. Loss of cranial waist on the lateral view, a PAS bulge on the ventrodorsal view and enlarged main pulmonary arteries are visible. A hypervascular lung field will be present if a left-to-right shunt predominates. When the shunt has become balanced or reversed, pulmonary vascularity tends to be normal, and electrocardiographic findings are compatible with RVH. These electrocardiographic changes are distinctly abnormal, since the majority of isolated and uncomplicated left-to-right shunts are associated with a left ventricular hypertrophy (LVH) pattern (Harpster, 1974). When shunt reversal occurs in the presence of severe pulmonary hypertension, systemic arterial hypoxemia will be present (arterial $O_2$ saturation <92 per cent; $PaO_2$ <80 mm. Hg). Cardiac catheterization will be required to establish a definitive diagnosis. This will often require the use of all available diagnostic methods, including pressure measurements, oxygen saturation (or $PaO_2$), pulmonary vascular resistance and angiocardiography.

Treatment of congenital left-to-right intracardiac shunts complicated by severe pulmonary hypertension is generally disappointing. Once pulmonary vascular resistance approaches or exceeds 50 per cent of systemic vascular resistance, closure of the defect is usually of negligible benefit and may prove disastrous. The ideal approach lies in early diagnosis and correction of the defect before the pulmonary vascular changes occur. In those patients in which the predominant clinical manifestations are right-sided heart failure, medical management of the heart failure may be temporarily beneficial. This will include exercise restriction, a low-sodium diet, digitalis drugs and diuretics.

**Pulmonary Venous Hypertension.** Left ventricular failure is by far the most common cause of pulmonary hypertension in the dog. While the hypertension observed is less severe than that from other causes, the pathophysiology is more complex. The initial abnormality is an elevation of the left ventricular end-diastolic pressure which results in increased left atrial pressure (LAP). LAP will be further altered when mitral valve insufficiency exists. Any change in LAP will be directly reflected upon the pulmonary circulation via the unvalved pulmonary veins. The resulting pulmonary venous hypertension causes a decrease in pulmonary artery compliance and an increase in pulmonary vascular resistance, leading to pulmonary arterial hypertension. In acute left-sided heart failure, pulmonary edema decreases oxygen diffusing capacity of the lungs and increases venous admixture. The resulting systemic hypoxemia further decreases pulmonary vascular compliance via increased sympathetic stimulation to vascular smooth muscle. In chronic left-sided heart failure, thickening and fibrosis of the alveolar-capillary interstitium increases the pulmonary vascular resistance. Both the decreased vascular compliance and increased resistance accentuate pulmonary hypertension.

The clinical signs of pulmonary venous hypertension are rarely related to the pulmonary artery hypertension that develops. The congestive heart failure state and accompanying pulmonary edema are the primary pathologic factors responsible for the clinical manifestations. Coughing, decreased activity and difficulty in breathing are the presenting complaints. In chronic left heart failure, pulmonary arterial hypertension may play a significant role in the development of right-sided heart failure.

The clinical findings vary considerably depending upon the severity of the pulmonary venous hypertension. Respiration may be normal, or severe dyspnea may be present at rest. Moist rales may be limited to the hilar areas or be widespread. A murmur of mitral insufficiency is most commonly found, but coexisting murmurs may be heard. When heart disease is advanced, cardiac arrhythmias and diastolic gallop rhythms are frequently present. Varying degrees of right-sided heart failure may be evident.

A diagnosis of left ventricular failure can usually be made on the basis of clinical findings, electrocardiograms and radiographs. On thoracic radiographs, left ventricular or biventricular enlargement predominates. Left atrial enlargement is, likewise, expected. This is seen on the lateral view as loss of caudal waist, and on the ventrodorsal view as a left auricular appendage bulge at the 3 o'clock position. Pulmonary edema can be visualized as diffuse alveolar densities extending outward from the hilum. The diaphragmatic lobes are the earliest and most severely involved. Electrocardiography reveals abnormalities compatible with left atrial enlargement ("P mitrale"), and an LVH or biventricular enlargement pattern. Cardiac arrhythmias are quite common, particularly when left heart disease is advanced. Supraventricular premature beats and atrial fibrillation are seen most frequently. Laboratory tests tend to be of limited value in differentiating between the various etiologies of left ventricular disease in the dog (Table 3). Cardiac catheterization studies will be useful in differentiating between congenital and acquired diseases.

The management of left-sided heart failure has been adequately discussed previously (Harpster, 1974), and an in-depth discussion will not be included here. Successful management lies in the restoration of cardiorespiratory stability by the use of digitalis glycosides, diuretics and sodium restriction. The potential benefits and hazards

*Table 3.   Etiologies of Left Ventricular Failure in the Dog*

1. Congenital
    (a) Patent ductus arteriosus
    (b) Interventricular septal defect
    (c) Subvalvular aortic stenosis
    (d) Endocardial fibroelastosis
    (e) Mitral valve anomalies
2. Acquired
    (a) Chronic valvular-myocardial heart disease
    (b) Cardiomyopathies
    (c) Bacterial endocarditis
    (d) Tachyarrhythmias
    (e) Bradyarrhythmias
    (f) Myocardial infarction
    (g) Traumatic injuries to the mitral valve apparatus

of the digitalis glycosides must be appreciated, and proper monitoring should accompany their use. Additional therapeutic measures may be required when left heart disease is advanced (Harpster, 1974).

**Primary Occlusive Pulmonary Vascular Disease.** Primary occlusive pulmonary vascular disease implies obstruction of pulmonary blood flow by a process which reduces the luminal diameter or functional patency of the pulmonary arterial vasculature. This may result from obstruction of the main pulmonary arteries by a large embolus or thrombus, or from diffuse small vessel disease.

Infestation by the parasite, *Dirofilaria immitis,* is the most common cause of primary occlusive pulmonary vascular disease in the dog. While major, acute obstructions may occur, the disease is more frequently of a gradual and insidious onset as a result of progressive small vessel disease. These changes are seen histologically as endothelial proliferation in the smaller pulmonary arterioles and medial hypertrophy of the larger pulmonary arterioles. The intimal villous proliferation of the major pulmonary arteries seen grossly at postmortem examination contributes minimally to the pulmonary hypertension occurring in heartworm disease. Additional contributions to pulmonary disease and hypertension can result from small pulmonary emboli, thrombi and the associated inflammatory reaction, as well as from superimposed bronchopneumonia. These latter changes are potentially reversible, whereas the small vessel changes tend to be irreversible.

Other causes of occlusive pulmonary vascular disease are rare in the dog. Pulmonary embolism with or without infarction is seen occasionally in association with malignant neoplasms. In the author's experience, pheochromocytoma and right atrial hemangiosarcoma are the most common malignancies in which this occurs. Massive pulmonary thrombosis of undetermined origin has been seen in a few dogs.

The clinical signs associated with progressive diffuse small vessel disease are similar to those previously discussed. Weight loss, lethargy and reduced exercise tolerance are the earliest and mildest signs noted. A cough may or may not be reported. When severe vascular obstruction exists, exertional dyspnea and collapsing spells may occur owing to "fixed" pulmonary blood flow. Sudden death can occur during these episodes. Abdominal enlargement may be the primary complaint when right heart failure is present. The signs reported in acute and massive pulmonary artery occlusion are usually of sudden onset and include heavy breathing and weakness, progressing to collapse. Death will occur within a short period of time unless the obstruction is relieved.

On physical examination, the findings will depend on the degree of pulmonary hypertension as well as on the presence or absence of superimposed pulmonary diseases. Weight loss, a harsh hair coat and dyspnea may be noted on casual observation. Harsh airway sounds and/or scattered rales are expected when a cough is part of the clinical history. A variety of abnormalities may be heard on cardiac auscultation, including irregularities of rhythm, murmurs and splitting of the second heart sound. Coarse, clicking, holosystolic murmurs over the mitral or tricuspid areas are especially common in toy breed dogs with symptomatic heartworm disease. A jugular pulse, hepatomegaly and ascites may all be present when right heart failure has occurred. In acute pulmonary artery occlusion, the physical findings tend to be much less rewarding. In the extreme situation, marked weakness, dyspnea and a shocklike state predominate. If sudden death does not occur, right heart failure will become manifest.

The majority of dogs with primary occlusive pulmonary artery disease have heartworm disease, which can be diagnosed by the detection of circulating microfilariae in the peripheral blood. These microfilariae must be differentiated morphologically from those of *Dipetalonema reconditum*. When heartworm disease does not exist, or is not accompanied by circulating microfilariae, the diagnosis is more difficult to establish. The thoracic radiographic findings in progressive small vessel disease are similar to those described under Clinical Recognition. In heartworm disease, pulmonary densities are common. These may be seen as poorly defined, patchy areas of increased interstitial density; more diffuse interstitial densities that appear to be distributed along the pulmonary arteries and their branches; and peribronchial thickening with associated patchy alveolar densities when superimposed bronchopneumonia is present. Interlobar fissure lines may be seen.

In acute pulmonary artery occlusion, radiographic findings are considerably less helpful. The cardiac silhouette will be within normal limits unless a chronic process preceded the acute event. Pulmonary vascularity may be diminished and pleural effusion is not uncommon.

The electrocardiogram in symptomatic heartworm disease will usually demonstrate abnormalities compatible with RVH. Singly occurring supraventricular and ventricular premature beats are not unexpected. Tachyarrhythmias are unusual, although both paroxysmal supraventricular tachycardia and atrial fibrillation have been recorded. Primary T-wave changes are frequently found.

Laboratory tests do not reveal consistent abnormalities, with the exception of circulating microfilariae. Anemia, eosinophilia, proteinuria, mild to moderate elevations in serum transaminase levels (especially SGPT) and elevations in the serum beta globulin fractions may all be seen in heartworm disease. These laboratory findings neither confirm nor substantiate the diagnosis, since they may be seen in a variety of other diseases. Pulmonary angiography and specific tests for the detection of serum antibodies to microfilariae have been advocated for the diagnosis of heartworm disease in the dog without circulating microfilariae (Wong et al., 1973).

Because of its rare occurrence and rapidly fatal clinical course, acute pulmonary artery occlusion is infrequently diagnosed ante mortem, except when associated with heartworm disease. Clinical consideration of the diagnosis followed by pulmonary angiography will be necessary for antemortem confirmation.

Once a diagnosis of symptomatic heartworm disease is firmly established, a substantial attempt to improve cardiorespiratory function should be made before treatment for the adult parasites. A thorough laboratory evaluation of the patient is indicated, with particular attention focused on liver and kidney function and for evidence of pulmonary infection. Corticosteroids are most useful in resolving the previously described interstitial pulmonary densities. Prednisolone is effective at an initial dose of 0.5 to 1.0 mg./kg. body weight. Reductions in the dose are made at 4- to 5-day intervals as long as clinical and radiographic improvement continues. If superimposed bronchopneumonia is present, culture of tracheobronchial secretions will allow selection of proper antibiotic therapy. Right-sided heart failure should be treated with digitalis glycosides and diuretics. Anticoagulants may be indicated for the thromboembolic complications that occur in this disease, although their use has not been properly investigated. Exercise restriction should be enforced during this "pretreatment" period. Supportive management is continued until heart failure is stabilized, clinical signs disappear and considerable clearing of interstitial and alveolar pulmonary densities is apparent on thoracic radiographs. A return of arterial $PaO_2$ measurements to normal during this pretreatment period is an encouraging finding. When the patient's condition is sufficiently stabilized, treatment against the adult parasites can proceed. For specific information on procedures for the treatment and prevention of canine heartworm disease, the reader should refer to the A.V.M.A. Council on Veterinary Service Report (1973).

Management of the pulmonary artery occlusion syndrome is most difficult and carries a high risk. Surgical removal of the obstructing process is the only available approach at this time. Thrombolytic drugs, such as urokinase, may be useful in the less critical patient when these drugs become available for clinical use.

**Diffuse Pulmonary Disease.** A wide variety of pulmonary diseases can result in an alteration of normal pulmonary function (i.e., interfere with gaseous exchange). While clinically significant pulmonary hypertension appears to be a rare complication of the primary pulmonary diseases, it has been recognized and tends to become overtly manifest during either acute exacerbations of the primary disorder or superimposed pulmonary infection. At least three separate factors contribute to the pulmonary hypertension. Pulmonary diseases cause a diminution of the pulmonary vascular bed by cellular infiltration and/or by destruction of pulmonary vasculature. Secondary fibroelastic intimal proliferation in the small pulmonary arterioles is an additional late complication in man, but one that the author has not seen in the dog. Systemic hypoxemia contributes to the pulmonary hypertension by decreasing pulmonary vascular compliance via smooth muscle constriction mediated by the sympathetic nervous system. Further interference with pulmonary blood flow may result from secondary polycythemia, resulting from chronic systemic hypoxemia.

The reader should refer to other articles in this section for clinical information and therapeutic approaches to the common diffuse pulmonary diseases. Secondary infection is a common complication with all these diseases and must be approached vigorously to minimize additional pulmonary damage.

## DIFFERENTIAL DIAGNOSIS

Differentiation of the various disorders causing pulmonary vascular disease is, indeed, a challenge. Pure pulmonary hypertension, although rarely present by itself, results in reduced exercise tolerance, typical thoracic radiographic findings and electrocardiographic abnormalities compatible with RVH. Complications of severe pulmonary hypertension include severe dyspnea, right-sided heart failure and exercise-related collapsing spells.

The above clinical manifestations are also compatible with a group of right-sided congenital cardiac anomalies including pulmonic stenosis, tetralogy of Fallot, Eisenmenger's complex, congenital tricuspid insufficiency and Ebstein's anomaly. Only the first three of these are typically associated with electrocardiographic evidence of RVH and the expected radiographic abnormalities. While age of the patient and position of cardiac murmurs may be helpful in making a distinction from pulmonary hypertension, cardiac catheterization will be necessary to establish a firm diagnosis. With the exception of Eisenmenger's complex, the pulmonary artery pressures will be normal in all the above conditions.

The collapsing spells associated with severe pulmonary hypertension are caused by a reduced left ventricular output, which is secondary to a fixed pulmonary blood flow. Similar exertion-related episodes may result from primary left ventricular disorders, including cardiac arrhythmias, the cardiomyopathies, aortic stenosis and myocardial infarction. Unless interventricular conduction abnormalities are present, elec-

trocardiographic findings compatible with RVH are lacking in these conditions, making differentiation from pulmonary hypertension more easily accomplished. The thoracic radiographic findings in these disorders also tend to differ considerably from those seen in pulmonary hypertension. When cardiac enlargement is present, isolated left ventricular or generalized cardiac enlargement is expected.

The pericardial diseases can also reduce cardiac output and cause a right-sided heart failure–like syndrome. Beyond these similarities, however, other analogous findings are usually lacking. In rare circumstances, cardiac catheterization may be required to establish a diagnosis. This is especially true when dealing with constrictive pericarditis.

## CONCLUSIONS

This discussion has dwelt upon a widely diverse group of diseases which can cause pulmonary vascular disease, pulmonary hypertension and cor pulmonale. The specific management of pulmonary hypertension, which in some of these disorders is responsible for the majority of the clinical signs, awaits the development of specific therapeutic measures. We must, therefore, manage the primary diseases in a manner that will prevent or minimize the secondary vascular changes. This can be accomplished only by early diagnosis and the utilization of effective therapeutic approaches.

### SUPPLEMENTAL READING

A.V.M.A. Council on Veterinary Service: Report on the procedures for the treatment and prevention of canine heartworm disease. J. Am. Vet. Med. Assn., *162*:660–661, 1973.

Baum, G. L.: Textbook of Pulmonary Diseases. Boston, Little, Brown and Co., 1965.

Harpster, N. K.: Chronic valvular-myocardial heart disease in dogs. In Kirk, R. W. (ed.): Current Veterinary Therapy V. Philadelphia, W. B. Saunders Co., 1974, pp. 282–295.

Harris, P., and Heath, D.: The Human Pulmonary Circulation. London, E. and S. Livingstone, Ltd., 1962.

Knight, D. H.: Effects of Chronic *Dirofilaria immitis* Infestations on Cardiopulmonary Dynamics and Right Ventricular Activation in the Dog. Gaines Veterinary Symposium, 1968, pp. 15–23.

Wong, M. M., et al.: Dirofilariasis without circulating microfilaria: A problem in diagnosis. J. Am. Vet. Med. Assn., *163*:133–139, 1973.

# THORACIC TUMORS

ROBERT S. BRODEY, D.V.M.
*Philadelphia, Pennsylvania*

Neoplasms of the thorax are more common than is generally realized. They can be diagnosed more frequently if the practitioner employs all the diagnostic tools available, in particular, radiography, bronchoscopy, cytology, exploratory thoracotomy and necropsy. The thorax of any older dog with signs of progressive cardiorespiratory disease should be examined radiographically after a careful history is taken and a thorough physical examination is performed. The important sites and types of thoracic neoplasms are outlined in Table 1.

## PRIMARY THORACIC TUMORS

### LUNGS

In cats, primary lung tumors make up from 2.4 to below 1 per cent of all neoplasms. In dogs, they make up 1 to 0.3 per cent of all neoplasms.

The differential diagnosis of primary tumors (which are uncommon) from metastatic lung tumors (which are common) can occasionally be difficult. The patient must be given a careful clinical examination to exclude a primary extrapulmonary neoplasm. This must be correlated with detailed radiographic, surgical and necropsy findings.

The three most common primary lung tumors in dogs are adenocarcinoma, squamous cell carcinoma and anaplastic carcinoma. In some instances, more than one histologic type is present in a single tumor. Adenocarcinoma may be less malignant than the other types, but more tumors need to be studied. In cats, adenocarcinoma appears to be the most common histologic type.

Primary lung tumors can metastasize to other portions of the lung via lymphatics and blood vessels, or by transmigration of tumor cells through the alveoli and bronchioles, particularly after coughing. In some instances, a unicentric lung tumor may become disseminated throughout the lung, resulting in nodules of similar size, thus making it difficult or impossible to determine the lobe of origin. Other causes of multiple lung tumors may be multicentric tumor origin in the lung or metastasis from an extrapulmonary site.

A study of dogs with primary lung tumors in the Philadelphia area showed no urban distribution of this disease. Lung carcinomas are rare in dogs under seven years of age and occur in dogs at the average age of 10 to 11 years. There is no sex predilection, but the boxer breed shows a predisposition to this neoplasm. In one study of 29 cases, the clinical signs ranged from one week to seven months in duration, with an

*Table 1. Thoracic Neoplasms*

| SITE | PRIMARY | METASTATIC |
|---|---|---|
| Lungs | Carcinoma | Carcinoma, sarcoma and melanoma |
| Pleura | Mesothelioma | Carcinoma, sarcoma and melanoma |
| Mediastinum | Lymphosarcoma (malignant lymphoma), heart base (aortic body) tumor and neuroblastoma | Carcinoma, sarcoma and melanoma |
| Heart | Hemangiosarcoma | Carcinoma, sarcoma and melanoma |
| Esophagus | Leiomyoma (osteosarcoma or fibrosarcoma in enzootic areas of *Spirocerca lupi*) | |
| Ribs | Osteosarcoma and chondrosarcoma (rarely plasma cell myeloma) | Carcinoma, sarcoma and melanoma |

251

average period of nine and a half weeks. The most common clinical sign was a nonproductive cough of increasing severity. Dyspnea was observed in the latter stages of the disease. Five of these 29 dogs had hypertrophic osteoarthropathy. Radiographically, a solitary lung mass with or without smaller lung nodules was usually visible. In three of the 29 dogs, multiple small lung nodules of uniform size, which were seen radiographically and at necropsy, were originally thought to represent metastatic rather than primary lung neoplasia.

Bronchoscopy and the collection of bronchial washings for cytologic examination are other important diagnostic aids.

If pleural effusion contains malignant cells, thoracotomy is contraindicated because seeding of the pleura has probably already occurred. Exploratory thoracotomy is indicated if a primary lung tumor is suspected, provided preoperative chest radiograms are negative for metastases and the dog's general condition is satisfactory. Grossly, a lung tumor usually appears as a firm grayish mass occupying all or part of the lobe(s). If hilar or mediastinal lymph node involvement is present, the prognosis is even more guarded. Pneumonectomy or lobectomy should be performed if no metastatic or inoperable local disease is found.

In general, the prognosis rests on two factors: the biologic behavior of the tumor and, to a lesser extent, the time of diagnosis. Early diagnosis and treatment are essential if some of these animals are to be salvaged. Many animals that are explored surgically weeks or months after clinical signs are first evident must be euthanatized because of metastases to the lung or regional lymph node, with or without inoperable local infiltration. In others, postoperative survival may be a matter of months. Cure is primarily restricted to the few carcinomas of lower grade malignancy or to those resected prior to the onset of clinical signs.

In man, some primary oat cell tumors of the lung have been associated with hormone production. Affected patients may develop Cushing's syndrome, hyperparathyroidism, carcinoid syndrome and gynecomastia. Similar changes should be looked for in dogs with primary lung tumors. It has already been observed that some dogs with lymphosarcoma have marked hypercalcemia, suggesting that a parathormone-like substance may be elaborated by the tumor cells.

## PLEURA

Now that cytologic examinations are being carried out more commonly than in former years, pleural mesotheliomas are being detected with greater frequency in our clinic. The typical patient is a middle aged or older dog with progressive dyspnea. Marked pleural effusion is the primary radiographic finding. Thoracentesis reveals a bloody pleural fluid containing cells that can usually be recognized as malignant and may appear to be of mesothelial (pleural) origin. Thoracentesis is often followed by rapid abatement of clinical signs until sufficient effusion recurs to cause severe atelectasis.

There is usually no surgical treatment for this rare neoplasm because it often involves both the parietal and the visceral pleura. Grossly, mesothelioma simulates a productive fibrinous pleuritis rather than a neoplasm. Surgical stripping of the involved pleura might be of value, particularly in cases in which the differential diagnosis (both gross and microscopic) between mesothelioma and chronic pleuritis is difficult or impossible. Intrapleural chemotherapeutic agents have not been evaluated.

## MEDIASTINUM

**Lymphosarcoma.** Cranial mediastinal involvement is common in feline lymphosarcoma. Such cases often occur in cats less than three years of age. The Siamese cat appears to have a special breed predilection for this disease. The clinical course is characterized by progressive dyspnea. Radiographically, a large homogenous mass in the cranial mediastinum displaces the trachea dorsally and the heart and lungs caudodorsally. Pleural effusion is often present by the time the cat shows clinical signs of respiratory insufficiency.

Gross enlargement of the sternal, mediastinal and hilar lymph nodes is seen in some dogs with generalized or visceral lymphosarcoma and may cause dyspnea, cough, dysphagia and regurgitation. On rare occasions, faciocervical edema secondary to cranial vena caval compression is also present. These mediastinal masses may be apparent on survey radiographs. In some instances radiographs of the barium-filled esophagus outline the lateral or dorsal displacement of the esophagus owing to the mediastinal lesions. If pleural effusion is present cytologic examination of the pleural fluid usually reveals atypical lymphocytes and increased numbers of lymphocytes.

In a few cases, percutaneous biopsy with a Vim-Silverman biopsy needle or exploratory thoracotomy may be necessary to make a definitive diagnosis.

Surgical treatment of canine lymphosarcoma is rarely indicated because of the multicentric nature of the disease, inoperable local involvement, or both. Palliative improvement may be obtained with corticosteroids, chemotherapeutic drugs and asparaginase. If the tumor appears to be localized, radiation therapy may be employed.

Because feline lymphosarcoma is due to a specific oncogenic virus that may be present in large amounts in the saliva, nasal secretions, urine and possibly feces of affected cats, such animals should be euthanatized until more definite information concerning host specificity of the virus is available. Furthermore, the blood of other cats in the household should be examined by immunofluorescence for the presence of the feline leukemia viral antigen, as this disease is readily spread horizontally. Virus-positive, clinically normal cats represent definite hazards to other virus-negative cats, as well as potential but as yet unproven hazards to man. Some of these virus-positive cats will develop lymphosarcoma in the ensuing months or years.

**Heart Base Tumor.**   Heart base tumors (most of which arise from the aortic body, a chemoreceptor organ) usually occur in middle-aged and older brachycephalic dogs, particularly boxers and Boston terriers. Some of these tumors are small, cause no clinical signs and are detected only as an incidental finding at necropsy. In the more extensive tumors, clinical signs, such as muffled heart sounds and congestive heart failure, are related to hemopericardium due to intrapericardial hemorrhage from the tumors(s). Further signs of passive venous congestion, i.e., edema of head, neck, forelegs and cranial sternal areas, are associated with neoplastic obstruction of the cranial vena cava, whereas ascites, hepatomegaly and often hind limb edema are observed with caudal vena caval obstruction. If both venae cavae are obstructed, quadrilateral limb edema may be present.

A mass at the base of the heart that displaces the tracheal bifurcation is often visible radiographically. In dogs with marked hemopericardium, the cardiac outline is greatly enlarged and almost uniformly rounded, particularly in the ventrodorsal projection. Pericardiocentesis (at the lower left third or fourth intercostal space) reveals a bloody fluid which, unlike blood, fails to clot when left standing. In the differential diagnosis of lesions causing hemopericardium, one should consider heart base tumor, hemangiosarcoma, idiopathic pericarditis with effusion and cracked left atrium.

In either of the two previously mentioned neoplasms, cytologic examination of the pericardial fluid may reveal malignant cells. However, non-neoplastic exfoliating mesothelial cells may take on bizarre appearances and may simulate malignant cells. This cellular differentiation can be made only by a competent cytologist.

If the clinical diagnosis is still not apparent after radiographic and cytologic studies, a left lateral thoracotomy at the fourth interspace should be performed. The heart base tumor appears as a firm, often nodular grayish mass between the aortic arch and pulmonary artery. It often invades the right atrial wall and thus may give rise to electrocardiographic abnormalities and detectable arrhythmias. The tumor may also implant over the epicardium and the inner surface of the fibrous pericardium. In a few instances, it metastasizes to the lungs and other distant sites. Complete surgical removal is rarely feasible after clinical signs have developed, because the lesion has usually infiltrated vital structures. Aspiration of the pericardial fluid or fenestration of the pericardium temporarily relieves the cardiac tamponade.

**Neuroblastoma.**   This rather rare neoplasm occurs most frequently in brachycephalic dogs. It may arise from the cranial mediastinal sympathetic ganglia and form a mass that gives rise to signs similar to those observed with other mediastinal neoplasms.

## HEART

Primary cardiac tumors, other than hemangiosarcomas, are rare. Hemangiosarcoma, although infrequent, should always be considered in the differential diagnosis of a tumor in the heart area. This tumor of vascular endothelial origin usually arises from the right atrial appendage. Because of its great vascularity and friability, hemopericardium is common. Presumptive diagnosis is based on the radiographic findings of pericardial effusion and the cytologic examination of the bloody pericardial aspirate. Definitive diagnosis is made after opening the pericardial sac at exploratory surgery or necropsy. Metastases to the lungs and other organs, including the spleen, are common.

## ESOPHAGUS

Tumors of the esophagus are rarely associated with clinical signs except for osteosarcomas and fibrosarcomas of the caudal thoracic esophagus, which are observed in dogs (primarily hunting breeds) of the southeastern United States. These sarcomas are related to the esophageal granulomas caused by the nematode parasite *Spirocerca lupi*. The resultant tumors are associated with progressive dysphagia, regurgitation, weight loss and, in many instances, hypertrophic osteoarthropathy. Radiographically, a large irregular filling defect in the caudal thoracic esophagus can be outlined after a barium meal is given. Metastatic lung nodules are common, and a characteristic ventral hypertrophic spondylosis is usually seen in the thoracic vertebrae directly above the esophageal sarcoma. Further confirmation of the diagnosis can be made by esophagoscopy and the detection of S. *lupi* ova in the feces or esophageal aspirate. If the diagnosis is still in doubt, an exploratory thoracotomy (left lateral) is indicated. Unfortunately, there is no satisfactory treatment for this lesion because of the extensive local involvement and the frequency of metastases.

Small submucosal leiomyomas are occasionally observed in the region of the esophagogastric junction, but they rarely become large enough to produce clinical signs. Gradual, progressive esophageal obstruction, associated with radiographic evidence of a smooth spherical mass in the distal region of the esophagus in an older dog (particularly in a nonenzootic area for S. *lupi*), should suggest the possibility of leiomyoma. Treatment is transthoracic esophagotomy and excision of the lesion. The prognosis should be excellent.

Epithelial tumors are rare in the dog, although a few squamous cell carcinomas have been observed. In Great Britain, squamous cell carcinoma of the cranial portion of the thoracic esophagus has been ob-

served in a number of cats. This lesion i either vary rare or nonexistent in Nort American cats.

## RIBS

Osteosarcomas, chondrosarcomas and less frequently, other sarcomas arise from the costochondral rib junctions, particularl of the more caudal ribs in large breed dog two to eight years of age. Osteosarcom grows rapidly, may infiltrate the adjacen ribs, diaphragm and pericardium and almos invariably metastasizes to the lungs. Al though the affected rib(s) may be excised the lungs are not grossly involved, th prognosis is poor because of early recui rence, metastasis, or both.

Chondrosarcoma usually grows moi slowly than osteosarcoma and metastasize much later in the course of the disease. Th histologic differentiation of chondrosai coma from chondroma may be very difficu and, in some cases, impossible. Most ca tilaginous rib tumors should be considere sarcomas until proved otherwise. Surgica excision of the involved rib(s) is often cura tive. If the tumor has broken through th parietal pleura, implantation metastases ai common.

Any dog having a rib tumor but not show ing lung metastases radiographically shoul be explored surgically in the hope that th lesion is chondrosarcoma. The surgeo should realize that the medial extension of rib tumor often greatly exceeds its later; swelling. A tumor in the shaft of the ri some distance from the costochondral junc tion probably is a metastatic rather than primary lesion.

## METASTATIC THORACIC NEOPLASMS

Metastatic lung disease is common an far exceeds primary lung neoplasia in fr quency of occurrence in both dogs and cat It is important to recognize that many dog with pulmonary metastases show no sigr referable to lung disease. Therefore preoperative chest radiograms (two view are indicated in animals with malignancie arising from sites that commonly produc lung metastases. Some important neoplasm in this category are: adenocarcinoma of th mammary gland; osteosarcoma of bone melanoma of the mouth and skin; carcinoma of the thyroid, tonsil and kidney; and hemangiosarcoma of the spleen. In general, lung lesions must exceed the diameters of the cross sections of the pulmonary vessels in order to be recognized radiographically. Typically, discrete, rounded nodular densities are observed. In some instances, diffuse miliary tumor infiltration of the lungs, associated with massive lymphangitic spread, may be confused with pneumonic consolidation. If the radiographs are considered suspicious but not conclusive, a second series several weeks later usually indicates an increase in size and number of neoplastic lesions.

Surgical treatment of lung metastases is rarely indicated because multiple lung lobes are usually involved. On rare occasions, however, a solitary lung metastasis detected radiographically may be an indication for exploratory surgery and possible lobectomy if the other lobes are free of tumors.

Metastases to the mediastinum, pleura, heart and ribs are more commonly detected by the pathologist than the clinician. However, changes such as greatly enlarged mediastinal or hilar lymph nodes or lytic rib shaft lesions can often be seen radiographically. Extensive pleural metastases may be manifested by marked (usually bloody) pleural effusion, which can be aspirated and examined cytologically.

### SUPPLEMENTAL READING

Craig, P. H., and Brodey, R. S.: Primary pulmonary neoplasms in the dog; a review of 29 cases. J. Am. Vet. Med. Assn., 147:1628–1643, 1965.
Moulton, J. E.: Tumors in Domestic Animals. Berkeley, Calif., University of California Press, 1961.
Nielson, S. W., and Horava, A.: Primary pulmonary tumors of the dogs, a report of sixteen cases. Am. J. Vet. Res., 21:813–830, 1960.

# PLEURAL EFFUSIONS

STANLEY R. CREIGHTON, D.V.M
W. Los Angeles, California

and ROBERT J. WILKINS, B.V.Sc.
New York, New York

## INTRODUCTION

Many diseases affect the pleura and result in the accumulation of abnormal volumes of fluid within the pleural space. In healthy animals, the pleural space is a potential space containing only a few milliliters of lubricating serous fluid. A constant volume of fluid is maintained because the rate of fluid formation is equal to the rate of fluid absorption. Abnormal pleural effusions occur when an underlying disease process upsets the normal homeostatic mechanisms of the pleura and allows increased volumes of fluid to collect in the pleural space. Pleural effusion is therefore a clinical sign and not a final diagnosis, and it is the clinician's duty to determine the exact underlying etiology of the effusion.

The pleura is a serous membrane composed of a single layer of flat mesothelial cells and a strong underlying fibroelastic layer containing the pleural lymphatics, arteries, veins and capillaries. The visceral pleura completely covers the lungs and continues onto the mediastinum and diaphragm, forming the mediastinal pleura. The thoracic wall is covered by the parietal pleura. In the normal animal, the visceral, parietal and mediastinal pleurae are separated by a thin film of normal pleural fluid which facilitates movement of the thoracic viscera during the respiratory and cardiac cycles. The mediastinum incompletely divides the pleural cavity into two compartments which communicate with each other in most dogs and cats, and therefore most effusions are bilateral. Abundant lymphatics and microscopic pores in the diaphragm allow communication between the peritoneal and pleural spaces. This feature may result in both pleural and peritoneal effusion from a single isolated lesion.

Normal fluid formation occurs through a transudative process and follows Starling's law. The majority of fluid originates from the parietal pleura, and the water and electrolytes are absorbed by capillaries and lymphatics of the visceral pleura. Absorption of protein occurs only through the lymphatics of the parietal and mediastinal pleura. Pleural lymphatics can also absorb water and electrolytes, and when abnormal quantities of fluid are present, this lymphatic reserve is mobilized to help remove fluid from the pleural cavities.

Abnormal fluids accumulate in the pleural space as a result of transudative and exudative processes. Most fluids accumulate as a result of increased fluid production rather than decreased absorption by the pleura. The increased production of fluid is usually caused by increased vascular hydrostatic pressure, decreased plasma osmotic pressure or inflammation of the pleura. The effusion undergoes a dynamic process of continuous formation and resorption. Because the fluid is not static, the physical, biochemical and cytologic features of the effusion change as the fluid remains in the pleural space. Results of fluid analysis will therefore vary depending on the rate of fluid formation, the duration of the illness and the response to treatment.

Cellular components which gain access to the pleural space through transudative processes such as increased hydrostatic pressure due to venous or lymphatic obstruction will eventually die and degenerate. This process releases cellular components which are chemotactic for neutrophils, macrophages and other inflammatory cells. The secondary inflammatory response which occurs in fluids that entered the pleural cavities through transudative processes is very common. These effusions are called modified transudates, because an inflammatory component (exudate) has been added to the original transudate. Modified transudates have many of the traditional characteristics of exudates, and cytologic evaluation is required if the nature of the effusion is to be determined.

## Clinical signs

The history and clinical signs are variable and depend upon the etiology of the effusion, the rate of fluid formation, the quantity of fluid and the type of fluid present. Small quantities of fluid usually do not produce signs and are difficult or impossible to detect radiographically. As the volume of fluid increases, the ability of the lungs to expand is compromised. This results in a decreased total lung capacity and tidal volume. In se vere effusions, the lungs may be partially or completely collapsed. These local areas of compression atelectasis result in a mis matching of ventilation and perfusion. Clin ical signs due to pleural effusion are usually a result of gas exchange abnormalities.

The most consistent sign is labored breathing. The animal's thorax may undergo a greater than normal excursion during the respiratory cycle. Abdominal breathing oc curs with severe effusions, and the whole animal may move during efforts to breathe Occasionally there is mouth-breathing, and the neck and head may be kept in an ex tended and elevated position. Some animal are reluctant to lie down and will stand with the elbows abducted. Others will rest only on their sternum with the head elevated. In general, animals with moderate to severe degrees of dyspnea and respiratory distress have very little remaining respiratory re serve, and even the slightest stress may re sult in respiratory arrest. The temperamen of the animal should be considered and minimal restraint used during physica examination or diagnostic procedures.

Coughing is sometimes seen and is usu ally nonproductive. It usually occurs with inflammatory diseases of the pleura but may result from lung involvement in the under lying disease process.

Auscultation of the lungs and heart ofter reveals muffled heart and lung sounds. In severe effusions the only functional lung tissue auscultated may be in the dorsal posterior portion of the thorax. Trapped pleural fluid may result in a local area o decreased or absent lung sounds.

Nonspecific extrathoracic signs are some times present and may be very helpful since they usually reflect the underlying etiology of the effusion. For example, a car diac arrhythmia may indicate that the effu sion is due to cardiac failure, or subcutane ous edema may indicate that hypoal buminemia is the etiology of the effusion Anorexia, weight loss, depression and de hydration may be complicating factors of wide variety of illnesses.

## Radiographic evaluation

Radiographic examination is an essentia part of the medical work-up when pleura effusion is suspected. Radiographs will an swer three important questions:

1. Is an effusion present?
2. Where is the most suitable site for thoracocentesis?
3. Is there any additional pathologic condition present which may indicate the source of the effusion?

Small quantities of fluid are usually not visible radiographically. When greater quantities of fluid are present, the most commonly observed changes are a loss of detail and increased density within the thorax. The cardiac silhouette may be obscured and the mediastinum widened. There is rounding of the lung borders at the costophrenic angles, and fluid-filled fissures may be present between lung lobes. The ventral lung lobe borders may appear scalloped. The visceral pleura may retract from the parietal pleura, making the pleural space visible.

Pleural thickening without effusion may be the result of active pleuritis or may be the sequela to prior episodes of effusion with scarring and fibrosis. Pleural thickening is sometimes an incidental finding in older animals.

Routine radiographic examination of the thorax should include both dorsoventral and lateral projections. Special techniques such as the standing lateral or lateral decubitus projections will demonstrate if the fluid is freely movable, trapped or encapsulated within fibrin adhesions. In dyspneic animals, careful restraint should be utilized to avoid any undue stress. It is better to postpone or cancel a procedure rather than risk the life of the animal by performing diagnostic tests.

In severe pleural effusions, there is usually little doubt radiographically that an effusion is present, but much of the detail within the thorax is obscured by the fluid. In these cases, as much fluid should be removed from the thorax as possible and the radiographs should be repeated. This will allow better visualization of the thoracic viscera and may indicate the underlying etiology of the effusion.

## LABORATORY EVALUATION

A routine hemogram, urinalysis and biochemical screen is indicated for every animal with pleural effusion because of the many diseases which can cause the condition. Biochemical tests should include BUN and total protein and albumin as well as liver function tests.

## THORACOCENTESIS AND CHEST DRAINAGE

In most cases of pleural effusion, complete laboratory evaluation of a fluid sample is necessary for a definitive diagnosis. Fluid can be obtained by means of thoracocentesis or closed chest tube drainage.

Thoracocentesis is a simple procedure which can also be used to drain the pleural cavity. Closed chest tube drainage is indicated (1) in severe or recurrent pleural effusions; (2) when the fluid is viscous, trapped or encapsulated; (3) following most thoracic surgery; and (4) as a route of therapy when lavage is used in the treatment of pyothorax.

The site of thoracocentesis is best determined after a careful review of the thoracic radiographs. If the fluid is diffuse, the seventh or eighth intercostal space is used. The size of the needle used will depend upon the size of the animal. An 18- to 20-gauge, 1″ sterile needle is satisfactory for average dogs. Suitable small flexible catheters which pass over or through a needle are sometimes used, especially if very small amounts of fluid are present.* A short, flexible tube placed between the needle and syringe makes thoracocentesis safer and easier, because the needle can be controlled and the syringe moved without fear of lacerating the thoracic viscera. A three-way valve attached to the syringe allows drainage without repeated chest aspirations.

The area to be aspirated should be clipped and scrubbed. Infiltration with a local anesthetic occasionally makes the procedure more acceptable to the animal. The needle should be placed below the level of the effusion and midway between the ribs to prevent damage to the intercostal vessels or nerves located posterior to each rib. Once the needle is under the skin, a small amount of negative pressure is placed on the syringe to prevent unnecessarily deep penetration by the needle and to allow fluid to flow into the syringe as soon as the pleural space is entered. Excessive movement of the needle or the animal should be avoided to prevent damage to the heart and lungs. Aspiration should be continued until 3 to 6 ml. of fluid is collected for laboratory evaluation or until the chest is completely drained. In order to drain both pleural

---

*Bardic Inside Needle Catheter, C. R. Bard Inc., Murray Hill, New Jersey 07974.

cavities completely it is usually necessary to aspirate both sides of the chest. Free fluid moves under the influence of gravity and gentle movement and lateral positioning before or during thoracocentesis sometimes increases the total fluid volume removed from each pleural cavity.

Various techniques for closed chest tube drainage have been described. In each case a large-bore, flexible catheter is placed within the pleural cavity and attached to a gravity flow or suction device for intermittent or continuous drainage of the chest.* These tubes can be left in place for days until the effusion has stopped. Closed chest tube drainage is well tolerated by both dogs and cats. The advantages of this technique over thoracocentesis are (1) repeated needle punctures can be avoided if large volumes of fluid are continuously being formed, (2) the volume and character of the fluid can be monitored each day and (3) it provides a route for the administration of various medications. In addition, fluid too viscous to be aspirated through a needle can sometimes be adequately removed through a large-bore chest drain.

Iatrogenic pneumothorax is a potential complication of both needle thoracocentesis and closed chest tube drainage. A small amount of air in the thorax of a normal animal is usually well tolerated. In an animal with pleural effusion, the effects of even small degrees of pneumothorax are more severe because cardiopulmonary function is already severely compromised. Needles, syringes, connectors and tubing should be carefully examined before the pleural space is entered to avoid this unnecessary complication.

## FLUID EVALUATION

Three to 6 ml. of fluid should be aseptically collected by thoracocentesis or closed chest tube drainage for laboratory evaluation. About 0.5 ml. of the aspirated effusion is immediately placed in a sterile container for subsequent bacteriologic evaluation. The remaining fluid is placed in an anticoagulant tube containing a small amount of EDTA. The physical appearance of the fluid is noted.

Laboratory testing should be performed as soon as possible. The total white blood cell and red blood cell counts are determined, and the myeloid:erythroid ratio calculated. The fluid is centrifuged at 300 RPM for five minutes to concentrate the cellular material. The supernatant is poured into a clean container, and the specific gravity and total protein are determined using Refractometer®.† A fluid volume equal to the approximate volume of the concentrated cellular material is left in the centrifuge tube so that the cells can be adequately resuspended. A small drop of the cell-rich fluid is placed on a glass slide and a thin smear is made. The smear is rapidly air dried and stained with a suitable stain, such as Wright's stain.

If the effusion is hemorrhagic, centrifugation will separate the red blood cells from the diagnostic inflammatory, mesothelial or neoplastic cells which form an upper white layer (buffy coat). In these cases, a sample of the buffy coat is aspirated with a capillary pipette before the supernatant is poured off. A drop of the buffy coat is placed on a glass slide and a smear is made as before.

When milky white effusions are aspirated, the presence of chylomicrons is detected by determining the degree of clearing of the lipid fraction of the fluid in a fat solvent such as ether. The supernatant fluid is divided into two equal aliquots. One to two drops of 1N sodium hydroxide is added to each tube to make the pH greater than 8.0. To one tube, an equal volume of ether is added, and to the other, an equal volume of water is added. The tubes are then mixed. The white color of the sample containing ether will clear completely when compared to the sample containing water if the effusion contains chylomicrons. A partial or lack of clearing of the white color indicates that the effusion does not contain chylomicrons and this is called a pseudochylous effusion. Milky white pleural effusions are not always pathognomonic of rupture of the thoracic duct, and further evaluation of these fluids is necessary if their source is to be determined.

## PATTERNS OF PLEURAL EFFUSION

Determination of the specific gravity and total protein of the effusion is an important part in the complete analysis of the fluid but this information alone can be misleading

---

*Brunswick Feeding Tube®, Brunswick Labs, 5836 W. 117th Place, Worth, Illinois 60482.

†American Optical Refractometer®, American Optical Co., Buffalo, New York.

ing and many times does not determine the etiology of the effusion. Traditionally, fluids are classified as transudates or exudates, based on the specific gravity and total protein content of the fluid, but this approach does not consider the important concept of dynamic fluid modification and the formation of modified transudates. Terms such as hydrothorax, hemothorax and pleuritis do not help in an understanding of the pathophysiology of the many different types of fluid formation. Cytologic evaluation of the fluid is the single most important step in fluid analysis. It is now apparent that diseases of specific organ systems produce characteristic patterns of effusion. By using the physical, biochemical and cytologic findings to classify the pattern of effusion, it is possible to predict which organ system and, in some cases, which disease is responsible for the effusion (Table 1).

The general cytologic features of pleural fluid should be evaluated before determining the pattern of effusion. This is done by determining the following:

1. Is the fluid inflammatory or non-inflammatory in nature? Inflammatory pleural effusions contain many neutrophils, macrophages, lymphocytes, plasma cells, mesothelial cells and, less commonly, eosinophils and mast cells. Acute inflammation is characterized by a predominance of granulocytes, while chronic inflammation features a dominance of mononuclear cells. Noninflammatory effusions have a very low cell content, specific gravity and total protein.

2. Is the fluid septic or sterile? Septic effusions contain microorganisms and evidence of active inflammation and phagocytosis. In nonseptic effusions, there is an absence of microorganisms but the fluid may be inflammatory or noninflammatory in nature.

3. Does the fluid contain neoplastic cells? If a tumor is responsible for the pleural effusion, the presence of neoplastic cells in the effusion will depend on the type of tumor and its location, the tendency for the tumor to exfoliate cells and the risk of a sampling error. Normal lining mesothelial cells are very sensitive and become reactive when any type of pleural effusion is present. Reactive mesothelial cells are large and have a basophilic cytoplasm. They may appear alone or in clusters and may be incorrectly called neoplastic cells. They must

be differentiated from true neoplastic conditions.

Once the general cytologic features are determined, the pleural effusion should be classified into one of seven different patterns of effusion. These are pure transudative, hemorrhagic, inflammatory, obstructive, chylous, neoplastic and pyogranulomatous.

**Pure Transudates.** These fluids are usually water clear and have a specific gravity of less than 1.013 and a very low total protein. The fluid usually contains very few cells. Long-standing pure transudative effusions may become modified transudates and contain more cells and protein than would be expected. A complete medical evaluation is necessary in these cases to document hypoalbuminemia. Severe hypoalbuminemia (serum albumin less than 1.0 gm. per 100 ml.) due to glomerulonephritis, renal amyloidosis, protein-losing enteropathy, hepatic failure or following major surgery is the most common etiology of pure transudative effusions.

Other physical findings which are sometimes seen with this type of pleural effusion include abdominal effusion and pitting edema of the limbs, face and scrotum. Laboratory evaluation will reveal hypoalbuminemia and possible alterations in liver or renal function. A urinalysis may reveal proteinuria.

**Hemorrhagic Effusions.** These effusions result from free hemorrhage into the pleural cavity. The cell counts, specific gravity, total protein, myeloid:erythroid ratio and cytologic evaluation are compatible with those in the peripheral blood. Long-standing hemorrhagic effusions may contain reactive mesothelial cells and a mild inflammatory component due to modification of the fluid. Blood-tinged fluids should not be classified as hemorrhagic effusions unless the packed cell volume approximates that of blood.

Blood within the pleural cavity undergoes rapid defibrination and does not remain clotted. It can be easily aspirated and has the same radiographic appearance as any pleural effusion. If an intercostal vessel or pulmonary vessel is accidentally tapped during thoracocentesis, the aspirated blood in this sample will clot, indicating that the blood is not from the pleural cavity. Platelets will be obvious in the latter case, a feature not seen in defibrinated effusions.

Table 1. *Classification and Etiologies of Pleural Effusions**

| DETERMINANTS OF CLASSIFICATION | PURE TRANSUDATE | OBSTRUCTIVE EFFUSION | INFLAMMATORY EFFUSION Septic | Sterile |
|---|---|---|---|---|
| Physical Appearance | Clear | Serous to serosanguineous | Serous, serosanguineous or purulent | |
| Specific Gravity | <1.013 | 1.013–1.040 | 1.021–1.033 | |
| Total Protein (gm./100 ml.)* | <1.0 | 1.0–7.2 | 2.8–5.1 | |
| Coagulation | None | May clot | None | Usually none |
| Common Causes | Severe hypo-albuminemia. | Heart failure: cardiomyopathy; cardiac anomalies; pulmonary atelectasis; lung torsion; diaphragmatic hernia; thromboemboli; mediastinal tumors; other tumors. | Pyothorax; extension of infection from lungs, trachea, esophagus, mediastinum; hematogenous; foreign bodies; idiopathic. | Pleuritis; diaphragmatic hernia; thoracic surgery, chest drains; steatitis; infection; idiopathic. |

*Modified from Creighton, S. R., and Wilkins, R. J.: Thoracic effusions in the cat. J. Am. Animal Hosp. Assn., 11:66–76, 1975.

Hemorrhagic effusions occur most commonly following thoracic trauma and occasionally following thoracic surgery. Trauma can rupture any of the systemic and pulmonary vessels near the pleural surface and allow blood to enter the pleural cavity. Rupture of a major vessel leads to significant hemothorax and systemic signs of blood loss such as tachycardia, pale mucous membranes, hypothermia and shock. Bleeding from rupture of pulmonary vessels tends to be self-limiting as the degree of hemothorax increases, owing to reduced blood pressure and increased hydrostatic pressure. The blood pressure in these vessels is lower than the systemic pressure, and as the lungs collapse owing to the hemorrhagic effusion, the active bleeding stops.

Animals with hemorrhagic effusions must be monitored closely to determine whether the condition is remaining stable or worsening. Systemic signs of blood loss should be monitored. Progressive respiratory distress and increasing amounts of pleural effusion will require thoracocentesis or closed chest tube drainage. Blood within the pleural cavity is rapidly reabsorbed, so that complete chest drainage may not be necessary in these cases. The advantages of autotransfusion and the possibility of a moderate degree of hemorrhagic effusion causing spontaneous hemostasis due to compression must be measured against the degree of dyspnea and respiratory distress when deciding how much of the fluid to remove from the pleural cavity. Severe or progressive blood loss will require blood transfusions and possibly an emergency exploratory thoracotomy.

Clotting defects such as occur in thrombocytopenia or warfarin poisoning can cause hemorrhagic effusions. Other causes include clotting defects; parasites, such as Dirofilaria; bleeding hemangiosarcomas of the heart, lungs or pleura; other tumors which may erode blood vessels; and lung lobe torsions. Treatment in these cases is directed toward the primary lesion as well as toward control and monitoring of the hemorrhagic effusion. (See article on "Lower Respiratory Tract Trauma.")

**Inflammatory Effusions.** Acute inflammatory effusions contain large numbers of neutrophils and moderate numbers of lymphocytes and macrophages. As the inflammatory component of the effusions becomes more chronic, the proportion of mononuclear inflammatory cells and reactive mesothelial cells increases. Septic inflammatory effusions contain visible microorganisms.

The severity of the inflammatory process can be estimated from the morphology of the cells present. In severe, overwhelming, suppurative pyothorax there are large numbers of free and phagocytized bacteria, toxic necrosis and degeneration of the neutrophils. The nuclei undergo karyolysis and karyorrhexis, which indicates rapid cell death, as opposed to nuclear pyknosis, which indicates a slower rate of death. The identity of many cells may be difficult to determine. In less severe cases, microorganisms may be absent or only within neutrophils, indicating that the infection is contained by the inflammatory response. In mild, nonseptic inflammatory effusions, toxic neutrophils are absent, nuclear mor-

**Table 1.**  *Classification and Etiologies of Pleural Effusions (Continued)*

| PYOGRANULOMATOUS EFFUSION | CHYLOUS EFFUSION | NEOPLASTIC EFFUSION | HEMORRHAGIC EFFUSION |
|---|---|---|---|
| Straw-colored | Milky white | Usually blood-tinged | Blood red |
| 1.027–1.045 | —— | 1.015–1.045 | 1.030–1.045 |
| 4.1–8.5 | —— | 1.5–7.5 | 4.5–7.5 |
| May clot | Usually none | May clot | None |
| Feline infectious peritonitis; other granulomatous diseases of the pleura. | Ruptured thoracic duct or other lymphatic abnormality; trauma; neoplasm; cardiomyopathy; chronic pleuritis. | Lymphosarcoma; metastatic carcinoma or adenocarcinoma; mesothelioma; other tumors. | Trauma; lung torsion; postoperative; thrombosis; tumors; coagulopathies. |

phology is intact and each cell is readily identifiable. Serial evaluation of inflammatory effusions is very helpful when assessing the animal's response to treatment. A favorable prognosis is indicated if an effusion originally containing large numbers of toxic neutrophils and many microorganisms changed to one containing normal intact neutrophils without microorganisms after appropriate therapy for pyothorax.

Infectious agents are the most common cause of inflammatory effusions, and the etiologic agent may be readily visible in smears of pleural fluid. Microorganisms isolated include *Pasteurella multocida, Streptococcus spp., E. coli, Pseudomonas spp., Staphylococcus spp., Actinomyces spp., Nocardia spp., Klebsiella spp., Proteus spp., Enterobacter spp., Corynebacterium spp., Bacterioides spp., Cryptococcus spp., Toxoplasma spp.* and *Aspergillus spp.* Many viral diseases affecting the respiratory tract of dogs and cats can, through extension of inflammation to the pleura, initiate an inflammatory effusion into the thoracic cavity.

The route of entry of the infecting agent is variable. Pleural involvement may be a result of (a) extension of infections from the lung, mediastinum or diaphragm; (b) penetrating wounds of the thorax, esophagus or neck; (c) hematogenous spread of the infectious agent to the pleura (e.g., feline infectious peritonitis); (d) contaminated foreign bodies such as grass awns or sticks; and (e) secondary infection of an already established pleural effusion. Finally, pyothorax can occur with no previous history of respiratory illness or thoracic trauma.

The clinical and radiographic findings are similar to those seen with any pleural effusion. Elevation of the body temperature is not a consistent finding and in chronically ill or debilitated animals the temperature may be subnormal.

Needle thoracocentesis will relieve respiratory distress and obtain a sample of fluid for laboratory evaluation. Treatment programs have included the use of broad-spectrum systemic and intrapleural antibiotics, intrapleural infusion of enzyme solutions containing chymotrypsis,* repeated thoracocentesis and thoracotomy. With the use of closed chest tube drainage the pleural cavities can be repeatedly lavaged with solutions containing saline, antibiotics and proteolytic enzymes. This aids in sterilization of the pleural cavities by dilution and removal of infected and necrotic material and breaks down fibrinous adhesions. The volume of lavage solution administered depends on the size of the animal. A volume of 100 ml. is administered twice daily in cats and small dogs. One-half the usual systemic dose of a broad-spectrum antibiotic such as chloromycetin or gentamicin and 5000 NF units of chymotrypsin per 100 ml. is added to the lavage solution. The same antibiotic used in the lavage solution should be used systemically at the recommended dose. Bacterial culture and sensitivity testing is essential for successful long-term management of pyothorax. For example, Nocardia pyothorax is best treated with penicillin and sulfadiazine. With la-

*Kymar Aqueous®, Armour and Co., Omaha, Nebraska 68103.

vage, pyothorax carries a reasonably fair prognosis. As with other forms of serosal lavage, careful monitoring of total serum protein, electrolytes, body temperature and cytology of the effusion is essential.

Therapy can be evaluated by progressive changes in the cytologic findings which include a decrease in the number of white blood cells, a change in cell type from predominately neutrophils to mononuclear cells, normal morphology of the inflammatory cells and a significant decrease in the number of bacteria. The duration of therapy is determined by the clinical response, radiographic and visual evidence of a decreasing rate of fluid formation and progressive improvement in the cytologic picture.

Complications of pyothorax include atelectasis, constrictive pleuritis, fibrous adhesions and sepsis.

Idiopathic inflammatory effusions are uncommon. There is no history of prior illness or trauma, and no obvious etiologic agents are seen microscopically. Treatment is symptomatic with routine broad-spectrum antibiotics and good supportive care. The prognosis is fair but the pleural inflammation tends to recur.

Closed chest tube drains and other such foreign objects in the pleural cavity will, by themselves, incite a mild sterile inflammatory effusion. The volume of fluid formed each day is usually less than 50 ml. in an average dog. This is a normal response of the pleura, and the fluid production will cease when the inciting agent is removed.

**Obstructive Effusions.** These effusions occur as a result of increased venous or lymphatic hydrostatic pressure due to obstruction, constriction or congestion of lymph or blood vessels. Initially these effusions contain a mixture of erythrocytes and lymphocytes with small numbers of neutrophils, eosinophils, macrophages and mesothelial cells. As the effusion becomes modified by the secondary inflammatory response of the pleura, the proportion of neutrophils and other inflammatory cells increases. Mesothelial cells may become very reactive and must be distinguished from neoplastic cells. These effusions are distinguished from pure nonseptic inflammatory effusions by the large number of erythrocytes and lymphocytes present.

The most common cause of obstructive effusions is heart failure. In the dog, this occurs when congenital anomalies or acquired heart disease results in right-sided heart failure or a combination of left- and right-sided congestive heart failure. In cats cardiomyopathy accounts for almost 80 per cent of obstructive effusions and congenital cardiac anomalies account for the remainder. Other causes include atelectasis of the lung with obstruction of blood and lymph vessels; diaphragmatic hernias, especially if the liver is herniated; constrictive pericarditis or pericardial effusion, which may occlude vessels near the heart and cause an increased hydrostatic pressure; and tumors which grow and compress vessels and lymphatics. Diagnosis depends on ruling out the various causes of obstructive effusions, and specific therapy depends upon the etiology.

**Chylous Effusions.** A complex network of lymphatic vessels and the thoracic duct transport intestinal lymph from the abdominal cavity to the systemic venous circulation near the heart. Any alteration in this lymphatic system which allows lymph to enter the pleural cavity results in a true chylous effusion. These effusions contain chylomicrons derived from intestinal lymph and have an opaque or translucent, white, milky appearance after centrifugation. When these effusions are alkalinized and mixed with an equal volume of ether, the chylomicrons dissolve and the white color clears completely, leaving a serous, straw-colored, clear fluid.

True chylous effusions contain large numbers of normal small and large lymphocytes mixed with small numbers of erythrocytes. Smudge cells, irregularly shaped free nucleoprotein from lysed lymphocytes, are consistently found in fluids containing large amounts of lymph. Neutrophils, eosinophils, macrophages and mesothelial cells are relatively few in number. When stained supravitally with Sudan III, the chylomicrons are easily recognized as small orange droplets.

When true chylous effusions remain in the pleural cavity for long periods of time, the fluid becomes modified. The relative number of neutrophils, plasma cells, macrophages and mesothelial cells increases. Secondary bacterial infection is rare because of the bacteriostatic properties of chyle.

True chylous effusions occur most commonly following thoracic trauma. Other important etiologies include tumors which in vade or obstruct the thoracic lymphatic system, thrombosis of the anterior vena cava near the termination of the thoracic duct due to thrombophlebitis, complications of intrathoracic surgery or congenital malformations of the thoracic duct.

The diagnosis of true chylothorax is based on the history, physical examination, radiology and the results of fluid analysis. Contrast lymphangiography is sometimes helpful in demonstrating the presence and location of defects in the lymphatic vessels.

A wide variety of metabolic abnormalities may occur in animals with chylous effusions. Chyle contains large amounts of lipid, lipoproteins, fat-soluble vitamins, electrolytes and lymphocytes. The thoracic duct system is the main pathway by which ingested fats and extravascular protein are transported to the general circulation. Deficiencies of these important nutrients and cells may occur quickly in animals with large volumes of pleural effusion or in those in which repeated thoracocentesis is necessary to relieve respiratory distress.

Treatment of true chylothorax is initially aimed at relieving respiratory distress by closed chest tube drainage and reducing the volume of lymph formed. This allows an opportunity for spontaneous healing to occur. In normal dogs the rate of flow in the thoracic duct is estimated to be 2 ml./kg./hr. Ninety-five per cent of this volume is from the liver and intestine. The rate of formation of intestinal lymph can be reduced by restricting oral intake of food and water. Complete fasting with intravenous maintenance of fluid and electrolyte balance for 4 to 7 days is indicated at the onset of therapy. After this period of time, small quantities of a diet low in fat and high in carbohydrate and protein are offered. These diets alter the fat content of chyle and reduce the rate of its formation, but they do not completely stop lymph production. Medium-chain triglyceride diets contain synthetic triglycerides which are absorbed directly into the portal circulation and bypass the lymphatic system.* Supplementation with these compounds may allow adequate ingestion of fat and energy without increasing the fat content of the chyle which is formed. In animals which become debilitated owing to removal of large volumes of chyle, par-

enteral hyperalimentation may offer a means of replacing essential nutrients over a long period of time.

If medical management fails to control the formation of true chylous effusions after 14 to 28 days, thoracotomy is indicated. The surgeon should attempt to remove any inciting agent and double-ligate the thoracic duct near the diaphragm. The procedure is at best difficult because of problems encountered in identifying the duct and successfully ligating it. A large number of animals continue to have chylous effusions after surgery and the prognosis in these cases is poor.

Milky white effusions without chylomicrons and the typical cytologic features of true chylous effusions are called pseudochylous effusions. The white color is due to cholesterol crystals, lecithin-globulin complexes or calcium phosphate crystals in the fluids. Cytologic examination of these fluids reveals chronic sterile inflammation, macrophages containing many fat droplets and degenerating fragmented cells. Lymphocytes and plasma cells may be seen. This fluid will not clear completely when ether is added, and chylomicrons are not seen when Sudan III is used to stain the sample.

In cats, acquired cardiomyopathy and lymphosarcoma are the most common underlying diseases resulting in pseudochylous effusions. In dogs, most cases are idiopathic. Occasionally tumors or infection may also be present. In idiopathic pseudochylous effusions, corticosteroids administered systemically and/or intrapleurally following chest drainage may halt the formation of fluid.

**Neoplastic Effusions.** These effusions may have an obstructive or inflammatory pattern but contain neoplastic cells. A diagnosis of tumor should not be made based on the cytologic evaluation alone unless confirmed by an experienced veterinary cytologist. Mesothelial cells and a wide variety of exfoliated normal cells may become reactive and undergo morphologic changes which are sometimes suggestive of neoplasia. Cytologic examination is used in conjunction with the history, physical exam, radiographic findings and other laboratory findings only to suggest a tumor in the pleural cavity. Any primary or metastatic tumor in the thoracic cavity is potentially capable of producing a neoplastic effusion.

*M.C.T. Oil, Mead Johnson Laboratories, Evansville, Indiana 47721.

Common examples include lympho-sarcoma, metastatic carcinomas and adeno-carcinomas and hemangiosarcomas.

**Pyogranulomatous Effusions.** These effusions are inflammatory in nature but occur specifically in feline infectious peritonitis. A vasculitis affects all serous membranes accompanied by a secondary pyogran-ulomatous serositis. Pyogranulomatous effusions are usually thick, viscous and straw-colored. The cytologic examination of these fluids reveals moderate numbers of neutrophils, plasma cells, lymphocytes, macrophages and erythrocytes. A coarse, granular background material, thought to be precipitated protein, stains pink with Wright's stain. These effusions are occasionally secondarily infected with bacteria which may be visible in the fluid, resulting in an active septic pleuritis.

Other additional information helpful in confirming the diagnosis of feline infectious peritonitis includes serosal inflammation and effusion in other body parts, elevation of the total serum protein and altered albu-min:globulin ratios or ocular lesions. The same cytologic pattern also occurs in the abdominal effusion. Treatment of feline infectious peritonitis is discussed elsewhere. To date, the disease usually carries a poor prognosis.

### SUPPLEMENTAL READING

Creighton, S. R., and Wilkins, R. J.: Thoracic effusions in the cat: Etiology and diagnostic features. J. Am. Animal Hosp. Assn., 11:66–76, 1975.
Perman, V.: Transudates and exudates. In Kaneko, J. J., and Cornelius, C. E. (eds.): Clinical Biochemistry of Domestic Animals, Vol. 2. 2nd ed. New York, Academic Press, 1971.
Perman, V., and Osborne, C.: Laboratory evaluation of abnormal body fluids. Vet. Clin. N. Am., 4:255–268, 1974.
Withrow, S., and Fenner, W.: Closed chest drainage and lavage in the treatment of pyothorax in the cat. J. Am. Animal Hosp. Assn., 11:90–94, 1975.

# PULMONARY EDEMA

NEIL K. HARPSTER, V.M.D.
*Boston, Massachusetts*

Pulmonary edema is the accumulation of an excessive amount of fluid within the lung. In the majority of clinical situations, this occurs only *or* in the early stages as an increase in the fluid content of the alveolar-capillary interstitial spaces (i.e., in-terstitial edema). As the process progresses, there is transudation of proteinaceous fluid into the alveoli and even into the respiratory bronchioles and more proximal portions of the tracheobronchial tree. The protein content of this fluid varies with the underlying etiology and the rapidity with which it develops.

Interstitial pulmonary edema, by itself, is usually not associated with clinical signs, unless other abnormalities of pulmonary ventilation or perfusion exist. Even with sophisticated tests and measurements, in-terstitial edema is diagnosed with difficulty. For these reasons, the following discussion will deal entirely with the symptomatic and more severe form, alveolar pulmonary edema.

## PATHOPHYSIOLOGY

### THE NORMAL LUNG

Even in the normal lung there is a small but significant movement of water and protein constituents of the blood across the pulmonary capillary membranes into the interstitial tissues. This movement is minimized by a precise balance of hydro-static and osmotic forces across the capillary walls. Those blood constituents that do accumulate in the alveolar-capillary interstitial spaces are removed primarily by an extensive and elaborate lymphatic system which returns them to the systemic veins.

The alveolar portion of the alveolar-capillary membrane is normally quite impermeable to the movement of water and other molecules. This resistance to movement is enhanced by surfactant (a lipoprotein complex locally synthesized by alveolar type II cells), which lines the alveoli and also exerts an antiatelectasis effect. Thus, in the normal lung there is a negligible movement of fluid and protein constituents into the alveoli.

## MECHANISMS RESPONSIBLE FOR PULMONARY EDEMA

Although certain clinical conditions exert their effect at one particular site, others are less clearly defined and may result in two or more abnormalities in the alveolar-capillary membrane. It should be mentioned here that once the formation of pulmonary edema is initiated, and despite the basic underlying etiologic agent(s), it tends to be self-propagating. This is a result of disruption of the fine balance between hydrostatic and osmotic forces across the pulmonary-capillary walls.

### HEMODYNAMIC PULMONARY EDEMA

In this type of pulmonary edema, the initiating factor is an abnormality in the capillary-interstitial pressure balance which favors a movement of fluids into the alveolar-capillary interstitial space.

#### Increased Pulmonary Capillary Hydrostatic Pressure

CARDIAC CAUSES. Left ventricular failure is by far the most common cause of pulmonary edema of cardiac origin in the dog. It occurs most commonly in association with chronic valvular-myocardial disease in the aged dog but is also seen with certain congenital cardiac defects ·that overwork the left ventricle. These include subvalvular aortic stenosis, patent ductus arteriosus, ventricular septal defect and endocardial fibroelastosis. Other, less common causes include cardiomyopathy of the giant breed dog and myocardial infarction, as well as tachyarrhythmias and bradyarrhythmias.

Whichever of the above causes is germane for a particular patient, the same sequence of hemodynamic abnormalities occurs. Elevation of the left ventricular end-diastolic pressure results in increased left atrial, pulmonary venous and pulmonary capillary pressures. In the presence of normal pulmonary capillary oncotic (colloidal osmotic) pressure, pulmonary edema occurs when the pulmonary capillary hydrostatic pressure is in a range of 25 to 30 mm. Hg.

There is a small group of other conditions that are exceedingly rare in the dog, but that have a similar hemodynamic effect on pulmonary capillary pressure. These include conditions that interfere with left atrial emptying, such as mitral stenosis and thrombotic or neoplastic masses in the left atrium, and pulmonary veno-occlusive disease. Here the initiating pressure elevation occurs proximal to the left ventricle; however, the end result is the same.

EXCESSIVE ADMINISTRATION OF FLUIDS. Overinfusion is particularly easy to accomplish in the small patient with a small circulatory volume. In the larger patient, it is more likely to occur when underlying heart disease or renal insufficiency (oliguria, anuria) exists. The mechanisms responsible for the development of pulmonary edema in this clinical setting appear to be a combination of increased pulmonary capillary hydrostatic pressure and decreased pulmonary capillary oncotic pressure, secondary to hemodilution.

#### Decreased Pulmonary Capillary Oncotic Pressure

A reduction in the colloidal osmotic pressure of the pulmonary capillaries likewise favors a movement of fluids into the alveolar-capillary interstitial space. This occurs most frequently in association with hypoproteinemia, and especially hypoalbuminemia, as seen with liver disease and protein-losing enteropathies and nephropathies. Although pulmonary edema is not usually a significant part of the clinical picture in these patients, it may be if underlying heart disease exists or fluid administration is attempted.

#### Pulmonary Lymphatic Insufficiency

Processes which interfere with pulmonary lymphatic drainage can result in pulmonary edema. This may occur as a patchy or diffuse involvement in the case of an inflammatory process, causing obstruction of peripheral lymphatic channels; or as a result of lymphatic spread of a neoplastic process. An anterior mediastinal mass may invade the major lymphatic ducts, resulting in partial or complete obstruction and the development of pulmonary edema.

### PERMEABILITY PULMONARY EDEMA

Here we are dealing with a large group of varying etiologic agents that superficially appear quite unrelated. The altered permeability effect that these agents share occurs on a basis of direct physical or chemical damage to either the alveolar epithelial or the pulmonary capillary cells. Most forms of noncardiac pulmonary edema belong in this group.

Those agents that alter alveolar epithelial cell permeability may directly damage these cells or may act by inhibition or inactivation of the alveolar surfactant substance. Specific causes include infectious agents such as bacterial and viral pneumonias, as well as inhalation of irritating gases, aspiration pneumonia, smoke inhalation and near drowning.

Alterations in pulmonary capillary permeability may result from direct damage to the endothelial cells as occurs with the canine infectious hepatitis virus but more commonly is a biochemical process that affects the metabolic functions of these cells and increases the size of intercellular pores that are normally present. This allows the passage of a larger quantity of blood constituents, including larger molecules, into the alveolar-capillary interstitial space. Specific causes include circulating toxins, as seen with endotoxic shock; $\alpha$-naphthylthiourea (ANTU) ingestion; and coralsnake venom. The release of circulating vasoactive substances (histamine, serotonin and others) has been postulated to cause endothelial cell contraction, with the formation of intercellular gaps. The release of these substances can be effected by a multitude of factors, including various types of shock and anaphylactic reactions.

## OTHER CAUSES OF PULMONARY EDEMA

The inclusion of specific causes in this group is usually due to an incomplete understanding of the mechanism(s) involved in the genesis of the pulmonary edema. Although mechanisms have been postulated for each of these, they are as yet unproven. High-altitude pulmonary edema, hypothalamic lesions, pulmonary embolism and chronic pulmonary disease all fall into this group.

Also included here is the severe pulmonary edema seen following electric shock. It appears most likely that this is an acute left-sided heart failure syndrome, as suggested by a diastolic gallop rhythm in

several patients. However, increased pulmonary capillary permeability secondary to electrical injury or release of vasoactive substances can also be postulated.

## BLOOD GAS ABNORMALITIES

Hypoxemia is generally the only abnormality present in the patient with interstitial and mild alveolar pulmonary edema. The defect here is one of impaired diffusion across the alveolar-capillary membrane. Carbon dioxide, because of its greater solubility, is usually unaffected; in fact, hypocapnia and respiratory alkalosis may exist owing to associated hyperventilation. Only when respiratory centers are depressed by either sedative drugs or coma will hypercapnia and respiratory acidosis come into play.

With more severe degrees of alveolar pulmonary edema, alveolar respiratory units, respiratory bronchioles and distal bronchioles become flooded. In addition, proteinaceous froth in the larger airways interferes with oxygen delivery to the bronchioles. Associated bronchoconstriction also interferes with ventilation. Now we are dealing with more than just a diffusion abnormality. Large respiratory units are receiving blood circulation without oxygen delivery; thus, a ventilation-perfusion abnormality exists. These patients frequently have severe degrees of hypoxia, as well as hypercapnia and respiratory acidosis.

## DIAGNOSTIC FEATURES

Most types of pulmonary edema are accompanied by a cough at some period in their clinical course. The cough is characteristically moist and productive. However, certain fulminating forms of pulmonary edema develop so rapidly that a cough is nonexistent or negligible. This occurs most frequently in acute left ventricular failure, secondary to ruptured chordae tendineae; electric shock; inhalation of smoke or other irritating gases; and anaphylactic reactions. These patients usually present with a history of progressive difficulty with respiration of short duration.

Physical examination will reveal a patient in varying degrees of respiratory distress. With severe pulmonary edema, as is notably seen with acute left-sided heart failure and electric shock, all efforts and energies are concentrated on the exchange of air. Cyanosis, restlessness and marked discomfort when lying down can be appreciated. Fine, moist, bubbling rales can be best heard over the hilar areas, bilaterally, but may be evident over all lung fields. Respiratory sounds may be so prominent as to make cardiac auscultation impossible. If cardiac function is severely compromised, the patient may present in varying degrees of shock (cold extremities, subnormal body temperature) or in a collapsed state.

Thoracic radiographs are often of considerable benefit in establishing the cause of the pulmonary edema. Those agents that disrupt alveolar epithelial permeability are characterized by diffuse, increased alveolar densities with marked airway prominence and peribronchial thickening. Overinfusion and decreased capillary oncotic pressure are typically seen as fine, diffuse, increased alveolar densities with little evidence of vascular prominence or airway involvement. Patchy areas of alveolar edema are most frequently seen with bacterial pneumonias and pulmonary embolism. Increased prominence of the pulmonary veins and pulmonary edema that radiates peripherally from the hilus are characteristic of left-sided heart failure.

In certain instances, the establishment of a specific etiology is not easily achieved. Here it is necessary closely to correlate a good history, respiratory and nonrespiratory physical findings, radiographic findings, plus laboratory and other diagnostic tests in order to arrive at a working diagnosis. In patients with severely embarrassed respiratory function, intensive treatment measures must often be instituted while a diagnosis is still being sought.

## TREATMENT

The basic goals of treatment are to improve the oxygenation of the blood, eliminate the pulmonary edema and return the patient to a stable condition. Specific methods to accomplish these results will be discussed below, using acute left-sided heart failure as an example. Specific and additional methods for the management of other forms of pulmonary edema will be discussed subsequently under their appropriate headings.

## HEMODYNAMIC PULMONARY EDEMA

### REDUCE WORKLOAD ON THE HEART

Hospitalization is an absolute necessity for the patient with acute left-sided heart failure. Complete cage rest in a quiet area is preferable to avoid patient stimulation and excitement. Treatment schedules should be arranged so as to disturb the patient minimally.

The administration of sedatives reduces apprehension and anxiety, allowing more complete rest. In addition, they permit slower, deeper and more efficient respiratory movements; curtail the dyspnea–pulmonary edema vicious circle; and reduce the physical activity of the patient. Morphine sulfate is the sedative of choice, administered at a dosage of 0.5 to 1.0 mg./kg. of body weight. Other sedatives can be used, such as hydrocodeinone bitartrate (Hycodan® [Endo]) at 1 to 2 mg./kg. orally, pentobarbital at 6 to 10 mg./kg. intramuscularly, and phenobarbital at 15 mg./5 to 7 kg. orally. These other agents appear to be less effective than morphine sulfate in this clinical setting.

### IMPROVE VENTILATION

Oxygen administration is extremely helpful in overcoming the existing hypoxemia. The ideal method of administration in severe pulmonary edema is by positive pressure via an endotracheal tube. This not only allows delivery of 100 per cent oxygen under increased pressure, but also reduces venous return by elevating the intrathoracic pressure. Unfortunately, this method is possible only in the collapsed patient. The most reasonable system for administering oxygen to a dog is a cage or tent in which oxygen concentrations of 50 to 60 per cent can be rapidly attained and maintained. Another advantage of the oxygen cage is that it obviates the need for handling, and the additional stress that this imposes on the patient.

Administration of bronchodilators is beneficial in relieving the bronchospasm that usually accompanies pulmonary edema from any cause. Aminophylline is the drug of choice, administered at a dosage of 6 to 10 mg./kg. of body weight slowly intravenously. The use of more potent bronchodilators, such as epinephrine and isoproterenol (Isuprel® [Winthrop]), may be of considerable benefit in pulmonary edema from other causes, but should be avoided in acute left-sided heart failure because their increased automaticity and excitability effects on the myocardium may induce serious and even fatal cardiac arrhythmias.

Maintenance of tracheobronchial airway patency is an absolute necessity if good results are to be realized. Brachiocephalic dogs with reduced laryngeal orifices and toy breeds with tracheal deformities are particularly difficult to manage. Dramatic improvement can frequently be accomplished with bypassing the area of luminal narrowing, as with endotracheal intubation or tracheotomy. Other upper airway obstructions in these patients occur in the form of edema fluid and tracheobronchial secretions, and as proteinaceous froth. The fluid accumulations should be removed whenever possible by suctioning. Proteinaceous froth can be reduced by vaporizing 40 to 50 per cent ethyl or isopropyl alcohol into the oxygen tent or cage. This lowers the surface tension of the froth bubbles, causing them to burst.

## REDUCE VENOUS RETURN AND EXCESSIVE BODY FLUIDS

The use of positive pressure ventilation has previously been mentioned as an effective method of reducing venous return by increasing intrathoracic pressure. Rotating limb tourniquets is a second method that is useful and effective in the treatment of the human patient with pulmonary edema. The difficulty in performing these procedures, as well as the additional stress and handling required, makes them generally irrational approaches in the dog, unless the patient is comatose.

**Diuretics.** The new, potent, intravenously administered diuretics are one of the most effective measures in overcoming the initial crisis. Both furosemide (Lasix® [Hoechst]) at 4 mg./kg. of body weight and ethacrynic acid (Edecrin® [Merck]) at 1 mg./kg. of body weight will usually result in a marked diuresis within 30 to 60 minutes. When the initial response is inadequate, an additional injection may be given in one to two hours. Both of these drugs are dose-dependent (i.e., higher doses result in greater diuresis). They are equal in potency to the mercurial diuretics but lack the renal toxic effects that prohibit the frequent administration of the mercurial diuretics.

**Phlebotomy.** This is one of the most direct methods of reducing venous return. Phlebotomy is usually reserved for those patients that have an inadequate response to the previously mentioned diuretics. It is performed by the initial removal of 10 per cent of the total blood volume (calculation is based on 80 ml./kg. of body weight as the approximate total blood volume). If required, additional 5 per cent increments of the total blood volume may be removed at one- to two-hour intervals until a satisfactory response is achieved, or a total of 20 per cent has been removed. All blood removed should be stored in an anticoagulant in the event that reinfusion is required, although this has never been necessary in our experience.

**Peritoneal Dialysis.** This procedure is particularly useful in the patient that is azotemic, or becomes azotemic during diuretic therapy, with persisting active heart failure (i.e., pulmonary edema). In this setting, peritoneal dialysis can serve the patient by removal of both excessive body fluids and retained renal waste products. A half-and-half mixture of the 7 per cent and 1.5 per cent dialyzing fluid should be used in order to have a mildly hypertonic solution. Only a moderate amount of the solution should be instilled, so as not to interfere with movement of the diaphragm and cause further embarrassment of respiration.

## STRENGTHEN MYOCARDIAL CONTRACTION—DIGITALIZATION

The intensive methods of digitalization are of less importance since the introduction of the potent, intravenous diuretics. In fact, the high incidence of digitalis intoxication, with associated cardiac arrhythmias which occur with these intensive methods, makes them potentially hazardous. This is especially true when active heart failure persists. Further reduction in cardiac output, associated with the toxic state and accompanying cardiac arrhythmias, makes heart failure even more difficult to control.

The method we prefer in dogs with acute left-sided heart failure is one we have named a semi-rapid method. This consists of initially giving 0.03 mg./kg. of body weight of digoxin (Lanoxin® [Burroughs Wellcome]) intravenously. This is followed in one to two hours with a maintenance dose of 0.02 mg./kg. of body weight daily, divided in two equal doses. This method

*Table 1.* *Summary of Treatment for Acute Left-Sided Heart Failure*

| TREATMENT | INITIALLY | 1 HOUR | 2 HOURS |
|---|---|---|---|
| Cage rest | Enforced | Continued | Continued |
| Sedation | Morphine sulfate (0.5 to 1.0 mg./kg. of body weight subcutaneously) | Repeat if inadequate | – |
| O₂ therapy | Plus vaporized alcohol (40 to 50%) | Continued | Continued |
| Aminophylline | (6 to 10 mg./kg. of body weight intravenously) | – | – |
| Reduce body fluids | Lasix® (4 mg./kg. of body weight intravenously) | Repeat Lasix® or phlebotomy* | Phlebotomy |
| Digitalis glycosides | Digoxin (½ T.D.D.† intravenously) | Digoxin (0.01 mg./kg. of body weight orally) | – |
| Antibiotics | Normal usage | – | – |

*See text for method of performing.
†T.D.D. = total digitalization dose. (The intravenous T.D.D. for digoxin is 0.06 mg./kg. of body weight.)

avoids toxicity, but gives the patient a full, calculated digitalization dose within the first 24 to 36 hours of treatment.

The digitalis glycosides should always be administered with care in the patient that has been receiving these preparations in the recent past. The best policy is to use only maintenance levels of digoxin, and to control the present crisis with other methods described.

Rapid and intensive methods of digitalization should not be carried out in patients with heart failure secondary to, or accompanied by, rapid ventricular arrhythmias. Even the use of maintenance doses in these instances should be followed carefully with electrocardiographic monitoring.

## ADDITIONAL METHODS

Table 1 lists a summary protocol for the treatment of acute left-sided heart failure. It can be appreciated that this method utilizes a program of constant monitoring. The goal is to relieve the pulmonary edema as rapidly as possible, but to avoid overtreatment and the creation of a situation worse than the one that currently exists. Additional medications are given at one and two hours only if an adequate response is not realized by the initial treatment. An attempt is made to get the patient on oral maintenance therapy as early as possible. Antibiotics are routinely added to the regimen to prevent secondary bacterial infection. This method has proved to be quite effective in a clinical setting.

In those patients in which reduced blood viscosity or decreased oncotic pressure exists, other methods which more specifically correct the underlying deficit may prove useful. As with other forms of pulmonary edema, one should avoid the administration of isotonic solutions which further expand the circulatory volume and contribute to the pulmonary edema. In the presence of anemia, the administration of packed red blood cells not only reduces the workload on the heart by an increase in blood viscosity, but also improves oxygen delivery to the tissues. In patients with decreased oncotic pressure, who are resistant to the measures previously discussed, the administration of hyperoncotic solutions such as plasma and dextran may result in dramatic diuresis. When methods such as these are being attempted, frequent monitoring of central venous pressure must be performed.

## PERMEABILITY PULMONARY EDEMA

In these forms of pulmonary edema, those measures discussed previously, with the exception of the digitalis glycosides, are routinely useful and of benefit. The digitalis glycosides are indicated only if right-heart function is compromised (i.e., right-heart failure exists). When the excessive production of bronchial secretions occurs, as is seen with the inhalation of certain irritating gases, the administration of anticholinergic agents such as atropine sulfate (0.4 mg./kg.)

in the early stages of onset may reduce the severity of the pulmonary edema considerably. However, as soon as the crisis has subsided, anticholinergic agents must be replaced with methods to liquefy the secretions so that expectoration is enhanced and the chance for bacterial superinfection is minimized.

When pulmonary edema occurs secondary to increased pulmonary capillary permeability, the administration of the adrenal corticosteroids may prove beneficial. The postulated mode of action is improvement in vascular integrity (i.e., decreased permeability). Those corticosteroids with a rapid onset of action, such as hydrocortisone sodium succinate (Solu-Cortef® [Upjohn]), are preferred.

Severe bacterial pneumonia, accompanied by pulmonary edema, can be successfully treated, consistently, only with antibiotics of laboratory-proven effectiveness. The best method of obtaining material for culture in these critically ill patients is by transtracheal aspiration. After material for culture is obtained, treatment with broad-spectrum, bactericidal antibiotics should be initiated while waiting for the culture results.

Pulmonary edema is a many faceted multi-etiologic problem of life-threatening magnitude. The specific cause is not always apparent from a cursory physical examination, and sometimes a very diligent and thorough search must be made. Fortunately for our patients, nonspecific general treatment is usually of benefit and buys us time to search for specific etiologies, which may permit more specific treatment. Almost without exception, pulmonary edema must be aggressively approached if a successful outcome is to be insured. The price paid for overtreatment is rarely as costly as the failure to treat adequately.

## SUPPLEMENTAL READING

Fishman, A. P.: Pulmonary edema: the water-exchanging function of the lung. Circulation, 46:390–408, 1972.

Luchi, R. J.: Pulmonary edema. In Conn, H. L., Jr., and Horwitz, O. (eds.): Cardiac and Vascular Diseases. Philadelphia, Lea & Febiger, 1971, pp. 503–508.

Robin, E. D., Cross, C. E., and Zelis, R.: Pulmonary edema. New England J. Med., 288:230–246, 1973.

Robin, E. D., Cross, C. E., and Zelis, R.: Pulmonary edema. New England J. Med., 288:293–304, 1973.

# PARASITIC DISEASES OF THE RESPIRATORY TRACT

J. F. WILLIAMS, M.R.C.V.S.
*East Lansing, Michigan*

A wide variety of clinical signs and pathologic lesions in dogs and cats results from invasion of the respiratory system by parasites. While the severity of the clinical manifestations depends largely on the number of organisms which arrive in the lungs, it is also determined by factors such as the site of predilection within the system and the nature of the host response. Further complicating the picture is the fact that not all the parasites which cause respiratory

disease live as adults in the lungs or associated structures; some (e.g., *Ancylostoma caninum*) merely pass through the lungs in the normal course of their migrations, while others intrude on the respiratory system only as a result of aberrant migration (e.g., *Spirocerca lupi*). Finally, parasites residing primarily in other systems may cause syndromes in which respiratory difficulty is one of the foremost presenting signs (e.g., *Dirofilaria immitis*). All these considerations have an important bearing on the diagnostic and therapeutic approaches to parasitic respiratory disease.

Individual clinical entities are best discussed in terms of the causative organisms involved. These can be grouped under some general headings, but an understanding of the biology of each parasite is necessary if rational bases are to be developed for the management of clinical cases and the prevention of further infections.

## PARASITES WHICH RESIDE IN THE RESPIRATORY SYSTEM

Most of the nematode helminths which reside as adults in the lungs of dogs and cats are metastrongyles. Their life cycles characteristically involve invertebrates, particularly slugs and snails, which act as obligatory intermediate hosts. Rodents and birds may prey on infected invertebrates and then act as transport hosts, conveying the parasite to domestic or wild carnivores. Clinical cases in domestic animals occur infrequently, but many authors suspect that undetected infections are widespread. However, lesions caused by these organisms are generally not common incidental findings at autopsy and it seems more likely that canine or feline lungworm infections are indeed rare and result from a casual spillover from sylvatic animal cycles.

### FILAROIDES OSLERI

This slender worm (up to 1 cm. long) lives in granulomatous nodules extending from the bifurcation of the trachea posteriorly into the bronchi.

**Clinical Signs.** Clinical cases occur in dogs in the first 1 to 2 years of life; the animal is presented with a history of a chronic deep cough which is sometimes productive of a foamy mucus. As the disease progresses and the granulomatous lesions protrude further into the bronchi, severe wheezing and dyspnea develop. During the early phases there is no effect on appetite and the dog eats well and maintains bodily condition. Later, as respiratory embarrassment becomes progressively worse, the animal may become emaciated. There is usually exacerbation of the respiratory difficulty after excitement or mild exercise. There is often a history of unresponsiveness to treatment with antibiotics, although there may be temporary remission after administration of steroids or antihistamines.

Physical examination of advanced cases usually reveals dyspnea with inflammation of the pharynx and larynx associated with abnormal lung sounds, particularly prominent rales, and increased thoracic resonance. Heart sounds may be difficult to detect above the noisy respiration.

**Diagnosis.** There are no characteristic blood changes. Although eosinophilia may be present, this is not sufficiently characteristic to distinguish the condition from chronic allergic states which must be considered in differential diagnosis.

Radiographic examination, particularly by bronchogram, is very helpful in detecting the obstructive granulomatous lesions in the trachea and bronchi. It also serves to rule out tracheal collapse or systemic mycotic infections as potential causes of this type of clinical condition. Bronchoscopy will reveal the raised nodules at the tracheal bifurcation. However, application of these types of diagnostic tools may be limited by the fact that anesthesia may be hazardous if severe respiratory distress is present and laryngeal edema following bronchoscopy could exacerbate the problem. Bronchial washings, if not obtainable by bronchoscopy, may be collected by puncture of the ventral trachea and aspiration through a cannula.

Washings or biopsies of bronchial nodules should be examined for the presence of embryonated eggs (80 $\mu$ long) or larvae (230 $\mu$ long). These larvae have a characteristically kinked tail. They are normally coughed up and swallowed but are hard to detect in fecal samples because they are few in number and easily distorted by flotation solutions. Microscopic examination of the sediment from fresh fecal samples diluted with a little saline is helpful. The larvae are slow in their movements. The only other larvae likely to be in fresh samples are those of *Strongyloides stercoralis* but they are stouter with a sharply pointed tail. Samples which are not fresh will often contain active hookworm larvae in a matter of hours.

**Treatment.** Temporary relief from respiratory distress can often be achieved with bronchodilators. Antihistamines are particularly appropriate, since the additional benefit of sedation may occur. Resolution of the lesions can be achieved with anthelmintic medication, but since cases are treated infrequently, it is difficult to assess the relative efficacy of drugs in clinical trials. An additional complication is that spontaneous remission may occur without anthelmintic treatment, and this also influences assessment of the value of chemotherapy.

Thioacetarsamide (Caparsolate ®, Abbott Laboratories, Chicago, Ill.) at the rate of 0.22 ml. of a 1 per cent solution/kg. body weight intravenously each day for 21 days appears to cause resolution of the nodules, beginning within 2 weeks. Bronchoscopic monitoring can be used to confirm this effect, but the clinical condition should be markedly improved by the end of the course. There is a report of successful treatment with thiabendazole (Thibenzole ® Merck, Sharp and Dohme Co., N.J.) (Bennett and Beresford-Jones, 1973). The drug was given daily at an initial rate of 32 mg./kg. body weight and was increased to 96 mg./kg. over a 23-day period. After 9 days, viable larvae were no longer present in the feces and the nodules decreased in size over the next several weeks. Thiabendazole must be introduced gradually to avoid vomiting. Levamisole (Tramisol ®, American Cyanamid, Princeton, N.J.) is effective against metastrongyles in all other domestic animals and, provided due care is taken, it is appropriate for use in the dog. High initial doses are very poorly tolerated in dogs, and it is best to increase the dose gradually from 2 mg./kg. daily per os to 8 mg./kg. over a 3-week period in order to avoid toxicosis. It has a bitter taste and dogs do not like it.

**Prevention.** The life cycle of *F. osleri* is unknown but it probably follows the pattern of other metastrongyles and involves mollusks as intermediate hosts. Although dogs might become infected by eating these, it seems more likely that rodents serve as transport hosts, since this has been shown to occur in other species of *Filaroides*. When snails or slugs are fed to dogs, the animals often vomit within minutes. If rodents are indeed responsible for transmission it would be difficult to prevent infection by interfering with the natural predatory habits of dogs. Other than instituting normal rodent control practices at breeding kennels there are no realistic preventive measures.

Efforts to control mollusks, although widely recommended, are of no proven value and might pose severe hazards if toxic agents are used.

### FILAROIDES MILKSI AND FILAROIDES HIRTHI

*F. osleri* has been discussed at length, since many of the biologic and medical characteristics of this parasite are common to other metastrongyles of dogs and cats. *F. milksi* and *F. hirthi* both occur in the parenchyma of the lungs in dogs.

*F. milksi* is a natural parasite of the skunk, and only a handful of cases have been recorded in dogs. The clinical signs typically reflect the interstitial pneumonia which results from the presence of adults and larvae in alveolar spaces. Progressive respiratory difficulty unresponsive to antibiotic therapy is generally observed.

There are no lesions visible on bronchoscopy, but bronchial washings contain embryonated eggs and larvae identical to those of *F. osleri*.

There is only one record of anthelmintic treatment of *F. milksi* and in that instance oral levamisole was used (Corwin et al., 1975). However, the dog was extremely dyspneic, requiring oxygen for maintenance, and died within 24 hours. It is worth noting that all the worms were dead at autopsy and that the massive release of foreign antigens may have contributed to the fatal outcome. Fatalities attributed to antigen release have been seen following levamisole treatment of sheep heavily infected with small metastrongyles. It seems wise to introduce the drug at low levels in order to avoid this complication.

*F. hirthi* is a recently discovered parasite which has apparently become well established in research beagle colonies (Hirth and Hottendorf, 1973). Like *F. milksi* it inhabits the alveoli and terminal bronchioles. However, no clinical signs have yet been described in infected animals, although focal granulomatous lesions occur around adult worms. It is not at all clear how transmission of this lungworm occurs in closed beagle colonies where intermediate and transport hosts are denied access. The small metastrongyles of sheep are capable of transuterine migration, and perhaps this mode of infection also occurs in dogs.

## CRENOSOMA VULPIS

This small metastrongyle (up to 1.5 cm. long) inhabits the bronchi and bronchioles of wild carnivores and occasionally domestic dogs. In severe cases bronchiolar occlusion may occur acutely owing to the arrival in the lungs of large numbers of larvae from the circulation. This may lead to emphysema and diffuse interstitial pneumonia. In the later stages of disease the adults reside principally in the bronchi and cause a persistent deep cough and chronic bronchitis. Diagnosis is based on the detection of straight-tailed larvae (250 to 300 $\mu$ long) in bronchial washings or in fresh feces. Anthelmintic treatment should be given as described for *F. osleri*.

## AELUROSTRONGYLUS ABSTRUSUS

This is the only metastrongyle of clinical importance in the domestic cat. Adult worms (up to 1 cm. long) live in the terminal bronchioles, and eggs and larvae pass up the bronchial tree.

**Clinical Signs.** The extensive interstitial pneumonia and bronchiolitis which develop result in a progression of clinical signs from an initial deep cough to severe dyspnea, accompanied by anorexia and marked wasting.

The severity of clinical cases depends on the number of organisms and, unlike the case with other lungworms, there is evidence that many cases go undetected. In one survey in the U.S.A. about 2 per cent of cats were shown to be infected. The life cycle involves snails as intermediate hosts but mice and birds are very effective transport hosts and, given the predatory habits of cats, infection by this means is probably commonplace.

Experimental infection in cats results in marked medial hypertrophy of the pulmonary arterial system, although the mechanism whereby this comes about is unknown. However, this type of lesion is commonly observed in feline lungs, and this observation has been interpreted as an indication that lungworm infection occurs at some stage in the life of many domestic cats.

**Diagnosis.** After an initial phase of patency, during which larvae may be found in bronchial washings or fresh feces, infections often become latent with few adults remaining in the lungs. There is evidence that reactivation may occur later, and this intermittent characteristic complicates the diagnosis. First-stage larvae have a kinked tail which bears a terminal spine. They measure 250 to 300 $\mu$ in the lungs but may be up to 400 $\mu$ in length by the time they appear in feces.

**Treatment.** There is very little information regarding suitable anthelmintic treatment. Severely affected cats require supportive treatment for the emaciation and dehydration which often accompany the chronic respiratory problem. Levamisole is undoubtedly effective in killing the parasites but care must be taken, since this drug is poorly tolerated by cats. The injectable form in particular is toxic, besides being highly irritating locally. Oral doses can be given, although cats dislike the taste. However, remission of clinical signs does occur in those which survive. The drug may be given at the rate of 25 mg./kg. every other day for five treatments.

There is no practical way to prevent outdoor cats from infecting themselves by hunting rodents or birds.

## CAPILLARIA AEROPHILA

This slender worm (up to 4 cm. long) inhabits the trachea and bronchi, and sometimes even the nasal passages, of wild carnivores and occasionally domestic dogs. It is not a metastrongyle but is closely related to the *Trichuroidea*, or whipworms. The life cycle is direct.

**Clinical Signs.** Clinical cases usually occur in young dogs which are presented with a chronic cough unresponsive to antibiotics. Severe bronchitis may lead to respiratory difficulty and mouth-breathing.

**Diagnosis.** Radiographic changes result from chronic inflammatory thickening of the bronchial mucosa. Bronchoscopic examination reveals an inflamed irregular bronchial epithelium, although the parasites themselves may be too deep in the bronchial tree to be seen with this instrument. Bronchial washings and fecal samples contain pale yellow, thick-walled unembryonated eggs (60 x 35 $\mu$) with bipolar plugs. However, egg output may be sparse even in severe cases, and repeated sampling is necessary in order to confirm a suspected case.

**Treatment.** There are no records of suc-

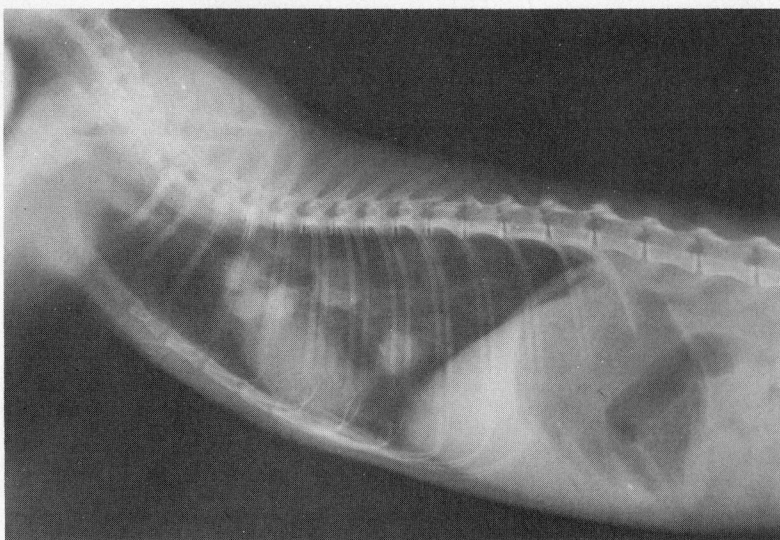

**Figure 1.** Lateral radiograph of cat showing well-circumscribed lesions caused by fibrous encapsulation of *Paragonimus kellicotti.*

cessful anthelmintic treatment in the literature but some promising results have been obtained in dogs treated with levamisole. Whether this proves to be of lasting value remains to be seen.

### PARAGONIMUS KELLICOTTI

*P. kellicotti* is a digenetic fluke (up to 1 x 0.5 cm.) which inhabits fibrous cysts in the lungs of wild carnivores and domestic cats and dogs. Although widely distributed in the U.S.A., the prevalence is greater in the north central region surrounding the Great Lakes. The life cycle involves two intermediate hosts, the first of which is an aquatic snail and the second a crayfish.

**Clinical Signs.**    Although light infections may occur without clinical consequences, heavy infections result in chronic coughing which progresses to extreme respiratory difficulty accompanied by severe emaciation, especially in cats. Often there is frequent gagging and sneezing of mucus which may contain blood. Secondary bacterial pneumonia is often superimposed in cats.

**Diagnosis.**    The dense, well-circumscribed cysts containing the flukes are visible radiographically (Fig. 1) but must be distinguished from tumor metastases which often assume a similar form. Confirmation of infection can be achieved by finding the eggs which are released into the bronchial tree through small openings in the cyst wall. Eggs are brownish-yellow in color and measure approximately 100 x 50 $\mu$. They are operculate and have a distinct shoulder at the opercular rim. On bronchoscopic examination the bronchial and tracheal mucus contains brown streaks when eggs are plentiful. However, microscopic examination of washings or fecal flotation samples may be necessary. The eggs float well in saturated sugar or salt solutions but tend to collapse and take on a distorted crescent shape.

**Treatment.**    There are no satisfactory anthelmintics for effective treatment of paragonimiasis. Bithionol has been recommended at the rate of 500 mg./kg. body weight for 7 days, but this drug is not well tolerated and may cause severe diarrhea. In an emaciated patient this is very undesirable. Antibiotic treatment combined with efforts to improve the quality and quantity of food intake appears to result in marked improvement. In the absence of any specific treatment, death of the flukes and resolution of the cysts sometimes occurs over a 6-month period.

**Control.**    Prevention of infection could only be achieved by curtailing the natural predatory habits of cats and dogs, and this is hardly feasible if the animals are allowed outdoors.

### NASAL ARTHROPODS

Infections of the nasal passages of dogs with nasal mites (*Pneumonyssus caninum*) or nasal pentastomids (*Linguatula serrata*) are occasionally manifested clinically. There are no adequate records of the prevalence of these infections, since they are more often casual findings rather than primary clinical problems.

Nasal mites swarm over the mucosal surfaces of the nasal passages and sometimes cause excessive mucous discharge and frequent sneezing. Unsuspected cases are often revealed during anesthesia of dogs with gaseous agents when the mites come streaming out of the nares and out onto the operating table. Diagnosis of suspected cases depends on demonstrating mites in mucous discharges, but there are no specific treatments known. The inhalation of vaporized organophosphate from a resinous fly-strip hung in the cage of hospitalized animals has been effective.

*L. serrata*, commonly known as the "tongue worm," also has a tendency to emerge from the nasal passages of dogs under anesthesia. The segmented adult pentastomids (up to 15 cm. long) attach to the mucosal surface of the nasal passages. Eggs are released which are either sneezed out or swallowed. Disseminated eggs are eaten by herbivores, especially rabbits, and larvae develop in viscera and lymph nodes. Larvae released from infected tissues in dogs migrate cranially up the esophagus to the nasal pharynx. Chronically infected animals may develop a foul-smelling nasal discharge in which eggs of the parasite are present. Surgical removal of parasites may be necessary in these instances.

## PARASITES WHICH MIGRATE THROUGH THE RESPIRATORY SYSTEM

The larval forms of several intestinal nematodes of dogs and cats pass through the lungs as a part of their normal migratory pattern. They are coughed up and then swallowed, maturing in the small intestine.

Larvae of *Toxocara canis* and *Toxocara cati* are often present in the lungs of newborn puppies and kittens, respectively, and heavy infections result in substantial hemorrhage into the alveoli during the first days of life. This may prove fatal. Further exposure of newborn and young animals to embryonated eggs contaminating the environment can result in severe pneumonia and extensive pulmonary consolidation. Although the pathogenesis of the lesions is undoubtedly attributable in part to the physical damage caused by larvae which rupture alveolar capillaries, ascarid infections are associated with the development of marked immediate hypersensitivity and allergic inflammatory responses to the worms in pulmonary tissues form an additional pathologic component.

Acute respiratory signs may appear in puppies a few days after exposure to larvae of *Strongyloides stercoralis*. These larvae penetrate the skin and pass from the pulmonary circulation into the airway and are coughed up. During this phase, a soft cough develops and the animal becomes anorexic before the onset of the alimentary phase. Although larvae of *Ancylostoma caninum* and other hookworms travel by a similar route, the respiratory signs are much less pronounced than with *S. stercoralis*. However, extremely heavy exposure to hookworm larvae can produce massive pulmonary hemorrhage and death.

Anthelmintics are ineffective against the migrating stages of these nematodes. Attention must be given to the elimination of adult parasites in the intestine in order to prevent environmental contamination by eggs or larvae.

## PARASITES WHICH MIGRATE ABERRANTLY INTO THE RESPIRATORY SYSTEM

### CUTEREBRA MACULATA

The larval stages of the rodent botfly quite commonly develop in the tissues of cats in rural areas. The eggs of the fly are deposited in the environment around burrows or holes made by rabbits or rodents. The larvae which hatch out can attach to the skin of many animals, including cats. They normally develop for several months in subcutaneous tissues around the face before emerging to pupate on the ground. However, the larvae quite often undergo an aberrant migration in cats and develop in the mucosa of the pharynx and occasionally even the trachea.

**Clinical Signs.** Signs usually occur in kittens in the late summer or fall. At this time the larvae have reached a size sufficient to obstruct the airway, causing dyspnea. This is sometimes preceded by loud snoring and gagging. Larvae which become dislodged may be coughed or sneezed up. Bacterial infection may develop in the pharyngeal lesions, leading to systemic signs of fever, anorexia and depression.

**Diagnosis and Treatment.** A thorough physical examination will reveal the obstruction which is usually visible in the pharyngeal region and may be palpable externally. Surgical removal of the larva is necessary but care must be taken to avoid rupturing the parasite, since this may precipitate systemic anaphylactic reactions. Antibiotics should be given postoperatively.

### SPIROCERCA LUPI

The esophageal worm of dogs occurs in the southern states of the U.S.A. The parasites generally inhabit granulomatous masses in the wall of the esophagus. Eggs released into the lumen through sinuses pass out in the feces. Coprophagous beetles act as intermediate hosts but rodents and birds serve as transport hosts. Larvae ingested in tissues migrate via the arterial system to the midthoracic region, where they move across to the esophagus.

**Diagnosis.** Respiratory signs result when aberrant larvae invade the trachea or bronchi. The resulting granulomatous mass interferes with respiration, and the severity of clinical signs depends on the size and site of the lesion. Radiographic and bronchoscopic examination will reveal the obstruction but definitive diagnosis can be achieved only if eggs ($38 \times 12\ \mu$) are present in bronchial washings.

**Treatment.** Anthelmintic therapy is unlikely to lead to complete resolution of long-standing lesions. Some success has been achieved with disophenol (D.N.P.®, American Cyanamid) at 1 ml./5 kg. body weight. Prevention is difficult because of the variety of transport hosts and the reservoir of infection in sylvatic carnivores.

## SYSTEMIC PARASITES WHICH CAUSE RESPIRATORY SIGNS

### DIROFILARIA IMMITIS

Canine heartworms, once associated only with the southern U.S. states, have become disseminated over a wide area in the eastern half of the country. This mosquito-borne filarial parasite inhabits the right heart and pulmonary artery of dogs and occasionally cats. A detailed account of the pathogenesis of heartworm disease and the associated clinical signs are presented elsewhere in this text. However, one of the cardinal signs of infection is coughing, and given the increasing frequency of *D. immitis* over such a large area, heartworm disease should always be considered in the differential diagnosis of persistent coughing and respiratory insufficiency.

### TOXOPLASMA GONDII

Infection with cystic forms of the protozoan parasite *T. gondii* is prevalent throughout the world in almost all species of animals and man. In recent years the complex pattern of transmission has been clarified by the identification of an intestinal coccidian phase in cats. Trophozoite and cystic stages in dogs and cats occur in a wide variety of tissues, and while infections are asymptomatic in the majority of cases, clinical toxoplasmosis does develop in some instances and the respiratory system is most often involved.

**Clinical Signs.** The clinical syndrome in both dogs and cats is variable in course but anorexia, fever and lethargy accompanied by dyspnea are the essential features. Proliferation of the organisms in the lungs leads to focal necrotic lesions, and these coalesce to form irregularly shaped areas of coagulative necrosis which are visible radiographically. Naturally occurring cases in dogs are often complicated by the simultaneous manifestation of distemper.

**Diagnosis.** A protracted syndrome characterized by the above signs and unresponsive to antibiotics is suggestive of toxoplasmosis, but definitive diagnosis is difficult. Rising titers in the indirect fluorescent antibody test over the course of the disease are strongly supportive.

**Treatment.** No specific treatment is known, but combinations of sulfadiazine (33 mg./kg. 4 times daily for 1 to 2 weeks) and pyrimethamine (2.2 mg./kg.) are used in humans. This regimen has not been tested adequately in dogs and cats but it is known to be very toxic and is at best likely only to relieve symptoms rather than eliminate infection.

## SUPPLEMENTAL READING

Bennett, D., and Beresford-Jones, W. P.: Treatment of *Filaroides osleri* infestation in a 16-month-old male Yorkshire Terrier with thiabendazole. Vet. Rec., 93:226–227, 1973.

Corwin, R. M., Legendre, A. M., and Dade, A. W.: Lungworm *(Filaroides milksi)* infection in a dog. J. Am. Vet. Med. Assn., 165:180–181, 1975.

Hirth, R. S., and Hottendorf, G. H.: Lesions produced by a new lungworm in Beagle dogs. Vet. Pathol., 10:385–407, 1973.

# SYSTEMIC MYCOTIC PNEUMONIAS

DANNY W. SCOTT, D.V.M.
*Ithaca, New York*

The systemic mycoses of small animals (blastomycosis, coccidioidomycosis, cryptococcosis and histoplasmosis) are caused by fungi that are basically saprophytic and live in soil or organic debris. Infections are usually contracted via inhalation of infectious spores or mycelial fragments. Thus, the respiratory system is a common location for these primary fungal diseases. The clinical signs associated with respiratory infection are similar in all the systemic mycoses. The enzootic occurrence of these diseases in well-defined geographic areas is diagnostically significant, as are the radiographic findings.

## NORTH AMERICAN BLASTOMYCOSIS

Blastomycosis is a chronic disease affecting dogs more commonly than cats. The most frequent sites of infection are the lungs and the bronchial and mediastinal lymph nodes. The respiratory form of blastomycosis is associated with chronic coughing (dry or moist), persistent or phasic pyrexia (103 to 105° F.), poor appetite, depression, wasting and purulent nasal discharge.

In enzootic areas, the following signs associated with a respiratory disease should suggest possible blastomycosis: (1) skin lesions (pyogranulomas, abscesses, fistulas); (2) lameness due to osteomyelitis; and (3) ocular lesions (uveitis, panophthalmitis). The fever in blastomycosis is not responsive to antibiotics.

Radiographically, multiple noncalcified nodules due to abscesses and/or granulomas are seen throughout the lung fields. Hilar lymphadenopathy is common but seems not to be as extensive as in histoplasmosis. Acute miliary, interstitial foci may be found throughout the lungs.

## COCCIDIOIDOMYCOSIS

Coccidioidomycosis is a chronic disease affecting dogs more commonly than cats. The most frequent sites of infection are the lungs and the bronchial and mediastinal lymph nodes. The respiratory form of coccidioidomycosis is associated with chronic coughing (dry), persistent or phasic pyrexia (103 to 105° F.), dyspnea, tachypnea, poor appetite, depression and wasting. In enzootic areas, the lack of response to antibiotics in respiratory disease is suggestive of coccidioidomycosis.

Radiographically visible pulmonary changes appeared after 8 to 21 days in dogs experimentally infected intratracheally with *Coccidioides immitis*. Hilar lymphadenopathy with encroachment on the trachea and main bronchi is common. The perihilar area of the lung contains an interstitial density that is usually very dense centrally where it blends with the radiodensity of the enlarged lymph nodes. Ill-defined, round or oval densities are seen in the peripheral lung fields, which are less lucent because of an increase in linear interstitial and peribronchial densities. Thin-walled cavitations can occur. Pleural thickening or small pleural effusions are commonly seen. A miliary, interstitial spreading to the lung is uncommon. Alveolar infiltrates or opacification of an entire hemithorax is also uncommon.

## CRYPTOCOCCOSIS

Cryptococcosis is a chronic disease affecting dogs and cats with equal frequency. The most common sites of infection are the central nervous system and the upper respiratory tract. Cryptococcosis only rarely causes granulomatous pulmonary lesions. Clinical and radiographic findings would be similar to those described for blastomycosis and coccidioidomycosis.

## HISTOPLASMOSIS

Histoplasmosis is a chronic disease affecting dogs more commonly than cats. The most common sites of infection are the lungs and the bronchial and mediastinal lymph nodes. The respiratory form of histoplasmosis is associated with chronic coughing (moist or dry), persistent or phasic pyrexia (103 to 106° F.), dyspnea, tachypnea, poor appetite, depression and wasting. In enzootic areas, the lack of response to antibiotics in respiratory disease is suggestive of histoplasmosis.

Radiographically, acute or chronic histoplasmosis often reveals multiple, granulomatous nodular lesions associated with diffuse interstitial consolidations in the perihilar areas. Massive hilar lymphadenopathy that causes narrowing of the terminal trachea and main bronchi is common. The bend in the terminal trachea is accentuated, and a lucent, horizontal, S-shaped curve is formed in the trachea and main bronchi. Bullae and thin-walled cavitations are rare. The remnants of benign histoplasmosis may be visible radiographically for the rest of the animal's life. They usually appear as multiple, miliary, calcified nodules, several millimeters in diameter, and as calcification of the hilar lymph nodes.

As is the case in so many diseases, the earlier the diagnosis of systemic mycosis can be made, and the more localized the infection, the greater are the chances for success. Prognosis also varies somewhat with the fungus involved. The primary respiratory forms of coccidioidomycosis and histoplasmosis are usually self-limiting, and patients recover spontaneously or with symptomatic and supportive therapy. However, the respiratory forms of blastomycosis and cryptococcosis are usually chronic and progressive, and fatal if not treated. For further information on etiopathogenesis, diagnosis and treatment of the systemic mycoses, see the article on "The Systemic Mycoses."

---

# LOWER RESPIRATORY TRACT TRAUMA

D. J. KRAHWINKEL, JR., D.V.M.
*Knoxville, Tennessee*

Damage to the thoracic cage and its contents occurs commonly following traumatic injury. Respiratory tract injuries may range from insignificant lesions to life-threatening conditions. Many animals die before veterinary care can be obtained because of the extensive nature of the injuries. Others require prompt attention and emergency therapy to sustain life. Owing to the frequency of respiratory tract injuries, all trauma cases should include a thorough physical examination and thoracic radiographs.

Evaluation of vital signs will determine the status of the patient. The color of the mucous membranes will help to ascertain the adequacy of respiration, while perfusion of the oral mucous membranes will reflect the status of circulation. Digital pressure is used to blanch the unpigmented gingiva which should refill within 1 to 2 seconds. The rate and quality of the peripheral pulse must be checked to evaluate cardiac function. Auscultation of the thorax is used to determine ventilation as well as cardiac rate and rhythm. Finally, the type and rate of respiration are noted to aid in the evaluation of pulmonary function. This should be done by listening for air flow rather than by observing the thoracic movement, since there is no good correlation between respiratory motions and ventilation.

For adequate tissue respiration the lungs must maintain $PaO_2$ at or above 60 mm. Hg and $PaCO_2$ at or below 48 mm. Hg. Otherwise, life is threatened because of increasing respiratory and metabolic acidosis and hypoxia of the central nervous system.

Emergency treatment is aimed at maintaining cardiopulmonary function until the primary problem can be diagnosed. Emergency procedures include

1. Maintenance of a patent airway (tracheostomy if needed).
2. Oxygen therapy by endotracheal tube, mask or cage.
3. Shock treatment by the intravenous administration of large volumes of lactated Ringer's solution, corticosteroids, antibiotics and sodium bicarbonate (best accomplished by inserting a large-bore jugular catheter).
4. Sealing any open chest wounds with ointment and bandage to prevent aspiration of air.
5. Close observation and monitoring of vital signs.

After emergency therapy has stabilized the patient, further diagnostic procedures should be performed. Lateral and dorsoventral thoracic radiographs are desirable if they can be taken without causing the animal stress. If this is not possible, other radiographic views such as standing laterals are substituted. Thoracocentesis may be performed if radiographs indicate the presence of fluids or free air in the thorax. Hematologic studies, especially serial hematocrits, are valuable to assess blood loss. If blood gas equipment is available, determinations of arterial $PO_2$, $PCO_2$ and pH are helpful in evaluating the ventilatory status.

Respiratory tract trauma may result in a single disease state or a combination of disease conditions. These disease states include

—Reduction of lung volume (pneumothorax, hemothorax, diaphragmatic hernia).
—Injury to the thoracic cage (fractured ribs, thoracic wounds).
—Reduction in number of functional alveoli (pulmonary contusion).
—Hypovolemic shock (hemothorax).
—Airway obstruction (hemorrhage, edema).

The above conditions will be discussed individually; however, the reader should remember that they commonly occur in various combinations. The specific injuries will depend on the type of trauma (i.e., blunt or penetrating) as well as the location of the trauma (i.e., directly to the thorax or indirectly to the thorax via the abdomen and diaphragm).

## DIAPHRAGMATIC HERNIA

### ETIOLOGY

Congenital diaphragmatic hernias occur in dogs and cats. The most common type is a peritoneopericardial hernia, which is due to a defect in the embryologic development of the septum transversum. The majority of diaphragmatic hernias are acquired as a result of trauma. When the animal experiences a traumatic blow to the abdomen (e.g., motor vehicle accident, kick or fall), there is a sudden rise in intraabdominal pressure. Since the most flexible portion of the abdominal boundary is the diaphragm, it suddenly domes cranially. If the glottis is open, the lungs deflate, leaving no counter pressure being applied to the diaphragm from the thoracic side. This results in a large pleuroperitoneal pressure gradient with disruption of the diaphragm and protrusion of abdominal organs into the thorax.

### PATHOPHYSIOLOGY

Even though the diaphragm is not essential for life, it is necessary for normal respiratory function. The inspiratory function of the diaphragm is assumed by other abdominal and thoracic muscles, resulting in accentuated abdominal and thoracic movement during respiration.

Loss of the intrathoracic negative pressure and entry of abdominal viscera into the thorax cause compression of the lungs, thereby reducing functional residual capacity. These compressed lung fields become atelectatic and are not ventilated but continue to be perfused, resulting in a ventilation-perfusion inequity and hypoxia. Hypercarbia with acidosis may result from hypoventilation. The herniated organs and lack of negative pressure also compress the great veins around the heart, thereby impeding venous return and reducing cardiac output.

The abdominal organs most commonly herniated are the liver, small intestine and stomach. These organs may move freely into and out of the thorax unless adhesions or strangulation develops. When the liver is involved and becomes strangulated, there may be transudation of large amounts of fluid that results in a hydrothorax as well as a diaphragmatic hernia. Obstruction of the small intestine may occur owing to adhesions or constriction of the hernia defect. When this occurs, the disease resembles a primary gastrointestinal problem. The most devastating problem occurs when the stomach becomes lodged within the thorax. The cardia and pylorus may both become occluded, and bloat develops. This rapidly compresses the remaining functional lung tissue as well as the vena cava. If not immediately corrected, the animal dies from respiratory failure and low cardiac output. Intrathoracic adhesions are not as common as one would expect, neither does there appear to be any correlation between the presence of adhesions and the contents or duration of the hernia.

No predilection for the site of tears has been observed, although the left side would appear to be more vulnerable, since the liver would buffer pressure applied to the right side. Tears have been observed to occur on the right and left, dorsally and ventrally, and at the costal insertion. It has been the author's observation that more tears occur in the muscular portion than in the tendinous portion of the diaphragm. The defect with congenital peritoneopericardial hernias is always ventral and near the diaphragmatic midline.

There may be little pathologic change associated with peritoneopericardial hernias, since the herniated organs enter the pericardial sac rather than the pleural space. Should the volume of herniated viscera become great, the compression of the heart and lungs would produce cardiovascular and respiratory problems. Cardiac murmurs may develop as a result of compression and distortion of the AV valves.

## SIGNS

The signs associated with diaphragmatic hernia depend on the content and volume of the herniated organs. Signs may be intermittent as organs move in and out of the thorax. In general, the signs are related to compression of the lungs and heart by the herniated organs or to obstruction of the gastrointestinal tract when it is occluded by the hernia ring.

Congenital peritoneopericardial hernias may manifest few or no signs, incidental discovery being common. It is usually observed in young dogs and cats; however, some animals may be several years of age. Many of these will have an associated defect in the ventral abdominal musculature. In these cases, there is only falciform fat between the heart and the skin of the abdomen. The animal may be smaller than its littermates, with low exercise tolerance. Anorexia, lethargy and vomiting are the most common symptoms, with dyspnea developing in severe cases. Auscultation may reveal muffled heart sounds and cardiac murmurs.

Acquired (or traumatic) diaphragmatic hernias may exhibit a variety of symptoms. The size and location of the tear determines which organs protrude and consequently which signs are seen. The history usually reveals a traumatic incident which may have been recent or long-standing. Hernias of two years' duration are not uncommon, with symptomatology apparent only when abdominal organs "slide" into the thorax. The most common symptoms are dyspnea, hyperpnea, fatigue and lethargy. The animal usually assumes a sitting position to relieve intrathoracic pressure. Abdominal breathing is common, especially in cats. The abdomen may have a "tucked-up" appearance in chronic cases where much of the abdominal viscera is located within the thorax. Anorexia and vomiting occur when the intestinal tract is obstructed. In acute hernias associated with a hemothorax (originating from a contused liver or rupture of diaphragmatic vessels), the mucous membranes will be pale owing to hemorrhagic shock. Gastric dilation within the thorax may produce cyanotic mucous membranes, while hepatic obstruction causes icterus.

Auscultation will usually reveal the heart sounds to be displaced and muffled by the herniated abdominal viscera. Respiratory sounds are commonly heard only in the dorsal thorax. If hemothorax or hydrothorax is present, muffling of the thoracic sounds is the predominate finding. Thoracic boryborygmi are not common partially as a result of ileus of the gut within a diaphragmatic hernia. Percussion reveals a reduced thoracic resonance.

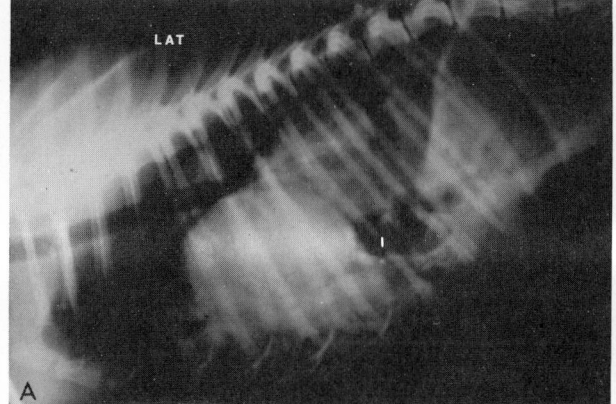

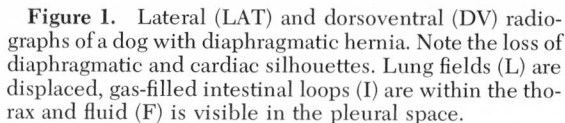

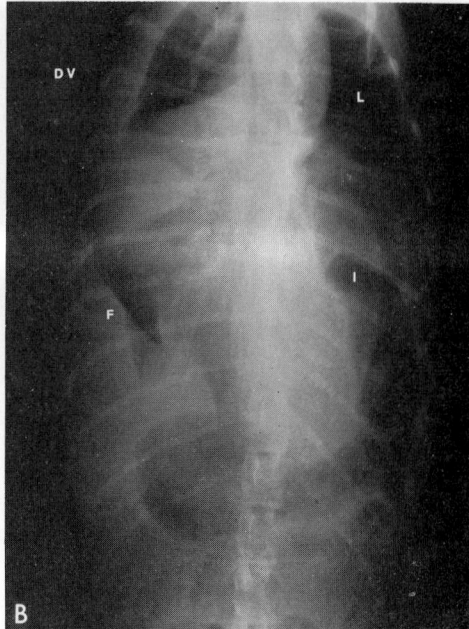

**Figure 1.** Lateral (LAT) and dorsoventral (DV) radiographs of a dog with diaphragmatic hernia. Note the loss of diaphragmatic and cardiac silhouettes. Lung fields (L) are displaced, gas-filled intestinal loops (I) are within the thorax and fluid (F) is visible in the pleural space.

## DIAGNOSIS

The tentative diagnosis is made on the basis of the history, symptoms and physical examination and is then confirmed by radiology. The animal should not be caused stress during the examination nor held in a head-down position in an attempt to accentuate the symptoms. This may greatly increase the volume of the hernia and prove to be fatal. Lateral and dorsoventral radiographs should be taken (Fig. 1). If these are not diagnostic, barium sulfate can be administered and additional radiographs can be taken in 30 minutes. Another diagnostic technique involves injecting 20 to 30 ml. of air into the abdominal cavity and holding the animal in an upright position for 5 minutes. A standing lateral radiograph is then taken which will show air in the dorsal pleural space in the case of a traumatic hernia or in the pericardial sac in the case of a peritoneopericardial hernia. In cases with associated hydrothorax or hemothorax, the fluid may have to be removed by thoracocentesis before diagnostic radiographs can be obtained.

Acquired diaphragmatic hernias can usually be confirmed by one or more of the following radiographic signs:

1. Loops of gas-filled or barium-filled intestine within the pleural space.

2. Loss of an intact diaphragmatic shadow.

3. Gas-filled stomach within the left hemithorax.

4. Loss of the cardiac silhouette.

5. Displacement of the lung fields dorsally and laterally.

6. Free fluid within the pleural space.

7. Free air in the pleural space following a pneumoperitoneogram.

Radiographs of a congenital peritoneopericardial hernia reveal an enlarged cardiac silhouette, loops of gas- or barium-filled gastrointestinal tract within the pericardial sac and loss of the ventral diaphragmatic contour (Fig. 2). The radiographic appearance of a diaphragmatic hernia can change as different abdominal organs move into and out of the thorax.

## TREATMENT

The surgical repair should be postponed until the animal has been treated for shock and stabilized unless respiration is severely compromised. If the stomach is dilated within the thorax, an emergency thoracocentesis should be performed to deflate the stomach. The presence of anemia, dehydration, infection, nephritis and hepatitis should be evaluated by the use of a complete blood count (CBC), serum glutamic-pyruvic transaminase (SGPT) and blood urea nitrogen (BUN). If a left-sided hernia is diagnosed, surgical correction must be accomplished as soon as possible because of

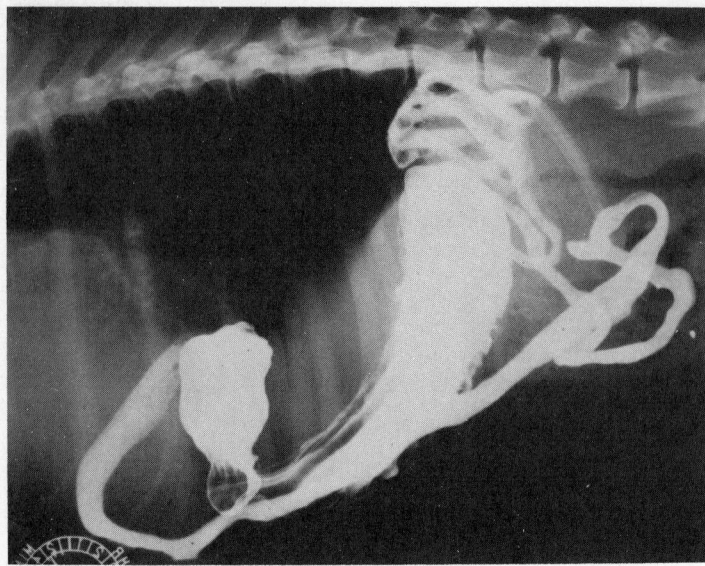

**Figure 2.** Lateral radiograph of a peritoneopericardial hernia following a barium swallow. The pyloric portion of the stomach and the duodenum are within the pericardial sac.

the possibility of intrathoracic gastric dilation. With this exception, surgery may be postponed until conditions are optimal. However, diaphragmatic herniorrhaphy should never be considered an elective procedure and unduly postponed.

An intravenous catheter should be inserted preoperatively for drug and fluid therapy. Except for shock treatment, large volumes of fluids should not be administered lest edema develop in damaged pulmonary tissue. Good anesthetic technique is imperative for proper management of diaphragmatic hernia. No respiratory depressant preanesthetic agent (e.g., narcotics) should be used. Atropine is used to reduce respiratory secretions and prevent brachycardia. Tranquilizers may be used to sedate nervous animals; however, it must be kept in mind that phenothiazine derivatives are hypotensive. A small dose of an ultrashort-acting barbiturate or halothane (Fluothane®) by mask is used for induction. The animal is quickly intubated and maintained on an inhalation anesthetic (e.g., halothane or methoxyflurane) and oxygen. Nitrous oxide should not be used because of the compromised pulmonary function. Ventilation should be assisted or controlled by manual or mechanical means until the hernia has been corrected and a negative intrathoracic pressure has been established. A balanced electrolyte solution should be administered during surgery, and a pad or

circulating warm water blanket* should be used to prevent hypothermia.

A ventral midline incision affords the most versatile surgical approach to diaphragmatic herniorrhaphy. A slight head-up positioning of the animal will assist in later reduction of the hernia. An incision is made on the abdominal midline from the xiphoid to the umbilicus. The anterior abdomen is opened and the falciform fat is removed. The abdominal wall is retracted and the abdominal viscera are displaced posteriorly to permit visualization of the diaphragm. The tear is observed or palpated to determine its location and which viscera are herniated. If the tear is in the ventral half of the diaphragm and intrathoracic adhesions are not present, repair can be accomplished without additional exposure. The herniated organs are reduced, and a thoracic drainage tube is inserted. The edges of the tear are grasped with Allis forceps and retracted upward while the repair is being made. If the tear is in the dorsal half of the diaphragm, or if there are adhesions within the thoracic cavity, this approach will usually not be adequate. In such a case, the posterior one-half of the sternum is split on the midline with heavy bone-cutting scissors, an osteotome or an oscillating bone saw. The sternum is retracted and the intact diaphragm is incised down to the hernia, care

---

*K-Pad, Gorman-Rupp Ind., Bellville, Ohio 44813.

being taken to avoid the phrenic nerves and the posterior vena cava (Fig. 3). The thoracic and abdominal organs are carefully inspected for perforations, torsions or other damage. Adhesions between the abdominal and thoracic organs are broken down by blunt dissection. The hernia is reduced and the abdominal organs are packed off posteriorly with a damp cloth. The edges of the diaphragm are grasped with Allis tissue forceps and are retracted upward. Suturing begins at the deepest end of the diaphragmatic tear with a sterile, nonabsorbable suture material. After the suture has been securely anchored at the deep end of the tear, a continuous suture pattern can be used to close the defect (Fig. 4). If the suture line is extremely long, the pattern should be interrupted in 2 or 3 places. In large active dogs, a two-layer closure is preferred. During the suturing process, special care should be taken to avoid damage to the phrenic nerves, vena cava, lungs and liver. If the diaphragm has been torn away from its costal attachment, it can be sutured to the intercostal space or around an adjacent rib. In a hernia of long duration, the edges of the diaphragm should be freshened before suturing. A thoracic drainage tube is inserted through the sternotomy. A stab wound is made in the skin over the lateral aspect of the 8th or 9th intercostal space, and a curved hemostat is inserted through the stab wound in the skin and tunneled subcutaneously forward one intercostal space (Fig. 5). The hemostat is then bluntly pushed through the intercostal space with the opposite hand protecting the heart and lungs. The end of a No. 18 French feeding tube is grasped with the hemostat within the thorax and is pulled retrograde through the tunnel, leaving 5 to 10 cm. inside the pleural space (Fig. 6). A purse-string suture is placed in the skin around the tube. The sternum is closed with 2 to 4 stainless steel wire sutures placed through the cut sternum rather than encircling it to avoid injury to the heart or lungs should a wire break (Fig. 7). The thoracic muscles, abdomen, subcutaneous tissue and skin are closed in a routine manner. The pleural space is evacuated of air and fluid by attaching a syringe or suction to the drainage tube. After negative pressure has been established within the pleural space, the chest tube is removed by placing the index finger

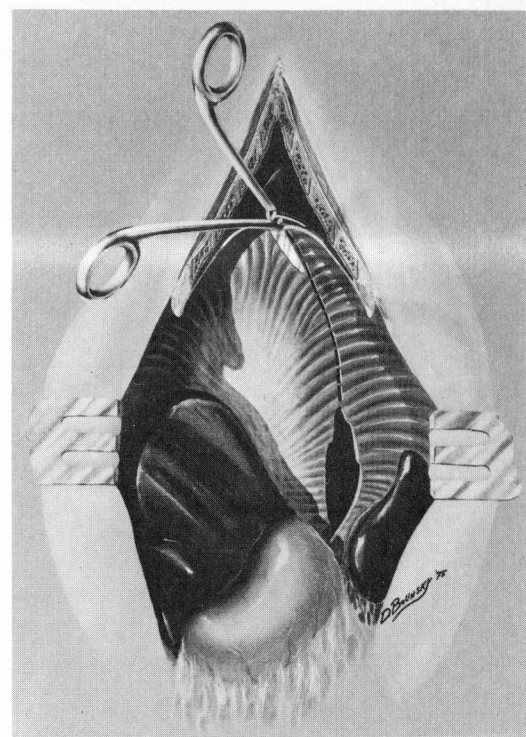

**Figure 3.** The intact diaphragm is incised down to the hernia defect for adequate retraction and exposure.

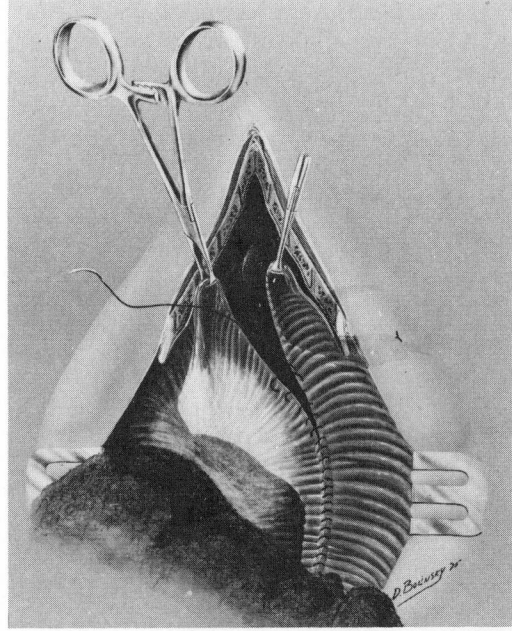

**Figure 4.** The edges of the diaphragm are retracted upward with Allis forceps and the abdominal viscera are "packed" posteriorly as suturing begins at the deep end of the hernia.

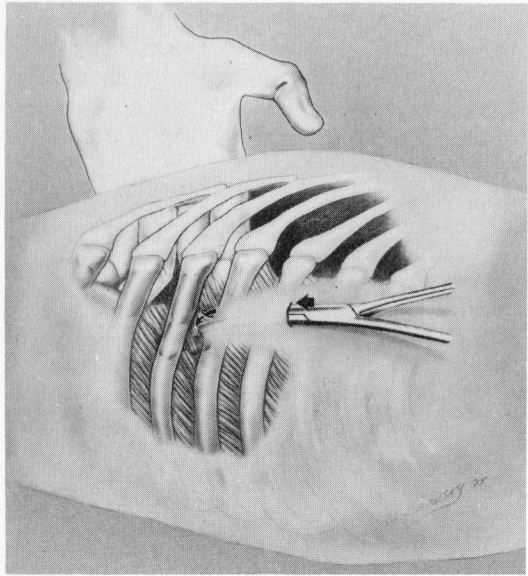

**Figure 5.** A subcutaneous tunnel is made through which to implant a thoracic drainage tube.

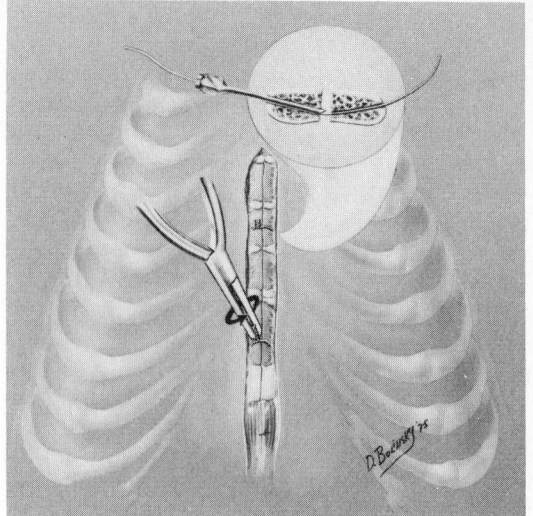

**Figure 7.** Stainless steel wire is used to close the sternotomy. Wires are passed through the sternebrae rather than encircling them.

of one hand over the subcutaneous tunnel and quickly withdrawing the tube with the opposite hand. The purse-string suture is tightened to prevent air from reentering the thorax. Respirations should be assisted (4 to 6/minute) until spontaneous respirations begin.

The animal should be maintained on oxygen by endotracheal tube until spontaneous ventilation is adequate and swallowing begins. The endotracheal tube is removed and

additional oxygen is administered by face mask or oxygen cage until the animal is able to maintain adequate oxygenation on room air. Antibiotics should be administered for 5 to 7 days, and intravenous fluids should be continued until the animal's appetite returns. At the time of discharge, the owner is advised to restrict the dog to leash exercise for a 30-day period. The skin sutures should be removed at 10 days, and the animal should be thoroughly examined to insure that there are no further complications.

## PNEUMOTHORAX

Pneumothorax is the accumulation of free air within the pleural space. This condition commonly occurs simultaneously with other injuries.

### ETIOLOGY

Air may gain access to the pleural space externally from a defect in the thoracic cage or internally from a leak in the lower respiratory tract. Causes of pneumothorax include the following:
Traumatic causes:
  —Penetrating wounds of the thoracic wall (e.g., missiles, surgery, fight wounds).
  —Laceration of tracheobronchial tree or pulmonary tissue (e.g., broken ribs, surgery).

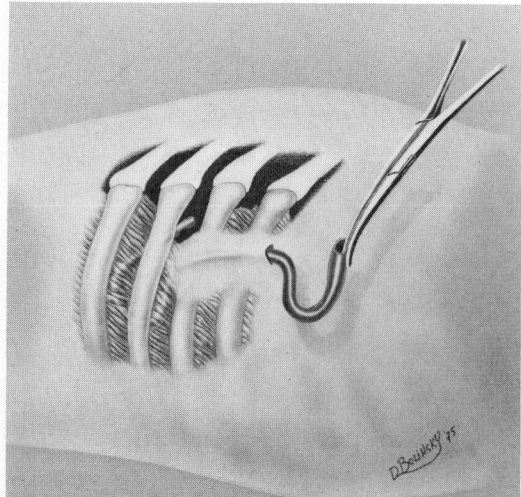

**Figure 6.** The thoracic drainage tube is inserted leaving 5 to 10 cm. within the pleural space.

—Blunt trauma with pulmonary contusion and alveolar rupture.
—Entry of air during thoracocentesis.
—Alveolar rupture due to vigorous mechanical or manual ventilation.
Nontraumatic causes:
  —Pulmonary rupture due to preexisting disease (e.g., neoplasia, pleuritis, pneumocele).
  —Spontaneous (rare except in racing greyhounds).

## PATHOPHYSIOLOGY

The pleural space normally contains no air. A small amount of pleural fluid provides for cohesion of the parietal and visceral pleura. The lungs remain inflated despite their elasticity because of a slight negative intrapleural pressure. When free air enters the pleural space, the negative intrapleural pressure is lost and the lung recoils away from the thoracic wall. Air entering one hemithorax will produce a bilateral pneumothorax due to the weakness of the mediastinum. In an effort to maintain tidal volume, the animal will expand the thoracic cage and increase respiratory effort. Dogs tolerate severe pneumothorax unless they are stressed.

Tension pneumothorax can be a rapidly fatal disease. This develops as a result of a valvelike defect in the pulmonary tissue. Air is sucked into the intrapleural space during inspiration but cannot escape during expiration. The condition is progressive, with intrapleural pressures quickly exceeding atmospheric pressures, thereby decreasing ventilation and venous return to the heart. Death results from hypoxia and reduced cardiac output.

## SIGNS

The signs associated with pneumothorax vary from none in mild cases to severe dyspnea in others. The more common signs include tachypnea, abduction of the forelegs and accentuated respiratory movements. Cyanosis may be seen in severe cases. Sucking thoracic wounds may be present in cases of penetrating trauma. Subcutaneous emphysema is sometimes evident over the thoracic and cervical areas. Broken ribs may be palpated or observed if much displacement is present.

Auscultation reveals reduced lung sounds in the ventral thorax. In addition, an increased resonance of heart sounds is noted in severe cases.

## DIAGNOSIS

The diagnosis is confirmed by radiography or thoracocentesis. Aspiration of free air from the pleural space is diagnostic of pneumothorax. Radiographs are a less hazardous diagnostic method. Lateral (Fig. 8) and dorsoventral views will reveal the following:
  —Elevation of the cardiac shadow off the sternum in recumbent lateral views.

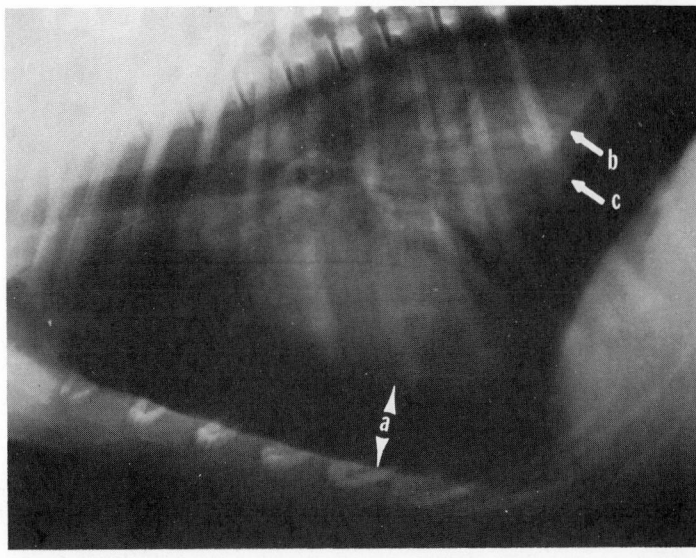

**Figure 8.** Lateral radiographs of a dog with pneumothorax. Note the elevation of the heart off the sternum (*a*) and the collapse of the lung lobes (*b,c*).

—Increased density of pulmonary tissue.

—Failure of pulmonary vessels to extend to the thoracic wall.

—Free air between the parietal and visceral pleura.

—In some cases, subcutaneous emphysema and fractured ribs.

Serial radiographs are useful in ascertaining the progress of the disease.

## TREATMENT

Most cases of pneumothorax can be successfully managed by nonsurgical methods. Mild cases respond to cage rest and observation. Non-narcotic sedatives may be used in active or excitable animals. If the leak has sealed, the air will be resorbed in a few days. Sucking wounds should be covered with a dressing and bandage to prevent further aspiration of air. Supplemental oxygen should be supplied in any case of pneumothorax with respiratory difficulty. Shock therapy may be required for those animals experiencing severe trauma. In cases with much air in the pleural space, evacuation is required by either thoracocentesis or tube drainage. Thoracocentesis is best performed with a large syringe, three-way stopcock and 20-gauge needle. For best results, both sides of the thorax should be aspirated, care being taken to avoid the intercostal and internal thoracic vessels. The thorax should be sufficiently evacuated to improve respiration. Total evacuation should not be attempted if there is an intrathoracic air leak, since this may reopen a sealed defect and cause worsening of the problem.

For repeated evacuation, a thoracic drainage tube should be implanted (Fig. 9), since it is more efficient and safer than repeated thoracocentesis. Local anesthetic is injected over 2 to 3 adjacent intercostal spaces of the lateral thorax. A stab wound is made in the skin and a curved hemostat is used to make a subcutaneous tunnel anteriorly 1 to 2 intercostal spaces. A No. 18 French feeding tube is carried through the tunnel with the curved hemostat and bluntly inserted through the intercostal space, leaving 5 to 10 cm. of the tube within the thorax. A purse-string suture is placed in the skin around the tube to prevent leakage, and a large syringe is used to evacuate the pleural space. The tube is covered with a light bandage to prevent mutilation by the animal,

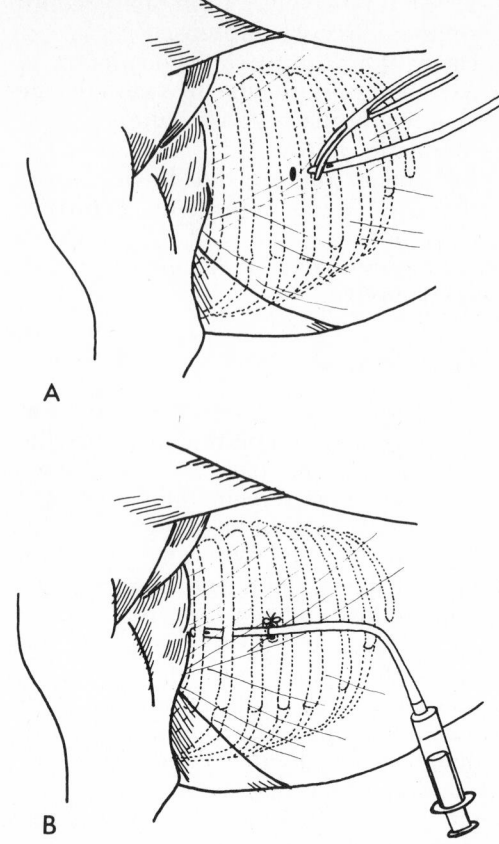

**Figure 9.** A thoracic drainage tube passed through a stab wound in the skin and into the thorax via a subcutaneous tunnel (*A*). A purse-string suture is placed around the tube, 5 to 10 cm. of which is left within the pleural space (*B*).

leaving the tip exposed for subsequent aspiration. The tube can be left in place for several days if needed. When removed, the purse-string suture is used to close the skin wound.

Tension pneumothorax requires immediate thoracocentesis or tube drainage and oxygen administration. After the animal has stabilized, surgical correction may be required.

Induction of anesthesia is accomplished by intravenous thiobarbiturate or halothane by mask. The trachea is immediately intubated and respiration is controlled manually or by mechanical ventilator. Anesthesia is maintained with minimal concentrations of halothane or methoxyflurane.

Wounds of the thoracic wall should be debrided and closed. If continued intrathoracic leakage occurs, exploratory surgery is indicated. A thoracotomy at the

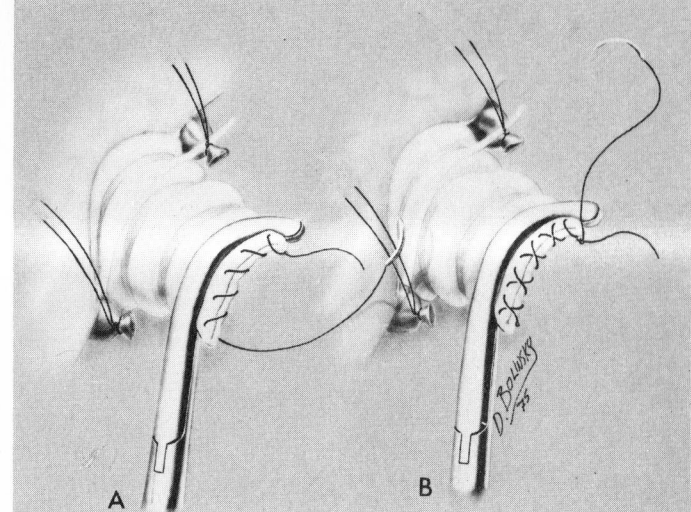

**Figure 10.** The bronchus is cross-clamped with a noncrushing clamp, and a row of continuous sutures is placed in the bronchus (A). The stump is oversewn with a second row of continuous sutures (B).

5th intercostal space of the affected side will give exposure to the entire hemithorax. If the affected side cannot be determined, a sternotomy is preferred in order to visualize all the thoracic organs. Severe damage to a lung lobe necessitates its removal. The pulmonary vessels can be ligated or clipped with hemostatic clips, and the bronchus is oversewn to prevent postoperative pneumothorax. Two rows of a continuous pattern utilizing 4-0 nonabsorbable suture and a small atraumatic tapered needle are used (Fig. 10). Portions of a lobe can be salvaged by cross-clamping above the injury with noncrushing forceps and amputating the damaged portion. A row of overlapping

mattress sutures is placed proximal to the clamps, and the end is oversewn with a simple continuous suture (Fig. 11). Small tears in the lung parenchyma near the lobe margin can be managed by ligating a portion of the lobe (Fig. 12). Tears in the central portions of the lobe can be sealed with an X-stitch placed across the defect (Fig. 13). Synthetic absorbable suture material of 5-0 size with a fine atraumatic tapered needle is used for all pulmonary suturing. Antibiotics should be administered for 5 to 7 days to prevent posttrauma infection, and activity should be restricted for two weeks. Sedatives can be used in the convalescent period if necessary.

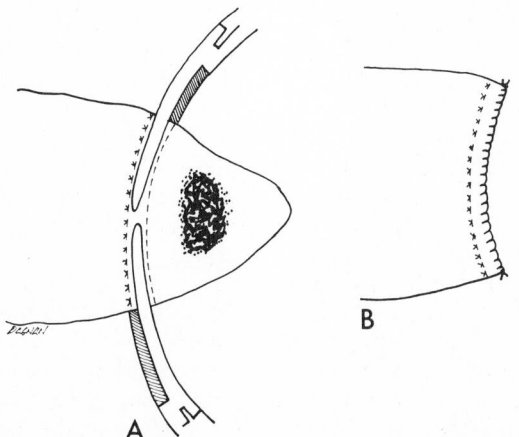

**Figure 11.** A portion of a lung lobe can be amputated by cross-clamping proximal to the injury and placing a row of overlapping mattress sutures above the clamps (A). The portion distal to the clamps is excised, the clamps are removed and the end is oversewn with a continuous suture (B).

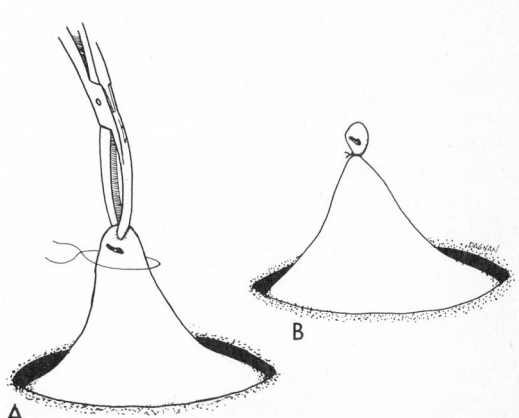

**Figure 12.** Small peripheral tears in the pulmonary tissue can be grasped with a hemostat (A) and ligated (B).

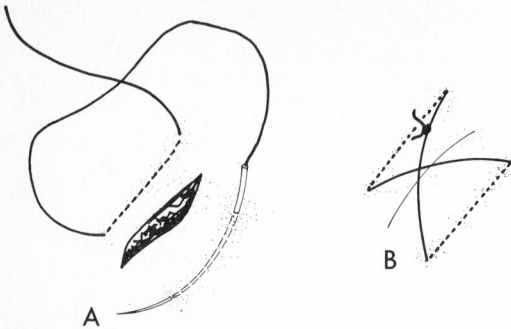

**Figure 13.** Small nonperipheral tears in the lung can be closed with an X-stitch placed across the defect (*A* and *B*).

## RIB FRACTURES

Rib fractures occur as a result of direct trauma to the thoracic cage. The trauma may be blunt (e.g., motor vehicle accident) or penetrating (e.g., high-velocity missile). These fractures constitute a small percentage of the fractures diagnosed in veterinary practice because the ribs are very flexible, especially in the young, and absorb trauma without fracturing. Many trauma cases with fractured ribs are not diagnosed because they either are asymptomatic or have other more serious injuries and the rib fractures are overlooked.

Other thoracic injuries are commonly associated with rib fractures. If the fractured ends of the rib are displaced into the thorax, puncture of a lung or major vessel may occur, resulting in pneumothorax and/or hemothorax. The intercostal vessels which lie immediately posterior to the rib may be severed, contributing to hemothorax. Any force sufficient to fracture a rib may also produce a pulmonary contusion as well as hemorrhage and edema of the thoracic wall.

When two or more adjacent ribs are broken in two places, a section of thoracic wall becomes free-floating and is termed "flail chest." The free-floating section is sucked inward with inspiration and pushed outward with expiration, resulting in ineffectual respiration.

## SIGNS

An animal with rib fractures may show few signs unless there are other associated intrathoracic problems. Painful respiration is one of the most common signs and results in hypoventilation and attempts to "splint" the thorax to reduce motion. Animals with "flail chest" may have severe respiratory embarrassment as the flail section moves independently of the remainder of the thoracic cage.

## DIAGNOSIS

Diagnosis is made by palpation and radiography. In some cases crepitation or distortion of the fracture site can be palpated, while in others subcutaneous emphysema is evident. The floating section of a "flail chest" is easily observed and palpated. Dorsoventral and lateral radiographs are usually diagnostic of rib fractures (Fig. 14). Although it results in a poorer quality film, the lateral view should be taken with the injured side up to reduce pain and prevent further intrathoracic damage. When radiography of the ribs is desired, the kvp must be increased over that for regular thoracic radiographs.

## TREATMENT

Animals with little respiratory difficulty or minor pain may be managed with cage rest and observation. Mild tranquilization

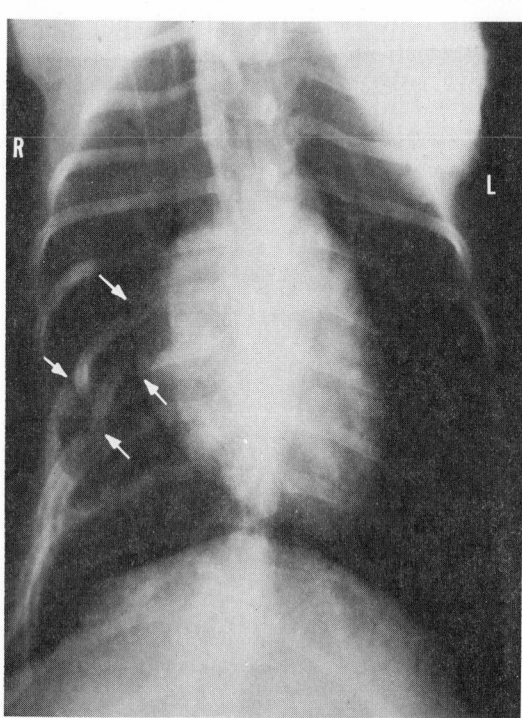

**Figure 14.** Dorsoventral radiograph of a dog with "flail chest." Note the adjacent ribs which are fractured in two places (arrows) and the sunken portion of the right thoracic rib cage.

can be used to quiet nervous individuals. If pain is severe, low doses of meperidine (2 to 4 mg./kg.) or pentazocine (1 to 2 mg./kg.) are beneficial. Supporting the thorax with a light, elastic support bandage is helpful in some cases to reduce fracture movement and pain. The benefits gained from the use of narcotic analgesics and bandaging must be weighed against their suppression of respiration. Animals with "flail chest" may require supplemental oxygen therapy.

Fractured ribs should be repaired when there is much displacement or the fractured ends project into the thorax as surgical repair hastens the recovery and prevents further damage. In addition, the fractures of "flail chest" must be repaired to maintain adequate respiration. Simple fracture repair may be postponed until the animal has stabilized; however, cases of "flail chest" may constitute an emergency and require immediate surgery. Inhalation anesthesia with positive pressure ventilation is essential for the repair, since the thoracic wall is not intact. Rib fractures may be repaired by several methods. Small intramedullary pins or Kirschner wires may be used to cross-pin the fracture site, with care being taken to be sure that the pins do not penetrate the medial cortex and enter the pleural space (Fig. 15A). Fractures can be repaired by wiring. Holes are drilled and the wires are placed in a craniocaudal direction to prevent a wire from injuring the lung should it fatigue and break (Fig. 15B). The most stable repair is accomplished by cross-pinning the fracture site and applying a tension band wire to compress the fracture site (Fig. 15C). A thoracic drainage tube is inserted when pneumothorax or hemothorax is present. Antibiotics are administered for 5 to 7 days and rest is enforced for two weeks. IM pins should be removed in 4 to 6 weeks.

## HEMOTHORAX

Hemothorax is defined as free blood in the pleural space. It may occur as a result of eroding lesions in the thorax or rarely as a result of a ruptured aneurysm. Traumatic causes include

— Missile penetration of heart, great vessels or lung.
— Lung laceration from a fractured rib.
— Rupture of intercostal vessels by a fractured rib.
— Iatrogenic causes resulting from vascular damage during thoracic surgery.
— Hepatic or diaphragmatic hemorrhage associated with a diaphragmatic hernia.

Traumatic hemothorax commonly occurs simultaneously with other conditions such as rib fractures, pneumothorax and pulmonary contusion. Death is rapid when large vessels or the heart is damaged. The free blood initially coagulates but then defibrinates and returns to a fluid state. The lungs are compressed by the encroaching pleural fluid, resulting in respiratory distress and hemorrhagic shock.

### SIGNS

The signs are attributable to pulmonary compression and shock. The animal may exhibit dyspnea, pale mucous membranes, weak thready pulses and weakness. Auscultation of the thorax reveals muffled heart sounds and dorsally displaced lung sounds. The clinical signs may vary with the rate and amount of hemorrhage.

### DIAGNOSIS

Radiographs will reveal the presence of free fluid in the pleural space. Lateral, dorsoventral and standing lateral views (Fig. 16) are all useful in determining the absence or presence of fluid as well as the amount. Serial radiographs are useful in ascertaining the progress of the disease. Depending on the amount of hemorrhage present, radiographs will show

— Ground-glass appearance of the thorax.

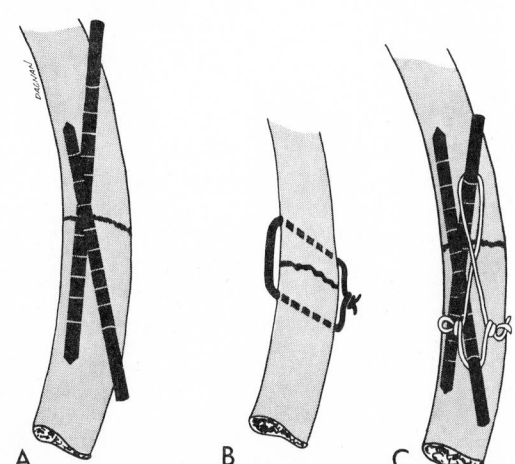

**Figure 15.** Rib fractures can be repaired by cross-pinning (*A*), wiring in a craniocaudal direction (*B*) or a combination of cross-pinning and a tension band wire (*C*).

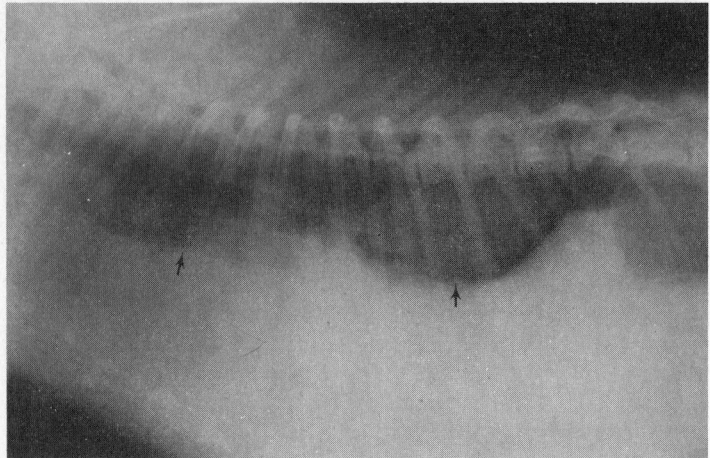

**Figure 16.** A standing lateral radiograph of a dog with hemothorax. Note the ground-glass appearance of the ventral thorax. A fluid line (arrows) is apparent, with lungs displaced dorsally.

—Radiodense fluid material between visceral and parietal pleura.

—Rounding of the costophrenic angle (dorsoventral view).

—Distinct interlobar fissures.

—Fluid line (standing lateral view).

Thoracocentesis is required to determine the type of fluid. This should be performed aseptically below the costochondral junction at the 4th or 5th intercostal space. An 18-gauge 1.5-inch needle is sufficient in most animals to penetrate the parietal pleura. Care must be taken to avoid damage to the heart, the intercostal vessels posterior to the rib and the internal thoracic vessels along the sternum. Each side of the thorax should be tapped two or three times and no aspirate obtained before ruling out hemothorax. With the use of a large syringe and stopcock, as much of the blood as possible is removed. It is usually necessary to tap both sides to evacuate the pleural space adequately. Examination of the fluid is useful in determining if other disease processes are involved. Serial packed cell volumes (PCV) on peripheral blood are helpful in evaluating whether or not hemorrhage is progressive.

### TREATMENT

Treatment for shock is the first consideration. The placement of a large-bore jugular catheter will greatly enhance subsequent treatment. Volume replacement with a balanced electrolyte solution (lactated Ringer's) is imperative along with intravenous corticosteroids, antibiotics and oxygen. Should vital signs not improve with the above therapy and the PCV continue to decline, fresh whole blood should be administered. If subsequent radiographs and PCV's indicate continued hemorrhage, emergency exploratory surgery must be performed. A lateral thoracotomy is preferred if the site of hemorrhage can be ascertained; otherwise, a sternotomy is used in order to explore the entire thorax.

## PULMONARY CONTUSION

Pulmonary contusion is a bruising of the lung manifested by hemorrhage and edema in the alveoli and interstitial spaces. Blunt trauma to the thorax is the usual cause of pulmonary contusion. The lungs are well protected by the rib cage; therefore, any force sufficient to bruise the lungs may simultaneously fracture ribs, creating a hemothorax or pneumothorax.

### SIGNS

The animal is usually dyspneic with rapid respirations. Hemoptysis is not a common finding but may occur in severely traumatized patients. Pulmonary rales may be ausculted. Severe pain, cyanosis or shock may be evident if rib fractures, pneumothorax or hemothorax is present.

### DIAGNOSIS

The diagnosis is made on the basis of a history of trauma, symptoms, physical findings and radiographs. Lateral and dorsoventral radiographs reveal irregular, patchy areas of consolidation and air bronchograms within lung lobes. Severe cases may be manifested by diffuse consolidation and collapse of an entire lobe. Some free air or blood may be present in the pleural space.

## TREATMENT

Supportive therapy is the treatment of choice for pulmonary contusion. Enforced rest and oxygen therapy are utilized to prevent hypoxia. Antibiotics are used to preclude infection in the devitalized lung tissue. To prevent additional edema in the damaged lung, fluid therapy must be limited. Diuretics aid in the removal of edematous fluid. Serial radiographs usually reveal much improvement in 24 to 48 hours and complete resolution in 3 to 10 days. Other concomitant disease conditions must be appropriately treated.

## PULMONARY HERNIA

Pulmonary hernias occur as a result of rib separation following traumatic laceration of the intercostal muscles and parietal pleura. This most commonly occurs following a dog fight and may be seen simultaneously with other thoracic injuries. If the skin is intact, subcutaneous inflation of the lung can be observed and a defect in the thoracic wall can be palpated. A lung lobe may protrude externally when the skin and underlying musculature are also lacerated.

If the skin is intact, a support bandage should be placed over the defect to prevent the lung lobe from entering the subcutaneous space and becoming strangulated. After the animal has been stabilized by symptomatic treatment, the problem can be corrected under general anesthesia and positive pressure ventilation. A thoracic drainage tube is implanted and the defect is closed by apposing the two adjacent ribs with large encircling sutures. The thoracic musculature is closed in a routine fashion.

If lung tissue is exposed externally, it should be covered with saline sponges to prevent desiccation and corrective surgery should be performed immediately. Damaged lung lobes are repaired or removed as described under pneumothorax and the defect is closed as outlined above. Rest should be enforced for two weeks, and prophylactic antibiotics should be administered for 5 to 7 days.

### SUPPLEMENTAL READING

Archibald, J., and Harvey, C. E.: Thorax. In Archibald, J. Canine Surgery. 2nd Archibald edition. Santa Barbara, American Veterinary Publications, 1974, pp. 381–427.
Berg, P.: Pneumothorax. In Kirk, R. W. (ed.): Current Veterinary Therapy V. Philadelphia, W. B. Saunders Co., 1974, pp. 243–245.
Carb, A.: Diaphragmatic hernia in the dog and cat. Vet. Clin. N. Am. 5:477–494, 1975.
Ticer, J. W., and Brown, S. G.: Thoracic trauma. In Ettinger, S. J. (ed.): Textbook of Veterinary Internal Medicine. Philadelphia, W. B. Saunders Co., 1975, pp. 629–648.
Wilson, G. P.: The diaphragm. In Bojrab, M. J. (ed.): Current Techniques in Small Animal Surgery. Vol. I. Philadelphia, Lea & Febiger, 1975, pp. 156–158.

# HYPERTROPHIC OSTEO-ARTHROPATHY

ROBERT S. BRODEY, D.V.M.
*Philadelphia, Pennsylvania*

This syndrome may be defined as a quadrilateral disease of the extremities, which in the dog is almost invariably a secondary manifestation of intrathoracic disease. If the initiating lesion is pulmonary, the condition is commonly referred to as hypertrophic pulmonary osteoarthropathy. This condition most commonly affects the dog and man, but it has rarely been reported in the cat. The pathophysiology is initially characterized by a rapid increase in peripheral blood flow in the distal half of the extremities. At the same time or very shortly thereafter, there is an extensive build-up of connective tissue around the distal bones and joints of the limbs, which extends proximally to the midshaft of the radius, ulna, tibia and fibula. This deposition of periarticular collagenous tissue causes the joints to appear swollen. Postmortem studies have shown that the articulations are essentially normal. The term osteoarthropathy is therefore a misnomer because there is no arthropathy associated with this disease. A third and very important component of the limb lesions is periosteal in nature and develops very shortly after the vascular and connective tissue changes.

The clinical picture is characterized by the sudden or gradual development of lameness, usually in all four limbs. In early cases, the affected extremities are painful, warm, pulsatile and swollen distally. The skin is taut because of the increase in thickness of the underlying tissues. This is particularly noticeable in the metacarpal and metatarsal areas. At no time is there pitting edema; therefore, hypertrophic osteoarthropathy should not be confused with generalized passive venous congestion, such as that observed with some heart base (aortic arch) tumors. As the condition becomes more chronic, pain may be less evident and the animal may walk with a stilted gait. The limbs appear less pulsatile and more indurated, suggesting that the vascular component has receded somewhat, whereas the connective tissue and periosteal new bone components have increased greatly. Much of the limb swelling is due to the soft tissue changes and not the periosteal new bone formation as was originally thought. It is often possible to palpate the irregular osteophytes, particularly along the caudal aspects of the ulna. Clinical signs of hypertrophic osteoarthropathy may precede, follow or develop at approximately the same time as signs relating to the intrathoracic lesion(s). The duration of osteoarthropathy in 53 dogs ranged from one day to one year. In 40 dogs, clinical signs had been observed from one day to four weeks. The signs of osteoarthropathy preceded those relating to intrathoracic disease in 37 dogs; signs of thoracic disease were observed initially in eight dogs, and signs of thoracic disease and osteoarthropathy were observed simultaneously in eight others.

Radiographically, periosteal new bone

formation and soft tissue swelling are very apparent and are usually bilaterally symmetrical. In early cases, periosteal new bone is detected along the shafts of the metatarsal and metacarpal bones. The periosteal new bone, characterized by the formation of coralliform osteophytes, develops distally on the shafts of the long bones and rapidly spreads proximally to the femora and humeri, occasionally to the pelvis and rarely to other flat bones. In a few chronic cases, the layer of periosteal new bone may greatly exceed the thickness of the original cortex. Whenever hypertrophic osteoarthropathy is suspected, lateral and dorsoventral radiograms of the thorax are indicated.

The differential diagnosis of this condition usually presents few problems. The clinical and radiographic changes are almost invariably present in all four extremities. The bilateral symmetry of the periosteal lesions, the absence of overlying pitting edema or destructive changes in the underlying cortices and the presence of one or more intrathoracic lesions are usually enough to allow the clinician to make the diagnosis of hypertrophic osteoarthropathy.

In the early European literature, hypertrophic osteoarthropathy in dogs was usually associated with pulmonary tuberculosis. Later workers postulated that peripheral anoxemia played a causative role, but this theory has yet to be proved. Recently, studies of hypertrophic osteoarthropathy in man and dogs have corroborated earlier evidence that the chest lesion(s) may stimulate afferent fibers of the vagus nerve and result in a reflex dilatation of peripheral vessels and subsequent increase in limb blood flow. Measurements of peripheral blood flow during surgery in man and dogs with hypertrophic osteoarthropathy demonstrate a dramatic decrease in the blood flow as soon as the main pedicle of the affected lung lobe(s) is severed. This sudden alteration of flow is not associated with any change in systemic blood pressure. In man, complete regression of hypertrophic osteoarthropathy has been brought about solely by section of the intrathoracic vagus nerve on the side of the lung lesion.

Neoplastic disease involving the lung is by far the commonest cause of hypertrophic osteoarthropathy. In a study of 60 dogs with osteoarthropathy seen at the University of

Pennsylvania from 1951 to 1970, the intrathoracic disease was neoplastic in 54 (90 per cent) of the cases. The neoplasms were metastatic in 35 dogs; the two commonest primary tumor sites were bone (15 dogs) and mammary gland (12 dogs).

In 17 dogs, osteoarthropathy developed after excision of a primary extrapulmonary tumor and coincided with subsequent development of lung metastases. Twelve of the 17 had amputations for limb osteosarcomas. They developed osteoarthropathy one to 14 months postoperatively; the mean and median times were five months. Primary lung tumors were present in 18 dogs and another had direct invasion of a bronchus by a rib sarcoma. Lesions seen in six dogs with non-neoplastic involvement of the chest were pneumonia (two dogs), subacute bacterial endocarditis (one dog), dirofilariasis (one dog), *Spirocerca lupi* granuloma of the esophagus (one dog) and rhabdomyosarcoma of the urinary bladder without lung metastasis (one dog).

Other non-neoplastic chest lesions that have been associated with hypertrophic osteoarthropathy include bronchiectasis, lung abscess, tuberculosis and other granulomatous diseases. In enzootic areas of *Spirocerca lupi* infection (the southeastern United States in particular), hypertrophic osteoarthropathy may be associated with either osteosarcoma or fibrosarcoma of the thoracic esophagus. It has been suggested that the sarcomatous invasion of the esophageal branches of the vagus nerve may play a role in the initiation of hypertrophic osteoarthropathy.

## TREATMENT

Treatment of hypertrophic osteoarthropathy depends upon the nature of the chest lesion. Most cases of the disease are associated with neoplastic chest disease. Multiple pulmonary metastases are usually present and treatment is not feasible. However, in five dogs, the lobectomy for primary tumor was performed for palliative reasons only, as small metastatic lesions were also present in the lungs. Mean survival in the four dogs that had regression of osteoarthropathy was only five weeks. The resection of a solitary primary lung tumor is associated with rapid regression of hypertrophic osteoarthropathy. Lameness and the increase in peripheral blood flow and periosteal connective tissue are usually greatly reduced or absent by the end of the first postoperative week. The periosteal lesions regress gradually but persist for many months. In eight other dogs, the lobectomy or pneumonectomy was done in the hope of effecting a cure. All animals showed regression of their osteoarthropathy. Their mean survival time was three months. Recurrence of osteoarthropathy in three of these dogs was associated with the development of metastatic lung tumors.

Non-neoplastic chest disease may be treated by resection of the lesion or by medical management. In one instance, a dog with pulmonary tuberculosis showed a rapid regression of hypertrophic osteoarthropathy following treatment with isoniazid and streptomycin.

### SUPPLEMENTAL READING

Brodey, R. S.: Hypertrophic osteoarthropathy in the dog: a clinicopathologic survey of 60 cases. J. Am. Vet. Med. Assn., *159*:1242–1256, 1971.

Flavel, G.: Reversal of pulmonary hypertrophic osteoarthropathy by vagotomy. The Lancet, *1*:260, 1956.

Holling, H. E., Brodey, R. S., and Boland, H. C.: Pulmonary hypertrophic osteoarthropathy. The Lancet, *2*:1269–1274, 1961.

# THERAPEUTIC PRINCIPLES IN RESPIRATORY DISEASE

JOAN A. O'BRIEN, V.M.D.
*Philadelphia, Pennsylvania*

The basic aim in the treatment of respiratory disease is restoration of normal function. This can require the use of one or many modalities of treatment. In general, the aims of therapy should be:

1. To treat infection.
2. To remove causes of irritation or bronchospasm.
3. To restore pleural integrity.
4. To maintain tracheobronchial clearance.
5. To insure adequate oxygenation.

## TREATMENT OF INFECTION

Sir William Osler has stated that man has an inborn craving for medicine! It has been our impression that this aphorism applies not only to taking medication, but to prescribing it—especially antibiotic therapy. Deciding whether infection is present is often difficult. Not all coughs are due to infection; many anatomic abnormalities may cause coughing, e.g., mild laryngeal incompetence, tracheal collapse, enlarged left atrium, or healed rib fractures with pleural adhesions. On the other hand, these abnormalities may predispose an animal to infection, and the decision to use antibiotics must be based on clinical judgment.

A dog which has been vaccinated with DHL and contracts "kennel cough" due to SV$_5$ virus does not require antibiotic therapy unless there is evidence of superimposed bacterial infection, i.e., persistent fever, rales, elevated white count. On the other hand, the pet shop "kennel cough" in an unvaccinated dog commonly has a bacterial as well as a viral component and requires antibiotic therapy. Since the bacteria isolated are commonly gram-negative, a broad-spectrum antibiotic is indicated (Head et al., 1975).

Antibiotic therapy in chronic bronchitis is a controversial subject. Recommendations have ranged from no antibiotic therapy through continuous antibiotic therapy. In our experience, chronic bronchitics will experience several exacerbations a year, usually manifested by a change in the "cough pattern." In these dogs, a 10-day course of tetracycline or ampicillin is used. The organisms grown from bronchial washings from these dogs are more commonly gram-negative, often with limited sensitivities, but the clinical response to this therapy has been encouraging. Failure to respond should prompt further evaluation.

It is in the dog with severe bronchopneumonia that prompt, appropriate and adequate antibiotic therapy is most needed. The organism should be identified and sensitivities determined, since prolonged therapy is often required. Before definitive results of culture have been obtained, Chloromycetin® is most useful for initial therapy. As a rule of thumb, if the fever does not start to drop after 48 hours of therapy, the antibiotic should be changed. It is important that antibiotics be administered by the proper route and at the correct dosage and intervals; it is also important that therapy be continued until objective evidence of resolution is documented by follow-up chest radiographs in order to prevent relapse and chronic sequelae. In some cases, this may mean antibiotic therapy of a month's duration.

Long-term antibiotic therapy is the only recourse in the palliative treatment of generalized bronchiectasis. Therapy does not alter the irreversible and progressive disease but helps by cutting down the bacterial load and associated systemic manifestations, so that the animal feels better.

If infection or, more properly, infestation is due to parasitic lung disease, then specific antihelmintic therapy, if such is available, is the prescription of choice. In many cases a superimposed bacterial infection can complicate the parasitic disease, and antibiotic therapy is required (see article on "Parasitic Diseases of the Respiratory Tract").

Persistent infection, localized to a particular lung segment or lobe as a result of lung abscess or localized bronchiectasis, requires surgical resection for cure (see article on "Lower Respiratory Tract Trauma").

## REMOVAL OF IRRITATION OR BRONCHOSPASM

AVOID TRIGGER SITUATIONS. Coughing can be a result of exposure to many irritant aerosols. Simple avoidance procedures such as changing to a nondusty kitty litter or avoiding use of perfumes (both doggie and people), cigarette smoke or spray insecticides may be effective in reducing the number and severity of coughing episodes.

DIMINISH RESPONSE TO IRRITATIONS. The list of cough preparations available is protean. Many of these preparations employ a shotgun approach and contain a barbiturate depressant, a narcotic or narcotic-like substance, an expectorant or an antihistamine-like agent. The ever-increasing proliferation of new products should suggest that the health professions are still looking for a panacea. While many of these products are relatively harmless and may be somewhat helpful, their routine and continued use, especially in chronic bronchial disease in an older patient, is not warranted. In the control of chronic bronchitic patients, we have found that low daily or alternate-day therapy with prednisolone (2.5 to 5.0 mg.) has been helpful. This therapy may often be given at intervals of 2 to 3 days, especially in cats with chronic allergic bronchitis. The owners should be aware of the potential hazards of increasing the dose indiscriminately and of the signs of a change in the cough pattern, which may indicate the need for antibiotic therapy.

Although antihistaminic drugs are widely used in cough preparations, it is the author's feeling that these are effective only when given in a tranquilizing dose, and that the effectiveness often ascribed to them in cough mixtures is due more to the other ingredients, e.g., prednisolone, in the mixture.

Bronchodilators. (Isoproterenol, theophylline, etc.) These are indicated in diseases characterized by bronchospasm (feline asthma, smoke inhalation, severe hypoxic disease). In most cases, these are acute diseases rather than chronic problems and call for short-term parenteral use rather than long-term oral administration. Indeed, the known duration of action of drugs like isoproterenol must make one view with skepticism their efficacy when administered orally 2 or 3 times a day.

Cough Suppressants. (Narcotic and narcotic-like drugs, e.g., codeine, dihydromorphinone). These drugs have a definite if restricted place in the treatment of painful, dry, unproductive cough. Such coughing is wasteful of energy and self-perpetuating by continual irritation of the tracheobronchial tree. The drugs are useful in the early stages of acute tracheobronchitis to break the irritating cycle. They should be used to effect only, and the client should be instructed that, unlike antibiotic therapy, these drugs are palliative only. Dosages and intervals should be based on signs, and while they may be required every 4 to 6 hours in the first few days, dosage intervals should be progressively lengthened as the paroxysms of coughing decrease. Their use may also be justified in the treatment of coughing due to inoperable lung tumor when comfort of the patient without hope of cure is the goal of management. These drugs are not recommended in the therapy of pneumonia or in the long-term management of chronic bronchitis.

## RESTORATION OF PLEURAL INTEGRITY

The restoration of normal intrapleural pressures necessary for ventilation may require simple or intricate intervention. These aspects are dealt with in detail in the articles on thoracic trauma and pleural diseases and will be only listed here.

(a) Thoracocentesis—simple needle aspiration.

(b) Chest tube—for removal of large or continually recurring amounts of fluid or air.

(c) Fixation of an unstable rib cage or flail chest causing paradoxical respiration.

(d) Diaphragmatic hernia repair.

## TRACHEOBRONCHIAL CLEARANCE

Expectorants. The saline expectorants are common ingredients in many cough mixtures. The irritant expectorants such as syrup of ipecac are very rarely used now.

Double-blind studies on people have demonstrated that saturated solution of potassium iodide (SSKI) is an effective expectorant. There is little difference between the therapeutic dose and that producing side effects, so that animals receiving this drug must be monitored closely. It is suggested that the dose start with one drop of SSKI/day (in milk to hide the bitter taste) and that the animal be observed closely for gastrointestinal signs. We have not used SSKI on cats. Alternatively, both calcium iodide and sodium iodide are ingredients in commercially available cough preparations. Expectorant action may also be obtained with humidification or aerosol therapy.

**Humidifiers or Nebulizers to Restore Normal Secretion Viscosity.**   Normally, inspired air is warmed and saturated by evaporation of water from the nasal, pharyngeal and tracheal mucosa by the time it reaches the tracheal bifurcation. This does not occur (1) with the administration of dry gases (with low relative humidity), (2) after tracheotomy, (3) in dehydrated animals and (4) with fever or hyperventilation from any cause.

If inspired air is dry, or if normal protective mechanisms are bypassed or the animal's liquid intake is inadequate for its demand, there is a tendency for drying of the mucosa of the bronchial tree. In addition, in the presence of infection or irritation, there is bronchial gland hypertrophy, proliferation of goblet cells and loss of ciliated epithelium which interfere with the normal function of the ciliary mucous pathway and impair drainage of secretions. Irritation and inflammation can cause repeated bouts of ineffective coughing which can cause bronchospasm and further retention of secretions. Rational uses of humidity or aerosolized water include (a) humidification of air or gases that bypass normal humidifying mechanisms of the nose and throat, (b) deposition of water in a liquid form in airways to allow function of the ciliary mucous blanket pathway and (c) prevention of discomfort due to irritated or inflamed airways.

The type of secretions presents problems in the management of bronchopulmonary disease. Secretions may be excessive, thick and tenacious (as in mucopurulent pneumonia) or insufficient (as in tracheobronchitis).

**Humidifiers.**   Steam humidifiers add water in gaseous form to inspired air. The principle is based on evaporation, and maximal water content is limited by temperature. Air saturated at 23° C. (room temperature) will be only 50 per cent saturated at 37° C. Air saturated at a higher temperature and cooled on delivery to a patient with lower temperature will "rain out" or condense in the upper airway.

If water is heated so that it provides saturated air at a temperature as high or higher than that of the patient, a major avenue of heat dispersal is blocked in the dog and cat, and heat retention with hyperpyrexia will result if steam humidification is prolonged.

An effective and safe means of providing highly humidified air to the small animal patient is the intermittent use of the bathroom shower to saturate the room. The animal is exposed to this humidity for 15-minute periods several times a day. Prevent chilling after exposure by drying and encourage coughing by coupage.

Bubble humidifiers pass a stream of gas through a liquid. These are ineffective in providing sufficient humidity for therapeutic use for hydration because of the low vapor pressure of water, but they have some use in anesthetic administration to prevent drying of mucosa.

**Nebulization.**   Nebulization is the dispersal of a bulk liquid in a mist of fine particles. Nebulizers add water by producing a fog of water droplets. The amount of water depends on the design of the nebulizer and is relatively independent of temperature. The stability of the fog depends on particle size. Droplets larger than 5 microns are deposited in the upper airway; those smaller than 0.5 microns are not deposited, but exhaled (Morrow, 1974).

PNEUMATIC NEBULIZER.   The commonly used jet nebulizer can be powered by oxygen but compressed air is a more common source. This nebulizer consists of a capillary tube submerged in the fluid to be nebulized and jet orifices which pass a gas stream across the tip of the capillary tube, creating negative pressure at this point (Venturi) and causing fluid to be sucked up the tube. The jet stream then propels the tiny droplets from the capillary tube tip, driving them against a baffle system, the design of which determines the size of the particles delivered. It is difficult to quantitate the amount of particulate water which is delivered to the patient with this type of nebulizer.

Such jet nebulizers are useful in providing hydration in upper airway problems but may be less effective in providing quantities of $H_2O$ particles in micron size that can reach the smaller bronchi.

ULTRASONIC NEBULIZER. The most effective nebulizer in use today is the ultrasonic nebulizer. This consists of a generator, which passes electrical energy to a piezoelectrical crystal which is vibrated at or near its own inherent frequency to generate large quantities of mist. The mist produced by the ultrasonic nebulizer is independent of gas flow. The air from the blower system can be filtered free of microorganisms and the fluid input can be varied from 0.5 ml. to 6 ml. per minute, so that therapy can be quantitated as well as qualitated. The efficiency of this unit is so great that overhydration in very small puppies may prove to be a consideration (Modell, 1967).

AEROSOLIZED DRUGS. In a report from the Committee on Therapy of the American Thoracic Society in 1967, the statement is made that many drugs including bronchodilators, antibiotics, detergents, ethyl alcohol, enzymes, adrenal corticosteroids, xanthines and mucolytic agents have been administered by aerosol. Of these agents, only isoproterenol, epinephrine and phenylephrine have been shown to decrease airway resistance. Further, it has been thought that many of the effects of nebulized medication with other than the ultrasonic nebulizer come from absorption of medication by the upper respiratory system with circulation of these agents to the lung rather than direct effect of delivery to the bronchi. There is some evidence that nebulized antibiotics such as gentamycin and kanamycin are useful in helping to sterilize mucopurulent secretions in pneumonia due to organisms sensitive to these drugs, but they do not supplant the need for parenteral antibiotics (Williams, 1974).

CONTAMINATION. There has been much discussion and concern about cross-infection with organisms from contaminated nebulizers because of the difficulty of complete sterilization. There have been varying reports of the efficacy of acetic acid in a 0.25 per cent solution in sterilizing and/or reducing the number of contaminating organisms present. It is suggested that this solution be nebulized in the thoroughly cleaned equipment if used daily and before each use

if the use is intermittent. If allowed to air out before patient use, no adverse effects of acetic acid have been reported. Scrupulous cleansing and sterilization is required of all nebulizing equipment. Prophylactic nebulization of antibiotics may cause overwhelming infection due to superinfection with resistant organisms.

ROUTE OF ADMINISTRATION. Although face mask nebulization can be utilized, it is time-consuming, and patients often will not tolerate this procedure.

We routinely use cage nebulization, with the bottom half of the cage shielded by plastic drape. Initially, the patient is placed in the cage for 30 minutes and observed for signs of discomfort or wheezing. Treatment durations have ranged from 30 minutes t.i.d. to 6 to 8 hours continually. Treatment periods must be followed by drying the animal and encouraging deep breathing and coughing, with mild exercise and chest-clapping to clear loosened secretions.

EFFICACY. There is continuous controversy over the benefits of aerosol therapy. Although particle size output is easily measured, the particle size and amount deposited in the lower airways is a matter of conjecture. It is the author's subjective view that aerosol therapy of half-strength saline has been helpful in the treatment of bronchopneumonia, that it should be coupled with chest-clapping and vibration to encourage coughing up of loose secretions. Humidifiers and aerosol therapy, although they may be soothing in upper airway disease or chronic bronchitis, do not appear to alter the course of the diseases themselves.

## OXYGENATION

Although central cyanosis is a reliable indicator of unsaturated hemoglobin, severe hypoxemia may be present in anemic animals without cyanosis. Arterial oxygen tensions ($PaO_2$) are a sensitive indicator of hypoxemia (see article on "Respiratory Function"). In any hypoxic animal, there is the possibility of acidosis. Respiratory acidosis is not often recognized, except in severe airway obstruction or in very severe pneumonia or heartworm disease with lung complications. Metabolic acidosis is seen more commonly due to the increased work of breathing in the presence of anoxia causing lactic acidosis. Although the $PaCO_2$ may be normal or low, bicarbonate is low, arterial pH is decreased and there is a need for bicarbonate replacement.

**Oxygen Therapy.** In many older cages, oxygen therapy was wasteful and expensive. Newer cages* with $CO_2$ absorber and temperature and humidity controls provide higher $O_2$ concentrations. Although initially more expensive, they are more economical to run. Oxygen may also be administered efficiently by transtracheal insufflation. The latter method in particular has been very useful (see article on "Shock: Pathophysiology and Management").

A severely anemic animal who is hypoxic from respiratory disease is in double jeopardy, since not only is its $PaO_2$ low, but its oxygen-carrying capacity is reduced and compatible blood tranfusions are in order to prevent tissue hypoxia.

Tracheotomy may be utilized to decrease dead space ventilation and to provide more direct access for loosening and suctioning secretions in an animal with severe bronchopneumonia. Scrupulous and aseptic techniques are necessary in the care of a tracheotomized patient (see article on "Upper Airway Obstruction Syndrome in Dogs").

### SUPPLEMENTAL READING

Head, J. R., Suter, P. F., and Ettinger, S.: Lower respiratory tract disease, Chapter 23. In Ettinger, S. J. (ed.): Textbook of Veterinary Internal Medicine, Vol. I. Philadelphia, W. B. Saunders Company, 1975.

Osler, W.: Aphorisms. Springfield, Illinois, Charles C Thomas, 1961.

Modell, J. H., Giammona, S. T., and Davis, J. H.: Effect of chronic exposure to ultrasonic aerosols on the lung. Anesthesiology, 28:680–688, 1967.

Morrow, P. E.: Aerosol characterization and disposition. Am. Rev. Resp. Dis., 110:88–99, 1974.

Williams, J., and Henry, M.: Steroid and antibiotic aerosols. Am. Rev. Resp. Dis., 110:122–127, 1974.

*Kirschner Cages, Seattle, Washington.

# INTERPRETATION OF PULMONARY RADIOGRAPHS

PETER F. SUTER, D.M.V.
*Davis, California*

Radiographic examination is an integral part of the diagnostic procedures in chest diseases of dogs and cats. The natural contrast provided by the pulmonary air facilitates the recognition of a large number of normal and pathologic structures of the thorax. It permits (1) exact anatomic location of a disease process at the gross and, occasionally, even at the subgross level; (2) documentation of the severity of involvement by disease; (3) screening for chest diseases in animals with obscure clinical signs or to relieve anxiety in concerned owners; (4) determination of the most likely etiologies (differential diagnoses) and sometimes determination of the final diagnosis; (5) following the progression or regression of disease over an extended period of time; and (6) evaluation of the effectiveness of therapy. Usually radiography serves to confirm a tentative clinical diagnosis and supplements it with additional information. Frequently, radiographs may provide new and unexpected findings (e.g., metastatic nodules or small quantities of pleural fluid) which were not anticipated clinically or are impossible to discern by other readily available methods of clinical investigation.

The interpretation of thoracic radiographs can be difficult because of the superimposition of normal and abnormal shadows and the subtlety of many abnormal densities. The variations between breeds in normal radiographic anatomy, the substantial overlap between normal and abnormal densities and the artifacts and density variations associated with inconsistencies in the radiographic technique and phase of respiration are substantial and require experience gained by looking at large numbers of

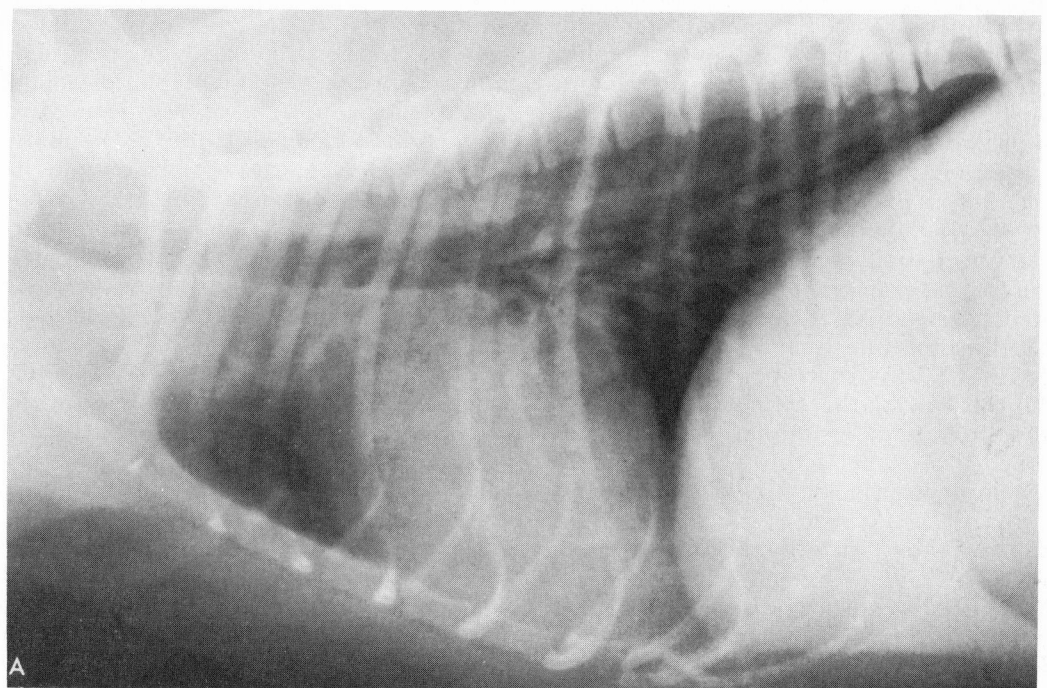

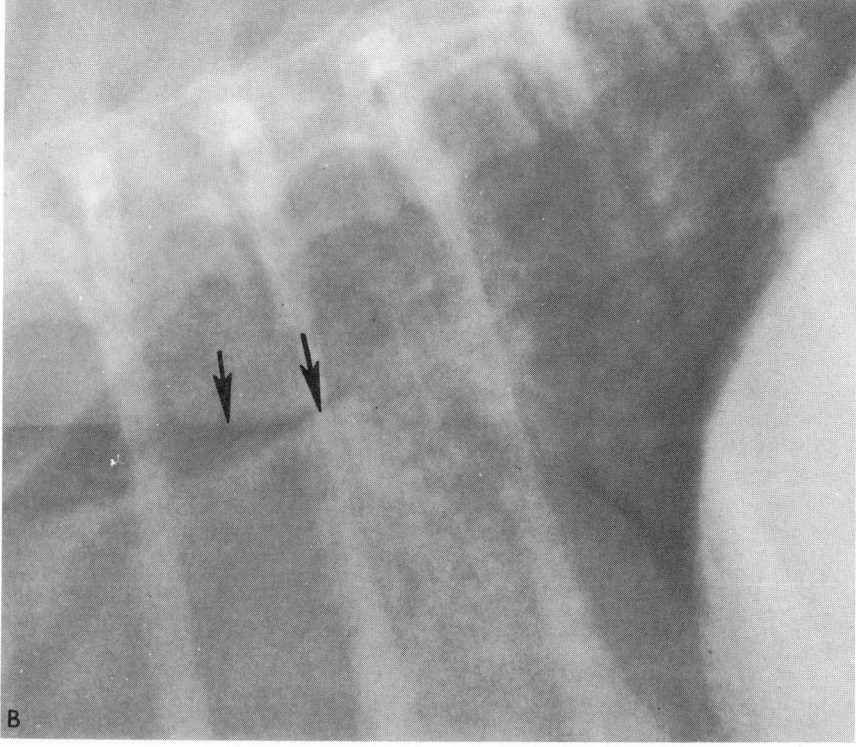

**Figure 2.**   Lateral recumbent radiograph of a female 7-year-old toy poodle with a dry, hacking cough and an inspiratory and expiratory wheeze. The inspiratory radiograph (A) contains no abnormality that would permit explanation of this animal's signs. On the expiratory radiograph (B), collapse of the lumen of the trachea at the bifurcation (arrow) is visible. The lumina of the main bronchi are also absent. A diagnosis of intrathoracic tracheal and bronchial collapse was made and confirmed by fluoroscopy. With only an inspiratory radiograph available, this dynamic type of obstructive intrathoracic disease would not have been diagnosed. This case illustrates that at times both inspiratory and expiratory radiographs are required.

by the spine in the dorsoventral radiograph or to bring thoracic wall lesions into profile. Ventrodorsal instead of dorsoventral radiographs, or positional radiographs made with a horizontal beam direction, may serve temporarily to visualize an area of interest obscured by pleural fluid.

Survey radiographs may have to be supplemented by special studies, such as fluoroscopic examination or bronchography. Intrathoracic airway diseases, such as early bronchiectasis or extramural or intraluminal bronchial obstruction, may require confirmation of the suspected lesion by bronchography. Pulmonary vascular abnormalities, such as dirofilariasis, pulmonary thrombosis or shunting with congenital heart disease, may require angiocardiography if the survey radiographs are equivocal. The nature and origin of lesions within or adjacent to the pulmonary hilus, mediastinum or diaphragm may have to be identified by esophagography.

For radiographic diagnostic purposes, lower respiratory tract diseases may be subdivided into two major groups:

1. Obstructive and nonobstructive lower airway disease (bronchitis, bronchiolitis, asthma).

2. Pulmonary parenchymal diseases (pneumonia, neoplasia, mass lesions).

## LOWER AIRWAY DISEASE

*Lower airway diseases* (collapsing intrathoracic trachea, tracheobronchitis, bronchiolitis, asthma, allergic bronchitis) can be difficult to diagnose radiographically because clinical signs and radiographic findings may not correspond; severe clinical signs such as fever, dyspnea, coughing and retching can be found in dogs or cats with normal-appearing radiographs.

Partial or total dynamic obstruction of the lower airways by collapse can only be recognized if the trachea or stem bronchi are involved. Small bronchi or bronchioli also collapse but do not cast individually recognizable shadows. A soft, poorly stabilized intrathoracic trachea or the stem bronchi collapse partially or totally during forced expiration or coughing, which can be seen as a marked narrowing of the airway lumen on expiratory radiographs (Fig. 2). On radiographs made during inspiration the lumina of these airways appear normal or

slightly dilated. In dogs with collapsing cervical trachea, the narrowing occurs during the opposite respiratory phases; namely, the trachea appears narrowed during inspiration and seems normal during expiration.

The degree of airway collapse is modified by breathing efforts and increased air flow resistance in the upper airways (nares, larynx, soft palate). These dynamic types of obstruction must be differentiated from morphologic obstructions due to hypoplastic trachea, tracheal stenosis, tracheobronchitis, intraluminal tracheal or bronchial blockage and extramural compression of the airways by an extrinsic mass. In the latter conditions any visible tracheal and bronchial narrowing is affected only slightly or not at all by the respiratory phase.

Uncomplicated, acute tracheobronchitis in dogs or cats rarely leads to radiographically recognizable changes. Visualization of tracheobronchitis is contingent on (1) substantial inflammatory thickening of the bronchial walls by severe mucosal edema, cellular infiltration of the bronchial wall or polypoid proliferation of the bronchial mucosa and submucosal glands; (2) extension of the inflammation into adjacent lung parenchyma; and (3) indirect or direct signs of airway obstruction. Severe inflammatory bronchial wall thickening is seen radiographically as an accentuation of the normal linear bronchial pattern (Fig. 3). Extension of inflammation into adjacent parenchyma makes the bronchial wall appear blurred. When looked at on-end, indistinct ring shadows, also referred to as "doughnut shadows," become visible in the central and middle portions of the lung. Concurrent inflammation in the pulmonary interstitium reduces the background density of the lung and the visibility of the vascular structures. These changes are particularly severe in chronic bronchitis or bronchiectasis. A progression of bronchitis to bronchopneumonia causes blotchy parenchymal densities (Fig. 4).

Individual shadows cast by the peripheral normal or inflamed small airways (bronchioli, terminal bronchi) cannot be seen radiographically. Nonetheless, some diseases affecting the peripheral airways can be assumed, based on the resulting change in the air content of the lung parenchyma. If the inflation of the alveoli and terminal bronchioli (end-air spaces) is altered significantly by airway obstruction, atelectasis

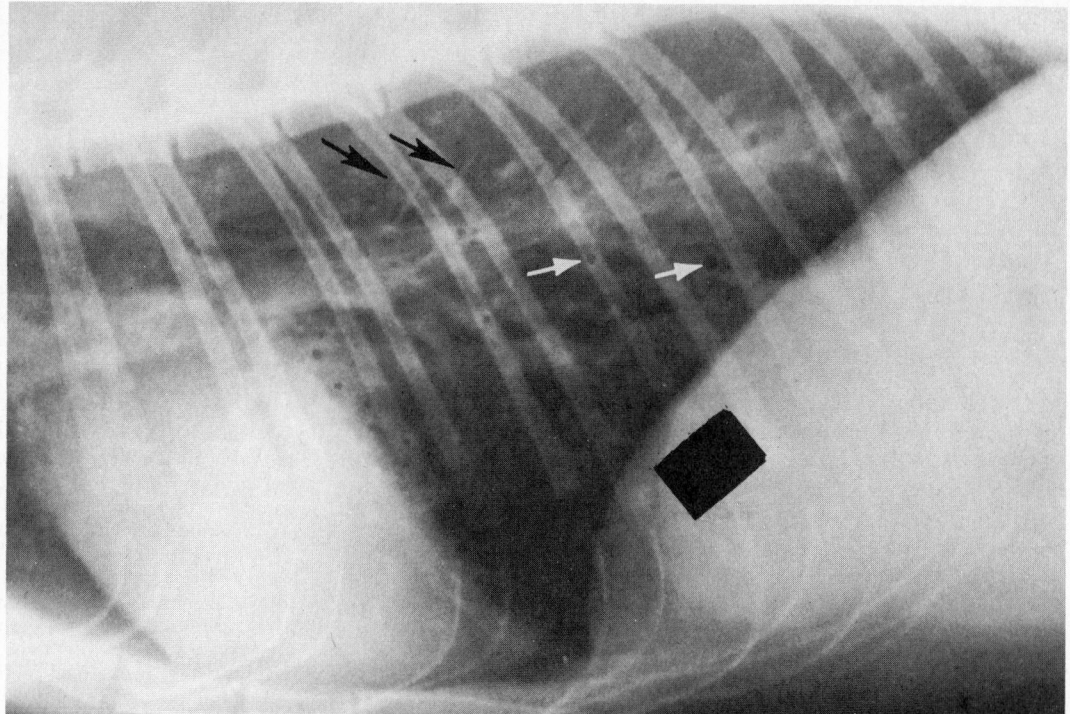

**Figure 3.**   Lateral recumbent radiograph of an adult female domestic shorthair cat with anorexia and dyspnea of four days' duration. The radiodensity of the lung is slightly increased and upon close inspection a large number of ill-defined linear shadows (black arrows) can be seen in the caudal lobes radiating toward the lung periphery. In some of the shadows small radiolucent centers (white arrows) representing bronchi seen end-on can be recognized. The arteries to the caudal lobe are poorly outlined. This radiograph is typical for a great many of the severe chronic bronchitis cases in the cat. The inflamed, thickened bronchial walls are responsible for an increased visibility of their walls. An increased bronchial pattern of this type can be seen with allergic, parasitic or secondary bacterial bronchitis.

hyperinflation or emphysema must be expected. Mucous plugs and mucosal swelling in asthma, obstructing bronchiolitis or microbronchitis can lead to *total obstruction* of the peripheral airways of one or more lung segments or an entire lung lobe, resulting in the resorption of the alveolar air and atelectasis. Radiographically, the collapsed lung areas become radiodense and smaller, which may induce a shifting of the mediastinum or heart toward the involved lobe(s) or may cause a substantial asymmetry of the diaphragm due to cranial displacement of the hemidiaphragm on the involved side.

Another alternative with asthma, obstructing bronchiolitis or microbronchitis is due to *incomplete blockage* of the small airways. Mucosal swelling, cellular infiltration, mucous plugs and bronchospasm in affected bronchioles may still allow air to enter the alveoli during inspiration. During expiration, however, the airway diameter is reduced, prolonging expiratory time and

trapping air in the pulmonary periphery. Trapping of air can induce emphysema, which in severe cases may be recognized radiographically by focal or generalized hypertranslucency of the involved areas, increased thoracic size (barrel chest), flattening and caudal displacement of the diaphragm and a small heart. Emphysematous lung lobes may displace and partially compress adjoining normal lung lobes. Openings between adjacent alveoli (pores of Kohn) or direct communications connecting bronchioles with surrounding alveoli (canals of Lambert) provide alternate ways for air to reach lung tissue distal to an obstruction of a bronchus, which is called collateral air drift and prevents atelectasis of obstructed lung segments.

Total obstruction of a major bronchus in the hilar area by intraluminal masses, such as foreign bodies or intraluminal tumors, or by extramural compression due to enlarged lymph nodes or neoplasms results in atelec-

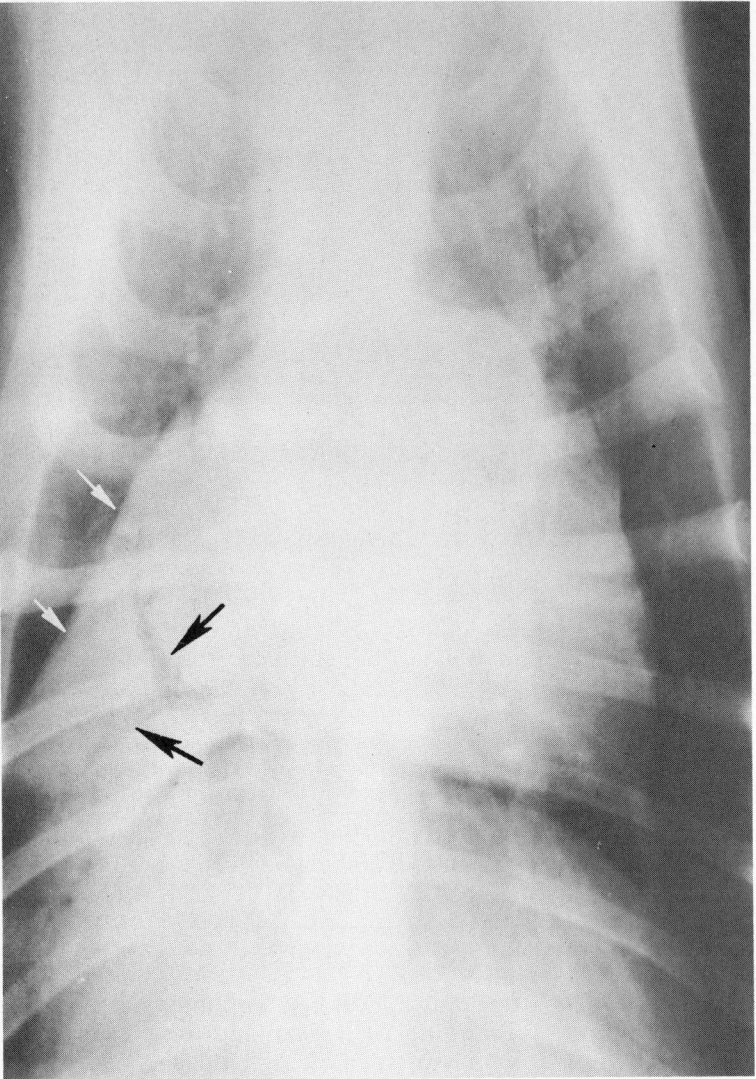

**Figure 4.** Dorsoventral radiograph of a male 6-year-old German shepherd dog that had sustained a fracture of the axis. The dog suffered a cardiac arrest and was resuscitated successfully. Since that event, however, the dog had a persistent fever. Contiguous with the right border of the cardiac shadow is a soft tissue-like, homogeneous radiodensity which contains two radiolucent tapering streaks (black arrows). The cranially well-demarcated, abnormal radiodensity represents a consolidated right middle (cardiac) lobe that contains radiolucent air bronchograms. The visualization of a lobar border (white arrows), the presence of air bronchograms and the absence of vascular markings within the radiodensity suggest an end-air space density (alveolar). The asymmetry of the lesion and the location are compatible with bronchopneumonia most likely due to aspiration of vomitus during resuscitation.

tasis which can be recognized as an increased lobar radiodensity. Often atelectasis may be followed by edema and interstitial pneumonia resulting from hypoxia and trapping of bronchial exudates distal to the obstruction. Partial bronchial obstruction, depending on its severity, may be unnoticed radiographically or may lead to air trapping and hyperlucency of the affected lobes.

## PULMONARY PARENCHYMAL DISEASE

Most *pulmonary parenchymal diseases* are recognized by an increased radiodensity of the lung. The increased radiodensity can be due to (1) replacement of the air in the end-air spaces (alveoli and terminal bronchioli) by exudates or transudates; (2) a loss of air from the end-air spaces; (3) an increased amount of interstitial tissue and blood in the capillaries; or (4) a combination of all three events. The majority of pulmonary parenchymal diseases induce a concurrent or consecutive change in air content, blood perfusion, interstitial tissue edema and cellular infiltration.

A small number of pulmonary conditions can be recognized because of a diminished pulmonary radiodensity (blacker than normal), which is commonly referred to as hypertranslucency and may be caused by (1) an increased air content (hyperinflation, airway disease, emphysema) or (2) a diminished pulmonary perfusion with blood (hypovolemia, cardiac shock, Addison's disease and right-to-left shunting of blood in congenital heart disease). Focal areas of hypertranslucency can be encountered with focal air trapping (focal emphysema), bullae, blebs, pulmonary cysts, pneumatoceles, cavitary lesions (abscesses), necrotizing neoplasms or infarcts.

It is advantageous to discriminate among the many diseases causing increased pulmonary radiodensity by grouping them into three basic categories according to easily recognizable radiographic criteria. This permits reducing the number of probable diagnoses to a more reasonable number of possibilities. The three basic categories are (1) disseminated, diffuse pulmonary disease with radiodensities in one or several lobes; (2) solitary focal densities; and (3) multiple focal densities.

A disseminated pulmonary disease is characterized by radiodensity spreading diffusely across one or several lung lobes and can be caused by a substantial loss of air from the end-air spaces (atelectasis) or by replacement of the alveolar air by fluid or cells (edema, pneumonia, hemorrhage). The resulting increased radiodensity is called alveolar density or end-air space pattern and is characterized by a confluent, mottled or homogeneous soft tissue-like radiodensity with fluffy borders where it merges with adjoining seemingly normal lung. Air-filled first- and second-order bronchi may be visible as dark branching streaks or stripes within the radiodense areas and are referred to as air bronchograms (Fig. 4). The vascular structures are obscured by the water-dense parenchyma. Borders of consolidated lobes become visible where they are in contact with a normal or less involved lobe. Air bronchograms are a valuable localizing sign for distinguishing between pulmonary and extrapulmonary intrathoracic densities, such as pleural fluid or mediastinal masses which do not contain air bronchograms. There are, however, a few diseases with end-air space pattern but without air bronchograms. Air bronchograms may be seen occasionally with severe interstitial disease.

The alveolar or end-air space pattern is compatible with diseases summarized in Table 1.

The predominant location of the radiodensities, the clinical signs, laboratory data and history are helpful in differentiating among the various alveolar diseases of Table 1. Bronchopneumonias are found

**Table 1. Disseminated Diseases With End-Air Space Pattern**

| ACUTE DISEASES | CHRONIC DISEASES (RARE) |
|---|---|
| Alveolar edema | Disseminated neoplasia |
| Bronchopneumonia | Granulomatous pneumonia |
| Aspiration pneumonia | |
| Hemorrhage | |
| Atelectasis | |

most often in the dependent portions of the cranial and middle lobes, whereas edemas are most often symmetrically distributed around the pulmonary hilus (Figs. 4 and 5). Hemorrhages have no local predilection but the history may provide the necessary clues for a diagnosis. Aspiration pneumonia is often seen in the dependent parts of the middle lobes, the accessory or the caudal lobes.

A disseminated, homogeneous (unstructured) increased radiodensity of the lung and loss of the normal contrast between the dense vascular structures and the radiolucent normal lung parenchyma can be caused by an increased amount of interstitial fluid (congestion), collagenous tissue or cellular interstitial infiltrates. These types of radiodensities are called interstitial densities and are encountered with diseases summarized in Table 2. The pattern is usually not radiodense enough to obscure the vascular markings totally; it merely smudges their borders. Diseases with interstitial pattern do not permit visualization of well-defined air bronchograms because the amount of air in the lumina of the alveoli is reduced but not totally eliminated as with an end-air space pattern (Fig. 6).

It is important, however, to be aware that radiographic recognition of interstitial disease may be elusive. Animals with severe clinical signs due to interstitial disease may show little or no concurrent radiographic changes. Regardless of the underlying disease, the homogeneous interstitial patterns

**Table 2. Disseminated Diseases With Homogeneous Interstitial Pattern**

Interstitial edema (congestion)
Interstitial pneumonia (pneumonitis)
Eosinophilic pneumonia
Interstitial hemorrhage
Pulmonary contusion (blunt trauma)
Fibrosis, scarring
Old age
Artifacts: expiratory radiographs, obesity

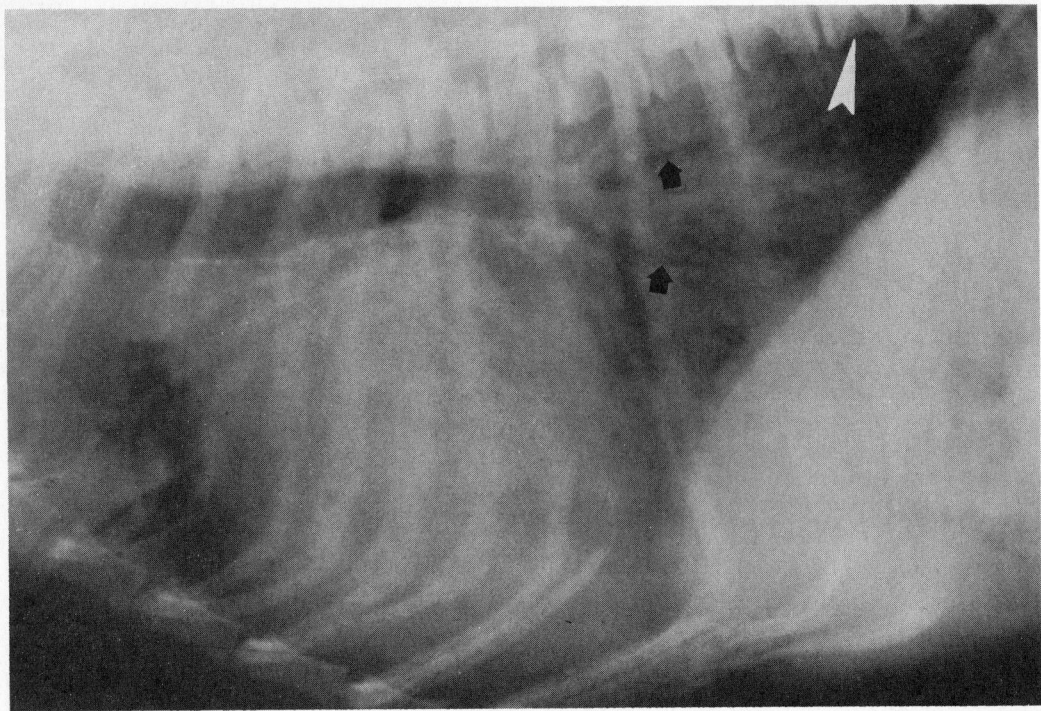

**Figure 5.** Lateral recumbent radiograph of a male 13-year-old miniature dachshund which was radiographed prior to anesthesia because of a loud holosystolic, mitral murmur. The increased radiodensity of the lung is real and could not be compatible with an expiratory radiograph because the wide trachea and the extension of the lung bodiaphragmatic recess caudal to the level of $T_{11}$ (white arrow) make such an assumption highly unlikely. The marked increase in the radiodensity of the caudal (diaphragmatic) lobe is thus a sign of a parenchymal pulmonary disease. The faintly visible air bronchograms within the radiodensity (black arrow) indicate an end–air space density. The associated cardiomegaly, the location of the lesion in the perihilar area and the auscultatory findings make pulmonary alveolar edema due to left-sided heart failure the most likely diagnosis.

look very much alike. There are usually few associated radiographic characteristics, such as preferred location or dissemination. Only the associated simultaneous lesions in other organs, such as cardiomegaly in cases of pulmonary congestion or rib fractures in cases of traumatic contusion, may assist in radiographically differentiating diseases with interstitial pattern.

Interstitial radiographic patterns can also be structured or inhomogeneous, namely, nodular, linear or reticular and nodular mixed (reticulonodular). Nodular densities are most commonly caused by multiple pulmonary metastases. Linear and reticulonodular interstitial patterns can be found with pulmonary fibrosis, old age, granulomatous disease, chronic congestion and disseminated pulmonary lymphosarcoma.

An abnormal vascular pattern of the lung is found with diseases which increase lung perfusion, reduce lung perfusion or cause dilatation of arteries or veins. It can be es-

sential to distinguish arteries from veins to make a diagnosis, i.e., differentiate dirofilariasis from left heart failure. In the lateral radiograph the vascular markings dorsal to the bronchial lumen are arteries. Pulmonary veins are located ventral to the bronchial lumen. In the dorsoventral or ventrodorsal radiograph, veins can be identified by their confluence in the area of the left atrium, whereas pulmonary arteries can be traced to their origin from the main pulmonary artery which is located in the cranial portion of the cardiac shadow. An intensified vascular pattern is characterized by an increased radiodensity of the pulmonary vascular markings (arteries and/or veins) because of their larger size and extension further into the periphery than normal. It can be associated with infection, inflammation, pulmonary congestion in left heart failure (veins enlarged) or shunting lesions such as left-to-right congenital heart diseases (patent ductus arteriosus, ventricular septal defect) or with peripheral arteriovenous

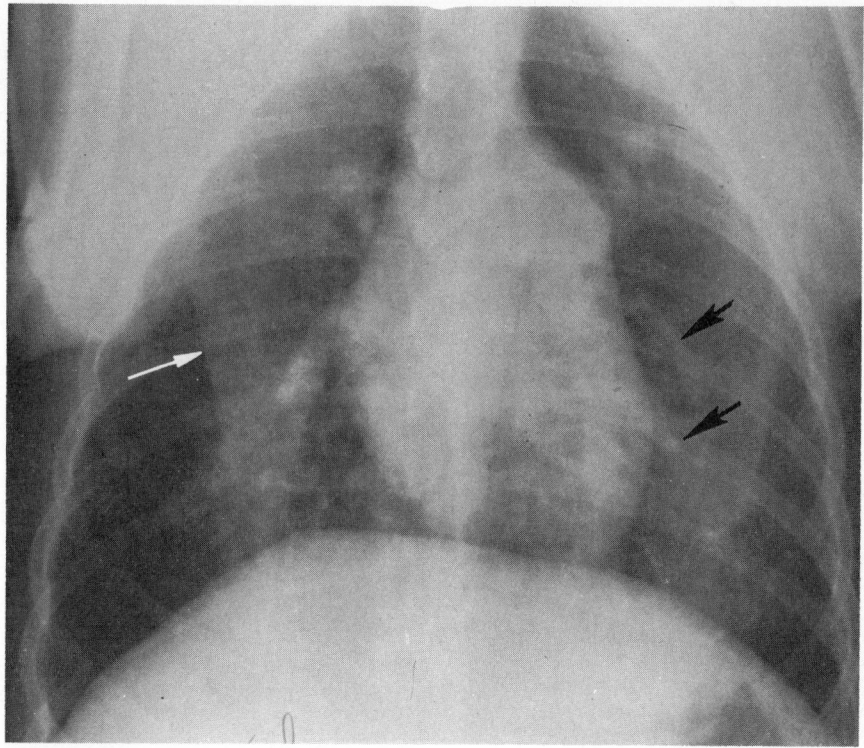

**Figure 6.** Dorsoventral radiograph of a female spayed 2-year-old terrier cross dog with dyspnea and gagging ersisting over one year. A homogeneous, hazy increased radiodensity of the lung markedly reduces the contrast etween it and the vascular structures in the caudal lobes; in particular, the outlines of the vascular structures in the ft caudal lobe (black arrows) are indistinct. The increased radiodensity is not intense enough to cause air ronchograms. This type of intermediate radiodensity is typical for an unstructured, disseminated interstitial type f radiodensity. Based on the clinical examination, a 23 per cent blood eosinophilia and the radiograph, the iagnosis of allergic pneumonia or pulmonary infiltrates with blood eosinophilia (PIE) was made. The dog re-ponded favorably to the administration of corticosteroids. The white arrow points to an artifactual density caused y a skin fold that is projected into the lung.

us fistulas. Enlarged vascular structures een on-end appear as nodular radioden-ities and can be confused with pulmonary arenchymal nodules (interstitial nodular attern). Dilated, distorted and/or truncated ulmonary vascular structures are a com-on abnormal vascular pattern with di-ofilariasis. A significant reduction in pul-onary perfusion, which can be recognized adiographically by the diminished size of e arteries and veins and a concurrent ypertranslucent lung, can be associated rith hypovolemic shock, severe dehydra-on, Addison's disease or reduced cardiac utput due to myocardial failure (cardiac hock).

*Focal pulmonary radiodensities* can be of ree types: (1) amorphous, blotchy densi-es with irregular shape, varying size and distinct borders; (2) round or oval adiodensities, over 4 cm. (1½ inches) in di-meter, with distinct borders, which are re-

ferred to as mass lesions; or (3) evenly rounded radiodensities less than 4 cm. in diameter which can be well or ill defined and are referred to as nodular lesions. All three types of densities can be solitary or multiple.

A small solitary nodule of 1 to 2 cm. in diameter is called a "coin lesion." Table 3 lists diseases which should be considered in the differential diagnosis of solitary le-

**Table 3.** *Solitary Pulmonary Radiodensities*

| AMORPHOUS, BLOTCHY DENSITY | MASS LESION OR NODULE (COIN LESION) |
|---|---|
| Focal pneumonic infiltrate | Abscess |
| Focal lung necrosis, infarct | Granuloma |
| Granuloma, abscess | Primary neoplasm |
| Focal hemorrhage, contusion | Metastatic neoplasm |
| Focal atelectasis | Hematoma |
| Neoplasm | Fluid-filled cyst |
| Infarct | |

sions. Solitary lesions quite often are incidental findings in clinically normal animals or in animals with vague clinical signs not referable to the respiratory system.

The differentiation of solitary pulmonary lesions is difficult and may require extensive clinical work-up, repeat radiographs, needle biopsy or exploratory thoracotomy.

*Multiple pulmonary, focal lesions* are among the most common radiographic findings. Breaking them down into groups with a common morphologic denominator is helpful. Tables 4, 5 and 6 can be used as a basis for differential diagnosis.

### Table 4.   Multifocal, Amorphous Pulmonary Radiodensities

Pneumonic infiltrates or necrosis (embolic spread of bacterial or fungal diseases; opportunistic pneumonias due to reduced host resistance)
Granulomas (fungal, parasitic toxoplasmosis, multiple foreign bodies)
Focal hemorrhage (coagulopathies, trauma, neoplasia)
Infarcts (dirofilariasis, trauma, neoplasia, heart failure)
Neoplasms (primary multicentric neoplasia, bronchiolar alveolar carcinoma, or complications of metastatic neoplasms)

Pinpoint nodules are the smallest, barely visible size of nodules; miliary nodules are nodules less than 3 mm. in diameter; both are only visible radiographically when present in large numbers. Their great number compensates for their small size and faint tissue density, which otherwise would make them invisible radiographically. Small densities which contain calcium, such as pulmonary osteomas or calcified dystrophic nodules, can be seen individually in spite of their small size. Pulmonary osteomas are small, focal pulmonary or pleural calcifications or ossifications (ectopic bone formation) commonly seen in dogs' lungs. Their significance is unknown.

### Table 6.   Diseases With Ill-Defined Nodules

Acute alveolar diseases (edema, hemorrhage, contusion)
Hemorrhage due to coagulopathies or severe trauma
Metastatic or disseminated primary neoplasia
Disseminated granulomatous diseases (parasitic, fungal, bacterial)
Pulmonary lymphosarcoma
Massive thromboembolic pneumonia
Aspiration pneumonia (small, 3-mm. nodules, alveolarization of barium in dysphagia)

Multiple nodular radiodensities can be well defined or ill defined. The probability is usually overwhelming that multiple well- to fairly well-defined nodular pulmonary lesions are a manifestation of metastatic disease. Nonetheless, fungal disease and the other diagnoses summarized in Table 5 should be carefully considered as differential diagnoses. The location of nodular lesions assists in their differentiation from vascular structures seen end-on. Nodules cast by vascular structures seen end-on are located in the central or middle portions of the lung field and are often superimposed onto another vascular structure running at approximately a 90-degree angle to the direction of the x-ray beam. These nodular shadows may be difficult to differentiate from true metastatic nodules superimposed onto a vessel. Nodular densities seen between vascular structures or in

### Table 5.   Disease With Well-Defined Nodular Radiodensities

| PINPOINT OR MILIARY NODULES (< 3 mm.) | LARGER NODULES (3 mm. to 40 mm.) |
|---|---|
| Hemic spread of: | Metastatic neoplasms |
| Fungal diseases | Fungal diseases |
| Bacterial diseases | Satellite nodules of primary neoplasia |
| Neoplasia | |
| Hematoma | Bacterial granuloma |
| Calcified, old, parasitic or fungal nodules | Fluid-filled cysts |
| Fibrotic nodules | Vascular structures projected end-on (hypervascular lung, dirofilariasis) |
| Alveolar microlithiasis | Bronchiectases filled with exudate |
| Artifacts: pulmonary osteomas | Artifacts: nipples, subcutaneous nodules |

he pulmonary periphery are highly suspicious for metastatic disease.

Radiographic recognition of metastatic pulmonary neoplasms depends on a favorable projection on the radiograph and on the number and absolute size of the nodules. The lower limit of visibility for small nodules is at 3 to 5 mm. in diameter, but one or two nodules of up to 12 mm. (½ inch) in diameter may often go unrecognized when located in the peripheral portions of the caudal lobes or when they are obscured by the shadows cast by the spine, vessels or diaphragm. Thus, a negative set of radiographs does not exclude the possibility of pulmonary metastatic disease. A second or sometimes third set of radiographs at an interval of three weeks to one month is often needed to confirm a negative result.

Ill-defined nodules are often mixed with well-defined nodules and can occur with both interstitial and alveolar types of lung disease. When present in large numbers, ill-defined nodules tend to coalesce and form amorphous, dense conglomerates of radiodensities. Poorly defined, small nodular radiodensities can also be associated with a diffusely increased background interstitial density or a reticular interstitial pattern (reticulonodular pattern). Lymphosarcoma and severe pulmonary parenchymal fibrosis are the most likely diagnoses associated with a reticulonodular pattern. Poorly defined, small nodules can also be seen owing to alveolar filling with dense aspirated material, i.e., barium.

Ill-defined, nodular radiodensities of 5 to mm. in diameter can be formed by exudates, transudates, granulation tissue or foreign material accumulating preferentially within the alveoli of one terminal bronchiole (acinus) while leaving adjacent areas relatively unaffected. Indistinct borders of a nodule can also be caused by pref-

erentially interstitially located disease spreading or spilling over into adjoining air spaces or extensively compressing them.

Although most pulmonary parenchymal diseases are characterized by one of the aforementioned categories of radiodensities, there are a few which defy classification. A variety of causes are responsible for these. In some cases it may be difficult to decide in which class a density fits because elements of various categories can be present simultaneously. This can be due to coexistence of two or more different disease processes within the lung; but it may also be caused by a simultaneous visualization of acute and chronic phases of the same disease. Associated lesions, such as cardiomegaly, pleural effusion or mediastinal or thoracic wall masses, may obscure some of the abnormal pulmonary densities and may interfere with their proper interpretation. Conclusions from radiographs as to the cause of the underlying disease should thus always be drawn only after careful consideration of the circumstances, the history, the physical examination and laboratory data.

## SUPPLEMENTAL READING

Biery, D. N.: Differentiation of lung diseases of inflammatory or neoplastic origin from lung disease in heart failure. Vet. Clin. N. Am., 4:711–721, 1974.

Silverman, S., and Suter, P. F.: Influence of inspiration and expiration on canine thoracic radiographs. J. Am. Vet. Med. Assn., 166:502–510, 1975.

Silverman, S., Poulos, P. W., and Suter, P. F.: Cavitary pulmonary lesions in animals. J. Am. Vet. Rad. Soc., 17:134–146, 1976.

Suter, P. F., and Lord, P. F.: Radiographic differentiation of disseminated pulmonary parenchymal diseases in dogs and cats. Vet. Clin. N. Am., 4:687–710, 1974.

Ticer, J. W.: Radiographic Technique in Small Animal Practice. Chapter 12, Thorax. Philadelphia, W. B. Saunders Co., 1975, p. 285.

# Section

# 4

# CARDIOVASCULAR
# DISEASES

STEPHEN J. ETTINGER, D.V.M.
*Consulting Editor*

# INTRODUCTION TO THE DIAGNOSIS AND MANAGEMENT OF HEART DISEASE*

STEPHEN J. ETTINGER, D.V.M.
*Berkeley, California*

## OVERVIEW

Heart disease in small animals may occur [at] any age. In the young, heart failure is most often associated with congenital cardiac defects and occasionally with inflammatory myocardial disease. In middle-aged animals, symptomatic heart disease is most likely to be the result of a progressive congenital heart disease, inflammatory myocardial disease, idiopathic cardiomyopathy, pericardial disease of varying etiology, heartworms or heart failure secondary to other organ malfunction. Chronic valvular heart disease principally affecting the mitral and occasionally the tricuspid valves is a most common cause of heart failure in older animals, although other cardiac conditions [do] occur which must be differentiated.

## TYPES OF HEART DISEASE

In veterinary medicine, we deal primarily with four major categories of heart disease: congestive heart failure, compensated prefailure states, arrhythmias and shock with hypotension.

Prodromal heart failure and congestive heart failure should be considered together because of their close interrelationship.

Arrhythmias may produce syncope, a prostrate or semiprostrate state, fatigue, hypotension and, if prolonged, congestive heart failure. Sudden death is a possible sequela to arrhythmias.

The hypotensive state may develop following the onset of an arrhythmia or may be the result of shock associated with decreased venous return, decreased cardiac filling or diminished cardiac emptying.

The articles in this section discuss current methods of recognizing and treating cardiovascular disease with the exception of hypotension due to shock. Shock and cardiac arrest are discussed elsewhere (see pages 26 to 44).

## RECOGNITION OF CONGESTIVE HEART FAILURE

Congestive heart failure describes the inability of the heart to pump blood adequately into the circulation. Such failure ultimately results in tachycardia, cardiac dilatation and/or hypertrophy and a retention or collection of edema fluid in one or more parts of the body.

Heart failure can result from either right heart disease or left heart disease. In right heart failure the end-diastolic pressures rise in the right ventricle. This increased pressure is transmitted backward, producing elevated right atrial pressures, increased vena caval and jugular pressures, increased peripheral venous pressures with venous engorgement, enlargement of the liver and spleen and, ultimately, ascites, subcutaneous edema and anasarca.

When the left side of the heart fails, there is a progression of signs beginning with coughing, dyspnea and tachypnea and progressing to exertional fatigue, paroxysmal

---

*This paper was supported by funds from the Berkeley Veterinary Research Foundation.

dyspnea, orthopnea, pulmonary edema and cyanosis.

Regardless of the etiology of the heart failure, the approaches to medical therapy remain similar. To appreciate the proper therapeutic approach to the treatment of heart failure it is necessary first to recognize the various phases of heart disease. Table 1 reviews the phases of congestive cardiac disease in the dog.

It is helpful to categorize heart disease further in terms of cardiac status and prognosis (Criteria Committee, New York Heart Association, 1974). The cardiac status may be determined to be *uncompromised, slightly compromised* or *moderately com-*

*promised.* Significantly the prognosi should be considered to be *good, good witl therapy, fair with therapy* or *guarded de spite therapy.*

The clinical description of heart diseas according to phase alone is useful, but i does not provide either the owner or th clinician with information regarding the se verity or prognosis of the condition. Thus while categorizing the clinical phase ( congestive heart disease, it is helpful to de termine the cardiac status and prognosis ; the same time, so that a rational approach t therapy may then be decided upon.

## METHODS OF THERAPY ACCORDING TO PHASE OF HEART DISEASE

The generally accepted methods, utilize individually or in combination, in th treatment of congestive heart failure ir clude exercise restriction; dietary restri tion of sodium; and the administration ( cardiac glycosides (digitalis), diureti agents, bronchodilators, sedatives and occ; sionally vasodilators, oxygen, narcotic sed; tives and defoaming agents.

In Phase I/IV cardiac disease, it is gene ally unnecessary to restrict exercise and di( or to provide specific drug therapy. This so because the patient has asymptomat heart disease and does not exhibit signs ( congestive heart disease. Exercise restri tion could be indicated to prevent ove stressing. Restriction of sodium intake probably contraindicated at this stage ( disease and the use of other therapeut agents is equivocal or unnecessary.

In Phase II/IV cardiac disease, exerci should be limited to walking or modera running. The sodium in the diet still nee not be restricted because congestive failu is not present. Digitalis and diuretics a not indicated, although bronchodilators a useful to relieve paroxysmal cardiac asthm Sedatives may be necessary for the mo excitable patient.

Phase III/IV heart disease is actually ; sociated with abnormal retention of sodiu and water in the body. Consequently tl dietary restriction of sodium to a modera degree would be indicated at this stag Exercise should be limited to walking a very limited running (if at all). Cardi glycosides are now indicated and diure therapy is indicated initially to help redu abnormal fluid accumulations. Where

### Table 1.  *Phases of Cardiac Disease**

| PHASE | DESCRIPTION |
|---|---|
| Phase I | Normal activity does not produce undue fatigue, dyspnea or coughing. Physical activity need not be limited in dogs in this phase of cardiac disease. |
| Phase II | The dog is comfortable at rest, but ordinary physical activity causes fatigue, dyspnea or coughing. In these dogs, exercise should be limited moderately; such activities as hunting and long periods of strenuous exercise should be avoided. |
| Phase III | The dog is comfortable at rest, but minimal exercise may produce fatigue, dyspnea or coughing. Signs may also develop while the dog is in a recumbent position (orthopnea). Physical activity must be limited, free running and stair climbing shoud be strictly avoided. Exercise should be limited to short walks and moderate house activity. |
| Phase IV | Congestive heart failure, dyspnea and coughing are present even when the dog is at rest. Signs are exaggerated by any physical activity. Total exercise restriction, i.e., absolute cage rest, is essential. |

CARDIAC STATUS**

1. Uncompromised
2. Slightly compromised
3. Moderately compromised

PROGNOSIS**

1. Good
2. Good with therapy
3. Fair with therapy
4. Guarded despite therapy

*Ettinger, S.J., and Suter, P.F.: Canine Cardiology. Philadelphia, W.B. Saunders Co., 1970.
**Criteria Committee, New York Heart Association, 1974.

diuretic therapy in early Phase III/IV heart disease may not need to be continued, in late Phase III/IV heart disease combined diuretic and digitalis therapy usually is necessary. Bronchodilators may also be indicated to supplement the clinical effects of digitalis and diuretics. Sedatives may be necessary in excitable or difficult to manage patients. The use of antitussive agents is indicated when the patient on optimal doses of digitalis, diuretics and bronchodilators continues to exhibit unproductive stressful coughing.

Phase IV/IV cardiac disease is overt congestive heart failure which demands marked exercise restriction (preferably cage rest). In addition the dietary restriction of sodium is essential. Therapeutic digitalization or readjustment of digitalis dosage levels is in order. Diuretics are indicated to help control abnormal fluid retention, and bronchodilators may be indicated to assist with the diuretic and antibronchospastic effects. Sedatives are necessary to reduce oxygen demands brought on by unnecessary excitement. They may help control central nervous system–mediated cardiac arrhythmias. When pulmonary edema develops, the use of alpha-adrenergic blocking agents, narcotic sedatives, oxygen therapy, defoaming agents and phlebotomy may be of value.

When properly treated, most cardiac patients are likely to respond as desired. The injudicious use of medication early in cardiac disease can be detrimental to the long-term well-being of the patient. The use of low-sodium diets in a noncongestive patient is not indicated and in fact may precipitate the onset of impending renal insufficiency.

Utilizing the knowledge of when specific cardiac therapeutic agents and management procedures are indicated, the clinician may consider on an individual basis each of the methods used in treating congestive cardiac disease. Table 2 is intended as a guide to the clinician in determining when to employ the various therapeutic techniques available.

## Arrhythmias

Abnormalities of cardiac conduction fall into two broad categories: (1) bradycardia, in which these abnormalities are responsible for a slower than normal rhythm; in-cluded in this group are the various forms of heart block; and (2) tachycardia, in which they cause a more rapid than normal rhythm.

Rhythm disturbances may result in reduced blood flow to the vital organs, thereby producing clinically detectable signs such as weakness, fainting, collapsing, a comatose state or death as well as congestive heart failure. Arrhythmias may be transient or long-standing. They may complicate congestive heart failure states or, if persistent, may induce congestive heart failure. The more commonly encountered cardiac rhythm disturbances are described and reviewed in the following articles.

The clinician must be alert for variations in the heart sounds and the peripheral pulse. When irregularities are apparent or a question exists about the cardiac rhythm, the definitive method of demonstrating the cardiac rhythm is to record an electrocardiogram. All leads and a long rhythm strip are necessary to evaluate the electrocardiogram properly.

Electrocardiographic monitoring of the surgical patient is an increasingly popular technique used in many hospitals. Abnormalities of the cardiac rhythm may be quickly recognized and treated prior to the development of cardiac arrest or ventricular fibrillation.

No one drug can be used to treat all rhythm disturbances. It is important to record the electrocardiogram first and recognize the irregularity when it occurs. Without the proper electrocardiographic interpretation, there is little value in memorizing the specific drugs indicated for treatment, since the choice of drugs to be used depends on the site of origin of the arrhythmia and the clinical severity of the problem. The following articles review the medications used for treating common cardiac arrhythmias.

## Summary

The diagnosis and management of heart disease requires more than a passing knowledge of the information given in Tables 1 and 2. Although treatment of the disease is the ultimate goal, the recognition of the cause or etiology is paramount.

Today, a cardiovascular examination cannot be considered complete without an ini-

*Table 2.* Recommended Therapeutic Schedule for Dogs and Cats With Chronic Heart Disease

| PHASE OF HEART DISEASE | EXERCISE RESTRICTION | LOW-SODIUM DIET | BRONCHO-DILATORS | DIGOXIN | DIURETICS | SEDATIVES | OTHER |
|---|---|---|---|---|---|---|---|
| I/IV | No | No | No | No | No | No | No |
| II/IV | Moderate | No | As needed | No | No | No | No |
| III/IV | Restricted | Early—moderate Late—strict | Yes | Yes | As needed | As needed | Occasional narcotic antitussives |
| IV/IV | Cage rest recommended | Yes | Yes | Yes | Yes | Yes, if required | Phlebotomy Vasodilators Oxygen |

tial thorough physical examination, radiographs of the thorax, a full lead electrocardiogram, and blood tests for routine counts, chemistries and microfilaria.

When additional studies are necessary to confirm or develop the diagnosis, cardiac catheterization for hemodynamic values and angiocardiography for structural visualization should be performed.

# NONCONTRAST RADIOLOGY OF THE CARDIO-VASCULAR SYSTEM

RICHARD T. DIXON, M.V.Sc.
*New South Wales, Australia*

Cardiac changes which are detectable on plain radiographs may be induced by three groups of disorders:

1. Congenital cardiac abnormalities, such as stenoses and defects.
2. Acquired cardiac disease, such as myocarditis, valvular endocarditis, etc.
3. Extracardiac interference with filling or emptying of the chambers. This interference may be pulmonary hypertension induced by congestion or heartworms or may be secondary to lung changes caused by pneumonia or neoplasia.

Detection of changes in the vascular system is confined to examination of the major pulmonary arteries and veins for evidence of overfilling or underfilling. If overfilled and distended, the vessels may have a clear outline, indicating vascular congestion, or may have a fuzzy, indistinct outline, indicating adjacent pulmonary edema.

To avoid production of spurious abnormalities caused by positioning and technical faults, strict attention should be paid to positioning the patient. Radiographs should be taken on peak inspiration to insure that the lungs are maximally inflated and that the diaphragm and abdominal viscera are displaced as far caudally as possible. If taking repeat radiographic series for comparison or evaluation, use the same techniques as those used initially to avoid the changes in density associated with changes in radiographic technique. It is not possible to insure that radiographs are taken at a particular phase of the cardiac cycle, so allowance should be made for size changes between systole and diastole.

## RADIOGRAPHIC POSITIONING

Two views should be taken to avoid the uncertainties and mistakes in interpretation when only one radiograph is examined. The two views usually taken are the recumbent lateral and the dorsoventral views.

The *lateral view* may be a right or left recumbent lateral view. The left side down is preferable, as there is less rotation, but the most important point is that any subsequent films should be taken with the same side down. The forelimbs should be pulled forward to uncover as much of the apical area as possible, and the hindlimbs should be pulled backward to diminish the pressure and forward movement of the abdominal viscera on the diaphragm. The upper limbs should be held horizontally, rather than pressed down on the table, in order to avoid rotation of the thorax; foam sponges placed between the limbs will help to maintain the limbs parallel to the table. The neck should be extended to avoid dorsal arching of the thoracic trachea. The primary beam should be directed over the widest part of the thorax, perpendicular to the 5th rib.

The *dorsoventral* view is taken so that the vertebral images will be superimposed on the sternebral images; any rotation will render the radiograph of doubtful diagnostic value for assessment of changes in cardiac size and position. The patient should be placed in sternal recumbency in the sphinx position, with the beam centered over the midline, level with the head of the 5th rib. Insure that the hind feet do not encroach on the thoracic field.

If the patient will not cooperate, even when tranquilized, use the *ventrodorsal position*, with the primary beam directed at the junction of the middle and posterior third of the sternum. It is most important that the animal be positioned so that it is exactly on its back, with no rotation. Even so, the heart will rotate so that the right ventricle and the pulmonary artery segment become more prominent; therefore, indiscriminate comparisons between radiographs taken in the two positions should not be made.

If there is a pleural effusion or free blood or pus in the thorax, as much of this should be aspirated as possible, and one or several of the following views should be taken, with the object of shifting the fluid to different locations in the thorax in order to obtain a composite view of all parts of the thorax:

*Standing transverse lateral view*, with the animal standing on all four feet and the primary beam directed horizontally through the 5th rib.

*Supine transverse lateral view*, with the patient lying on its back and a horizontal beam directed at the 5th rib.

*Erect transverse lateral view*, with the animal standing erect on its hind feet and the primary beam directed horizontally through the 5th rib.

*Erect transverse ventrodorsal view*, with the animal positioned as before and the primary beam directed at the junction of the middle and posterior third of the sternum.

## RADIOGRAPHIC INTERPRETATION

Assessment of changes in the cardiovascular system depends on detection of changes in size, shape and position of the structures. For this reason the radiographs must be of sufficient quality for these changes to be seen.

**The Lateral View.** Depending on breed and species, the angle that the cardiac axis forms with the sternum varies considerably from the average of 45 degrees—from the almost vertical heart of the greyhound to the almost horizontal hearts of the Pomeranian and Chihuahua. The degree of sternal contact with the right ventricle also varies, but if one measures the distance from the posterior dorsal edge of the second sternebra to the most anterior point of contact between heart shadow and sternum ($f$) and the distance from this contact point to the posterior dorsal edge of the seventh sternebra ($e$), the ratio $f/e$ is $1.17 \pm 0.66$, with no differences attributable to breed, sex or right or left lateral positioning. Likewise, if the distance is measured from the anterior ventral edge of the sixth thoracic vertebra to the anterior dorsal edge of the sixth sternebra, and the portion proximal to the tracheal bifurcation is called $c$ and the distal portion is called $d$, the ratio of $d/c$ is $3.01 \pm 0.69$, with no difference attributable to breed, sex or right or left lateral positioning.

The cardiac silhouette on the lateral view consists of a triangle, with a base that is craniodorsal, and comprises the right and left atria and the pulmonary artery and veins. At the cranial angle is the cranial "waist" caused by the junction of the anterior vena cava with the right atrium. The anterior side of the triangle comprises the base of the aorta, the right auricle and the right ventricle. The posterior side is somewhat straighter and is made up of the left ventricle and the left auricle.

The lateral radiograph should be placed on the illuminator, with the cranial end to the observer's right, and assessed as follows:

(1) Enlargements in the 1 o'clock to 3 o'clock position may be caused by a heart-base tumor, a poststenotic dilatation of the aorta if there is a valvular aortic stenosis (not if the stenosis is subvalvular) or a right auricular enlargement.

(2) Enlargement in the 4 o'clock to 7 o'clock position, giving an increase in sternal contact with the right ventricle, indicates right ventricular enlargement and results in a decrease in the numerical value of $f$. The ventricular enlargement may be associated with any congenital abnormality causing right ventricular engorgement or hypertrophy, with heartworm infestation or with pulmonary hypertension occasioned by pneumonia or neoplasia. It will occur also in terminal heart failure from any cause. It may be accompanied by a damming back of blood into the liver, causing that organ to appear rounded and engorged

and there may be associated ascites, with consequent loss of abdominal detail.

(3) Enlargement of the silhouette from 7 o'clock to 10 o'clock indicates left ventricular enlargement. The border may become straighter and more vertical, but one should not rely on its overlapping the diaphragmatic shadow, as the latter can vary widely in position relative to the left ventricle, especially in late expiration and early inspiration. Left ventricular hypertrophy (as distinct from enlargement) is usually concentric rather than eccentric and so can be visualized only by contrast radiographic techniques. Enlargement usually occurs in the later stages of changes caused by septal defects and may occur in terminal heart failure from any cause.

(4) Enlargement at the 11 o'clock position is due to left atrial and auricular enlargement and shows as squaring or bulging of the dorsocaudal angle of the triangle. It occurs with aortic stenosis and with left AV insufficiency.

(5) Total cardiac silhouette enlargement may occur with pericardial sac distention by effusion (pericarditis) or hemorrhage (tamponade). It will also occur in terminal uncompensated heart failure. In cases of distention by fluid, the enlargement may be slightly more related to the right or left sides.

(6) Elevation of the tracheal *bifurcation*, with a decrease in the numerical value of $c$, is associated with enlargement of the left ventricle. It may also be seen in the later stages of enlargement of the right ventricle.

(7) Elevation of the left main stem bronchus to form an angle with the right bronchus rather than a superimposed image will occur with enlargement of the left atrium.

(8) Elevation of the terminal portion of the trachea (as distinct from the bifurcation) may be due to right atrial enlargement, to the presence of a heart-base tumor or to enlargement of the cranial mediastinal lymph nodes. Extreme care is needed in evaluating this change if the neck was not extended when radiograph was taken, as flexure of the neck can result in dorsal displacement and arching of the thoracic trachea.

(9) Changes in size and position of the lobar pulmonary arteries and veins may also be detected. The artery lies dorsal to the associated bronchus, and the vein lies ventral. Increase in arterial size occurs with engorgement associated with left-to-right shunts associated with septal defects, with heartworm infestation, with chronic anemia and with pulmonary hypertension. Increase in the venous size is associated with aortic stenosis, left AV incompetence and the later stages of septal defect changes, when the shunt becomes a right-to-left one. Decrease in size of the pulmonary arteries is associated with pulmonic stenosis, tetralogy of Fallot and right-to-left shunts. It may occur in shock and may be produced artificially by overinflating the lungs, especially when taking radiographs using temporary positive pressure in an intubated patient.

**The Dorsoventral View.** Regardless of whether the dorsoventral or ventrodorsal position is preferred, the radiograph should be placed on the illuminator and viewed as if the animal were lying on its back. In the dorsoventral view, using the vertebral column as a dividing line, the ratio of the left side of the silhouette (LH) compared to the right side (RH) should not be greater than 3/2. At the same time the width of the cardiac silhouette (LH + RH) should not be greater than two thirds of the total thoracic width. Additional work indicates that these ratios can be applied to the ventrodorsal view and that they are not affected by breed or sex.

The cardiac silhouette appears as a lopsided egg and should be examined for the following changes:

(1) Enlargement at the 12 o'clock position indicates enlargement of the ascending aorta, associated with a poststenotic knob, where the stenosis is valvular rather than subvalvular.

(2) Enlargement at the 1 o'clock position is due to enlargement of the main stem pulmonary artery (pulmonary conus, pulmonic knob). It occurs as a poststenotic dilatation resulting from a valvular pulmonic stenosis, either singly or as part of a tetralogy of Fallot, or it may be associated with heartworm infestation or may occur with severe pulmonary hypertension.

(3) Enlargement at the 2 o'clock position may be seen in cases of left auricular enlargement.

(4) Enlargement from 3 o'clock to 5 o'clock occurs with left ventricular enlargement. Remember that quite severe concentric hypertrophy can occur in the left ventricle, with decrease in left ventricular volume, with a small or undetectable

*Table 1.*  *Radiographic Changes Seen in Various Cardiovascular Abnormalities*

| CONDITION | RADIOGRAPHIC CHANGE | | | | | | | |
|---|---|---|---|---|---|---|---|---|
| | Right Atrial Enlargement | Right Ventricular Enlargement | Left Atrial Enlargement | Left Ventricular Enlargement | Main Pulmonary Artery | Lobar Pulmonary Artery | Lobar Pulmonary Vein | Aorta |
| Aortic Stenosis | | | ++ | | | Left artery elevated | ++ | +Valvular −Infundibular |
| Heartworm infestation | | + | | | + | Enlarged and tortuous | | |
| Left AV insufficiency | | Secondary | + | | | Secondary | ++ | |
| Patent ductus arteriosus | Secondary | Secondary | Secondary | | Prominent | Engorged | | Sometimes a left lateral bulge |
| Pulmonary hypertension | | + | | | Enlarged if severe | + | | |
| Pulmonic stenosis | | + | | | Knob if valvular stenosis | Undercirculation | | |
| Right AV insufficiency | + | + | | | | | | |
| Septal defects | | + | Secondary | Secondary | Rare | + | | |
| Tetralogy of Fallot | | ++ | | | Knob if valvular stenosis | Undercirculation | | |

change in the size of the overall silhouette, so that a change in the left ventricular size is usually a late change.

(5) Enlargement from 5 o'clock to 10 o'clock (inverted D) indicates an enlarged right ventricle. This frequently results in the silhouette being displaced to the left, so that the initial impression is that of left ventricular enlargement. If in doubt, examine the silhouette to determine if the apex of the heart has been shifted to the 4 o'clock position from its normal position at 5 o'clock.

(6) Enlargement at the 11 o'clock position may indicate right atrial enlargement, but the superimposition of the cranial vena cava, pulmonary artery and aorta can make this change a difficult one to detect.

(7) The pulmonary arteries lie lateral to their respective bronchi, with the veins lying medially. Enlargement with truncation and tortuosity is usually a sure indication of heartworm infestation, whereas enlargement without tortuosity occurs with left-to-right shunts, chronic anemia and pulmonary hypertension. Venous engorgement occurs with aortic stenosis, right-to-left shunts, left AV insufficiency and left ventricular failure.

## CONCLUSION

Any one radiographic change can be seen accompanying a number of congenital or acquired cardiovascular problems (see Table 1), and it may well be that changes are occurring (such as concentric left ventricular hypertrophy) which can not be detected by noncontrast radiography. For this reason, noncontrast radiography of the cardiovascular system should always be considered as an aid to diagnosis; after the radiographs have been examined and the changes assessed, they should be further evaluated together with the history, clinical signs and ECG changes, and then reevaluated to insure that any subtle changes have not been overlooked that could be of value in both diagnosis and prognosis.

## SUPPLEMENTAL READING

American Animal Hospital Association: A Manual of Clinical Cardiology, 1972. 3612 East Jefferson Boulevard, South Bend, Indiana 46615.
Ettinger, S. J., and Suter, P. F.: Canine Cardiology. Philadelphia, W. B. Saunders Co., 1970.
Hamlyn, R. L.: Analysis of the cardiac silhouette in dorsoventral radiographs from dogs with heart disease. J. Am. Vet. Med. Assn., 153:1446, 1968.
Olsson, S. E.: The Radiological Diagnosis in Canine and Feline Emergencies. Philadelphia, Lea & Febiger, 1973.
Ticer, J. W.: Radiographic Technique in Small Animal Practice. Philadelphia, W. B. Saunders Co., 1975.
Wood, A. K. W.: The use of a small mobile X-ray generator and contrast techniques for the radiographic examination of the canine thorax. M. V. Sc. Thesis, University of Sydney, 1971.
Wyburn, R. S., and Lawson, D. D.: Simple radiography as an aid to the diagnosis of heart disease in the dog. J. Small Animal Pract., 8:163, 1967.

# EVALUATION OF THORACIC, PERICARDIAL AND ABDOMINAL EFFUSIONS

ROBERT J. WILKINS, B. V. Sc.
New York, New York

The accumulation of fluid within the thoracic cavity, pericardial sac or abdomen is a clinical sign that can be a manifestation of a variety of disease processes (Table 1). These serous cavities are lined by a single layer of flattened mesothelial cells and connective tissue which emcompass the viscera and cavity walls. Normally, a small amount of fluid is present within each cavity, lubricating the opposing surfaces of visceral and

*Table 1.  Types of Fluid Effusions*

| | PURE TRANSUDATES | MODIFIED TRANSUDATE (OBSTRUCTIVE) | INFLAMMATORY EFFUSIONS | | | CHYLOUS EFFUSIONS | NEOPLASTIC EFFUSIONS | HEMORRHAGIC EFFUSIONS |
| --- | --- | --- | --- | --- | --- | --- | --- | --- |
| | | | *Sterile* | *Septic* | *Pyogranulomatous* | | | |
| *Characteristics* | | | | | | | | |
| Physical Appearance | Clear to straw-colored | Serous to serosanguineous | Serosanguineous → blood-tinged to port-wine colored | | Serous to serosanguineous | Milky after centrifugation | Usually blood-tinged | Blood red |
| Specific Gravity | < 1.013 | 1.013–1.032 | 1.021 – 1.036 | | 1.027 – 1.048 | — | 1.015–1.045 | 1.030–1.048 |
| Total Protein (gm. %) | < 1.0 | 1.0–5.0 | 2.8 – 6.0 | | 3.5 – 8.5 | — | 1.5–7.5 | 4.5–8.0 |
| Coagulation | None | May clot | None | | Fine precipitate | Usually none | May clot | May clot |
| Cytology | Few cells | Blood and lymph cells | Acute-chronic Nontoxic Nonseptic inflammation | Acute-chronic Toxic Septic inflammation | Chronic Nontoxic Active inflammation | Lymphorrhage ± sterile inflammation | Neoplastic cells present | Blood cells M:E <1:200 |
| *Common Causes* | | | | | | | | |
| All Cavities | Hypoalbuminemia; overhydration; nephrotic syndrome | Congestive or obstructive heart failure; thrombosis; neoplasms obstructing lymphatics and blood vessels | Steatitis; postsurgical drains or implants | Empyema; penetrating wounds; ruptured abscess; extension of local adjacent infection | Feline infectious peritonitis | | Lymphosarcoma; metastatic carcinoma; adenocarcinomas; mesothelioma; hemangiosarcoma | Trauma; thrombocytopenia; postsurgical bleeding diathesis |
| Pleural | | Cardiomyopathy; cardiac anomalies; pulmonary atelectasis; lung torsion; pulmonary neoplasia; diaphragmatic hernia; mediastinal tumors | Pleuritis; diaphragmatic hernia; pneumonia | Pyothorax; extension of infection from lungs, trachea and esophagus | | Acute chylothorax; chronic chylothorax; chronic pleuritis | Thymoma | Lung torsion |
| Pericardial | | Heart-base tumors; peritoneopericardial diaphragmatic hernia | Benign idiopathic pericardial effusion; heart-base tumor; other metastatic tumors | Pericarditis (bacterial or fungal) | | Uncommon | Heart-base tumors | Atrial rupture; erosive neoplasms at heart base (e.g., hemangiosarcoma) |
| Peritoneal | Intestinal malabsorption | Portal venous obstruction; hepatopathies; cirrhosis; bile duct carcinoma; sclerotic carcinomatosis | Urine peritonitis; bile peritonitis; pancreatic peritonitis; gastric peritonitis; chronic active hepatitis; diaphragmatic hernia; long-standing obstruction to | Intestinal perforation; ruptured pyometra | | Obstruction of mesenteric lymphatics (postprandial) | Gastrointestinal and genitourinary tumors | Acute rupture of hemangiosarcoma; torsion of stomach or spleen; pheochromocytoma (eroding vena cava) |

parietal pleura, pericardium or peritoneum. The fluid is considered to be dialyzed from plasma, its flow and composition regulated by the lining mesothelial cells.

The pleural and peritoneal cavities are drained by the lymphatic system, particularly the large lymphatics located on the perimeter of the diaphragm. Here most macromolecules and cellular elements pass via the lymphatic drainage to the cisterna and thoracic duct into the blood circulation. Reabsorption from the pericardial sac is much more restrictive; generally the cells do not recirculate from this cavity.

Excessive fluid accumulation may be either a passive transudate or an active exudate, related to the underlying disease process. The cause of transudation, i.e., the passive passage of fluid from blood or lymphatics through the interstitium and lining membrane into these body cavities, is varied and complex. There are, however, several factors common to its occurrence, and these are related to the direction of movement of fluids and constituents between blood and interstitial tissues. These factors include (1) changes in hydrostatic forces such as increased capillary or lymphatic resistance to flow, (2) increased permeability and (3) decreased hydrostatic interstitial pressure. The most common cause of increased hydrostatic pressure is partial or complete distal obstruction to venous or lymphatic drainage. Typical examples are seen in heart failure, cirrhosis and tumor obstruction. The other factors of importance are the osmotic pressure effects. Transudation of water from blood to tissues occurs when the plasma oncotic pressure falls; it is most often seen in severe hypoalbuminemic states or when the interstitial oncotic pressure rises.

These factors also operate in the case of exudates, but the greater component operating is the active process, usually inflammatory in nature, resulting in the effusion of larger amounts of proteins, macromolecules and cellular elements from the blood. Long-standing effusions, whether initially transudative or exudative in type, can become modified, a factor which must be considered in evaluating the effusion.

The differential diagnoses in cases where effusion is one of the clinical signs can be made on the basis of a thorough history and clinical examination, routine radiographs and laboratory testing, including hemogram, biochemical analysis and urinalysis. Collection and examination of the effusion play an important role in diagnosis of the condition. Physical appearance, chemical analysis and cytologic evaluation should be included in the analysis. Unless one is experienced at examining cytologic preparations, it is advised that both stained and unstained smears and an aliquot of the fluid specimen (3 cc. in EDTA anticoagulant) be submitted to a veterinary cytologist or clinical pathologist for interpretation.

Table 1 outlines the most common types of fluid specimens obtained from the three body cavities. The physical, biophysical and chemical properties and commonly encountered causes for the fluid accumulation are also outlined.

# PRINCIPLES OF CARDIAC CATHETERIZATION

GARY L. WOOD, D.V.M.,
*and* PETER F. SUTER, D.M.V.
*Davis, California*

Cardiac catheterization involves the placing of catheters in the great vessels and chambers of the heart to obtain diagnostic information. Data commonly collected are blood pressures, pressure gradients across valves, oxygen tensions in the heart chambers and great vessels, and indicator dye dilution or thermodilution concentration curves. In addition, the production of angiocardiograms is usually a part of cardiac catheterization.

Small animal practitioners should be

familiar with the potential usefulness and limitations of cardiac catheterization to help best those animals that may benefit from it. This will permit them to select appropriate cases for referral to a catheterization laboratory. Although it is neither difficult nor expensive to pass a catheter from a peripheral vein to the heart, data collected and angiocardiograms produced by this nonselective method are frequently of limited value. Because the expense of equipment needed for proper selective catheterization is prohibitive and its indications are limited, this type of procedure is confined to specialty hospitals, institutions or veterinary schools.

This article discusses the principles of cardiac catheterization, including the indications, contraindications, procedures and complications. For additional information readers are encouraged to consult the references listed at the end of this article.

## Indications

There are three indications for cardiac catheterization: (1) to obtain a specific diagnosis when routine methods have failed; (2) to gather quantitative data and detailed morphologic information for prognosis and planning of therapy, especially surgical treatment; and (3) to collect scientifically valuable information for the study of a particular disease, defect or drug.

Routine clinical methods may permit the clinician to arrive at a specific diagnosis in congenital heart diseases such as uncomplicated patent ductus arteriosus or vascular ring anomalies. However, the definitive diagnosis of many congenital heart defects, such as atrial or ventricular septal defects, aortic stenosis, tetralogy of Fallot or complex malformations, is frequently incomplete or impossible by routine methods alone. Cardiac catheterization may confirm a suspected lesion, point out additional defects or complications or occasionally refute the clinical diagnosis altogether.

In heart failure due to congenital heart disease, clinical and survey radiographic findings can be equivocal or provide insufficient information to select the most appropriate therapy. In pulmonic or aortic stenosis, the pressure gradient (difference in systolic pressures) across the narrowed valve area and the specific location of the stricture (valvular, subvalvular or supravalvular) offer valuable prognostic and presurgical information that can be provided only

by cardiac catheterization. In addition, a combination of two or more congenital heart defects can occur. For instance, cardiac catheterization in pulmonic stenosis may detect complications such as tricuspid insufficiency or atrial or ventricular septal defects. A specific intravitam diagnosis in cyanotic heart disease such as tetralogy of Fallot, Eisenmenger's complex or reversed patent ductus arteriosus is obtainable only by cardiac catheterization.

Our knowledge of most congenital heart diseases has been greatly advanced by cardiac catheterization. It continues to be the most useful diagnostic procedure in these cases. Our knowledge of the hemodynamic events in normal hearts, in those altered by specific drug agents, and those with acquired heart diseases has also been greatly advanced by catheterization, even though it may not be essential for the clinical management of most animals. Conditions such as canine and feline cardiomyopathies, heartworm disease and chronic valvular fibrosis have been more precisely defined through cardiac catheterization. In addition, catheterization procedures can be indicated in the diagnosis of heartworm disease without circulating microfilariae. The diagnosis in animals with suspected cardiac tumors, atrial thrombosis or pericardial diseases may require selective or nonselective catheterization.

## Contraindications

Cardiac catheterization should be performed only if there is adequate indication. It is not a short cut to a definitive diagnosis. There are several potential contraindications to cardiac catheterization: (1) moderately severe to severe congestive heart failure, (2) serious respiratory disease, (3) life-threatening arrhythmias, (4) foci of infection (especially cardiovascular or respiratory) and (5) known hypersensitivity to any contrast agent used. Some contraindications are relative, because complications resulting from them may be prevented or controlled by appropriate measures. Heart failure due to a congenital defect may be temporarily controlled with digitalis, diuretics and a low-sodium diet to permit anesthesia and catheterization. Arrhythmias may be controlled by antiarrhythmic drugs; respiratory infections can be influenced by antibiotics.

Catheterization must be planned by using the cumulative information obtained in arriving at the tentative clinical diagnosis. Prior to cardiac catheterization, all animals must undergo a careful cardiovascular examination, including complete physical examination, electrocardiogram, thoracic radiographs, complete blood count, urinalysis and tests for renal and hepatic dysfunction. Special procedures such as phonocardiography, vectorcardiography or blood gas studies should sometimes precede catheterization. The relative advantages versus the risks and expenses of catheterization must be weighed fully and carefully explained to the client.

## PROCEDURE

Catheterization performed by a trained team with adequate equipment produces most consistent results. Equipment and protocol vary widely depending on the institution carrying out the procedure. However, four basic functions must be provided for: (1) preparation and surgical catheterization of the animal, (2) monitoring the animal and recording the hemodynamic data, (3) producing angiocardiographic recordings and (4) being prepared for emergencies.

Lists of instruments and equipment for performing aseptic vascular surgery and of radiopaque catheters and guide wires commonly used have been published (Wood *et al.*, 1975). Equipment for general anesthesia is also needed. The apparatus used for monitoring the animal includes a multichannel medical recorder adapted for electrocardiography and blood pressure measurements, strain gauge pressure transducers and a blood gas analyzer. For indicator dye dilution studies, a detectable dye is injected upstream from the sampling point. A sampling device which draws dye-containing blood from the heart, great vessel or peripheral vessel through a densitometer or other instrument that determines indicator concentration is needed. In thermodilution studies, a cold solution is injected and a thermistor is used to detect changes in blood temperature at the catheter tip. A minicomputer may determine hemodynamic parameters directly from the data.

Angiocardiography requires at least a conventional x-ray machine which permits multiple short-interval exposures and fluoroscopy. Image intensification is essential to reduce radiation hazards to all persons involved. An automatic rapid film or cassette changer is needed, although it is possible to obtain serial radiographs at a slower rate by changing cassettes manually through a simple cassette tunnel. For recording dynamic events, a cinefluoroscopic unit or video tape recorder is essential. A power injector is needed to deliver the contrast medium at the appropriate time and as a bolus into the heart or great vessels. The preferred contrast media are sodium or methylglucamine salts of diatrizoate*,** or iothalamate.† An automatic film processor facilitates rapid development and evaluation of the radiographs during the procedure. This allows immediate repeat or complementary studies while the animal is still under anesthesia.

For handling cardiovascular emergencies that may arise, a direct current defibrillator and emergency drugs must be on hand at all times. A list of current drugs for cardiac emergencies has been published (Wood *et al.*, 1975). Continuous monitoring of the animal, especially constant display of the electrocardiogram, enables recognition of minor complications while they still can be prevented from developing into major complications.

Anesthetic programs for animals with cardiovascular disease vary widely. Care must be taken to minimize doses of cardiotoxic agents. This becomes particularly important when pressure data are critical to the diagnosis or prognosis. An approach that leaves myocardial function nearly unimpaired and alters hemodynamic data little is use of a "balanced" anesthesia, using the synthetic analgesic fentanyl citrate‡ with the muscle relaxant pancuronium bromide.§ This combination requires artificial respiration and close anesthetic monitoring.

After induction of anesthesia and preparation of the surgical site, a cutdown on the jugular vein and carotid artery or femoral artery and vein is performed. Direct puncture of either ventricle should be reserved for animals in whom a selective antegrade or retrograde approach through a peripheral vessel is impossible. Using the

---

*Hypaque-M-75%® and Hypaque 50%®, Winthrop Laboratories, New York, New York 10016.

**Renografin-76®, and Renovist®, E. R. Squibb and Sons, Inc., New York, New York 10016.

†Conray 60%®, Mallinckrodt Chemical Works, St. Louis, Missouri 63160.

‡Sublimaze®, McNeil Laboratories, Fort Washington, Pennsylvania 19034.

§Pavalon®, Organon, Inc., West Orange, New Jersey 07052.

fluoroscopic image and/or pressure tracings as a guide, radiopaque catheters are passed through the artery and vein to the desired positions in the heart or great vessels. A flexible metal guide wire may be useful in accomplishing proper placement of the catheter tip. The position of the inserted catheter tip must be monitored at all times, preferably by direct fluoroscopic control or indirectly by pressure recordings displayed on an oscilloscope. Without exact knowledge of the catheter tip location, interpretation of the recorded data or injection of contrast medium or indicator dye at the desired location is difficult. Frequent flushes of heparinized dextrose or saline are necessary to prevent clotting within catheters.

With the catheters in place, the hemodynamic data are collected. Pressures, blood gases from different locations or indicator dye dilution curves may substantiate a diagnosis. Abnormal pressures are important in the evaluation of cases with stenotic lesions or hypertension of the pulmonary vascular bed. The size of the systolic pressure gradient across a stenotic pulmonic or aortic valve area provides valuable information concerning the severity and prognosis of the condition. Shunting lesions, valvular insufficiencies or myocardial failure may also alter pressures. Pressure data are prone to numerous artifacts, and experience is required to record and interpret them accurately.

Measurement of blood gas tensions at various sites through the heart and great vessels is of value in determining the location and severity of shunting defects. In addition, these data aid in the anesthetic management of the animal. Indicator dye dilution or thermodilution studies are useful in the qualitative and quantitative evaluation of shunting or regurgitating lesions and for determining cardiac index and peripheral or pulmonary vascular resistance.

After data collection has been completed, angiocardiography is performed. In selective angiocardiography, contrast medium is injected as close to the expected lesion as possible and its flow is recorded on rapid-sequence radiographs, cinefluoroscopic film or video tape. Proper dose of contrast medium, shape of the catheter tip, timing and pressure of the injection and appropriate film sequence to demonstrate the exact morphology of the lesion are important. Hand injection is usually unsatisfactory because the entire dose of contrast medium

should be delivered as a bolus, momentarily replacing the nonopacified blood in the area of interest. This is facilitated by using the largest diameter catheter which can be advanced through the peripheral vessel and by using an injection pressure obtainable only by a power injector. Relative to blood flow, stenotic and shunting defects are best demonstrated by selective injection proximal to the lesion. Regurgitating defects are delineated by injecting distal to the lesion. Nonselective angiocardiography, which is done by injecting contrast medium into a peripheral vein, is not as valuable as selective procedures, owing to superimposition of opacified structures and dilution of contrast medium by blood. Before removing the catheters and closing the surgical site, the films and data should be reviewed for completeness.

## COMPLICATIONS

If the animal is carefully examined before the procedure, and if contraindications are observed, complications can be kept to a minimum. Animals with cardiac disease must be expected to respond with more serious complications than would normal animals. The most important consideration is to recognize and correct minor problems before they can progress into major complications.

The most common minor complications are cardiac arrhythmias. These are usually single atrial or ventricular premature contractions caused by the catheter tip rubbing against the endocardium. Withdrawal of the catheter tip from the sensitive area will usually result in return of normal sinus rhythm. If minor arrhythmias are allowed to persist, they may advance to more serious disturbances such as ventricular tachycardia. If this occurs, additional steps should be taken before further deterioration can occur. Myocardial sensitivity and depression should be minimized by reducing the anesthetic level and increasing oxygenation with assisted respiration and increased oxygen flow. If necessary, short-acting antiarrhythmic drugs such as lidocaine should be injected directly into cardiac chambers. Ventricular fibrillation requires immediate external cardiac massage and direct current defibrillation while adequate oxygenation is maintained by positive pressure ventilation.

Additional complications may arise from too vigorous manipulation of catheters.

Gentleness is required to avoid damaging valve leaflets or causing cardiac tamponade by perforating the walls of the atria, ventricles or great vessels. During pressure injection of contrast medium, the catheter tip must not be lodged between trabeculae or against the endocardium. Subendocardial or even pericardial injection of contrast medium may occur, resulting in persistent arrhythmias or cardiac tamponade.

Other complications, such as hemorrhage, congestive heart failure, cardiogenic shock, infection, thrombosis or embolism, are avoided by prudent technique. Adverse effects of contrast medium can be minimized by careful attention to dose. Sometimes knowing when to terminate a procedure prematurely in cases in which severe complications have developed can be crucial to the animal's welfare, even if data collection is considered incomplete.

## CONCLUSIONS

Because cardiac catheterization is expensive and requires special training, it is limited to institutions or specialty practices. It can provide valuable data for the differential diagnosis and prognosis of many cardiovascular diseases, particularly congenital defects. It is most rewarding when it is used to confirm a diagnosis established by a complete routine cardiovascular exam. Careful planning and execution of each procedure is a prerequisite for successful cardiac catheterization.

## SUPPLEMENTAL READING

Buchanan, J. W.: Selective angiography and angiocardiography in dogs with acquired cardiovascular disease. J. Am. Vet. Radiol. Soc., 6:5, 1965.

Buchanan, J. W., and Patterson, D. F.: Selective angiography and angiocardiography in dogs with congenital cardiovascular disease. J. Am. Vet. Radiol. Soc., 6:21, 1965.

Ettinger, S. J., and Suter, P. F.: Canine Cardiology. Philadelphia, W. B. Saunders Co., 1970.

Knight, H. D.: Principles of cardiac catheterization. In Kirk, R. W. (ed.): Current Veterinary Therapy V. Philadelphia, W. B. Saunders Co., 1974.

Wood, G. L., Ettinger, S. J., and Rhode, E. A.: Angiocardiography. In Ticer, J. W.: Radiographic Technique in Small Animal Practice. Philadelphia, W. B. Saunders Co., 1975.

# DIURETICS

A. D. J. WATSON, B.V.Sc.
*Sydney, Australia*

The intravascular and extravascular fluid compartments are normally in a state of flux, with a continual movement of water and diffusible solutes from vessels at the arteriolar end of the microcirculation and back into the vascular compartment at the venous end. This exchange is controlled by a number of forces, the most significant of which are the hydrostatic pressure within vessels and the colloid oncotic pressure exerted by the plasma proteins, particularly albumin.

When the balance between these forces is upset by hypoalbuminemia (as in hepatopathy, glomerulonephropathy and protein-losing enteropathy) or by obstructive conditions (e.g., congestive heart failure or hepatic fibrosis), there is a net loss of fluid from vessels into tissues and a diminished arterial volume. The resulting decrease in renal perfusion causes reduced glomerular filtration and increased secretion of aldosterone (through the renin-angiotensin mechanism). These factors, together with other adaptive changes, produce increased retention of sodium and water, which causes expansion of the volume of extracellular fluid, including plasma.

In mild heart failure, the expansion of blood volume may be a useful compensation, since it tends to increase venous return to the heart and maintain cardiac output. However, in more severe heart failure, fluid retention cannot repair the arterial volume deficit, because much of the retained fluid is lost from vessels and accumulates in tissues and body cavities. The edema fluid in lungs and other tissues, together with venous congestion, causes cellular hypoxia and hinders organ function.

Diuretic agents are useful in the treatment of congestive heart failure because they reduce fluid retention and congestive changes; in this way, they may limit the clinical manifestations of heart failure and improve the overall cardiac status of the patient. However, diuretic therapy represents only one aspect of the management of congestive heart failure; it should be considered in conjunction with other measures intended to limit salt and fluid retention (low-sodium diet); to decrease cardiac workload (rest, sedation); to improve cardiac output (cardiac glycosides); or otherwise to support the patient (bronchodilators, antitussives, oxygen, paracentesis).

While a large number of diuretic agents have been used in the past, furosemide and the thiazide derivatives are generally regarded as the most useful of the agents currently available. These drugs inhibit the active resorption of sodium, and consequently the passive resorption of water, in the renal tubules. The resulting diuresis is often accompanied by augmented potassium loss, because the high concentration of sodium in tubular fluid promotes potassium-sodium exchange in the distal nephron.

*Furosemide (frusemide)* is a potent diuretic which can be given orally or parenterally. Diuresis begins within one hour of oral administration and persists for approximately four hours. After intravenous or intramuscular injection, diuresis commences in five to twenty minutes, and continues for about two hours. Furosemide is given by mouth in doses of 2 to 5 mg./kg. (repeated one to three times daily) or parenterally at 1 to 2 mg./kg. (may be repeated in two hours, or increased if diuresis is inadequate). Once the desired response is achieved, subsequent dosage and frequency of administration should be adjusted according to individual patient requirements.

In addition to its action in removing edema fluid, furosemide increases renal blood flow and may therefore be of value in treating ischemic renal failure. Furthermore, studies in people have revealed extrarenal hemodynamic effects which could be particularly beneficial in the treatment of pulmonary congestion and edema.

Unlike some other diuretics, furosemide remains effective even when excessive extravascular fluid has been removed. Overdosage may therefore cause hypovolemia and circulatory collapse, as well as depletion of various ions. For this reason, it is suggested that, whenever possible, furosemide should be given intermittently as required rather than continuously. Furthermore, the concurrent use of furosemide with some antibiotics may be inadvisable:

there is evidence that the drug enhances the nephrotoxic potential of aminoglycosides, cephalosporins and polymyxins and increases the ototoxic effects of aminoglycosides.

The *thiazide diuretics* are less potent than furosemide and are generally given orally. Diuresis begins within an hour of administration and continues for 12 to 24 hours, so they are usually given once or twice daily. The total daily doses suggested by Ettinger and Suter (1970) for the thiazides are chlorthiazide, 20 to 45 mg./kg.; hydrochlorthiazide, 2 to 4 mg./kg.; and benzydroflumethiazide (bendrofluazide), 0.2 to 0.4 mg./kg. These dosages should be reduced and intermittent therapy adopted whenever possible to avoid excessive depletion of potassium and other ions. Thiazide derivatives should probably be avoided in patients with impaired renal function, because they tend to decrease renal blood flow and glomerular filtration rate.

The thiazides and furosemide promote urinary potassium loss, which may already be increased in edematous states because of secondary hyperaldosteronism. Prolonged, continuous diuretic therapy may therefore cause hypokalemia, which in turn can induce digitalis intoxication. Consequently, supplementation of the diet with potassium-rich foods (fruit, nuts) or liquid potassium chloride may be advisable with long-term, intensive diuretic treatment. This complication can be avoided, however, with intermittent therapy.

[*Editor's Note*: In addition to hypokalemia, electrolyte depletion of sodium and potassium may develop, as may azotemia and/or alkalosis. These factors need to be considered whenever untoward reactions occur in an animal receiving diuretics.]

### SUPPLEMENTAL READING

Dikshit, K., *et al.*: Renal and extrarenal hemodynamic effects of furosemide in congestive heart failure after acute myocardial infarction. New Engl. J. Med., 288:1087–1090, 1973.

Ettinger, S. J., and Suter, P. F.: Diuretics. *In* Canine Cardiology. Philadelphia, W. B. Saunders Co., 1970.

Frazier, H. S., and Yager, H.: The clinical use of diuretics. New Engl. J. Med., 288:246–249 and 455–457, 1973.

Hardy, R. M.: Diuretics. *In* Kirk, R. W. (ed): Current Veterinary Therapy V. Philadelphia, W. B. Saunders Co., 1974.

# DIGITALIS GLYCOSIDES IN CANINE MEDICINE

ALLEN W. HAHN, D.V.M.
*Columbia, Missouri*

One approach to the problem of improving poor myocardial performance in congestive heart failure is to use drugs to improve myocardial contractility. The class of drugs known as cardiac or digitalis glycosides has a long history of being useful (and also toxic) in this respect. Only in the last 20 years, however, has a more thorough understanding of the action of these drugs become clarified—much still has to be learned and applied. While there are large amounts of data available on the chronic use of these drugs in man and significant studies in experimental animals, especially the dog, there is much less information available in clinical canine cardiology. There is also considerable controversy about the usefulness of these drugs in canine medicine. In a study done on comparisons of treatment regimes for canine congestive heart failure, Hamlin *et al.* (1973) found that dogs that received neither digoxin nor digitoxin as part of a treatment regime for failure lived longer than dogs receiving either glycoside. The reason for this was not explored in depth and while the study was soundly criticized (Patterson *et al.*, 1973), it does point out that our knowledge of therapy in clinical cardiac failure is far from complete.

This article will review some of the current knowledge that has been made available by research in this field and will point out how this knowledge can be applied to the problem of improvement of myocardial contractility in the failing canine heart.

## HISTORICAL ASPECTS

The use of the powdered leaves of the purple foxglove plant, *Digitalis purpurea*, was first described in 1542 by Leonard Fuchs, who recommended digitalis as both a purgative and an emetic drug. Some 119 years later, it was included in the London Pharmacopoeia, where it was recommended in the treatment of epilepsy and consumption and as a sedative drug. It was widely misused during the 17th and 18th centuries and gained a reputation as a poison. It remained for William Withering, an English physician practicing first in Shropshire-Stafford and later in Birmingham, England, to document its clinical usefulness in what has become a classic in the field of clinical pharmacology. Withering carefully documented the use of several forms of digitalis leaves in over 150 patients and published, in 1785, his "Account of the Foxglove and Some of its Medical Uses: with Practical Remarks on Dropsy and Other Diseases." The drug again fell into misuse and during the 19th century was considered too poisonous for use in patients. By the early 20th century, with the advent of more rational medical practice, it then became more widely and wisely used on patients in congestive heart failure. A further account of the history of digitalis can be found in the article by Estes and White (1965).

It is interesting that even today various preparations available for use in both man and animal still use the same formulation used by Withering. Many of the myths that surround the use of the digitalis glycosides are those that were propagated during the late 19th and early 20th century. Nonetheless, the drug remains today at the pinnacle of popularity for the treatment of congestive heart failure in man and, likewise, in both the dog and the cat. Many improvements have been made in formulations of products available, but the principle of their usage still remains essentially the same.

## ACTIVE PRINCIPLE

The class of drugs that were referred to earlier as cardiac glycosides are characterized by a general chemical formulation as

329

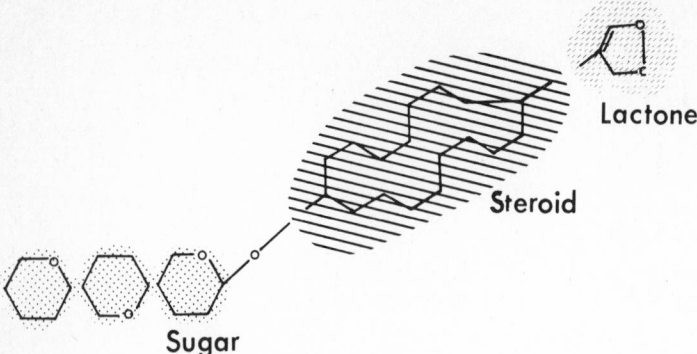

**Figure 1.** The general structural formula for the digitalis glycosides. The lactone-steroid "complex" is known as a genin (i.e., digoxigenin, digitoxigenin, etc.) or an aglycone. When the sugar is added, the molecule is known as a glycoside.

shown in Fig. 1. There is a central steroid nucleus with an attached lactone ring and sugar molecule. The basic ring structure (steroid and lactone) is known as a genin, or sometimes as an aglycone. When a sugar molecule is added to the steroid ring (in position 3) the entire molecule is then known as a cardiac glycoside, cardioactive glycoside or digitalis glycoside. Some 400 glycosides have been isolated from many natural sources, primarily the leaves of several species of plants and also from seeds, toad skins and recently from several species of insects that feed on plants that synthesize the active glycosides (Rothschild *et al.*, 1970; Scudder and Duffey, 1972; von Euw *et al.*, 1967).

A glycoside known as *ouabain* is obtained from the seeds of the African arrow-poison plant, *Strophanthus gratus*. The structural formula of ouabain is shown in Fig. 2A. The glycoside is strongly hydrophilic and is available for parenteral injection only. It is poorly absorbed from the gastrointestinal tract, probably because of destruction in either the stomach or the duodenum. After intravenous administration it is rapidly distributed to tissue. Ouabain is one of the more rapidly eliminated of the cardiac glycosides, elimination being primarily by the renal route with a plasma half-life of 18 hours (Selden and Smith, 1972). This particular glycoside is useful in emergency situations and must be given by the parenteral (preferably intravenous) route.

One of the most common and popular glycosides is digoxin. Digoxin is obtained from the leaves of the Grecian foxglove plant, *Digitalis lanata*. The plant is grown at present in commercial quantities specifically for the pharmaceutical industry, primarily in the Netherlands and in

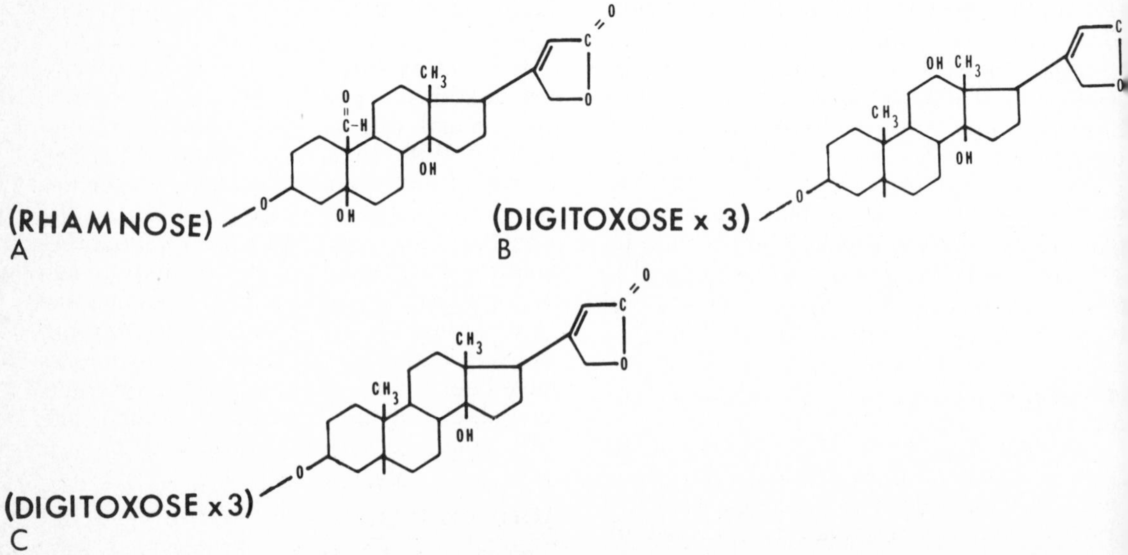

(RHAMNOSE)
A

(DIGITOXOSE x 3)
B

(DIGITOXOSE x 3)
C

**Figure 2.** The general structural formula of *A*, ouabain; *B*, digoxin; *C*, digitoxin. *Note:* The digoxin and digitoxin differ only in the presence of OH at the C12 position.

Ecuador. Its structural formula is shown in Fig. 2*B*, and it is intermediate in its hydrophilic/hydrophobic properties. It is available as an elixir and in pill and injectable forms. Note that the chemical structure shows a hydroxyl molecule at the C12 position in the steroid ring. Apparently, because of this molecule (which causes it to be known as a polar molecule), its absorption, distribution and elimination are more rapid than its sister compound, digitoxin.

Digitoxin is obtained from the leaves of the purple foxglove plant, *Digitalis purpurea*. Its structural formula is shown in Fig. 2*C*. Note that there is no hydroxyl molecule at the C12 position in the steroid ring. This is the *only* chemical difference between it and digoxin. Apparently, however, this sole difference is responsible for many of the differing features of digitoxin. The drug is available as an elixir and in pill and injectable forms. It is strongly hydrophobic and is also bound quite strongly to plasma proteins (about 90 per cent in the dog). Digoxin is bound to plasma proteins at about the 20 to 25 per cent level in the dog.

The formulation of cardiac glycoside administered is of singular importance. Use of whole-leaf digitalis preparations is difficult to justify for two reasons. First, the amount and proportion of active glycosides in these preparations is a function of the region where the plant was grown, the amount of rainfall and sun the plant received and the amount of soil nutrients available. Doherty (1968) has termed them "polyglots" of digitalis glycosides. A clinician never knows which of many cardioactive glycosides may be producing an effect, and uniformity can never be guaranteed. Secondly, and probably more importantly for canine cardiology, whole-leaf digitalis (from *D. purpurea*) has as its principal glycoside digitoxin. Oral forms (except for tinctures) of this glycoside have been shown to have highly variable absorption rates from the gut in the dog and to be strongly bound to plasma proteins. It is for these reasons that clinicians should concentrate their efforts on purified glycosides for use in a digitalis therapy regime.

An order form of preparation is still available for use in veterinary medical cardiac treatment regimes. This is one which contains Digitaline, Strophanthus and sparteine. These oral formulations, holdovers from less definitive days in human medicine, contain such small amounts of Digitaline (a semipurified digitoxin) as to be essentially ineffective. Strophanthus is a close relative of ouabain and probably not absorbed from the gut. Sparteine is from the squill family and likewise is probably poorly or erratically absorbed. In any case, the are *no* objective data available showing that these drugs have a positive inotropic or chronotropic effect on the failing canine myocardium. Other formulations closely akin to the above also contain nitroglycerin (a coronary vasodilator for anginal attacks due to coronary atherosclerosis in man— hardly a significant problem in the dog) and cactus extract. The pharmacologic basis for cactus extract escapes most Western world clinicians. The clinical use of either of these preparations has no rational basis.

## MECHANISM OF ACTION

Study of the effects of the cardiac glycosides at the myocardial muscle cell receptor sites is an area of intense activity in the research laboratory. The precise mechanism remains undefined, but present evidence suggests that the glycosides inhibit the sodium-potassium-ATPase system and mobilize calcium at the sarcomere level (Lüllman and Peters, 1973; Repke *et al.*, 1973). Calcium, of course, is crucial to the contractile process, and by being available in greater quantities for release to contractile proteins, contractility is enhanced. This increase in contractility of the myocardium itself is known as positive inotropy. Contractility is generally taken to imply an increase in stroke work of the ventricle when both end-diastolic volume and arterial pressure are held constant.

One of the compensatory mechanisms of the failing myocardium is its attempt to conserve its energy. This is done often at the expense of cardiac performance (Katz, 1975). The cardiac glycosides, while increasing myocardial contractility to enhance performance, do so at the expense of increased energy expenditure in the myocardium.

The concentration of cardiac glycosides in myocardial tissue necessary to effect positive inotropy appears to be linearly related to dose. Recent studies in anesthetized dogs by Kim, Noble and Zipes (1975) have established this linear dose response in regard to contractility, but their studies also showed a nonlinear response of conducting tissue to the glycosides.

The clinician is interested in the positive inotropic actions of the drugs but with this he must take the toxic effects that occur with the administration of the glycosides. It is these toxic effects, primarily neural in nature, which are responsible for a large portion of the toxic response accorded to cardiac glycosides. Were this toxic effect easily predictable, one could approach the problem accurately and scientifically. The use of the digitalis glycosides, however, remains very much an art, because the toxic effects seem to be related to a state of the autonomic nervous system at the time of administration, and it is this state which is still impossible to predict for a given patient.

The effects on the central nervous system of the cardiac glycosides are predominantly threefold (Gillias *et al.*, 1975). The primary and best known of these is a vagomimetic effect, that is, stimulation of the vagus nerve. This stimulation results in cardiac slowing and delayed conduction at the atrioventricular (AV) node. In addition, the glycosides also sensitize the arterial baroreceptors to increase their afferent tone. This, then, also enhances the vagomimetic effect. In low doses, the glycosides inhibit sympathetic outflow, but larger doses excite the autonomic nervous system, resulting in enhanced sympathetic outflow and cardiac arrhythmias.

It has been postulated that these effects may, in part at least, be responsible for the extracardiac toxicities that are observed in many patients. These are anorexia, vomiting, diarrhea and muscular weakness. In man, additional extracardiac effects also include diplopia, confusion and certain psychiatric symptoms.

An increase in contractility, caused by the glycosides, results in an increase in cardiac output in the failing heart. This increase is also observed in the hearts of normal intact animals but appears to be quickly readjusted by functional operating control mechanisms. The heart rate is slowed by the vagal effect. This cardiac slowing is not present in either atropinized animals or transplanted hearts (Leachman *et al.*, 1971). The neural effects are also accompanied by toxic effects which include depression of the AV nodal conduction and the development of heart blocks, as previously mentioned. Also, increased irritability of the ventricular myocardium causes the development of ventricular tachyarrhythmias (premature ventricular contractions, ventricular tachycardia and possibly ventricular fibrillation).

The digitalis glycosides are not drugs to be trifled with. Their margin of safety is extremely narrow. While they remain the cornerstone of therapy for heart failure in human medicine, a recent survey has shown that approximately 20 per cent of patients receiving digoxin were toxic upon admission to hospitals (Ogilvie and Ruedy, 1972).

## ABSORPTION, DISTRIBUTION AND EXCRETION OF THE GLYCOSIDES

The above three factors determine how fast a particular glycoside will reach a myocardial receptor site. Videbaek and Brock (1974) found that in the nonfailing myocardium of anesthetized dogs a maximal increase in contractility was proportional to the accumulated dose and achieved at a concentration of 140 nanograms of digoxin per gram of myocardial tissue. Other than acute experiments, of course, there is no way to measure the precise amount of glycosides available in the myocardium. Nonetheless, by knowledge of how the drug is absorbed, distributed to the tissue and excreted, it is possible to make a semiquantitative approach to the use of the glycosides. Since digoxin is the most commonly used glycoside and since many nonuniformities have been attributed to digitoxin, the following discussion will concentrate on digoxin.

Perhaps we simply think we know more about the kinetics and transformation of digoxin, but it does appear at this time to be the most predictable of the three most commonly used cardiac glycosides. As mentioned earlier, chemically it is a polar molecule, with the hydroxyl group at the C12 position. It appears to be absorbed uniformly when given in alcoholic elixir, approximately 75 to 90 per cent of the administered dose being absorbed (Krasula *et al.*, 1976). In pill form, absorption depends on gastrointestinal motility and also upon how the particular tablet has been compacted by the manufacturer. Several near tragedies in human medicine have stimulated extensive studies on bioavailability. Several manufacturers with long-term reputations for careful formulation of their products have been spared much of the trauma accorded to other formulations. In this instance, cheap drugs are not necessarily the most cost effective nor the safest.

Absorption of digoxin is uniform and rapid with peak plasma concentrations occurring approximately 40 to 60 minutes after administration. Distribution to body tissues is completed in approximately 10 hours. The initial half-life of this distribution through tissues is approximately 0.5 to 1.5 hours. Elimination of digoxin appears to be primarily by the renal route with plasma half-lives of 24 to 40 hours. This plasma half-life is variable among dogs, with Breznock (1972) reporting mean half-lives of 38.9 hours, studies in our laboratory showing half-lives of approximately 30 hours and the work of Doherty (1973) showing half-lives of approximately 24 hours. There is some binding of digoxin to plasma proteins (about 25 per cent), but this is far less than the 90 per cent attributed to digitoxin (Baggot and Davis, 1973). There appears to be some degradation of digoxin and biotransformation by the liver. Breznock (1975) has recently found that the plasma half-life may be significantly shortened in dogs medicated with phenobarbital. These factors are quite interesting because phenobarbital does not shorten the half-life of digoxin in man but does shorten the half-life of digitoxin. These studies demonstrate that there is a marked species difference in the metabolism of the glycosides, particularly between man and the dog. This was pointed out by earlier studies of Detweiler (1966).

## DOSAGE AND REGIMES

The process of giving an amount of digitalis glycoside that achieves adequate body stores to correct cardiac contractile deficits is known as "digitalization." Dosage schedules are calculated to reach this point and hopefully will not reach toxicity. It has been assumed that a large initial amount of drug should be given in order to arrive at the therapeutic level as soon as possible. This is known as a loading-dose regime and has been given in both intensive and rapid schedules. Marcus (1975) has shown, however, that steady-state levels can be achieved in about five excretion half-lives and that these levels are the same as those achieved with a loading-dose schedule

without the potential (and very real) problem of toxicity.

Armed with the preceding information about absorption, distribution and elimination of digoxin, it is now possible to take a comparative look at various dosage regimes which have been recommended. Certainly the precise dose capable of producing an inotropic effect and not a toxic effect is yet to be established. Recent studies of Fillmore and Detweiler (1973) have shown that it is possible to maintain normal dogs on a subacute toxic level, without death for a period up to 10 days. With this as a guideline, we can now begin to look at the application of some of the pharmacokinetic data available in dogs (Breznock, 1973).

In order to examine the relative accumulation of digoxin in tissues, we chose to simulate the effects of different dosage regimes by means of a mathematical model which describes the kinetics of the drug in the body. While such a technique has many drawbacks in terms of absolute quantitation, it provides a ready means to study the *relative* effects of these regimes. Using a small laboratory digital computer to solve the equations describing the kinetics of the drug, we were able to graph the amount of drug in the body at any particular time after the first dose.* To simplify the problem further, we chose to assume that 70 per cent of any orally administered digoxin dose was absorbed and distributed to tissues. This absorption half-life was simulated at 0.5 hour. Excretion by the kidney was allowed to proceed with a half-life of 30 hours. The difference between the amount of drug absorbed and the amount of drug excreted at any given time is plotted as body stores.

This formulation says nothing about where in the body the drug is stored and does not take into account any biotransformation of the drug. Nevertheless, by comparing the body stores to those of the previously cited known toxic nonfatal regime given to normal dogs, some valid *comparisons* can be made.

Figure 3A is a plot of the relative body stores of digoxin ($\mu$g./kg. body mass) obtained with this known toxic intravenous dose. The × symbols show the dose and the

---

*Thanks are due to Mr. Jesse W. Hartley of the Computer/Electronics Laboratory, Dalton Research Center, who programmed the model for the computer simulation.

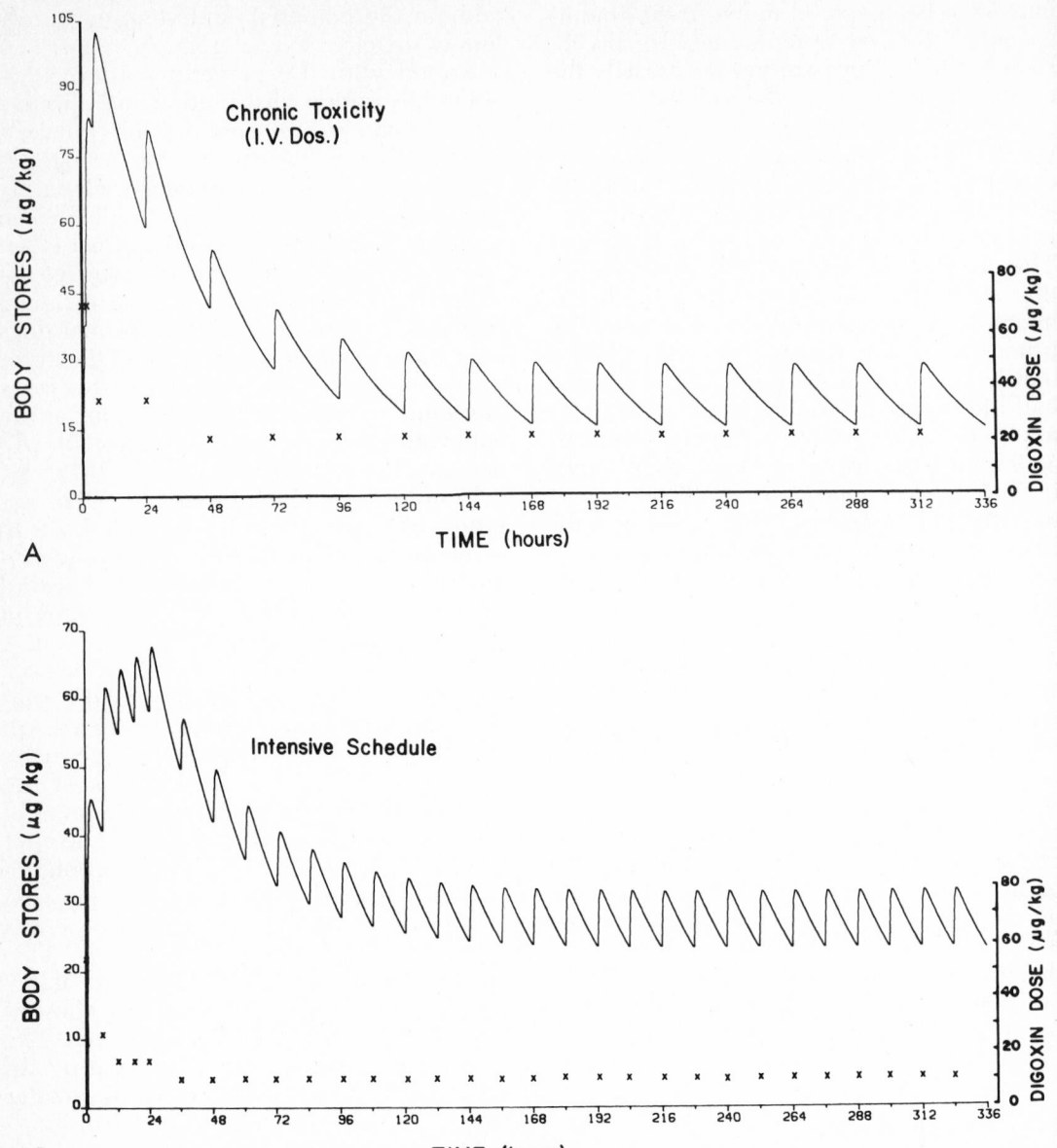

**Figure 3.**    Simulation of the kinetics of body stores of digoxin administered under various dosage regimes. The dose(s) of digoxin are denoted with "×". *A*, Body stores calculated with a known toxic dose (IV). *B*, Body stores calculated with an intensive-method loading dose. One half of a calculated digitalizing dose is given initially, one fourth in 6 hours, one sixth at 12, 18, 24 hours and finally a maintenance dose. *C*, Body stores calculated with a rapid-method loading dose. One sixth of the calculated "digitalizing" dose is given t.i.d. for 2 days and then a maintenance dose is given. *D*, Body stores calculated with a slow maintenance schedule of 0.005 mg. (5 μg.)/lb. b.i.d.

Rapid Schedule
BODY STORES (μg/kg)
DIGOXIN DOSE (μg/kg)
TIME (hours)

C

Slow Maintenance Schedule
BODY STORES (μg/kg)
DIGOXIN DOSE (μg/kg)
TIME (hours)

D

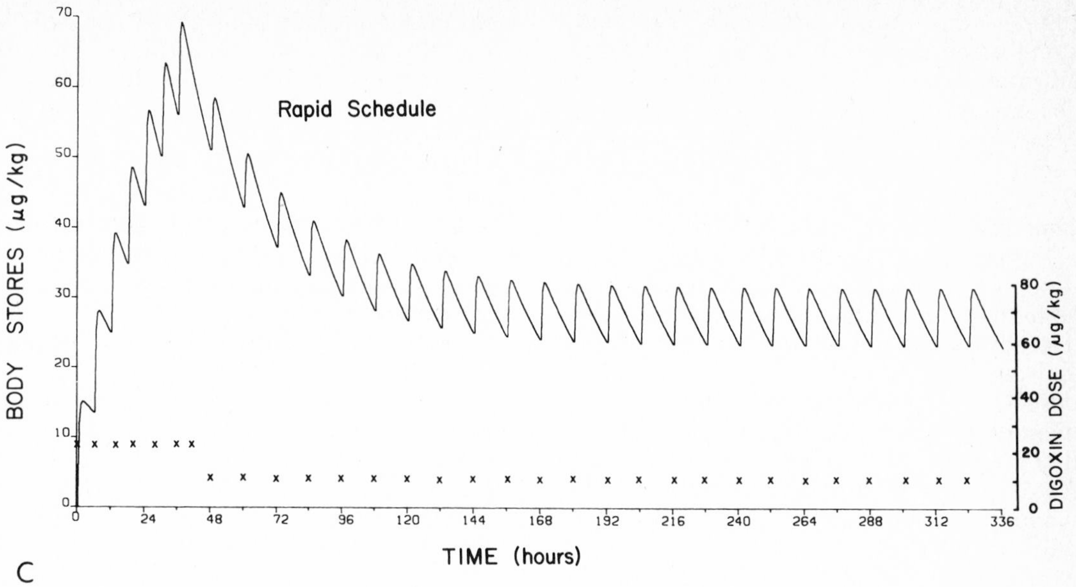

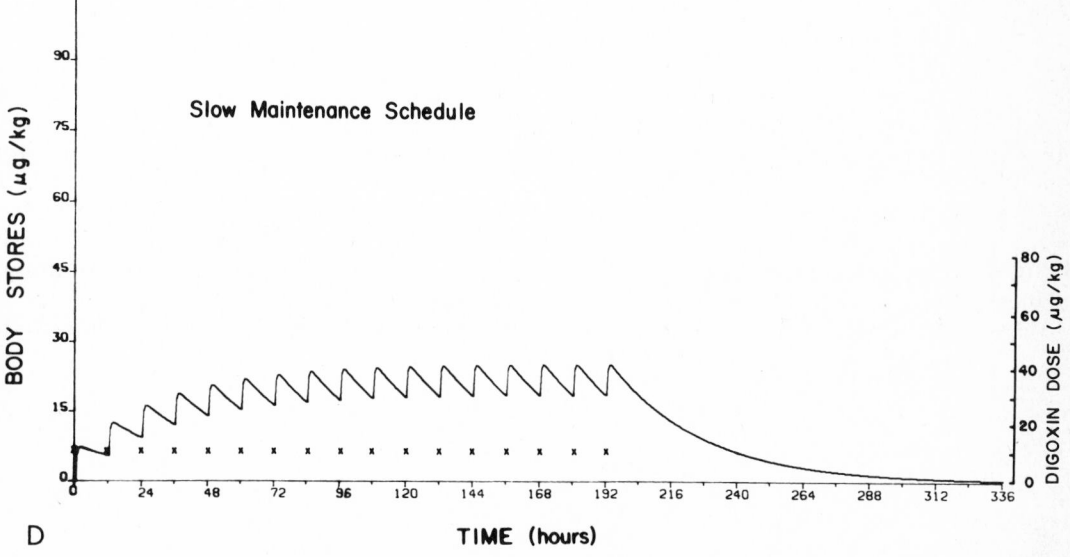

time given. Figure 3*B* shows the body stores when an intensive oral method of digitalization is used. Note that there is a large "overshoot" present and that the final value lies not far from that of the toxic regime. Figure 3*C* is a simulation of the rapid method of digitalization and, again, the same problems are present.

Figure 3*D* shows the body stores when a dose of 5 $\mu$g./lb. (11 $\mu$g./kg.) is given b.i.d. Note that while it takes five days to achieve a steady-state level, there is no "overshoot" and certainly less chance of toxicity. This dose of 11 $\mu$g./kg. b.i.d. has been recommended by Harris (1974) and has, in the author's experience, been quite satisfactory. Note, also, in Figure 3*D* that after 8 days, when the dosage is stopped, it takes 5 more days for the body stores to approach zero. This is true regardless of the dose regime used.

All the above curves assumed normal renal function. Note what happens if renal excretion rate is halved (Fig. 4). This will occur when BUN rises to about 50 mg./dl. This increases the excretion time of digoxin to approximately two and a half days. Given the same dosage as in Figure 3*D*, observe that steady-state levels of digoxin in Figure 4 now rise to much higher (and possibly toxic) levels. The regime was halted on day 8. Significant quantities of the drug still remained when the plotting was stopped.

These data represent average values for dogs and are highly simplified. Yet they do show the merits of a nonloading dose regime and also remind us of the profound effect that renal function can have on the kinetics of the drug.

There appears, then, to be very little rationale for the use of a loading-dose schedule to achieve a state of increased myocardial contractility. Certainly, the practice of administering digoxin until toxic effects appear cannot be condoned.

In summarizing dosage regimes, one still is left with the fact that the extremely narrow margin of safety with the use of any cardiac glycoside makes dosage considerations for this drug a clinical experiment. Certainly, however, the guidelines presented by Harris seem, at the present time, to be the most successful, if success is measured by clinical improvement and lack of toxic signs.

There are limited observations that larger dogs require a smaller dose *rate* of digoxin than smaller dogs for digitalization (Ettinger, 1966). Studies have shown that puppies can tolerate higher dose rates than mature dogs without becoming toxic. The same findings have been observed in children (Vargo *et al.*, 1975). These observations might be explained on the basis of higher myocardial mass to body mass ratios and in smaller apparent volumes of distribution of the drug.

The above dosage formulations are predi-

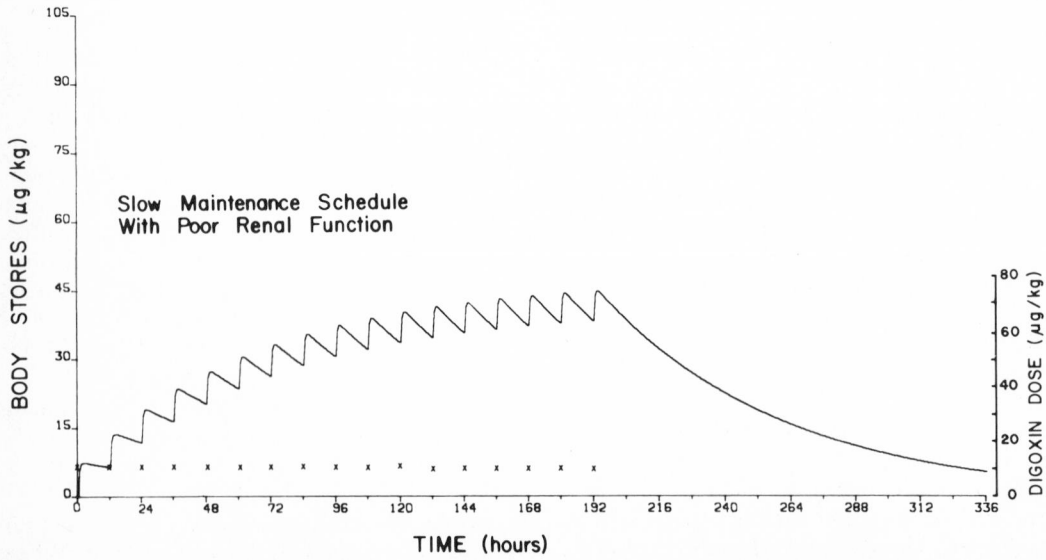

**Figure 4.** Body stores calculated with a slow maintenance regime as in Figure 3*D*, but with renal function (digoxin clearance) one half of normal (i.e., digoxin half-life is now 60 hours). Note the higher level of steady-state stores which might be inferred to approach toxic levels. This type of excretion pattern would occur in renal failure due to any cause.

cated on the fact that the particular patient has normal renal function (BUN less than 20 mg./dl.), normal thyroid function and normal values of serum electrolytes. Dosage rate is calculated on the basis of *lean* body mass and must be readjusted for fat animals and animals with large amounts of ascitic fluid. The above recommended dose of 11 μg. (0.011 mg.)/kg. can be incremented in quantities of 2 μg./kg. for greater concentrations and decremented by the same amount for dosage control.

While these schedules hold for dogs, they should *not* be applied to the cat. A study of toxicity and tolerance in feline congestive failure is just beginning to emerge (Tilley and Liu, 1975). At present a safe guideline is probably 50 per cent of the canine dose.

The management of a digitalization regime requires constant "feedback" cues to which the clinician must be ever alert. At an indication of toxicity, dosage should cease for 24 hours and then be resumed at a decremented rate. When treating failure cases on an outpatient basis, the clinician should request, at least, phone contact with the client every 48 hours during the first week of therapy. Clients should also be instructed to notify the doctor when *any* of the toxic signs appear and to stop medication with the glycosides.

One of the significant advances in the field of digitalis therapy has been the development of a sensitive, and relatively simple to perform, assay method for digoxin and digitoxin in serum and other body fluids. The technique is known as radioimmunoassay (RIA) and uses an isotopically tagged antigen (digoxin or digitoxin) and antibodies to these to measure the competitive binding of nonlabeled drug in serum. The method measures concentration in nanograms per milliliter of serum (parts per million). Although sophisticated isotope counting equipment and careful chemical techniques are required, many laboratories, especially in metropolitan areas, offer the services at modest costs.

It has been through the application of this assay method, after its introduction by Smith and colleagues in 1969, that enormous advances have been made in the identification and management of digitalis toxic status and in the pharmacokinetics of the drug (Smith, 1971). Limited studies in dogs with spontaneous congestive heart failure seem to indicate that serum concentrations above 2.5 to 3 ng./ml. (8 to 10 hours *after* the last administration of the drug) have a better probability of being toxic (Hahn *et al.*, 1975–1976). This is about the same concentration seen in man with digitalis toxicosis.

[*Editor's Note:* Most practicing cardiologists recommend the approximate dosage of 0.022 mg./kg. (0.01 mg./lb.) body weight daily as a maintenance dose of digoxin. As discussed, this varies with the dog's size, condition and renal function. Cats require lower dosages than do dogs.

Although Dr. Hahn prefers not to use the loading-dose method, some clinicians still prefer this technique for animals presented in congestive heart failure when intravenous glycoside infusions are not used.]

## INDICATIONS FOR USE OF THE CARDIAC GLYCOSIDES

The predominant indication for use of the digitalis glycosides is in congestive heart failure. This has been discussed in great detail in this volume and elsewhere. The glycosides are useful regardless of the cause of congestive failure but certainly are less effective when the failure is caused by the myocardiopathies and may be harmful in severe hypertrophic forms of myocardial disease. The reason for this is apparently that the glycosides cause obstruction of the aortic outflow tract in the hypertrophic myocardiopathies and must be used with extreme caution here. They are most effective when used in congestive failure due to mitral or tricuspid insufficiency.

Other indications are in supraventricular tachyarrhythmias, but here the usefulness is usually through a vagomimetic action rather than through an enhancement of myocardial contractility.

These drugs must be used with great caution, if at all, in the presence of ventricular arrhythmias, since they tend to increase the irritability of the ventricular myocardium.

They should be given with extreme caution in the presence of compromised renal function. A guideline is to cut the dosage level in half for each 30 mg./dl. that BUN is elevated over 20. Poor renal function, as mentioned earlier, decreases body store elimination, and hence less drug must be given.

Diuretic therapy almost always accompanies a digitalis glycoside regime. While there appears to be no direct interaction of the two forms of drugs, most diuretics increase renal potassium loss and thus tend to lower serum potassium. Lowered potassium values *potentiate* the inotropic *and* toxic effects of the glycosides, and the management of a digitalis regime calls for monitoring of potassium levels.

If a low potassium level is present, the action of the glycosides is potentiated and, in particular, the toxic effect appears to be accentuated. Hypokalemia should be corrected with potassium supplementation.

It is difficult to predict precisely how much the dosage should be cut if hypothyroidism is present, although Doherty (1968) has found that in man the half-life of the drug is significantly prolonged with poor thyroid function.

## EFFECT OF DIGITALIS GLYCOSIDES ON THE ELECTROCARDIOGRAM

While the electrocardiogram is extremely useful in monitoring the effects of the drug, it is by no means a *sine qua non* in establishing toxicity. One of the effects that the drug has on the electrocardiogram is a marked coving of the ST segment. This is illustrated in Figure 5. It was mentioned also that the AV nodal tissue was affected so that impulse conduction is slowed. This will cause prolongation of the P-R interval. This is illustrated in Figure 6. More severe effects begin to show up as toxicity approaches.

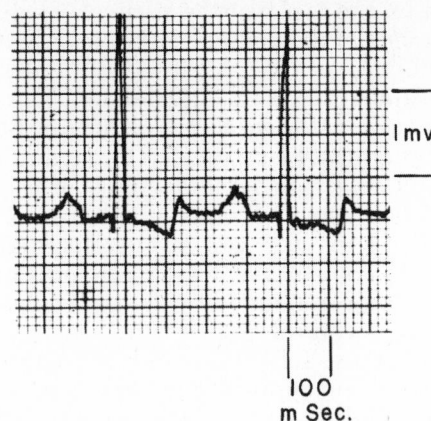

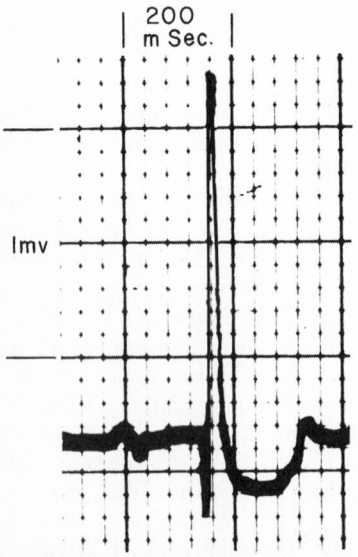

**Figure 5.** A "typical" ST segment showing marked "coving" is a result of digoxin. This does not always occur in a "digitalized" patient and, in fact, is relatively rare. (25 mm./sec. and 1 cm. = 1 mV.)

**Figure 6.** First-degree AV block (prolonged P-R interval) in a dog receiving digoxin. While occurring with some regularity in dogs on digoxin, it is by no means a constant finding. (50 mm./sec. and 1 cm. = mV.)

These are generally, first, conduction disturbances such as complete atrioventricular block and junctional rhythm. Life-threatening arrhythmias (those of ventricular origin) usually start with single premature ventricular contractions (Fig. 7) and may progress to a bigeminal rhythm (i.e., a normally conducted beat followed by a premature ventricular beat as shown in Figure 8). These can then lead to paroxysmal ventricular tachycardia and finally to fatal ventricular fibrillation.

These electrocardiographic changes are not constant for every case of toxicity and vary widely from patient to patient. The above are only representative samples of what can occur. When either ST segment changes or P-R interval changes begin to

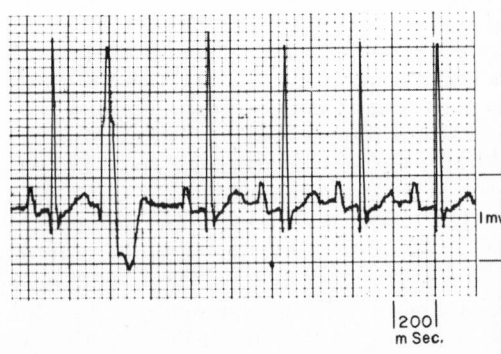

**Figure 7.** A premature ventricular contraction in dog receiving digoxin. This arrhythmia started after the initiation of therapy and represents one of the toxic signs that may signal further toxicity. (25 mm./sec. and 1 cm. = 1 mV.)

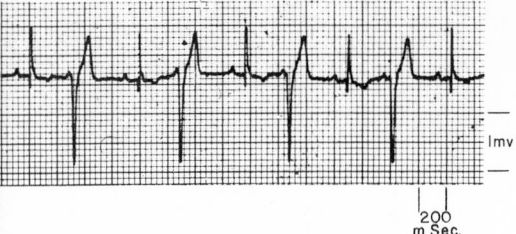

Figure 8.   A bigeminal rhythm in digoxin toxicosis. This is a more severe ventricular arrhythmia and needs to be closely monitored to preclude even more severe ventricular arrhythmias. (25 mm./sec. and 1 cm. = 1 mV.)

occur in a patient, the clinician should be alerted that the level of the drug is approaching toxicity, and the dosage regime should be modified carefully.

## SUPPLEMENTAL READING

Baggot, J. D., and Davis, L. E.: Plasma protein binding of digitoxin and digoxin in several mammalian species. Res. Vet. Sci., 15:81–87, 1973.

Breznock, E. M.: Pharmacokinetics of the Cardiac Glycosides, Digoxin and Digitoxin in the Dog. Ph.D. Dissertation, Ohio State University, Columbus, Ohio, 1972.

Breznock, E. M.: Application of canine plasma kinetics of digoxin and digitoxin to therapeutic digitalization in the dog. Am. J. Vet. Res., 34:993–999, 1973.

Breznock, E. M.: Effects of phenobarbital on digitoxin and digoxin elimination in the dog. Am. J. Vet. Res., 36:371–373, 1975.

Detweiler, D. K.: Comparative pharmacology of cardiac glycosides. Fed. Proc., 26:1119–1124, 1966.

Doherty, J. E.: The clinical pharmacology of digitalis glycosides: A review. Am. J. Med. Sci., 255:382–414, 1968.

Doherty, J. E.: Digitalis glycosides—Pharmacokinetics and their clinical implications. Ann. Int. Med., 79:229–238, 1973.

Estes, J. W., and White, P. D.: William Withering and the purple foxglove. Sci. Am., 212(June):110–119, 1965.

Ettinger, S.: Therapeutic digitalization in dog in congestive heart failure. J.A.V.M.A., 148:525–531, 1966.

Fillmore, G. E., and Detweiler, D. K.: Maintenance of subacute digoxin toxicosis in normal beagles. Toxicol. Appl. Pharmacol., 25:418–429, 1973.

Gillis, R. A., Pearle, D. L., and Levitt, B.: Digitalis: A neuroexcitatory drug. Circulation, 52:739–742, 1975.

Hahn, A. W., Ettinger, S. J., and Pensinger, R. R.: Unpublished observations, 1975–1976.

Hamlin, R. L., Pipers, F. S., Carter, K. L., and Lederer, H.: Treatment of heart failure in dogs without use of digitalis glycosides. Vet. Med./Small Animal Clin., 68:349–356, 1973.

Harris, S. G.: Digitalis glycosides. In Kirk, R. W. (ed.): Current Veterinary Therapy V. Philadelphia, W. B. Saunders Co., 1974, pp. 320–323.

Katz, A. M.: Congestive heart failure: Role of altered myocardial cellular control. New Engl. J. Med., 293:1184–1191, 1975.

Kim, Y. I., Noble, R. J., and Zipes, D. P.: Dissociation of the inotropic effects of digitalis from its effects on atrioventricular conduction. Am. J. Cardiol., 36:459–467, 1975.

Krasula, R. W., Gardella, L. A., Zaroslinsk, J. F., and Morris, R. N.: Comparative bioavailability of four dosage forms of digoxin in dogs. Fed. Proc. (Abs), 35:327, 1976.

Leachman, R. D., Cokkinos, D. V. P., Cabrera, R., Leutherman, L. L., and Rochielle, D. G.: Response of the transplanted denervated human heart to cardiovascular drugs. Am. J. Cardiol., 27:272, 1971.

Lüllman, H., and Peters, T.: Storstein, O. (ed.): Studies on the Site of Action of Cardiac Glycosides. Symposium on Digitalis. Forlag, Oslo, 1973, pp. 125–131.

Marcus, F. I.: Digitalis pharmacokinetics and metabolism. Am. J. Med., 58:452–459, 1975.

Ogilvie, R. I., and Ruedy, J.: An educational program in digitalis therapy. J.A.M.A., 222:50–55, 1972.

Patterson, D. F., Abt, D. A., Detweiler, D. K., Buchanan, J. W., Knight, D. H., and Pyle, R. L.: On digitalis glycosides in treatment of heart failure: Criticism and reply. Vet. Med./Small Animal Clin., 68:708–717, 1973.

Repke, D. R. H., Herrmann, I., Kunze, R., Portius, H. J., Schön, R., and Schöfeld, W.: Mechanism of digitalis action and the importance of the kinetics of the formation and decomposition of glycoside-receptor complex for understanding of overall pharmacokinetics of digitalis compounds. Symposium on Digitalis. Forlag, Oslo, 1973, pp. 143–157.

Rothschild, M., von Euw, J., and Reichstein, T.: Cardiac glycosides in the oleander aphid, *Aphis nerii*. J. Insect. Physiol., 16:1141–1145, 1970.

Scudder, G. G. E., and Duffey, S. S.: Cardiac glycosides in the lygaeidae. Canadian J. Zoo., 50:35–42, 1972.

Selden, R., and Smith, T. W.: Ouabain pharmacokinetics in dog and man. Circulation, 45:1176–1182, 1972.

Smith, T. W.: The clinical use of serum cardiac glycoside concentration measurements. Am. Heart J., 82:833–837, 1971.

Tilley, L. P., and Liu, S.-K.: Cardiomyopathy and thromboembolism in the cat. Feline Pract., 1:32–41, 1975.

Vargo, T., Lewis, R., Purdine, J., and Schwartz, A.: Comparison between puppies and adult dogs following infusion of digoxin. Pediat. Res., 8:355, 1975.

Videbaek, J., and Brock, A.: The relationship between myocardial content of digoxin and increase in myocardial contractility. Acta Pharmed. Toxicol., 35:212–222, 1974.

von Euw, J., Rishelson, L., Parsons, J. A., Reichstein, T., and Rothschild, M.: Acrodenolides (heart poisons) in a grasshopper feeding on milkweed. Nature, 214:35–39, 1967.

# THE ROLE OF BRONCHO-DILATORS IN THE TREATMENT OF CONGESTIVE HEART FAILURE

GARY R. BOLTON, D.V.M.
*Ithaca, New York*

Theophylline and aminophylline are xanthine derivatives having specific actions which make them beneficial in the treatment of congestive heart failure.

## Mechanism of action

The xanthines are potent bronchodilators, but they also stimulate the myocardium and have diuretic and vasodilator effects. Their beneficial effects in the treatment of congestive heart failure are given in Table 1.

The cardiac effects include increases in heart rate, force of contraction, cardiac output and blood pressure. Venous filling pressure is decreased owing to more efficient emptying of the ventricles. The augmentation of cardiac output increases blood pressure and, combined with vasodilation of coronary, pulmonary and systemic arteries and veins, leads to a more rapid blood flow and more efficient circulation.

The xanthines also have a mild diuretic action. This is partially due to an increase in cardiac output and renal perfusion, but there is also an inhibitory effect on sodium reabsorption in the renal tubules. These agents are used clinically for their cardiac stimulant and bronchodilator effects rather than for their diuretic action, since diuresis is mild and inconsistent. They may be used in conjunction with the mercurial diuretics which they potentiate by improving cardiac output and renal perfusion.

Bronchodilation is also beneficial in the treatment of congestive heart failure. The xanthines increase vital capacity by relaxing the bronchospasm that accompanies cardiac dyspnea. This affords the patient relief from the coughing and dyspnea that occur with pulmonary congestion and edema.

## Therapeutic uses

Aminophylline and theophylline are effective in controlling the clinical signs of congestive heart failure. In the early stages of heart failure, when coughing, dyspnea and exercise intolerance are mild, aminophylline and a low-sodium diet alone will be effective in alleviating the clinical signs (Table 2). When signs become more severe, the xanthines may be used in combination with drugs such as digoxin, other diuretics or narcotic cough suppressants (Table 2). When used in conjunction with the digitalis glycosides, their actions on cardiac output are complementary.

Intravenously, aminophylline produces a marked increase in cardiac output which begins immediately and persists for 30 minutes or more. This makes it useful in the

**Table 1.** *Beneficial Actions of Aminophylline and Theophylline*

Increase cardiac output
Decrease venous filling pressure
Increase blood pressure and renal perfusion
Increase blood flow; promote more efficient circulation
Dilate coronary, pulmonary and systemic vasculature
Promote diuresis
Effect bronchodilation

340

**Table 2.** *Therapeutic Regimes for Use of Bronchodilators in Treatment of Congestive Heart Failure*

| MILD HEART FAILURE | MODERATE TO SEVERE HEART FAILURE | EMERGENCY HEART FAILURE |
|---|---|---|
| Aminophylline | Digoxin (alone if possible) | Digoxin (IV or IM) |
| Low-sodium diet | Aminophylline (if needed) | Lasix® (IV or IM) |
| Rest | Diuretics (if needed) | Aminophylline (IV or IM) Mercuhydrin® (SC) |
| | Narcotics (if needed) | Morphine (SC) |
| | Low-sodium diet | Oxygen |
| | Rest | Adjunctive therapy Rotating tourniquets Venoclysis |

treatment of pulmonary edema and emergency congestive heart failure (Table 2).

## ROUTES OF ADMINISTRATION, PREPARATIONS AND DOSAGES

Therapeutic doses are usually given orally, in the form of aminophylline tablets or theophylline elixir (Table 3). Other preparations are available, and some combine a xanthine derivative and a narcotic cough suppressant (Table 3). Aminophylline contains theophylline and ethylenediamine. The latter enhances the absorption of theophylline. The injectable products are reserved for emergency therapy or for intractable animals. Intravenous administration of aminophylline must be slow to avoid the undesirable development of headache, dizziness, nausea, palpitation, precordial pain and hypotension. Intramuscular injection causes pain which can persist for hours after the injection.

## UNWANTED SIDE EFFECTS

Although the xanthines are safe drugs, occasional side effects may occur. The most frequent is gastric irritation, with nausea

**Table 3.** *Preparations and Dosages*

| GENERIC NAME/STRENGTH | TRADE NAME | DOSAGE |
|---|---|---|
| Aminophylline: tablets—1.5 grain injectable—250 mg./cc. | Aminophylline Injection® (Searle) | 10 mg./kg. oral b.i.d. or t.i.d. 10 mg./kg. IV or IM, b.i.d. or t.i.d. (For IV use, dilute in 10 to 20 cc. of physiologic saline or 5% dextrose in water, and *inject slowly*.) |
| Theophylline elixir: 80 mg./tbs. | Elixophylline® (Sherman) | 10 mg./kg. oral b.i.d. or t.i.d. |
| Theophylline: 2- and 4-grain capsules | Aerolate® (Flemming) | 10 mg./kg. oral b.i.d. or t.i.d. |
| Diphylline: tablets—100* and 200 mg. elixir—100† and 160‡ mg./Tbs. | Luffylin® (Mallinckrodt) Neothylline® (Lemmon) | 10 mg./kg. oral b.i.d. or t.i.d. |
| Theophylline and glyceryl guaiacolate: capsules—100 mg. theo, 90 mg. guaiac elixir—100 mg./Tbs. theo, 90 mg./Tbs. guaiac | Quibron® (Mead-Johnson) | capsule—1 cap./15 kg. b.i.d. or t.i.d. elixir—1 Tbs./15 kg. b.i.d. or t.i.d. |
| Aminophylline and phenobarbital: tablets—100 mg. amino, ¼ grain pheno tablets—100 mg. amino, ½ grain pheno | | 1 tab./15 kg. b.i.d. or t.i.d., as needed for desired sedation |
| Theophylline and noscapine: 100 mg. theo, 15 mg. nosc | Half-strength Theo-Nar® (Key) | 1 tab./15 kg. b.i.d. or t.i.d. |

*Luffylin® only.
†Luffylin® only.
‡Neothylline® only.

and vomiting. Preparations such as Elixophylline®, Neothylline® and Aerolate® are less irritating and may be used if aminophylline tablets cannot be tolerated. Occasionally, use of the xanthines must be discontinued when gastric upset cannot be avoided.

Additional side effects are due to CNS stimulation and include dizziness, restlessness, hyperexcitability and insomnia. Severe cases of seizures, shock and death have been recorded in man, but at therapeutic levels these side reactions are uncommon.

Arrhythmias may occasionally develop because of the stimulatory effects on the myocardium, but this is also an unusual occurrence.

## SUMMARY

The xanthine derivative bronchodilators are safe, effective, reliable agents for use in treating all stages of congestive heart failure. Their major effects are stimulation of the myocardium and relaxation of bronchial smooth muscle.

## SUPPLEMENTAL READING

Ettinger, S. J., and Suter, P. F.: Canine Cardiology. Philadelphia, W. B. Saunders Co., 1970.

Friedberg, C. K.: Diseases of the Heart. Philadelphia, W. B. Saunders Co., 1966.

Goldberg, L. I.: Pharmacology of cardiovascular drugs. In Hurst, J. W., Logne, R. B., Schlant, R. D., and Wenger, N. R. (eds.): The Heart. 3rd ed. New York, McGraw-Hill Book Co., 1974.

Mudge, G. H.: Diuretics and other agents employed in the mobilization of edema fluid. In Goodman, L. S., and Gilman, A. (eds.): The Pharmacological Basis of Therapeutics. 4th ed. New York, The Macmillan Co., 1970.

Ritchie, J. M.: Central nervous system stimulants. Part II: The xanthines. In Goodman, L. S., and Gilman, A. (eds.): The Pharmacological Basis of Therapeutics. 4th ed. New York, The Macmillan Co., 1970.

# LOW-SODIUM DIETS

WILLIAM P. THOMAS, D.V.M.
*Philadelphia, Pennsylvania*

## ROLE OF SODIUM RETENTION IN THE PATHOPHYSIOLOGY OF CONGESTIVE HEART FAILURE

In the complex pathogenesis of congestive heart failure, retention of sodium and water by the kidneys plays a central role. While reduction in effective cardiac output is the initiating event, retention of sodium and water is largely responsible for the clinical signs of congestion and edema which characterize cardiac failure from nearly all types of cardiac disease.

The normal cardiovascular system has a considerable reserve capacity that enables it to maintain effective cardiac output under a variety of normal physiologic and pathologic conditions. When cardiac output becomes inadequate for total body requirements, several compensatory mechanisms involving nervous, cardiovascular, renal and endocrine systems are activated. Acute reductions in effective cardiac output are countered by several short-term compensatory (reserve) mechanisms. Under the influence of sympathoadrenal stimulation, tachycardia, increased myocardial contractility, peripheral arterial vasoconstriction and central venous vasoconstriction combine to improve venous return, maintain cardiac output and redistribute blood flow to more vital organs (heart, brain) at the expense of visceral and peripheral circulations, including the kidney. Persistent reduction of effective cardiac output, as occurs with most clinically important types of heart disease, also stimulates long-term compensatory mechanisms, including cardiac hypertrophy and renal sodium and water retention, to maintain cardiac output and reestablish normal blood flow distribution.

In this regard, renal sodium retention must be viewed as a normal compensatory mechanism. The obligatory water retention which accompanies sodium retention increases plasma and extracellular fluid volumes, augmenting venous return to the heart. The increased diastolic filling of the ventricles stretches the myocardial fibers, invoking the Frank-Starling mechanism to increase the force of contraction and the stroke volume. As long as the ventricles can increase their output by this mechanism, sodium retention is compensatory and advantageous. When cardiac reserve is exceeded, however, the increasing plasma volume and venous pressure places a greater load on the already maximally stressed ventricles, reducing cardiac efficiency and cardiac output. Further sodium retention occurs and a vicious cycle is created, with sodium retention contributing to the decline in cardiac function and ultimately to pulmonary and/or systemic congestion and edema.

The mechanisms that appear to contribute to renal sodium retention in heart disease are summarized in Figure 1. Renal arterial vasoconstriction and diminished renal blood flow reduce glomerular filtration rate (GFR) while the filtration fraction increases. The resulting increased oncotic pressure and decreased hydrostatic pressure (Starling forces) in peritubular capillaries enhance proximal tubular sodium reabsorption. In addition, the reduced pressure and

volume of blood perfusing the kidney stimulates the release of renin from the juxtaglomerular cells of the afferent arterioles. Renin acts enzymatically on circulating angiotensinogen to produce angiotensin I, which is converted to the physiologically active angiotensin II. Besides its potent vasoactive properties, angiotensin II stimulates the release of aldosterone from the zona glomerulosa of the adrenal cortex. Aldosterone acts on the distal renal tubules to increase active sodium reabsorption. Water is reabsorbed both passively along with sodium and under the influence of increased ADH secretion from the posterior pituitary gland. The result is an increase in total body sodium and extracellular and plasma fluid volumes.

The role of sodium retention in cardiac compensation and congestive heart failure has been confirmed in dogs with surgically induced heart lesions and in dogs with spontaneous congenital and acquired heart disease. Dogs in congestive heart failure (based on clinical evaluation) have increased plasma and extracellular fluid vol-

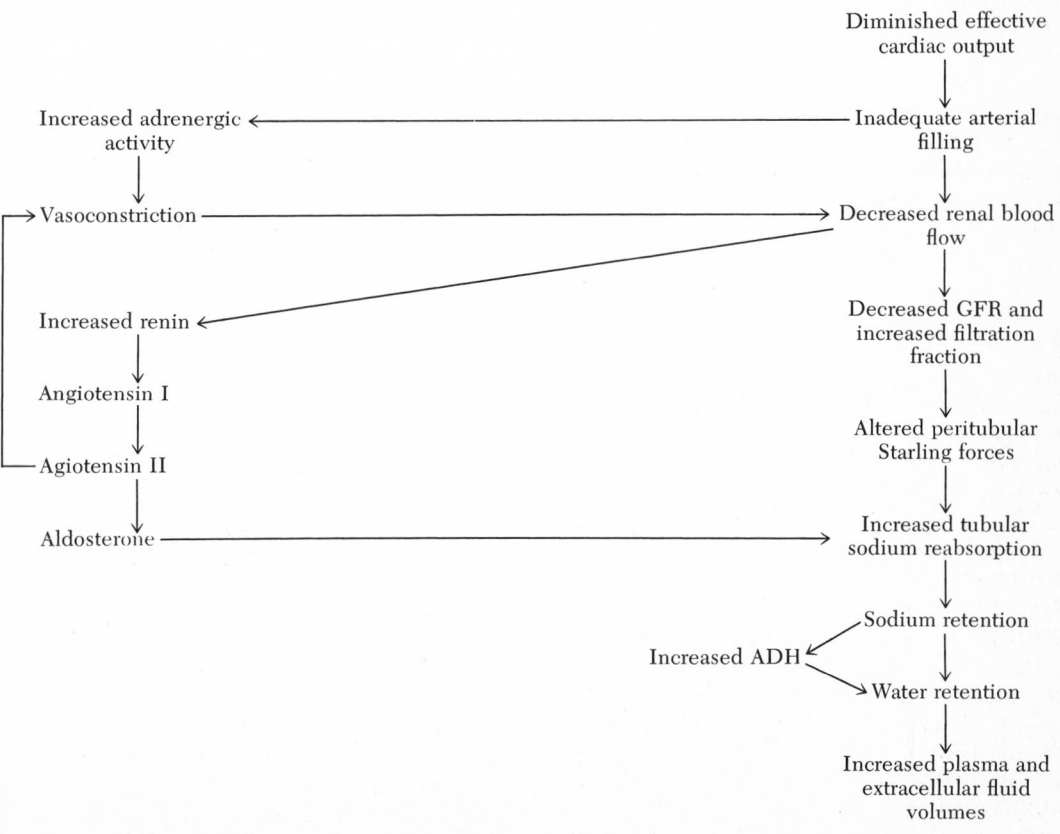

**Figure 1.**   Pathogenesis of compensatory sodium and water retention in heart disease.

umes, increased total body sodium content (with *normal* plasma sodium concentrations) and increased aldosterone production. In addition, when compared with normal dogs whose daily sodium excretion closely parallels intake, these dogs demonstrate markedly impaired ability to excrete a sodium load, with intake always exceeding excretion. Dogs with spontaneous or experimental heart lesions but without objective clinical signs of congestive heart failure excrete a sodium load at a reduced rate. Thus, there is evidence for sodium retention during all stages of heart disease.

## The low-sodium diet

The effect of feeding a diet low in sodium has been studied both in normal dogs and in dogs with spontaneous and experimental heart lesions. In normal dogs and in compensated affected dogs, total body sodium and extracellular fluid volume remain unchanged, as sodium excretion decreases in proportion to the reduced intake. (Sodium depletion by dietary restriction alone is very difficult to achieve in normal dogs without almost total elimination of sodium from the diet.) In affected dogs with signs of congestive heart failure, substantial reductions in these variables occur, even though percentage sodium retention by the kidney remains elevated. Clearly, there is value in the use of a low-sodium diet to help reduce sodium retention in the therapy of congestive heart failure. Its use in the prodromal stages to delay the onset of edema may be warranted in some patients. However, sodium restriction should always be considered an adjunctive measure with primary therapy directed toward improvement of the underlying cardiac dysfunction. The positive inotropic effects of the cardiac glycosides alone will often sufficiently improve renal perfusion to promote a diuresis and reduce sodium retention.

When the response to improvement of cardiac function with the digitalis glycosides is not sufficient for the patient's comfort, reduction of excess total body sodium and extracellular fluid may be accomplished by promoting sodium excretion and/or reducing sodium intake. Cardiac glycosides and natriuretic diuretics accomplish the former, while the latter is achieved by the low-sodium diet. The relative importance of diet versus diuretics in reducing sodium retention remains a source of controversy. In human medicine, the current trend is toward increased reliance on diuretics to allow the patient more dietary freedom. Because low-sodium diets are unpalatable to most people, many patients prefer the quality of life on a less restricted diet. In small animals, sodium content may be less important than habit and familiarity in determining the patient's dietary preferences. The main obstacle to successful implementation of a restricted diet is usually the client, and the clinician must have the client's understanding and cooperation for the dietary therapy to be successful. Since the majority of cardiac patients in small animal practice are middle-aged and older, established feeding habits may be difficult to overcome. Many clients prefer the administration of diuretics and the inconvenience of frequent urination to upsetting their established owner-pet relationship by a strict, inflexible diet.

The prime objective in the dietary management of heart disease is the reduction of sodium intake. In addition, proper caloric and vitamin content is important, and ingredients of high digestibility and biologic value should be used to maximize absorption and utilization, while minimizing metabolic wastes produced, since the function of the liver, kidneys and gastrointestinal tract is compromised during congestive heart failure. A diet high in calories and protein is especially important in patients with advanced cardiac failure and cardiac cachexia. Sodium restriction may be moderate (16 to 20 mg./kg. body wt./day) or severe (6 to 8 mg./kg. body wt./day), depending on the severity of the condition, response to other concurrent therapy and acceptance of the diet by both patient and client. Obviously salty foods, especially treats such as potato chips and cured meats, should be strictly avoided. Low-sodium treats such as unsalted nuts or crackers can be purchased in most supermarkets or health food stores. Most processed canned and frozen foods should also be avoided. No salt or salt-containing spices should be used in preparing the diet. Sodium is the critical element to be avoided, and many foods not obviously salty to the taste may contain substantial amounts of sodium. Commercial canned, semimoist and dry dog and cat foods have moderate to high sodium contents (350 to 800 mg./100 gm. dry wt.), and

hould not be used when strict sodium re-
triction is necessary. Commercial prescrip-
ion diets with moderately low (250 mg./100
;m. dry wt.) and very low (30 to 50 mg./100
;m. dry wt.) sodium contents are convenient
nd provide balanced nutrition. The very
ow-sodium preparations, when used with-
ut supplementation, severely restrict
odium intake and may be required only in
atients with advanced chronic congestive
eart failure. The expense of such diets may
e prohibitive to clients with large dogs.

Owners of older animals may prefer to
repare a homemade diet, although nutri-
ional balance may be questionable. The
American Heart Association and its chapters
ave prepared several booklets for human
eart patients which provide detailed
;uidelines for preparation, lists of allowed
nd restricted foods and sample recipes and
nenus. These are available from local heart
ssociations and can be quite useful for
lient education. In addition, the sodium
nd caloric content of a wide variety of foods
an be found in Composition of Foods, Ag-
iculture Handbook #8, U.S.D.A. Table 1
s provided as a very general guide for
electing ingredients low in sodium. In
;eneral, the diet should contain allowable
ean meats, vegetables and cereals in com-
ination to minimize sodium content and
rovide balanced nutrition. A multivitamin
reparation without sodium can be added.
Organ meats (heart, liver, kidney) should be
voided in favor of lean skeletal meats
white meat chicken, beef, lamb), and al-
owable vegetables should be used liber-
lly, as they are the ingredients lowest in
odium. Palatability may be improved using
onsodium-containing spices (Table 1) or a
ommercial salt substitute (usually potas-
ium chloride). The salt substitute is espe-
ially recommended when the patient is
lso taking diuretics. The transition to the
ew diet is usually easier if the usual diet is
eplaced by gradually increasing the per-
entage of the low-sodium diet over several
ays or weeks.

In advanced cases where strict sodium re-
triction becomes important, other sources
f sodium ingestion may become sig-
ificant. If the local water supply is high in
odium content, or if a sodium-exchange
ype of water softener is used, low-sodium
ottled water should be considered.
odium-containing medications should be
eplaced, where possible. In all but the

**Table 1.  Guide to Selection of Foods for Low-Sodium Diet***

| RECOMMENDED | TO BE AVOIDED |
|---|---|
| *Meat, Fish, Fowl* ||
| Beef | Ham |
| Pork (uncured) | Bacon |
| Lamb | Shellfish (crab, shrimp, lobster) |
| Chicken (light meat) | Frankfurters |
| Turkey (light meat) | Brains, beef |
| Veal | Liver, beef |
| Fresh-water fish | Kidney, beef |
| Rabbit | Heart, beef |
| Duck | Sausage |
|  | Bologna and other luncheon meats |
| *Vegetables* ||
| Most fresh vegetables | Frozen or canned vegetables |
| Beans | Celery |
| Broccoli | Spinach |
| Cabbage | Beets |
| Corn | Chard |
| Lettuce | Mushrooms, canned |
| Onions | Olives |
| Peas | Pickles |
| Potatoes | Sauerkraut |
| Rice | Kale |
| Squash | Vegetable juices |
| Tomatoes | |
| *Fruits* ||
| All fresh fruits | Dried fruits |
| *Cereals, Breads, Nuts* ||
| Unsalted nuts (walnuts, peanuts, cashews) | Salted nuts |
| Low-sodium bread | Bread (white, wheat, rye, etc.) |
| Cornmeal | Most dry breakfast cereals |
| Flour | Crackers |
| Oats | Peanut butter |
| Puffed Rice | Pastries and cakes |
| Wheat germ | Potato chips, pretzels |
| Puffed Wheat | |
| Shredded Wheat | |
| Macaroni | |
| Spaghetti | |
| Popcorn (unsalted) | |
| *Dairy Foods* ||
| Unsalted butter or margarine | Whole, evaporated or dry milk |
| Cream | Sour cream |
| Low-sodium milk | Buttermilk |
| Egg yolks | Cheeses |
|  | Cottage or cream cheese |
|  | Ice cream |
|  | Salted butter or margarine |
|  | Egg whites |
|  | Yogurt |

*Continued on next page*

*More complete lists may be found in Composition of Foods, Agriculture Handbook #8, U.S.D.A. and in booklets available from local heart associations.

**Table 1.** *Guide to Selection of Foods for Low-Sodium Diet (Continued)*

| RECOMMENDED | TO BE AVOIDED |
|---|---|
| *Other* | |
| Sugar | Rawhide chew strips |
| Honey | Most candy bars |
| Lard | Molasses |
| Shortening and salad | Garlic salt |
|   oils | Onion salt |
| Salt substitutes | Celery salt |
| Garlic | Mustard and other |
| Pepper |   prepared dressings |
| Chili powder | Baking powder |
| Onion powder | Baking soda |

most severe cases, these steps should be unnecessary.

Adherence to a low-sodium diet in advanced congestive heart failure may reduce the diuretic dosage required to maintain sodium and fluid balance and thereby becomes a valuable adjunct to digitalis therapy. Caution must be used in prescribing a strict low-sodium diet to patients with other sodium-depleting conditions, including chronic renal disease, chronic vomiting or diarrhea, desalting dehydration and adrenal insufficiency.

## SUMMARY

While the use of cardiac glycosides remains the most valuable therapy in congestive heart failure, restriction of sodium intake to help reduce total body sodium content and extracellular fluid volume is valuable, especially in advanced cases, and may minimize the need for diuretics. The degree of sodium restriction required is based upon the patient's condition and response to medical therapy. Depending upon the preference of the client and patient, commercial or homemade diets can be used. A balance between medicinal and dietary therapy

which is acceptable to both client and patient and gives the patient the greatest continuous relief should be the ultimate therapeutic objective.

## SUPPLEMENTAL READING

Barger, A. C., Ross, R. S., and Price, H. L.: Reduced sodium excretion in dogs with mild valvular lesion of the heart, and in dogs with congestive heart failure. Am. J. Physiol., *180*:249–260, 1955.

Barger, A. C., Rudolph, A. M., and Yates, F. E.: Sodium retention in heart disease. Mod. Conc. Card. Dis. 23:226–227, 1954.

Barger, A. C., Wilson, G. M., Price, H. L., Ross, R. S., Brooks, L., and Boling, E. A.: Relationship between exchangeable sodium and rate of sodium excretion in dogs with experimental valvular lesions of the heart Am. J. Physiol., *180*:387–391, 1955.

Bojs, G. E., and Conn, H. L.: Distribution of body sodium, potassium, and water and the excretion of aldosterone in dogs with spontaneous heart failure Am. Heart J., *69*:72–82, 1965.

del Greco, F.: The kidney in congestive heart failure Mod. Conc. Card. Dis., *44*:47–52, 1975.

Ettinger, S. J., and Suter, P. F.: Canine Cardiology Chap. 10. Philadelphia, W. B. Saunders Co., 1971.

Genest, J., Granger, P., de Champlain, J., and Boucher R.: Endocrine factors in congestive heart failure. Am J. Cardiol., *22*:35–42, 1968.

Hamlin, R. L., Smith, C. R., and Ross, J. N.: Detection and quantification of subclinical heart failure in dog J. Am. Vet. Med. Assn., *150*:1513–1515, 1967.

Hamlin, R. L., Smith, R. C., Smith, C. R., and Power T. E.: Effects of a controlled electrolyte diet, low in sodium, on healthy dogs. Vet. Med./Small Animal Clin., *59*:748–751, 1964.

Knapp, W. A.: Nutritional management of chronic congestive heart failure in the dog. Proceedings of the 101st Annual Meeting, A.V.M.A., 1965, pp. 148–151.

Knight, D. H.: Influence of diet on the pathogenesis and treatment of congestive heart failure in the dog. In Kronfeld, D. S.: Canine Nutrition. Philadelphia University of Pennsylvania Press, 1972.

Morris, M. L., and Collins, D. R.: Heart failure—commentary on nutritional management of small animals. Topeka, Mark Morris Assoc., 1969.

Pensinger, R. R.: Dietary control of sodium intake in spontaneous congestive heart failure in dogs. Vet. Med./Small Animal Clin., *59*:752, 1964.

Wallace, C. R., and Hamilton, W. F.: Study of spontaneous congestive heart failure in the dog. Circ. Res., *11*:301–314, 1962.

# TACHYAR-
# RHYTHMIAS

RONALD W. HILWIG, D.V.M.
*Tucson, Arizona*

Tachyarrhythmia is the collective term which signifies a rapid and often irregular heart rate. Many dogs and cats in the examination room exhibit a relative tachycardia due to anxiety but the rate and rhythm are usually quite uniform. After becoming accustomed to the surroundings and to handling during the examination, most animals' heart rates will not be excessive. Rates exceeding 140 beats per minute or rhythms with a definite irregularity, excluding normal sinus arrhythmia, should be viewed with suspicion and evaluated via the electrocardiogram. An accurate history should be obtained *and the current medications determined* in those cases where an arrhythmia or tachycardia is discovered.

It is the purpose of this article to present typical ECG's of the common tachyarrhythmias in dogs and cats and to suggest possible maneuvers or medications to control the abnormal rhythms. All ECG's were from dogs, using lead II at a paper speed of 25 mm./sec., for illustrative uniformity.

## ELECTROCARDIOGRAPHIC FINDINGS

Figure 1 is an ECG from a normal dog with normal sinus rhythm. The P-P interval is quite constant throughout the recording.

Figure 2 is an ECG from a dog with advanced heartworm disease and evidence of right ventricular enlargement (S wave amplitude greater than that of R wave). A variation in the origin and pathway of atrial depolarization (wandering pacemaker) is evident by the change in P wave contour. This by itself is not very significant if the rhythm remains normal. In this instance, however, atrial (or junctional) premature beats (PB) are seen frequently and must be considered as a pathogenic condition. Ventricular depolarization occurs over normal pathways as evidenced by the minimal changes in the QRS complex. A compensatory pause (resetting or resetting with pause) frequently, but not always, follows the supraventricular premature beat.

Figure 3 is an ECG from a dog with paroxysmal atrial tachycardia (PAT), an arrhythmia that frequently accompanies atrial premature beats (APB). Rapid bursts of depolarization impulses which originate in the atrium or the AV junction are carried over the normal conduction pathways to the ventricles. The P waves may be superimposed on the preceding T wave or be unobservable. Discrete P waves, with an abbreviated PQ (P-R) interval, may be observed during the tachycardia. Reversion to normal rhythm for a short time, with an abrupt slowing of heart rate, is usually spontaneous.

Figure 4 is an ECG from a dog which illustrates a therapeutic dilemma. This continuous recording shows left ventricular

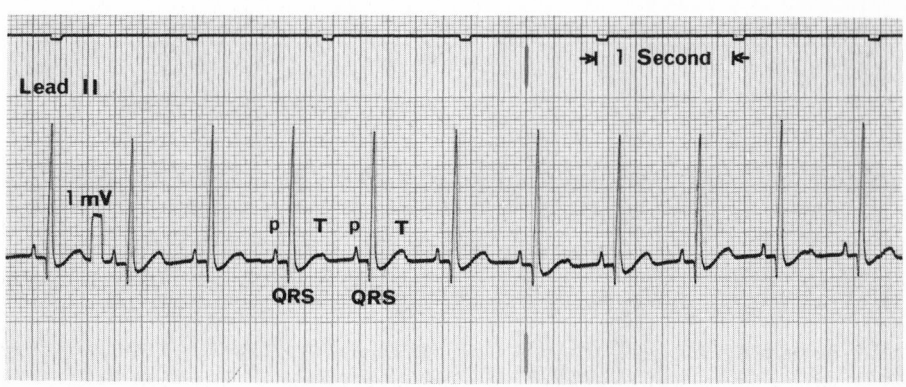

**Figure 1.** Normal sinus rhythm.

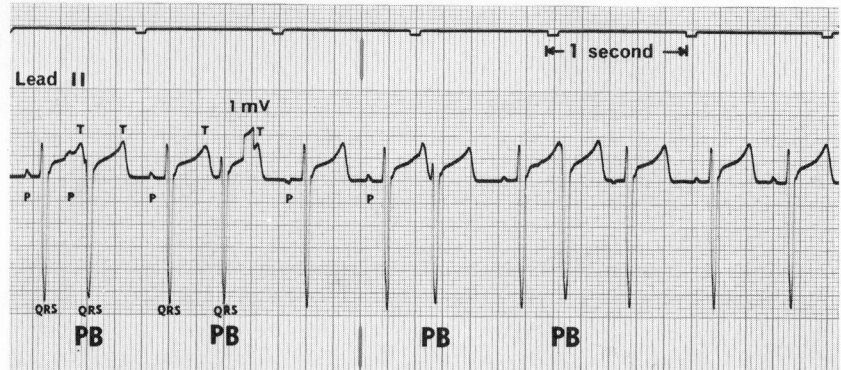

**Figure 2.**   Atrial (or AV junctional) premature beats (PB). Waveforms are also indicative of right ventricular enlargement and a wandering atrial pacemaker.

premature beats (LV), right ventricular premature beats (RV), atrial premature beats (A), paroxysmal atrial tachycardia (PAT) and, by chance, a fusion beat (FB) (i.e., two beats originating from different loci are superimposed for that beat). A definite tachycardia, which should be treated, exists, but the therapeutic agent of choice has inherent dangers as discussed below.

Figure 5 is an ECG from a dog with advanced AV valve regurgitation and illustrates the ominous rhythm of atrial fibrillation. No productive and synchronous contractions of the atria exist (no P waves are seen), and blood is pooled in the atria and great vessels drained by them. The ventricular rate is rapid and irregular, and many ventricular beats are not sufficiently productive to eject blood from the heart. The ventricular depolarization occurs over the normal pathways, and the QRS complex thus remains quite normal.

Figure 6 is an ECG from a dog with frequent and often paired left ventricular premature beats (large letters). The abnormal QRS complexes are elongated in time, are inverted in polarity and have larger voltages than the normal conducted beats. A large,

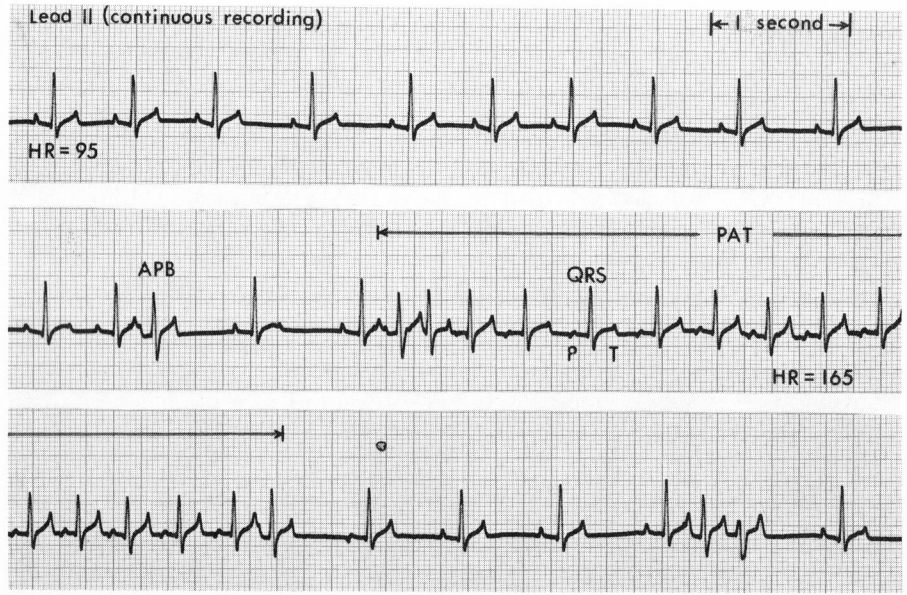

**Figure 3.**   *Top tracing:* Normal segment with sinus arrhythmia. *Bottom tracings:* Paroxysmal atrial (or AV junctional) tachycardia (PAT) and atrial (or AV junctional) premature beats (APB).

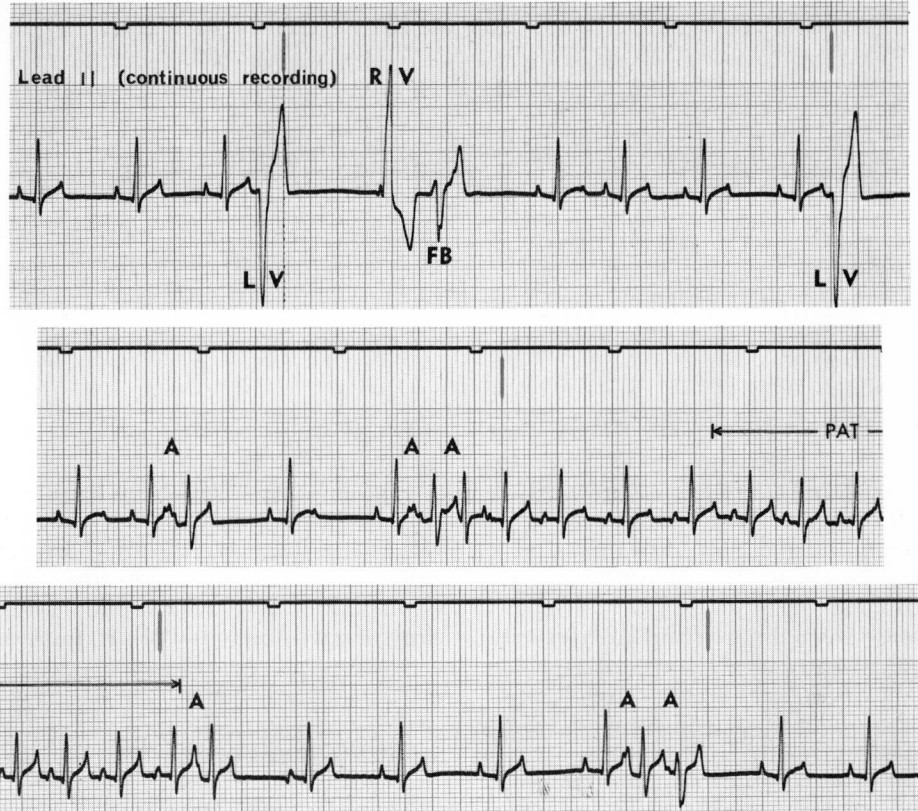

**Figure 4.** Continuous recording with left ventricular (LV) and right ventricular (RV) premature beats, atrial (or AV junctional) premature beats (A) and paroxysmal atrial (or AV junctional) tachycardia (PAT). A fusion beat (FB) also appears by chance.

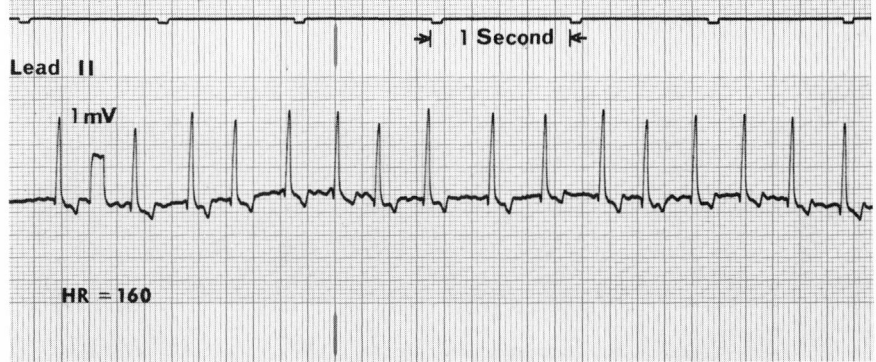

**Figure 5.** Atrial fibrillation. An absence of P waves and a fast, irregular ventricular rate typify this tachyarrhythmia.

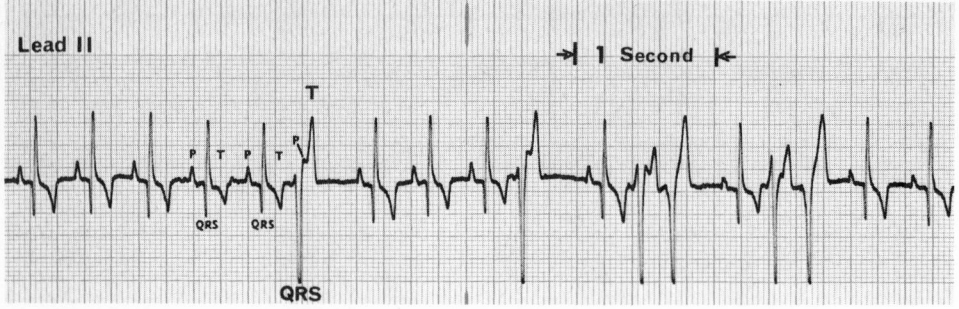

**Figure 6.** Left ventricular premature beats (large letters) appearing singly and in pairs.

opposite-polarity T wave with ST-segment elevation follows the abnormal QRS complex. An occasional ventricular premature beat in an otherwise healthy dog is of equivocal significance, but if frequent or in short burst, as illustrated, it must be considered pathologic.

Figure 7 is an ECG from a dog with paroxysmal ventricular tachycardia (PVT) from a left ventricular focus of excitation. Long bursts of ventricular beats at an excessively high rate are interspersed with periods of relatively normal heart rhythm. The abnormal QRS complexes are inverted and elongated and are followed by ST-segment elevation and large, opposite-polarity T waves. This condition is exceedingly hazardous and must be treated, since it frequently progresses into ventricular fibrillation.

Figure 8 is an ECG from a dog with ventricular tachycardia from a right ventricular focus. The QRS complexes are very large and elongated followed by a slurring of the ST segment into the large, opposite-polarity T wave. An occasional P wave (p) may be seen superimposed on the tachycardia, giving evidence that the supraventricular

pacemaker was active but overridden by the faster ventricular focus.

Figure 9 is an ECG from a dog with ventricular fibrillation, a rapidly fatal arrhythmia if it is not reverted to another rhythm that is compatible with life. Electrical defibrillation is the most successful procedure, if anything will work, to terminate this arrhythmia.

## SUGGESTED TREATMENT

Treatment of tachyarrhythmias is aimed at returning the rhythm to normal or reducing the ventricular contraction rate to below 100 beats per minute.

The tachyarrhythmias, and the relative therapeutic measures used to arrest them, may be placed in two broad categories, namely, supraventricular (atrial premature beats, paroxysmal atrial or junctional tachycardia and atrial fibrillation) and ventricular (frequent ventricular premature beats, paroxysmal ventricular tachycardia and ventricular tachycardia).

The current medications being administered should always be considered when as-

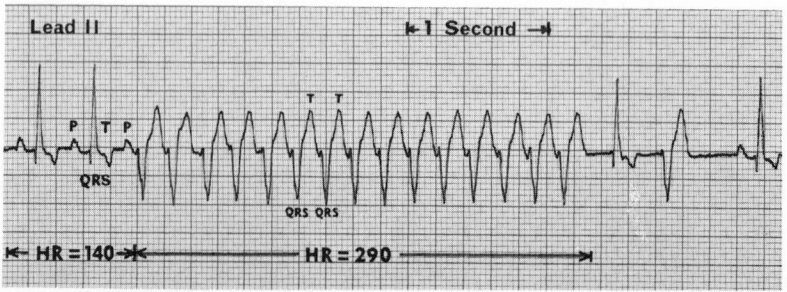

**Figure 7.** Paroxysmal ventricular tachycardia (PVT) from a left ventricular focus.

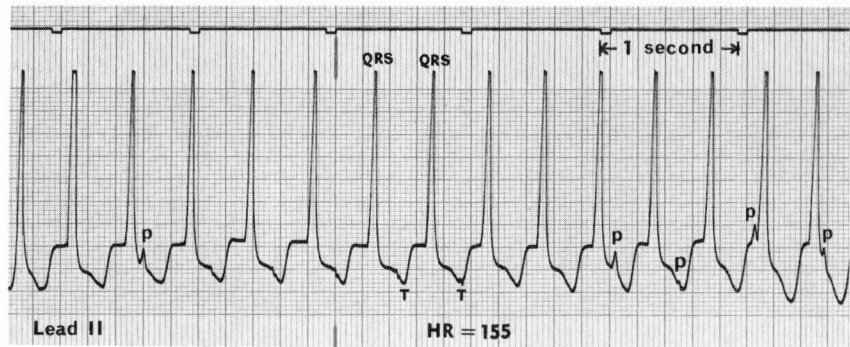

**Figure 8.** Ventricular tachycardia from a right ventricular focus. Some P waves are superimposed on the basic rhythm, indicating that the normal pacemaker was still active but overridden by the faster ventricular pacemaker.

sessing an arrhythmia, since these are frequently the cause of the abnormality in electrical conduction. The greatest offender in this respect is digitalis glycoside; its overdosage may produce arrhythmias that include, among others, all the tachyarrhythmias discussed above. Constant reevaluation and adjustment of glycoside therapy should be effected over the course of treatment.

Quinidine is another potential genitor of arrhythmias and electrical dissociation of the heart. Occasionally, owing to anticholinergic properties, a tachycardia may develop prior to the desired cardiac slowing effect of this drug.

Treatment of supraventricular tachyarrhythmias is aimed at stimulating vagal reflexes such as applying digital pressure to the eyeballs or carotid sinus or administration of vasopressors, digitalis glycoside or beta-adrenergic blocking drugs. Some drugs are used to delay conduction time or to increase the refractory period of the tissue for conduction of electrical impulses. Care must be used when giving negative ino-

tropic drugs such as quinidine or propranolol in the presence of congestive heart failure.

Treatment of ventricular tachyarrhythmias is aimed at slowing the ventricular rate by making it less excitable and less responsive to stimuli which may otherwise stimulate it to depolarize. Drugs which increase excitability or shorten the refractory period of ventricular tissue are contraindicated under these conditions.

Table 1 below illustrates various therapeutic regimens used to terminate supraventricular and ventricular tachyarrhythmias. Not all regimens will work in all animals, and in some arrhythmias, especially the ventricular tachyarrhythmias, no currently used drug may be corrective. Ventricular fibrillation does not respond favorably to drug administration but stopping contractions with potassium chloride or acetylcholine and restimulating the myocardium with calcium chloride and manual massage have been attempted when an electrical defibrillator has been unavailable.

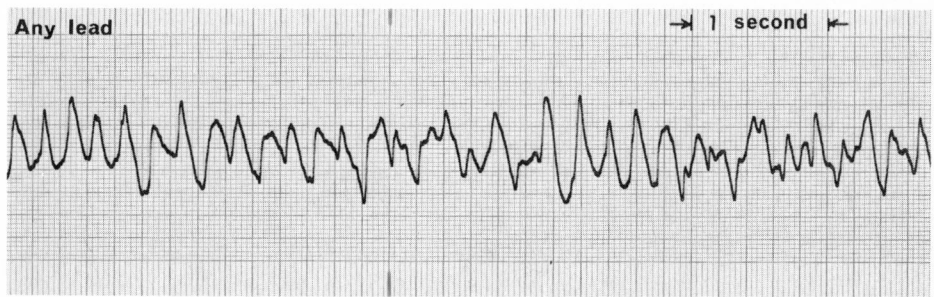

**Figure 9.** Ventricular fibrillation with complete dissociation of all electrical activity; a terminal arrhythmia.

*Table 1.*  *Tachyarrhythmia Drugs*

| ARRHYTHMIA | DRUG | DOSE AND ROUTE* | INTERVAL | REMARKS |
|---|---|---|---|---|
| Supraventricular (atrial premature beats, paroxysmal atrial tachycardia, atrial fibrillation) | Digitalis glycoside | 0.02 to 0.04 mg./kg. total dose IV (in ¼ doses) | Each 30 minutes | Intoxication rapidly attained. Reserved for urgent cases. Drug of choice for atrial fibrillation to slow ventricular rate. |
| | | 0.02 to 0.04 mg./kg. PO (Adjust upward as required) | Twice daily | Preferred route of administration. May increase ventricular rate if arrhythmia is ventricular in origin. Dosage depends upon product used and clinical response. |
| | Propranolol | 2.0 to 40 mg. P.O. | 2 to 3 times daily | Not predictable in action. Not recommended if congestive heart failure is present. Good for digitalis-induced tachyarrhythmias. |
| | Quinidine | 0.6 to 2.0 mg./kg. IM | 6 to 8 hours | Rarely used. Not predictable in action. Not recommended if congestive heart failure is present. Unreliable in converting atrial fibrillation to sinus rhythm in dogs. |
| | | 6 to 20 mg./kg. PO | 6 to 8 hours | Preferred route of administration. Preferred drug in the presence of both supraventricular and ventricular tachyarrhythmias. Do not use if AV block is present. |
| | Phenylephrine | 0.15 to 0.8 mg. IV, slowly to effect or 3 to 6 times this dose. IM or SC | As required | Indicated for sinus tachycardia. ECG monitoring required during administration. Antagonized by atropine. Do not use if ventricular tachycardia is present. |
| | Methoxamine | 1 to 5 mg. IV slowly or 2 to 10 mg. IM | As required | Same as phenylephrine |
| Ventricular (Frequent ventricular beats, paroxysmal ventricular tachycardia and ventricular tachycardia) | Lidocaine (2% without epinephrine) | 2 mg./kg. IV as a bolus | Do not exceed 2 or 3 doses | Convulsions if dose exceeds 4 mg./kg. Drug of choice to differentiate between atrial fibrillation and ventricular tachycardia. Effective duration of action is 10 to 20 minutes. Use in emergencies only. ECG monitoring advised. |

| Drug | Dosage | Frequency | Comments |
|---|---|---|---|
| Procainamide | 4 to 8 mg./kg. IV or 25 to 50 mg./minute by IV drip | Do not exceed 2 or 3 doses | Hypotension may follow IV administration. Use in emergencies only. ECG monitoring advised. |
|  | 8 to 16 mg./kg. IM | As required | Rarely used. |
|  | 125 to 500 mg. PO | 6 to 8 hours | Preferred route of administration. Supplied in 250 mg. capsules only. Agranulocytosis may develop with continuous usage. |
| Quinidine | 0.6 to 2.0 mg./kg. IM | 6 to 8 hours | Rarely used. |
|  | 6 to 20 mg./kg. PO | 6 to 8 hours | Preferred route of administration. Frequent ECG evaluation advised. Discontinue if QRS complex elongates more than 25%. Caution recommended in presence of congestive heart failure. Do not use in presence of AV block. |
| Diphenylhydantoin | 4 mg./kg. slowly IV | Once | Administer orally after first dose. Good for digitalis intoxication, if this is cause of arrhythmia. |
|  | 30 to 100 mg. PO | 3 to 4 times daily | Discontinue after 2 days of withholding digitalis administration. |
| Potassium chloride | 1 to 5 ml. of a 4% solution slowly IV | Once | ECG monitoring advised. Discontinue digitalis if this is cause of arrhythmia. Cardiac arrest may result from overdosage or rapid IV administration. |
| Propranolol | 10 to 40 mg. PO | 2 to 3 times | Actions unpredictable and may not be corrective. Do not use in presence of congestive heart failure. |
|  | 1 to 3 mg. slowly IV | Once; repeat only if no effect is seen | ECG monitoring required. Reserved for emergencies. |

*IV = intravenously
IM = intramuscularly
SC = subcutaneously
PO = per OS

# BRADYAR-RHYTHMIAS AND PACEMAKER THERAPY

KATHY KEATING BROWN, D.V.M.
*Irmo, South Carolina*

In the normal individual with a heart rate of 40 to 160 beats per minute, hemodynamic parameters are maintained by compensatory mechanisms. Above 160 beats per minute, cardiac output and systemic blood pressure fall rapidly. In diseased hearts, there may not be sufficient reserve to tolerate rate extremes. At 20 to 40 beats per minute, there is a decrease in cerebral blood flow. Convulsions and coronary insufficiency can result in death if medical or surgical intervention does not follow.

Impulse formation occurs in the pacemaker cells of the sinoatrial node owing to spontaneous diastolic depolarization. Excitation spreads through the atria via three internodal tracts and Bachman's bundle to the atrioventricular node. The function of the AV node is to delay impulses from the SA node to allow sufficient time for ventricular filling. The AV junction can also function as a secondary pacemaker site in the absence of SA node activity. The specialized conduction system is continued as the common bundle of His which divides into a right bundle branch and left anterior and posterior bundle branches. These branches arborize to form the subendocardial Purkinje network. A decrease in the rate of impulse formation from the sinus node to the Purkinje network enables more distal tissues of the conduction system to assume pacemaker function in the event of SA or AV node dysfunction. The normal sinus rate is 60 to 200 cycles per minute, the lower AV junction rate 40 to 60 per minute and the Purkinje network and ventricles rate 20 to 40 per minute.

The mechanisms of arrhythmias are abnormal automaticity, abnormal conduction or a combination of both. Disturbances in impulse formation can result in sinus bradycardia or ectopic rhythms such as nodal or idioventricular rhythm. Conduction disturbances result in sinoatrial block, atrioventricular block of varying degrees or bundle-branch blocks.

Sinus bradycardia, defined as a heart rate less than 50 beats per minute, can be physiologic owing to excessive parasympathetic tone. Pathologic states which contribute are cerebral lesions, increased intracranial pressure, coronary heart disease and hypertension in man, congenital lesions, drug effects, electrolyte imbalances and a variety of infectious diseases. The presence or absence of symptoms generally relates to the extent of hemodynamic impairment and is clinically manifested as dizziness, weakness or syncope. The electrocardiogram in sinus bradycardia shows each P wave followed by a QRS complex. Prolonged diastolic pauses represent periods of sinus pause, sinus arrest or atrial standstill which are responsible for the troublesome symptomatology. Commonly reversible causes of sinus bradycardia are digitalis or quinidine intoxication, hyperkalemia and hypoxia. Treatment is directed at removal of the underlying cause. Atropine (0.6 to 2.0 mg. parenterally) should rapidly produce a rate increase. Isoproterenol given as a bolus (0.05 mg.) or diluted 1 mg./200 cc. 5% dextrose in water and administered by intravenous drip can be useful. If drug therapy does not produce a demonstrable improvement within minutes, pacemaker intervention can be considered.

One clinically recognizable condition caused by a slow sinus rhythmicity is known as "sick sinus node syndrome." The actual stimulus for a decreased rate of firing is often not determined. Infiltrative or inflammatory lesions around the SA node prevent synchronous atrial activity and delay or interrupt conduction to the AV node. The likelihood of emergence of ectopic atrial activity, paroxysmal junctional tachycardia and ventricular tachyarrhythmias is enhanced. This complex, referred to as bradycardia-tachycardia, is generally refractory to medical therapy and responds best to pacemaker intervention.

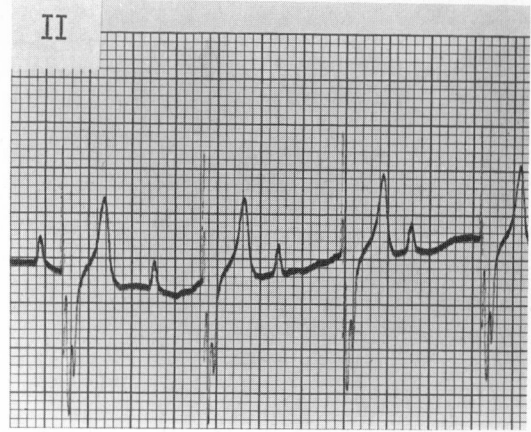

**Figure 1.** Lead II ECG of dog in complete heart block. Note the "pacemaker spike" occurring regularly every 16.5 boxes which just precedes the QRS complex.

## ATRIOVENTRICULAR HEART BLOCK

Atrioventricular block is defined as partial delay or complete interruption of impulse transmission from the atria to the ventricles. First-degree AV block is a relatively benign conduction disturbance. Electrocardiographic diagnosis is made on the basis of an increased duration of the P-R interval (normal P-R interval = 0.12 sec.). Treatment is often unnecessary unless digitalis or propranolol intoxication is present. Atropine and isoproterenol enhance AV nodal conduction and decrease the P-R interval.

Second-degree AV block is a more ominous conduction disturbance. It can be recognized on an ECG as an occasional P wave not followed by a QRS complex (sometimes called Mobitz Type II). There may be a regular sequence of unconducted to conducted beats resulting in 2:1, 3:1 pattern. This can be a forerunner of complete AV block. A variant form of second-degree block is seen as progressive prolongation of the P-R interval until ventricular depolarization fails to follow the longest P-R interval. This arrhythmia is commonly seen with digitalis intoxication.

If depolarization occurs in the atria at a rapid rate, impulses may reach the AV node during the refractory period and fail to reach the ventricles. This produces a physiologic atrioventricular block and can cause a slow ventricular rhythm.

Complete heart block or third-degree AV block occurs when there is total failure of impulse transmission through the AV node. The atria and ventricles have pacemaking sites independent of each other. Generally the ventricular rate is slower than the atrial rate. The appearance of the QRS complex depends on the pacemaker for ventricular depolarization. Wide, bizzare complexes result from an escape focus below the common bundle. Relatively normal complexes result from a junctional pacemaker. In complete heart block there is no consistent P-R interval and the rate is generally less than 40 beats per minute.

Complete AV block is not a common finding in the dog. It occurs in man subsequent to myocardial infarctions in chronic ischemic heart disease. Chronic valvular disease, myocardial and endocardial fibrosis, congenital cardiac lesions, drug intoxication and many acute infectious diseases interrupt conduction through the bundle branches.

Clinical findings associated with the bradycardia relate to a decreased cardiac output and hypotension. Cerebral circulatory deficits produce listlessness, confusion, drowsiness and syncope. Decreased renal blood flow results in a decline in urine production and azotemia. Stokes-Adams seizures are seen in at least half the cases of complete heart block, ventricular asystole and ventricular flutter-fibrillation. The first heart sound varies in intensity because of the changing relationship between atrial and ventricular contractions and change in position of valve cusps. Soft-pitched fourth heart sounds (atrial contractions) may be heard.

Treatment is usually symptomatic because removal of the basic underlying cause may not be possible. Isoproterenol is the medical treatment of choice. It can be administered in a 0.05-mg. bolus or as an intravenous drip (1 mg./200 cc. 5% dextrose in water) to produce a ventricular rate between 80 and 120 beats per minute (Ettinger, 1969). Long-term management with oral isoproterenol or atropine is not consistently effective. There are several reported cases of spontaneous regression of complete heart block in the dog (Dear, 1970) but the treatment of choice is pacemaker intervention.

The earliest work on electrical stimulation was done on surgically created heart blocks in the dog. Zoll (1951) first demonstrated that electrical stimulation was safe and feasible in man. The decision to pace is based on the presence of symptoms and the type of block present. Currently, there are 16 companies which manufacture over 100 pacemaker models. Asynchronous or fixed-rate units can be used for atrial or ventricular pacing. This mode delivers a predetermined number of stimuli per minute irrespective of the inherent cardiac rate. Synchronous pacemakers have a sensing circuit which can be inhibited or triggered by a detected signal. A P-synchronous unit senses atrial depolarization and acts as an artificial AV conduction system which paces the ventricles after an appropriate delay. The R-synchronous pulse generator adjusts its output with the ventricular electrogram. A bifocal demand unit can sense either chamber and paces the ventricle as needed.

Application of electrical stimuli to the myocardium is accomplished by several methods, each with inherent advantages and disadvantages. Transvenous pacing is currently most popular in man because it eliminates the need for a thoracotomy. The external jugular vein is most frequently used in the dog but the femoral vein can be used for temporary pacing. Positioning of the electrode in either the right atrium or the right ventricle generally requires the use of fluoroscopy. Some balloon-tipped catheters are available for temporary pacing and may be positioned blindly; however, this is accomplished with difficulty in the dog. The electrode is then connected to an external stimulus source or an implantable generator, depending on the intended duration of pacing. For permanent positioning of the electrode, a loop is passed through the tricuspid valve and out into the pulmonary artery. The electrode is withdrawn slowly and the tip is positioned in the apex of the right ventricle. In the immediate postoperative period, electrode instability, fracture or perforation can cause loss of capture. Threshold required for stimulation varies over a range from 0.3 ma. to 10 to 15 ma. Threshold is low initially, rises and then declines and reaches a plateau at approximately 30 days. The pulse generator is usually set at 2 to 4 times threshold. Most manufacturers have sales and service personnel available to assist in threshold measurements and to advise on techniques. It is often possible to obtain used pacemakers at lower cost. Most of the cost incurred is for purchase of a suitable lead (about $75 to $100).

Transthoracic pacing requires a thoracotomy and placement of electrodes directly on the epicardial surface. "Cobra-head" electrodes are sutured to myocardium through an incision in the pericardium at the apex of the heart. A strain-relieving loop is made to avoid tension on sutures. A "corkscrew" electrode is available which twists into the myocardium and is also held in place by fibrous attachment to polyester netting on the electrode above the tip. Fibrous tissue does not build up on the electrode-myocardial interface.

The pulse generator is placed in a pocket created between muscle layers wherever the lead length will allow. Sites used are between the abdominal oblique muscles, dorsal to the scapulae and retroperitoneal areas. A Dacron pouch is available which is useful in preventing pulse generator migration and aids in ease of pacemaker replacement. The leads are tunneled subcutaneously from either the transvenous incision or the thorax to the pulse generator. Excessive tension on the skin overlying the battery is to be avoided so that pressure necrosis and extrusion of the pacemaker cannot occur.

For most exacting measurements of pacemaker functioning, special diagnostic equipment is necessary. Some of the more common problems can be recognized on the ECG. Exit block from a rise in threshold may occur and the pacing stimulus would fail to elicit a ventricular response (loss of capture). Battery depletion is a troublesome problem stemming from the necessity to use outdated and donated units to keep the cost in a feasible range. Impending failures may be seen as a change in the shape of the QRS complex or a rate change. The amplitude of the pacing spike will usually decrease.

Abnormal or erratic firing will change the spike-to-spike interval, indicating a sensing problem or malfunctioning electrode. A competitive rhythm between the intrinsic heart rate and pacemaker rate results in ventricular tachyarrhythmias or ventricular fibrillation.

Available energy sources dictate the longevity of the power source. The improved conventional mercury-zinc cell can often be used for approximately 44 to 63 months without replacement. Other sources are lithium-iodide or nickel-cadmium. New energy sources including plutonium-238 batteries may increase the longevity to over 79 months and may indeed outlive the patient. Many factors influence the life span of both the power source and the electrode but such a discussion is beyond the scope of this chapter.

The use of pacemakers in veterinary medicine for arrhythmias which do not easily lend themselves to medical management is not an economic impossibility. Since the dog was used as the original experimental model, techniques are well suited for animal use clinically and may prove to be a valuable addition to progressive veterinary medicine.

## SUPPLEMENTAL READING

Buchanan, J., Dear, M., Pyle, R., and Berg, P.: Medical and pacemaker therapy of complete heart block and congestive failure in a dog. J. Am. Vet. Med. Assn., 152(8):1099, 1968.

Dear, M. G.: Spontaneous reversion of complete A-V block to sinus rhythm in the dog. J. Small Animal Pract., 11:17–26, 1970.
El-Sherif, N., Scherlag, B., and Lazzava, R.: Pathophysiology of second degree atrioventricular block: A unified hypothesis. Am. J. Cardiol., 35:421, 1975.
Ettinger, S.: Isoproterenol treatment of atrioventricular block in the dog. J. Am. Vet. Med. Assn., 154(4):398, 1969.
Ettinger, S., and Suter, P.: Canine Cardiology. Philadelphia, W. B. Saunders Co., 1970, pp. 271–309.
Friedberg, C.: Diseases of the Heart. 3rd ed. Philadelphia, W. B. Saunders Co., 1966, pp. 468–600.
Furman, S., and Escher, D.: Modern Cardiac Pacing. A Clinical Overview. Bowie, Missouri, Charles Press, 1975.
Haft, D.: Treatment of arrhythmias by intracardiac electrical stimulation. Progr. Cardiovasc. Dis., 16(6):539, 1974.
Hurst, J., Logue, B., Schlant, R., and Wanger, N.: The Heart. Arteries and Veins. 3rd ed. New York, McGraw-Hill Book Co., 1974, pp. 495–585.
Moss, A., and Davis, R.: Brady-Tachy Syndrome. Progr. Cardiovasc. Dis., 16(5):439, 1974.
Scherlag, B., Samet, P., and Helfant, R.: His bundle electrogram. Circulation, 46:601, 1972.
Zoll, P. M.: Resuscitation of the heart in ventricular standstill by external electric stimulation. N. Engl. J. Med., 247:768, 1952.

# BACTERIAL ENDOCARDITIS

MICHAEL G. DEAR, M.R.C.V.S.
*British Columbia, Canada*

Endocarditis is an inflammation of the endocardium. The cause may be infectious or noninfectious and morphologically may be mural or valvular. Mural (or parietal) endocarditis is frequently a manifestation of other systemic diseases (e.g., uremia and acute renal insufficiency), although it also occurs as an extension of valvular endocarditis. The term infectious endocarditis will be used in recognition of the increasing awareness of nonbacterial infectious agents, their possible public health significance and the similarity of presenting signs for endocarditis independent of its cause.

Viral endomyocarditis in children has been associated with coxsackie (especially type B), ECHO, rubella, varicella and adenoviruses. In animals, experimental endomyocarditis infections have been induced in mice (adenovirus, reovirus, vaccinia, coxsackie B) and in rabbits (poxvirus

III). Encephalomyocarditis virus (EMCV) has caused disease in mice, rats, hamsters, pigs and chimpanzees. For the latter virus to produce clinical disease an activating stimulus or agent is usually necessary. Such agents include the trauma of needle puncture, digitalis, cortisone, antibiotics such as chloramphenicol or streptomycin, metals, stress, exercise, etc. EMCV is a picornavirus with a worldwide distribution. This information merits clinical consideration because of the suggested implication of viruses in the pathogenesis of the congestive forms of cardiomyopathy in cats. The role of viruses in the vascular pathology of equine viral arteritis, the necrotizing arteritis of Aleutian disease of minks and the myocarditis of cattle infected with foot and mouth virus is well known.

The public health aspect of these infectious agents should be considered. *Rickett-*

*sia burnetii* (in Q fever) and *Bedsonia* or *Chlamydia psittaci* (in psittacosis) have both been isolated as the cause of infective endocarditis in man where routine blood cultures failed to reveal the causative organism.

## INCIDENCE

The incidence of endocarditis in dogs is variable probably because of the variability of the criteria used to make the diagnosis. The reported incidence of endocarditis demonstrated at necropsy varied from 0.58 per cent (on over 11,000 necropsies) through 0.74 per cent, 2.27 per cent, 5.8 per cent to 6.6 per cent (on 600 necropsies). The highest incidence of valvular involvement appears to correlate with that which sustains the greatest closed pressure. In order of decreasing frequency of involvement are the mitral, aortic, pulmonic and tricuspid valves.

## ETIOLOGY AND PATHOGENESIS

Infectious endocarditis may result from viral, bacterial or fungal causative agents, the most common of which are bacteria as far as is known. Gram-positive nonhemolytic streptococci are isolated most frequently but hemolytic streptococci and staphylococci occur regularly with occasional reports of infection with *Pseudomonas aeruginosa, Escherichia coli* and *Erysipelothrix rhusiopathiae*.

Bacteria are deposited on the valves not via capillaries but from the blood in the cardiac chambers. Preexisting damage to the valves or mural endocardium facilitates bacterial deposition presumably on platelet thrombi or valvular vegetations. Thus dogs with acquired or congenital heart disease are predisposed to infectious endocarditis. In man, the implantation of prosthetic valves facilitates the induction of bacterial endocarditis. Any animal which has a source of infection, e.g., abscesses and paradontal disease, and concurrent heart disease is highly susceptible to infectious endocarditis, with subsequent valvular deformity or cardiac arrhythmias resulting in congestive heart failure. Bacteria and microemboli are released from the vegetations, and metastatic embolization may produce abscesses in the kidney, liver and brain.

## CLINICAL RECOGNITION

As a result of multiple organ involvement and the possibility of metastatic embolization, patients having infectious endocarditis may present with cardiac, neurologic, renal or other signs. It is helpful, therefore, to adopt the approach of problem-oriented medical records. Problems are resolved through four phases of action: (1) data base collection, (2) problem definition, (3) plan formulation and (4) follow-up (progress notes).

## DATA BASE COLLECTION (HISTORY AND PHYSICAL EXAMINATION)

Both acute and chronic forms of infectious endocarditis present with nonspecific signs such as lethargy, weakness, inappetence and weight loss. Emboli may lodge in specific sites, causing lameness, dyspnea and neurologic, renal and gastrointestinal disturbances. There is no breed or sex incidence, although the condition is seen more in middle-aged and older dogs. The history may reveal a previous infection or traumatic incident.

Fever is not a consistent feature but may occur recurrently. Septicemia, pallor, a systolic heart murmur of recent origin in the mitral or aortic area, possibly a cardiac arrhythmia and sometimes a localized infection (anal sacculitis, bronchopneumonia, prostatitis) may be found on physical examination. Embolization to the eyes may produce petechiation, to the kidneys will show paralumbar pain and to the brain will show encephalitic signs.

## INITIAL PROBLEM LIST AND PLAN FORMATION

The problem list may contain several diverse clinical signs which require an expanded data base collection for resolution.

**Diagnostic Plan (Dx).** This includes a complete blood cell count, blood biochemistry (an SMA-12), an electrocardiogram and thoracic radiographs, probably in that order of clinical and economic importance. A blood culture is an expedient diagnostic aid if it is positive. Its clinical value must be assessed in terms of the severity of the animal's condition and economics. Antibiotic therapy should be withdrawn for one week prior to sampling the blood, and the patient's temperature should be recorded frequently, blood samples being taken every hour for four or more cultures during peak pyrexic periods. At least 5 to 10 ml. of blood is required per sample, with good aseptic preparation of the skin prior to venipuncture. Negative cultures do not negate the possibility of the syndrome.

Leukocytosis may or may not be present, neutrophilia usually exists during bacteremic phases and monocytosis may occur. Blood biochemistry may suggest embolization to other organs. Electrocardiography and radiography are helpful in differentiating primary cardiomyopathies from bacterial endocarditis. Viral endocarditis may lead to cardiomyopathy. In the early stages of endocarditis there may be no electrocardiographic changes, but as coronary emboli occur, a secondary myocarditis manifested by cardiac arrhythmias and congestive heart failure results. One 3-year-old Irish setter with atrial fibrillation, pyrexia and a positive blood culture reverted to sinus rhythm on antibiotic therapy and cage rest.

**Therapeutic Plan (Rx).** The therapeutic plan varies with the clinical situation.

(1) When there is a serious cardiac arrhythmia with or without signs of heart failure, therapy is directed at correcting the arrhythmia and combating the infection concomitantly.

    (a) Antiarrhythmic treatment.

    (b) The use of vitamin E for its anti-thrombogenic properties where embolization of the coronary vessels is suspected.

    (c) Antibiotic therapy (procaine penicillin G, 1 to 2 million units twice daily IM and dihydrostreptomycin at 10 mg./kg. twice daily IM).

(2) Where less serious clinical signs are present, antibiotic therapy may be delayed for one week to permit blood cultures to be performed. An in-vitro assay of the cultured organism's sensitivity to various serum concentrations of the appropriate antibiotic may be made. Even where there is a negative culture but where the clinical signs are consistent with endocarditis, it is advisable to treat intensively, as if the diagnosis were proven. Treatment should be prompt, intensive and prolonged. Fibrin deposits on the valves and the relative avascularity of the valves limit the host's ability to overcome the infection. Bacteriostatic drugs are not recommended.

    (a) For penicillin-sensitive organisms, intramuscular procaine penicillin G in doses of 1 to 2 million units every 12 hours for 3 weeks are recommended. It is more economical and practical to have the owner maintain the medication at home using oral penicillins (e.g., ampicillin). The timing and duration of the therapy must be stressed if resistant strains of bacteria are to be avoided. Staphylococcal infections frequently respond well to synthetic penicillins such as cloxacillin and dicloxacillin.

    (b) For gram-negative organisms, bactericidal drugs such as streptomycin, gentamicin and kanamycin may be used. Overdosage of these agents produces toxicity and it is important to use the dosage and duration recommendations of the manufacturers.

(3) Exercise should be restricted and elective surgery should be postponed.

## FOLLOW-UP (PROGNOSIS AND CONVALESCENCE)

The prognosis on cases of infectious endocarditis is very much dependent on the precipitating causes and the response to therapy. Endocarditis is one cardiac condition where complete clinical resolution may be achieved.

## PROPHYLAXIS

Any animal with preexisting heart disease should receive antibiotic therapy pre- and postoperatively for both surgical procedures and dentistry.

# HEARTWORM DISEASE

J. GREGG BORING, D.V.M.
*Auburn, Alabama*

## INTRODUCTION

Heartworm disease has received much attention as a clinical problem. In dogs, this infectious disease is caused by *Dirofilaria immitis* and is so named because the adult parasites lodge in the venous return, right ventricle and pulmonary outflow tracts of the cardiovascular system

The disease has a cosmopolitan distribution. The highest incidence occurs in coastal areas because the parasites' transmission vector is the mosquito. In many inland states dogs exhibit a high incidence of infection and the disease is progressively spreading. In some areas of the United States, evaluation for internal parasites should routinely include a test for *Dirofilaria immitis* microfilariae.

Owing to public awareness and routine blood examinations by veterinarians, the disease is now generally diagnosed earlier and more animals are successfully treated. Of recent interest is the fact that numerous heartworm-infected dogs do not exhibit a microfilaremia. It is known that numbers of circulating microfilariae do not indicate the adult parasite population.

## DIAGNOSIS

Blood samples are the generally accepted method for detecting heartworm disease. Characteristic microfilariae, borne live by the adult parasite, circulate in the peripheral vasculature and are microscopically visible. The microfilariae are usually isolated and identified either in a fresh blood smear or by centrifugation or are filtered out by millipore filters.

Proper identification of microfilariae is imperative, since a subcutaneous adult parasite, *Dipetalonema reconditum*, also produces a small number of circulating microfilariae. Identification is essential because the subcutaneous parasite is considered nonpathogenic at the present time and is usually not treated. The present treatment for heartworms is toxic and an injustice would be done to animals treated as a result of improper identification of microfilariae.

Microfilariae are identified by size and shape, by movement in fresh blood smears as well as by special staining procedures, such as acid phosphatase. In general, microfilariae belonging to *Dirofilaria immitis* have "snakelike" motions without forward movement in fresh blood smears. They measure 300 to 320 microns in length by 6 to 8 microns in width and have "cigar-shaped" or tapered heads and straight tails. Microfilariae belonging to *Dipetalonema reconditum* have definite forward movement across the microscopic field in fresh blood smears, measure 260 to 280 microns in length by 6 to 7 microns in width and have parallel sides and a blunt head. The tails have a "button-hooked" appearance in 30 per cent of the microfilariae. The most distinguishing features to most practicing veterinarians are the shape of the head and the movement in blood smears.

Accurate diagnosis is complicated by the fact that some 15 to 20 per cent of the dogs do not exhibit circulating microfilariae. The reasons may be immature adults, all male or female adult population, immune responses, overcrowding of adult population and use of drugs for other parasitic infections which causes a secondary microfilaricidal effect. Three blood tests on different days should be run, preferably between the hours of 3 and 10 p.m., as microfilariae appear in larger concentrations in the late afternoons and after dogs have received food. If microfilariae still are not present, then diagnosis will have to be based on clinical examination, history and radiologic findings.

Obviously, physical examination and a thorough history should preclude microscopic and radiographic evaluations. History of an affected dog will usually indicate the following order of events: gradual weight loss, loss of endurance when exercised, coughing, accumulation of abdominal fluid, labored breathing, increased temperature and cyanotic mucous membranes. The signs will depend on the time and severity of parasitic infection and the individual dog.

Survey thoracic radiographs are the tests for diagnosing and treating microfilaria-free dogs. Typical changes occur in the cardiac silhouette and pulmonary arteries secondary to pulmonary hypertension. Enlargement of the pulmonary arterial segment and right ventricle is the major change on the cardiac silhouette. The lungs exhibit enlarged, tortuous pulmonary arteries secondary to thromboembolization.

## PREVENTION AND CONTROL

Controlling heartworm disease is a matter of breaking the life cycle of the heartworm at one point. However, the principle of breaking the life cycle with chemical or surgical procedures often leads to serious sequelae or even death. Therefore, prevention of the disease is the preferable treatment.

Today, the most accepted prevention is daily oral doses of diethylcarbamazine (DEC).* The drug is given in low doses (5.0 mg./kg. body weight) and is well tolerated by dogs. In the hyperendemic tropical areas where dogs have year-long mosquito exposure, the drug treatment must extend throughout the full year. If the mosquito population is seasonal or exposure is limited to visiting dogs in mosquito areas, the treatment should begin 15 days prior to exposure and extend 60 days after exposure.

Irreversible shock and death following administration of diethylcarbamazine has been reported in dogs with large numbers of circulating microfilariae. For this reason, caution should be exercised in examining blood samples for microfilariae prior to preventive procedures with DEC.

Diethylcarbamazine has been incriminated as the possible cause of sterility in some breeding animals. Further investigations in controlled studies have been unable to produce this problem and no evidence of abnormal sperm quality has been exhibited at present.

Prior to the discovery and use of DEC, preventive therapy consisted of a two-day series of intravenous treatment of thiacetarsamide* at 6-month intervals in tropical areas and 4- to 6-month intervals following mosquito seasons in nontropical areas. Other control and preventive methods are related to vector elimination, which is controlling the mosquito population by insecticides, repellents and screening of kennels.

## TREATMENT

It is important to note that heartworms can be successfully treated. Each heartworm case should receive an individual evaluation prior to treatment. Limitations of treatment depend on the amount of irreparable damage done to major organs from mechanical impairment of blood flow and toxic products released from live and dying adult heartworms. Treatment varies between the chronically infected animal and the asymptomatic animal.

At present arsenical drugs are used to reduce or eliminate adult heartworms. The current regimen favors divided daily doses of 0.2 mg./kg. of body weight of thiacetarsamide. This is given twice daily by the intravenous route for 2 or 3 days. Arsenic is a heavy metal and will cause damage to major organs when given in levels sufficient enough to kill adult heartworms. The liver and kidneys appear to be most severely affected. Since these organs are already embarrassed by poor circulation from adult heartworms, they should be closely monitored by clinical pathologic studies before, during and after treatment. The asymptomatic dogs usually exhibit minimal clinical signs secondary to death of adult heartworms and damage done by arsenical compounds. The chronically infected dog may exhibit more severe signs, with treatment success depending on adequate rest and posttreatment recuperation.

Some dogs cannot tolerate arsenical therapy and are poor surgical candidates. Long-term low doses of levamisole HCl is now a popular and widely used alternative adulticidal and microfilaricidal drug. This compound at present is not FDA-approved for use in dogs and cats and is potentially toxic, causing both liver and brain lesions. Owing to recently observed drug-induced

---

*Caricide® and Styrid-Caricide®, American Cyanamid Company, Princeton, New Jersey; Dirocide®, E. R. Squibb & Sons, Inc., New Brunswick, New Jersey.

*Caparsolate Sodium®, Diamond Laboratories, Des Moines, Iowa, and Abbott Laboratories, North Chicago, Illinois; Filaranide®, Fromm Laboratories, Grafton, Wisconsin.

lesions, the author cannot recommend the use of this drug at present as either an adulticidal or microfilaricidal agent.

Survey thoracic radiographs are essential in the asymptomatic and the chronically affected dog. Adult heartworms killed during treatment are filtered by the lungs, causing a thromboembolic pneumonia. In the chronically infected dog the lungs and pulmonary arteries are already damaged by naturally dying heartworms. Survey radiographs will exhibit the degree of pretreatment damage, thus allowing a clinical prognosis as to whether the lungs can withstand the pulmonary shock created by dying adult heartworms following arsenical treatment.

Good nursing care and careful posttreatment management will make the difference between success and failure. In the author's opinion, body temperatures should be taken twice daily following treatment. A rise in body temperature usually indicates pneumonia created by showers of emboli to the lungs. Therefore, at the first signs of increased temperatures, high doses of antibiotics should be initiated. Steroids are helpful in reducing the pulmonary inflammation which is probably an allergic protein reaction created by the dying adult heartworm fragments.

Following adulticidal treatment, microfilariae must be removed from the circulating blood. The microfilariae exist in the circulating blood 18 to 36 months following removal of adult heartworms. There are three important reasons for eliminating the microfilariae. First, the dog with circulating microfilariae is in a carrier state and is a potential threat to uninfected dogs. Secondly, recent studies have indicated pathologic changes associated with large numbers of circulating microfilariae. Thirdly, a prevention program using diethylcarbamazine may cause a shock reaction followed by death of the animal.

Microfilariae therapy is initiated 3 to 6 weeks following adulticidal therapy. At present two compounds being used for elimination of microfilariae are dithiazine iodide* and levamisole.†

Dithiazine iodide is approved by FDA for use as a microfilaricide. Dose varies from 4 to 20 mg./kg. of body weight daily given orally. The drug will cause vomiting and diarrhea and is potentially nephrotoxic in the high dose ranges. Dithiazine iodide should be given until microfilariae are cleared from the blood, which is usually within 7 to 10 days.

Levamisole is FDA-approved for parasite control in cattle, sheep and hogs at the present time. It is an accepted practice to use this drug as a microfilaricide, but until it has FDA approval, it must be considered an experimental drug. The dose is 10 mg. of active ingredient per kg. of body weight given daily until the blood is free from microfilariae. The microfilariae are usually cleared in 6 to 12 days.

After adult heartworms are killed and the microfilariae are cleared from the circulating blood, preventive therapy should be initiated. Dogs in endemic areas should be checked for microfilariae every 4 to 6 months regardless of preventive therapy.

Animals introduced into heartworm-free kennels in endemic areas or animals transported from endemic areas to other kennels should be isolated and repeatedly tested for 60 days prior to exposure to resident animals via mosquitoes.

## SUPPLEMENTAL READING

Bradley, R. E.: Canine Heartworm Disease: The Current Knowledge. Department of Veterinary Science, Institute of Food and Agriculture Sciences, University of Florida, Gainesville, 1972.

Jackson, R. F.: Canine dirofilariasis. In Kirk, R. W. (ed.): Current Veterinary Therapy III. Philadelphia, W. B. Saunders Co., 1968, pp. 216–220.

Jackson, R. F.: Complications during and following chemotherapy of heartworm diseases. J. Am. Vet Med. Assn. *154*:393–395, 1969.

Jackson, R. F., Morgan, H. C., Otto, G. F., and Jackson W. F.: Heartworm disease in the dog—Report of a symposium. J. Am. Vet. Med. Assn., *154*:369–397 1969.

Jackson, W. F.: Radiographic examination of the heartworm infected patient. J. Am. Vet. Med. Assn. *154*:380–382, 1969.

Knight, D. H.: Heartworm infestation. In Kirk, R. W (ed.): Current Veterinary Therapy IV. Philadelphia, W. B. Saunders Co., 1971, pp. 196–200.

Mills, J. N., and Amis, T. C.: Levamisole as a microfilaricidal agent in the control of canine dirofilariasis. Aust. Vet. J., *51*:310–314, 1975.

Morgan, H. C.: Laboratory examination of the heartworm infected patient. J. Am. Vet. Med. Assn *154*:378–380, 1969.

Newton, W. L., and Wright, W. H.: The occurrence of a dog filarioid other than *Dirofilaria immitis* in the United States. J. Parasitol., *42*:246–258, 1956.

---

*Dizan®, Elanco Products Company, Indianapolis, Indiana.

†Ripercole®, American Cyanamid Company, Princeton, New Jersey; Levasole®, Pitman-Moore, Inc., Washington's Crossing, Pennsylvania.

Otto, G. F., *et al.*: Variability in the ratio between the numbers of microfilariae and adult heartworms. J. Am. Vet. Med. Assn., *168*:605–607, 1976.

Proceedings of the Heartworm Symposium 1974. Compiled by the American Heartworm Society. H. C. Morgan, Editor. Bonner Springs, Kansas, VM Publishing, Inc.

Simpson, C. F., Bradley, R. E., and Jackson, R. F.: Crystalloid inclusions in hepatocyte mitochondria of dogs treated with levamisole. Vet. Path., *11*:129–137, 1974.

Wong, M. M., Suter, P. F., Rhode, A. E., and Guest, M. F.: Dirofilariasis without circulating microfilariae: A problem in diagnosis. J. Am. Vet. Med. Assn., *163*:133–139, 1973.

Wylie, J. P.: Detection of microfilariae by a filter technique. J. Am. Vet. Med. Assn., *156*:1403–1405, 1970.

# PERICARDIAL EFFUSION

K. W. KNAUER, D.V.M.
*College Station, Texas*

The pericardium, consisting primarily of fibrous connective tissue, is a protective sac that envelops the heart. The space between the epicardial surface of the heart and the visceral surface of the pericardial sac normally contains 1 to 2 ml. of serous fluid, which helps to lubricate these surfaces and to stabilize the heart. Accumulation of excess fluid in the pericardial sac is termed pericardial effusion and, in cases of acute filling, can result in cardiac tamponade. In cardiac tamponade, the pericardial sac is unable to distend rapidly and the resultant compressing effect on the heart impairs diastolic filling. The prognosis in acute cardiac tamponade is often grave. With slow accumulation, the pericardium will stretch and its fluid content may exceed a capacity of one liter in a large dog.

Pericardial effusion is infrequently seen in the dog; however, this syndrome constitutes an entity which may figure high in the list of differential diagnoses of those dogs presented with signs of heart failure. Most of the effusions seen will be serous in nature, these being followed by a lesser incidence of hemorrhagic and exudative effusions. About half the reported cases of pericardial effusion are due to heart-base tumors and other neoplasms. Primary pericardial disease is rare, with most pericardial effusions occurring secondarily to diseases of the heart and adjacent structures or as the result of generalized systemic disease.

## CLASSIFICATION AND ETIOLOGY

Pericardial effusions may be classified on the basis of their physical properties: hemorrhagic, serosanguineous, transudates or exudates.

Hemorrhagic effusions which clot upon withdrawal are seen in cardiac rupture, especially left atrial tear, which is most often seen in small male dogs over 8 years of age and having chronic mitral insufficiency. Iatrogenic laceration of coronary vessels and heart-wall puncture during cardiac catheterization produce hemorrhagic effusions. Inadvertent puncture of the myocardial wall during pericardiocentesis may give a false positive finding of hemorrhagic effusion. Trauma, primary cardiac neoplasms, metastatic neoplasms and heart-base tumors may cause hemorrhagic effusions. However, the effusions accompanying tumors may not clot after withdrawal.

Serosanguineous pericardial effusion may occur with pericardial cysts or may occur as a benign, unexplained phenomenon, while pericarditis associated with uremia may produce an effusion varying from serofibrinous to sanguineous. Congestive heart failure, hypoproteinemia, overhydration and peritoneopericardial hernias usually produce a serous pericardial effusion. Exudative effusions may result from systemic infections such as leptospirosis, toxoplasmosis, distemper, nocardiosis, coccidioidomycosis, tuberculosis and actinomycosis.

Pericardial effusion in congestive heart failure, myocardiopathies and cases of myopericarditis results from varying degrees of obstruction of the venous and lymphatic drainage of the myocardium itself. Myocardial interstitial fluid increases and is essentially "massaged out" to the epicardial surface and into the pericardial sac. The pressure gradient of high endocardial pressure and low epicardial pressure favors this direction of flow. This mechanism may be a method by which the myocardium protects itself from excessive tissue fluid that would alter its contractility. Pericardial effusion in these instances is actually "myocardial effusion" and would be similar to the method by which ascites forms, being an effusion from liver and intestinal surfaces rather than from the parietal peritoneum.

## DIAGNOSIS

If the amount of pericardial effusion is small, the diagnosis may be very difficult. Only when larger amounts of fluid accumulate, or when they appear very acutely such as in left atrial rupture, are diagnostic signs present. The classic signs of pericardial effusion include muffling of the heart sounds; peripheral venous engorgement; poor mucous membrane perfusion; and a weak, rapid femoral pulse. The jugular and lateral saphenous veins are distended and the jugular vein may also have a prominent pulsation. A jugular catheter placed with its tip in the anterior vena cava will record a moderate to severe elevation in central venous pressure. Venous back pressure due to the cardiac tamponade induced by large effusions will also congest and enlarge the liver. Mild elevations in SGPT and BUN values due to venous congestion will also be seen. Impairment of diastolic filling accounts for the lowered cardiac output and poor membrane perfusion. A lowering of peripheral blood pressure may be evaluated by a slow capillary filling time and a weak femoral pulse. Systemic blood pressure also may be measured by direct percutaneous needle puncture of the femoral artery while recording the pressure on a hand-held manometer, connected by tubing to the needle. External noninvasive blood pressure measuring devices that utilize the principle of reflected ultrasound to measure blood pressure in the tibial artery are also available to detect the peripheral hypotension. Circulation time in moderate-to-large effusions is usually markedly increased and often is in the 20- to 30-second range, with a very diffuse end point. Evidence of primary disease should be evaluated by complete physical examination, since pericardial effusion is often secondary to another process, and signs such as

fever may be present in effusions of infectious etiology, uremia in uremic pericarditis, concurrent neoplasia in metastatic tumor effusions, etc.

As the effusion becomes more progressive, signs such as general debility, weakness, ascites, dyspnea, pulmonary edema, pleural effusion and eventually death occur. In acute effusions, progression to death may occur very rapidly.

**Electrocardiography.** Dogs with pericardial effusions have no pathognomonic electrocardiographic signs. Often the ECG is normal. Heart rate is sometimes increased to compensate for the decreased stroke volume. Occasionally the electrocardiogram in pericardial effusion will show low QRS-complex voltages (less than 0.7 mv. in all leads, frontal plane and horizontal plane) and elevations or depressions of the ST segment from the isoelectric baseline. These changes are nonspecific and may be present in obese dogs, in those with pleural effusions or diaphragmatic hernias and sometimes in normal animals. However, when the low-voltage, ST-segment deviation ECG is seen, lateral and DV radiographs of the chest are always warranted.

**Radiography.** Characteristic roentgenographic signs are usually present when there is a large amount of pericardial effusion; however, small quantities are difficult to diagnose from cardiac chamber enlargement. Even when the diagnosis of pericardial effusion is confirmed, the amount of fluid present is difficult to estimate radiographically owing to the variability of cardiac chamber size relative to the external silhouette. Severe pericardial effusion is characterized by a massively enlarged, globular, cardiac silhouette in the lateral and dorsoventral projections. The borders of the silhouette are very uniform, giving the typical appearance of the "basketball heart." When the silhouette touches the thoracic wall, the former may be flattened or scalloped by the ribs. Where the pericardium touches the diaphragm, it is usually the diaphragm that is flattened, but the diaphragmatic continuity is uninterrupted in contradistinction to peritoneopericardial diaphragmatic hernia.

The hilar area is displaced dorsally, but the structures remain visible except in those cases where effusion is secondary to heart-base tumors or left atrial rupture. The lung field is usually clear.

In the lateral view the posterior cardiac

border becomes distinctly rounded. The caudal vena cava is usually dilated and denser than normal and may become obscured as it enters the posterior cardiac shadow.

If pleural effusion is also present it will obscure the cardiac silhouette and should be removed by thoracocentesis before exposing further radiographs.

Fluoroscopic examination in suspected pericardial effusion may be diagnostically valuable. Weak or absent pulsations are seen in the ventral portions of the heart shadow, being replaced by fluid wave undulations. The dorsal border, or base of the heart, will usually pulsate normally. Pneumopericardiography using plain film or fluoroscopic examination may be helpful to delineate lesions such as cysts and neoplasms. For convenience, air contrast can be placed in the pericardial sac after pericardiocentesis is performed.

Angiocardiographic studies using positive (radiopaque dye) or negative (carbon dioxide) contrast studies may be performed by injections of either medium into the jugular or cephalic veins, followed in 2 to 3 seconds by a plain film lateral radiograph of the thorax. The presence of the contrast in the right atrium and right ventricle will permit an estimation of intracavitary volume compared to overall cardiac silhouette and size. In pericardial effusion, the intracavitary volume is ordinarily normal even though the cardiac silhouette is massive. However, in gross cardiac dilatation cases the intracavitary volume is large, with a corresponding large silhouette.

At specialized diagnostic centers which have heart stations and nuclear medicine departments, two other techniques may be available for diagnosis of pericardial effusions. Radioactive trace elements which have short half-lives such as sodium pertechnetate (technetium-99 m) may be injected intravenously, and the heart-liver area may be imaged with a scintillation camera for radioactivity. Normal dogs will have cardiac blood pools and liver blood pools that are confluent, while animals with pericardial effusion will have a clear area of separation between the heart and liver pools. This test is limited in that effusion volumes of less than 150 ml. are difficult to detect.

A more sensitive technique is the use of reflected ultrasound to differentiate the ventricular wall from the pericardial sac. Echocardiography utilizes a transducer that is placed in the left lower fifth intercostal space. Ultrasound waves being transmitted through the heart are partially reflected by ventricular wall-fluid interfaces and are picked up by the transducer. The signals are displayed on an oscilloscope, with the ventricular free wall appearing as a pulsating line. In pericardial effusion another line appears outside the pulsating ventricular free-wall line, this line representing the nonpulsating pericardial sac. The technique is highly sensitive for small quantities of pericardial effusion, and hollow transducers are made which allow pericardiocentesis under precise echocardiographic control.

## TREATMENT

**Pericardiocentesis.** Pericardiocentesis is both a diagnostic technique and a treatment for pericardial effusion. Pericardiocentesis may be used to establish or exclude the presence of pericardial effusion, to relieve the symptoms of cardiac compression and, by clinical pathologic examination, to aid in determining the etiology of effusions that are drained. Ideally, pericardiocentesis should be performed as a confirmatory procedure, after the likelihood of pericardial effusion has been established by thorough physical and supportive examinations.

Dogs in severe congestive heart failure with pulmonary edema and respiratory distress should be treated prior to pericardiocentesis. Oxygen may be supplied by face mask or $O_2$ cage, and rapid intravenous digitalization and diuresis may also be initiated. Low doses of morphine may reduce pulmonary edema and dyspnea while also relieving the apprehension attending the pericardiocentesis. Normally premedication is not required for pericardiocentesis in dogs not in congestive heart failure. Acepromazine® or Demerol® may be used in the apprehensive patient that is not in congestive heart failure.

Prior to performing pericardiocentesis, a small sample of blood should be withdrawn from a peripheral vein. This sample is divided and placed in two tubes, only one of which contains an anticoagulant. The sample without anticoagulant should be noted for length of time until clotting occurs. This will be compared to the fluid removed from the pericardial sac. If the pericardial fluid coagulates in approximately the same amount of time as the untreated blood sample, the effusion fluid is probably blood, and a cardiac tamponade may exist. The peripheral sample with anticoagulant and a pericardial effusion sample with anticoagulant can be examined in the laboratory for the purpose of comparison. If the effusion is pure hemorrhage, the proportion of cellular elements will be similar to that of the peripheral blood sample.

In restraining the dog for pericardiocentesis, the right lateral recumbency position similar to that used for electrocardiography is recommended, except that the front legs are pulled farther cranially. Simultaneous electrocardiographic monitoring is desirable if available.

The lower half of the left hemithorax from the 3rd rib to the costal arch should be clipped and surgically prepared. The site of needle introduction for pericardiocentesis is between the 4th and 6th intercostal spaces on the left at the costochondral junction. Review of the lateral radiograph will be useful in determining which space to use. A 16-gauge Venocath® is usually ideal for making the tap. After infiltrating the puncture site with lidocaine, the Venocath® is disassembled and the plastic wings covering the needle are opened. The needle is attached to a 30- to 60-cc. syringe and the needle is inserted through the posterior part of the intercostal space, care being taken to avoid the costal artery, vein and nerve. The needle is directed at a 45-degree angle, medially and dorsally. Resistance will be felt as the pericardial sac is contacted, and a decided short thrusting motion may be needed to penetrate it.

If the electrocardiogram is being monitored, there will be no abnormalities noted when the needle punctures the pericardium. However, if the myocardium is punctured or the epicardium is encountered, a ventricular premature contraction (VPC) or a series of VPC's will occur. If ectopic beats occur and the needle can be felt to touch the epicardial surface, and no effusion is obtained on aspiration, the existence of gross cardiomegaly rather than pericardial effusion should be considered. If fluid is obtained, enough should be removed so that it can be divided into three samples for examination. One sample should be placed in a sterile tube for culture to determine the presence of infectious agents. Another sample should be placed in a plain tube and

observed for clotting. If clotting readily occurs, or if the third sample, placed in a tube with anticoagulant, resembles the previously drawn peripheral blood sample, the pericardiocentesis should be terminated. If it is evidently not pure blood, the third tube should be submitted for clinical pathological examination, specifically for cytologic examination of the sediment.

The polyethylene catheter, with its guide wire in place, may be inserted through the needle into the pericardial sac if the fluid is not whole blood. The guide wire is removed and the needle is pulled out of the thorax. The plastic wings of the Venocath® are reclosed around the needle to prevent damage to the catheter. A three-way valve is inserted between the syringe and the Venocath® to facilitate removal of large volumes of fluid.

Fluid removal is typically slow through the small-diameter catheter. Changing the dog's body position may be necessary to remove as much fluid as possible. The pericardiocentesis catheter may be used to instill an equal quantity of air for negative contrast pneumopericardiography when as much of the fluid as possible has been removed. By taking lateral, standing lateral and dorsoventral projections, the degree of fluid relief can be assessed and the presence of neoplasia or cysts may be evaluated. The catheter may be removed and prophylactic antibiotics should be administered for several days. Treatment of congestive failure should continue whenever significant dysfunction exists. Reexamination should be performed every 2 to 3 days to determine if the effusion is tending to recur.

**Surgery.**  After one or two repeat pericardiocenteses have failed to correct the accumulation of a nonsanguineous, sterile effusion, surgical intervention may be indicated. Surgery affords the opportunity for exploration of the pericardial sac and thorax as well as for obtaining biopsy material of any abnormal structures found. Creation of a pericardial window of sufficient size to discourage spontaneous closure will allow the pericardial effusion to drain into the pleural space, where it will usually be more readily reabsorbed.

Surgery is the treatment of choice in constrictive pericarditis in which the pericardial space is obliterated by scar tissue, which interferes significantly with cardiac function. Complete pericardiectomy should be performed in these cases. Pericardial cysts may be completely excised. Specific medical therapy should be given if pericardial fluid cultures are positive.

## PROGNOSIS

Pericardial effusion secondary to congestive heart failure responds well to medical management of the primary problem. Benign idiopathic pericardial effusion tends to recur but may respond to repeat pericardiocentesis or a surgically created pericardial window. Effusions due to infection respond depending on the ability to manage the etiologic agent medically. Bloody effusions may disappear spontaneously or may sometimes be surgically corrected; however, most are fatal. Pericardial cysts may respond to surgical intervention. Constrictive pericarditis requires a guarded to poor prognosis. Traumatic rupture of the pericardium and either primary or metastatic neoplasia causing effusions are usually fatal.

### SUPPLEMENTAL READING

Bolton, G. R.: Pericardial diseases. In Ettinger, S. J.: Textbook of Veterinary Internal Medicine. Philadelphia, W. B. Saunders Co., 1975, pp. 1039-1043.
Ettinger, S. J.: Pericardiocentesis. In Symposium on Biopsy Techniques. Vet. Clin. N. Am. 4:403-412, 1974.
Ettinger, S. J., and Suter, P. F.: Canine Cardiology. Philadelphia, W. B. Saunders Co., 1970.
Friedberg, C. K.: Diseases of the Heart. 3rd ed. Philadelphia, W. B. Saunders Co., 1966.

# CANINE MITRAL VALVE DISEASE

N. JOEL EDWARDS, D.V.M.
*Latham, New York*

Of all the conditions producing clinical canine heart disease, those that involve the mitral valve are the most common. If only the acquired cardiovascular diseases are considered, mitral valve disease can be found in approximately 75 per cent of all those patients exhibiting signs of congestive heart failure. The usual cycle of events is the development of mitral valvular insufficiency over a 2- to 6-year period, beginning at 2 to 5 years of age and causing signs of left ventricular failure. This can then proceed to generalized congestive heart failure.

Numerous reports in the veterinary literature have referred to this condition as mitral insufficiency, chronic valvular fibrosis, chronic valvular myxomatosis, valvular endocardiosis, nodular valvitis, warty valve disease or leaky valve disease. In the mid 1960's, Detweiler *et al.* reported the presence of microscopic intramural myocardial arteriosclerosis in association with valvular pathology (fibrosis). These lesions appeared to progress to myocardial necrosis and fibrosis in conjunction with the development of congestive heart failure. The etiology of this syndrome has yet to be defined, and confusion continues to exist over whether the insufficiency of the mitral valve is the result of primary valvular disease or the result of primary myocardial disease affecting the ventricular myocardium, in particular the papillary muscles leading to secondary mitral imcompetence.

Regardless of this confusion, it is possible further to define the problem, its symptomatology and its clinical importance to the practicing veterinarian. It must be kept in mind that this disease condition can involve both the left (mitral) and right (tricuspid) atrioventricular valves and, rarely, the semilunar valves. However, in the dog the mitral valve is by far the most commonly involved, usually becoming insufficient and rarely becoming stenotic. Mitral insufficiency is also seen as a congenital defect due to abnormal leaflet formation and has been reported by Hamlin *et al.* in Afghan and Great Dane pups.

The genetic basis of the congenital type and the predisposition for the acquired type have yet to be determined. Most veterinarians, however, recognize the tendency for acquired mitral valvular insufficiency to occur much more frequently in the smaller breeds, while most larger breeds with mitral insufficiency appear to have primary disease of the myocardium (cardiomyopathy).

Although most acquired mitral insufficiencies are related to chronic valvular fibrosis, other noncongenital alterations of the mitral apparatus must also be considered. These include severe left ventricular enlargement, particularly dilatation, causing dilation of the valve annulus and resulting insufficiency; ruptured chordae tendineae; bacterial endocarditis; ventricular and atrial dysrhythmias; and papillary muscle dysfunction.

To appreciate the action of the mitral valve it is necessary to understand not only the valve leaflets but the entire valve apparatus. This includes the posterior left atrial wall, the mitral valve annulus, the valve leaflets, the chordae tendineae, the papillary muscles and the left ventricular wall (Fig. 1).

The function of each of these components can be visualized if we consider the valve leaflets as being suspended by the annulus between the atrium and ventricle connected by chordae tendineae to the papillary muscles below, which are an extension of the left ventricle wall. During systole, as ventricular pressure rises, the valve leaflets close by overlapping and are in apposition, stopping the flow of blood from regurgitating into the left atrium. The leaflets are prevented from prolapsing up into the atrium by the chordae tendineae which are being kept taut by the papillary muscles. It can be seen that mitral valve action becomes a coordinated effort involving the entire apparatus and that alterations in the function of any part of the apparatus have the potential to produce a "leaky valve." This leakage of blood retrograde into the left atrium produces turbulence which is heard as a murmur on the examination table.

The advent of echocardiography utilizing sound waves has made it possible to evaluate accurately valve leaflet motion during the cardiac cycle. Angiocardiography is also useful in evaluating leaflet motion.

Each of the mitral apparatus components is involved in the pathology of the chronic valvular fibrosis–intramural myocardial heart disease complex resulting in mitral insufficiency. The mitral *valve leaflets* are primarily affected by collagen and myxomatous deposits that result in fibrosis, which causes thickening, nodularity, stiffness and shortening of the valves, making it difficult for the leaflets to overlap and "seal off" the atrium. The *chordae tendineae* undergo this same process, which results in either shortened chordae that restrict valve apposition or elongated weakened chordae that allow the leaflets to prolapse into the atrium or that do not adequately control valve motion, resulting in the "floppy valve" syndrome. As the volume of regurgitant blood increases, dilation of the *left atrium* draws the posterior mitral leaflet further posteriorly and dorsally, making it more difficult to appose the anterior or septal leaflet. As the *left ventricle* begins to enlarge, it causes a dilatation of the annular ring, further pulling the leaflet margins apart. Also as the left ventricle enlarges, the angle at which the papillary muscles anchor the leaflets changes, altering the mobility and direction of the leaflets. As Detweiler *et al.* described in advancing cases of congestive heart failure, myocardial necrosis and fibrosis are seen as sequelae to intramural coronary arteriosclerosis. These changes occur earliest in the papillary muscles and

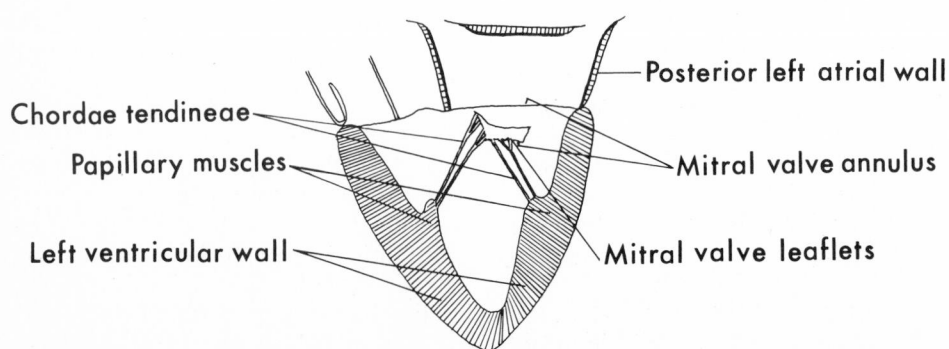

**Figure 1.** The mitral valve apparatus of the heart. (Adapted from Perloff, J. K., and Roberts, W. C.: Circulation 46:227, 1972.)

adjacent left ventricular wall, further compromising their roles in the normal action of the entire valvular apparatus. The extent to which these vascular lesions influence papillary muscle and left ventricular muscle function is yet to be determined.

## CLINICAL FINDINGS

What is observed clinically depends on the stage of development of the previously described process. Problems identified on the physical examination with mitral insufficiency patients include the following:
1. Systolic heart murmur loudest over the 5th–6th intercostal space on the left side of the thorax and frequently radiating over much of the left thorax.
2. Venous distention.
3. Rapid jerky pulse.
4. Pulsus alternans.
5. Nocturnal dyspnea.
6. Tachypnea at rest.
7. Cough.
8. Orthopnea (difficult breathing while lying down).
9. Decreased tolerance to exercise.
10. Cyanosis at rest or on exercise.
11. Enlarged abdomen (as right heart failure becomes part of the syndrome).
12. Rales indicative of pulmonary edema.
13. "Pounding" heartbeat on palpation of thorax.

Radiographic findings may include the following:
1. Normal cardiac silhouette and lung field.
2. Left atrial enlargement.
3. Left ventricular enlargement.
4. Loss of caudal waistline of the cardiac silhouette.
5. Dorsal elevation of the trachea.
6. "Forked" bronchi sign.
7. Dilated pulmonary veins.
8. Pulmonary edema.
9. Pleural effusion. ⎫ As right heart fail-
10. Ascites.          ⎬ ure becomes part
11. Hepatomegaly.  ⎭ of the syndrome.

Electrocardiographic findings may include the following:
1. Within normal limits.
2. Increased heart rate > (180/min.)
3. Left ventricular hypertrophy (LVH).
   a. QRS > 0.05 sec. small breeds.
      > 0.06 sec. large breeds.
   b. $R_{II}$ > 2.5 mv. small breeds.
      > 3.0 mv. large breeds.
   c. MEA* < +40 degrees in frontal plane.
4. P mitrale
   a. $P_{II}$ > 0.04 sec.
5. ST segment repolarization changes.
6. Supraventricular arrhythmias.
7. Ventricular arrhythmias.
8. Development of right ventricular hypertrophy (RVH) later on in the course of the disease.
   a. May shift MEA* to normal.
   b. $Q_{I, II, III, aVF}$ > 0.5 mv.
9. P pulmonale
   $P_{II}$ > 0.4 mv. particularly in toy breeds.

Laboratory findings may include the following:
1. Normal CBC.
2. Slightly increased total RBC.
3. Slightly increased hemoglobin.
4. BUN—Normal or elevated.
5. SGPT—Normal or elevated.
6. SGOT—Normal or elevated.
7. Increased LDH— ⎫ If significant
isoenzymes 1 + 2.    ⎪ myocardial
8. Increased CPK—  ⎬ disease is
isoenzyme MB.          ⎭ present.
9. Decreased total protein.
10. Normal electrolytes (may be altered by treatment).

### Rule-out List
1. Primary respiratory tract disease.
   a. Chronic obstructive respiratory disease (CORD).
   b. Collapsed trachea.
   c. Bronchopneumonia.
   d. Pulmonary neoplasia.
   e. Cor pulmonale.
   f. Heartworm disease.
   g. Tracheobronchitis.
2. Bacterial endocarditis.
3. Congenital heart disease.
   a. PDA with mitral insufficiency.
   b. Aortic stenosis with mitral insufficiency.
   c. Ventricular septal defect (VSD).
   d. Pulmonic stenosis (occasionally).
   e. Congenital mitral insufficiency.
4. Tricuspid insufficiency.
5. Traumatic rupture of chordae tendineae.
6. Canine congestive cardiomyopathy with mitral insufficiency.

---

*MEA = mean electrical activity

7. Pericardial effusion.

8. Neoplasia with metastasis to myocardium.

The differential diagnoses for such a rule-out list are adequately explored elsewhere. The minimal data base should include the following:

1. Signalment: Age, sex, breed.
2. Careful physical examination and classification of the murmur.
3. CBC, urinalysis, fecal exam.
4. Thoracic radiographs.
5. ECG.

## CLASSIFICATION

For purposes of management of the clinical patient with chronic valvular fibrosis–intramural myocardial disease the condition is classified according to clinical signs and physical, radiographic and electrocardiographic findings. There are four classes, and each class correlates with the progressive order of the syndrome discussed earlier.

Young puppies occasionally have vanishing, "innocent" or "physiologic" murmurs. These patients are asymptomatic, have grade 1 to 3/6 early to midsystolic murmurs that can be intermittently present but should disappear by 4 to 6 months of age. The murmurs are best heard around the 5th intercostal space, at or just above the costochondral junction. No therapy is required. If the murmur does not disappear at 6 months of age, these patients should be reevaluated and reclassified accordingly.

Table 1 summarizes the characteristics of these classes of patients seen with mitral insufficiency and the maintenance of each.

**Class I.** Patients in this class are generally 2 years of age or older and have a grade 1 to 3/6 midsystolic or holosystolic murmur that can be heard best at the left 5th intercostal space (ICS), at or just above the costochondral junction. The murmur does not usually radiate very far, and the dogs are asymptomatic. Thoracic radiographs and routine electrocardiograms are usually normal, and no therapy is needed. Follow-up examination should be scheduled in 6 to 12 months, and the client should be advised of the condition.

**Class II.** The class II patient has a grade 2 to 4/6 mid- or holosystolic murmur heard loudest at the left 5th intercostal space, at or slightly below the costochondral junction.

The murmur also tends to radiate downward toward the sternum and may be heard on the right side of the thorax as well as dorsally on the left side of the thorax. They are usually well compensated unless heavily stressed. A mild, persistent, nonresponsive cough may be present, but the class II patient does not experience orthopnea and therefore sleeps well at night. Thoracic radiography usually reveals early left atrial enlargement, mild pulmonary congestion, beginning loss of the caudal waistline of the cardiac silhouette, early left ventricular enlargement and some dorsal elevation of the trachea. The electrocardiogram may be normal or may show some evidence of early left ventricular hypertrophy and ST segment repolarization changes. The mean electrical axis (MEA) in the frontal plane is usually normal. Management of these patients generally includes possible use of a low-sodium diet and of aminophylline 6 to 10 mg./kg. and reevaluation in 3 to 4 months.

**Class III.** The class III patient is beginning to show significant signs of cardiac embarrassment, namely, recurrent cough that does not respond to "home remedies," nocturnal dyspnea, decreased exercise tolerance, panting at rest and decreased activity. The murmur heard is usually grade 3 to 5/6 and is holosystolic and harsh in character. It is heard loudest at the left 6th intercostal space and radiates in all directions over the left thorax. Frequently a left precordial thrill is present. Some signs of pulmonary embarrassment are usually heard as increased vesicular sounds or rales, particularly in the hilar area. Hepatomegaly and splenomegaly may be present. Pulse quality is usually poor, with a jerky pulse most common. Radiography usually reveals tracheal elevation, left atrial and ventricular enlargement and loss of the caudal waistline of the cardiac silhouette. Some rounding of the cardiac silhouette may be present. Pulmonary venous congestion and early or moderate hilar edema will usually be present. Electrocardiography will usually indicate biventricular enlargement, P mitrale and P pulmonale. Occasionally, supraventricular and/or ventricular arrhythmias may also be present.

Management of the class III patient consists of digitalization using digoxin 0.06 to 0.2 mg./kg. divided by four and admin-

*Table 1.*  *Classification of Patients With Mitral Insufficiency*

| CLASS | CLINICAL SIGNS | MURMUR | PULMONARY SYSTEM | X-RAY | ECG | INITIAL Rx | MAINTENANCE | FOLLOW-UP EXAM | PROGNOSIS (LIFE SPAN) |
|---|---|---|---|---|---|---|---|---|---|
| I | None | 1 to 3/6 left 5th ICS, usually 2 years of age or older | Normal | Normal | Normal | None | None | 6 to 12 months | Greater than 4 years |
| II | None unless severely stressed; may have slight cough without orthopnea | 2 to 4/6 left 5th–6th ICS, may have thrill, may radiate | Normal | LVE, slight dorsal elevation of trachea, slight pulmonary congestion | Normal or LVH, ST segment repolarization changes | Outpatient Possible low-sodium diet, aminophylline 6 to 10 mg./kg. t.i.d. | Possible low-sodium diet; be prepared to digitalize as symptoms progress, aminophylline | 3 to 4 months | Greater than 2 years |
| III | Cough, nocturnal dyspnea, decreased exercise tolerance, panting at rest, enlarged abdomen, weak pulse | 3 to 5/6 left 6th ICS, usually has thrill, radiates well | Increased vesicular murmur, hilar rales | Tracheal elevation, LVE, RVE, LAE, loss of caudal cardiac waistline, pulmonary venous congestion, hilar edema | Biventricular enlargement, P mitrale, sometimes P pulmonale, occasional arrhythmia | Hospitalize or outpatient, restrict exercise, low-sodium diet, digitalization, diuretics as needed | Digitalization, low-sodium diet, diuretics as needed, decreased exercise, periodic monitoring of BUN and electrolytes | 14 to 60 days (initial should be in 14 days) | 1 to 2 years |
| IV | Dyspnea usually severe at rest, cough, cyanosis, collapse, weak pulse, enlarged abdomen, hemoptysis | Sometimes difficult to hear heart because of pulmonary sounds, 4 to 6/6 at left 6th–7th ICS | Diffuse rales and loud harsh pulmonary sound heard throughout thorax | LVE, RVE, RAE, LAE, pulmonary edema, elevation of trachea, pleural effusion | As class III with greater prevalence of arrhythmias; take ECG in comfortable position | In hospital emergency $O_2$, cage rest, morphine, rapid digitalization, diuretics, possible phlebotomy | Digitalization, diuretics as needed, restrict exercise, low-sodium diet, watch for organ disease and treat | 14 days, if survive initial class IV crisis | 6 to 12 months, usually less than 6 months |

LVH = left ventricular hypertrophy
LVE = left ventricular enlargement
LAE = left atrial enlargement
RVE = right ventricular enlargement
RAE = right atrial enlargement

istered b.i.d. over 48 hours in the hospital. A maintenance dosage is then calculated as 1/6 to 1/8 of the total dose *used*, and the patient is maintained on the maintenance dosage split b.i.d. Digitalization is determined by an extension of the P-R interval 0.02 second beyond the predigitalization interval or until toxic signs develop, whichever occurs *first*. If the patient cannot be hospitalized, digitalization should consist of administering digoxin at 0.02 mg./kg. split b.i.d., and the owner should be advised to watch for toxic signs. In either case, the patient should return in 14 days from the start of the digitalization period for a follow-up examination and electrocardiogram. Return visits should be scheduled at 30- to 60-day intervals. Adequate clinical work-up *before* digitalization with particular emphasis on liver, kidney and electrolyte status is imperative. As digoxin is thought to be bound to albumin by the liver and excreted as the unchanged glycoside by the kidneys, impairment of either of these organs will alter the removal of digoxin from the body and potentiate toxicity.

In addition, limitation of exercise and low-salt diets are usually necessary for the class III patient. Diuretics used initially and then periodically as needed may be necessary to control pulmonary edema or ascites. Periodic monitoring of electrolytes is advisable while the patient is on both digoxin and diuretics, as decreased serum potassium levels increase myocardial sensitivity to the digitalis glycosides. Cough depressants may also be needed to control excessive coughing spasms.

**Class IV.** The class IV patient is in emergency status with dyspnea, hemoptysis, cyanosis, pulmonary edema and collapse as the presenting signs resulting from uncompensated heart failure. These patients should be placed immediately into an oxygen cage and given therapy with a minimum of handling. Morphine sulfate, 0.5 to 1.0 mg./kg. SC, is administered initially followed by furosemide (Lasix®), 4.0 mg./kg. IV or IM. Intravenous digoxin, 0.01 to 0.02 mg./kg., can be administered slowly with constant monitoring and a maintenance dosage of 0.01 mg./kg. orally b.i.d. initiated in two hours. When monitoring the class IV patient, do not force him to remain recumbent but take the electrocardiogram in the standing or sitting position. If the initial therapy is inadequate, phlebotomy to remove a blood volume of 8 to 10 ml./kg. of body weight may be indicated. Radiography and further physical examination are withheld until stabilization is achieved, at which point the patient is handled like the class III patient. When examined, the class IV patient will exhibit varying degrees of respiratory distress. It is difficult to auscultate cardiac sounds owing to pulmonary edema, and the pulse is usually very weak and rapid. Radiographically, extensive pulmonary edema and cardiomegaly are usually present. Electrocardiograms show class III patterns with frequent arrhythmias, particularly supraventricular arrhythmias.

In working with the chronic mitral fibrosis–myocardial syndrome it is important not to condemn the class I and II dog to an early death while at the same time keeping in mind the severity of the possible progressive development to classes III and IV. It is also imperative to consider the hemodynamic consequences of pump (heart) failure with respect to coexisting disease states that may present therapeutic or dietary enigmas or that may alter an initial therapeutic regime that was previously adequate.

## SUPPLEMENTAL READING

Bolton, G. R.: Handbook of Canine Electrocardiography. Philadelphia, W. B. Saunders Co., 1975.

Detweiler, D. K., *et al.*: The natural history of acquired cardiac disability of the dog. Ann. N.Y. Acad. Sci., *147*:318, 1968.

Ettinger, S. J., and Suter, P. F.: Canine Cardiology. Philadelphia, W. B. Saunders Co., 1970.

Fisher, G. C., Wessel, H. U., and Sommers, H. M.: Mitral insufficiency following experimental papillary muscle infarction. Am. Heart J., *83*:382–388.

Frater, R. W. M., and Ellis, F. H.: The anatomy of the canine mitral valve. J. Surg. Res., *1*:171–179, 1961.

Hamlin, R. L., *et al.*: Congenital mitral insufficiency in the dog. J. Am. Vet. Med. Assn., *146*:1088–1100, 1965.

Harpster, N. K.: Chronic valvular myocardial heart disease in dogs. In Kirk, R. W. (ed.): Current Veterinary Therapy V. Philadelphia, W. B. Saunders Co., 1974.

Liu, S., and Tilley, L. P.: Malformation of the canine mitral valve complex. J. Am. Vet. Med. Assn., *167*:465–471, 1975.

Perloff, J. K., and Roberts, W. C.: The mitral apparatus. Circulation, *46*:227–239, 1972.

# MYOCARDIAL DISEASES IN DOGS

PHILLIP N. OGBURN, D.V.M.
*St. Paul, Minnesota*

The cardiomyopathies or diseases of the myocardium recently have received widespread attention in veterinary medicine because of their presence in certain systemic disorders as an apparent intrinsic idiopathic or primary disease and because of similarities to the spectrum of disease occurring in man.

Attempts to classify or categorize these diseases in dogs have paralleled the development of cardiomyopathy classification in man. Cardiomyopathies may be best classified for clinical purposes into those diseases which develop for unknown reasons, primary cardiomyopathy, and those which develop from known causes, secondary cardiomyopathies (Table 1). There are two basic types of primary cardiomyopathy in dogs: a congestive and a hypertrophic form. Congestive cardiomyopathy is the most common form of primary cardiomyopathy and is characterized by an idiopathic dilatation of all cardiac chambers. The hypertrophic form, possibly analogous to idiopathic subaortic stenosis in man and hypertrophic cardiomyopathy in cats, is manifest as a pronounced thickening of the left ventricular wall. This disease, which alters the size and configuration of the ventricular lumen, has only recently been recognized.

Secondary cardiomyopathies are often myocardial diseases of complex etiology which may be caused by specific infectious agents or by severe noninfectious systemic disease. The myocardial involvement, while secondary to the initiating disease, may complicate the clinical course and may require specific treatment. The diseases listed in Table 1, while not inclusive of all diseases which may secondarily involve the myocardium, include the ones most likely to be encountered in practice. Not enough data have been accumulated to allow a detailed consideration of hypertrophic cardiomyopathy.

The clinical features produced by myocardial disease may be extremely diverse because of the differing pathophysiologic mechanisms involved in the development of these diseases and because of the variable extent of anatomic or biochemical injury to the myocardium. A positive diagnosis of myocardial disease can be made only from the development of signs and symptoms of heart failure in the absence of preexisting heart disease which may occur during the course of an infectious disease or major systemic disorder or from unknown causes.

The initial manifestations of myocardial disease may be acute or may develop slowly. Frequently, myocardial disease is suspected because one or more of the following clinical signs is observed:

1. Arrhythmias.
2. Intracardiac conduction abnormalities, i.e., bundle-branch block, AV block, ST segment deviation.
3. Cardiac chamber enlargement (atrial or ventricular).
4. Pericardial effusion, cardiac tamponade, pericardial friction rubs.
5. Murmurs.
6. Congestive heart failure (right and/or left).

Because of differences in the clinical syndrome, breeds affected, incidence and pathophysiology, the primary and secondary cardiomyopathies will be considered separately.

*Table 1.  Etiologic Classification of Cardiomyopathy in Dogs*

| |
|---|
| *Primary Myocardial Disease* |
|    Canine congestive cardiomyopathy |
|      (idiopathic cardiomyopathy) |
|    Canine hypertrophic cardiomyopathy |
| *Secondary Myocardial Disease* |
|    Ischemic—Microscopic intramural myocardial |
|      infarction |
|    Infectious—Bacterial, protozoan, viral |
|    Neoplastic—Aortic-body tumors, |
|      hemangiosarcoma, etc. |
|    Metabolic—Uremia, hypothyroidism |
|    Toxic—Digitalis, anesthetics |

## PRIMARY MYOCARDIAL DISEASE

### CONGESTIVE CARDIOMYOPATHY (Idiopathic)

Canine congestive cardiomyopathy is considered to be an idiopathic myocardial disease of large or giant breed dogs in which primary myocardial weakness results in marked atrial and ventricular dilatation, secondary atrioventricular valve incompetence and congestive heart failure accompanied by atrial fibrillation. The disease usually develops in male dogs between the ages of 1 and 5 years; however, diagnosis has been made in animals as young as 4 months and as old as 11 years. The breeds with the highest frequency of occurrence are, in order of their prevalence: the Great Dane, St. Bernard, German shepherd and Irish wolfhound. Other breeds in which the diagnosis has been made include the Newfoundland, Afghan hound, English bulldog, Great Pyrenees, English setter, Doberman pinscher, Scottish deerhound, collie, bouvier des Flandres and standard poodle.

The disease is progressive and signs of right heart failure usually develop before symptoms of left heart failure occur. In contrast to chronic atrioventricular valvular disease, dogs with congestive cardiomyopathy do not have significant valvular fibrosis. Figure 1 provides a schematic overview of the associated factors in this disease.

The life expectancy of the affected animal depends on the degree of myocardial damage. Although some dogs die suddenly even after failure has been effectively controlled, most dogs will experience a disease process which may last from 6 months to 1½ years. An occasional animal may live longer.

### CLINICAL SYNDROME

Affected dogs in early stages of the disease may show no outward clinical signs. More often nonspecific signs of illness, such as lethargy, anorexia, weight loss and fatigue, are initial indicators of disease. With advanced deterioration the dog may show emaciation, labored breathing, cough, a distended abdomen, limb edema, weakness and collapse.

Although this disease affects the entire myocardium, signs of right heart failure usually predominate. Ascites, systemic venous engorgement and prominent jugular pulses are common.

Characteristically, physical examination reveals the presence of severe tachyarrhythmias, commonly atrial fibrillation which causes a wide variation in the rate and amplitude of the heart sounds. The first heart sound may be the only sound of the cardiac cycle which can be heard consistently. While systolic murmurs of AV valvular insufficiency occur in this disease, they are often not fully appreciated because of ventricular rates in excess of 180 beats per

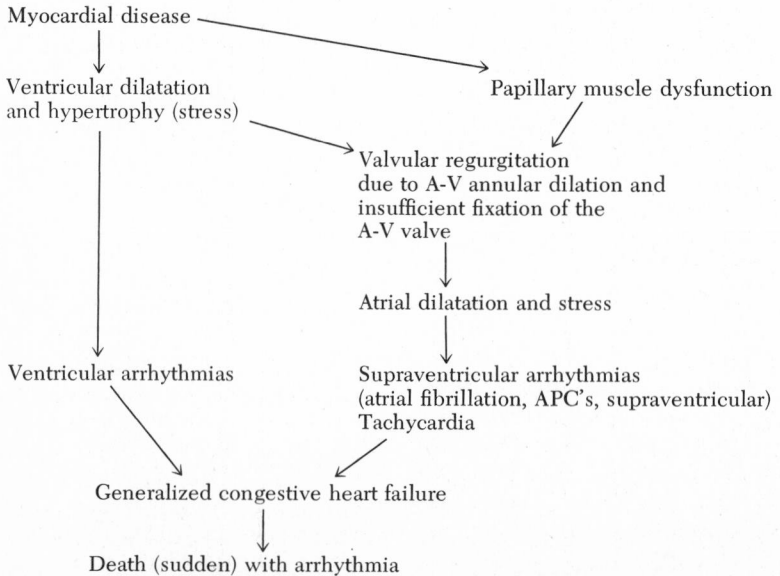

**Figure 1.** Proposed pathogenetic mechanism of congestive cardiomyopathy. (Modified from Ettinger, 1975.)

ninute. Diastolic gallops may appear prior o the development of arrhythmias and are a ign of ventricular dilatation. Pleural and pericardial effusion may muffle respiratory and cardiac sounds in addition to compromising pulmonary and cardiac function.

Radiographically, typical signs of bilateral congestive heart failure are present. Right and left heart enlargement accompanied by interstitial pulmonary edema, pleural effusion, hepatomegaly and ascites is usually observed. The cardiac silhouette, although enlarged because of cardiac dilatation and possible pericardial effusion, is, however, often indistinct because of hydrothorax and pulmonary edema. The left atrial border is usually prominent, displacing the left main bronchus dorsally. The posterior vena cava may become widened and elevated.

Although electrocardiographic parameters in giant breed dogs are slightly different from those in other breeds, patterns which suggest left ventricular enlargement, biventricular enlargement, generalized atrial enlargement and rhythm disturbances are often found. Atrial fibrillation is the most common arrhythmia and is characterized by a loss of normal P waves, irregular baseline undulations and rapid, irregularly spaced ventricular (QRS) complexes. Atrial and ventricular premature contractions occur in approximately 20 per cent of the cases.

Clinical blood chemistries are usually unchanged except that low serum protein levels, hypoalbuminemia and slight rises in BUN and SGPT may be found. Urinalysis does not usually reveal abnormalities, although occasional dogs may have proteinuria. Total urinary output may be reduced. Selective angiography may demonstrate secondary mitral and tricuspid valvular incompetence which occurs coincident with atrial and ventricular dilatation.

### DIFFERENTIAL DIAGNOSIS

Congestive cardiomyopathy should be distinguished from other diseases which may have similar clinical signs. Because congenital atrioventricular valvular complex anomalies and endocardial fibroelastosis have been confirmed in some of the involved breeds, notably the Great Dane, caution must be exercised when making the diagnosis of congestive cardiomyopathy in young animals. The differentiation of these diseases in young dogs is difficult, and even

with cardiac catheterization and angiography one may not be certain of the diagnosis. Frequently the diagnosis is made at necropsy.

Primary acquired atrioventricular valve fibrosis which results in mitral or tricuspid insufficiency in many large and small breeds is usually detected in older animals before clinical evidence of heart failure occurs. Mitral insufficiency, which is usually the most severe of the two, is characterized by a left apical holosystolic murmur. The resulting left heart failure from mitral insufficiency brings on clinical signs such as cough and dyspnea. Although most older dogs with acquired valvular disease have a normal sinus rhythm, arrhythmias such as atrial and ventricular premature contractions are frequently observed. Atrial fibrillation is not as commonly identified in AV valvular disease as it is in congestive cardiomyopathy.

Bacterial endocarditis, pericarditis, dirofilariasis and diseases which produce secondary cardiomyopathy are other conditions which must be considered when making a diagnosis of congestive cardiomyopathy.

### GROSS PATHOLOGY

The heart appears to be enlarged with all chambers dilated and relatively thin-walled. The total cardiac mass does not seem appreciably greater than normal. Significant AV valvular fibrosis is uncommon and AV annular dilatation is consistently present. Although most hearts show no gross myocardial changes, myocardial fibrosis, small intramural myocardial infarcts, ruptured chordae tendineae and endocardial jet lesions may be noted.

### THERAPY

In all cases of heart failure the primary objective of treatment is to restore cardiac capacity to near normal levels, i.e., to restore cardiac compensation. Relief of congestive signs may occur following the use of digitalis glycosides alone. Digitalis increases ventricular contractility, prolongs atrioventricular conduction and slows the heart rate. Prolongation of AV conduction is very important in patients with atrial fibrillation, in which ventricular rates may be so rapid that the time for ventricular filling is severely shortened. Digitalis, through its nodal effect, may effectively reduce the ventricular rate. Digoxin is the most effective digitalis glycoside for the treatment of this condition. Because most animals are presented in severe congestive heart failure, a regimen of rapid digitalization is usually initiated following hospitalization (see pp. 329 to 339).

In certain cases, the use of digoxin alone may not be adequate to control heart failure. Diuretics which reduce blood volume by promoting sodium diuresis may be required to improve circulatory capability. The thiazide diuretics are preferred in the less acute case in which rapid diuresis is not necessary (see p. 328). Furosemide is a particularly rapid-acting and potent diuretic and is best reserved for severe congestive states in which a rapid diuresis is necessary. During intensive treatment with Lasix®, dehydration may occur even though pulmonary edema or ascites persists. The serum electrolytes, sodium and potassium, may become depleted during the use of diuretics and therefore electrolyte concentrations should be routinely monitored, particularly when the use of high levels of diuretics is necessary. Signs of electrolyte depletion include weakness, trembling, stupor and vomition and develop more rapidly when animals are fully digitalized.

Antiarrhythmic agents, such as propranolol (Inderal®) quinidine sulfate (Quinidex®, Quinaglute®), procainamide (Pronestyl®) and lidocaine, may be necessary to control various rhythm disturbances. Propranolol, a beta-adrenergic blocking agent, given orally every 4 to 6 hours at a dose of 10 to 80 mg. depending on the animal's size and response, may aid in controlling extremely rapid ventricular rates which cannot be controlled with digoxin alone. Propranolol prolongs the AV conduction time, thereby reducing the ventricular rate. The *negative* inotropic function of this compound does not seem to have a serious effect on fully digitalized patients at normal therapeutic doses but caution should still be exercised when its use is contemplated. Propranolol is also particularly effective in controlling digitalis-induced arrhythmias.

Quinidine, procainamide and lidocaine may be employed to control serious ventricular arrhythmias. Although quinidine is particularly effective in converting atrial fibrillation to normal sinus rhythm, it frequently is necessary to use such high levels

that toxicity is a problem. More commonly reversal of atrial fibrillation is achieved with external DC cardioversion in conjunction with quinidine therapy. Unfortunately conversion to normal sinus rhythm is usually temporary, and electrical cardioversion should be reserved for those patients who radiographically show little cardiomegaly and therefore have the best chance for long-term survival.

## SECONDARY MYOCARDIAL DISEASE

Many clinical cases of secondary myocardial disease are not recognized by clinicians because the symptoms are masked or compounded by the initial disease. More frequent diagnoses of myocardial involvement come from the knowledge of disease syndromes which may affect the heart and of their distinguishing factors.

The electrocardiogram, which may provide evidence of myocardial disease by showing arrhythmias, conduction disorders and ST segment changes, still does not provide clues to the etiology. Other specialized examinations such as radiography, hematology, organ biochemistry, culture, biopsy and cardiac catheterization can provide important information which may be employed in addition to a careful physical and history to yield a more definitive diagnosis.

### ISCHEMIC MYOCARDIAL DISEASE

Dogs are afflicted with arteriosclerotic disease involving the small intramural myocardial arteries of the heart. This pathologic condition involves hyalinization of the arterial intima and media, thereby reducing the arterial lumina and progressively limiting blood flow to the adjacent myocardium. Ischemic changes may be detected electrocardiographically as arrhythmias or as ST-segment deviations.

The parallel development of valvular and myocardial disease in aging dogs depresses the hemodynamic efficiency of the heart and allows the development of congestive heart failure. Major arteriolar disease has also been reported in congenital aortic and pulmonic stenosis.

Specific therapy for this form of disease has not been developed in dogs, since there are no clinical means to determine its sever ity. The use of digitalis glycosides which reduce heart rate and ventricular end-diastolic pressure indirectly augments ventricular myocardial blood flow.

## INFECTIOUS MYOCARDIAL DISEASE (MYOCARDITIS)

Myocarditis is an inflammatory myocardial disease which may have acute or chronic stages. Myocarditis may be caused by bacterial (Staphylococcus, Streptococcus, *E. coli*, etc.), protozoan (Toxoplasma, Trypanosoma) and unknown viral agents. It is frequently observed in conjunction with bacterial endocarditis and generalized septicemias.

The physical signs of disease in myocarditis are similar to those found in any myocardial disorder. The severity of signs usually depends upon whether the disease is acute or chronic and upon the severity of the primary disease. In cases of acute myocarditis there may be no symptoms other than fever or depression, and no abnormality of the heart may be disclosed on physical examination. Presenting symptoms related to myocarditis may be labored breathing, gagging, weakness, recurrent fever, signs of pulmonary congestion or pneumonia, failure to thrive or obvious congestive heart failure. Congestive heart failure may be of sudden onset and may be refractory to treatment. Sudden death may be observed.

Next to electrocardiographic evidence of myocardial disease, thoracic radiography may reveal signs of chamber enlargement. Most radiographic changes in myocarditis are minimal and do not allow appreciable differentiation from other cardiac-related diseases. Systolic murmurs and diastolic gallop rhythms of sudden onset are significant when they are auscultated in dogs that previously had no detectable auscultatory abnormalities.

When symptoms of cardiac involvement occur during any infection or systemic disease, myocarditis must be suspected. The appearance of congestive heart failure during the course of an acute or chronic infection in an animal without previous heart disease is virtually pathognomonic of myocarditis.

Laboratory tests which identify specific myocardial involvement are not available; the use of blood cultures and sensitivity testing are advised when evidence of bacteremia exists.

Chagas' disease is a chronic protozoan disease caused by *Trypanosoma cruzi*, which is transmitted, at least in man, by an insect vector. The organism invades many tissues but it shows a predilection for the myocardium. The clinical features are usually associated with a chronic myocarditis resulting in congestive heart failure. The disease in the United States is confined to the Southwest. Electrocardiographic abnormalities and heart failure may be the only features clinically observed.

Myocardial involvement is frequently noted pathologically in Toxoplasma infections but rarely does the disease result in clinically detectable myocardial damage. Toxoplasmosis should be considered when other common causes of myocarditis have been ruled out.

The primary objective of treatment is to eliminate the source of infection or toxemia while treating failure and controlling signs of disease, such as arrhythmias. In bacterial myocarditis, specific antibiotic therapy is indicated, with concomitant use of digitalis, diuretics and antiarrhythmic drugs as indicated for each individual condition. Prolonged treatment of several weeks to months with appropriate antibiotic therapy and symptomatic support is sometimes necessary to control the condition. Relapses after cessation of treatment are not uncommon. Repeat CBC's, blood culture, electrocardiograms and radiographs are helpful in judging the course of the disease and the dog's response to treatment.

## NEOPLASTIC MYOCARDIAL DISEASE

Neoplastic involvement of the heart, whether primary or secondary, is reported to occur in 5.5 per cent of all cases of cardiovascular disease in the dog. The clinical features of cardiac neoplasia will vary depending on the extent of myocardial involvement or on the degree of chamber or vessel obstruction. Neoplasms of the heart may be classified as either primary or secondary (metastatic) tumors.

Tumors originating from cardiac structures, i.e., primary tumors of the heart, are uncommon. The most frequently observed primary tumors are aortic-body tumors, sarcomas, fibromas and rhabdomyomas.

Aortic-body tumors (chemodectomas) arise from specialized chemoreceptor tissue in the aortic arch. The site of the tumor in the periadventitial tissue between the aorta and the pulmonary artery often gives rise to the general diagnosis of heart-base tumor. It should be remembered that other tumors such as malignant lymphoma and aberrant thyroid and parathyroid tissue may be identified in a similar location. Although the tumor is slow-growing, it may invade the right atrium and metastasize to the lung and thoracic lymph nodes.

Male dogs over 8 years of age of the brachycephalic breeds—Boston terrier, boxer and English bulldog—are especially predisposed to this tumor, although it is certainly not confined to those breeds. Clinical signs of the disease are manifest as alterations resulting from pericardial effusion, vascular obstruction and congestive heart failure.

Large masses encroaching on the anterior mediastinum may displace the esophagus and trachea. Selective angiography may demonstrate the tumor indirectly by showing alteration of chamber and vessel configuration or may illustrate the tumor directly by opacifying the mass with contrast media. Attempts at surgical correction are generally unsuccessful.

Cardiac fibromas may arise from valves, where they appear as small, nonmalignant papillary tumor masses, or they may arise from the stroma of the myocardium. Accurate diagnosis depends largely on angiographic filling defects within the heart.

Sarcomas are the most common malignant primary cardiac tumors in dogs. In contrast to other tumors of the heart such as fibromas and aortic-body tumors, which are largely nonmalignant, sarcomas are predominantly intramural, i.e., they arise from the stroma and invade the myocardium of the atria or ventricles. The clinical features of invasive tumors of the myocardium involve congestive heart failure, pulmonary disease and rapidly progressive deterioration. Metastasis is primarily to the lung.

Hemangiosarcomas frequently arise from primary sites in the spleen and metastasize to the heart in older dogs, particularly the German shepherd. Primary hemangiosarcomas may originate in the right atrium near the coronary groove at the entrance to the right auricle. Widespread metastasis to other organs, especially to the lung, have been observed in tumors originating from the heart and the spleen.

Lymphosarcomas may invade the myocardium and result in reduction of cardiac performance, culminating in congestive heart failure. The deterioration of cardiac performance may alter the course of proposed therapy for the malignancy.

Carcinomas arising from various organs in the body may metastasize to the heart, particularly the right atrium.

## METABOLIC MYOCARDITIS ASSOCIATED WITH SYSTEMIC DISEASE

Pericarditis and myocarditis resulting in congestive heart failure without evidence of valvular disease have been recognized in dogs with systemic lupus erythematosus. The typical dog with SLE develops autoimmune hemolytic anemia, thrombocytopenic purpura and glomerulonephritis. Dermatitis, polyarthritis and thyroiditis may also be noted. The diagnosis of SLE is made upon finding positive LE cells on serial tests along with the presence of antinuclear antibodies (LE prep). Additionally Coombs' test or a test for complement fixing antibodies to DNA-histone complexes or the rheumatoid factor may prove diagnostic. Low levels of corticosteroids have been effective in controlling the disease in most cases.

Severe kidney disease may result in secondary myocardial and valvular degeneration, fibrosis and mineralization. The manifestations of such involvement vary from mild myocardial degeneration with cardiac enlargement to severe mineralization of the myocardium and valves (usually aortic and mitral). The onset of systolic murmurs which may change in quality and intensity with increasing valvular damage signals the involvement of cardiac structures in the disease. Congestive heart failure is a frequent complication of major myocardial and valvular disease.

Hypothyroidism may cause a nonspecific cardiomegaly and symptoms of congestive heart failure. Those animals in whom T-values have been 1.0 μg. or less have responded to l-thyroxine with resolution of their congestive patterns. These animals had largely been unresponsive to digitalization before thyroid therapy.

## TOXIC CARDIOMYOPATHY

Toxic cardiomyopathies, or myocardial disease caused by drugs, endotoxins, electrolyte imbalance, etc., constitute a group in which it is difficult to show direct evidence of myocardial involvement. In many cases myocardial depression is detected only by careful analysis of sequential electrocardiograms or by careful monitoring of ventricular contractility or cardiac output. When death occurs as a result of this type of myocardial disease, there are no detectable gross or microscopic myocardial lesions.

Digitalis intoxication, Addison's disease (hyperkalemia), hypokalemia, anesthetic overdose, shock and many other similar conditions can severely compromise cardiac performance. The signs of these conditions—AV block and premature ventricular contractions in digitalis toxicity; bradycardia, atrial standstill and tall peaked T waves in hyperkalemia; prolongation of the Q-T interval, small biphasic T waves and muscular weakness in hypokalemia; reduction of heart sounds, bradycardia and a decline in arterial pressure in anesthetic overdose; pallor, poor perfusion even though fluid volume has been restored and weakened heart sounds in shock—may help to differentiate the cause of myocardial depression.

### SUPPLEMENTAL READING

Dear, M. G.: Myocardial diseases. In Kirk, R. W. (ed.): Current Veterinary Therapy V. Philadelphia, W. B. Saunders Co., 1974.

Ettinger, S. J., and Suter, P. F.: Canine Cardiology. Philadelphia, W. B. Saunders Co., 1970.

Ettinger, S. J.: Diseases of the myocardium. In Ettinger, S. J. (ed.): Textbook of Veterinary Internal Medicine. Philadelphia, W. B. Saunders Co., 1975.

Fregin, G. F., Luginbuhl, H., and Guarda, F.: Myocardial infarction in a dog with bacterial endocarditis. J. Am. Vet. Med. Assn., 160:956, 1972.

Goodwin, J. F.: Congestive and hypertrophic cardiomyopathies. A decade of study. Lancet, 1:731, 1970.

Luginbuhl, H., and Detweiler, D. K.: Cardiovascular lesions in dogs. Ann. N.Y. Acad. Sci., 127:517, 1965.

Perloff, J. K.: The cardiomyopathies–Current perspectives. Circulation, 44:942, 1971.

# FELINE CARDIO-MYOPATHY

LAWRENCE P. TILLEY, D.V.M.
New York, New York

A review of clinical experience and the necropsy records at The Animal Medical Center in New York revealed that heart disease is an important clinical entity in the cat. Cardiomyopathy, in which the basic abnormality is in the heart muscle rather than in the valves or some other part of the heart, accounts for approximately 95 per cent of acquired heart disease in cats. This paper will consider the etiology, classification, clinical features, electrocardiography and thoracic radiography of two forms of cardiomyopathy. Its main purpose will be to establish firm criteria for diagnosis and a firm basis for therapy of cardiomyopathy.

## ETIOLOGIC AND CLINICAL CLASSIFICATION

Cardiomyopathy may be either primary or secondary. The primary cardiomyopathies are myocardial diseases of unknown causes. Secondary cardiomyopathies are those in which the myocardial involvement is secondary to a systemic illness. Table 1 outlines a combined etiologic and clinical classification of cardiomyopathy in the cat.

Primary cardiomyopathy, both "congestive" and "hypertrophic," represents the most common forms of the disease in the cat. Both these forms can also be classified according to the combined nature of the hemodynamic fault and accompanying pathology (Fig. 1). Congestive cardiomyopathy is manifested by a dilated flabby heart with resultant failure of the heart as a pump. The important features in the hypertrophic form of cardiomyopathy are massive hypertrophy, resistance to filling of the ventricles, small ventricular size and often obstruction to the outflow tract from the left ventricle.

Primary cardiomyopathy was diagnosed

**Table 1.**  *Known Etiologic and Clinical Classification of Feline Cardiomyopathies*

*Primary Cardiomyopathy*
  Congestive
    Idiopathic
  Hypertrophic (familial? and nonfamilial)
    Obstructive
    Nonobstructive
*Secondary Cardiomyopathy*
  Myocarditis
    Viral, suspected on the basis of clinical
      evidence and histopathology
  Vascular disease (ischemic cardiomyopathy),
    association seen with diabetes mellitus
  Hypertrophic cardiomyopathy
    Secondary to chronic renal disease and
      associated arterial hypertension
    Secondary to chronic anemia
  Neoplastic diseases (myocardial infiltration,
    mass compression of major vessels)

in 251 of 3745 cats examined at necropsy at The Animal Medical Center from January, 1962, to April, 1974; 182 of 251 cats (73 per cent) had the hypertrophic form and 69 of 251 cats (27 per cent) had the congestive form. Over 40 per cent of the cats affected with either form of the disease had thromboembolism at necropsy.

## HYPERTROPHIC CARDIOMYOPATHY

### CLINICAL FEATURES

Cats in this group have left ventricular hypertrophy with or without muscular ventricular outflow obstruction. Cats can be affected at any age, but hypertrophic cardiomyopathy is most common in young (over one year) and middle-aged adults. More male than female cats are affected. Based on present clinical evaluations, the Persian cat appears to be one of the breeds for which this disease shows a predilection. Dyspnea is the most frequently occurring clinical sign, because of either pain from thromboemboli or pulmonary edema due to heart failure. Other signs include acute posterior paralysis, lethargy and anorexia. Sudden death is also frequent.

On physical examination, cats with severe left ventricular hypertrophy will often have an exaggeration of the normal left ventricular thrust on palpation of the thorax. Moist rales, cardiac murmurs, gallop rhythms and arrhythmias are frequently auscultated. A fourth heart sound or atrial gallop is a common finding and is often direct evidence of the hemodynamic features of this disease. The stiffness or reduced distensibility of the greatly thickened ventricles will interfere with passive ventricular filling. A vigorous atrial contraction is then required for proper ventricular filling.

### ELECTROCARDIOGRAPHY

The electrocardiogram is helpful in the diagnosis of hypertrophic cardiomyopathy, since a normal tracing is unusual. Many of the tracings have axis deviations with abnormalities of duration and amplitude of the QRS complexes, indicating left ventricular hypertrophy. The most important electrocardiographic feature is the frequent occurrence of intraventricular conduction defects. Conduction disturbances include left bundle-branch block, Wolff-Parkinson-White syndrome and left anterior hemiblock. Left anterior hemiblock, a block of the anterior division of the left bundle, is the most frequently occurring conduction disturbance in the hypertrophic form of cardiomyopathy (Fig. 2).

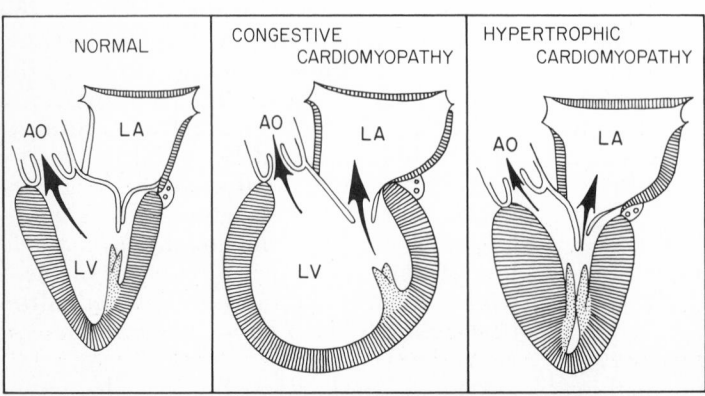

**Figure 1.**  *Left,* normal left ventricle is shown for comparison. *Center,* congestive cardiomyopathy is represented by poor myocardial contractility with dilatation of heart chambers. *Right,* hypertrophic cardiomyopathy represents severe left ventricular hypertrophy, resulting in impaired ventricular distensibility and compliance. (From Tilley, L. P., and Liu, S.-K.: Feline Pract., 5:33, 1975. Illustration by Loretta Tilley.)

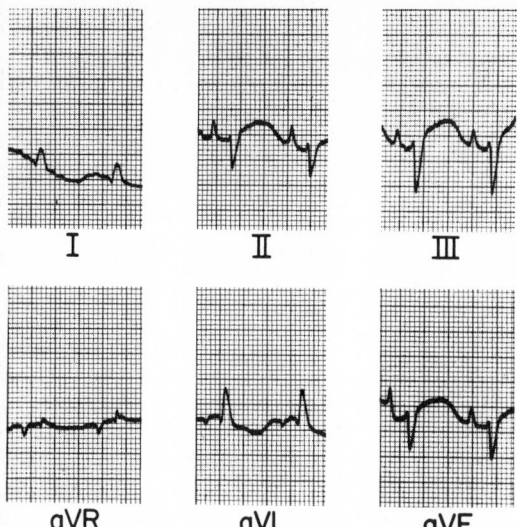

I            II            III

aVR            aVL            aVF

**Figure 2.** Electrocardiogram recorded from a 5-year-old Persian cat with acute dyspnea. The mean electrical axis illustrates a severe left axis deviation. This is consistent with a complete block of the anterior fascicle of the left bundle. This results in a qR in leads I and aVL and S in leads II, III and aVF to complete the criteria. This pattern is commonly associated with hypertrophic cardiomyopathy. (Paper speed = 50 mm./sec.; 1 cm. = 1 mv.)

## RADIOGRAPHY

Cardiomegaly is evident on thoracic radiographs in almost all cats with hypertrophic cardiomyopathy. Left and right atrial enlargement is predominantly seen, because of the resistance of the ventricles to distention due to hypertrophy. In cats with cardiac decompensation, extracardiac signs of left-sided heart failure are primarily represented by pulmonary congestion or edema.

## TREATMENT

**Therapeutic Principles.** The primary hemodynamic disturbance in hypertrophic cardiomyopathy is a resistance to left ventricular filling, causing clinical signs in most cats. Figure 3B illustrates the hemodynamics in a 3-year-old cat with hypertrophic cardiomyopathy who had an obstruction to left ventricular filling. The left ventricular end-diastolic pressure (EDP) is elevated to 40 mm. Hg, more than 8 times normal (mean = 4.5 mm. Hg) (Fig. 3A). An elevated EDP has been a consistent finding in cats with hypertrophic cardiomyopathy. Two factors are mainly responsible for the impeded diastolic filling of the ventricles. First, the severe hypertrophy of the left ventricle causes a reduction in the size of the lumen. Second, there is a loss in the distensibility of the ventricular myocardium, impeding the normal relaxation of the ventricle in diastole and interfering with the inflow of blood from the atria.

Based on these findings, the natural history of hypertrophic cardiomyopathy can be constructed (Fig. 4). Stress and tachycardia appear to be important precipitating factors in producing acute dyspnea and pulmonary edema. Owing to the thick hypertrophied left ventricle, an obstruction to left ventricu-

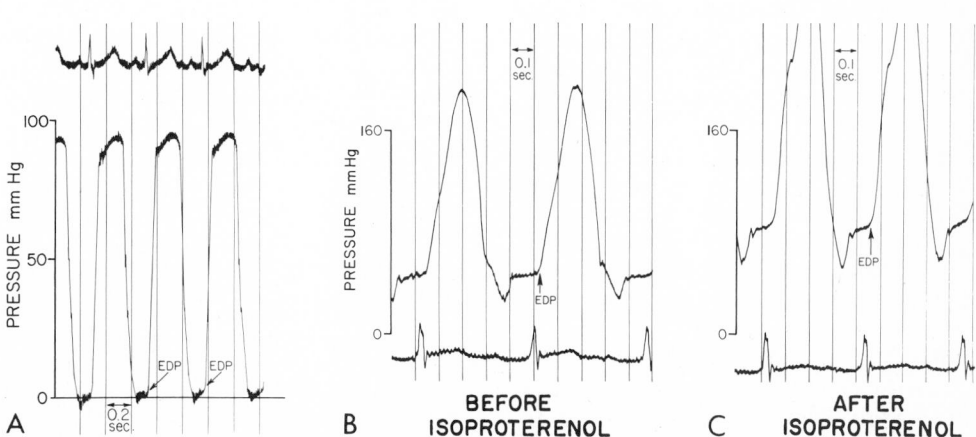

A            B  BEFORE ISOPROTERENOL            C  AFTER ISOPROTERENOL

**Figure 3.** Left ventricular pressure tracing (A) from a normal 2-year-old cat. The end-diastolic pressure (EDP) is less than 5 mm. Hg. Left ventricular pressure tracing in a cat with hypertrophic cardiomyopathy before (B) and after (C) the infusion of isoproterenol (Isuprel®). Isoproterenol (a beta-adrenergic stimulating agent) simulates a stress situation and causes a rise in left ventricular end-diastolic pressure. This drug response is an almost unique feature of hypertrophic cardiomyopathy.

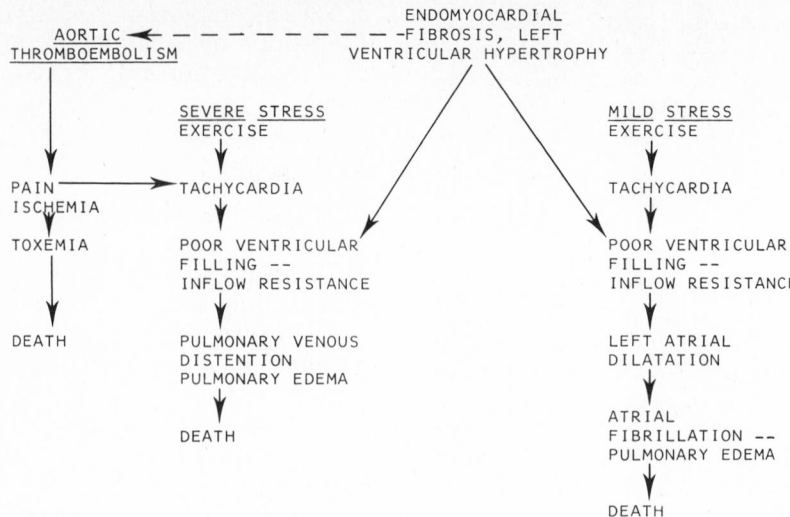

**Figure 4.** Proposed natural history of hypertrophic cardiomyopathy with or without aortic thromboembolism.

lar filling exists. A tachycardia produced by stress or exercise shortens diastolic filling time and further limits diastolic filling. Cardiac output decreases because the tachycardia is insufficient to compensate for the drop in stroke volume caused by poor filling. Pulmonary congestion and edema with dyspnea result from mitral regurgitation. If the disease progresses gradually, the left atrium will enlarge to increase its reservoir capacity. Atrial fibrillation with subsequent pulmonary edema and death may eventually occur. Aortic thromboembolism itself is a cause of stress and tachycardia because of the pain and shock produced. Dyspnea, pulmonary congestion and edema are often quickly reversed with rest and medication aimed at slowing the heart rate. This reflects the flexible nature of the EDP, depending on the momentary hemodynamic condition.

**Hemodynamic Studies.** The elevated left EDP not only reflects the severity of the disease but is the main determinant of clinical signs and prognosis. With this in mind, drug studies were done to establish a treatment regimen for the reduction of left ventricular inflow resistance and to increase the rate of filling of the left ventricle.

Isoproterenol (Isuprel®, Winthrop), a beta-adrenergic stimulating agent, simulates a stress situation and causes a rise in left ventricular EDP (Fig. 3C). This drug response is an almost unique feature of hypertrophic cardiomyopathy. There should be a decrease or an absence of change in the EDP, as seen both in the

normal left ventricle and in other forms of left ventricular disease. The principal circulatory effects of isoproterenol are a lowering of the peripheral vascular resistance, an increase in the heart rate and its action as a potent inotropic agent on the heart muscle. With hypertrophic cardiomyopathy, the inotropic action due to sympathetic stimulation has an adverse effect on diastolic function and appears to increase the rigidity and reduce the distensibility of the ventricular muscle. This finding supports the proposed natural history in Figure 4. Such effects of stress and the accompanying increase in the level of catecholamines can be blocked by pretreatment with beta-adrenergic blocking agents.

Propranolol (a beta-adrenergic blocking agent) (Inderal®, Ayerst) is the drug of choice to counteract stress with accompanying tachycardia and rise in catecholamines. After the use of propranolol in a cat with hypertrophic cardiomyopathy, the EDP was significantly reduced. Beta-adrenergic blockade has little effect on the resting state, but the increase in inflow obstruction (EDP) from the administration of isoproterenol is decreased by the use of propranolol.

Exercise, atropine-induced tachycardia and digitalis glycosides will also serve to increase the ventricular inflow resistance and decrease the rate of filling of the left ventricle. In our laboratory, ouabain has been shown to cause a rise in the left EDP and an increase in obstruction of the left ventricular outflow tract in cats with hypertrophic cardiomyopathy. This action of oua-bain is believed to result from a sustained increase in the force of left ventricular con-traction. Digitalis glycosides are known to increase the force of myocardial contraction in compensated as well as failing hearts. It appears that the muscular outflow tracts of these cats participate in this inotropic re-sponse. Ouabain therefore intensifies the systolic obstruction with subsequent eleva-tion of the already elevated EDP despite its positive inotropic effect. Accordingly, digi-talis glycosides should be administered with caution in cats with hypertrophic car-diomyopathy. Digoxin is not contraindi-cated in atrial fibrillation. Digoxin together with propranolol can sometimes be very valuable in the control of the ventricular rate.

**Congestive Heart Failure.** Treatment is symptomatic with therapy similar to that for heart failure in the dog. Treatment should include rest, a low-sodium diet, slowing of the heart rate, improvement of cardiac ef-ficiency and relief of pulmonary congestion and edema. Cage rest is the most important part of the therapy. Furosemide (Lasix®, Hoechst) in the injectable form at a dosage of 2 to 4 mg./kg. of body weight can be used at first for the acute stages of left-sided heart failure. This diuretic in tablet form can then be used at a dosage of 2 mg./kg. of body weight every second or third day for main-tenance.

**Aortic Thromboembolism.** Throm-boembolism may occur at any stage of the disease or may be the presenting sign. The surgical removal of the aortic thromboem-boli should be considered within a few hours of onset. The underlying heart dis-ease and any other sites of embolization should first be evaluated. Propranolol and propranolol with aspirin are under clinical trial at present for their platelet aggregation effects and appear to be effective in preven-tion of arterial thromboemboli. A dose of 0.3 gm. of aspirin with Maalox® (Ascriptin®, Rorer) is given every 5 to 7 days to the average-sized cat (or ¼ tablet every second day).

## PREVENTION

Prevention of heart disease is best for cats that are asymptomatic or completely re-lieved of the aortic thromboemboli and/or left-sided congestive heart failure. As a re-sult of the previously cited hemodynamic

studies and the preliminary results of a double-blind trial, propranolol is advised for all cats with hypertrophic cardiomy-opathy. As discussed in the proposed natu-ral history (Fig. 4), pulmonary edema and sudden death are thought to follow an episode of tachycardia which has brought about even greater curtailment of left ven-tricular filling. Propranolol should serve to prevent these fatal complications of hyper-trophic cardiomyopathy.

Propranolol serves to slow the heart rate, to lower left EDP, to improve the ventricu-lar filling time, to decrease oxygen demand of the myocardium, to act as an antiar-rhythmic agent and to reduce outflow pres-sure gradients in the obstructive form and is especially important in counteracting a rise in the left EDP when this is increased with stress and accompanying tachycardia. Re-cent reports have also shown propranolol to have an effect on platelet aggregation, with resultant prevention of arterial thromboem-boli. Propranolol is *contraindicated in the presence of arterial thromboemboli* be-cause of its peripheral vasoconstrictive properties. It is important that the clinician be familiar with the basic concept of ad-renergic receptors and the pharmacology of propranolol. Propranolol is used now at an approximate dosage of 2.5 to 5.0 mg. (¼ to ½ of a 10-mg. tablet) two to three times a day for the average-sized cat. For each patient that is given propranolol the drug dosage should be adjusted toward specific individual end points. The dose must be progressively increased to evaluate whether propranolol is effective, ineffective or toxic. The end points should be a definite thera-peutic effect, a resting sinus rhythm, and suppression of stress-induced tachycardia (Fig. 5) or of side effects such as lethargy or progression of signs of congestive heart failure.

## CONGESTIVE CARDIOMYOPATHY

As illustrated in Figure 1, congestive car-diomyopathy is manifested by a dilated flabby heart with resultant failure of the heart as a pump. The clinical presentation primarily reflects severe congestive heart failure with right-sided heart failure being predominant. Dyspnea, orthopnea, severe depression and weight loss are the common clinical signs; sudden death is very fre-quent. Auscultation will often reveal a gal-

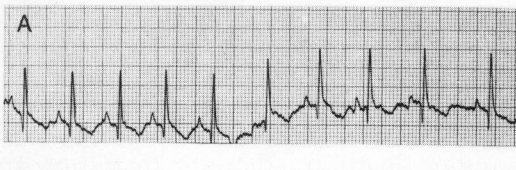

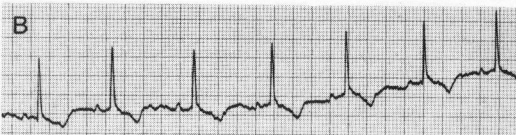

**Figure 5.** Lead II electrocardiogram representing the effect of two weeks' administration of propranolol to a cat with hypertrophic cardiomyopathy. The increase in heart rate during the stress of the electrocardiogram (B) is less than before therapy (A). The heart rate has dropped from approximately 220 to 140 beats per minute. Note tall and wide QRS complexes, an indication of left ventricular hypertrophy. (Paper speed = 50 mm./sec.; 1 cm. = 1 mv.)

lop rhythm, systolic murmurs of mitral regurgitation and muffled heart sounds due to pleural effusion. The electrocardiogram is almost always abnormal, showing tall and wide QRS complexes, ventricular premature contraction and atrioventricular dissociation. Thoracic radiographs reveal enlargement of all chambers, noted best in the dorsoventral position. Pleural effusion and hepatomegaly, signs of right-sided heart failure, are common with congestive cardiomyopathy.

The prognosis for cats with congestive cardiomyopathy is very poor. Only a few days to a few weeks elapse between the onset of clinical signs and death from congestive heart failure. Therapy includes cage rest, a low-sodium diet, digoxin and furosemide (Lasix®). Cats are extremely sensitive to digoxin and should never be rapidly digitalized. They should be monitored on a maintenance dose in correlation with their weight, stage of heart failure and toxic side effects. The average maintenance dosage is approximately 0.008 to 0.010 mg./kg. body weight/day in two divided doses for the average cat (e.g., ¼ of a 0.125 mg. digoxin [Lanoxin®, Burroughs-

Wellcome] tablet, two times a day for a 6-kg. cat).

## CRITERIA FOR THE DIAGNOSIS OF CARDIOMYOPATHY

1. Cardiac enlargement with or without cardiac decompensation on thoracic radiographs.
2. Presence of an abnormal electrocardiogram.
3. Presence of a third or fourth heart sound, gallop rhythm or both.
4. Recent (acquired) murmurs of mitral insufficiency in the adult cat in the absence of infection, anemia (PCV less than 20 per cent) and other hyperkinetic states of the circulatory system.
5. Exclusion of other causes of heart disease: primary valvular disease (acquired or congenital), pericardial effusion and sufficient pulmonary dysfunction to cause cor pulmonale.
6. Presence of systemic arterial thromboemboli.

Criteria 1 and 5 are considered essential, while criteria 2, 3 and 4 are not considered essential. Criterion 6 is almost always correlated with cardiomyopathy.

### SUPPLEMENTAL READING

Goodwin, J. F.: The congestive and hypertrophic cardiomyopathies. A decade of study. Lancet, 1:731–739, 1970.

Harris, S. G., and Ogburn, P. N.: The cardiovascular system. In Catcott, E. J. (ed.): Feline Medicine and Surgery. 2nd ed. Santa Barbara, California, American Veterinary Publications, 1975.

Hurst, J. W.: The Heart. 3rd ed. New York, McGraw-Hill Book Co., 1974.

Oakley, C. N.: Clinical recognition of the cardiomyopathies. Circ. Res., Suppl. II, 34 and 35: 152, 1974.

Tilley, L. P.: Feline cardiology. Vet. Clin. N. Am., 1976 (in press).

Tilley, L. P., and Liu, S.-K. Cardiomyopathy and thromboembolism in the cat. Feline Pract., 5:32, 1975.

Wolstenholme, G. E. W., and O'Connor, M.: Hypertrophic obstructive cardiomyopathy. Ciba Foundation Study Group, #37. London, J. & A. Churchill, 1971.

# THE ELECTROCARDIOGRAPHIC CHANGES ASSOCIATED WITH ELECTROLYTE DISTURBANCES

EDWARD C. FELDMAN, D.V.M., *and* STEPHEN J. ETTINGER, D.V.M.
*Berkeley, California*

Several electrolytes play a major role in the genesis of the transmembrane action potential. Action potentials, when of sufficient intensity, promote impulse formation and subsequently conduction across cardiac tissue. The electrolyte composition of serum normally remains within well-defined limits. Deviation from the normal concentration of one or more of the serum electrolytes occurs in a variety of disease states. Such deviations of serum electrolyte concentrations may have a marked effect on impulse conduction and thus on cardiac rate and/or rhythm.

In the clinical veterinary setting alterations in serum potassium are responsible for the vast majority of cardiac irregularities that occur with electrolyte imbalances. Although calcium, sodium, hydrogen and magnesium imbalances may also induce variations in cardiac conductivity, it has been our clinical experience that only potassium and calcium alterations are seen with enough frequency to warrant discussion.

The variability of criteria employed in interpreting the electrocardiogram (ECG) and of the normal range of serum electrolyte concentrations accounts for some degree of difficulty in correlating ECG and serum electrolyte alterations. It is unwise to predict the serum level of potassium or calcium from ECG changes, particularly when the abnormal concentrations are only slightly outside the normal range. This does not diminish the usefulness of the ECG in detecting the cardiotoxic effects of electrolyte abnormalities.

The accuracy of the electrocardiographic diagnosis improves when the interpreter is alert to the possibility of an electrolyte imbalance, when control tracings are available for comparison and when the patient is followed with serial tracings. Monitoring of the ECG during the intravenous administration of potassium and calcium salts or of agents which alter the concentrations of these ions contributes significantly to the effectiveness and safety of such therapy.

## HYPOKALEMIA

Lowered extracellular potassium concentrations are associated with various disease states as well as with commonly utilized therapeutic regimens in veterinary practice. The following include the most frequently encountered instances of hypokalemia in our practice: (1) loss from the gastrointestinal tract during bouts of chronic and severe vomiting and/or diarrhea; (2) urinary loss in the diuresis phase of renal disease; (3) loss secondary to diuresis stimulated by the use of drugs; (4) loss associated with excessive use of diuretic agents such as the thiazides and furosemide*; (5) rarely, loss associated with excessive administra-

---

*Electrolyte alterations are most likely to occur when the diuresis is prolonged, unmonitored or associated with the concomitant use of low-sodium and low-chloride diets.

tion of corticosteroids or in Cushing's syndrome; (6) loss following the development of alkalosis associated with the use of alkalinizing agents such as sodium bicarbonate; and (7) in diabetic animals, loss secondary to the use of insulin, which shifts potassium from the extracellular to the intracellular fluid compartment of the body.

Hypokalemia can be reflected on the electrocardiogram as a progressive sagging of the ST segment and decreased amplitude of the T wave. The basic electrophysiologic alteration is a gradual shift of the repolarization wave from systole into diastole. Therefore, accompanying the decreased amplitude of the T wave is a repolarization wave occurring after the T wave (U wave). The merging of a flat or positive T wave with a positive U wave may erroneously be interpreted as a prolonged T wave and therefore a prolonged Q-T interval. In advanced hypokalemia the amplitude and duration of the QRS interval are increased. It is believed that the QRS complex is widened diffusely secondary to a generalized slowing of conduction in the ventricular myocardium and/or Purkinje fibers. The amplitude and the duration of the P wave increase and the P-R interval is slightly prolonged.

Atrial and ventricular premature contractions are seen frequently in hypokalemic animals. Animals receiving digitalis and also suffering from low extracellular potassium concentrations are prone to the above-mentioned arrhythmias as well as to supraventricular tachycardia with block and ventricular tachycardia. The normal level of serum potassium in our laboratory ranges between 3.5 and 4.8 mEq./l. Changes in the electrocardiogram have not been observed in animals which have serum potassium concentrations in the 3.0 to 3.5 mEq./l. range. Changes have been recorded when the serum potassium level was between 2.5 and 3.0 mEq./l. ECG alterations occur in almost all dogs and cats with serum potassium levels below 2.5 mEq./l.

Treatment is directed toward the correction of the underlying clinical problem as well as potassium supplementation. Ideally, potassium is supplemented orally. When this route is contraindicated, the potassium salt can be administered subcutaneously or intravenously, after being diluted in the parenteral fluids. Generally, we begin potassium therapy with 7 mEq. added to each 250 ml. of intravenous fluids. Adjustments in this dose are based on serial ECG's and frequent monitoring of serum electrolyte concentrations.

## HYPERKALEMIA

Hyperpotassemia is not an uncommonly encountered clinical problem. It is attributed most frequently to renal failure associated with oliguria or anuria. Endocrine causes of high serum potassium concentrations include the moderate or occasionally severe elevations seen in adrenal insufficiency as well as the mild elevations which may occur in untreated ketoacidotic diabetic animals. Acidosis alone, which tends to shift potassium from within the cells to the extracellular fluid, may also inhibit renal potassium excretion, thereby promoting hyperkalemia. The rapid infusion of potassium-containing fluids is another cause of hyperkalemia. Potassium-sparing diuretic compounds such as triamterene and spironolactone may be responsible for a build-up of extracellular potassium levels which, if unaltered, may be critical.

The importance of hyperpotassemia is the severe and potentially lethal cardiotoxic effect of the imbalance. Hyperkalemia can be readily diagnosed, and prompt therapeutic measures, which may be life-saving, will rapidly reverse the imbalance to within normal limits.

The clinical syndrome of hyperpotassemia is manifested by general muscle weakness, listlessness, bradycardia and peripheral vascular collapse. The effects on the heart are in many ways similar to those of quinidine and procainamide. They consist of a decrease in excitability, an increase of the refractory period of the heart muscle and a slowing of conduction.

Clinically, the most prominent manifestations of hyperkalemia are found on the ECG, which is a vital tool for estimating its functional severity. The earliest electrocardiographic alteration is peaking of the T wave, which occurs when the serum potassium concentration exceeds 5.5 mEq./l. This change is frequently associated with shortening of the Q-T interval. The characteristic tall, steep, narrow and pointed T waves occur before the ECG shows any measurable alteration of the QRS complex. T-wave changes are not seen in all cases of mild hyperkalemia. As the serum potassium concentration continues to rise, the T wave may lose its classic "peaked" shape because the T-wave abnormalities secondary to intraventricular conduction disturbances obscure the primary T-wave changes.

Slowing of the intraventricular impulse conduction is responsible for the QRS complex alterations which occur as the serum potassium concentration exceeds 6.5 mEq./l. At this juncture the T-wave abnormalities and the uniformly widened QRS complex allow the presumptive diagnosis to be made. With increasing serum potassium concentrations the QRS duration increases progressively. There is a rough correlation between duration of the QRS complex and the degree of hyperpotassemia.

As serum potassium levels rise above 7 mEq./l. the P-wave amplitude decreases and its duration becomes prolonged secondary to slowing of conduction through the atria. The P-R interval also increases in duration as a result of slower atrioventricular transmission. When serum potassium concentrations exceed 8.5 mEq./l. the P wave frequently becomes invisible. When P waves are absent, an erroneous diagnosis of atrial fibrillation or atrial asystole may be made, particularly when the ventricular rate is irregular.

Continued elevation of serum potassium can be associated with deviation from the baseline of the ST segment. With concentrations reaching the magnitude of 11 to 14 mEq./l. the electrocardiographer may see ventricular asystole or ventricular fibrillation.

Therapy in the hyperkalemic patient is threefold. First, one must lower the serum potassium; second, the serum sodium and/or calcium concentration must be raised; and third, the etiology of the electrolyte imbalance must be determined so that specific therapy may be instituted. Therapy need not be overzealous when potassium concentrations are below 6.5 mEq./l., whereas intensive therapy must be instituted in animals with serum potassium concentrations greater than 8 to 8.5 mEq./l.

Lowering of the serum potassium can be accomplished by the intravenous infusion of a 10 per cent glucose solution. Five to 10 cc./kg. body weight should be given in the first 30 to 60 minutes and then the drip may be slowed. Glucose causes a potassium shift from the serum into the cells, apparently by altering cell membrane characteristics and

by promoting deposition of glycogen. Subcutaneous or intravenous infusions of regular insulin at a dose of 0.5 to 1.0 U./kg. body weight will enhance the cellular uptake of glucose. For each unit of regular insulin one should administer at least 20 cc. of 10 per cent dextrose to avoid hypoglycemia.

Sodium bicarbonate also rapidly lowers serum potassium by causing a shift of the potassium ion into the cells secondary to alkalinization of the serum. Eighty to 100 mEq. of sodium bicarbonate should be added to each liter of glucose containing intravenous fluids. This maneuver is especially valuable when acidosis is present but is also effective in animals with normal acid-base status.

Sodium and calcium antagonize the cardiotoxic effects of potassium. In animals with extreme hyperkalemia the intravenous infusion of 5 to 20 cc. of calcium gluconate within a 5-minute period and under electrocardiographic monitoring will rapidly reverse the ECG and clinical evidence of cardiac toxicity without affecting the serum level of potassium. This effect is transient and must be accompanied by other means of lowering the potassium concentration. Infusion of saline intravenously dilutes serum potassium and may aid in monitoring a lowered serum level of the cation.

## HYPOCALCEMIA

Hypocalcemia is not a frequently encountered entity in veterinary practice other than in the lactating bitch. Hypocalcemia may also be attributed to idiopathic hypoparathyroidism, high intestinal fluid loss secondary to diarrhea and chronic renal failure in association with retention of phosphorus. It may also develop in association with paralytic ileus.

Symptoms associated with hypocalcemia include increased nervous excitability, tetany and convulsions.

Hypocalcemia prolongs the duration of the action potential in cardiac cells. This results in an increased duration of the ST segment and of the Q-T segment. There is a good correlation seen between the severity of the hypocalcemia and the time duration of the ST segment. The duration of the T wave in animals with hypocalcemia is not altered. The combination of hypocalcemia and hyperpotassemia which can occur in animals with uremia can be recognized by the presence of a prolonged ST segment and a narrow, peaked T wave.

Treatment of hypocalcemia includes calcium gluconate infusion intravenously and determination of, as well as initiation of therapy for, the underlying cause of the disturbance.

## HYPERCALCEMIA

Hypercalcemia is observed in primary hyperparathyroidism, multiple myeloma, bone metastasis, some lymphomas, in selected cases of carcinoma and transiently with the intravenous administration of calcium.

Electrocardiographically hypercalcemia is associated with an ST segment which is short or absent. Occasionally, particularly in heart disease, premature beats, paroxysmal tachycardia and even death may result from hypercalcemia.

Treatment is directed toward finding the etiology of the alteration. Parathyroid tumors must be surgically removed. Attempts at reducing serum calcium concentration through intensive fluid therapy and diuresis may be tried. Use of drugs such as mithramycin has not been described in the dog or cat.

## SODIUM AND CHLORIDE

Hypernatremia can be encountered with decreased or absent fluid intake, diabetes insipidus or osmotic diuresis. Hyponatremia is seen in functional disorders lead-ing to the defective excretion of water, such as the inappropriate secretion of antidiuretic hormone or in hypoadrenocorticism; in renal disease with defective excretion of water, such as acute renal failure with oliguria or in chronic renal failure; in psychogenic polydipsia; and in congestive heart failure. It may also occur following sodium-depleting diuretic compounds. Hypochloremia is encountered most often following excessive diuresis by drugs and after prolonged vomiting and/or diarrhea.

Electrocardiographically the alterations in serum sodium and chloride concentrations are of little clinical significance because the levels necessary to alter the action potential are usually incompatible with life. Arrhythmias related to hyper- or hyponatremia are not seen in clinical medicine. The interrelationship of sodium and potassium is of some therapeutic usefulness. The depression of conduction induced by potassium can be reversed by administration of sodium and is exaggerated by lowering the sodium concentration.

### SUPPLEMENTAL READING

Bellet, S.: Essentials of Cardiac Arrhythmias. Philadelphia, W. B. Saunders Co., 1972.
Ettinger, P. O., Regan, T. J., Oldewurtel, H. A., and Kahn, M. I.: Ventricular conduction delay and asystole during systemic hyperkalemia. Am. J. Cardiol., 33:876–886, 1974.
Fisch, C.: Relation of electrolyte disturbances to cardiac arrhythmias. Circulation, 47:408–419, 1973.
Surawicz, B.: Relationship between electrocardiogram and electrolytes. Am. Heart J., 73:814–832, 1967.

# ANESTHESIA FOR THE DOG WITH HEART DISEASE

WILLIAM MUIR, D.V.M.
Columbus, Ohio

The ability safely to anesthetize the small animal patient with either congenital or acquired cardiac disease requires a thorough knowledge of the patient's medical history and an understanding of the basic phar-macophysiologic effects of the drugs to be used. This knowledge combined with clinical experience with a particular drug or combination of drugs is oftentimes far safer than attempting a new anesthetic technique on the presumptive basis of negligible cardiopulmonary effects. To date, although newer drugs are continually being developed, there is no anesthetic technique which surpasses all others for the clinical management of anesthesia for the cardiac patient.

A calm and effortless transition to an anesthetic state is mandatory in the patient with cardiac disease. Struggling, gagging and coughing reduce cardiac output and result in the appearance of cardiac dysrhythmias in the normal dog and could seriously affect the patient with reduced cardiac reserve. The preceding statement generally implies the use of a preanesthetic ataractic or sedative in dogs. In selecting the proper drug for this purpose, a drug's potential depressant effects upon myocardial function must be assessed in addition to the drug's influence upon the autonomic nervous system. Excessive sympathetic or parasympathetic activity due to the drug's direct effects or indirect effects (respiratory depression and hypercarbia) may induce cardiac dysrhythmias during anesthetic induction and maintenance. Furthermore, reflex dysrhythmias from tracheal intubation, surgical stimulation, ocular manipulation, sudden changes in blood pressure, etc., may be accentuated in the compensated cardiac patient.

*Diazepam* (Valium®) has proved to be a very effective and safe premedicant, particularly in the aged dog with cardiac disease. Doses of 0.2 to 0.6 mg./kg. administered intramuscularly or intravenously produce minimal effects upon ventricular function or arterial blood pressure and may impart an antidysrhythmic effect.

The narcotic analgesic *morphine* is also recommended as a preanesthetic in patients with cardiac disease. Low doses of morphine (0.8 to 0.16 mg./kg.) have little effect upon cardiac output or arterial blood pressure while producing a significant degree of analgesia and sedation. Respiratory depression may be evident, however, and if larger dosages than those recommended are used, arterial hypotension can be expected. When extremely low doses (0.2 to 0.6 mg./kg.) of morphine are administered intramuscularly or intravenously, cardiac output may actually increase in dogs with valvular heart disease. The previous observation combined with morphine's ability to redistribute fluid to peripheral tissue beds in patients with pulmonary edema makes it an excellent premedicant.

*Fentanyl* (Sublimaze®), a new short-acting synthetic narcotic, has been shown to produce significantly less cardiac depression and more analgesia than morphine when administered intravenously in dogs. Fentanyl administered alone, however, produces a mild excitatory response and involuntary muscle contractions in the unanesthetized dog. The combination of fentanyl with the tranquilizer droperidol produces a neuroleptanalgesic (narcotic plus a tranquilizer). The intravenous administration of 1 ml./12 kg. of a 50:1 ratio of the commercially available product (Innovar-Vet®, 0.4 mg./ml. fentanyl and 20.0 mg./ml. droperidol, Pitman-Moore) provides an excellent state of unconsciousness and analgesia with minimal cardiovascular depression. If atropine is administered prior to the administration of this combination, hemodynamic variables (cardiac output, heart rate and arterial blood pressure) actually increase. The benefits of these effects in the normal or diseased cardiac patient are questionable and will be discussed later. Although this neuroleptanalgesic appears to be clinically beneficial to the cardiovascular system when administered according to the aforementioned dosage, it depresses respiration, predisposing the animal to both respiratory and metabolic acidosis. Acidosis during the anesthetic period could be potentially harmful to the dog with reduced cardiac reserve. When administered intramuscularly alone at 0.5 ml./12 kg., Innovar-Vet® will produce excellent tranquilization with a minimum of respiratory depression. An advantage of the use of any narcotic (morphine, fentanyl) is the potential reversibility of the agent. Either nalorphine (Nalline®), 0.4 mg./kg., or naloxone (Narcan®), a narcotic antagonist, purported partially to reverse narcotic-induced respiratory depression, may be used.

The use of *atropine* for routine preanesthetic medication in the dog with either congenital or acquired heart disease is not recommended. This drug has been advocated and indiscriminately used in almost all dogs to be anesthetized for one of two reasons: (1) the reduction of excessive salivary secretion and (2) the prevention of excessively slow heart rates (<60 beats per minute). Dogs with cardiac disease, particularly those in a moderate to severe degree of decompensation, are generally extremely dependent upon hemodynamic reflex mechanisms and the autonomic nervous system for maintenance of ventricular function. A parasympatholytic drug not only increases heart rate—which in turn increases myocardial work and oxygen consumption, further increasing the stress upon an already compromised heart—but also predisposes to tachycardia-dependent dysrhythmias by increasing electrical inhomogeneity of electrical recovery within the myocardium. Although atropine's value in purely parasympathetically induced bradycardias is appreciated and well-known, there is considerable doubt as to its efficacy in slow heart rates induced by "vagal-vagal" reflexes. The beneficial effect of atropine in depressing salivary secretions is also questionable in that the secretions, although reduced, are generally much more viscous and could predispose to small airway occlusion and atelectasis. Atropine has also been shown to increase anatomic dead space and prolong anesthesia time; both effects must be considered potentially harmful in the dog with cardiac disease. Atropine should never be used routinely on the supposition that it cannot hurt and may help. The drug should be reserved for those patients in which there is a definite therapeutic indication for its administration. The dosage recommended for atropine is 0.2 to 0.4 mg./kg. subcutaneously or intravenously in emergency situations.

The time-honored and time-tested drugs for induction to anesthesia are the ultrashort-acting barbiturates *thiamylal* and *thiopental* (Surital® and Pentothal®, respectively). When used in anesthetic doses (12 to 20 mg./kg.), these drugs produce a dose-related depression of cardiac output, arterial blood pressure and contractility. The *thiobarbiturates* are also said to possess direct cardiotoxic effects and are known to predispose to premature ventricular depolarization and bigeminy. Periods of apnea lasting several minutes are not uncommon when these drugs are administered in large doses or to extremely depressed or debilitated patients. Regardless of this knowledge, the thiobarbiturates remain the most popular means for induction to anesthesia in veterinary medicine for two reasons: (1) no safer agents are available at present, albeit newer, less hemodynamically depressant drugs are available in Europe (althesin,

etomidate); and (2) when judiciously used with watchful monitoring and careful titration of drug dosage versus patient response, these drugs remain well within the expected safety expectations of any anesthetic available. When the cardiac patient with acquired heart disease has been properly preanesthetized, the dosage needed to induce the patient to anesthesia should rarely exceed 8 mg./kg. administered intravenously. Extreme care must be implemented in patients with congenital heart disease and a right-to-left shunt, in which case an intravenous drug may bypass the pulmonary circulation and speed the onset of systemic effects and reduce the amount of drug needed to induce anesthesia. The reverse is true for a left-to-right shunt.

Another drug which is increasing in popularity because of the absence of cardiovascular depression is *ketamine hydrochloride* (Vetalar®, Ketaset®). When used alone or in excessive dosages, this drug produces extreme excitement, muscle rigor and occasionally convulsions in the dog. Endotracheal intubation is difficult, if possible at all, owing to the maintenance of the swallowing reflex. Because of these excitatory effects and the increases in cardiac work imposed, it is not recommended when administered singularly in the dog with cardiac disease. Ketamine in combination with low dosages of a tranquilizer or sedative produces fairly rapid excitement-free anesthetic induction in the dog with a minimum of cardiorespiratory depression. Ketamine (6 mg./kg.) and xylazine (0.5 mg./kg.) or acetylpromazine (0.4 mg./kg.) have been safely administered intravenously in the dog for purposes of induction to anesthesia. However, this anesthetic induction technique awaits further research and clinical justification in the dog with heart disease.

Two types of drugs which have gained a great deal of popularity and acceptance in severely debilitated, high-risk patients with heart diseases are *nitrous oxide* ($N_2O$) and the *neuromuscular blocking agents*. Nitrous oxide is not an anesthetic in dogs but does improve analgesia and muscle relaxation with minimal cardiovascular changes. Pancuronium bromide (Pavulon®), a steroid-based, long-acting nondepolarizing neuromuscular blocking agent, when administered intravenously to dogs (0.04 mg./kg.) produces about 20 minutes of paralysis with slight increases in heart rate, arterial blood pressure and cardiac contractility. The combination of 50:50 per cent $N_2O:O_2$, a neuromuscular blocking agent (pancuronium) and a narcotic (fentanyl, 0.04 mg.) is referred to as "balanced anesthesia." Provided that ventilation is adequately controlled, this anesthetic technique is the basis for what is believed to be the best method for maintaining stable hemodynamics in patients with normal or decreased cardiac function. Both pancuronium and fentanyl may be readministered at reduced dosages after induction to anesthesia for maintenance of anesthesia without fear of significant cardiac depression. A further advantage of this technique is the ability, if necessary, to reverse the effects of both drugs. Fentanyl may be reversed, as previously described, with Naline® and pancuronium with neostigmine sulfate (Prostigmine®) or edrophonium (Tensilon®) after the patient has been atropinized. This anesthetic technique requires careful monitoring and experience with its usage if its true value is to be appreciated and taken advantage of clinically.

*Inhalation anesthetics* are being widely used in veterinary practices today. They are also used in the majority of clinical cases involving cardiac catheterization and cardiac surgery. Although these drugs act as potent depressants of cardiac function, this effect is dose-related, thereby implying that when used in low concentrations, they can be safely used with other less depressant anesthetic or preanesthetic drugs to produce anesthesia in the cardiac patient. This implies that mask induction to an anesthetic state with high concentrations (>2 per cent) of an inhalation anesthetic (enflurane, halothane, methoxyflurane) is to be avoided in the patient with heart disease.

In order of their ability to decrease cardiac contractility and arterial blood pressure at equal depths of anesthesia (from most to least depressant) they are enflurane (Ethrane®), halothane (Fluothane®), methoxyflurane (Metofane®) and diethyl ether (Ether®). It has been argued that the resultant myocardial depression will cause a decrease in cardiac work and oxygen consumption and, provided that the hypotensive effective is not severe, that the effects of inhalation anesthetics may in fact rest an overworked heart. Because of the possible beneficial effects of a decreased cardiac workload and the opposite effects and potential for dysrhythmia formation invoked with digitalis, it is not recommended that digitalis therapy be initiated or increased in the dog with suspected or known heart disease immediately prior to anesthesia. If it is ascertained that benefit can be gained by the administration of digitalis, blood levels should be established and stabilized at least one week prior to anesthesia. Furthermore, at light planes of anesthesia, the cardiac depressive effects of the inhalation anesthetics are minimal in normal dogs; the effect in dogs with impaired cardiac function has not been adequately investigated.

In addition to a dose-dependent negative effect upon cardiac contractility, the inhalation anesthetics sensitize the myocardium to dysrhythmias; this is particularly true of enflurane and halothane. The dysrhythmias produced are generally easily controlled with intravenously administered lidocaine (Xylocaine®), 4 to 8 mg./kg. Most compensated cardiac patients with acquired heart disease tolerate inhalation anesthesia surprisingly well, provided that anesthetic induction has been smooth. It should be noted, however, that inhalation anesthetics are taken up by the blood from the lungs much more slowly in patients with congenital heart disease and a right-to-left intracardiac shunt; this prolongs induction and recovery from anesthesia. The reverse is true in a left-to-right shunt.

In summary, there is currently little evidence to recommend one inhalation anesthetic over another for use in the dog with heart disease, provided that low concentrations are used and adequate patient monitoring is carried out.

In conclusion, all patients with heart disease, whether acquired or congenital, must be adequately ventilated. Whether this is accomplished manually or mechanically is not important, provided that it is done properly. Ventilation is of paramount importance in patients with right-to-left intracardiac shunts. Close patient monitoring is also of extreme importance. Ideally, for most clinical practices this would include an electrocardiogram and central venous pressure monitoring. If possible, arterial pressure monitoring would be greatly beneficial (Physiometric). At the present time, it appears that familiarity with a balanced anesthetic technique is ideal for severely compromised cardiac patients that must undergo anesthesia. For those dogs that are not as stressed, morphine or diazepam pre-anesthesia, a thiobarbiturate, $N_2O/O_2$ and a low concentration of an inhalation anesthetic may be used. If only minimal cardiac impairment is suspected, the clinician's ex-

perience and the patient's medical history should predict the anesthetic drugs used. The safest way to administer any anesthetic to the dog with heart disease is to perform attentive patient monitoring and titration of the potentially least toxic anesthetics against the desired effect.

# COMMON CONGENITAL HEART DEFECTS

## Aortic Stenosis

R. LEE PYLE, V.M.D.
*Fort Collins, Colorado*

Aortic stenosis is a congenital cardiac defect characterized by a narrowing or constriction in the left ventricular outflow tract-aortic valve region. It is the third most commonly occurring congenital heart defect in the dog and has also been reported in the cat. Three distinct types of aortic stenosis are recognized in the dog. The supravalvular type (rarest) has been reported in one dog and is characterized by a narrowing just above the aortic valve. Valvular aortic stenosis is also a relatively rare condition, in that less than 10 cases are reported in the literature. This type is characterized by thickened and deformed aortic cusps which cause obstruction at the valvular level. The third, and by far the most common type is subvalvular (subaortic) stenosis (SAS), which is recognized as various degrees of fibrous ring formation in the left ventricular outflow tract below the aortic valve (Fig. 1.).

### PATHOPHYSIOLOGY

The fibrous ring in the outflow tract acts to narrow the orifice through which blood must pass when flowing from the left ventricle to the aorta. The heart, in order to maintain an adequate output, compensates by increasing left ventricular pressure so that blood can pass through the narrowed orifice with greater velocity. However, the increased velocity results in turbulent blood flow which clinically translates into a

systolic murmur. Since the left ventricle must work harder to generate a greater ventricular pressure, the myocardium hypertrophies. The hypertrophy may be manifested electrocardiographically and/or radiographically.

### DIAGNOSIS

Aortic stenosis occurs predominantly in the younger members of three breeds—Newfoundland, boxer and German shepherd. There is substantial evidence that subvalvular stenosis has a hereditary basis in the Newfoundland.

The history is often unremarkable. In the typical situation, an apparently healthy pup is presented for the first routine examination. It is not until the veterinarian auscultates the heart that any signs of heart disease are noted. If heart failure is present, it is usually manifested initially as left heart failure, i.e., coughing and dyspnea. In very advanced cases, ascites and limb edema (right heart failure) may be evident. In very severely affected dogs, syncope and sudden death are common events.

Palpation of the thorax often reveals a thrill that is strongest in the lower left fourth to fifth intercostal spaces. In severe cases, the femoral pulse may be weak because of obstruction to blood flow from the left ventricle and, in addition, a thrill may be palpated over the carotid arteries. A

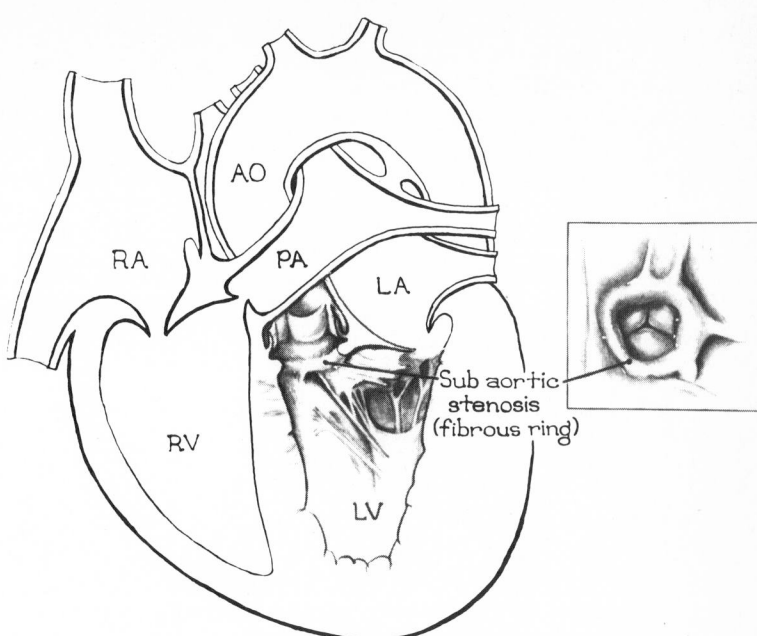

**Figure 1.** Drawing to show the appearance of the fibrous ring in the left ventricular outflow tract and its relationship to major structures of the heart. The insert depicts the fibrous ring as viewed from the ventricular side. The three aortic valve leaflets can be seen beyond the fibrous ring. *RA*, right atrium; *RV*, right ventricle; *AO*, aorta; *PA*, pulmonary artery; *LA*, left atrium; *LV*, left ventricle. (Courtesy of Dr. D. F. Patterson and the American Animal Hospital Association.)

crescendo-decrescendo or decrescendo low-pitched systolic murmur is heard best in the lower left fourth to fifth intercostal spaces. Occasionally, a decrescendo diastolic murmur accompanies the systolic murmur. Depending on the intensity, the murmur is often heard well in the lower right second to fourth intercostal spaces and over the carotid arteries at the thoracic inlet.

The electrocardiogram is frequently normal. This is true even in dogs which, at postmortem examination, have significant left ventricular hypertrophy. Some of the very severely affected individuals may have ECG changes indicative of left ventricular hypertrophy and ischemia. These changes include high amplitude R waves (greater than 3 mv.) in lead II and ST segment depression. In advanced cases, with secondary mitral insufficiency, atrial fibrillation may be present.

One of the earliest and most reliable radiographic signs is poststenotic dilatation of the aorta. This is most easily visualized in the lateral view in which the dilated ascending aorta creates a bulge in the cranial cardiac silhouette. Enlargement and cranial extension of the aorta may also be visible in the dorsoventral view. The left ventricular hypertrophy that accompanies "pure" aortic stenosis may not be readily apparent in conventional thoracic radiographs because the hypertrophy is concentric. However, in advanced cases with concomitant mitral insufficiency, the left ventricle and left atrium may be greatly enlarged. Angiocardiograms made by injection of contrast material into the left ventricle (via an arterial catheter) demonstrate varying degrees of narrowing of the left ventricular outflow tract. Poststenotic dilatation of the ascending aorta and mitral regurgitation may also be seen.

Measurement of the left ventricular-aortic gradient, using a catheter and a pressure transducer, can provide useful diagnostic evidence. When the catheter is withdrawn from the left ventricle to the aorta, there is a drop in the peak systolic pressure as the tip of the catheter traverses the region of the stenosis in the left ventricular outflow tract. This reduced peak systolic pressure is also reflected in the aorta. The magnitude of the gradient is a rough indicator of the severity of the disease. In normal dogs, there is essentially no difference between peak left ventricular and peak aortic pressure.

## TREATMENT

Surgical removal of the fibrous ring is the treatment of choice for this problem; however, the need for cardiac bypass does not make this a very practical procedure in veterinary medicine. Furthermore, the diffuse nature of the fibrous lesion in certain dogs would make total correction quite difficult.

The alternative approach is to handle the problem medically, using digitalis and diuretics when congestive heart failure occurs. (See articles on therapy for congestive heart failure, pages 327 to 346.) Unfortunately, once congestive heart failure supervenes, the prognosis is grave.

**SUPPLEMENTAL READING**

Ettinger, S. J., and Suter, P. F.: Canine Cardiology. Philadelphia. W. B. Saunders Co., 1970.

Patterson, D. F.: Epidemiologic and genetic studies of congenital heart disease in the dog. Circ. Res., 23:171–202, 1968.

Pyle, R. L.: Aortic stenosis. *In* A Manual of Clinical Cardiology. Elkhart, Ind., American Animal Hospital Association, 1972.

Pyle, R. L., Patterson, D. F., and Chacko, S.: The genetics and pathology of discrete subaortic stenosis in the Newfoundland dog. Am. Heart J., 92:324–334, 1976.

# Atrial Septal Defect

Congenital atrial septal defect (ASD) is a hole or opening in the septum which divides the left and right atrium. The defect has been reported in the dog and cat.

There are two important types of ASD. If the defect is situated low in the atrial septum and there is no normal septal tissue between the defect and the atrioventricular valve, it is referred to as a primum type. By far the most common defect is the secundum type in which the defect is located in the fossa ovalis region of the atrial septum. In this type, there is normal septal tissue between the defect and the atrioventricular valves.

Isolated ASD's are quite rare. This may be due to the fact that, as isolated defects, they generate relatively mild clinical findings and, as a result, they are not recognized clinically. Usually a case comes to the attention of a veterinarian for some type of heart disease other than ASD and it is only through special laboratory studies and/or postmortem examination that the ASD is detected. In a family of boxer dogs, secundum type ASD was frequently associated with aortic and/or pulmonic stenosis.

## PATHOPHYSIOLOGY

The defect in the atrial septum allows blood to shunt from the left atrium to the right atrium because pressure in the left atrium is higher than pressure in the right atrium. The shunting causes a volume overload in the right side of the heart, the lungs, and the left atrium. As a result, the right atrium, right ventricle and left atrium may enlarge and there may be various clinical signs of pulmonary congestion.

If for any reason (e.g. tricuspid insufficiency) right atrial pressure is higher than left atrial pressure, then venous blood will shunt across the defect to the arterial side. The outstanding clinical finding resulting from a right to left shunt would be cyanosis.

## DIAGNOSIS

In considering a diagnosis, one must remember that an animal with an ASD usually presents as some other type of congenital heart disease, and it is only through subsequent study that one finds an ASD; however, in this discussion, "pure" ASD will be considered.

The history may be unremarkable. Some animals may evidence dyspnea, weakness and other nonspecific signs. Ascites may be present if the dog is in right-sided heart failure.

On auscultation, a grade 1 to 3 ejection murmur is heard best in the pulmonic area. The murmur is related to the relative pulmonic stenosis caused by the increased volume of blood in the pulmonary artery. Splitting of the second heart may be heard due to delayed closure of the pulmonary valve. Auscultation of the lungs may reveal rales.

The electrocardiogram may be normal; however, right axis deviation compatible with right ventricular enlargement is sometimes present.

Radiographically, one may see right atrial enlargement, right ventricular enlargement, main pulmonary artery enlargement, as well as increased vascularity and congestion in the lung fields. An angiocardiogram made by injecting contrast medium (via a venous catheter) into the left atrium will demonstrate left to right shunting at the atrial level. It is often possible to advance the same venous catheter into the left ventricle. The knowledge of having manipulated a venous catheter into the left atrium as well as into the left ventricle supports a diagnosis of ASD.

Measurement of the blood oxygen content in the right atrium can provide valuable information. An increase in oxygen content over normal venous levels would be expected.

Indicator-dilution curves may also be employed. In this procedure, a dye is injected into a vein, and dye decay is recorded on the arterial side. Due to the atrial shunt, the decay slope is decreased when compared to normal.

## TREATMENT

In man, ASD's are frequently closed surgically, using heart-lung bypass. The same technique could be applied to animals, although no significant efforts along this line have been made to date.

Short of surgical treatment, medical management using digitalis and diuretics should be used when congestive heart failure supervenes (see articles on therapy for congestive heart failure, pp. 327 to 346).

### SUPPLEMENTAL READING

Ettinger, S. J., and Suter, P. F.: Canine Cardiology. Philadelphia, W. B. Saunders Co., 1970.
Pyle, R. L., and Patterson, D. F.: Multiple cardiovascular malformations in a family of Boxer dogs. J. Am. Vet. Med. Assn., *160*:965–976, 1972.

# Ventricular Septal Defect

Ventricular septal defect (VSD) is a congenital heart defect in young dogs and cats in which there is an opening in the septum that separates the left ventricle from the right ventricle (Fig. 2). A defect occurs whenever normal septation patterns are disturbed during embryonic development. A VSD can be situated just about anywhere in the ventricular septum; however, in most cases it is located in the basilar portion of the ventricular septum—the so-called membranous portion of the ventricular septum. The opening of the defect in the right ventricle is usually located under the septal leaflet of the tricuspid valve, and in the left ventricle the opening is in the left ventricular outflow tract below the aortic valve.

## PATHOPHYSIOLOGY

In isolated VSD there is a shunting of blood from the left ventricle across the VSD to the right ventricle during systole. Such shunting occurs because the pressure in the left ventricle is four to five times higher than the pressure in the right ventricle. Flow across the VSD creates turbulent blood flow which translates clinically into a systolic murmur. Furthermore, such shunting creates a volume overload in a circuit which includes the right ventricle, lungs,

left atrium and left ventricle. The volume overload can induce a stress on the right ventricle, which in turn responds by enlarging. Occasionally the shunt is so large that pulmonary hypertension develops. This leads to an increase in right ventricular pressure that is equal to or greater than left ventricular pressure. When this occurs, venous blood is shunted into the systemic circulation, resulting in cyanosis.

## DIAGNOSIS

In isolated VSD, the defect is frequently so small that the animal is asymptomatic and it is only when the heart is specifically examined that any sign of disease is detected. Occasionally, an animal may present with signs of pulmonary congestion (coughing, dyspnea). In cases with pulmonary hypertension, ascites and cyanosis may be evident.

On auscultation, a harsh, holosystolic murmur is heard best on the right thoracic wall just above the sternum at the third and fourth intercostal spaces. The murmur is significantly less intense over most of the left thorax (an important differential feature). The intensity of the murmur on the right thoracic wall is not necessarily an indication of the size of the VSD. Splitting of

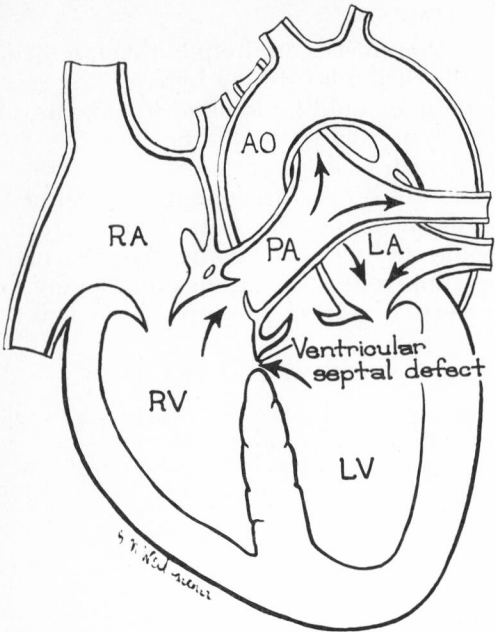

**Figure 2.** This diagram shows a ventricular septal defect located in the basilar portion of the ventricular septum. Blood usually flows across the defect from the left ventricle *(LV)* to the right ventricle *(RV)* because of the higher systolic pressure in the left ventricle. *RA,* right atrium; *AO,* aorta; *PA,* pulmonary artery; *LA,* left atrium. (Courtesy of Dr. D. F. Patterson.)

enlarged as is the main pulmonary artery. The lungs are hypervascularized and congested. The left atrium may also appear enlarged.

Definitive diagnosis can be established through angiocardiographic study. By injecting contrast material into the left ventricle (via an arterial catheter), the left to right shunt across the VSD can be appreciated. With pulmonary hypertension and a right to left shunt, an additional injection of contrast material would be made in the right ventricle.

Increased $O_2$ content in the blood from the outflow tract of the right ventricle is another means of achieving information helpful in making a diagnosis. Blood oxygen measurements made near the apex of the right ventricle would be expected to be normal, since the septal defect is located toward the base of the heart.

the second heart sound due to delayed closure of the pulmonary valve may be noted. If pulmonary hypertension is present, the murmur may be considerably reduced in intensity or may even be absent.

The electrocardiogram is frequently normal. In severely affected dogs, various degrees of right axis deviation may be observed. In the very early stages of right ventricular hypertrophy, only late terminal forces (S waves) in the left chest leads may be observed.

The radiographic findings depend on the severity of the defect. Radiographs from the mildly affected animals are normal. In severely affected cases, the right ventricle is

## TREATMENT

No treatment is necessary in asymptomatic cases or in ones in which the shunt is known to be small. Total surgical correction of the defect is possible; however, heart-lung bypass is required. Banding of the pulmonary artery has been used to treat VSD. This basically involves a constriction of the main pulmonary artery. The banding increases right ventricular pressure and reduces the amount of blood shunting across the VSD.

In cases where surgical intervention is not done, medical therapy with digitalis and diuretics is indicated when congestive heart failure occurs (see articles on therapy for congestive heart failure, pp. 327 to 346).

### SUPPLEMENTAL READING

Ettinger, S. J., and Suter, P. F.: Canine Cardiology. Philadelphia, W. B. Saunders Co., 1970.

Knauer, K. W.: Interventricular septal defect. *In* A Manual of Clinical Cardiology. Elkhart, Ind., American Animal Hospital Association, 1972.

# Tetralogy of Fallot

Tetralogy of Fallot is a complex congenital heart malformation in the dog and cat. It occurs more frequently in the keeshond than in other breeds. The complex is composed of a ventricular septal defect, varying degrees of aortic overriding, and pulmonary stenosis. The fourth feature, right ventricular hypertrophy, occurs as a secondary effect (Fig. 3).

## PATHOPHYSIOLOGY

The hemodynamics in tetralogy relate to the severity of the underlying defects. In the severe form, the so-called typical case, there is moderate to severe pulmonic stenosis which generates a crescendo-decrescendo systolic murmur. In addition, there is an increase in right ventricular pressure which equals or exceeds left ventricular pressure. The increased pressure, in combination with the ventricular septal de-

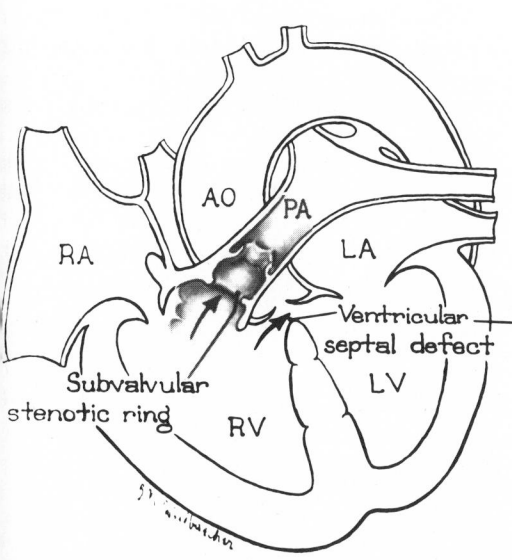

**Figure 3.** Diagram of the heart of a dog with a typical tetralogy of Fallot. There is a ventricular septal defect which is overridden by a rightwardly displaced aorta (AO). There is a subvalvular pulmonic stenosis represented by a ring of tissue in the right ventricular outflow tract. The pulmonary valve and artery (PA) are hypoplastic. The right ventricle (RV) is hypertrophied. RA, right atrium; LV, left ventricle. (Courtesy of Dr. D. F. Patterson and the American Animal Hospital Association.)

fect and overriding aorta, results in a portion of the venous blood entering directly into the aorta and the remainder of the systemic circulation. The clinical result of the venous admixture is a marked cyanosis which worsens with stress.

Since a significant portion of right ventricular blood enters the systemic circulation without ever passing through the lungs, there is actually low pulmonary blood flow. This low flow is manifested radiographically as hypovascular lung fields.

In milder forms of tetralogy, the pulmonic stenosis is not as severe and, as a result, the right ventricular pressure may be considerably below the left ventricular pressure. In this instance, a left to right shunt would exist and the animal would not be cyanotic.

## DIAGNOSIS

In severely affected dogs, dyspnea is quite evident. Cyanosis is usually present from about the time of weaning or even earlier. Other findings associated with tetralogy include stunting and secondary polycythemia. Death sometimes results from embolic damage secondary to bacterial endocarditis. Congestive heart failure is very uncommon.

Auscultation reveals a loud ejection murmur (pulmonic stenosis) heard best in the left third intercostal space near the costo-chondral junction. The murmur may also be heard well on the right side. If the murmur is of great enough intensity, a thrill may be palpable in the same areas.

The electrocardiogram is usually indicative of severe right ventricular hypertrophy—i.e., a marked rightward and cranial displacement of the ventricular depolarization forces.

Radiographs of the thorax reveal characteristic features of tetralogy. There is usually marked right ventricular hypertrophy which is most evident in the dorsoventral view. Perhaps the most characteristic radiographic feature is "coving" of the pulmonary artery segment—i.e., the portion of cardiac silhouette in the dorsoventral view associated with the main pulmonary artery is "coved" or "empty" due to hypoplasia of the vessel. In the lateral and dorsoventral views, the lungs often appear hypovascular because of decreased pulmonary blood flow. The ascending aorta frequently appears enlarged in the lateral view.

An angiocardiogram made by injection of contrast material into the right ventricle reveals a thickened right ventricle, valvular or subvalvular pulmonic stenosis, a right to left shunt through a ventricular septal defect, and hypoplastic pulmonary arteries. The ascending aorta is dilated and overrides the ventricular septal defect.

## TREATMENT

The treatment of choice is total surgical correction, including closing the ventricular septal defect and eliminating the pulmonic stenosis. This procedure requires heart-lung bypass. A less involved and less satis-

factory surgical technique is to create a shunt between the aorta or subclavian artery and the pulmonary artery. This serves to increase pulmonary blood flow and improve the oxygen status of the animal.

It is rare that dogs with tetralogy develop congestive heart failure; however, should this occur, standard medical therapy would be indicated (see articles on therapy for congestive heart failure, pp. 327 to 346).

### SUPPLEMENTAL READING

Ettinger, S. J., and Suter, P. F.: Canine Cardiology. Philadelphia, W. B. Saunders Co., 1970.
Patterson, D. F.: Tetralogy of Fallot. *In* A Manual of Clinical Cardiology. Elkhart, Ind., American Animal Hospital Association, 1972.
Patterson, D. F., Pyle, R. L., Van Mierop, L. V., Melbin, J., and Olson, M.: Hereditary defects of the conotruneal septum in keeshond dogs: Pathologic and genetic studies. Am. J. Cardiol., 34:187–205, 1974.

# Persistent Right Aortic Arch

Persistent right aortic arch (PRAA) is a congenital vascular malformation which results from abnormal development of the aortic arch system. There is no cardiac disease associated with isolated PRAA; therefore, one would not expect to hear any heart

murmurs or detect any other sign of heart disease.

Specifically, PRAA occurs when the aorta originates from the right fourth aortic arch rather than from the left fourth aortic arch (Fig. 4). As a result of the aorta arising to the

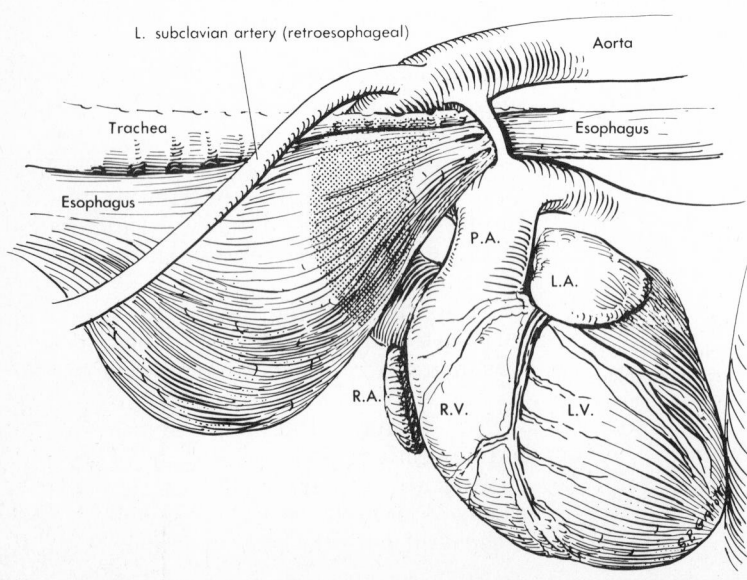

**Figure 4.** Drawing of the heart and related structures in a dog with persistent right aortic arch as viewed from the left side. The esophagus and trachea are incarcerated in a vascular ring which includes the aorta to the right, the ligamentum arteriosum dorsolaterally, the pulmonary artery to the left and the base of the heart ventrally. (Courtesy of Dr. J. W. Buchanan.)

right and coursing through the thorax to the right of the esophagus, a vascular ring is formed around the esophagus. The vascular ring is located at the level of the ligamentum arteriosum where the ligamentum arteriosum forms the dorsolateral aspect of the ring, the pulmonary artery is to the left, the aorta is to the right, and the base of the heart forms the ventral aspect of the ring. Occasionally, a retroesophageal left subclavian artery may occur which contributes to the esophageal constriction.

## DIAGNOSIS

PRAA has been recognized in many breeds; however, it occurs more frequently in the German shepherd and Irish setter. The outstanding clinical feature is regurgitation of solid food shortly after eating. The food appears undigested and, if retained for a period of time, may have a foul smell. The vomiting commences when the animal begins eating solid food; therefore, these cases usually come to the attention of a verterinarian between four and eight weeks of age. Other findings in severely affected dogs may include emaciation, dehydration, stunting and aspiration pneumonia. Dilatation of the cervical esophagus can be demonstrated by closing off the nose and mouth and then gently compressing the thorax. This manipulation causes the esophagus to balloon markedly in the cervical region.

Definitive diagnosis can be obtained through barium contrast study of the esophagus and angiography. A barium swallow will demonstrate a dilated esophagus from the cervical region down to the base of the heart. A dorsoventral radiograph or angiogram can be made by injecting contrast material into the ascending aorta via a catheter introduced into the carotid artery. Such a study will demonstrate the aorta's arising to the right of the trachea and esophagus.

In considering a diagnosis, the most important esophageal disease which must be differentiated from PRAA is achalasia. In contrast to PRAA, the esophagus in achalasia is usually dilated throughout its length.

## TREATMENT

Basically, treatment consists of relieving the stricture around the esophagus by dividing the ligamentum arteriosum. The surgery should be done as early as practical so as to reduce the degree of permanent esophageal disease. The area of concern is approached through a left fourth intercostal space incision. After entering the thorax, an incision is made in the mediastinal pleura above the left vagus nerve at the edge of the bulging esophagus. The incision is extended caudally parallel to the aorta. Gentle dissection is employed until the entire esophageal constriction area can be visualized. The ligamentum arteriosum grossly appears as a fibrous ligament; however, occasionally it may be patent, creating a need for a ligature to be placed around both ends of the ligamentum arteriosum before dividing. The left recurrent laryngeal nerve which loops around the ligamentum arteriosum should be identified so as to prevent injury to the nerve. Not infrequently, a persistent left vena cava is seen with PRAA. This vein, if large, can course directly over the area of the ligamentum arteriosum. The vein must be dissected free and reflected so that the surgery can be completed.

Following division of the ligamentum arteriosum, the esophagus is dissected free of the surrounding tissue above and below the stenotic segment. This assures that fibrous bands and adhesions will not interfere with esophageal function.

Immediate postoperative care is primarily concerned with food management. Initially, soft baby foods are fed several times a day for two weeks. Liquid oral vitamins are also given. Starting the third week, the animal is titrated against various types of food and feeding intervals until an acceptable regimen is established.

Regurgitation can be minimized by training the animal to eat in a semi-erect position. This is done by placing the food on a table or some similar object so that the dog must place his forefeet on the object in order to eat. This position assists in moving food down the esophagus.

### SUPPLEMENTAL READING

Buchanan, J. W.: Persistent left cranial vena cava in dogs: Angiocardiography, significance, and coexisting anomalies. J. Am. Vet. Rad. Soc., 4:1–8, 1963.
Buchanan, J. W.: Symposium: thoracic surgery in the dog and cat, III. Patent ductus and persistent right aortic arch surgery in dogs. J. Small Animal Pract., 9:409–428, 1968.
Ettinger, S. J., and Suter, P. F.: Canine Cardiology. Philadelphia, W. B. Saunders Co., 1970.
Mulnix, J. A., and Severin, G. A.: Persistent right aortic arch. *In* A Manual of Clinical Cardiology. Ekhart, Ind., American Animal Hospital Association, 1972.

# PATENT DUCTUS ARTERIOSUS

E. M. BREZNOCK, D.V.M.
*Davis, California*

## ANATOMY

The ductus arteriosus, the distal portion of the sixth left aortic arch, is a thick-walled arterial channel connecting the pulmonary artery to the aorta. This channel bypasses the lungs during the fetal period and closes spontaneously shortly after birth. Although species variability occurs, the ductus in the canine and feline species is probably completely closed by the end of the second week of life. The mechanism of closure is still debated, but it is probably a combination of hemodynamic, neurologic, humoral and gas tension effects initiated with the onset of respiration and the drop in pulmonary vascular resistance.

## INCIDENCE AND ETIOLOGY

Patent ductus is an isolated defect, but occasionally is associated with other cardiac anomalies. Genetic factors are significant. Respiratory difficulty at birth has been suspected in man and animals of being a cause of incomplete closure. A breed and sex predilection exists (poodle, German shepherd, keeshond, cocker spaniel), with a preponderance of cases being females (70 per cent).

## SYMPTOMS AND PHYSICAL SIGNS

The uncomplicated patent ductus in animals produces no symptoms. Serious, life-threatening symptoms develop in a high percentage of patients with patent ductus arteriosus. Failure to thrive with respiratory infections is always a potential problem. Dyspnea and cardiac failure develop not infrequently in pups 8 to 10 weeks of age. The most striking sign is the continuous machinery murmur. The murmur is rough and thrilling and increases in intensity at the beginning of the second cardiac sound. In animals with a small thoracic cage, the murmur and thrill can usually be perceived anywhere on the chest wall; in large dogs it may be perceived only on the left hemithorax at the level of the cardiac base. The development of severe pulmonary hypertension (75 torr) with reversal of shunt blood flow may cause this murmur to disappear. A wide pulse pressure at rest is usually found in the normal ductus.

## ELECTROCARDIOGRAPHY AND RADIOGRAPHY

In less than 5 per cent of the cases, electrocardiographic tracings are normal, and in 95 per cent left ventricular enlargement is present (indicated by >3.5 mv. R wave in leads II, III and aVF). Radiographically, there will be an increase in lung vascularity, prominent pulmonary artery segments and a typical bulge to the aortic root at the level of the patent ductus.

## CLINICAL COURSE

Untreated patent ductus arteriosus may lead to complications and to premature death. Few animals with PDA (<10 per cent) have been observed to be older than 4 years of age. If left untreated, most patients will probably die from subacute cardiac failure with fulminating pulmonary edema before they become adults.

## DIFFERENTIAL DIAGNOSIS

The continuous murmur in the area of the left cardiac base in an acyanotic asymptomatic patient is almost pathognomonic of patent ductus arteriosus. Other conditions producing a continuous murmur may have to be considered among the diagnostic possibilities. Pulmonary arteriovenous fistulas may produce a continuous murmur over the site of the fistula in the lung. Aorticopulmonary window is the lesion most frequently confused with patent ductus arteriosus. Auscultation and angiocardiography or exploratory thoracotomy will help in differentiation. Ventricular septal defect with aortic insufficiency may be difficult to separate from patent ductus arteriosus, especially if the ductus has a concomitant ventricular septal defect. The continuous murmur auscultated in dogs with a ventricular septal defect with aortic insufficiency is usually loudest over the right base and much lower in intensity with minimal thrill. Electrocardiographic findings do not show the typical left ventricular enlargement pattern of patent ductus.

## Associated Congenital Cardiovascular Lesions

In pulmonic stenosis, tetralogy of Fallot, pulmonary atresia and single ventricle, the presence of an associated patent ductus is fortunate, and the shunt may be responsible for keeping the neonate alive. With ventricular or atrial septal defects, a patent ductus is actually harmful, and surgical closure of the ductus alone may be life-saving. In three cases with ventricular septal defect and patent ductus, the septal defect closed spontaneously following surgical closure of the ductus.

## Atypical Ductus

Pulmonary hypertension associated with patent ductus may be due to increased flow, to secondary lesions which are the result of increased flow or to irreversible alterations in pulmonary vessels. Electrocardiograms will usually illustrate right ventricular enlargement. These patients are frequently suspected of having a large interatrial or ventricular septal defect because of the clinical resemblance to the more common lesions of septal defect.

## Anesthesia

Some patients with asymptomatic patent ductus arteriosus can be safely anesthetized with thiobarbiturate induction and halogenated hydrocarbon gaseous anesthesia. This protocol may prove life-threatening in cardiac decompensated patients with compensated cardiovascular reflexes because of negative inotropic and hypotensive effects of the halogenated hydrocarbon anesthetics. For this reason most patent ductus patients are preanesthetized with intramuscular atropine (0.04 mg./kg. body weight), preoxygenated and induced with intravenous fentanyl (0.02 mg./kg. body weight) for analgesia and pancuronium (0.06 mg./kg. body weight) for muscle relaxation. Because the induction dose of fentanyl and pancuronium lasts 25 and 45 minutes, respectively, pancuronium is repeatedly given as needed; fentanyl in a lactate drip is given at a rate of 0.8 $\mu$g./kg./minute. Fentanyl is reversed with intramuscular naloxone (0.006 mg./kg. body weight); pancuronium is reversed with intravenous neostigmine (0.03 mg./kg. body weight) and atropine (0.02 mg./kg. body weight).*

## Treatment

Although a chemotherapeutic approach to closure of patent ductus arteriosus may soon be a reality, the nonoperative treatment of patent ductus is currently limited to the temporary treatment of such complications as cardiac failure, respiratory infections and pulmonary edema. Some difference of opinion concerning the role of operative and nonoperative treatment of patent ductus exists. Increasing evidence and agreement suggest that early surgical intervention not only is advisable but may be life-saving. If radiogram evaluation confirms cardiac enlargement and the ductus has been proved to be the sole cause of this enlargement or the major contributing cause, the ductus should be interrupted after appropriate preparation. If the patient is in acute cardiac failure, an attempt at pharmaceutical stabilization (viz., diuretics, cage rest) of the patient prior to surgical intervention is recommended. However, critical delays in surgery may prove fatal and should be avoided. The neonatal patient (4 to 6 weeks of age) withstands the surgical procedure as well as older animals, and there is no justifiable reason for withholding operation. Puppies as young as 4 to 6 days of age in acute cardiac failure from patent ductus have responded rapidly and favorably to thoracotomy and surgical interruption of the patent ductus.

The ductus closes spontaneously early in life or not at all. Because the operation is technically simple, is quickly performed and carries a quite low morbidity it should be performed as soon as the diagnosis is confirmed. Early operation eliminates the danger of subsequent development of pul-

---

*Anesthesia protocol prepared by I. McLeish, B. Hart and S. Haskins.

monary hypertension, respiratory complications and changes in vessel character (viz., compliance, distortion, elasticity), all of which may result in increased morbidity.

The question of ligation of the ductus versus division in animals is equivocal at this time. Recanalization of the ductus in man rarely occurs (<0.05 per cent) following surgical ligation of the patent ductus. Few cases of recanalization have been seen in animals following interruption of the patent ductus by ligation with suture or hemostatic clip application. The much shorter life span of animal species probably minimizes the likelihood of this complication.

**Surgical Techniques.** Only the important aspects of the surgical techniques for interruption of patent ductus will be presented here. An extrapericardial approach is in most instances all that is needed for adequate exposure. Blunt dissection anteriorly (between the main pulmonary artery and aorta) and posteriorly (between the aorta and the afferent pulmonary artery feeding the left cranial lung lobe) is performed following retraction of the vagus nerve either dorsad or ventrad. Care should be taken to avoid severe trauma to the left recurrent laryngeal nerve as it passes behind the ductus. The aorta may be freed sufficiently so that it may be cross-clamped if necessary to avoid catastrophe in the event of injury to the ductus or great vessels. Once anterior and posterior dissection is complete and adequate, a hemostatic vessel clip or two can be applied (with a fold of ductus tissue between), if this is the method of interruption chosen.

If ligation is selected as the method of interruption, minimal careful medial dissection may be performed before attempting to pass a right-angle mixter behind the ductus. A curved hemostat may be used for medial blunt dissection, but under no circumstances should the curved hemostat be used in place of the right-angle mixter for passage behind the ductus (for carriage of the ligation silks). Only a right-angle mixter of the correct size should be utilized (and this depends on the size of the patient). Placement of the right-angle mixter is most safely and most easily accomplished by positioning the instrument deep into the dissected area posterior to the ductus. Next, advance the jaws of the mixter anteriorly on the medial aspect of the ductus until the tips can be visualized in the dissected area anterior to the ductus. Tissues remaining on the medial side of the ductus will be carried to the anterior dissection area by the tips of the mixter and must be bluntly or sharply removed before silk ligatures can be placed between the mixter jaws. Deep seating of the mixter jaws prior to advancement behind the ductus will add greatly in prevention of puncture or tearing any vessel. Hypotensive or hypothermic anesthesia in special instances may be indicated, but in the vast majority of cases it is not recommended unless the surgeon (or anesthetist) is thoroughly familiar with these methods. Ligation with two silk sutures is recommended with a fold of ductus tissue between. Transection and oversewing of ductus ends is technically more difficult, carries a higher morbidity and mortality and requires costly pediatric ductus clamps for successful repair. If this technique is attempted, an intrapericardial approach makes dissection and isolation of the ductus easier for application of the ductus clamps. Following interruption of the ductus, palpation of the epicardial surface should be performed for identification of concomitant cardiac defects.

If pulmonary hypertension is suspected or present, pulmonary artery pressure readings should be taken while the ductus is temporarily occluded. Maintenance of high pulmonary artery pressure or an elevation of the pressure upon occlusion of the ductus is usually indicative of inability to withstand interruption of the ductus. A fall in the pulmonary artery pressure during temporary occlusion of the ductus indicates that the procedure can safely be completed. Although interruption of patent ductus with concomitant pulmonary hypertension in man has resulted in a not infrequent successful ligation with survival of the patient, occlusion of patent ductus in dogs has repeatedly proved fatal. Even when performed as a two-stage interruptive procedure, the results have been unfavorable.

**Postoperative Care.** Following thoracotomy, the pneumothorax is usually eliminated in dogs over 5 kg. in body weight with three-way stopcock, syringe and needle after closure of the thoracotomy incision. In smaller patients, an intercostal catheter is left in place until adequate tidal volume is observed, with stabilization of the patient following reversal of the pancuronium. Digitalis is infrequently needed for pharmaceutical cardiac assistance.

**Complications.** Injury to the recurrent laryngeal nerve may occur, with potential paralysis of the left vocal cord and phonetic changes. No permanent damage has been seen.

## PROGNOSIS

After successful closure of the ductus, whether by division, suture or clip interruption, in the absence of any other cardiac defects, restitution to a physiologically normal state is complete. Asculted murmurs which result as a sequela of the patent ductus (viz., mitral insufficiency) should in most instances spontaneously regress following ligation of the patent ductus. The incidence of late complications (viz., infection, recanalization, heart failure) is minute.

### SUPPLEMENTAL READING

Breznock, E. M.: Patent ductus arteriosus. In Bojrab, J. (ed.): Current Techniques in Small Animal Surgery I. Philadelphia, Lea & Febiger, 1975, pp. 296–301.

Elliott, R. B., and Starling, M. B.: The effects of prostaglandins, prostaglandin inhibitors, and oxygen on the closure of the ductus arteriosus, pulmonary arteries, and umbilical vessels *in vitro*. Prostaglandins, 8:187–203, 1974.

Eyster, G. E., Eyster, J. T., Cords, G. B., and Johnston, J.: Patent ductus arteriosus in the dog: Characteristics of occurrence and results in one hundred consecutive cases. J. Am. Vet. Med. Assn., 168:435–438, 1976.

Heymann, M. A., and Rudolph, A. M.: Control of the ductus arteriosus. Physiol. Rev., 55:62–78, 1975.

Tsuji, H., Shapiro, M., Magidson, O., Dunne, E., Dykstra, P., and Kay, J. H.: Surgical treatment of high pressure patent ductus arteriosus. Circulation, 27:652–657, 1963.

# PULMONIC STENOSIS

JAMES W. BUCHANAN, D.V.M.
*Philadelphia, Pennsylvania*

The term pulmonic stenosis encompasses all forms of obstruction to blood flow from the right ventricle to the pulmonary artery. Thus, it may be supravalvular, valvular, immediately subvalvular or infundibular in location (Fig. 1). Branch stenosis, as described in man, has not been recognized in dogs. The valvular type may be caused by fusion of the valve commissures, leaving a small, usually centrally located orifice, or by thickened, immobile valve leaflets without fusion. The latter is usually associated with hypoplasia of the pulmonic root.

A second type of obstruction has been observed immediately below the valve leaflets. In this form, a complete or partial fibrous ring occurs adjacent to and sometimes involving the base of the pulmonary valve leaflets. Not infrequently, this type is associated with thickened, but not fused, myxomatous valve leaflets and a hypoplastic pulmonic root.

A third site of obstruction is lower in the right ventricular outflow tract. In this region, hypertrophy of the crista supraventricularis muscle band or the entire right ventricular outflow tract may cause significant obstruction. In some instances, only a long, narrow channel exists through which blood flows out of the right ventricle. Either type of infundibular hypertrophy may occur as a primary lesion, but more often it appears to be secondary to valvular or immediately subvalvular stenosis.

Pulmonic stenosis occurs about as frequently as patent ductus arteriosus in a hospital clinic population and has been found in a variety of breeds, but more commonly

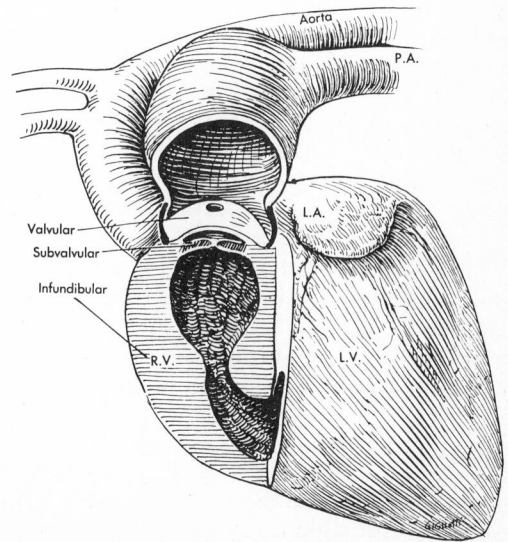

**Figure 1.** Locations of different forms of pulmonic stenosis.

than expected in English bulldogs, Chihuahuas and terrier type dogs. Experimental breeding of affected beagles has shown that it can be inherited (Patterson, 1968).

## DIAGNOSIS

A diagnosis of pulmonic stenosis in moderate and severe cases usually can be made on the basis of age, breed, history, auscultation, palpation, electrocardiography and survey radiography. In mild cases, cardiac catheterization and angiocardiography usually are necessary to confirm the diagnosis. These studies also should be performed in moderate and severe cases for preoperative evaluation.

Many dogs with pulmonic stenosis are asymptomatic, and the abnormality is detected incidentally during a routine physical examination. When the abnormality is more obstructive, excessive tiring with exercise and occasional fainting may be reported. In dogs with severe stenosis, right-sided congestive heart failure may occur in the first few months of life. Cyanosis is not seen in dogs with isolated pulmonic stenosis except in terminal stages.

Pulmonic stenosis ordinarily causes a systolic murmur heard best in the ventral portion of the left third intercostal space. Often a precordial thrill can be palpated in the same area. The apex beat may be more palpable on the right side. Descriptive characteristics of the murmur, such as separation from the first heart sound and mid-systolic accentuation, may be evident in a phonocardiogram but often are not sufficiently obvious to warrant a confirming diagnosis by auscultation alone, even by experienced persons. Delayed closure of the pulmonary valve evidenced by splitting of the second heart sound may be audible.

Right ventricular hypertrophy occurs in response to outflow obstruction. This is ordinarily manifested in electrocardiograms by right axis deviation in the frontal plane (large S waves in leads II and aVF) and large S waves in unipolar exploring chest leads over the region of the left ventricle.

## RADIOGRAPHY

Dorsoventral radiographic changes associated with right ventricular hypertrophy include increased right-sided convexity and sometimes rightward deviation of the cardiac silhouette if enlargement occurs with concentric hypertrophy. Poststenotic dilatation of the main pulmonary artery also occurs and may be seen as a prominence in the left cranial segment of the cardiac silhouette. Although main pulmonary artery enlargement occurs, the branches distal to the primary right and left branches are not enlarged and may appear smaller than normal. This helps to distinguish pulmonic stenosis from dirofilariasis and left-to-right shunting congenital defects in which the peripheral pulmonary artery branches may be enlarged. In lateral radiograms, right ventricular enlargement and poststenotic dilatation of the main pulmonary artery may cause loss of the cranial waist and elevation of the trachea cranial to its bifurcation.

Angiocardiography should be performed routinely in dogs suspected of having pulmonic stenosis. In the absence of specialized equipment, the diagnosis may be confirmed in some cases by a single lateral radiogram made immediately upon completion of an intravenous injection of radiopaque contrast material, such as sodium meglumine diatrizoate (Cardiografin®), 1.0 ml./kg. of body weight. This must be injected into a jugular vein as rapidly as possible through an 18-gauge needle.

It is preferable and often essential to make a selective angiocardiogram by injection directly into the right ventricle. This avoids superimposition of the right atrium on the right ventricular outflow tract area. A right ventricular injection may be made by direct cardiac puncture; however, I prefer to insert a catheter through the jugular vein, cranial vena cava and right atrium into the right ventricle. With only a little practice, this can be done under a fluoroscope.

If blood pressure recording equipment is available, the systolic pressure in the right ventricle should be compared with that in the pulmonary artery. Normally, the two should be the same. The degree of difference between the two (pressure gradient) is a useful indicator of the degree of obstruction. Pressure tracings recorded while the catheter is being withdrawn from the pulmonary artery into the right ventricle demonstrate the pressure gradient and the "pull-out pattern." More detailed explanations of these can be found in texts on clinical cardiology.

## SURGERY

**Indications.** The indications for surgery are not always clear, even when cardiac catheterization has been performed. In man, if the gradient is less than 50 mm. Hg, surgery is not recommended. If the gradient is between 50 and 100 mm. Hg, surgery is recommended if any clinical signs are evident. If the gradient exceeds 100 mm. Hg, surgery is always recommended.

A sufficient number of dogs with pulmonic stenosis have not been studied under normal environmental conditions to establish whether similar or different gradients should be used as indications for or against surgery. It seems reasonable, however, on the basis of cases studied with and without signs of cardiac disability, to suggest that the values used as guidelines for recommending surgery in man can be used in dogs. In the absence of cardiac catheterization data, surgery appears to be indicated in any dog having signs of cardiac disability, regardless of age. It is also indicated in dogs less than one year of age without signs of disability but in which radiographic evidence of cardiac enlargement is present. Asymptomatic young dogs should be examined radiographically at 3- to 4-month intervals, until they are over one year of age, before a decision is made about whether surgery is indicated. It is unlikely that a dog reaching 6 months of age without radiographic evidence of cardiac enlargement or electrocardiographic evidence of right ventricular hypertrophy will ever require surgery.

**Principles.** Surgical correction of pulmonic stenosis necessarily has to be approached in different ways, depending upon the type of obstruction present, the equipment available and the experience of the surgeon. In some instances simple valvulotomy is sufficient, and this is essentially a one-man operation. In other cases temporary venous occlusion and an open right ventriculotomy or pulmonary arteriotomy are needed to alleviate the stenosis effectively. In a third category, cardiopulmonary bypass and major remodeling or patch-grafting of the right ventricular outflow tract are indicated.

Most dogs with pulmonic stenosis have either the valvular fusion type or an immediately subvalvular fibrous ring. In some instances, both types are present. It is usually not possible to distinguish between these forms by any means other than direct vision. Of more importance is the angiocardiographic recognition of the occasional dog with marked hypertrophy of the right ventricular outflow tract resulting in a long, very narrow channel in which improvement following simple valvulotomy and dilatation is highly unlikely, and in which an attempt to correct the condition without the use of cardiopulmonary bypass or temporary venous occlusion probably is not justifiable. The more common types of valvular and immediately subvalvular pulmonic stenosis may be approached by the relatively simple technique of inserting a valvulotome into the right ventricle through a pursestring-controlled stab incision. However, I prefer to use temporary venous occlusion and an open pulmonary arteriotomy for the advantage of direct visual examination of the valve and the type and degree of correction required. More detailed descriptions of the surgery are given elsewhere (Buchanan and Lawson, 1974).

### SUPPLEMENTAL READING

Buchanan, J. W., and Lawson, D. D.: Cardiovascular system. In Canine Surgery. 2nd Archibald ed. Santa Barbara, California, American Veterinary Publications, Inc., 1974.

Patterson, D. F.: Epidemiologic and genetic studies of congenital heart disease in the dog. Circ. Res., 23:171–202, 1968.

# OPEN-HEART SURGERY IN THE DOG*

GEORGE E. EYSTER, V.M.D.,
and A. THOMAS EVANS, D.V.M.
*East Lansing, Michigan*

The first reported clinical open-heart surgical success in the dog occurred in 1966. Since that time, periodic and occasionally successful surgical procedures have been performed on clinic cases in the dog. However, owing to the considerable time, equipment expense and instrumentation, these procedures have been limited to large medical centers and universities.

## PREOPERATIVE CONSIDERATIONS

The dog, which has been most frequently used as a bypass animal, is perhaps one of the more difficult animals for extracorporeal circulation or cardiopulmonary bypass. This is probably related to the extreme fragility of the canine red cell and to its subsequent destruction. If a hemic prime is used, blood incompatibilities are seen, and even in matched blood, homologous blood syndrome can cause death in a high percentage of dogs. In addition, whenever an animal used for bypass is affected with heartworm disease, there appears to be an anaphylactic type reaction associated with the destruction of microfilaria in the extracorporeal pump system.

Many of these problems can be alleviated by the use of (1) nonhemic prime, (2) previously demonstrated heartworm-free dogs or high levels of steroid in the prime solution and (3) wetting agents added to the prime solution to decrease red cell destruction due to red cell fragility. Nonhemic prime has been popular since 1960 as a method of diluting the blood and alleviating the problems associated with transfusion when donor blood is used in the bypass procedure. Many solutions have been used; however, we feel that lactated Ringer's is probably the ideal solution.

In the experimental laboratory, heartworm-free dogs should be used. However, the reaction to the microfilaria is alleviated or eliminated if a high level of steroid is administered in the prime solution. Approximately 100 mg. of prednisolone will eliminate the majority of the heartworm-induced reactions. Survival is also improved if the dog has been prophylactically treated for 5 days with antibiotics that tend to sterilize the gastrointestinal tract.

Pluronic F-68, a pluronic polyol, approximately 4 gm./liter of prime solution, has a protective effect on red cells. With this protective mechanism, both the osmotic and the mechanical fragility of the red cells are decreased, and bypass time can be extended to three to four times that of the nonpluronic procedures.

Before cardiopulmonary bypass or corrective open-heart surgery can be considered diagnosis is imperative. Complete cardiac catheterization is performed, including pressure monitoring, selective angiography indicator dilution techniques for cardiac output studies and shunt determinations intracardiac oxygen monitoring and occasionally intracardiac electrocardiography The importance of these preoperative considerations cannot be overemphasized. The techniques involved in preparation for open-heart surgery and the occasional differences in approach require that the surgeon be prepared to enter at the correct location and be acquainted with all the possible ramifications of the disease process *Open-heart surgery must not be an exploratory procedure.*

In order to accomplish successful cardiopulmonary bypass, monitoring equipment must be obtained. Included are ar electrocardiogram and at least two pressure monitors, all of which can be visualized on a large oscilloscope. Preparatory to and throughout the procedure and in the post

---

*The authors acknowledge with appreciation the help and cooperation of the following staff members of Michigan State University who are members of the cardiac surgical team: L. K. Anderson, D.V.M.; G. L. Blanchard, D.V.M.; David DeYoung, D.V.M.; and Mark Zimmer, B.S.

406

operative period, electrocardiograms and arterial and venous pressures are important in the total management of the patient. Success of the procedure requires understanding of abnormalities and correction of these abnormalities as they develop. In addition, a DC defibrillator is mandatory, since cardiac arrest and fibrillation are not infrequent sequelae of bypass. The operating room team must have available blood gas monitoring equipment (pH, $PaO_2$ and $PaCO_2$). This equipment provides the surgical team with the ability to monitor and control the efficiency of the cardiopulmonary heart-lung equipment. Metabolic acidosis is a usual sequela of cardiopulmonary bypass, and bicarbonate should be administered as needed.

## ANESTHETIC MANAGEMENT

The anesthetic management of a patient during cardiopulmonary bypass is similar to management of a patient with cardiac disease or shock. For the relatively mild case, the method of anesthesia should not be different from already established anesthetic principles. For the critically ill patient, greater care is needed because of compromised cardiovascular function and vastly diminished physiologic reserves.

The patient's preanesthetic evaluation should include the appropriate clinical pathology tests to evaluate the organ systems effectively. Preanesthetic medication consists of atropine sulfate (0.08 mg./kg.) administered subcutaneously 20 minutes prior to induction of anesthesia. The choice of induction agent is governed by the severity of the patient's illness. An ultrashort-acting thiobarbiturate (Surital®) is administered slowly in a dose sufficient to enable intubation in those patients that are mildly affected. In critically ill patients, a mask induction with halothane (Fluothane®) is preferred. In comatose animals, nitrous oxide and oxygen administered by mask may be sufficient for intubation. In all cases, especially those critically ill, preoxygenation with 100 per cent oxygen is advisable.

During surgical preparation for total bypass, anesthesia is maintained with 0.5 to 1.0 per cent halothane, nitrous oxide and oxygen. Nitrous oxide is discontinued if oxygen saturation of hemoglobin becomes 85 per cent or less. In addition, the surgeon should reposition lung packs to allow a greater pulmonary exchange area and decrease arterial-venous shunting. Intermittent positive pressure breathing is used to ventilate the patient during preparation for total bypass. Inspiratory pressure and volume are regimented by maintaining $PaCO_2$ at 40 mm. Hg. Gross hyperventilation should be avoided in order to prevent reductions in cardiac output and cerebral blood flow.

Monitoring of physiologic variables greatly increases the anesthetist's control of anesthesia depth. Routinely monitored are central venous pressure, arterial pressure, ECG, blood pH, blood gases and hemoglobin saturation with oxygen. Knowledge of these parameters enables the anesthetist to monitor cardiac function, cardiac irritability, pulmonary function and tissue perfusion. Blood gas values and pH are monitored at 30-minute intervals, with appropriate therapy instituted. If surgical electrocautery is used to control hemorrhage, a muscle relaxant, gallamine triethiodide (Flaxedil®) (0.5 mg./kg.) or succinylcholine (Sucostrin®) (0.5 mg./kg.) is given to control muscle twitching from electrical stimulation of nerve fibers. The elimination of vigorous twitching prevents unnecessary muscle trauma and consequently reduces sites of hemorrhage. Reduced supplemental doses of a muscle relaxant may be used to provide continued relaxation during the surgical procedure, thus enabling the anesthetist to use low concentrations of halothane. During the period of total bypass, 0.5 to 1.5 per cent halothane is used to maintain anesthesia. A vaporizer is situated between the oxygen source and the oxygenator allowing vaporization of halothane. Normal $PaCO_2$ is maintained by using a mixture of 95 per cent oxygen and 5 per cent carbon dioxide to oxygenate the blood. The lungs are sustained in a partially expanded state by means of continuous positive pressure (30 to 40 mm. Hg) and by an artificial "sigh" at 15-minute intervals.

Close supervision of the patient is required in the postanesthetic period. Intravenous fluids should be continued 24 hours postoperatively (2.5 per cent dextrose in half-strength Ringer's) or until the animal begins oral alimentation. Central venous pressure monitoring during this period will help in assessing volume replacement of fluids. Cardiac irritability is most severe in the postoperative period and may require treatment with lidocaine (Xylocaine®) administered to effect. The patient should remain in an oxygen-enriched environment until the effects of anesthesia have abated. Blood gas measurements are helpful in evaluating success of oxygen therapy and treatment of acidosis. Chest drainage tubes, one on either side of the mediastinum, remain in place for 24 hours or until postoperative hemorrhage has stopped. Hemorrhage is usually severe because of the administration of herparin during bypass. In our experience, the administration of the heparin antagonist protamine (protamine sulfate) is difficult to monitor, and consequently hemorrhage may continue postoperatively for several hours. The gradual decline in blood platelet numbers observed during cardiopulmonary bypass probably also contributes to the increased tendency to hemorrhage. Depending on available ancillary services, administration of whole blood or blood components (packed cells, platelets) should be considered.

Supplemental drug therapy is kept to a minimum during the postoperative period in order to assess the patient's cardiovascular and respiratory function more accurately.

## SURGICAL TECHNIQUES

Cardiopulmonary bypass is accomplished by connecting venous drainage lines from the right atrium and vena cava to a pump oxygenator system. The oxygenator is lower than the patient, and flow to the oxygenator is by gravity. From the oxygenator, the blood flows through a pump and is returned to the dog usually by way of the femoral artery.

Surgery is generally accomplished through right lateral thoracotomy in the fourth or fifth space. The venae cavae are isolated and the azygos vein is ligated. Heparin, 350 units/kg., is administered intravenously and repeated at a half-dose/hour. The cannulae are slipped into the posterior and anterior vena caval openings and are sewn by pursestring ligatures in the right atrium and right atrial appendage. Usually a femoral artery is exposed, and a cannula is placed in the artery. The cannulae are then connected by sterile tubing to the cardiopulmonary heart-lung bypass equipment, and bypass is begun by removing the clamps. Total cardiopulmonary bypass is accomplished by constricting the vena cava with tourniquets around the cannulae. In the dog, bypass requires a relatively large volume flow. Ninety to 100 ml./kg./minute is advisable, and success is much improved if procedures last less than one hour. The heart may now be opened, and internal cardiac manipulations can be accomplished.

In veterinary medicine today, open-heart surgical procedures include correction of large ventricular septal defects, atrial septal defects, pulmonic stenosis, subvalvular aortic stenosis, tetralogy of Fallot, heartworms and, in a few cases, mitral valve replacement.

*Atrial septal defects* are only rarely encountered. Only if the animal presents with evidence of heart failure is surgery indicated. Surgery for atrial septal defect correction is accomplished through a simple atriotomy and by a direct closure of the opening. Only rarely is the hole so large that a patch is necessary. Results with this procedure have been excellent in veterinary medicine.

*Pulmonic stenosis*, generally of the muscular or infundibular type, is best corrected by open-heart surgery. However, like an atrial septal defect, only when the animal is showing signs and symptoms of failure is surgery indicated. As a general rule, animals with gradients between the right ventricle and pulmonary artery exceeding 80 mm. Hg are surgical candidates. The right ventricular outflow tract is opened from 5 mm. below the pulmonic valve to the apex of the heart. Offending muscular tissue is excised. If subvalvular pulmonic stenosis is also present, the subvalvular ring is removed. If valvular stenosis is present, it too can be repaired at this time. The reopened, rechanneled right ventricular outflow tract is then closed.

Only a small percentage (less than 25 per cent) of *ventricular septal defects* have a large blood flow across the defect. When this occurs, or if the animal is in failure, surgery is indicated. The ideal correction for ventricular septal defect is total correction using direct suture or a patch repair of the defect. The right ventricle is opened perpendicular to the pulmonary outflow tract, and the ventricular septal defect is visualized. In most cases, direct closure can be accomplished. Care must be taken not to include the right bundle branch in the sutures.

A few successful clinical *mitral valve replacements* have been accomplished in the dog. The approach to the mitral valve is from the right side, over the base of the heart, parallel to the right atrium and to the right of the pulmonary veins. The old valve is removed, a prosthetic valve is inserted and placed and the left atrium is closed. Many postoperative complications are seen with this disease, not the least of which revolves around the preoperative pulmonary failure. Because of the expense of prosthetic devices in the dog, clinical repairs have infrequently been accomplished.

At the conclusion of the cardiac procedure, the cannulae are removed and atrial pursestring sutures are drawn tight. Heparin is neutralized by no more than 1 mg. protamine/1 mg. heparin. The chest is closed after placement of the drainage tubes.

In our experience, animals surviving for the first 12 hours will recover.

## SUMMARY

Open-heart surgery is being accomplished in veterinary medicine, but it is an infrequent clinical procedure. Not only are the diseases (excluding mitral regurgitation) relatively uncommon, but the equipment costs and technique development, surgical time, anesthesia time and medical care preclude this procedure for most dog owners. The surgical team must accept the realization that the cost of this procedure cannot be borne by the client. In spite of these financial considerations, it is assumed that open-heart surgery in the dog will continue at medical institutions and schools. More frequently, universities and some large medical hospitals are developing the instrumentation and techniques of open-heart surgery. Most are used in experimental studies and have, on occasion, been adapted for clinical use. It is likely that this trend will continue.

## SUPPLEMENTAL READING

Bernstein, E. F., *et al.*: Sublethal damage to the red blood cell from pumping. Circulation, *35, 36* (Suppl. 1):1226–1233, 1967.

Braden, T. D., *et al.*: Correction of a ventricular septal defect in a dog. J. Am. Vet. Med. Assn., *161*:507–512, 1972.

Godfrey, W. D., *et al.*: Canine heart worms in experimental cardiac and pulmonary surgery. J. Surg. Res., 6:331–336, 1966.

Miyauchi, Y., Inoue, T., and Patton, B. C.: Adjunctive use of a surface-active agent in extracorporeal circulation. Circulation, *33, 34* (Suppl. 1):71–77, 1966.

Neville, W. G.: Extracorporeal Circulation. Chicago, Year Book Medical Publishers, Inc., 1967.

Neville, W. G.: Superiority of buffered Ringer's lactate to heparinized blood as total prime of the large volume disc oxygenator. Ann. Surg., *165*:206–216, 1967.

Wylie, W. D., and Churchill-Davidson, H. C.: A Practice of Anesthesia. 3rd ed. Chicago, Year Book Medical Publishers, Inc., 1972, pp. 651–715.

# GENERAL GUIDELINES FOR CLINICAL EXAMINATION OF THE CARDIO-VASCULAR SYSTEM IN LARGE ANIMALS

G. F. FREGIN, V.M.D.
*Kennett Square, Pennsylvania*

*Editor's Note:* Equine cardiology is rapidly becoming part of the "pet practice" considered in the past to include principally dogs and cats. This brief chapter should serve as an outline for the companion pet practitioner who is periodically called upon to examine the pet horse.

Clinical examination of the cardiopulmonary (heart/lungs) system in the horse is an extremely important aspect of a soundness examination. Diseases of the heart and lungs as a cause of unsoundness in the horse are second in importance only to diseases of the musculoskeletal system. There are at the present time no studies on the prevalence of cardiovascular disease in the horse; however, cardiac arrhythmias and murmurs occur more frequently in this species than in any other domestic animal.

The following general guidelines are suggested for use in the physical examination of the cardiovascular system in large animals.

## DIAGNOSIS

### History

1. Onset of clinical signs—dyspnea, cough, decreased performance.
2. Previous illness—inoculation and worming.
3. Intended use—past, present and future.

### Inspection (Animal as a Whole)

1. Mucous membranes—color and capillary refill time.
2. Degree of filling of peripheral veins.
3. Jugular pulse.
4. Presence or absence of edema in dependent areas.
5. Apex beat—3rd to 5th left intercostal space in the middle of the lower one third of the thorax.

### Palpation

1. Lower one third of the thorax—3rd to 5th left intercostal space.
2. Hand corresponding to side—palm at 5th intercostal space with fingers extended forward under shoulder musculature and downward toward sternal margin.
3. Thrill.
4. Displacement of cardiac impulse.
5. Intensity of cardiac impulse.

### Percussion (Area of Cardiac Dullness)

1. Gross enlargement only.
2. Left side—edge of sternum ventrally, 3rd left intercostal space anteriorly, dorsally and caudally, 4th rib approximately 5 to 6 inches dorsal to sternum, through 5th left intercostal space at a distance 1 to 2 inches above the sternal border to reach sternum in the 6th left intercostal space.
3. Right side—3rd to 4th right intercostal space to a distance 1 to 2 inches above the sternal border.
4. Increase dorsally and caudally to 6th

left intercostal space with cardiac enlargement. With pulmonary emphysema, decreased area of cardiac dullness, disappearing first in the 5th left intercostal space and becoming lower in the 4th left intercostal space. May disappear entirely on the right.

### Arterial Pulse

Assess volume and contour and pulse pressure in
  1. Submaxillary.
  2. Coccygeal.
  3. Transverse facial.
  4. Common digital.
  5. Abdominal aorta and iliacs (rectal) exam.

### Venous Pulse

1. Jugular—reflects right atrial pressure, fills to approximately 10 cm. above level of right atrium point of shoulder.
  a. A wave—positive with right atrial contraction.
  b. C wave—positive with upward movement of atrioventricular valve and with carotid artery pulsation in early systole.
  c. X wave—negative with downward pull of atrioventricular valves in late systole.
  d. V wave—positive as atrium and veins fill with blood during ventricular systole.
  e. Y wave—negative with rapid flow of blood into ventricles.
2. Fills during expiration, empties during inspiration.

### Blood Pressure

1. The specific gravity of blood is about 1.050 to 1.060 and that of mercury is about 13.6, so that for every 13 mm. above or below the heart a pressure of 1 mm. Hg is added to or subtracted from the weight of the blood.
2. Coccygeal artery—86 to 137/40 to 72 mm. Hg
Median artery—108 to 150/144 to 194 mm. Hg

### Auscultation

1. Mitral area—5th left intercostal space one half the distance between point of shoulder and sternum.
2. Aortic area—4th left intercostal space 1 inch below point of shoulder.

3. Pulmonic area—3rd or 4th left intercostal space in the middle of the lower one third of the thorax.
4. Tricuspid area—3rd to 4th right intercostal space in the lower one half of the ventral one third of the thorax.

Auscultation is the most important part of the physical examination of the heart, requiring patience, a quiet environment and an understanding of the events of the cardiac cycle. Electrocardiography, however, must also be considered as an adjunct in the diagnosis of cardiovascular disease in large animals. Normal electrocardiographic data are available for the horse and to a lesser degree for the bovine. This information is of even greater value when previous recordings are available for comparison.

### Electrocardiogram

1. Left and right arm electrodes on respective limbs, approximately 8 cm. below level of the olecranon.
2. Right and left leg electrodes—may be placed over stifles.
3. Precordial leads (C or V leads):
  a. CV6LL—6th left intercostal space—level of costochondral junction
  b. CV6LU—6th left intercostal space—level of point of shoulder
  c. V 10—over spine of 6th thoracic vertebrae
  d. CV6RL—6th right intercostal space level of costochondral junction
  e. CV6RU—6th right intercostal space level of point of shoulder
4. The following leads should be recorded:

| I | aVR | $CV_6LL$ | $CV_6RL$ |
|---|-----|----------|----------|
| II | aVL | $CV_6LU$ | $CV_6RU$ |
| III | aVF | $V_{10}$ | |

### Cardiac Auscultation (The Stethoscope)

1. Ear pieces—rostrally.
2. Head piece.
3. Flexible tubing—18 inches in length, ⅛ inch in diameter.
4. Chest piece.
  a. Open bell—placed on skin loosely to hear low frequency sounds; on skin stretched to attenuate lower frequencies.
  b. Diaphragm—passes high frequency sounds and attenuates lower frequencies.

*Table 1.  Typical Signs of the Most Important Congenital Cardiovascular Lesions in Large Animals*

| | VENTRICULAR SEPTAL DEFECT | TETRALOGY OF FALLOT | PATENT DUCTUS ARTERIOSUS |
|---|---|---|---|
| Auscultation | Harsh, pansystolic murmur often overriding $S_2$, usually loudest in 2–4 right intercostal space or occasionally pulmonic area. Radiates and may be heard in 5-6 left intercostal space. Thrill usually present. | Systolic murmur transmitted widely over right and left thoracic wall. Character and intensity of murmur are variable. | In foals a grade II to III (out of V) continuous murmur usually sharply localized to 3rd–4th left intercostal space at level of point of shoulder. Disappears normally by 4th day. Little information available for adult. With pulmonary hypertension, murmur may not be continuous; some disappear and accentuation and splitting of $S_2$ may be present. |
| Electrocardiogram | Most often within normal limits. | Right ventricular enlargement pattern. | Insufficient data available. Right ventricular enlargement pattern possible in right-to-left type. |
| Radiographs | Cardiac silhouette often normal with small defects. Generalized cardiac enlargement, with prominence of main pulmonary artery segment; increased pulmonary vascular markings and left atrial prominence may be present with large defects. | Right ventricular enlargement without prominence of pulmonary artery segment. Prominence of ascending aorta. | Insufficient data available. |
| Angiocardiogram | Selective injection into pulmonary artery is usually satisfactory to demonstrate flow of contrast media from left to right ventricle (in foals). | Contrast medium passes from right ventricle into left ventricle and aorta (right-left shunt). Aorta and hypoplastic pulmonary artery simultaneously opacified. | |
| Cardiac Catheterization | Increase in blood oxygen saturation often minimal and pressures normal with small ventricular septal defects. Right ventricular and pulmonary arterial pressures elevated with large defects and pulmonary hypertension. | Elevated right ventricular pressure and lower pulmonary arterial pressure. (R.V. 90 to 160/10 and P.A. 30 to 40/5 to 10 mm. Hg.) | With left-right shunt, oxygen saturation of pulmonary blood may be elevated and blood pressure elevated in pulmonary artery and right ventricle. In right-to-left type, pulmonary artery pressure equal to or greater than aortic pressure. |
| Miscellaneous | Small defects are compatible with normal longevity. Racing performance has been adversely affected, although showing and hunting may be tolerated. | Stunting of growth, cyanosis and dyspnea with exertion. | |

5. More pressure does not amplify sounds; it only attenuates certain frequencies.

## DEPENDABLE SIGNS OF CARDIOVASCULAR DISEASE IN THE HORSE

1. Grade 4 or greater systolic murmur at resting heart rate in the absence of anemia. (Systolic ejection murmurs may appear with accelerated heart rate.)

2. Grade 3 or greater prolonged diastolic murmur at resting heart rate. (Presystolic and early diastolic flow murmurs are physiologic and may appear with elevated heart rates, excitement and exercise.)

3. Precordial thrill (in the absence of anemia).

4. Generalized venous distention.

5. Pericardial friction rub.

6. Atrial fibrillation or flutter.

7. Complete heart block.

8. Intermittent claudication with loss of arterial pulse.

9. Atrial and ventricular extrasystoles consistently present and of frequent occurrence.

## SIGNS SUGGESTIVE OF HEART DISEASE IN THE HORSE

1. Low-intensity systolic murmurs in animals in which not previously heard, in older animals and in areas in which flow murmurs are not usually audible.

2. Occasional atrial or ventricular premature beats.

3. Arrhythmias developing after exercise.

4. Minor deviations of ST segment of T wave.

5. Increased area of cardiac dullness.

6. Cough—left heart failure
Dyspnea
Ascites or edema
Generalized weakness (decreased cardiac output and low oxygen)
Cyanosis

7. Fainting—rupture of vessel (aortic-pulmonic-uterine), arrhythmia and decreased cardiac output.

**Table 2.** *Typical Signs of the More Important Acquired Cardiovascular Lesions in Large Animals*

| CONDITION | GENERAL SIGNS | AUSCULTATION | ETIOLOGY |
|---|---|---|---|
| Semilunar Valve Regurgitation | Insufficiency of aortic or pulmonic valve allows regurgitation of blood into corresponding ventricle during diastole. Uncommon on right side in horse. Water-hammer pulse (Corrigan) with significant degree of aortic insufficiency (A.I.). | Prolonged decrescendo diastolic murmur of A.I. beginning with or shortly after $S_2$. Best heard over heart base and usually transmitted well to the cardiac apex. May have variable intensity. | Bacterial endocarditis. Chronic valvular fibrosis associated with aging. Dilatation of valve rings. Congenital (fenestration). |
| Atrioventricular Valve Regurgitation | Deformity of the mitral and tricuspid valve cusps, dilatation of the valve ring or rupture of the chordae tendineae may result in regurgitation of blood into atrium during ventricular systole. Left side more commonly affected in equine, right side in bovine. Systolic pulsation in jugular vein with tricuspid insufficiency. | Grade III (in absence of anemia) or louder holosystolic murmur in mitral and/or tricuspid areas. | Acquired a. Bacterial endocarditis b. Chronic valvular disease c. Myocarditis Congenital |

*Continued on next page*

*Table 2.* *Typical Signs of the More Important Acquired Cardiovascular Lesions in Large Animals (Continued)*

| CONDITION | GENERAL SIGNS | AUSCULTATION | ETIOLOGY |
|---|---|---|---|
| Pericardial Disease | Usually secondary to pneumonia and pleuritis. Pericardial effusion following equine influenza or equine viral arteritis. Leukemia. Traumatic a. Ingestion with perforation (most common form in cattle—second only to leukemia, causing problem in both species) b. Rupture following violent activity | Pericardial friction rub. Muffling of heart sounds from fluid accumulation within pericardium. If acute and severe, cardiac tamponade may develop. | Infectious Allergic Traumatic Generalized congestive heart failure Acquired—secondary to leukemia |
| Myocardial Disease | Inflammation, degeneration or other pathologic process affecting the myocardium. Congestive heart failure may develop. Sudden death due to fatal arrhythmia. | Tachycardias Murmurs or gallop sounds Cardiac arrhythmias a. Premature systoles b. Paroxysmal tachycardia c. Atrial fibrillation | Infectious a. Bacterial b. Influenza c. Purpura hemorrhagica d. Equine infectious anemia Allergic Migration of Strongylus larvae Paralytic myoglobinuria Embolism a. Bacterial b. Parasitic endarteritis Acquired—secondary to leukemia |
| Endocardial Disease (Bacterial Endocarditis) | Inflammatory lesions affecting cardiac valves and mural endocardium. Embolic phenomena with or without accompanying signs. Recent infection with prolonged fever, weakness, weight loss and development of cardiac murmur. Aortic valves most frequently affected followed by mitral, tricuspid and pulmonary valves in equine. | May be within normal limits. Tachycardia Murmur or gallop sounds | Allergic (streptococci) Bacterial |

*Table 3. Condensed Listing of the More Important Arrhythmias in Large Animals*

| IRREGULARITY | CLINICAL OCCURRENCE | HEART RATE USUALLY OBSERVED (BEATS/MINUTE) | DIAGNOSIS | CLINICAL SIGNIFICANCE |
|---|---|---|---|---|
| Sinus Arrhythmia | Horses at rest; always present in incomplete atrioventricular block with dropped beats. | 25 to 40 (25 to 50) | Interval between heart beats progressively decreases for a series of beats, then lengthens again. Often difficult to detect by auscultation unless stopwatch or watch with second hand employed. | None, unless associated with acute infectious process (i.e., strangles). Disappears with adequate exercise, excitement or atropine. (Decrease in vagal tone.) |
| Atrial Fibrillation | Congestive heart failure. Mitral and tricuspid insufficiency. Degenerative or inflammatory myocardial diseases. Rare instances of paroxysmal atrial fibrillation. | 40 to 70 Although bradycardias and tachycardias may be seen (20 to 150). | Irregular heart rate. Pulse deficit. Irregularity increases with excitement or exercise. Heart sounds of varying intensity. Absence of atrial heart sound. Absence of P waves on electrocardiogram (F waves 300 to 500) | Atrial myocardial disease. Ability to perform strenuous work limited and stamina reduced. Prognosis more favorable in those with relatively slow rates at rest and no other detectable signs of cardiovascular disease. These animals are candidates for treatment to abolish the arrhythmia. (i.e., quinidine sulfate). Prognosis grave in those with rapid irregular rates at rest and with the development of congestive heart failure. In cattle usually secondary to gastrointestinal problems arrhythmias often revert to normal sinus rhythm without further therapy. |
| Atrial Flutter | Atrial myocardial disease. May occur during treatment for atrial fibrillation. | 100 and up Depends on degree of AV block. | Definite diagnosis impossible without electrocardiogram (F waves 200 to 250). | Rarely reported. Thought to be a sign of serious cardiac disease. |

*Continued on next page*

*Table 3.  Condensed Listing of the More Important Arrhythmias in Large Animals  (Continued)*

| IRREGULARITY | CLINICAL OCCURRENCE | HEART RATE USUALLY OBSERVED (BEATS/MINUTE) | DIAGNOSIS | CLINICAL SIGNIFICANCE |
|---|---|---|---|---|
| Premature Contractions | Inflammatory, degenerative or neoplastic myocardial disease. Reflexes from gastrointestinal tract. Congestive heart failure. Drugs or toxins, acute infections. | 40 to 70 (25 to 80) Sometimes near normal rate. Heart rate often not affected. | Heart beat occurs early and diastole is prolonged. Second heart sound and peripheral pulse may be absent or reduced in intensity. Irregularity may decrease with an increase in heart rate. | Atrial systoles suggest atrial myocardial disease. Ventricular premature systoles may occur in the absence of other signs of heart disease. Myocardial disease should be suspected, however, if they are frequent at rest, multifocal in origin or induced or increased in frequency following exercise. |
| Paroxysmal Tachycardia | Congestive heart failure, myocarditis. (Septicemia or toxemia.) Severe digestive disturbances. | 80 to 140 One case reported up to 240. | Rapid regular rate, sudden onset and abrupt termination. Duration variable. | Ventricular tachycardia usually indicates serious cardiac disease, such as myocarditis, myocardial degeneration and metastatic neoplasms. Atrial tachycardia occurs less frequently and may be associated with less serious signs (primary or secondary). |
| Incomplete AV Block With Dropped Beats | High vagal tone in the absence of heart disease. | 20 to 40 (25 to 50) | Slow, irregular rate. Atrial sound often audible. | A functional phenomenon resulting from vagal activity at rest. Normally disappears with excitement or exercise. Any factor increasing vagal tone may favor AV block. Cardiac lesions such as myocarditis or myocardial degeneration. |
| Complete AV Block | Severe myocardial disease. | 10 to 20 | Usually regular, slow ventricular rate. Atrial sounds at a more rapid rate may be heard. Bruit de canon (intermittently loud $S_1$) may be heard when atrial contraction occurs immediately before ventricular contraction. | Severe myocardial disease. |

## THERAPY

**Digitalization.**   Ventricular slowing may be accomplished through digitalization, and this should be carried out in horses in congestive heart failure.

The following digitalization and maintenance doses are recommended:

| PREPARATION | DIGITALIZATION DOSE | DAILY MAINTENANCE DOSE* |
|---|---|---|
| *Oral* | | |
| Digitalis | 1.5–3.0 gm./50 kg./day | 1/8 to 1/5 the digitalization dose |
| Digitalis Tincture | 15–30  ml./50 kg. | |
| Digitoxin | 1.5–3.0 to 1.5 mg./50 kg. | |
| Digoxin | 1.0 to 1.5 mg./50 kg. | |
| *Parenteral* | | |
| Ouabain | 0.6–0.9 mg./50 kg. | 0.5 to 0.8 mg./50 kg. |
| Digoxin | 0.5 to 0.75 mg./50 kg. | 0.25 to 0.40 mg./50 kg. |

*The total daily dose should be divided into equal amounts to be administered every 12 hours.

**Quinidine Sulfate Therapy.**   Quinidine therapy of atrial fibrillation is highly effective in horses. The following dose schedule for oral administration may be used:

| | |
|---|---|
| 1st day | 10 gm. (test dose) |
| 2nd day | 10 gm., 4 times daily |
| 3rd and 4th day | 10 gm., 6 times daily |

Only in exceptional cases has it been necessary to give higher doses, as follows:

| | |
|---|---|
| 5th and 6th day | 10 gm., 7 times daily |
| 7th and 8th day | 10 gm., 8 times daily |

These doses are to be given at 2-hour intervals. The quinidine sulfate powder is suspended in water and administered by stomach tube. In most cases (80 per cent), it is not necessary to exceed a dose of 60 gm. daily. Doses at levels higher than this are dangerous. Side effects of quinidine in horses include erythema and edema of the nasal mucosa, gastrointestinal disturbances, urticarial wheals and laminitis. The swelling of nasal mucosa occurs to a greater or lesser extent in most treated animals. It may become severe enough seriously to interfere with breathing and may require an emergency tracheotomy. However, this is seldom necessary, since the reaction is related to dosage and usually subsides if the drug is stopped or the dose is reduced to the level tolerated on previous days. Laminitis should be treated early and vigorously with cortisone to avoid permanent damage to the feet. After the arrhythmia is abolished, the treatment should continue for two or three days at a dose of 10 gm. twice daily. Two to three months' rest is desirable before exercise is resumed.

# Section

# 5

# HEMOLYMPHATIC DISORDERS AND ONCOLOGY

JACK E. HATHAWAY, D.V.M.
*Consulting Editor*

# MANAGEMENT OF ANEMIA IN THE DOG AND CAT

HUGH BILSON LEWIS, B.V.M.S.
*Lafayette, Indiana*

## GENERAL DISCUSSION

An animal is said to be anemic when the oxygen-carrying capacity of the blood is reduced below the normal for the age, sex, breed and species in question. In almost all cases there is a decrease in the total number of circulating erythrocytes, hemoglobin concentration and packed cell volume when compared to the normal group. It is important to understand that anemia is rarely a primary disease in small animals and usually reflects a more generalized disease process. Thus, a diagnosis of anemia without some etiologic or pathophysiologic explanation is inadequate.

### CLINICAL SIGNS

The clinical signs of anemia result from both the decreased oxygen-carrying capacity of the blood and the various physiologic adjustments made to increase the efficiency of the shrunken erythron, thereby reducing the workload of the heart. These physiologic compensatory adjustments include increased cardiac output, shunting of blood away from the superficial and splanchnic areas and increased blood flow to reduce the circulating time of the erythrocyte. The extent of the compensatory adjustments varies with the severity of the anemia, the rapidity of its development, the blood volume change and the cardiovascular status of the animal. In the dog, and to a lesser extent in the cat, there is also a compensatory shift to the right in the oxygen dissociation curve, permitting the extraction of increased amounts of oxygen without a decrease in oxygen pressure. This effect may play a substantial role in minimizing cellular hypoxia in anemic states.

The general clinical signs are noted in Table 1. Other signs referable to the patho-physiologic mechanism involved may also be seen, e.g., icterus, hemorrhage, hemoglobinuria, splenomegaly, hepatomegaly, etc.

### LABORATORY PROCEDURES AND EVALUATIONS

The initial laboratory procedures used to establish the presence of anemia are hematocrit, red cell count and hemoglobin concentration. Of these procedures, the microhematocrit technique is the most accurate and useful. Besides measuring the PCV, the color and character of the plasma (icteric, hemoglobinemic) and the size and color of the buffy coat (pink in the presence of reticulocytosis) can be noted. The spun-down microhematocrit can be retained in case there is reason later to make a smear of the buffy coat cells (RBC parasites, RBC morphology, erythrophagocytosis, LE cell preparation, etc.). The plasma portion can be used to measure the plasma protein concentration using the refractometer, information that can sometimes be useful in distinguishing blood loss from hemolytic anemias.

*The Wintrobe red cell indices\** can be calculated from the above laboratory evaluations, and a morphologic characterization can be made. The mean cell volume (MCV) is a very precise parameter that is unaffected by many common biologic variables, such as excitement. The mean cell hemoglobin concentration (MCHC) is the most accurate and precise index. These two cell constants are very useful in the initial clas-

---

$$*MCV = \frac{PCV \times 10}{RBC \ (millions)} = cubic \ microns$$

$$MCHC = \frac{HgB \times 100}{PCV} = \%$$

421

**Table 1.** *Common Clinical Signs of Anemia*

| REFERABLE TO DECREASED RBC MASS AND TISSUE HYPOXIA | REFERABLE TO PHYSIOLOGIC COMPENSATORY CHANGES |
|---|---|
| Muscular weakness:<br>  Lassitude, increased fatigability,<br>  unsteady gait, etc. | Tachycardia, tachypnea. |
| | Cardiac enlargement (chronic). |
| Cardiac murmur:<br>  Soft, systolic, waxes and wanes. | Cold extremities, vomiting, anorexia,<br>  postprandial fainting, pallor of mucous<br>  membranes, etc.—all are effects of<br>  redistribution of blood. |
| Fainting on exertion.<br>Behavior changes:<br>  Aggressive⟷Nonaggressive | |

sification of anemias and should be calculated in all suspected anemias in which the PCV, RBC and Hgb have been measured accurately. The indices should be interpreted as macrocytic, normocytic or microcytic (MCV) and either normochromic or hypochromic (MCHC). These interpretations should always be checked, however, by careful inspection of a stained blood smear for red cell morphology.

The red cell indices provide a measurement of the *average* change in size and hemoglobin content of the circulating red cells: the smear permits identification of individual cellular abnormalities and therefore can provide some indication of the pathophysiologic process involved in the anemia. The stained smear should be inspected for cell size, shape, hemoglobin content, color, inclusion bodies, etc. Such findings, together with their interpretations, are listed in Table 2.

Although the blood smear may provide evidence of increased red cell production (polychromasia, macrocytosis, Howell-Jolly bodies, nucleated RBC, etc.), it is best to perform a reticulocyte count (new methylene blue stain) as part of the initial laboratory work-up in anemic animals. The number of reticulocytes per 1000 red cells should be counted and expressed as a percentage. (Counting can be made easier by using a gridlike insert in the microscope eyepiece.)

## CLASSIFICATION OF ANEMIAS

The initial evaluation allows differentiation of an anemia into *responsive* or *nonresponsive* type. It may also allow for further classification into the four basic categories of *blood loss, increased destruction, maturation abnormalities* and *decreased production* (Fig. 1).

In a responsive anemia, there is no problem with red cell production. The erythroid

**Table 2.** *Interpretation of Blood Smear Observations in Anemia*

| | |
|---|---|
| Normocytosis, normochromia | Nonresponsive |
| Macrocytosis with polychromasia | Responsive anemia |
| Macrocytosis without polychromasia | Maturation arrest—nuclear:<br>  $B_{12}$ and folate deficiencies |
| Nucleated RBC with polychromasia | Very responsive—marked left shift |
| Nucleated RBC without polychromasia | Marrow damage—release defect |
| Howell-Jolly bodies | Responsive/splenectomy |
| Microcytosis | Maturation arrest—cytoplasmic<br>  Fe, Cu and $B_6$ deficiencies |
| RBC fragmentation | Hemolytic—membrane abnormality, vasculitis,<br>  marrow/splenic problem |
| Basophilic stippling with nucleated RBC<br>  but no polychromasia | Lead poisoning |
| Heinz bodies | Hemolysis—oxidant stress |
| "Smooth" spherocytosis | Autoimmune hemolysis |
| "Spiky" spherocytosis | Membrane/enzyme defect |
| RBC agglutination | Possibly autoimmune, particularly IgM type<br>  (complete antibodies) |
| Reticulocyte clumping in the cat | Possibly autoimmune and FeLV + |
| Erythrophagocytosis | Autoimmune, toxemias, RBC parasites |
| Lymphocyte clumping | Possibly autoimmune |

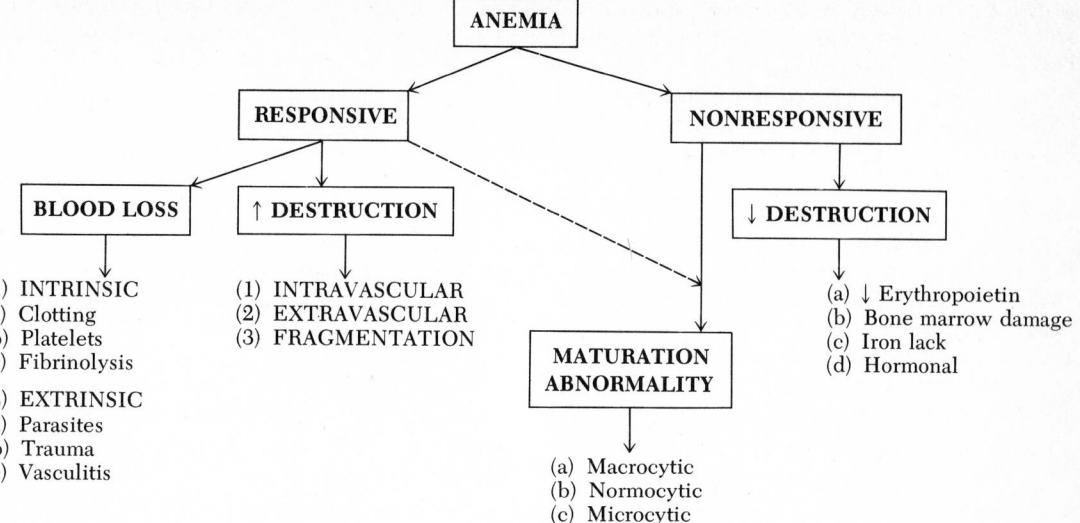

**Figure 1.** Pathophysiologic classification of anemia.

marrow responds to the decreased red cell mass by accelerating erythropoiesis. This is reflected in the peripheral blood by the appearance of macroreticulocytes, polychromasia, Howell-Jolly bodies, nucleated red cells, macrocytosis, etc., and by the associated findings of leukocytosis (neutrophilia) and the appearance of reticuloplatelets. Examination of bone marrow would reveal a decreased M:E ratio. Anemias of this type are caused by either *blood loss* or *hemolysis.*

In a nonresponsive anemia there is clearly a red cell production problem. The erythroid marrow is unable to produce enough red cells to replace those lost by normal attrition. This can result from a deficiency of a factor necessary for red cell production (e.g., iron), from toxic inhibition (chemicals, infection, neoplasia) or from a deficiency of erythropoietic stem cells. The peripheral blood shows none of the typical signs of accelerated erythropoiesis.

The group of anemias characterized by abnormalities of maturation show erythroid marrow hyperproliferation sufficient to maintain the circulating RBC mass but have no accompanying increase in the number of reticulocytes delivered to the blood. (The M:E ratio is decreased, and there is sometimes evidence of increased red cell destruction due to the destruction of defective cells.) Further subdivision of this group can be made on the basis of changes in cell size and hemoglobin concentration. Macrocytic anemia reflects an abnormality in nuclear development with failure of cell division, giving rise to larger cells. Hypochromic microcytic anemias, on the other hand, reflect abnormalities in hemoglobin synthesis. Erythrocytes apparently need a full complement of hemoglobin before they are normally released from the bone marrow; thus, in the early stages of iron deficiency, for example, the developing cells are held back by the marrow longer than is normal, and as the disease progresses, they may even undergo extra cell divisions, producing the typical microcyte.

In Figure 1 this group is classed as both responsive and nonresponsive. This is because, although few of the typical signs of increased erythropoiesis are seen in the blood in the advanced stages, they are seen during the earlier stages. Also, at all stages the bone marrow shows erythroid hyperplasia.

The classification of anemias by pathophysiologic mechanisms is useful because it promotes an understanding of the disease processes. The major shortcoming is that some anemias are due to more than one pathophysiologic mechanism. Often, one mechanism predominates early in the course but another supervenes.

## RETICULOCYTE COUNT

Before going on to discuss the mechanisms leading to anemia it is worthwhile to consider the reticulocyte count more carefully, since this measurement is of pivotal importance in the classification of anemias and can sometimes be difficult to interpret.

Since the life span of erythrocytes in the dog is about 100 days, about 1 per cent of the cells are turned over each day. These appear in the peripheral blood as reticulocytes, i.e., about 1 per cent of the total red cells circulating are reticulocytes. In the cat, the cell turnover is greater than 1 per cent, and hence the normal reticulocyte count is greater than 1 per cent. Also, the reticulocytes have a longer life span than in the dog. In the analysis of an anemia, one should compare the elevated reticulocyte count to this normal value. This is then called the *reticulocyte production index* (RPI).

The observed reticulocyte count depends not only on the level of marrow production but also on the total number of adult cells diluting each day's reticulocyte production. Thus, an animal whose PCV has fallen from 50 to 25 will have an observed reticulocyte count of 2 with a normal production index. In this situation a normal number of reticulocytes are diluted in only half the normal number of circulating erythrocytes, effectively doubling the count. Therefore, with a lower than normal packed cell volume, the reticulocyte count must first be corrected to a normal cell volume (45 in the dog) before the production index can be calculated. For example,

PCV = 15
Reticulocyte count = 12 %

Corrected count = $12 \times \dfrac{15}{45} = 4\%$

This is called the *"absolute" reticulocyte count*. A further correction is made for the presence of "shift" reticulocytes. In anemias with high erythropoietin stimulation, marrow reticulocytes will be delivered to the circulation one or more days before their usual maturation stage. This prolongs the time for maturation in the circulation; reticulum remains visible in these cells for more than one day. Approximate reticulocyte maturation time prolongations for normal individuals at specific PCV levels are as follows*:

---

| PCV | BLOOD RETICULOCYTE MATURATION (DAYS) |
|---|---|
| 45 | 1.0 |
| 35 | 1.5 |
| 25 | 2.0 |
| 15 | 2.5 |

To obtain an accurate index of daily reticulocyte production, the "absolute" reticulocyte count must be corrected for this phenomenon. These shift cells are identified on the blood smear as pale blue macrocytes (Wright's stain). Using the previous example, the correction now becomes

$$12 \times \frac{15}{45} \times \frac{4.0}{2.5} = 1.6$$

This value is known as the *reticulocyte index* and indicates that erythrocyte production is 1.6 times normal. High values (above 3.0) are characteristic of hemolytic anemias, whereas low values are characteristic of hypoproliferative anemias.

Although these figures have been derived for man, we have found them also to be applicable to the dog, but not to the cat. This is because of the similarity between the RBC life spans, normal reticulocyte counts and types of erythroid response in man and dog.

## BLOOD LOSS ANEMIAS

Blood loss can be acute, subacute or chronic. The character of the peripheral blood picture varies markedly, the degree of response depending on the severity and rapidity of blood loss, while the persistence of the response is related to the duration of the blood loss: if signs of increased erythropoiesis are still present after 10 to 14 days, continued hemorrhage must be considered.

Up to about the first 12 hours after acute blood loss, all the red cell parameters are normal, i.e., PCV, RBC, Hgb, reticulocyte count, reticulocyte index, MCV, MCHC, etc. Subsequently, hemodilution occurs, owing to mobilization of extravascular fluids and to salt and water intake. The full extent of the red cell deficit may not be evident from the PCV for one or more days. At this time the anemia is *normocytic, normochromic* and apparently *nonresponsive*. After 4 to 5 days, the reticulocyte count increases, and the anemia becomes obviously *responsive* and slightly *macrocytic*.

---

*Adapted from Finch, C. A.: The Red Cell Manual. Seattle, University of Washington, 1969.

If bleeding continues, sufficient iron (in hemoglobin) will eventually be lost to produce *iron depletion*. At this point the anemia becomes progressively less responsive, the reticulocyte count falls and the RBCs become *normocytic* and *normochromic*. The shortage of iron severely limits erythropoiesis. If bleeding continues, a state of absolute iron deficiency will result, and the cells will become progressively smaller (microcytic) and deficient in hemoglobin (hypochromic). This is the classic *iron deficiency anemia*. In pet animals the diet is usually rich in iron, so that iron deficiency anemia is almost always due to *chronic blood loss*.

In those cases presented as iron deficiency anemia, strenuous efforts should be made to establish a site of blood loss. This often turns out to be the G.I. tract. Occasionally, this type of anemia is the first sign of an intestinal neoplasm. It is obviously not sufficient simply to diagnose iron deficiency anemia and to correct the condition with oral or parenteral iron.

## HEMOLYTIC ANEMIAS

Survival of the red cell depends on its ability to maintain membrane integrity and pliability despite continued exposure to noxious forces in the circulation. A hemolytic state exists when the life span of the red cell is decreased. If this decrease is balanced by increased erythropoiesis, there is full compensation and no anemia. Hemolytic anemia occurs when decreased red cell survival is not balanced by increased erythropoiesis.

Red cell damage can be caused by a variety of mechanisms intrinsic and/or extrinsic to the red cell. The red cell may be lysed or fragmented by trauma, may lose membrane because of metabolic abnormalities or may undergo "coagulation necrosis" of a portion of its contents. Damage, if it does not result in immediate destruction, leads either to a rigid deformed cell or to a symmetrical spherocyte. Whichever shape deformity occurs, the cell has lost pliability and is susceptible to destruction.

Most pathologic destruction occurs through interaction between the red cell and the RE cell. Either there is total engulfment by the RE cell or fragments of cell membrane are broken off, making the cell more susceptible to subsequent destruction. The by-products of hemoglobin catabolism, as expected, are increased (e.g., bilirubin).

The process of *red cell phagocytosis* is particularly well developed in the spleen, where special anatomic relationships provide a monitor for testing the "normalcy" of the red cell. When discharged through the splenic arterioles into the pulp, red cells squeeze back into active circulation through small clefts in the venous sinusoids. These clefts are probably the smallest orifices through which the red cell must pass in the entire vascular system. During this passage, the red cell is examined for intercellular debris such as nuclear fragments or denatured hemoglobin (Heinz bodies); if present, this debris is removed. Stasis within the unfavorable environment of the spleen leads to red cell sphering and therefore has been said to "condition" the red cell for destruction. While normal cells survive this passage, cells that are abnormal owing to increased rigidity or globulin- or complement-coating are often preferentially destroyed.

The RE system in the spleen not only is the most sensitive detector of defective cells but also, when hypertrophied, may develop the capacity to destroy normal cells. This acquired hemolytic capacity of unknown cause is called primary hypersplenism. Continuous increased intrasplenic red cell destruction in hemolytic conditions may lead to work hypertrophy and secondary hypersplenism.

Severe membrane damage causes spherocytosis and/or rupture of the red cell with release of its contents into the circulation. While small amounts of hemoglobin may simply deplete the haptoglobin-hemopexin systems, producing hemosiderinuria, large amounts are associated with overt hemoglobinemia and hemoglobinuria, and very severe cases can cause renal damage.

*Fragmentation* of red cells in the circulation results in both phagocytosis of the pieces and intravascular lysis. With depletion of plasma haptoglobin and hemopexin, methemalbumin appears in the circulation, and hemosiderin is found in the urine sediment (Prussian blue stain). Overt hemoglobinemia and hemoglobinuria rarely occur. Red cell fragmentation can be identified on the blood smear. Abnormalities in the red cell or the vasculature or the presence of impediments to blood flow can produce this combined pattern of breakdown, e.g., membrane abnormalities associated with liver disease, vasculitis, heartworm disease, splenic or bone marrow disease.

The compensatory increase in erythropoiesis in hemolytic anemia occurs after a lag period of a few days. If hemolysis is sudden in onset and phagocytic in type, its presence may be reflected only by a rapid drop in the PCV and hyperbilirubinemia. In a few days, however, the combination of anemia and abundant supply of iron from catabolized red cells accelerates erythropoiesis to rates of three or more times normal. (Red cell production in hemolytic anemia is higher than in other anemias, presumably because catabolized red cells provide the best source of iron.)

Hemolytic anemias associated with RE destruction are by far the largest and most difficult group to understand. Splenomegaly suggests abnormal erythrocyte sequestration and destruction in that organ.

Laboratory tests separate four important groups of hemolytic conditions associated with RE destruction:

1. The antiglobulin or *Coombs' test* identifies *immune hemolytic anemias*. These may appear *de novo* or may be associated with other conditions (e.g., lupus erythematosus and lymphatic leukemia), and also perhaps with certain drugs, viruses, bacteria and parasites (e.g., penicillin, distemper virus, FeLV, *Leptospira*, *Babesia*, *Haemobartonella* and *Dirofilaria*).

2. *Heinz body anemias* are associated with excessive denaturation of hemoglobin within the red cell. They can be demonstrated after staining with new methylene blue or Nat's stain. The spleen is very efficient at removing these structures from the circulating red cells as they pass through its sinusoids. Heinz bodies are frequently observed in the red cells of cats with a variety of complaints, but a primary Heinz body hemolytic anemia occurs only after exposure to excessive oxidant stress, as seen in cats treated with urinary antiseptics containing methylene blue. It is also a possibility that an animal with an enzyme defect in the hexose monophosphate shunt might present with a primary Heinz body hemolytic anemia or at least have an increased susceptibility to oxidant compounds.

3. *Membrane and metabolic lesions* are difficult to diagnose. No comprehensive screening tests are available, and the precise nature of the defect is rarely classified until a specific assay demonstrates the abnormality. Pyruvate kinase deficiency has been described in basenjis and more recently in beagles. There is little doubt that other metabolic abnormalities will be described in the future.

4. *Infestation of red cells by parasites* can predispose the cells to removal by the spleen, the best known example of this being haemobartonellosis in cats. The mechanism is not clear, but in some parasitic hemolytic anemias (e.g., *Anaplasma* in cattle) antibodies have been demonstrated. *Babesia canis* causes a hemolytic anemia very similar to some types of autoimmune hemolytic anemia, i.e., predominantly intravascular and Coombs' positive in some cases.

## INDICATORS OF HEMOLYTIC DISEASE

1. Signs of a regenerative anemia; hyperbilirubinemia; hyperbilirubinuria; occasionally hemoglobinemia or even hemoglobinuria.

2. In some cases increased red cell osmotic fragility (autoimmune, red cell enzymopathy, babesiosis).

3. Hemosiderinuria. This is a very sensitive detector of occult intravascular hemolysis or of a past hemolytic episode.

4. Splenomegaly, particularly evident in extravascular hemolytic states.

5. Signs seen on the blood smear. *Spherocytes* are prehemolytic red cells usually associated with autoimmune hemolytic anemia. In stained smears they appear as deeply stained cells with no central pallor. They are spherical instead of discoid and therefore have less reserve volume. Consequently, they have increased osmotic fragility. Recently we observed spherocytes on a blood smear collected from a young beagle with a very severe responsive anemia. Instead of having a smooth membrane as in autoimmune hemolytic anemia, the spherocytes were spiked or rough. This dog was later demonstrated to have pyruvate kinase deficiency. Similar cells were also seen on a blood smear from a basenji with PK deficiency. The finding of such cells may therefore be suggestive of an enzymopathy or similar intrinsic red cell abnormality.

*Fragments* and distorted cells are partially destroyed cells with an increased osmotic fragility, predisposing them to an early demise. *Erythrophagocytosis* is seen in those cases in which antibody is capable of fixing complement to the red cell membrane. The chance of observing this phenomenon may be increased by heating blood to 37° C. for an hour or so. It is seen in some autoimmune hemolytic anemias but also in septicemias, toxemias and some parasitic infections (*Haemobartonella, Babesia*).

## MATURATION ABNORMALITIES

In conditions typified by vitamin $B_{12}$ and folate deficiencies there is a defect in DNA production due to enzymatic abnormalities in the pathway of pyrimidine and purine synthesis. Most dogs and cats have diets rich in vitamin $B_{12}$, and stores are usually good; it is therefore unlikely that $B_{12}$ deficiency would be associated with anemia in the dog and cat. Folate balance is theroretically more marginal in most species, and a poor diet or increased requirement may create a negative balance leading to deficiency. Increased requirements for folate may result from pregnancy, prolonged erythroid hyperplasia or infections. We have seen a few cases of folate-responsive macrocytic anemia in dogs on anticonvulsant therapy.

Vitamin $B_{12}$ and folate deficiencies produce morphologically identical abnormalities in the erythron. Red cell precursors are enlarged, nuclear chromatin is of fine texture, the evolution of the nucleus lags behind hemoglobin synthesis and the period of hemoglobin synthesis is prolonged. These changes in the nucleated red cells are referred to as *megaloblastic* changes. The cytoplasmic reticulum is usually lost before the nucleus is extruded from the cell, so that the reticulocyte count is inappropriately low. Circulating red cells are macrocytic and often irregular in shape. The major lesion is cell death during maturation (ineffective erythropoiesis). Response to specific therapy is dramatic; reversion to normal erythropoiesis occurs within two to three days.

The presence of hypochromic, microcytic red cells indicates a disturbance in hemoglobin production that may be due to impaired availability of any component of the hemoglobin molecule. Iron deficiency is the usual cause. Such a deficiency imposes a limitation on cellular proliferation, and marrow erythroid hyperplasia is only moderate. Pyridoxal phosphate ($B_6$) deficiency also impairs hemoglobin synthesis. It appears to be not so much a deficiency as a specific manifestation of a marrow defect. The result is the accumulation of iron within the red cell precursor cells. We have seen one such possible case in a cocker spaniel.

## HYPOPROLIFERATIVE ANEMIAS

All degrees of marrow failure can occur, from complete aplasia to a suboptimal response to an anemia of different cause, e.g., blood loss. There are three basic causes of hypoproliferation: marrow damage, impaired erythropoietin production and iron deficiency. **For diagnosis, it is necessary to examine a bone marrow sample.**

### MARROW DAMAGE OR FAILURE

Marrow incompetence may result from disorders intrinsic to the red cell precursors, from damage caused by myelotoxic drugs or from replacement by malignant cells or fibrous tissue. With generalized marrow damage, all the cells normally produced in the marrow are decreased, i.e., red cells, white cells and platelets. The degree of anemia is dependent on the severity of the marrow involvement.

Erythropoietin levels are usually elevated in this condition, and if some erythropoiesis is possible, reticulocytes and even nucleated red cells may be seen in the blood. This response, however, is obviously inappropriate with the degree of anemia present. When calculated, the reticulocyte index would be close to or below basal levels.

Inappropriate numbers of nucleated red cells (metarubricytes and rubricytes) are also seen in disorders that alter the stromal architecture of the marrow (myelophthisic anemias). Immature granulocytes and macroreticuloplatelets can also be seen in the peripheral blood.

### IMPAIRED ERYTHROPOIETIN PRODUCTION

**Anemia of renal disease.** In severe kidney disease there is usually failure of eryth-

*Table 3.*   *Definitive Diagnosis of Anemia*

| CONDITION | SPECIAL/DIAGNOSTIC FEATURES | ETIOLOGY | TREATMENT |
|---|---|---|---|
| 1. *Blood Loss* | | | |
| a. Acute | Normal PCV; normal total protein. Nonresponsive: normocytic, normochromic. Normal reticulocyte count. | Trauma. Coagulopathy. | Blood/fluid replacement. |
| b. Subacute | Anemic; decreased total protein. Responsive picture: elevated reticulocyte count. | Trauma. G.I. parasites. Thrombocytopenia. | As above. |
| c. Chronic | Microcytic, hypochromic anemia. Few reticulocytes; many platelets. Hyperplastic bone marrow. No storage iron in bone marrow. Low serum iron; low percentage saturation. | G.I. parasites. G.I. ulceration. Neoplasia. Urinary tract. Ectoparasites. | Treat primary disease and replace iron. |
| 2. *Hemolytic* | | | |
| a. Intravascular | Responsive signs; high reticulocyte index. Hyperplastic bone marrow. Hyperbilirubinemia/=uria. Hemoglobinemia; hemoglobinuria; hemosiderinuria. ± spherocytosis; ± Coombs' test. ± autoagglutination. Fragmentation. Inclusion bodies. Increased osmotic fragility. | Autoimmune (IgM and /or complement). ? FeLV in cats. Toxins, drugs, *Dirofilariae*. *Babesia canis*. | Immunosuppressants (e.g., prednisolone). Supportive. |
| b. Extravascular | Responsive signs; high reticulocyte index. Splenomegaly. Hyperbilirubinemia/=uria. ± spherocytosis; ± Coombs' test (IgG). Spiky spherocytosis—young animal. Heinz bodies. Inclusion bodies. | Autoimmune (IgG). Membrane-ATP lesions. Oxidant stress. Haemobartonella. ? FeLV. | As above and/or splenectomy. Remove oxidant. Tetracycline *per os*—3 weeks 1% thioacetarsamide sodium (0–5 ml./ 5 kg. on 2 alternate days) |
| c. Fragmentation | Fragments on blood smear. Poikilocytes. Microspherocytes. Rarely, hemoglobinemia. | Vasculitis; D.I.C. *Dirofilariae*. Myelofibrosis. Marrow/spleen disease. | See later. Supportive. Further diagnostic work. |

| 3. *Maturation Defect* | | | |
|---|---|---|---|
| a. Nuclear | Nonresponsive but marrow hyperplastic. Macrocytosis without polychromasia. High MCV. Active bone marrow with megaloblastic changes. | $B_{12}$ and folate deficiencies. Antifolate drugs (e.g., anticonvulsants). Malabsorption states. | $B_{12}$, folic acid. Withdraw drug. Correct underlying problem; multivitamins. |
| b. Cytoplasmic | Microcytic, hypochromic anemia. Active bone marrow with many metarubricytes. No stainable iron; low serum iron. | Iron deficiency. | Replace iron. |
| | Large masses of iron and "ringed" sideroblasts; high serum iron. | $B_6$ deficiency/dependency. | Vitamin $B_6$. |
| 4. *Hypoplastic* | Nonresponsive blood picture. Marrow hypoplastic or aplastic; bone marrow examination necessary for diagnosis. | | |
| a. ↓ Erythropoietin | Mild to moderate anemia. Marrow fairly cellular but no sign of response. | Chronic kidney disease. | Supportive. Anabolic steroids (e.g., oxymetholone 1–2 mg./kg./day). |
| b. Bone marrow damage | Often see nucleated RBC in the blood in the absence of other responsive signs. Marrow can be hypoplastic or aplastic. Cells occasionally vacuolated. Primary tumor or metastasis. | Toxins: Chemical, bacterial, drug, viral. FeLV. Panleukopenia. The leukemias: carcinomas, etc. | As above. See later. |
| c. Iron lack | Signs of iron deficiency. Masses of iron in the RE cells, but unavailable for RBC production. RBC normocytic, normochromic. Anemia mild to moderate. | Blood loss. Diet. Inflammation, chronic disease, neoplasia. | Replace iron. Supportive. |
| d. Hormonal | Mild normocytic, normochromic anemia. Marrow hypoplastic. | Hypothyroid. Anterior pituitary insufficiency. Hypoadrenocorticism. | Thyroid hormone. |

ropoietin production as well as excretory function. The degree of kidney damage correlates well with the severity of the resulting anemia. The anemia is normocytic and normochromic, and the reticulocyte count is usually close to normal. A hemolytic component has been described, but the major defect is in the production of erythropoietin. In dogs with chronic interstitial nephritis the packed cell volume often remains steady in the 18 to 25 per cent range.

**Anemias associated with endocrine disturbances.** Animals with hypothyroidism and hypopituitarism have a decreased tissue metabolic rate. Thus, there is less demand for oxygen, resulting in shrinkage of the oxygen delivery apparatus, i.e., fall in hemoglobin, red cell count and packed cell volume. Eventually a new equilibrium is established whereby red cell production is maintained at a level sufficient to maintain the reduced red cell mass. The anemia is usually only moderate and is normocytic and normochromic. The reticulocyte count is, of course, normal or below.

### IRON DEFICIENCY

As mentioned previously, an inadequate supply of iron limits erythropoiesis. Iron deficiency at the red cell precursor level can arise as the result of the following:

1. A block in the RE cell function which inhibits the normal recirculating of iron to the erythroid marrow.

2. Loss of body iron stores, so that erythropoiesis is dependent on the turnover of iron in the existing red cell mass (no storage iron).

3. Blood loss. Erythropoiesis would be dependent on mobilization of iron from tissue stores and from intestinal absorption. The iron released from normal red cell attrition is not sufficient to support accelerated red cell production.

### THE ANEMIA OF INFLAMMATION

Anemia is frequently associated with inflammation due to infection, immune disease, neoplastic disease, etc. The anemia is usually mild, and the red cells are normocytic and without regenerative signs. *Target cells* or *leptocytes* are frequently a prominent feature in the peripheral blood. There are at least three components in the pathogenesis of this type of anemia.

1. The iron supply delivered to the erythroid marrow is decreased. This is due to interference in its release from the RE cells.

2. There is some increase in the destruction of circulating erythrocytes. This is apparently due in some cases to intravascular fragmentation associated with vasculitis and/or intravascular coagulation. This effect produces an added demand for iron.

3. It is reported that inflammation causes a decrease in erythropoietin production.

In hypoproliferative anemias associated with iron deficiency, no stainable iron (Prussian blue) is demonstrable in bone marrow sections or smears. In those hypoproliferative anemias due to marrow damage or failure, decreased erythropoietin production or inflammation, some bone marrow stores will be demonstrable. In many cases, excess iron stores are present because iron is not used in erythropoiesis.

In all anemias in which hypoproliferation is suspected, bone marrow aspiration or biopsy should be performed, and the section of smear should be evaluated for cellularity, M:E ratio and the presence of storage iron.

If the above outline is followed, it is not difficult to determine whether an anemia is responsive or nonresponsive and is due to blood loss, hemolysis, a maturation abnormality or marrow hypoplasia. Table 3 illustrates how this scheme can be used in order to arrive at a more definitive diagnosis. Some of the conditions listed are rare, and care and restraint must be exercised before such a diagnosis is made (preferably with a second opinion from a clinical pathologist). Some of these conditions are dealt with more fully later in this section.

The various treatments listed are also covered in appropriate detail elsewhere in this and other sections.

# AUTOIMMUNE HEMOLYTIC ANEMIA

ROBERT W. BULL, D.V.M.
*East Lansing, Michigan*

Autoimmune diseases are a group of diseases in which tissue injury is mediated by self-destructive autoantibodies. This is a paradox with respect to the understood functions of the immune system. Immunoresponsiveness is usually a temporary proliferation of immunocompetent cells for the production of a specific antibody to a foreign antigen for the protection of the host. Activation of the immune system by an autologous determinant causes a continuous self-perpetuating type of proliferation of the system that is destructive rather than protective for the organism. The mechanism leading to immune recognition of a self-component is not known. Theories range from viral modification of cell membranes, so that they appear different, to the establishment of foreign clones of immunocompetent cells that are not tolerant of the host. Some lesions are caused by the direct action of autoantibodies, while others result from tissue deposition of antigen-antibody complexes. This article will focus on one autoimmune disease, autoimmune hemolytic anemia (AIHA).

There are two distinct forms of AIHA: Secondary or symptomatic AIHA is associated with systemic lupus erythematosus, lymphosarcoma, lymphogenous or myelogenous leukemia and histoplasmosis. Primary or idiopathic AIHA involves only the red cells themselves. It is an acquired immunohematologic state in which an unknown element has activated the animal's immune system to produce an autoantibody (gamma globulin) that has specific immunologic affinity for its own red cells. The majority of antibodies are the incomplete "warm" type, with 37° C. the optimal temperature of activity, but it is possible to have a "cold" antibody which is most active in a temperature range of 4° to 24° C. In either case, binding of the autoantibody to the red cells causes severe hemolytic anemia.

## CLINICAL FINDINGS

The disease more frequently affects 2- to 8-year-old females. Presenting signs are weakness, dyspnea, fever, pallor and possible collapse, all of acute onset. The feces and urine may be darkly pigmented, suggestive of excessive red cell destruction. Icterus is not a prominent feature. Upon palpation, most dogs have splenomegaly and slight to moderate peripheral lymphadenopathy. Hepatomegaly may occasionally be observed. In animals with severe anemia, tachycardia and holosystolic cardiac murmur may be present. Animals with cold-type antibody generally present with gangrenous lesions of the dependent portion of the body after exposure to cold.

## LABORATORY FINDINGS

Hematologic findings are indicative of an acute hemolytic anemia caused by splenic cell entrapment and destruction rather than by intravascular hemolysis. Hemoglobinemia and hemoglobinuria are not general features. The hematocrit and hemoglobin levels are well below normal values, and morphologically the red cells exhibit polychromasia, anisocytosis and poikilocytosis. Spherocytes are frequently the predominant cell type. Coating of the red cells with autoantibody causes them to lose their biconcave disc shape and become spherical. Marked reticulocytosis and moderate to marked leukocytosis with an absolute neutrophilia and a shift to the left provide evidence of an active bone marrow response. During a hemolytic crisis, azotemia, proteinuria and bilirubinuria may occur.

Special techniques are needed to confirm the diagnosis of AIHA. The *direct antiglobulin test* (Coombs' test) substantiates the diagnosis of AIHA. The basis of the antiglobulin test is immunologic (Fig. 1). The autoantibodies most frequently involved

Immunologic Basis of the Antiglobulin Test

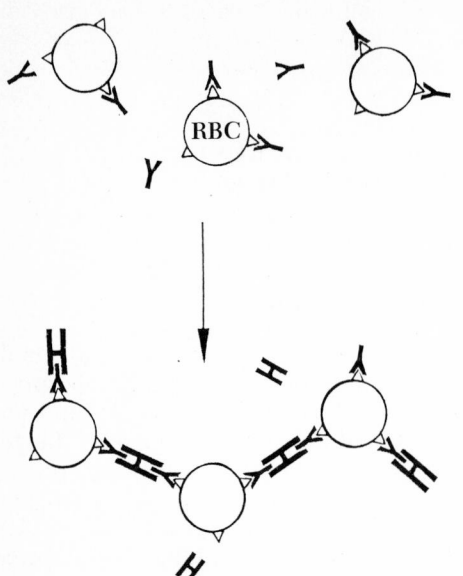

**Figure 1.** Incomplete autoantibody **Y** binds to specific red cell determinants but cannot couple two or more red cells. The addition of antiglobulin **⊥** forms the link to cause agglutination.

are of the "incomplete" or single binding site type of antibody. The antibody attaches to the red cell membrane but is not capable of binding two or more red cells together, so its presence is not detectable by the routine method of red cell–antibody interaction, i.e., agglutination. The antiglobulin provides a link between the antibody-coated red cells, causing them then to agglutinate. The antiglobulin must be species-specific in order for the test to be valid. Antiglobulin is prepared by means of immunization of another species with gamma globulin of the species for which the antiglobulin is desired. Various species-specific antiglobulins are commercially available but must be absorbed with washed, normal, homologous red cells to remove naturally occurring heteroagglutinins. If this is not done, false positive reactions occur.

A clotted blood sample is obtained from the patient for the direct antiglobulin test. The serum is removed and saved for the indirect test. Sufficient red cells are washed from the clot to prepare a cell suspension. The cells must be thoroughly washed with saline to remove all plasma proteins except those bound to the cell membrane. A 2 per cent cell suspension is made in saline. Equal volumes, 0.1 ml., of the cell suspen-

sion and the antiglobulin are combined in test tubes, set up in triplicate and incubated at 37° C., at room temperature and at 4° C. for 15 minutes. After incubation, the tubes are centrifuged at 1500 rpm for 15 seconds and then shaken to check for agglutination. Appropriate negative controls, i.e., cells minus the antiglobulin, must be included for comparison. A positive reaction is agglutination, or the irreversible clumping of red cells, indicating autoantibody coating. Occasionally the autoantibody is the complete type. In this case, autoagglutination substantiates the antibody coating of the patient's red cells.

The *indirect antiglobulin test* determines whether autoantibodies in the patient's serum have affinity for a determinant on the red cells of normal dogs. Washed saline cell suspensions are prepared from several normal, healthy dogs. The test is done in two steps: First, the cells are sensitized by combining an equal volume of cell suspension with the patient's serum and incubating for 30 minutes at the three temperatures, as for the direct test. The cells are then washed several times to remove unbound protein. Antiglobulin is added to the washed, sensitized cells and incubated again for 15 minutes at the various temperatures, centrifuged and checked for agglutination. A positive indirect antiglobulin test in conjunction with a positive direct antiglobulin test confirms that the red cell destruction is antibody-mediated. The combination of a positive indirect and a negative direct antiglobulin test is not indicative of AIHA but rather identifies an incomplete anti–red cell antibody, invoked by a foreign stimulus and not related to the observed anemia.

The presence of spherocytes can be affirmed by the *osmotic fragility test* (Fig. 2). Washed cells are exposed to various concentrations of NaCL solutions. Decreasing salt concentrations result in increased water uptake by the cells, causing them to swell and eventually to rupture. Spherocytic cells have reduced swelling capability, and rupture occurs in the more isotonic concentrations. Normal cells do not hemolyze until approximately half isotonic-strength solutions are reached.

## DIAGNOSIS

A positive direct antiglobulin test in an animal with acute hemolytic anemia confirms the diagnosis of AIHA. It is impor-

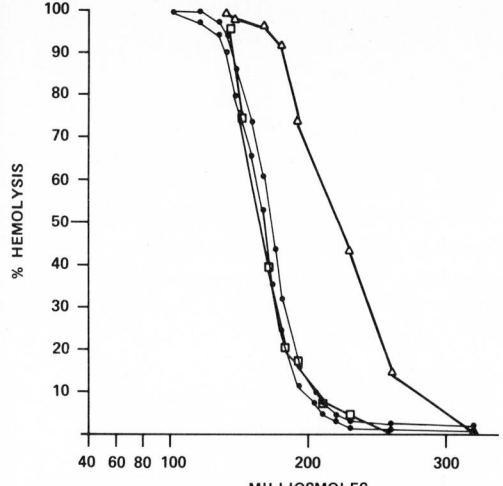

**Figure 2.** Osmotic fragility curve. The normal curve is represented by the ● and □. A typical curve of spherocytic red cell is depicted by △.

tant to determine whether the immune-mediated anemia is primary or secondary to another disease state, since this will influence the management of the patient. Secondary AIHA is most frequently associated with systemic lupus erythematosus (SLE). This is a multisystem autoimmune disorder that can be differentiated from primary AIHA by the presence of thrombocytopenia, glomerulonephritis and systemic polyarthritis. It is not within the scope of this article to deal with SLE, which is covered in greater detail in another article in this section.

The clinician must realize that immune-mediated anemia can result from modification of the red cell membrane induced by certain infectious agents or drugs. The attachment of the offending agent serves as the antigenic stimulus for antibody production. Complete history and physical examination allow differentiation of this group of immune-mediated anemias from the true autoimmune type.

## THERAPY

The unknown etiology of AIHA necessitates a therapeutic plan aimed at inducing a temporary remission of the disease state. Extended remissions are frequent, even without medication, but the owner should be alerted to the recurrent nature of the disease and the fact that AIHA may be the first manifestation of a more complex autoimmune or lymphoproliferative disorder.

The general approach is directed toward inhibition of autoantibody production and/or removal of the major site of red cell destruction, the spleen. Immunosuppressive agents, prednisone or prednisolone, are generally effective in suppressing autoantibody production. For the first 5 to 10 days, the usual dosage is 2 mg./kg./day in divided doses, which is then lowered to 1 mg./kg./day for maintenance. In most dogs, the direct antiglobulin test becomes negative during corticosteroid administration and is potentially an indication for termination of immunosuppressive therapy. However, in one dog in which remission was achieved and immunosuppressive therapy was terminated, the direct antiglobulin test remained positive. Therefore, rather than a negative direct antiglobulin test, correction of the anemia, as assessed according to hematocrit and hemoglobin levels, is suggested as the cirterion to determine whether corticosteroid therapy should be discontinued.

It is impossible to predict the duration of remission. Some patients experience extended periods of remission without therapy, whereas others have recurrent hemolytic episodes while on maintenance therapy. In patients nonresponsive to corticosteroids, splenectomy is recommended. The rationale is (1) it removes one of the major lymphoid organs of the body, thereby reducing the autoantibody production, and (2) it eliminates the primary organ of red cell destruction. In most instances, splenectomy and supplemental immunosuppression will induce extended remissions, but proper management of the patient requires a program of regular examinations for the early detection of recurrent anemia and immunologic disorders.

### SUPPLEMENTAL READING

Bull, R. W., *et al*: Autoimmune hemolytic disease in the dog. J. Am. Vet. Med. Assn., *159*:880–884, 1971.

Lewis, R. M., *et al*: A Syndrome of Autoimmune Hemolytic Anemia and Thrombocytopenia in Dogs. In Scientific Proceedings of the 100th Annual Meeting of the American Veterinary Medicine Association, 1963, pp. 140–163.

Pirofsky, B.: Autoimmunization and the Autoimmune Hemolytic Anemias. Baltimore, The Williams and Wilkins Co., 1969.

Schalm, O. W., *et al*.: Veterinary Hematology. 3rd ed. Philadelphia, Lea & Febiger, 1975.

Sodikoff, C. H., and Custer, M. A.: Secondary autoimmune hemolytic anemia in cats. Animal Hosp., 2:20–23, 1966.

# PYRUVATE KINASE DEFICIENCY ANEMIA

K. W. PRASSE, D.V.M.
*Athens, Georgia*

Pyruvate kinase (PK) deficiency anemia is a congenital hemolytic disease transmitted as an autosomal recessive trait (Brown and Yao-sheng, 1975). Heterozygote carriers are not anemic but can be detected by means of their reduced erythrocytic PK activity. Erythrocytic PK deficiency should be considered in the young dog with unremitting anemia and extreme reticulocytosis (15 to 70 per cent) and when other more common causes of regenerative anemia, especially hemolytic causes, have been eliminated. It has been described in basenjis (Ewing, 1969; Searcy *et al.*, 1971; Tasker *et al.*, 1969) and beagles (Prasse *et al.*, 1975) but should be suspected in other breeds as well. The PK deficiency results in impaired erythrocytic glucose metabolism, reduced cell deformability, shortened erythrocyte life span and progressive anemia within the first year of life.

## CLINICAL FINDINGS

Affected dogs are usually presented between 2 months and 1 year of age and usually die by 3 years of age. Presenting signs include syncope during exercise, weakness, easy fatigability or excessive sleeping. Littermates may also be affected. Frequently, dogs over 6 months old have been previously treated for an anemic disorder. Physical findings include pallor, tachycardia, splenomegaly and, sometimes, orange feces. Icterus is not usually apparent. Clinical signs do not seem as severe as might be expected based on the degree of anemia. This is evidence of a chronic insidious anemia in which physiologic adaptation has occurred.

## LABORATORY FINDINGS

The primary step in diagnosis of PK deficiency is to establish that the anemia is regenerative (reticulocytosis or polychromasia). Both hemolysis and hemorrhage cause regenerative anemia, and their differentiation is necessary. Overt hemorrhage may be subtle or absent as with ancylostomiasis or external blood-sucking parasites. Furthermore, these agents may be concomitant conditions in the PK-deficient patient and may be misdiagnosed as the primary etiology. Hemolysis generally yields high reticulocyte counts (over 10 per cent) and is associated with normal plasma protein concentration. Hemorrhage, in contrast, yields more moderate reticulocyte counts (2 to 10 per cent) and hypoproteinemia. Occasionally hyperbilirubinemia and icterus occur as evidence of hemolysis (or liver disease), but many cases of chronic hemolytic disease are without these findings. Marked urobilinogenuria and orange discoloration of feces are evidence of increased bilirubin formation from hemolysis even in the absence of icterus.

Evaluation of specific causes is conducted when a hemolytic mechanism is strongly suspected. Direct Coombs' and lupus erythematosus tests should be conducted and are consistently negative in PK-deficient dogs. Examination for erythrocytic parasites should be made and drug incompatibilities should be considered as possible causes of the hemolytic disease.

Several findings are characteristic, but not specific, for PK deficiency anemia. Reticulocytosis is usually extreme (15 to 70 per cent). MCV and MCHC indicate macrocytosis and hypochromia, but the values simply reflect the presence of large numbers of reticulocytes in the blood. Metarubricytosis is common, and its presence necessitates correction of WBC counts. Spiculated erythrocytes may be observed on stained blood films. Osmotic fragility of PK-deficient erythrocytes is normal but may be increased with incubation for 24 hours at 37° C.

The autohemolysis test on PK-deficient erythrocytes yields abnormal results which reflect an abnormality of erythrocytic glycolysis. In man, enzyme deficiency anemias have been subdivided into Type I, in which autohemolysis *in vitro* is reduced by the addition of glucose, or Type II, in which autohemolysis is retarded only by the addition of ATP. PK-deficient erythrocytes should yield Type II autohemolysis. However, the test should be used only as a screening procedure to detect an intracellular metabolic defect and should not be considered specific for PK deficiency.

Bone marrow examination is seldom indicated in regenerative anemias, but if conducted in the anemic PK-deficient dog, a reduced M/E ratio and erythroid hyperplasia should be anticipated. In the PK-deficient dog over 1 year of age, difficulty may be experienced either in penetrating the bone with the aspiration needle or in aspirating an adequate bone marrow sample. Radiographic examination is then indicated for possible detection of osteosclerosis and myelofibrosis, obliterative marrow lesions which are progressive and ultimately lead to hematopoietic failure and death. Osseous lesions are consistent findings in PK-deficient dogs during the second or third year of life. The normal radiographic soft tissue density of bone marrow is replaced by thickening of trabecular bone (osteosclerosis) and replacement of hematopoietic tissue by fibrous connective tissue (myelofibrosis). The pathogenesis of these lesions is obscure.

**Erythrocytic Pyruvate Kinase Assay.**

The definitive diagnosis is dependent upon an assay for erythrocytic PK activity. Laboratories experienced with canine samples and knowledgeable about values typical of the normal or carrier status in dogs should be used. Addresses for these laboratories* may be acquired from the Hemolytic Anemia Committee of the Basenji Club of America. Details of sample collection, shipping procedures and other required information should be obtained from the laboratory prior to sample collection. The testing laboratory will report results as numerical values, but, more importantly, an interpretation of the values, i.e., normal, carrier or affected, will be provided. Numerical values for PK activity are not interchangeable between laboratories. Likewise, normal and abnormal values cannot be transposed from the literature and applied to those of a commercial laboratory.

## MANAGEMENT

Treatment of affected dogs is limited to supportive care. The life expectancy may be increased with periodic blood transfusions, good nutrition and strict limitation of the dog's physical activities. Hematinics are not beneficial.

Splenectomy has resulted in some benefit in affected children—the anemia is somewhat diminished but hemolysis persists, transfusion requirements decline and osseous changes may revert to normal. However, experience has been far too limited to make any recommendation for dogs.

Once diagnosis of PK deficiency anemia has been established in a dog, parents and littermates should be tested for the enzyme deficiency. It is recommended that carriers be neutered to prevent the persistence of this hereditary defect.

### SUPPLEMENTAL READING

Brown, R. V., and Yao-sheng, T.: Studies of inherited pyruvate kinase deficiency in the basenji. J.A.A.H.A., *11*:362–365, 1975.

Ewing, G. E.: Familial nonspherocytic hemolytic anemia of basenji dogs. J. Am. Vet. Med. Assn., *154*:503–507, 1969.

Prasse, K. W., Crouser, D., Beutler, E., Walker, M., and Schall, W. D.: Pyruvate kinase deficiency anemia with terminal myelofibrosis and osteosclerosis in a beagle. J. Am. Vet. Med. Assn., *166*:1170–1175, 1975.

Searcy, G. P., Miller, D. R., and Tasker, J. B.: Congenital hemolytic anemia in the basenji dog due to erythrocyte pyruvate kinase deficiency. Can. J. Comp. Med., *35*:67–70, 1971.

Tasker, J. B., Severin, G. A., Young, S., and Gillette, E. L.: Familial anemia in the basenji dog. J. Am. Vet. Med. Assn., *154*:158–165, 1969.

---

*At present the only available testing laboratory is: Dr. R. V. Brown, Department of Biology, Virginia Commonwealth University, 701 W. Franklin, Richmond, Virginia 23220.

# POLYCYTHEMIA

JACK E. HATHAWAY, D.V.M.
*St. Louis, Missouri*

Polycythemia signifies an increase in the number of circulating erythrocytes. This increase may be of a relative or absolute nature. Relative polycythemia is the result of a reduction in plasma volume following fluid loss or dehydration. The actual red cell mass remains normal. Relative polycythemia (hemoconcentration) is a common feature of many diseases and is characterized by a modest increase in the packed cell volume (PCV 55 to 65 per cent). Absolute polycythemia refers to an increased red cell mass from increased erythropoiesis in the presence of a normal erythrocyte life span. There are two major groups of absolute polycythemia, primary and secondary (Table 1). This discussion concerns the differential diagnosis and management of absolute polycythemia.

Absolute polycythemia is characterized by a major increase in the packed cell volume (PCV 69 to 80 per cent) dependent on the underlying cause. Cardiovascular signs predominate because the increased blood viscosity slows its passage in the circulation. Secondary polycythemia or erythrocytosis is a response to an extramedullary stimulus and is hormone-dependent. The principal stimulating factor is increased production of erythropoietin (erythrocyte stimulating factor) as a result of hypoxia, renal neoplasms or cysts and, occasionally, other tumors. In contrast, primary polycythemia, also known as polycythemia vera or erythremia, is independent of hormonal control. Erythropoietin blood levels are not elevated in this myeloproliferative disease. Another feature of importance in the pathogenesis and differentiation of primary from secondary polycythemia is that all the cellular components of the marrow (leukocytes, erythrocytes and platelets) are

*Table 1.   Types of Polycythemia*

---

1. Relative polycythemia
2. Absolute polycythemia
   A. Primary (erythremia, polycythemia vera)
   B. Secondary (erythrocytosis)
      (1) Hypoxia
      (2) Renal mass
      (3) Methemoglobinemia

---

generally present in increased numbers in the blood with primary polycythemia, whereas the erythroid elements alone are hyperplastic in secondary polycythemia.

Polycythemia vera is a myeloproliferative disorder of dogs, cats, cattle and man. It appears to be an uncommon disease in animals, as compared to man. The characteristic triad of signs is a brick red discoloration of the mucous membranes (plethora), splenomegaly and a marked increase in the circulating red cell mass. A wide variety of vasomotor and neurologic signs are observed, because the increased blood viscosity slows the rate of blood flow. Thrombosis and hemorrhage are frequent complications of this disorder.

## DIAGNOSIS

The management of the polycythemic patient is dependent on establishing the pathogenesis of the disease. The salient features to be considered when differentiating polycythemia vera from erythrocytosis are depicted in Table 2. The anamnesis and the physical examination should be directed toward establishing the presence or absence of heart or lung disease and splenomegaly, and the demonstration of a mass in the region of the kidney. The coloration of the mucous membranes may prove useful, particularly in hypoxic patients. The presence of hypoxia can be confirmed by measuring the oxygen saturation of arterial blood. Levels below 95 per cent saturation are found in hypoxia. It has been our experience that extensive pulmonary disease is the most frequent cause of secondary polycythemia in the dog, although congenital cardiac anomalies such as pulmonic stenosis and patent ductus arteriosus should be considered in young dogs. Erythropoietin blood levels are increased in all cases of secondary polycythemia. An intravenous pyelogram or arteriogram may be helpful in dogs with polycythemia secondary to renal carcinoma (Scott, 1972). The presence of leukocytosis, thrombocythemia and increased numbers of immature erythrocytes in the circulating

*Table 2.*   *Differential Diagnosis of Polycythemia**

| | POLYCYTHEMIA VERA | HYPOXIA | RENAL |
|---|---|---|---|
| *History* | Multiple symptoms, dyspnea, vertigo | Heart or lung disease | None or renal disease |
| *Examination* | | | |
| Mucous membranes | Plethora | Cyanosis | Congestion |
| Spleen | ↑ (75%) | N | N |
| Liver | ↑ (50%) | N | N |
| *Hemogram* | | | |
| PCV (%) | 60 to 80% | 50 to 80% | 50 to 60% |
| WBC | ↑ | N | N |
| Platelets | ↑ | N | N |
| Nucl. RBC | + | − | − |
| *Bone marrow* | | | |
| Erythroid | ↑ | ↑ | ↑ |
| Myeloid | ↑ | N | N |
| Megakaryocytes | ↑ | N | N |
| *Special tests* | | | |
| Arterial oxygen sat. | N | ↓ | N |
| Erythropoietin | N | ↑ | ↑ |
| Pyelogram | N | N | A |

↑ = increased, ↓ = decreased, N = normal, A = abnormal, + = present, − = absent.
*The features of polycythemia vera and erythrocytosis secondary to hypoxia or renal disease.

blood is indicative of generalized marrow hyperplasia. These changes are typical of polycythemia vera in man. The leukocytosis and thrombocythemia are not always seen in dogs, however.

## THERAPY

Once the diagnosis of polycythemia vera has been established, the major purpose is to decrease the circulating red cell mass, thereby alleviating the signs of this myeloproliferative disorder. This is accomplished by the use of periodic phlebotomy and myelosuppressive drugs. The aim of treatment is to keep the packed cell volume under the upper limits of normal for the patient (PCV 48 to 55 per cent). Phlebotomy simply removes the end product (mature erythrocyte) of this proliferative process. In our experience the withdrawal of 250 to 500 ml. of whole blood (10 to 20 ml./kg.) every 48 hours has been well tolerated by the dog. Replacement therapy with plasma or plasma substitutes is not necessary. Phlebotomy to achieve a normovolemic state is essential prior to surgical procedures to avoid thrombosis and/or hemorrhage.

A combination of phlebotomy and a myelosuppressive agent appears to be the best approach to successful management. The myelosuppressive agent attacks the proliferative process at its origin. Alkylating agents such as uracil mustard (Urical®) and cyclophosphamide (Cytoxan®) have been used for this purpose (Carb, 1969). Radioactive phosphorus, $^{32}$P, at a dose of 2 to 5 mCi. given intravenously, has resulted in prolonged remissions in the dog in our experience and that of others (Bush, 1972). Radioactive phosphorus acts as a form of localized ionizing radiation and should be used with caution. Since a latent period follows the administration of a myelosuppressive agent, a longer time is required to reduce the red cell mass than with phlebotomy. Overdoses of myelosuppressive agents may lead to aplastic anemia.

Polycythemia vera in the dog has been effectively managed in the above manner for five years. This chronic myeloproliferative disorder is, therefore, relatively benign and the prognosis is fair to good. Animals can be effectively controlled for several years if the packed cell volume is kept under 55 per cent. Thrombosis and infarction may occur if this is not done. The natural course of polycythemia vera in man may terminate in bone marrow failure (myelofibrosis, aplastic anemia) or chronic myelogenous leukemia. This has not yet been observed in the dog, since the majority of animals died or were euthanatized prematurely.

SUPPLEMENTAL READING

Bush, B. M., and Fankhauser, R.: Polycythemia vera in a bitch. J. Small Animal Pract., 13:75–89, 1972.
Carb, A. V.: Polycythemia vera in a dog. J. Am. Vet. Med. Assn., 154:289–297, 1969.
Scott, R. C., and Patnaik, A. K.: Renal carcinoma with secondary polycythemia in the dog. J. A. Animal Hosp. Assn., 8:275–283, 1972.

# INHERITED HEMORRHAGIC DEFECTS

W. JEAN DODDS, D.V.M.
*Albany, New York*

Inherited defects of blood coagulation and platelet function in animals are not as rare as was once believed. It is difficult to determine the actual numbers of affected animals, since some die at birth or before veterinary attention is sought, while others, especially the mildly affected or carrier animals, remain undiagnosed. Within the last decade, the veterinary profession has become increasingly aware of bleeding syndromes. Animals with inherited and acquired bleeding diseases are now being recognized, diagnosed, treated and referred to hematology specialty groups.

The incidence of human hemostatic defects is one in every 2000 live births. The frequency is probably higher in some animal species, especially within purebred lines, because of the inbreeding and line breeding commonly practiced. Canine hemophilia is more frequently observed in rare breeds that are inbred by necessity or in bloodlines in which a particular animal of superior quality is extensively bred to improve the breed type.

## DIAGNOSIS

To identify bleeding defects in individual animals, one must understand the principles and the interpretation of various diagnostic tests. It is also necessary to know which tests can feasibly be performed by

Supported in part by NIH Grant HL09902, awarded by the National Heart and Lung Institute, PHS/DHEW.

the practitioner and which tests require specialized expertise, reagents and equipment available only in hemostasis laboratories.

The laboratory screening tests commonly used for diagnosis of bleeding diseases are listed in Table 1. Specific details about these and other, more specialized tests can be found in the references listed at the end of this article. The following tests are uncomplicated and can be performed by the practitioner and/or local clinical or hospital laboratory:

Whole blood clotting time
Partial thromboplastin time
Prothrombin time

**Table 1.** *Diagnostic Tests for Screening Hemorrhagic Defects*

*Intrinsic System Coagulation Tests*
　Whole blood clotting time
　Recalcification time
　Partial thromboplastin time
　Prothrombin consumption time
　Fibrinogen concentration
　Clot solubility time
*Extrinsic System Coagulation Tests*
　Prothrombin time
　Stypven time
*Platelet Function Tests*
　Platelet count
　Clot retraction time
　Bleeding time
　Platelet aggregation
　Platelet retention or adhesiveness
　Stypven time
*Fibrinolytic System Tests*
　Clot lysis time
　Fibrinogen-fibrin degradation (split) products

Stypven time
Platelet count
Clot retraction time
Clot lysis time
Fibrinogen-fibrin degradation products

More complex or specialized tests, such as those for quantitating the activity and antigen of specific coagulation factors or for determining plasminogen levels are performed only in large clinical or research hemostasis laboratories. Practitioners should use these laboratories for further diagnostic or confirmatory tests. The Thrombo-Wellcotest®* is a sensitive latex-agglutination commercial test for measuring fibrinogen-fibrin degradation products (FDP) in human blood. The test antibody to human FDP cross-reacts sufficiently with canine FDP to permit its use for detection of canine disseminated intravascular coagulation.

An important consideration when assaying for coagulation factors or platelet function is that these measurements are meaningless without parallel tests from normal animals of the same species. Normal values for these tests vary considerably between species, especially in comparison to humans, who have relatively less active coagulation and fibrinolytic systems. Coagulation tests also vary between laboratories, since different types of reagents, methods and standards may be used. For these reasons, a control of homologous normal blood or plasma (preferably a pool of homologous samples) must be run simultaneously with the patient sample.

## PRINCIPLES OF TREATMENT

The same general principles apply in treating each different type of bleeding disorder. To control moderate or severe hemostatic defects, adequate replacement therapy of the correct type is needed. Coagulation factors and platelets are quite labile, so that whole blood, plasma or its concentrates must be transfused as soon as possible after collection or must be stored frozen at $-40°$ C. or more preferably at $-70°$ C. Household freezers maintain temperatures of only $-15$ to $-20°$ C. and are not

satisfactory for preserving coagulation factor activity. Techniques for freezing and storing animal platelets are currently being adapted from those recently perfected for human platelets.

Maximal utilization of blood products can be achieved by removing and freezing the plasma from fresh units of whole blood soon after collection, then storing the packed red cells at $3°$ C. for up to 6 weeks. For transfusion, the packed cells are readily reconstituted with an equal volume of fresh-frozen plasma, saline-dextrose or a similar type of infusion fluid relating to the specific needs of the patient. Whole blood and packed red cells are best collected in plastic bags rather than vacuum bottles, and the red cells are better preserved for longer periods in citrate phosphate dextrose anticoagulant than in acid citrate dextrose.

Another important consideration is the use of typed and crossmatched blood, since animals with moderate or severe bleeding defects will most likely require repeat transfusions during their lifetimes. Unfortunately, blood-typing sera for animal species are not yet available from commercial sources, so the profession must rely on the few veterinary immunohematology groups that offer this service.

The importance of animal blood-typing can best be illustrated in dogs. About 60 per cent of the random canine population is positive for the strongly hemagglutinating A antigen (CEA-1 in the new nomenclature) and 40 per cent is negative. The risk of transfusion incompatibilities must not be overlooked. Another canine red cell antigen, Tr (CEA-7), should also be considered when transfusing blood, since it exists in half the random dog population. The ideal canine blood donor is both A-negative and Tr-negative. Several research groups, practitioners and veterinary institutions now maintain banks of A-negative universal-donor dog blood. Other ways to avoid mismatched transfusions include typing the recipients to determine their specific needs and, alternatively, using red cells only when absolutely necessary (packed cell volumes [PCV] below 20 per cent).

For treatment of platelet defects, whole blood should be used within 8 hours of collection or, preferably, processed into platelet-rich plasma concentrates and infused immediately. If platelets are not needed, the blood is centrifuged for

---

*Thrombo-Wellcotest® for fibrinogen-fibrin degradation products, 20-test kit, Burroughs-Wellcome Co., Wellcome Research Division, 3030 Cornwallis Rd., Research Triangle Park, North Carolina 27709.

platelet-poor plasma, which is removed and either used immediately or frozen at $-40°$ C. or below in sterile plastic containers. Plasma can be stored for a year in this manner and should be thawed only once before use.

Fresh-frozen plasma transfusions given at appropriately spaced intervals are the treatment of choice for all nonplatelet bleeding disorders except hemophilia, von Willebrand's disease (VWD) and fibrinogen defects. These three conditions will respond to plasma transfusions but are preferably treated with plasma-concentrate therapy. The standard dose of fresh-frozen plasma for all types of bleeding is 6 to 10 ml./kg. of body weight, infused at a rate of 4 to 6 ml./min. In severe bleeding diseases this dose is given 2 or 3 times daily at regular intervals for 3 to 5 days or until bleeding is controlled. The frequency and duration of transfusions depend on the coagulation defect. For example, the *in-vivo* half-life of coagulation factors VIII and IX is short (10 to 18 hours), and transfusions should be given frequently. Fibrinogen and prothrombin deficiencies can be treated once a day or every other day, since the half-life of these clotting factors is about 3 days.

In the treatment of hemophiliacs and patients with VWD or fibrinogen defects, plasma-concentrate therapy has obvious advantages. It provides large amounts of coagulation factors in small volumes, which are more effective in controlling bleeding; it is less time-consuming; and it avoids the risk of circulatory overload. The most practical method of preparing concentrates of animal plasma is cryoprecipitation. The more potent, specialized coagulation factor concentrates used in humans are not yet available for animals.

Cryoprecipitates of whole fresh-frozen plasma contain 5 to 15 times (average 10) the concentration of factor VIII and fibrinogen, an average yield of about 50 per cent, and traces of other clotting factors. Cryoprecipitates are easily prepared by slow thawing of frozen homologous plasma at 4° C., centrifuging the precipitate at 4° C., pooling, and refreezing at $-40°$ C. or preferably at $-70°$ C. They can be stored for a year at these temperatures. This procedure provides two products: the cryoprecipitate and its supernatant ("cryo-super"). Most of the prothrombin-complex coagulation activity and albumin remain in the cryo-super, which is saved and stored for treatment of hypoproteinemic states, prothrombin-complex deficiencies such as hemophilia B (factor IX deficiency) and warfarin poisoning and for use as a plasma expander.

The cryoprecipitate is carefully thawed for use, dissolved in a small volume of 5 per cent saline-dextrose or cryo-super and infused at a rate of 4 to 6 ml./min. For hemophilia A (factor VIII deficiency), the cryoprecipitate prepared from 12 to 20 ml. of whole plasma per kg. of body weight is given *twice* daily for 3 to 5 days or until bleeding stops. For fibrinogen deficiencies, the same amount is given *once* daily. The dose of VWD varies with the severity of the defect and with the degree of bleeding; usually the regimen for hemophilia A is followed for 1 or 2 days.

Proper management of bleeding disorders also requires the best physiologic environment for hemostasis, tissue repair and prevention of subsequent hemorrhage. Several commonly prescribed drugs interfere with hemostasis and must be avoided or used with extreme caution. Most of these drugs—aspirin, promazine-type tranquilizers, phenylbutazone, sulfonamides, nitrofurans, local anesthetics and antihistamines—act by impairing platelet function and are contraindicated in patients with moderate to severe coagulation defects because they further compromise the stability of the hemostatic plug. Even small doses of aspirin can alter platelet function and prolong bleeding time for 5 to 7 days. A hemophiliac depends upon platelets as the only normally functioning portion of his hemostatic process, and impairment of their function abolishes his only defense against spontaneous hemorrhage.

Another consideration is the effect of live-virus vaccines and viral diseases on platelet and endothelial functions. The viremia following vaccination or exposure usually at 5 to 10 days, often produces a relative thrombocytopenia (decreases of up to 100,000 platelets/mm.$^3$). During this period individuals with hemostatic defects should be watched for bleeding, and elective surgical procedures should be avoided. These procedures can safely be performed either within the first 48 hours after vaccination or after 10 to 14 days.

Large hematomas heal best if left undisturbed, provided that the bleeding has been controlled with transfusions. We usually do not attempt to drain hematomas, and healing and resorption can take several weeks. The area may eventually rupture or become necrotic and drain; this lesion is best left to heal as an open wound. If the wound becomes badly infected or is bleeding profusely, it should be packed with topical thrombin and antibiotic ointment and bandaged tightly. However, most animals will attempt to remove these bandages, especially when healing begins, reinjuring themselves in the process. Oral systemic antibiotics should be given in high doses for 7 to 10 days.

All medication for hemophiliacs and other severely affected bleeders should be administered orally, intravenously or subcutaneously with a small-gauge needle. Intramuscular injections should never be given because large hematomas frequently develop at the injection site. Affected animals are best housed individually in pens or cages with smooth sides and vertical bars to minimize trauma. It is important to eradicate external and internal parasites to prevent anemia and debilitation. Oral iron and vitamin supplements are useful during and after bleeding episodes. The diet should be of high quality and be softened to avoid injury to the gums and intestinal tract. Bones or biscuits are not advisable.

## RECOGNITION AND TREATMENT OF SPECIFIC DEFECTS

The major types of inherited hemorrhagic defects are listed in Table 2. Those currently recognized in animals are described briefly below. More detailed information about these conditions can be found in the references.

**Fibrinogen (Factor I) Deficiencies (Afibrinogenemia, Hypofibrinogenemia).** Inherited fibrinogen disorders, which are rare in humans, occur in goats (afibrinogenemia) and dogs (hypofibrinogenemia). Both disorders have an autosomal, incompletely dominant inheritance. They are less common than acquired fibrogen deficiencies that occur with intravascular coagulation. Family studies are necessary to establish the hereditary nature of suspected cases. The canine disorder, reported in a family of St. Bernards, was characterized by *subnormal* fibrinogen levels, or hypofibrinogenemia. This condition leads to severe or lethal hemorrhage.

**Table 2.** *Types of Inherited Hemorrhagic Defects in Animals*

Fibrinogen (factor I) deficiencies
  (afibrinogenemia, hypofibrinogenemia)
Prothrombin (factor II) deficiency
  (hypoprothrombinemia)
Factor VII deficiency
Hemophilia A (factor VIII or AHF deficiency,
  classic hemophilia)
Christmas disease (factor IX deficiency,
  hemophilia B)
Factor X (Stuart factor) deficiency
Factor XI (PTA) deficiency
Factor XII deficiency (Hageman trait)
Von Willebrand's disease (pseudohemophilia,
  vascular hemophilia)
Platelet function defects (thrombasthenia or
  Glanzmann's disease, thrombopathia)
Multiple defects (double hemophilia, hemophilia
  AB)
Miscellaneous defects (Ehlers-Danlos syndrome)

Fibrinogen deficiency states are diagnosed by marked prolongation of all clotting tests, since these tests depend on fibrinogen for formation of the fibrin end point. The bleeding time may be prolonged. The defect is corrected *in vitro* by addition of purified fibrinogen but not thrombin. Bioassays of fibrinogen in affected patients vary from zero to subnormal ($< 150$ mg./dl.). Low levels of fibrinogen are found by immunologic methods and when plasma is heated to 56° C. or treated with 25 per cent ammonium sulfate. Erythrocyte sedimentation and plasma viscosity are low.

The severity of these diseases necessitates large daily doses of fresh-frozen plasma or, preferably, homologous fibrinogen concentrates (cryoprecipitates) to control bleeding episodes. Heterologous fibrinogen concentrates are commercially available but should be avoided because of their potential immunogenicity.

**Prothrombin (Factor II) Deficiency (Hypoprothrombinemia).** Hereditary prothrombin deficiency is characterized by moderately low (10 per cent of normal) levels of prothrombin. We have studied a family of boxers with hypoprothrombinemia, in which all but three puppies of a litter bled to death from massive epistaxis.

The disease is inherited as an autosomal trait and produces a mild to moderately severe bleeding tendency. Prothrombin times are prolonged, as is the Stypven time; thrombin times are normal. Bleeding episodes are usually controlled by daily transfusions of fresh-frozen plasma, prothrombin-complex concentrates or cryo-super.

**Factor VII Deficiency.** Deficiency of clotting factor VII has an autosomal, incompletely dominant inheritance and has been recognized in Alaskan malamutes and in beagles. The disorder was discovered fortuitously in Canada, Great Britain and New York State during routine laboratory screening of commercial beagle colonies. The coincidence probably reflects the widespread use of this breed for biologic research. Affected animals exhibit a mild bleeding tendency or are asymptomatic, although easy bruisability and an apparent susceptibility to demodicidosis have been noted. Demodex infestation could result from the defective extrinsic clotting system in factor VII deficiency, which provides a warm and moist tissue environment that is ideal for the mange site.

Factor VII deficiency can be definitely diagnosed by a prolonged prothrombin time and a normal Stypven time. Homozygotes have 1 to 4 per cent of normal factor VII levels, whereas heterozygotes have slightly prolonged prothrombin times and about 50 per cent factor VII. Surgical procedures can safely be performed on affected dogs, although the patients may require transfusions with fresh-frozen plasma. The half-life of factor VII is very short (4 to 6 hours), so treatment should be given at frequent intervals. Fortunately, affected beagles rarely require therapy.

**Hemophilia A (Factor VIII or AHF Deficiency, Classic Hemophilia).** Hemophilia A, a sex-linked recessive trait, is the most commonly reported inherited coagulation defect of humans and animals, affecting about 80 per cent of these patients. It occurs in dogs, horses and cats. Most breeds of dogs and mongrels have been reported to have hemophilia A. The breeds include Irish setters, German shepherds, collies, Labrador retrievers, golden retrievers, beagles, Shetland sheepdogs, greyhounds, Weimaraners, Chihuahuas, Samoyeds, Vizslas, English bulldogs, miniature and standard poodles, miniature and standard schnauzers, St. Bernards, Brittany spaniels and Alaskan malamutes. One family of cats with hemophilia A has been studied, as have four other isolated cases that were diagnosed after protracted postsurgical hemorrhage.

The disease can be severe, moderate or mild, depending on the frequency and extent of clinical problems and the degree of factor VIII deficiency. Bleeding problems are more frequent and severe in large breeds of dogs, which may reflect a predisposition to spontaneous hemarthroses because of the greater weight bearing on their joint surfaces. Bleeding episodes usually begin after affected puppies are weaned, especially during the periods of live-virus vaccination, and as they start to play more aggressively with their littermates. Puppies may also bleed from the umbilicus at birth or from the gums during teething. One of the first indications of an underlying hemorrhagic disorder is hematoma formation after an intramuscular injection. Bleeding into the gastrointestinal tract discolors the feces with fresh or digested blood, and internal hemorrhage can be suspected when the hemophiliac becomes anorectic and/or listless. Hematemesis may occur, but epistaxis is uncommon.

The most frequently encountered bleeding problems involve the limbs and joints and are often misdiagnosed in puppies as fractures or sprains. Large body-surface or muscle-mass hematomas may develop. Dogs with mild or moderately severe hemophilia can survive tail-docking and ear-cropping without alarming bleeding and may not be diagnosed until young adulthood. Frequently the owner or clinician does not recognize the earlier symptoms of intermittent lameness or small swellings that disappear without treatment.

The disease is transmitted as an X chromosome–linked recessive trait by asymptomatic (carrier) females; 50 per cent of their sons will be affected, and 50 per cent of their daughters will be carriers like themselves. However, the misconception that females cannot be "bleeders" has led to confusion and misdiagnosis. Mating of hemophilic males with carrier females can produce affected hemophilic females. Several severe autosomal bleeding diseases exist in which animals of both sexes are equally affected.

Hemophiliacs have defective intrinsic clotting but normal extrinsic clotting and platelet function. The prothrombin consumption (serum clot) time is very short. In hemophilia A the clotting defect is corrected by normal plasma, which contains factor VIII, but not by normal serum, which does not. The primary bleeding time, dependent on functional platelets, is normal but the secondary bleeding time is markedly prolonged because of defective fibrin formation.

The diagnosis is confirmed by specific factor VIII assays. Severely affected animals have less than 1 per cent of normal, homologous factor VIII activity; moderately affected patients have 1 to 5 per cent; and mildly affected patients have 5 to 20 per cent. Immunologic assays recently developed to measure factor VIII-related antigen (FVIII-RA) show that hemophiliacs have normal or higher than normal FVIII-RA levels. The low factor VIII activity in this disorder is evidently caused by a factor VIII molecule that is present in normal amounts but is mutant and nonfunctional. This finding has made possible a relatively high degree of accuracy in the detection of carriers among female relatives of hemophiliacs. Carrier females have reduced factor VIII activity levels (40 to 60 per cent of normal) but normal or high FVIII-RA levels.

The treatment of choice for bleeding episodes is homologous plasma concentrates, such as cryoprecipitates, given 2 or 3 times daily, with or without matched red blood cells, as required. It is especially important to withhold drugs that impair hemostasis.

**Christmas Disease (Factor IX Deficiency, Hemophilia B).** The severe bleeding disorder called Christmas disease is much less common than hemophilia A. It has been reported only in four breeds of dogs: Cairn terriers, black and tan coonhounds, St. Bernards and cocker spaniels. The inheritance and types of bleeding episodes are the same as for hemophilia A. All affected dogs have severe deficiencies, with factor IX levels less than 1 per cent of normal. The St. Bernards with Christmas disease are especially difficult to maintain because of their size and the large volume of homologous plasma or concentrates required to control bleeding episodes.

Similar to hemophilia A, there is defective intrinsic clotting and a normal primary bleeding time. However, the clotting defect in Christmas disease is corrected by both normal plasma and normal serum because serum does contain factor IX activity. Female carriers are detected by their low levels of homologous factor IX activity (40 to 60 per cent of normal).

The half-life of factor IX is slightly longer than that of factor VIII, so transfusions to control bleeding need be given only twice daily. Specific treatment with fresh-frozen plasma or cryo-super has been discussed. Factor IX concentrates have been recently developed for human use but are not yet available for animals.

**Factor X (Stuart Factor) Deficiency.** Factor X deficiency has been reported to occur in humans and in cocker spaniels. The disease is inherited as an autosomal, incompletely dominant trait and occurs with variable clinical severity in both sexes. Bleeding problems are often serious or lethal in newborn and young adult dogs, but affected mature dogs rarely bleed unless subjected to surgical procedures. Affected newborns show bruising of the skin, umbilical bleeding and massive internal abdominal or thoracic hemorrhage. Young adults may have prolonged estrual bleeding, hematuria and intrathoracic, gastrointestinal or gingival bleeding.

It appears to be lethal in the homozygous state. This probably reflects the central role of factor X in both the intrinsic and the extrinsic clotting systems. Affected dogs that survive are presumably heterozygotes and exhibit a mild coagulation defect. Both the prothrombin and Stypven times are slightly prolonged; the partial thromboplastin time is moderately prolonged. Factor X levels are 18 to 65 per cent of normal. Platelet function, bleeding times and other clotting factors are normal.

Treatment is given once daily and should consist of either fresh-frozen homologous plasma or prothrombin-complex concentrates, when they become available for animals. Feeding vitamin $K_1$ to pregnant bitches and to newborns of affected parents has not been successful in ameliorating the fatal bleeding episodes of affected puppies. It had been hoped that this would compensate for the physiologic hypoprothrombinemia common to all newborn mammals and thus relieve another insult to the hemostatic function of factor X-deficient pups.

**Factor XI (PTA) Deficiency.** A bleeding disease similar to human factor XI deficiency has been reported in Holstein cattle, springer spaniels and Great Pyrenees. This condition has an autosomal, incompletely dominant inheritance. It produces minor spontaneous bleeding episodes, such as hematuria and subcutaneous hematomas, as well as severe, protracted or lethal hemorrhage within 24 hours of any type of surgical procedure. Bleeding does not usually occur during the surgery. In an affected canine family, the propositus experienced life-threatening hemorrhage after a routine ovariohysterectomy and then 3 years later when her foreleg was fractured by an automobile. Each time more than 2 months of extensive, intermittent blood component and antibiotic therapy was required to control bleeding and secondary infection.

Diagnosis is based on defective intrinsic but normal extrinsic clotting. Platelet function and bleeding times are normal. Factor XI levels are from less than 1 to 10 per cent of normal in homozygotes and from 25 to 60 per cent in heterozygotes. Relatively small volumes of fresh-frozen plasma given before surgery will usually prevent bleeding in affected individuals, but massive daily therapy is required once bleeding starts.

**Factor XII Deficiency (Hageman Trait).** Deficiency of factor XII (Hageman factor) does not cause a bleeding tendency. The defect is a hereditary disease in humans and has recently been recognized in a cat. On the other hand, several species—including marine mammals, fowl and reptiles—are normally born without factor XII activity or antigen. The deficiency is usually discovered fortuitously. It is manifested by very long whole blood clotting and plasma recalcification times and a short prothrombin consumption time.

**Von Willebrand's Disease (Pseudohemophilia, Vascular Hemophilia).** Like hemophilia A, von Willebrand's disease (VWD) is characterized by factor VIII deficiency. There are several important differences, however, including autosomal, incompletely dominant inheritance; prolonged primary bleeding times; reduced platelet retention (adhesiveness in a glass-bead column); abnormal ristocetin-induced platelet aggregation; low levels or variant forms of factor VIII-related antigen (FVIII-RA); and a paradoxical increase in circulatory factor VIII activity after transfusion with normal or hemophilia A plasma. Until the advent of immunologic assays for FVIII-RA, the last phenomenon was considered diagnostic of VWD.

In addition to affecting humans, von Willebrand's disease has been observed in a family of Poland-China swine, a family of inbred rabbits and five families of dogs: German shepherds, golden retrievers, miniature schnauzers, Scottish terriers, and Doberman pinschers. Isolated instances have involved a Cairn terrier, a Shih Tsu, a Siberian husky and a miniature poodle.

The factor VIII deficiency in VWD has variable expression within affected families but is usually mild (1 to 20 per cent of normal) or moderately severe (20 to 60 per cent). Severely affected (less than 1 per cent) homozygotes are rare and have clinical bleeding problems more like those of hemophilia A. In contrast to hemophiliacs, patients with VWD usually have low levels of FVIII-RA in parallel with their factor VIII activity. Recent studies in humans, however, have identified variant types of VWD with normal levels of a mutant factor VIII antigen. In these instances, family studies to determine the inheritance pattern and other diagnostic criteria must be included for a definitive diagnosis.

The bleeding diathesis in VWD varies from mild to moderate and tends to cause high morbidity and low mortality. Surgical procedures or trauma exacerbates bleeding and may result in lethal hemorrhage. Other signs include recurrent hematuria and melena; serosanguineous otitis externa; protracted bloody diarrhea initiated by stress, parasites or infections; prolonged estrual bleeding; and subcutaneous hematomas. Dogs with this disease may appear to have eosinophilic gastroenteritis, since both states are marked by eosinophilia, shifting leg lameness and similar radiographic changes. The clinical severity of VWD decreases with successive pregnancies in females and with age in both sexes.

Because VWD is usually less severe than hemophilia A, affected animals frequently survive to reproduce. Affected canine families come from excellent-quality show stock, and consequently VWD is becoming more prevalent in certain lines of German shepherds, golden retrievers, miniature schnauzers and Doberman pinschers. Our profession has an increasing responsibility to inform dog owner-breeders about these defects and to encourage blood-testing of their breeding stock in order to avoid perpetuating these inherited traits.

Because individuals with VWD can synthesize their own factor VIII activity for about 24 hours after transfusion, treatment of bleeding episodes need not be as vigorous as in hemophilia A. Cryoprecipitate given twice daily for 1 or 2 days are the treatment of choice. While the factor VIII deficiency of VWD is readily corrected by transfusion, correction of the bleeding time and platelet retention is usually transient; the reasons for this are not fully understood.

**Platelet Function Defects (Thrombasthenia or Glanzmann's Disease, Thrombopathia).** Quantitative platelet-function defects with a hereditary basis have been described in humans, a family of fawn-hooded rats and two families of dogs: otterhounds and basset hounds. Isolated cases have been reported in a horse, foxhound, Scottish terrier, golden retriever and German short-haired pointer. These disorders have an autosomal dominant or incompletely dominant inheritance and are manifested as a moderately severe bleeding diathesis in homozygotes and a mild or inapparent disease in heterozygotes. Bleeding is aggravated by trauma or surgery. Other signs include surface bruising, gastrointestinal or urogenital bleeding and hemarthroses.

Diagnostic findings depend on the specific type of platelet dysfunction. A spectrum of these diseases exists in humans, each with its own characteristics. The defect in otterhounds is mixed, with abnormalities similar to both thrombasthenia (Glanzmann's disease) and thrombopathia (Bernard-Soulier syndrome). In basset hounds the defect is more thrombopathic than thrombosthenic. Affected dogs from both families have abnormal platelet aggregation with ADP and thrombin. The otterhounds have abnormal collagen aggregation, clot retraction, Stypven times, platelet factor 3 release, platelet fibrinogen levels and platelet survival and morphology. Giant, bizarre platelets are observed by phase-contrast and electron microscopy.

Animals with these diseases usually do not require treatment for their spontaneous bleeding episodes, if they are properly managed and housed individually. Control of serious hemorrhagic episodes or presurgical treatment requires transfusions of fresh platelet-rich plasma, platelet concentrates and/or matched fresh whole blood. Drugs that further compromise platelet function are contraindicated.

### SUPPLEMENTAL READING

Dodds, W. J.: Hereditary and acquired hemorrhagic disorders in animals. In Spaet, T. H. (ed.): Progress in Hemostasis and Thrombosis, Vol. 2. New York, Grune and Stratton, 1972.

Dodds, W. J.: Blood coagulation, hemostasis and thrombosis. In Melby, E. C., Jr., and Altman, N. H. (eds.): Handbook of Laboratory Animal Science, Vol. 2. Cleveland, CRC Press, Inc., 1974.

Dodds, W. J.: Bleeding disorders. In Ettinger, S. J. (ed.): Textbook of Veterinary Internal Medicine, Vol. 2. Philadelphia, W. B. Saunders Co., 1975.

Owen, C. A., Jr., Bowie, E. J. W., and Thompson, J. H., Jr. (eds.): The Diagnosis of Bleeding Disorders. 2nd ed. Boston, Little, Brown and Co., 1975.

# THROMBO-CYTOPENIC PURPURA

ROBERT J. WILKINS, B.V.Sc.
*New York, New York*

Thrombocytopenia is the reduction of circulating blood platelets to below the minimum normal number for a particular species. In the dog and cat, this would be a platelet count of less than 200,000 / cu. mm. The platelets function in hemostasis. Platelets are required to maintain the integrity of vascular endothelial cells and to plug small gaps in the capillaries when endothelial cells age, die and are being replaced. Spontaneous hemorrhages into tissues will not occur unless there are insufficient platelets to comply with this normal physiologic function. Clinical signs of bleeding, the hallmark of severe thrombocytopenia, do not usually occur until the platelet count drops below 50,000 to 70,000/cu. mm.

## CLINICAL SIGNS

When severe thrombocytopenia does occur, spontaneous hemorrhages into tissue in the form of pinpoint extravasations of blood (petechiae) or larger spreading-type hemorrhages (ecchymoses) occur. This type of hemorrhage is most prominent within the mucous membranes of the oral cavity, conjunctiva, sclera, penis and prepuce and in vulvar and vaginal mucosa. Hemorrhages may be noted in the skin in areas where the hair coat is sparse, such as the abdomen, axilla, inguinal region or inside the ear. Overt bleeding from any of the body orifices—the mouth, penis, anus, vulva or nose—and seeping hemorrhages of the gums adjacent to the teeth are not uncommon. Hemorrhage can be easily induced in thrombocytopenic animals by comparatively light trauma. A head shake, bite or scratch may induce significant bleeding. Injections or even use of a hair clipper is sufficient to traumatize local vessels and cause subcutaneous and cutaneous bruising and hemorrhage.

## CAUSES OF THROMBOCYTOPENIA

Thrombocytopenic disorders, although presenting with clinical similarities, have many underlying causes and are generally classified according to the physiologic disturbance of platelet production, distribution or destruction.

**Disorders of Production.** The blood platelet is derived from the bone marrow megakaryocyte by a process of fragmentation of these polypoid cells, with the release of preformed platelet subunits into the circulation. Approximately 150 to 200 platelets are derived from one mature megakaryocyte. Production defects within the bone marrow affecting the megakaryocytic series ultimately lead to peripheral thrombocytopenia. Under these circumstances, platelet survival is relatively normal, but platelet turnover is decreased. Examples of conditions seen in animals include hypoplastic marrow damage caused by drug idiosyncrasies to sulfonamides, estrogens and phenylbutazone, or bone marrow suppression due to cytotoxic drugs such as melphalan, vincristine and cyclophosphamide.

Aplasia, hypoplasia and myelofibrosis of the bone marrow producing thrombocytopenia may occur as the result of irradiation, chemical toxicity, chronic infection and ehrlichiosis. Bone marrow displacement as a result of cellular infiltration or neoplastic myeloproliferation is often ac-

companied by thrombocytopenia. Lymphosarcoma, lymphocytic leukemia, myelogenous leukemias and multiple myeloma are the most common examples of bone marrow displacement in dogs and cats. Ineffective thrombopoiesis has also been described in some of these conditions. There is an increased megakaryocytic mass without proportional increase in platelet turnover. The defect may involve disorderly platelet formation, abnormal release or intramedullary destruction of platelets.

**Disorders of Distribution.** Once released from the bone marrow, the platelet survives in the circulation 6 to 7 days. This time period is variable depending on physiologic requirements. Approximately two thirds of the total platelets are in the general circulation, while the remaining one third is sequestered in the spleen, forming a reserve pool that exchanges freely with the general circulation. Thrombocytopenia has been observed in dogs with splenomegaly and hypersplenism.

**Disorders of Utilization.** Acute massive or chronic protracted hemorrhage, regardless of the cause, can often deplete the vasculature of platelets until bone marrow production can replace this loss. This process usually takes several days from the onset of the initial reduction in peripheral blood platelet numbers. Platelets may also be consumed within the circulation, as may occur in disseminated intravascular coagulation. One classic and common cause of depletion of platelets is seen in older dogs with metastatic disseminated hemangiosarcoma as a result of the local vascular abnormalities and hemorrhage. Widespread or severe vascular injury (vasculitis) can also cause thrombocytopenia due to direct consumption of platelets by damaged endothelium. This mechanism is considered to be operative in animals with thrombotic thrombocytopenic purpura.

**Disorders of Destruction.** Immune injury to platelets following antigen-antibody reactions on the platelet surface membrane results in accelerated removal by the reticuloendothelial system, particularly the spleen and liver. Immune-mediated platelet destruction is usually unaccompanied by other diseases; is commonly found in middle-aged female dogs, especially poodles; and has been recognized, although rarely, in the cat. This disease entity is most frequently referred to as idiopathic thrombocytopenic purpura. In these cases, antibodies are thought to be directed against structurally altered platelet membranes, an expression of an autoimmune disease similar to and occasionally occurring in conjunction with autoimmune hemolytic anemia.

The pathogenesis of other cases of immune-mediated thrombocytopenia (IMTP) includes the attachment of antibodies to platelets with adsorbed viral, bacterial or drug antigens, and the absorption by platelets of circulating antigen-antibody complexes. In all these cases, the presence of the antigen-antibody complex on the platelet membrane results in the accelerated reticuloendothelial removal of the platelet from the circulation. Drugs that have been incriminated as causing IMTP in the dog include certain antibiotics, sulfonamides, phenylbutazone, thiazides and their derivatives, digitoxin, estrogens, quinidines, diphenylhydantoin and dinitrophenol.

## DIAGNOSIS

The differentiation of thrombocytopenic states requires a thorough clinicopathologic examination. Hematologic screening should include a complete blood count, examination of the peripheral blood smear, platelet count, reticulocyte count, Coomb's test, prothrombin time, partial thromboplastin time, clot retraction time, fibrinogen, and test for fibrin split products. A bone marrow biopsy is advised when hypoplastic or myeloproliferative disease is suspected. Adequate or increased marrow megakaryocytes along with active erythropoiesis help eliminate a primary bone marrow problem. Biochemical parameters and blood culture may also help differentiate some of the causes of thrombocytopenia. Studies of platelet kinetics using chromium-54–labeled platlets may be helpful but are generally restricted to research laboratories.

Confirmation of immune-mediated thrombocytopenia is possible using the platelet factor 3 (PF-3) release assay for detection of platelet isoantibodies. Several recent modifications of this test have enabled it to be used clinically as a rapid screening test. The test serum is heated to 56° C. for 30 minutes. Citrated platelet-rich plasma (PRP) and platelet-poor plasma (PPP) are prepared from a normal animal. A mixture of 0.1 ml. test serum and 0.1 ml. PRP is incubated at 37° C. for 10 minutes. A 0.1 ml. aliquot of the reaction mixture is then added to 0.1 ml. PPP and, after 30 minutes at 37° C., 0.2 ml. of 0.025 M calcium chloride is added. Clotting time is recorded with a stopwatch. The test is positive if the clotting time is shortened by more than 10 seconds from the control.

## TREATMENT

Therapy for thrombocytopenia should be directed toward the control of bleeding, reestablishing higher numbers of circulating blood platelets, and eliminating any underlying disease process.

A transfusion of fresh whole blood, platelet-rich plasma or platelet concentrate may be necessary in severely thrombocytopenic animals temporarily to arrest an acute, life-threatening hemorrhage or to prepare the animal for surgery. Platelet-rich plasma can be prepared by centrifuging fresh A.C.D. blood at 1500 rpm for 3 to 5 minutes and then separating the platelet-rich plasma from the cells. Platelet concentrate may be prepared by further centrifugation of the platelet-rich plasma. Generally, the platelets from a 250-ml. pack of whole blood will provide about 50 million platelets. For an average 60-kg. dog, this number of platelets, whether given in blood, PRP or platelet concentrate, would theoretically raise the platelet count by 40,000/cu. mm. Generally, occult bleeding stops if the platelet count is greater than 70,000/cu. mm. It is important to use fresh platelets for transfusion. Platelets stored for more than 12 hours rapidly lose their hemostatic activity. Repeat transfusions are indicated if uncontrolled hemorrhage and persistent or recurrent severe thrombocytopenia occur.

Corticosteroid therapy is indicated when an immune mechanism is thought to be responsible for the thrombocytopenia. The effects of steroid therapy include (1) inhibiting sequestration of platelets by the reticuloendothelial system, (2) reducing the titer of antiplatelet antibody and (3) stimulating platelet production from marrow megakaryocytes. Prednisone is the steroid most widely used, and the dosage ranges from 1 to 3 mg./kg. body weight/day as a divided dose. Other forms of adrenocortical steroids have proved effective but offer no special advantage over prednisone. Steroids are maintained at this dose rate for 1 to 2 weeks and are then progressively reduced to a low maintenance dose, e.g., 2.5 to 5.0 mg./day. Alternate-day administration of corticosteroids may also be used. Complete withdrawal can be contemplated when platelet levels have been stabilized. Often, platelet counts may remain slightly below normal (100,000 to 200,000/cu. mm.). This may reflect a compensated thrombocytolytic state, while other animals may respond with a temporary overproduction of platelets (responsive thrombocythemia). Prolonged therapy with high doses of steroids for more than 4 weeks is not recommended, since this in itself may cause thrombocytopenia.

Splenectomy is indicated in those cases where hypersplenism and splenomegaly are responsible for the thrombocytopenia. In immunologically mediated thrombocytopenia, splenectomy should be considered in acute cases unresponsive to transfusions and high-dose corticosteroid therapy and in chronic recurrent thrombocytopenic states refractory to prednisone.

In these situations, the spleen is primarily responsible for removal of platelets, since it is the main site of antiplatelet antibody synthesis. Bone marrow biopsy must be done to establish a functional hematopoietic reserve before splenectomy is performed.

Chronic recurrent IMTP resistant to steroid therapy and splenectomy may respond to immunosuppressive agents such as cyclophosphamide (Cytoxan®) at a dosage of 5 to 6 mg./kg. body weight or azathioprine (Imuran®) at a dosage of 2 mg./kg. body weight. These drugs are given for 3 days, and the dose is then decreased by one third for maintenance. Care should be exercised because of their myelosuppressive effects.

Any drug administered prior to the onset of thrombocytopenia is a potential cause and therefore should be suspended. Control of infection, if present, is accomplished with appropriate broad-spectrum antibiotic therapy.

In patients with primary marrow disease, whether aplastic or myeloproliferative, transfusions are indicated until alternate therapy is effective at reestablishing bone marrow function.

# DISSEMINATED INTRAVASCULAR COAGULATION

GARY J. KOCIBA, D.V.M.
*Columbus, Ohio*

Intravascular coagulation and activated fibrinolytic mechanisms are present to varying degrees in a variety of diseases. These hemostatic changes are referred to as disseminated intravascular coagulation (DIC), intravascular coagulation-fibrinolysis syndrome or consumption coagulopathy. DIC is always secondary to an underlying disease and should not be interpreted as a specific disease. It is an intermediary mechanism of disease. DIC might be compared to a process such as inflammation in that the term describes a series of changes that are associated with a wide variety of diseases. In DIC simultaneous activation of the coagulation and fibrinolytic mechanisms

causes intravascular fibrin thrombus formation and a bleeding tendency. The bleeding defect in DIC is usually related to thrombocytopenia and a deficiency of some clotting factors. The platelets and clotting factors are depleted by consumption during the active hemostatic process and fibrinolytic digestion of clotting proteins. The digestion of fibrin and fibrinogen by the active fibrinolytic mechanism generates increased levels of circulating fibrinolytic split products. Fibrinolytic split products may act as anticoagulants and also induce a severe platelet function defect, thereby potentiating the bleeding tendency. Organ dysfunction may occur in DIC either from the primary disease or secondary to capillary obstruction by fibrin thrombi.

Factors which contribute to the development of DIC include hypotension, stasis of blood flow, release of tissue thromboplastin from degenerating cells, vasculitis, exposure of blood to abnormal surfaces and reticuloendothelial cell blockade. These factors provide maximal opportunity for activation of the coagulation mechanism or decreased clearance of activated coagulation factors. Therefore, severe systemic diseases are more likely to be associated with clinically detectable DIC. Diseases that have been associated with DIC in the dog and cat are presented in Table 1. It should be emphasized that increased awareness and improved diagnostic capabilities will undoubtedly lengthen this list.

## CLINICAL SIGNS

The variety of causes and variable degrees of DIC may make recognition of the process difficult. Clinical signs in animals with DIC are frequently attributable to the primary disease. Clinical evidence of DIC includes petechial and ecchymotic hemorrhages, abnormal bleeding from venipuncture sites, epistaxis, gastrointestinal bleeding and hematuria. Large intramuscular hemorrhages and bleeding into body cavities are occasionally observed. Some animals with DIC have very few hemorrhages in spite of severe abnormalities in clotting tests.

## LABORATORY DIAGNOSIS

Since DIC is a complex syndrome, the changes that are associated with the process

**Table 1.** *Diseases Associated with DIC in Dogs or Cats*

| Infections | Miscellaneous |
|---|---|
| Septicemia | Shock |
| Infectious canine | Endotoxemia |
|   hepatitis | Heat stroke |
| Leptospirosis | Hemorrhagic |
| Panleukopenia |   pancreatitis |
| Trypanosomiasis | Hemolytic disease |
| Rocky Mountain spotted | Gastric torsion |
|   fever | Heartworm disease |
| | Hemorrhagic enteritis |
| *Neoplasia* | Hepatic necrosis |
| Carcinoma | Extracorporeal |
| Lymphosarcoma |   circulation |
| Hemangiosarcoma | Surgical trauma |
| Granulocytic leukemia | Diaphragmatic hernia |

are not always spectacular nor all present simultaneously. The changes that are helpful for the diagnosis of DIC include

—Prolonged one-stage prothrombin time
—Prolonged partial thromboplastin time
—Thrombocytopenia
—Increased levels of fibrinolytic split products
—Petechial hemorrhages
—Abnormal bleeding from venipuncture sites
—Fragmented erythrocytes (schistocytes)
—Decreased levels of coagulation factors (I, II, V, VIII, X)

The most consistent changes associated with DIC are prolonged partial thromboplastin time, thrombocytopenia and increased levels of circulating fibrinolytic split products. A latex agglutination test is available for detection of human fibrinolytic split products. The Thrombo-Wellcotest®* is simple to perform and appears to be reliable for detecting increased levels of fibrinolytic split products in dogs and cats. Fibrinolytic split products are present in very low concentrations in normal animals. In our laboratory, a positive Thrombo-Wellcotest® at a serum dilution of 1/25 or greater is evidence for enhanced fibrinolysis.

## TREATMENT

**Aims.** Since DIC is always secondary to some primary disease, specific therapy must be directed toward correction of the underlying disease. Until this is accomplished, one must attempt to prevent both excessive intravascular fibrin strand formation and life-threatening hemorrhages.

**Specific Treatment.** Impaired tissue perfusion is an important contributing factor in DIC; therefore, the most critical measures in the management of acute syndromes of DIC usually are the treatments for shock, acidosis, hypoxia and hemoconcentration. Fluid and electrolyte therapy may be sufficient if the primary disease is easily recognized and treated.

The use of heparin anticoagulation for arresting the intravascular fibrin deposition and clotting factor consumption may be helpful in selected instances. Heparin is not

---

*Thrombo-Wellcotest®, Burroughs Wellcome Co., Wellcome Research Division, 3030 Cornwallis Road, Research Triangle Park, North Carolina 27709.

always necessary or desirable. However, there are instances in which heparin administration is indicated. One instance is when DIC is severe and life-threatening (hemorrhage or organ dysfunction) and the underlying disease is treatable but requires time for correction. An example of this is septicemia, in which heparin therapy may inhibit the progression of DIC until the antibiotic and fluid therapy is effective in controlling the disease. Another instance in which heparin may be beneficial is in the treatment of patients with DIC and severe anemia due to blood loss or hemolysis. The administration of blood or plasma to such patients may provide the precursors (clotting factors and platelets) for further intravascular fibrin strand formation and cause death. Heparinization of the patient prior to administration of blood or plasma decreases this possibility. A third instance in which heparinization may be valuable is when DIC is recognized in a bleeding patient but the underlying disease process has not been diagnosed. Heparin therapy may keep the animal alive while additional diagnostic procedures are performed.

The dosage of heparin for dogs and cats is not well established. Normal dogs very rapidly clear intravenously administered heparin (150 units/kg. is cleared in less than 2 hours). The treatment of choice is an initial intravenous injection of 75 units/kg. followed by a continuous intravenous drip containing heparin at a dosage of 600 units/kg./day. If continuous intravenous infusion is not practical, 1000 units/kg. can be administered subcutaneously at 12-hour intervals. With either treatment schedule, the one-stage prothrombin time, activated partial thromboplastin time or activated coagulation time* should be performed on samples collected at 12- to 24-hour intervals. Optimal heparin therapy should maintain a prolongation of the clotting tests to 2 to 3 times normal. The dosage should be adjusted accordingly to correct for variations in heparin clearance rates. It is not advisable to administer heparin on a dosage schedule which allows the coagulation mechanism to fluctuate between normal

and abnormal. This fluctuation may allow the replenishment of clotting factors and platelets which then are consumed when the anticoagulant is cleared from the circulation. It should also be emphasized that heparin is not an innocuous drug. Intramuscular injections should be avoided to decrease the risk of intramuscular hemorrhage. Patients that are receiving heparin should be carefully monitored for evidence of bleeding. Severe hemorrhages that develop while patients are on anticoagulant therapy should be treated by discontinuing the heparin and giving blood or plasma if needed.

The response to heparin therapy is difficult to monitor. Desirable signs include the arrest of hemorrhage from venipuncture sites or of hematuria and an overall clinical improvement in the patient. If hypofibrinogenemia is present, fibrinogen levels should be increased within 12 hours after heparin administration is started. Platelet numbers increase at a slower pace, taking at least 24 to 48 hours to return to normal in successfully treated patients. Fibrinolytic split products may be detectable at high levels for 24 to 48 hours after initiation of treatment.

The heparin therapy should be continued for as long as needed to suppress the DIC. However, this can only be determined by discontinuing treatment and judging the patient's response. If the hemostatic defect recurs when heparin is discontinued, the heparin therapy may have to be resumed. Acute forms of DIC generally require treatment only for 2 to 3 days.

The use of adrenal corticosteroids in patients with DIC is controversial. Potential deleterious effects of corticosteroids include blockade of the reticuloendothelial system, inhibition of fibrinolysis and potentiation of catecholamine effects on blood vessels. The disadvantages of steroid therapy may be outweighed by the beneficial effects in patients with shock. The use of other anticoagulants, platelet aggregation inhibitors, alpha-adrenergic blockers and fibrinolytic agents has not been adequately evaluated. Inhibitors of the fibrinolytic mechanism such as epsilon-aminocaproic acid should never be used alone in patients with DIC, since fibrinolytic digestion of intravascular fibrin is protective and blockade may complicate the disease.

*Activated Coagulation Time, Vacutainer® 3206XF534, Becton-Dickinson and Co., Rutherford, New Jersey 07070.

SUPPLEMENTAL READING

Bowie, E. J. W., and Owen, C. A., Jr. (chairmen): Symposium on the diagnosis and treatment of intravascular coagulation-fibrinolysis (ICF) syndrome, with special emphasis on this syndrome in patients with cancer. Mayo Clin. Proc., 49:635–679, 1975.
Deykin, D.: The clinical challenge of disseminated intravascular coagulation. N. Eng. J. Med., 283:636–644, 1970.
Greene, C. E.: Disseminated intravascular coagulation in the dog: A review. J.A.A.H.A., 11:674–687, 1975.
Kociba, G. J., and Hathaway, J. E.: Disseminated intravascular coagulation associated with heartworm disease in the dog. J.A.A.H.A., 10:373–378, 1974.

# GAMMOPATHIES

ARTHUR I. HURVITZ, D.V.M.
*New York, New York*

Electrophoretic separation of serum protein defines the albumin and alpha, beta and gamma globulin components. Antibodies or immunoglobulins are found primarily in the beta and gamma globulin fractions in dogs and cats. Abnormalities in the immunoglobulins are termed gammopathies. They can be classified as follows:

1. Decreased immunoglobulin levels (deficiencies)
2. Increased immunoglobulin levels
   a. Polyclonal (heterogenous)
   b. Monoclonal (homogenous)

Serum electrophoresis is a useful technique for the screening of gammopathies. Alterations in serum albumin/globulin ratio, especially elevated globulin levels, warrant electrophoresis to determine which globulin fraction is altered, its configuration and its size. Decreased immunoglobulin levels are characterized by low beta and gamma globulin levels. The electrophoretic pattern provides a clinically useful grouping of those gammopathies associated with elevated levels of immunoglobulins. An electrophoretic broad band of diffuse hyperglobulinemia is characteristic of polyclonal gammopathies, which arise from persistent stimulation of the immune system. The presence of a narrow, homogenous band giving a "spikelike" deformation of the electrophoretic pattern characterizes monoclonal gammopathies. This abnormal, dense, sharply defined electrophoretic band is composed of a homogenous monoclonal protein termed M-component, or paraprotein. The M-component is thought to be the product of a single clone of immunoproliferative cells which synthesizes and secretes abnormal quantities of a normal immunoglobulin and/or excess free light chains of this immunoglobulin into the blood. The light chains, being small enough to pass through the renal glomerulus, are concentrated in the urine and are called Bence Jones proteins.

## DECREASED IMMUNOGLOBULIN LEVELS

A variety of immunologic deficiency states are recognized in man. These deficiency gammopathies may be either congenital or acquired. Hereditary immunologic deficiency diseases have not been satisfactorily described in dogs and cats. Pneumonia caused by *Pneumocystis carinii* has been reported in several miniature dachshunds in Australia. Preliminary investigations indicated an inheritable immune deficiency state which allowed the organisms to become pathogenic.

Acquired deficiencies can occur secondarily to a number of disease states affecting the lymphoid tissue, such as monoclonal gammopathies and lymphoid neoplasms. There is an excessive loss of immunoglobulins in subjects with the nephrotic syndrome or with protein-losing enteropathy.

## INCREASED IMMUNOGLOBULIN LEVELS

### POLYCLONAL GAMMOPATHIES

In general, a polyclonal gammopathy is a nonspecific serum protein abnormality observed with many diseases. It does not permit a specific disease diagnosis. The disorders which may produce polyclonal gammopathy are listed in Table 1. Most of

**Table 1.** *Conditions Exhibiting Polyclonal Gammopathies*

*Protracted Infections*
    Pyoderma
    Feline infectious peritonitis
    Pyometra
    Granulomatous Disorders
*Parasitism*
    Heartworm disease
    Ascariasis
    Ancylostomiasis
    Ehrlichiosis (canine tropical pancytopenia)
*Immunologically Mediated Disease*
    Systemic lupus erythematosus
    Rheumatoid arthritis
    Immune-mediated thrombocytopenia
    Eosinophilic myositis
*Idiopathic*

these disease entities are described in other articles in this text under the appropriate organ system involved.

## MONOCLONAL GAMMOPATHIES

Monoclonal gammopathies are most commonly associated with neoplasms involving the immunoglobulin-forming cells (multiple myeloma, macroglobulinemia, L-chain disease, lymphosarcoma). Sometimes, monoclonal immunoglobulin increases are associated with diseases other than multiple myeloma and lymphoproliferative diseases, such as nonreticular neoplasms, liver disease and cold agglutinin disease. A monoclonal globulin spike in the electrophoretic patterns of normal individuals is occasionally detected; this condition has been designated "essential benign monoclonal gammopathy." A substantial portion of these benign gammopathies convert to symptomatic cases. Since life expectancy may be related to the time of recognition of the abnormality, early differential diagnosis is important in proper disease management.

### CLINICAL SIGNS

The clinical features are attributable to the proliferation of neoplastic cells and/or their protein product (M-component). The most common manifestations directly related to the presence of the M-component include infection, bleeding diathesis and the hyperviscosity syndrome. Animals with monoclonal gammopathies should be considered immunologic cripples, since they often develop an acquired immunologic deficiency. The lowered resistance to infection has a complex etiology, often involving both cellular and humoral factors. Death due to infection is common in patients with monoclonal gammopathies. The combined effects of anoxia, clotting abnormalities and thrombocytopenia are thought to cause the bleeding tendency. Increased viscosity of the plasma (hyperviscosity syndrome) is often produced when the M-component is high molecular weight IgM macroglobulin (macroglobulinemia) and, rarely, by aggregative forms of other immunoglobulin classes, such as polymeric IgA. Because of their increased size and shape, these proteins can increase plasma viscosity up to 7 times normal values. This results in mental depression, visual disturbance and other neurologic manifestations. Diagnosis of the hyperviscosity syndrome may be confirmed by demonstration of increased serum viscosity with an Ostwald viscometer.

### AIMS OF TREATMENT

1. Reduce the population of proliferating cells (mass size) as determined by palpation or visualized on radiographs.
2. Decrease serum paraprotein level to 50 per cent or less of pretreatment value and to less than 4 per cent/100 ml. of serum.
3. In the presence of urinary Bence Jones protein, the excretion should be decreased to less than 50 per cent of pretreatment value.
4. Lower serum viscosity if hyperviscosity is present.
5. Control infections, hemorrhaging and other signs associated with the monoclonal immunoglobulin.

### TREATMENT

Treatment is based on a combination of surgery, radiation therapy, chemotherapy and supportive measures. Surgical intervention is done when an operable lesion will improve the clinical condition and well-being of the animal. Surgical procedures may therefore include repair of a pathologic fracture or removal of an encroaching tumor mass near the spinal cord.

Radiation therapy of localized lesions is often employed in human medicine. Myelomatous cells are moderately susceptible to radiation which is used to reduce the size of lytic bone lesions and relieve the pain associated with the neoplasm. Cobalt radiation is most commonly used, the dose varying with the location, depth and extent of the lesion.

Corticosteroids, alone or in combination with alkylating agents, are used to depress the elaboration of M-component. Corticosteroids are also beneficial in the presence of thrombocytopenia and anemia; these complications arise from the disease or from the administration of cytotoxic or alkylating agents.

In man, the systemic treatment of choice is cytotoxic drugs such as 1-phenylalanine mustard (melphalan, Alkeran®), cyclophosphamide (Cytoxan®) or chlorambucil (Leukeran®). In dogs, combined therapy with Alkeran® (0.05 mg./kg./day) and prednisone (0.5 mg./kg./day) has been effective in reducing the population of proliferating cells and lowering the M-component. Hemograms should be performed frequently to determine optimal dosage and avoid bone marrow depression. Plasmapheresis is the method of choice for the treatment of hyperviscosity syndrome. Plasmapheresis is a technique whereby the offending protein is partially removed by bleeding the animal and then replacing its red blood cells. Plasmapheresis is also helpful in handling hemorrhagic complications due to the influence of M-components. Plasmapheresis temporarily removes the offending protein that may be coating platelets, inhibiting thrombin activity with delayed fibrin promotion, or absorbing clotting factors. When plasmapheresis is not possible, withdrawal of large amounts of blood is probably also beneficial if the animal is not severely anemic.

Coverage with broad-spectrum antibiotics is recommended, and the introduction of pathogens during the performance of routine procedures should be avoided.

## PROGNOSIS

The prognosis for patients with monoclonal gammopathies is still unfavorable, particularly in widely disseminated multiple myeloma. Nevertheless, treatment does offer some hope in delaying the progression of the disease. Most patients die of secondary complications, with intercurrent infection being the most common factor. The animals are immunologically crippled and are therefore unable to overcome infection. Immunologic embarrassment may explain the widespread dissemination of other types of neoplasms observed in some animals with monoclonal gammopathies. Protracted bleeding, pathologic fractures and cord lesions are other complications encountered.

### SUPPLEMENTAL READING

Farrow, B. R. H., Watson, A. D., Hartley, W. J., and Huxtable, C. R. R.: *Pneumocystis* pneumonia in the dog. J. Comp. Pathol., 82:447, 1972.
Hurvitz, A. I., Haskins, S. C., and Fischer, C. A.: Macroglobulinemia with hyperviscosity syndrome in a dog. J. Am. Vet. Med. Assn., 157:455–460, 1970.
Hurvitz, A. I., *et al.*: Bence Jones proteinemia and proteinuria in a dog. J. Am. Vet. Med. Assn., 159:1112–1116, 1971.
Osborne, C. A., *et al.*: Multiple myeloma in the dog. J. Am. Vet. Med. Assn., 153:1300–1319, 1968.
Shepard, V. J., Dodds-Laffin, W. J., and Laffin, R. J.: Gamma A myeloma in a dog with defective hemostasis. J. Am. Vet. Med. Assn., 160:1121–1127, 1972.

# LABORATORY DIAGNOSIS OF IMMUNOLOGIC DISORDERS

RONALD D. SCHULTZ, Ph.D.
*Ithaca, New York*

An increased awareness of immunology and the rapid progress in immunologic technology during the past decade have led to the development of clinical immunology in veterinary medicine. As a result, immunologic methods of laboratory diagnoses have become increasingly important in all aspects of veterinary clinical medicine. In considering any animal whose condition presents a diagnostic problem, or who presents with a recognized disease but of an as yet unknown etiology (e.g., granulomatous colitis of boxers, generalized demodectic mange), an immunologic aspect should be considered. To test the patient for an immunologic disorder—allergic, autoimmune, immunodeficiency or immunoproliferative—a minimal understanding of the laboratory tests available and the samples required for these tests is essential. It is the purpose of this article to provide the basic information of methods in use by immunologists which may be applicable to clinical diagnosis. For the challenges of modern veterinary medicine to be met it will be necessary for the clinician to come into the laboratory and the laboratory scientist to go into the clinic; when this happens, progress is inevitable.

A possible approach to the clinical and laboratory evaluation of an animal suspected of having a disease or disorder in which at least some of the signs are immunologically based is presented in Figure 1.

## IMMUNE-MEDIATED DISORDERS

### AUTOIMMUNE HEMOLYTIC ANEMIA (AIHA)

Autoimmune hemolytic anemia is a hemolytic state in which antibody and/or complement can be demonstrated on the erythrocytes (see article earlier in this section for the description and characteristics of the disease). Laboratory diagnosis would include a CBC, bone marrow biopsy, autoagglutination test and the antiglobulin (Coombs') test. The direct antiglobulin test is essentially as follows:

1. Erythrocytes are obtained from a blood clot or from blood collected in EDTA.

2. A small quantity of erythrocytes are washed 3 to 4 times in physiologic saline solution (PSS) or phosphate-buffered saline (PBS).

3. The washed erythrocytes are suspended in PSS or PBS to a final concentration of 2 per cent.

4. In small tubes or wells of a microtiter plate, equal quantities of the 2 per cent erythrocytes and antiglobulin reagent at various dilutions are mixed together and incubated at 37° C. for 30 minutes, then

at room temperature for 30 minutes. The erythrocytes are also added to autologous serum or plasma to detect autoagglutinins.

5. Agglutination is observed macroscopically or microscopically.

*Note:* For the test to be valid, cells from a normal dog should be run simultaneously and they should not agglutinate.

The antiglobulin reagent to test for canine AIHA should have reactivity to canine IgG and C3 (a complement component) and should not agglutinate normal canine erythrocytes. A canine Coombs' reagent is commercially available from Miles Laboratories, Elkhart, Indiana.

The indirect antiglobulin (Coombs') test which determines the presence of antibodies to erythrocytes in the serum of a patient suspected of having AIHA appears to be of little or no value in the diagnosis of canine or feline AIHA.

*Sample required:* Clotted blood and EDTA tube (lavender stopper) of blood.

### RHEUMATOID ARTHRITIS (RA)

Rheumatoid arthritis is often a severe, progressive polyarthritis affecting numerous organ systems, the most frequent site of injury being the synovial lining of the joints (see article on "Canine Polyarthritis").

The laboratory diagnosis would always include a rheumatoid factor (RF) test. RF is IgM, IgG or IgA with antibody activity to altered IgG. Most of the tests for RF detect predominantly IgM rather than IgG or IgA. A canine or feline rheumatoid latex reagent is not available commercially and the human reagent is unsatisfactory. The test we find most satisfactory for detection of RF is the Rose-Waaler test.

The Rose-Waaler test is essentially an antiglobulin test using red cells (usually sheep) sensitized with a subagglutinating dose of rabbit or canine anti-SRBC antibodies. In our experience approximately 60 to 75 per cent of dogs with clinical signs of RA show positive results in the Rose-Waaler test. We have arbitrarily stated that the serum has to have a titer of 1/16 or greater to be considered positive.

Poor mucin precipitation of synovial fluid can also be used as a diagnostic aid for RA. The test is performed as follows: Glacial acetic acid is added dropwise to a test tube containing synovial fluid from the patient and one from a control dog (if available). In

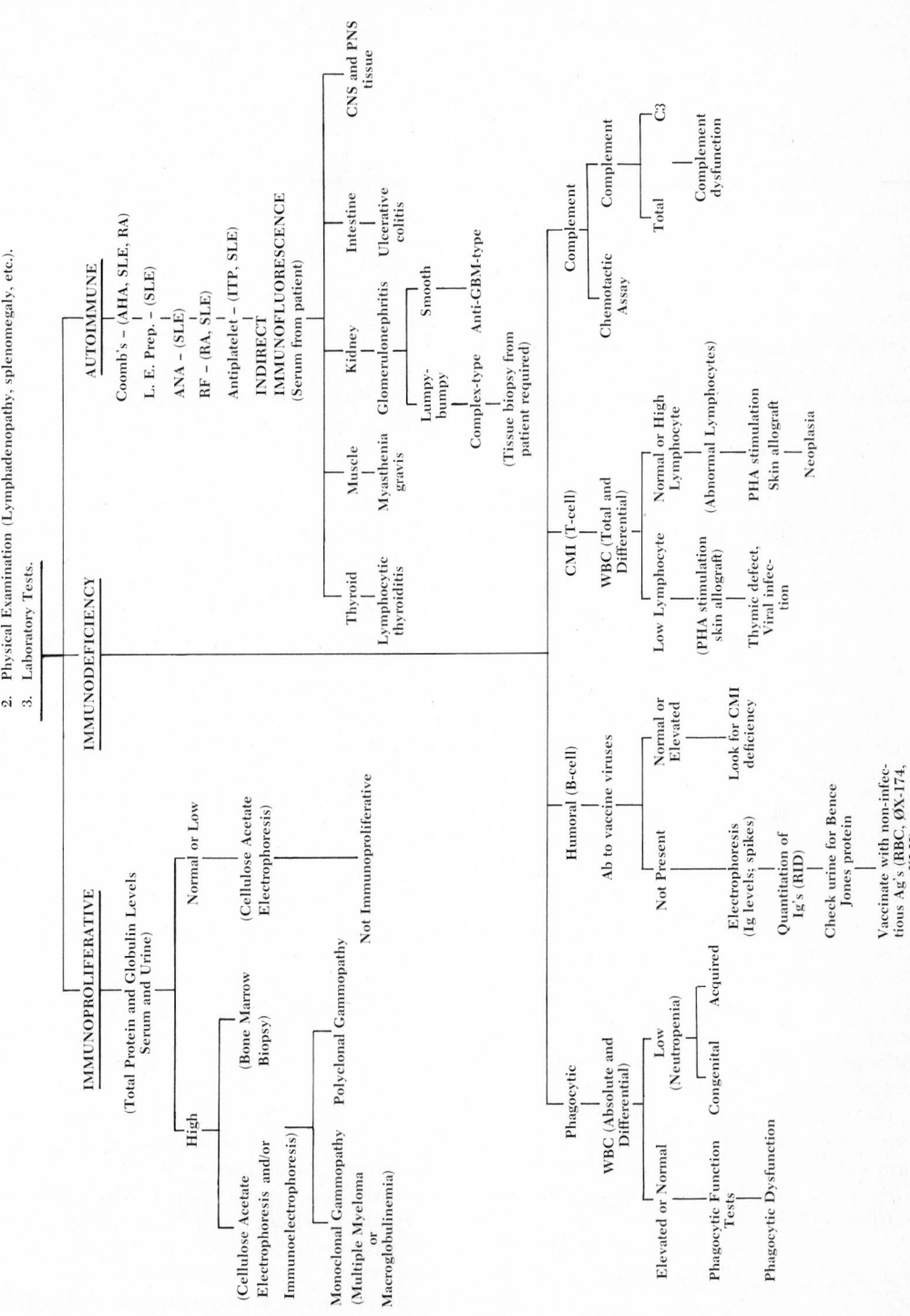

Figure 1.

dogs with RA or septic arthritis, loose and friable clots or only a flocculent precipitate will form, whereas in normal dogs or dogs with SLE or degenerative joint disease, a firm, hard, ropy, nonfriable clot will form. Complement, particularly the C3 component, is low or depleted in the synovial fluid of many human patients with RA. Similar tests for reduction or depletion of C3 in canine RA have not been reported, therefore these tests are currently not used routinely.

*Sample required:* Serum and synovial fluid (if available).

*Note:* We are currently studying canine rheumatoid arthritis and would appreciate receiving serum samples, synovial fluid and history from dogs in which at least six of the following nine criteria are positive findings:

1. Morning stiffness.
2. Pain on motion or tenderness of joint.
3. Soft tissue swelling.
4. Similar swelling within past 3 months.
5. Symmetrical onset of joint symptoms and swelling.
6. Radiographic changes.
7. Poor mucin precipitate consistent with RA.
8. Histologic changes consistent with RA.
9. Rheumatoid factor.

We will test the serum for RF and send the results as promptly as possible.

## IMMUNOLOGIC THROMBOCYTOPENIC PURPURA (IMTP)

Immunologic thrombocytopenic purpura occurs when antibody and/or sensitized T cells cause the number of platelets to fall below that number essential for maintenance of vascular integrity and normal hemostasis.

Laboratory diagnosis would include a CBC and an assay for antiplatelet antibody (i.e., platelet factor 3 test). (See article on "Thrombocytopenic Purpura" earlier in this section.)

*Sample required:* CBC and blood collected for serum.

## SYSTEMIC LUPUS ERYTHEMATOSUS (SLE)

Systemic lupus erythematosus is a generalized disorder which involves many organ systems. It is frequently characterized by the presence of antinuclear antibody (ANA) and lupus erythematosus (LE) cells and the simultaneous occurrence of two or more of the following disorders: AIHA, IMTP, RA (presence of RF) or immune-complex glomerulonephritis (see article on "Systemic Lupus Erythematosus" later in this section).

The LE cell test is the most reliable indicator of SLE; however, it is only positive in about 75 per cent of dogs with SLE. The antinuclear antibody (ANA) immunofluorescence test is a reliable screening test but is not specific for SLE.

**LE Cell Test.** The direct LE cell test can be performed as follows: the clot from a 5-ml. blood sample is incubated for 2 hours at 37° C., strained through a fine wire mesh into a tube and centrifuged. Smears are made from the buffy coat and are stained and examined for LE cells. LE cells are polymorphonuclear neutrophils which have phagocytized nuclear material. An indirect procedure is also available which requires serum from the patient and a blood sample from a normal dog. The technique is basically the same as above.

**ANA Immunofluorescence Test.** The antinuclear antibody (ANA) immunofluorescence test in our laboratory is performed as follows:

1. Serum from the patient diluted 1:5 placed on Vero cells and incubated for 30 minutes. *Note:* The Vero cells are grown on 8-chamber slides (Lab-Tek®) until 50 per cent of the cell layer is grown in. The cells are then fixed for 10 minutes with cold (4° C.) methanol or acetone.

2. The cells are washed in PBS for 10 minutes with at least three changes of PBS.

3. The slides are flipped to remove as much buffer as possible, and anti-canine IgG labeled with fluorescein isothiocyanate (FITC) is placed on the sections of the slide and incubated for 30 minutes.

4. Step 2 is repeated. The slides are dipped in distilled water and then air-dried.

5. A suitable solution such as phosphate-buffered glycerol or elvanol is placed on the slide, a coverslip is applied and the slides are viewed for fluorescence with a microscope equipped for fluorescence microscopy.

An ANA kit which contains the substrate slide, FITC-labeled anti-canine IgG and a positive control serum is available from Miles Laboratories, Elkhart, Indiana.

Additional tests available to detect anti-

DNA antibody and antinuclear antibody include the radioimmunoassay (RIA) and the latex assay, respectively. The RIA procedure is an excellent test but it is not satisfactory for routine screening of clinical samples because of cost and equipment necessary. The latex particles sensitized with calf-thymus DNA in our experience does not compare favorably with the presence of ANA by immunofluorescence or LE cells; therefore we cannot recommend it at this time.

*Samples required:* Clotted blood sample for LE cell test and serum for ANA immunofluorescence test.

## AUTOIMMUNE THYROIDITIS (LYMPHOCYTIC)

Hypothyroidism mediated by antibody and/or cells is characterized by lethargy, easy fatigability, patchy alopecia, infertility and intolerance to cold. Antibody to thyroglobulin or microsomal antigen can be detected by the tanned red cell hemagglutination test. The indirect immunofluorescence test is also used to detect anitbody to thyroid antigens.

Recently we have used the lymphocyte blastogenesis test and a thyroid extract as antigen to detect antigen-responsive lymphocytes in dogs with autoimmune thyroiditis.

**Agar-Gel Diffusion Test.** This simple test can be used to detect antibody (predominantly IgG) to certain soluble tissue or serum antigens (i.e., altered IgG, lens protein). It is performed by punching holes (wells) in agar and allowing antigen and antisera to diffuse toward each other. In the region where optimal concentrations of antigen and antibody exist, precipitin lines will form. The major disadvantage of the test is its lack of sensitivity.

**Immunofluorescence.** Antibody to numerous tissues, including thyroid, muscle, intestine, intercellular cement substances (pemphigus), central and peripheral nervous tissue and others, can sometimes be detected by indirect immunofluorescence. The technique is essentially the same as that described for the ANA immunofluorescence test, with the specific tissue (usually cryostat section) substituted for the tissue culture (Vero) cells. An FITC-conjugated anti-canine or anti-feline IgG is

necessary for the test and is available from several commercial sources.

*Sample required :* Serum.

## IMMUNE-COMPLEX GLOMERULONEPHRITIS

(See article on "Glomerulonephropathy and the Nephrotic Syndrome.")

Immune-complex glomerulonephritis requires a needle or wedge biopsy of kidney for clinical diagnosis. The immunofluorescence test and electron microscopy are the techniques of choice. For the immunofluorescence test, an anti-canine IgG and anti-canine C3 labeled with FITC are used to detect immune complexes in the mesangium and/or on the glomerular basement membrane (GBM). A lumpy-bumpy pattern of fluorescence is indicative of immune-complex glomerulonephritis. A second immune-mediated, anti-GBM glomerulonephritis has not been reported to date for the dog or cat but if present would be characterized by a smooth pattern of fluorescence on the GBM.

# IMMUNOPROLIFERATIVE DISORDERS (GAMMOPATHIES)

The techniques of cellulose acetate electrophoresis, immunoelectrophoresis, radial immunodiffusion (RID), bone marrow smear and the thermal test for Bence Jones proteins in urine are the laboratory tests most frequently used specifically to diagnose multiple myeloma, macroglobulinemia (monoclonal gammopathies) or polyclonal gammopathies (see article on "Gammopathies"). In addition, the routine techniques to determine total protein (i.e., refractometer, biuret) and A/G ratios frequently alert the clinician to the possibility of a gammopathy.

Cellulose acetate electrophoresis is a quantitative electrophoretic technique available in most human and veterinary clinical laboratories. We find the Beckman Microzone® technique very satisfactory. With this technique, eight samples of serum can be simultaneously separated into at least five or six fractions: albumin (most anodal), $\alpha_1$, $\alpha_2$, $\beta_1$, $\beta_2$ and $\gamma$ globulin. IgG myeloma proteins are generally, but not always, found in the $\gamma$ globulin region, and

IgA myeloma and macroglobulinemia (IgM) are generally found in the $\beta$ regions.

Immunoelectrophoresis differs from cellulose acetate electrophoresis in that serum is separated in an electric field, and then an agar-gel diffusion reaction with antisera to serum proteins is performed. This technique can separate serum into 20 or more fractions and is principally a qualitative technique. It is useful for demonstrating abnormalities in proteins such as myeloma globulins and Bence Jones proteins in urine. RID performed in agar containing antisera is a sensitive quantitative technique used to determine the amount of immunoglobulin or specific complement component present in serum. It requires antisera specific for the particular protein to be quantitated as well as antigens which can be used as specific protein standards. RID kits are available commercially from Miles Laboratories, Elkhart, Indiana, for the quantitation of several canine immunoglobulins. Antisera to canine IgG and IgM are available from Cappel Laboratories, Downingtown, Pennsylvania.

The thermal solubility test for Bence Jones protein in urine is performed by adjusting the pH to 5 and heating the urine slowly to boiling. Most Bence Jones proteins will precipitate at temperatures between 50° and 60° C. and will redissolve on boiling. When the urine is allowed to cool, the proteins reprecipitate. If albumin is present in the urine, the precipitate will not redissolve at high temperatures. Urostix®* are specific for albumin and will not detect the presence of Bence Jones proteins.

In certain chronic diseases (i.e., brucellosis, pyometra) and autoimmune diseases (SLE), an elevation of gamma globulin will occur which can be recognized on cellulose acetate electrophoresis as a polyclonal gammopathy (heterogenous $\gamma$-globulin elevation). This elevation results from constant antigenic stimulation and perhaps a defect in suppressor T-cell activity.

*Samples required:* Serum and urine.

## IMMUNODEFICIENCY DISORDERS

Immunodeficiency disorders reflect an impairment in one or more of the major components of immunity: *nonspecific immunity*, including (1) phagocytic cells (e.g., PMN and macrophages) and (2) effector substances (i.e., complement); and/or *specific immunity*, including (1) humoral (antibody) immunity (the B-cell system) and (2) cell-mediated immunity (CMI) (the T-cell system). Immunodeficiencies are classified as primary or secondary deficiencies. The primary deficiency diseases are genetically defined inborn errors of the body's defense mechanisms and can affect nonspecific as well as specific components of the immune response. Primary deficiencies are very uncommon in the dog and cat, but they do occur.

Secondary immunodeficiencies are acquired as a consequence of numerous conditions, including infectious disease, neoplasia, aging, drug therapy, failure to receive colostrum and certain nutritional deficiencies. Secondary immunodeficiencies are more common than primary deficiencies. We, as well as others, have reported secondary immunodeficiencies or immunosuppression associated with canine distemper infections, canine generalized demodectic mange, nutritional deficiencies, feline panleukopenia, feline leukemia, age (see article on "Canine Vaccines and Immunity"), and perhaps numerous other as yet unrecognized conditions.

Clinicians should consider immunodeficiency or immunosuppression when an animal is presented with a history of chronic infection, autoimmune disease or neoplastic disease.

Deficiencies of the humoral immune system would most often be characterized by infections with extracellular pyogenic pathogens (e.g., streptococci). Selective IgA deficiencies may be characterized by chronic respiratory or gastrointestinal infections. The presence of microbes normally not pathogenic for the animal is often a clue to immunodeficiency disorders (e.g., *Pneumocystis carinii* or streptococci isolated from the lung or *Giardia* in the gut). Deficiencies of cell-mediated immunity are associated with infections caused by facultative intracellular pyogenic pathogens (e.g., acid-fast organisms, Brucella, Salmonella, certain viruses and fungi).

A suggested approach to the clinical and laboratory diagnosis of an animal suspected of an immunodeficiency disease is presented in Figure 1.

---

*Ames Co., Elkhart, Indiana.

## NONSPECIFIC IMMUNITY

If a deficiency in nonspecific immunity is suspected, such as cyclic neutropenia or chronic granulomatous disease, the following laboratory tests may be used as an aid to diagnosis.

**Phagocytic and Bactericidal Function Tests.** Phagocytic index and bactericidal activity tests measure the ability of cells to phagocytize and subsequently kill bacteria, a function of the lysozomal enzymes. The test is performed by mixing a suspension of bacteria (e.g., staphylococci or *E. coli*) with a suspension of leukocytes from the patient and a normal control in the presence of fresh serum. After an appropriate period of time the number of viable bacteria is determined for patient and control by direct bacterial plate count techniques. The inability to phagocytize and/or kill bacteria is indicative of a deficiency in neutrophil function and rarely monocyte or macrophage function.

**Nitroblue Tetrazolium Test (NBT).** This test is particularly useful to detect nonfunctional neutrophils in chronic granulomatous disease (CGD). Neutrophils from normal dogs or cats rapidly reduce nitroblue tetrazolium (NBT) during *in-vitro* phagocytosis. Neutrophils from animals with CGD are unable to reduce NBT. A kit for the NBT test is available from Sigma Chemical Co., St. Louis, Missouri.

*Sample required:* Blood collected in preservative-free heparin; 50 units/ml. of blood is ideal for the above tests. Large quantities of heparin can affect the NBT test.

**Total Hemolytic Complement.** $CH_{50}$ can be detected in dogs by adding fresh serum to sheep red blood cells sensitized with rabbit antibody. For the cat, chicken or rabbit red blood cells sensitized with cat antibody can be used. Sensitized cells mixed with serial dilutions of the patient's and a control animal's serum are incubated, and the highest dilution of serum giving 50 per cent hemolysis is recorded. A difference of 3 or more dilutions from the control would suggest a complement deficiency in the patient. Total hemolytic complement assays measure all components of the complement system.

**Quantitation of C3 Component by RID.** The C3 component of complement as well as other individual components can be purified, and antisera to them can be made. These antisera can be used to quantitate the complement component in serum. If purified complement standards are not available for standardization, serum from normal dogs can be used to compare values with dogs suspected of having complement deficiencies. We have recognized depletion of C3 in dogs with autoimmune thyroiditis and in some dogs with immune-complex glomerulonephritis. We also currently use this assay to measure C3 in joint fluid of dogs suspected of having rheumatoid arthritis.

## SPECIFIC IMMUNITY

### DEFICIENCIES IN THE HUMORAL IMMUNE RESPONSE (B-CELL SYSTEMS)

These should be considered if an animal does not produce antibody to vaccine viruses after proper immunization, has very low gamma globulin levels or suffers from chronic infection with extracellular pathogens. In dogs, antibody to canine distemper virus (CDV) and canine adenovirus 1 (CAV-1) should develop within three to four weeks after vaccination and will persist for long periods of time. Antibody to the parainfluenza virus $SV_5$ could also be used as an indication of humoral immunocompetence if this virus is included in the routine vaccine schedule. In the cat, feline panleukopenia, feline herpes virus or calicivirus vaccine virus antibody can be used as an indication of immune responsiveness. If, after proper and repeated vaccination, antibody to these viruses is not present, a humoral immunodeficiency should be suspected.

During the early neonatal period a humoral immunodeficiency exists in pups and kittens which do not receive colostrum, for whatever reason, since 95 to 98 per cent of their immunoglobulins are obtained by means of absorption of colostrum.

Numerous other antigen preparations (i.e., foreign red blood cells, keyhole-limpet hemocyanin, $\phi$X-174) can be used to determine immunocompetence in the dog and cat. Tests such as cellulose acetate electrophoresis, immunoelectrophoresis and radial immunodiffusion to quantitate the various classes of immunoglobulin can also be used to detect humoral immunodeficiencies (see description of techniques above).

## DEFICIENCIES IN CELL-MEDIATED IMMUNITY (T-CELL SYSTEM)

These provide the greatest challenge to the clinician and immunologist. Recently a number of *in-vitro* correlates of CMI have been developed for clinical diagnosis; however, none of them completely correlates with CMI *in vivo*. An approach to the patient with CMI deficiency would include a CBC to determine the presence of lymphopenia. Approximately 60 to 75 per cent of the peripheral blood lymphocytes are T cells; therefore, any significant reduction (less than 1000 lymphocytes/mm.$^3$) could suggest a CMI deficiency. The presence of normal numbers of lymphocytes *does not*, however, indicate that CMI is normal.

Delayed type dermal hypersensitivity (DTH) to most antigens is minimal or absent in dogs and cats; therefore this test cannot be used routinely to determine T-cell function.

Skin allograft transplants, on the other hand, are a reliable and simple-to-perform *in-vivo* method to check CMI in dogs and cats. Normal rejection time for both dogs and cats is 12 ± 2 days. Delays of one week or more from normal would be significant and indicate impairment of T-cell function.

Skin sensitization with chemicals like dinitrochlorobenzene (DNCB) has been suggested as a measure of CMI in man; however, DNCB sensitization in the dog and cat has proved less than satisfactory, even when biopsies are obtained for microscopic evaluation.

**The Lymphocyte Blastogenesis (Transformation) Technique.** This test has proved extremely helpful in the laboratory diagnosis of CMI deficiency in the dog and cat. The technique is subject to a variety of trials and tribulations; however, after optimal conditions for the test are established, it is an excellent immunodiagnostic tool in a variety of clinical conditions and promises to have wider applicability in the future.

Modifications of the technique were evaluated, and tests currently in use in our laboratory are outlined below:

Optimal conditions established for mitogenic stimulation of canine and feline peripheral blood cells in the macro test were as follows: Heparinized blood was centrifuged at 400 xg. for 10 minutes to obtain a buffy coat and leukocyte-rich plasma fraction, devoid of as many erythrocytes as possible. The white cell suspension was diluted, so that 0.1 ml. contained between 5 x 10$^5$ and 5 x 10$^6$ leukocytes. Cells were placed into 21 x 70-mm. screw-capped glass vials which contained 1 ml. of RPMI-1640 media with 100 units of penicillin, 100 $\mu$g. of streptomycin, 10 per cent fetal bovine serum (FBS) and an optimal amount of mitogen.

Optimal conditions for the micro test differed slightly from those of the macro test: Heparinized blood was centrifuged on a ficoll-isopaque gradient for 15 minutes at 1300 xg. The mononuclear cell layer was removed, and the cell suspension was adjusted, so that 0.1 ml. contained between 5 x 10$^4$ and 5 x 10$^5$ cells. Cells were placed in wells of a flat-bottomed 96-well microtiter tissue culture plate which contained 0.1 ml. of the media used in the macro test. The mitogens included phytohemagglutinin (PHA), concanavallin A (Con-A), pokeweed mitogen (PWM) and *E. coli* lipopolysaccharide (LPS). Culture tubes with loosened caps and microtiter plates were incubated for 72 hours at 39° C. in 5 per cent $CO_2$ and air. Two $\mu$Ci. of $^3$H thymidine was added in a volume of 0.5 ml. to the tubes and 1 $\mu$Ci. in 0.1 ml. was added to the wells. For the macro test the cells were centrifuged, washed, precipitated with trichloroacetic acid (TCA) and dissolved in formic acid, and the radioactivity was determined by scintillation spectrophotometry. The cells in the micro-plate test were harvested with a MASH II (Microbiological Associates, Bethesda, Maryland).

With one or both of the above techniques we have evaluated a large number of dogs and cats admitted to the Small Animal Clinic of the New York State College of Veterinary Medicine, as well as dogs and cats from various research experiments at the James A. Baker Institute for Animal Health. The following should be used as a guideline when performing the test on clinical samples: Samples should be run in duplicate or triplicate and repeated at least one time on another day before any conclusions are drawn from results. Lymphocytes should be cultured in autologous serum or plasma in addition to FBS to detect immunosuppressive factors (e.g., generalized demodectic mange). Values should be compared to normal mean values established for a large number of control animals but, more importantly, should be compared to normal control samples run simultaneously with the animal being evaluated.

Under the conditions outlined, the test has been found to be a very useful diagnostic tool. Clinical and experimental conditions in which we have found significant suppression of canine lymphocyte responses to phytomitogens have been canine distemper, generalized demodectic mange (autologous serum or plasma present), certain nutritional deficiencies, a percentage of dogs with lymphosarcoma, a small number of dogs with aspergillosis and a percentage of dogs older than 9 years of age. Suppression in the cat has been associated with feline leukemia virus infection, clinical leukemia, panleukopenia virus infection and an occasional animal without specific disease. It is our experience that feline lymphocytes in general respond more poorly to PHA than do those of the dog or other species. The cat lymphocytes respond well to Con-A and PWM. It is not currently known whether this reflects a difference in lymphocyte subpopulations of the cat as compared to those of other species, or if it is a technical artifact. It is also of interest to note that steroid treatment of the dog does not affect the lymphocyte response to phytomitogens. Based on a number of experimental studies, numerous cell manipulations and drug treatment of dogs and cats, we would suggest that the following populations of cells are stimulated by mitogens:

PHA—T cells.

Con-A—T cells (perhaps more than one subpopulation).

PWM—T and B cells (early response 2 and 3 days after stimulation is predominantly in T cells).

LPS—B cells (in many dogs and cats peripheral blood lymphocytes do not respond to *E. coli* LPS).

**Inhibition of Cell Migration (MIF).** This test measures the production of the lymphokine, migration inhibition factor (MIF). If this factor inhibits the migration of macrophages it is called "macrophage migration inhibition factor," and the factor that inhibits the migration of blood monocytes and neutrophils is called "leukocyte migration inhibition factor." The basic technique we have found suitable for the dog is one in which peripheral blood cells are packed into a capillary tube or placed in a well of an agarose plate, and antigen or mitogen is added to the cells. If MIF is produced, little or no migration occurs. If the lymphocytes are unable to produce MIF, normal migration occurs. The inability to produce MIF would be correlated with a lymphocyte

deficiency and presumably a deficiency of CMI. There are also modifications of the technique in use for the dog and cat which utilize guinea pig peritoneal macrophages as the target cells. Our experience with the technique as a clinical immunodiagnostic test has been unrewarding, and the test is not routinely used in our laboratory.

**Cytotoxicity Tests.** A number of cytotoxicity tests are available to measure lymphocyte cytotoxicity, antibody-complement cytotoxicity or antibody-dependent K-cell cytotoxicity. The cytopathic activity of lymphocytes against target cells (i.e., tumor cells, viral infected cells, erythrocytes) in cell culture is assumed to have its *in vivo* counterpart in some of tissue-damaging reactions associated with CMI. In the test, target cells are labeled with $^{14}C$ or $^{3}H$ thymidine, $^{125}IUDR$ or $^{51}Cr$. These labeled cells are then mixed with lymphocytes and incubated for 12 to 24 hours. At the end of incubation the amount of cell damage is expressed as a percentage of radiolabel released. The cell damage is due to a lymphokine (T-cell product) known as a cytotoxic factor or lymphotoxin.

Antibody-dependent K-cell cytotoxicity presumably is achieved by the K cell damaging the target cell in the presence of antibody. No complement is added. Antibody with specific activity for the target cell in the presence of complement will cause cell damage. Both assays also utilize a radioisotope-labeled cell to determine the amount of cell damage.

These assays have particular application for the measurement of specific cellular or humoral activity to antigens (i.e., viral or bacterial) or tumor cells.

**Specific Assay for T and B Cells.** The assay currently in routine use to identify the B cell would be the membrane immunofluorescence test for immunoglobulin. The test for T cells in man is the erythrocyte rosette-forming assay (E-RFC). However, further research is required to establish the significance and validity of erythrocyte rosette-forming assays to detect T cells in the dog. The circumstances in which the T- and B-cell assays are of definite clinical value are rather limited at the present time and they remain a research tool.

**Transfer Factor.** This is another lymphokine (product) that can be released or extracted from human lymphocytes. This remarkable and somewhat mysterious material can apparently transfer the information necessary for specific CMI. Although transfer factor is being used therapeutically in man for a number of disorders, currently there are no definitive studies to suggest that a similar substance exists in dogs or cats. Therefore, therapy in dogs or cats with preparations termed "transfer factor" would appear premature.

### ADDITIONAL IMMUNODIAGNOSTIC TESTS

**Radioallergosorbent Test (RAST).** Immunoglobulin E, the antibody involved in the immediate hypersensitivity reaction (type I) as well as in immune responses to vermin infections, is difficult to detect with conventional tests because serum concentrations are very low. A number of laboratories interested in immediate hypersensitivity (atopy) are currently attempting to modify the RAST to measure specific IgE in dogs. In the technique, serum IgE is measured by adding the dog's serum to allergen-linked cyanogen bromide–activated sepharose (dextran). After thorough washing, the absorbed IgE antibodies are measured by the uptake of radioisotope-labeled purified anti-canine IgE. The reaction is extremely sensitive, as are other radioimmunoassay (RIA) procedures, but it does require a specialized laboratory. The test could be considered an *in-vitro* correlate of skin testing for type I hypersensitivity.

Another test which is an RIA test to measure IgE is the radioimmunosorbent test (RIST). This test is used to measure only the quantity of IgE in serum and is not a measure of the activity of IgE with regard to a specific allergen (antigen).

Total IgE levels in the serum are also measured by a radioactive single RID procedure. Rabbit anti-canine IgE is incorporated into agar and standards or unknown sera placed in wells (see discussion of RID earlier in this article). An invisible precipitin ring forms, which is visualized by incubating with $^{125}I$-labeled goat anti-rabbit IgG followed by radioautography. The concentration of IgE is determined by measuring the diameter of the ring and comparing it to the standard preparations.

The clinical significance of quantitation of IgE is currently not known, because the range of values for normal dogs is large and because intestinal parasitic infections greatly increase the levels of IgE, making it difficult to relate values to allergic conditions. In addition, the IgE level does not identify offending allergens; therefore, skin tests or the RAST must be used for that purpose.

**Organ Transplant Histocompatibility Testing.** Dog leukocyte antigens (DLA), like human leukocyte antigens (HLA), are histocompatibility antigens found on the membrane of numerous cells, including the lymphocytes. These antigens are specific markers or fingerprints for an individual dog and can be used to determine compatibility for possible organ transplant. A number of laboratories in the United States, Canada and Europe have typing antisera for DLA. Another immunologic test to determine compatibility between recipient and potential donor animals for organ transplant is the mixed leukocyte culture (MLC) test. This test is very similar to the lymphocyte blastogenesis test (see discussion earlier in this article). Lymphocytes from the recipient are mixed with lymphocytes from the donor that have been treated with mitomycin C or irradiated to prevent DNA synthesis. The procedure that then follows is essentially that outlined for the lymphocyte blastogenesis test. With the use of both tests (leukocyte typing and MLC) identification of a potential donor for organ or bone marrow transplant that would likely be more compatible could be made, and chances for survival of the allograft would be greatly improved.

With the immunologic technology and typing sera currently available as well as the surgical expertise for organ transplant in the dog, it is anticipated that this procedure will become more common in the future. One area of particular interest in clinical practice will be kidney transplants, because of the high percentage of older dogs developing chronic renal diseases. The opportunity for prolonged survival in these animals may be significant, since kidney transplantation in man is at present very successful.

### SUMMARY

A significant number of immunodiagnostic tests are currently available to the clinician through cooperative studies between the immunology research laboratory and the clinic. We have found this marriage between basic research and clinical science a very rewarding and worthwhile relationship at the New York State College of Veterinary Medicine and the James A. Baker nstitute for Animal Health. We anticipate hat new and improved clinical immunodiagnostic tests will be conceived as a esult of the relationship.

## SUPPLEMENTAL READING

Bloom, B. R., and Glade, P. R. (ed.): In Vitro Methods in Cell-Mediated Immunity. New York, Academic Press, 1971.

Gell, P. G. H., Coombs, R. R. A., and Lachmann, P. J. (ed.): Clinical Aspects of Immunology. 3rd ed. Oxford, Blackwell Scientific Publications, 1975.

Rose, N. R., and Bigazzi, P. E. (ed.): Methods in Immunodiagnosis. New York, John Wiley and Sons, 1973.

Schultz, R. D.: Immunologic disorders in the dog and cat. Vet. Clin. N. Am., 4:153–174, 1974.

Vyas, G. N., Stites, D. P., and Brecher, G. (ed.): Laboratory Diagnosis of Immunologic Disorders. New York, Grune and Stratton, 1975.

# CANINE SYSTEMIC LUPUS ERYTHEMATOSUS

ROBERT M. LEWIS, D.V.M.
*Ithaca, New York*

Systemic lupus erythematosus in dogs is a complex, multisystem disorder characterized by the simultaneous or sequential development of four distinct clinical syndromes: autoimmune hemolytic anemia, idiopathic thrombocytopenic purpura, glomerulonephritis and symmetrical (rheumatoid) polyarthritis. Accompanying, or in some cases preceding, the development of these clinical abnormalities are a variety of autoantibodies, which may play an important role in the disease by reacting against the patient's own tissues.

Seventy-five per cent of affected dogs are young adult females between two and eight years of age. No breed predisposition has been found, nor have instigating factors, such as exposure to drugs, chemicals, sunlight or infectious disease, been evident in the histories of affected dogs. The most striking clinical features of this canine malady are the hematologic components—autoimmune hemolytic anemia and thrombocytopenic purpura.

Autoimmune hemolytic anemia in dogs is characterized by acute hemolytic crises, during which the significant signs of disease are those related to anemia (pallor, weakness, shortness of breath and loss of stamina), those due to increased red blood cell destruction (icterus and heavily pigmented stools and urine) and those related to an acute systemic disease (anorexia, fever, malaise, polydipsia, vomiting and diarrhea).

Laboratory abnormalities include severe anemia, with hemoglobin levels as low as 2.0 gm./100 ml., leukocytosis with a shift to the left, reticulocytosis, spherocytosis, positive direct and indirect antiglobulin (Coombs') tests, bilirubinemia and urobilinuria. Eluates prepared from erythrocytes of affected dogs sensitize normal canine red blood cells to the indirect antiglobulin test, thereby establishing that the antierythrocyte antibody is an autoantibody.

Dogs with autoimmune hemolytic anemia usually respond favorably to large doses of corticosteroids. The remissions that ensue may be prolonged; however, recurrent crises are frequent. Splenectomy has been of use in refractory cases, producing long-term remissions in approximately 50 per cent of dogs treated in this fashion.

Thrombocytopenic purpura is the most frequent hemorrhagic disorder seen in dogs and may be prominent in canine systemic lupus erythematosus. It is characterized by the sudden onset of petechiae and ecchymoses in the skin and mucous membranes, hematuria, epistaxis and melena. Platelet levels fall below 100,000/cu. mm.

and, although circulating platelets may be virtually absent, numerous megakaryocytes are present in the bone marrow. Corticosteroids in large doses (2 mg./kg. of body weight daily) are effective in relieving the symptoms. Platelet levels can be expected to return to normal within 10 days, and bleeding usually stops within 48 hours after adequate treatment is started. Continual treatment with low levels of corticosteroids is occasionally required to maintain longterm remission in some dogs. The results of splenectomy in refractory cases have been variable.

Although less dramatic than the hematologic components, of equal importance to the host are the lesions in the kidneys and joints. The renal lesion, clinically detected by persistent proteinuria, plays a significant role in the course of the disease, and uremia is a frequent cause of death. Histologically, the lesion is membranous glomerulonephritis. The basement membranes of glomerular capillaries are thickened, and affected capillary walls have a wire loop appearance. Not all glomeruli are affected to the same degree within a given kidney. Eventual sclerosis and hyalinization of glomeruli lead to progressive renal failure.

The outstanding feature of glomerulonephritis is persistent proteinuria, usually with urine of high specific gravity. Treatment of chronic glomerulonephritis is directed toward preventing development of the nephrotic syndrome (hypoproteinemia, proteinuria, edema, ascites, hypercholesterolemia) by maintaining the animal on a low-sodium, high-quality protein diet. If azotemia develops, additional treatment for renal failure must be instituted.

The lesions responsible for the intermittent, salicylate-responsive polyarthritis commonly observed in affected dogs may become severe enough to contribute significantly to the debilitation of the host. Histologically, severely affected joint capsules have congested arterioles, capillaries and venules, diffuse infiltrations of lymphocytes and plasma cells, foci of necrotic collagen, focal deposition of fibrin and necrotizing vasculitis. Villous proliferation of synovium and fibrovascular connective tissue into the joint space contributes to pannus formation between opposing articular surfaces and leads to ankylosis and permanent deformity of the joint. Focal necrosis of cartilage produces a pitted articular surface to which fibrin tags are adherent, and subchondral bone resorption is associated with intraosseous fibrosis. The synovium is generally thickened and contains discrete nests of mature plasma cells.

Clinically, the peripheral joints are affected, with thickened joint capsules and mild pain. The animals usually show more discomfort when first getting up in the morning, and there is bilateral symmetry to the affected joints.

Treatment of the arthritis is palliative, a great deal of reliance being placed on the intermittent use of buffered aspirin and enforced rest because the lesions are progressive.

Serologic abnormalities make up an interesting portion of canine systemic lupus erythematosus. Hyperglobulinemia is common. Antibodies to nucleoprotein, DNA, RNA, thyroglobulin, erythrocytes and 7S gamma globulin (rheumatoid factor) can be found in various combinations in affected dogs. A serum factor responsible for the production of lupus erythematosus (LE) cells is consistently present. The value of these autoantibodies as markers of increased susceptibility to immunologic disease in dogs is not yet known. However, abnormal antibodies, such as those mentioned previously, have been observed in asymptomatic offspring of dogs known to have systemic lupus erythematosus. Consequently, the diagnosis of systemic lupus erythematosus is warranted when an animal is found to have one or more of the previously described clinical entities, in conjunction with a positive lupus erythematosus (LE) cell test. Usually, additional serologic abnormalities will also be found.

Treatment is directed toward alleviating the signs of the prominent clinical syndrome. The disease tends to recur by crisis and each exacerbation should be treated vigorously. During periods of remission, the animal often requires no medication, despite continual signs of persistent tissue damage, e.g., proteinuria and morning stiffness. Although the disease is progressive and the prognosis guarded, many affected animals can be maintained in relatively good health if the owners are observant and conscientious in the home treatment of the patient.

Genetic analysis of breeding experiments in a closed colony of dogs derived from parents affected with systemic lupus erythematosus indicates that genetic mechanisms alone cannot account for the abnormalities which characterize the canine form of this disease. Rather, the results of these experiments indicate the possibility of a replicating infectious agent (virus?) as the etiologic factor responsible for canine systemic lupus erythematosus. Studies to characterize the transmissibility of the disease in dogs are currently under way in an effort to answer this important question.

In addition to the major organ involvements mentioned above, canine patients with SLE have also manifested erosive skin lesions (discoid lupus) and neuromuscular signs associated with seizure, polymyositis and abnormal behavior (psychosis). The extent to which immunologically mediated

vascular lesions contribute to these less common symptoms is a subject of current investigation.

## SUPPLEMENTAL READING

Lewis, R. M.: Models of autoimmunity: canine systemic lupus erythematosus. Proceedings of a symposium: Animal Models for Biomedical Research. Washington, D.C., National Academy of Sciences, 1968, pp. 21–34.
Lewis, R. M., and Hathaway, J. E.: Canine systemic lupus erythematosus; presenting with symmetrical polyarthritis. J. Small Animal Pract., 8:273–284, 1967.
Lewis, R. M., and Schwartz, R. S.: Canine systemic lupus erythematosus. Genetic analysis of an established breeding colony. J. Exper. Med., 134:417–438, 1971.

# FELINE LEUKEMIA VIRUS–ASSOCIATED DISEASES

SUSAN M. COTTER, D.V.M.
*Boston, Massachusetts*

Feline lymphosarcoma is a contagious disease caused by a single-stranded, enveloped RNA virus, classed as an oncornavirus. The term "lymphosarcoma" (LSA) refers to solid lymphoid tumors and "leukemia" refers to primary involvement of blood and bone marrow. The feline leukemia virus (FeLV) causes LSA, lymphocytic leukemia, the myeloproliferative diseases and aplastic anemia and is implicated indirectly in other infectious diseases. The feline sarcoma virus (FeSV) is serologically indistinguishable from FeLV and causes fibrosarcoma.

## CLINICAL MANIFESTATIONS OF LYMPHOSARCOMA

Lymphosarcoma can affect any organ of the body, with clinical signs dependent on the area of involvement. Diagnosis rests on demonstration of malignant cells in tumor

biopsy, in pleural or peritoneal effusions, in peripheral blood or in marrow aspirates.

Mediastinal LSA is more common in young cats, with dyspnea being the customary complaint. Physical findings include dull lung sounds ventrally, an incompressible anterior thorax and posterior displacement of the apex heart beat. Other less frequent signs are wheezing, coughing and dysphagia. A widened anterior mediastinum may be present radiographically, but visualization of thoracic structures may be obliterated by pleural effusion. The trachea is usually deviated dorsally. Diagnosis is made by microscopic examination of pleural fluid containing large numbers of immature lymphocytes. Examination of pleural fluid will differentiate LSA from other conditions causing hydrothorax. In the presence of a mediastinal mass, thoracocentesis is indicated, since small amounts of fluid are not visible radiographically.

Alimentary LSA is uncommon in the Boston area but is the most common form in Scotland, possibly reflecting differences in virus strains. Single or multiple mesenteric lymph nodes are frequently enlarged. The stomach or intestines may be diffusely thickened or contain a single mass. Renal lymphoma is usually bilateral, resulting in large irregular kidneys. The granulomatous form of feline infectious peritonitis (FIP) frequently causes irregular kidneys and is indistinguishable from renal lymphoma on palpation. Chronic pyelonephritis and renal infarction may lead to irregular kidneys without significant enlargement. Generalized peripheral lymphadenopathy is occasionally seen with feline LSA.

A small number of cats with LSA have lesions in a single location not classified in the above categories. Epidural LSA may cause posterior paralysis. This must be differentiated from spinal trauma, meningeal FIP and aortic embolism. Cats with spinal LSA, as opposed to other forms, frequently have marrow involvement, so that an aspirate may provide a diagnosis. An early manifestation of spinal LSA may be irritation of dorsal spinal nerve roots with signs similar to those seen in steatitis. The cat may bite at the area and appear to be in pain. There may be rippling of the skin of the dorsal lumbar area.

Retrobulbar LSA may cause the globe to protrude. This must be differentiated from an abscess or other tumors. Intraocular LSA often invades the iris, causing anterior uveitis. Raised skin lesions may be caused by LSA and must be differentiated from mast cell tumor and various inflammatory or neoplastic processes of the skin.

The final classification is that of true leukemia. Cats with solid tumors of LSA usually have normal blood counts. In recent years there has been an apparent increase in the incidence of primary leukemia involving blood and marrow without solid tumors. Almost 50 per cent of 144 cases of LSA at Angell Memorial Animal Hospital from 1972 to 1975 were of this type.

The reasons for this increase include the following: (1) a specific strain of FeLV may prevail in Boston, predisposing to this form of the disease; (2) more extensive diagnostic procedures are being done in cases of aplastic anemia and have shown that the bone marrow may contain malignant cells when the blood does not; (3) anemic cats which are given supportive treatment and moni-

tored over a period of time may ultimately develop leukemia.

Clinical signs and physical findings in leukemic cats are usually vague and include lethargy, anorexia, weight loss, anemia and sometimes fever. Splenomegaly and hepatomegaly are inconsistent findings in lymphocytic leukemia. The packed cell volume (PCV) usually ranges from 8 to 15 per cent. The anemia is usually nonregenerative, with low reticulocyte counts often in the presence of circulating nucleated red blood cells, including occasional rubricytes and prorubricytes.

The total white blood count (WBC) is usually normal or below normal, although cases do occur in which the total WBC is over 400,000/cu. mm. Neutropenia is often present, predisposing to infection. The total lymphocyte count may be high or low, with variable numbers of abnormal cells from atypical lymphocytes to blasts. Immature lymphocytes may appear transiently in the circulation in other infectious diseases and indicate reaction to antigenic stimulation rather than leukemia. Platelet numbers are variable.

The persistence of immature lymphocytes in the blood, particularly in an anemic cat, warrants examination of the bone marrow. A bone marrow aspirate may confirm a diagnosis of leukemia when the blood contains only a few abnormal cells. Normal cats have less than 20 per cent normal lymphocytes (most have less than 10 per cent). A positive diagnosis of leukemia can be made if over 40 per cent of the nucleated marrow cells are lymphocytes and the majority of these are prolymphocytes and blasts. Caution is advised in interpretation of hypocellular marrow samples, since relative lymphocytosis may occur.

Cats in a preleukemic state have vague or occasionally no signs of illness except mild anemia (PCV 25 to 30 per cent) with a few atypical lymphocytes. No specific treatment is indicated except to treat any coexisting problems such as infection. These cats should be closely monitored for signs of leukemia or other diseases.

## MYELOPROLIFERATIVE DISEASE

Myeloproliferative disease encompasses such disorders as erythroleukemia, granulocytic leukemia, thrombocythemia, reticuloendotheliosis and myelofibrosis. Although these diseases are classified according to the cell line primarily affected, the distinction is difficult because multiple abnormalities may be present in a single cat over a period of time or at the same time. Lymphoblasts may be found in the blood or marrow associated with primitive red cell precursors. Myelofibrosis may be regarded as another proliferative manifestation of pluripotential marrow cells forming fibroblasts and later fibrous connective tissue. Myelofibrosis may be the terminal phase in cats with myeloproliferative disease who have been kept alive for several months with supportive treatment.

As in lymphocytic leukemia, the primary presenting sign of myeloproliferative disease is anemia. Splenomegaly and hepatomegaly are more striking in this disease than in lymphoid malignancy. Both organs are usually heavily infiltrated with hematopoietic cells. This phenomenon is called myeloid metaplasia. Chemotherapy in these diseases is unlikely to produce complete remission, although some cats may be maintained for several months with supportive treatment and periodic transfusions.

Mast cell leukemia (mastocytosis) is apparently unrelated to FeLV. Cats with this disease are usually anemic with massive splenomegaly. Mast cells may sometimes be found in the blood or marrow. Solid tumors may be localized to the skin or may occur as an intestinal mass, previously called argentaffinoma. A terminal event in mastocytosis may be a perforated duodenal ulcer thought to occur because of histamine release by mast cells. Some cats with mast cell tumors will go into long remissions with corticosteroid therapy alone. Initial treatment should consist of prednisone, 2 mg./kg. daily for two weeks, followed by 5 mg. prednisone every 48 hours, continued indefinitely. Splenectomy is indicated if splenomegaly is present.

## OTHER DISEASES ASSOCIATED WITH FeLV

Table 1 lists disorders that have occurred in association with FeLV. The FeLV is not the primary cause of the infectious diseases but is a predisposing cause because of virus-induced immunosuppression. FeLV suppresses the cell-mediated immune response, and humoral antibody may also be suppressed. Therefore, a cat infected with FeLV is highly susceptible to many infectious diseases.

The relationship of FeLV to absorption or abortion of fetuses is not clear. There may be a direct effect of FeLV on the placenta or fetus, or some additional infectious agent may be involved. Neonatal deaths in kittens have been attributed to FeLV-induced thymic atrophy. Glomerulonephritis of the immune-complex type is related to damage caused by deposition of FeLV-associated antigen-antibody complexes on the basement membrane.

**Table 1.**  *Disorders Seen in Association with FeLV in Boston Cats*

| DISEASE | NO. OF POSITIVE/ TOTAL NO.* | % POSITIVE* |
|---|---|---|
| Lymphosarcoma | 97/144 | 70 |
| Myeloproliferative disease | 8/11 | 72 |
| Nonregenerative anemia | 89/128 | 70 |
| Haemobartonellosis | 13/23 | 57 |
| Feline infectious peritonitis (FIP) | 34/57 | 60 |
| Infertility, uterine disease | 13/26 | 50 |
| Glomerulonephritis | 4/8 | 50 |
| Toxoplasmosis | 3/4 | 75 |
| Fever, unknown origin | 5/14 | 36 |
| Bacterial septicemia | 15/16 | 94 |
| Stomatitis | 13/26 | 50 |
| Chronic respiratory infections, sinusitis | 6/18 | 33 |
| Poorly healing abscess | 5/8 | 62 |
| Atypical panleukopenia† | 5/7 | 71 |
| Iritis | 2/4 | 50 |

*Positive for FeLV by immunofluorescence.
†Atypical is defined as clinical signs and histologic lesions of panleukopenia occurring in an adult vaccinated cat.

Bacterial infections such as bite-wound abscesses and necrotic stomatitis associated with leukopenia rather than the expected leukocytosis may indicate FeLV immunosuppression. Poor response to treatment also characterizes these disorders when they occur in the FeLV-positive cat.

## SEROLOGIC TESTS FOR FeLV AND IMMUNE RESPONSE

A fluorescent antibody test is commercially available which will detect the presence of FeLV in peripheral white blood cells and platelets. Malignant cells need not be present because the virus can replicate in normal cells. The test is simple and practical for the practitioner, since it requires only an unstained, unfixed blood film. The test is accurate in detecting viremia if the test antiserum is prepared carefully to be sure it is specific for FeLV and run with adequate controls. A positive test indicates that the cat is viremic (infected with FeLV) but is *not* a diagnostic test for leukemia or any other disease. Up to 1 per cent of healthy cats tested at random are positive for FeLV. Healthy cats living in close association with an FeLV-positive cat have a 30 to 50 per cent chance of being positive. Seventy to 90 per cent of cats with LSA are positive, so that a negative test does *not* exclude LSA as a diagnostic possibility. Cats with infectious diseases as listed in Table 1 are also likely to be positive.

Many healthy cats exposed to FeLV are able to develop neutralizing antibody and thus eliminate the virus. When the virus transforms a host cell, an antigen is induced on the cell membrane (feline oncornavirus cell-membrane antigen, FOCMA). The immune system may then be able to recognize the transformed cell as foreign and produce antibody directed against the cell-membrane antigen (FOCMA antibody). If FOCMA antibody is produced, the cat will be resistant to development of LSA and will remain healthy even in the presence of persistent viremia. One cannot assume that the FeLV-positive cat is doomed to develop a fatal illness in the near future. Studies involving 128 cats in cluster households indicate that 69 FeLV-positive cats had a 38 per cent mortality in two years as compared to 8 per cent for FeLV-negative cats in the same environment (Essex *et al.*, 1975). For this reason, the diagnostic work-up in a cat with signs of illness must not stop with receipt of a positive test for FeLV, assuming that the owner wishes to treat the cat if a curable illness is found.

## EPIDEMIOLOGY AND PUBLIC HEALTH CONSIDERATIONS

Feline leukemia is contagious from one cat to another. It appears to be most easily spread to young cats, but cats of all ages are susceptible. Spread of virus probably occurs by means of respiratory secretions, saliva and possibly urine. Exposed cats will become infected or immune, depending on degree of exposure and immune response.

Cats separated by individual caging or separate rooms are less likely to become infected. It is difficult to isolate FeLV-positive cats within a veterinary hospital, since many cats with severe infectious diseases also have FeLV. The best prevention is good ventilation, individual caging with small numbers of cats per room and having attendants wash their hands after handling each cat.

In a multiple-cat household, the diagnosis of LSA in a single FeLV-positive cat means that the other cats in the house have already been exposed. Elimination of this cat for the protection of the others is of no value unless other FeLV-positive cats in the house are also eliminated. Hardy (1974) has shown that isolation or elimination of FeLV-positive cats is effective in preventing spread of FeLV to other cats in the house.

FeLV-positive cats should be kept indoors to protect other cats and to protect the FeLV-positive cat from exposure to other infections to which he is susceptible. The virus does not live long outside the cat. After an FeLV-positive cat leaves the house, it should be safe to bring in a new cat after one month.

The FeLV will grow in human cells in tissue culture. Although serologic surveys have shown antibodies to various FeLV-associated antigens in human serum, there is no positive association of FeLV with leukemia in man. No instances of human leukemia have ever been traced to cats and there is no increased incidence of leukemia in veterinarians or in families who have owned cats with LSA. There is currently no sound basis for advising euthanasia of

FeLV-positive cats on the basis of danger to man. This information should be discussed with owners of an FeLV-positive cat.

## TREATMENT OF LYMPHOSARCOMA

### AIMS OF TREATMENT

LSA should still be considered an incurable disease at this time. Although an occasional cat will actually be cured, the vast majority will eventually die of their disease. The goal of therapy is remission, a state in which clinical and laboratory signs of leukemia have disappeared. Even when a "complete" remission is achieved, there is almost certainly hidden disease which remains. When a positive diagnosis of LSA has been made, the clinician must consider several factors in making recommendations to an owner regarding treatment of the cat.

### CLIENT CONSIDERATIONS

The decision to treat a cat with LSA must ultimately rest with the owner, given enough information and emotional support by the veterinarian to help him make a rational decision. It may be difficult psychologically to live with a pet that has a terminal illness. For this reason the entire family should be involved, and the decision should not be made abruptly in the rushed atmosphere of an examination room. The owner should have an understanding of the disease, potential danger to other cats, prognosis, potential side effects of treatment, frequency of clinic visits and cost. The owner should not be made to feel guilty if he does not desire to pursue treatment. Owners who proceed reluctantly are often dissatisfied and quit at the first complication. Most owners who desire treatment are grateful to the veterinarian for the help and extended time given to the cat. The relationship with these people can be close and rewarding for both doctor and client. When assuming responsibility for treatment, the veterinarian must be certain that emergency care is available, since serious problems may arise abruptly during the course of treatment. The patient should be treated on an outpatient basis to give the owner and the cat as much time together as possible. In a metropolitan area, a clinician should consider referring the patient to a colleague with a specialty interest in oncology.

### PATIENT EVALUATION PRIOR TO THERAPY

When the diagnosis of LSA is made, further evaluation is still required to determine the extent of the disease and whether secondary problems are present. Problems referable to the primary disease include organ dysfunction such as renal failure, dyspnea, vomiting or posterior paralysis. The clinician must attempt to predict whether the dysfunction would be reversible if chemotherapy were effective. Paralysis due to spinal lymphoma may be permanent. A laminectomy may be needed in cats with acute and complete paralysis.

Myelosuppression predisposes the cat to infection and severely limits chemotherapy. Anemia is frequently present in leukemia with bone marrow involvement, but it is generally mild or absent in cats with solid tumors. Myelosuppressive drugs should only be used in anemic cats if supportive measures including blood transfusions are available. Leukopenia and thrombocytopenia are more serious complications, since routine replacement of white cells and platelets is not a practical procedure in cats. Myelosuppressive agents should not be given to a cat with WBC's less than 5000/cu. mm. or platelet counts less than 100,000/cu. mm. Low absolute neutrophil counts predispose to infection. Thrombocytopenia occurs less frequently than leukopenia and is a grave prognostic sign.

Although the fever may be directly associated with the LSA, infection may be present. Ideally, blood and urine cultures should be done. Any infection must be treated aggressively, and antibiotics are indicated in the febrile cat. In the rare instances of apparently localized lymphomas (alimentary mass or a single enlarged kidney), excision should be carried out followed by chemotherapy. The prognosis may be better in these cats, particularly if they are FeLV-negative.

In summary, the ideal cat to treat is afebrile with normal or near normal blood parameters, no coexisting infection and normal liver or kidney function.

### SPECIFIC THERAPY

The percentage and length of remissions are greater when multiple chemotherapeutic agents are used in combination. The combination chosen should include drugs which act differently on the malignant cell and have different toxicities. The effect on the malignant cell may then be additive while toxicity is not. Conservative treatment schedules with low doses or single agents are safe, but the degree and duration of remission are not likely to be good. Treatment must be aggressive, risking some side effects to obtain longer remissions. Drugs and schedules listed here are intended to serve as a guide. They must be modified according to patient response. Table 2 outlines medication and monitoring schedules. Frequent monitoring of the hemogram is critical to avoid excessive myelosuppression. The most effective combination to date is cyclophosphamide,* vincristine† and prednisone (COP).

When initiating treatment, COP should be used if the WBC, PCV and platelet counts are adequate, there is no severe organ dysfunction and infection is absent or at least is being controlled with antibiotics. In the presence of myelosuppression, only vincristine and prednisone should be used initially. In the presence of organ dysfunction or cachexia, initial doses of cyclophosphamide and vincristine should be decreased.

*Cytoxan®, Mead Johnson, Evansville, Indiana.
†Oncovin®, Lilly, Indianapolis, Indiana.

Cyclophosphamide is an alkylating agent which inhibits cell division by causing irreversible cross-linkages of DNA chains. This drug is well absorbed and well tolerated orally but may be given intravenously. In man, there is evidence that cyclophosphamide is more effective and less toxic when given in intermittent high doses than when given on a daily basis. Preliminary results suggest that this is true in cats. Dose-limiting myelosuppression is the primary side effect, usually first seen as leukopenia. Hemorrhagic cystitis caused by the metabolites of cyclophosphamide in the urine is uncommon in the cat. The owner should be made aware of this possibility, however, and cyclophosphamide should be discontinued if signs of cystitis occur. Alopecia is not a common problem in the cat, although clipped hair may not regrow.

The initial dose of cyclophosphamide is 300 mg./m.²* as a single dose. This dose is repeated every three weeks and is adjusted depending on weekly blood count changes. The WBC usually drops in 7 to 10 days and rises to normal in 14 days, but delayed leukopenias may occur. Ideally, the WBC should drop to 2000 to 4000/cu. mm. the week after administration. If the WBC does

*Surface area in square meters (m.²) $= \dfrac{4W + 7}{W + 90}$

where W = wt. in kg. (See also page 477.)

**Table 2.**    *Schedule of Treatment for Feline LSA with COAP\**

| | WEEK | | | | | | | | | | | | | | |
|---|---|---|---|---|---|---|---|---|---|---|---|---|---|---|---|
| | 1 | 2 | 3 | 4 | 5 | 6 | 7 | 8 | 9 | 10 | 11 | 12 | 13 | 14 | 15 |
| *Medication Schedule* | | | | | | | | | | | | | | | |
| Cyclophosphamide** (300 mg./m.²) P.O. | x | | | x | | | x | | | x | | | x | | |
| Vincristine (0.75 mg./m.²) I.V. | x | x | x | x | | | x | | | x | | | x | | |
| Prednisone (2 mg./kg.) P.O. | Daily | | | | | | | | | | | | | | |
| *Monitoring Schedule* | | | | | | | | | | | | | | | |
| CBC | x | x | x | x | x | x | x | x | | x | x | | x | x | |
| Platelet count | x | x | | | | | | x | | | x | | | x | |
| Urinalysis† | x | | | | | | | | | | | | | | |
| BUN† | x | | | | | | | | | | | | | | |
| SGPT† | x | | | | | | | | | | | | | | |
| Bone marrow‡ | x | | | | | | | | | | | | | | |
| Chest x-rays (mediastinal mass) | x | | | x | | | x | x | | | | | x | | |

*COAP = Cyclophosphamide, Oncovin® (vincristine), prednisone.
**Dose adjusted to provide WBC of 2000 to 4000/cu. mm. and granulocytes of 1000 to 2000/cu. mm. at nadir.
†To be repeated if indicated by clinical signs.
‡To be examined in cases of leukemia or anemia.
NOTE: Continue this medication program for minimum of one year.

not decrease to this range, the dose of cyclophosphamide should be increased three weeks later to 400 mg./m.$^2$

A more conservative approach may be used in the poor-risk patient. The poor-risk patient has persistent anemia, leukopenia or thrombocytopenia and does not respond to vincristine and prednisone alone. In this approach, cyclophosphamide is administered at a dose of 12.5 mg. (¼ tablet) daily for 4 days, withdrawn for 7 days and then repeated for 4 days. In anemic cats that do not respond to vincristine and prednisone, this schedule of cyclophosphamide may be used as long as supportive transfusions are available.

Vincristine is a plant alkaloid that interferes with the mitotic spindle, arresting mitosis in metaphase. When used with cyclophosphamide, cells in various phases of cell division are attacked. Vincristine is given intravenously at a dose of 0.75 mg./m.$^2$ weekly for four injections and then every three weeks on the same day as cyclophosphamide. Vincristine is not significantly myelosuppressive and may be used in cats with leukopenia, anemia or thrombocytopenia. The primary side effects reported in man are constipation and peripheral neuropathy with tingling or discomfort in the extremities and decreased segmental reflexes. Vomiting on the day of the injection has been observed in dogs. While one must be aware of these effects, they have not been noted in cats. Vincristine is expensive and is stable with refrigeration for only two weeks after reconstitution.

Prednisone is not myelosuppressive and has a direct toxic effect on lymphocytes. Cats tolerate long-term prednisone well, with owners seldom reporting cushingoid signs. Prednisone is used orally at a dose of 2 mg./kg. per day.

Most cats treated with COP will go into remission. The length of remission varies greatly, with a median of about four months. It is not unusual for cats to do well from six to ten months and rarely a cat will be cured. However, some cats, particularly those with leukemia, anemia or leukopenia, may not respond. Treatment may be stopped after continuous complete remission for one year. Causes of death include relapses, anemia refractory to transfusion therapy and infection caused by myelosuppression due to chemotherapy or direct immunosuppression of FeLV. Once relapse occurs, secondary remission is difficult to achieve; if remission does occur, it is usually of short duration. Several drugs have been used, usually as single agents, but results to date have been disappointing.

Adriamycin* is an anthracycline antibiotic which reacts with DNA to form complexes. Side effects include myelosuppression, gastroenteritis and myocardial damage. It can be used in the cat at an initial dose of 30 mg./m.$^2$ every three weeks IV with careful monitoring of the hemogram. The dose should be increased until the WBC drops to 2000 to 4000/cu. mm. seven days after injection. A partial response was noted in one of four cats. The maximum cumulative dose should be 400 mg./m.$^2$ to prevent cardiac toxicity.

Cytosine arabinoside (Ara-C)** is a pyrimidine antagonist, acting against DNA synthesis. It has been used in combination with cyclophosphamide, vincristine and prednisone (COAP). If used as a single agent, the dosage of Ara-C is 50 mg./m.$^2$ SC b.i.d. for 5 days, every three weeks. Since this drug is myelosuppressive, a blood count should be done one week after completing the course of injections.

L-asparaginase has been quite effective in dogs with LSA but has been less effective in cats. It is not myelosuppressive. The primary toxicities are anaphylaxis and hepatotoxicity. This drug is not yet commercially available, but if used in the cat should be given at an initial dose of 8000 units/m.$^2$ IV daily for 5 days, then once weekly.

Bleomycin† reacts with DNA to prevent cell division. It is not myelosuppressive and occurs in highest concentration in lungs and skin. The major toxicity is pulmonary fibrosis. Partial short-term remission was obtained in two cats at a dose of 10 to 15 mg./m.$^2$ IM weekly with no obvious side effects. Periodic thoracic radiographs are indicated.

## SUPPORTIVE TREATMENT

Blood transfusions may be necessary prior to treatment or periodically in cats

---

*Adriamycin®, Adria Laboratories, Wilmington, Delaware.
**Cytosar®, Upjohn Co., Kalamazoo, Michigan.
†Blenoxane®, Bristol Laboratories, Syracuse, New York.

which remain anemic during treatment. Chronically anemic cats may live relatively normal lives as house cats with a PCV as low as 10 per cent. Transfusions (100 cc. for the average cat) may be given on an outpatient basis every two to three weeks as needed to maintain the PCV above this value. Cats tolerate repeated transfusions well without crossmatching; however, the life span of transfused cells is apparently shorter after multiple transfusions. A transfusion supplies about 0.5 mg. of iron per ml. of blood. Iron or other hematinics are not indicated, since serum iron is normal or often elevated in these cats.

Anabolic steroids may help prevent negative nitrogen balance in animals receiving long-term corticosteroids. Testosterone derivatives have been reported to stimulate erythropoietin production in aplastic anemias and facilitate oxygen unloading to tissues by hemoglobin, but a clinical response is not often observed in the anemic cat. Erythropoietin levels are often elevated in aplastic anemia of man, so that the bone marrow may not be capable of responding. Testosterone propionate in oil* may be given at a dose of 2 mg./kg. IM weekly.

Antibiotics should not be used prophylactically but should be started at the first sign of infection, preferably after appropriate cultures are taken. Bactericidal drugs are more likely to be effective than bacteriostatic drugs because of decreased ability of the host to respond to infection.

Immunotherapy has not been used at this institution. It may become an important adjunct to treatment in the future. It is most likely to be useful in cats in remission, since the immune system has the best chance of responding when minimal tumor is present.

## TREATMENT OF APLASTIC ANEMIA

Approximately 70 per cent of cats with aplastic anemia are infected with FeLV, and some eventually develop leukemia if kept alive with supportive treatment. Periodic reticulocyte counts can be monitored for signs of marrow regeneration. The marrow should be examined to search for leukemic infiltration. Treatment includes periodic transfusions and testosterone derivatives as outlined for the anemic cat with LSA. If there is no response to this treatment after 4

to 6 weeks, prednisone may be added at a dose of 2 mg./kg. per day. Prednisone is not used initially, since it would interfere with the ability to make a diagnosis of early leukemia. The mode of action of prednisone in feline aplastic anemia is not well understood, since it does not appear to stimulate erythropoiesis. It may act to lengthen the life span of those RBC's present by inhibiting destruction by the reticuloendothelial system. The long-term prognosis for cats with aplastic anemia is poor, but an occasional cat will recover after receiving supportive treatment for a period of time.

## TREATMENT OF OTHER FeLV-POSITIVE CATS

Healthy FeLV-positive cats will not benefit from any treatment known at this time. In a protected environment they may remain healthy for years, and an occasional FeLV-positive cat will revert to negative.

The FeLV-positive cat with signs of illness is a difficult problem. The prognosis must be guarded in these cats but their illness may be treatable, and a diagnostic work-up should proceed in the same manner as it would if the cat were FeLV-negative. Treatment for seemingly minor problems must be more aggressive and prolonged than for the same problem in the FeLV-negative cat. Chemotherapy is not indicated in the absence of a positive diagnosis of malignancy, since it will cause further immunosuppression.

### SUPPLEMENTAL READING

Cotter, S. M., Hardy, W. D., Jr., and Essex, M. E.: Association of feline leukemia virus with lymphosarcoma and other disorders in the cat. J. Am. Vet. Med. Assn. *166*:449–454, 1975.
Cotter, S. M.: Feline leukemia virus induced disorders. Vet. Clin. N. Am., Philadelphia, W. B. Saunders Co. 6:367–378, 1976.
Essex, M.: Horizontally and vertically transmitted oncornaviruses of cats. Adv. Cancer Res., *21*:175–248, 1975.
Essex, M., Hardy, W. D., Cotter, S. M., Jakowski, R. M. and Sliski, A.: Naturally occurring persistent oncornavirus infections in the absence of disease. Infect Immunol., *11*:470–475, 1975.
Gilmore, C. E., and Holzworth, J.: Naturally occurring feline leukemia: Clinical, pathologic and differential diagnostic features. J. Am. Vet. Med. Assn. *158*:1013–1025, 1971.
Hardy, W. D., Jr.: Management of lymphosarcoma. In Kirk, R. W. (ed.): Current Veterinary Therapy V Philadelphia, W. B. Saunders Co., 1974, pp. 381–387

*Oreton®, Schering, Kenilworth, New Jersey.

# CANINE LYMPHO-SARCOMA AND LEUKEMIA

E. GREGORY MacEWEN, V.M.D.,
*New York, New York*

*and* PAUL W. HESS, D.V.M.
*St. Thomas, U.S. Virgin Islands*

Malignancies of the hematopoietic system account for 8 to 10 per cent of the canine malignant tumors and are the third most common tumor type seen in the dog. Unlike feline hematopoietic malignancies, there is no known viral etiology. The different types of neoplastic diseases of the hematopoietic system are listed in Table 1. The major disease categories presented in Table 1 differ with respect to morphology, clinical signs and often response to therapy.

## LYMPHOPROLIFERATIVE DISORDERS

Lymphoproliferative neoplasm is a neoplasm arising from the lymphoid tissue, lymphosarcoma being the most common.

### CANINE LYMPHOSARCOMA

Lymphosarcoma (LSA), the most common canine hematopoietic neoplasm, accounts for 5 to 7 per cent of all tumors seen in the dog. LSA may occur in dogs of any age but is seen most frequently in dogs over 5 years of age. There is no known breed or sex predilection, although boxers, Dobermans, golden retrievers and Scottish terriers are most frequently affected in our clinics. Recent work has shown that both humoral and cellular immunity is suppressed in dogs with LSA.

CLINICAL SIGNS

Lymphosarcoma can develop in any organ, but there are four clinically recognized forms, based on the gross distribution of disease. In order of decreasing occurrence, they are (1) multicentric, (2) alimentary, (3) anterior mediastinal and (4) the unclassified form which includes cutaneous LSA.

Dogs often present with nonspecific signs of illness, such as fever, weight loss and anorexia. Specific clinical signs depend on extent and location of disease. Most dogs with multicentric LSA have painless enlargement of the lymph nodes. The tonsils may be enlarged, and as the disease progresses, the enlarged nodes can cause lymphatic obstruction, resulting in edema of the face and extremities. Hepatosplenomegaly may be present in advanced cases. Ten to 15 per cent of our patients have hypercalcemia (pseudohyper-

*Table 1.  Hematopoietic Neoplasms*

I. Lymphoproliferative Disorders
  A.  Lymphocytes
    1. Lymphosarcoma
      a.  Multicentric (most common)
      b.  Alimentary
      c.  Anterior mediastinal
      d.  Cutaneous
    2. Lymphocytic leukemia
      a.  Chronic (well differentiated lymphocytic) leukemia
      b.  Acute (stem cell lymphoblastic) leukemia
  B.  Immunoglobulin-secreting cells (plasma cells)
    1. Myeloma
    2. Macroglobulinemia
  C.  Reticulum cell
    1. Reticulum cell sarcoma
II. Myeloproliferative Disorders
  A.  Erythrocyte
    1. Erythremic myelosis, erythroleukemia
  B.  Granulocyte
    1. Eosinophilic leukemia (well differentiated, poorly differentiated)
    2. Basophilic leukemia (well differentiated, poorly differentiated)
    3. Myelocytic leukemia (well differentiated, poorly differentiated)
  C.  Reticuloendothelial cells
    1. Reticuloendotheliosis
  D.  Megakaryocyte
    1. Megakaryocytic leukemia

parathyroidism). These patients are presented with polydipsia and polyuria.

Dogs with the alimentary form may be extremely emaciated when presented and have a history of vomiting and chronic diarrhea. They may be suffering from protein-losing enteropathy.

The mediastinal form of LSA, which is rare, is associated with respiratory dyspnea. Our studies indicate that about 50 per cent of the dogs with hypercalcemia have had mediastinal involvement.

The cutaneous form of LSA, which may involve the skin alone or the skin and peripheral lymph nodes, has a number of clinical appearances. The most common form is characterized by multiple raised erythematous or pale plaques that are firm and invasive to the skin. They may be ulcerated and oozing serum. Another type of cutaneous LSA is moist erythematous, patches of indurated skin, usually arising from an adjacent lymph node. The lesions are usually nonpruritic and may be complicated by secondary bacterial infection.

## Diagnosis

Hematologic findings are variable and frequently within normal ranges. Approximately 40 per cent of our patients have a leukocytosis of 20,000 to 30,000 white blood cells per cubic millimeter. As the disease progresses, the bone marrow may become involved and neoplastic lymphocytes may be detected in the blood. Progressive bone marrow involvement leads to anemia. Coombs'-positive hemolytic anemia may rarely occur. Significant thrombocytopenia is not often seen in the dog. Bone marrow aspiration should be performed in LSA patients with abnormal circulating lymphocytes or significant anemia. The actual incidence of bone marrow involvement is unknown, but our findings indicate about 20 to 30 per cent will have infiltration of lymphocytes into the marrow.

A knowledge of the functional status of the liver and kidney and serum calcium level is important in prognosis, especially if chemotherapy is desired. Monoclonal paraprotein spikes, seen on the serum protein electrophoresis, occur in about 5 to 6 per cent of our patients with lymphoproliferative diseases. The paraneoplastic conditions associated with monoclonal paraprotein increases are discussed in the article on gammopathies. Monoclonal protein is a product of functional malignant lymphoid cells or bursa-equivalent cells (B cells).

The extent of disease should be determined by radiography of the thorax and abdomen. Diffuse lymphatic spread of tumor cells to the lungs is characterized by a mixed linear and alveolar pattern. In dogs with the mediastinal form, pleural effusions may be present. Cytologic examination of the fluid will usually reveal atypical lymphocytes and lymphoblasts, whereas chylothorax is characterized by mature lymphocytes.

The final diagnosis is made histologically by the characteristic pathologic patterns in the biopsy sample, usually from an excised lymph node or occasionally other sites such as tonsils, liver, bowel or skin. It is difficult to make the diagnosis relying on needle aspiration of the lymph node. The entire lymph node should be removed, capsule intact, and carefully sectioned, and fresh imprints should be made. The impression smear can be used to help establish a diagnosis and allow therapy to be started while awaiting the final histopathologic report. Submandibular lymph nodes should not be removed because they are usually reactive and make the histologic interpretation difficult.

## Treatment

The aim of therapy is to control the disease process and extend the life of the dog with as few undesirable side effects as possible. There is no known cure, but the disease can be controlled. LSA is a rapidly fatal disease; without treatment, dogs have an average survival time of less than one month after diagnosis. There are two basic methods of treating canine LSA: (1) single, sequential drug therapy and (2) combination drug therapy. (The principles of cancer chemotherapy are discussed in another article in the section.)

**Single, Sequential Chemotherapy.** Many drugs have been studied and found to be effective for the treatment of LSA (Table 2). Drugs are used until drug resistance supervenes or toxicity occurs.

**Combination Chemotherapy.** Combination chemotherapy has been shown to be more effective than the sequential use of single agents in human lymphoma patients and most veterinary oncologists have expe-

*Table 2.  Suggested Dosage Schedule for Single Agent Therapy in Canine LSA*

| DRUG | DOSE AND ROUTE | SIDE EFFECTS |
|---|---|---|
| Prednisone | 1-2 mg./kg. orally once daily | Polydipsia, polyuria |
| Vincristine (Oncovin®, Lilly) 1-mg. and 5-mg. vials | 0.025-0.05 mg./kg. IV weekly or biweekly | Perivascular irritation, constipation |
| Cyclophosphamide (Cytoxan®, Mead Johnson) 25-mg. and 50-mg. tablets; injectable | 2 mg./kg. orally daily 10 mg./kg. IV weekly | Myelosuppression, hemorrhagic cystitis |
| Cytosine Arbinoside Cytosar®, Upjohn) 100-mg. and 500-mg. vials | 30-50 mg./kg. SC weekly | Myelosuppression |
| 6-Thioguanine (Tabloid, Burroughs Wellcome) 40-mg. tablets | 1.5 mg./kg. orally daily | Myelosuppression |
| L-asparaginase (experimental) | 200-400 I.U./kg. IP weekly | Anaphylaxis |

rienced similar results in dogs. The advantages of combination chemotherapy are (1) the fraction of tumor cells killed by each drug is independent of the other agents, (2) different classes of drugs have different toxic effects on normal tissues, (3) different classes of drugs act on different phases of the cell growth cycle and (4) there is a delay in the emergence of drug-resistant cells.

Combinations of drugs for the treatment of canine lymphosarcoma are summarized in Table 3. The combination protocol which we have been evaluating in our clinics causes minimal bone marrow suppression and is well tolerated by the patients. Early indications are that this protocol is effective in the treatment of canine LSA. The drug combination is vincristine (a mitotic inhibitor), cyclophosphamide (a DNA inhibitor) and cytosine arabinoside or methotrexate (antimetabolites). The drugs are given at weekly or biweekly intervals. This protocol eliminates the necessity of relying on the client to administer the drugs at home. Orally administered prednisone (0.5 to 2.0 mg./kg. of body weight) daily or on alternate days can also be added to the protocol. Splenectomy does not enhance survival time or response to chemotherapy and, in fact, may worsen the prognosis. Therefore, we do not advise splenectomy.

The alimentary form of LSA may be limited to one area of the gastrointestinal tract (solitary) or it may be diffuse and involve the entire small and large bowel. The combined drug protocol can be used for those patients with diffuse tumor involvement. Solitary bowel lymphomas can be managed by surgical resection. The gastrointestinal lymphomas usually do not respond to chemotherapy. Alkylating agents such as cyclophosphamide (2 mg./kg. of body weight daily, orally) and intralesional steroids (triamcinolone, 2 to 6 mg.) have been used to treat cutaneous LSA but with very little success.

## HYPERCALCEMIA

Hypercalcemia may be seen in association with various types of malignant conditions. Our studies indicate that approximately 10 per cent of the dogs with lymphosarcoma have a concurrent hypercalcemia (serum calcium greater than 12 mg./100 ml.). The usual presenting signs of these dogs are polydipsia, polyuria and muscle weakness. Approximately 50 per cent of the lymphoma patients with hypercalcemia had mediastinal involvement. Any dog with suspected or proven mediastinal lymphosarcoma should be evaluated for hypercalcemia.

Hypercalcemia is caused by the production of physiologically active substances which stimulate bone resorption. These substances are parathyroid hormone–like peptides. The hypercalcemia can cause degeneration and necrosis of the renal tubules and eventual calcification or nephrocalcinosis. This results in loss of renal concentrating capability, progressive renal dysfunction and eventual renal failure.

Therapy for hypercalcemia is directed

*Table 3.*   *Drug Combinations Used in Canine LSA*

| DRUGS | DOSAGE* | | REFERENCE |
|---|---|---|---|
| Vincristine (Oncovin®)<br>Cyclophosphamide (Cytoxan®)<br>Vincristine (Oncovin®)<br>Cytosine Arabinoside (Cytosar®)<br>*or*<br>Methotrexate (Lederle) | 0.025–0.05 mg./kg. IV<br>10 mg./kg. IV<br>As before<br>30–50 mg./kg. SC<br><br>0.8 mg./kg. IV | Week #1<br>Week #2<br>Week #3<br>Week #4<br><br>Week #4 | Repeat cycle,<br>starting on week #5 | MacEwen and Hess |
| Prednisone<br>Cyclophosphamide (Cytoxan®)<br>Vincristine (Oncovin®) | 2.0 mg./kg. orally x 7 days, then 1.0 mg./kg. daily<br>5.0 mg./kg./day orally x 7, then 2.5 mg./kg. daily<br>0.03 mg./kg. IV every 14 days | | Squire (1973) |
| Prednisone<br>Cyclophosphamide (Cytoxan®)<br>Vincristine (Oncovin®) | 10 mg./m.² BSA    twice daily for 7 days<br>50 mg./m.² BSA    4 consecutive days weekly<br>0.5 mg./m.² BSA    single dose | Induction of remission | Madewell (1975) |
| Cyclophosphamide (Cytoxan®)<br>6-Mercaptopurine (Purinethol®)<br>Methotrexate (Lederle) | As above<br>50 mg./m.² BSA daily<br>2.5 mg./m.² BSA b.i.d. once weekly | Maintenance therapy | |

*The usual method of expressing drug dosages is by body weight (i.e., mg./kg.). Dosage based on body-surface area (BSA) in square meters (m.²) may be a more reliable method to administer chemotherapeutic agents in the dog because of the wide variation in body sizes. Table 4 is a conversion table of weight to BSA for dogs.

**Table 4.** *Conversion Table of Weight to Body-Surface Area in Meters for Dogs*

| KG. | M.$^2$ | KG. | M.$^2$ |
|---|---|---|---|
| 0.5 | 0.06 | 26.0 | 0.88 |
| 1.0 | 0.10 | 27.0 | 0.90 |
| 2.0 | 0.15 | 28.0 | 0.92 |
| 3.0 | 0.20 | 29.0 | 0.94 |
| 4.0 | 0.25 | 30.0 | 0.96 |
| 5.0 | 0.29 | 31.0 | 0.99 |
| 6.0 | 0.33 | 32.0 | 1.01 |
| 7.0 | 0.36 | 33.0 | 1.03 |
| 8.0 | 0.40 | 34.0 | 1.05 |
| 9.0 | 0.43 | 35.0 | 1.07 |
| 10.0 | 0.46 | 36.0 | 1.09 |
| 11.0 | 0.49 | 37.0 | 1.11 |
| 12.0 | 0.52 | 38.0 | 1.13 |
| 13.0 | 0.55 | 39.0 | 1.15 |
| 14.0 | 0.58 | 40.0 | 1.17 |
| 15.0 | 0.60 | 41.0 | 1.19 |
| 16.0 | 0.63 | 42.0 | 1.21 |
| 17.0 | 0.66 | 43.0 | 1.23 |
| 18.0 | 0.69 | 44.0 | 1.25 |
| 19.0 | 0.71 | 45.0 | 1.26 |
| 20.0 | 0.74 | 46.0 | 1.28 |
| 21.0 | 0.76 | 47.0 | 1.30 |
| 22.0 | 0.78 | 48.0 | 1.32 |
| 23.0 | 0.81 | 49.0 | 1.34 |
| 24.0 | 0.83 | 50.0 | 1.36 |
| 25.0 | 0.85 | | |

(From Ettinger, S. J.: Textbook of Veterinary Internal Medicine. Philadelphia, W. B. Saunders Co., 1975.)

toward (1) restoring hydration, (2) maintaining urine flow, (3) reducing intake of calcium and (4) eradicating the source of the parathyroid-like hormone (malignant lymphocytes). Fluid replacement should be achieved with saline, since increased sodium excretion is accompanied by increased calcium excretion. Intravenous administration of furosemide (Lasix®) will result in calcium diuresis, but serious depletion of $Na^+$ and $K^+$ can occur, so these electrolytes should be monitored closely. Glucocorticoids are highly effective for the treatment of hypercalcemia. The primary mechanism of action appears to be related to inhibition of tumor growth. Prednisone, in doses of 1 to 2 mg./kg. divided b.i.d., has been effective in causing tumor cell inhibition.

Dogs with hypercalcemia secondary to LSA have not responded to chemotherapy as well as those with normal calcium levels. If severe renal insufficiency has occurred, renal biopsy may be necessary to evaluate the extent of damage and aid in the prognosis.

## SUPPORTIVE CARE

Proper monitoring of the toxic effects of chemotherapeutic agents is essential to successful management of lymphoma patients. A complete blood count should be performed every 7 to 14 days, and liver and kidney function tests should be performed periodically. Antibiotics are indicated to protect the dog against infection if the leukocyte count drops below 4000/cu. mm. or there is evidence of an infection. The use of prophylactic antibiotics is usually not needed. It may be necessary to administer blood transfusions when severe anemia develops. Anabolic steroids can be used to help prevent bone marrow depression.

## PROGNOSIS

Canine LSA is a fatal disease; without treatment, it will rapidly lead to the death of the animal. The response of the disease to chemotherapy varies with each individual animal. Although chemotherapy is not curative, the life of many animals can be prolonged to a significant degree. With appropriate chemotherapy in a patient without advanced disease, one can expect an average survival time of 8 months after diagnosis (with a range of 4 to 18 months). A clinical staging system based on gross tumor localization, hematologic findings and constitutional signs can be used as a prognostic aid. Essentially, as the disease becomes more advanced, the prognosis becomes poorer.

### LYMPHOCYTIC LEUKEMIA

Lymphocytic leukemia originates in the bone marrow, has different presenting signs and is managed differently from lymphosarcoma. There are two basic types of lymphocytic leukemia. The well differentiated type is characterized by mature lymphocytes as the predominant cellular component of the peripheral blood and bone marrow and seems to be similar to its human counterpart, chronic lymphocytic leukemia. The other form of lymphocytic leukemia is characterized by poorly differentiated lymphocytes (lymphoblasts) in the peripheral blood and bone marrow and seems to resemble the acute lymphoblastic leukemia seen in humans. It is important that these leukemias not be confused with the leukemia that can occur in advanced lymphosarcoma patients, since these patients have a different prognosis and are treated differently.

## LYMPHOCYTIC (WELL DIFFERENTIATED) LEUKEMIA

This rare condition of middle-aged dogs is characterized clinically by intense splenomegaly but only slight peripheral lymphadenopathy. Characteristically, the hemogram reveals large numbers of small lymphocytes in the blood and bone marrow. The leukocyte counts usually vary from 30,000 to 50,000/cu. mm., with a high proportion (60 to 80 per cent) of lymphocytes. Bone marrow aspiration reveals a high percentage of lymphocytes (60 to 80 per cent) with a few lymphoblasts.

Canine patients with this form of leukemia may exhibit hyperproteinemia which on serum electrophoresis is a monoclonal gammopathy. The nature and amount of the protein (globulin) resulted in an increase in the serum viscosity (the hyperviscosity syndrome).

Chlorambucil (Leukeran®, Burroughs Wellcome, 2-mg. tablets) is an alkylating agent effective against lymphocytic leukemia. A dosage of 0.2 mg./kg. body weight is usually administered orally for 7 to 10 days; then the dose is reduced to 0.1 mg./kg. orally, daily. Although the number of patients we have treated with chlorambucil is low, one dog was treated for a period of only 5½ months before the chlorambucil was stopped and this dog is still in remission some 18 months later. Thus, the prognosis for dogs with this leukemia may be good.

## LYMPHOBLASTIC (POORLY DIFFERENTIATED) LEUKEMIA

This is a leukemia of immature or poorly differentiated lymphocytes (lymphoblasts). Lymphoblastic leukemia may account for 5 to 10 per cent of the hematopoietic tumors seen in the dog. It is usually seen in dogs under 4 years of age but can occur in older dogs. This form of leukemia is characterized by weight loss, weakness and febrile episodes. Clinical signs are normally present for only 2 weeks before presentation. The common physical findings are pale mucous membranes (anemia) and splenomegaly with or without peripheral lymphadenopathy. The hemogram will usually reveal a high white blood cell count (>60,000/cu. mm.), with lymphoblasts accounting for as many as 80 per cent of the cells. Bone marrow aspiration often reveals hypercellular marrow with many lymphoblasts. There will usually be depression or replacement of normal bone marrow precursors.

We have seen 16 cases of this form of leukemia in the past three years. The first 10 cases were treated with cyclophosphamide and no dogs lived longer than 2 weeks. The last six dogs have been treated with a combination of vincristine (0.025 mg./kg. body weight intravenously, weekly) and prednisone (1 mg./kg. orally, daily), and all six achieved remission. Remission is defined as less than 15 per cent lymphocytes in the bone marrow. Once remission is achieved, the vincristine is given every other week. The prognosis for this type of leukemia is still very poor, and in those dogs put into remission, the average survival time was only 5 months.

## MYELOPROLIFERATIVE DISORDERS

Neoplasms originating in the nonlymphoid cells of the bone marrow are uncommon in the dog. The total number of myeloproliferative diseases probably represents 1 per cent of the total number of canine hematopoietic neoplasms. There is no known etiology in domestic animals, but in man, radiation is known to induce this type of leukemia. In cats, the feline leukemia virus is associated with the development of myeloproliferative tumors.

The clinical and pathologic manifestations include lethargy, fever, splenomegaly, mild peripheral lymphadenopathy, anemia and leukocytosis. These disorders can originate from any stem-cell precursor in the bone marrow. Cell types in which the disease originates include granulocytic, eosinophilic, basophilic and megakaryocytic leukemias.

The most definitive way to establish a diagnosis is thorough examination of the blood and bone marrow. The leukocyte count is usually elevated and the granulocytes vary in maturity from "stem cells" to mature granulocytes. Occasionally, cells may be so immature that the identification of the immature (blast) cells can only be sustained by "the company they keep" (i.e., by the presence of intermediate and more mature forms of the same leukocyte series).

The differential diagnosis is complicated by problems of differentiating between leukemoid reactions and true leukemia. The typical hemogram of granulocytic leukemia is a neutrophilia or basophilia with a left shift to myeloblasts. When immature or bizarre neoplastic cells cannot be classified unequivocally as granulocytes, their granulocytic origin can be verified by the use of a peroxidase stain. In leukemoid reactions, myeloblasts are rarely seen in the peripheral blood.

Anemia is generally present because of the massive displacement of normal bone marrow cells (myelophthisis). The platelet count can be either elevated or depressed.

There are few reports describing the management of these types of leukemia in the dog. We have treated two cases of granulocytic leukemia, one of basophilic leukemia and one of eosinophilic leukemia, very successfully with hydroxyurea (Hydrea®, Squibb) at 50 mg./kg., divided b.i.d. The dog with basophilic leukemia is alive after 3 years of periodic hydroxyurea therapy. Another chemotherapeutic drug which has been used successfully in man is busulfan (Myleran®, Burroughs Wellcome, 2-mg. tablets), an alkylating agent. Its effectiveness in the dog has not been determined.

## SUPPLEMENTAL READING

Hardy, W. D., Jr.: Management of lymphosarcoma. In Kirk, R. W. (ed.): Current Veterinary Therapy V. Philadelphia, W. B. Saunders Co., 1974, pp. 381–387.
Madewell, B. R.: Chemotherapy for canine lymphosarcoma. Am. J. Vet. Res., 36:1525–1528, 1975.
Nielsen, S. W.: Myeloproliferative disorders in animals. In Myeloproliferative Disorders of Animals and Man. U.S. Atomic Energy Commission, Oak Ridge, Tenn., 1970, pp. 297–313.
Squire, R. A.: Spontaneous hematopoietic tumors of dogs. Natl. Cancer Inst. Monograph, 32:97–116, 1969.
Squire, R. A., Bush, M., Melby, E. C., Neely, L. M., and Yarbrough, B.: Clinical and pathologic study of canine lymphoma: Clinical staging, cell classification, and therapy. J. Natl. Cancer Inst., 51:565–572, 1973.

# RADIATION THERAPY

EDWARD L. GILLETTE, D.V.M.
*Fort Collins, Colorado*

This discussion will be limited to malignant tumors occurring primarily in the head and neck region of dogs. Radiation therapy of skin cancer is discussed in the section of Dermatologic Diseases. Tumors occurring in the head and neck region are often difficult to excise surgically. Radiation therapy can be useful either alone or in combination with surgery for localized tumors. Squamous cell carcinomas are the most frequently irradiated tumors of the head and neck at Colorado State University. Other tumors frequently irradiated are adamantinomas, fibrosarcomas and adenocarcinomas. Radiation facilities are available at a number of the larger veterinary institutions and may be offered by radiation oncologists at human medical institutions.

Cancer incidence increases with age, and increasing numbers of cancer patients are being seen in veterinary practices. The actual incidence of cancer in dogs is probably not rising, but companion animals are receiving continually improved medical care. This medical care and the fact that animals are increasingly protected within the home may contribute to longer life spans. Because these animals have been a part of a family for long periods of time, owners are demanding that their pets receive effective therapy for these diseases.

If the dog is in good physical condition and has no other serious medical problems it is often appropriate to suggest extensive therapy for cancer as long as the probability for control seems reasonable to the owner.

Histologic diagnosis is essential for better prognosis and to aid in determining the extent of the disease.

## STAGES OF THE DISEASE

Radiation therapy is most effective for localized disease. It is sometimes useful to irradiate regional lymph nodes if they are suspected to be involved. Radiation therapy is not ordinarily done if the disease has metastasized to distant organs unless there is some effective method for treating the metastatic lesion.

Most patients treated at Colorado State University had advanced localized disease. Tumors of the head and neck are sometimes difficult to detect early by the owner. Early signs include bleeding, pain associated with eating or foul breath. Occasionally tumors are found on physical examination by a veterinarian or when an animal is brought in specifically for teeth cleaning.

The veterinary profession should encourage animal owners to arrange periodic physical examinations for their older animals, specifically to evaluate for the presence of cancer and other diseases associated with old age. In animals, as in man, the probability for control of cancer is much greater if the disease can be detected and treated early. Cancer of the oral cavity has commonly invaded beyond the primary tissue into adjacent bone. Although this can be treated effectively with ionizing radiations of high energy, the probability for control is reduced.

Tumors of the nose usually are very advanced by the time of diagnosis. Epistaxis or difficulty in breathing may be the clinical signs which alert the owner to the problem. Radiographs may reveal extensive damage of the nasal bones or turbinates. Occasionally there is invasion into the frontal sinuses at the time of the initial diagnosis.

## AIMS OF TREATMENT

The aim of radiation therapy is to control the tumor without causing excessive normal tissue damage. This is difficult to accomplish because tumor-controlling radiation doses are usually at the highest level tolerated by normal tissue. Radiation can kill normal proliferating cells as effectively as it can tumor cells. In the course of protracted or fractionated irradiation, several doses are given over an extended period of time. With this technique, normal tissues have an opportunity to repopulate and repair most radiation damage during the intervals between treatments. This provides normal tissues with a certain advantage over tumor cells, and at the end of the course of treatment the normal tissues in the irradiated tumor bed may be sufficiently spared so that serious complications do not result.

The main purpose of radiation therapy is to control local disease which cannot effectively be surgically removed because of the size, invasiveness or location of the tumor.

## SPECIFIC TREATMENT

At Colorado State University cancer of dogs is treated either with an orthovoltage x-ray machine or with a cobalt-60 teletherapy unit. The cobalt-60 unit is used primarily for head and neck tumors because of the presence of bone in the irradiated field. Bone absorbs low-energy radiations 4 to 5 times more effectively than soft tissue. For this reason the surface of the bone may receive exceedingly high doses, but the penetration dose reaching deeper bone will be very low. X or gamma rays with energies exceeding 500 KeV. are equally absorbed in bone and soft tissue. Therefore, if the tumor has invaded bone it can be treated effectively with cobalt-60 gamma radiation, which has an energy of 1.25 MeV. If the tumor is over bone but not invading it, the bone will be protected by the higher energy radiation because it does not receive a higher dose even at the surface than does the soft tissue.

The protocol used at Colorado State University is based on 10 equal fractions given on a Monday-Wednesday-Friday schedule. The total doses vary from 3500 to 4500 rads. Recent studies of dose response indicate that a high percentage of radiation necroses may occur with doses in excess of 4500 rads given according to that schedule. However, if the dose is much lower than 4000 rads the percentage of tumor control is decreased.

## ADDITIONAL OR ANCILLARY TREATMENT

Radiation therapy often can be used effectively with surgery. Our practice has been to irradiate tumors in locations other than the head and neck following surgery. This is currently being done for fibrosarcomas in man. Postoperative radiation therapy allows the surgeon to be quite aggressive. The radiation therapist can then follow up with a full course of irradiation. In this manner both modalities are used to their greatest effect.

In the head and neck region there is usually no advantage to prior surgery if high-energy radiation beams are available. However, a biopsy is essential to determine the type of tumor. If it seems appropriate, excisional biopsy can be done. This will reduce the tumor volume and the number of cells to be destroyed by radiation.

## COMPLICATIONS

The greatest limitation to radiation therapy is the overall medical condition of the animal. It is particularly important to evaluate liver function prior to initiation of radiation therapy. Knowledge of the status of the cardiovascular and urinary systems is also needed.

Dogs are lightly anesthetized to immobilize them during therapy. They are anesthetized 10 times in a 3-week interval in our program. Although short-acting anesthetics such as pentothal are used, the anesthetic risk is significant. However, only one patient has died during therapy in our experience.

The most serious complication following radiation is radionecrosis. This usually occurs at the center of the radiation field at higher doses. Although the precise mechanism of radiation necrosis is still in doubt, it may be due to late developing damage of the microvasculature supporting dependent tissue. Radiation death of cells is usually linked to mitosis. Capillary endothelial cells turn over at a relatively slow rate, and it may take several weeks for these cells to divide and exhibit radiation damage. Radiation necrosis may be seen from a few weeks to 6 months following irradiation.

## FOLLOW-UP

In most cases, follow-up care is relatively simple. A moist desquamation may occur within 1 to 2 weeks following completion of radiation therapy. Usually this is not excessively irritating. Occasionally dogs will begin scratching or licking at the irradiated

area and cause additional damage. In these cases it is necessary to prevent traumatic injury with bandages, side bars or Elizabethan collars. Topical skin ointments can be used to alleviate the irritation. If the dog is prevented from injuring the radiation field, the moist desquamation usually heals in approximately 2 weeks. Hair loss over the irradiated field will occur, and new hair growth is usually depigmented.

Our practice is to evaluate tumor and normal tissue responses 1, 3 and 6 months following radiation therapy. At 1 month acute radiation damage should be over and normal tissues are beginning to heal. At 3 months the normal tissue reaction should have subsided and the tumor should have regressed completely. If canine tumors recur it is usually within 6 months following radiation therapy. If the tumor has not recurred after 6 months, the probability for recurrence is small. Cancer patients receiving radiation therapy at Colorado State University are followed at 6-month intervals by means of questionnaires mailed to the animal owners for their evaluation. These are sent to the owners until the tumor recurs or the animal is lost to follow-up for other reasons.

Table 1 shows the percentage of control of canine tumors for at least one year following radiation therapy. All the squamous cell carcinomas, fibrosarcomas and adenocarcinomas treated in dogs over the past 18 years are included. Although not all tumors were of the head and neck, the majority were located in that region. The table shows the effect of total dose on probability of control. The overall control rate for squamous cell carcinomas was 34 per cent. This control rate could be increased to 46 per cent if doses in excess of 4000 rads were given. Greater dose response effects were seen for fibrosarcomas and adenocarcinomas. If

**Table 1.** *Percentage of Control of Canine Tumors for at Least One Year After Radiation Therapy*

| TUMOR TYPE | 2000-5000 RADS | 3000-5000 RADS | 4000-5000 RADS |
|---|---|---|---|
| Squamous cell carcinoma | 34% (52)* | 34% (44) | 46% (26) |
| Fibrosarcoma | 27% (26) | 35% (20) | 44% (9) |
| Adenocarcinoma | 50% (10) | 66% (6) | 100% (2) |
| TOTAL | 34% (88) | 37% (70) | 49% (37) |

*Numbers in parentheses are the number of tumors in the group.

doses in excess of 4000 rads were given for fibrosarcomas, a 44 per cent control rate was achieved as compared to only 27 per cent for the full range of doses, which varied from 2000 to 4500 rads. Very few adenocarcinomas were treated; however, 50 per cent of these were controlled with radiation doses varying from 2500 to 4000 rads. Only two dogs were irradiated with doses greater than 4000 rads, both of which are surviving free of disease at least one year following therapy.

The objective of radiation therapy is to control the disease and maintain function without causing serious complications. In many cases this can be accomplished with the proper use of equipment capable of delivering an effective radiation beam. It is essential that adequate radiation physics support be available to those treating tumors. The dosimetry is critical because the latitude between tumor control and excessive normal tissue damage is very small. From a review of cases treated at Colorado State University it appears that serious normal tissue complications, especially radionecrosis, will occur with high frequency following doses of 4500 rads or greater. The probability for control of

tumors at less than 3000 rads is very low. Therefore, the acceptable tumor dose/ normal tissue response range is between 3500 and 4500 rads.

## PREVENTION

The precise causes of cancer are as yet unknown. It is probable that a combination of factors are involved, including immunologic status, viral agents, chronic irritation or exposure to chemical or physical carcinogens. It is important that veterinarians encourage those clients with animals in the older age group to bring their pets for regular checkups. Cancer occurs with greatest frequency in dogs between 8 and 10 years of age. If cancer can be detected early, it can be more effectively treated by either surgery or radiation.

### SUPPLEMENTAL READING

Batsakis, J. G.: Tumors of the Head and Neck. Baltimore, The Williams and Wilkins Company, 1974.
Fletcher, G. H.: Textbook of Radiotherapy. 2nd ed. Philadelphia, Lea & Febiger, 1973.
Hall, E. J.: Radiobiology for the Radiologist. New York, Harper and Row, 1973.

# CANCER CHEMOTHERAPY

PAUL W. HESS, D.V.M.
*St. Thomas, U.S. Virgin Islands*

Cancer chemotherapy drugs are very potent and toxic and cause injury to normal as well as malignant cells. Several guidelines must be followed by the clinician if their use is to benefit the patient and satisfy the client with good quality extended survival. The practicing veterinarian should meet the following standards in order to utilize cancer chemotherapy safely:

1. Establish histologic diagnosis of malignancy.
2. Be familiar with the drugs and their potential toxicity.
3. Use therapeutic dosages established for dogs and cats.
4. Monitor for toxicity at regular intervals.
5. Evaluate an adequate response.

6. Carry out the therapeutic program according to your own best judgment and not that of the client.
7. Obtain willing and full cooperation of the client.
8. Inform the client of all aspects of the therapy, i.e., toxicity of the drugs, frequency of visits and desired final results.

## GENERAL CONSIDERATIONS

Chemotherapy is the primary mode of therapy for those neoplasms that are multicentric in origin, such as lymphosarcoma, multiple myeloma and leukemia, or for those animals with generalized disease or widespread metastasis. Antineoplastic agents are also used as adjuncts to surgery, radiotherapy or immunotherapy. With this method, one mode of therapy is used to reduce the total number of tumor cells, and chemotherapy drugs may be used to kill the residual neoplastic cells. This approach is best suited for solid tumors which are likely to metastasize rapidly.

Non-neoplastic diseases such as canine pemphigus and polycythemia vera respond to the immunosuppressive or myelosuppressive activity of chemotherapy drugs. In man, diseases such as rheumatoid arthritis, systemic lupus erythematosus, autoimmune hemolytic anemia, idiopathic thrombocytopenic purpura and various renal diseases including the nephrotic syndrome and immune glomerulonephritis are managed with cancer chemotherapy because of the drugs' immunosuppressive properties. Finally, these drugs may be palliative in the relief of pain and discomfort caused by widespread neoplastic disease.

## MODE OF ACTION

Knowledge of the cell life cycle is important for understanding the cytotoxic effects of antineoplastic drugs. The cell cycle can be defined as that time interval from one mitosis to the next. This interval can be divided into several phases:

1. $G_1$—RNA and protein synthesis prior to DNA synthesis.
2. S—DNA synthesis.
3. $G_2$—RNA and protein synthesis prior to mitosis.
4. M—Mitosis.
5. $G_0$—Resting or nonproliferating.

Generally, the response of cells to drugs varies depending on their position in the cell cycle and whether they are cycling or resting. The cells most sensitive to cytotoxic agents are those which proliferate rapidly. Anticancer drugs either combine with the DNA macromolecule or interrupt DNA synthesis. Normal rapidly growing tissues, particularly bone marrow, gastrointestinal tract epithelium and hair follicles, are extremely sensitive to cytotoxic drugs and often limit the amount of chemotherapy that can be administered.

A summary of the classes of anticancer drugs and their mechanism of action is presented in Table 1. This table also lists whether they are specific (S) or nonspecific (NS) with respect to cell cycle phase, i.e., at what point the drugs damage proliferating cells.

## FACTORS AFFECTING USEFULNESS

Several factors determine the clinical usefulness of chemotherapeutic drugs. Cancer cells may be resistant to the effect of these drugs owing to anatomic location (central nervous system) or stage of proliferation (resting). Pharmacologic factors influence a drug's concentration at its primary site of action or the time period during which drugs are available for activity.

The route of administration may improve the antitumor effect of a given drug by allowing it to reach high concentrations in the area of greatest need. The distribution of drugs is important, because drugs may accumulate in certain areas as a result of binding or active transport and thus may not be available. Certain drugs are inactive and must be metabolized to achieve their active form, such as cyclophosphamide, which requires metabolism by the liver in order to be effective. The excretion of some drugs is

*Table 1.* *Classes of Anticancer Drugs and Their Mechanisms of Action*

| CLASS OF AGENTS | MECHANISM OF ACTION | CELL CYCLE PHASE SPECIFIC/NONSPECIFIC |
|---|---|---|
| Alkylating Agents | Cross-linkage of DNA helical chain | NS |
| Antimetabolites | Interruption of purine, pyrimidine and folic acid metabolism | S |
| Antibiotics | Binding to DNA to inhibit DNA and RNA synthesis | NS |
| Plant Alkaloids | Interference with spindle proteins necessary for mitosis | S |
| Corticosteroids | Unclear | NS |
| Hormones | ——— | NS |
| Miscellaneous Hydroxyurea | Inhibition of nucleotide enzyme | S |

critical, since some drugs may accumulate and produce severe toxicity if organ function is not adequate.

Combinations of anticancer drugs may be synergistic or antagonistic. For example, vincristine improves the transport of methotrexate, while hydrocortisone inhibits methotrexate transport. For these reasons, the clinician should become thoroughly familiar with each drug prior to clinical use.

## PRETREATMENT EVALUATION

Prior to administering these drugs, the veterinarian should obtain a complete history to establish if any previous therapy has been given, or if there has been any other recent illness which may influence the effectiveness of the drugs. A complete physical examination along with baseline laboratory data, including a hemogram and liver and kidney function tests, is mandatory. Other special tests such as bone marrow examination or special radiographic procedures may be needed in order to evaluate completely the extent of disease or underlying complications. The results of these examinations often influence the decision to initiate therapy or the selection of the most effective drugs to be used.

## ANTICANCER DRUGS

Currently there are over 20 anticancer agents commercially available to the veterinarian for cancer therapy in animals. Sometimes dosages are listed on the basis of body-surface area; however, this author prefers the use of body weight to calculate dosage. In Table 2, these drugs are listed according to class with the following information: generic and brand names, manufacturer, types of preparations available, sensitive neoplasms, suggested dosages and frequency of administration. The dosages suggested for each drug have been calculated for maximal effectiveness and minimal toxicity. However, doses should be altered according to the individual animal's sensitivity to the drug and overall physical condition.

## TOXICITY AND COMPLICATIONS

Anticancer drugs kill normal as well as malignant cells. The toxic side effects sometimes limit the use of a single drug or combination of drugs. The side effects most commonly encountered include alopecia, anorexia, vomiting, diarrhea, thrombocytopenia, leukopenia, anemia and oral mucosal ulceration. If toxicity is slight to moderate, temporary dosage reduction or withdrawal of the drugs will allow the body to retain normal function while cellular regeneration takes place. However, if severe toxicity occurs, the drugs may have to be permanently discontinued.

Certain agents usually given by the intravenous route are very irritating and cause local reactions when they are allowed inadvertently to leak into the extravascular tissue during administration. Severe pain, erythema and erosion of tissue will occur. Therefore, great care should be taken when administering vincristine, vinblastine, actinomycid D and Adriamycin®.

Toxic side effects directly related to the use of anticancer drugs are monitored routinely by means of physical examination and hemograms every 7 to 10 days. A few of the drugs have unique side effects: cyclophosphamide—hemorrhagic cystitis; 5-fluorouracil—severe neurotoxicity (this drug cannot be given to cats); vincristine—neuromuscular weakness and severe constipation. Drugs should be discontinued if bone marrow depression results in leukocyte counts below 3000/cu. mm. and platelet counts below 75,000/cu. mm.

Side effects indirectly related to the drugs are those due to rapid tumor-cell breakdown. Abnormal liver and renal function often accompanies tumor-cell breakdown along with the possible local reactions of pain, edema, inflammation and abscess formation or tissue necrosis.

## TREATMENT OF TOXICITY

It is very important for the veterinarian to remember that once a drug has been administered there is nothing (with the exception of methotrexate) that can neutralize its action or prevent serious delayed side effects. A thorough explanation to the client about toxic side effects before the use of anticancer drugs will allow the client to observe the patient at home to detect the earliest signs of complications. This may result in earlier treatment of complications.

Treatment of severe bone marrow depression is directed toward protecting the body against severe endotoxemia, bleeding

**Table 2.** *Antineoplastic Agents*

| DRUG | SENSITIVE NEOPLASMS | SUGGESTED DOSAGE |
|---|---|---|
| *Alkylating Agents* | | |
| Cyclophosphamide (Cytoxan®, Mead Johnson) 25-mg. and 50-mg. tablets; 100-mg., 200-mg. and 500-mg. vials | LSA*, lymphoreticular leukemias, reticulum cell sarcoma, mast cell tumors, transmissible venereal tumor, miscellaneous solid tumors | 6 mg./kg. for 3 days, then 2 mg./kg. daily orally or 10 mg./kg. IV every 7 to 10 days |
| Nitrogen mustard (Mustargen®, Merck Sharp and Dohme) 10-mg. vials | LSA, mast cell tumors | 0.1-0.5 mg./kg. IV daily |
| Chlorambucil (Leukeran®, Burroughs Wellcome) 2-mg. tablets | Chronic lymphocytic leukemia, macroglobulinemia | 0.2 mg./kg. daily orally |
| Thiotepa® (Lederle) 15-mg. vials | Mast cell tumors, miscellaneous sarcomas and carcinomas | 0.5 mg./kg. daily for 10 days intralesionally or IV |
| Busulfan (Myleran®, Burroughs Wellcome) 2-mg. tablets | Granulocytic leukemias, Myeloproliferative disorders | 1 mg./kg. daily orally |
| Melphalan (Alkeran®, Burroughs Wellcome) 2-mg. tablets | Multiple myeloma, monoclonal gammopathies | 0.05 mg.-0.10 mg./kg. daily orally |
| *Antimetabolites* | | |
| Methotrexate (Lederle) 2.5-mg. tablets 5-mg. and 50-mg. vials | LSA, acute lymphocytic leukemia, transmissible venereal tumor | 0.06 mg./kg. daily orally or 0.3 mg./kg. weekly IV |
| 6-Mercaptopurine (Purinethol®, 6-MP, Burroughs Wellcome) 50-mg. tablets | LSA, acute lymphoblastic leukemia, myelogenous leukemia | 2 mg./kg. daily orally. |
| 6-Thioguanine (Tabloid, Burroughs Wellcome) 40-mg. tablets | LSA, mast cell tumor | 2.5 mg./kg. daily orally |
| 5-Fluorouracil (5-FU, Fluorouracil®, Roche Laboratories) 500-mg. vials | Miscellaneous carcinomas and sarcomas | *Do NOT use in cats* Dog: 5 mg./kg. every 5 to 7 days IV |
| Efudex (5 FU Cream and Solution 2% and 5%, Roche Laboratories) | Cutaneous tumors | Apply topically b.i.d. for 2 to 4 weeks |
| Cytosine arabinoside (Ara-C®, Cytosar®, Upjohn) 100-mg. and 500-mg. vials | LSA, granulocytic leukemia, mast cell tumors | 5-10 mg./kg. IM daily for 2 weeks or 30 - 50 mg./kg. IM weekly |
| *Antibiotics* | | |
| Actinomycin D (Cosmegen®, Merck Sharp and Dohme) 500 μg./vial | LSA, miscellaneous sarcomas and carcinomas | 0.015 mg./kg. IV for 3 to 5 days, then wait 3 weeks for marrow recovery |
| Doxorubicin HCl (Adriamycin®, Adria) 10-mg. vials | Osteosarcoma, miscellaneous sarcomas and carcinomas | N.A.† for dogs or cats 2 mg./kg. every 3 weeks, IV in humans |

---

*LSA = lymphosarcoma.
†N.A. = not available.

*Continued on next page*

*Table 2.*   *Antineoplastic Agents (Continued)*

| DRUG | SENSITIVE NEOPLASMS | SUGGESTED DOSAGE |
|---|---|---|
| Bleomycin (Blenoxane®, Bristol) 15 units/vial | Squamous cell carcinoma, miscellaneous carcinomas | N.A. for dogs or cats<br><br>0.3-0.5 units/kg. once or twice weekly, IV or IM in humans |
| *Plant Alkaloids* Vincristine (Oncovin®, Eli Lilly) 1-mg. and 5-mg. vials | LSA, acute lymphoblastic leukemia, reticulum cell sarcoma, mast cell tumor, transmissible venereal tumor | 0.025-0.05 mg./kg. IV every 7 to 10 days |
| Vinblastine (Velban®, Eli Lilly) 10 mg./vial | LSA, mast cell tumor | 0.1-0.4 mg./kg. IV every 7 to 10 days |
| *Hormones* Adrenal corticosteroids (Prednisone) | LSA, acute lymphoblastic leukemia, mast cell tumors, multiple myeloma, miscellaneous tumors | 1–2 mg./kg. daily orally, divided b.i.d. |
| Estrogens (DES, ECP) | Perianal adenomas, advanced carcinomas of prostate | DES: 1 mg. every other day orally ECP: 1-2 mg. IM every 2 to 4 weeks |
| Testosterone | Mammary tumors, bone marrow depression | 2 mg./kg. IM 3 times weekly |
| *Miscellaneous* Hydroxyurea (Hydrea®, Squibb) 500-mg. capsules | Myelogenous leukemia, mast cell tumor | 80 mg./kg. every 3 days or 40-50 mg./kg. daily orally |
| Ortho, para prime DDD (opDDD) (Mitotane®, Lysodren®, Calbio) 500-mg. tablets | Adrenal cortical adenomas and carcinomas | 46 mg./kg. daily orally to effect |

or septicemia. Blood transfusions, massive antibiotic therapy and other intensive care procedures are used to support the animal during this critical period. Mild vomiting and diarrhea can generally be controlled by routine means.

### DRUG COMBINATIONS

It has been stated that the optimal method of using cancer chemotherapy is by combinations of drugs. Combinations of drugs can suppress or delay the eventual existence of drug-resistant cells and prolong the time necessary for these cells to produce clinically apparent disease. If combination chemotherapy is given intermittently (a different drug every few weeks) rather than continuously (all drugs at the same time on a weekly basis), there tend to be greater tumor-cell death and less immunosuppression. When drugs are selected for combination therapy, a better response may be expected if the following guidelines are used: (1) only drugs with known activity against a specific neoplasm should be used, (2) drugs should have different mechanisms of action and (3) drugs should have different ranges of toxicity.

Currently, several combinations of drugs are used to control various neoplastic diseases in animals. Canine lymphosarcoma has been treated with various combinations of prednisone, cyclophosphamide, vincristine, cytosine arabinoside and L-asparaginase (University of California at Davis). Canine transmissible venereal tumor can be very effectively treated with a combination of vincristine, cyclophosphamide and methotrexate. In the future, newer combinations of drugs may prove more effective in controlling other neoplastic diseases.

## SUMMARY

Newer information concerning advances in pharmacology, toxicity, indications for use or prolonged survival of animals with cancer is being discovered daily. Public awareness of the beneficial aspects of chemotherapy along with advances in other forms of therapy has placed additional responsibility on the veterinarian to offer these drugs or other newer techniques to the client whose pet has developed cancer. At a slower rate, we are able to predict accurately the biologic behavior of certain tumors. Therefore, we can honestly say that treatment does prolong the survival of cats and dogs with malignant tumors, and we should not be inclined toward euthanasia.

## SUPPLEMENTAL READING

Chabner, B. A., Myers, C. E., *et al.*: The clinical pharmacology of antineoplastic agents. N. Eng. J. Med. 292:1107–1113 and 1159–1168, May, 1975.
Cline, M. J., and Haskell, C. M.: Cancer Chemotherapy. Philadelphia, W. B. Saunders Co., 1975.
Hess, P. W.: Basic Principles of Cancer Chemotherapy, AAHA Scientific Proceedings, Vol. II, 1975, pp. 102–106.
Hess, P. W.: Principles of cancer chemotherapy in a symposium of veterinary clinical oncology. Vet. Clin. N. Am., 7: in press, February, 1977.
Thielen, G. H.: Veterinary medical oncology. *In* Ettinger, S. J. (ed.): Textbook of Veterinary Internal Medicine. Philadelphia, W. B. Saunders Co., 1975, pp. 127–149.

# IMMUNO-THERAPY OF CANCER

E. GREGORY MacEWEN, V.M.D.
*New York, New York*

The most commonly used methods of treating cancer are surgical excision, cryosurgery, radiation therapy and chemotherapy. Another form of therapy which cannot be considered conventional therapy at this time is immunotherapy. Immunotherapy of cancer is an attempt to initiate or augment the immune system of a patient to obtain an immune response which will inhibit the growth or spread of an existing tumor. The conventional methods of cancer therapy do not kill all the patient's tumor cells. These cells can therefore proliferate and form another tumor. Immunotherapy, in combination with conventional therapy, may destroy the tumor cells remaining after conventional therapy and thus reduce the possibility of tumor recurrence.

## THE IMMUNE SYSTEM

The immune system is a highly complex array of components (defense cells and biologically active substances) which provide protection against invading foreign antigens such as bacteria, particulate material and tumor-associated antigens. The immune system consists of granulocytes, the reticuloendothelial system, the lymphoid system and the complement system. The lymphoid system is made up of both cellular and humoral (antibody) components and is thought to be very important in preventing tumor development. Lymphocytes which are associated with the thymus in their development are termed T lymphocytes. Lymphoid cells which are influenced by the mammalian equivalent of the bursa of Fabricius are known as B cells. The T cells or "killer cells" are important in graft vs. host reactions, delayed hypersensitivity skin reactions and tumor cell rejection. The B cells produce immunoglobulins (cytolytic antibody) which together with complement can cause tumor cell destruction. When activated, macrophages play an important role in the inhibition of tumor cells. The recent and rapid growth of our knowledge concerning the immune system in general and tumor immunology in particular has provided a sound basis for clinical trials of immunotherapy in cancer patients.

## THE IMMUNE SYSTEM AND CANCER

The rationale for the use of immunotherapy against tumors is based on a number of clinical and experimental observations. For instance, tumor-specific antigens (TSA) can be demonstrated on the surface of many tumor cells. In humans, they have been reported in melanomas, sarcomas, intestinal carcinomas and Burkitt's lymphoma. Tumor-specific antigens are found in feline leukemia virus–positive cats with lymphosarcoma, and strong evidence exists for TSA in canine osteosarcoma cells. These unique tumor antigens are not found on normal cells, so an immune response will be directed against the tumor cells but not against the normal cells. There is evidence that an immune response against tumor cells can be mounted in both man and animals. In man, the histologic appearance of mononuclear cellular infiltration around the tumor or in the lymph nodes draining tumors often resembles the classic delayed hypersensitivity reactions and is associated with an improved prognosis. In cats, the feline leukemia virus–transformed lymphocytes produce a new antigen in the cell surface called the feline oncornavirus-associated cell-membrane antigen (FOCMA). Antibodies directed against the FOCMA cause lysis of the transformed or cancerous cells and will prevent the development of lymphosarcoma. Preliminary evidence indicates that approximately one third of the cats infected with the feline leukemia virus produce antibodies against FOCMA.

Other evidence for the involvement of the immune system in the development of tumors is the high incidence of cancer associated with naturally occurring and acquired immunodeficiency conditions. This has been well documented in humans with congenital immunodeficiencies and in iatrogenically immunosuppressed organ transplantation patients. Similar studies to define the extent of immunodeficiency conditions are now under way in veterinary medicine. A recent study of dogs with spontaneous neoplasms and lymphoproliferative and solid tumors revealed that both the humoral and the cellular components of the immune system were depressed to some degree.

The growth of established tumors can be either halted or enhanced by immunologic manipulations. *In-vitro* experiments have shown that the serum of cancer patients may have circulating antigen-antibody complexes which can block the ability of sensitized lymphocytes to destroy tumor cells in tissue culture. These immune complexes have been termed "blocking factors." Brodey and Fidler have demonstrated that blocking factors are present in dogs with osteosarcoma and that after amputation the amount of these factors decreases. The amount of these factors increases when tumor recurrence or metastasis occurs. Therapeutic methods of reducing the amounts of blocking factors in the blood have been attempted (plasmapheresis and low-dose chemotherapy), but little clinical benefit occurs.

## METHODS OF IMMUNOTHERAPY

The methods currently under investigation for immunotherapy can be divided into three categories: (1) passive immunotherapy, (2) specific active immunotherapy and (3) nonspecific active immunotherapy.

**Passive Immunotherapy.** Passive immunotherapy involves the administration of immune mediators such as lymphocytes, antibodies, complement and transfer factor.

Attempts to transfer lymphocytes from a healthy donor to a recipient with cancer have met with little success. The disadvantages to this form of therapy are (1) elaborate cell separation equipment and tissue typing procedures are necessary and (2) rejection of transfused lymphocytes and even graft vs. host reactions can occur. This form of therapy is impractical for routine veterinary use.

The use of blood constituents, such as circulating antibody and complement, has been under evaluation in our clinic for the last three years. We have found that intravenous administration of fresh heparinized blood and plasma from healthy cats and dogs in doses of 15 to 20 ml. per kg. of body weight every 3 days will cause destruction of the tumor cells. In contrast, plasma or blood from cats with leukemia does not have any antitumor effect. The active factor in cat and dog blood has not yet

*Table 1.* Nonspecific Immunopotentiators

| AGENT | MECHANISM OF ACTION | POTENTIAL CLINICAL USES | UNIQUE FEATURES |
|---|---|---|---|
| *Biologic Potentiators* | | | |
| Bacillus Calmette-Guerin (BCG)* | Stimulates macrophages and lymphocytes<br>Delayed hypersensitivity reaction (T cell) | Melanoma (man)<br>Lymphosarcoma (with chemotherapy<br>Osteosarcoma (with amputations) | Living, attenuated *Mycobacterium bovis* organism (public health hazard?) |
| *Corynebacterium parvum*** | Stimulates macrophages and phagocytosis<br>Acts primarily through B cells | Lung carcinoma (man)<br>Wide variety of tumors in experimental animals | Formalin killed<br>No exo- or endotoxins<br>Safe |
| Mixed bacterial vaccine (MBV) † | Stimulates macrophages and T cells<br>Endotoxic effect | Wide variety of solid tumors, sarcomas and feline mammary carcinomas | Mixture of *Serratia marcescens* and *Streptococcus pyogenes* |
| *Chemical Potentiators* | | | |
| Imidothiazoles (Levamisole®)‡ | Stimulates delayed hypersensitivity (T cells) | In leukemia, may have some anti-tumor effects<br>May augment chemotherapy in treated leukemia patients<br>Immune recovery after chemotherapy<br>Granulomatous disease (feline eosinophilic granulomas)<br>Chronic pyodermas | Oral administration safe at 5 mg./kg. body weight (3x week) |
| Polynucleotides (polyadenylic acid, PolyA; polyuidylic acid, PolyU) | T-cell stimulator<br>Antibody response<br>Action similar to transfer factor | Immune restoration | |

*BCG. Tice Strain, Research Foundation, 70 West Hubbard Street, Chicago, Illinois 60610.
**C. *parvum*. Burroughs Wellcome (7 mg./cc.). 3030 Cornwallis Road, Research Triangle Park, North Carolina 27709.
†MBV. Farbenfabriken Bayer, Wuppertal, Germany.
‡Levamisole HCl. Pitman-Moore, Inc., Washington's Crossing, New Jersey 08560.

been isolated, but based on similar studies in leukemic AKR mice, it is thought that the factor is a component of complement. It is speculated that antibody directed toward antigens in the leukemic cell membrane is present, but because of a deficiency in the level of complement or complement components, tumor destruction cannot occur. Based on the observation that serum causes leukemic cell destruction in AKR mice, we have been attempting this in cats and dogs with lymphosarcoma. This form of therapy must be considered experimental even though we have treated 40 cats and 5 dogs with lymphosarcoma and documented 100 per cent regression in 50 per cent of the patients treated. Partial regression (25 to 75 per cent reduction of tumor volume) was seen in the remaining 50 per cent of the patients. If the active factor was identified, it could be extracted, purified and administered to cats and dogs with lymphosarcoma.

Transfer factor is derived from lymphocytes and is capable of transferring immunity from a sensitized host to an unsensitized host. This factor is under investigation and is being used to treat cancer patients and patients with certain granulomatous diseases.

**Specific Active Immunotherapy.** In this form of immunotherapy, attempts are made to immunize the host against specific tumor antigens. Various vaccine preparations made from killed tumor cells are modified to increase their immunogenicity. It is speculated that when these vaccines are administered at different sites in the body (intradermally), different components of the immune system are stimulated (e.g., cellular immunity). These vaccines are usually given in combination with other forms of therapy, such as surgery or chemotherapy, in an attempt to elicit a new or stronger immune response against the tumor. The disadvantange of this type of immunotherapy is the difficulty in adequate preparation and inactivation of the tumor cells. One method of specific active immunotherapy which has shown some promise in experimentally transplanted tumors and in spontaneous mammary tumors in the dog involves reacting inactivated tumor cells with an enzyme called neuraminidase. Neuraminidase removes sialic acid (a glycoprotein) from the cell surfaces of malignant cells and renders the cell more immunogenic. This form of therapy may be useful in veterinary medicine, and further investigations are in progress.

**Nonspecific Active Immunotherapy.** This form of immunotherapy is based on the observation that infections, both local or systemic, are associated with tumor regression and an improved prognosis. It is thought that nonspecific stimulation of the immune system by certain antigens will result in an increased response to tumor-associated antigens. A number of agents are under investigation as nonspecific immunopotentiators, but they can all be classified as either biologic or chemical agents. A summary of the properties of the most widely used nonspecific immunostimulators, together with their potential clinical uses, is given in Table 1.

## SUMMARY

Cancer immunotherapy is a relatively new field of clinical investigation. At present, immunotherapy should be restricted to those patients with small amounts of tumor. Further clinical studies are needed, together with quantitative measurements of the patient's antitumor immune responses, to demonstrate the conditions under which immunotherapy can be safe and effective as a form of cancer therapy.

## SUPPLEMENTAL READING

Brodey, R. S., Fidler, I. J., and Beck-Nielsen, S.: Correlation of *in vitro* response with clinical course of malignant neoplasia in dogs. Am. J. Vet. Res., *36*: 75-80, 1975.

Currie, G. A.: Eighty years of immunotherapy. A review of immunological methods used for the treatment of human cancer. Brit. J. Cancer, *26*:141-153, 172.

Essex, M., Sliski, A., Cotter, S. M., Jakowski, R. M., and Hardy, W. D., Jr.: Immunosurveillance of naturally occurring feline leukemia. Science, *190*:790-791, 1975.

MacEwen, E. G.: General concepts of immunotherapy of tumors. J. Am. Anim. Hosp. Assn., *12*:363-373, 1976.

Morton, D. L.: Immunotherapy of cancer, Cancer, *30*:1647-1655, 1972.

# DERMATOLOGIC DISEASES

Richard E. W. Halliwell
*Consulting Editor*

# NEOPLASIA OF THE SKIN AND MAMMARY GLANDS IN DOGS AND CATS

D. E. BOSTOCK, M.R.C.V.S.
*Cambridge, England*

The correct management of tumors is an important part of small animal practice. The incidence of malignant neoplasms in California has been estimated by Dorn and his colleagues to be 381 per 100,000 dogs and 156 per 100,000 cats per year. In dogs, clinically significant benign tumors are at least as common as malignant tumors, giving an overall incidence of 780 per 100,000. In cats, however, malignant neoplasms occur with four times the frequency of benign tumors, so that the total annual incidence of all neoplasms in this species is about 195 per 100,000.

Many authors have reported the relative frequency of the different histologic types of tumor based upon study of biopsy material that is prone to artificial selection. Nevertheless, their findings are of great interest, since they bear some relationship to the field situation.

In these surveys, tumors of skin, subcutaneous tissues and mammary glands form the majority of all neoplasms in dogs, accounting for 58 per cent of the total, while in cats they provide 36 per cent, being second in importance to the lymphoid malignancies in this species.

In Table 1, the relative frequency of the various types of skin tumors in dogs and cats in America is compared to that in Great Britain, showing a close similarity in incidence. In dogs, the only notable variations between the two areas occur with anal adenomas, which are apparently twice as common in the U.S.A. as in the U.K., and with histiocytomas, which are more common in Britain. In cats, the most obvious difference is in the relative distribution of fibromas and fibrosarcomas. In the U.S.A.,

these two tumors arise with the same frequency, but in Britain the malignant type is 10 times as common as the benign. Since the distribution in dogs does not reveal this variation, it cannot be easily explained by differences in diagnostic criteria and may be due to different strains of the feline sarcoma virus in the two countries.

## MAMMARY TUMORS

Mammary tumors alone account for about 52 per cent of all neoplasms in female dogs and for less than 3 per cent in male dogs. They are extremely rare in male cats but provide about 22 per cent of the total number of tumors in female cats.

In addition to being obviously sex-linked, the incidence of mammary neoplasia is closely age-associated. The rate is very low until 6 years of age, after which it rises rapidly to a peak of 2,400 per 100,000 dogs and 250 per 100,000 cats between 9.5 and 10.5 years of age. After this, the total incidence begins to decline, although the relative proportion of highly malignant mammary cancers continues to increase.

### CANINE MAMMARY TUMORS

There is little obvious breed predisposition to mammary neoplasia, although some evidence suggests that there is a decreased incidence in Chihuahuas as compared to other purebred dogs.

In spite of their being such common tumors, canine mammary neoplasms present a major prognostic problem owing to their marked pleomorphism and to the

493

**Table 1.** *Distribution of Skin Tumors in the Dog and Cat Based on Histologic Examination of Surgically Excised Material*

| TUMOR TYPE | RELATIVE FREQUENCY OF ALL TUMORS IN DOGS (%) | | RELATIVE FREQUENCY OF ALL TUMORS IN CATS (%) | |
|---|---|---|---|---|
| | U.S.A.* | U.K.† | U.S.A.* | U.K.† |
| Mastocytoma | 21.34 | 19.15 | 7.33 | 7.69 |
| Hepatoid adenoma | 18.29 | 9.82 | — | — |
| Lipoma | 8.64 | 8.49 | 6.02 | 2.34 |
| Sebaceous adenoma | N/S | 8.22 | N/S | 2.34 |
| Fibrosarcoma | 5.89 | 7.42 | 12.05 | 25.42 |
| Melanoma | 5.01 | 6.27 | 1.20 | 2.68 |
| Squamous cell carcinoma | 3.86 | 5.39 | 16.28 | 17.39 |
| Fibroma | 3.15 | 2.29 | 12.05 | 2.68 |
| Hemangiopericytoma | 3.15 | 4.24 | 1.20 | — |
| Hemangioma | 3.00 | 2.44 | 2.27 | 0.33 |
| Histiocytoma | 2.54 | 6.04 | — | — |
| Basal cell tumor | N/S | 4.13 | N/S | 14.72 |
| Reticulum cell sarcoma | N/S | 3.33 | N/S | 2.68 |
| Papilloma | 2.54 | 2.26 | — | — |
| Perineural fibroblastoma | N/S | 1.64 | N/S | 0.33 |
| Hepatoid adenocarcinoma | N/S | 1.53 | — | — |
| Malignant hemangioendothelioma | 1.52 | 1.30 | 1.20 | 1.00 |
| Sweat gland adenocarcinoma | N/S | 1.17 | N/S | |
| Myxosarcoma | N/S | 0.99 | N/S | 0.67 |
| Leiomyoma | N/S | 0.88 | N/S | 0.33 |
| Sweat gland adenoma | N/S | 0.73 | N/S | 0.33 |
| Sebaceous adenocarcinoma | N/S | 0.45 | N/S | — |
| Trichoepithelioma | N/S | 0.44 | N/S | 0.33 |
| Liposarcoma | 0.41 | 0.38 | 1.20 | — |
| Calcifying epithelioma | N/S | 0.34 | — | — |
| Ceruminous gland adenocarcinoma | N/S | 0.29 | N/S | 13.04 |
| Lymphosarcoma | N/S | 0.27 | N/S | 1.00 |
| Leiomyosarcoma | N/S | 0.15 | N/S | 0.67 |
| Myxoma | N/S | 0.15 | N/S | — |
| Ceruminous gland adenoma | N/S | 0.05 | N/S | 1.67 |

N/S = Not separately specified.
*Figures for U.S.A. based on a series of 984 canine and 83 feline tumors reported by Brodey.
†Figures for U.K. obtained from a study of 2616 canine and 288 feline skin neoplasms received from veterinarian for histologic diagnosis at the Department of Clinical Veterinary Medicine, Cambridge, England.

lack of follow-up data following surgical excision. In the past, inconsistency of nomenclature has made direct comparisons of the results of different workers difficult; however, WHO has recently published an internationally agreed upon classification of these and many other neoplasms in animals that should eliminate this problem.

In bitches, the inguinal mammary glands are involved in neoplastic transformation three to four times more often than are any of the anterior glands. Table 2 lists the different types of mammary tumors that may arise, with their relative frequencies; it can be seen that 51 per cent of tumors received as surgical biopsy material are histologically benign (fibroadenomas and simple adenomas). Although this may be an artificially low figure, because obviously benign tumors are not referred for histologic

**Table 2.** *Distribution of Canine Mammary Neoplasms Based on Histologic Examination of Surgically Excised Material**

| TUMOR TYPE | RELATIVE FREQUENCY (% |
|---|---|
| Fibroadenomas (benign mixed tumors and complex adenomas) | 45.5 |
| Solid carcinomas | 16.9 |
| Tubular adenocarcinomas | 15.4 |
| Papillary adenocarcinomas | 8.6 |
| Simple adenomas | 5.0 |
| Anaplastic carcinomas | 4.0 |
| Sarcomas | 3.1 |
| Carcinosarcomas | 0.6 |
| Benign mesenchymal tumors | 0.5 |

*Figures were obtained from an unselected series 1625 canine mammary tumors submitted by gener practitioners to the Department of Clinical Veterina Medicine, Cambridge, England, for diagnosis.

**Table 3.**  *Postmastectomy Survival Time of Bitches With Histologically Confirmed Mammary Carcinomas\**

| TUMOR TYPE | ONE-YEAR SURVIVAL (%) | | MEDIAN SURVIVAL TIME (WEEKS) | |
| --- | --- | --- | --- | --- |
| | *Invasive* | *Well-Defined* | *Invasive* | *Well-Defined* |
| Papillary | 50 | 86 | 65 | 128 |
| Tubular | 44 | 74 | 38 | 110 |
| Solid | 26 | 73 | 26 | 82 |
| Anaplastic | 24 | — | 11 | — |

\*Tumors were apparently completely excised and there was no clinical evidence of metastasis at the time of surgery, based on biopsy material from 220 mammary carcinomas.

examination, several different series have revealed a remarkably similar distribution.

At present, surgical excision of mammary neoplasms is the treatment of choice. It is the dog with a histologically malignant but apparently completely excised lesion that presents the greatest challenge with respect to an accurate prognosis. Most tumors in this category are carcinomas that can be divided into four distinctive histologic types and further classified as well defined or locally invasive tumors (Table 2). In Table 3, the percentage of one-year survival and median survival time are shown for dogs with each carcinoma subtype, from which it can be seen that the criterion of local infiltration is more important for prognosis than is tumor morphology. Well-defined lesions carry a similar prognosis, regardless of their architectural pattern, although there is some difference between the behavior of the invasive carcinomas, in which solid and anaplastic types carry a significantly poorer prognosis than that of papillary or tubular carcinomas.

The percentage of survival at one year is important, because most animals that are still alive after one year can be considered cured; they eventually die from causes unrelated to the original neoplasm. This is illustrated in Figure 1, in which deaths from all causes are shown to increase in a linear fashion with time after surgery, but tumor deaths show an obvious plateau at about 60 weeks.

These figures apply only to carcinomas that measured less than 5 cm. in diameter at surgery; tumors larger than this always carry

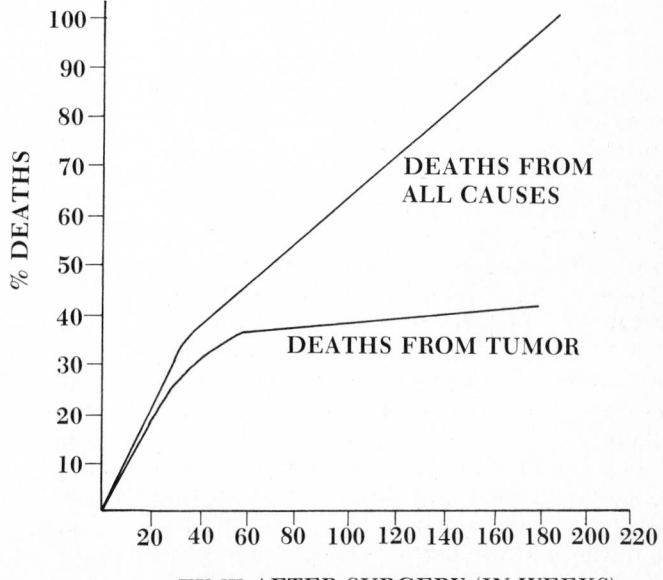

**Figure 1.**  Deaths from mammary carcinomas compared with deaths from all causes in bitches with a surgically excised tubular or solid mammary carcinoma.

DEATHS FROM ALL CAUSES

DEATHS FROM TUMOR

% DEATHS

TIME AFTER SURGERY (IN WEEKS)

a poor prognosis, regardless of morphology. On the other hand, the length of time a tumor is reported to have been present before diagnosis has little effect on the outcome of surgical excision.

The other important class of malignant mammary tumors is the sarcomas, which include osteosarcomas, chondrosarcomas and fibrosarcomas. These tumors all carry a similar, guarded prognosis, with a 40 per cent one-year survival rate following surgery.

Malignant mammary tumors may sometimes metastasize to the skin lymphatics, leading to a rapidly spreading, ulcerative lesion that clinically resembles hidradenitis suppurativa. The prognosis for such cases is hopeless. The cause of death from mammary cancer is generally pulmonary metastasis, with the regional lymph nodes being involved in the majority of animals. Spread to the liver, bone and CNS is unusual in dogs. Local recurrence is common following removal of invasive tumors and is generally the cause of death in dogs with fibrosarcomas, which rarely metastasize.

It is difficult to be certain of the most effective form of surgical intervention, owing to lack of controlled comparisons between different methods. It seems likely, by analogy with the results of treatment in human patients, that a wide excision of the tumor to include surrounding normal tissue is essential if local recurrence is to be prevented. Extensive dissection of adjacent glands and regional lymph nodes may not be necessary, however, unless they are clinically involved. If there is already clinical evidence of invasion of the superficial lymph nodes, the deeper nodes and lungs will probably contain tumor deposits, and the prognosis must be guarded, whatever form of treatment is adopted.

This raises the problem of what should be done for the dog that shows no clinical evidence of metastasis after complete excision of an invasive carcinoma. It is most unsatisfactory to inform the owner that the dog has a 50 to 70 per cent chance of dying within the year if no postsurgical therapy is attempted, although what form this therapy should take is far from clear at present. For women, in whom a similar situation can arise, some surgeons are now instituting routine, postoperative multiple chemotherapy. Although this has not yet been used in dogs, some institutes are studying the value of postsurgical immunotherapy in animals with minimal residual tumor in an attempt to delay the growth of metastatic lesions.

There have been reports that testosterone derivatives, such as drostanolone propionate, or testosterone itself will delay the growth or even cause regression of inoperable canine mammary carcinomas. In addition, antiestrogens such as Tamoxifen (Nolvadex® [I.C.I.]) have been used. In the absence of well-controlled trials, it is difficult to evaluate the results of this type of therapy, but there is little doubt that the dramatic regressions sometimes encountered in women are rarely seen in dogs. There is similarly no evidence that spaying at the time of mastectomy will improve the prognosis.

## FELINE MAMMARY TUMORS

Feline mammary neoplasms do not show the variety of morphologic types or predilection for the inguinal glands seen in dogs. They appear clinically as multinodular, invasive tumors, more than 90 per cent having the histologic appearance of tubular or papillary adenocarcinomas. The mixed tumors seen commonly in dogs do not occur.

Compared with tumors of similar morphology in dogs, cat mammary carcinomas have a more malignant behavior pattern and carry a worse prognosis. Thus, Weijer and his colleagues found that the overall one year survival rate following surgery was only 10 per cent, although for animals with small tumors (less than 8 cu. cm. in volume) this rose to 50 per cent. The cause of about 80 per cent of postsurgical deaths in this species is pulmonary metastasis, with local recurrence accounting for the remainder.

## ETIOLOGY OF MAMMARY TUMORS

The cause of mammary neoplasms in carnivores is unknown. There have been several reports of oncornaviruses associated with the feline disease, but no causal relationship has been established. Dorn and his colleagues have demonstrated that in dogs and cats without oophorectomy there is a sevenfold increase in incidence of mammary cancer, indicating that hormonal factors are of great importance in their genesis.

## TUMORS OF THE SKIN AND SUBCUTANEOUS TISSUES

These tumors will be considered, for the most part, in the order of frequency in which they occur in the dog in the United States.

### MASTOCYTOMAS

Mastocytomas are undoubtedly the most clinically significant skin tumor in dogs but are much less important in cats. In dogs, they have a very pronounced breed incidence, occurring with about twice the expected frequency in boxers, Boston terriers and Labrador retrievers and six times less frequently in Chihuahuas. They may arise anywhere in the skin, occur usually in middle-aged or older animals and can be divided clinically into two main types: In the more common type, the mass appears as a rapidly enlarging, ulcerated and sometimes multinodular tumor, with a firm, whitish cut surface mottled by areas of hemorrhage. The less common clinical type consists of a fairly well defined, slowly growing, soft and flabby tumor that shows little tendency toward ulceration through the overlying tissue and has a rubbery, pale-yellowish cut surface.

Rapidly growing tumors are revealed histologically as highly invasive cellular lesions composed of cells with large, immature nuclei and sparse cytoplasm. Mitotic figures are very common, and lymphatic infiltration may be conspicuous. Histologically, the slowly growing type is a well-differentiated tumor consisting of a fibrous stroma that contains a diffuse infiltrate of discrete mast cells, separated by edema fluid. Variable numbers of eosinophil polymorphs are also present, and mitotic figures are very rare. A type with an intermediate degree of differentiation, in which the cells, although having abundant cytoplasm, are fusing together to form solid sheets, is also discernible histologically.

These different morphologic types of mastocytoma are of considerable prognostic significance (Table 4). The percentage of 6-month survival is of importance, because the majority of dogs that survive for this length of time after surgery subsequently die from unrelated causes. Tumor deaths are generally due to massive metastasis to the regional lymph nodes, with inoperable

**Table 4.** *Postsurgical Survival Time of Dogs With Apparently Completely Excised Mastocytomas**

| TUMOR TYPE | DEAD FROM TUMOR AT 6 MONTHS (%) | MEDIAN SURVIVAL TIME (WEEKS) |
|---|---|---|
| Well-differentiated | 12 | 54 |
| Intermediate | 17 | 26 |
| Poorly Differentiated | 77 | 14 |

*Based on biopsy material from 114 cases.

local recurrence frequently complicating the condition. More distant metastasis, with tumors in the solid viscera and lungs, is unusual. The treatment of choice is therefore early radical excision of the primary tumor and regional lymph nodes, followed, in the case of intermediate and poorly differentiated tumors, by a course of radiotherapy to these sites as soon as the skin has healed. Total doses of up to 3500 rads given in five weekly fractions will give very useful palliation, although total cures, especially in the more malignant tumors, should not be expected.

Inoperable primary tumors may be treated directly by radiotherapy or multiple chemotherapy, as discussed for lymphosarcomas, following which temporary remissions lasting a few months can be expected.

In cats, mastocytomas appear as firm, whitish, dome-shaped nodules that measure less than ½ cm. in diameter. They frequently arise on the head, although multiple lesions all over the body do occur. Histologically, they resemble the intermediate type seen in dogs, without the eosinophil infiltration. Despite the straightforward nature of surgical excision of solitary nodules, the prognosis should always be guarded. The majority of cats develop a generalized disease, with widespread infiltration of the subcutaneous tissues, spleen, liver and bone marrow a few months after the initial surgery.

A rapid clinical diagnosis is made possible in most cases of mastocytoma by staining a touch preparation of the scarified surface, either following removal or *in situ*, with 1 per cent toluidine blue solution at pH 3.1 for 30 seconds. Following this procedure, all but the most poorly differentiated cells will show the presence of multiple intracytoplasmic red granules.

The cause of skin mastocytoma is not known but a related disease, mast cell leukemia, has been shown by Lombard, Moloney and Rickard to be caused by a transmissible agent in dogs.

## HEPATOID (PERIANAL) ADENOMAS

These neoplasms arise only in dogs, usually over 10 years of age, and are derived from the hepatoid cells found in the subcutaneous tissues around the anal ring, lateral to the prepuce, and on the dorsal and ventral surfaces on the root of the tail. The commonest site for neoplastic transformation is undoubtedly the perianal region. There is a marked sex predisposition—both American and British researchers have found the male/female ratio to be 8.8/1. Cocker spaniels may be more prone to the disease than are other breeds, and the marked difference in relative frequency of this neoplasm between the U.S.A. and the U.K., noted previously, could be due to a difference in breed distribution in the two areas. Anal adenomas are frequently multiple and appear as slowly growing, rubbery tumors that eventually ulcerate and bleed. The cut surface is pinkish and divided into numerous tiny lobules that can be seen histologically to consist of large, clearly defined epithelial cells with central, round nuclei and abundant eosinophilic cytoplasm. Mitoses are rare, although squamous metaplasia is a common finding.

Following wide surgical excision, the prognosis is good; however, owing to the nature of the site, complete removal is not always feasible, especially with large tumors. Local recurrence can therefore present a problem in up to 30 per cent of cases, although it is sometimes difficult to be certain whether these are recurrent tumors or new primary tumors arising from adjacent glands.

Since the majority of anal adenomas are under the influence of testosterone, castration or the administration of estrogens will often lead to marked, albeit temporary, regression. Intralesional injection of 10 to 20 mg of a long-acting preparation of diethylstilbestrol every 2 to 3 weeks for 3 to 5 injections will usually induce dramatic shrinkage. This type of treatment is especially valuable in reducing the size of large tumors prior to surgery but cannot be relied upon as the sole therapeutic regimen. Prolonged administration of estrogens must also be avoided because of the secondary effects on the prostate. Treatment by radiotherapy or cryosurgery can also be effective, although with both these methods there is considerable danger of fibrosis of the anal sphincter, with consequent intractable constipation if the entire anal ring is involved.

## HEPATOID ADENOCARCINOMAS

The malignant counterpart of the hepatoid adenoma is relatively uncommon and, surprisingly, occurs with equal frequency in male and female dogs. It appears as a rapidly growing, invasive and ulcerated mass composed of small, hyperchromatic cells with less cytoplasm than in adenomas. Although the cells are still arranged in solid lobules, small clumps can be seen invading the surrounding connective tissues and lymphatic vessels, with mitotic figures being common.

Because of the invasive nature of these tumors, total excision is difficult, and most hepatoid adenocarcinomas will recur locally within a few months. Metastasis to the deep inguinal lymph nodes and, less often, to the lungs, is also a common sequel, so that the prognosis must always be guarded. Hormonal therapy is of little value, but radiotherapy will induce temporary remissions.

## LIPOMAS

The incidence of lipomas in dogs is probably much greater than surveys based on surgically excised material would indicate since many of these tumors are detected only incidentally at postmortem examination. Clinically significant lesions arise about twice as frequently in female as in male dogs and are especially common in Labrador retrievers and small terriers. Predilection sites are the subcutaneous fat of the flanks, of the medial aspect of the thigh and of the sternal region in chronically overweight animals. Lipomas grow very slowly and on gross palpation feel soft and almost cystic in structure. They are mobile over the surrounding tissues, and the skin does not ulcerate or lose its hair. Although lipomas may be very large at diagnosis, lesions with a diameter of 10 cm. or more being common, surgical excision is simple in most cases.

Occasionally, especially with tumors in the groin, the mass will infiltrate between muscle bellies, rendering total removal impossible. Local recurrence is to be expected in these cases, and postoperative radiotherapy is of little value.

Grossly, lipomas are surrounded by a thin capsule and have a homogeneous cut surface composed of apparently normal fat. Histologically, this consists of a completely uniform sheet of large, clearly defined, fat-filled cells with tiny pyknotic nuclei. Some tumors also contain bundles of mature collagen.

Since affected dogs are usually obese, it seems likely that hyperplasia of the adipose tissue predisposes these tumors, which can be prevented by instituting sensible dietary habits. Even after diagnosis, an extremely strict diet is of great value for a few weeks prior to surgery, since this tends to reduce the size of the lesion and improve its definition from surrounding tissues. However, it may be difficult for the owner to appreciate the degree of calorie restriction necessary, and such attempts are doomed to failure unless supervised closely by the veterinarian.

### LIPOSARCOMAS

These are uncommon neoplasms that do not arise from lipomas but are rapidly growing and invasive from the start. The cut surface is firm, white and homogeneous, the histologic appearance being of a closely packed sheet of large cells with pale-staining nuclei and abundant cytoplasm. Mitoses may be common, and some cells contain one or more variably sized intracytoplasmic fat droplets.

If the site of the mass makes complete surgical excision feasible, the prognosis is fair. Although local recurrence does occur in a minority of cases, metastasis is unusual.

### SEBACEOUS ADENOMAS

These tumors are found mainly in elderly dogs and are less common in cats. There is no sex predisposition, but spaniels and Boston terriers are more commonly affected than are other dog breeds. Common predilection sites include the eyelids, face and head, although the back and limbs can also be involved. Multiple lesions are common and appear as small (less than 1 cm.), superficial, rubbery nodules covered by a thin,

shiny, hairless epithelium. Histologically, they consist of numerous, well-defined "packets" of mature sebaceous cells with abundant pale-staining and foamy cytoplasm, surrounded by a narrow rim of small, hyperchromatic "reserve" cells. In the less well-differentiated types, these reserve cells tend to predominate.

Sebaceous adenomas, which are often referred to as "warts," are usually of little clinical significance, although some may ulcerate and become infected while those on the eyelids can cause epiphora. The treatment of choice is surgical excision, which is straightforward and leads to a complete cure. Cryosurgery is also useful, especially for multiple lesions on the face.

### SEBACEOUS GLAND ADENOCARCINOMAS

Malignant sebaceous gland tumors are seen occasionally in dogs. They arise mainly on the face or neck and can be distinguished from their benign counterpart by their larger size, rapid rate of growth and early ulceration through the skin. Histologically, they consist almost entirely of active reserve cells, with a few differentiated cells among them. Mitotic figures and infiltration into surrounding tissues are conspicuous. Even in these malignant tumors, the prognosis is fair following adequate surgery, but about half will recur locally and metastasize to regional lymph nodes and lungs.

### FIBROSARCOMAS

Fibrosarcomas are the commonest skin tumors in cats in Britain, although in America they are not as important as squamous cell carcinomas, as previously noted. In both dogs and cats, there is a definite predisposition for the distal extremities, including the ears and nose in cats, although tumors on the flanks and back are also seen. The tumor appears clinically as a rapidly growing, invasive, ulcerated solitary mass closely attached to surrounding tissues. It is very firm in consistency and has a white, fibrous cut surface, consisting of haphazardly arranged, parallel bundles of fibroblasts that produce a variable amount of intercellular collagen. The edge of the lesion is indistinct, but there is no evidence of vascular infiltration.

The treatment of choice is radical surgical

excision. When this can be performed extensively enough, the prognosis is good, since metastasis is rare in both dog and cat. The main problem following surgery is local recurrence, which must be expected in tumors of the legs and face, especially in cats. In these cases, cures can be effected by amputation of the limb or tail, but when this is not possible, postoperative prophylactic radiotherapy is always a wise precaution and can delay recurrence for months or even years. The inoperable tumor is not particularly sensitive to radiotherapy or chemotherapy, and in these cases, the prognosis is hopeless.

The cause of fibrosarcomas in dogs is unknown, but American researchers have shown the feline disease to be transmissible and caused by a specific oncornavirus (feline sarcoma virus).

## MELANOMAS

Skin melanomas may be seen in most dog breeds but are rare in cats. They tend to occur more frequently in Scottish terriers than would be expected from the distribution of this breed in the general population.

These tumors can arise anywhere in the skin, although predilection sites include the eyelids, distal limbs, interdigital spaces and oral mucosa. They have a variable gross appearance and clinical behavior. Many are slowly growing, rubbery lesions, clearly demarcated from surrounding tissues and having an intensely, pigmented, black cut surface, while a smaller proportion grow rapidly, invade surrounding tissues and ulcerate through the overlying skin. The latter tend to have a less pigmented cut surface and may contain completely amelanotic areas.

These gross differences are reflected in the histologic appearance. Although no melanoma is encapsulated, the smaller, slowly growing tumors are well defined and composed of a loose stroma, heavily infiltrated by polygonal cells, the internal structure of which is obscured by masses of intracytoplasmic melanin. The more rapidly growing types are invasive and composed of spindle-shaped cells, with oval, hyperchromatic nuclei, often arranged in bundles or whorls. Only a proportion contain pigment, and mitoses may be common.

After treatment, about 25 per cent of dogs with skin melanomas develop widespread visceral metastases, usually within six months of the original surgery. Tumor-related deaths are rare after a year has elapsed. Well-defined, heavily pigmented lesions carry a much better prognosis than invasive, rapidly proliferating tumors, but there is little evidence that the site of the tumor affects the outcome of treatment. Well-differentiated tumors can occasionally metastasize but tend to do so many months after surgery.

Forms of treatment other than surgery have been employed infrequently. Localized tumors are usually radiosensitive, but the visceral metastases present a major therapeutic problem that prevents use of conventional techniques.

## SQUAMOUS CELL CARCINOMAS

Relatively, cats are affected much more frequently than dogs. Predilection sites in cats include the ear tips, eyelids and external nares (nearly always when these areas are white), but in dogs, lesions may be found anywhere on the head, flanks or limbs. In cats, squamous cell carcinomas usually appear as small, highly erosive lesions, with a firm fibrous base closely attached to the underlying tissues. They become covered with crusts of dried brownish exudate and initially may be confused with inflammatory reactions.

Histologically, they are composed of a fibrous stroma containing irregularly shaped, solid foci of prickle cells. Cells toward the center of each focus tend to undergo keratinization, and tumors can be graded into prognostically significant types on this basis (Table 5). Following radical surgery, the prognosis is favorable for well-differentiated tumors but very poor for poorly differentiated tumors, because of the frequency of regional lymph node and pulmonary metastasis in addition to local recurrence.

White cats may develop a precancerous hyperkeratosis of the ear tips, often present for some years before malignant transformation supervenes. Removal of the pinna in these cases is a valuable prophylactic procedure.

Fortunately, the majority of squamous cell carcinomas in dogs are well differentiated, and following surgery, the prognosis is favorable. Behavior of the unusual poorly differentiated lesions is similar to

**Table 5.** *Prognosis Following Surgical Excision of Feline Squamous Cell Carcinoma of the Skin\**

| TUMOR TYPE | 6-MONTH SURVIVAL (%) | MEDIAN SURVIVAL TIME (WEEKS) |
|---|---|---|
| Well-differentiated | 100 | 42 |
| Poorly Differentiated | 0 | 17 |

\*Based on biopsy material from 21 cases.

that in cats, and the same considerations apply.

The cause of squamous cell carcinomas in dogs is not known, but the propensity for cats to develop them in unpigmented areas has been ascribed to the carcinogenic effect of sunlight.

## FIBROMAS

Fibromas occur about four times more frequently in female than in male dogs in Great Britain, although this is apparently not the case in America. They are unusual in cats in Britain, as previously noted. The gross appearance is of a slowly growing, well-defined tumor that does not infiltrate the surrounding tissues and is often seen in the groin and vulvar region in bitches, other predilection sites being the limbs and flanks. The cut surface is yellowish-white, rubbery and obviously fibrous. The overlying skin does not ulcerate but may lose its hair. The histologic appearance is mature collagenous fibers laid down in parallel bundles or large whorls by small, oval cells with densely staining nuclei and sparse cytoplasm. Mitotic figures are rare, and the mass is clearly separated from the surrounding connective tissues.

Following complete excision, the prognosis is good.

## HEMANGIOPERICYTOMAS

The great majority of hemangiopericytomas arise in dogs, nearly always on the limbs. There is no strong breed association, although some authors have suggested an increased frequency in boxers and spaniels, with most affected animals over 10 years of age.

These tumors are believed to arise from the supporting cells of blood vessels and are usually slowly growing, multinodular masses, tightly fixed to the skin and underlying fascia and having a firm fibrous, yellowish cut surface. Histologically, they are nonencapsulated and are composed of small, spindle-shaped cells, with active hyperchromatic nuclei, producing a sparse intercellular collagenous stroma. The characteristic appearance is of tight whorls, a few cells wide, arranged around a central capillary; however, in the more rapidly growing lesions, this appearance is lost, at which point differentiation from fibrosarcoma can be difficult.

Hemangiopericytomas are often neglected, since they cause little discomfort to the dog, and may thus be very large when advice is finally sought. Large tumors on the distal extremities can present a considerable surgical problem, so that in these cases, local recurrence is frequent. Metastasis is rare from all but the most poorly differentiated lesions, however, and a cure can be expected following amputation of the limb when multiple local recurrence has proved impossible to control by more conservative therapy.

## HEMANGIOMAS

Hemangiomas are well-defined, slowly growing neoplasms which in Great Britain are seen mainly in dogs. They generally arise in the loose skin of the trunk or neck but can be found on the legs, are rarely more than 1 to 2 cm. in diameter and have a dark purple cut surface. On gross examination they may be difficult to distinguish from melanomas, but if gently washed, hemangiomas develop a characteristic "honeycomb" or lacy appearance. Histologically, the neoplasm is sharply demarcated from the surrounding tissues and consists of large blood-filled spaces separated by a thin, mature fibrous wall that is lined by a single layer of flattened, well-differentiated endothelium.

Following surgical excision, the prognosis is good; local recurrence is most unusual.

## HISTIOCYTOMAS

These tumors are confined to dogs and appear to be more common in Britain than in America (Table 1). They can arise in most breeds, although there is some indication that boxers and Labradors are more frequently affected, and have a characteristic age distribution, most affected dogs being between 4 months and 4 years old, with a peak incidence at about 18 months. Predilection sites include the face, ears and feet; on gross examination the lesion appears as a solitary, dome-shaped, painful mass that grows rapidly to a maximum diameter of 1 to 2 cm. in a few weeks. The overlying skin loses its hair and then ulcerates, but the tumor is freely mobile over the subcutaneous tissues, and the regional lymph nodes are not involved. Histologically, the appearance is of a closely packed and homogeneous sheet of large histiocytic cells with oval, pale-staining, indented nuclei and indistinct cytoplasmic boundaries. Mitotic figures are common, and the tumor has a highly malignant appearance. In older lesions, a diffuse infiltration by lymphocytes becomes conspicuous, and in longstanding tumors these cells predominate.

Treatment by either conventional surgery or cryosurgery will result in a complete cure, with local recurrence being rare and metastasis unknown. Indeed, if histiocytomas are not treated, they will regress spontaneously within a few weeks. This type of behavior is suggestive of a virus-induced tumor, but attempts at cell-free transmission have so far failed.

## BASAL CELL TUMORS

Basal cell tumors are believed to arise from the stratum germinativum and are relatively much more common in cats than in dogs. In both species, they arise mainly on the head and neck; in dogs, they show a marked breed predisposition, with spaniels being most frequently affected. The gross appearance is of a well-defined mobile tumor, with a firm, whitish cut surface, which may reach several centimeters in diameter before diagnosis is made. The histologic appearance is variable, the majority of tumors consisting of a dense, mature collagenous stroma that contains numerous clearly defined solid foci of epithelial cells. These are often brick-shaped, with the outer layer of cells arranged radially. In rare cases, a few of the central cells are keratinized and the term "basosquamous" tumor can be employed, while some tumors, called trichoepitheliomas, produce structures resembling mature hair follicles. Other morphologic types in which the cells

form loops or chains are also seen. Some basal cell tumors are heavily pigmented, owing to the accumulation of intracytoplasmic melanin granules, and these may be confused with melanomas on gross inspection.

There is no prognostic significance related to the different morphologic types. Surgical excision is generally uncomplicated and local recurrence unusual, although there have been a few reports of metastasis, probably from poorly differentiated tumors.

## RETICULUM CELL SARCOMAS

These tumors present a considerable diagnostic problem, especially in dogs, because they must be distinguished from histiocytomas, poorly differentiated mastocytomas, histiocytic lymphosarcomas and chronic inflammatory lesions. Unlike histiocytomas, reticulum cell sarcomas arise in middle-aged or older animals, in which they appear as a solitary, rapidly growing dome-shaped lesion on the feet, face or flanks. This is not self-limiting and soon ulcerates through the skin. The owner usually presents the animal at a relatively early stage, for the tumors cause considerable irritation. Histologically, the appearance is of a diffuse infiltration of the dermal connective tissues by cells with oval, indented nuclei and indistinct cytoplasmic boundaries. The cells are not arranged in any definite pattern, and mitoses are fairly common. Staining for reticulin may reveal a network of fine fibers surrounding individual cells, but this is lost in the less well-differentiated tumors.

Following surgical excision, the prognosis is fair, with a small proportion of dogs subsequently experiencing local recurrence and metastasis to the regional lymph nodes. Figures are not available for the prognosis in cats, but it is probably worse than that for dogs. Reticulum cell sarcomas are extremely radiosensitive, and useful palliation can be obtained in dogs with metastatic tumors by this means or by the use of combination chemotherapy, as for lymphosarcoma.

## PAPILLOMAS

Papillomas are almost invariably seen in dogs and, apart from the multiple intraoral masses caused by a host-specific papo vavirus, are small, solitary lesions found mainly on the head, eyelids and feet.

They are between four and five times more common in male than in female dogs, although there is no breed predisposition, and appear as raised, crusty lesions that rarely measure more than 1 cm. in diameter. They are clinically insignificant, and therefore the tendency is to remove them only following traumatic injury or secondary infection.

Histologically, the appearance is of multiple, finger-like projections of the dermal connective tissues, covered by an extremely hyperkeratotic stratified squamous epithelium. The rete pegs are long and branching, but there is no tendency for isolated cell nests to penetrate the mesodermal tissues.

Following surgical excision or cryosurgery, the prognosis is excellent.

## PERINEURAL FIBROBLASTOMAS (NEURILEMOMA, SCHWANNOMA)

Perineural fibroblastomas arise occasionally in the subcutaneous tissues in dogs but very rarely in cats. They are similar, both morphologically and behaviorally, to hemangiopericytomas and may be a variation of this tumor, although on histologic examination they are seen to contain large, solid whorls of spindle-shaped cells. The central zone is amorphous and hyaline in appearance, resembling the pacinian corpuscles from which they are considered to arise.

## SWEAT GLAND ADENOMAS

Most of these tumors arise on the back or flanks in old dogs, especially spaniels, and appear as well-defined, slowly growing lesions that are rarely more than 2 cm. in diameter at diagnosis. They have a fibrous cut surface that frequently contains a number of cysts, is lined by a thin, shiny membrane and is filled with a watery, yellowish secretion. Histologically, the cysts are lined by a flattened cuboidal epithelium that sometimes forms papillary ingrowths into the lumen, while solid tumors are composed of mature fibrous stroma that contains small, discrete tubules.

Surgical excision is straightforward, and following this, the prognosis should be good.

## SWEAT GLAND ADENOCARCINOMAS

Sweat gland adenocarcinomas arise on the back, flanks and feet. They usually enlarge quite slowly but are adherent to the surrounding tissues and skin, which eventually ulcerates. They may measure several centimeters in diameter and have a pale, fibrous cut surface that is seen to contain multiple irregular tubules separated by a collagenous stroma on histologic examination. The tubules are lined by a columnar epithelium that may be arranged as branching papillary structures within the lumen. Infiltration into the surrounding tissues is usual, but vascular invasion is seen only in poorly differentiated carcinomas.

Following wide surgical excision, the prognosis should be favorable, although poorly differentiated tumors can recur locally and will, rarely, metastasize.

## MALIGNANT HEMANGIOENDOTHELIOMAS (HEMANGIOSARCOMAS)

Fortunately, these highly malignant neoplasms are uncommon in both cats and dogs, but among the latter they are usually seen in German shepherds.

They can arise anywhere in the skin, are rapidly growing and usually ulcerate through the overlying epidermis at an early stage. There is no definite edge, and the tumor is firmly attached to surrounding tissues, making total removal very difficult. The cut surface is firm, sometimes mottled by hemorrhage, and in the larger masses contains areas of necrosis. Histologically, the appearance is of numerous plump, oval cells that may be lining small, flattened, blood-filled spaces or merely arranged in a closely packed sheet. Mitotic figures are common, and there is obvious infiltration of surrounding connective tissue. Great care must be taken to distinguish between these tumors and exuberant granulation tissue, in which the capillary proliferation can resemble a neoplastic change, although in the latter mitotic figures are unusual and there is generally an accompanying fibroblastic proliferation.

Following any form of treatment, the prognosis for animals with malignant hemangioendothelioma must be poor, with local recurrence and widespread metastasis almost invariable.

## Myxosarcomas

These tumors are seen about twice as frequently in female as in male dogs but are unusual in cats. They are a variant of the fibrosarcoma and usually arise in the subcutaneous tissue of the groin, back or limbs. The gross appearance is of a poorly defined, soft and spreading mass composed of whitish, translucent, gelatinous material that is very difficult to excise surgically. Histologically, myxosarcomas are relatively acellular, consisting mainly of an abundant mucinous matrix that separates small numbers of polygonal cells with long, filamentous cytoplasmic processes. Mitoses are rare, and vascular invasion is absent.

These tumors do not metastasize, so that radical surgical excision should lead to a complete cure. Unfortunately, however, because of their spreading nature, removal is rarely complete unless the mass is situated in a limb that can be amputated. For lesions in other sites, the prognosis must always be poor, with multiple local recurrence to be expected.

Well-defined benign tumors (myxomas) can be encountered, but these are much less common than their malignant counterpart.

## Leiomyomas

These tumors are unusual in dogs and rare in cats. Four times more common in bitches than in male dogs, they are often found in the vulvar lips and the groin but can also be encountered on the back and flanks. Leiomyomas grow slowly and appear as well-defined, hard nodules with a pale, homogeneous cut surface that is seen, microscopically, to consist of mature smooth muscle cells arranged as interdigitating parallel bundles, producing a "herringbone" pattern.

Surgical excision is generally straightforward, and the prognosis should be favorable.

The rare malignant tumors, leiomyosarcomas, closely resemble fibrosarcomas in both appearance and behavior. They can be distinguished from leiomyomas histologically by their invasive nature and poorly differentiated constituent cells, many of which contain mitotic figures.

## Calcifying epitheliomas

These are unusual tumors that arise on the back and flanks of old dogs, where they are slowly growing but tend to become superficially ulcerated and secondarily infected. The cut surface is firm and fibrous and contains large dry, crumbly areas with a chalky center, which on histologic examination are seen to consist of solid foci of heavily keratinized prickle cells. The central cells have lost their structure and are being replaced by calcified, structureless debris, while there is a thin zone of small, hyperchromatic prickle cells at the rim of each focus.

The prognosis is good, since these tumors do not metastasize and local recurrence is rare following surgical excision.

## Ceruminous gland adenocarcinomas

Although rare in dogs, ceruminous gland tumors are among the commonest skin neoplasms of cats. They arise from the wax-secreting glands of the external auditory canal and, unlike other adnexal tumors, are usually malignant, appearing as a solitary, quite rapidly growing, dome-shaped fleshy mass that protrudes from the canal. Histologically, the degree of differentiation is variable, the commonest type consisting of a loose, fibrous stroma that contains closely packed, irregularly shaped tubular structures lined by one or more layers of columnar epithelial cells. Vascular infiltration is not common, and the diagnosis of malignancy is based upon invasion of the surrounding connective tissues by neoplastic cells.

Because of the inaccessible nature of the site and the invasiveness of the tumor, total excision is difficult, and the usual sequel is local recurrence. In a minority of cases, metastasis to the parotid lymph node is also seen, but cures can be effected in early cases by radical excision. This type of tumor may also respond well to cryosurgery.

The less common benign tumors or ceruminous adenomas are small, circumscribed, slowly growing masses that consist histologically of mature acini lined by well-differentiated columnar cells and containing an eosinophilic secretion. Following surgical excision of these lesions the prognosis is good.

## Lymphosarcomas

Although lymphosarcomas are very common neoplasms in dogs and cats, primary skin manifestations are rare in both species. When they do occur, the appearance is quite typical: nodules develop simultaneously in many areas, with a predilection for the abdomen, face and ears. The lesions begin as small, dome-shaped masses, about 5 mm. in diameter, which ulcerate and enlarge to produce irregular, plaquelike erosions, each with a red, weeping and painful surface and a raised, firm edge. Adjacent lesions will often coalesce to produce extensive ulcers, especially on the abdomen.

In some animals, the skin lesions are the only ones present at diagnosis, although many animals will have grossly enlarged superficial lymph nodes. Dogs may also show an associated leukemia, with total white cell counts in excess of 50,000 cu. mm.

Examination of a biopsy specimen from the edge of the ulcerated area will reveal heavy infiltration of the dermis by a homogeneous sheet of cells, which in dogs are often histiocytic in type. These have large, pale-staining, indented nuclei and a moderate amount of cytoplasm, while lymphocytic or lymphoblastic types predominate in cats.

The prognosis is always very poor, and even with treatment, survival for longer than 15 weeks is unusual. However, useful palliation and alleviation of the clinical signs can be obtained by chemotherapy. A combination of vincristine sulfate, cytosine arabinoside, prednisone and cyclophosphamide used simultaneously is especially effective. The dosage schedule for this is as follows:

Vincristine sulfate: 0.5 mg./M$^2$ by IV injection. Once weekly for 4 to 6 weeks, then once every 2 weeks.

Cytosine arabinoside: 100 mg./M$^2$ by IV injection. Once daily for the first 4 days of treatment. Repeat every 2 months if necessary.

Cyclophosphamide: 50 mg./M$^2$ orally every other day for one month, then every other day on alternate weeks.

Prednisone: 20 mg./M$^2$ orally daily for 1 week, then every other day. This treatment will probably need to be continued indefinitely, with a monthly check on total WBC.

The body-surface area of an animal can be calculated from the following formula: Surface area = 2.268 × Weight in kg.$^{0.367}$ × Length in cm. (taken ventrally from the tip of the nose to the base of the tail). (See also conversion table in Appendix.)

[*Editor's Note:* In the last few years, there have been a few reports of canine mycosis fungoides. Clinically, this presents as ulcerative lesions that tend to heal with some resultant crusting and scaling. As some lesions heal, others will appear. There is some predilection for the mucocutaneous junctions, but the lesion may become generalized.

Histologically, two forms are distinguished: the preneoplastic stage and the tumor stage. In the former, there is a dermal infiltrate with mononuclear cells— lymphocytes, histiocytes and some larger cells. In the later stage, the large mononuclear cells predominate and invade the epidermis, forming microabscesses of Pautrier.

Topical nitrogen mustards are of therapeutic value in man, but to date there are no reports of their use in dogs.]

## SUPPLEMENTAL READING

Bostock, D. E.: The prognosis in cats bearing squamous cell carcinoma. J. Small Animal Pract., 13:119–125, 1972.

Bostock, D. E.: The prognosis following surgical removal of mastocytomas in dogs. J. Small Animal Pract., 14:27–40, 1973.

Bostock, D. E.: The prognosis following the surgical excision of canine mammary neoplasms. Europ. J. Cancer, 11:389–396, 1975.

Bostock, D. E., and Owen, L. N.: An Atlas of Neoplasia in the Cat, Dog and Horse. London, Wolfe Medical Publications, 1975.

Brodey, R. S.: Canine and feline neoplasia. Adv. Vet. Sci. Comp. Med., 14:309–354, 1970.

Dorn, C. R., Taylor, D. O. N., Schneider, R., Hibbard, H. H., and Klauber, M. R.: Survey of animal neoplasms in Alameda and Contra Costa Counties, California. II. Cancer morbidity in dogs and cats from Alameda County. J. Natl. Cancer Inst., 40:307–318, 1968.

Lombard, L. S., Moloney, J. B., and Rickard, C. G.: Transmissible canine mastocytoma. Ann. N.Y. Acad. Sci., 108:1086–1105, 1963.

Weijer, K., Head, K. W., Misdorp, W., and Hampe, J. F.: Feline malignant mammary tumors. I. Morphology and biology: Some comparisons with human and canine mammary carcinomas. J. Natl. Cancer Inst., 49:1697–1705, 1972.

World Health Organization Bulletin: International Histological Classification of Tumors of Domestic Animals. 50:1–142, 1974.

# TOPICAL DERMATOLOGIC THERAPY

R. M. SCHWARTZMAN, V.M.D.
*Philadelphia, Pennsylvania*

## INTRODUCTION

Although the discussion in this chapter centers on local or topical therapy, systemic treatment should be of equal importance in the management of the patient with a dermatologic problem. The influence of other systems on the skin often demands that treatment be internal as well as topical. It would be irrational to treat a dermatosis related to a Sertoli cell tumor or atopic disease by means of external application of medicaments when the correct therapeutic approaches are the surgical removal of the testes and hyposensitization, respectively. As in all branches of medicine, the patient must be considered as a whole—one cannot separate the integumentary system from the other systems of the animal. Furthermore, correct treatment depends upon the definitive diagnosis.

Dermatologic therapy is as much an art as it is a science. This chapter will serve to instruct the reader in general terms concerning when to apply a particular agent and vehicle; however, knowledge in handling the dermatologic patient will be best gained through experience.

Although topical therapy may be utilized for specific treatment of a patient (as in the case of an animal with scabies), in the main it more often serves to (1) abate or control a dermatosis until specific measures can be employed, (2) facilitate healing in conjunction with that afforded by specific internal medication or (3) control or cure a problem of unknown cause.

There are particular difficulties related to the practice of understanding topical dermatologic therapy. Today, the modes of action of many drugs employed in the practice of dermatology are not known. Tar and sulfur are used extensively and with remarkable success in the management of skin diseases despite the fact that the molecular mechanism involved in their activity is not known. Veterinarians face additional problems in the practice of topical dermatologic therapy in that most of the veterinary literature dealing with the subject has not been related to in-depth studies that allow critical evaluation of the particular medicament. Also, information dealing with species idiosyncrasies to drugs rarely finds its way into the veterinary literature. The most intensive investigative work dealing with dermatologic agents has been done in man and small laboratory animals, and this information, though useful, does not necessarily apply to the domestic animal. Investigations dealing with the stratum corneum and the composition of the epidermal lipid film and sebaceous glands in domestic animals must be undertaken to provide background information for an understanding of percutaneous absorption of drugs.

## GENERAL PRINCIPLES

1. Certainty of diagnosis is almost always necessary for proper treatment. However, in the absence of etiologic information, topical therapy is an important aspect of the therapeutic management of the patient. In addition, topical therapy is of value as an adjunct to systemic treatment and will hasten the recovery to a normal state.

2. The choice of topical measures is determined largely by the presenting morphologic characteristics and the stage and site of the eruption. One should be able to recognize the nature of a dermatosis—acute or chronic, dry or exudative, infected or noninfected, superficial or deep—and treat it accordingly.

3. Topical remedies are chosen to produce specific effects according to the characteristics of the lesion. Practice and study can lead to mastery. It is strongly suggested that one use a few remedies and know everything that there is to know about them rather than be confused by the vast ocean of available dermatologic drugs.

4. A remedy may harm rather than help. When in doubt, begin with the mildest and most indifferent agent; when using a new medicament, observe the effect on a small area before proceeding to a larger area. Do not change to a new remedy as long as the dermatosis is improving satisfactorily with the older one.

5. When a remedy disagrees with the patient, discontinue its use at once and try to find the cause of the disagreement.

6. The action of topical remedies will depend to some degree on the mode of application and removal. One must give adequate instructions to the client and often demonstrate exactly the correct manner of use, application and removal of each preparation.

## TYPES OF VEHICLE

As mentioned previously, the choice of a particular remedy is largely dependent upon the morphologic characteristics of an eruption. It is therefore important to be able to recognize a particular type of eruption before choosing a particular medical program.

An acute eruption is one in which weeping, exudation, erythema, edema or vesiculation and crusting are evident. The eruption is sore, hot to the touch and tender or painful to the patient. The subacute eruption is characterized by infiltration and thickening of the skin, minimal erythema and edema and varying degrees of pigmentation and is warm to the touch. The chronic eruption is one in which pigmentation and thickening of the skin are marked; scaling and crusting are evident; there is little or no erythema, weeping or vesiculation; and the lesion is cold to the touch and not tender to the patient.

Wet dressings, medicated baths and lotions are indicated for treatment of the acute eruption (listed in order of preference). Shake lotions and pastes are most applicable to the subacute eruption. Ointments and creams are indicated for the chronic eruption.

*Cleansing baths* are used to remove dirt, debris, scale, etc. Usually the temperature of the water should be between 95 and 100° F. Soap which is alkaline in reaction may be used in the more chronic type of dermatoses but is contraindicated in acutely irritated eruptions. Neutral soaps or soaps formed of corn oil, tallow, coconut oil, olive oil, whale oil and sesame oil are less irritating and may be employed in the more acute eruptions. After being bathed, the patient should be dried by patting with soft towels rather than by vigorous rubbing.

*Medicated baths* achieve a number of results, depending on the particular ingredient incorporated in them. For example, sulfur and tar baths are antiseborrheic in their effect, tar baths are antipruritic and antieczematous, colloidal baths (corn starch and baking soda) are soothing and antipruritic and oil baths serve to lubricate and hydrate the skin. In general, medicated baths are soothing in their effect and are particularly applicable to veterinary medicine, in which dermatoses involve large areas of the animal's integumentary system. It is obvious that a cow with a generalized eruption may not be treated economically with topical applications of antibiotic cream or ointment. A medicated bath is applied either as a shampoo (as with antiseborrheic agents) or by pouring the medicament on the animal and allowing it to remain on the patient for a varying period of time. The individual response to the medicated bath usually determines the frequency of medication required.

*Moist compresses* (wet dressings) are particularly soothing and are indicated for the acute eruption. They maintain drainage, are efficient in cleansing and prevent rapid changes in the temperature of the skin. In general, they are antiphlogistic, antipruritic and mildly antiseptic. The compresses should be sufficiently thick (20 layers of gauze or turkish towel pinned snugly above the affected part, with or without an impermeable wrapping—plastic wrap, oil cloth, etc.), kept constantly wet and changed frequently (every two hours if possible). Moist compresses represent the most satisfactory method of handling an acute eruption. However, their use in veterinary medicine may be impractical, since they require extensive nursing care, which is often not available, and a reasonable degree of cooperation from the patient, which one cannot always obtain. Among common solutions used for wet dressings are saline, Burow's solution (aluminum acetate diluted 1 part to 10 or 20) for its anti-inflammatory effect, boric acid solution (4 teaspoons to 1 pint of water) as an antiseptic and potassium permanganate solution (1 part to 4,000 or 10,000) for mycotic infections.

*Powders* are most conveniently used in the treatment of intertriginous areas. They protect from the irritating action of friction and from maceration and also exert a cooling effect. Different powders are selected because of particular characteristics. Zinc oxide and talc are white and are somewhat absorbent. Kaolin is highly absorbent. Boric acid powder has antiseptic properties. Powdered tannic acid is an astringent. Undecylenics and other fatty acid powders are fungistatic in effect. Menthol is cooling, and powdered sulfur is antiparasitic.

*Shake lotions* (or lotions) are liquid preparations usually having water (with suspending agents such as methylcellulose), alcohol or both as a base, with active ingredients in solution or suspension. As the liquid evaporates, a cooling effect is achieved at the inflamed site, and the ingredient remains in contact with the lesion. Lotions are especially useful in extensive dermatoses, since they may be painted or dabbed on. They should not be used in exudative dermatoses, because they block oozing or weeping. Various medications, such as antipruritics, keratolytics and antiseptics, are added to the solutions and affect the eruption accordingly. In general, lotions have certain advantages; they are easy to apply, cooling, drying and protective. Their disadvantages are that they are not penetrating and usually have a superficial action.

*Liniments* are oily or fatty substances emulsified or suspended in an aqueous medium or other liquid solutions suspended in an oily medium (e.g., carron oil, which is an emulsion of linseed oil and limewater). Liniments constitute a transition medicament between lotions and ointments. Their advantages are that they are easy to apply, protective, soothing and softening. They are fairly penetrating. Their disadvantages are that they are occlusive, heating, greasy and messy.

*Ointments* or salves, creams and oils are perhaps the oldest form of topical dermatologic preparations. They are fatty substances, the base of which is animal, vegetable or mineral fats (petrolatum); emulsion bases; or inert oils (Carbowax®). Ointments in general have the following advantages or indications: they are softening and protective and facilitate the removal of scale and crusts; many have good penetrating activity.

In addition, they usually can absorb large quantities of moisture, and significant amounts of active medicaments may be incorporated into them. Their major disadvantages are that they may be greasy and are heating and occlusive. Surface-active agents such as Span® (sorbitan esters) and Tween® (a sorbitan polyoxyalkalene derivative) are often incorporated in ointment bases to increase the penetration of drugs.

**Emulsions.** The oil-in-water emulsion bases (washable bases) appear to improve the penetration of active medicaments by facilitating intimate contact between the drug and the cellular structure of the skin. The water-in-oil type of emulsion and inert oils tend to occlude the skin surface, thereby inhibiting evaporation and leading to swelling and hydration of the stratum corneum, which in itself leads to greater penetration of medicaments.

OIL-IN-WATER EMULSIONS. As indicated by the name, these emulsions contain oil droplets dispersed in a continuous phase of water. A variety of lipid materials and emulsifiers are employed: higher fatty alcohols, petrolatum, glycerine, water and an emulsifying agent (Unibase®, Parke-Davis); stearyl alcohol, glyceryl monostearate, spermaceti, propylene glycol, mineral oil, water, a preservative and an emulsifying agent (Dermabase®, Mancelle); saturated aliphatic alcohols, polyhydric alcohol, lauric acid esters, petrolatum, water and an emulsifying agent (Multibase® Ar-Ex).

Since the bases are freely miscible in water, they provide two immediate advantages: they may be used successfully in exudative lesions, and they are not greasy to the touch and can easily be washed out of the hair coat. In general, the oil-in-water emulsions are quite penetrating and are preferred as vehicles for protective agents against ultraviolet light. In veterinary practice, the oil-in-water emulsions are highly desirable, because of the ease with which they may be washed out of the pelage and because they do not stain rugs, upholstery, clothing, etc.

WATER-IN-OIL EMULSIONS. In this vehicle form, water is dispersed in a continuous phase of oil. These emulsions are useful in lubricating the skin surface and are particularly suitable for incorporation of antibiotics. They are reasonably penetrating in their action. As mentioned previously, the water-in-oil emulsions tend to occlude the skin surface, leading to suppression of evaporation and swelling of the stratum corneum, which in itself allows for greater penetration of drugs incorporated in the ointment.

A variety of lipid materials are employed in the synthesis of water-in-oil bases. Hydrosorb® (Abbott) is a mixture of oleic acid ester and amide of diethanolamine, oleic acid and white petrolatum; Aquaphor® (Duke) is a mixture of esters and alcohols or cholesterol and petrolatum; lanolin is wool fat with 25 to 30 per cent water; Polysorb® (Fougera) contains sorbitan sesquioleate in a wax petrolatum mixture.

The *inert oils* (including petrolatum, mineral oil, Carbowax® and polyethylene glycol) are in general more occlusive than the previously mentioned ointments. They are particularly indicated when retention of heat is desired and for the incorporation of antibiotics. Their action tends to be more superficial than the emulsion bases, although through suppression of evaporation and swelling of the stratum corneum, some degree of penetration of incorporated drugs is allowed.

Petrolatum is a purified mixture of semi-solid hydrocarbons obtained from petroleum, and mineral oil or liquid petrolatum is a mixture of liquid hydrocarbons.

Carbowax and polyethylene glycols are miscible in water and are mixtures of polymers with the formula $HOCH_2$ $(CH_2OCH_2)_n$ $CH_2OH$. The number (n) placed after Carbowax or polyethylene glycol is indicative of the approximate molecular weight. The range of molecular weight for polyethylene glycol is 200 to 700 and for Carbowax is 1000 to 6000. The viscosity of the polyethylene glycols and the melting point of Carbowax are directly proportional to the molecular weight.

*Vanishing creams* are oil-in-water emulsions containing stearic acid and a large quantity of water. They disappear when rubbed into the integument. The cold creams are employed for their cosmetic effect (cleansing and emollient). They are water-in-oil or oil-in-water emulsions and usually consist of beeswax, mineral oil, borax and water.

*Pastes* are semisolid preparations consisting of mixtures of greases and finely dispersed powder in varying proportions (usually 50:50). Pastes provide the skin's surface with a protective layer, tend to absorb secretions to a certain degree and in general have a milder effect and are less macerating, occlusive and heating when compared with ointments.

*Propylene glycol* (1,2-propanediol) has become increasingly popular as a dermatologic vehicle in recent years. It is a clear, colorless, viscous and odorless liquid. It absorbs moisture when exposed to air and is completely miscible in all proportions in water, chloroform and acetone. It is soluble in ether and will dissolve in many essential oils. Propylene glycol is bacteriostatic, capable of inhibiting the growth of certain organisms (staphylococci, streptococci and *E. coli*).

Studies dealing with the toxicity of propylene glycol have shown it to be a relatively innocuous material. The single oral $LD_{50}$ for dogs is 0.5 gm./kg. of body weight. When administered parenterally, high doses of propylene glycol produce a tranquilizing or depressant effect. Intramuscular injections of propylene glycol result in a local irritation reaction. Topical applications of propylene glycol produce little to no toxicity, sensitization or irritation.

As a dermatologic vehicle, propylene glycol serves as an excellent solvent for many active dermatologic medicaments and usually does not react with them. It spreads evenly on the cutaneous surface and penetrates the lesions on which it is applied. Prolonged contact of the active agent with the diseased skin is afforded by propylene glycol because of its slow evaporation rate. It is nongreasy and freely washable from the hair coat and does not stain clothing, rugs, upholstery, etc. In general, it serves to soften and humidify the skin. It appears to be an ideal vehicle in veterinary medicine (when one is dealing with an entirely scalped animal) because of its miscibility in water and nonocclusive action. It can be used in intertriginous areas and with exudative lesions, where an aqueous vehicle might add too much moisture to an already wet area and oils or greasy vehicles might aggravate a situation already present.

## DIMETHYL SULFOXIDE

Dimethyl sulfoxide (DMSO), a derivative of lignin, is a highly polar, stable, hydroscopic organic liquid with remarkable solvent properties. It is freely miscible with lipids, organic solvents and water.

DMSO possesses a number of interesting

pharmacologic actions: (1) antiinflammatory activity; (2) bacteriostatic activity; (3) diuretic activity (in dogs); (4) local analgesia; (5) as a penetrant-carrier, with enhanced absorption of heparin, insulin and sulfadiazine through the intact bladder; (6) potentiation of insulin in the dog; and (7) as a tranquilizer, when applied topically.

It has been shown by a number of investigators that DMSO promotes the cutaneous penetration of a number of substances: (1) vasoconstrictors, (2) antiperspirants and (3) corticosteroids. Additionally, studies have shown that DMSO has no effect on potentiating topically applied anesthetic agents, and with some materials it may have the paradoxical effect of interfering with penetration. The mechanism by which DMSO promotes skin penetration has not been established. It is known, however, that it does not disrupt the horny membrane or affect the stress-strain capacity of the stratum corneum and has little effect on the water-holding capacity of the horny layer.

It is generally accepted that rather high concentrations of DMSO are necessary to achieve promotion of penetration of an active agent. Usually a concentration of at least 70 per cent is necessary before the effectiveness of DMSO to enhance penetration is realized.

# MISCELLANEOUS TOPICAL AGENTS

## SILICONES

Silicones such as Silicote® ointment and Silicote® liquid spray (Anar-Stone) are polymers of dimethyl siloxan. They impart a chemically inert protective film when applied to the skin's surface. They are not miscible with water and therefore are of value in protecting the skin from draining wounds or exposure to unusually moist or humid environmental conditions. They are less resistant to oils and organic solvents.

## SOAPS

Ordinary soap is a sodium or potassium salt of fatty acids. As soaps emulsify lipids with water, they help to remove dirt from the skin. The ordinary soap hydrolyzes in water and produces an alkaline reaction, which in itself may be irritating to the skin.

The neutral soaps or soap substitutes usually consist of long-chain esters with a sul-

fate salt at the end of the molecule. In an aqueous medium they yield a pH of approximately 7. Examples of neutral soaps are Lowela® (Westwood), which contains sodium lauryl sulfoacetate in a corn dextrin base acidified with lactic acid, and Dove® (Lever), which contains acyl isothionate.

Germistatic soaps are used in veterinary medicine and are of value as an adjuvant in the treatment of bacterial infections of the skin. In general, the germistatic soaps are effective against gram-positive organisms (staphylococci and streptococci) and are less effective against gram-negative bacteria. Germistatic soaps such as pHisoHex® (Winthrop), Dial® (Dial) and Ceptacol® (Vestal) contain hexachlorophene, tetramethylthiuram disulfide or 3,4,4'-trichlorocarbanilide as bacteriostatic agents.

## DEMULCENTS

The demulcent drugs are a group of water-soluble compounds having a high molecular weight. Most of the demulcent drugs are gums, mucilages or starches. They tend to coat over irritated or abraded tissue surfaces to protect the underlying cells from irritating contacts. A demulcent can be applied to the skin as a lotion or as a wet dressing and can be applied to the mucous membranes of the body as electuaries, nebulae or enemas, or as a drench. They are often used as vehicles to mask the taste of obnoxious drugs and particularly to form more stable suspensions or emulsions of drugs in aqueous vehicles.

*Acacia, U.S.P.* (gum arabic) and *tragacanth, U.S.P.* (gum tragacanth) are dried, gummy exudates from the respective plants. These gums readily dissolve in water to form mucilages. *Glycyrrhiza, U.S.P.* (licorice root) consists of the ground, dried rhizome and roots of the *Glycyrrhiza glabra* plant. Glycyrrhiza also is employed as a flavoring agent, especially for swine.

## ASTRINGENTS

Astringents are drugs that are used locally to precipitate proteins. These drugs do not penetrate deeply. Their precipitant action is exerted only on the surface cells and is relatively weak. As a result of the action of an astringent upon the surface tissue cells, the permeability of the cell membrane is greatly reduced but there is no loss of cell viability. Many germicidal preparations possess an astringent action even in high dilution. Astringent drugs include the salts of heavy metals such as silver, mercury, zinc and aluminum.

Another group of astringent compounds is of vegetable origin. Nearly all of these owe their activity to the presence of tannic acid. Other vegetable astringents are gallic acid, kino, gambir (pale catechu), *Quercus* (oak bark), *Rubus* (blackberry) and sumac.

A large number of tannic acids occur naturally. The most common one is gallotannic acid, which is obtained from nutgalls on oak trees. The tannic acids are hydrolyzed from glycosides consisting of several molecules of tannic acid combined with glucose. These glycosides are correctly called tannins. Most of the astringent action of plants comes from their tannin content. The astringent activity of different compounds depends upon the rate of release of the tannic acid content. The tannic acid from oak galls is released rapidly as compared with *Krameria*.

The most important pharmacologic activity of tannic acid is its ability to precipitate proteins. It also forms insoluble complexes with many of the heavy metals, alkaloids and glycosides. Tannic acid has therefore been used in treatment of certain types of poisonings. Tannins have found numerous uses in industry, particularly in the leather industry, in which they are used to precipitate the proteins in animal hides during the process of tanning. The same effect is produced when tannic acid is applied to the sore foot pads of dogs unaccustomed to rough concrete or other coarse surfaces.

## PERCUTANEOUS ABSORPTION

In general, gases and substances that are lipid-soluble are capable of penetrating the skin, whereas water and electrolytes are not able to pass through the integumentary system. Lipid-soluble substances appear to penetrate the skin rapidly and completely, and if the substance is also soluble in water, its absorption is increased. The following factors are considered to facilitate percutaneous absorption: hydration, hyperemia, increased cutaneous temperature and keratolytics or other agents which disrupt the stratum corneum or irritate the integument.

There are two routes of passage by which an agent may penetrate the skin: (1) transepidermal and (2) transappendageal. In the transepidermal route, the barrier to the penetration of an agent through the skin is the stratum corneum. It is generally accepted that the entire stratum corneum acts as the barrier and that once the stratum corneum is removed (in toto), the agent is capable of freely penetrating the integument. The role of the surface lipid film in percutaneous absorption is uncertain at this time. In the transappendageal route, it is proposed that the agent enters a follicle and passes through the follicular wall (which is less resistant than the surface epidermis) and/or the sebaceous gland and thence to the dermis itself.

The actual ability to penetrate the skin is an inherent quality of the particular agent itself. A vehicle may facilitate absorption but it cannot force penetration of an agent which is not capable of passing through the skin.

It is important to emphasize that, although comments on percutaneous absorption are probably applicable to most species, the ability of any agent to penetrate the skin should really be established for each agent and for each species of animal.

Lipid-soluble substances, phenolic compounds, salicylic acid, hormones (testosterone, estrogens, steroids) and lipid-soluble vitamins are absorbed freely through the skin. Of the heavy metals, copper and metallic mercury (in ointment vehicle) are absorbed through the hair follicles and sebaceous glands. Salts of lead, tin, copper, arsenic, bismuth, antimony and mercury may conjugate with fatty acids from the sebum or hydrolytic products of keratin to form lipid-soluble salts that may be absorbed through the skin. The penetration of any of these heavy metals as salts is increased if they are applied in ointment form. Animal and vegetable fats and mineral oils enter the pilosebaceous apparatus and penetrate the sebaceous glands. It is questionable, however, whether they enter the dermis from the epidermal appendage.

Organic solvents such as ether, benzene, alcohol and chloroform appear to enhance absorption of substances through the skin. Ethanol (70 per cent) serves as an excellent penetrating vehicle for a number of compounds. Of particular importance is its use as a vehicle for rotenone in the treatment of demodectic mange: a 1 per cent solution of the latter in 70 per cent ethanol has proved acaricidal and beneficial in the treatment of this disease.

Increasing the concentration of a particular medicament does not facilitate penetration. Occlusion has a marked effect on cutaneous absorption in that it leads to hydration of the stratum corneum, which promotes softening and maceration of the epidermal barrier. When the stratum corneum is so affected, favorable conditions are created for the retention of substances in close contact with the skin. Ointments, pastes and lotions tend to increase the absorption of an active agent in decreasing order of their occlusive potential (as listed). Oil-in-water (washable-base) ointments owe their ability to facilitate penetration of the medicament to their miscibility with an exuding lesion. This makes for intimate and prolonged contact with the skin surface.

## CLEANSING METHODS

Before initiation of specific dermatotherapy, the presenting lesion should be cleaned. Hair, crusts, dirt and the like must be removed, since they tend to retain or trap inflammatory debris and/or infectious material (both of which may intensify the dermatitis). They also may absorb an active agent applied to the skin and thus inactivate the desired effect or prevent necessary intimate contact of the agent with the skin surface.

Hair should be removed from the lesion proper and from the adjoining normal areas. If the lesion is dry, clippers may be employed; if exudative and crusty, curved scissors are preferred for the removal of hair.

The more acute lesion should be treated in the most sympathetic manner, wet dressings being most desirable. Ordinary soaps should be avoided, because of their potential irritating effect; neutral soaps are applicable if the patient is not unduly sensitive to them. For subacute dermatoses, cleaning may be accomplished with mineral oil, olive oil or cleansing cream. In chronic conditions in which massive scales or crusts or medicaments are present, organic solvents such as carbon tetrachloride or benzene can be used for cleansing.

Ulcerative lesions which contain necrotic tissue or purulent crusts should be cleaned in such a manner as to remove the debris surgically or with proteolytic enzymes. Trypsin and chymotrypsin in ointment form or in solution (as a spray) have been reported to produce favorable results. Both enzymes are derived from extracts of bovine pancreas. They are effective over a pH range of 5 to 7, hydrolyzing naturally occurring proteins without injury to living tissue. Trypsin catalyzes hydrolysis of peptide bonds after the basic amino acids lysine, arginine and histidine. Chymotrypsin catalyzes hydrolysis of peptide bonds after the aromatic amino acids phenylalanine, tryosine and tryptophan. The incorporation of an antibiotic such as neomycin appears to have a synergistic effect. The frequency of application depends upon the degree of contamination of the ulcer; the more contaminated, necrotic, etc., lesion requires application as many as four times daily.

## ACTIVE DERMATOLOGIC AGENTS

The following classification of dermatologic agents is based on their mode of action, and examples are given for each group.

1. Antipruritics. Pruritus is usually relieved by substitution of some other sensation such as cold or heat for the itching, by induction of anesthesia or by protection from external influences or their antiinflammatory action.
   a. Menthol—0.125 to 1 per cent
   b. Phenol—0.5 to 2 per cent
   c. Camphor—0.125 to 1 per cent
   d. Liquor carbonis detergens—3 to 10 per cent (a 20 per cent alcoholic solution of crude coal tar)
   e. Hydrocortisone 1 to 2.5 per cent and other steroids (see article on "Steroid Therapy in Skin Disease")

2. Keratoplastics. These agents tend to increase the thickness of stratum corneum.
   a. Salicylic acid—0.5 to 3 per cent
   b. Various tars
   c. Resorcin

3. Keratolytics and Antiseborrheics. These agents tend to remove or reduce the thickness of stratum corneum.
   a. Salicylic acid—5 to 20 per cent
   b. Resorcin—5 to 20 per cent
   c. Sulfur
   d. Selenium sulfide

4. Antieczematous Agents. These may act in several ways, such as antipruritics, "reducing" agents (extraction of oxygen from the tissues) or simple protectants. They are

classified here on the basis of practical experience as to their usefulness in eczematous dermatoses.

*Mild in action:*
   a. Ichthyol® (ichthammol)—3 to 10 per cent
   b. Liquor carbonis detergens—3 to 10 per cent
   c. Naftalan or ali-naph-zone—5 to 25 per cent (derived from Russian crude oil refined in Germany)

*Moderate to strong in action:*
   d. Crude coal tar—1 to 10 per cent
   e. Chrysarobin—0.125 to 10 per cent

*Strong in action:*
   f. Anthralin (Cignolin®)—0.1 to 5 per cent

5. Antiseptics and Antibiotics
   a. Ammoniated mercury—3 to 20 per cent
   b. Cinnabar, purified (red sulfide of mercury)—1 to 10 per cent
   c. Vioform® (iodochlorhydroxyquin)—1 to 3 per cent
   d. Furacin® (nitrofurazone)
   e. Quinolor® (halquinols)
   f. Penicillin—500 $\mu$/gm.
   g. Tyrothricin
   h. Aureomycin® (chlortetracycline)—3 per cent
   i. Bacitracin—500 $\mu$/gm.
   j. Terramycin® (oxytetracycline)—3 per cent
   k. Neomycin—0.5 per cent
   l. Polymyxin B sulfate—8000 $\mu$/gm.

6. Parasiticides
   a. Sulfur (ppt.)—3 to 30 per cent
   b. Benzyl benzoate—25 per cent emulsion
   c. DDT—10 per cent powder

7. Fungicides
   a. Acid salicylic—5 to 20 per cent
   b. Acid benzoic—5 to 10 per cent
   c. Resorcin—1 to 10 per cent
   d. Unsaturated fatty acids
   e. Vioform® (iodochlorhydroxyquin)—3 per cent
   f. Sterosan® (chlorquinaldol)—3 per cent
   g. Nystatin
   h. Cuprimyxin (Unitop®, Roche)—0.5 per cent
   i. Tolnaftate (Tinavet®, Schering)—1 per cent

8. Astringents
   a. Tannic acid—3 to 10 per cent
   b. Zinc oxide—15 to 25 per cent
   c. Alum—0.5 to 5 per cent
   d. Aluminum chloride solutions—20 to 30 per cent

9. Corticosteroids
   a. Hydrocortisone—1 per cent
   b. Hydrocortamate (Ulcortar®, Ulmer)—0.5 per cent
   c. Prednisolone—0.5 per cent
   d. Methylprednisolone (Medrol®, Upjohn)—0.25 per cent
   e. Triamcinolone—0.1 per cent
   f. Dexamethasone—0.1 per cent
   g. Betamethasone valerate (Valisone®, Schering)—0.1 per cent
   h. Fluorometholone (Oxylone®, Upjohn)—0.025 per cent
   i. Fluocinolone acetonide (Synalar®, Syntex)—0.025 per cent
   j. Flurandrenolide (Cordran®, Lilly)—0.03 per cent
   k. Flumethasone pivalate (Locorten®, CIBA)—0.03 per cent

# CANINE PYODERMA

P. J. IHRKE, V.M.D.,
R. E. W. HALLIWELL, M.R.C.V.S.,
*and* M. J. DEUBLER, V.M.D.
*Philadelphia, Pennsylvania*

## INTRODUCTION

Cutaneous pyogenic bacterial infection is termed pyoderma. A number of classifications may be used to describe pyodermas dependent on etiology, site and depth within the integument. They may further be subdivided into primary and secondary pyodermas. The latter may result from a variety of cutaneous insults or in association with a number of disease processes both cutaneous and systemic.

Site predilection at interdigital and intertriginous areas (axilla and groin), pressure points, anatomic defects and mucocutaneous junctions is known to occur. These pyodermas may be classified according to their site (e.g., interdigital pyoderma). In addition, they may be classified as surface, superficial or deep. Classification as to the depth of infection is perhaps most useful in therapeutic considerations, since rational therapy is contingent upon depth of involvement.

### ETIOLOGY

An understanding of cutaneous bacterial ecology is important; a dynamic balance exists among the resident skin organisms that form the stable bacterial community. Normal canine skin is colonized primarily by micrococci with lesser numbers of diphtheroids and clostridia. Occasionally, *Staphylococcus aureus*, Proteus species and gram-negative rods may be present as transient organisms in the total skin population. Almost any cutaneous insult, either external or internal, may initiate an ecologic shift in resident populations, permitting S. *aureus* or some other potential pathogen, such as Proteus or Pseudomonas species, to colonize the skin in significant numbers. At this point, pyoderma may occur. External trauma, self-trauma due to pruritus, poor grooming, dry skin, ectoparasitism and internal endocrinologic changes may all act as precipitating factors that lead to the establishment of bacterial infection. Once infection is established, factors such as nutrition, immunologic competence, allergic hypersensitivity reactions and initial therapy influence prognosis.

In our view, S. *aureus* is the major bacterial pathogen of canine skin. However, its isolation from a lesion does not necessarily imply that it is involved in the pathogenesis of the lesion, since S. *aureus* has a tendency to colonize any abnormal skin. In addition, the isolation of a micrococcus (such as *Staphylococcus epidermidis)* from a pustule is usually not significant and implies that (a) S. *aureus* was indeed present but was not isolated or (b) the pustule is not bacterial in origin (e.g., dermatitis herpetiformis).

## SURFACE PYODERMAS

This term may be used to describe very superficial erosions of the skin. Although S. *aureus* may frequently be cultured from these lesions, bacterial involvement is probably only secondary. Pyotraumatic dermatitis (hot spots, acute moist eczema) and the various skin fold pyodermas (lip fold, facial fold, vulvar fold, tail fold) are included in this category.

### PYOTRAUMATIC DERMATITIS

Pyotraumatic dermatitis is one of the more common canine skin diseases. It is most often seen in thick-coated, long-haired breeds and is more prevalent during the summer months. The lesion is usually erythematous, swollen, alopecic and exudative, with a rapid onset and progression. The exact etiology is unknown, but any factor that can initiate an itch-scratch cycle may predispose to the condition. Clinically, the lesions appear to be secondary to trauma. However, extreme self-trauma in some dogs will not initiate a hot spot, whereas surprisingly minimal self-trauma may do so in another animal. Ectoparasites, allergy, irritants, impacted anal sacs, otitis externa, foreign bodies and poor grooming seem to be contributing factors.

Treatment should include, if possible, correction of the predisposing factor. The involved area should be clipped and gently cleansed with a dilute, mild, antiseptic such as hexachlorophene (pHisoHex®, Winthrop). Moderate dosages of parenteral corticosteroids (e.g., prednisolone, 5 to 25 mg., dependent upon size of animal, in divided doses) for 5 days are indicated. In addition, a steroid-antibiotic cream such as Neosynalar® (Diamond) or a steroid aerosol (e.g., Valisone® [Schering]) may be used topically. In early cases, astringents (e.g., Domeboro® [Miles]) may be used instead of topical creams.

### SKIN FOLD PYODERMAS

Skin fold pyodermas are seen in a number of breeds in association with anatomic defects that create a moist, dark, warm environment. All are characterized by exudative, odoriferous, erythematous lesions within skin folds.

Lip fold pyodermas are seen in breeds such as cocker and springer spaniels and occasionally in setters. Halitosis is a frequent owner complaint. Facial fold pyodermas are seen in brachycephalic dogs. In these cases, corneal ulceration is a frequent sequela resulting from self-trauma. Vulvar fold pyodermas are seen in obese bitches that have been spayed before the first estrus. Breeds with corkscrew tails such as Boston terriers or English bulldogs are susceptible to tail fold pyodermas.

Palliative medical therapy consists of clipping the hair, gentle cleansing daily with an antiseptic solution such as pHisoHex® (Winthrop) or hydrogen peroxide and the topical application of a steroid antibiotic cream (Neosynalar®, Diamond) or ointment (Cortisporin®, Burroughs Wellcome). Diethylstilbestrol may be tried in the treatment of vulvar fold pyodermas. However, in all these conditions, surgical ablation of the anatomic defect offers the only permanent cure.

## SUPERFICIAL PYODERMAS

A superficial pyoderma is a bacterial infection in which multiple abscesses are present either subcorneally or in intact hair follicles.

### IMPETIGO

Impetigo, or "puppy pyoderma," is a relatively benign condition usually seen in young dogs and characterized by obvious pustules in the hairless areas of the groin. Poor nutrition and a dirty environment have been implicated as contributing factors. Occasionally, impetigo may appear as a minor complication of a more severe systemic illness such as distemper.

Correction of any predisposing causes and gentle cleansing with a product such as pHisoHex®, Betadine® (Purdue-Frederick) or Domeboro® (Miles) may be the only therapy required. For more severe cases, 7 to 10 days of antibiotic therapy is indicated.

### SUPERFICIAL FOLLICULITIS

Superficial folliculitis is a more severe disease than impetigo, and diagnosis often presents a challenge. The pustular stage may be quite transient, and frequently the visible lesions consist of multiple papules and crusts. The degree of pruritus ranges from extreme to nonexistent, and patchy or widespread hair loss with hyperpigmentation may occur.

Several forms of this disease are encountered. The most benign form occurs in the groin area of pubescent dogs and is probably hormonally related. The follicular orientation of the pustules differentiates this condition from impetigo.

"Short-haired dog pyoderma" presents as a rather benign disease in smooth-coated dogs such as great Danes, dobermans, Dalmatians, weimaraners and dachshunds. Clinically, the condition presents as small "bumps" diffusely affecting the trunk. Discrete patches of alopecia and hyperpigmentation may occur, mimicking ringworm. Rarely, a mixed bacterial-fungal infection may be present. Miniature schnauzers manifest a rather characteristic folliculitis in association with a discrete band of dorsal midline seborrhea. The condition has been termed "schnauzer bumps."

Lastly, a superficial folliculitis may present as a very pruritic disease. This is probably due to a bacterial hypersensitivity phenomenon. Rapidly expanding circular patches of alopecia with peripheral erythema and scaling usually occur on the ventrum of the animal. Frequently, since the pustular phase is very short, this disease is misdiagnosed as ringworm.

Treatment of any superficial folliculitis should include attention to possible underlying causes such as seborrhea (either sicca or oleosa), which is the most commonly associated skin disease. Keratolytic or antiseborrheic shampoos used in conjunction with emollient rinses may be necessary (see article on "Canine Seborrhea"). Generally, long-term (4 to 6 weeks) use of an antibiotic with a gram-positive spectrum is required. Corticosteroids are contraindicated in this disease in spite of more rapid initial visible improvement. The clinical improvement seen, even when corticosteroids are used as sole therapy, makes it very difficult to assess the efficacy of any antibiotic used concomitantly. Furthermore, when the folliculitis has developed as a result of seborrhea sicca, corticosteroids will further suppress sebum production, leading to the eventual worsening of the problem upon cessation of therapy.

## DEEP PYODERMAS

A deep pyoderma is a bacterial infection involving structures beneath and beyond the hair follicle. Suppuration, necrosis and fistula formation are frequently present. Often, the involved areas are hot and painful. Deep pyodermas may be divided into three categories: furunculosis, cellulitis and hidradenitis suppurativa.

## FURUNCULOSIS

Furunculosis usually develops from the extension of a folliculitis as a result of a follicular rupture and the subsequent spread of bacterial infection. Consequently, the lesions are larger than those associated with folliculitis, and pus can often be expressed from them. Thus, furunculosis presents as a much more obvious pyoderma than does folliculitis.

Perhaps the most common type of furunculosis is the muzzle pyoderma seen in young, short-haired breeds. Usually this is a benign and transient condition that rarely warrants extensive antibiotic therapy. It often resolves spontaneously upon sexual maturity. Gentle scrubs with pHisoHex® or hot packs using water, Domeboro® or other astringents are helpful. Parenteral antibiotic therapy for several weeks is recommended in cases that show extensive involvement or persist beyond puberty. Occasionally, this disease may exhibit a tendency to spread and act as a nidus for distant infections on calluses and other body sites. If this occurs, vigorous therapy (4 to 8 weeks) with an appropriate antibiotic determined by means of a culture and sensitivity test should be instituted.

Nasal pyoderma, which is a rare disease, presents as a painful, swollen furunculosis on the bridge of the nose. Shepherds and pointers appear to have an increased incidence of this condition. Gentle handling is the key to successful therapy, because severe scarring is a common sequela of either the disease itself or overzealous therapy. Gentle cleansing with a product such as pHisoHex® may be necessary if sufficient debris is present to prevent adequate drainage. Appropriate systemic antibiotic therapy should be instituted for at least one month. Topical use of products such as Cortisporin® or Toptic® (Lilly) ointment is recommended. If self-trauma is a problem, either tranquilization or use of an Elizabethan collar may be required to prevent further trauma. In refractory cases, the dermatophyte *Trichophyton mentagrophytes* should be suspected of participating in a mixed infection, and fungal cultures should be taken.

Furunculosis is also seen as a frequent secondary complication of generalized demodectic mange. Vigorous, prolonged (1 to 2 months) systemic antibiotic therapy is usually necessary.

## CELLULITIS

Cellulitis is a deep pyoderma characterized by diffuse, spreading, edematous and sometimes suppurative inflammation. Unlike furunculosis or focal abscess formation, cellulitis is poorly defined and tends to dissect widely along and through tissue planes. Cellulitis is most frequently seen in association with generalized demodectic mange but may occur as a primary disease entity, either in a generalized form, interdigitally, or in association with a callus. It should be noted that interdigital pyodermas may result from continual foot chewing associated with atopic disease. Although *S. aureus* is probably the initiating organism in most cases, Proteus and Pseudomonas species are frequently seen as secondary invaders. In addition, the possibility of a concomitant *Candida* infection should be considered.

Cellulitis presents a therapeutic challenge and recurrence is common. Bacterial isolation and identification with antibiotic sensitivity tests are essential, and long-term (1 to 3 months) antibiotic therapy is indicated. Ideally, an antibiotic should be chosen to which all the pathogens are sensitive. If this is not feasible, success may sometimes be achieved by treating only the *S. aureus* infection.

As an adjunct to the above-mentioned therapy, symptomatic treatment with hot antiseptic soaks or whirlpool baths may be helpful. Betadine® or magnesium sulfate may be added to the water. Callus pyoderma also requires correction of predisposing environmental factors. Dogs should be encouraged to sleep on a mattress or other cushioning substance such as Astroturf®.

Specific and nonspecific immune defects are sometimes noted in cases of cellulitis. In some of these cases, a partial deficit of *in vitro* phagocytic performance has been demonstrated, and autogenous bacterins have proved efficacious. Such therapy is not universally successful, and it either should be restricted to those animals in which there is a defect demonstrated by laboratory tests or should be instituted as a last resort when all other therapy fails.

## HIDRADENITIS SUPPURATIVA

Hidradenitis suppurativa is recognized as a rare, bacterial infection involving the apocrine sweat glands and adjacent deep structures. Since the histologic criteria for this disease are quite specific and infrequently met, many cases showing gross similarities to the disease are probably improperly diagnosed as a type of hidradenitis. Histologic confirmation of apocrine sweat gland infection is essential in order to establish the diagnosis.

Hidradenitis suppurativa is most often seen in collies and Shetland sheep dogs. Erythematous, suppurative, granulating, sharply demarcated plaques with serpiginous borders are seen primarily in the groin and axilla and occasionally on the head. Three sequential months of therapy with different antibiotics should be instituted as dictated by bacterial cultures and sensitivity tests. Cultures should be taken from macerated biopsy material, since superficial cultures retrieve contaminant organisms. A guarded prognosis should always be given, since this condition is often refractory to therapy.

## JUVENILE PYODERMA

Juvenile pyoderma is the name generally given to a poorly understood condition usually seen in puppies less than 4 months of age. Characteristic lesions include acute, severe swellings of the lips and eyelids, with variable involvement of other mucocutaneous junctions. A regional lymphadenopathy is present, and abscess formation with suppuration may result. Cellulitis, deep folliculitis and focal abscesses are frequently seen, with crusting and suppuration. Paradoxically, single members of a litter or entire litters may be affected.

This disease entity may or may not be associated with a staphylococcal infection. Although frequently staphylococci may be isolated from characteristic lesions, occasionally sterile material is obtained. A hypersensitivity phenomenon or other as yet undetermined factors may be responsible for the pathogenesis of the disease.

Despite the fact that pathogenic bacteria may not be causative in the disease, antibiotic therapy is still recommended to control or prevent secondary infection. Treatment with a broad-spectrum antibiotic is recommended, and short-acting corticosteroids (prednisolone, 5 to 15 mg. daily, depending upon animal size, in divided dosages) may be given concomitantly with antibiotics.

## ANTIBIOTIC THERAPY

Once the diagnosis of pyoderma has been made, proper antibiotic therapy should be initiated. Proper therapy implies the choice of an antibiotic with a known spectrum of activity directed against organisms which are common cutaneous pathogens. Secondly, the establishment and maintenance of effective therapeutic dosages are of utmost importance. Once the animal is receiving adequate doses of an effective antibiotic, therapy must be maintained long enough to insure cure rather than transient remission.

### ANTIBIOTIC SELECTION

Antibiotic selection may be either empirical or based upon a culture and sensitivity test. If an empirical selection is to be made, certain principles must be followed. Since *S. aureus* is most frequently the only isolate in infections of the skin, obviously an antibiotic should be chosen with activity against gram-positive cocci. In addition, the antibiotic should not be inactivated by penicillinase, since most cutaneous pathogenic *S. aureus* organisms elaborate penicillinase.

During the past several months, cultures were taken of 83 cases of superficial and deep pyodermas in canines seen at the Small Animal Hospital of the University of Pennsylvania. Cultures in which only a micrococcus was isolated were discarded, and the only cultures recorded in Tables 1 and 2 were those in which *S. aureus* with and without gram-negative cultures (either Proteus or Pseudomonas) was isolated. When more than one organism was isolated, sensitivity tests were run on a composite of isolates and on each isolate separately. Sometimes the sensitivities of the composite were not the sum total of those of the constituents. The Kirby-Bauer method was used to determine bacterial sensitivity or resistance to 25 antibiotics, and results were recorded as sensitive or resistant. Cases which official protocol would denote as intermediate sensitivity were recorded as resistant.

These antibiotics were chosen because of known usefulness, common usage or potential value in veterinary medicine. It will be seen from Tables 1 and 2 that ampicillin, penicillin, tetracycline and sulfa drugs are

### Table 1. Antibiotic Sensitivities– No Previous Therapy

| Systemic Antibiotics | STAPH. AUREUS (34 CASES) | COMPOSITE (6 CASES) | GRAM-NEGATIVE (3 CASES) |
|---|---|---|---|
| Ampicillin | 7 | 1 | 1 |
| Carbenicillin | 30 | 2 | 1 |
| Caphalothin | 33 | 2 | 1 |
| Chloramphenicol | 30 | 4 | 1 |
| Clindamycin | 27 | 2 | — |
| Lincomycin | 25 | 1 | — |
| Cloxacillin | 32 | 2 | — |
| Erythromycin | 29 | 3 | — |
| Gentamycin | 34 | 3 | 2 |
| Kanamycin | 33 | 2 | 1 |
| Nafcillin | 31 | 1 | — |
| Novobiocin | 31 | 2 | — |
| Oleandomycin | 29 | 1 | — |
| Oxacillin | 32 | 1 | — |
| Penicillin | 7 | 1 | — |
| Streptomycin | 22 | 1 | 1 |
| Tetracycline | 13 | — | 1 |
| Tobramycin | 34 | 4 | 2 |
| Trimethoprim-sulfadiazine | 18 | 2 | 1 |
| Triple Sulfa | 10 | 2 | 1 |
| *Topical Antibiotics* | | | |
| Bacitracin | 25 | 4 | — |
| Cuprimyxin | 32 | 6 | 3 |
| Furacin® (nitrofurazone) | 33 | 2 | 1 |
| Neomycin | 33 | 2 | 1 |
| Polymyxin B | 24 | 3 | 2 |

### Table 2. Antibiotic Sensitivities– Previous Antibiotic Therapy

| Systemic Antibiotics | STAPH. AUREUS (28 CASES) | COMPOSITE (5 CASES ) | GRAM-NEGATIVE (8 CASES) |
|---|---|---|---|
| Ampicillin | 4 | 1 | 4 |
| Carbenicillin | 18 | 3 | 2 |
| Cephalothin | 26 | 1 | 2 |
| Chloramphenicol | 23 | 2 | 3 |
| Clindamycin | 16 | — | 1 |
| Lincomycin | 13 | — | 1 |
| Cloxacillin | 22 | 1 | 1 |
| Erythromycin | 12 | — | 1 |
| Gentamycin | 27 | 4 | 7 |
| Kanamycin | 27 | 3 | 3 |
| Nafcillin | 26 | 1 | — |
| Novobiocin | 28 | 3 | 4 |
| Oleandomycin | 17 | — | — |
| Oxacillin | 25 | — | — |
| Penicillin | 5 | — | 1 |
| Streptomycin | 15 | — | 2 |
| Tetracycline | 5 | 1 | 3 |
| Tobramycin | 28 | 4 | 7 |
| Trimethoprim-sulfadiazine | 14 | 3 | 3 |
| Triple Sulfa | 8 | 2 | 2 |
| *Topical Antibiotics* | | | |
| Bacitracin | 19 | — | 3 |
| Cuprimyxin | 25 | 4 | 4 |
| Furacin | 25 | 3 | 4 |
| Neomycin | 28 | 3 | 4 |
| Polymyxin B | 23 | 3 | 5 |

poor choices in the treatment of any pyoderma. In cases in which previous antibiotic therapy has been given, a rather precipitous drop in sensitivities occurs. It may well be that cross-resistance is developing, and when therapy with an appropriate antibiotic has proved ineffective, a culture and sensitivity test is advisable before proceeding. Additionally, a culture and sensitivity test should be done in lieu of empirical treatment in long-standing infections, deep infections and cases in which a mixed bacterial infection is suspected. Toxicity, ease of administration, bacteriostatic versus bactericidal activity and expense of the drug should be considered in selection of the antibiotic after sensitivity test results are obtained. For example, if good sensitivity is obtained to a safe, less expensive generic drug, such as erythromycin, it should be used in preference to a potentially toxic drug, such as gentamycin. In addition, if only *S. aureus* is isolated from a lesion, a narrow-spectrum antibiotic, such as erythromycin, Lincocin® (Upjohn) or TAO® (Roerig [Pfizer]), should be used rather than a broad-spectrum antibiotic, such as Keflex® (Lilly). When interpreting bacterial sensitivities, it should be noted that *in-vitro* laboratory sensitivity does not always guarantee *in-vivo* results. Less than ideal results that are sometimes encountered when using chloramphenicol in deep pyodermas are an example of this phenomenon.

In mixed cultures in which gram-negative bacteria are isolated in addition to *Staphylococcus*, ideally a composite sensitivity test should determine the choice of the antibiotic. If no single antibiotic is effective against all pathogenic isolates, success may sometimes be obtained by simply treating the *S. aureus* infection. In our laboratories, coagulase-positive *S. aureus*, Pseudomonas and Proteus are the only commonly isolated pathogens. Generally, *S. epidermidis*, micrococcus and other less common isolates are usually considered to be saprophytic.

### DOSAGE (SEE TABLE 3)

All animals receiving systemic antibiotics should be weighed and given the proper number of milligrams per kilogram of body

*Table 3.* *Systemic Antibiotic Dosages*

| GENERIC NAME | TRADE NAME AND MANUFACTURER (IF NOT AVAILABLE GENERICALLY) | ROUTE OF ADMINISTRATION | SUGGESTED DOSAGE |
|---|---|---|---|
| Ampicillin | ——— | PO, SC, IM, IV | 20 mg./kg. b.i.d. |
| Carbenicillin | Geopen® Geocillin®(Roerig) | IM, IV, PO | *† |
| Cephalothin | Keflex®(Lilly) | PO | 20-30 mg./kg. b.i.d. |
| Chloramphenicol | ——— | PO, SC, IV | 20-50 mg./kg. t.i.d. |
| Clindamycin | Cleocin®(Upjohn) | PO | *† |
| Lincomycin | Lincocin® (Upjohn) | PO | 20 mg./kg. b.i.d. |
| Cloxacillin | Tegopen® (Bristol) | PO | *20 mg./kg. b.i.d. or t.i.d. |
| Erythromycin | ——— | PO | 10-15 mg./kg. t.i.d. |
| Gentamycin | Gentacin® (Schering) | SC | 4 mg./kg. b.i.d. s.i.d. |
| Kanamycin | Kantrim® (Bristol) | SC | 6-8 mg./kg. b.i.d. |
| Nafcillin | Unipen® (Wyeth) | PO | *20 mg./kg. b.i.d. or t.i.d. |
| Oleandomycin | TAO® (Roerig [Pfizer]) | PO | *20 mg./kg. t.i.d. |
| Oxacillin | Prostaphlin® (Bristol) | PO, IM, IV | *20 mg./kg. b.i.d. or t.i.d. |
| Penicillin | ——— | PO | 20,000 units/kg. q.i.d. |
| Streptomycin | ——— | IM | 10-20 mg./kg. t.i.d. |
| Tetracycline | ——— | PO | 15-20 mg./kg. t.i.d. |
| Tobramycin | Nebcin® (Lilly) | IV, IM, SC | *† |
| Trimethoprim- sulfadiazine | Tribrissen® (Burroughs Wellcome) | PO | 30 mg./kg. s.i.d. |
| Triple Sulfa | ——— | PO | 60 mg./kg. b.i.d. |

*Not approved for veterinary use.
†Dosage not determined.

weight. Improper dosage is probably the most common error in the treatment of pyodermas. Recommended dosages should be strictly adhered to in 75-kg. Great Danes as well as in 3-kg. poodles. The creation of resistant bacterial strains is not a "shortcut" to proper therapy! Another common error is administering antibiotics for too short a period of time. In general, the longer an infection has been present and the deeper the infection, the longer the therapy required to cure the condition.

## TOPICAL THERAPY

Ordinarily, topical antibiotics are unnecessary in the treatment of most canine pyodermas. An exception would be their use in surface pyodermas such as pyo-traumatic dermatitis or skin fold infections. Occasionally, topical antibiotics may be useful as adjunctive therapy in localized deep pyodermas such as hidradenitis suppurativa. However, under no circumstances should topical antibiotics be used as the sole therapy in deep pyodermas.

# CANINE SEBORRHEA

L. N. HORWITZ, V.M.D.,
*and* P. J. IHRKE, V.M.D.
*Philadelphia, Pennsylvania*

## INTRODUCTION

Seborrhea can be defined as an abnormal increase of secretions from the oil glands of the skin. This definition stems from the greasy appearance of the surface of the skin found in some types of seborrheic disease. However, this definition is incomplete. The pathogenesis of seborrhea is probably more complex, involving both quantitative and qualitative changes in sebaceous secretion and perhaps a defect in the keratinization process of the epidermis. Additionally, the term seborrhea sicca is used to imply reduced sebum secretion.

Mild scaling of the stratum corneum, commonly referred to as dandruff, differs in degree and possibly in type from that seen in seborrhea. Most normal skin exhibits some degree of scaling. This can be increased by such factors as low relative humidity in the environment and excessive washing, which removes the natural lipid film from the skin surface.

The seborrheic disease complex is a major problem in canine dermatology. In the dermatology clinic of the University of Pennsylvania School of Veterinary Medicine, 10 per cent of the cases presented are diagnosed as having seborrhea. Unfortunately, our knowledge of the etiology and pathogenesis of seborrhea is incomplete, but investigations are being conducted to enhance our understanding of the disease. Meanwhile, seborrhea continues to present to the veterinarian a diagnostic and therapeutic challenge.

Seborrheic dermatitis in man is a chronic scaling eruption frequently seen with oily skin and with or without inflammation. The primary sites of involvement are intertriginous regions and hairy regions rich in sebaceous glands. These regions include the scalp, eyebrows, nasal folds and presternal area. Blepharitis frequently accompanies the disease.

The histopathology of seborrheic dermatitis is not diagnostic. The stratum corneum shows focal areas of parakeratosis which indicates an increase in epidermal turnover. The epidermis shows moderate acanthosis and spongiosis, and there is a mild inflammatory infiltrate in the dermis.

It is not certain that any of the seborrheic diseases in the dog are truly analogous to human seborrheic dermatitis. Nonetheless, seborrheic disease in the dog, as in man, is characterized by excessive desquamation of the stratum corneum. The regions most frequently affected are also similar and involve those areas containing high concentrations of sebaceous glands: the perioral region, the periocular region, the dorsal trunk and the preen area of the tail.

## CLINICAL CLASSIFICATION

The disease may be divided into seborrhea sicca and seborrhea oleosa, based on the rather subjective evaluation of oil content of the pelage. Seborrhea sicca is the dry, scaling form of the disease. Usually fine, white scales are seen in association with a dry, dull pelage. Irish setters, German shepherds and dachshunds frequently exhibit this type of seborrhea. The oily, odoriferous form with yellowish, greasy deposits matting the pelage is termed seborrhea oleosa. Pruritus, erythema, ventral keratin accumulations and a concomitant ceruminous otitis are often noted. This clinical picture closely parallels seborrheic dermatitis in man. Blonde cocker spaniels and springer spaniels are commonly affected with this disease.

## ETIOLOGIC CLASSIFICATION

On the basis of etiology, canine seborrhea may be divided into primary and secondary forms (see Table 1). Primary may be further divided into primary idiopathic and primary metabolic. Primary idiopathic is that form for which an underlying cause cannot be determined. A cure is most difficult in these cases, but with proper treatment the condition can be symptomatically controlled. However, with primary endocrine dysfunctions and secondary seborrhea, we are presented with seborrheic disease for which an underlying cause can be determined. A thorough history and physical examination and judicious use of clinical pathology are essential in determining the etiology of a secondary seborrhea. After proper diagnosis, a cure can then be effected.

## CUTANEOUS BACTERIOLOGY

Superficial pyodermas, such as impetigo or superficial folliculitis, frequently accompany seborrheic disease in the dog. Normal canine skin contains a surprisingly low number of bacteria. The total number of organisms is between 100 and 200 per square centimeter and is made up almost exclu-

**Table 1.** *Classification of Seborrhea*

I. Primary Idiopathic Seborrhea
II. Primary Metabolic Seborrhea
  A. Endocrine-related
    1. Hypothyroidism
    2. Gonadal aberrations
  B. Aberrations in Lipid Availability
    1. Dietary deficiency
    2. Malabsorption
    3. Defects in fat metabolism
III. Secondary Seborrhea
    1. Ectoparasitic
    2. Allergic
    3. Dermatomycosis
    4. Autoimmune

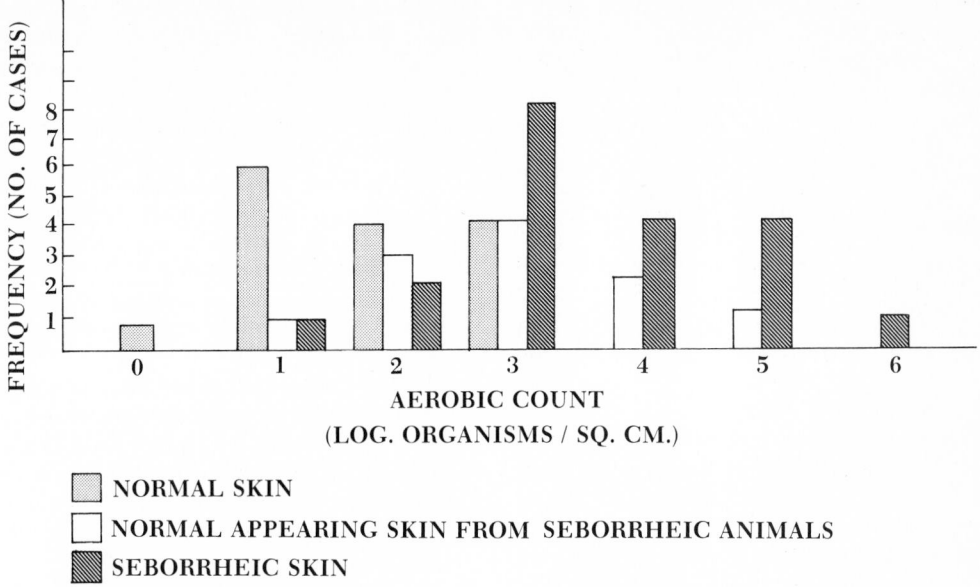

**Figure 1.** Frequency distribution of aerobic organisms per square centimeter.

sively of micrococci. In seborrheic skin there is a significant increase in the numbers of bacteria (Fig. 1). The total numbers range between 10 and 100,000. This increase is in aerobic organisms, with coagulase-positive staphylococcus having replaced the micrococcus (Table 2). The presence of large numbers of pathogenic staphylococci along with a probable decrease in the natural resistance in seborrheic skin would account for the pyoderma that accompanies canine seborrhea.

## CUTANEOUS LIPIDS

In an attempt to determine the etiology and pathogenesis of seborrhea, the basic question arises as to whether the defect is epidermal and/or sebaceous in origin. The increase in epidermal turnover may result in inadequate maturation of the cells of the stratum corneum, possibly leading to excessive desquamation. Differences are noted in the skin lipid pattern when normal and seborrheic skin are compared. The skin lipid film, a secretory product of the sebaceous gland, is the lipid-aqueous emulsion that covers the skin and hair coat. In normal canine skin the lipid film is made up primarily of sterol and wax esters (Table 3). There are small amounts of free cholesterol and triglycerides, but little or no free fatty acids are present. In seborrheic skin there is a significant increase in the relative amounts of free fatty acids and a decrease in the relative amount of diester waxes.

These data seem to indicate major differences in sebum between normal and seborrheic animals. Interestingly, in seborrheic animals, the aberrant lipid pattern appears consistent in cases of both seborrhea sicca and seborrhea oleosa. Furthermore, in

**Table 2.** *Quantitative and Qualitative Bacteriology of Normal and Seborrheic Canine Skin*

| | AEROBIC ORGANISMS | | |
|---|---|---|---|
| TYPE OF SKIN | *Mean Value/ Sq. Cm.* | *Major Components* | *Minor Components* |
| Normal skin (10 animals) | 148 | Micrococcus | Diphtheroids Bacillus species |
| Seborrheic skin (10 animals) | 10,113 | *Staphylococcus aureus* | Diphtheroids Bacillus species |

**Table 3.** *Skin Lipid Components—Mean Percentages*

| | TOTAL LABILE FATTY ACIDS* | TOTAL CHOLES-TEROL† | DIESTER WAX |
|---|---|---|---|
| Normal skin | 3.45 | 48.45 | 48.19 |
| Seborrhea sicca | 12.20 | 54.82 | 32.20 |
| Seborrhea oleosa | 7.57 | 54.31 | 38.05 |

*Total labile fatty acids = fatty acids + mono-, di- and triglycerides.

†Total cholesterol = free cholesterol and cholesterol ester.

all breeds studied, a similar pattern is noted. This suggests that the two clinical forms of seborrhea may in fact be the same disease with a range of clinical expressions due to breed variations.

## PATHOGENESIS

As indicated earlier, seborrhea is divided into three major categories based on causation: secondary, primary metabolic and primary idiopathic. Correct categorization is of utmost importance, since proper therapy varies widely among these three groupings.

**Secondary Seborrhea.** Seborrhea may occur secondarily as a clinical sign in association with a number of unrelated disease processes. This is not surprising, since desquamation and inflammation are among the more common cutaneous responses to insults, either internal or external. Clinical signs of scaling, crusting and alopecia often occur secondary to ectoparasitic dermatoses, allergic disease, ringworm or autoimmune disease.

Perhaps the most commonly observed secondary seborrhea is associated with flea infestation and concomitant allergic hypersensitivity reactions. Scaling, especially in the dorsal-lumbar-sacral area, is frequently misdiagnosed as a primary seborrhea. Many other parasitic diseases may also mimic primary seborrhea.

Generalized crusting and scaling in association with secondary pyoderma is usually noted in cases of generalized demodectic mange. The differential diagnosis of sarcoptic mange should not present a major problem, since, a primary maculopapular rash coupled with site predilection on the margins of the pinna, lateral elbows and ventral midline thorax aids in differentiation. The secondary seborrhea seen with Cheyletiella infestation is usually dorsal in involvement, and a history of contagion can often be elicited. Careful history, a good physical examination and judicious skin scrapings will usually reveal an underlying parasitic problem.

Generalized scaling, perhaps associated with continuous low-grade self-trauma, is sometimes seen in animals with atopic disease. A history compatible with allergic disease, digital and facial self-trauma and positive intradermal skin testing substantiates this diagnosis.

Occasionally, ringworm may mimic seborrhea. However, in most instances, dermatophyte lesions are more discrete and localized than primary seborrhea. A history of contagion, involvement of the owners, skin scrapings and fungal cultures are all useful in the diagnosis of dermatomycosis.

Somewhat symmetrical facial and distal extremity scaling may be seen in association with autoimmune diseases such as lupus erythematosus. Since skin lesions seen in autoimmune diseases are often rather bizarre and characteristic, differential diagnosis is not a major problem.

**Primary Metabolic Seborrhea.** Seborrhea that occurs in association with a metabolic disease process which directly affects skin lipids may be termed primary metabolic seborrhea. Either aberrations in lipid availability to the skin or hormonal changes leading to deranged sebaceous flow may be responsible for this type of seborrhea.

ENDOCRINE-RELATED. Since both thyroidal and gonadal hormones profoundly affect the physiology of the skin and particularly sebum production, variations in the production, the utilization or the delicate dynamic balance of these hormones may contribute to seborrheic disease. Seborrheic animals with underlying hypothyroidism do not always present as typical obese, lethargic heat-seekers. Generally history and clinical signs suggestive of hypothyroidism are rather subtle in this group. In our laboratory a T4 value of less than 1.5 $\mu$g./100 ml. (Nuclear Medical Kit) is considered definitive for hypothyroidism. Values between 1.5 and 2.0 are considered to be in a "gray area" and as such are handled according to clinical impression. Frequently, animals with only a mildly depressed T4 value will respond rather dramatically to replacement therapy. Irish setters, Dobermans and Afghans appear to be overrepresented in this category.

In male dogs, intransigent seborrhea may occasionally be seen in association with abnormally aggressive behavior. Histories of indiscriminate mounting or fighting with either male or female dogs may offer a clue to categorization. Bitches with a history of irregular estrus, prolonged anestrus or pseudocyesis may have an associated, somewhat cyclical seborrhea.

ABBERATIONS IN LIPID AVAILABILITY. A deficiency in fat or other improper dietary management is probably the most common type of primary metabolic seborrhea. Semi-moist commercial dog foods and unusual table food combinations are most often implicated in this form of seborrhea. Occasionally, malabsorption of nutrients (especially fat) in a good diet may lead to seborrhea. In these cases, the possibility of underlying intestinal or pancreatic problems should be investigated. Since the liver is of utmost importance in lipid metabolism, hepatic disease has also been implicated in the pathogenesis of seborrhea.

**Primary Idiopathic Seborrhea.** Seborrhea may also exist as a discrete disease entity in which no contributing external or internal causation can be determined. Unfortunately, many seborrheas must be placed in this category. The breed incidence of primary idiopathic seborrhea in German shepherds, cocker spaniels, Irish setters, Dobermans and dachshunds suggests a hereditary basis for the disease.

It should be reemphasized that in primary seborrhea, clinical signs are usually gradual in onset. Site predilection is mainly dorsal, and more severe involvement is often noted on the dorsum of the tail in the preen body region, on pressure points and diffusely on the pinna of the ear, with or without a concomitant ceruminous otitis. A penetrating "rancid-fat" odor is also often associated with seborrhea.

## THERAPY

Again, it should be emphasized that rational therapy must be based upon the proper categorization of the seborrheic patient. Attempts must be made to investigate the possibility of each type of secondary and primary metabolic seborrhea before conventional palliative antiseborrheic therapy is initiated.

**Secondary Seborrhea.** Therapy should center on treatment of the primary disease entity. Although antiseborrheic shampoos may facilitate the eradication of ectoparasites or afford the animal some relief in atopic disease or autoimmune disease, the use of antiseborrheic therapy should be considered as an adjunct to more specific treatment.

**Primary Metabolic Seborrhea** Normalization of the lipid components of sebum is the desired effect of all types of metabolic manipulation.

ENDOCRINE-RELATED. Hypothyroid seborrheic dogs are placed on oral sodium levothyroxine (Synthroid,® Flint). Dosages are obviously contingent upon the degree of hypothyroidism present and individual animal variations. However, therapeutic regimens commonly vary between 0.1 mg. and 0.3 mg. given either 2 or 3 times daily. It is important to note that since the half-life of L-thyroxine is no more than 12 hours, it is essential to give this drug at *least* twice daily. (A 15-kg. dog is usually given 0.2 mg. twice daily.) Owners are told to expect personality changes (increased activity and playfulness) within 2 weeks and beneficial cutaneous changes within 6 weeks. At 6 weeks, a reexamination is indicated and a second T4 assay is performed. Owing to fluctuations in serum thyroxine levels, it is imperative to obtain a sample in the middle of the day, approximately 3 hours after administration of the dose. Either the animal is maintained on the initial dosage or the dosage is increased, depending on the elevation in T4. Obviously, hypothyroid animals should probably remain on Synthroid for the rest of their lives. If an animal with a slightly depressed T4 assay does not respond to supplementation, thyroid medication should be withdrawn after the 6-week trial period.

Seborrheic male dogs exhibiting abnormally aggressive behavior may respond to castration. In the future, antiandrogen drugs may prove useful as an alternative to surgery. Concomitantly, bitches with cyclical seborrheic problems often respond dramatically to ovariohysterectomy.

ABERRATIONS IN LIPID AVAILABILITY. Animals suspected of having seborrhea related to fat deficiency are placed on an adequate basic diet. (We prefer commercial dry and canned food in a ratio of about 3:1.) Both polyunsaturated (peanut, corn or safflower) oils and saturated (pork, beef or chicken) fats are added to the dog's diet on a regular daily basis. Specific recommendations vary between 1 teaspoon and 2 tablespoons daily of each type of fat, depending upon the animal's size. Commercial fat supplements do not appear to offer any advantage over the above-mentioned fats.

In malabsorption cases, therapy is directed toward alleviating the cause of the malabsorption. Likewise, in hepatic disease, the underlying cause must be treated medically.

**Primary Idiopathic Seborrhea.** If no underlying cause can be determined, the goal of control instead of cure must be stressed to the owner. Proper client education is critical with a disease such as seborrhea, in which client frustration may be high. Owners of animals with severe idiopathic seborrhea should be dissuaded from breeding these dogs because of the likelihood of genetic predilection. Fat supplementation, as mentioned previously, should be initiated. Keratolytic, antiseborrheic shampoos are often quite beneficial. Commercial canine and human products such as Pentrax® (Texas Pharmacal), Sebutone® (Westwood), Thiomar® (Evsco), Ionil-T® (Owen), Seleen® (Diamond), Selsen-Blue® (Abbott), Domerine® (Miles Veterinary Division),

and Sebulex® (Westwood) have all proved useful. Shampoos must be individualized to each animal; no one ideal product exists. Since coal tar shampoos may noticeably darken certain white dogs, products such as Seleen, Selsen-Blue or Domerine are recommended for such animals. In most instances, weekly use of the shampoo is indicated. After thorough lathering, the shampoo must be left on the animal for 10 to 15 minutes before rinsing. The importance of shampoo contact time should be stressed to the owners. In animals with seborrhea sicca, an emollient bath oil rinse is desirable following the shampoo. Products such as Alpha-Keri® (Westwood), Domol® (Miles), Shamp-Aid® (Miles Veterinary Division) bath oils may be used. Two capfuls of oil placed in ½ gallon of warm water provides a good emulsion. This mixture is then poured over the animal and rubbed in thoroughly. The animal should then be toweldried without rinsing. In most cases, primary idiopathic seborrhea may at least be controlled by a conscientious owner following a regular regimen of dietary supplementation and frequent shampoos.

---

# DIAGNOSIS AND MANAGEMENT OF IMMUNE-MEDIATED MUCO-CUTANEOUS DISORDERS IN THE DOG

ANTHONY A. STANNARD, D.V.M.,
*and* SHARON G. YASKULSKI,
D.V.M.
*Davis, California*

## INTRODUCTION

Several disease syndromes in the dog affect the oral mucosa, various mucocutaneous junctions and the skin itself. Of primary concern in this section are those diseases thought to be immune-related, including

pemphigus vulgaris and systemic lupus erythematosus (SLE), both of which have been fairly well characterized. In addition, disease syndromes have been observed in the dog that are identical to or that strongly resemble pemphigus foliaceus and bullous pemphigoid in man.

Since many of the above syndromes have not been well characterized in the dog and since their clinical appearance and management are similar in most respects, they will be discussed as a group.

## CLINICAL SIGNS

The onset of clinical signs in the immune-mediated mucocutaneous disorders may be slow and insidious or abrupt and fulminating. With the exception of systemic lupus erythematosus, most cases do not exhibit signs of systemic illness such as depression, fever, etc., unless the disease process is severe and widespread. The lesions that may be observed in the immune-mediated mucocutaneous disorders exhibit considerable variation in their appearance and distribution. Ulcers, erosions, focal crusting, vesicles, bullae and pustules can be present. Within the oral cavity, the tongue, gingivae, palate and buccal mucosa may be affected. The oral lesions usually consist of erosions and ulcers, although remnants of ruptured bullae can occasionally be observed. The mucocutaneous junctions that are commonly affected include the lips, eyelids, anus, vulvar margins and preputial orifice. In addition, the nipples, external ear canals, nail beds and junction of the skin and footpads may be involved. The most common types of lesions observed at these sites are erosions, ulcers and focal crusting. The greatest variety of lesions occur when the skin itself is involved. A characteristic distribution pattern for lesions involving the skin has not been recognized.

It should be stressed that gross evidence of vesiculation or bulla formation is extremely rare in dogs with the various immune-mediated mucocutaneous disorders, even though many of the human counterparts (especially pemphigus vulgaris and bullous pemphigoid) are characterized by bulla formation. This fact probably relates to the anatomic differences between the skin of the dog and that of man—in particular, to the thinner epidermis of the former.

## DIAGNOSIS

Although an immune-mediated mucocutaneous disorder could be considered in the differential diagnosis of any dog with lesions involving the oral mucosa, mucocutaneous junctions or the skin itself, a dog with involvement of all three areas or two of the three areas (i.e., oral cavity and mucocutaneous junctions, oral cavity and the skin, skin and mucocutaneous junctions) is the most likely candidate.

As far as differential diagnosis of immune-mediated mucocutaneous disorders on a clinical basis is concerned, the most problematic is the dog with lesions limited to either the oral cavity or the skin. In dogs with lesions limited to the skin, a thorough history and physical examination combined with basic diagnostic aids such as a Wood's light exam, skin scrapings, gram-stained smears of any exudate present, bacterial and fungal cultures, etc., should eliminate many of the differential diagnoses. In dogs with lesions limited to the oral cavity, such etiologic considerations as bacterial infections, trauma, caustic chemicals, severe dental disease and chronic uremia should be eliminated.

At the present time, microscopic examination of biopsy material is the only readily available method for definitively diagnosing the immune-mediated mucocutaneous disorders. Although the histologic lesions are somewhat subtle and difficult to demonstrate, they are highly diagnostic when present. Biopsy specimens of several lesions in various stages of development should be obtained and fixed in formalin. Biopsy of a minimum of three and preferably five to six sites greatly increases the chances for a definitive diagnosis. The tissues should be submitted to a dermatopathologist or a pathologist with an interest in dermatology. The pathologist should be made aware that you are considering one of the immune-mediated mucocutaneous disorders as a possible diagnosis and what the comparable diseases in man are.

Both direct (looking for tissue fixed immunoglobulin) and indirect (looking for circulating autoantibodies) immunofluorescence studies are extremely valuable in the diagnosis of these disorders in man. Preliminary work indicates that they are of value in the dog as well. At present, these tests are being performed in only a few institutions. Hopefully, the techniques will soon be standardized and more readily available. The LE preparation and/or the antinuclear antibody test are frequently positive in SLE.

## THERAPY AND MANAGEMENT

Obviously, once a definitive diagnosis of one of the immune-mediated mucocutaneous disorders has been made, therapy should be instituted immediately. It should be stressed that because it is frequently difficult to make a definitive diagnosis, therapy is often instituted on the basis of a tentative diagnosis alone.

The treatment of choice for the mucocutaneous disorders is the systemic administration of glucocorticoids. The initial dose of glucocorticoids that is required to bring the eruption under control may be quite high. After the disease is in remission, the dose may be gradually reduced until a maintenance dose is determined. The course of most mucocutaneous disorders is chronic and usually requires lifelong treatment.

Initially, prednisone at a dosage of 2 mg./kg./day is given orally in two divided doses. If the patient shows little or no improvement in 48 to 72 hours, the dose of prednisone should be increased to 6 to 12 mg./kg./day. Once an effective dose of glucocorticoids has been established, most dogs show a dramatic improvement in the lesions. Individual judgment determines the advisability of initially administering a broad-spectrum antibiotic concurrently with the glucocorticoids.

After the lesions have resolved, the dose of prednisone should be *gradually* reduced until a maintenance dose is determined. It should be stressed that premature or too rapid a reduction in the dose of glucocorticoids may result in an acute exacerbation of the clinical signs. For long-term maintenance, an alternate-day regimen of glucocorticoid administration (i.e., every other morning) is probably the method of choice.

In some dogs with mucocutaneous disorders the disease process may be refractory to even high doses of glucocorticoids. In such cases the addition of a cytotoxic drug, cyclophosphamide, may be necessary. Cyclophosphamide is given at a dosage of 1.5 to 2.5 mg./kg. orally once daily on four consecutive days of each week. Dogs weighing less than 10 kg. should receive 2.5 mg./kg. daily, dogs 10 to 25 kg. should receive 2.0 mg./kg. daily, and dogs over 25 kg. should receive 1.5 mg./kg. daily. The dose of prednisone when combined with cyclophosphamide is lower when prednisone is used alone and should be given at an initial dose of 1.0 to 1.5 mg./kg. orally daily with dogs over 25 kg. receiving the lower dose. Once the disease is in remission, the dose of both drugs should be gradually decreased and given at increasing intervals.

Since cyclophosphamide may cause bone marrow depression, gastrointestinal disturbances, hemorrhagic cystitis, nephrotoxity and hepatotoxicity, there is a need for weekly laboratory tests initially and periodically thereafter. Cyclophosphamide should be temporarily discontinued if clinical signs of toxicity develop, if the white blood cell count falls below 5000 cells/cu. mm., if the platelet count falls below 100,000 cells/cu. mm. or if a rising BUN level is detected. The administration of prednisone may be maintained unless toxic signs continue or worsen. Cyclophosphamide may be reinstituted when signs of toxicity have ceased unless hematuria has occurred.

In summary, the use of cytotoxic drugs such as cyclophosphamide should be reserved for difficult cases, and the clinician should be thoroughly familiar with the drug's actions, side effects, toxicities, etc., before utilizing them.

[*Editor's Note*: It is usually possible to differentiate histologically between the immune-mediated mucocutaneous diseases, although as is emphasized in this article, a number of biopsies and a competent and patient pathologist are prerequisites. Bullous pemphigoid is the more benign disease, and direct and indirect fluorescent antibody tests may be helpful in diagnosis. SLE is more severe and usually is accompanied by other organ system involvement. Pemphigus is usually fatal unless treated, and, again, both direct and indirect fluorescent antibody tests may be helpful in diagnosis.

The reader is reminded that not all mucocutaneous diseases are immune-mediated. Care must be taken to exclude mucocutaneous candidiasis (see article in *Current Veterinary Therapy V*) and also mycosis fungoides and some lymphoreticular neoplasms, which can have a mucocutaneous distribution (see Muller and Kirk, 1976.)]

## SUPPLEMENTAL READING

Hurvitz, A. I., and Feldman, E.: A disease in dogs resembling human pemphigus vulgaris; case reports. J Am. Vet. Med. Assn., *166*:585, 1975.

Muller, G. H., and Kirk, R. W.: Small Animal Dermatology. 2nd ed. Philadelphia, W. B. Saunders Co. 1976.

Stannard, A. A., Gribble, D. H., and Baker, B. B.: A mucocutaneous disease in the dog, resembling pemphigus vulgaris in man. J. Am. Vet. Med. Assn. *166*:575, 1975.

# RADIATION THERAPY IN DERMATOLOGY

DARRYL N. BIERY, D.V.M.
*Philadelphia, Pennsylvania*

Radiation therapy is a useful modality for treating selected benign and malignant skin diseases of dogs and cats. The skin neoplasms most radioresponsive are squamous cell carcinoma, anaplastic carcinoma, mast cell sarcoma, perianal adenoma and perianal adenocarcinoma. Malignant melanoma and fibrosarcoma are less radioresponsive but may be controlled effectively with radiation. Benign lesions, such as acropruritic granuloma and eosinophilic granuloma, which fail to respond to conventional medical treatment may be treated effectively with radiation therapy.

## PRINCIPLES

Biologically, radiation effectively kills both normal and neoplastic mammalian cells and theoretically could be used to control any tumor. The major limitation, however, to controlling a tumor *in vivo* with irradiation is the response of the adjacent normal tissue. Excessive irradiation of normal tissues may lead to severe desquamation and necrosis of skin or underlying structures. To minimize these complications the radiotherapist should limit the maximal dose of radiation to that which can be tolerated by normal tissue within the treatment portal.

Complications caused by excess irradiation of normal tissues may be difficult to manage, discouraging to the animal owner and veterinarian and possibly life-threatening to the animal, even though the maximal dose may not be tumoricidal. Irradiation may be given by one of two methods: (1) teletherapy, in which the X or gamma rays are produced some distance from the lesion; or (2) brachytherapy, in which radon or cobalt is either implanted in a lesion or used as a surface pack. Today most veterinary radiotherapy in dogs and cats is done with teletherapy using 200- to 300-kilovolt x-ray machines (orthovoltage), cobalt-60 or cesium-127. Orthovoltage

therapy is adequate for skin lesions less than 4 cm. thick or for lesions less than 4 cm. below the skin surface. The quality of the radiation (half-value layer) must be determined in each instance by the radiotherapist. The half-value layer is selected on the basis of size, involvement and type of lesion. Generally, benign and malignant skin lesions are treated with 1 to 4 mm. of aluminum or 1 mm. of copper half-value layer radiations, depending on the depth or thickness of the lesion. A *diagnostic x-ray machine can not and should not be used as a therapeutic unit.*

## MALIGNANT SKIN LESIONS

Radiotherapy of skin neoplasms should be considered, especially if the tumor is inoperable or has recurred following previous surgical excision. Prior to the decision to treat an animal with radiation therapy, a thorough medical examination of the patient should be done, including biopsy of the lesion, palpation of the lymph nodes and radiographs of the thorax and primary lesion site. The animal should have a reasonable life expectancy if radiation therapy is to be given, although in some animals short-term palliation may be as important as a cure to the client. Many neoplasms such as sarcomas can be treated with less than curative doses to produce regression, stasis of tumor growth or relief of pain, thus making the animal more comfortable for a slightly prolonged life span.

There is a paucity of data concerning the effectiveness of radiotherapy in the treatment of skin neoplasms. The probability of cure, therefore, cannot be stated precisely. Following radiotherapy in dogs and cats at the University of Pennsylvania, one-year survival data without clinical evidence of tumor recurrence are approximately 50 per cent for squamous cell carcinoma and 40 per cent for mast cell tumor. Of the tumors which recurred within one year, almost all

527

decreased in size following radiation therapy. The rate of tumor regression has not proved helpful prognostically. Approximately 50 per cent of the fibrosarcomas decreased in size following radiation therapy and did not recur for approximately 6 to 14 months. These data are similar to those reported by Dr. E. L. Gillette at Colorado State University. The tumors treated with radiation therapy either were difficult to remove surgically or had recurred following previous surgery. The histologic and clinical staging of the tumors and radiation therapy protocols were not uniform. Even though an insufficient amount of quantitative data are available in veterinary medicine, it is obvious clinically that cure rates differ for the individual tumor based on numerous factors, such as general patient health and location and clinical staging of the tumor. If tumors are treated for cure, they must be treated aggressively with a maximal irradiation dose.

Ideally 4000 to 5000 rads (absorbed dose) should be given to achieve a cure. The total radiation dose is divided into equal fractions of approximately 400 rads and is given on alternate days for approximately three weeks. For some tumors, such as transmissible venereal tumor and perianal adenoma, smaller doses of approximately 1500 to 2500 rads may be adequate to control the lesion.

## BENIGN SKIN DISEASE

Benign skin lesions that respond favorably to radiation therapy are acropruritic granuloma in the dog and eosinophilic granuloma in the cat. Radiation therapy should not be given unless all other conventional therapeutic treatments have failed. Following radiation therapy, approximately 50 per cent of the acropruritic granulomas in dogs have healed without recurrence. The radiation doses are usually fractionated into equal doses of 300 to 500 rads and are given once weekly until improvement is ob-

served. Improvement is usually observed within four weeks, but occasionally therapy must be protracted from six to eight weeks. Total doses that have been effective range from 800 to 3000 rads.

It appears helpful to prevent or discourage the dog from licking or chewing the lesion at least between the first several radiation treatments by (1) bandaging the lesion and (2) using a liquid dressing such as Obtundia,®* which may be applied to either the lesion or the bandage.

Approximately 30 to 50 per cent of the eosinophilic granulomas that do not improve with conventional medical therapy will heal following radiation therapy. Once-weekly fractions of 300 to 500 rads given over a period of four to eight weeks for total doses ranging from 500 to 4000 rads have been effective. Solitary eosinophilic granulomas respond more favorably than do multifocal lesions. Dr. Donald Thrall at the University of Georgia has successfully treated multifocal lesions of eosinophilic granuloma with strontium-90 beta-ray therapy. We have not used radiation therapy for the treatment of other benign skin lesions such as chronic dermatitis, otitis externa and elbow granulation as reported in the veterinary literature.

## SUPPLEMENTAL READING

Biery, D. N.: Radiation therapy in small animals. Pennsylvania Vet., June, 1971, pp. 4–6.

Gillette, E. L.: Indications and selection of patients for radiation therapy. Vet. Clin. N. Am., 4:889–896, November, 1974.

Gillette, E. L.: Radiation Therapy . (See p. 479 of this text.)

Silver, I. A.: Use of radiotherapy for the treatment of malignant neoplasms. J. Small Animal Pract., 13:351, 1972.

Von Essen, C. F.: Roentgen therapy of skin and lip carcinoma: Factors influencing success and failure. Am. J. Roentgenol., 83:556, 1960.

---

*Obtundia®, Otis Clapp and Son, Inc., Cambridge, Massachusetts.

# DEMODICOSIS (DEMODECTIC MANGE, FOLLICULAR MANGE, RED MANGE)

DANNY W. SCOTT, D.V.M.
*Ithaca, New York*

Demodicosis is an inflammatory, parasitic skin disease of dogs in which a larger than normal number of demodectic mites inhabit visible skin lesions. Why this normal skin resident produces disease in some dogs and not in others has intrigued clinicians and investigators for years. Current evidence suggests that demodicosis is an immunodeficiency disease, with probable hereditary predisposition in most cases.

## ETIOLOGY

*Demodex canis (D. folliculorum* var. *canis)* is a normal inhabitant of canine skin and is found in small numbers in most healthy dogs. The life cycle of the mite is apparently spent entirely on the host, but this cycle is incompletely understood. The parasite resides within the hair follicles and occasionally the sebaceous glands and apocrine sweat glands of the skin.

Four stages of *D. canis* may be demonstrated in skin scrapings. Fusiform eggs hatch into small, six-legged larvae, which molt into eight-legged nymphs and then into eight-legged adults. The male adult measures $40 \times 250 \mu$, the female $40 \times 300 \mu$. Mites (all stages) may sometimes be found in the lymph nodes, intestinal wall, blood, spleen, liver, kidney, urinary bladder, lung, urine and feces. However, mites found in these extracutaneous sites are usually dead and degenerate and probably represent simple drainage to these areas via the bloodstream or lymphatics.

## EPIDEMIOLOGY

*D. canis* is a normal resident of canine skin. Transmission occurs by direct contact from bitch to nursing neonates during the first two to three days of neonatal life. Attempts to transmit the disease by feeding dogs mites, by injecting mites intraperitoneally or by placing diseased animals in direct contact with non-neonate animals have failed. Puppies taken by cesarean section and raised away from the bitch do not harbor mites, indicating that *in-utero* transmission does not occur and emphasizing the importance of direct contact during the neonatal period.

It has been suggested that, in susceptible dogs, the skin is ecologically favorable for the reproduction and growth of the mites, allowing colonization of the hair follicles by thousands of mites, with subsequent development of demodicosis. Predisposing factors that have been suggested include age, short hair, inadequate diet, rapid growth, stress, accidents, boarding, estrus, nursing puppies, hunting or work, heartworms, nervousness, abnormally high or low environmental temperature, serum protein abnormalities, vaccinations, surgery, parturition, endoparasitism, poor condition, debilitating diseases and inherited or genetic factors. Most of these factors are difficult to evaluate and, at best, are highly unlikely. Some of these factors, such as hair coat length, sebaceous gland size and activity, sex, hypothyroidism and biotin deficiency, have been shown to have no effect on the development or progression of demodicosis.

The importance of heredity and immunodeficiency is firmly established. Demodicosis is most commonly seen in purebred dogs. The disease frequently occurs on a litter basis, or in related dogs. Frequently, the same bitch, though clinically normal her-

529

self, will produce litter after litter that becomes totally or in part affected with demodicosis. Elimination of such "carriers" greatly reduces the incidence of demodicosis in that population or kennel of dogs. This would certainly suggest a hereditary predisposition to demodicosis.

Demodicosis has been produced in dogs by treatment with antilymphocyte serum or long-term, high-dosage corticosteroids. Dogs with generalized demodicosis exhibit marked T-cell suppression (cell-mediated immunodeficiency) as assessed by *in-vitro* lymphocyte blastogenesis to various mitogens. This T-cell suppression is corrected as the mite population is eradicated, which suggests that T-cell suppression is associated with the presence of large numbers of mites. The serum from dogs with generalized demodicosis markedly suppresses the T-cell responses of normal dog lymphocytes. This serum immunosuppressive factor also disappears as the mites are eradicated. Serum protein electrophoresis in dogs with generalized demodicosis has revealed constant elevations in the $alpha_2$- and beta-globulin fractions.

The above information has served as the basis for a current hypothesis concerning the pathogenesis of generalized demodicosis in the dog: Generalized demodicosis is a manifestation of a specific T-cell defect, probably hereditary in nature, wherein the mite *Demodex canis* is allowed to multiply to large numbers and induce a humoral substance (in the $alpha_2$- or beta-globulin fraction?) that causes generalized T-cell suppression (cell-mediated immunodeficiency).

Although the preceding hypothesis explains the great majority of demodicosis cases, it certainly does not explain how an older dog can suddenly develop demodicosis. When this occurs, a thorough search is in order to determine the underlying endogenous or exogenous immunosuppressive factor(s). Examples of such factors are corticosteroid therapy, anticancer therapy, lymphosarcoma and malignant neoplasia.

## CLINICAL SIGNS

Demodicosis is manifested in two very distinct and vastly different clinical forms. The *localized or squamous form* typically presents as one to five small, well-circumscribed, erythematous, scaly, nonpruritic areas of alopecia around the eyes, lips or forelegs in a 3- to 10-month-old dog.

The *generalized or pustular form* is usually a severe disease and can terminate fatally. It is characterized by alopecia, erythema, edema, seborrhea, pyoderma and pruritus affecting large areas of the body. Marked peripheral lymphadenopathy is a constant finding. The skin possesses a very rancid or "mousy" odor due to bacterial action on surface lipids. The skin is quite tender and bleeds easily. Dogs with severe deep pyoderma are frequently febrile, depressed, lethargic, and partially anorectic. Demodicosis may sometimes become generalized without development of pyoderma.

## DIAGNOSIS

Skin scrapings, properly made and interpreted, are diagnostic. The affected skin should be squeezed to help extrude the mites from the hair follicles, and skin scrapings should draw blood. Diagnosis is made either by the demonstration of large numbers of adult mites or by finding an increased ratio of immatures to adults. The demonstration of an occasional adult mite in skin scrapings is consistent with a diagnosis of normal, *not* demodicosis.

Histopathologic studies reveal two stages of generalized demodicosis: (1) a stage of minimal to absent cellular response, when mites are confined to hair follicles; and (2) a stage of extensive cellular response, probably foreign body in nature, when follicular rupture occurs and mites are released into the dermis. These histologic findings, combined with the absence or presence in very small numbers of lymphocytes, are consistent with the proven state of cell-mediated immunodeficiency. They are certainly not consistent with former suggestions that generalized demodicosis was a manifestation of a delayed-type hypersensitivity reaction.

## TREATMENT

Just as the prognosis and course of the localized and generalized forms of demodicosis differ vastly, so do the therapeutic measures. Most dogs with *localized* demodicosis recover in three to eight weeks. An acaricidal preparation such as rotenone (Goodwinol®, Goodwinol Co.; Canex® Pitman-Moore), benzyl benzoate (Benzyl

**Table 1.** *Agents Used With Little Success in Treatment of Generalized Demodicosis*

| | |
|---|---|
| Acetarsonic acid | Mercuric sublimate |
| Acetone | Mineral oil |
| Alcohol | Nicotine |
| Arsenicals | Normal serum |
| Benzyl benzoate | Oil of thuja |
| Caraway oil | Peruvian balsam |
| Cashew nut oil | Phenamidine |
| Castor oil | Phenol |
| Chaulmoogra oil | Phenothiazine |
| Chlordane | Pine tar |
| Chlorox | Radiation |
| Cottonseed oil | Raw meat |
| Cresol | Riboflavin |
| Cythioate (Proban®) | Ronnel (Ectoral® orally and/or 1–2* aqueous dips) |
| DDT | Rotenone |
| Dichlorvos (orally and topically) | Salicylic acid |
| Disophenol (D.N.P.) | Sea water |
| Ether | Selenium sulfide |
| Fenthion (Talodex®, Neguvon®) | Sesame oil |
| Formalin | Sodium hyposulfite |
| Garlic | Sodium iodide |
| Gasoline | Sterile extract of fetal tissue |
| Green soap | Sterile milk |
| Griseofulvin (Fulvicin®) | Sulfur dioxide |
| Hexachlorocyclohexane | Sulfurated potash |
| Hydrochloric acid | Tar |
| Iodine | Thiabendazole |
| Iontophoresis | Thiocyanates |
| Kerosene | Trichlorfon |
| Lard | Trypan blue |
| Levamisole (Tramisol®, Ripercol®) | Turpentine |
| Lime sulfur | Xylol |
| Lindane | Zinc oxide |

Hex®, Evsco) or benzoyl peroxide gel (OxyDex® gel, DVM) should be applied to affected areas once daily and rubbed in well. The daily rubbing required to apply topical medications frequently causes more hair to fall out of parasitized follicles. Thus, the owner should be warned that the lesions may at first appear more hairless and larger after a few days of treatment. Topical treatment should be continued until hair regrowth is evident (average 4 to 8 weeks).

The results of treatment of *generalized* demodicosis have, in the past, been frustrating and inconsistent. The plethora of therapeutic claims and recommendations attests to the inconsistency of the results obtained. The two major shortcomings of most reports are (1) failure to indicate what form of demodicosis was being treated (localized or generalized) and (2) failure to allow for the fact that (because of small numbers of dogs treated) some cases of generalized demodicosis spontaneously regress with symptomatic therapy (especially in dogs less than one year of age). Virtually every drug ever developed has probably, at one time or another, been tried in the treatment of generalized demodicosis. Table 1 contains a list of the drugs that have been used with little or no success, on generalized demodicosis. One must regard all claims of therapeutic efficacy in generalized demodicosis with skepticism. Only one therapeutic regimen has been shown to be of consistent benefit in the treatment of generalized demodicosis.

Treatment must be directed at both the demodicosis and the secondary deep pyoderma. Deep pyoderma develops in over 50 per cent of cases of generalized demodicosis and is likely to occur secondary to the immunodeficiency state induced by the mites. Bacteriologic culture and antibiotic sensitivity testing must always be done to insure proper antibiotic therapy in these severe pyodermas. The major organisms involved are *Staphylococcus* spp. (58 per cent of cases), *Proteus* spp. (23 per cent) and *Pseudomonas* spp. (19 per cent). The presence of severe *Pseudomonas* pyoderma indicates a poorer prognosis, since deaths have been directly attributable to

*Pseudomonas* septicemia and abscess formation in multiple organs.

Antibiotics should be administered for a minimum of three weeks when deep pyoderma is present. A bactericidal agent should be chosen, again, in consideration of the established state of immune suppression. When deep pyoderma is severe and large areas of skin are ulcerated and fistulous, antiseptic (Betadine®, Purdue-Frederick) whirlpool bath therapy is indicated for 20 minutes daily until such denuded areas are healed. This is to prevent excessive percutaneous absorption of the acaricidal agent and potential toxicosis.

The miticidal agent of choice is topical ronnel. An approximate 4 per cent ronnel solution is prepared by adding 180 ml. of Ectoral® (Pitman-Moore) Emulsifiable Concentrate (33 per cent ronnel) or 250 ml. of Korlan-E® (Dow) (24 per cent ronnel) to 1000 ml. propylene glycol. This solution is apparently stable and effective for at least four weeks, whereas aqueous ronnel solutions become inactivated within 24 to 48 hours (the organophosphate is hydrolyzed). The solution should be shaken before application, since the two ingredients tend to separate. The treatment schedule is as follows:

1. The dog is clipped to remove body hair and facilitate application of the miticide. This may have to be repeated in long-haired breeds in 4 to 6 weeks.
2. The solution is applied to one third of the dog's body daily. Plastic or rubber gloves must be worn when applying this solution. The third of the body being treated must be thoroughly covered. The solution should be used liberally, rubbed in well and allowed to dry on. Ophthalmic ointment is used to protect the dog's eyes when the anterior one third of the body is being treated. *It is essential that every square inch of skin be treated!* One *cannot* simply treat visibly affected areas of skin. Attempts to treat more than one third of the body daily have resulted in rapid organophosphate poisoning.
3. Weekly skin scrapings are begun after five weeks of therapy. At this time, mites are often found to be dead and decreasing in number. Treatment is continued for three to four weeks *beyond* the finding of multiple (6 to 10) negative skin scrapings. Average duration of therapy is 12 to 15 weeks.

Expected side effects are mild to moderate erythema, marked scaling of the skin and mild to moderate weight loss. No attempt is made to control these, since they are self-limiting upon cessation of therapy. Occasional side effects are signs of organophosphate poisoning—anorexia, vomition, diarrhea and trembling—especially in small breeds. If these are seen, discontinue treatment, bathe the dog and treat with atropine until recovery occurs (24 to 48 hours). Therapy is then reinstituted, with one third of the dog's body being treated *every other day*.

The most alarming possible side effect has been hepatotoxicity. Four out of 65 dogs have, after variable intervals of therapy, developed signs referable to hepatic necrosis, with moderate to striking elevations in SGPT levels. Unfortunately, these dogs either had recently been on or at the time were on other drugs. Three of the four dogs recovered with symptomatic therapy and cessation of therapy. One dog died within 48 hours. Whether or not these reactions were associated with the miticidal solution, with the other drugs or with a combination thereof is not known. However, until this question is answered, one must be aware of the possible hepatotoxic side effects of the topical ronnel solution.

It must be emphasized that this treatment is harsh, rigorous, messy and somewhat expensive. Also, it is not totally free of hazard. It is neither indicated nor needed in the localized form of demodicosis. It is, however, the only consistently effective treatment regimen in the chronic, generalized case. This therapeutic regimen has been effective in over 90 per cent of such cases.

The use of corticosteriods in demodicosis is contraindicated. The author has seen cases of localized demodicosis apparently abruptly converted to severe, fulminating generalized demodicosis with the use of corticosteroids, including the most severe cases of demodicosis ever seen by the author. *Corticosteroids* suppress the specific and nonspecific immune response in an already immunosuppressed patient and *have no place in the treatment of demodicosis of any type!*

## PROGNOSIS

The prognosis for the *localized* form of demodicosis in young dogs is very good. Over 90 per cent of these cases recover in 3 to 8 weeks, probably in spite of therapy rather than because of it. These cases rarely relapse. However, it must be made clear to the owner that about 10 per cent of these localized cases will go on to generalize, again, in spite of treatment.

The prognosis for the *generalized* form is poor unless treated. Some of these dogs, especially those less than one year of age, will make spontaneous recoveries if treated symptomatically (control deep pyoderma and seborrhea, etc.). If treated as described above, a 90 per cent chance of recovery may be expected. Again, the presence of severe *Pseudomonas* deep pyoderma probably warrants a poorer prognosis. The potential of possible drug-related hepatic necrosis must be kept in mind.

The appearance of demodicosis in *any* form in an older dog warrants a guarded to poor prognosis. As mentioned previously, an underlying endogenous or exogenous immunosuppressive factor must be suspected.

Additionally, 7 of 65 (11 per cent) dogs with generalized demodicosis have developed bronchopneumonia, usually in the absence of concurrent pyoderma. The bacteria involved have been normal residents (*Aerobacter* spp., *E. coli*, *Proteus* spp.) in pure culture. This incidence of bronchopneumonia is certainly in excess of that usually seen in other dog populations and probably reflects the state of immunodeficiency present in dogs with generalized demodicosis.

## PROPHYLAXIS

Because of the strong probability that most cases of generalized demodicosis involve hereditary predisposition, it is suggested that dogs with generalized demodicosis, or dogs having produced litters affected with generalized demodicosis, not be used for breeding. Since demodicosis is not thought to be a contagious disease, it seems unlikely that a treated dog, truly relieved of its mite population, could ever contract the disease again.

[*Editor's Note*: A rotenone concentrate designed to be used as a 0.8 per cent solution in an alcoholic vehicle has been marketed all over the world except in the U.S.A. by Coopers for many years. Owing to stringent E.P.A. requirements, it is highly unlikely that this product will be available in this country in the foreseeable future. There are indeed rotenone products available here, but they are generally marketed in poorly penetrating bases and/or concentrations too weak to be effective. Studies at the University of Pennsylvania confirm that this is a highly effective therapy, and some 90 to 100 per cent of mites are killed by a single application.

A home-made rotenone solution has been used at the University of Pennsylvania for some years and is prepared as follows: 35.5 gm. powdered rotenone (e.g., Pennick and Co., New York) is taken up in a pint of chloroform and added to 3400 cc. of 70 per cent ethyl alcohol. A chemical hood should be used for the preparation.

This is a useful product for demodicosis, but we have not been able to compare its efficacy critically to the commercial product. Neither of these products should be applied to over one fourth of the body in a 24-hour period.]

## SUPPLEMENTAL READING

Scott, D. W., Farrow, B. R. H., and Schultz, R. D.: Studies on the therapeutic and immunologic aspects of generalized demodectic mange in the dog. J. Am. Anim. Hosp. Assn., *10*:233–244, 1974.

Scott, D. W., Schultz, R. D., and Baker, E.: Further studies on the therapeutic and immunologic aspects of generalized demodectic mange in the dog. J. Am. Anim. Hosp. Assn., *12*:203–213, 1976.

# FELINE EOSINOPHILIC GRANULOMA

PAUL W. HESS, D.V.M.
*St. Thomas, U.S. Virgin Islands*

*and* E. GREGORY MacEWEN, V.M.D.
*New York, New York*

Feline eosinophilic granuloma (FEG) is a frequently encountered skin disease of cats, one form of which is commonly referred to as "rodent ulcer." The actual incidence of this disease in cats is unknown, but we have treated and evaluated 140 cats with various forms of FEG over the past 4 years, in our respective clinics. The disease is characterized by chronic, progressive skin lesions, involving the lips, oral cavity, skin of the trunk and extremities.

## ETIOLOGY

The etiology is unknown; however, clustering of cases has been reported. We have observed multiple cases in some households, indicating that the disease could be spread between cats by an infectious agent. Attempts to identify an infectious bacterial or viral agent have been unsuccessful. We have been able to transmit the disease from one area of the skin to another area on the same cat with autologous tissue.

Eosinophilia refers to an increase in the number of eosinophilic leukocytes above normal. The eosinophil is thought to be associated with allergic disorders and parasitic infections. Recently it has been shown that eosinophils are attracted by insoluble or soluble antigen antibody complexes, which they will phagocytize. The relationship between the eosinophil and the immune complexes and the evidence that identical lesions can be induced in experimental animals with intradermal injections of antigen-antibody complexes suggest that FEG may be an immunologically related disease.

We have observed an interesting phenomenon associated with cats with chronic granulomas who were unresponsive to all forms of therapy attempted. Five cats were placed in cage confinement in our respective hospitals, and within a 6- to 10-week period the lesions regressed. No therapy was attempted and none of these cats has since developed granulomas. This has made us speculate on the possibility that an environmental factor or perhaps stress (cage confinement) has allowed some endogenous substance to be released to cause regression of the lesions.

## CLINICAL SIGNS

Clinically, cats with FEG are presented with ulcerated and sometimes proliferative lesions which can occur on the lips, tongue, palate, skin of the trunk, inguinal region and rear legs and between digital pads. The oral lesions are usually raised plaquelike masses that are red and ulcerative. The other lesions are usually proliferative and ulcerated and ooze serum. The cats are normally presented with a history of excessive licking and pruritus of particular areas of the body. The gross appearance of the lesions and clinical signs vary with the anatomic location and extent of involvement (Table 1).

FEG is seen most frequently in domestic short-haired cats. The average age of cats with FEG in our studies was 3 years. In our series of cases, 72 per cent of the cats were female, most of which (65 per cent) had undergone ovariohysterectomy.

## DIAGNOSIS

The diagnosis of FEG is usually based on the characteristic clinical appearance and location of the lesions. Clinical pathologic findings include a mild eosinophilia (greater than 8 per cent) in approximately 60 per cent of our cases. The eosinophilia varied depending on the previous therapy given (e.g., corticosteroids). About one half the cases had a higher than normal serum protein content and an altered albumin to globulin ratio. Serum protein electro

534

**Table 1.**   *Clinical Features of Eosinophilic Granuloma*

| SITE | CLINICAL APPEARANCE AND SIGNS |
|---|---|
| Lips | Generally bilateral ulceration with erosion of tissue. Licking of lips with varying degrees of erythema and hemorrhage. |
| Oral cavity (tongue, palate, pharynx) | Raised to slightly raised nodules with very little erosion or ulcerations but with whitish plaques and erythema of the borders. Difficulty eating and swallowing, with excessive salivation. |
| Skin of trunk and extremities | Raised nodular areas with definite borders. Erythema and/or ulceration may be present. Excess licking with alopecia are presenting signs. |
| Paws | Edema with moist clear or slightly purulent exudate. Painful for the cat to walk. |

phoresis revealed an increase in the total protein and a broad-based elevation in the beta- and gamma-globulin fraction. We have found that the increase in the level of gamma globulins is correlated with a longer duration of disease.

The histopathologic appearance of the lesions is similar no matter where their location but will vary with the duration of disease and according to any previous therapy which may have been given. Microscopic infiltration of the dermis with eosinophils, lymphocytes, plasma cells and histiocytes can be seen. Frequently, extensive mast cell infiltration has been seen and may confuse the histologic diagnosis. Also, there may be collagen necrosis with giant cells and epithelial cells present. Ulceration of the epidermis is common.

Eosinophilic granuloma must be differentiated from neurogenic dermatitis, which usually results from excessive licking and superficial ulceration of the skin in the flanks and dorsum of the back. The linear or intradermal granuloma, which is rare in our experience, usually occurs in young cats (1 year old) and is characterized by an erythematous, well-circumscribed, linear thickening in the skin of the extremities. Licking will cause ulceration, and the condition can then be readily confused with an eosinophilic granuloma. These cats usually will not have eosinophilia. The linear granuloma has been known to undergo spontaneous regression. The eosinophilic granuloma that can occur on the tongue or hard palate is often clinically diagnosed as squamous cell carcinoma and can only be differentiated by means of histologic examination.

## STAGING

We have developed a staging system to aid in our approach to the medical management of the patient. Stage I patients are those cats that have received no previous therapy. The Stage II patients have received previous therapy and responded but have recurrent disease. Finally, Stage III patients are those who are refractory to the conventional therapy (corticosteroids). In our experience this staging system is more accurate as a prognostic indicator than the extent or location of the lesions and the duration of the clinical signs.

## THERAPY

In the past, radiation was the usual treatment for cats with FEG. However, radiation therapy is limited by the availability of facilities, proper equipment and economic factors. Medical and surgical intervention are best suited to the practitioner with limited facilities. Surgery generally is used only as an adjunct to medical therapy or to aid in the diagnosis (biopsy). Early aggressive therapy of Stage I patients with frequent follow-up is the most important approach, because Stage II and III patients have a higher rate of recurrence even though they usually respond to most therapeutic regimens. Based on the results obtained in treating a large series of cases we advise the use of the following drugs. The actual drug, dosage and frequency of administration will depend on stage of disease and previous therapy (Table 2). All patients must be followed closely and observed for recurrent disease. Agents which have been shown to be effective are the following:

*Table 2.*   *Stages of Eosinophilic Granulomas*

| STAGE OF DISEASE | THERAPY | EXPECTED RECURRENCE AT 6 MONTHS |
|---|---|---|
| *Stage I*<br>Primary—no previous therapy | Intralesional triamcinolone,<br>megestrol acetate (Ovaban®)<br>(spayed females) | 10–25% |
| *Stage II*<br>Recurrent granuloma—<br>previously responsive<br>to steroids | Intralesional triamcinolone,<br>megestrol acetate (Ovaban®)<br>(spayed females) | 50% |
| *Stage III*<br>Refractory to intralesional<br>steroids | Single agents:<br>Levamisole-thiabendazole<br>Megestrol acetate<br>Radiation therapy<br>Experimental immunoadjuvants<br>Combination therapy:<br>Steroids plus levamisole or<br>thiabendazole<br>Megestrol acetate plus<br>Levamisole or thiabendazole<br>Steroids plus megestrol acetate (Ovaban®) | 50% |

**Corticosteroids.** This form of therapy has been the most commonly used and is still considered the best choice for treating FEG.

1. Triamcinolone (Vetalog®, Squibb) 6 mg./cc., is given by intralesional injection weekly until the lesion regresses completely, usually in 3 to 4 weeks. The intralesional dose is 3 mg. per treatment, and after regression of the lesion, 3 mg. can be given subcutaneously for 2 weeks.

2. Prednisone (5-mg. tablets) is given at a dosage of 2 mg./kg. divided BID, orally, until total regression; dosage should then be tapered gradually over the next two weeks. (Our experience with this therapy is limited.)

**Hormones.** Recently there have been a few case reports in the veterinary literature on the use of megestrol acetate (Ovaban®, Schering) for the treatment of FEG. The rationale for this approach is obscure, but preliminary studies indicate that this is effective.

Megestrol acetate (Ovaban, 5-mg. tablets) has been administered to 20 animals with eosinophilic granulomas (Stage II, 11 cases; Stage III, 9 cases). The drug was administered at a dose of 1 mg./kg. given intermittently every other day until 100 per cent regression was obtained (usually in 4 to 6 weeks). Then megestrol acetate was given once a week for 2 months, after which the

patient was given a maintenance dose of 1 tablet every other week. This produced complete regression in 5 of the 11 Stage II and 6 of the 9 Stage III patients, producing a response to the drug in about 55 per cent of cases. Spayed females seem to respond best to the drug. Side effects, which can be severe, included polydipsia, polyuria, polyphagia and weight increase. We caution the practitioner about the use of megestrol acetate in other than spayed females, because of the possible side effect of prolonged progesterone therapy on the uterus.

**Immunopotentiating Agents.** Evidence based on the histologic appearance and the possible role of the eosinophil has led us to believe that FEG may be an immunologically mediated disease. Immunopotentiation, or immunostimulation, is an attempt to initiate or augment an immune response toward a disease process. Immunostimulation has been shown to be effective in the treatment of some neoplastic conditions (see article on "Immunotherapy of Cancer"). We have been studying the effectiveness of both the chemical and the biologic immunopotentiators. The chemical immunostimulants include the common anthelmintics levamisole and thiabendazole. The biologic immunostimulant which we have studied and found to be effective is a mixture of killed *Serratia marcescens* and *Streptococcus pyogenes*. This preparation is under study and is still considered too experimental to warrant routine clinical use. We have found both types of immuno-adjuvants to be effective in the treatment of Stage III eosinophilic granuloma patients.

### Agents Available

1. Levamisole (Pitman-Moore, 100-mg. tablets) was administered in the dosage of 5 mg./kg. three times weekly (Monday-Wednesday-Friday) until 75 to 100 per cent regression had occurred (4 to 6 weeks) and then weekly thereafter for at least 2 weeks.

2. Thiabendazole (Mintezol®, Merck) 5 to 10 mg./kg. was given in a manner similar to that for levamisole.

The expected response rate with either of these agents is around 50 per cent, that is, one half of those treated regress at least 75 per cent.

We advise that the immunopotentiators be used only if the cat fails to respond either to intralesionally administered corticosteroids or to megestrol acetate. Further clinical investigations are necessary before the actual effectiveness of the agents can be determined.

Combination therapy may also be an effective way to approach the treatment of Stage III patients. We have found that granulomas which were unresponsive to steroids would then respond to steroids after a treatment course of levamisole.

Adjuvant methods of therapy include surgical removal of oral lesions to relieve mechanical problems associated with swallowing or mastication. Broad-spectrum antibiotics may be helpful to control the secondary bacterial infection.

Topical antibiotic-steroid combination ointments may also be used but are generally not that effective in our experience.

### PROGNOSIS

Stage I patients will usually completely respond to corticosteroid therapy, with an expected recurrence rate of 10 to 25 per cent within 6 months. The Stage II and Stage III patients respond to most therapy regimens if the treatment is administered for a prolonged period, but they usually have a 50 per cent recurrence within 6 months. Seventy-five per cent of the altered females respond to megestrol acetate (Ovaban). We have not followed enough patients to give an accurate recurrence percentage. FEG should be treated for a minimum of 3 to 6 weeks with an agent before another drug is tried. Many of the cases with chronic extensive lesions are slow to respond and do not show significant improvement for at least 4 weeks.

### SUPPLEMENTAL READING

Muller, G.H., and Kirk, R.W.: Eosinophilic ulcer. In Small Animal Dermatology. Philadelphia, W.B. Saunders Co. 1969, p. 264–266.
Scott, D. W.: Observations on the eosinophilic granuloma complex in cats. J.A.A.H.A., *11*: 261–270, 1975.

# HYPO-SENSITIZATION IN THE TREATMENT OF ATOPIC DISEASE

RICHARD E.W. HALLIWELL, M.R.C.V.S.
*Philadelphia, Pennsylvania*

### INTRODUCTION

Atopic disease can be defined as an inherited predisposition to develop IgE antibodies to the environmental allergens that gain access by being inhaled. The IgE antibodies attach to mast cells in the skin and to blood basophils in the circulation. Upon access, the allergen is carried via the bloodstream to the mast cells, where degranulation occurs with the release of pharmacologically active substances, including histamine and proteolytic enzymes. The main manifestation of the disease in the dog is pruritus, in contrast to asthma and hay fever, which are the major manifestations in man. The condition accounts for 3 to 4 per cent of dermatologic cases seen in canine practice.

Hyposensitization, which involves the injection of gradually increasing amounts of antigen, has been practiced in man since the 1920's. The classic concept of the therapeutic mechanism assumes that the beneficial effect is due to the formation of so-called blocking antibodies. These are protective, circulating IgG antibodies that have the effect of binding any inhaled antigen before it can reach the site of fixation of IgE in the skin. Few studies, however, have shown a good correlation between the titer of blocking antibodies and the clinical results. It may be that there is a more centrally acting mechanism that involves lymphocyte reactivity to the antigen.

## DIAGNOSIS

It is beyond the scope of this chapter to give an extensive description of the clinical signs of atopic disease. For this, the reader is referred to the supplemental reading list. However, a brief outline will be given, since a correct diagnosis is a prerequisite for successful hyposensitization therapy. The diagnosis can be derived from (a) the clinical signs and (b) intradermal skin testing.

**Clinical Signs.** The hallmark of atopic disease is pruritus. The pruritus often has a characteristic distribution involving the feet, the axilla and the face, but it may become generalized. It is questionable as to whether there is a primary eruptive process in atopic disease, but a variety of dermatologic changes are induced by self-inflicted trauma. A number of secondary changes may result, which include seborrhea and a predilection to pyoderma.

The pruritus is usually seasonal, coincident with the animal's sensitivities. In about 50 per cent of cases, however, the animal develops perennial pruritus as it becomes sensitized to dust and mold in its internal environment. In a small number of cases, the sensitivities are restricted to such allergens, and the problem exacerbates in the winter.

The clinical signs of atopic disease may be characteristic, but a definitive diagnosis cannot be made without confirmation by means of intradermal skin tests.

**Intradermal Skin Tests.** This method is preferable to scratch or prick tests because it is easier to perform and more sensitive. The animal is restrained in lateral recumbency without tranquilization or anesthesia. The hair on the lateral chest area is clipped and 0.05 cc. of a 1000 PNU or a 1:1000 W/V solution is injected. House dust extract, which tends to be irritant, is used at 250 PNU (1:4000 W/V). Positive and negative controls are included in the form of phosphate-buffered saline and a 1:100,000 dilution of histamine phosphate. A positive skin test is denoted by a wheal which exceeds that of the saline control by 3 mm. or more. It is essential that the animal not be given antihistamines for at least three days prior to skin testing. Corticosteroids have a more prolonged effect upon skin reactivity and additionally are immunosuppressive. If the animal has been given corticosteroid for a short period (1 to 3 months), it is recommended that three weeks elapse before skin testing is carried out. When more prolonged steroid therapy has been employed, up to three months may be required before a valid skin test is obtained. The ability to respond to an intradermal injection of histamine phosphate will return on cessation of steroid therapy well before reactivity to antigens. Thus, absence of a histamine wheal certainly implies that it is useless to proceed with a skin test, but its presence does not necessarily imply that a valid test will ensue.

It is important to remember that a positive skin test is merely an indication that the animal has skin sensitizing (IgE) antibodies to the allergens under investigation. It does not necessarily imply that the symptoms are caused by atopic disease. The skin test results must be considered in light of the clinical signs and the history of the patient.

The selection of allergens for skin testing must depend upon the geographic location, since not all allergens have a country-wide distribution. It has become more convenient and expeditious to use groups of antigens for skin testing, and although this can be reliable, it has some limitations. In general, the grass pollen antigens cross-react and, thus, it is unnecessary to test with individual grasses. The tree pollens cross-react less well, but then tree pollen allergy is not among the commonest allergies contributing to atopic disease, and adequate results are usually obtained by using a mixture. In this context, it should be remembered that a highly allergic animal will give a positive skin test to a very high dilution (even down to 1 PNU) of antigen. Thus, a seven-tree mix of 1000 PNU which contains 140 PNU of each type of pollen is probably adequate for diagnosis. The molds and the weeds likewise do not cross-react well. The latter are of great clinical significance; it is not recommended that weed mixes be used for skin testing. Obviously, the ideal skin testing regimen has to be devised with many factors in mind. It may be theoretically ideal to test with a large number of allergens, but there is a limitation to the number of injections which can be given to the average dog at any one time, and instituting a number of testing sessions will preclude participation of many clients because of financial considerations. A compromise protocol is thus usually adopted. The allergens used at the University of Pennsylvania are listed in Table 1.

## ALTERNATIVE FORMS OF THERAPY

Corticosteroids are highly effective in atopic disease. They represent the treatment of choice when the involvement is for a short period each year. However, the undesirability of maintaining animals on long-term corticosteroids has led to the search for other forms of therapy for animals affected perennially or for long periods of the year.

Antihistamines may be effective in selected cases, but even if they are effective, they may end up being far more expensive than hyposensitization.

## METHODS OF HYPOSENSITIZATION

Essentially, there are two main approaches: (1) aqueous extracts, which are rapidly absorbed and require a large number of injections; and (2) alum-precipitated extracts, which are more slowly absorbed, thus requiring fewer injections.

**Selection of Allergens.** There is a limit to the number of allergens that can be included in a vaccine in a highly allergic dog. Increasing the number can result in either (1) administering an allergenic load so large as to be potentially dangerous, or (2) diluting each one to such an extent that it may not be therapeutically effective. The vaccine is thus usually restricted to a maximum of 10 allergens.

In selecting these, three considerations are important, namely, the size of the skin test response, the animal's environment and the season of involvement. In considering the skin test response, the time of year that testing is carried out is important. Thus, antiragweed antibodies may have fallen to a low level by July, and, if testing is performed at that time, a reduced significance from a weak skin test may be falsely attributed to this allergen. Environmental considerations are also relevant. For example, if there is a strong response to feather mix, and the owner has recently disposed of all the feather pillows, it is unnecessary to include this allergen. Equally, if there is a response to tree pollens, and the animal's problem does not commence until June of each year, tree antigens can be left out if other considerations do not readily permit their inclusion.

Ideally, the schedule should commence in time to permit the dose to reach 1 cc. of the maintenance vial at least a month before the clinical signs commence. In the case of

## Table 1. *Allergens Used for Skin Testing**

| | | |
|---|---|---|
| House dust | Mold mix #2 | Marsh elder |
| Sheep wool |    (*Curvularia, Fusarium, Pullularia,* | Eastern tree mix |
| Kapok |      *Mucor, Rhizopus*) | Eastern grass mix |
| Cottonseed | Mold mix #3 | Ragweed (tall and short) |
| Human epithelium |    (*Alternaria, Aspergillus, Hormodendrum,* | Kochia |
| Cat epithelium |      *Penicillium*) | Goldenrod |
| Tobacco | English plantain | Yellow dock |
| Feather mix | Bayberry | Lamb's-quarters |
| | Pigweed | Sheep sorrel |
| | | Dandelion |

*Testing conducted at the University of Pennsylvania.

perennially affected dogs, this clearly cannot be achieved, but it is wise to commence therapy when the environmental allergic load is at its lowest.

PREPARATION AND USE OF AQUEOUS EXTRACTS. The third (maintenance) vial is made up to contain 10 cc. of allergen mixture of between 10,000 and 20,000 PNU/ml. This will usually mean 1 cc. of 20,000 PNU solution of each allergen when 10 are employed, but possibly 2 to 3 ml. when only a small number of allergens are used. Vial #2 is a 10-fold dilution of #3 and, likewise, #1 is a 10-fold dilution of #2. Each vial is made up to 10 cc., and the schedule given in Table 2 is followed.

Rush hyposensitization with aqueous extracts is a new approach that was begun in Scandinavia for the treatment of children with allergic asthma. Injections are given at 2- to 6-hour intervals for the first 4 to 7 days, enabling a maintenance level to be built up within that period of time. Initial studies at the University of Pennsylvania have shown that this appears to be a safe and efficacious technique, but further work is necessary before this is tried in the field.

PREPARATION AND USE OF ALUM-PRECIPITATED EXTRACTS. Exactly the same considerations are followed in mixing the extract except that only two vial strengths are used. The slower release of the allergen permits commencing at a higher strength. Vial #2 will contain the same amount of strength of allergens as vial #3 in the aqueous extract, and vial #1 will be a 10-fold dilution. The injection schedule for alum-precipitated extracts used at the University of Pennsylvania is shown in Table 3.

When additional season's therapy is planned with aqueous extract, it is quite safe to recommence therapy with vial #2. Alternatively, therapy can be maintained year round with 1-cc. doses of vial #3 administered every 4 to 8 weeks. Giving such large doses at greater intervals could carry a risk of anaphylaxis. Booster injections at maintenance dosage can probably be safely given at 2- to 4-month intervals using alum-precipitated extracts, but if a greater interval elapses, it would be wise to drop to a smaller dose and work up again.

**Results.** Experience over the last 10 years at the University of Pennsylvania has shown that hyposensitization is a safe and efficacious therapy for atopic disease. Approximately 75 per cent of patients obtain complete or substantial relief. The remaining 25 per cent respond less well or not at all. A proportion of the poor responders will respond better to a second year of therapy than to the first.

An unanswered question is the length of therapy required. Some animals appear to

***Table 2.*** *Schedule for Hyposensitization—Aqueous Extracts**

| | VIAL #1 (100–200 PNU/ml.) | VIAL #2 (1000–2000 PNU/ml.) | VIAL #3 (10,000–20,000 PNU/ml.) |
|---|---|---|---|
| Day 1 | 0.1 cc. | | |
| 3 | 0.2 | | |
| 5 | 0.4 | | |
| 7 | 0.8 | | |
| 9 | 1.0 | | |
| 11 | | 0.1 cc. | |
| 13 | | 0.2 | |
| 15 | | 0.4 | |
| 17 | | 0.8 | |
| 19 | | 1.0 | |
| 21 | | | 0.1 cc. |
| 23 | | | 0.2 |
| 25 | | | 0.4 |
| 27 | | | 0.8 |
| 29 | | | 1.0 |
| 39 | | | 1.0 |
| 49 | | | 1.0 |
| 69 | | | 1.0 |
| 89 | | | 1.0 |
| 119 | | | 1.0 |
| 149 | | | 1.0 |
| 179 | | | 1.0 |
| and so on, as required | | | |

*Subcutaneous injection.

***Table 3.*** *Schedule for Hyposensitization—Alum-Precipitated Extracts**

| | VIAL #1 (1000–2000 PNU/ml.) | VIAL #2 (10,000–20,000 PNU/ml.) |
|---|---|---|
| Day 1 | 0.1 cc. | |
| 8 | 0.2 | |
| 15 | 0.4 | |
| 22 | 0.8 | |
| 29 | 1.0 | |
| 36 | | 0.1 cc. |
| 43 | | 0.2 |
| 50 | | 0.4 |
| 57 | | 0.8 |
| 64 | | 1.0 |
| 84 | | 1.0 |
| 104 | | 1.0 |
| 134 | | 1.0 |
| 164 | | 1.0 |
| 194 | | 1.0 |
| and so on, as required | | |

*Subcutaneous injection.

be cured after one year's therapy. In other animals, two years' therapy seems to effect a cure, whereas some cases appear to require indefinite maintenance therapy. In all events, even if perennial therapy is required, our current evidence suggests that it is safer to be giving perennial hyposensitization than perennial corticosteroids. Side effects from injections of allergen are extremely rare and usually consist merely of pruritus following injection. This can be prevented by prior antihistamine therapy.

Allergenic extracts are not expensive, and a large volume practice can readily turn hyposensitization into a profitable specialty. Alum-precipitated extracts are more costly, but this evens out as fewer injections are required. It must be emphasized, however, that this is not something that should be commenced without proper reading and preparation. Not only will poor results ensue, but in unskilled hands, the technique can be potentially hazardous.

### SUPPLEMENTAL READING

Anderson, W. A.: Canine allergic inhalant dermatitis. Ralston-Purina Co., 1975.
Baker, E.: The management of allergic disease by hyposensitization. J. Am. Vet. Med. Assn., 154:491–494, 1969.
Chamberlain, K. W.: Biological management of the allergic patient. Vet. Clin. N. Am., 4(1):65–77, 1974.
Halliwell, R. E. W., and Schwartzman, R. M.: Atopic disease in the dog. Vet. Rec., 89:209–214, 1971.

# STEROID THERAPY IN SKIN DISEASE

RICHARD E. W. HALLIWELL, M.R.C.V.S.
*Philadelphia, Pennsylvania*

## INTRODUCTION

Steroids are organic molecules with a structure based upon the perhydrocyclopentophenanthrene nucleus (Fig. 1). They are related to, and often derived from, sterols that are found abundantly in nature—particularly as constituents of animal and plant fats. They also occur in vegetable oils and animal nervous tissue; others are from yeasts and other microbiologic sources.

Advances in steroid chemistry and therapy have been one of the most outstanding achievements in modern medicine. There is now available a vast range of steroid derivatives with an amazingly broad spectrum of biologic activity. Most remarkable is the fact that a minor substitution or configurational change in the molecule may produce a compound with an entirely different biologic activity.

Although initially these compounds were derived primarily through isolation of the biologically active steroid from animal tissues, chemical processes were later developed by which comparatively cheap starting materials of both animal and plant origin could be employed in a wide range of synthetic processes, thus producing the enormous range of steroid compounds that are now available synthetically. The chemical structures of some major steroid compounds are shown in Figure 1.

The compounds to be considered in this chapter are the corticosteroids, androgenic steroids, estrogenic steroids, antiandrogenic steroids and progesteronal steroids.

## CORTICOSTEROIDS

These compounds have their main value as highly effective therapeutic agents in the treatment of allergic skin diseases. They are also of value in the treatment of autoimmune skin diseases and in many inflammatory skin conditions of unknown etiology. The anti-inflammatory action of cortisone was known many years ago, but it was in use as a routine anti-inflammatory agent for a short time only. It was rapidly superseded by the synthetic analogues which proved much more potent with fewer undesirable

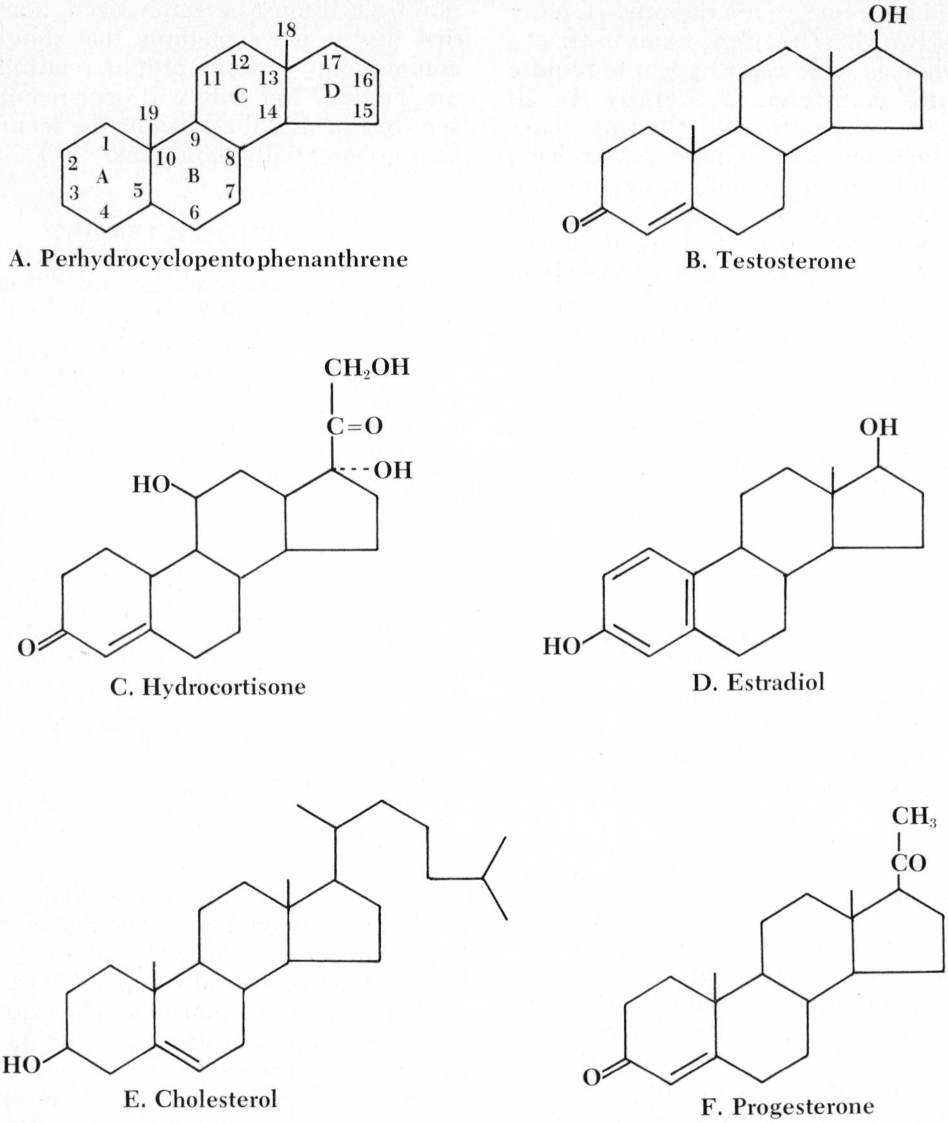

A. Perhydrocyclopentophenanthrene

B. Testosterone

C. Hydrocortisone

D. Estradiol

E. Cholesterol

F. Progesterone

**Figure 1.** Structures of some steroid compounds.

side effects. The relative anti-inflammatory potency of some of the common corticosteroids is indicated in Table 1.

## MODE OF ACTION OF ADRENAL CORTICOSTEROIDS

Despite continuing intensive research, little is known about the means by which corticosteroids exert their anti-inflammatory action. Some concepts, however, have received support in recent years.

If one considers the pathway of a type I (IgE-mediated) allergic reaction, corticosteroids can moderate the reaction as fol-

lows: (1) they are immunosuppressive and will tend to deplete lymphoid tissue and hence prevent the formation of antibodies—both protective (IgG) and IgE; (2) IgE antibody exerts its influence by attaching to mast cells, and there is evidence that corticosteroids depress the number of mast cells in the skin; (3) corticosteroids stabilize membranes and are antienzymic and thus will have an inhibitory effect on mast cell degranulation; (4) in a way that is not fully understood, corticosteroids inhibit the mediators of inflammation that result from mast cell degranulation.

In a type III allergic reaction (mediated

*Table 1.* *Approximate Relative Anti-inflammatory Activity of Common Corticosteroids*

| | |
|---|---|
| Cortisone | 0.8 |
| Hydrocortisone | 1.0 |
| Triamcinolone | 3.0 |
| Prednisone | 3.5 |
| Prednisolone | 4.0 |
| Methylprednisolone | 5.0 |
| Dexamethasone | 29.0 |
| Flumethasone | 30.0 |
| Betamethasone | 30.0 |

by complement-fixing antibody) corticosteroids can also act at various stages in the pathway. They are immunosuppressive, but more important, they are anticomplementary. That is to say, they inhibit the complement sequence that is the central mechanism in the pathogenesis of this type of allergic reaction.

Corticosteroids are also highly effective in cell-mediated hypersensitivity (type IV reaction). They are immunosuppressive in cell-mediated immunity just as they are in humoral immunity, and they also inhibit the mediators of cell-mediated hypersensitivity.

Corticosteroids reduce the inflammation associated with bacterial infections. There is a recently described polymorph dispersal factor, which has the effect of dispersing polymorphs from the site of a bacterial invasion. This explains why staphylococcal pyoderma will often clinically improve very dramatically with the use of corticosteroids alone. Clearly, however, this is not the treatment of choice.

Another important mechanism by which corticosteroids act is through stabilization of lysosomal membranes. Lysosomes contain proteolytic enzymes which, upon release, cause cell damage. This in turn releases more lysosomal enzymes, and the sequence becomes self-perpetuating. This type of mechanism can follow any sort of inflammatory response. Corticosteroids, by their membrane-stabilizing action, thus abort this sequence of events.

## INDICATIONS

Short-term corticosteroids are indicated in a wide range of dermatologic disorders, including parasitic allergies (together, of course, with parasiticidal therapy) and atopic disease when the involvement is for a limited period each year. They may be employed to reduce sebum production and as anti-inflammatory agents in seborrhea oleosa. They may be used both intralesionally and parenterally in lick granulomas. Long-term corticosteroids are indicated in autoimmune skin diseases once a specific diagnosis has been made.

Corticosteroids are contraindicated in demodectic mange and in superficial and deep pyodermas. Although they may be effective antipruritics, they are also contraindicated in seborrhea sicca, since they will further suppress sebum production and compound the problem over the long term.

## TYPES OF PREPARATIONS AVAILABLE

Corticosteroids are available for oral and parenteral administration, and there is marked variation in the length of action of a single dose of individual steroids. Conventionally, the length of action is taken to be the time during which the individual's endogenous corticosteroid release is depressed. Short-acting corticosteroids (with suppression of the adrenal glands for less than one and one-half days) include prednisone, prednisolone and methylprednisolone (Medrol®, Upjohn). Long-acting corticosteroids (with an action greater than two and one-half days) include dexamethasone and betamethasone. It is quite possible, however, that in some instances the anti-inflammatory effect of a single dose may persist longer than the measurable physiologic effect. A number of repository corticosteroid preparations are available which have a much longer duration of action. Thus the effect of methylprednisolone acetate (Depo-medrol®, Upjohn) is probably two to three weeks and that of triamcinolone acetonide (Vetalog®, Squibb) and betamethasone diproprionate (Betasone®, Schering [also contains betamethasone sodium phosphate]) is up to 30 days. It must be emphasized that the criteria for judging the length of action of a corticosteroid are imprecise, and clinical effects may be noted for a much longer time than are the apparent physiologic effects. It is clearly unnecessary for the practitioner to acquaint himself with all the products available. It is more rational for him to familiarize himself thoroughly with a limited number and get to know the advantages and limitations of each.

## SELECTION OF CORTICOSTEROIDS

The factors that must be taken into account when selecting a corticosteroid include the following:

1. The species. A preferred corticosteroid in one animal is not necessarily the preferred drug in another animal. For example, methylprednisolone acetate (Depo-medrol®, Upjohn) seems to be a preferred steroid in the cat because of its profound anti-inflammatory action and very few side effects, whereas it does not appear to offer any advantages over other corticosteroids in the dog.

2. The price of the drug. Many of the newer corticosteroids are expensive and offer little advantage in many instances over the cheaper, older steroids, such as prednisolone and prednisone. Cushingoid effects can occur as readily with triamcinolone as with prednisolone.

3. The nature of the condition. A clinician may opt for one course of therapy when short-term therapy only is required (e.g., acute moist eczema, hot spot) and another when a longer-lasting effect is desired. It is quite unnecessary to use a long-acting steroid (e.g., methylprednisolone acetate) in the former case. Remember that it is never wrong to use a short-acting corticosteroid, because you can add to it as required.

4. The nature of the animal. Injectable long-acting steroids may be preferred with an intractable animal that is difficult to treat.

## DOSAGES

It is impossible to lay down hard and fast rules concerning corticosteroid dosages. An effective dose for a specific condition in one animal may be quite inappropriate for a different condition in another animal. The clinician must become thoroughly familiar with the actions—both desired and otherwise—of a limited number of steroids in a wide range of diseases. However, some generalizations can and should be made.

1. The dosage of prednisolone or prednisone required to control an allergic skin disease is from 0.5 to 1.0 mg./kg. daily. In general, such problems are usually controllable by the lower mg./kg. dose in larger animals, higher relative doses being required for smaller animals.

2. The dosage of other steroids producing an equivalent anti-inflammatory effect can be computed by reference to Table 1.

3. Chronic inflammatory skin disease in which much secondary change has occurred will usually require higher doses.

4. Exercise extreme caution when treating sick and aged animals. Remember that liver damage may increase duration of action, and impaired renal function may heighten any potential electrolyte imbalances.

**Alternate-Day Therapy.** Special considerations apply to the case that requires long-term corticosteroid therapy. Such cases will most often be autoimmune diseases or cases in which a diligent search for etiology has failed and the clinician is forced to treat symptomatically. Such an approach must also be used when the client is unable or unwilling to subject the animal to a work-up which may provide a diagnosis and lead to specific therapy. These clients must be informed that they are jeopardizing their animals' lives and that side effects are to be expected sooner or later.

There is abundant evidence that because of the diurnal variation in endogenous corticosteroid secretion, a less deleterious effect on the body can be produced by giving a short-acting corticosteroid on day 1 at 9 A.M. (this would be prednisone, prednisolone or methylprednisolone acetate) and no additional therapy until 9 A.M. on day 3. This gives the adrenal gland time to recover and results in an almost complete recovery in the blood picture (eosinopenia and lymphopenia) by 9 A.M. on day 3. Clinically, the approach should be to reduce the patient to a minimal maintenance dosage on a daily basis and then double the dosage for administration at 9 A.M. on the first day of the alternate-day therapy.

**Withdrawal from Corticosteroids.** An animal that has been on corticosteroids for a long time (six months or more) may go into an adrenal crisis if therapy is stopped suddenly. This is particularly likely if some stressful condition is superimposed, such as surgery or intercurrent disease. It must be remembered that extreme suppression of adrenocortical function will follow long-term corticosteroid therapy, although this can be minimized by alternate-day therapy. In general, two approaches are used:

1. Gradual weaning of the steroids over a period of four to six weeks. In general, this would mean halving the dose each week and then converting to alternate-day therapy, and perhaps therapy every third day.

2. A quicker withdrawal can be achieved using ACTH to stimulate the adrenals. In this context it must be remembered that the length of action of a gel preparation of ACTH is little more than 12 hours, and thus it should be administered twice daily. Although it may take many weeks for the adrenal glands to return completely to normal even with this approach, it appears to be safe to administer ACTH for three weeks, while at the same time gradually lowering and stopping the steroid. It is wise to determine the total eosinophil count once a week for 2 to 3 weeks after the drug has been discontinued, since this will provide advance warning of impending adrenal crisis. Should an animal require some surgery or enter any other stressful situation in the weaning period, it is advisable to recommence steroids for a short while.

*Remember that the best way to achieve withdrawal from long-term corticosteroids is never to start them.*

## ESTROGENS

Estrogenic therapy of skin diseases of small animals is at best empirical. We are not yet at the stage where estrogenic assays are routinely available, and whether or not the so-called estrogen deficiencies are real entities is a matter of debate. Certainly conditions are seen which respond to estrogenic therapy, but these compounds are potent substances with profound pharmacologic effects, and their value in therapy of selected conditions does not necessarily imply that the original condition was due to estrogen insufficiency.

Estrogens have two major actions on the skin: they suppress sebum production and they promote keratinization. Many estrogenic substances are commercially available, but all have a significant incidence of side effects and the newer ones offer little material advantage over diethylstilbestrol.

### INDICATIONS

Low doses of estrogens are of value in therapy of seborrhea oleosa provided that the clinician is absolutely certain that increased sebum production is involved.

Pruritic conditions are sometimes encountered in spayed bitches and may present as a papular eruption (ventral) or as a predisposition to a pyoderma. Low doses of estrogens may be employed if they are not contraindicated for any other reason and if care has been taken to rule out any other possible etiology. They may also be of value in vulvar dermatitis of spayed bitches, but surgical reconstruction offers the only permanent cure for this condition.

Estrogens are highly effective when given by local injection in reducing the size of anal adenoma prior to surgery. Acanthosis nigricans in the spayed bitch will sometimes respond well to low doses of estrogens, particularly when accompanied by low doses of corticosteroids.

In the cat, estrogens may be tried in the therapy of feline endocrine alopecia and also in miliary dermatitis—both in spayed females only.

### SIDE EFFECTS

The clinician must remember that estrogens are highly potent substances and should be used with extreme caution. Excessive doses in the dog will cause profound bone marrow depression, the initial manifestation of which is often thrombocytopenic purpura. Some individual animals will show an unpredictable individual idiosyncrasy to the drug and will show toxicity at a much lower dosage than would be toxic to the general population.

Unspayed bitches may show signs of estrus, and spayed animals may become attractive to males. In general, the potential uterine side effects mean that use of estrogenic drugs should be restricted to males and spayed females.

In the cat, estrogens appear to be hepatotoxic, and they should be used with great caution in this species. This is reversible and the drug should be discontinued at the first sign of trouble.

If estrogens are to be of value in skin diseases, they will exert their influence in low doses. A cat should never receive more than 0.1 mg. of diethylstilbestrol daily, and therapy should be changed to alternate days with the same dosage after 2 weeks. If maintenance therapy is required, it is dangerous to exceed 0.2 mg. total dosage per week.

In the dog, dosage of diethylstilbestrol should not ordinarily exceed 0.1 mg./5 kg. body weight per day. For long-term therapy (over a month) this dosage should be halved or given on alternate days. Ten milligrams of repository diethylstilbestrol can safely be injected intralesionally in anal adenomas on three to five occasions at 2-week intervals in all but small dogs (less than 10 kg.).

## ANDROGENS

The major effects of androgens on the skin can be ascribed to their anabolic action and to their stimulatory effect on sebaceous glands.

As is the case with estrogens, androgenic therapy in skin diseases is highly empirical. Clinicians describe patterned hair loss and hyperpigmentation in intact males, termed hypoandrogenism; however, there are vast numbers of dogs that maintain perfectly normal hair coats following castration. The problem is, of course, that androgens are secreted by the adrenals as well as by the testes, and estrogens are secreted by the testes in addition to androgens. Until we have accurate methods applicable to the routine laboratory measurement of all these steroids, we are left in the unhappy situation of theorizing that some skin problems may arise from a relative imbalance of androgens and estrogens and must proceed somewhat blindly from that point.

### INDICATIONS

The major indications for androgens are in conditions of the dog and cat in which castration has resulted in a dermatologic disorder.

Castrated male dogs occasionally present with patterned symmetrical hair loss. There is often seborrhea sicca and sometimes some generalized hyperkeratosis. Methyltestosterone in a dosage of 0.5 mg./kg. body weight daily may be tried in such cases, and a brisk response is usually seen. A slightly lower dosage will usually suffice for maintenance.

Castrated male cats will sometimes develop symmetrical alopecia, and there may be an associated miliary dermatitis. Two to 5 mg. of methyltestosterone may be helpful, but megestrol acetate (see later) is usually more effective.

### SIDE EFFECTS

Androgens, in the dosages mentioned, are relatively free from side effects, the main problem being a resumption of the male characteristics for which the animal was neutered in the first place.

## ANTIANDROGENS

A number of antiandrogenic drugs have been tried in the past in the treatment of seborrhea oleosa associated (as by definition it should be) with increased sebum production. The somewhat waxy feel to the hair coat in some cases of seborrhea sicca in fact makes it quite difficult to distinguish between the two types of seborrhea in some instances. Antiandrogens may be of benefit in this condition in both sexes owing to their suppressive action on sebum production. One such compound is currently undergoing clinical trials, the results of which are awaited with interest.

## PROGESTERONES

Progesteronal agents may have a direct stimulatory effect on sebaceous glands, but additionally they may have profound effects on other hormones, including antiestrogenic and/or antiandrogenic activity. Despite their broad physiologic effects, these agents have been disappointing in dermatologic therapy until the advent of megestrol acetate (Ovaban®, Schering). The original reports from England of its value in feline dermatology have been confirmed by many clinicians in the United States.

The mode of action is far from clear. Antiinflammatory properties of a drug are normally judged by (1) its ability to induce lymphopenia and eosinopenia and/or (2) its effect upon induced granulomas. There is no evidence based on either criterion that megestrol acetate has any direct antiinflammatory action. It does have antiestrogenic and antigonadotropic activity and also mild glucocorticoid properties, as judged by its effect on liver glycogen, but it is hard to ascribe its therapeutic efficacy to any of these properties.

It is of course noteworthy that most of the conditions in which it is helpful are of unknown etiology. Also of great interest, and quite inexplicable, is the fact that its therapeutic efficacy is confined almost exclusively to the feline.

### INDICATIONS

Initial reports commented on its value in feline miliary dermatitis, in which it is highly efficacious. In most cases, the animal responds within a week, but maintenance dosage is usually required to keep the animal asymptomatic. Many possible etiologies have been ascribed to this condition, but it is important to distinguish it from flea-bite dermatitis, which it resembles clinically. The former, however, is seen exclusively in spayed or castrated animals. The drug will in fact help flea-bite dermatitis, but higher doses are required for complete control.

Feline endocrine alopecia, another condition of unknown etiology, is also responsive to the drug. It is of value in treating eosinophilic granulomas (see article on "Feline Eosinophilic Granuloma"), and its action here appears to be complementary to that of corticosteroids. Dramatic results are often seen with use of a combination of methylprednisolone acetate (Depo-Medrol®, Upjohn) (4 mg./kg. every 2 weeks) and megestrol acetate.

The dosage of megestrol acetate employed at the University of Pennsylvania is usually 0.5 mg./kg. body weight daily for 2 weeks, and then every other day for 2 weeks. Miliary dermatitis and feline endocrine alopecia may require maintenance therapy at 0.5 mg./kg. every 3 to 5 days.

In the dog, its value appears to be limited according to reports to date. Some cases of pruritic seborrhea sicca are responsive but rather large doses are required (e.g., about 1 mg./kg. body weight daily).

## SIDE EFFECTS

Since it is a progesteronal agent, megestrol acetate should probably not be used for long-term therapy in intact females. Some veterinarians do not remove the uterine body when spaying cats, and there have been reports of development of endometritis in the remaining uterine body following long-term therapy. Such occurrences are very rare but can prove difficult to handle. The mild glucocorticoid activity means that megestrol acetate is contraindicated in diabetics.

Side effects encountered have included polyphagia and occasional personality changes, the animal in most cases becoming more docile. Occasionally the reverse has been noted. Essentially, however, it seems to be a very safe drug that will quickly find its way into the dermatologic armory of the practicing veterinarian.

---

# ECTOPARASITES

LLOYD REEDY, D.V.M.
*Dallas, Texas*

Ectoparasites are a major cause of dermatologic problems in both dogs and cats. They should be considered first in the dermatologic examination. Proper diagnosis is essential to good results. It is very embarrassing to overlook a case of scabies to diagnose it as an allergy. A thorough clinical history; close, careful examination of the lesions and the entire body with good lighting and magnification; and proper skin scrapings will do much to eliminate error. When insecticides are dispensed or recommended, directions should be written down and the potential dangers of overdosage or improper use should be discussed. Ophthalmic ointments should be used in the animal's eyes and the animal's ears should be plugged with cotton before dips are applied. Idiosyncrasies to insecticides can occur, and this is especially true in

young or debilitated animals. The owners should also be cautioned as to possible reactions in man, and it is wise to advise that rubber gloves be worn.

## FLEAS

Fleas (Siphonaptera) are brown, wingless insects with laterally compressed bodies and strong legs adapted for leaping. In the adult stage, all are blood-sucking ectoparasites of endothermal animals. Two species, *Ctenocephalides felis* and *C. canis*, are most commonly found in dogs and cats. *C. felis* is usually found on both dogs and cats and occasionally on the mouse, rat, chicken, baboon and man. When the two species occur together, *C. felis* competes more favorably than *C. canis*.

## LIFE CYCLE

Only adult fleas are found on the host, where mating and oviposition generally occur. The eggs, which are small, white and spherical, fall quickly from the pelage and often collect in the bedding. Under optimal conditions (25° C. and 80 per cent relative humidity) the incubation period is two to four days. The larvae are small, white, maggot-like and legless. Caudal processes called anal struts assist in movement. There are three larval stages, called instars, but active feeding takes place only during the first two stages. The larvae ingest organic material, especially blood-containing fecal pellets of the adults. This material falls off the host with the eggs and collects in the bedding. Shortly after molting, the third instar larva spins a cocoon, which is oval and inconspicuous. A pupa forms in a few days, and this stage lasts about two weeks, during which time the adult is formed. The life cycle from eggs to adult, under optimal conditions of temperature and humidity, is completed in 18 to 21 days, but in nature it probably is longer. Life span depends on temperature, humidity and the presence of a suitable host. Desiccation from low humidity can shorten the life of adults sooner than starvation, since they can live for a year or longer without food if humidity is high but die in a few days if humidity is low. Fleas are more prevalent in the summer on outside dogs and cats but may be found all year on house pets.

## CLINICAL EFFECTS

Affected dogs and cats may show only mild responses to fleas, but more frequently, restlessness, biting, scratching, ruffled hair coat and self-induced trauma are seen. Erythema with a papular reaction occurs at the site of the bite. Self-excoriation, resulting from the pruritus, can produce hair breaking and local alopecia. These lesions are usually located on the posterior half of the animal's body, primarily at the base of the tail, along the dorsum, on the flanks and in the inguinal area. In chronic cases, the skin becomes thickened and indurated.

Flea bites can cause an allergic dermatitis. The sensitization occurs when a chemical substance in the flea saliva is introduced during feeding. This is believed to be a hapten (incomplete antigen) which

*Table 1.  Major Types of Parasiticides*

1. *Natural or Botanical*—Chemicals found in plants used since prehistoric times.
   Some earth compounds still in use today—sulfur and arsenic.
   Botanical compounds—rotenone, pyrethrins and nicotine.
   Generally, natural compounds act by either contact or stomach activity; most offer quick kill but have little residual activity.
   Pyrethrin is derived from the flower of the chrysanthemum. It is less toxic to warm-blooded animals but very toxic to insects and other cold-blooded animals. Controls primarily horseflies, fleas, lice and mosquitoes.
2. *Chlorinated Hydrocarbons*—Developed primarily during World War II.
   Those which tend not to persist offer fairly long-term residual control but are not mobile in the environment (do not accumulate in food chains and are relatively nonpersistent).
   Examples: Toxaphene, methoxychlor, lindane.
3. *Carbamates*—Effective against insects developing resistance to certain other insecticides.
   Inhibitor of cholinesterase activity at a lower level than many commonly used organophosphates.
   No marked tendency to attack central nervous system of higher animals. Since it is a crystalline solid, it is one of the safer pesticides to handle. It has a low order of toxicity toward mammals.
   In the dust form, it is not readily absorbed through the skin.
4. *Organophosphate Compounds*—Developed after World War II.
   Inhibit production of cholinesterase, which is essential to normal nerve function.

combines with a dermal collagen to form a complete antigen. Both delayed (cell-mediated) and immediate (humoral-mediated) reactions have been found to occur. Severe reactions result in an area of acute moist or serous dermatitis ("hot spot") that is most common on the posterior parts of the body but may occur anywhere, including the head and neck. Cats may react with numerous small, crusted miliary papules in the same areas.

## DIAGNOSIS

Infestation is diagnosed by finding either fleas or flea excrement on the host. The excrement is seen as small, dark, gritty particles in the pelage which turn brownish red on white filter paper when moistened. Since the fleas may carry the intermediate form of the common dog and cat tapeworm, *Dipylidium caninum*, the presence of tapeworm segments on the perianal area would also confirm the presence of fleas.

Sometimes the clinician is presented with cases that appear to be related to flea-bite hypersensitivity, but fleas or evidence of fleas cannot be found. Intradermal test blebs (0.03 to 0.05 cc.) of dilute antigen (1:10 or 1:20) may be made on the shaved lateral thorax. Appearance of wheal within 15 or 20 minutes would support the diagnosis of flea-bite hypersensitivity. Alternatively, delayed reactions may occur (24 to 48 hours) which are equally significant.

## CONTROL

Most of the commercial insecticide sprays, dips and powders will kill adult fleas on the host. The most common cause of reinfestation is failure to treat the premises properly, especially the animal's bedding. Flea eggs and cocoons are very resistant to therapy, and the premises should therefore be treated at least twice. Most topical preparations have very short residual action. All dogs and cats in the household should be treated at the same time.

## DOGS

Most veterinarians prefer dippings at 2-week intervals supplemented with applications of flea powder once or twice weekly. Kem Dip® (Thuron) is very effective against both fleas and ticks. It contains 5 per cent Delnav, 1 per cent DDVP and 10 per cent penthane. It is diluted 2.5 to 5.0 ounces per gallon for topical use on dogs only. Five per cent methylcarbamate dust (Sevin®, Thuron) is satisfactory for between dippings.

## CATS

Only preparations approved for use on cats should be used. Since cats object to sprays and dips, 5 per cent Sevin dust applied two or three times weekly is very useful. When applying dusts, it is necessary to apply it along the back, around the neck and on the ventral body, fluffing the hair back and forth to cause the powder to penetrate the hair coat.

## FLEA COLLARS AND FLEA TAGS

Most of the pets presented to veterinary offices have flea collars or flea tags. Very few of the practitioners questioned by the author recommend their use in flea control. There are two basic types of flea collars in the United States. One releases a vapor of insecticide (Vapona®, Shell) and the other releases a powder which is spread over the animal's body by normal activity (Baygon® and Sevin®, Thuron). There are precautions with these products, especially with their use on cats and certain breeds of dogs (e.g., greyhounds), so the directions should be read and followed.

## PREMISES

It is necessary to coordinate treatment of the premises with topical applications of insecticides to all pets in the household. Special care must be given to areas where the pets sleep or spend most of their time. Since the eggs and cocoons are resistant to therapy, several applications at 2- to 4-week intervals are recommended. Vacuuming these areas before and after treatment is helpful. Injudicious use of insecticides in the home must be avoided to prevent staining the carpets and furniture. Most veterinarians recommend the use of a professional exterminator. This is still probably the best approach, but most clients consider it expensive. An alternative is the use of premise flea fogger bombs, a good example of which is Vet Fog® (Thuron). Directions for their use are on the can and should be read and followed carefully. Doghouses, kennels, yards and runs should be cleaned thoroughly and then sprayed with Kem Dip (12 ounces per gallon) every 14 to 28 days.

## OTHERS

Oral organophosphates are not recommended for the control of fleas because of their potential toxicity. Care must be taken when topical insecticides are used with other organophosphates such as Task® (Shell). Flea antigen (Haver-Lockhart) has been used with some success in flea-bite hypersensitivity, but flea control measures should not be ignored.

## TICKS

Ticks are divided into two major families: hard ticks (ixodids) and soft ticks (argasids). All pass through four stages: egg, larva (seed

## Table 2.   *Common Parasiticides**

| NAME | MANUFAC-TURER | INGREDIENTS | ADVANTAGES | DISADVANTAGES |
|---|---|---|---|---|
| **SPRAYS** Pet Spray | Vet Kem | 0.5% Carbaryl 0.05% Pyrethrins | Quick kill against fleas, ticks and lice. Easy to apply. | Must be applied to insect. Low concentration and rapid evaporation cause poor repellent and residual action. |
| Norsect | Norden | 0.50% Carbaryl 0.075% Pyrethrins 0.15% Piperonyl butoxide (tech) | As above. | As above. |
| Sect-a-Spray | Evsco | 0.50% Pyrethrins 0.50% Piperonyl butoxide (tech) 0.05% Carbaryl | As above. | As above. |
| **POWDERS** Flea and Tick Powder | Vet Kem | 5% Carbaryl | Low skin absorption. Effective against ticks, fleas and lice. Evaporation slow and therefore fairly long residual action. | Difficult to apply to long-haired animals. |
| **DIPS** Kem Dip | Vet Kem | 5% Delnav 1% Vapona® 10% Penthane | Effective against ticks, fleas and lice. Can also be used as premise spray (yards, kennels, etc.). | Involves wetting the dog. Not to be used on cats. Should not be used more often than 7-14 days. Long-term effectiveness against fleas, but not as good as powders. |
| Dermaton | Burroughs Wellcome | 24.5% 2-chloro-1-(2,4-dichlorophenyl) vinyl diethyl phosphate | Good against resistant fleas. Some veterinarians use one teaspoon to a pint as a "wipe," applying sparingly every other day in severe cases. | Use on dogs only. |
| Gamma R-X | Carson Chemicals | 8.82% Lindane | Effective scabicide. | Do not use on cats. |
| Lime sulfur | | | Effective against scabies mites. Can be used on cats. | Bad odor. Not as effective against ticks and fleas. |

| | Manufacturer | Active Ingredients | Effective against scabies. | Do not use on cats. |
|---|---|---|---|---|
| Para-Dip | Haver-Lockhart | 8% Carbaryl 3.9% Gamma Benzene Hexachloride (from lindane) 1% Captan | Effective against scabies. | Do not use on cats. |
| **SHAMPOOS** | | | | |
| Mycodex with lindane | Beecham-Massengill | 0.30% Lindane | Quick kill against fleas and lice. | Since the product is rinsed off, no residual action. Not to be used on cats or nursing puppies. Not effective against ticks. |
| Fleavol | Norden | 0.05% Pyrethrins 0.5% Piperonyl butoxide (tech) | As above. | As above, but can be used on cats. |
| KFL Shampoo | Pitman-Moore | 0.05% Pyrethrins | Can be used on cats. Quick kill against fleas and lice. | Not effective against ticks. Animal must be wet to use and rinsed off, so no residual action. |
| **COLLARS AND TAGS** | | | | |
| Tick collar | Vet Kem | 9.4% Carbaryl | Simple to apply. Very low skin absorption. Normal activity of day causes dispersion of insecticide. Does not depend on vaporization. Kills both ticks and fleas. Long residual action (up to five months). | Should not be used on cats. May not be as effective in dogs with flea-bite hypersensitivity, since concentration of insecticide on rear of body may not be high enough to repel fleas. Read precautions on the label. Some owners find odor offensive. |
| Flea Medallion (for dogs) | Vet Kem | 18.6% Vapona | Simple to apply. | Not to be used on cats. Not effective against ticks. Since this product works by vaporization, it may not be as effective as other products applied directly. This is especially true in flea-bite hypersensitivity. Read precautions on the label. |
| Flea Collars (for dogs and cats) | Vet Kem | 9% Vapona (Dogs) 4.7% Vapona (Cats) | Same as Flea Medallion. | Same as Flea Medallion. |

*Space does not permit the listing of all common parasiticides and their manufacturers. This list includes examples of the types commonly available to most veterinarians. Other manufacturers may have similar ingredients. Consult your veterinary drug supplier. Read and follow the directions carefully, especially the precautions for use.

tick), nymph and adult. The larva has six legs; the nymph and adult have eight. The larva, nymph and adults of both sexes are parasites and feed on blood and lymph. All stages of the hard ticks have a heavy chitinous shield or scutum on the dorsal surface. In the adult male, the scutum extends almost to the posterior margin of the body. In the larva, nymph and adult female, it is restricted to the anterior half of the dorsal surface. The female, nymph and larva distend when engorged with blood. Ticks may hibernate through the winter.

The brown dog tick or kennel tick (*Rhipicephalus sanguineus*) is found in tropical and temperate regions of the world and is especially common in the southwestern United States, Central America, Southern Europe and Africa. The dog and several wild carnivores are the primary hosts, but cats and man can be affected.

## LIFE CYCLE

The brown dog tick is a three-host tick. Its life cycle can be as short as two months but often is much longer. After feeding and mating on the final host, the female detaches, drops off and moves in a horizontal direction until it encounters a vertical object. It then climbs this object, often a wall or fence, and begins to lay 1000 to 5000 eggs in a protected crack or crevice. The eggs hatch in about three weeks, depending on temperature, and the larvae seek a new host. They feed for 3 to 8 days, detach, drop to the ground and in about a week molt to nymphs. Nymphs find a new host, feed for 3 to 11 days, drop off and in 11 to 15 days molt to adults. Adult females feed for about a week; males remain attached for weeks or months. Under ideal conditions ticks can survive unfed for up to one year, but usually survival over 2 months is rare.

## CLINICAL EFFECTS

Ticks may attach almost anywhere on the body but are especially common around the neck, in the ears and between the toes. Tick bites may cause inflammation and irritation as well as anemia from blood loss. They may also serve as vectors of bacterial, rickettsial, viral and protozoal diseases. Engorging females may produce a toxin which can cause a posterior paralysis followed by total motor paralysis. Removal of the tick is usually curative. Surprisingly large nodular allergic reactions may sometimes occur.

## CONTROL

Owners should be warned not to pick ticks off their dogs because of the danger of anaphylactic reactions. Instead, tick sprays should be applied directly to the tick. The brown dog tick is the only tick species in the United States that has developed well-defined resistance to insecticides. The organophosphate Diazinon® (Ciba-Geigy) is reported to be effective against resistant strains, but there is danger that resistance is now developing to this insecticide.

## DOGS

Affected dogs should be dipped every two weeks in Kem Dip® (Thuron) (2.5 to 5.0 ounces per gallon). Dead ticks may not drop off for several days, and blood-engorged ticks may take longer to die than those at other stages in the cycle. The newer tick collars (e.g., the Vet Kem collar, which contains 9.4 per cent methylcarbamate) may be tried, but it is not yet clear how effective these are in practice.

## PREMISES

It would be best to refer those clients who have problems with ticks in the home to a professional exterminator. Vet Fog® (Thuron) has been found to be effective. Treatments should be repeated every two weeks. Yards and kennels should be treated every two weeks through the summer with Kem Dip (12 ounces per gallon). Special care must be taken to apply the insecticide to vertical objects such as walls and especially cracks and protected areas.

## SARCOPTIC MANGE

*Sarcoptes scabiei canis* is the mite which causes scabies or sarcoptic mange in the dog. Interhost transmission to man is usually transient and mild but is a valuable diagnostic aid as well as a potential source of embarrassment to the veterinarian if the diagnosis is missed.

## LIFE CYCLE

The sarcoptic mite spends its entire life cycle on the host, and transmission is by direct contact. The entire life cycle takes 10 to 14 days. Mating occurs on the surface of the skin, and fertilized females as well as males and unfertilized females burrow into the epidermis. The fertilized female deposits eggs in the tunnel behind her. Eggs hatch in 3 to 8 days, and larvae migrate to the skin and molt through protonymphs and tritonymphs to adults. The adult stage is reached 4 to 6 days after the eggs hatch. The mite cannot survive much over 24 hours away from the host, so that reinfection from the premises is not a problem.

## CLINICAL EFFECTS

Since transmission is by direct contact, the typical case is a new puppy from a pound or commercial supplier. An intensely pruritic papular eruption with crusting and scaling, especially along the margins of the ears, on the elbows and on the lower thorax, are noted. The skin appears dry, rough and thickened. Alopecia and secondary infections are not uncommon.

## DIAGNOSIS

Ideally the characteristic mites and/or eggs should be demonstrated on skin scrapings. Pruritic areas, especially the tips of the ears, should always be scraped. Sometimes the mites may not be found whether or not the owner has bathed the dog or applied topical medication. If there is a history of dog-to-dog transmission or dog-to-human transmission, all dogs in the household should be treated for sarcoptic mange. Although human infections with animal scabies are generally believed to be mild and self-limiting, severe pruritus and prolonged papular eruptions have been reported. When the disease is suspected, the clinician should warn the owners of the possible animal-to-human transmission. If clinical evidence is strong, the case should be treated whether or not the mite can be demonstrated.

## TREATMENT

Since the mite prefers the dog and will only reproduce on the dog, it is essential to treat all dogs in the household repeatedly until the disease is under control. Bathing with an antiseborrheic shampoo (Thiomar®, Evsco) to remove the scale is recommended before dipping. Bathing and dipping every 5 days for eight treatments seems to give the best results. Most commercial dips will kill the mite but 0.03 to 0.06 per cent lindane with or without organophosphates (e.g., Para-Dip®, Haver-Lockhart) is for resistant cases. Dips should be mixed fresh each time before application and not stored, since they deteriorate.

## LICE

Lice are wingless insects that are dorsoventrally flattened. They are divided into two groups: sucking lice (anoplurans) and biting lice (mallophagans). Lice are host-specific and spend their entire life on the host, surviving only a few days if separated. They are spread by direct contact or through contaminated brushes and combs. The eggs (nits) are connected to the host hairs, and the entire life cycle takes 14 to 21 days. *Trichodectes canis* is the common biting louse of dogs and may act as the intermediate host of the dog tapeworm, *Dipylidium caninum*. It is much more active and causes more irritation than *Linognathus setosus*, the only sucking louse found on the dog. Lice are found primarily on the neck and shoulders, especially under the collar. They can cause restlessness, pruritus, skin inflammation and alopecia. Diagnosis is based on the clinical signs plus the demonstration of the parasite or its eggs. Although common in Europe, lice are still rare in the United States.

## CONTROL

Five per cent Sevin® (methylcarbamate) dust or Kem Dip® (Thuron) should be applied every 7 to 14 days until all stages of the parasite are eradicated. All dogs on the premises should be treated.

## HEAD MANGE IN CATS

*Notoedres cati* is an epidermal mite which causes head mange in cats. It has been reported in rabbits and dogs, but this is rare. Animal-to-man transmission has also been reported. It resembles *Sarcoptes scabiei* and has a similar life cycle. Transmission is by direct contact. The mite causes persistent pruritus, alopecia and excessive scaling and crusting of the ears, face and neck. The skin may become thickened and wrinkled. The entire body can be involved. The condition must be differentiated from dermatomycosis, superficial pyoderma and seborrhea. Skin scrapings should demonstrate the presence of the mite or its eggs. The condition is becoming very rare, particularly in the United States.

## CONTROL

Lime sulfur (2.5 per cent) or malathion (0.5 per cent) dips applied weekly for at least six treatments are reported to be effective. It usually is not necessary to treat the premises, since the mite is an obligatory parasite and cannot survive away from the host. Treating all the cats in the household is essential if good results are to be obtained.

## CHEYLETIELLA

*Cheyletiella yasguri* has only recently been recognized on the dog in North America, and previous reports of *C. parasitovorax* from the dog may have been *C. yasguri. C. parasitovorax* is commonly found in the pelage of rabbits, rarely in the cat and occasionally in the dog. Both are large mites, nonburrowing and obligatory parasites. All stages—the egg, larva, first and second nymph and adult—occur on the host, and transmission is by direct contact. Both dogs and cats can be infested with these mites. Animal-to-man transmission is believed to be less common than sarcoptic

mange, but the condition is clinically similar.

## CLINICAL EFFECTS

Mild pruritus with abundant yellow-gray scales along the dorsum and on the rump, top of the head and nose are common. The mite should be demonstrated on skin scrapings. Puppies appear to be more commonly affected, but any age may be susceptible. Remember that the mite is a surface dweller, and only a shallow scraping is required after the skin is moistened with mineral oil.

## TREATMENT

Antiseborrheic shampoos (Thiomar®, Evsco) to remove the scale, followed by insecticide dips every 5 to 7 days for eight treatments (0.5 per cent malathion), are usually effective. All dogs in the household, as well as cats and rabbits, should be treated. The problem of reinfestation from the premises should be considered. Kennel areas should be cleaned and treated with a good insecticide spray (Kem Dip, 12 ounces per gallon). Bedding should be destroyed or thoroughly sprayed. Households may require the use of a professional exterminator or Vet Fog® bombs (Thuron). Treatments should be repeated in two to four weeks. Precautions on the label should be followed carefully.

### SUPPLEMENTAL READING

Flynn, R. J.: Parasites of Laboratory Animals. Columbus, Ohio State University Press, 1973.
Hazeltine, W.: Chemical resistance of the brown tick. J. Econ. Entomol., 52:332, 1959.
Muller, G. H., and Kirk, R. W.: Small Animal Dermatology. 2nd ed. Philadelphia, W. B. Saunders Co., 1976.

# SKIN MANIFESTATIONS OF DEEP MYCOSES

GEORGE H. MULLER, D.V.M.
*Walnut Creek, California*

While some deep mycoses infect only internal organs, such as lungs, liver and spleen, others produce skin lesions directly or through fistulization. Such lesions and the fungal diseases that cause them will be discussed here. In contrast to some dermatomycoses, deep fungal infections are not contagious. They are often acquired through inoculation of the fungus into the wound. The actual development of a deep mycosis depends on the site and manner of inoculation and the specific immunologic resistance of the host. Some deep fungi are so pathogenic that almost all inoculated animals can be infected, while others can cause disease only in individuals with low resistance. The type and location of the lesion vary also with each species of fungus. One form of *Sporothrix* infection forms round cutaneous nodules that may spread along lymphatics; *Nocardia asteroides* can cause ulcers, fistulas and abscesses of the paws; *Aspergillus niger* may prefer mucous membranes and *Curvularia geniculata* commonly produces fistulas of the paw with purulent exudate–containing granules.

In general, systemic mycoses are relatively rare except in specific geographic areas where certain mycoses are endemic. As with any rare disease, the diagnosis of deep mycoses can be overlooked if it occurs in a region where it is not expected. It is advisable to keep this in mind for skin diseases that fail to respond to treatment and cause the lesions described in this article.

## Sporotrichosis

The skin lesions of sporotrichosis occur first at the site of entry of the causative fungus *Sporothrix schenckii*, and this site is usually one of the extremities. Puncture wounds from thorns, wood slivers or bites provide a channel of entry for the organism. Sporotrichosis is most common in climates of high humidity and warmth, namely, the coastal regions and river valleys of the southern United States or in other countries with similar climates.

It is advisable to look for the classic lesions, which are multiple round, firm, nontender nodules with a raised border that can become ulcerated and discharge a thick, brownish-red exudate. Whenever such lesions are seen and do not respond to antibiotic therapy, diagnostic procedures should be performed that may reveal the presence of the fungus.

In practice, culture of the purulent exudate is the best method of diagnosis. Inoculation of Sabouraud's medium at 25° C. or of brain-heart infusion agar at 37° C. will result in rapid growth of *Sporothrix* in positive cases. Biopsy of the affected tissue with periodic acid-Schiff (PAS) or Gomori's

methenamine silver (GMS) stains reveals the organism in the form of small, ovoid or cigar-shaped pleomorphic bodies.

Sporotrichosis can be classified into three types. The *cutaneous form* remains localized in the skin and consists of many slowly multiplying firm nodules. When these lesions also invade the lymphatic system, it is called the *cutaneolymphatic type*, which is the most common form of the disease. When the fungus invades other tissues, such as the bone, lung, liver, spleen, kidney, testes and gastrointestinal and central nervous systems, it is called the *disseminated form* of sporotrichosis.

Fortunately, the undisseminated forms respond well to sodium iodide solution (20 per cent) given orally at a daily dose of 0.05 mg./kg. body weight. Within one week, initial clinical response occurs, but treatment should be continued for 30 days after the disappearance of lesions. The disseminated form is usually unresponsive to inorganic iodides. On the basis of reports of disseminated sporotrichosis in man, amphotericin B should be considered for therapy of similar cases in the dog.

## Nocardiosis

Although nocardiosis is best known for its invasion of the respiratory system and other internal organs, it is capable of producing skin lesions in dogs and cats. Such lesions consist of nodules, ulcers, fistulas and abscesses with an affinity for the legs. Cutaneous hypertrophy is common, and mycetoma-like enlargement of the feet occurs. The individual lesions are often circular, consisting of a central zone of necrosis surrounded by a halo of granulation tissue. A brownish-red exudate drains from the center of such lesions. In cats, *Nocardia asteroides* is one of the causes of pyothorax. It is advisable to examine the external lymph nodes, which are usually swollen and can even have draining fistulas. (See page 261.)

Diagnosis is made by culturing the causative organism, *Nocardia asteroides*, on Sabouraud's agar at 25° C. The colony is smooth, soft and orange, with a wrinkled surface and long, thin mycelia. Direct smear stained by Gram and acid-fast methods may be useful. Biopsy material stained with PAS, GMS or Brown and Breen (B & B) gram tissue stains may also be diagnostic. It is normally a soil saprophyte and belongs to the group of pathogenic actinomycetes.

Treatment of nocardiosis has been somewhat successful with sulfonamides. Sulfadimethoxyine, 24 mg./kg. orally s.i.d., or sulfadiazine at a dose of 1 to 6 gm. daily for 2 to 3 months has been used. In addition, penicillin can be given simultaneously for short periods of time. Recently, a new antibiotic, clindamycin, has been used for actinomycosis in man and may also be useful in animals. Nocardial mycetoma in man has also recently been reported to respond to a combination of trimethoprim and sulfamethoxazole (Tribrissin®, Burroughs Wellcome). (See also the combination treatment by surgery and chemotherapy described in Section 13, "Infectious Diseases.")

## NORTH AMERICAN BLASTOMYCOSIS

Although rare in dogs and cats, *Blastomyces dermatitidis* can cause skin lesions. These consist of papules, pustules, ulcers and subcutaneous abscesses. When skin lesions are seen, they are often only external manifestations of the presence of the disease internally, especially in the lungs and lymph nodes. The disease has a rapid course and is often fatal. Therefore, immediate laboratory diagnosis is indicated. Pus from the abscesses should be examined microscopically for characteristic budding, yeastlike cells and should be cultured on blood agar at 37° C. and on Sabouraud's agar containing cycloheximide and chloramphenicol at room temperature. The colony is moist and glabrous at the beginning and later develops a fluffy, white mycelium, which turns light brown. Serologic tests are also useful for diagnosis as is biopsy of material stained with PAS and GMS.

North American blastomycosis occurs mostly in the eastern half of the United States and Canada but has been reported as far west as Texas.

Treatment with amphotericin B can be attempted, but the prognosis may be poor, especially if the patient is debilitated.

## MYCETOMA

Mycetoma is a rare disease that affects the skin and subcutaneous tissue anywhere but is especially common on one of the feet. Lesions consist of draining fistulas, and the exudate contains small granules. Characteristically, there is much granulation tissue and swelling until the entire foot is hard and grotesquely swollen. Its failure to respond to antibiotic treatment differentiates this disease from abscesses and other infections.

There are a number of possible causative organisms. *Curvularia geniculata* and *Allescheria boydii* are the most common. Although *Helminthosporium* spp. have been reported as causative organisms of mycetoma, they may have been erroneously identified and the actual agent may belong to the genus *Drechslera*. In that case, the condition is not a true mycetoma but phaeohyphomycosis. *Nocardia asteroides* can also cause mycetoma-like changes in the feet of dogs and cats.

Diagnosis is made by culturing the exudate on plain Sabouraud's dextrose agar, because media used routinely for dermatomycosis will inhibit these fungi. Biopsy and staining with PAS and GMS are often useful.

Treatment for mycetoma is very difficult, and surgical removal of some of the fibrinous mass is temporarily helpful. Amputation of the affected paw can be used as a last resort and is usually curative.

## PHAEOHYPHOMYCOSIS

Phaeohyphomycosis is caused by the dematiacious fungus *Drechslera spicifera*, which has a preference for subcutaneous tissue. The typical lesion is a subcutaneous nodule that gradually enlarges and develops one or more fistulas from which a yellow, pink or purulent-looking exudate drains. The opening of the fistula appears ulcerated but seems to be relatively painless.

The lesions usually are located on the leg and chest. So far, the infection has been confirmed only in the cat and the horse; however, it is possible that some reported mycetomas of dogs may have actually been phaeohyphomycosis caused by *D. spicifera*, which resembles the mycetoma fungi of the genus *Curvularia* or *Helminthosporium*.

Diagnosis can be established by culture and biopsy. Exudates from fistulas or pieces of biopsy tissue are planted on plain

Sabouraud's dextrose agar without cyclo-heximide or antibiotics. The colonies grow rapidly at room temperature and progress in color from white to black, with a flat, velvety surface. Positive identification is made by microscopic appearance of the conidiophores and conidia. The biopsy specimen stained with periodic acid-Schiff (PAS) reveals typical fungal elements.

It is necessary to differentiate phaeohyphomycosis from chronic abscesses, mycetoma, feline leprosy, foreign body fistulas and tumors. Treatment can be accomplished by surgically excising all affected tissue and surrounding adipose layers. For recurrences, excise all newly affected tissue again. Specific systemic drugs have not yet shown effectiveness, but the same oral medications outlined for nocardiosis can be tried in resistant cases.

## OTHER MYCOSES

Several other systemic fungal infections affect dogs and cats but they rarely affect the skin. These include *Cryptococcus neoformans*, *Coccidioides immitis*, *Aspergillus fumigatus*, *Histoplasma capsulatum* and organisms belonging to Phycomycetes.

[*Editor's Note*: There is no evidence to suggest that the deep mycotic infections represent a zoonotic health hazard. However, it is recommended that simple precautions be taken, such as disposing of contaminated exudates and avoiding contact with open wounds.]

### SUPPLEMENTAL READING

Nitidandhaprabhas, P., and Sittapairochana, D.: Treatment of nocardial mycetoma with trimethoprim and sulfamethoxazole. Arch. Derm., Vol. 3, October, 1975.

---

# SPOROTRICHOSIS

DANNY W. SCOTT, D.V.M.
*Ithaca, New York*

Sporotrichosis is a chronic granulomatous and usually cutaneolymphatic infection caused by the dimorphic fungus, *Sporothrix schenckii*. It has been reported in horses, mules, dogs, cats, cattle, camels, fowl, swine, rats, mice, hamsters, chimpanzees and man. The geographic distribution is probably universal, although the fungus requires high humidity and a relatively warm climate and is therefore thought to be more common along the coastal regions and river valleys of the southern United States. The disease is usually endemic and rarely epidemic. The fungus is thought to be a ubiquitous saprophyte in nature, which attains pathogenicity primarily by wound contamination. In man, the disease is considered to be an occupational hazard, affecting laborers, farmers and florists most frequently.

*S. schenckii* has been isolated from soil, humus, plants, fertilizer, sphagnum moss, water, the mouth of normal rats and humans and the human gastrointestinal tract and tracheobronchial tree. Most commonly, wound contamination is the mode of infection. Sporotrichosis is not thought to be a contagious disease.

Three clinical forms of sporotrichosis have been described. The first and most common presentation is the cutaneolymphatic form, wherein the infection is limited to the skin, subcutaneous tissues and lymphatics. Classically, firm, round, tender nodules form at the site of entry, usually an extremity, and spread along the lymphatics. The nodules may be ulcerative and/or suppurative, discharging a thick, brownish-red exudate.

The second form is the disseminated case. This usually follows the primary cutaneolymphatic form or, rarely, a primary respiratory infection. Tissues reported to be involved include bone, eye, lung, gastrointestinal tract, central nervous system, liver, spleen, kidneys, mammary gland, testes and epididymis.

The third form is a primary cutaneous form, in which the lesions begin dorsally and do not appear to follow lymphatic channels as they spread. The lesions are multiple, diffusely scattered, circular, raised, alopecic, ulcerated, crusted, nonpainful, nonpruritic, varying in size from 0.5 to 3.5 cm. in diameter, and scattered over the head, ears, neck, trunk and extremities.

The primary lesion is a granuloma. Demonstration of the organisms in biopsy material is usually difficult and unrewarding. The use of specific fungal stains (periodic acid-Schiff, Gomori's methenamine silver or specific fluorescent antibody) is more helpful in attempts to demonstrate the organisms than is the usual hematoxylin and eosin. In tissues, the organism is pleomorphic (oval, rounded or cigar-shaped). Direct microscopic examination of exudate from lesions is usually unrewarding because of the paucity of organisms in exudates or tissues.

Culture of exudates or tissues is thought to be a very reliable procedure. Sabouraud's agar, Francis' glucose cystine agar or brain-heart infusion glucose blood agar may be used. *S. schenckii* is a dimorphic fungus, a budding yeast in tissues and on media at 37° C., and a mycelium at room temperature. Because there are several nonpathogenic *Sporotrichum* spp., it is essential that the tissue form be demonstrated to identify positively the pathogenic fungus. Two-tenths milliliter of a dense mycelial suspension is injected intratesticularly in mice. A purulent orchitis develops, from which pus may be expressed, gram-stained and examined for the characteristic "cigar bodies."

The treatment of choice for sporotrichosis is sodium iodide. This drug is very effective in the cutaneolymphatic forms. A 20 per cent aqueous solution is administered orally to dogs at a dosage of 1.0 ml./5 kg. every 8 to 12 hours. A good response is usually obtained within 30 days, but therapy must be continued for three to four weeks beyond the apparent "cure" to prevent relapses. If signs of iodism should appear, treatment should be halted until signs regress and then reinstituted at a lower dosage.

The cat is very sensitive to the toxic effects of iodine compounds. Signs of iodism in the cat include vomiting, anorexia, depression, muscular twitching, hypothermia, cardiovascular collapse and death. The suggested dosage for the 20% sodium iodide solution for cats is 0.5 ml./5 kg. orally every 12 to 24 hours.

The disseminated form of sporotrichosis is often resistant to sodium iodide. Dramatic improvement in human cases has been obtained with amphotericin B. This highly nephrotoxic drug has not been evaluated in canine sporotrichosis and should be used with caution.

Surgical incision, excision and cauterization of cutaneolymphatic lesions are often followed by increased suppuration and ulceration.

Sporotrichosis is potentially hazardous to man. Handling of infected animals should be minimal. Protective clothing, especially gloves, should be worn to decrease the chance of transmission through open wounds.

### SUPPLEMENTAL READING

Scott, D. W., Bentinck-Smith, J., and Haggerty, G. F.: Sporotrichosis in three dogs. Cornell Vet., 64:416–426, 1974.

# DERMATO-PHYTE INFECTIONS

ROBERT W. KIRK, D.V.M.
*Ithaca, New York*

Dermatophytes cause a superficial infection of the skin that involves the keratinized cells of the skin, hair and nails. Dermatomycosis is a broad term for fungal disease, which may include the deeper mycotic infections.

Saprophytic fungi are omnipresent in our environment. Of the thousands of species, only a handful have acquired pathogenicity in animals. Fungi, however, are not nearly as common a cause of skin disease as supposed, and many nonspecific, pruritic dermatoses are diagnosed as dermatomycosis on the basis of inadequate evidence. Some clinicians use "grass fungus" as a catchall term for these problems when, in fact, allergic contact dermatitis or factors other than fungi are involved.

Fungi are plants and are typically parasites of plants or saprophytes of plant products. Some fungi are also pathogenic in animals and man, although bacterial diseases usually capture a large share of the clinician's attention.

The host-parasite relationship in dermatophytosis is unusual. The fungi are efficient parasites which live on, not in, the skin. Their growth takes place only in dead, keratinized structures, and they avoid living tissue completely.

Dermatophytosis can be transmitted from animals to man, from animals to other animals and from man to animals. Zoophilic fungi prefer animals as hosts and often cause acute inflammatory reactions when they invade man. This inflammation is unfavorable to the invading fungus, thereby limiting the progress of the infection. Zoophilic fungus infections rarely cause an inflammatory reaction in animals, so that much of the time the dermatophyte is able to exist in a symbiotic relationship with the host.

## DIAGNOSTIC PROCEDURES

*Skin scrapings* may be useful in confirming a suspicion of fungal infection, but it is usually desirable to expand the laboratory investigation to fungal cultures for definitive results. To make a proper scraping, wet the scalpel blade with water, select an area near the margin of a lesion that is growing rapidly and scrape to accumulate hair, scales and other keratin debris. Deep scrapings are not needed.

This material may be dense with the hair and debris. It can be "cleared" by adding a few drops of 10 per cent KOH to the slide and either allowing it to stand for 30 minutes or heating it very gently (avoid boiling) for 15 to 20 seconds over a flame. High degrees of heat should be avoided.

Zaias and Taplin (1966) report that the direct demonstration of fungi in skin, nail or hair scrapings is facilitated by dissolving the alkaline clearing agent KOH (20 per cent by weight) in a solvent of 60 per cent water and 40 per cent DMSO. With this reagent, hyphae can often be seen as well in one minute without heating as in 20 minutes or more with the classic plain aqueous alkaline solution described above. The DMSO-containing reagent must not be used if more than 20 minutes will elapse between preparation of the specimen and microscropic examination or all hyphae will be dissolved. The DMSO increases transport of the KOH through the keratin tissues, and its high refractive index (like xylene) enhances optical clearing. Increasing the proportion of DMSO above 50 per cent decreases the clearing properties.

Because heat is generated during preparation of the stock DMSO-KOH solution, it is *imperative* that the following procedure be used in formulation of the mixture!

1. Place 20 gm. of KOH in a 200- or 250-ml. Erlenmeyer flask submerged halfway in an ice water bath.

2. Slowly add about 50 ml. of distilled water to the KOH and gently rotate the flask until the mixture is clear. The flask should remain ice cold.

3. Slowly add 36.6 ml. of 100 per cent DMSO while rotating the flask.

4. When the flask has again cooled, carefully pour the contents into a 100-ml. graduated cylinder. Bring the volume to 100 ml. with distilled water. Insert stopper tightly, and mix gently by inverting the cylinder several times. If the contents become warm, place the cylinder in the ice water bath again.

5. Hold the cylinder and stopper firmly, and shake vigorously until interfaces disappear and the solution becomes clear.

6. Transfer contents immediately to screw-top bottles or dropper bottles, as the solution will corrode rubber and will seal ground-glass stoppers permanently in place.

Identification of a mycotic infection, especially on glabrous skin, can be made by finding the branching mycelia. Generally, brown-colored hyphae are nonpathogenic species. The mycelial filaments are uniform in diameter (2 to 6 microns), septate and variable in length and degree of branching. Older hyphae are usually wider and may be divided into beadlike chains of rounded cells (arthrospores). It is possible to confuse hyphae with artifacts such as threads, wisps of cotton, fiberglass or elastic fibers and early KOH crystal formations from overheated or dried-out slide preparations. Keratinized cell wall "skeletons" and cholesterol crystals which make up the so-called mosaic fungus may be the most difficult to differentiate from fungal hyphae.

Hair shafts should be carefully examined for spores. Ectothrix spores form a prominent sheath on the outside of the hair as well as growing inside the hair shaft. They are found in *Microsporum* and in *Trichophyton mentagrophytes* infections. Endothrix spores are found growing inside the hair shaft without a conspicuous external sheath. Endothrix spores are found in some common human dermatophyte species, but almost all the zoophilic species have ectothrix spores. Occasionally, spores of nonpathogens may be found associated with hair shafts.

The *Wood's light* is ultraviolet light filtered through nickel oxide. In addition to its use in diagnosis and to obtain infected material for culture, the Wood's light is helpful in determination of the progress of therapy. However, it has several limitations.

All examinations must be made in a dark room. The only common dermatophyte of dogs and cats which causes hair to fluoresce is *Microsporum canis*, but even here, less than half the positive cultured cases also show fluorescence. A positive response to Wood's light for this fungus is a bright yellow-green, not unlike that seen by shining the light on the numerals of a fluorescent watch face. Many factors influence fluorescence. It may not begin all at once; it may be destroyed by medication (iodides); and other substances such as keratin, dyes, soap, petroleum and medicaments may also fluoresce and give false positive reactions. One must be certain that short stubs of hair in infected areas are actually producing the fluorescence. This can be proved by using forceps to extract some of them from their follicles and noting under the Wood's light that the portion of the hair that was within the follicle also fluoresces brightly. If these hairs are used for inoculating cultures, one can almost always get a positive, readily identifiable colony.

The usefulness of the Wood's light can be summarized—a positive response is highly suggestive, but a negative response is not conclusive, since the patient may be either free of infection or affected by a nonfluorescing dermatophyte.

The *fungal culture* is the most reliable method for diagnosis and identification of dermatomycosis. It requires only a few minutes to inoculate media, and most pathogens grow into distinctive colonies in one to three weeks at room temperature.

The suspected lesion is cleansed with 70 per cent alcohol to reduce contamination. The sample for inoculation should be obtained from the periphery of a rapidly growing lesion. A small scraping of superficial keratin and hair should be obtained and deposited carefully but firmly on the center of the culture medium surface. The culture bottle should be closed, but the cap unscrewed a quarter turn to allow aerobic growth. Ideally, the bottle is placed on a cabinet shelf to incubate at room temperature. A pan containing water should be placed in the cabinet to assure relatively high humidity for growth and to prevent dehydration of the medium.

Because an adequate sample is vital, there are two additional techniques which may help assure a positive culture. If the case involves a dermatophyte that causes hair to fluoresce, the sample should be obtained from an area which is positive to the test. Often, single hairs may be plucked from an area because of their brilliant fluorescence. This makes an ideal inoculum. Another technique has the advantage of accumulating much keratin debris as the inoculum. In this procedure, a sterile toothbrush is rubbed vigorously over the suspected lesion. The bristles trap scaly material and hair which can be shaken out of the brush into a sterile Petri dish for transfer to the culture bottle, or shaken directly onto the surface of the medium in a Petri dish. Alternately, a sterile scalpel blade can be used to scrape dry scales onto a piece of paper or the Petri dish.

In recent years, Sabouraud's agar has been modified by the addition of agents designed to inhibit growth of extraneous bacteria, yeasts and fungi. Indicator agents have also been included in some media to show pH changes, a factor which may help differentiate pathogens from saprophytes. When carefully used, the method is accurate in a high percentage of cases. However, these media tend to oversimplify the identification of fungi and may cause serious diagnostic errors.

Sabouraud's dextrose agar is slightly acidic and thus deters growth of many bacteria. This effect is enhanced by the addition of chloramphenicol. Cycloheximide is added to inhibit growth of saprophytic (contaminant) fungi and all yeasts except *Candida*. This fortified medium has been popular for many years. However, the restrictive agents delay colony growth and early development of typical pigments. Taplin et al. (1969) modified Sabouraud's agar by adding cycloheximide, with gentamicin and chlortetracycline as antibacterial agents and phenol red as a pH indicator. They called it dermatophyte test medium (DTM). Dermatophytes utilize protein in the medium first with an output of alkaline metabolites (hence, a red color forms in the medium). When protein is exhausted, the dermatophytes utilize carbohydrates, giving off acid metabolites (so the medium color returns to yellow). Contaminant fungi utilize carbohydrate first, and only later, protein; so they too may produce a red color in DTM —but only after a prolonged incubation (14 days or more). Consequently, DTM cultures should be no older than 14 days when read. In come cases, DTM may depress development of spores and the red color hides colony pigmentation, so dual inoculation in DTM and plain Sabouraud's medium may be advisable, since this allows evaluation of colony type. Halliwell has noted that *Aspergillus, Alternaria* and *Penicillium* are saprophytes that occasionally turn DTM red within 10 days. Colony color and type will easily help make the differential diagnosis.

Rinaldi *et al.* (1973 have developed a new, rapid sporulation medium (RSM). This uses bromothymol blue as the color indicator (yellow at pH below 6.0, blue-green at higher pH). Although bromothymol has been slightly inhibitory to some dermatophytes, the balance of nutrients (like potato dextrose agar) in the medium seems to encourage early sporulation, and the light blue-green color does not completely mask typical colony pigmentation.

*Stained slide preparations* allow detailed structure of fungi to be determined rather simply. Specimens of mycelia (and spores) from mature colonies can be teased apart and spread on a microscope slide, flooded with lactophenol cotton blue stain, covered with a coverslip and examined.

An alternative and often more successful method is the "acetate tape slide." Preparations for this purpose are easily made with pressure-sensitive tape from stationery stores. No. 800 acetate-backed tape preserves the preparation longer, but other tapes are adequate for most purposes. To make the preparation, a "flag of tape," 0.5 inch by 0.5 inch, is fastened to the end of a wooden applicator stick or wire needle or grasped in forceps, and the sticky surface of the flag is touched to the surface of the colony just proximal to the advancing periphery. The tape is then pressed, sticky side down, on a slide with a drop of lactophenol cotton blue stain and examined under the microscope. The tape selectively removes the upper branches of hyphae-bearing conidia and avoids the taxonomically valueless vegetative mycelium. The details of microscopic evaluation for recognition of specific fungi are given in Figure 1.

## CLASSIFICATION AND INCIDENCE OF SUPERFICIAL MYCOTIC INFECTIONS

The terminology used to classify dermatophytes is exceedingly complex because of the large number of synonyms. Dermatophytes can be categorized as zoophilic, those whose normal host is mammals other than man; anthropophilic, those whose normal host is man; and geophilic, those whose normal habitat is soil. Of the dermatophytes affecting animals, almost all are of the genus *Microsporum* or *Trichophyton*. Three fungi cause 99 per cent of all clinical cases of ringworm in dogs and cats in the United States. These are *M. canis, M. gypseum* and *T. mentagrophytes* (var. *granulare*). In cats, 98 per cent of cases are caused by *M. canis*, with 1 per cent due to *M. gypseum* and 1 per cent to *T. mentagrophytes*. In dogs, 70 per cent of cases are due to *M. canis*, 20 per cent to *M. gypseum* and 10 per cent to *T. mentagrophytes*. Bone and Jackson (1971) report a much higher incidence of *T. mentagrophytes* in the Florida area and speculate on the possible importance of "contaminant fungi" as a factor in the etiology of skin disease of dogs and cats.

The literature reporting the incidence of dermatomycosis is confusing, since there is a high incidence in hot, humid climates (Florida, northeastern Australia) but a low incidence in cold, dry climates. There is also great regional variation in the frequency of the specific fungus cultured.

Kaplan and Ivens (1961) reported that the seasonal incidence of ringworm in dogs and cats in the United States varies with the species of the fungus. This may be somewhat dependent on the climate, on the animals' habits of being outdoors and thus more exposed to geophilic species, and so on.

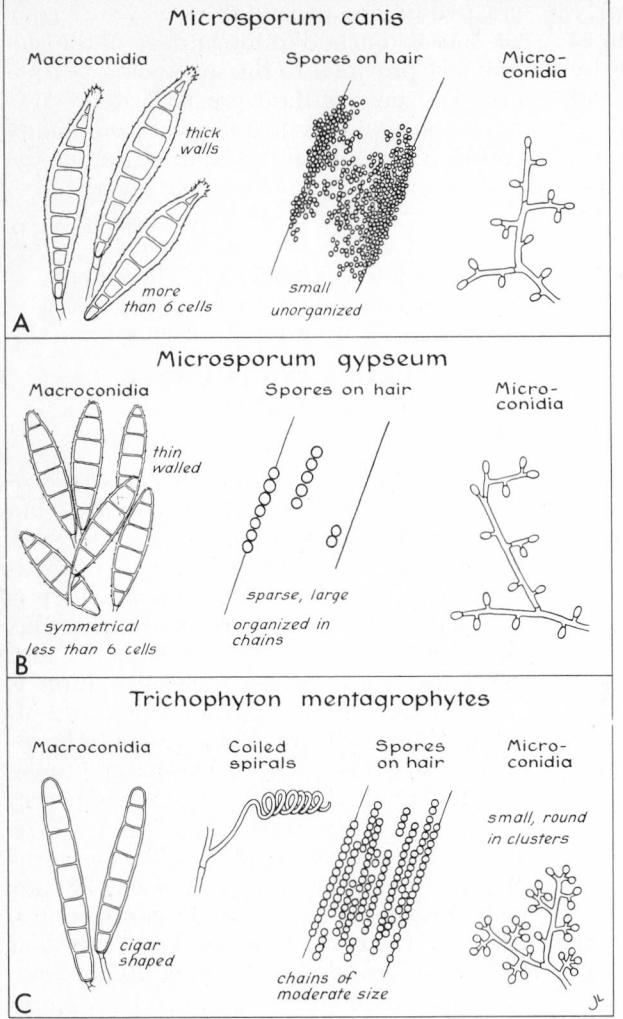

**Figure 1.** Characteristic microscopic morphology of (A) *M. canis*, (B) *M. gypseum* and (C) *T. mentagrophytes*.

In general, the incidence for dogs was as follows:

*M. canis* was high in the period from October to February and low from March to September.

*M. gypseum* was high in the period from July to November and low from December to June.

*T. mentagrophytes* was present all year, with the peak occurring in November and December.

In general, the incidence for cats was as follows:

*M. canis* varied little all year.

*M. gypseum* and *T. mentagrophytes* were rarely reported in cats, but there may be a slight increase during the summer and fall months.

Other dermatophytes, seen more rarely in small animal practice, are listed in Table 1.

Additional information about dermatophytes, subcutaneous mycoses and systemic mycoses that attack man and animals is presented in Table 2.

The three major small animal dermatophytes will be discussed here.

**Microsporum canis.** This zoophilic fungus is by far the most common dermatophyte of dogs and cats. It also commonly produces disease in man, in whom it causes a more severe inflammatory reaction than anthropophilic species. *M. canis* is worldwide in distribution. It is endemic in catteries, where all the young may be affected clinically. Adult cats may be asymptomatic carriers. Spores are small and present in masses on the hair shaft. The affected hairs frequently, but not always, fluoresce to a bright yellow-green because of a tryptophane metabolite produced by

**Table 1.** *Dermatophytes Causing Natural Infection*

| DERMATOPHYTE | RESERVOIR* | FREQUENCY† Dog | Cat | Monkeys | Wild and Domestic Rodents | Birds |
|---|---|---|---|---|---|---|
| **Common** | | | | | | |
| M. canis | Z | U | U | U | F | — |
| T. mentagrophytes | Z | F | F | U | U | — |
| M. gypseum | G | F | F | F | F | — |
| T. simii | A | R | — | U | — | F |
| M. gallinae | Z | — | R | — | R | U |
| **Rare, but reported** | | | | | | |
| M. audouinii | A | R | — | R | — | — |
| M. cookeii | G | R | — | R | — | — |
| M. distortum | ? | R | R | R | — | — |
| M. persicolor | Z | R | — | — | U | — |
| M. vanbreuseghemi | G | R | — | — | R | — |
| T. equinum | Z | R | — | — | — | — |
| T. erinacei | Z | R | — | — | U | — |
| T. megninii | A | R | — | — | — | — |
| T. rubrum | A | R | — | R | — | — |
| T. schoenleinii | A | R | R | — | — | R |
| T. verrucosum | Z | R | R | — | — | — |
| T. violaceum | A | R | R | — | — | — |
| E. floccosum | A | R | — | — | — | — |

*Z, Zoophilic; A, anthropophilic; G, geophilic.
†U, Usual; F, frequent; R, rare, but reported.
From Muller, G. H., and Kirk, R. W.: Small Animal Dermatology. 2nd ed. Philadelphia, W. B. Saunders Co., 1976.

**Table 2.** *Fungi That Attack Man and Animals*

| DERMATOPHYTE | RESERVOIR | INCIDENCE IN ANIMALS | INCIDENCE IN MAN |
|---|---|---|---|
| Microsporum canis | Cats (head, especially nose area and feet) | Frequent: cats, dogs, monkeys; Occasional: sheep, horses, rodents; Reported: cattle, pigs | Very common |
| Microsporum distortum | Unknown | Reported: cats, dogs, horses, monkeys | Uncommon |
| Microsporum audouinii | Man | Reported: dogs, monkeys | Rapidly decreased from epidemic status to sporadic |
| Microsporum gypseum | Soil | Frequent: dogs, horses, rodents; Occasional: cats, monkeys; Reported: cattle, pigs | Occasional |
| Microsporum nanum | Pigs (body, frequently behind ears) | Frequent: pigs | Rare |
| Microsporum persicolor | Bank vole (tail) | Frequent: the bank vole; Reported: dogs | Uncommon |
| Microsporum cookeii | Soil | Reported: dogs, monkeys | Reported |
| Microsporum vanbreuseghemi | Soil | Reported: dogs, rodents | Rare |
| Trichophyton gallinae | Poultry (combs and wattles: "chicken comb favus") | Frequent: chickens; Reported: cats, dogs, rodents, monkeys | Rare |

*Continued on next page*

From Muller, G. H., and Kirk, R. W.: Small Animal Dermatology. 2nd ed. Philadelphia, W. B. Saunders Co., 1976.

**Table 2.** *Fungi That Attack Man and Animals (Continued)*

| DERMATOPHYTE | RESERVOIR | INCIDENCE IN ANIMALS | INCIDENCE IN MAN |
|---|---|---|---|
| *Trichophyton ajelloi* | Soil | Questionable: dogs, cattle, horses | (One possible infection reported) |
| *Trichophyton simii* | Soil or simians (face) or poultry (combs, wattles) | Frequent: monkeys and chickens in India<br>Reported: dogs, small mammals in India | Occasional to frequent in India |
| *Trichophyton mentagrophytes* | Dogs (body and/or face only) or rodents | Frequent: dogs, monkeys, rodents<br>Occasional: cats, cattle, pigs, sheep, horses | Frequent |
| *Trichophyton equinum* | Horses (flank) | Frequent: horses<br>Reported: dogs | Rare |
| *Trichophyton erinacei* | Hedgehogs (nose) | Frequent: hedgehogs<br>Reported: guinea pigs | Frequent, but sporadic |
| *Trichophyton verrucosum* | Cattle (head) | Frequent: cattle<br>Occasional: sheep, horses<br>Reported: cats, dogs, pigs | Common |
| *Trichophyton megninii* | Man | Reported: dogs | Very common in Europe and North Africa |
| *Trichophyton rubrum* | Man | Reported: dogs, monkeys | Very frequent |
| *Trichophyton violaceum* | Man | Reported: cats, dogs | Very frequent (in the Old World and Asia) |
| *Trichophyton schoenleinii* | Man | Reported: animals, birds | Common in the Old World |
| *Epidermophyton floccosum* | Man | Reported: dogs | Common |

| SUBCUTANEOUS MYCOSES | RESERVOIR | INCIDENCE IN ANIMALS | INCIDENCE IN MAN |
|---|---|---|---|
| *Sporothrix schenckii* | Soil, vegetation, timber | Frequent: horses<br>Reported: fowl, cattle, rodents | Sporadic; infrequent |
| *Mycetoma (eumycotic)* | Soil, vegetation | Reported: dogs, cats, horses | Rare |
| Chromomycosis | Soil | Reported: dogs, horses | Rare |

| ACTINOMYCETOUS INFECTIONS | RESERVOIR | INCIDENCE IN ANIMALS | INCIDENCE IN MAN |
|---|---|---|---|
| *Dermatophilus congolensis* | Dried crusts of skin from infected animals | Frequent in endemic regions: cattle, sheep<br>Reported: goats, horses, antelopes, deer, swine, foxes, cats | Infrequent |
| *Nocardia asteroides* | Soil | Frequent: cattle and dogs<br>Occasional: cats, horses, goats, pigs, rabbits, trout | Infrequent |
| *Actinomyces bovis, A. israelii* | Endogenous; normal flora mouth, tonsils | Incidence 0.2–2% in cattle in the United States<br>Occasional: pigs<br>Reported: cats, sheep, dogs, horses, deer | Infrequent |

the fungus. This metabolite is only produced by fungi which have invaded actively growing hair and cannot be elicited from an *in-vitro* infection of hair. Fluorescence is not present in scales or crusts or in cultures of *Microsporum* grown on laboratory media. The green fluorescent material can be extracted by hot water or by cold 2 N sodium bromide solution. The fluorescence changes color at various pH's, and it can be quenched by various ions—especially iodides. Many soaps, medications and so on produce fluorescence, so the clinician must be certain that the color he observes is an indicator of hair pathology. It is interesting to note that these metabolites are agents which may produce a "biologic contact dermatitis"—the inflammatory reaction that is seen in some patients.

The colony on Sabouraud's dextrose agar develops fairly rapidly, forming a white cottony or woolly aerial mycelium. The pigment on the undersurface is yellowish-orange, later changing to a reddish-brown.

Macroconidia are usually produced in fair numbers and are long, spindle-shaped and thick-walled, with an asymmetric knob. The rough surface is particularly evident at the knob, and each macroconidium is composed of more than six compartments (Fig. 1*A*).

**Microsporum gypseum.** *Microsporum gypseum* is a soil-inhabiting fungus which occasionally infects man and animals. It is worldwide in distribution. Sporulation on the hair shaft is mainly ectothrix, but the spores are sparse and in chains. Fluorescence is rare, but if present, it is very dull. In animals, thick, well-circumscribed, tightly adherent gray crusts are typical in clinical lesions. Chronic cases in the dog respond to treatment slowly.

The colony grows rapidly, with a surface texture like chamois because of the multitudes of macroconidia. The surface is rich cinnamon buff in color centrally, but it terminates in a border of downy, white mycelium. The pigment on the undersurface is cream to tan in color.

Macroconidia are present in enormous numbers. They are large, thin-walled, ellipsoid structures the shape of cucumbers. The surface is rough and up to six compartments may be present (Fig. 1*B*).

**Trichophyton mentagrophytes.** This dermatophyte has many variants. Its zoophilic form (var. *granulare*) is highly infectious and may transfer to man, in whom it causes an inflammatory form of ringworm. It is more common in laboratory animals and horses than in dogs and cats. In the generalized form in the dog and cat, it presents dry, scaly, diffuse lesions which are exceedingly resistant to treatment. It may also cause localized infections of canine nails (onychomycosis). Another form (var. *erinacei*, also called *T. erinacei*) affects hedgehogs in England and New Zealand. Dogs contacting the hedgehog may contract the disease. Ectothrix chains of spores are found in the hair. There is no fluorescence. The distribution of *T. mentagrophytes* is worldwide.

The zoophilic form characteristically produces a flat colony with a white to cream-colored, powdery surface. The powder, which has the appearance of face powder sprinkled in concentric rings and rays, consists mainly of enormous clusters of microconidia. Some strains develop dark red pigment on the reverse side of the colony.

The zoophilic form of *T. mentagrophytes* has more numerous microscopic structures than anthropophilic or pleomorphic strains. Macroconidia are present in association with microconidia early in the life of the colony. Many strains also produce numerous coiled spirals.

The macroconidia are cigar- or club-shaped with thin, smooth walls. They have narrow attachments to the vegetative hyphae (Fig. 1*C*).

## TRANSMISSION OF DERMATOPHYTES

When an animal is exposed to a dermatophyte, infection may or may not be established, and even if it is, disease in the form of skin lesions may not result. This situation has already been alluded to in *M. canis* infections in cats, but similar carrier states exist with many dermatophytes. It often appears that young animals (including man) are more susceptible to infection and are more likely to show clinical lesions than are adults. This difference may be caused by physiologic variation in the skin at different ages, or it may be from acquired immunity or hypersensitivity. There is some clinical and experimental evidence that infection may be enhanced or lesions intensified if the host is nutritionally debilitated (i.e., vitamin A or otherwise deficient). Once the disease is established, it runs a course that may be uninfluenced by treatment and may resolve spontaneously. Following recovery, a resistance to infection has been noted, and it is probable that acquired immunity plays a part in the epidemiology. There is no evidence of cross-immunity between species of fungi.

Dermatomycosis has been transmitted by rubbing infected tissue into gently abraded skin, and it is assumed that natural infection is by contact. Contaminated brushes, combs and clippers may be important fomites. Dawson and Noodle (1968) report that some fungal elements may remain viable in the dry state for as long as five to seven years, and *M. canis* may live at least 13 months. Carrier cats may spread infection for short periods, but the real long-term reservoir in a cattery is the cat with minimal clinical lesions. Control measures in a cattery are difficult but crucial (see Prophylaxis).

## THE SKIN'S RESPONSE TO DERMATOPHYTES

One of the confusing aspects of fungal disease is the variable clinical picture that is presented. In mild infections on glabrous skin, the response is minor and easily missed. It causes mild hypertrophy of the horny layer. There is scant fungal growth, and special stains may be needed to demonstrate fungi. As fungal growth becomes more prolific, the entire epidermis may hypertrophy. These same hypertrophic changes occur in the hair follicles, but the root sheath is well cornified so the hairs become surrounded by wide collars of keratinized scales and hyphae. The bulge may produce a conical dilation of the opening of the hair follicle, a process which gives a false impression of papillomatous swelling. Mycotic infections invade hairs only in anagen and grow down the follicle to the "critical level" or fringe of Adamson, where mitotic activity is evident. (Dermatophytes do not survive in living cells.)

The invasion of hair by *Microsporum* spp. has been studied by Kligman (1956). Hair is always invaded in both ectothrix and endothrix infections. The endothrix fungi are those that do not form masses of external spores. Fungal elements deposited on the skin reach the follicle orifice by the second day; they penetrate the hair shaft by working under the cuticle, lifting it away from the shaft and growing downward. Fungal elements reach Adamson's fringe by the seventh to eighth day. Growing hair has carbohydrates, nitrogenous substances and nucleoprotein derivatives in addition to keratin, and one of these may meet the metabolic needs of the fungus to support growth. As stated previously, the metabolic wastes from fungal growth may produce a contact dermatitis reaction in the host. Fungi do not penetrate hairs *in vitro*; when hair growth terminates, fungal growth terminates, and the clinical infection resolves spontaneously. A "patch of ringworm" is a community of more or less independent hair infections, as each follicle is in its own stage of the hair cycle. In addition, Kligman has found that for some unknown reason a few hairs are resistant to fungal invasion even while they are growing. All "club" or dead hairs are always resistant, however. The reaction in the viable follicle cells consists of mild congestion and edema of the dermal papilla together with a mild lymphocytic infiltration. If secondary bacterial infection occurs, microabscesses form in the superficial epidermis together with a suppurative folliculitis. A localized severe inflammation accompanied by swelling, with a deep, boggy ulcerative area exuding pus, is known as a kerion.

The gross appearance of dermatomycosis varies even in infections produced by the same organism. There are usually different degrees of scaling and encrustation of epithelial debris and loss of hair. The hair loss is not permanent unless the follicle is destroyed by secondary bacterial infection. Usually the hairs become brittle and break off near the skin surface, leaving a short stubby hair shaft which can be seen emerging through scales and crusts.

In the course of some "ringworm" infections, the organisms tend to die out in the center of the lesions, and the skin then returns to normal. Those organisms at the periphery of the lesion remain active. The reason for this phenomenon is unknown.

## DIFFERENTIAL DIAGNOSIS

Seborrheic lesions frequently mimic the circular lesions of ringworm. Differentiation is made by noting the course of the lesions and by evaluating the entire skin of the body rather than the individual lesions. Demodicosis, especially its localized form, also develops circular lesions. A skin scraping quickly differentiates the two conditions. Abrasions of circular shape may resemble ringworm lesions. Contact dermatitis of the paws is often mistakenly called a "fungal infection." Bacterial hypersensitivity also produces crusted circular lesions which may have central clearing. These can be diagnosed by skin culture and by intradermal skin tests with bacterial antigens.

## CLINICAL MANAGEMENT

**Systemic Treatment.** Griseofulvin is the drug of choice. The dose of the microcrystalline form (Fulvicin-U/F®, Schering) is up to 50 mg./kg. of body weight daily. This can be administered once daily with food. The drug may cause vomiting if given on an empty stomach, and absorption is greatly enhanced if the drug is administered with a high-fat meal. The drug should be continued for four to six weeks, or longer in severe cases. It is important to continue treatment until mycologic cultures are negative or until two weeks beyond clinical recovery (Kaplan). When response is evident, the dosage shoud be reduced to 25 mg./kg. of body weight once daily. Good results have been reported with massive doses given once weekly (150 mg./kg.). In cases of onychomycosis, the course is long, and griseofulvin may be necessary for four to six months. Even then, treatment is sometimes disappointing. Avulsion of affected nails or shaving affected skin may remove the infective spores and be worth considering as part of the treatment.

Griseofulvin is contraindicated during pregnancy (especially the first three weeks), since it is highly teratogenic. It also tastes bitter and may produce nausea as a side effect in a high percentage of patients.

Contrary to earlier beliefs, Epstein *et al.* (1972) have shown that levels of griseofulvin appear in the outer stratum corneum of human skin within eight hours of dosage, and the levels decrease within 24 hours of cessation of medication. The drug may enter the stratum corneum with sweat by the "wick" effect. Similar studies have not been reported in other species, however.

**Topical Treatment.** The affected areas, or even the entire patient, should be shaved to avoid reinfestation from infected hairs. Gentle cleansing with Betadine® (Purdue-Frederick) or Weladol® (Pitman-Moore) is useful to prevent secondary bacterial infection and for its antifungal effect.

Dipping or rinsing with Captan® is a useful adjunct to griseofulvin treatment. A dip prepared from a 1:200 dilution of 45 per cent technical Captan is safe for dogs and cats. One or two dips a week can be given until clinical improvement appears. A 2 per cent solution of 38 per cent commercial lime sulfur orchard spray can be used topically in the same manner with excellent effect.

Numerous topical fungicidal and fungistatic ointments are in common use. Many of these are keratolytic agents (salicylic acid, undecylenic acid) that remove the keratin "soil" which the fungus needs to grow in. Clinicians should use great care when applying irritating preparations. They are usually not recommended, since they may encourage secondary pyoderma.

Many new, relatively nontoxic and nonirritating preparations have come on the market recently. Tolnaftate preparations (Tinactin®, Schering) are fungistatic but have been consistently ineffective in animal dermatomycosis—especially in areas of hairy skin. A new 2 per cent topical cream or solution of miconazole nitrate (Micotin [Conofite,® Pitman-Moore]) gives promise for topical use, particularly because of its low toxicity and wide fungicidal spectrum. Haloprogin (Halotex®, Westwood) is also a new fungicidal, broad-spectrum topical agent which is a halogenated phenol derivative. Available in 1 per cent cream or solution, it gives promise for treatment of dermatophyte and *Candida* infections in dogs. Clotrimazole (Lotrimin®, Schering) is another new, broad-spectrum, fungicidal agent available in 1 per cent cream or solution. It too has promise for effective use in animal dermatomycosis and candidiasis. Cuprimyxin (Unitop®, Hoffman, LaRoche) is also effective topically.

Knudsen (1975) has shown (in dermatophyte infections of man) that fungi can be cultured not only from the visible lesion but also from the normal-looking skin up to 6 cm. from the margin of the lesion. This emphasizes the need to extend topical treatments well into the areas of normal skin surrounding obvious lesions.

## PROPHYLAXIS

Griseofulvin can be used prophylactically on exposed animals. One massive, single dose (200 mg./kg. of body weight) may be effective. Infected animals should be isolated to prevent contact with people or other pets. It is necessary to sterilize or destroy bedding, leashes and other contaminated equipment.

Control measures in cat colonies have been well documented by Dawson and Noodle (1968). They showed that many normal cats have dermatophytes. However, the disease is most common in kittens, less so in adult females and least common in adult males. The infection can be airborne or spread by direct contact. Carrier cats may spread the infection for a short time, but the long-term reservoir is the cat with minimal clinical lesions. Cats in the home are potent sources of infection to children, and hospital treatment is advisable, at least initially.

An infected cattery should be surveyed by examining each cat carefully under a Wood's light and by culturing the hairs of each cat, using Mackenzie's brush technique. Cats with fluorescent hairs or with positive cultures should be isolated, especially in regard to the ventilation system. They should be treated with full doses of griseofulvin for at least six weeks and managed so that they do not change cages. Attendants should wear gloves and protective clothes and caps; walls, benches, cages and so on should be washed down once weekly with iodophor or some effective iodine cleansing solution. Over a period of weeks these procedures usually result in satisfactory control. However, one should remember that *M. canis* persists in the dry premises for at least 13 months.

When new cats are added to a colony they should be examined carefully under Wood's light, hairs should be cultured using the brush technique and the cats should be held in strict isolation for 14 days until culture results are known. Under no circumstances should new cats be added to the colony unless the tests are negative.

## SUPPLEMENTAL READING

Ajello, A., George, L. K., Kaplan, W., and Kaufman, C.: Laboratory Manual for Medical Mycology, P.H.S. Pub. No. 994. Washington, D.C., U.S. Government Printing Office, 1963.

Al-Doory, Y., Vice, T. E., and Olin, F.: A survey of ringworm in dogs and cats. J. Am. Vet. Med. Assn., 153:429, 1968.

Baxter, M.: Ringworm due to *M. canis* in cats and dogs in New Zealand, N.Z. Vet. J., 21:33, 1973.

Bibel, D. J., and LeBrun, J. R.: Effect of experimental dermatophyte infection on cutaneous flora. J. Invest. Derm., 64 (No. 2):119–123, 1975.

Blakemore, J. C.: Dermatomycosis. *In* Kirk, R. W. (ed.): Current Veterinary Therapy V. Philadelphia, W. B. Saunders Co., 1974.

Bone, W. J., and Jackson, W. F.: Pathogenic fungi in dermatitis. Vet. Med. Small Animal, 66:140–142, 1971.

Butler, A. A.: Topical treatment of nail and skin infections with miconazole—A new broad-spectrum antimycotic. Mykosen, 14:187, 1971.

Connole, M. D.: Ringworm due to *T. mentagrophytes* in a dog. Aust. Vet. J., 44:528, 1968.

Dawson, C. O., and Noodle, B. M.: Treatment of *Microsporum canis* ringworm in a cat colony. J. Small Animal Pract., 9:613, 1968.

Easton, K. L.; cutaneous North American blastomycosis in a Siamese cat. Canad. Vet. J., 2:350, 1961.

Epstein, W. L., Shah, V. P., and Riegelman, S.: Griseofulvin levels in stratum corneum. Arch. Derm., 106:344, 1972.

Felsher, Z.: Observations on the fluorescent material in hairs infected by Microsporum in tinea capitis. J. Invest. Derm., 12:139, 1949.

Gip, L.: Topical treatment with clotrimazole in dermatomycosis. Curr. Ther. Res., 16:27, 1974.

Halliwell, R. E. W.: Personal communication, 1976.

Jackson, W. F.: Personal communication, 1975.

Jungeman, P. F., and Schwartzman, R. M.: Veterinary Medical Mycology. Philadelphia, Lea & Febiger, 1972.

Kaplan, W., and Ivens, M. S.: Observations on seasonal variations in incidence of ringworm in dogs and cats in the U.S.A. Sabouraudia, 1:91, 1961.

Kligman, A. M.: Pathophysiology of ringworm infections in animals with skin infections. J. Invest. Derm., 27:171, 1956.

Knudsen, E. A.: The real extent of dermatophyte infection. Brit. J. Derm., 92:413–416, 1975.

Mackenzie, D. W. R.: The extra-human occurrence of *T. tonsurans* var. *sulfureum* in a residential school. Sabouraudia, 1:58, 1961.

Okoshi, S., and Hasegawa, A.: *Microsporum gypseum* isolated from feline ringworm. Jap. J. Vet. Sci., 29:195, 1967.

Rebell, G., and Taplin, D.: Dermatophytes, Their Recognition and Identification. Coral Gables, Florida, University of Miami Press, 1970.

Rinaldi, M. G., Stevens, V. J., and Holde, C.: A new sporulation medium for primary isolation and identification of dermatophytes. Abstract, Am. Soc. Micro. Meeting, Miami, 1973.

Taplin, D., Zaias, N., Rebell, X., and Blank, H.: Isolation and recognition of dermatophytes on a new medium (DTM). Arch. Derm., 99:203, 1969.

Wilson, J. W., and Plunkett, O. A.: The Fungus Diseases of Man. Berkeley and Los Angeles, University of California Press, 1967.

Wright, A. I.: Some observations on ringworm in dogs and cats. Vet. Annual, 14:148, 1973.

Zaias, N., and Taplin, D.: Improved preparation for the diagnosis of mycologic disease. Arch. Derm., 93:608, 1966.

# FELINE LEPROSY

GEORGE T. WILKINSON,
M.R.C.V.S.
*Brisbane, Australia*

Feline or cat leprosy is the term used to denote a condition occurring in the cat in which single or multiple granulomas form in the skin and which is associated with the presence of large numbers of acid-fast bacilli. The disease was first described in New Zealand but has since been reported in Australia, the United States, Canada and the United Kingdom and probably has a worldwide distribution.

## ETIOLOGIC AGENT

The acid-fast bacilli appear as long, slender rods, between 3 and 6 microns in length, and are morphologically similar to the tubercle bacillus. They tend to stain with Ziehl-Neelsen in a somewhat beaded fashion, which has been considered by some workers to be an indication of degenerative changes in the organism. Australian workers in a study of the bacilli attempted to culture the organisms on Löwenstein-Jensen and Dorset egg media, but no growth occurred after an incubation period exceeding 8 months at 37° C. When injected into rats, the bacilli produced the typical infection of experimental rat leprosy, and similarly when inoculated into guinea pigs, the characteristic reaction of rat leprosy infection in this species occurred. In the guinea pig infection, a local lesion extends to the regional lymph node from the site of injection and is then eliminated by the immune response of the host, so that bacilli are not recoverable at necropsy. These studies strongly suggested that the causative organism of feline leprosy is *Mycobacterium lepraemurium,* the rat leprosy bacillus.

This bacillus has received a good deal of attention in medical research, since the disease it evokes in rats and mice provides a very good animal model for the study of human leprosy. Unlike the tubercle bacillus, the organism cannot be cultured on artificial media but can be grown on tissue cultures of rat cells.

## CLINICAL SYNDROME

Affected cats are usually in good general health. The lesions show a predilection for the head and limbs and develop quite rapidly, taking the form of soft, fleshy, spherical, tan-colored nodules in the skin and subcutis. These nodules may be single or multiple, more commonly the latter, and range in size from 1 to 3 cm. in diameter. They are painless, nonfluctuant to palpation and usually quite freely movable over the underlying tissues. In some cases the overlying skin remains intact but frequently there is quite extensive superficial ulceration of the skin, revealing a red, raw, finely granular surface with a slight, serosanguineous exudate. The regional lymph nodes are usually enlarged and firm but not tender to palpation.

In rare cases the condition may become generalized, with large numbers of skin lesions over the entire body surface. Such cats show a progressive loss of bodily condition, and necropsy reveals a systemic infection with granulomatous lesions in the internal organs, particularly the spleen, liver and lungs.

An impression smear taken from an ulcerated lesion and stained with Ziehl-Neelsen stain reveals the presence of very large numbers of acid-fast bacilli mainly contained within the cytoplasm of histiocytes, although some may be lying free in the exudate.

## HISTOLOGY

Histologically there is an extensive granulomatous inflammatory process involving both the dermis and the subcutis. Often there is ulceration of the epidermis, with granulation tissue forming the base of the ulcerated area. Large numbers of histiocytes are present, mostly with quite voluminous cytoplasm that occasionally contains what appear to be lipid droplets, imparting a foamy appearance to the cells. The lesions are infiltrated with polymorphonuclear leukocytes, lymphocytes and plasma cells, with occasional multinucleated giant cells of the Langhans type being present.

The majority of lesions are noncaseating, but in the occasional case when caseation occurs it takes the form of a structural necrosis with the formation of lightly staining areas, similar to those seen in tuberculosis. The granulomatous lesions are not encapsulated and tend to spread into the deeper tissues. One report described the envelopment of subcutaneous nerve tissues by the granulomatous process with invasion of the nerves by inflammatory cells.

Very large numbers of acid-fast bacilli are present throughout the lesions, being so numerous that a section stained with Ziehl-Neelsen shows large areas of pink color when held up to the light. The bacilli are packed into parallel bundles within the cytoplasm of the histiocytes, particularly of the giant cells when these are present. The bundles of bacilli tend to displace the nucleus of the histiocyte against the cell membrane. The regional lymph nodes exhibit a granulomatous type of reaction, but actual lesions may be difficult to find. A smear of the node, however, will usually reveal numerous acid-fast bacilli.

Histologically the condition resembles that seen in the lepromatous form of human leprosy, in rat leprosy and in the skin condition associated with the presence of *M. ulcerans* in man. Human lepromatous leprosy is characterized by the presence of large numbers of histiocytes, many with foamy cytoplasm, containing numerous acid-fast bacilli arranged in parallel bundles. There is a tendency for the inflammatory process and the bacilli to invade subcutaneous nerve tissue, and a similar process has been reported in feline leprosy but not in rat leprosy.

Human leprosy is thought to be associated with some impairment of the immunologic defense mechanisms of the body, and the same may be true of cats affected with feline leprosy. This may be the reason for the lack of success in reproducing the disease experimentally by injection of *M. lepraemurium* into cats.

## TRANSMISSION

Transmission is thought to occur via the bites of infected rats, and this probably accounts for the predilection sites being the head and limbs. Another possibility is via the bites of infected cats, but a survey conducted by this author on the mouth flora of 100 cats failed to reveal any acid-fast organisms.

## DIAGNOSIS

Diagnosis is based on the fairly characteristic appearance of the skin lesions at the predilection sites, plus the finding of very large numbers of acid-fast bacilli in parallel bundles within the cytoplasm of the histiocytes in impression smears of the lesions stained with Ziehl-Neelsen.

Differential diagnosis must include the lesions of skin tuberculosis. This condition is not common in the cat, occurring with a somewhat lower frequency than feline leprosy. The lesions probably arise following the bite of cats affected with open pulmonary tuberculosis. Lesions may be single or multiple, occurring mainly on the head and limbs and present as flattened circular areas that are firmly adherent to the underlying subcutis. They are rather plaquelike to the touch and often show superficial ulceration with a raw, finely granular surface. As with feline leprosy, a Ziehl-Neelsen–stained impression smear of a lesion will reveal the presence of acid-fast bacilli. In the case of skin tuberculosis, however, bacilli are never very numerous. They may be difficult to find and do not show the characteristic arrangement in parallel bundles within the histiocytes that is seen in feline leprosy. Tubercle bacilli can be cultured on artificial media and produce characteristic lesions when injected into guinea pigs. Finally, the two conditions may be distinguished histologically. In skin tuberculosis, caseation is much more frequent and the bacilli are usually rather sparsely scattered throughout the center of the lesion. In feline leprosy, caseation is rare and the bacilli are present in massive numbers throughout the lesion.

Generalized cryptococcosis may present a picture somewhat similar to that of feline leprosy but the conditions can readily be distinguished by examination of smears of the lesions. Chronically infected cat bites may also resemble feline leprosy occasionally, but, again, smear examination will provide a correct diagnosis.

## TREATMENT

When accessible, the lesions can be removed surgically and will not recur at the same site. Cases in which surgical excision is impracticable may be treated with the human antileprosy agent, diaminodiphenylsulfone (Dapsone, [Avlosulfon®, Ayerst]) given orally at a dose rate of 50 to 100 mg./kg. body weight daily. The bacillus is sensitive to streptomycin, but in view of the susceptibility of the cat to the toxic effects of this antibiotic, systemic adminstration is not recommended in this species. However, it may be practicable to inject small doses of streptomycin intralesionally without provoking serious side effects. The antibiotic rifampicin has been shown to possess bactericidal effects on the human leprosy bacillus and has been tried in cats with mixed results. If other therapeutic agents prove ineffective, however, it may be tried at a dose rate of 5 mg./kg. body weight daily.

### SUPPLEMENTAL READING

Brown, L. R., May, C. D., and Williams, S. E.: A non-tuberculous granuloma in cats. New Zealand Vet. J., 10:7–9, 1962.

Lawrence, W. E., and Wickham, N.: Cat leprosy: Infection by a bacillus resembling *Mycobacterium lepraemurium*. Aust. Vet. J., 39:390–393, 1963.

Robinson, J.: Skin granuloma of cats associated with acid-fast bacilli. J. Small Animal Pract., 16:563–567, 1975.

Schiefer, B., Gee, B. R., and Ward, G. E.: A disease resembling feline leprosy in western Canada. J. Am. Vet. Med. Assn., 165:1085–1087, 1974.

Wilkinson, G. T.: A nontuberculous granuloma of the cat associated with an acid-fast bacillus. Vet. Rec., 76:777–778, 1964.

# ALLERGIC CONTACT DERMATITIS

G. S. WALTON, M.R.C.V.S.
*Liverpool, England*

## INTRODUCTION

Many agents coming into direct contact with the skin will produce either physical or chemical damage. Others, after repeated application, may induce an allergic hypersensitivity response in individual animals. Although the majority of sensitizing agents within a home environment are nonirritant, certain substances, such as phenolic agents, can produce chemical damage if present in sufficient concentration and may later induce allergic changes, which further heighten the degree of skin damage. The skin response is characterized by irritation, tissue damage and self-trauma. If the challenge is prolonged, secondary skin changes, such as skin thickening, hyperkeratosis and hyperpigmentation, may occur and secondary bacterial infection may ensue. Although on cursory examination it may be impossible to differentiate between the different types of responses, careful study will reveal a number of differences which are of fundamental importance as aids in diagnosis.

A survey of the incidence of allergic contact sensitivity in dogs brought to the author's clinic in Great Britain revealed that this condition accounted for approximately one per cent of skin conditions.

## PHYSICAL CONTACT REACTIONS

The severity of the physical damage produced by such agents as sand, gravel, coarse vegetation or incompetently used clipper blades will depend on the mode of application of the individual agent, the intrinsic pattern of skin reactivity displayed by the individual animal and the degree of protection afforded by the coat.

Physical contact dermatitis occurs most frequently on the feet and pressure areas. When produced elsewhere on the body, it often displays an irregular, asymmetric pattern of damage.

The response is usually apparent within a few hours of initial contact.

## CHEMICAL CONTACT REACTIONS

The nature and severity of the skin changes produced by chemical irritants will vary with that chemical's state, concentration, volume and corrosive capacity.

Powerful corrosive agents will produce skin changes which become obvious immediately following initial application.

Weak irritants or more powerful corrosive agents present in low concentration often produce little macroscopic evidence of skin damage following initial application, but on repeated application, an escalation of skin changes occurs, which in time leads to irritation, inflammation and later a variety of secondary skin changes. Unlike contact allergies, subsequent application of this group of agents in dilute form will not produce evidence of skin change when applied to a normal area of skin of the sufferer.

## ALLERGIC CONTACT DERMATITIS

### The allergic mechanism

Allergic contact dermatitis is caused by a delayed, cell-mediated response (type IV reaction). Unlike physical or chemical contact reactions, a response is never observed following initial exposure and may not occur until repeated or continuous challenge has occurred over some years. On the other hand, of course, most animals are subjected to repeated or continuous challenge by a large number of potential contact allergens throughout their lives without ever developing a hypersensitivity response.

The factors determining whether or not contact allergy develops are obscure. There is evidence that certain strains of laboratory animals do possess a genetic predisposition to this type of response (Polak and Turk, 1969), but there are, as yet, no conclusive data suggesting that such factors are operative in either man or the domestic pet. It is noteworthy, however, that over 20 per cent of cases of contact allergy seen at the University of Liverpool Dermatology Clinic in a recent series were Golden Labradors. Abrasions and repeated minor trauma appear

to aid initiation of this type of response both in the laboratory animal and in man, and this may also be important in the dog.

Once an allergic reaction to a chemical has been established, the severity of the ensuing changes associated with continuing antigenic challenge will be enhanced by irritants, skin alkalinity, perspiration, abrasives and a wide variety of other agents.

The response has been divided into three phases. The first is the refractory phase, during which time there is no evidence of skin change or of immunologic activity. Next there will be an incubation phase, during which application of the antigen produces no clinical evidence of a contact reaction, but during which an immunologic mechanism is being initiated and is detectable by *in-vitro* methods. This phase lasts a minimum of five days and possibly up to three weeks. This fact explains why clinically apparent responses are not noted in less than five days after the initial exposure. Finally, there is the period of hypersensitivity, during which application of the sensitizing agent will produce evidence of skin change; this stage remains for many years.

It is important to remember that because allergic contact allergy is cell-mediated, the response of a sensitized animal to the allergens is not immediate. This latent period varies from a few hours to up to five days. Furthermore, the time taken for the skin lesions to resolve is likewise not immediate. If no further allergen is applied and all excess allergen is removed from the skin surface, the skin takes at least seven to ten days to return to normal. In severe, chronic contact allergies this period may be much longer.

Observations carried out in the dog have shown that the total length of the refractory and sensitizing periods is in excess of two years in over 70 per cent of cases and is rarely less than six months. It is thus unwise immediately to incriminate new factors in the contact environment.

There appears to be no age predisposition, but because of the relatively long refractory period observed in most cases, the prevalence of this type of allergy in the author's clinic is very low in animals under six months of age.

Once sensitization has occurred, possibly following repeated challenge to one small, confined area of the body, application of the allergen to any part of the skin will produce a skin reaction. The reaction will occur in response to low concentration of the appropriate allergen, and its severity will not be related directly to the concentration of the allergen.

## NATURE OF ALLERGENS

Contact allergens may be single ions, such as cobalt, nickel or iodine; slightly larger compounds of relatively low molecular weight, such as formaldehyde; or substances such as oleoresins, which have a more complex formulation. Most are haptenic in nature and must be linked to a skin fraction before they reach full antigenicity (Calnan, 1968).

The power of a substance to induce allergic contact reactions is variable and believed to be related to its chemical reactivity and reaction constant (Calnan, 1968). Certain allergens, such as poison ivy, are classed as being powerful sensitizers because of their capacity to produce allergic responses in the skin of a high percentage of any population repeatedly exposed to their action. Within such populations, however, certain individuals will be encountered who fail to become sensitized. Conversely, other substances are classed as weak sensitizers, since they produce hypersensitivity responses only infrequently within a population.

No explanation is available as to why an animal will develop a sensitivity to only one particular sensitizing agent and will fail to produce a similar response to any one of the many other sensitizing agents within its environment and with which it comes into repeated contact.

Allergic contact dermatitis in the dog, and less frequently in the cat, has been associated with agents in the external environment, such as plants and plant pollens. Contact allergies to the fibers of wool, nylon or other synthetic or natural furnishings appear to be extremely rare, but they may frequently occur in response to dyes, mordants or finishes used in the manufacture of carpeting, blankets and other forms of soft furnishing. They may also be associated with floor polishes and cleansers, preservatives or the accelerators or antioxidants used in rubber products.

It must also be remembered that allergic responses may suddenly develop to pharmaceutical agents or their bases following prolonged or repeated application into the ear or onto other parts of the body.

## CLINICAL PICTURE

Application of the appropriate allergen following sensitization will produce evidence of a local irritation. The skin color will appear to be normal, with no evidence of edema in some animals, while in others there will be evidence of hyperemia and even bulla formation or exfoliation over the contact sites.

Irritation, when contact is prolonged, will often lead to the production of self-inflicted skin damage, which may be confined to only one or two contact sites or may involve all contact areas. When an animal indulges in rubbing or drags its body across rough surfaces in an attempt to gain relief, lesions may be produced on sites other than the contact areas.

Small items such as rugs and blankets will produce lesions that are confined to the abdomen and axillae and may also involve the anterior parts of the face, the perineal area and the area below the accessory pads. In animals that have been clipped, lesions may additionally be found over other areas where hair cover is sparse.

If the animal walks over a surface containing the allergen but does not lie on that surface, lesions will be found to involve only the skin between the foot pads. If the animal both lies on and walks over the allergenic surface, all potential contact sites will be affected. The irritation may be seasonal when plant allergens are involved.

No regional pattern will be observed in responses produced to allergens which are present in large amounts and in fluid form (e.g., shampoos), the response occurring whenever and wherever the agent manages to penetrate the coat or come into direct contact with the skin.

## DIAGNOSIS

One must rely on the case history, clinical picture and isolation procedures to diagnose allergic contact dermatitis in the dog. It may be confirmed by provocative exposure or by patch testing.

There is usually a history of a fairly sudden onset of irritation, with or without evidence of other skin changes, involving but confined to contact areas, and it is unlikely that more than one animal within the same environment will be similarly affected at one time.

Hyperemia, scaling, skin thickening and hyperpigmentation may be noted in the long-standing case, and this may be accompanied by some peripheral spreading of the lesions around the contact areas. It is important to assess whether there is evidence of a seasonal pattern of response, which may be associated with a plant contact allergy to either the pollen or the foliage. Similarly, it is relevant to assess whether there is evidence of continuous irritation throughout the year, indicating that the allergen is in daily contact with the subject's skin, or whether the irritation occurs intermittently, indicating that the animal's skin encounters the allergen only on sporadic occasions. It may then be possible, with the help of a cooperative owner or handler, to compile a list of potential allergens and to decide on a method of elimination.

If the skin changes are minimal, removal of the inciting cause will bring about resolution of lesions within seven to ten days. If secondary changes are severe, it may be necessary to isolate the subject for a longer period of time and to treat the animal empirically with steroids and antibiotics, and on occasion to administer sedation, until resolution has taken place. The animal's environment may then be enlarged slowly, adding one item every seven days until a response is noted. To confirm the diagnosis it is advisable to remove the suspected allergen for a few days before repeating the challenge to allow the skin changes to resolve.

## PATCH TESTING

Patch testing with potential allergens can be carried out by applying a suitable concentration and formulation of the allergen to a previously selected area of "normal" skin on a hair-covered area of the body (open patch test) (Table 1). The use of occlusive dressings (closed patch test) is unsatisfactory in the dog, and the allergen should merely be rubbed into the test site, which is then suitably marked. The test sites are then examined daily over a five-day period for evidence of erythema. In many cases the test animal will draw attention to the response by attempting to scratch or nibble. It is therefore essential that the number of test sites used be kept to a minimum, with not more than four substances being tested per side at any one time.

Patch testing is extremely useful for discovering the particular allergen concerned. When confronted with a response to a substance present in carpeting or furnishings, however, it may be of limited value in determining which item contains that particular allergen, since a list of the substances used during the manufacture, dyeing, mordanting or finishing of individual items is often not freely available from the manufacturers. In this situation, when a limited number of internal contactants, such as area rugs, are implicated, a closed patch test may be attempted. In addition, the investigator may still be forced to carry out elimination procedures followed by provocative challenge using individual items.

## HYPOSENSITIZATION

Attempts at hyposensitizing animals using both oral and intravenous challenge have proved disappointing to date. Reliance must be placed on prevention of further contact with the relevant allergen.

### SUPPLEMENTAL READING

Calnan, C. D.: Allergic contact dermatitis. In Gell, P. G., and Coombs, R. R. (eds.): Clinical Aspects of Immunology. 2nd ed. Oxford, Blackwell Scientific Publications, 1968.
Polak, L., and Turk, J. L.: Genetic background of certain immunological phenomena with particular reference to the skin. J. Invest. Derm., 52:219–232, 1969.

*Table 1.* Suggested Concentrations and Vehicles for Canine Patch Testing

| SUBSTANCE | CONCENTRATION AND VEHICLE |
|---|---|
| *Dyes* | |
| Acetanilide, acridine, alizarin red 1034, aniline black, aniline brilliant green, anthraquinone, anthraquinone blue, chrome yellow | Powder |
| Alizarin red, hair dyes, naphthol yellow, nigrosine, Nile blue, pontamine black, rhodamine B, safranine, tartrazine blue, Victoria blue | Undiluted |
| Fuchsin, methylaniline, indigo | 10% solution |
| Alizarin 778, methyl violet | 2% solution |
| Aniline dyes | 2% in olive oil or paraffin |
| Diazonium salts | 1% in paraffin wax |
| Fluorescein | 1% in 70% alcohol |
| *Mordants and Intermediates* | |
| Chrome alum | Undiluted |
| Cobalt oxide, naphthalene | Undiluted |
| Chromium potassium sulfate, formaldehyde naphthol | 10% aqueous |
| Copper sulfate, pyrogallol, sodium thiosulfate | 2% aqueous |
| Chromium chloride, chromium sulfate, picric acid | 2% aqueous |
| Hydroxymercurichlorphenol, tannic acid | 0.5% aqueous |
| *Miscellaneous* | |
| Floor cleaners, detergents, dirt repellents, aluminum chloride | 1% aqueous* |
| Nickel sulfate | 5% aqueous |
| Floor polishes and waxes | 5% in olive oil or 70% alcohol* |
| Medicaments | At therapeutic dose* |
| Oleoresins | As instructed |
| Dyed objects | Attempt to extract with water, alcohol, olive oil, acetone, chloroform |

*If in doubt, or following a positive reaction, carry out control tests on normal animals to exclude possible irritant reactions.

# ALLERGIC RESPONSES TO INGESTED ALLERGENS

G. S. WALTON, M.R.C.V.S.
*Liverpool, England*

## INTRODUCTION

Allergic responses to ingested allergens may produce inflammation and tissue damage manifested by skin irritation, gastrointestinal signs or, rarely, respiratory embarrassment. Such symptoms are not pathognomonic of an allergic response and may be stimulated by nonallergic mechanisms in individual animals possessing an intolerance or idiosyncrasy to a particular food or ingested agent. The symptoms may also be mimicked during the course of other disease states.

Changes may also occur within body tissues following the ingestion of toxic quantities of certain substances, or conversely when an animal has been fed over a variable period of time on a diet which is deficient in one or several nutritional factors.

Dermatologic responses to ingested allergens have been found to account for less than 1 per cent of skin conditions, and it is thus essential that the possibility of other allergic or nonallergic mechanisms that may be responsible for the presenting symptoms be investigated and ruled out before proceeding further.

## ALLERGIC MECHANISMS

Ingested allergens may, following repeated challenge, stimulate the production of an IgE-mediated (type I) response and/or an Arthus type (type III) response within one or more organs of the body. The possibility that delayed cell-mediated responses to ingested allergens are produced in the dog and cat is still being investigated, since it is known that on rare occasions this type of response occurs in man in association with ingestion of certain contact sensitizers.

The mechanisms by which sensitization is initiated are incompletely understood. All animals ingest a large number and wide variety of potential allergens daily throughout their lives, but the majority of animals remain refractory, never displaying any clinical evidence of sensitization.

When sensitization does occur, it is subject to marked individual variation. Investigations carried out in the dog and cat (Walton, 1967) have revealed that although in theory animals may produce a clinical response within seven days of first being exposed to a given allergen, in practice sensitization is invariably preceded by a long refractory period. In 68 per cent of cases, animals had been exposed to the allergen concerned for periods in excess of two years before clinical evidence of an allergic response became apparent. Symptoms then occurred suddenly and recurred following every subsequent challenge by that allergen, even when the allergen was present in only minute amounts.

It has been found that allergic responses to ingested allergens are precise and that alterations to an allergen, by cooking or processing, can profoundly affect its capacity to evoke a hypersensitivity response in the previously sensitized animal. Multiple sensitivities to ingested allergens appear to be rare in the dog and cat and were noted in only 12 instances of a series of 500 cases diagnosed in the author's clinic. In these animals, the subsequent sensitivities tended to affect the original organ of shock and developed singly over several years. There was no evidence of genetic predisposition.

No satisfactory explanation exists as to why an individual animal suddenly develops a sensitivity to only one specific allergen and fails to produce a similar response to the many other potential allergens within its diet. Similarly, little is known of the factors that determine why an allergic hypersensitivity response to an ingested allergen is localized preferentially to one organ of the body, such as the skin, bowel or lungs, with responses involving more than one organ probably occurring in less than 10 per cent of cases.

## ALLERGENS INVOLVED

Responses to ingested allergens are most frequently encountered to food and food products, but whether the weight or pattern of exposure influences the development of this type of response is not known. In the United Kingdom, allergic responses to cow's milk, which is included in a number of commercial dog foods and is also fed separately to many animals, account for approximately 25 per cent of allergic responses to ingested allergens. The allergic response may be highly specific and restricted to one antigenic determinant, or cross-reaction may occur. For example, the response to cow's milk may cross-react with beef proteins and vice versa. Usually, however, reactions to a protein of one species do not cross-react with that same protein of another species.

Responses to mutton allergens appear to occur more frequently in Great Britain than in the United States, accounting for approximately 10 per cent of cases; a possible explanation for this is that mutton is fed more frequently to animals in Britain. The clinician must assume, however, that any item within an animal's diet is a potential allergen, and an item cannot be ignored because it is being fed in small quantities or intermittently.

Reactions to sugars and minerals, unless they are of animal origin, are very rare, but reactions to cereals can occur and are precise; in Great Britain they are most frequently associated with wheat meal and wheat meal products and account for approximately 14 per cent of cases.

## CLINICAL SIGNS

The clinical features of allergic responses to ingested allergens in the dog and cat are subject to individual variation. Onset of symptoms is usually sudden and affects only one member within an animal population. It can occur for the first time at any age and may be noted for the first time in an aged animal which has received that allergen daily throughout its life. The changes may then be very severe, involving the skin, alimentary tract and/or, rarely, the respiratory system; the nervous system and kidney have also been suggested as possible "organs of shock" in man but to date have not been proved to occur in the dog or cat.

**Skin Responses.** Skin responses to ingested allergens in the sensitized animal may produce symptoms of generalized pruritus, urticaria, self-inflicted skin damage and a variety of cutaneous changes.

Generalized pruritus is evident in over 98 per cent of cases and is characterized by excessive scratching, licking or rubbing by the subject. It is often possible to demonstrate an exaggerated scratch reflex, and there may be evidence of spontaneous skin twitching. When the response has been present over a period of time, and the animal has been subjected to repeated allergenic challenge, the presenting feature may be self-inflicted skin damage, which may be generalized or manifest as regionalized areas of rubbing or precisely localized lesions over areas of convenience, that show marked individual variation. In over 30 per cent of cases, the skin appears to be of normal color and texture on macroscopic examination, excluding those areas that had been subjected to self-inflicted damage.

Sometimes cases show a generalized hyperemia, which may be accompanied by edema and skin thickening and may lead to seborrheic changes and a diffuse thinning of the coat. Cases may also show a bilateral otitis and on some occasions a secondary entropion as a result of long-standing facial edema. Alternatively, some dogs may present with a generalized papular eruption or with irregular plaques of edema over the trunk and limbs. In both types of case there may also be edema of the face and/or the ear flaps.

Symptoms often appear within 4 to 24 hours of challenge in the previously sensitized animal. If no further allergen is ingested, the skin will return to normal within the next 24 to 48 hours, unless self-inflicted damage or secondary changes have been severe.

Following repeated allergenic challenge, there will be an escalation of the condition due to secondary skin thickening, scale formation and possibly secondary infection. The skin may develop a musty or rancid odor, coat growth may be affected and skin pigmentation may be increased. All these latter changes result from skin inflammation and are not pathognomonic of cutaneous allergy.

**Alimentary Responses.** Alimentary responses to ingested allergens may involve all or only part of the tract.

Gastric involvement will be typified by vomiting or abdominal discomfort, occurring immediately following or within two hours of ingestion of the appropriate allergen.

Lower alimentary involvement may affect the whole or part of the small intestine and/or the large intestine and may cause abdominal discomfort with the passage of watery, mucoid or hemorrhagic feces within 12 to 24 hours of allergen ingestion. Symptoms usually persist for up to 12 hours and then resolve unless further allergenic challenge takes place.

When repeated allergic reactions involving the small and/or large intestine have continued over a long period of time, resolution of symptoms may be delayed and may require the use of steroid therapy for a variable period of time following removal of the allergenic challenge.

**Respiratory Responses.** Respiratory symptoms, which are very rare, may follow either the swallowing or possibly the inhalation of the appropriate ingested allergen during feeding. The symptoms of respiratory involvement are those of acute bronchial constriction, which, unless treated with steroids, persist for several hours. Symptoms may be noted either immediately following feeding or following a delay of up to 12 hours after allergen ingestion.

## DIAGNOSIS

Only when all other possible causes of inflammation, skin irritation or altered gut motility either of infective or noninfective etiology have been investigated and eliminated should the possibility of an allergic response to ingested allergens be considered. Particular care must be given to excluding the possibility of other types of cutaneous allergy. Remember that internal parasites may also be responsible for both gastrointestinal signs and pruritus.

An accurate case history is invaluable. It may reveal the following:

1. A sudden onset of symptoms occurring at any age, involving only one animal within a closed community;

2. No evidence of subsequent spread of symptoms to other animals within that community or to other in-contact animals;

3. Transitory improvement following the use of steroids or other anti-inflammatory drugs, with recurrence of symptoms following their withdrawal.

The history may also expose a correlation between the ingestion of an individual agent and the onset of symptoms. If no such correlation is apparent and an ingested allergen is still suspected, it is essential that a test meal investigation be carried out.

## TEST MEAL INVESTIGATION

Before commencing a test meal investigation, it is important to obtain a complete list of all potential ingested allergens that the subject may have received, appreciating that a severe response may follow ingestion of minute amounts of allergen by the previously sensitized animal. Other items that the animal chews, such as rawhide bones, should also be considered.

It must be remembered that commercial foods contain conglomerations of many potential allergens that may be common to different brands. Many animals also receive or obtain tidbits or food from other sources, and such sources must be investigated and the potential allergens obtained established; pastry, for instance, may contain wheat meal, egg and milk.

Examination of the completed list should then reveal possible foods which, because they have not been present in the previous diet, could be fed to the subject, excluding the previously employed potential allergens.

If a suitable diet cannot be formulated, the animal should be placed on a restricted diet containing only one or two potential allergens, such as meat from a known animal source (e.g., chicken or lamb) and vegetables and rice for three weeks.

When secondary changes are marked, it may be necessary to maintain an animal on the original test diet for three or four weeks and also to give steroids, antibiotics and, on some occasions, sedation. This applies particularly to the chronic skin problem. Evidence of clinical improvement may be difficult to find during the earlier parts of such investigations, but if the allergen has been removed, it is usually possible to reduce steroid dosage after seven to ten days without an exacerbation of symptoms.

A more radical approach is to place the animal on a sugar and water diet or glucose and water. This approach is of value when dealing with alimentary allergies, in which removal of the relevant allergen will usually bring about improvement within a few days, but is too drastic in the long-standing cutaneous allergy, which may require not only removal of the cause but also empirical therapy to bring about resolution of secondary changes.

If improvement does not follow the use of a restricted diet, steps should be taken to insure that the diet is being adhered to strictly, and having obtained satisfaction on this point, the possibility that the restricted diet actually contains the relevant allergen should be explored and appropriate changes made.

Once improvement has been achieved, one allergen at a time should be readmitted to the basic diet for a period of seven to ten days; if a response occurs, the latest inclusion should be removed and then reintroduced some days later to confirm the diagnosis. If no response occurs to an agent after its inclusion in the diet for seven to ten days, that substance can be assumed to be of no importance.

## OTHER DIAGNOSTIC TESTS

Intradermal, scratch and prick tests are of little value in diagnosis because the available antigens at present, despite careful preparation, often bear little relationship to the substances producing the response within the organ of shock. It is possible to obtain a true positive reaction in a minority of cases, but in many animals a false negative reaction can occur, since the animal's response is not to the pure allergen but to a digestion breakdown product, which may then possibly be linked to a tissue or serum complex.

Serologic tests are also limited because of the nonavailability of a suitable battery of antigenic substances for routine diagnosis.

In certain cases an elevated eosinophil count may be found, but this is not pathognomonic of an allergic response and is encountered in many other conditions, such as parasitic infections or infestations and chronic diseases of the alimentary tract or skin. Dietary allergies are usually corticosteroid-responsive, and some relief may be obtained with antihistamines. Neither, however, are suitable for long-term therapy.

## THERAPY

Hyposensitization techniques for this type of allergy are in their infancy, and although it has been suggested that the feeding of minute amounts of allergen may be of value in certain cases, the procedure is hazardous and can produce serious side effects, as can the injection of dietary allergens. Until knowledge increases, the aim is still to eliminate the relevant allergen from the diet.

### SUPPLEMENTAL READING

Walton, G. S.: Skin manifestations of allergic response in domestic animals. Observations on one hundred confirmed cases. Vet. Rec., *81*:709–713, 1967.

# Section
# 7

# DISEASES
# OF THE
# EYE

STEPHEN I. BISTNER, D.V.M.
*Consulting Editor*

# EXAMINATION OF THE EYE

STEPHEN I. BISTNER, D.V.M.
*New York, New York*

Because of its anatomic structure and transparent media, the eye permits the examiner to observe directly many pathologic processes as they develop. The development of many refined techniques has made ophthalmology one of the most exacting, interesting and rewarding of the clinical specialties.

As in any type of medical examination, the detailed examination of the eyes should be preceded by a careful history. The following categories should be included in the history: (1) chief complaint (C.C.); (2) present illness (P.I.); (3) review of systems (R.S.); and (4) past history (P.H.).

## EXTERNAL EXAMINATION

### INSPECTION OF THE GLOBE AND NEUROMUSCULAR EXAMINATION

A careful, systematic scheme of examination should be used when examining the eyes. A general inspection of the globe and external ocular structures should be conducted before any detailed examination of the eye is undertaken. Inspect the globe in normal daylight or room light and observe the relationship of the globe to the orbit and the eyelids. Note whether the eyes are in the same visual axis or whether a tropia is present. Note any undue prominence of either or both eyes. Note the presence of any other facial lesions (e.g., facial paralysis) which may affect the symmetry of the orbit. Inspect the external ocular structures (lids, conjunctiva, cornea, sclera and lacrimal apparatus). Note the position of the eyelids, the size of the palpebral aperture, the position of the membrana nictitans, the presence of nystagmus, unequal pupils, blepharospasm, lagophthalmos or ocular discharges.

The tonic eye reflexes are used in the determination of extraocular muscle function and localization of lesions in the central nervous system. The dog and cat have seven extraocular muscles: (1) rectus medialis; (2) rectus lateralis; (3) rectus dorsalis; (4) rectus ventralis; (5) obliquus dorsalis; (6) obliquus ventralis; and (7) retractor bulbi. Cranial nerves 3, 4 and 6 (oculomotorius, trochlearis, abducens) innervate the extraocular striated muscles and are examined together. Nerve 4 innervates the obliquus dorsalis, nerve 6 innervates the rectus lateralis and part of the retractor bulbi and nerve 3 innervates the rectus medialis, the rectus ventralis, the obliquus ventralis and the levator palpebrae superioris. Pupillary dilatation is controlled by preganglionic neurons in the first three thoracic spinal cord segments, the cranial thoracic and cervical sympathetic trunks, and by postganglionic neurons in the cranial cervical and sympathetic nerves that course through the middle ear to reach the orbit and dilator pupillae. Parasympathetic fibers in nerve 3 innervate the sphincter pupillae muscle.

The integrity of cranial nerve 3 may be evaluated by examining: (1) the size of the pupil; (2) the reaction of the pupil to light; (3) the presence or absence of ptosis or drooping of the upper eyelid because of paralysis of the levator palpebrae superioris muscle; and (4) deviation of the eye which has been reported as being medial, while others have reported the characteristic lateral deviation as seen in man. In oculomotor nerve palsy with a normal pupillary response, if all the extraocular muscles innervated by the third nerve are affected, then an intracranial lesion should be suspected. If individual extraocular muscles are involved, then a peripheral nerve lesion may exist. If an oculomotor nerve palsy exists in association with a dilated pupil, an intraorbital and/or intracranial lesion should be suspected.

Paralysis of the trochlear nerve produces a transient strabismus, resulting in a slight upward deviation of the eye (rarely seen). The affected animal may compensate for this by developing a head tilt.

583

Paralysis of the abducens nerve results in a medial deviation of the affected eye with inability to gaze laterally.

It is important to check tonic neck and eye reflexes when evaluating the extraocular muscles. When the nose is elevated, the forelimbs extend and the hindlimbs flex. As the nose is elevated, the eye should remain focused within the center of the palpebral fissure. Deviating the head to one side results in increased extensor tonus on that side. Normally, nystagmus should be observed on lateral deviation of the head (with the quick phase toward the side of the deviation).

Strabismus is observed in dogs with disease of their vestibular system. With the head in certain positions, interference with the normal vestibular mechanism that maintains the eyeball position in adjustment with the position of the head causes the eyeball on the affected side to deviate ventrolaterally. Unlike the similar strabismus with oculomotor nerve palsy, this is transient, occurring only with the head in certain positions. Movement of the head will alleviate the strabismus. Strabismus of this type is referred to as vestibular strabismus.

A bilateral ventrolateral position of the eyeballs is commonly encountered in severely hydrocephalic dogs with an enlarged cranial cavity. This is assumed to result from the associated deformity of the orbit and not to be due to bilateral oculomotor nerve compression. This is supported by the fact that the eyeballs can move in all directions and there is no associated mydriasis or ptosis.

The size of the palpebral fissure is controlled by the following muscles of the eyelids. The orbicularis oculi is innervated by the auriculopalpebral branch of the facial nerve—cranial nerve 7. Contraction of this muscle closes the palpebral fissure. The levator palpebrarum is innervated by the oculomotor nerve—cranial nerve 3. When this muscle contracts, it elevates the upper eyelid, enlarging the palpebral fissure. Smooth muscle present in both eyelids is innervated by sympathetic postganglionic axons that enter the orbit with the ophthalmic nerve. Contraction of this smooth muscle enlarges the palpebral fissure. Disease of the facial nerve or its auriculopalpebral branch causes failure of the fissure to close in response to any stimulus. Usually the fissure on the affected side is slightly larger than that on the normal side. Disease of the oculomotor nerve paralyzes the levator palpebrarum and the upper eyelid will droop—ptosis. Defects in the other structures innervated by the oculomotor nerve will also be observed—strabismus and mydriasis. Disease of the sympathetic innervation to the smooth muscle of the eyelids causes the palpebral fissure to be slightly narrowed—one of the components of Horner's syndrome.

The third eyelid's position in reference to the eyeball depends on the position of the eyeball in the orbit and the tone in the smooth muscle of the third eyelid. If the eyeball is retracted, the third eyelid passively protrudes. This is seen in some cases of tetanus. Normal tone is maintained in the smooth muscle by its sympathetic innervation which is similar to that of the eyelids. This tonic mechanism keeps the third eyelid retracted in its normal position. Disease of this sympathetic innervation causes the third eyelid to protrude slightly across the medial aspect of the eyeball—another component of Horner's syndrome.

## PUPILS

Normal pupillary response requires that nerves 2 and 3 be intact, and involves only brainstem connections. When light directed toward the lateral retina is shone into the eye, the visual impulse created passes through the optic nerve to the optic chiasm where an opportunity for crossing to the opposite side occurs. In the cat, about 66 per cent of the optic nerve fibers and, in the dog, about 75 per cent decussate at the optic chiasm. Optic nerve axons conducting impulses initiated in the medial retina will cross in the chiasm to the contralateral optic tract. Impulses originating from the lateral retina mostly enter the ipsilateral optic tract from the chiasm. The optic nerve has two components: one is composed of those fibers that pass to the pupillary centers within the brainstem; the second is composed of those fibers that synapse in the thalamus, which in turn project the impulses to the visual cortex of the brain. The pupillary fibers leave the optic tract and synapse in the midbrain, where crossing occurs. Impulses reach the rostral portion of the oculomotor nucleus, which contains cell bodies of preganglionic parasympathetic axons. Axons from the oculomotor nucleus project in the oculomotor nerve through the orbital fissure and periorbita, where synapse in the ciliary ganglion occurs between the preganglionic parasympathetic axons and the cell bodies of the postganglionic parasympathetic axons. The postganglionic nerves are continued as the short ciliary nerves to the eye supplying the constrictor pupillary muscle.

Because of the numerous opportunities for crossing of light-stimulated axons, stimulation of the retina of one eyeball affects the preganglionic parasympathetic neurons of each oculomotor nerve and thus induces pupillary constriction in both eyeballs. The response in the nonstimulated eyeball is called the consensual or indirect response.

Disease that interferes with the light-sensitive neurons between the retina and the optic chiasm will cause failure of the pupillary reflex to occur in either eyeball when light is directed into the eyeball on the side of the lesion. However, light directed into the contralateral eyeball will elicit pupillary constriction in both eyeballs. In room light, the pupil of the eyeball on the side of the lesion will be dilated more than normal. If the entire optic chiasm or both optic tracts were totally destroyed, no response would occur to light directed into either eyeball and both pupils would be dilated. Unilateral optic tract lesions do not usually disturb the pupillary reflex.

If the parasympathetic (oculomotor nerve) pathway is interrupted on one side, the pupil will be widely dilated on that side. Light directed into either eyeball will elicit pupillary constriction only in the eyeball contralateral to the parasympathetic pathway lesion. If a retrobulbar lesion destroyed the function of the optic nerve and the ciliary ganglion, the pupil on that side would be widely dilated and unresponsive to light directed into either eyeball. Light directed into the unaffected eyeball would induce pupillary constriction only in that same eyeball.

The pathway for the sympathetic innervation of the dilator pupillae muscle involves both central and peripheral components. Centrally, the sympathetic component involves the hypothalamus and rostral midbrain with projections through the pons, medulla and descending lateral tectosegmentospinal system. The preganglionic neurons of the peripheral sympathetic pathway are located within the first three thoracic spinal cord segments. The axons from the thoracic and cervical sympathetic trunk course cranially to reach the cranial cervical ganglion ventromedial to the tympanic bulla. Synapse occurs and postganglionic nerves travel via the long ciliary nerves to innervate the dilator pupillae muscle. Additionally, this same pathway provides innervation of the smooth muscle of the periorbita, eyelids and membrana nictitans.

A lesion anywhere in the pathway of this nerve could produce sympathetic denervation and the characteristic Horner's syndrome (miosis, ptosis, prolapse of the membrana nictitans and apparent enophthalmos). In general, experience shows that central nervous system lesions cranial to the first thoracic segment rarely produce Horner's syndrome, with the exception of intracranial injury with contusion of the midbrain structures involving the origin of the lateral tectosegmentospinal system.

Horner's syndrome is usually involved with a component of the lower motor neuron pathway, beginning possibly at the level of the first three thoracic segments. Table 1 may be helpful in differentiating the most common lesions that may be associated with Horner's syndrome.

## ASSESSMENT OF VISUAL FUNCTION

Assessment of visual function in pet animals presents a difficult problem, and the veterinarian must depend on objective signs and reflexes to estimate vision. A common test often used to assess vision is the "menace reaction." This involves passing the hand or an object in front of the animal's eyes and noticing the presence or absence of a blink reflex.

The response of the pupil to light also can be used to evaluate function of the visual system. Each pupil should be tested individually using a bright focal source of illumination, and the opposite eye should be covered. The consensual pupillary response also should be tested. An obstacle course also can be very valuable in assessing visual function. Styrofoam cylinders mounted on a platform can be used to create the course. The light intensity in the examining room can be varied, and alternate patching of the eyes can be helpful in detecting lesions.

*Table 1.  Common Lesions Associated with Horner's Syndrome*

| LOCATION | LESION | ASSOCIATED NEUROLOGIC DEFICIT |
|---|---|---|
| T1–T3 spinal cord | External injury<br>Neoplasm | Pelvic and thoracic limb paresis or paralysis, with lower motor neuron deficit in thoracic limbs and upper motor neuron deficit in pelvic limbs |
| T1–T3 ventral roots—proximal spinal nerves | Avulsion of roots of brachial plexus | Brachial plexus paresis or paralysis of the thoracic limb on the same side |
| Cranial thoracic sympathetic trunk | Lymphosarcoma<br>Neurofibroma | None if confined to the trunk |
| Cervical sympathetic trunk | Injury from surgical intervention in the area or from dog bites<br>Neoplasm | None if unilateral; bilateral lesions interfere with esophageal function |
| Middle ear cavity | Otitis media | Signs of peripheral vestibular disturbance—ipsilateral ataxia, head tilt and nystagmus; facial palsy |
| Retrobulbar | Contusion | Varies with degree of contusion to the optic and oculomotor nerves which also influence pupillary size |

## EXAMINATION OF THE ORBIT

Observe the orbits for size. Look for swelling, depression, fistula or laceration of the orbital margin. If the orbit is enlarged, note whether the swelling is hard or soft, painful or nonpainful. Retrobulbar abscesses produce exophthalmos attended by pain, immobility of the eye, chemosis, edema of the eyelids, and pain on opening the mouth. Orbital tumors may not be painful. Orbital retrobulbar hemorrhage or orbital fracture may occur following severe head trauma from automobile accidents. Enophthalmos may result from shrinkage of orbital contents (as in phthisis bulbi following ocular injury), from paralysis of the sympathetic nerve in Horner's syndrome or from loss of retrobulbar fat in emaciation and dehydration.

## EXAMINATION OF THE EYELIDS

Note any inflammation along the margins of the eyelids and any inability to close the lids (lagophthalmos). The eyelids should touch the globe, thus preventing an accumulation of tears and debris. The cilia or eyelashes on the dog's upper eyelids are arranged in three irregular rows. The lower eyelids of dogs and both eyelids of cats are devoid of cilia. When examining the lids for the presence of entropion or ectropion, it is best not to manipulate the head, as this may distort the normal lid-globe relationship. The lids of dogs and cats have a very poorly developed tarsal plate, making manipulation relatively easy. Observe the edges of the lids for signs of entropion, ectropion, trichiasis or distichiasis. Observe the eyelids for symblepharon or for swelling, edema, redness or a localized inflammation, which may indicate an internal or external hordeolum. Examine the lid margins for indication of any growths.

## EXAMINATION OF THE EYE USING FOCAL ILLUMINATION

In examining the anterior segment of the eye, the use of a simple optical system combining a focal source of illumination and condensing lens with an ophthalmic loupe or magnifying glass enables the observer to illuminate and examine various structures of the eye. The most highly refined source of focal illumination and magnification is the biomicroscope.

The combination of the slit lamp providing a source of focal illumination and the corneal microscope provides a method for careful and detailed examination of the eye, especially the anterior segment. The slit lamp enables the clinician accurately to locate the depth of a lesion in the cornea and lens. The major advantage of the biomicroscope is the ability to view pathologic processes in the living structure with great detail, and therefore more accurately diagnose, treat and formulate prognosis about diseases of the eye.

## EXAMINATION OF THE CONJUNCTIVA

Note whether the conjunctiva is pale, injected, pigmented, hemorrhagic or jaundiced. The inferior or ventral conjunctiva usually is more hyperemic than the upper. Pigmentation occasionally is present, especially on the superior bulbar conjunctiva. Usually a few follicles are present on the conjunctival surface, especially that of the third eyelid.

Note whether the conjunctiva is relatively smooth and dry, or excessively moist. Note any lacerations or erosions of the conjunctiva. These may be demonstrated using fluorescein. After initial inspection of the conjunctiva, additional tests may be required, such as the Schirmer tear test, culture, cytologic examination or the use of stains.

It is important to recognize pathologic congestion of the bulbar conjunctiva. There are two forms: superficial and deep. Superficial congestion usually is characteristic of external ocular irritation from foreign bodies, bacteria, trauma or allergic reactions. Deep congestion indicates an involvement of the cornea or the deeper structures within the eye. Normally, the deeper vessels around the limbus are difficult to see; however, when congested, they produce a distinctive "red flush" around the eye.

The palpebral (outer) and bulbar (inner) surfaces of the nictitating membrane should be inspected. The anterior surface of the membrane normally is smooth, and the leading edge frequently is pigmented. The bulbar surface can be examined by placing a few drops of topical anesthetic (proparacaine HCl) in the eye, and gently using a small, atraumatic thumb forceps to evert the third eyelid. The bulbar surface usually contains a few small follicles. The following are frequently found abnormalities that may be associated with the third eyelid: eversion of the cartilage; hypertrophy; protrusion; inflammation and hypertrophy of the gland of the third eyelid; foreign bodies; and hyperplasia.

**Conjunctival Smears, Scrapings and Cultures.** Conjunctival scrapings and cytologic examination can be very helpful in establishing an etiology and outlining an effective treatment regimen in conjunctivitis. In performing conjunctival scrapings, use a platinum spatula (Kimura spatula) whose tip has previously been sterilized in the flame of an alcohol lamp. Scrape the inferior conjunctival cul-de-sac, preferably without prior topical anesthesia, since anesthetics may distort the cells. Place the material on two glass slides, and fix one in acetone-free 95 percent methanol for 5 to 10 minutes; then stain with Giemsa stain. Heat fix the other slide and apply Gram stain.

Culturing the conjunctiva also can be a valuable aid, especially in chronic conjunctivitis. Sterile cotton applicators, fluid thioglycollate media and blood agar media are needed to perform cultures. Evert the palpebral conjunctiva of the lower lid, and pass one side of a sterile cotton applicator, previously moistened with sterile broth or thioglycollate media, over the palpebral conjunctival surface. Streak the swab onto a sterile blood agar plate; then place it into a tube of thioglycollate broth. No topical anesthesia is used prior to culturing, since preservatives present in anesthetics can inhibit the growth of bacteria.

## EXAMINATION OF THE LACRIMAL SYSTEM

Look for excessive tearing or a hypofunction of tear secretion. Note any swelling, redness or pain in the area of the lacrimal puncta and the lacrimal "sac." The nasolacrimal system can be evaluated by several basic tests. When excessive tearing exists, it must be determined if the tearing is due to: (1) partial or complete obstruction of the excretory mechanism; (2) increased lacrimal secretion from chronic ocular irritation, as in distichiasis or trichiasis; (3) physiologic increase in tear production as may occur with uveitis. The first diagnostic step is the use of the primary dye test. To perform this test, place a drop of fluorescein dye from a sterile fluorostrip into the eye. After two to five minutes, the external nares are examined with the aid of a Wood's light for the presence or absence of fluorescein dye. If dye is present, one can conclude that the lacrimal excretory system is patent and functioning. If epiphora exists yet the primary dye test indicates that the lacrimal excretory system is patent, then hypersecretion of tear fluid may be implicated as the cause for the epiphora.

If no stain appears at the external nares, the primary dye test is negative, demonstrating an obstruction to normal tear flow in the excretory mechanism. Irrigation of the nasolacrimal system is then indicated.

The production of normal lacrimal secretion can be tested by using the Schirmer tear test. This test is performed by placing a strip of filter paper (Whatman N. 40, 35 mm. long and 5 mm. wide, with a 5 mm. flap turned back at one end) in the inferior conjunctival cul-de-sac. The amount of wetting is measured in millimeters after a period of one minute. No topical anesthesia or drops of any kind should be used prior to conducting the test. The tear flow response in the dog, as measured with the Schirmer tear test, is a measure of corneal sensitivity and the animal's ability to produce tears. In normal dogs, wetting of the Schirmer test papers ranges from 10 to 25 mm. in one minute.

## EXAMINATION OF THE SCLERA

Note the color of the sclera and look for nodules, hemorrhage, lacerations, cysts or tumors. Normal sclera is white to blue-white. The sclera may appear blue because it is abnormally thinned and the uveal tract shows through. Look for staphylomas. Look for any injection of the scleral vessels and accompanying edema. Episcleritis can produce local scleral inflammation, whereas deep-seated ocular diseases such as glaucoma and uveitis produce generalized scleral vessel injection.

## EXAMINATION OF THE CORNEA

The cornea should be smooth, moist, free of blood vessels and transparent. Note any ulceration or opacity of the cornea. Slight opacities are termed nebulae; dense ones, leukomas. The canine cornea is oval, with a diameter of 12.5 to 17 mm. The horizontal measurement is 1 to 2 mm. greater than the vertical axis. Measurement of the corneal diameter with calipers may prove valuable when evaluating glaucoma and buphthalmia. In puppies, the cornea tends to be hazy, thus restricting ophthalmoscopic examination until four to six weeks of age.

Such diseases of the cornea as corneal inflammation, pigmentation, degeneration, trauma and neoplasia frequently may alter its transparency.

Test the corneal sensitivity by touching the cornea with a wisp of dry cotton. Instill a topical anesthetic—proparacaine hydrochloride, 0.5 per cent (Ophthaine,® Squibb)—into the conjunctival sac of each eye. Use a small forceps to pull the third eyelid gently away from the corneal surface and examine its inner surface for foreign bodies, hyperplastic tissue, inflammation, follicle formation or parasites (*Thelazia*). Observe the corneal surface for the presence of foreign bodies.

External ophthalmic stains can be very helpful in diagnosing lesions of the cornea. Fluorescein does not actually stain tissues. Being somewhat acid, the normal precorneal tear film stains yellow or orange with fluorescein. The intact corneal epithelium, having a high lipid content, resists penetration of water-soluble fluorescein and is not colored by it. Any break in the epithelial barrier permits rapid fluorescein penetration into the stroma, or even into the anterior chamber. When the epithelial surface has regenerated, the green color disappears, regardless of whether the underlying stroma is thickened, thinned, scarred or irregular.

Fluorescein may be applied by placing a strip of fluorescein-impregnated filter paper into the conjunctival sac until it is moistened by the tears. Excess dyes should be irrigated away with the saline solution. Fluorescein staining of the eye is transient and usually disappears in 30 to 45 minutes.

Unlike fluorescein, rose bengal actually stains cells and their nuclei. It selectively stains devitalized corneal and conjunctival epithelium a readily visible red. Its main use has been identification of corneal and conjunctival lesions due to keratitis sicca.

Rose bengal is instilled as a 1 per cent aqueous solution. Application causes irritation to the cornea, and one drop of topical anesthesia prior to instillation of the dye is helpful in preventing irritation. Excess rose bengal should be removed by irrigation.

If an ulcer is present, note whether the borders are regular or irregular and whether the ulcer is superficial or deep. Ulcers that are progressive and deep present a guarded prognosis. It is advisable to culture deep ulcers and to make a scraping of their borders.

The scrapings should be stained with Giemsa, and the type of cells determined. If the ulcer appears to be deep, look for evidence of anterior synechia, prolapsed iris, iridocyclitis, cataract, extrusion of the lens, fistula or hemorrhage.

Look for deposits on the posterior surface of the cornea (keratitic precipitates). These precipitates vary in size and shape, but they are indicative of a disease of the uveal tract.

## INTERNAL EXAMINATION

### EXAMINATION OF THE ANTERIOR CHAMBER

Examine the anterior chamber, and observe its depth; note changes in the transparency of the ocular media, such as hypopyon, hyphema, fibrin, or foreign bodies. Look for anterior synechiae.

### EXAMINATION OF THE IRIS

The color of the iris in each eye may vary. Observe the shape or size of the iris; an iris that is thickened and muddy in color indicates an infiltration of the uveal tract. Look for the presence of atrophy, tears, synechiae, persistent pupillary membranes, iridodonesis, iridodialysis, nodules, tumors, cysts or colobomas. Examine the pupillary border of the iris for signs of atrophy or posterior synechiae to the anterior lens capsule. Complete posterior synechia results in iris bombe and secondary glaucoma.

### EXAMINATION OF THE LENS

Complete examination of the lens requires that the pupil be dilated. The lens may be examined with a focal source of illumination and a loupe, with an opthalmoscope, or with a biomicroscope. Examine the lens for the presence of pigment, adhesions, opacities, the position of the lens (subluxation or luxation) or the absence of the lens (aphakia).

### OPHTHALMOSCOPY

**Examination of the Retina.** Examination of the retina with an ophthalmoscope is an essential part of every complete eye examination. For adequate visualization of the fundus, dilate the iris with tropicamide solution, 1 per cent.

Examine each patient's eye grounds in a dark room. To examine the right fundus, hold the ophthalmoscope in the right hand and view the fundus with the right eye. Keep both eyes open when using the ophthalmoscope; it causes less strain to accommodation. Starting with the ophthalmoscope at 0 setting, hold the ophthalmoscope about 20 inches from the patient's eye. Observe the pupil and the tapetal reflex. Bring the ophthalmoscope to within 1 inch of the patient's eye and place the setting on −1 to 3 to view the optic disk and retina. If the disk is not immediately seen, follow the retinal vessels back to the disk. Find the setting at which the retina can be seen most clearly. Inserting more plus lenses into the ophthalmoscope focuses the lens on more anterior structures within the eye.

Direct ophthalmoscopy provides a highly magnified view of the fundus in which the image is real and upright. The magnification is 15× in an emmetropic eye, less in hyperopia, and more in myopia. The area of visualization is usually about two disk diameters. The extent to which the peripheral retina may be examined in dogs varies with the degree of dilatation of the pupil and the length of the muzzle. In dolichocephalic breeds, the peripheral, medial aspect of the fundus can be examined in greater detail using direct ophthalmoscopy. Indirect ophthalmoscopy permits good visualization of all areas of the fundus.

The fundus is that portion of the inner eye which includes the optic disk or papilla, the retinal vessels, tapetum lucidum and nigrum.

Examine the optic disk and note its shape and color, and the presence of a physiologic cup. The optic disk may assume various shapes—round to triangular—and its periphery may be pigmented. The disk itself should be flat with distinct margins, and ranges from pink to gray-white. In larger dogs, the disk usually is located within the tapetum lucidum and in smaller dogs, within the nontapetal area.

The retinal vessels can be divided into primary veins, secondary veins and arterioles. The primary veins are the two to five largest vessels in the retina. The blood in the veins is dark red to purple. The retinal vessels should be flat as they run across the edge of the disk. Note whether the disk is depressed (cupped) or elevated as in papilledema or papillitis. If cupped, the disk may appear larger than normal, and the vessels disappear at its periphery.

The veins of the retina can be distinguished from the arteries by virtue of their larger diameters. The veins are dark red to purple in color, whereas the arteries are somewhat lighter. The cilioretinal arterioles are five to nine in number. They are bright red in color, of smaller diameter, and more tortuous than the veins, and do not anastomose within the disk. The dog does not have a central artery and vein.

The tapetum lucidum is located in the superior half of the fundus and is roughly triangular in shape. The tapetum may vary in color from blue and green to orange or yellow. The mosaic appearance is caused by the underlying pigment epithelium and choroid, which can be seen through the tapetal layer. The nontapetal fundus (nigrum) occupies the inferior portion of the fundus and usually is brown to black in color.

The fundus of the cat differs from the dog's in that the optic disk is smaller, the tapetum lucidum occupies a much larger area, the veins and arterioles enter and leave the optic disk circumferentially, and no definite physiologic cup is visible.

The optic disk should be flat. In the dog, it normally measures about 1.5 mm. in diameter. If the disk has to be viewed by placing more convex (+) lenses in the ophthalmoscope, it probably is elevated. Papilledema is a swelling of the optic disk, is usually bilateral, and may be caused by passive congestion within the disk. The disk edges usually are blurred, the veins full and tortuous, and the arterioles smaller than normal. Papilledema need not be caused by conditions in which the intracranial pressure is elevated.

Inflammation of the optic disk is termed papillitis. It may be difficult to distinguish between papillitis and papilledema; however, in papillitis there is usually less swelling than in papilledema, often loss of vision, inflammation of surrounding retina and vitreous, and hermorrhages in the disk. Note whether the disk appears to be depressed or cupped. A small cup in the center of the disk is normal; marked depression that extends to the periphery of the disk is abnormal. Glaucoma is the most common cause of cupping of the optic disk. Both typical and atypical colobomas may cause defects of the optic disk. The optic disk may appear whiter than normal in progressive retinal atrophy, optic atrophy, glaucoma and anemia.

Observe the retina for signs of hemorrhage. Flame-shaped hemorrhages usually are situated in the superficial parts of the retina, and round hemorrhages, in the deeper parts. Preretinal hemorrhage usually obliterates the retinal vessels.

Pigmentation of the retina may be congenital or pathologic. Pigment usually is present in old hemorrhages, and exudates and pigment spots are present in certain types of hereditary retinal atrophy. Pigment migration may occur in retinitis and in chorioretinitic scars. Depigmentation of the fundus exposes the choroid and choroidal circulation.

Most retinal detachments in animals are associated with giant retinal tears, and the retinal tissue can be seen as a wavy, white sheet in the vitreous chamber. Bullous localized detachment of the retina may be caused by exudative choroiditis or hemorrhage. Spontaneous reattachment may occur when the exudate is reabsorbed. The retina may be completely detached from the ora serrata and resemble a tent when viewed with the ophthalmoscope. In retinal detachment, the underlying tapetum, choroid and pigment epithelium are frequently visible.

**Examination of the Vitreous.** The normal vitreous is clear and homogeneous. Examine the vitreous with lenses−1 to +8. Check for cloudiness, discoloration or the presence of masses. Cloudiness may be due to hemorrhage, uveitis or choroiditis. Small opacities in the vitreous may appear as "snowflakes" and move when the eye is moved. If the opacities remain stationary, the condition is asteroid hyalosis. Larger masses in the vitreous may indicate retinal detachment, vitreous abscesses or organized areas of inflammation.

Because of the constant movement of the animal's eye, scanning of the fundus by direct ophthalmoscopy is simplified; however, fixation on one portion of the fundus may be very difficult. It is important when using the direct ophthalmoscope to utilize ocular movements as an advantage and not attempt to "chase and fixate on small ocular lesions."

Indirect ophthalmoscopy has been used increasingly in veterinary medicine. It has several distinct advantages. The intense illumination is of value in cases with hazy ocular media. The indirect image with less magnification allows less distortion and a much larger field of view than that obtained with direct ophthalmoscopy (35 degrees compared to 9 degrees with direct ophthalmoscopy). Indirect ophthalmoscopy permits examination at a safe distance from fractious animals. The binocular, stereoscopic indirect headsets permit the examiner to manipulate the animal's head while, at the same time, holding the condensing lens.

The condensing lens which supplies the greatest versatility in indirect ophthalmoscopy is the + 20 diopter plano-convex lens with a diameter of 35 mm. The working distance of this lens is about 2 to 3 inches from the patient's eye. The convex side of the lens should be held toward the observer in order to minimize light reflections and image distortion. Right-handed examiners can hold the lens in the left hand, thus leaving the right hand free to draw pictures; or the examiner can hold the lens in the right hand and manipulate the animal's head with the left hand. Good mydriasis is essential for good indirect ophthalmoscopy. One per cent tropicamide or a combination of 2 per cent Cyclogyl® (cyclopentolate hydrochloride) and 10 per cent phenylepherine has proved satisfactory as dilating agents.

When using the condensing lens in indirect ophthalmoscopy, the image that is formed is real and inverted.

## SPECIALIZED DIAGNOSTIC TECHNIQUES IN OPHTHALMOLOGY

### TONOMETRY

Glaucoma is an increase in intraocular pressure incompatible with normal ocular and visual functions. It is therefore important to be able to record changes in ocular tension in order to diagnose and treat glaucoma.

**Digital Tonometry.** This method involves estimating ocular tension by judging the impressibility of the ocular coats when pressure is applied to the globe by the index fingers, which are placed on the upper eyelids of the animal. The sensation of ocular fluxation from the normal eye is learned with practice, and variations can be detected as experience is gained. This method requires much practice, is inaccurate and

usually it is possible to detect less than 5 mm. Hg change in intraocular tension.

**Schiötz Tonometry.** This tonometer has been widely used in veterinary medicine to determine ocular tension in small animals. The instrument consists of a corneal foot plate, plunger, holding bracket, recording scale and 5.5-, 7.5-, 10.0- and 15.0-gm. weights. The principle of the Schiötz tonometer is that the amount which the plunger protrudes from the footplate is related to the indentability of the cornea, which in turn is related to the intraocular pressure. The plunger is connected to a scale, so that 0.05 mm. protrusion of the plunger equals one scale unit. In order to transfer the readings on the Schiötz tonometer in terms of intraocular tension, it is necessary to calibrate them against absolute readings of the intraocular pressure manometrically measured. These readings (based on measurements in humans) are available in tables which come with each tonometer.

The technique of Schiötz tonometry in dogs and cats is not very difficult. The dog is placed in the sitting or dorsal recumbent position. Topical anesthesia is instilled, and the eyelids are held open by the fingers, which are placed quite far away from the lid margins. The footplate must be placed vertically on the central aspect of the cornea. Three readings are taken in each eye and then averaged. Normal intraocular tension with the Schiötz tonometer in dogs is 15 to 25 mm. Hg.

There are many inherent defects built into the use of Schiötz tonometry in small animals: (1) the instrument itself, which must be kept clean and in good functioning order; (2) extraocular muscle contraction and manipulation of the eyelids artificially raises intraocular tension; (3) differences in ocular rigidity between animal eyes and those of man can greatly alter the interpretation of ocular tension; (4) differences in curvature of the globe between man and animals can greatly affect the interpretation of readings with the Schiötz tonometer.

**Applanation Tonometry.** In applanation tonometry, a known, very small area of the cornea is flattened by a known force. The advantage of this technique over the indentation method (Schiötz) is that the errors due to ocular rigidity and corneal curvature are greatly reduced. In dogs, we have used two types of applanation tonometers. One of the oldest types was that developed by Maklakov and modified into the Tonomat®* tonometer. The instrument, although not expensive, requires time and skill to develop a good technique for its use. The Tonair®* tonometer is a hand-held applanation tonometer of constant weight that measures the intraocular tension in terms of the amount of air pressure required to flatten a small area of the cornea. The instrument is not difficult to use; however, if possible, it should be used by the same individual so that the results obtained are repeatable.

## GONIOSCOPY

Glaucoma is an increase in intraocular pressure incompatible with normal ocular visual functions. Glaucoma can be caused by many different disorders—all elevating intraocular pressure. In many types of glaucoma, there is an abnormality in the anterior angle of the eye (filtration angle). Gonioscopy permits one to visualize and examine the iridocorneal angle, which cannot be seen without the use of the contact lens.

The Koeppe gonioscopic lens seems to be well suited to domestic animals. It is available in a 17-, 19-, and 21-mm. size. The lens can be inserted into the eye following the application of topical anesthesia. In fractious animals, a tranquilizer may be needed. The lens can be filled with 1 per cent methylcellulose or can be filled with saline. Avoid having air bubbles present, as this distorts the view. The inside of the lens is illuminated with a Barkan lamp, otoscope head or binocular indirect ophthalmoscope. Magnification suitable to visualize the angle can be provided with an otoscope head, indirect ophthalmoscope or a Haag-Streit goniomicroscope.

### TRANSILLUMINATION OF THE EYE

If an intense light (Finoff ocular transilluminator) is placed on the sclera behind the ciliary body, the light will be transmitted to the interior of the eye and will produce a tapetal reflex in the pupil. If the light is placed over a solid mass in the eye, the light will not be scattered, and a light reflex

will not be produced in the pupil. If the light is placed over a cystic area in the eye, the rays of light will not be interfered with and the light will diffuse throughout the eye. Thus, transillumination can be used to aid in differentiating solid tumor masses in the eye as opposed to cystic lesions. Transillumination also may be used to diagnose atrophy of the pigment layer of the iris. This layer normally prevents transilluminated light from going through the iris. In iris atrophy, the transilluminated light will appear in the areas of iris atrophy. To utilize the principles of transillumination, the examining room should be completely dark and the observer should be partially dark adapted.

### OCULAR ULTRASONOGRAPHY

The technique of exploring the eye with high frequency sound waves uses the principles of ultrasonography. The advantages of high frequency ultrasonographic waves (500 megacycles/second) are that they can penetrate tissues that are opaque to light (such as the sclera, edematous cornea cataractous lens, etc.) and can delineate structures that are transparent to x-rays.

In A-mode ultrasonography, an ultrasonic probe is placed in contact with the cornea. As the sound pulse traverses the eye, it is partly reflected as it passes through tissues of different acoustic density until, eventually, the transmitted energy is absorbed. The reflected sound waves are received by a microphone and converted into electrical impulses, which are then converted by an oscilloscope into light impulses. The technique has proved very valuable in veterinary medicine when used in selected cases.

### ELECTRORETINOGRAPHY

The retina, like other nervous tissue generates electrical currents. An electrical potential exists between the retina and the cornea, with the cornea being more positive. When a flash of light strikes the retina, rapid changes in retinal potentials occur and are recorded as the electroretinogram.

The electroretinogram represents the mass-response of the retina to a stimulus. The pattern of the electroretinogram can vary among different species of animals depending on whether retinal photoreceptors are predominantly rods or cones.

---

*Computer Instruments Corp., Hempstead, New York.

Essentially, the electroretinogram in the dog consists of three major components. The A wave is a negative potential whose origin and significance is not yet completely understood. It probably originates from the photoreceptor layer. The B wave is the most important element. Its origins are probably from the Müller (glial) cells of the retina. Inactivation of the ganglion cell layer or damage to the optic nerve has no effect on the configuration of the B wave. The major component of the B wave is associated with scotopic activity, and the B wave becomes progressively larger in the dark-adapted state. The C wave may be unrelated to the actual processes of vision and appears to be associated with metabolism in the pigment epithelium.

As a clinical tool, the single flash ERG, which depends upon mass retinal response, may be of value in several ways: (1) It can be used in cases of unexplained visual loss where the fundus appears normal and where the ERG may permit differentiation between retinal disease or disease affecting the nerve fiber layer or central visual pathways. (2) When the fundus cannot be visualized because of opacification of the ocular media, the possibility of retinal degenera-tion can be ruled out by the use of the electroretinogram.

In interpreting the significance of electroretinography, as used at the present time clinically in veterinary medicine, it must be realized that the single-flash ERG gives very little indication of the physiologic processes taking place in the retina. With the single-flash technique testing mass retinal response, one can show whether the waves present are normal, depressed in amplitude, absent or irregular in morphology. The investigator must be aware that selective disorders of the rod and cone system in dogs will not be detected by the single-flash ERG. To obtain information of selective damage to rods and cones, "dynamic electroretinography" must be applied.

### SUPPLEMENTAL READING

Aguirre, G. D., and Rubin, L. F.: Progressive retinal atrophy in the miniature poodle: An electrophysiologic study. J. Am. Vet. Med. Assn., *160*:191-201, 1972.

Bistner, S. I.: Examination of the eye. Vet. Clin. N. Am., *1*:29-52, 1971.

deLahunta, A.: Small animal neurophthalmology. Vet. Clin. N. Am., 3:491-501, 1973.

# PRACTICAL OCULAR THERAPEUTICS

STEPHEN I. BISTNER, D.V.M.
*New York, New York*

Medications used in treating ocular disorders of animals may be divided into categories based on pharmacologic action. The purpose of this section will be to describe a series of drugs which the author feels are practical to maintain as a basic armamentarium of ophthalmic agents used in diagnosing and treating the common ocular disorders seen in animals. Whenever possible, tables will be used to simplify understanding. It should be emphasized from the outset that a large number of ophthalmic agents do not have to be stocked in a veterinary hospital. Many of the special products mentioned here can be prescribed and will obviate maintaining inventories of drugs.

Other articles in this text dealing with specific ocular disease should also be consulted.

## PRINCIPLES OF OPHTHALMIC DRUG ABSORPTION AND ADMINISTRATION

Before discussing routes of administration of ophthalmic pharmaceuticals, one should understand several basic principles pertaining to absorption of logical ophthalmic drugs. The rate of delivery of an ophthalmic drug to the desired site is dependent on numerous factors:

1. The vehicle in which the drug is sus-

pended and the nature of the drug itself, including toxicity, pH and stability. The cornea is covered by a precorneal tear film, and the cornea itself has variable permeability, the corneal epithelium being more permeable to fat soluble compounds and the stroma being more permeable to water-soluble compounds. If the corneal epithelium is damaged, a much higher level of drug may be achieved in the corneal stroma. Ophthalmic drugs should possess biphasic solubility to maximal corneal penetration.

2. The degree of vascularization and inflammation present in the eye can affect the level of drug present. A highly inflamed eye will carry away drugs more rapidly.

3. Drainage of ophthalmic agents through the nasolacrimal system can also influence the rate of disappearance of agents.

There are numerous ways in which ophthalmic agents can be delivered to the eye:

1. Topical solutions are easily instilled into the eye but do not remain in the eye for long periods of time. Therefore, if solutions are used, increased frequency of dosage is recommended. Solutions may be suspended in vehicles such as polyvinyl alcohol or methylcellulose to increase their contact time.

2. Ointments have advantages over solutions in that a longer ocular contact time is maintained and they are carried away through the nasolacrimal system less rapidly.

3. Subconjunctival injections are a very effective way of achieving high levels of medication into the anterior ocular segment. The injections can be made using a tuberculin syringe, and a 25- or 26-gauge needle and topical anesthesia is usually all that is required.

4. Subpalpebral lavage with ocular medication can be performed by placing a polyethylene tube in the superior conjunctival fornix through the upper lid and delivering medication either through a continuous drip or by injecting medication into the polyethylene tube. A commercial subpalpebral lavage set is available.*

5. Retrobulbar injections can be given for local anesthetic blocks or to deliver steroids such as might be needed in retro-orbital

optic neuritis. For dogs and cats, a 1.5 inch, 20-gauge needle is inserted at the caudal angle formed by the junction of the lateral orbital ligament and the zygomatic arch and is directed toward the lateral canthus of the opposite eye.

6. Agents may also be injected directly into the eye in cases of severe infection (intracameral injections—see Table 5).

7. Finally, newer developments in drug delivery systems have produced methods for the slow release of medication by sustained release devices (Ocusert®†). Although these devices are currently being developed and used in people, all tests performed would indicate that they will have equally good potential for sustained drug delivery in animals.

## DRUGS AFFECTING THE AUTONOMIC NERVOUS SYSTEM

Manipulation of the autonomic nervous system involves the use of agents that stimulate the adrenergic or cholinergic receptor sites.

### ADRENERGIC DRUGS

Adrenergic agents are used for their mydriatic effects, which may also include cycloplegia. Mydriasis (dilatation of the pupil) may be produced by sympathomimetic or parasympatholytic mechanisms.

Clinically, mydriatics are used to dilate the pupil to permit fundus and lens examination. Tropicamide, 0.5 to 1.0 per cent, is used for this purpose. The longer-acting mydriatics are used most routinely in the therapy of anterior uveitis. Because of the cycloplegic action of these agents, the ciliary body is relaxed and ciliary spasm is relieved. Mydriatics are also used when dense, central nuclear or cortical cataracts make it difficult for animals to see around the cataractous lens. Dilation of the pupil permits the animal to see around the obstructed direct visual axis.

Administration of parasympatholytic agents in dogs and especially in cats induces salivation and excessive drooling. In cats, I prefer 0.5 per cent Mydriacil (tropicamide, Alcon) drops or atropine ointment when possible to eliminate the undesirable side effect.

---

*Subpalpebral Lavage Apparatus, Becton-Dickinson, Rutherford, New Jersey.

†ALZA Pharmaceuticals, Palo Alto, California.

## Sympathomimetic Drugs

| | PER CENT | MYDRIASIS | DURATION OF ACTION |
|---|---|---|---|
| Phenylephrine | 10% | 20 to 30 min. | 2 to 3 hours |

May produce conjunctival irritation with prolonged use. Major use is in achieving maximal mydriasis when used in conjunction with a parasympatholytic drug such as atropine.

## Parasympatholytic Drugs

| | PER CENT | MYDRIASIS—CYCLOPLEGIA | DURATION OF ACTION |
|---|---|---|---|
| Atropine | 1 to 4% | 30 to 40 min. | 5 to 7 days or longer |
| Cyclopentolate HCl | 0.5 to 2% | 30 to 45 min. | 3 to 5 days |

(Will produce severe chemosis if not combined with phenylephrine 10%.)

| | | | |
|---|---|---|---|
| Tropicamide | 0.5 to 1% | 30 min. | 4 to 6 hours |

(Short-acting dilating agent—author's choice for fundus examination.)

Adrenergic agents are contraindicated in narrow-angle glaucoma. However, the prolonged use of atropine will not produce undesirable side effects, and adrenergics are frequently used for long periods of time in uveitis cases.

### Cholinergic drugs

Cholinergic agents are used for their miotic effects. They produce pupillary constriction, ciliary muscle contraction, dilatation of conjunctival and iris blood vessels and increased aqueous outflow. Miotics can be classified into two groups based on their mechanism of action (direct or indirect):

1. Cholinomimetic agents act directly on muscle end plates and resemble acetylcholine. Pilocarpine, available in solution of 0.5 to 4 percent is the agent most frequently used. Pilocarpine may be used in treating initial attacks of glaucoma (see article on "Treatment of Glaucoma in Dogs"); however, prolonged use of pilocarpine in animals frequently produces ocular irritation.

2. Miotics of longer duration of action may be used. These agents inhibit the enzyme cholinesterase and prolong the locally produced acetylcholine at the motor end plates. Longer-acting miotics are very potent and must be used with caution to avoid cholinergic side effects. The miotic that I use is Phospholine Iodide ® (echothiophate iodide, Ayerst) because of its low irritant properties over a prolonged period of time. Dosage frequency is one drop every 12 to 24 hours.

All miotics may have serious side effects, both ocular and systemic: the use of miotics in glaucoma therapy will not be discussed here, but the article on glaucoma should be consulted. Systemic cholinergic side effects such as vomiting, diarrhea, bradycardia and salivation can be observed, especially with the stronger anticholinesterase miotics.

### Topical Miotics for Canine Glaucoma Therapy

| | STRENGTHS USED | USUAL REGIMEN | KEEPING QUALITY OF EYE DROPS | RELATIVE DURATION OF ACTION |
|---|---|---|---|---|
| Parasympathomimetics—Direct acetylcholine-like action on nerve endings: | | | | |
| Pilocarpine | 0.5 to 4% | q. 4 to 6 hr. | Satisfactory | Short |
| Cholinesterase inhibitors—Indirect action by accumulation of acetylcholine: | | | | |
| Eserine®* (physostigmine) | 0.25% to 1% | q. 4 to 6 hr. | Unsatisfactory | Moderate |
| Isoflurophate®(DFP) | 0.1%(oil) | q.d. to b.i.d. | Unsatisfactory | Long |
| Phospholine iodide® (echothiophate iodide) | 0.125 to 0.25% | q.d. to b.i.d. | Satisfactory | Long |
| Humorsol®† (demecarium bromide) | 0.125 to 0.25% | q.d. to b.i.d. | Satisfactory | Long |
| Drug with both direct and indirect actions: | | | | |
| Carbachol | 0.75 to 3% | q. 4 to 8 hr. | Satisfactory | Short |

*Abbott Laboratories, North Chicago, Illinois.
†Merck Sharp and Dohme, West Point, Pennsylvania.

## TOPICAL ANESTHETIC AGENTS

There are numerous topical ophthalmic anesthetic agents available. The choice of which agent is best suited to a particular condition is left to the individual's discretion. I prefer proparacaine hydrochloride,* 0.5 per cent; however, it should be refrigerated to prevent breakdown and discoloration of the product. Topical anesthetics are used primarily for diagnostic and minor surgical procedures. Prolonged use of topical anesthetics may retard corneal healing and produce systemic toxicity.

*Onset and Duration of Topical Anesthetics in Man*

| SINGLE ADMINISTRATION | ONSET | DURATION (minutes) |
|---|---|---|
| 0.4% Benoxinate HCl | 15 seconds | 20 |
| 1.0% Butacaine sulfate | 2 to 3 min. | 30 to 60 |
| 1.4% Cocaine HCl | 2 min. | 10 |
| 0.5% Dyclonine HCl | 2 to 4 min. | 30 to 50 |
| 1.4% Lidocaine HCl | 4 to 5 min. | 30 |
| 0.5% Proparacaine HCl | 15 sec. | 15 |
| 0.5% Tetracaine HCL | 2 to 3 min. | 20 to 30 |

## CORTICOSTEROIDS

Ocular inflammation is one of the most serious of all ocular diseases. If inflammation is not treated early and with effective therapy, ocular function can be lost. Corticosteroids in ocular disease produce generalized suppression of ocular inflammatory disorders and help to maintain ocular structure and physiology.

### ACTION OF ANTI-INFLAMMATORY AGENTS

The beneficial effects of corticosteroids in treating ocular disease can be summarized as follows: (1) they reduce cellular and fibrinous exudation and decease tissue exudation, (2) they diminish the formation of scar tissue, (3) they limit neovascularization and (4) they reduce capillary permeability.

In order to achieve maximal beneficial effects from corticosteroids in ocular disease, several very important principles of treatment must be understood:

1. Determine what route of administration will best treat the ocular disorder, i.e., topical, subconjunctival or systemic.

2. Use high levels of steroids early and long enough to suppress inflammation.

3. Do not discontinue steroid therapy too early, especially in treating the more chronic cases of uveitis.

A low dose of steroid therapy may have to be continuously used in order to maintain ocular comfort.

### INDICATIONS

**External Ocular Disease.** Allergic blepharitis, conjunctivitis, irritant conjunctivitis, superficial punctate keratitis, infiltrative corneal disease, chronic neovascularization, deep interstitial keratitis.

**Uveitis.** Anterior uveitis, posterior uveitis, iritis, iridocyclytis, scleritis, episcleritis.

**Orbital Disease.** Optic neuritis, pseudotumor of orbit.

### SELECTION OF STEROIDS

The choice of corticosteroids may seem confusing to the practitioner, but several important points must be kept in mind: (1) the ocular bioavailability of the drug (penetration of the steroid into the tissues desired), (2) the anti-inflammatory activity desired and (3) the duration of effect.

Following the topical administration of corticosteroids in the eye, the highest levels are found in the cornea and conjunctiva. The penetration of topically applied steroids is determined by differential solubility characteristics and tissue factors. The derivative used in the corticosteroid preparation is significant because it increases corneal penetration and achieves the necessary levels in the aqueous humor. Changing the steroid derivative from the alcohol to the acetate greatly increases the penetrative ability of the steroid. As an example, 1 per cent prednisolone acetate* provides higher concentrations of corticosteroids in the aqueous and corneal stroma than 0.1 per cent dexamethasone alcohol, 0.1 per cent dexamethasone phosphate and 1.0 per cent prednisolone phosphate. However, if the corneal epithelium is severely damaged, other forms of steroids, especially prednisolone phosphate, may penetrate just as well.

Knowing the anti-inflammatory activity of various steroid compounds can also be help-

---

*Ophthaine® drops, E. R. Squibb Co., Princeton, New Jersey.

*Prednefrin Forte Drops® Allergan Pharmaceuticals, Irvine, California.

ful in selecting agents for treating ocular disease:

| STEROID | RELATIVE ANTI-INFLAMMATORY ACTIVITY |
|---|---|
| Hydrocortisone | 1 |
| Prednisolone | 4 |
| Methylprednisolone | 5 |
| Bethamethasone | 25 |
| Dexamethasone | 25 |
| Fluorometholone | 40 |

Corticosteroids have their most dramatic effect in those diseases affecting the cornea, uveal tract and external structures of the eye. They are ineffective in degenerative diseases of the cornea, retina or uveal tract.

The route of administration is quite important when considering steroid administration. If the lesion is superficial, involving the lids, conjunctiva or cornea, topical steroid drugs or ointments are usually effective. On the other hand, if the lesion is posterior to the iris, e.g., in chorioretinitis or optic neuritis, systemic steroid therapy may be utilized to effect (see Table 1).

**Topical Therapy with Steroids.** When drops are used, they should be applied frequently, usually 6 to 8 times a day during the first 24 to 48 hours. In general, I prefer to use the ointments in treating animals because of the longer contact time and decreased frequency of administration. Topical therapy should in general be continued for 2 weeks after all signs of disease have disappeared.

**Injection.** Local injection of corticosteroids refers to subconjunctival injections, which provide a rapid way of delivering high concentrations of corticosteroids. The repository forms of injections, such as methyprednisolone acetate, may provide a source of steroid that lasts for up to 2 weeks.

## CONTRAINDICATIONS

Purulent bacterial infections and ulcerations should not be treated with corticosteroids for a prolonged period of time because of the danger of superinfection with other bacterial or fungal agents. When severe corneal disease threatens to cause extensive visual loss, corticosteroids can be combined with effective antimicrobial therapy to prevent permanent visual alteration associated with scar tissue.

## ANTIBIOTICS AND SULFONAMIDES

It would be impossible in the space allotted to give a detailed description of each antibiotic or sulfonamide that is available for treating ocular diseases. Individual articles dealing with specific ocular disorders should be consulted. However, several basic points can be very important for understanding the use of topical and systemic antibiotics in ocular disease:

1. In external ocular disease infections, the use of conjunctival and corneal scrapings and of bacterial culture and sensitivity tests is important.

2. For most noncomplicated external ocular disease problems, an antibiotic having a combination of neomycin, polymyxin B and bacitracin will suffice.

3. For gram-negative infections, particularly *Pseudomonas* infections, I prefer the use of gentamicin ophthalmic ointment (Garamycin® ointment [Schering]) coupled with subconjunctival gentamicin. Additional treatment for *Pseudomonas* infections should include the topical use of disodium EDTA, $10^{-2}$ molar solution, which serves as an antagonist for the proteolytic enzymes released by the *Pseudomonas* organisms. Disodium EDTA is available from Abbott Laboratories* in the form of Endrate® solution (150 mg./ml.). To formulate the solution for topical administration, add 0.4 ml. of Endrate solution to 14.6 ml. of Adapt®solution (Burton, Parsons). Apply the mixture to the affected cornea 5 to 6 times a day.

Rapidly progressing corneal ulcers may be spreading because of the production of collagenase enzyme in the cornea. This enzyme can be inhibited by the use of acetylcysteine (Mucomyst® [Mead Johnson], 4-ml. vials). Although not approved for use in the eye, topical application of acetylcysteine drops 4 times a day helps to evert further spread of corneal ulcers associated with collagenase.

4. The penetration of various antibiotics applied topically is summarized in Table 2:

5. One of the best ways of delivering high concentrations of antibiotics to the eye is by way of subconjunctival injections. Subconjunctival injections of antibiotics are useful in treating severe corneal ulcers, anterior uveitis, panophthalmitis and endophthalmitis. Care must be taken in ad-

---

*Abbott Laboratories, North Chicago, Illinois.

### Table 1.　Glucocorticoid Therapy*

TOPICAL GLUCOCORTICOID OPHTHALMIC PREPARATIONS

| Generic Name | Trade Name | Strengths Available |
|---|---|---|
| Cortisone acetate ointments | Cortone acetate | 1.5% |
| Hydrocortisone acetate suspensions | Hydrocortone acetate | 2.5% |
| Hydrocortisone solution | Optef drops | 0.2% |
| Hydrocortisone acetate ointment | Hydrocortone acetate | 1.5% |
| Hydrocortisone ointment | Cortril | 0.5% and 2.5% |
| Hydrocortisone phosphate solution (as the disodium salt) | Corphos | 0.5% |
| Prednisolone phosphate solution (as the disodium salt) | Hydeltrasol, Optival | 0.5% |
| Prednisolone phosphate ointment (as the disodium salt) | Hydeltrasol | 0.25% |
| Prednisolone alcohol solution | Prednefrin S | 0.2% |
| Prednisolone acetate suspension | Prednefrin Forte | 1.0% |
| Prednisolone acetate suspension | Prednefrin | 0.12% |
| Prednisolone sodium phosphate | Inflamase | 0.125% |
| Prednisolone sodium phosphate | Inflamase Forte | 1.0% |
| Dexamethasone phosphate solution (as the disodium salt) | Decadron | 0.1% |
| Dexamethasone phosphate ointment | Decadron | 0.05% |
| Dexamethasone suspension | Maxidex | 0.1% |
| Fludrocortisone hemisuccinate solution | Florinef hemisuccinate | 0.1% |
| Betamethasone | Celestone | 0.1% |
| Triamcinolone acetonide | Kenalog | 0.1% |
| Fluorometholone | FML | 0.1% |
| Medrysone (hydroxymesterone) | HMS | 1.0% |

INJECTABLE GLUCOCORTICOIDS

| Generic Name | Trade Name | Strengths Available |
|---|---|---|
| Cortisone acetate suspension U.S.P. | Cortone acetate | 25 mg. and 50 mg./ml. |
| Dexamethasone phosphate (as the disodium salt) | Decadron phosphate | 4 mg./ml. |
| | Hexadrol phosphate | 4 mg./ml. |
| Hydrocortisone for injection (as the sodium succinate) | Solu-Cortef | 100 mg., 250 mg., 500 mg. and 1000 mg. vials |
| Hydrocortisone injection | Cortef sterile solution | 5 mg./ml. |
| | Infusion hydrocortisone | 5 mg./ml. |
| Hydrocortisone suspension | Cortef intramuscular | 50 mg./ml. |
| Hydrocortisone acetate | Cortef acetate | 50 mg./ml. |
| | Hydrocortone acetate | 25 mg. and 50 mg./ml. |
| | Cortril acetate | 25 mg./ml. |
| Hydrocortisone butylacetate suspension | Hydrocortone-TBA | 25 mg./ml. |
| Methylprednisolone acetate suspension | Depo-Medrol | 20 mg., 40 mg. and 80 mg./ml. |
| Methylprednisolone sodium succinate | Solu-Medrol | 40 mg., 125 mg., 500 mg. and 1000 mg. vials |
| Prednisolone acetate suspension | Meticortelone soluble | 25 mg./ml. |
| | Nisolone aqueous | 25 mg./ml. |
| | Sterane intramuscular and intra-articular | 25 mg./ml. |
| Prednisolone butylacetate suspension | Hydeltra-TBA | 20 mg./ml. |
| Prednisolone phosphate | Hydeltrasol | 20 mg./ml. |
| Triamcinolone diacetate suspension | Aristocort parenteral | 25 mg./ml. |
| Triamcinolone acetonide suspension | Kenalog parenteral | 10 mg./ml. 40 mg./ml. |
| Betamethasone (acetate and disodium phosphate combination) | Celestone Soluspan | 6 mg./ml. |

*From Ellis, P. P., and Smith, D. L.: The Handbook of Ocular Therapeutics and Pharmacology. 4th ed. St. Louis. The C. V. Mosby Co., 1973, pp. 22 and 23.

**Table 2.** *Intraocular Penetration of Antibiotics in the Normal Eye\**

| AGENT | ROUTE OF ADMINISTRATION | | |
| | *Systemic* | *Topical* | *Subconjunctival* |
| --- | --- | --- | --- |
| Ampicillin | Fair | Fair-Good | Good |
| Bacitracin | None | Fair | Good |
| Chloramphenicol | Good | Good | Good |
| Colistin | Poor | Poor | Good |
| Erythromycin | Poor | Poor | Fair |
| Gentamicin | Poor | Poor | Fair |
| Kanamycin | Poor | Poor | Fair-Good |
| Neomycin | Poor | Fair | Good |
| Novobiocin | None | None | Good |
| Penicillin | Fair (high doses necessary) | Fair-Good | Good |
| Polymyxin B | Poor | Fair | Good |
| Streptomycin | None | None if cornea is intact | Fair-Good |
| Tetracyclines | Poor | Poor | Poor |

*\*These data represent only general estimations because of limited investigations in domestic animals.*

ministering subconjunctival injections so that minimal amounts (less than 1 cc.) are administered (Tables 3 and 4). Some agents used for subconjunctival injections are quite irritating and may produce pain and even conjunctival sloughing. In general, subconjunctival (subtenons) injections can be given using topical anesthetics and a tuberculin syringe with a 25- or 26-gauge needle.

In recent months, numerous articles, both investigational and clinical, have been published about the intracameral injection of antibiotic and antibiotic-steroid preparations. In general this form of treatment has been reserved for very severe cases of endophthalmitis or panophthalmitis. Anterior chamber or vitreous aspiration with small needles may precede injection of antibiotics or steroids. Aspirated material is submitted for culture and sensitivity. Intravitreal injections are usually made through the pars plana and anterior chamber injections at the limbus, utilizing a tuberculin syringe and a 26-gauge needle. Care must be taken in performing intracameral injections, since excessive concentrations of antibiotics may produce damage to the corneal endothelium or to the retina. Table 5 gives some of the recommended dosages for intracameral injections based on experimental studies.

In preparing gentamicin for anterior chamber injection, gentamicin solution 40 mg./cc. can be used. Steroid can be added to the injection by using soluble dexamethasone with a concentration of 4 mg./cc. Draw 0.1 cc. of gentamicin into a tuberculin syringe, add 0.9 cc. of dexamethasone to the same syringe and allow the solutions to mix. Using a 26-gauge needle, withdraw some aqueous fluid for culture and cytologic examination and inject 0.6 cc. of the solution mixture into the anterior chamber.

**Table 3.** *Antibiotics and Dosages for Subconjunctival Administration*

| ANTIBIOTIC | DOSAGE |
| --- | --- |
| Neomycin | 100 to 500 mg. |
| Bacitracin | 10,000 units |
| Plus Polymyxin B | 5 to 10 mg. |
| Erythromycin | 100 mg. |
| Novobiocin | 15 mg. |
| Plus Polymyxin B | 5 to 10 mg. |
| Penicillin G | 500,000 units |
| Plus Streptomycin | 50 mg. |
| Soframycin | 250 to 500 mg. |

*Other Agents* (listed alphabetically):

| | |
| --- | --- |
| Amphotericin B | 15 to 125 $\mu$g. |
| Carbomycin | 2.5 mg. |
| Chloramphenicol sodium succinate | 50-100 mg. |
| Kanamycin | 10 to 20 mg. |
| Oleandomycin | 1.25 mg. |
| Spiramycin | 10 to 20 mg. |
| Tetracyclines | 2.5 mg. |

## TEAR SUBSTITUTES

The precorneal tear film has been described in the article on "Diseases of the Cornea." Recent developments have indicated that the mucous layer of the corneal tear film is equally as important as the aqueous layer in maintaining health of the

**Table 4.** *Preparation of Antibiotics for Subconjunctival Injection**

| PROCESS | AMPICILLIN | GENTAMICIN | PENICILLIN G | METHICILLIN |
|---|---|---|---|---|
| Amount in commercially prepared vial | 1000 mg. | 80 mg./2 ml. | 5.0 megaunits | 1000 mg. |
| Number of vials needed | 1 | 1 | 1 | 1 |
| Diluent volume to be added to each vial | 5.0 ml. | —— | 2.5 ml. | 5.0 ml. |
| Volume to remove for injection | 0.5 mg. | 0.5 ml. | 0.5 mg. | 0.5 ml. |
| Antibiotic dose in injection volume | 100 mg. | 20 mg. | 1.0 megaunits | 100 mg. |

*From Jones, D. B.: External Ocular Diseases: Diagnosis and Current Therapy. Internat. Ophthalmol. Clin. *13*:21, Winter, 1973.

cornea. Numerous artificial tear preparations have been developed that have characteristics which resemble mucous secretion. Most of these preparations contain either polyvinyl alcohol or various forms of high molecular weight water-soluble polymer mucins that resemble material produced by conjunctival goblet cells. In all cases, these artificial tear film products must be used frequently to maintain their effect. Some of the products that are commercially available are listed in the table below.

| TRADE NAME | PREPARATION | MANUFACTURER |
|---|---|---|
| Adapt Drops }<br>Adsorbotear } | High molecular weight water-soluble polymer | Burton Parsons and Company |
| Isopto Tears | Hydroxypropyl methylcellulose | Alcon Labs |
| Liquifilm Tears | Polyvinyl alcohol | Allergan Pharmaceuticals |
| Tearisol | Hydroxypropyl methylcellulose | Smith, Miller, Patch |
| Tears Naturale | Water-soluble polymeric system | Alcon Labs |

In addition to the products described above, there is another ocular lubricant which is marketed as a sterile ophthalmic ointment, Lacri-lube® ocular lubricant. This bland ointment is basically a white petrolatum base with mineral oil.

I have administered Adapt Drops® 5 to 7 times a day, in cases of keratitis sicca. Recently, I have increased the use of Lacri-lube ointment (Allergan) because of the longer contact time that it provides. Lacri-lube ointment is especially good for evening treatments, although it is also used during the day.

## ANTIVIRAL AGENTS

The use of antiviral agents has limited application in veterinary medicine. Idoxuridine ointment (0.5 per cent)* at 4-hour intervals, has been used to treat

*Stoxil Ophthalmic Ointment®, Smith, Kline and French, Philadelphia, Pennsylvania.

keratitis associated with feline viral rhinotracheitis–induced keratitis and conjunctivitis in cats.

## ANTIFUNGAL AGENTS

Keratomycoses have proved to be some of the most difficult medical cases to treat successfully. The incidence of this problem has increased, especially with better aids for recognition and with the continued use of steroid therapy over long periods of time.

Organisms most frequently isolated in keratomycosis include *Aspergillus, Mucor* and *Candida* species.

Various forms of treatment for mycotic keratitis are available; however, if a confirming diagnosis of mycotic keratitis is made, it is recommended that a veterinary ophthalmologist be consulted to assist in treatment. Additionally, cultures and sensitivity tests of mycotic organisms are very important in establishing effective therapy.

Treatment of keratomycosis can include the following:

1. Chemical cautery with 2 to 7 per cent tincture of iodine, 30 per cent sodium sulfacetamide and 5 per cent *topical* nystatin.

2. Amphotericin B can be used topically. The lyophilized preparation is reconstituted so that 5 mg. of amphotericin B is available in each ml. of 5% dextrose solution. This preparation is refrigerated and used topically 4 to 5 times a day.

3. The most effective class of drugs in treating keratomycosis and mycotic en

**Table 5.** *Antibiotic Treatment of Endophthalmitis**

| ANTIBIOTIC | DOSAGE | USUAL SENSITIVITY SPECTRUM |
|---|---|---|
| Gentamicin** | 0.4 mg. | Broad spectrum of gram-positive and gram-negative organisms: especially effective against S. *aureus, Proteus, Pseudomonas* and other Enterobacteriaceae. |
| Lincomycin† | 1.5 mg. | Group A strep, *D. pneumoniae S. aureus, Corynebacteria, Clostridia,* Bacteroides. |
| Kanamycin | 0.5 mg. | Includes both gram-positive and gram-negative organisms, esp. *E. coli,* Proteus species, *Salmonella, Shigella, Neisseria* and some staphylococci. |
| Tobramycin | 0.5 mg. | Similar to gentamicin; especially effective against *Pseudomonas aeruginosa* and Enterobacteriaceae. |
| Methicillin | 2 mg. | Gram-positive organisms, esp. coagulase-positive staphylococci. |
| Cephaloridine | 0.25 mg. | Broad spectrum including S. *aureus* and gram-negative organisms, but not *Pseudomonas*. |
| BBK-8 | 0.4 mg. | Broad spectrum of gram-positive and gram-negative organisms, esp. *Pseudomonas*. |
| Carbenicillin | 2 mg. | Gram-negative organisms, esp. *Pseudomonas*. |
| Clindamycin | 1 mg. | Gram-positive organisms, esp. resistant coagulase-positive staphylococci |
| Amphotericin B | 5 to 10 μg! | Fungal endophthalmitis such as *Candida albicans* and Aspergillus |
| Chloramphenicol | 2 mg. | Broad spectrum of gram-positive and gram-negative organisms: effectiveness determined by specific sensitivity data |

*Dosage recommended for intravitreal injection.

**0.4 mg. (400 μg.) of gentamicin can be used safely in anterior chamber.

†A mixture of 1 mg. of lincomycin and 0.2 mg. (200 μg.) gentamicin has been used clinically and experimentally without toxic effects.

dophthalmitis is the polyene antibiotics. In the tetraene class, pimaricin ointment (Natamycin®) 1 per cent is the drug of choice.

Two drugs in the imidazole class of antifungal drugs, namely miconazole ointment (Conofite®, Pitman-Moore) and clotrimazole, are currently being investigated in cases of keratomycosis. All the aforementioned drugs are not readily available, and it is strongly recommended that if a diagnosis of keratomycosis is made, additional help in treatment should be sought from a veterinary ophthalmologist.

## CARBONIC ANHYDRASE INHIBITORS AND HYPEROSMOTIC AGENTS

Carbonic anhydrase inhibitors in the form of diuretics are used as synergistic medication along with miotics and hypertonic agents in lowering intraocular pressure. Various types of carbonic anhydrase inhibitors are available; however, the exact cause of the ocular hypotensive effect is not exactly known. In general, it must be remembered that the carbonic anhydrase inhibitors decrease aqueous outflow by 60 per cent, thus leaving 40 per cent aqueous humor formation.

If the anterior drainage angles are severely compensated (see article on glaucoma), other agents such as intravenous urea or mannitol or oral glycerin (glycerol) may have to be administered.

*Carbonic Anhydrase Inhibitors*

| U.S.P. OR N.F. NAME | DOSAGE | ACTION: ONSET (DURATION) |
|---|---|---|
| Acetazolamide (oral) | 125 to 250 mg. 1 to 4 times daily | 2 hr. (4 to 6 hr.) |
| Acetazolamide (intravenous) | 250 to 500 mg. in 5 to 10 ml. distilled H₂O | 5 to 10 min. (2 hr.) |
| Dichlorphenamide (oral) | 50 mg. 1 to 4 times daily | 30 min. (6 hr.) |
| Ethoxzolamide (oral) | 125 mg. 1 to 4 times daily | 2 hr. (5 hr.) |
| Methazolamide (oral) | 50 to 100 mg. 3 times daily | 2 hr. (4 to 6 hr.) |

*Hyperosmotic Agents*

| U.S.P. OR N.F. NAME (SOLUTION) | DOSAGE | ACTION: ONSET (DURATION) |
|---|---|---|
| Glycerol (50%) | 1 to 1.5 gm/kg. body weight | 10 to 30 min. (4 to 5 hr.) |
| Mannitol (20%) | 1 to 2 gm/kg. body weight | 30 to 60 min. (6 hr.) |
| Urea (30%) | 1 to 2 gm./kg. body weight | 30 to 45 min. (5 to 6 hr.) |

Side effects with carbonic anhydrase agents are variable and depend on the agent being used. The following side effects may be noted: (1) polydipsia and polyuria, (2) anorexia, (3) weakness and ataxia, (4) panting, (5) vomiting and (6) diarrhea. If any of these signs develop, reduction in dosage of medication is indicated. Dichlorphenamide (Daranide®, Merck Sharp and Dohme) seems clinically to cause fewer side effects in dogs than does acetazolamide (Diamox®, Lederle).

## PRACTICAL DIAGNOSTIC AIDS

1. Fluorescein and rose bengal are two of the more commonly used dyes that aid in the diagnosis of external ocular disorders. Fluorescein is used primarily in the form of impregnated paper strips. Corneal epithelial lesions stain green and conjunctival lesions stain orange-yellow. Fluorescein can also be used to test nasolacrimal patency by observing the passage of dye through the nasolacrimal system and its exit at the external nares. The use of ultraviolet light can be quite helpful in assessing the passage of dye.

2. Rose bengal is a vital stain for dead and degenerating corneoconjunctival epithelium and mucus. A topical anesthetic should be placed in the eye before the use of rose bengal, because of the irritative nature of the dye. Dead and degenerating epithelial cells can be demonstrated by rose bengal in keratoconjunctivitis sicca, pannus of German shepherds, corneal lipoidosis and pigmentary keratitis.

3. The Schirmer tear test is used to evaluate tear production. Prepared filter paper strips, 5 x 30 mm., are used.* The notched end of the strip is placed in the inferior conjunctival cul-de-sac for one minute. No topical anesthesia is used. Normal wetting is 10 to 25 mm. in one minute. (See article on "Examination of the Eye" for further details.)

### SUPPLEMENTAL READING

Ellis, P. Q., and Smith, D. L.: Handbook of Ocular Therapeutics and Pharmacology. 4th ed. St. Louis, The C. V. Mosby Co. 1973.

---

*Schirmer Tear Test Papers, SMP Division, Cooper Laboratories, Cedar Knolls, New Jersey.

## Basic Ophthalmic Pharmaceuticals and Diagnostic Aids Stocked in Veterinary Pharmacy

---

*Adrenergics*
½ and 1% Mydriacil® (tropicamide drops)—Alcon Laboratories Inc., Fort Worth, Texas
1-4% Atropine drops (ointment)
10% Neo-Synephrine Hydrochloride® drops—Winthrop Laboratories, New York, New York

*Cholinergics*
2 and 4% Pilocarpine drops

*Antibiotics*
Neomycin, polymyxin B, bacitracin—ointment of choice
Garamycin® ophthalmic ointment (gentamicin sulfate)—Schering Corporation, Kenilworth, New Jersey
Terramycin-polymyxin B sulfate ophthalmic ointment®—Pfizer Laboratories, New York, New York
Chloromycetin® ophthalmic ointment—Parke Davis and Company, Detroit, Michigan

*Antibiotic-Steroid Combinations*
Maxitrol® ophthalmic ointment—Alcon Laboratories

*Steroid-Decongestant*
Prednefrin mild drops—Allergan Pharmaceuticals, Irvine, California

*Artificial Tear Preparations*
Adapt Drops®—Burton Parsons and Company, Inc. Washington, D.C.
Lacri-lube® ophthalmic ointment—Allergan Pharmaceuticals

*Topical Anesthetic*
Proparacaine HCl drop, 0.5% (Ophthaine®)—E. R. Squibb Company, Princeton, New Jersey

*Ophthalmic Irrigating Solution*
Dacriose® solution, 4 oz.—Smith, Miller & Patch Division, (Cedar Knolls, New Jersey), Cooper Laboratories, San German, Puerto Rico

*Steroids*
Maxidex® ophthalmic ointment—Alcon Laboratories
Prednefrin Forte®ophthalmic drops—Allergan Pharmaceuticals

*Glaucoma Therapy*
Cardrase® tablets (ethoxzolamide), 62.5 mg. tablets—Upjohn Company, Kalamazoo, Michigan
Diamox® (acetazolamide) parenteral injection, 500-mg. vial—Lederle Company, Pearl River, New York
Glycerin 75% (Glyrol®), aqueous solution—Smith, Miller and Patch Division, Cooper Laboratories.

Gelatt, K. N.: Applied Veterinary Ocular Pharmacology. American Animal Hospital Asociation Home Study Course, Ophthalmology.
Havener, W.: *Ocular Pharmacology*, St. Louis, The C V. Mosby Company, 1974.
Henkind, P., Friedman, A. H., and Berger, A. W., (eds) Physicians' Desk Reference for Ophthalmology 1975, Medical Economics Company, Oradell, New Jersey 07649.

# DISEASES OF THE EYELIDS

GRETCHEN M. SCHMIDT, D.V.M.

*East Lansing, Michigan*

Diseases of the eyelids may account for the following ophthalmic problems: chronic conjunctivitis, chronic superficial keratitis or ulcerative keratitis. Inspection of the anatomy and function of the eyelids should be part of the diagnostic plan for each of these problems. See article on "Examination of the Eye" for details concerning inspection of the eyelids.

The following discussion on diseases of the eyelids is divided into two categories: abnormal eyelid opening (palpebral fissure) and enlargement of the eyelid. The palpebral fissure may be abnormally small or narrow or it may be abnormally large or wide. An enlargement of the eyelid may be localized or generalized.

## NARROW PALPEBRAL FISSURE

An abnormally narrow or small palpebral fissure may be due to blepharospasm, entropion or ptosis. Blepharospasm is constant contraction of the orbicularis oculi muscle, usually occurring because of ocular pain. If prolonged, blepharospasm can cause spastic anatomic entropion. Entropion (turning inward of the eyelid) can be an anatomic defect or a functional problem due to pain. Topical anesthesia of the external ocular structures with proparacaine HCl will alleviate the blepharospasm due to pain so as to differentiate anatomic entropion from functional entropion due to blepharospasm. Entropion of the upper eyelid in dogs results in trichiasis (the turning inward of the normal lid cilia). Trichiasis may cause keratitis, conjunctivitis or pain.

### ANATOMIC ENTROPION

Anatomic entropion of the lower or upper eyelid alone is corrected surgically, as described in standard surgery texts. Entropion of the lateral canthus is caused by absent or weak lateral canthal support. The palpebral fissure is shortened owing to the lack of lateral support, and the upper and lower eyelids become "wrinkled" with both entropion and ectropion. Lateral canthal entropion commonly occurs in St. Bernards, Norwegian elkhounds, and chows. The procedure for correction of lateral canthal entropion is Wyman's lateral canthoplasty, which straightens the eyelids by lengthening the palpebral fissure.

Anatomic entropion that is not usually surgically corrected is that due to loss of orbital contents. Enophthalmos, phthisis bulbi and microphthalmos may have associated entropion owing to lack of global support of the eyelids. (See article on "Diseases of the Orbit.")

### FUNCTIONAL ENTROPION— BLEPHAROSPASM

Entropion caused by blepharospasm is treated by correcting the cause of the blepharospasm. Eyelid problems to be ruled out as causes of blepharospasm are distichiasis (an abnormal row of cilia) and ectopic cilia in the palpebral conjunctiva. Both conditions should be corrected surgically by excision of the cilia with the hair follicles. Diseases of the conjunctiva, cornea and anterior uvea and glaucoma should also be ruled out as causes of blepharospasm.

### PTOSIS

Ptosis is drooping of the upper eyelid and results in a narrow palpebral fissure. Neurologic deficits of the oculomotor nerve and sympathetic nervous system should be considered as causes of ptosis. Loss of orbital contents and swelling of the eyelid may also result in ptosis. Ptosis is not usually treated specifically in animals.

## WIDE PALPEBRAL FISSURE

If the palpebral fissure is too large, the eyelids do not close completely or effectively (lagophthalmos). To maintain the health and protection of the cornea, the eyelids must blink normally or keratitis results. (See article on "Diseases of the Cornea.")

## ANATOMIC LAGOPHTHALMOS

Ectropion (turning outward of the eyelid) can be due to excessive length of the eyelid, loss of lateral canthal support or, as the result of scar tissue, contraction in the eyelid. If the ectropion is severe enough to result in keratitis, surgical correction is indicated. Blepharoplasty procedures used to correct ectropion include triangular excision of the lid, lateral canthoplasty and V-Y plasty.

Partial agenesis of the upper eyelid, a congenital defect of cats, may result in partial lagophthalmos in the region of the absent eyelid. If keratitis results, the surgical correction described by Roberts and Bistner is indicated.

## FUNCTIONAL LAGOPHTHALMOS

Normal eyelids may be lagophthalmic because the orbital structures are enlarged. Orbital structures may be enlarged owing to a retrobulbar mass or buphthalmos from glaucoma. Congenital lagophthalmos is often present in brachycephalic breeds with prominent eyes, such as the Pekingese. This partly accounts for the high incidence of corneal problems in these animals.

Symptomatic therapy for functional lagophthalmos is aimed at protection of the cornea and replacement of the tear film. Tarsorrhaphies (suturing the lids closed) or artificial tear medication (Adapt®, Burton, Parsons) are temporary means to accomplish these aims. Shortening of the palpebral fissure by excising the lateral one eighth to one fourth of the lid margins and closing the wound with skin and tension sutures is a permanent correction of the enlarged palpebral fissure.

# EYELID ENLARGEMENT

Generalized enlargement of the eyelids is usually due to edema and/or inflammation. Chemosis of the palpebral conjunctiva often accompanies blepharitis and may not allow complete closure of the eyelids. Symptomatic therapy for protection of the cornea as in functional lagophthalmos is indicated until the lids return to normal. Blepharitis may be secondary to a dermatologic problem or a conjunctivitis, in which case the primary disease is treated. If no other cause for the blepharitis can be found, secretions expressed from the eyelid glands, which open at the lid margin, should be cultured and examined cytologically. Bacterial blepharitis is commonly caused by staphylococcal infections. Symptomatic therapy for blepharitis includes daily applications of hot packs to the eyelids to cleanse them and expression of infected glandular material. Broad-spectrum antibiotics administered systemically may be indicated if bacterial infection is suspected.

Localized enlargement of an eyelid can be caused by neoplasia, inflammation or infection. Abscesses of the eyelid glands (chalazions) or cilia follicles (hordeolums) are treated with hot packs, expression or curettage of the inflammatory exudate and, if extensive, systemic broad-spectrum antibiotics.

Slow-growing pedunculated masses on the eyelids should be removed if they cause blepharospasm or keratitis. Electrocautery at the base of the tumor is one means of excision. Suturing is usually not necessary. Histopathologic evaluation is indicated to determine the nature of the tumor. Broad-based tumors of the eyelids require wide excision and extensive reconstructive surgery if more than one third of the eyelid margin is involved. If one third or less of the eyelid margin is removed, closure of the defect can be accomplished without additional tissue. Reconstructive techniques for full-thickness lid resections have been described by Gelatt. Histopathologic examination is indicated to determine the nature of the tumor and whether excision was complete.

## SUPPLEMENTAL READING

Gelatt, K. N.: Resection of the cilia bearing tarsoconjunctiva for correction of canine distichia. J. Am. Vet. Med. Assn., *155*:892, 1969.

Gelatt, K. N., and Blogg, J. R.: Blepharoplastic procedures in small animals. J. Am. Animal Hosp. Assn., *5*:67-78, 1969.

Helper, L. C., and Magrane, W. G.: Ectopic cilia of the canine eyelid. J. Small Animal Pract., *11*:185-189, 1970.

Roberts, S. R., and Bistner, S. I.: Surgical correction of eyelid agenesis in the feline. Proc. Am. Soc. Vet. Ophthalmol., pp. 18-20a, 1968.

Wyman, M.: Lateral canthoplasty. J. Am. Animal Hosp. Assn., 7:196-201, 1971.

# DISEASES OF THE CONJUNCTIVA

RON C. RIIS, D.V.M.
*Ithaca, New York*

Diseases of the conjunctiva are common but may go unnoticed by both the owner and the clinician. If the chief complaint is conjunctivitis, the etiology may vary widely. A systematic evaluation of each case of conjunctivitis is necessary. It is based upon ocular examination, cytology, biopsy, culture and a general physical examination.

## NORMAL ANATOMY

The conjunctiva is a tissue layer attached to the lid margins and the corneal limbus. At these attachment points, a smooth and consistent transition in cell morphology takes place.

The lid margin is a mucocutaneous junction at which pigmentation consistently diminishes. The total cell layers decrease, while the basal cells become less compact and rounder; the superficial cells become vacuolated and elongated but never cornified.

The cells of the dorsal palpebral conjunctival surface become a mixture of cuboidal epithelial and goblet cells. Goblet cells become more abundant in the upper fornix area, varying in shape from columnar within the folds to cuboidal on the exposed surface. In the dog, goblet cell contents consist of sulfate mucin and alpha sialic acid mucin that histochemically stain as both neutral and acid mucopolysaccharide (Borisevich, 1971). Each goblet cell functions as a unicellular apocrine mucous gland, its contents contributing an essential component of the precorneal tear film.

In the fornix area, the subepithelial tissue is highly vascular. Mononuclear cells may be extravascular, depending upon the stimulus that causes their presence.

The bulbar conjunctiva has a characteristic superficial cell transition from the orderly layers of epithelial cells and goblet cells in the fornix to polygonal cells and mononuclear cells with macrophage characteristics at the limbus. The conjunctival epithelium thins to a few cell layers. These cells are noncornified, with or without the reappearance of melanin pigment. The subepithelial tissue is loosely arranged with a rich supply of vessels and lymphatics within a few millimeters of the limbus.

The posterior bulbar surface of the nictitans has a cellular morphology capable of many changes, depending upon the animal's immunologic stimulation. Epithelioid cell types predominate in this area. Focal elevations of these cells by accumulations of lymphocytes are the origin of follicles that hypertrophy with stimulation. The goblet cell is present near the dorsal one third of the nictitating membrane but decreases in frequency near the margin.

The anterior palpebral surface of the membrana nictitans is covered with stratified squamous epithelial cells and goblet cells. The abundance of goblet cells increases toward the fornix, where folds of conjunctiva permit mobility of the nictitating membrane. These folds are lined with crypts of goblet cells and small concentrations of lymphocytes. The presence of focal lymphocyte proliferations can be observed clinically as follicles or papillae.

The ventral palpebral conjunctiva is a continuation of goblet surface cells from the fornix to within a few millimeters of the margin. More folds and crypts characterize this area from the dorsal palpebral surface. This characteristic lends itself to excisional biopsy with rare complications. The cell morphology expected in this area varies from the elongated goblet cell in the fornix to the cuboidal or polyhedral epithelial cell toward the margin. Macrophages and mononuclear cells are found throughout the epithelial layer. Melanocytes are more plentiful closer to the margin. The subepithelial tissue may contain small numbers of mast cells and mononuclear cells (primarily lymphocytes and plasma cells).

605

Normal cell morphology has been emphasized because it is useful in the systematic evaluation of conjunctival disease.

## CLINICAL SIGNS AND EVALUATION OF CONJUNCTIVAL DISEASE

Most uncomplicated conjunctivitis cases have an insidious onset. Pain is minimal and may be manifested by blepharospasm or lagophthalmos. A discharge may vary from serous to mucopurulent to suppurative. Vision is usually unaffected, since the cornea, anterior chamber, iris and pupil all remain normal. Digital manipulation of the lid surface allows the visualization of the conjunctival surfaces. A good light source with or without the aid of magnification allows the examiner to evaluate the vasculature. The surface tissue is homogeneously reddened, indicating superficial congestion and extravasation of blood. Deep congestion that is seen in the circumcorneal inflammation of acute iritis and the episcleral inflammation of acute glaucoma will not disappear within 30 seconds after topical application of 10 per cent phenylephrine; however, superficial conjunctival congestion blanches readily.

The most valuable aid to intelligent treatment for conjunctival disease is the evaluation of a smear of the exudate, mucous thread or surface cells obtained by scraping. The exudate or mucous thread may be picked up with a sterile cotton swab and rolled gently on several slides. A conjunctival scraping can be easily performed without topical anesthetic or excessive restraint. Cells from the conjunctival surface can be obtained by using a small "Kimura"® platinum spatula* that has previously been sterilized in an alcohol flame. Alternatively, a sterile D & C plastic disposable cytology spatula can be used. The spatula is held at right angles to the surface one wishes to examine cytologically. Light scraping pressure is applied to the surface without causing bleeding. Several scrapings provide adequate cells to be transferred gently to the slides containing the exudate or mucous thread.

Three slides should be made, one each for new methylene blue, Giemsa and Gram stains. The recommended permanent stain

for cytologic evaluation is the Giemsa stain. The slide for this stain should be fixed immediately in 95 per cent methanol (acetone-free) for a minimum of 5 minutes or until the slide can be stained conventionally with Giemsa. The Gram-stained slide allows one to categorize organisms as gram-positive or gram-negative. The most valuable slide is the one stained with new methylene blue, because it is a simple, rapid and informative procedure. The stain is applied to the air-dried slide, and a coverslip is placed over the specimen. If excessive stain is applied, the material to be examined will be dark blue and opaque. By using absorbent paper, draw enough stain from the edge of the coverslip to stabilize the coverslip and allow visualization of the material.

Consider what you find cytologically in light of the normal cellular morphology. An acute inflammatory process will show abnormal numbers of PMNs. This population may be further classed as septic, if the cells appear degenerate and accompanied by organisms, or nonseptic, if neither of these two characteristics is present.

A chronic inflammatory process will have primarily mononuclear cells made up of lymphocytes, plasma cells and reactive epithelioid cells. Allergic conjunctival reactions in animals are unlike those in man, which show eosinophils. Plasma cells, Russell body cells and mast cells are present in animals. If a population of mononuclear cells characteristic of chronic antigen-antibody stimulation is found, antibiotics alone will not achieve results without the incorporation of steroids.

It is important to note the presence of intracytoplasmic inclusions which may reflect the primary etiology or secondary complications. The information gained can direct the clinician to further diagnostic cultures or the best choice of medications. The type of organisms present should help determine whether drugs effective against rods or cocci should be used. At the other end of the spectrum, a population of lymphocytes and monocytes is found in the viral diseases of cats.

## CONJUNCTIVAL BIOPSY PROCEDURE

Lidocaine topical anesthesia instilled into the fornix every 15 seconds over a 3-minute period gives ample desensitization for

---

*#11–390, Sparta Instrument Corporation, 305 Fairfield Ave., Fairfield, New Jersey 07006.

biopsy. Good restraint is required to immobilize the head and evert the lower lid to expose the ventral palpebral area. A fine-toothed forceps and blunt (Stevens tenotomy) scissors are needed to elevate and excise a 2 mm. x 4 mm. sample of conjunctiva. Bleeding is generally minimal if the sample is removed superficially and with its long axis parallel to the lid margin. A disposable portable ophthalmic cautery pencil* can be used if hemorrhage is encountered. The tissue sample removed should be placed gently on a piece of paper with the conjunctival surface up to prevent curling before fixation in 10 per cent formalin or Bouin's.

## BACTERIAL CONJUNCTIVITIS

Numerous factors protect the conjunctiva from bacterial infection, including the continuous flushing mechanism of tears, epithelial cell phagocytosis, the mechanical barrier of an intact mucous membrane and the immune complexes present (Riis, 1975).

The inflamed conjunctiva responds to infection basically by exudation (discharge) or proliferation (follicular or papillary hypertrophy).

Culture studies of normal canine conjunctiva show that many pathogens are considered normal flora (Bistner et al., 1969). The criterion used in clinical judgment of their significance should be whether they are causing an inflammatory reaction that is septic, as evaluated cytologically. The cellular response is usually predominantly polymorphonuclear, with phagocytosis of the organisms and resultant toxic changes of either the organisms or the cell.

Once a bacterial agent is suspected the clinician must re-evaluate the process according to its clinical characteristics. A suppurative inflammatory process generally displays a mucoid to purulent discharge. A mucoid discharge is common in keratoconjunctivitis sicca but is not necessarily suppurative. The production of mucus by the goblet cells is inversely proportional to the amount of aqueous tear production. Nonsuppurative mucoid accumulations usually are clear. As the mucous thread changes from colorless to yellow-green or red, it reflects pathologic changes.

A Schirmer tear test is mandatory in the evaluation of conjunctivitis with mucoid discharge characteristics. The mucus should be gently removed prior to the test with the aid of a dry cottonball or absorbent paper. A tear test less than 5 mm./60 seconds could indicate a primary sicca problem resulting in the mucoid discharge or a conjunctival inflammation that temporarily occludes lacrimal duct patency. Antibiotics compatible with the choice of the corneal wetting agent should be used. In other words, if an antibiotic ointment is used for the bacterial infection, use Lacri-lube® ointment* for the wetting agent; if an antibiotic solution is desired, the wetting agent solution should be methylcellulose or polyvinyl alcohol. Ointments offer the advantage of less frequent instillation, but the absorption is less than with solutions, which must be instilled up to 6 times per day.

**Conjunctival Complications.** Consider more than the bacterial conjunctivitis when a diagnosis is being formulated. Related lid problems, nasolacrimal obstructions, skin conditions, mouth diseases, foreign bodies, urogenital or anal diseases and systemic disease may contribute to conjunctival disease. Occasionally a purulent discharge is seen with panophthalmitis or endophthalmitis. It is important to be aware of this more serious inflammatory involvement, so that more vigorous treatment such as systemic and/or subconjunctival antibiotics can be administered.

Chronic conjunctivitis usually reflects its long-standing involvement with characteristic periorbital alopecia, marginal depigmentation and thick, dull membranes. The cornea may also become reactive. Fine vessels may cross the limbus superficially, causing the cornea to appear hazy. A scraping of the conjunctiva would yield many macrophages laden with cellular components and bacteria. The likelihood that previous antibiotics have been used dictates only nursing care for 48 hours prior to culture and sensitivity testing in order for meaningful results to be obtained.

In the initial evaluation, if fluorescein stain is not taken up focally by the conjunctiva or cornea, an antibiotic along with a topical steroid is indicated. Hot packs during the topical treatment as well as systemic

---

*#74493, Pitman-Moore, Inc., Washington Crossing, New Jersey 08560.

*Allergan Pharmaceuticals, 2525 Dupont Drive, Irvine, California 92664.

antibiotics may be beneficial. Good results have also been obtained by using repositol steroids. Betasone-Vet®*, 0.1 to 0.2 cc. injected into the bulbar subconjunctiva gives anti-inflammatory action for approximately 2 to 3 weeks. This steroid preparation does not produce undesirable granulomas, as some steroid preparations do; however, like other repositol steroids, it is not reversible.

**Mycotic Conjunctivitis.** The prolonged use of antibiotic steroids may allow complication by a fungal opportunist, in which case a dry exudate is usually noted on the lid margins and the conjunctival surfaces are hyperemic. In some cases, the organisms produce a pigment that is outstanding. *Aspergillus niger* produces a black exudate and *Candida* produces a white-to-yellow exudate. Smears and scrapings stained with new methylene blue readily provide the diagnosis.

Cytologically, the mycotic organisms fall into broad categories of nonseptate hyphae (*Mucor* spp.), septate hyphae (*Aspergillus* spp. and *Penicillium* spp.), arthrospores (*Geotrichum* spp.), budding cells (*Candida* spp., *Cryptococcus*, *Blastomyces* spp., *Pityrosporum* spp.) or filamentous mycelial fragments (*Actinomyces* spp., *Nocardia* spp.).

Few drugs with antifungal actions are mild enough to use within the conjunctiva. Nystatin ointment (100,000 units per gm.) is most effective against the *Candida* spp. This ointment should be instilled b.i.d. for 4 weeks. The nystatin solution can be mixed with methylcellulose drops, 100,000 units/ml. Miconazole** ointment is well tolerated in the eye, but it may be useless against *Aspergillus* spp. Amphotericin B† has the broadest spectrum but is the most toxic to the conjunctival tissues. Hydrate and dilute as directed for a concentration of 125 micrograms to be instilled as a subconjunctival injection. The injection can be repeated every other day for 2 weeks.

**Membranous Conjunctivitis.** Clinically this conjunctivitis is characterized by the formation of a membranous exudate that adheres to the conjunctival surface (Firat,

1974). Well-circumscribed oral lesions may coexist. This condition is very difficult to treat because diagnostic tests are often inconclusive. Conjunctival scrapings usually yield high numbers of PMNs in homogeneous strands of hyaline material. Biopsy specimens of the conjunctiva may help differentiate the condition. An immunologic work-up is necessary.

Many times only a fibrinous mass containing PMNs is adherent to a necrotic, reactive conjunctival surface. Plasma cells and Russell body cells predominate in the subepithelial layers. Culture usually yields a variety of organisms, none of which is influential in the condition. Steroids actually aggravate this condition. The surgical removal of the irritating membrane may be necessary. The partial control of the membrane can be brought about with the topical application of enzymes t.i.d. Over a prolonged period, enzymes that are proteolytic* or fibrinolytic** or active against hyaluronic acid† have been used. Combinations of enzymes with a broad-spectrum antibiotic‡ may achieve satisfactory control (Firat, 1974). This condition and a good response have been reported in young animals.

If the diagnostic data lead toward a pemphigus-like condition, the treatment is entirely different. The treatment of mucocutaneous pemphigus in dogs has been somewhat successful with oral steroids or cytotoxic drugs used at immunosuppressive dosages (Hurvitz).

**Dacryocystitis.** Inflammation leading to obstruction of the nasolacrimal duct systems may present as conjunctivitis. Demonstration of an obstruction by the failure of fluorescent dye to appear at the nasal opening or on the tongue within 2 to 3 minutes following ocular administration verifies the need for mechanical flushing of the ducts.

Cytology and culture of the material forced from the nasolacrimal system may incriminate the etiologic agent responsible for the inflammation. The frequent use of

---

*Schering Corporation, Kenilworth, New Jersey 07033.

**Conofite®, Pitman-Moore, Inc., Washington Crossing, New Jersey 08560.

†Fungizone®, Squibb Pharmaceuticals, Box 4000, Princeton, New Jersey 08540.

*Alpha-chymotrypsin (Chymar®), Armour Pharmaceutical Co., Box 1022, Chicago, Illinois 60690.

**Streptokinase-dornase (Varizyme®), American Cyanamid Co., Box 400, Princeton, New Jersey 08540.

†Hyaluronidase—(Wyadase®), Wyeth Laboratories, Box 8299, Philadelphia, Pennsylvania 19101.

‡Elase with Chloromycetin, Parke, Davis Co., Joseph-Campau-At-The-River, Detroit, Michigan 48232.

topical antibiotic solutions and a broad-spectrum parenteral antibiotic for 7 to 10 days is indicated. If the infection does not respond under medical management, surgical procedures are necessary.

**Parasitic Conjunctivitis.** Conjunctivitis is the presenting complaint that may ultimately incriminate a parasite residing adjacent to or within the conjunctival membranes. Puppies with demodectic mange showing substantial lid involvement may have large numbers of mites in the mucoid strands of the lower conjunctival fornix. Topical methylcellulose drops mixed with 0.03 per cent phospholine iodide* both protects the ocular tissues and destroys the mite while the focal or generalized demodicosis is being treated with conventional procedures.

*Cuterebra* larvae have been removed from cat, dog and rodent eyelids that show focal swelling and inflammation of the conjunctiva. Differential diagnosis of a hordeolum or chalazion is made easy by noting the small hole leading to the surface from the larvae. Surgical enlargement of the hole is necessary to remove the larvae without rupturing its cuticle. Topical antibiotic treatment is used following the removal.

A nematode, *Thelazia californiensis* or *callipaeda*, can be deposited by an arthropod vector onto or near the mucous membranes. These nematodes produce a mild follicular conjunctivitis. If the parasite is mechanically removed and the irritated surfaces are treated topically with an organic phosphate drop (phospholine iodide, 0.03 per cent*) and a steroid antibiotic b.i.d. for several days, the condition generally clears.

**Chlamydia Conjunctivitis.** This agent has also been called *Bedsonia* and *Miyagawanella felis*. Chlamydiae appear to be closely related to true bacteria, since they possess both DNA and RNA; are sensitive to the action of antibiotics; and may contain muramic acid, a component unique to bacterial cell walls.

*Chlamydia psittaci* includes agents of psittacosis, bovine abortion, feline pneumonitis and guinea pig, hamster, mouse and rabbit inclusion conjunctivitis.

The disease may be enzootic in catteries and laboratory animals. Infection of newborn or newly introduced animals may range in clinical signs from occasional sneezing and naso-ocular discharge to a chronic respiratory disease complicated by secondary invaders.

In cats, the marked clinical sign in the acute stage is a unilateral chemotic conjunctiva with increased lacrimation. The unilateral ocular signs usually affect the opposite eye within one week. At this stage of the disease, a conjunctival scraping will yield epithelial cells that contain the cytoplasmic perinuclear inclusion bodies. With new methylene blue, Wright or Giemsa stains, the Chlamydia inclusions appear as a mass or a packet of individual particles of distinct blue or purple.

A mucoid exudate begins to appear within several days after the onset. This brings more inflammatory cells into the cytologic picture, making it more difficult to demonstrate the inclusion bodies. The clinical picture develops into the more chronic characteristic form of conjunctivitis that may persist for months if untreated.

To isolate Chlamydia, exudate from the conjunctiva should be collected with a spatula or swab and the specimen should be placed into sterile broth containing antibiotics (streptomycin) to which Chlamydia is insensitive. This material is then inoculated into the yolk sac of 6- to 8-day-old embryonated chicken eggs.

Chlamydia conjunctivitis responds well to chloramphenicol and/or tetracycline topical application in the acute stages. If the original unilateral involvement is treated as a bilateral problem, the other eye is usually spared the course of infection.

In the chronic systemic diseases, the topical treatment is supplemented with alternating chloramphenicol-tetracycline systemic antibiotics for a minimum of 2 weeks.

Instruct all individuals in contact with these cases that human infection has been reported several times. Good nursing care and cleanliness are indicated to prevent infection.

**Allergic Conjunctivitis.** This conjunctivitis most commonly accompanies atopy. The ocular irritation may begin with a seasonal manifestation and with age may become continuous with the generalized skin condition. A sign that owners may observe is the itching and rubbing of the eyes and ears with the front feet. The conjunctival surfaces usually appear hyperemic.

---

*Ayerst Laboratories, Inc., 685 Third Avenue, New York, New York 10017.

The conjunctival scraping has been the most informative aid in diagnosing allergic conjunctivitis. Unlike man, animals react with abundant plasma cells, Russell body cells and lymphocytes. A biopsy of the conjunctiva will demonstrate these cells in abnormal numbers infiltrating the epithelial layers and congesting the extravascular connective tissue adjacent to the basement membrane. Perivascular cuffing is prominent as well.

The diagnosis and treatment of the ocular manifestation of allergic disease require pursuit of the systemic antigen, including skin testing. A change in the environment or feeding practices may give some relief. Many animals are relieved with low, alternate-day steroid administration, either topically or systemically. Ophthalmic medications with sympathomimetics are helpful in temporarily constricting the hyperemic vasculature. Antihistamines have not provided noticeable relief. Some of the ingredients in ophthalmic medications that have caused ocular irritations are neomycin, gentamicin, methylcellulose and sulfa derivatives. The prolonged use of these drugs may cause hyperemic changes or other reactions upon instillation.

## VIRAL CONJUNCTIVITIS

Viral diseases that produce conjunctivitis have several common characteristics. The conjunctiva is usually hyperemic, with some chemosis. The discharge may vary from serous to seromucous in cases uncomplicated by bacteria. A history of each case may reveal that the animal has been anorexic, febrile, coughing, sneezing or showing a nasal discharge. Epiphora may be present.

Among the viral diseases known to manifest conjunctivitis in dogs is canine distemper. The young, unvaccinated dog is the most readily infected. Once infected, the viremia causes a febrile response within 7 to 12 days. At this time the examination may show mild inflammation of the conjunctiva, tonsils and pharynx. A conjunctival scraping may be helpful in diagnosis. The cellular response is primarily mononuclear, made up of lymphocytes and monocytes. The epithelial cells may contain inclusions within the cytoplasm. As the disease progresses, these cytologic findings change to those characteristic of a bacterial infection. By the time the animal has progressed through a second febrile episode with diarrhea and respiratory complications, the pursuit of inclusions in the conjunctival cells is fruitless. If the nursing care of an infected dog attempts medically to support the conjunctivitis, bacterial complications can be minimized by applying broad-spectrum antibiotic ointments topically t.i.d.

The viral diseases in cats that produce conjunctival signs may be difficult to document. The herpes virus has presented problems for many breeders with newborn kittens, young cats and older active adult cats. Conjunctival scrapings seldom yield intranuclear inclusions but always yield a typical mononuclear response. Viral cultures from the conjunctiva or infected cornea usually show cytopathic effects on feline kidney cells within a few days of the first passage. The diagnosis is made easy by means of positive cultures; without these, the clinician must rely on the clinical signs, conjunctival scrapings and a response to antiviral ointments.

Good results have been achieved by applying 5-iodo-2-deoxyuridine (IDU) ointment* q.i.d. for 5 days. Antibiotic ointments can be used in combination with the antiviral ointments, since no antagonistic reactions have been reported.

A rhinotracheitis booster vaccination rapidly elevates the herpes titer many fold as a clinical aid to the recovery of the infected animal.

## TUMORS OF THE CONJUNCTIVA

Conjunctival tumors are most frequently found at either the margin of the lid or the limbus. The locally invasive properties of these tumors usually attract the owner's attention fairly early in their development.

Biopsy, needle aspiration or impressions of the tumors will yield cells characteristic of lipomas, lymphomas, histiocytomas, papillomas, adenomas, melanomas, sarcomas and carcinomas. Usually the tumor is excised and submitted for histopathologic evaluation.

Large tumors that challenge the plastic

---

*Stoxil®, Smith Kline and French Laboratories, 1500 Spring Garden St., Philadelphia, Pennsylvania 19101.

surgeon should also be evaluated for cryotherapy response. By twice freezing a tumor to −25° C., antigenic changes of the tumor incite reactive inflammatory rejection of the tumor, which ultimately achieves both correction and nonrecurrence.

A tumor that has recently been seen with increasing frequency has characteristics of inflammation among a stromal network of histiocytes and fibrocytes (Smith *et al.*, 1976). This tumor begins in the limbal sub-conjunctival area and invades the cornea. Both early and invading forms of this tumor has responded to intratumor or adjacent subconjunctival steroid therapy. Advanced forms have been surgically removed and treated postoperatively with steroids.

## SUPPLEMENTAL READING

Bistner, S. I., Roberts, S. R., and Anderson, R. P.: Conjunctival bacteria—Clinical appearances can be deceiving. Mod. Vet. Pract., December, 1969, pp. 45–47.

Borisevich, V. B.: Histochemical data on the study of mucin of conjunctival basket cells in dogs. Arkh. Anat. Gistol. Embriol., *61*:39–44, 1971.

Firat, T.: Ligneous conjunctivitis. Am. J. Ophthalmol. 78:679–688, October, 1974.

Hurvitz, A.: Veterinary Clinical Immunology Seminar 1975 (personal communication). Animal Medical Center, New York, New York.

Riis, R. C.: The Normal Canine Conjunctiva: Thesis. New York State College of Veterinary Medicine, 1975.

Smith, J., Bistner, S., and Riis, R. C.: Infiltrative corneal lesions resembling fibrous histiocytomas: Clinical and pathologic findings in six dogs and one cat. J. Am. Vet. Med. Assn., *169*:722-726, 1976.

---

# DISEASES OF THE CORNEA

PAUL F. DICE II, V.M.D.
*Seattle, Washington*

The cornea is the avascular, transparent anterior portion of the ocular fibrous tunic. Its two main functions are permitting passage of light into the interior of the eye and being the first refractive surface of the ocular system. This discussion will update views on anatomy, with clinical pertinence, and causes of pathologic changes in this transparent structure.

## ANATOMY AND PATHOPHYSIOLOGY

The classic histologic outline of the cornea demonstrates a deceptively simple four-layered structure in the dog and cat. In the past several years, attempts to detail the corneal anatomy using modern ultrastructural techniques have been made. These studies have helped toward understanding a few of the keratopathies.

### EPITHELIUM

Although the tear film is smooth and the appearance of the epithelium is smooth on light microscopy, scanning electron microscopy reveals the surface to be covered by a blanket of minute folds called microplicae.

The consensus to date is that these folds are covered by acid mucopolysaccharides, the major components of the deep layer of the tear film. There is some evidence that the number of microplicae decreases in "dry eyes" and in human and feline herpes keratitis. There appear to be various cell types, one of which is the inactivated melanoblast. This cell, when activated by injury or vascularization, becomes a clinical problem, particularly in the dog.

### BASEMENT MEMBRANE

This membrane is actually a part of the epithelium. The corneal epithelium rests on a basement membrane composed of a glycoprotein matrix that contains embedded collagenous material. Fibrils from the basement membrane penetrate this stromal matrix, thus acting as anchors. The epithelial cells are in turn attached to the basement membrane by hemidesmosomes. The basement membrane as such is a product of the epithelial cells.

It is interesting to note that when the epithelium is removed, as in surgical débridement or superficial abrasions, the basal cells are usually torn, leaving a portion of the cell adhering to the basement membrane. In this instance, the basal epithelial cells slide and migrate over the old basement membrane and quickly bond to it. A good bond appears to occur rapidly only if the basement membrane is not altered. Clinical trials in dogs usually 5 years old and older indicate that a mechanical disturbance tips this delicate bonding and causes "buckling" of the surface epithelium, allowing breaks to occur, with resultant fluid, ointment and debris accumulation under the epithelial edges. If a superficial keratectomy is performed, a new epithelial layer regenerates to cover the defect without an underlying basement membrane. In this instance, a new membrane is synthesized by the epithelium, but it appears that several months are required to complete the epithelial-stromal bond.

## STROMA

The stroma forms the bulk of the cornea and comprises mainly collagen fibrils and their surrounding matrix. The fibers of the stroma are composed of collagen coated with a layer of glycoprotein and mucopolysaccharides. The fibrils are straight, lying parallel to one another. Groups of fibrils are gathered together to form lamellae. The corneal cells lie in the lamellar interspaces in a flattened appearance. There are various opinions as to the reason for normal corneal transparency, but most agree that a combination of small fibril diameter and regular arrangement is necessary.

## DESCEMET'S MEMBRANE

The posterior portion of the stroma is covered by a thin, transparent, elastic structure called Descemet's membrane. Although very elastic, this membrane is composed of collagen rather than elastin. It is formed by the endothelium and apparently grows slowly throughout life. This layer does not retain fluorescein stain, but the stroma does.

## ENDOTHELIUM

Endothelial cells are large, flattened, mesodermal cells that line the internal surface of the cornea. They are continuous with the anterior uvea. This layer is most impor-

tant in the maintenance of corneal deturgescence (Mishima and Hadlys, 1968), when the endothelium must overcome the innate tendency of the stroma to become edematous. The so-called "metabolic pump" is an active process that requires energy. When endothelial cells are damaged, the pump mechanism fails, and aqueous humor enters the stroma. This causes swelling directly above the defective cells and, if prolonged, can cause diffuse swelling.

## CONGENITAL LESIONS

### DERMOID

This is the term given to an aberrant growth of skin and hair on the cornea and/or conjunctiva. The aberrant growth varies in size, pigmentation, and location but is usually near the temporal limbus area and can be observed soon after the eyelids open. There is a suggestion of hereditary transmission in the St. Bernard, but otherwise these lesions are believed to be nonfamilial. Clinical signs include mucinous discharge, particularly around the aberrant tissue, blepharospasm and occasionally ulceration. Treatment consists of surgical extirpation by means of a superficial keratectomy to include conjunctival involvement. Results are excellent.

### MICROCORNEA

This is a smaller than normal cornea, often associated with microphthalmos. No visual impairment is observed, and there is no treatment. The breeds most often afflicted are miniature schnauzers, collies and poodles (toy and miniature). Hereditary transmission is suggested in the first two breeds.

### CORNEAL OPACITY (DEEP)

Deep corneal opacities and/or pigmentation are observed soon after the eyelids open. On close examination, persistent pupillary strands can be observed attached to the internal corneal surface. This abnormality is considered a nonfamilial defect except in the basenji and old English sheepdog. The embryonal strands usually atrophy by 4 to 6 months of age. A periodic exacerbation of corneal edema may occur owing to pulling of the strands on the deep corneal tissue during the normal pupillary movement if the strands remain beyond 6 months. Cutting these strands near the corneal attachment has improved the corneal edema in a few cases.

## INFLAMMATION (KERATITIS) AND ULCERS

### SUPERFICIAL KERATITIS (NONULCERATIVE)

A superficial corneal inflammation without fluorescein stain uptake may evidence diffuse or focal edema and vascularization with pigmentation in the more chronic form. It may be due to corneal irritation from adnexal abnormalities (aberrant cilia, eyelid malformations and neoplasms), foreign bodies, exposure keratitis and keratoconjunctivitis sicca.

**Eyelid Abnormalities.**    (See article on Diseases of the Eyelids.)

**Foreign Bodies.**    Foreign bodies adhering to the corneal surface are often overlooked by the examiner owing to surrounding pathologic changes and lack of fluorescein stain uptake (if the foreign body is on the surface). The most common foreign bodies in the dog and cat are paint flakes, vegetative material and metal shavings. Most can be removed with topical anesthesia (0.5 per cent proparacaine HCl). If the exact depth of the foreign body is not known, I suggest removal be performed under a short-acting anesthetic. A foreign body spud or tip of a 26-gauge needle can often be used for this purpose.

**Exposure Keratitis (Neurologic).**    We are concerned here with cranial nerve denervation, namely V (maxillary nerve) and VII (facial nerve). Clinical signs with fifth nerve damage, whether traumatic or degenerative, may be superficial edema and vascularization. Ulcers are often a part of the pathologic condition and tend to become chronic. Tearing becomes diminished but not totally absent, resulting in accumulation of mucinous material. Diagnosis is made when touching the corneal surface elicits no corneal reflex. It is important not to contact the eyelids while trying to elicit the corneal reflex. Paralysis of the seventh cranial nerve causes an inability of the eyelids to close. In this condition, the cornea and eyelids retain their sensation. The cornea usually becomes cloudy on the exposed portion. There are usually other signs of facial paralysis, such as drooping of the face on the affected side. Therapy in both conditions is palliative and is directed toward keeping the cornea moist by lacrimomimetics (Adapt®, Burton, Parsons; methylcellulose) or by a lubricating ointment (Lacri-lube®, Allergan) and symptomatic therapy.

**Exposure Keratitis (Non-neurologic).** This category includes exposure due to proptosis, exophthalmos, buphthalmos, nasal folds, prolonged anesthesia and occasionally severe lower ectropion. Corneal treatment again is symptomatic, while specific therapy is directed toward the etiology. A marginal tarsorrhaphy may be most beneficial if the globe is threatened.

**Keratoconjunctivitis Sicca (KCS).** One of the most common superficial corneal disease complexes in the canine population is related to changes in the precorneal film. It is very important that the corneal wetting by the Schirmer Tear Test® be determined in keratitis cases. Not all cases of KCS have zero tear readings. As clinicians, we must be able to recognize the disease entity dealing with wetting recordings of 0 to 10 mm./minute. Clinical signs may include a mucinous to thick mucopurulent discharge, corneal vascularization, opacity and pigmentation. Ulceration occurs in approximately 25 per cent of KCS cases. Treatment is directed toward keeping the cornea moist (lacrimomimetics), alleviating symptoms (antibiotics and/or steroids), determining residual functional lacrimal tissue by the use of systemic pilocarpine and, if the medical approach is inadequate, surgery. Surgery ranges from closing the lower canaliculi to conserve tears when the readings are from 5 to 10 mm./minute to parotid duct transposition with readings of 0 to 5 mm./minute. (See article on "Diseases of the Nasolacrimal System" for further discussion.)

### SUPERFICIAL KERATITIS (ULCERATIVE)

All the above conditions could result in ulceration if they are extensive or prolonged. In this section, we will describe two additional categories—burns and infections.

**Burns.**    Alkali burns to the globe from detergents, lime or plaster are generally much more devastating than acid or thermal burns. Mild alkali burns result in patchy or total epithelial loss and edema. Mild to severe burns can cause severe stromal opacification, increase in corneal thickness and heavy aqueous exudation. It has been demonstrated that collagenase is produced by regenerating corneal epithelium and polymorphonuclear neutrophils in alkali burns. Treatment consists of immediate irrigation of the injured globe with tap water or saline for at least 15 minutes, or, if available, weak neutralizing solutions may be used. For alkali burns, boric acid or 0.5 per cent acetic acid solutions are advised. For acid burns, 3 per cent sodium bicarbonate solution is recommended (Ellis and Smith, 1973). To chelate calcium in lime burns, 0.3 per cent solution of EDTA is beneficial. Twenty per cent acetylcysteine (Mucomyst®, Mead Johnson) mixed in equal parts with Adapt® (Burton, Parsons) is very useful for its anticollagenase properties, and administration every three hours is recommended. Topical antibiotic solution should be used to prevent secondary bacterial invasion. A cycloplegic such as 1 per cent atropine is beneficial to control anterior uveal irritation (ciliary spasm). The author has utilized a therapeutic soft contact lens in two patients after lime burns and observed that patients were more comfortable than patients treated without their use.

In acid, thermal and tear gas burns (including Mace®), treatment is symptomatic mainly to keep the cornea lubricated and prevent secondary bacterial infection. Acids precipitate stromal proteins and seldom go further than the anterior stroma.

## Infections

BACTERIAL. A bacterial infection can usually be detected because of its purulent discharge, stromal ulceration and gross adjacent inflammatory reaction. The superficial form may spread across the cornea but seldom causes perforation. Cellular infiltration, vascularization and associated edema are usually present. The organisms cultured in our clinic have predominantly been *Staphylococcus, Streptococcus, Proteus, Escherichia coli* and *Pseudomonas*, in that order. Our initial choice of medication for superficial ulceration is Neosporin solution® (Burroughs Wellcome) every 3 hours. Ciliary spasm may be controlled with 1 per cent atropine ointment t.i.d. If reexamina-

tion in 48 hours does not indicate improvement, a corneal scraping (Gram and Giemsa stains) and culture into blood agar and sensitivity tests should be performed. If Gram stain indicates gram-negative rods, the medication should be changed to topical gentamicin ointment (Garamycin®, Schering) every 3 hours. I do not apply conjunctival flaps to superficial infections (acute). A rapidly destructive keratitis may be due to *Pseudomonas*, often associated with anterior uveitis, with resultant hypopyon. Suggested treatment is collyrium to clear debris, 10 per cent acetylcysteine (Mucomyst®) every 2 hours as an anticollagenase, gentamicin ointment every 2 hours and 25 to 40 mg. subconjunctivally, cycloplegics and prevention of self-mutilation to the globe. Topical therapy may be changed to every 3 to 4 hours in 36 hours if there is improvement but should be continued for 10 to 14 days.

VIRAL. *Feline herpesvirus* is responsible for an active epithelial and anterior stromal disease. It is usually observed in cats over one year of age with some upper respiratory clinical signs. However, it has not been unusual in our clinic to observe this keratitis as a unilateral finding in seemingly normal cats. The epithelial lesion is often most helpful in the diagnosis, with the central cornea evidencing dendritic ulcers that appear much like cracks in a window pane. These discrete ulcers may coalesce in a week or two to form large superficial ulcers with vessels. Often the dendritic ulcers are without vessels. Diagnosis is based on clinical signs and, if available, fluorescent antibody localization from corneal and conjunctival scrapings. Treatment is very specific; the most readily available drug is idoxuridine (Stoxil®, Smith Kline and French, or Herplex®, Allergan). The 0.1 per cent solution hourly for the first 10 to 12 hours and then every 2 to 3 hours is recommended. The 0.5 per cent ointment should be applied every 2 to 3 hours for 10 days. Steroids should not be used until epithelialization is complete and then to decrease vascularization and/or scarring.

*Canine distemper*, a pantrophic virus, is the most common virus known to cause keratitis. There is direct epithelial destruction in the acute stage and secondary keratoconjunctivitis from the lacrimal gland involvement (dacryoadenitis). Treatment for the general disease is of paramount importance, but symptomatic therapy for the eyes must be continued as needed.

*Canine herpes virus* has been described in a few cases of superficial keratitis in the dog, but further work remains to be reported on as it is available.

FUNGAL (KERATOMYCOSIS). Keratomycosis must be suspect in a slowly progressive corneal ulcer previously treated with a variety of antibiotics and/or steroids. The two fungi observed most frequently are *Aspergillus* and *Candida*. There may be accompanying stromal vascularization, blepharospasm, iridocyclitis, corneal opacity and photophobia. *Aspergillus* causes more diffuse malacia of the anterior stroma with less tendency to ulcerate. *Candida* is quite often the cause of multifocal plaques in the anterior layers, surrounded in the early stage with ulcerative edges.

For specific diagnosis, the organism must be identified by scrapings stained with Giemsa and Gram as well as cultured on Sabouraud's agar. Antimycotic therapy includes nystatin (Mycostatin®, Squibb) in the powder form, made up in a solution of 100,000 units/cc. Recommended dose is two drops every 3 hours. It is effective against *Candida*. Amphotericin B (Fungizone®, Squibb) in a prepared concentration of 0.5 per cent solution is employed topically every hour for 6 to 8 hours and then every 2 hours. A 0.5 cc. subconjunctival injection of this concentration is recommended initially. Amphotericin B has limited effectiveness against most agents involved in oculomycoses. Recommended dosages of amphotericin B have been 150 micrograms subconjunctivally every 2 days. Two new drugs in the imidazole class of antifungal agents, namely miconazole (Conofite®, Pitman-Moore) ointment and clotrimazole, are currently under investigation. A pyrimidine antifungal agent, flurocytosine (Ancobon®, Roche) has been used to treat cryptococcal fungal infections and also keratomycosis. The drug most reliably effective against most keratomycoses appears to be pimafucin (Natamycin®), a drug made in the Netherlands and not readily available in the United States (DeVoe, 1972). It is used as a 5 per cent solution every 2 hours topically. A cycloplegic should be used to relieve the iridocyclitis that usually accompanies the keratomycosis. Broad-spectrum antibiotics should also be used to prevent secondary bacterial infection.

## SUPERFICIAL KERATITIS (DEGENERATIVE)

**Recurrent Erosions.** Recurrent superficial erosions are usually initiated by infection or trauma. In both types, loss of or injury to the basement membrane interferes with the tight bond between regenerating epithelial cells and the basement membrane formed by hemidesmosomes. They are observed in all breeds of dogs and may be the cause of the long described "boxer ulcer." It occurs mainly in dogs 5 years old and older, male or female (spayed and intact). Clinical signs may include lacrimation, evidence of little pain to severe blepharospasm and basically a clear cornea below the surface defect in the early stages. Treatment consists of surgical débridement of the loosely adherent epithelium with a curved blade perpendicular to the surface. This can be performed under topical anesthesia in most cases. Prevention of self-mutilation is of paramount importance, since newly formed epithelium is not firmly attached to the basement membrane for up to three weeks, and any corneal contact (including rubbing of the lids) may prevent a good bond. If the corneal defect persists, débridement may be repeated. Topical antibiotic solutions mixed with or without acetylcysteine 20 per cent in equal parts 4 to 5 times daily are recommended. I prefer no ointments in treatment of this defect. Estrogen has been advocated as part of the therapeutic regime for this condition. We have been extremely pleased with the use of a hydrophilic contact lens (Plano-T® by Bausch and Lomb) to protect this type of cornea after débridement. Its use has given a number of patients more relief and shortened the "bonding" time. We have a hypertonic sodium chloride solution (Adsorbon$_a$ C, 2 per cent, Burton, Parsons) in conjunction with the lens.

**Collagenase-Associated Keratopathy.** When stressed, epithelial cells, leukocytes, fibroblasts and certain bacteria can produce collagenase and cause a "melting" of the cornea. There appears to be a high incidence among brachycephalic breeds. In any corneal ulcer that appears to "melt" rapidly, this phenomenon should be considered in the therapy.

Treatment is directed toward the specific cause of the ulcer with the addition of an anticollagenase. These compounds work by binding the calcium essential for the enzyme activity. The irreversible compound most readily available is cysteine in the form of acetylcysteine (Mucomyst®). This drug was designed as a mucolytic agent. We use 20 per cent Mucomyst mixed equal parts with Adapt®, and this combination appears to prolong shelf life, but it still must be refrigerated once it is opened. Instillation is 2 to 3 drops every 2 to 3 hours. Serum also contains anticollagenase properties. In the case of a pending corneal breakdown, a 360-degree bulbar conjunctival flap may be applied after abnormal corneal tissue is trimmed away.

**Corneal Sequestration.** This degenerative disease is observed in cats, namely Persians, and less frequently in Siamese and shorthairs. The cats are presented with central dark brown or black corneal plaques. The plaques are composed of necrotic epithelial and anterior stromal tissue and do not retain fluorescein stain. Moderate to severe discomfort is observed with epiphora. Etiology is at present unknown. Every effort should be made to correct any obvious predisposing problems, such as entropion or chronic keratoconjunctivitis.

Treatment consists of symptomatic therapy, such as steroid therapy, to decrease the vascularization in the absence of surrounding ulceration. Once the cornea appears "quiet," superficial keratectomy is the treatment of choice. We have performed several partial penetrating keratoplasty procedures with excellent results in those corneas involving deep stromal tissue. Keratoplasty is extremely rewarding in the cat.

**Degenerative Pannus.** This disease is present mainly in the German shepherd, shepherd-type dogs and occasionally in any breed. It is usually observed in dogs 3 years old and older and in either sex. The exact etiology is unknown. Theoretical causes include hypersensitivity, environmental influences, heredity and virus. Clinically, there is subepithelial vascularization, scarring and accompanying pigmentation. It usually begins in the inferior-temporal limbal quadrants and may encompass the entire cornea if not treated. The epithelium is intact. Therapy is directed toward minimizing vascularization by use of topical corticosteroids. There is no "cure" for this disease, but in the majority of cases it can be controlled. Our therapy of choice consists of topical dexamethasone ointment every 3 hours for three to five days, and then main-

tenance once or twice daily for three to four weeks, after which most cases can be maintained on a regimen of one application daily on alternate days, indefinitely. Reexaminations are weekly for three weeks, then every three months. Corticosteroid cautions are described to the owner. Radiation therapy or cauterization have not been successful in our experience. Surgical therapy is not recommended for the vascular component of this disease.

### INTERSTITIAL KERATITIS

This type of keratitis is usually associated with anterior uveal disease and less often with pericorneal lesions such as scleritis and neoplasms. Clinical signs may include corneal edema, photophobia, blepharospasm and deep stromal vascularization. The vessels radiate in an even fashion, from the limbus toward the center of the cornea, and in a short time assume a "brushlike" pattern. These vessels are straight and less red than are superficial ones. Probably the most common cause of interstitial keratitis in the young dog is postvaccinal reaction to immunization against canine hepatitis. Other causes include any insult to the anterior segment, such as trauma, infection and neoplasms. Therapy of anterior uveitis will be discussed in the article on "Diseases of the Uveal Tract, Uveitis and Immunologically Mediated Ocular Disorders."

### CORNEAL EDEMA

Corneal edema may result from a variety of abnormalities (Dohlman, 1968). In cases of moderate epithelial and anterior stromal edema, topical hypertonic solutions or ointments such as 2 or 5 per cent sodium chloride or 40 per cent glucose may provide some relief. Moderate to severe edema may best be handled with a membrana nictitans or bulbar conjunctival flap for 10 to 14 days to act as a bandage. This may be another indication for hydrophilic contact lenses in some patients.

### DEGENERATION

#### FATTY DEGENERATION

Corneal opacities due to fat infiltration vary in shape, size and density, particularly in the dog. Such degenerative changes may follow any type of corneal injury or degeneration. It is also reported to be found in humans in certain lipid metabolic disorders. Occasionally a 360-degree perilimbal fatty infiltration may be observed in cats 6 to 7 years old and older. Fatty degeneration of the cornea cannot be treated satisfactorily. Keratectomy or keratoplasty may be of value in superficial forms when vision is limited.

## BAND KERATOPATHY

The calcium present in band keratopathy may be successfully removed with the use of topical 0.03 M EDTA solution. After the epithelium is removed, the solution may be applied to the cornea soaked in a Weckcel sponge for 10 to 15 minutes. The calcium is then scraped or wiped away. Unfortunately, the calcium may recur.

# DYSTROPHY

There is much controversy as to the definitions concerning corneal degenerations and dystrophies. A degeneration usually pertains to a variety of histological and chemical changes in the corneal periphery, and may be unilateral or bilateral. It is more often observed in the older patient. Corneal dystrophy implies a developmental and frequently hereditary condition. Dystrophic pathology is frequently in the corneal axis, bilateral, and often begins early in life. Treatment is usually not rewarding.

## CORNEAL DYSTROPHY IN THE MANX CAT

A familial dystrophy has been described in the Manx (Bistner *et al.*, 1976). The report describes marked corneal edema, disintegration of collagen and severe bullous keratopathy. The epithelium and stroma were mainly involved, while the endothelium appeared normal.

## CORNEAL DYSTROPHY IN THE AIREDALE

We have observed and described a corneal opacity in three related Airedales which involved 80 to 90 per cent of the cornea, bilaterally symmetrical. The immediate perilimbal area was clear. Histochemistry revealed fatty acids. The opacity involved the anterior half of the stroma. Recurrence was evident two years after a successful partial penetrating keratoplasty.

## CORNEAL DYSTROPHY IN THE BOSTON TERRIER AND CHIHUAHUA

This might also be listed as a degenerative condition. A corneal opacity has been observed in these breeds, usually over 4 years of age; its course is insidious. Initially, the central cornea becomes opaque from what appears to be edema. The central corneal tissue then thins and becomes conical. The edema may then progress toward the limbus. There is no effective medical therapy. Penetrating keratoplasties have been performed with little success. Prognosis is grave if the central cornea becomes extremely conical. Tarsorrhaphy is palliative but is not successful, owing to the progressive nature of the disease.

### SUPPLEMENTAL READING

Bistner, S. I., Aguirre, G. D., and Shively, J.: Corneal dystrophy in the Manx cat. Invest. Ophthalmol, 15:15–26, 1976.

DeVoe, A. G.: Symposium on the Cornea. St. Louis, The C. V. Mosby Co., 1972, p.46.

Dohlman, C. H., (ed.): Corneal edema. Int. Ophthalmol. Clin., 8: entire issue, 1968.

Ellis, P. P., and Smith, D. L.: Ocular Therapeutics and Pharmacology (Handbook). 4th ed. St. Louis, The C. V. Mosby Co., 1973, p.87.

Mishima, S., and Hadlys, B.: Physiology of the cornea. Int. Ophthalmol. Clin., 8:527–560, 1968.

# DISEASES OF THE NASOLACRIMAL SYSTEM

GARY M. BRYAN, D.V.M.
*Pullman, Washington*

The maintenance of an adequate tear film is essential for both visual acuity and comfort of the eye. Disorders of the lacrimal system may result in irritation and unsightly blemish to the patient and occasional blindness.

## ANATOMY AND PHYSIOLOGY

Tears serve three basic functions. As a lubricant they are essential for maintaining both the optical integrity of the cornea and the comfort of the anterior portion of the globe and conjunctiva. They are vital in aiding corneal metabolism, supplying both nutrients and oxygen and carrying away waste products. In addition, they aid in protecting and healing by flushing away and diluting foreign material, by exerting antibacterial activity and by serving as a vehicle for cell migration from the limbus during corneal wound healing.

These functions are performed by a tear film consisting of three layers: an inner mucoid layer on the surface of the cornea and conjunctiva, a middle aqueous layer and an outer oily layer. Each layer has its own function and is secreted by different glands. The very thin mucin layer is secreted by conjunctival goblet cells. Its function is primarily supportive, serving as an interface to allow the aqueous portion to adhere to the corneal and conjunctival surfaces. The outer lipid layer also serves a supportive role, helping to retard evaporation and preventing overflow from the lid margins. It is a secretion primarily of the meibomian glands of the eyelids.

The middle or aqueous layer is responsible for all the primary functions of the tear film. Keratoconjunctivitis sicca (KCS) results when this layer is markedly diminished or lost. The term "tears" will be used primarily to refer to this portion of the film. These tears are secreted from both the lacrimal and the nictitans glands. In both cases they enter the conjunctival sac through multiple ductules. Recent work in the dog has shown that the lacrimal gland supplies approximately 60 per cent of the tears and the nictitans gland approximately 40 per cent. Of clinical importance is that either gland is able to maintain the integrity of the tear film without help from the other. This "double safe" system may indicate how vital tears are to vision. Dogs also have small accessory lacrimal glands in the conjunctiva, but by themselves they are unable to maintain a functional tear film. Removal of both the lacrimal and nictitans glands leads rapidly to KCS.

Tear secretion in small animals is primarily of two types, basal or continuous and reflex. The psychogenic tearing of the human is not seen in our patients. Reflex tearing is just an exaggeration of the normal process, brought about by factors such as corneal or conjunctival irritation, strong smells and certain compounds either ingested or given parenterally. In humans it is thought that the accessory lacrimal glands are responsible for the basal or continuous tear secretion. This is not true in the dog.

The neurologic stimulus for tear secretion is parasympathetic, the degree of tear flow being proportional to the number of stimuli rather than to any sympathetic-parasympathetic interplay. Stimuli are always present to maintain the basal flow. When the surface of the eye is irritated, reflex lacrimation is initiated by sensory fibers of the ophthalmic branch of the trigeminal nerve. Parasympathetic motor fibers to the tear glands emerge from the brain stem with the facial nerve. Within the facial canal these fibers leave the seventh nerve and travel to the orbit via the greater petrosal nerve. This separation may be of localizing value in facial nerve paralysis. Central nerve damage will result in KCS while more peripheral problems will not affect tear secretion.

Many drugs will affect tear secretion. Topical anesthetics will lower it approximately 50 per cent. Pilocarpine, topically, orally or parenterally, will increase it. Subcutaneous pilocarpine can increase secretion up to 50 per cent, but at this level the effect on salivation is even greater. Atropine, topically, orally and parenterally, can lower tear secretion to 50 per cent.

The tear film is spread over the surface of the cornea by blinking, which the dog does much less frequently than man, and by movement of the third eyelid from contractions of the retractor muscle. The tear film in a dog with a facial paralysis is not affected if the quantity of tears is adequate. Tears, even at the basal secretory level, are produced faster than they can evaporate, necessitating the nasolacrimal drainage system. The flow of tears goes from lateral to medial across the eye, ending at the lacrimal puncta. The mucus layer is also continually changing and a "mucous thread" forms in the conjunctival cul-de-sac and moves across the eye to accumulate at the medial canthus. This "sleep" accumulation will often increase in inflammatory conditions. The tears both flow and are pumped through the puncta into the lacrimal canaliculi. The dorsal and ventral canaliculi soon converge deep to the medial canthus into a very small lacrimal sac and on into the nasolacrimal duct which will empty into the ventral region of the nasal cavity at a level near the upper canine tooth. Either punctum and canaliculus can usually handle the drainage, and this is necessary if one is congenitally stenotic or becomes injured. The nasal opening of the duct, unlike that of the horse, is very difficult to find, so all flushing and cannulation of the system is done from the upper end.

Although the tears may play a role in maintaining the moisture of the nasal cavity mucosa, it is probably minor. Small nasal glands line the cavity and appear capable of supplying moisture without help from the tears. It is of interest, however, that these nasal glands are also under parasympathetic control and their fibers travel with the same nerve and synapse at the same ganglion as do those stimulating tear secretion.

## EVALUATION OF THE SYSTEM

Specific tests are available in the diagnosis of disorders of the nasolacrimal system. They are used to measure the tear secretion, evaluate the results of corneal and conjunctival drying and determine the patency of the drainage system.

The Schirmer Tear Test® is inexpensive, easy to perform and gives a fairly accurate and reproducible estimate of tear secretion. Following dry cleaning of any mucous accumulations on the lids, the strip is placed under the middle of the lower eyelid. Topical anesthesia should not be used prior to the test, since the results will thus be falsely lowered. The lids may have to be held shut to prevent the patient from working the strip free. In one minute the average dog and cat will show approximately 20 mm. of wetting. If the value is less than 10 mm., one should suspect KCS; readings under 5 mm. are usually accompanied by signs of dryness. Evaluation of the result, however, must always include comparison with the patient's clinical signs.

Both eyes should always be checked when the Schirmer test is performed, even though only one appears to be clinically involved. A marked irritation in one eye, such as resulting from KCS, may initiate a reduction in tear secretion in the otherwise normal opposite eye. The reason for this is not known. In addition, the patients should be kept fairly quiet while the test is run, since excitement may stimulate reflex secretion and falsely elevate the readings, at least in the normal eye.

Rose bengal dye has been used to stain the mucus and dead epithelial cells that accumulate on the cornea and conjunctiva in KCS. Since this dye is irritating, a topical anesthetic should be used first. One drop of dye is placed on the eye and allowed to remain for 15 to 20 seconds. The excess is then rinsed away. The mucus and epithelial accumulations will stain a pale red. The test is not widely used, since it adds little to the clinical examination and Schirmer tear test.

Fluorescein dye is used to test for the patency of the nasolacrimal duct. One drop of the standard ophthalmic solution is placed in each eye. It should appear in the nasal orifice within 5 minutes. Cotton-tipped applicators should be inserted gently up the nostrils at one-minute intervals to detect the dye, since in some dogs it will enter the nose but not appear at the nostril opening. If the dye does appear, the nasolacrimal duct is patent, and flushing is not necessary. Should the dye not appear, there is at least a functional closure of the system, and flushing is indicated. If flushing is necessary, a topical anesthetic is usually all that is required to facilitate insertion of the lacrimal needle and flushing with saline or collyrium. Both puncta should be cannulated; the solution should emerge from both the opposite punctum and the nose. The ability to flush fluid through to the nose does not mean that the duct is physiologically open, only that under pressure it is patent. An inflammatory condition could still be present, causing a functional blockage.

Occasionally there are blockages or other abnormalities of the nasolacrimal duct that can only be demonstrated by means of contrast studies, so techniques for dacryocystography have been developed in dogs. This is especially beneficial where foreign bodies or neoplasms have occluded the duct. With the animal under general anesthesia, dye is injected into one punctum while the other is occluded. Both lateral and dorsoventral films are taken, but the latter are difficult to evaluate because the dental arcade overlaps the ducts. The technique has not worked well in brachycephalic breeds, owing to the short length of the ducts.

## DISEASES OF THE SYSTEM

In general, disorders of the nasolacrimal system fall into two categories: either a diminished or absent tear flow, with resultant keratoconjunctivitis sicca (KCS), or interference with tear drainage, with resultant epiphora. Congenital defects, infections, tumors, injuries and foreign bodies in the drainage system form a miscellaneous category.

### KERATOCONJUNCTIVITIS SICCA

When secretion from both the lacrimal and nictitans glands is significantly impaired, KCS is the result. It is seen more commonly in older dogs. A proportionately higher number of dachshunds, cocker spaniels, pugs and English bulldogs are affected, but any breed at any age may be affected.

One of three conditions must be present for the problem to occur: (1) the parasympathetic stimulation is not reaching the glands, (2) the glands are incapable of responding to the stimulation or (3) the secretion is unable to reach the conjunctival sac via the small outflow ducts. A combination of these factors may exist.

An attempt should be made to determine the specific etiology. Careful and detailed history-taking is important. Neurogenic loss can occur in many ways, the most obvious being injury with nerve damage. If the central portion of the facial nerve is involved, the typical muscle paralysis will accompany the KCS. Problems can also occur with damage to the ophthalmic branch of nerve V, since decreased corneal and conjunctival sensation results in loss of the lacrimal reflex. Depending on the type and extent of damage, these could be permanent. A transient neurogenic KCS is commonly seen with many debilitating systemic diseases, such as pyometra, end-stage kidney disease and bacteremias. If these patients survive, tear secretion will usually return to normal. Other cases in this category are idiopathic—the animal will seem healthy, but tear secretion can be maintained only with continual drug stimulation.

Glandular injury with resultant KCS can occur in several ways. Canine distemper can cause a transient adenitis of both tear-secreting glands, with diminished bilateral tear flow. This is the most common cause of KCS in the younger dog and can be an aid in the diagnosis of distemper. If the dog recovers, the tear flow usually returns to normal. Owing to their direct effect on the tear-secreting glands, two drugs may cause KCS by significantly decreasing tear secretion: sulfadiazine in long-term dosage and phenazopyridine in even short-term dosage may have this effect and should not be used in dogs. It is also possible for the tear glands to become infected retrograde from a severe bacterial conjunctivitis. The resultant drop in tear secretion will further aggravate the initial problem.

Chronic conjunctivitis can also cause scarring around the ductules, interfering with the discharge of tears into the conjunctival sac. Vitamin A deficiency, with its resultant epithelial dysgenesis, can cause similar problems, but such nutritional deficiencies are now rare in clinical practice.

Whatever the cause, the effect of the dryness results in a typical clinical picture. The eye loses its glistening appearance, with the cornea appearing dull and the conjunctiva thick and reddened. There is a thick, sticky, ropy discharge that is difficult to clean away. Corneal ulcers are frequently a sequela. Schirmer tear test readings are usually below 5 mm., and fluorescein staining may reveal superficial corneal excoriations even when no true ulcers are present. Blepharospasms are common, and secondary spastic entropion may occur. In time, corneal vascularization and pigmentation occur. This eventually results in vision impairment, and if untreated, permanent blindness can result.

If the problem is bilateral, the possibility of canine distemper, a drug reaction or, in an older dog, a generalized metabolic disorder should be considered. If the condition is unilateral, look for evidence of preexisting infections or possible neurogenic problems. If the nostril on that side is also dry, the parasympathetic supply may be missing. Swabs for culture and sensitivity testing should always be obtained, since bacterial activity is usually present, even if not the primary cause. The cornea should be stained with fluorescein; if staining indicates that there are no ulcers or severe excoriations, corticosteroids should be used in conjunction with the antibiotics.

The primary medical treatment is to supply needed moisture to the eye. Mucus should be cleaned away with collyrium, saline or even warm water as often as necessary. An artificial tear such as Adsorbotear® (Burton, Parsons) should be used initially several times daily. An ointment such as Lacri-lube® (Allergan) can be used at bedtime for a more prolonged action. An antibiotic-corticosteroid ointment should be used at least three times daily. In addition to the pharmacologic effect, the ointment vehicle aids in lubrication. I have not found mucolytic agents like acetylcysteine (Mucomyst®, Mead Johnson) to be worthwhile. If there are no contraindications, steroids such as triamcinolone or methylprednisolone can be injected subconjunctivally near both the lacrimal and nictitans glands to aid in reducing any adenitis and in opening up the drainage channels.

The effectiveness of pilocarpine in stimulating tear secretion in clinical cases of KCS is variable, depending on the etiology of the problem, which is not always clear-cut. A pilocarpine stimulation test is used to evaluate the patient's response to the drug. This is not done if a preexisting cardiac or respiratory problem renders use of the drug dangerous. A generic solution of 4 per cent pilocarpine hydrochloride (4 mg./ml.) is used. After a bilateral Schirmer test is performed, the patient is given 1 ml. of the solution per 10 kg. of body weight subcutaneously. The Schirmer test is repeated in 20 to 30 minutes. Normally, in addition to profuse salivation, tear secretion will increase an average of 50 per cent. If there is little response in a KCS eye, there is little value in using pilocarpine as therapy. However, often the KCS eye will show a relatively greater response than the normal eye, indicating that pilocarpine may be of value in therapy.

Pilocarpine may be used either topically or orally, and the standard ophthalmic preparations are most convenient. Topically it may be used either undiluted or mixed with collyrium or artificial tear preparation to give a final concentration of pilocarpine between 0.25 and 0.50 per cent. This solution can be applied several times daily without any systemic toxicity and usually without intraocular effects. Oral pilocarpine is also effective but requires more careful observation to avoid toxicity. The 3 per cent ophthalmic preparation contains approximately 1 mg. per drop. Initially the dog is given 1 drop per 5 kg. of body weight mixed with food twice daily. Every two or three days this is increased by 1 drop until he starts showing signs of excessive lacrimation, the first sign of pilocarpine overdosage. This usually precedes vomiting and diarrhea. The highest level possible without producing toxicity should be maintained.

After two or three weeks of extensive medical treatment, most of the early clinical signs should have abated. Antibiotics may no longer be necessary. Topical steroids may still be used if conjunctival thickening and corneal cloudiness persist. At this time you should determine if the patient is starting to produce his own tears or whether continuing medication is needed. If further medication is necessary but is easily handled by the owner, this method should be followed. However, if the natural tear secretion has not returned within a month and the patient is difficult to maintain, surgery should be considered.

The technique of parotid duct transposition is well described in the veterinary literature. If successful, the procedure gives excellent and gratifying results, and the patient becomes a conversation topic in his neighborhood. Frequently, no further medication will be needed other than routine cleaning. The dog should be evaluated for surgery by determining first that a parotid duct is present (they are missing in some English bulldogs) and that there is an adequate salivary flow. A drop of a bitter drug like atropine placed on the tongue will enable one to determine salivary flow. In this examination do not mistake the zygomatic papilla for the parotid. Assuming adequate salivary flow is present, the primary postoperative complication is the formation of concretions or precipitates on the eye. This may occur to some degree in as many as 25 per cent of cases. The exact composition of these formations is unknown, but they do contain triple phosphates. Their presence requires that the eye be cleaned daily, but normal solutions may not be effective. Calcium EDTA solutions have been partially effective in dissolving the material, and Lacri-lube used daily helps to keep them soft, so that they can be washed away more easily. This complication will be permanent.

## CONGENITAL STENOSIS OF LACRIMAL PUNCTA

Occasionally there will be a thin film of tissue covering a lacrimal punctum. Usually only the lower punctum is involved, and if the rest of the system is open and normal, there may be no clinical signs. Should both be affected or the remaining canaliculus become blocked, a marked epiphora will result. Atresia of one or both canaliculi is described but appears less commonly than congenital blockage of the puncta.

Dogs with one punctum blocked are more prone to dacryocystitis, so that, if possible, correction should be attempted. Under anesthesia, the opposite canaliculus should be flushed with saline. This will usually cause the thin veil of tissue to bulge, and it can be nicked with a #65 Beaver blade or sharply pointed iris scissors. Once cut, the tissue

contracts, leaving an adequate punctum. If an antibiotic-steroid ointment is used for several days, catheterization or cannulation usually is not necessary.

## HYPERTROPHY OF NICTITANS GLANDS

A spontaneous enlargement of the nictitans glands is seen in young dogs. An inherited defect is suspect, for although many breeds are affected, there is a high incidence in some lines of Boston terriers and English bulldogs. As the glands enlarge, they cause the third eyelid to evert, making the enlarged reddened structure easily visible. The condition is always bilateral but only one side may have everted at the time of the initial examination. There is some conjunctivitis present, and the dog's appearance is displeasing.

Topical use of an antibiotic steroid ointment affords temporary relief; the eversion may even reverse itself. However, when treatment is stopped, the problem rapidly returns. Injecting steroids such as triamcinolone subconjunctivally into the nictitans glands usually has the same effect. Surgical removal of both glands is indicated, even if only one has everted. This is easily done under short-acting anesthesia, with 1:1000 epinephrine infiltration into the area to control hemostasis. A possible complication of this surgery would be development of KCS at a later date. If tear flow is adequate, as usually is the case in puppies, the value of surgery is worth the small risk. Following surgery, an antibiotic steroid ointment is used at least three times daily for a week. No sutures are necessary, and if the surgeon has not left a window in the third eyelid, the patient's postoperative appearance is normal.

## DACRYOCYSTITIS

Virtually all inflammatory conditions along the lacrimal drainage system are called dacryocystitis, even though the lacrimal sac portion is small. The most common etiology is bacterial infection, which may have either descended from the conjunctival sac or ascended from the nasal cavity. Small grass awns or seeds will occasionally slip into a canaliculus and cause a chronic nonresponsive problem. Nasal tumors can either invade the duct or occlude it from external pressure.

Even a small amount of inflammation will cause the duct to swell shut and result in epiphora. It is often associated with conjunctivitis, so that the dacryocystitis may initially be missed. The conjunctiva is usually reddened and a mucopurulent discharge is present, but close examination and palpation will reveal a stringy discharge emerging from one or both puncta, and the medial canthal area may be slightly swollen. The fluorescein test will be negative, and when the canaliculi are flushed, additional exudate will be forced through. Most ducts can be flushed open, but excessive pressure should not be used.

If the condition is suspected, a swab for culture and sensitivity should be taken from the canalicular exudate before any topical anesthetic is used. Either a liquid antibiotic-steroid preparation or an ointment that has been warmed until liquefied should be flushed through the system with a syringe and lacrimal needle. If the problem is severe, the duct should be flushed daily with such a preparation, in addition to topical treatment. Systemic antibiotics and corticosteroids are usually not necessary, but topical therapy should be continued for two or three weeks.

If there is difficulty in keeping the nasolacrimal duct open, it can be cannulated through the upper punctum with a small-gauge polyethylene tube. The tubing is run out through the nostril and then sutured in place to both the upper eyelid and the side of the nose. The system can then be flushed through the lower punctum. In medium-sized and larger dogs, a number 3½ French urinary catheter works well for this.

If medical treatment fails to open a plugged duct and a canula cannot be passed completely through the system, the patient should be anesthetized for a more complete exam. The upper portion of the duct should again be flushed gently and visually inspected under low-power magnification for any foreign bodies. The head and mouth should first be examined, radiographs should be taken for evidence of dental or nasal disease affecting the duct and then dacryocystography should be performed. This should at least give the location of the blockage, so that a surgical correction can be evaluated.

## EPIPHORA (TEAR STAINING) OF POODLES

A particular form of epiphora is commonly seen in poodles, Maltese and occasionally other breeds. The eyes are usually not irritated, but there is a flow of tears over the medial canthus and down the sides of the face. In light-colored dogs this leads to an objectionable staining. Whether the etiology is anatomic or inflammatory is still debated by some, but the evidence leans toward an inflammatory closure of the nasolacrimal ducts.

The discharge is aqueous, with little evidence of an accompanying conjunctivitis. Although occasionally a lid abnormality such as distichiasis is seen, anatomic defects do not seem to play a role in the problem. The Schirmer tear test may initially seem elevated as the cul-de-sac is filled, yet after the initial rapid rise, it levels off, and one-minute readings are rarely over 25 mm. and often much less. Therefore, excessive secretion of tears does not seem to be a factor. The fluorescein test is usually negative or very slow, yet the ducts can be flushed easily, indicating a functional but not complete blockage. Examination of the throat and regional lymph nodes usually reveals some tonsillitis-pharyngitis, and when questioned, the owner can often recall signs compatible with this problem.

The condition is treated as a low-grade chronic infection in the nasopharynx, with subsequent inflammation of the nasolacrimal ducts interfering with the drainage of tears. Harrison showed a decade ago that low levels of tetracycline mixed with the food for a month would control the problem. This has been verified by others, and additional antibiotics also have proved to be effective. Systemic corticosteroids added to the antibiotic seem to enhance the effect, and if an antibiotic-steroid preparation is also used topically in the eye the result is even more reliable. I use a systemic oral preparation containing tetracycline, novobiocin and prednisolone (Delta Albaplex® [Upjohn]) for 12 to 14 days in standard dosage. A topical antibiotic-steroid of choice, either liquid or light ointment, is also used t.i.d. for three weeks.

Most cases will clear completely within the treatment time, but an occasional recurrence is to be expected. Should this happen, the tonsils should be evaluated for possible removal. Even if the tonsils are removed, the medical treatment should be repeated. If the throat is normal and the nasolacrimal ducts can still be flushed, the medical treatment can be repeated or the nictitans glands can be removed. Surgery should not be done unless tear flow is adequate (at least over 10 mm. on the Schirmer test). The surgery is performed as in hypertrophy of the nictitans glands in puppies. The exact reason why most cases of epiphora will respond to this surgery is unknown. When the glands are removed, medical treatment, both topical and systemic, should be re-peated for 7 to 10 days. Surgical failures are usually associated with recurring attacks of tonsillitis.

## SUPPLEMENTAL READING

Aguirre, G. D., Rubin, L. F., and Harvey, C. E.: Keratoconjunctivitis sicca in dogs. J. Am. Vet. Med. Assn., *158*:1566–1579, 1971.
Gelatt, K. N., *et al.*: Evaluation of tear formation in the dog. J. Am. Vet. Med. Assn., *166*:368–370, 1975.
Severin, G. A.: Nasolacrimal duct catheterization in the dog. J. Am. Animal Hosp. Assn., 8:13–16, 1972.
Yakely, W. L., and Alexander, J. E.: Dacryocys-torhinography in the dog. J. Am. Vet. Med. Assn., *159*:1417–1421, 1971.

# DISEASES OF THE ORBIT

JEFFREY S. SMITH, M.R.C.V.S.
*Ithaca, New York*

Diseases of the orbit are not infrequently seen in small animals. Before considering the diagnostic signs and etiology involved in orbital disease, a review of normal orbital anatomy is important.

## ANATOMY

The orbital space is an irregular cavity, the components of which take the shape of a cone, accommodating the globe anteriorly. The long axis of this cone is directed ventroposteriorly and medially.

The following structures outline the orbit, thereby protecting the globe and the retrobulbar soft tissues: (1) Dorsally, the frontal bone protects the eyeball anteriorly and the temporal muscle lies in contact with the posteromedial orbital structures. (2) Medially, the frontal bone, the palatine bone, the temporal muscle and the pterygoid muscles line the orbit. (3) The bony anterior orbital margin is formed by the lacrimal, maxillary and zygomatic bones. (4) Laterally, the anterior orbital margin is ligamentous; this strong band is the orbital ligament. Posterior to this, the zygomatic arch, the vertical ramus of mandible and the thick masseter muscle combine to reinforce the lateral boundaries. (5) The posterior limit of the orbital cone is the sphenoid bone. (6) The ventral floor of the orbital cavity is supportive soft tissue; the bulk of this is medial pterygoid muscle, the zygomatic salivary gland (dog only) and adipose tissue. Vital vessels such as the maxillary artery and the maxillary and buccal branches of the fifth nerve lie between the medial pterygoid and the ventral portion of temporal muscle in this region.

Retrobulbar tissues include the seven extraocular skeletal muscles; cranial nerves II, III, IV, VI and a branch of V; sympathetic nerves; arteries and veins; smooth muscle and fat. The tunica bulbi or Tenon's capsule (which envelopes the globe and the retrobulbar tissues) is a fascial reflection of the periosteum lining the skull. Smooth muscle fibers, under sympathetic stimulation, ramify in the fascial cone and impart an inherent tone to the supporting tissue, contributing to normal ocular position. Also contributing is the periorbital fat which fills all unoccupied portions of the orbit and supports the suspended eyeball. Eyeball movement is under the control of the extraocular muscles, the origin of which is the sphenoid apex of the orbital cone. The primary lacrimal gland occupies a fossa beneath the supraorbital process of the frontal bone within the confines of the orbital fascia. Peribulbar adnexa in the form of the conjunctivae, nictitating membrane and eyelids compose the most rostral of the pro-

*Table 1.* Disorders of the Orbit

| DISORDERS | CLINICAL SIGNS |
|---|---|
| **Developmental Abnormalities** | |
| 1. Hydrocephalus with malformation | 1. Lateral strabismus. |
| 2. Anophthalmia or microphthalmia | 2. Absent or smaller than normal eyeball; narrow palpebral fissure. |
| 3. Shallow bony orbit (considered acceptable in brachycephalics) | 3. Exophthalmos; exposure keratoconjunctivitis. |
| 4. Orbital vascular anomaly | 4. Exophthalmos; pulse or fremitus detectable through the globe. |
| **Trauma** | |
| 1. Orbital fractures | 1. Depression fracture with soft globe, suggesting penetrating bone fragment; ocular positional displacement. |
| 2. Hemorrhages | 2. Episcleral hemorrhage; retrobulbar hemorrhage with proptosis. |
| 3. Penetrating foreign bodies (e.g., darning needle or sharp bone lodged in the roof of the mouth, grass awn) | 3. Discharging sinus through the conjunctiva, skin or buccal mucosa; pain upon opening the mouth. |
| **Infection** | |
| 1. Viral | 1. Enophthalmos may be seen secondary to debilitation. |
| 2. Bacterial; fungal | 2. Ocular discharge; usually secondary via a penetrating object through the oropharynx or conjunctiva, or via sinusitis. |
| 3. Parasitic (e.g., Dirofilaria) | 3. Granulomatous lesions caused by wandering larvae, seldom manifest as a problem. |
| **Neoplasia** | |
| 1. Primary sarcomas or carcinomas (e.g., zygomatic salivary gland adenomas [dog only]) | 1. Strabismus; exophthalmos; exposure keratoconjunctivitis discharges. |
| 2. Metastases or local extensions (e.g., squamous cell carcinoma originating in the anterior ocular segment) | 2. Neurologic deficits. |
| **Miscellaneous Conditions** | |
| 1. Zygomatic sialocele | 1. Abnormal swelling of ventral orbit; possible strabismus, swelling in the dorsal oral vestibule. |
| 2. Horner's syndrome | 2. Enophthalmos; nictitans protrusion; miosis; ptosis. |
| 3. Myositis | 3. Exophthalmos; pain with dysphagia in acute stage; enophthalmos and sinking of the globe upon opening the mouth when muscles of the head have atrophied. |

tective barriers. The nasal cavity and paranasal sinuses are air-filled cavities in close proximity to the orbit. The ethmoid labyrinth lies between the medial walls of the orbits. The frontal sinus lies dorsal and the maxillary sinus ventral to the orbital cavity.

## CLINICAL SIGNS

Abnormal position of the globe is a cardinal sign associated with a variety of diseases involving the orbit. Displacement in *any* direction may follow orbital fractures. Exophthalmos or anterior protrusion of the globe may superficially mimic glaucoma and must be differentiated from this by assessment of intraocular pressure. Exophthalmos is suggestive of any retrobulbar mass such as an abscess or granuloma, a neoplasm or perhaps a hematoma following trauma. Zygomatic salivary gland inflammation or tumor and vascular anomalies must also be considered. Exposure keratitis is a common sequela to exophthalmos. Strabismus, or deviation of the globe, suggests imbalance in extraocular muscle tone. Causes may include traumatic extraocular muscle rupture; damage to one or more of cranial nerves III, IV and VI, which innervate the extraocular muscles; or space-occupying lesions. (An abnormal swelling would suggest the last.)

Enophthalmos, or sinking of the globe into the orbit, is usually accompanied by secondary nictitans protrusion. Causes may include (1) loss of tone in the retrobulbar cone or (2) interference with one or more of the components of sympathetic orbital innervation (Horner's syndrome). In cases of chronic inflammation, such as periorbital muscular degenerative diseases, and debilitation in which retrobulbar fat is lost, enophthalmos also develops. The action of the mandible will exacerbate the enophthalmos when the jaws are opened. Additionally, discharges may appear anywhere around the globe, through the conjunctivae or through the periorbital skin. In such cases a draining tract can usually be found with the use of a blunt probe.

It is essential to examine the posterior buccal cavity when orbital disease is suspected, since discharges or proliferative tissue often follows the line of least resistance ventrad to enter the oral cavity immediately posterior to the last dorsal molar tooth.

Causes of orbital inflammation include (1) penetrating foreign bodies via the pharynx or periorbita (e.g., grass seeds), which tend to migrate retrobulbarly if lodged in the conjunctiva; (2) paranasal sinusitis, or tooth abscess, with bone lysis and secondary orbital involvement; and (3) invasive neoplasia.

Pain upon opening the mouth and dysphagia may exist in orbital inflammation. Pain exhibited upon opening the mouth occurs because of the downward pressure applied to the retrobulbar tissues by the vertical ramus of the mandible. The animal may yawn to one side and be reluctant to eat food. Temporomandibular or periorbital muscle disease will also induce these signs.

Some ocular signs of orbital disease are consistent with disruption of vital vessels and nerves. Neurologic manifestations not yet mentioned include adnexal and corneal hypalgesia (sensory branches of the fifth nerve); optic neuritis leading to blindness with dilated, unresponsive pupils (second nerve); and papilledema. Vascular disturbances may lead to orbital venous congestion and edema or ischemic degenerative changes. Space-occupying vascular anomalies are rare but must be considered.

Chorioretinal degeneration may be a secondary complication of orbital disease either by direct extension or owing to retrobulbar pressure effects. Hemorrhage may be seen on fundus examination.

## DIAGNOSTIC PROCEDURES

1. Cytologic examination of discharge or tissue material from the retro-orbital space can be helpful in achieving a diagnosis. An 18-gauge needle is slowly inserted into the retro-orbital space via a point immediately posterior to the middle of the lateral orbital ligament. Surgical biopsy of a space-occupying lesion of of the orbital musculature may be necessary.

2. When a discharging sinus is suspected, exploration of the area with a blunt probe may disclose the tract and the site of origin (e.g., paranasal sinus). This may require general anesthesia.

3. Examination of the oral cavity requires general anesthesia for critical evaluation. Hard and soft palates, masseter ridges and upper molar teeth should be checked for abnormalities.

4. Three radiographic views should be taken: (a) dorsoventral, (b) lateral and (c) an-

teroposterior through an open mouth. A fine metal ring placed in the conjunctival fornices is beneficial in outlining the anterior orbital borders and eyeball position. Such a ring can be hand-made from the metal stilette of an intravenous catheter (Bardic*), or a suitable ring can be purchased (Flieringa ring†). Contrast radiography may be desirable in outlining a suspected radiolucent retro-orbital mass. A curved 25-gauge needle and a three-way valve are used to inject 5 to 15 ml. of air *slowly* into the bulbar subconjunctival space. Films are taken with the needle and a ring in place. Should the zygomatic salivary gland and ducts need to be outlined, 1 to 2 ml. of Renografin-60®‡ are injected via the zygomatic papilla, utilizing a blunted 23-gauge needle. When orbital extension of a primary intracranial space-occupying lesion is suspected, cavernous sinus venography should be contemplated.

## TREATMENT OF ORBITAL INFECTIONS

Retro-orbital inflammation usually requires a drainage procedure for resolution. A suitable drainage tract opening into the oral cavity can be created in the following manner: Under general anesthesia, a small stab incision is made ½ to 1 cm. posterior to the last upper molar tooth. A closed hemostat is slowly inserted via this incision dorsally through pterygoid muscle. Once in position behind the globe, the instrument is opened. Fluid will begin to drain immediately. The retrobulbar space may then be irrigated with an antiseptic solution. An alternate site for drainage is via the medial canthus. A curved hemostat is inserted through the bulbar conjunctiva following the bony medial wall of the orbit into the retrobulbar space.

Recurrence of the orbital infections suggests the possible presence of a foreign body. In cases of chronic orbital inflammation in which a discharging sinus is evident, the sinus is demarcated with a malleable probe and followed surgically. The approach to the orbit for this procedure may be along the tract (conjunctival) or via a vertical incision made posterior to the lateral orbital ligament over the zygomatic arch. Once the inciting cause has been removed, a Penrose drain is placed so that it is continuous with the ventral aspect of the incision and the roof of the mouth via the incision described above. The drain is then tied to form a loop via the commissure of the lips. It should be removed 1 to 4 days later via the mouth. Topical and systemic antibiotics are administered.

The possibility of an exposure keratitis must be considered and temporary tarsorrhaphy or a nictitans flap may be utilized until the proptosis subsides.

## TREATMENT OF ORBITAL TRAUMA

Emergency treatment of traumatic proptosis: Clean the globe gently and reduce edema by application of a sponge saturated with hypertonic solution (10 per cent dextrose, 15 per cent mannitol). The cornea should be kept moist with artificial tears. Attempt to replace the globe, provided that there has not been extrusion of intraocular contents. Lateral canthotomy is often necessary to provide adequate space to replace the globe. Make the lateral canthotomy incision large enough to allow replacement of the congested eyeball. Venous congestion will be relieved by a lateral canthotomy because of reduced lid pressure upon vortex and ciliary veins. Fractures and/or retrobulbar hemorrhage may make replacement difficult or even impossible. Should it be necessary to cut the lateral orbital ligament, this should be sutured separately once the eyeball has been replaced. *Never* aspirate fluid from the orbit or anterior ocular segment in an attempt to relieve pressure. Cover the eyeball with a nictitans flap *and* temporary tarsorrhaphy if possible. The flap and tarsorrhaphy should be kept in place for two weeks, after which time the globe should be reevaluated.

Postoperative therapy following traumatic proptosis involves the use of systemic and topical antibiotics, preferably broad-spectrum with bactericidal action, e.g., gentamicin (Garamycin ointment®*) topically and ampicillin systemically. Systemic corticosteroids should be utilized to minimize uveitis induced by traumatic

---

*C. R. Bard, Inc., Murray Hill, New Jersey.

†Sparta Instruments Co., Fairfield, New Jersey 07006.

‡E. R. Squibb and Sons, Inc., Princeton, New Jersey.

---

*Garamycin Ophthalmic Solution®, Schering Corp., Kenilworth, New Jersey 07033.

28

DISEASES OF THE LENS

proptosis. A repository corticosteroid (i.e., methylprednisolone acetate, 10 mg.) can be given retrobulbarly to reduce inflammation. Topical 1 per cent atropine ointment twice daily is administered to minimize pain associated with intraocular muscular spasm and to minimize iris adhesions.

Complications following orbital trauma may include (1) retrobulbar hematoma, which usually regresses in approximately two weeks; (2) permanent damage to ocular contents (e.g., retinal detachment, synechiae or cataract formation); (3) ocular strabismus, which often spontaneously corrects itself within several months; (4) keratoconjunctivitis sicca; (5) nasolacrimal duct stenosis leading to epiphora; and (6) glaucoma associated with a compromised drainage angle.

In various ocular conditions an indwelling subpalpebral catheter may be implanted with the following advantages: (1) it facilitates continuous treatment of the affected globe; (2) it minimizes the handling and excitement of fractious animals; and (3) it facilitates application of medication to an eye over which a nictitans flap and/or tarsorrhaphy has been placed.

In placing a subpalpebral lavage apparatus, a 14-gauge needle is inserted through the dorsolateral conjunctival fornix to emerge from the skin of the upper eyelid. A PE 190 Silastic®* catheter of desired length is fed retrograde down through the lumen of the needle and the latter is withdrawn. The tip of the catheter is flared by holding it over a flame, and the flared portion of the catheter is pulled superiorly so that it lies in the fornix. Adhesive bandage is wrapped around the catheter as it passes over the zygomatic arch, and a nylon suture is placed through the bandage, skin and underlying periosteum to fix the position of the tube. Controlled liquid administration may then be given via a drip set or syringe from outside the cage. It may be necessary to apply a covering bandage to insure the integrity of the catheter. Once the catheter has been placed, a nictitans flap and tarsorrhaphy can be completed if required.

SUPPLEMENTAL READING

Buyukmihci, N.: Exophthalmos secondary to zygomatic adenocarcinoma in the dog. J. Am. Vet. Med. Assn. 167:162, 1975.
Koch, S. A.: Differential diagnosis of exophthalmos in the dog. J.A.A.H.A., 5:229, 1969.
Oliver, J. E.: Cranial sinus venography in the dog. J. Am. Vet. Radiol. Soc., 10:66, 1969.
Rosenthal, J.: Surgical treatment of chronic retrobulbar abscess. Vet. Med./Small Animal Clin., 68:663, 1973.

*Dow Corning Company, Midland, Michigan 48640.

# DISEASES OF THE LENS

CHARLES J. PARSHALL, JR., D.V.M.
Akron, Ohio

The overall functions of the lens in the dog and cat are similar to those of the human being. However, data suggesting poor accommodative capability of the lens system in animals indicate less emphasis on visual acuity and more on peripheral vision. This is perhaps the reason cataract lens extraction in the animal restores vision without the use of corrective artificial lenses. In animals, the lens is considered diseased when opacities obstruct the transmission of light or when the lens is dislocated. These conditions may be present as a primary disease (intrinsic lesions) or secondary disease (systemic or other ocular regional disease affecting the lens). Details of lens disease treatment and surgery are found in several references.

This discussion is directed to the general practitioner whom the author believes seeks information on the recognition of eye disease in order to advise his clients. Since authors of previous editions of this publication have adequately described the cataract and lens extraction, this discussion will attempt to augment these references in order to relate principles in approach to disease of the lens and to highlight concurrent dis eases which bear a possible relationship to lens pathology.

The lens can be considered a fairly uncomplicated structure. It is unique, being avascular and reacting passively to inflammation. It is a compact, biconvex, nearly optically pure structure surrounded by a thin elastic hyalinized membrane, the capsule. The adult lens is acellular except for anterior subcapsular columnar epithelial cells populating the region of the vertical equator. Embryologically, cellular activity is also found in the anterior central subcapsular region.

The lens is held in position by two supportive structures adherent to the lens capsule: the zonules and the hyaloid ligament. The zonules are tough fibrils connecting the equator of the lens capsule to the ciliary body. The hyaloid ligament is the region of firm (semisolid) vitreous adherent to the posterior lens capsule. The concave space filled by the lens in the region of the hyaloid ligament is the hyaloid fossa. In younger animals, the capsular-vitreous adhesion is more firm than in older animals (a fact of importance in lens extraction technique). Early in embryogenesis, the hyaloid region contains primary vitreous and hyaloid vasculature. Occasionally, remnants of these structures are visible in the adult animal.

Within the lens capsule, there are regions (the cortex and the nucleus). Instrumentation enables one to delineate zones within the lens: embryonic, fetal and adult nuclei as well as slight linear opacities called sutures within the fetal and adult nucleus and cortex. The lens is a laminated, slightly flattened sphere. The laminations are produced by elongated epithelial cells which eventually lose their cell nuclei and become fibers. The individual cell nuclei are lost except in the active subcapsular centers, i.e., the equatorial and anterior subcapsular regions of the fetal animal and the equatorial regions of the neonate and adult. The fibers extend from specific geometric centers of activity and are of uniform length.

The lens sutures are formed by the junction of the ends of the elongated cells or fibers. The sutures appear as an orderly geometric configuration, especially within the lens nucleus. With magnification, the suture appears to be two parallel lines with a clear space between them. The opaque lines are considered to be light reflected from the tips of the linear arrangement of fibers. In the fetal and adult nucleus, the sutures anterior to the center of the lens appear as an erect Y. The sutures posterior to the center of the lens appear as an inverted Y. In the adult animal, the sutures of the cortex have many variations, perhaps because of the shifting center of cellular activity and increased size of the lens. In the aged animal, one can recognize a hazy zone in the center of the lens which can be transilluminated to visualize the fundus. This condition is called nuclear sclerosis and is the result of normal physiologic compression of the lens, which must take place during life or the lens would become a huge structure because of continued lamellar growth of the lens.

## EXAMINATION OF THE LENS

The position of the lens and its transparent biconvex nature create several prerequisites for examination of the total structure *in vivo*. To eliminate reflections, a dark room is required. To visualize the equatorial and zonular regions, mydriasis is required. Short-acting agents to dilate the pupil are preferred, such as 1 per cent tropicamide (Mydriacyl®, Alcon). Mydriatics are contraindicated in preglaucomatous and glaucomatous patients. The regions and structures of each eye to be examined include the lens (nucleus, cortex), capsule, zonules and hyaloid fossa.

The general practitioner cannot be expected to have a slit lamp biomicroscope for detailed examination. However, a reasonable examination can be achieved with a magnifying loupe (common 4 × magnification) and a focusing penlight. The principle is to obliquely observe the pathway of focused light which is an optical section of the lens. Opacities are reflected in varying sizes, shapes and positions. Normal zonules, capsule, nuclear zones and sutures are visible by varying the inspection and light source angles in the course of examining the entire lens and supportive structures.

It is important to examine eye structures other than the lens to reveal concurrent relevant pathology. One must also consider the animal's systemic condition. Examination of the lens should account for the position, stability, size and clarity of the lens, the capsule and hyaloid fossa, the zonule attachments, pupil shape and size, synechia, depth of the anterior chamber, clarity of the aqueous and evidence of systemic or other regional disease. Slit-lamp biomicroscopy is important in examination for potential hereditary lens defects.

## DISEASE CONDITIONS

The lens may be altered by four basic processes: biologic, immunologic, local disturbances and systemic disturbances. Biologic processes would include senility changes (nonpathologic), congenital (perhaps hereditary) cataracts and other such disorders (congenital absence of the lens, posterior lenticonus, etc.). Immunologic processes would include some forms of phacolytic uveitis (phacoanaphylaxis). Local disturbances would include trauma, irradiation injury, chemical injury, glaucoma, uveitis and iritis. Systemic disturbances would include diabetes and toxemias. Lens disease can be a passive response to outside forces such as disturbances of normal metabolism or surrounding tissue disease. Cataract development may, indeed, be the lens' only reacting sign of disease (abnormal metabolism, cellular develpment). True inflammation and neoplasia of the intact lens are practically unheard of. The cataract and the dislocated lens with or without concurrent disease will be the subject of the following discussion.

**Lens Opacities (Cataract) Without Concurrent Disease.** Any opacity of the intact lens may be suspected as being a primary form of cataract when not found concurrently with other signs of disease. Cataracts must be suspected as being secondary when certain concurrent disease is present. Classification of cataracts is helpful only when referable to progress of the condition. Description of location, size, structure affected, age of onset and clarity are, therefore, useful for future reference. Transillumination and ophthalmoscopy are important to detect function and concurrent disease of the fundus. Cataracts are important to the animal as the cause of visual loss or of inflammation or participation in other disease processes. In addition, cataracts are important to the owner and the veterinarian as indications of primary and potential underlying disease. The owner of a breeding animal must consider the hereditary potential of cataracts. It is impossible to differentiate hereditary and nonhereditary cataracts solely from the charanter of the lens. Breed predisposition

and line history are more suggestive. Test breeding systems, although costly, may yield the only definite proof.

Cataracts may be focal, cortical, nuclear or diffuse. They may develop rapidly or slowly, unilaterally or bilaterally. In the adult, cataracts may be seen in three phases of development. First, there is a general diffuse haze and swelling (imbibition aqueous). Second, the lens becomes very opaque with consolidations of lens material (perhaps altered metabolism, accumulation of insoluble metabolites, osmotic changes). Third, the lens appears to become consolidated and dense, with shrinkage of the lens mass and wrinkling of the anterior capsule (soluble and diffusible lens material is released back into the aqueous). The third phase is better known as the resorption phase. A peculiar form of cataract, the Morgagnian cataract, is characterized by a dense consolidated nucleus freely gravitating in liquefied cortex within an intact lens capsule. (This form of cataract has potentially serious sequelae.)

Cataracts are usually brought to the veterinarian's attention by the owner who recognizes visual problems or some description of a white pupil. The most significant service a general practitioner can render to that owner is a thorough ophthalmologic and physical evaluation of his pet. To render this service, the practitioner must have considerable expertise in ophthalmology or should refer the case to an experienced colleague.

The only treatment, lens extraction, is a procedure demanding experience and attended by potentially serious complications. The only way to determine structural change which may reduce the effectiveness of extraction is to examine the eyes before dense lenses preclude fundus evaluation. Good pupillary light reflexes require functioning photoreceptor cells, optic nerve, optic tract pathways to midbrain and nerve pathways to the iris but not the central visual center of the brain. Therefore, the presence or absence of the pupil reflex is not necessarily an indication of either vision or blindness. At times, the decision for or against surgery may have to be based on the condition of visible ocular structures and the reaction of the pupil to light. The decision based on the suggestion: "What have you got to lose?" may also be logical as long as the owner is aware of the uncertainties.

Electrophysiologic inspection (elec

troretinography, ERG) to gain additional information is available in several institutions. The ERG is not a diagnostic panacea. The ERG relates only the function of a segment of the optic pathway (cells of the neural retina) and has no direct bearing on the function of vision. Cataract extraction is only recommended in the blind animal which, preferably, has been favorably evaluated. Exceptions might be made in the "What have you got to lose?" instance and the unilateral cataract case in which the diseased lens is thought to contribute to other concurrent disease.

Spontaneous resorption of the lens does occur in varying degrees in about 25 per cent of dogs with cataracts under three to five years of age. A significant percentage of such cases can regain partial vision once the process is completed. During the interim between recognition of the cataract and potential surgery, one may consider dilating the pupil to increase the amount of light passing to the retina.

**Lens Opacities with Concurrent Disease.** There is no clear clinical distinction between primary and most secondary lens cataracts. Cataracts can exist with concurrent ocular or systemic disease. Disease conditions commonly concurrent with cataracts are uveitis, iritis, diabetes, glaucoma, trauma, persistent pupillary membrane and persistent hyaloid plaque, systemic or regional diseases which give rise to intraocular inflammation. It must be made clear that cataracts are not always present in these disease conditions. The altered ocular environment present in these conditions, which may contribute to cataract development, can include rupture of the lens capsule, kinetic injury of ocular tissue, blood and aqueous chemistry changes, inflammation and multiple congenital anomalies. In contrast to the conditions surrounding the simple cataract, the above conditions described may require immediate treatment of the concurrent disease and not necessarily removal of the cataractous lens. The exception is the occasional cataract process that contributes to intraocular disease.

**Anterior Uveitis.** Cataracts can be a part of inflammation in two basic instances: cataracts resulting from inflammation of surrounding tissue, and cataract development causing inflammation. In the former condition, the aqueous transudate or exudate, synechia or altered aqueous may induce abnormal metabolic changes leading to cataract formation. In the latter condition, antigenic or otherwise toxic lens material diffuses into the aqueous and stimulates inflammation within the surrounding tissue. In both situations, once intraocular inflammation is in progress, the signs appear to be the same: photophobia and blepharospasm. In addition, the signs of the active state include conjunctival and episcleral congestion, conjunctival and corneal edema, cloudy aqueous, iris swelling, hyper-reactive pupil, cellular precipitates on the corneal endothelium, transudates on the anterior lens capsule, synechia and cloudy lens. In the quiescent, previously inflamed eye, one may recognize anterior capsule pigmentation, synechia, pupil irregularities and focal to diffuse cataract formation. Occasionally, complete pupil synechia (pupil obstruction to aqueous flow) is found with iris bombé and glaucoma.

During the lens resorption phase, animals respond with varying degrees of inflammation which is thought to be the reaction to the toxic or antigenic nature of the released lens material. In severe cases, engorged macrophages may not readily pass through the trabecular meshwork of the aqueous draining regions of the eye, obstructing aqueous outflow, setting up conditions for glaucoma, i.e., phacolytic glaucoma and potentially phacolytic anaphylaxis (the latter has not been reported in animals). The Morgagnian cataract produces potentially dangerous sequelae, because of the possibility of large volumes of liquefied lens proteins leaking from the lens capsule, causing a severe immunologic reaction.

The treatment of this type of lens disease involves control of inflammation. Occasionally, the inflammation cannot be controlled medically until the lens is extracted. Whether or not the lens is recommended for extraction in the quiescent eye depends upon the same factors described for the simple cataract. The condition may be unilateral or bilateral and is treated both systemically and topically. Antibiotics are used, as the etiology is often unknown. Corticosteroids are used to control the inflammation rapidly. Parasympatholytic agents (atropine, 1 to 4 per cent) are used to control ciliarispasm. Severe cases may receive one or more subconjunctival antibiotic/steroid injections.

**Diabetes.** Diabetes is common in the

dog. Cataracts develop secondarily to diabetes usually in the older animal. The diagnostic problem is to determine the presence and cause of hyperglycemia. It is important to recognize the possibility of diabetes in the dog before recommending cataract extraction. Cataract extraction in the controlled diabetic dog usually is successful. However, surgery in the uncontrolled diabetic dog may result in postoperative complications such as poor to slow healing of surgical wounds, hemorrhage and severe postoperative inflammation.

**Trauma.** Forceful injury to the region of the eye can affect the lens in several ways: zonular rupture (lens luxation), kinetic nonpenetrating wounds and penetrating foreign body. Luxations do not necessarily result in cataract formation. Kinetic trauma and foreign body trauma usually result in degrees of lens opacity. The best example of kinetic, nonpenetrating trauma resulting in cataract development is the eye hit by BB shot. The shot is often reflected from the corneal surface, producing kinetic and thermal injury to the cornea and kinetic injury to all intraocular tissue. It may take 7 to 10 days for signs of cataract development to appear. Foreign body penetration of the lens is seen less commonly, but the result may be focal to diffuse cataract development and inflammation elsewhere in the eye.

Treatment of the kinetic nonpenetrating injury is often unsuccessful, and a poor prognosis must be given if hemorrhage persists or if vision is absent 7 to 10 days after treatment. Treatment is established initially to correct problems of tissue damage and edema (especially retinitis and optic neuritis). Systemic antibiotics and corticosteriods and osmotic agents are used. (Be aware of dangers of osmotic agents in presence of hemorrhage.) Depending upon the degree of lens opacity and vision of the opposite eye, cataract extraction may be indicated after the eye becomes quiescent.

Treatment of conditions caused by penetrating foreign material requires systemic antibiotics, topical antibiotics and parasympatholytic agents, and preparation for intraocular surgery to repair wounds, remove foreign material and possibly extract the lens. If the foreign body has caused minor focal lens damage, the subsequent cataract may be small and of minor concern.

**Persistent Pupillary Membrane.** This anomaly is not uncommon and is hereditary in some breeds of dogs. In cases with posterior synechia, the lens may develop an anterior capsular cataract. Unless the condition is extensive, treatment is not considered. The treatment is either excision of the membrane strands or lens extraction. There is a distinct possibility that other anomalies are concurrent (persistent hyaloid, retinal dysplasia).

**Persistent Hyaloid.** When this embryonic structure does not resorb before birth, a plaque may develop with or without persistent hyaloid vessels in the region of the hyaloid fossa. The persistent hyaloid is difficult to differentiate from a posterior subcapsular cataract. A truly focal plaque without overlying cataract will probably not progress. Surgical excision requires intracapsular extraction and excision of the hyaloid plaque. One case was attempted by extracapsular extraction, and later simple incision of the plaque to provide a light pathway was successful. All too often, plaques are found following extracapsular extraction. Although considered rare, there exists the distinct possibility that behind a dense cataractic lens, along with other persistent structures of the hyaloid apparatus, functional hyaloid vessels may remain.

**Lens Opacities Induced by Irradiation and Chemical Toxicity.** Ultraviolet, infrared and x-irradiation in high doses can induce lens changes and other eye lesions. There are probably more iatrogenic cataracts produced than is currently recognized. An especially critical period in the development of the lens is the first few days of gestation. During this period, certain drugs used in the pregnant animal may produce lenticular changes. When the young are born and examined at several weeks of age, such lesions may mistakenly be attributed to herditary defects. Cataractogenic agents have been described in many species of animals. Such agents include alloxan, cobalt chloride, several of the dinitrophenol and related compounds, galactose, triparanol and many others. The author has recognized one situation which developed in all pups of one litter born of a bitch treated with dinitrophenol (DNP) during the first week of pregnancy. High doses of continued corticosteroid agents may also result in cataract formation. There is emerging evidence of transient cataract development in young puppies fed protein-deficient diets.

**Lens Luxation and Subluxation.** Com

plete luxation of the lens is a complete dislocation from the hyaloid fossa with total zonule rupture. The lens, therefore, may gravitate to any chamber. There are several important points to consider, since the dislocated lens has mass which can be put into motion with abrupt head and eye movement. Kinetic energy transmitted from the lens mass through the vitreous can exert traction on the retina. The retina can be detached with resultant blindness. The subluxated lens is also subject to the forces of kinetic energy. Not uncommonly, the lens luxation (complete or incomplete) is unrecognized until one or more of the following signs develop: glaucoma, corneal edema, iritis/uveitis, pupillary blockage or blindness.

The most common cause of lens luxation is severe traumatic injury. The condition should be sought after any trauma to the head. Often lens luxation by zonule rupture occurs with glaucoma after secondary enlargement of the globe. Severe iritis, uveitis, iridocyclitis or ciliary neoplasia may also cause zonule degeneration and subsequent lens displacement. Spontaneous lens luxation has been reported in several breeds of dogs. However, one must consider factors related to the excitability and head-shaking habits of these animals at play. The terrier breeds are the type of dog usually affected. One cannot ignore the potential kinetic energy contributing to zonule damage and subsequent lens luxation in these animals.

Because of the conditions usually present at the time of recognition, treatment is initiated to attack concurrent disease rather than the lens luxation. Although some of these conditions are causes of lens luxation, they also may be sequelae of luxation. The dislocated lens occupies other chambers, interferes with aqueous drainage, irritates tissues and can set up kinetic detachment of the retina. Treatment will be discussed relative to the lens location, mobility and concurrent disease.

VITREOUS CHAMBER. Removal of the lens in the vitreous chamber is somewhat like trying to retrieve a clear marble from the bottom of a dish of gelatin. The lens may be difficult to see and, once grasped, the traction created can lead to immediate retinal detachment. In general, the lens in this position rarely creates problems except in the highly excitable dog which constantly creates kinetic injury.

POSTERIOR AQUEOUS CHAMBER. Since this is the approximate normal position of the lens, no correction is necessary unless recurrent luxation or associated inflammation is noted. Without any known trauma, one might be wise to search for evidence of glaucoma as the cause of luxation.

PUPILLARY SPACE. This condition is fortunately not common. It can be a transient situation with movement of the dislocated lens between chambers. Pupillary blockade is an emergency condition existing when the lens becomes locked within the pupil space by spastic contraction of the iris. The condition is extremely painful. Glaucoma usually develops rapidly as the flow of aqueous is acutely obstructed. The signs are acute severe pain, photophobia and blepharospasm of both eyes. The signs of the acute case prior to glaucoma are congestion and recognition of the lens in the pupillary space. Rapid treatment is necessary. Examination may demand anesthesia (general) in extremely painful cases. Miotic agents are contraindicated even in the presence of glaucoma, because of the already spastic iris contracting around the lens. Systemic osmotic agents (mannitol) followed by oral carbonic anhydrase inhibitors (dichlorphenamide, acetazolamide) may have to be used to control glaucoma. Topical and perhaps subconjunctival injections of atropine are necessary to relieve the ciliarispasm and miosis. Surgical extraction of the lens is necessary if the lens migrates into the anterior chamber or remains in the pupillary space. Spontaneous relocation in the hyaloid fossa may relieve signs and temporarily postpone lens extraction.

ANTERIOR CHAMBER. Because the lens moving about the chamber leads to considerable tissue damage and inflammation, and because of the possibility of pupillary blockade, the lens should be surgically removed. The inflammatory reaction produced by the lens, along with occupation of the drainage angle, predisposes the animal to glaucoma. Prolonged irritation increases the opportunity for corneal endothelial scarring. Besides being prepared for surgery, the animal is treated for possible concurrent conditions including inflammation and glaucoma. There is some danger in using miotic agents to trap the lens in the anterior chamber; however, the practice is effective and used often.

**Glaucoma.** Lens luxation present in many cases of glaucoma is probably secondary to stretching and rupture of the zonules due to enlargement of the globe. However, glaucoma can develop in several ways in relation to lens disease: phacolytic uveitis, obstruction of the drainage angle, ciliary body luxation (concurrent with lens dislocation), pupillary blockade and inflammation due to lens irritation of ocular tissue. Treatment is established for one or for combinations of inflammation, glaucoma and lens luxation. Treatment for inflammation is the same as for uveitis. Treatment for glaucoma is standard: carbonic anhydrase inhibitors (dichlorphenamide, acetazolamide) orally, possibly rapid-acting intravenous osmotic agents (mannitol) in very congestive cases, and topical miotic agents or drugs effecting a decrease in aqueous production (pilocarpine, echothiophate, physostigmine, etc.). As mentioned above, there is a distinct reason for not using miotic preparations in the case of pupillary blockade. Ultimate control of lens-induced glaucoma may be by lens extraction combined with specific glaucoma surgery (cyclodialysis, sector iridectomy, etc.).

## SUPPLEMENTAL READING

Duke-Elder, S.: Diseases of the lens and vitreous glaucoma and hypotony. In System of Ophthalmology. Vol. 11. St. Louis, The C. V. Mosby Co., 1969.
Havener, W. H.: Ocular Pharmacology. St. Louis, The C. V. Mosby Co., 1966.
Jensen, H. E.: Stereoscopic Atlas of Clinical Ophthalmology of Domestic Animals. St. Louis, The C. V. Mosby Co., 1971.
Magrane, W. G.: Canine Ophthalmology. Philadelphia, Lea & Febiger, 1968.
Prince, J. H., et al.: Anatomy and Histology of the Eye and Orbit in Domestic Animals. Springfield, Ill., Charles C Thomas, 1960.

# RETINOPATHIES

GUSTAVO AGUIRRE, V.M.D.
*Philadelphia, Pennsylvania*

Retinal diseases (retinopathies) can be hereditary, metabolic, infectious, inflammatory or the result of retinotoxic drugs, vitamin deficiencies, traumatic injuries and nonhereditary developmental defects. Evaluation and diagnosis of retinal diseases necessitates familiarity with the many ophthalmoscopic variations present in the normal canine and feline retina. Additional tests, such as the pupillary light reflex and behavior (vision) testing, and retinal function studies such as electroretinography can aid in localizing the lesion site and in determining the extent of the visual deficit.

## INFLAMMATORY RETINOPATHY

The close apposition of the retina and pigment epithelium to the choroid makes it very difficult, in some cases, to differentiate retinal from choroidal inflammations. Active retinitis and/or chorioretinitis is characterized ophthalmoscopically by cellular infiltrates, edema, retinal exudates, focal granulomas and bullous retinal detachments. Cellular infiltrates, the hallmark of inflammatory retinopathy, appear as dull gray, slightly raised areas with indistinct borders in the tapetal retina and as white to gray areas with indistinct borders in the nontapetal retina. Excessive accumulation of inflammatory exudates about retinal blood vessels will result in perivascular cuffing. Progression of the inflammatory retinal and/or retinochoroidal disease is characterized by enlargement of the lesion, the presence of satellite lesions with active inflammation and/or the extension of the lesion into the vitreous.

Healed or inactive retinitis results in focal to diffuse retinal atrophy, appearing as bright hyperreflective areas in the tapetal retina and as flat, pale to light brown areas of depigmentation in the nontapetal retina. Clusters of pigment within the hyperreflective foci are commonly seen and indicate the proliferation and migration of pigment epithelial cells. Attenuation and thinning of the retinal vascular tree are usually present following widespread retinal inflammatory disease.

Diffuse multifocal retinitis is most commonly seen with canine distemper infection. Widespread exudative retinitis and choroiditis are seen in cats with feline infectious peritonitis, as well as in some cases lymphosarcoma and toxoplasmosis. In toxoplasmosis, the lesions most often appear as small, multifocal granulomas. Granulomatous chorioretinitis is characteristic of the systemic mycosis. In many cases of inflammatory retinopathy, however, no known etiologic agent is recognizable.

The treatment of inflammatory retinal disease is frequently unrewarding. Specific therapy should be utilized when possible. In those cases in which corticosteroids are indicated, high levels can be administered systemically or by the retrobulbar route. Topical medication is not effective in treating inflammatory diseases of the posterior pole.

## RETINAL HEMORRHAGE

Retinal hemorrhages can be the result of trauma, inflammation, anemia, blood dyscrasias, lymphosarcoma and other lymphoproliferative malignancies. In a small number of collies affected with the collie ectasia syndrome, preretinal and vitreal hemorrhages are not uncommonly seen during routine ophthalmoscopic examination. The visual prognosis in these cases is poor, because extensive vitreal hemorrhages with secondary retinal detachments frequently occur.

Retinal hemorrhages are a common presenting sign of generalized hypertension in the dog. These hemorrhages occur perivascularly and intraretinally as well as superficially. Several dogs with hypertensive disease have presented with these signs unilaterally, the fellow eye having a complete intraocular hemorrhage. Clinical diagnosis of hypertension in the dog has been difficult because the blood pressure measuring instruments available for use in man cannot be used with any degree of reliability in the dog. Accurate diagnosis has been possible only by measuring the arterial blood pressure directly. Treatment of the hypertension with methyldopa (Aldomet®, Merck Sharp and Dohme, 80 mg./15 kg. given 2 times a day) in a small number of cases has been encouraging.

In general, retinal hemorrhages in small animals are most frequently seen following blunt trauma to the head and are located deep within the retinal layers (appearing as "dots") or more superficially within the nerve fiber layer (appearing flame-shaped). There is no treatment for retinal hemorrhages. Dot and flame-shaped hemorrhages reabsorb rather quickly, leaving almost no detectable ophthalmoscopic abnormalities. Preretinal and vitreal hemorrhages, especially the latter, are usually more extensive and have a poorer prognosis.

## NUTRITIONAL RETINOPATHY

Vitamin A deficiency in small animals results in night blindness followed by a widespread retinal degeneration. Except under very carefully controlled laboratory conditions, it is nearly impossible to produce vitamin A deficiency in a clinical situation. Vitamin A deficiency as a cause of retinal degeneration should be suspected only in animals with impaired fat absorption.

Cats fed purified experimental diets deficient in taurine, an aminosulfonic acid, develop retinal degeneration. The retinal lesions are similar, although progressive, to the ones seen in feline central retinal degeneration (see the section on Retinal Atrophy of the Cat, later in this article). They begin as focal lesions in the center of the area centralis and, as the animal continues to be fed the experimental diet, progress to band-shaped retinal lesions to be followed by complete retinal degeneration.

An analogous situation occurs clinically in cats whose diet consists exclusively of commercial dog food preparations. Many of these dog food diets are completely deficient in taurine, and cats fed on these diets develop a progressive retinal degeneration like that seen experimentally.

## RETINAL DETACHMENT

Retinal detachment is a separation of the retina from the overlying pigment epithelium. It can be partial or complete, the latter usually associated with a disinsertion of the retina at the ora serrata. The completely detached retina can appear to be funnel-shaped and located behind the lens, or can be folded and lying over and obscuring the optic nerve head.

Partial retinal detachments are exudative or solid. Solid or flat detachments can be the result of primary or metastatic tumors, while exudative detachments can be cystic or bullous and associated with retinal inflammation.

In animals, unlike man, surgical correction of retinal detachments is not recommended. Medical therapy for retinal detachments is also unsuccessful except in cases of exudative detachments associated with retinal inflammation.

Hereditary retinal detachments are present in several dog breeds. A retinal developmental defect (retinal dysplasia) occurs in the Bedlington terrier, Labrador retriever and Sealyham terrier and is characterized by blindness secondary to retinal detachments. The immature retina usually lies behind the lens in a funnel-shaped retinal detachment. Similarly, retinal detachments occur in some Australian shepherd dogs with hereditary microphthalmia, equatorial scleral staphylomas and abnormalities in the shape and position of the pupil. In the Old English sheepdog, retinal dysplasia can occur in association with congenital cataracts. In those breeds in which the heredity of retinal dysplasia has been investigated, a simple recessive inheritance occurs.

Hereditary retinal detachments occur in approximately 10 per cent of collies affected with the collie ectasia syndrome, a recessively inherited ocular disease which affects about 80 per cent of the breed. The lesions of the collie ectasia syndrome consist of avascularity and hypoplasia of the temporal choroid, peripapillary or posterior polar scleral ectasia and retinal detachments. An ophthalmoscopic diagnosis is possible at 5 to 6 weeks of age, and most of the dogs with retinal detachments are recognized at this time. In many cases, however, retinal detachments occur only in the affected adult collie. A disease similar to the collie ectasia syndrome is recognized in the Shetland sheepdog. Retinal detachments, however, are rare, and the exact mode of inheritance is unknown.

### RETINAL ATROPHY IN THE DOG

Hereditary retinal degenerations are the most common retinopathies recognized in dogs.

*Progressive retinal atrophy* (PRA) is a general term describing a number of outer retinal degenerations affecting a large variety of purebred as well as mongrel dogs. In general, the term PRA defines an end-stage retinal disease characterized ophthalmoscopically by retinal thinning, resulting in tapetal hyperreflectivity, marked retinal vascular attenuation and secondary atrophy

of the optic nerve head. These changes often appear most prominent in the equatorial and peripheral retinal regions where the caliber of the vessels is narrower than in the central regions.

At the time the dog is presented with the classic ophthalmoscopic abnormalities, there is invariably some degree of visual impairment, especially defective night vision. With progression of the disease, day vision deteriorates, and the dog ultimately becomes blind. In some dogs, especially the miniature and toy poodles, vision can be further impaired by the presence of cataracts, which frequently begin in dogs over 3 to 4 years of age. With time, these progress to affect the entire lens cortex, resulting in a complete, mature cataract.

PRA is recognized in a number of breeds. The following are some of the breeds affected with PRA and the age at which ophthalmoscopic abnormalities are present (taken in part from Barnett, 1969):

| BREED | AGE AFFECTED |
|---|---|
| Irish setter | 6 months |
| Cairn terrier | Under 1 year |
| Miniature long-haired dachshund | Under 1 year |
| Cardigan Welsh corgi | 6 months |
| Norwegian elkhound | 2 to 3 years |
| English cocker spaniel | 3 to 5 years |
| Miniature and toy poodles | 3 to 5 years |
| Collie | 1 year |
| Samoyed | About 3 years |
| Miniature schnauzer | 5 to 6 years |

In contrast to ophthalmoscopic diagnosis, a definitive diagnosis of PRA can be made with electroretinography by 6 weeks of age in Irish setters and Norwegian elkhounds and by 9.5 weeks of age in miniature poodles.

The inheritance of PRA has been thoroughly investigated only in the Irish setter, Norwegian elkhound and miniature and toy poodle, in which it is a simple recessive disorder. Although the inheritance pattern has not been investigated in the other breeds, it is most likely that the diseases are also inherited as simple recessive traits. As a general rule, dogs with PRA should be suspected of having an inheritable disorder, and owners should be advised against breeding.

At the present time, there is no known treatment for PRA. By the time the ophthalmoscopic abnormalities are recognized, widespread retinal degeneration has occurred.

Unlike PRA, *central progressive retinal*

*atrophy* (CPRA) is a specific pigment epithelial dystrophy. Pigment epithelial cells become hypertrophied and hyperplastic and cause a secondary retinal degeneration.

These abnormalities initially are present in the posterior pole just temporal to, and slightly above, the level of the optic disk. Ophthalmoscopically, these lesions are seen in dogs two to three years of age and appear as distinct focal areas of pigmentation. With progression of the disease, the zone of pigmentation spreads from the posterior pole into the retinal periphery. Thinning of the retinal vessels, although present, is not as marked as in PRA and occurs at a much later stage of the disease. An ophthalmoscopic finding present in many dogs with advanced CPRA is a "sheen" over the retinal surface, which interferes with critical focusing of retinal structures.

Although dogs with CPRA are able to see both at night and in the daytime, they are unable to see objects clearly, because the central retina—the area responsible for the best vision—is initially destroyed. Dogs affected with CPRA are able to see moving objects because movement of an object stimulates the normal peripheral visual fields. It is only when the object becomes stationary that the dog is unable to locate it.

CPRA is recognized in the Labrador and Golden retriever, Shetland sheepdog, Border collie, redboned coon hound and others. As with PRA, almost any breed can be affected.

Breeding studies which would detail the inheritance of CPRA are lacking. However, in the Labrador retriever it appears that the disease is inherited as dominant with variable penetrance (K. C. Barnett, personal communication). Until more is known about the inheritance of CPRA, it would be advisable not to use affected dogs or their progeny in a breeding program.

## RETINAL ATROPHY IN THE CAT

Retinal degeneration in cats is a frequently observed clinical entity. The disease is inherited as a simple recessive trait in the Persian breed, but in other breeds, as well as in domestic cats, sporadic cases of unknown etiology are usually the rule rather than the exception.

Retinal atrophy has been produced experimentally in the cat by feeding certain purified diets deficient in taurine. Whether or not dietary as well as "toxic" influences or even inflammatory diseases play a role in most clinical cases is unknown at this time. Regardless of cause, the ophthalmoscopic features of the disease are characterized, in the early cases, by tapetal granularity and retinal vascular thinning. With progression of the disease, there is a marked increase in tapetal reflectivity and loss of the retinal vessels. This latter finding can be so extensive that the retinal vessels may appear to be completely absent. At this stage of the disease, the cats are completely blind.

The age of onset is variable and may be entirely dependent on the actual cause of the disease. In Persian kittens, for example, definite ophthalmoscopic abnormalities are present by 10 to 12 weeks of age. Most sporadic cases, on the other hand, are usually seen after 6 to 12 months of age.

A specific disease of the area centralis is *feline central retinal degeneration* (FCRD). The ophthalmoscopic features of this disease are usually variable between animals, although the lesions are bilaterally symmetrical. The lesions can be small and rounded, involving only the center of the area centralis. In some cats, however, the lesions can be elliptically shaped, with prominent nasal extension or nasal satellites. Rarely, one can see a band-shaped atrophy of the retina in the posterior pole associated with an area centralis lesion. Regardless of the size or shape of the lesion, the center is always hyperreflective, while the periphery appears to have a more darkly "pigmented ridge." As the angle of the incident light changes, the reflectivity of the different areas in the lesion also appears to change.

It is probable that most if not all cases of feline central retinal degeneration result from taurine deficiency (see earlier under "Nutritional Retinopathy"). Cats with this retinal disease should be fed exclusively with cat food diets to arrest the progression of the disease.

An interesting feature of FCRD is that affected animals appear normal and usually show no obvious signs of visual deficit. When the electroretinogram is recorded, however, cone function abnormalities are present. This indicates that, although the ophthalmoscopic lesion is localized, the cone disease is present throughout the retina.

## SUPPLEMENTAL READING

Aguirre, G. D.: Progressive retinal atrophy in the miniature poodle: an electrophysiologic study. J. Am. Vet. Med. Assn., *160*:191–201, 1972.

Aguirre, G. D., and Rubin, L. F.: Progressive retinal atrophy (rod dysplasia) in the Norwegian elkhound. J. Am. Vet. Med. Assn., *158*:208–218, 1971.

Barnett, K. C.: Primary retinal dystrophies in the dog. J. Am. Vet. Med. Assn., *154*:804, 1969.

Rubin, L. F.: Atlas of Veterinary Ophthalmoscopy. Philadelphia, Lea & Febiger, 1974.

# DISEASES OF THE UVEAL TRACT, UVEITIS AND IMMUNO-LOGICALLY MEDIATED OCULAR DISORDERS

CRAIG A. FISCHER, D.V.M.
*St. Petersburg, Florida*

The anterior uveal tract is inflamed frequently and, because of its structure and function, it is involved in almost all intraocular inflammatory conditions. Of the three layers of the eye, the uveal tract lies between the external collagenous sclera and the internal and posteriorly situated retina. The majority of the intraocular tissues are nourished by blood or its derivatives, such as aqueous fluid formed from serum proteins, which eventually leads from the major and minor vascular channels of the uveal tract. Therefore, when uveal damage is prolonged and extensive, regardless of cause, there is extended intraocular hypotension, vascular compromise and hypoxic tissue degeneration resulting in phthisis bulbi.

Inflammatory processes of the anterior uveal tract (anterior uveitis or iridocyclitis) usually involve both the iris (iritis) and ciliary body (cyclitis), while those of the posterior uveal tract involve the choroid (choroiditis). Total uveal inflammation is termed panuveitis. Although not fully agreed upon, the terms ophthalmitis and panophthalmitis are reserved for those conditions in which all three layers of the eye, but particularly the uveal tract, are part of a septic inflammatory process highlighted by abscess formation in the vitreous body. The retina and choroid often share nonspecific inflammatory processes because of their close proximity, but retinochoroiditis and chorioretinitis are not interchangeable terms, as each points out the particular tissue which is thought to be initially and more severely affected.

## SIGNS AND SYMPTOMS

**Anterior Uveitis.** Obvious signs of ocular irritation, such as blepharospasm, photophobia, excessive lacrimation and follicular hyperplasia of the conjunctiva with discharge, are associated with many inflammatory conditions of either the anterior uveal tract or the cornea.

Pupillary constriction of the affected eye (miosis) is seen in both anterior uveitis and Horner's syndrome; the latter also has enophthalmos with protrusion of the nictitating membrane, ptosis but normal intraocular pressure. Concomitant central lens opacities coupled with miosis in anterior uveitis often result in a visual deficit in the affected eye. Less obvious manifestations of anterior uveitis are congestion of the short, brush-like deep circumcorneal vessels (ciliary injection), congestion and swelling of the iris stroma, sedimented exudates (hypopyon), and cellular and proteinaceous precipitates adhered to the posterior surface of the cornea (keratic precipitates). Similar precipitates may be seen on the anterior face of the iris. Fibrinocellular conglomerates in addition to pigment often adhere to the anterior surface of the lens. Irregularity of the outline of the pupil and mild to moderate anterior displacement of the face of the iris (iris bombé) are often overlooked. A head loupe to provide magnification and the use of a source of focal illumination are very helpful in performing an examination. The slit lamp biomicroscope is, however, the preferred instrument for examination.

A relatively easy but sensitive method of evaluating the presence of subtle or early anterior uveal inflammation is the determination of intraocular pressures (IOP). A decrease in IOP in the affected eye develops because of inhibition of the aqueous output by the ciliary body and increased aqueous uptake by the iridic vasculature. A decrease in IOP from normal (dog, 18 to 24 mm. Hg; cat, 20 to 25 mm. Hg) of 8 mm. Hg or more is indicative of anterior uveitis–induced intraocular hypotension. Just as important, quantitative tonometry gives the investigator a fixed value which one can use as a measure for therapeutic and/or spontaneous changes in condition (Table 1).

**Posterior Uveitis.** Disorders of the posterior uveal tract (choroid) are slightly less common in comparison with anterior uveal disease. Inflammatory processes adjacent to the ciliary body (peripheral uveitis) often produce exudates in the anterior vitreous, including fibrin strands, cells and pigment. There are usually concomitant signs of minimal anterior uveal involvement, such as mild ocular hypotony detectable by tonometry, conjunctival congestion, and pigment, fibrin and cells adhered to the anterior and posterior lens capsule. The peripheral fundus is best visualized by indirect ophthalmoscopy. In most cases, choroidal inflammatory disorders in their active stage are manifested by subretinal fluid accumulation, resulting in focal to diffuse cystic retinal detachment. Less frequently, focal, slightly elevated yellow (nontapetum) and gray (tapetum) lesions are observed in the fundus, indicating full thickness choroidal inflammation. Noticeable visual deficits associated with choroiditis depend on the extent and severity of the process. When the process subsides, chorioretinal adhesions are formed, usually with marked pigment redistribution in the adjacent retina (Table 1).

## PATHOGENESIS OF UVEITIS

In the past, inflammatory ocular diseases, directly initiated and mediated by known biologic agents and diagnosed and monitored by various testing procedures, have been emphasized. More frequent, however, and equally devastating to the eye, are those inflammatory disorders with less definable etiologic factors and, for many reasons, no demonstrable causative agent. Neverthe-

***Table 1.*** *Signs of Uveitis*

|  | ANTERIOR (IRITIS, IRIDOCYCLITIS) | POSTERIOR (CHRONIC CYCLITIS, CHORIORETINITIS) |
|---|---|---|
| Subjective | Pain, sensitivity to light, tearing, redness (ciliary injection), visual loss | Visual loss |
| Objective | Decreased intraocular pressure, fibrin, cells in anterior chamber | Vitreous opacities (cells, fibrin) |
|  | Congestion and swelling of the iris | Infiltration and membrane formation in pars ciliaris retinae |
|  | Hemorrhages in iris stroma | Chorioretinal foci; central near optic disk; peripheral near pars ciliaris retinae, or disseminated |
|  | Hypopyon, hyphema | |
|  | Keratitis | |
|  | Posterior synechiae | Chorioretinal scars |
|  | Nodules in iris stroma or at the pupillary border | Exudative detachment of the retina |
|  | Iris bombé | Intrabulbar optic neuritis |
|  | Iris atrophy at pupillary border in the stroma | Vasculitis (retina) |
|  | Secondary glaucoma | |

less, there appear to be certain pathobiologic processes which are common to all inflammatory reactions, and it is the understanding of these factors that has brought about new and more effective therapy.

Factors which influence intraocular inflammation are: (1) stimulus, (2) host response and, most important, (3) integrity of ocular structures (Fig. 1). The degree of severity and duration of the inflammatory cycle are governed largely by the potency, quantity and duration of the stimulus. The cumulative effect of these factors determines the degree of intraocular vascular compromise, fibrosis and tissue structural alteration. The greater the degree of structural alteration of the ocular tissues, the greater the probability of continuation or recurrence of inflammation and eventual total loss of function.

The ability of the uveal tract to manifest dramatic, prolonged, immunologically mediated inflammatory reactions may be rationalized if the uveal tract is equated with lymph nodes, with the overlying sclera as its capsule. In early life, lymph nodes are seeded with two types of potential immunocytes (lymphocytes and their precursors). Those lymphocytes derived from the bone marrow are short-lived, produce circulating antibody and initiate and mediate immediate hypersensitivity responses. Thymus-derived lymphocytes are long-lived, become sensitized and actively initiate and regulate local delayed hypersensitivity responses. When one and especially both immune systems are activated by antigenic stimuli, there is a resultant local inflammation and lymphoid hyperplasia in the lymph node.

Because of its intimate contact with systemic circulation and favorable microstructure, the uveal tract of the eye is similarly seeded with the two types of immune mediators which can activate and/or mediate local intraocular inflammation in the presence of a variety of antigens. Furthermore, it appears that, once the eye is seeded with the immunocytes, the potential for reactivation of immune processes, in the presence of antigen, remains for long periods and increases with age. Regardless of the initiating cause and once the immune process begins, there is subsequent cell death, intensification of the inflammatory process and tissue structural alteration (Fig. 1). Whereas fibrosis, as part of the healing reaction in other organs, is a benign result of inflammation, in the eye it often leads to loss of tissue function and blindness. There-

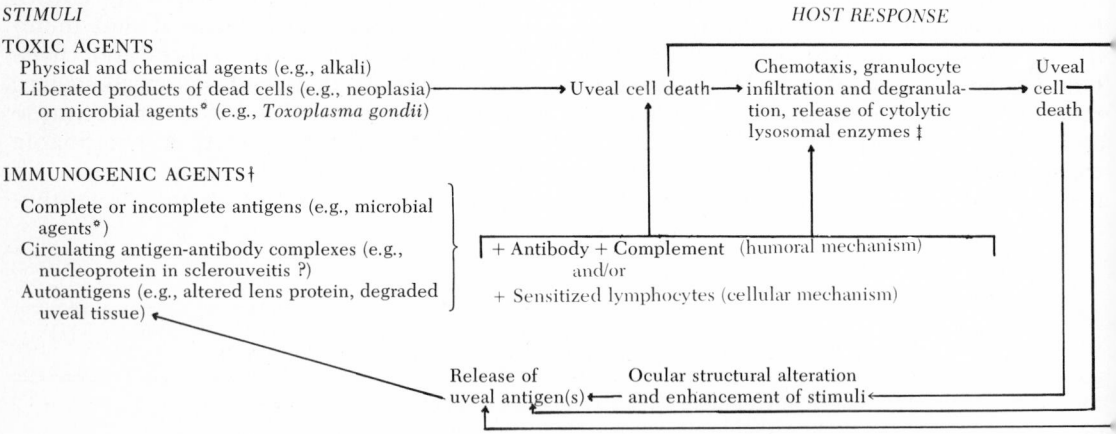

*STIMULI*                                                                                           *HOST RESPONSE*

TOXIC AGENTS
 Physical and chemical agents (e.g., alkali)
 Liberated products of dead cells (e.g., neoplasia) ———→ Uveal cell death ——→ Chemotaxis, granulocyte      Uveal
  or microbial agents° (e.g., *Toxoplasma gondii*)                              infiltration and degranula- ——→ cell
                                                                               tion, release of cytolytic       death
                                                                               lysosomal enzymes ‡

IMMUNOGENIC AGENTS†
 Complete or incomplete antigens (e.g., microbial
  agents°)
 Circulating antigen-antibody complexes (e.g.,            + Antibody + Complement  (humoral mechanism)
  nucleoprotein in sclerouveitis ?)                           and/or
 Autoantigens (e.g., altered lens protein, degraded       + Sensitized lymphocytes (cellular mechanism)
  uveal tissue)

                                    Release of          Ocular structural alteration
                                    uveal antigen(s) ←— and enhancement of stimuli ←

*STRUCTURAL ALTERATION*

*CHRONIC (RECURRENT) INFLAMMATORY PHASE*

The degree of severity and the final outcome of the uveal inflammatory episode, defined in terms of structural alteration, depend on the *potency, quantity* and *duration* of the stimulus (e.g., nonreplicating agents generally lead to less structural alteration than replicating agents).

°Antimicrobial intervention inhibits this step.
†Immunosuppressive intervention inhibits this step.
‡Corticosteroid intervention inhibits this step.

**Figure 1.**   The common inflammatory pathway of uveitis with therapeutic intervention.

fore, the significant theme in the treatment of most uveal inflammatory conditions is to quickly and effectively suppress the inflammatory cycle by inhibiting as many of the separate steps, including the immune reaction, as possible.

Nonimmunologic host responses, such as the release of certain forms of prostaglandins, are now also known to play significant roles in intensifying intraocular inflammatory reactions.

Stimuli in the form of toxic agents may be necrotizing, such as chemical or physical agents. For example, strong alkaline chemicals placed on the corneal surface will be absorbed into the anterior chamber, thus altering the pH which results in lysis of cells lining the anterior and posterior chamber, with resultant iridocyclitis. Other necrotizing toxic agents, such as degenerating neoplastic cells, release cytolytic products resulting again in iridocyclitis (Fig. 1). Toxic factors, which in themselves are non-necrotizing but trigger the acute inflammatory pathway (Fig. 1), are materials such as starch, gut sutures and silk sutures.

Exogenous antigens may be complete, such as organic pollens, or incomplete, such as certain drugs which require further molecular change before activating the immune system. Endogenous antigens may be autoantigens, which are certain normal cellular or cell-derived components such as lens protein which the immune system failed to recognized as "self." The immune system recognizes these "new" molecules as "foreign" and reacts accordingly, and is exemplified in the lens induced uveitis reaction. Circulating antigen-antibody complexes formed from combinations of humoral antibody with exogenous stimuli such as streptococcal antigen or endogenous antigens have the potential of triggering events in the common inflammatory pathway once these complexes reach the uveal tract via the circulatory system. Regardless of the stimuli, however, uveal cell death is initiated and its products trigger the infiltration of granulocytes, particularly polymorphonuclear cells, which release toxic lysosomal enzymes; these, in turn, perpetuate further cytolysis, resulting in the liberation of degraded uveal tissue which, in itself, is potentially immunogenic (Fig. 1).

Until recently, much emphasis has been placed on the classification of uveal reactions as being suppurative or nonsuppurative, granulomatous or nongranulomatous. Certain criteria are assigned to each category and, in some cases, the type of inflammatory pattern is clearcut and is beneficial in defining certain etiologic factors (e.g., suppurative keratouveitis caused by *Pseudomonas aeruginosa* and granulomatous panuveitis caused by the feline infectious peritonitis agent). This approach, however, is less than satisfactory in the majority of uveal inflammatory disorders presented clinically to the general practitioner, because the criteria for this classification are often difficult, if not impossible, to recognize. More satisfactory is the unifying concept of the uveal inflammatory cycle presented in Figure 1, as it incorporates the rationale that almost any stimulus, if potent and in large quantities, will set off an acute inflammatory response which will be initially suppurative in clinical appearance.

Trauma (Table 2), particularly direct blows to and about the head, often results in one or both eyes with subconjunctival and intraocular hemorrhage, either in the anterior segment and/or posterior segment of the eye. On occasion, the base of the iris and the adjacent ciliary body become disinserted from their fibrous scleral base and become anteriorly displaced, obliterating the aqueous outflow channels. There is usually pooling of blood in and subjacent to the ciliary body and, when extensive, the entire complex (disinsertion and hemorrhage) can lead to intractable secondary glaucoma.

Hemorrhage due to trauma into the anterior chamber, which is always accompanied by uveal inflammation, is treated with topical corticosteroids (1 per cent Inflammase Forte® [Smith, Miller and Patch] or 1 per cent Prednefrin Forte® [Allergan]) and 0.3 to 0.5 ml. subconjunctival corticosteroids (Depo-Medrol®, 40 mg./ml., or Vetalog® [Upjohn], 6 mg./ml.) and mydriatics such as 1 per cent to 4 per cent atropine sulfate ophthalmic solutions. Hemorrhage into the vitreous is treated with 0.3 ml. corticosteroids (Depo-Medrol, 40 mg./ml.) deposited in the sclera under the capsule of Tenon and near the equator of the eye, plus topical mydriatics. Optic nerve contusion with loss of vision is treated with retrobulbarly administered 0.5 to 0.7 ml. corticosteroids (Depo-Medrol, 40

**Table 2.** *Specific and Nonspecific Uveal Disorders*

Traumatic disorders*

Microbial diseases
  Bacteria
  Viruses
    Infectious canine hepatitis (ICH), postvaccinal anterior uveitis*
    Feline infectious peritonitis* (cats)
    Herpes keratouveitis (cats and dogs)
    Canine distemper
  Fungi
    Cryptococcosis*
    Coccidioidomycosis
    Blastomycosis*
    Nocardiosis
    Histoplasmosis
    Candidiasis
    Paecilomycosis
    Aspergillosis
Parasites
  Toxoplasmosis (cats)
  Ascariasis
  Filariasis
Microbial and parasitic hypersensitivity diseases
  Toxoplasmosis (dogs and cats)
  Leptospirosis
  Streptococcosis
  Histoplasmosis
Auto-immune diseases
  Lens induced uveitis
  Necrogranulomatous sclerouveitis
Neoplastic diseases
  Primary uveal neoplasms
  Secondary uveal neoplasms
Idiopathic clinical and histopathologic syndromes of uveitis associated with other systemic diseases

*Probably the most common disorder in some etiologic categories in dogs and cats.

mg./ml.). This anti-inflammatory therapy rationale persists through most uveal inflammatory conditions and is the principal means of inhibiting the possibility of intractable structural alteration of the eye. Mydriatics are used to prevent adhesion-forming blood clots which can obliterate the pupillary space. Fibrinolytic enzymes administered subconjunctivally or otherwise have questionable effect.

Bacteria in animals generally have no unusual intraocular affinity. They affect the uveal tract in conditions of penetrating ocular injuries, in overwhelmong septicemias and when certain agents, particularly *Pseudomonas aeruginosa*, liberate diffusible toxins in deep progressive keratitis.

Viral agents directly affecting the uveal tract are far more common than bacteria. The infectious canine hepatitis (ICH) adenovirus type 1 initially attacks the endothelial cells of the uveal vascular channels in addition to those on the posterior surface of the cornea. There is an intense inflammatory reaction initiated by widespread endothelial cytolysis. Circulating antibody adhering to viral antigen, with subsequent complement-binding and release of lysosomal enzymes with further cellular destruction (Fig. 1), increases the inflammatory response. Damage to the endothelial cells of the cornea causes inhibition of the normal corneal hydration balance, resulting in corneal edema and the "blue eye" appearance.

The initial inflammatory reaction, with marked exudation and structural alteration, is so intense that secondary complications, despite quick and intense therapy, occur with disturbing frequency. These complications include: (1) persistent corneal edema with bullous keratopathy; (2) secondary glaucoma caused by either diffuse peripheral anterior synechia or pupillary seclusion leading to iris bombé; or (3) phthisis bulbi. Anterior uveitis usually develops 7 to 10 days after the animal is initially vaccinated with modified live canine hepatitis virus and rarely occurs on subsequent vaccinations with the same virus.

Therapy of adenovirus type 1 (ICH) uveitis must be quick, intense and persistent. Corticosteroids given subconjunctivally and topically are used, but the intensity of the inflammatory response is often overwhelming and surpasses the effect of corticosteroids. Dilatation of the pupil with mydriatics is most important and is the greatest deterrent against the complication of secondary glaucoma. In most cases, topical atropine sulfate ophthalmic solutions in concentrations greater than 1 per cent are needed. Atropine sulfate (a parasympatholytic drug) may be combined with other mydriatics such as phenylephrine hydrochloride, 10 per cent (a direct-acting sympathomimetic drug), to create an additive effect. Initially, mydriatic drops may be required every two hours to produce dilatation.

The most common cause of unilateral or bilateral granulomatous uveitis in cats is the feline infectious peritonitis (FIP) agent which is thought to be a virus. Immunologic intervention in the perpetuation of the dramatic vascular lesions appears to be a major factor, and the ocular changes may very well progress without the direct presence of the agent. Generally, the anterior chamber becomes cloudy with cells and fibrin early in the process. Dilated vascular channels on the surface of the iris, along with intense iridal swelling, are easily observable. The conglomeration of fibrin, concentrated serum protein and acute and chronic inflammatory cells may present as hypopyon or, more commonly, as large "mutton fat" keratic precipitates. These ocular manifestations, along with hyperproteinemia (>8.0 gm./100 ml.) and a reversed A/G ratio with or without peritoneal or thoracic effusions, are rather diagnostic of FIP. There may be, however, no anterior uveal involvement early in the disease but rather lesions confined to the posterior segment of the eye. These include focal choroidal pyogranulomas with or without retinal vasculitis, with perivascular exudates. Generally, when the hyperproteinemia exceeds 9.0 gm./100 ml., the retinal vessels appear dilated and assume unusually straight patterns. In over 50 per cent of those cases of FIP with ocular involvement, there is clinical and/or histopathologic evidence of meningitis.

Whereas exposure rates to systemic fungal agents may be quite high in certain areas of the United States, clinical disease appears only in those animals that have been excessively exposed or in those with defective immune responses. Once these agents reach the vascular system, usually through the respiratory tract, anterior and/or posterior uveitis is quite common and is often observed prior to manifestations of disorders in other organs. The inflammatory response to these agents is granulomatous or pyogranulomatous, with the formation of keratic precipitates anteriorly and cystic retinal detachments and subretinal granulomas posteriorly. Cryptococcosis found in dogs, cats and most other species of animals is one of the most common systemic fungal disease affecting the eye and may be treated systemically (see article on "Systemic Mycotic Pneumonias") and locally with mydriatics. There is generally a concomitant diffuse pyogranulomatous pneumonia and meningitis. Uveal involvement may occur in systemic blastomycosis, nocardiosis, coccidioidomycosis, aspergillosis, paecilomycosis and candidiasis. The *Histoplasma* agent may be directly found in the choroid or may be related to uveal hypersensitivity reactions without the direct presence of the organism.

*Toxoplasma gondii* appears to incite intraocular inflammation either by being present in the ocular tissues or by stimulating a uveal tract-oriented immunogenic response while being present elsewhere in the body (brain, heart, liver, diaphragmatic and extraocular muscles and lymph nodes). In cats, the direct presence of the organism in intraocular tissue may cause a multifocal fulminating retinochoroiditis, optic neuritis and granulomatous anterior uveitis.

Paired serologic examinations five weeks apart in the face of intraocular inflammation are essential for the diagnosis of toxoplasmosis. Early in the disease, a serum sample may reveal a substantial raise (>1:256) in antibody titer against *Toxoplasma gondii* on the Sabin-Feldman (S-F) dye test or on the more recent hemagglutination test. Complement-fixing antibody titers are absent in this stage. Five to six weeks later, the S-F dye test or hemagglutinating antibody titers show at least a fourfold rise and often exceed dilutions of 1:1026, and complement-fixation antibody titers are generally 1:8 to 1:64. In those animals with defective immune systems (e.g., puppies with concomitant canine distemper infections or adult animals with lymphoma), the serologic tests for *Toxoplasma gondii* are often negative because of immunosuppression.

## TREATMENT

Treatment in most cases of ocular toxoplasmosis is subconjunctival, systemic and topical corticosteroids, depending on the severity and location of the inflammation. In cats with fulminating retinochoroiditis and optic neuritis, one may choose to deal directly with the organism by administering pyrimethamine (Daraprim®, Burroughs Wellcome), an antimetabolite and folic acid inhibitor administered orally at 2 mg./lb./day in two divided doses for three days. This is followed by 1 mg./kg./day in two divided doses every other day for 10 to 21 days, depending on the clinical response.

Sulfadiazine should be administered concomitantly with pyrimethamine orally at 2 mg./kg./day, four times daily for 14 to 21 days, until reevaluation of therapy has been undertaken. Sulfadiazine is a powerful paraaminobenzoic acid (P.A.B.A.) inhibitor, a substance critical for the growth and multiplication of the toxoplasmosis agent.

Signs of toxicity, such as anorexia, emesis, diarrhea and malaise, are to be expected but may be effectively counteracted with folinic acid (calcium leucovorin) given intramuscularly at 1 mg. (0.35 ml.)/day during pyrimethamine therapy. Hospitalization is advised during the course of this treatment regimen, as complete blood counts including total platelet counts are indicated every fifth day because bone marrow depression may be another complicating factor. Chlortetracycline hydrochloride (Aureomycin®, Lederle) given orally at 30 mg./kg./day in four divided doses for 14 to 21 days may be substituted for pyrimethamine, although its mechanism of action with protozoa is not well understood.

The anti-inflammatory effects of corticosteroids are necessary, along with the antiparasitic therapy, to preserve ocular structural integrity during active infection. Oral administration of prednisone at 2 mg./kg./day is usually effective and should be slowly decreased as the inflammatory process subsides. Owners of affected animals should be warned of the possible zoonotic hazards of toxoplasmosis.

Focal choroidal and retinal lesions caused by ascarid larval migrations are more common than most investigators suspect, although clinical manifestations are rare because of their usual confinement of activity to the posterior segment of the eye. Filarial worms are present in many species of animals but are uncommon. Tropical birds, however, should be suspected of having filarial uveitis when intraocular inflammation is mild but persistent. Close observation often reveals the filarial worm to be alive and moving in the anterior chamber or dead and sedimented to the inferior chamber angle area.

Neoplastic diseases should be suspected in uveal inflammatory disorders which tend to be granulomatous in character. In other words, the ignition of the common inflammatory pathway in the uveal tract (Fig. 1) due to lysis of neoplastic and degraded healthy cells often overshadows the space-occupying feature of the neoplastic mass.

Melanomas, either slowly developing or rapidly growing, are the most common primary intraocular tumor in small animals and appear to originate solely in the anterior uveal tract. Rarely do they invade the immediate extraocular tissues, but systemic metastasis must be suspected. Ciliary body adenomas and adenocarcinomas, as with all primary intraocular neoplasms, are generally unilateral and are second to melanomas in frequency but rarely metastasize. Usually intraocular neoplasms are presented in an advanced state, and enucleation, with rapid histopathologic confirmation, is the treatment of choice. If primary uveal neoplasms are focal, however, excision biopsy procedures may be considered. If the choroid is suspected of being involved in a neoplastic process, then systemic metastasis or rarely extraocular invasive tumorous processes must be considered.

Ocular metastasis, involving both eyes in more than 25 per cent of cases, is quite common and generally involves the anterior uveal tract with or without choroidal invasion. Lymphoreticular neoplasms (lymphoma, etc.) are the most common metastasizing tumors, although the ocular adnexa and globe may be a primary site, and often appear similar to granulomatous diseases. Carcinomas (mammary gland, prostate, etc.) are second and hemangiomatous tumors are third in frequency. Diagnostically, cytologic examination of aqueous, vitreous or subretinal fluid is a rapid method of classifying intraocular neoplasms and provides a framework for prognosis or therapy.

Many cases of uveitis have no apparent etiologic factor(s), although there may appear to be some pattern of clinical relationship with concomitant nonocular disorders. Persistent anterior and/or posterior uveitis or focal retinal degeneration may be associated with destruction of tissue of the central nervous system (CNS) by primary or secondary CNS neoplasms or by inflammatory encephalitic or encephalomyelitic disorders. Uveitis may also be related to clinical and subclinical urinary infections and transient idiopathic peripheral lymphadenopathy appear to be uveitis-related.

One possibility of relationship is in "antigen sharing," in which certain tissues of the body (e.g., neuronal material, myelin and pigment of the CNS), when altered by various means, release large amounts of antigenic factors, some of which may be identical to components normally found in the uveal tract. When the immune system becomes sensitized and mounts its response against this overwhelming amount of "foreign material," the antigen-antibody interaction with subsequent inflammation (Fig. 1) takes place not only at the primary source of antigenic pooling (e.g., CNS) but also in the uveal tract where certain components, previously considered normal, are now attacked by sensitized immunologic mediators.

## IMMUNOLOGICALLY MEDIATED OCULAR DISORDERS

Besides the presence of immune mechanisms specific in certain steps of the common inflammatory cycle, there are certain ocular diseases which appear to be primarily initiated and predominantly mediated by events intrinsic to and surrounding the antigen-antibody reaction. One example in which immunologic factors dominate the promotion and prolongation of ocular inflammation is in the case of lens induced uveitis (LIU). The sequence of events in LIU is as follows: (1) cataract formation; (2) solubilization of lens protein and diffusion of this material through the altered lens capsule into the general circulation via the uveal vasculature and outflow channels; (3) recognition and sensitization of immunocytes to the "foreign" lens protein; (4) infiltration of sensitized immunocytes into the uveal tract, some with the potential of participating in cellular immune reactions and others capable of producing soluble (humoral) antibody; and (5) initiation and mediation of the inflammatory cycle when antibody and sensitized lympocytes interact with antigen (lens protein) with local lymphoid hyperplasia.

Unless the antigenic substance (lens protein) is removed, the immune reaction remains stimulated and inflammation progresses. Therefore, intracapsular lens extraction, thorough flushing of the anterior and posterior chambers and liberal administration of topical and subconjunctival corticosteroids are the treatment of choice.

The immune system may also recognize normal tissue, which has been altered by various means (microbial invasion, trauma, anoxia, etc.), as being "foreign" and subsequently reacts, which may be the mechanism of necrogranulomatous sclerouveitis in dogs. This condition is a persistent intractable inflammatory disease, usually appearing bilaterally but not necessarily at the same time, of the deep sclera in which the adjacent uveal inflammation is dominated by lymphoid proliferation. The sclera is focally or diffusely thickened and appears light brown. The adjacent circumlimbal cornea is usually gray owing to edema and cellular infiltration. Systemic and intralesional corticosteroids may relieve the inflammation for a short period, but eventually intractable secondary glaucoma and/or suspicion of a malignant neoplasm leads to loss of the eye.

One or more immune parameters such as anti-DNA antibody, positive direct Coombs' test, positive canine rheumatoid factor and positive LE preparations are often present, indicating that canine necrogranulomatous sclerouveitis is one manifestation of a systemic rejection of certain tissues. In this case, circulating antigen-antibody complexes may also enter into the initiation of scleral inflammation (Fig. 1). Signs of shifting lameness with joint effusions (rheumatoid arthritis), albuminuria and renal casts (glomerulonephritis), anemia (hemolytic anemia), acquired heart murmurs (cardiac valvular disease), etc. should be evaluated.

Necrogranulomatous sclerouveitis is not to be confused with benign lymphoid hyperplasia which occurs in the subconjunctival tissues adjacent to the cornea. Sclerouveitis is now treated with a combination of corticosteroids and immunosuppressive drugs after partial excision biopsy is performed and the diagnosis is confirmed. Cyclophosphamide (Cytoxan®, Mead Johnson), a cytotoxic alkylating agent, is administered orally at 2.5 mg./kg./day in two divided doses for the first week, and 2.5 mg./kg./day in two divided doses thereafter, and may be continued as a maintenance dose until full remission of the lesion is achieved. Hematocrit and leukocyte counts, including total platelet counts, are necessary as a weekly surveillance of bone marrow depression. Cyclophosphamide should be temporarily withdrawn if the total leukocyte count falls below 4000/cu. mm., if anemia becomes severe or if the total platelet count falls below 50,000/cu. mm. Other complications may be anorexia, emesis, diarrhea, hemorrhagic cystitis and hair loss.

Oral prednisone administered orally at 2 mg./kg./day in two to three divided doses is initiated along with cyclophosphamide. This is gradually reduced to 0.5 mg./kg./day, which may be continued as a maintenance dose level. ACTH (Acthar®, Armour), 80 units intramuscularly, is given after the third week of therapy and every third week thereafter if high levels of corticosteroids are continued.

## SUPPLEMENTAL READING

Aronson, S. B., and Elliott, J. H.: Ocular Inflammation. St. Louis, The C. V. Mosby Co., 1972.

Henkind, P., and Friedman, A. H. (eds.): Physician's Desk Reference for Ophthalmology. Oradell, N.J., Medical Economics Co., 1972.

Kaufman, H. (ed.): Ocular Anti-Inflammatory Therapy. Springfield, Ill., Charles C Thomas, 1970.

Maumenee, E. A., and Silverstein, A. M. (eds.): Immunopathology of Uveitis. Baltimore, The Williams & Wilkins Co., 1964.

# TREATMENT OF GLAUCOMAS IN THE DOG

KIRK N. GELATT, V.M.D.,
ROBERT L. PEIFFER, JR., D.V.M.,
and ROBERT M. GWIN, D.V.M.
Gainesville, Florida

Glaucomas include ocular diseases that exhibit increased levels of intraocular pressure which are detrimental to the maintenance of ocular health and vision. For convenience, glaucomas are divided clinically into three main types: (1) primary, (2) secondary and (3) congenital. In primary glaucoma, no overt abnormalities for the elevated intraocular pressure can be detected. Secondary glaucomas represent the largest group, with causes varying from iridocyclitis, intumescent cataracts and hyphemas to intraocular neoplasms. The congenital glaucomas usually exhibit goniodysgenesis.

## CLINICAL SIGNS

For optimal clinical management of the glaucomas, clinical signs should be analyzed individually and collectively and, if at all possible, the most likely cause of the glaucoma should be determined. Reliance on only 1 or 2 clinical signs for the diagnosis of glaucoma will invariably confuse the process with other diseases of the cornea, anterior uvea and ocular fundi. The diagnosis of glaucoma must be timely, since the elevated intraocular pressure can produce irreversible damage to the optic disk and ocular fundus. Once the disease process has been sufficiently analyzed, vigorous medical treatment should be initiated.

The clinical signs of glaucomas in the dog include all or some of the following: mydriasis, corneal edema, congestion of the conjunctival and episcleral veins, buphthalmia, ocular pain, lens luxation (e.g., subluxation, anterior and posterior luxation) and retinal and optic disk changes. The intensity of these clinical signs will vary based on the duration of the disease and the contributing factors. We believe that many glaucomas actually represent a chronic process that usually presents clinically at an advanced stage, not infrequently as one of the congestive types (Table 1).

**Table 1.** Breeds of Dogs Reported With Glaucoma

American cocker spaniel
Basset hound
Beagle
Brittany spaniel
Cairn terrier
Chihuahua
English cocker spaniel
Fox terrier (smooth and wire-haired)
Jack Russell terrier
Manchester terrier
Norwegian elkhound
Miniature and toy poodle
Sealyham terrier
Springer spaniel
Welsh corgi

This work was supported in part by U.S.P.H.S. Grant #EY 01465-02, and Special U.S.P.H.S. Fellowships #EY 01977-02 (Peiffer) and #EY 05100-01 (Gwin).

## DIAGNOSTIC METHODS

Adequate management of the glaucomatous patient requires consecutive examinations with tonometry, gonioscopy, ophthalmoscopy and slit lamp biomicroscopy.

**Tonometry.** Both indentation and applanation tonometric instruments may be used to estimate intraocular pressure (intraocular tension) in the dog. The less expensive Schiötz tonometer provides a reasonable estimation of intraocular pressure using a standard method with proper positioning of the instrument on the center of the cornea. The normal range of intraocular pressure in the dog is 15 to 25 mm. Hg (Schiötz). The upper range of normalcy in the dog may even extend to 30 mm. Hg (Schiötz) using the human calibration tables for the instrument.

**Gonioscopy.** Gonioscopic examination of the anterior chamber angle is essential for determination of the type of glaucoma and of the best methods of treatment. The clinical classification of glaucoma is based on gonioscopy, since only gonioscopy allows the following observations: open angle, narrow angle, closed angle, recessed angle, anomalous angle, peripheral anterior synechiae, and so on. The intraocular pressure of many glaucomatous globes not infrequently necessitates immediate medical treatment to reduce intraocular pressure and corneal edema sufficiently to permit detailed gonioscopic examinations. The Franklin, Troncoso, Koeppe or Cardona direct goniolenses can be used in the dog. Both eyes should be examined.

**Ophthalmoscopy.** Ophthalmoscopy (direct and/or indirect) is imperative for analysis of the tapetal and nontapetal fundi, retinal blood vessels and the optic disk. Cupping of the optic disk occurs, in our opinion, more frequently than is reported but is difficult to recognize in its early stages because of the wide anatomic variations of the normal optic disk. In a laboratory environment and by means of consecutive fundus photographs of beagles bred for glaucoma, cupping of the optic disk can be detected in early to moderate stages of the disease. The cupping is evident with gradual progressive enlargement and excavation of the normal physiologic cup.

**Other Methods.** We should not be satisfied with the existing diagnostic procedures for the canine glaucomas. Although still very new, the different provocative tests (water, mydriatic) and tonography offer additional parameters with which the state of aqueous humor dynamics can be analyzed. Our limited experience shows that these tests may be more useful for certain types of glaucoma than for others. The water provocative tests in primary glaucoma of the beagle can distinguish the control dogs from early glaucomatous dogs at 1 year of age.

## EFFECTS IN SPECIFIC BREEDS

Most forms of glaucoma in the dog occur in association with reduced rate of outflow of aqueous humor through the anterior chamber angle. The uveoscleral outflow channels in the dog have not been studied. Glaucoma in the American cocker spaniel has been generally believed to be a narrow-to-closed angle type; however, a recent report described a cocker with goniodysgenesis, i.e., a pigmented, partial to complete sheet of mesodermal tissue superimposed above or dispersed among the pectinate ligaments. To enter the filtration angle, aqueous humor would need to traverse "flow holes" within the sheets or other areas of seemingly normal angle. Glaucoma in the basset hound is also characterized by goniodysgenesis, with the persistence of broad sheets of mesodermal tissues bridging the inner limbus. In both breeds with these angle anomalies a direct relationship between the deformities and reduced aqueous humor outflow has not been established. Frequently, the acute congestive glaucoma in the basset hound is complicated by concurrent iridocyclitis.

Primary glaucoma in the beagle is characterized by an open iridocorneal angle. In its advanced stages the anterior chamber angle may be open, narrow or closed, influenced by the degree of buphthalmia, position(s) of the luxated lens and alterations and/or displacement of the vitreous humor.

Glaucomas in toy and miniature poodles may be either open- or closed-angle, so that gonioscopy is necessary in order to differentiate the two types. Although goniodysgenesis has been described in the wire-haired fox terrier, lens removal in the early stages of glaucoma in this breed may successfully prevent recurrence of elevated pressures.

The frequency of glaucoma may be increasing in selected breeds because of their popularity. Frequency is also influenced by improved veterinary diagnostic abilities, increased number of referral patients and continued pressure by the public for better veterinary services and care.

The clinical signs of glaucoma may vary depending on the antecedent disease(s). Based on the classification depicted in Table 2, the various types of glaucoma, clinical signs and medical and/or surgical treatments can be divided into a number of categories to permit some generalizations.

## PRIMARY GLAUCOMA

**Open-angle.** Primary open-angle glaucoma in the beagle is characterized by an insidious, chronic increase in intraocular pressure (30 to 40 mm. Hg, Mackay-Marg tonometry), with resulting buphthalmia, mild mydriasis, elongation of the ciliary processes and mild episcleral and conjunctival congestion. The disease is usually apparent bilaterally in beagles from 6 to 18 months of age. The zonules eventually tear with subluxation that may progress to anterior or posterior luxation. Cupping and atrophy of the optic disk are evident in most glaucomatous dogs, with blindness occurring by 3 to 4 years of age without therapy. Intraocular pressure rises progressively above normal and after lens luxation can

vary markedly, probably influenced by the position of the lens and vitreous body.

Glaucoma in the beagle can be controlled satisfactorily by miotics, such as demecarium bromide or echothiophate iodide, before lens luxation. However, after lens luxation, because the iridocorneal angle may be either open or closed, removal of the lens and miotic therapy are recommended when the angle is open. If the iridocorneal angle is closed, the lens is removed, and an iridencleisis or cyclodialysis is recommended. The prognosis is more favorable if the angle is open.

**Narrow- or Closed-angle.** Glaucoma in the American cocker spaniel is generally accepted as a narrow- to closed-angle type. However, in at least one cocker, persistent mesodermal sheets of tissue bridged the iridocorneal angle. In some dogs, several episodes of transient corneal edema may precede presentation of the dog with acute congestive glaucoma.

The signs of acute glaucoma in the cocker include corneal edema, mydriasis and intense congestion of the conjunctival and episcleral vessels, and intraocular pressure frequently exceeds 80 mm. Hg (Mackay-Marg). Because of the corneal edema, the iridocorneal angle, position of the lens and the ocular fundus cannot be adequately examined. Intraocular pressure is usually rapidly reduced by intravenous mannitol and acetazolamide (Table 3) and topical 2

*Table 2.* *Classification of Glaucomas in the Dog*

I. Primary Glaucoma
  A. Open-angle (beagle)
  B. Narrow-angle (American cocker spaniel)
II. Secondary Glaucoma
  A. Lens-Induced
    1. Luxation (subluxation, anterior and posterior luxation (wire-haired fox terrier)
    2. Phacolytic glaucoma
    3. Lens-induced uveitis
    4. Intumescent cataract
  B. Traumatic
    1. Intraocular hemorrhage (hyphema)
    2. Intraocular foreign bodies
  C. Inflammatory
    1. Angle obstruction with inflammatory cells and fibrin
    2. Peripheral anterior synechiae
    3. Pupillary obstruction with iris bombé
  D. Intraocular Tumors
    1. Primary
    2. Secondary
III. Congenital Glaucoma
  A. Mesodermal goniodysgenesis (basset hound)
  B. Other anterior segment anomalies

*Table 3.* *Recommended Drugs and Dosages for the Treatment of Glaucomas in the Dog*

I. Miotics
  A. 2-4% Pilocarpine hydrochloride or nitrate—b.i.d. to q.i.d.
  B. 0.75-3.0% Carbachol—b.i.d. to q.i.d.
  C. 0.125-0.25% Echothiophate iodide—s.i.d. to b.i.d.
  D. 0.125-0.25% Demecarium bromide—s.i.d. to b.i.d.
II. Osmotic Agents
  A. Glycerol—1-2 ml./kg. orally preop to b.i.d.
  B. Mannitol—1-2 gm./kg. IV preop
III. Diuretics
  A. Acetazolamide—10 mg./kg. b.i.d. orally (10 mg./kg. IV)
  B. Dichlorphenamide—10 mg./kg. b.i.d. to t.i.d. orally
  C. Ethoxzolamide—4 mg./kg. b.i.d. orally
  D. Methazolamide—10 mg./kg. b.i.d. orally
IV. Sympathomimetics
  A. 1-2% Epinephrine bitartrate, hydrochloride or borate

per cent pilocarpine instilled every 15 minutes.

If the corneal edema is not excessive, gonioscopy is recommended to estimate angle width before initiation of therapy. Once intraocular pressure has been reduced, the iridocorneal angles of both eyes are evaluated. If the angle is narrow but opens somewhat with therapy, we recommend continuation of miotics and, if necessary, low doses of ocular hypotensive diuretics (supplemented with potassium). If the iridocorneal angle is narrow to closed, we prefer to perform an iridencleisis. Miotics may be initiated after cessation of the postoperative inflammation, and the opposite eye is treated prophylactically with miotics.

As the glaucoma progresses in the American cocker spaniel, the lens may subluxate and buphthalmia may occur. With lens subluxation to luxation (anteriorly or posteriorly), medical control is difficult, and usually lens removal and iridencleisis are recommended. Medical control of advanced cocker glaucoma is usually impossible because of angle closure and extensive peripheral anterior synechiae.

## SECONDARY GLAUCOMA

**Lens-induced.** Glaucomas associated with abnormalities of the lens occur frequently in dogs, especially the terrier breed. The role of *lens luxations* in the development of glaucoma in the dog is controversial. In our experience with beagle glaucoma, lens luxations simply aggravate the preexisting glaucoma. Lens luxation appears to occur early in the glaucoma in the smooth and wire-haired fox terrier and the Sealyham terrier.

The luxated lens may contribute to glaucoma through a number of mechanisms. The loose lens may produce a moderate iridocyclitis, and the inflammatory cells and aqueous fibrin may further embarrass the outflow of aqueous humor. Production of aqueous humor may be increased as a result of traumatization of the ciliary body by the lens. The loose lens itself may totally occlude the pupil, resulting in an immediate elevation of intraocular pressure and iris bombé. The disturbance of the vitreous humor by the luxated lens may be sufficient to move the vitreous forward and obstruct the pupil. The lens may also tear the anterior hyaloid membrane, migrate into the vitreous and even displace the vitreous into the pupil and anterior chamber.

Removal of the luxated lens in the fox terrier in the early stages of glaucoma may result in the cessation of glaucoma. However, in cases of lens luxation and buphthalmia, iridencleisis or cyclodialysis is combined with lens removal. Miotic and diuretic treatment is necessary preoperatively to lower intraocular pressure and may be indicated at lower doses postoperatively.

*Phacolytic glaucoma* in the dog is infrequent in our experience and is associated with spontaneous cataract resorption. The lens capsules are usually intact, and cytology will reveal macrophages containing presumed lens material. Treatment includes diuretics, osmotic agents and topical and systemic corticosteroids. Once intraocular pressure is reduced, the lens is removed, preferably intracapsularly.

Glaucoma related to *lens-induced uveitis* may occur in association with spontaneous cataract resorption through an intact capsule, after traumatic rupture of the lens capsule or after extracapsular cataract extraction. The uveitis associated with spontaneous cataract resorption in the dog in our experience is not usually severe and can usually be adequately controlled by topical and systemic corticosteroids and mydriatics. In the event that the uveitis intensifies or glaucoma develops, removal of the intact cataractous lens is essential.

Glaucoma associated with *intumescent cataracts* is usually mild and appears to be due to a relative pupillary block caused by the swollen lens and the angle closure associated with the forward movement of the basal iris caused by the accumulation of aqueous humor. Once intraocular pressure is reduced (usually with osmotic diuretics), the cataract should be removed.

**Traumatic.** We have not observed glaucoma associated with trauma with the frequency it occurs in man. The more common sequela to traumatic *hyphema* and *intraocular foreign bodies* in the dog is usually severe inflammation. If intraocular pressure becomes elevated with an associated hyphema, blood staining of the cornea may result. We prefer osmotic agents and intravenous acetazolamide to reduce intraocular pressure in the presence of hyphema. Once satisfactory ocular hypotony is achieved, the anterior chamber is opened through a limbal incision, and the blood clot is gently removed by irrigation and suction.

**Inflammatory.** The glaucomas associated with anterior uveitis invariably involve the formation of posterior synechiae and/or peripheral anterior synechiae. The anterior uveitis associated with reaction to attenuated canine hepatitis vaccination may be complicated by glaucoma. The iridocorneal angle and associated structures are usually extensively infiltrated, with inflammatory cells severely compromising the outflow of aqueous humor. The clinical signs include those of both iridocyclitis and glaucoma, with the pupil frequently normal in size. Because most patients are pups, buphthalmia rapidly develops. Prognosis for this condition should be guarded because of the not infrequent, severe damage to the filtration angle. Treatment is directed toward rapid reduction of intraocular pressure by intravenous mannitol and acetazolamide, and the inflammation is suppressed by topical and systemic corticosteroids. If the damage to the angle is not irreversible, the condition may respond and resolve in 14 to 21 days. The buphthalmia may decrease as the intraocular pressure returns to within normal limits.

Glaucoma may also result from iridocyclitis when the pupil becomes obstructed either by adhering to itself (occlusion) or by annular posterior synechiae (seclusion) with the lens or vitreous. Because aqueous humor cannot pass through the pupil and therefore accumulates in the posterior chamber, the iris bulges forward (iris bombé) and concurrently may produce acute angle closure, with formation of peripheral anterior synechiae. Upon examination, the cornea is not usually opaque, thereby permitting detection of the iris bombé, a small frozen pupil and a very shallow anterior chamber. Although the intraocular pressure as measured on the cornea may be normal or even low, the pressure posterior to the iris is elevated.

Medical therapy is directed toward reducing intraocular pressure with intravenous acetazolamide and mannitol and intensive topical mydriatics to break some of the posterior synechiae and relieve the pupil blockage. If the pupil blockage cannot be broken within 4 to 6 hours, an iridencleisis or iridectomy is performed. We prefer the iridencleisis because of the extensive peripheral anterior synechiae frequently associated with this type of glaucoma.

Diuretics, topical and systemic corticosteroids and mydriatics are continued postoperatively. If the iridocyclitis can be rapidly suppressed, management of the glaucoma is not difficult, and within the next 1 to 3 months all medications may be stopped. Occasionally phthisis bulbi may occur, associated with extensive ciliary body destruction due to the inflammation and pressure atrophy.

**Intraocular Tumors.** Glaucoma may develop secondary to primary and secondary intraocular tumors related to rapid growth of the mass, invasion of the iridocorneal angle, obstruction of the angle with metastatic tumor cells, hemorrhage or even inflammatory cells. A tumor should be suspected in glaucoma presenting with concurrent hyphema.

For the not infrequent extensive intraocular tumors with glaucoma, enucleation is recommended. In selected eyes in which the mass is not extensive and can be satisfactorily localized, iridectomy, iridocyclectomy or iridocyclosclerectomy with a scleral graft can be performed.

## CONGENITAL GLAUCOMA

Glaucoma in the basset hound is classified as a congenital glaucoma because of a concurrent *goniodysgenesis*. The glaucoma usually develops after 1 year of age. Although heavily pigmented mesodermal sheets of tissue may bridge the iridocorneal angle rather than the pectinate ligaments, a direct relationship between the angle anomaly and reduced outflow of aqueous humor has not been demonstrated.

Glaucoma in the basset hound is usually presented as an acute congestive glaucoma not infrequently with a concurrent iridocyclitis. The disease is usually bilateral, although 1 to 3 years may elapse before the second eye is affected. Like the other breed-related glaucoma, basset glaucoma may also represent a chronic process in which the advanced stage presents clinically as an acute attack.

The clinical signs of basset glaucoma include severe corneal edema, mydriasis, intense episcleral and conjunctival congestion, blepharospasm, lacrimation and aqueous humor flare. Intraocular pressure is frequently 50 to 60 mm. Hg (Mackay-Marg), and buphthalmia rapidly progresses. The lens may be subluxated, but usually the aphakic crescent is small. Fundus changes, including those of the optic disk, are variable.

Gonioscopy through those corneas that are at least translucent usually reveals narrow-to-closed angles. Detailed examination of the glaucomatous angle is not usually possible; however, gonioscopy of the opposite eye frequently detects persistent mesodermal sheets for one half to two thirds of the angle's circumference as well as a narrow angle.

We believe prognosis for glaucoma in the basset hound should be guarded because of the difficulty in controlling the disease medically and/or surgically and the need for intensive therapy. The not infrequent iridocyclitis may compromise further management of the glaucoma because it contributes to the angle closure and because the inflammatory cells and fibrin occlude the "flow holes" in the mesodermal sheets.

Medical treatment for acute basset glaucoma includes intravenous acetazolamide and mannitol and 2 per cent pilocarpine topically every 10 to 15 minutes until the attack is relieved. Maintenance medical therapy includes topical 0.125 to 0.250 per cent echothiophate iodide or demecarium bromide two times a day and dichlorphenamide (50 mg. three times a day).

In the event that medical therapy is not adequate or must be maintained at unusually high levels for control, cyclodialysis or other filtering procedures are recommended. If the lens is subluxated, lens removal should be considered. Even after surgery, continued medical therapy, often at lower levels, must be maintained. Potassium (1 gm./day) may be given as a supplement to the diet.

## TREATMENT

No single regimen of treatment for glaucoma in the dog is possible because of the number of different causes. Similarly the treatment of one type in its acute phase may differ from that in its advanced and chronic stages. In most patients glaucomas are presented in fairly advanced stages, thereby requiring intensive treatment with a more guarded prognosis. Surgical procedures, such as iridencleisis, cyclodialysis and other procedures, are used frequently in conjunction with medical treatments.

Miotics, diuretics, osmotic agents and epinephrine derivatives are used singly and in combination for the medical treatment of canine glaucomas (Table 3). Because of the advanced stages of glaucoma, combinations of drugs are frequently essential to reduce intraocular pressure satisfactorily. Miotics improve aqueous humor outflow, probably owing to stimulation of the ciliary body musculature. We prefer 2 to 4 per cent pilocarpine on a short-term basis, since the drug not infrequently becomes quite irritating and is apt to produce intense conjunctival hyperemia. Pilocarpine is instilled 3 to 4 times daily. The long-acting miotics, i.e., demecarium bromide and echothiophate iodide, are instilled two times a day. As these strong miotics may produce an iritis or initially increase intraocular pressure, concurrent diuretic therapy is recommended for at least a few days or for longer periods of time. The 0.125 per cent concentrations of these drugs are used initially, and the 0.250 per cent concentrations are used later.

Sympathomimetics, such as 1 to 2 per cent epinephrine, once or twice daily, are useful in the medical management of glaucoma in the dog but may be somewhat irritating. Epinephrine is thought to reduce intraocular pressure by both reducing aqueous humor secretion and improving aqueous outflow. Preliminary work in glaucomatous beagles with 2 per cent epinephrine suggests that intraocular pressure may decrease from 10 to 20 per cent.

Diuretics such as acetazolamide, ethoxzolamide and dichlorphenamide reduce aqueous humor formation 40 to 60 per cent and lower intraocular pressure accordingly. Acetazolamide is frequently used intravenously for acute glaucoma. Oral acetazolamide is also useful in the long-term treatment of canine glaucoma; however, vomiting and diarrhea are occasional complications. Ethoxzolamide and dichlorphenamide are used for long-term management; our preference is dichlorphenamide. Occasional side effects from dichlorphenamide include vomiting, diarrhea, depression, hyperventilation and paresthesias (dog licks its paws). With long-term diuretic therapy, we also recommend diet supplementation with potassium.

Mydriatics are generally contraindicated

for the glaucomas except for those associated with iridocyclitis. Atropine (1 per cent) and phenylephrine (10 per cent) are used for these cases. Phenylephrine (10 per cent) may also be used to relieve pupillary blockages associated with lens luxations.

## LIST OF SOURCES OF DRUGS:

Acetazolamide—American Cyanamid (Vetamox)
          Lederle Laboratories (Diamox)
Antibiotics—Corticosteroids—Alcon Laboratories (Maxitrol)
          Diamond Laboratories (Anaprime)
Carbachol—Alcon Laboratories (Isopto Carbachol)
          Allergan Pharmaceuticals (P.V. Carbachol)
Dichlorphenamide—Alcon Laboratories (Oratrol)
          Merck Sharp and Dohme (Daranide)
Epinephrine—Alcon Laboratories (Glaucon and Epinal)
          Allergan Pharmaceuticals (Epifrin)
          Barnes-Hind (Eppy)
          Person and Covey ($E_1$)
          Professional Pharmacal (Mytrate)
Ethoxzolamide—Allergan Pharmaceuticals (Ethamide)
          Upjohn (Cardrase)
Glycerol—Mallinckrodt Chemical
Mannitol—Abbott (Mannitol, IV, 15%)
          Merck Sharp and Dohme (12.5 gm. in 50 ml.)

Methazolamide—Lederle Laboratories (Neptazane)
Phenylephrine—Professional Pharmacal (Efricel)
          Winthrop (Neo-Synephrine)
Pilocarpine—Alcon Laboratories (Isopto Carpine)
          Allergan Pharmaceuticals (P.V. Carpine and Pilofrin)
          Barnes-Hind (Mi-Pilo)
          Professional Pharmacal (Pilocel)
          Smith, Miller and Patch (Pilocar)
Potassium—Eli Lilly (Potassium Triplex)

## SUPPLEMENTAL READING

Bedford, P. G. C.: The aetiology of primary glaucoma in the dog. J. Small Animal Pract., 16:217-239, 1975.
Gelatt, K. N.: Familial glaucoma in the beagle dog. J.A.A.H.A., 8:23-28, 1972.
Gelatt, K. N., Peiffer, R. L., Jr., Gwin, R. M., and Sauk, J. J.: Glaucoma in the beagle. Trans. Am. Acad. Ophthalmol. Otolaryngol., 81:636–643, 1976.
Gelatt, K. N., Peiffer, R. L., Jr., Jessen, C. R., and Gum, G. G.: Consecutive water provocative tests in normal and glaucomatous beagles. Am. J. Vet. Res., 37:269–273, 1976.
Lovekin, L. G.: Primary glaucoma in dogs. J. Am. Vet. Med. Assn., 145:1081-1091, 1964.
Magrane, W. G.: Canine glaucoma. II. Primary classification. J. Am. Vet. Med. Assn., 131:372-374, 1957.
Magrane, W. G.: Canine glaucoma. III. Secondary classification. J. Am. Vet. Med. Assn., 131:374-378, 1957.
Martin, C. L.: Scanning electron microscopic examination of selected canine iridocorneal angle abnormalities. 11:300-306, 1975.
Martin, C. L., and Wyman, M.: Glaucoma in the basset hound. J. Am. Vet. Med. Assn., 153:1320-1327, 1968.

# OCULAR NEOPLASIA

ROY W. BELLHORN, D.V.M.
*Bronx, New York*

## GENERAL CONSIDERATIONS

If ocular neoplasia or paraocular neoplasia is suspected, answers to the following questions are significant in order to handle the case properly: (1) Is the tumor primary to the eye and/or orbit, or is it secondary? (2) If primary, is it malignant or benign? and (3) If malignant, what is the prognosis for the animal? While neoplasia is a relatively rare cause of ocular disease, it may have a pro-

found effect upon the fate not only of the eye but of the animal. The following procedures should be followed in order to answer the above questions as fully as possible.

## MEDICAL WORK-UP

A thorough *history* may provide evidence of a general deterioration of the animal's health status, suggesting the presence of leukemia or other widespread neoplastic disease. If there is a history of previous neoplastic disease, such as the removal of a mammary gland tumor, what were the histopathologic characteristics of that tumor? It is also important to know the behavior of the current tumor, i.e., whether it has been noticed for a long time and whether there has been any recent or marked change in its appearance.

A thorough *physical examination* may disclose palpable tumor elsewhere, such as in the mammary glands, lymph nodes or even thyroid. Auscultation of the chest may provide evidence of pulmonary abnormalities suggestive of metastatic tumor. Although the animal was presented because of an obvious or suspected tumor in one eye, careful examination of the fellow eye may reveal a similar condition. Bilaterality is suggestive of either metastatic tumor or a leukemic process.

*Radiographic examination* of the skull may provide evidence that the orbital tumor is malignant. Thoracic and/or abdominal radiographs may indicate either a primary tumor away from the eye or metastasis of the ocular tumor to lung or liver, for example.

### BIOPSY AND EXCISION

The decision to biopsy or to excise a lid or orbital mass completely is dependent upon the size and location of the tumor. A diffusely infiltrative lid tumor or an extensive orbital tumor should be biopsied in order to ascertain the characteristics of the tumor. Surgical excision may not be a consideration if, for example, the biopsy reveals that the lid tumor is a lymphosarcoma and therefore probably represents only one of a number of tumor foci in the animal. Surgical excision would also be unnecessary if the tumor proved to be a histiocytoma, which has a tendency to regress spontaneously. Biopsy of an orbital tumor may demonstrate a highly malignant process, and because of its extensiveness, a successful surgical outcome would be questionable. Biopsy of an intraocular tumor would be a very rare consideration, and usually one must decide whether to attempt to excise the tumor or to enucleate the globe. In general, I prefer enucleation of a globe containing tumor. Excision (e.g., iridectomy or iridocyclectomy) can be considered in those cases in which the tumor is readily accessible and

relatively small. However, the attendant risk of incomplete excision and the possible enhancement of metastasis must be considered.

### HISTOLOGIC EXAMINATION

All tissue suspected to be tumorous should be submitted for histologic examination. Solid tissue (e.g., lid) should be placed into 10 per cent formalin using a volume of formalin equivalent to 10 times the volume of the tissue sample. If the tissue sample is quite large (e.g., orbital tumor), the sample may be cut into smaller pieces in order to enhance fixation.

Enucleated eyes may be placed into approximately 200 cc. of 10 per cent neutral buffered formalin and submitted for histologic examination. It is very important not to cut into the eye prior to submitting it to the pathologist, inasmuch as the fixation process under these circumstances causes the eye to become markedly shrunken and distorted. This distortion can create great difficulty in ascertaining the origin and extent of the pathologic process. Zenker's or Bouin's solution for fixation of eyes is superior to formalin, since artifactual defects are minimized. If these solutions are used, it is necessary that certain postfixation steps be taken at certain time intervals in order to prepare these globes properly for the pathologist (Saunders and Rubin, 1975). If practitioners do not have adequate time to perform these steps or if they do not wish to keep several types of fixatives on hand, the use of formalin is certainly to be recommended, since it does allow good histologic examination. A detailed history and detailed results of the clinical examination should accompany the specimen, since this frequently is helpful to the pathologist evaluating the pathologic process.

### CYTOTOXIC THERAPY

Radiation and/or chemical cytotoxic therapy has merit in selected cases; in fact, the results of the biopsy could suggest it to be the therapy of choice (e.g., conditions such as leukemia). Histologic examination of the excised tumor may suggest that postoperative radiation is indicated because the tumor was incompletely excised. Inasmuch as this field is a specialty in itself, it is recommended that the help of colleagues who have expertise in this area be sought when cases of this nature are encountered.

## FOLLOW-UP INFORMATION

In order that we may better understand the biologic behavior of the various tumors encountered in the eye and adnexa of animals, follow-up information is very desirable. This information should be solicited from the owners and forwarded to persons involved in the case, such as the pathologist. Information of value would be whether or not the tumor recurred, whether the animal died of metastatic disease, and whether there was a postmortem examination, as recommended for any animal with a history of neoplastic disease.

## EXTRAOCULAR TUMORS

### LIDS AND ADNEXA

Surgical excision of benign tumors such as papillomas or adnexomas is recommended whenever there is evidence that the tumor is increasing in size or that its presence is bothersome to the animal (e.g., irritative conjunctivitis). Histopathologic examination will reveal whether the tumor was of a benign nature and also whether it was completely excised. If incomplete excision is evident, reoperation is not always necessary in the case of benign tumors, since they usually do not continue to grow; the fact that it was incompletely excised is useful information to the clinician, inasmuch as any postoperative swelling in that region may be an indication of regrowth rather than, for example, a suture abscess. In this way, immediate reoperation may be considered, rather than medical treatment for a possible infection.

If the lid tumor is found on initial palpation to be diffusely infiltrative rather than sharply demarcated, a wide surgical excision is advisable to insure that all the tumor is removed. If the histopathologic examination shows the tumor to be malignant, invasive and/or incompletely excised, postoperative radiation may be a consideration.

If the tumor is quite large and rapidly growing, biopsy may be the procedure of choice, in that it may show radiation to be an acceptable alternate form of therapy rather than surgery. In some instances, such as in histiocytoma, the biopsy may suggest that nothing need be done, since this form of tumor frequently regresses spontaneously.

Sebaceous gland adenomas are commonly encountered in the lids of dogs and may be mistaken clinically for a chalazion. Thus, whenever a "chalazion" is removed by curettage and the mass recurs, adnexal tumor should be suspected, and excisional removal and, of course, histopathologic confirmation of the suspected disease process are recommended.

## CONJUNCTIVA AND CORNEA

Dermoids of the cornea and/or conjunctiva are encountered in both dogs and cats and, if not bothersome to the animal or its owner, need not be removed, since they are stationary masses. If surgical excision of a corneal dermoid is decided upon, the client should be advised that a scar in that region may result. This is especially true if the dermoid is deep into the corneal tissue, and a conjunctival flap is employed to enhance healing of that weakened area. In my experience, some owners are just as upset about the visual presence of the scar as they were with the dermoid.

All tumors or tumorous-appearing masses surgically excised from the cornea and/or conjunctiva should be submitted for histopathologic diagnosis. In certain types of neoplastic processes, postoperative radiation may be advisable. There are certain inflammatory conditions that may closely resemble a tumor, such as nodular fasciitis or fibrous histiocytoma, and if recurrence were to be observed, they could be treated with subconjunctival steroids rather than a second surgical procedure. Melanomas at the limbus must be carefully assessed. Gonioscopic examination of the anterior chamber angle in that region should be performed to ascertain whether or not the melanoma is an extension of an intraocular melanoma or whether it is invading the eye. In either of these instances, it might be wise to consider enucleation rather than to attempt surgically to remove that black mass at the limbus.

In some instances a tumor presenting as a subconjunctival mass may, in reality, be only an extension of an orbital tumor. Thus, surgical dissection of subconjunctival tumors should be performed carefully and thoroughly to insure that all tumorous tissue has been removed.

## ORBIT

Since there is a wide variety of tissues in the orbit, the tumor types encountered may originate from bone, muscle, blood vessels, nerves, fat or glands. Because cats and dogs possess an open orbit, most orbital tumors are quite extensive before becoming evident. Skull radiographs are recommended to ascertain any evidence of malignancy, (e.g., osteolytic and/or osteogenic factors). In those instances, surgical intervention may be only a futile gesture. A biopsy of the tumor may be preferable to total excision, since, again, the histopathologic diagnosis may indicate that the prognosis is already quite grave. The biopsy may also suggest that radiation therapy could offer a meaningful alternative to surgery in some instances.

In my experience, complete removal of an orbital tumor without having to remove the eye as well has not been the usual situation. This point should be discussed with the owner prior to surgery.

Rather than representing a distant metastasis, secondary orbital tumors are usually the result of invasion. Adenocarcinoma or epidermoid carcinoma from adjacent glands, sinuses or nasal passages; osteogenic sarcoma arising from the bony walls of the orbit; and oral malignant melanomas have all been observed to invade the orbit. These examples of secondary orbital tumors further point out the need for skull radiographs and thorough examinations prior to consideration of surgery.

## INTRAOCULAR TUMORS

Both primary and secondary intraocular tumors are encountered and in almost all instances involve portions of the uveal tract. If the tumor is bilateral, it is suggestive of either a leukemic type or a secondary type. However, if the tumor is unilateral, it is not possible by means of ocular examination alone to tell if it is primary or secondary. Thus, again, thorough examination of the animal and detailed history are important as well as thoracic and abdominal x-rays.

Primary intraocular tumors are usually melanomas, adenomas or adenocarcinomas. In the dog and cat, malignant melanoma occurs far more commonly in the iris and ciliary body than in the choroid; this situation is the reverse in man. Malignant melanomas of the eye in cats and dogs have a tendency to metastasize to either the lungs or the liver; this is similar to their behavior in man. Radiographic evidence of tumor in the lungs and/or liver therefore suggests that the intraocular tumor could be malignant melanoma. To date, metastasis of lung carcinoma or hepatic carcinoma to the eye has not been reported; however, one instance of a bronchogenic carcinoma metastasizing to both eyes has been encountered. If one suspects that a unilateral tumor is a malignant melanoma, enucleation of the eye rather than removal of the tumor is recommended, even if the tumor appears to be small and readily accessible. It is not uncommon histologically to observe small foci of tumor in areas separate from the large, more obvious melanoma. Also, since malignant melanomas spread via the bloodstream, surgical manipulation of the globe could enhance metastasis. If a small, focal, pigmented mass is observed in the iris of one eye, one could consider treatment with systemic antibiotics and corticosteroids and observe the behavior of the mass for a short period of time (7 to 14 days), inasmuch as focal iritis or a focal iris hemorrhage may sometimes appear as a black mass and would possibly diminish in size during the treatment period. If, however, the small focal mass either remains the same size or enlarges only slightly, the possibility of iridectomy can be considered. But, again, one must be very cautious in this approach, since there are potential postoperative complications, including metastasis.

Pigmented cysts of the iris epithelium may clinically simulate an iris melanoma by displacing a portion of the iris anteriorly. Dilating the pupil and transillumination with a bright, focal beam of light will demonstrate the cystic nature of these masses. Free-floating iris epithelial cysts are observed on occasion in the anterior chamber. In general, these cysts cause no problems, but if they should mechanically block the angle and create a secondary glaucoma, they can be ruptured with a needle knife or removed surgically.

Cysts of the ciliary body processes may be encountered and, again, be evidenced clinically by displacement of the lens and/or iris. Their cystic nature can also be demonstrated by transillumination after pupil dilatation. If the cysts continue to enlarge or if they are already creating an intraocular problem, they also can be ruptured with a needle knife.

Adenomas and adenocarcinomas of the ciliary body are the second most commonly encountered primary tumors of the eye, and they too may present clinically as a displacement of the iris and lens, with subsequent glaucoma and/or intraocular hemorrhage and/or retinal detachment. They have been removed surgically; however, the overall results have usually not been rewarding, in that postoperative complications led to loss of vision or the tumor recurred. Because these tumors have been known on several occasions to metastasize and also because they are locally invasive, I feel it is better to consider enucleation of the eye rather than surgical excision of the tumor.

Secondary intraocular tumors, as noted earlier, usually involve the uveal tract; however, they may involve just the retina and/or the optic nerve. In many instances, the presenting clinical signs are intraocular hemorrhage, retinal detachment and/or glaucoma. In these instances, the possibility of malignant lymphoma or a primary tumor elsewhere in the body should be thoroughly investigated, especially if the ocular signs are bilateral. Mammary gland adenocarcinoma metastasizing to the eye is at present the most commonly encountered metastatic ocular tumor; however, thyroid adenocarcinoma, bronchogenic carcinoma and uterine adenocarcinoma, for example, have also been encountered.

### SUPPLEMENTAL READING

Saunders, L., and Rubin, L.: Ophthalmic Pathology of Animals. Basel, S. Karger, 1975.

# FELINE OCULAR DISORDERS

ALAN D. MacMILLAN, D.V.M.
*Davis, California*

The following aspects of feline ophthalmology were selected for discussion because these are the most frequently encountered conditions in our referral clinic and because conversations with practitioners treating feline disease indicate that these particular disorders are often perplexing.

## CONJUNCTIVITIS

The most frequently encountered ocular disorder of cats is conjunctivitis. In most instances, the etiology is not obvious at the time of initial examination, and it is a challenge to determine the precise cause and to prescribe the proper therapy.

In our clinic the majority of cases of feline conjunctivitis, if not directly caused by infectious agents, are at least complicated by their presence. Chlamydia, feline herpesvirus, Mycoplasma, picornavirus (calicivirus), reovirus and assorted bacteria have all been isolated from the conjunctivae of cats. It is not practical to attempt to describe the clinical ocular signs produced by one agent versus those of another, because each of these agents may produce a variety of clinical signs that may appear similar to those of another agent, depending on the stage of the disease.

Fluorescent antibody testing of conjunctival scrapings and/or direct isolation of the causative agent are definitive diagnostic procedures that are not available to most practitioners, nor are they used in most instances in our clinic.

A helpful diagnostic procedure that should be done on all cats with conjunctivitis is the microscopic examination of conjunctival scrapings. The microscopic appearance of conjunctival scrapings taken from cats infected with either Chlamydia, Mycoplasma or feline herpesvirus has previously been described.

The diagnostic approach taken in this clinic, after a history and physical examination have been completed, is to take a conjunctival scraping initially to evaluate the types of cellular response and the presence or absence of intracytoplasmic inclusions and bacteria. Scrapings should be taken from the upper palpebral conjunctiva with a Kimura (or similar rounded) spatula. A gentle scraping, which in most cases will not require topical anesthesia, is sufficient. Scrapings are spread onto glass slides and allowed to air dry.

In the laboratory, the slides are fixed in Bouin's fixative for 30 minutes, stained with dilute Giemsa stain for 30 minutes, dipped quickly into 95 per cent alcohol and air dried. The slides should be examined at a low power to identify the cell types and then oil immersion should be used to identify inclusions in the cytoplasm of the epithelial cells.

To summarize the result of conjunctival scraping in cats, we examine the scrapings for the following:

*Chlamydia*—Intracytoplasmic inclusions, usually in groups or clusters, that are in focus in the same plane as the nucleus of the epithelial cells. These are observed most frequently in the first two weeks after onset of signs. After this time, one may observe homogeneous "blue bodies" 1 to 3 $\mu$ in diameter. The accompanying inflammatory cell response is primarily polymorphonuclear, with a few large and small lymphocytes.

*Mycoplasma*—Basophilic intracytoplasmic "inclusions" that are in focus not at the level of the nucleus but at or near the cell wall. Oftentimes a portion of the inclusion can be seen to overlie the nucleus. The accompanying inflammatory cell response is primarily polymorphonuclear, with a few lymphocytes.

*Herpesvirus*—Inclusions are usually not seen. The presence of large mononuclear cells with basophilic cytoplasm is a characteristic cell type often seen. The accompanying inflammatory cells are predominantly lymphocytes, with a few polymorphs.

*Reovirus and Calicivirus*—Definitely diagnosed best by isolation in feline cell cultures.

*Bacteria*—The presence of large numbers of bacteria in the scraping should suggest that a culture be taken of the conjunctival sac. A mixture of polymorphs and lymphocytes is generally seen.

Therapy in our clinic for any given case of feline conjunctivitis, when examined for the first time, consists of topical oxytetracycline-polymyxin B ointment*, since Chlamydia, Mycoplasma and a wide variety of bacteria are sensitive to this antibiotic combination.

## ENTROPION

Entropion (inversion of an eyelid) is included here because in cats this condition is most frequently seen in association with, or following, conjunctivitis. The entropion is frequently bilateral and occasionally affects both the upper and lower eyelids. The cornea is invariably irritated, and the associated discomfort is manifested by blepharospasm and epiphora.

To determine whether or not a particular entropion will require surgical correction, a drop or two of topical anesthetic may be instilled onto the involved eye. If the eyelids return to their normal position once the pain is relieved, the entropion is considered secondary. Continued instillation of topical anesthetic to relieve the cat's discomfort is not recommended, since corneal healing may be significantly retarded and normal epithelium may be damaged. The cornea should be protected from further eyelid irritation by either a nictitating membrane flap or a temporary partial tarsorrhaphy, in which a single suture (4-0 or 5-0) is utilized to oppose the eyelids laterally. This temporary shortening of the intercanthal length by one third will prevent inversion of the eyelids and at the same time allow the cornea to be medicated directly. When the cornea has healed and there is no evidence of discomfort, the single suture is removed.

If topical anesthesia does not relieve the entropion, surgical correction will be required. One should search carefully for adhesions between the conjunctival surfaces of the nictitating membrane and the lower eyelid. If adhesions are present, these should be broken down with a blunt spatula. Surgical techniques to evert an eyelid properly are described in any of several texts on feline or canine surgery.

---

*Terramycin®, Pfizer, Inc., New York, New York.

## CORNEAL SEQUESTRATION

Corneal sequestration is a specific corneal disease of cats. The breeds most often affected are the Persian and the Siamese. It is characterized by the formation on the cornea of a dark brown or black plaque that is usually unilateral. The plaque is usually associated with marked superficial corneal vascularization, although avascular cases have been observed. A variety of causes have been postulated including trauma, exposure, infection and metabolic disorders; however, the etiology remains unknown.

Treatment should be directed toward first correcting any obvious accompanying abnormalities, such as conjunctivitis or entropion. In certain cases the plaque will spontaneously slough off; however, most cases will require surgical removal of the plaque. A superficial keratectomy extending slightly beyond the area of the plaque is the procedure of choice. Occasionally, the sequestration will return as the keratectomy heals, in which case a second keratectomy should be performed. The surgically created ulcer should be treated with antibiotics prophylactically and a cycloplegic to minimize ciliary spasm and secondary photophobia.

[*Editor's Note*: Partial penetrating (lamellar) corneal grafting has also proved to be of value in cases of corneal sequestration and may be considered in treatment.]

## CORNEAL ULCERS

In general, the diagnosis, therapy and prognosis of corneal ulcers in the cat are similar to those in other species; however, the ulcerative keratitis associated with feline herpesvirus infection deserves special attention.

All the cases thus far described in the veterinary literature have emphasized the branching, dendritic form of herpetic ulcers. While a staining dendritic ulcer is considered pathognomonic, we have isolated feline herpesvirus from cats with multiple punctate and fusiform superficial ulcers. In man at least six different sizes and shapes of corneal ulcers are attributed to herpesvirus. In our experience, proven cases of herpetic keratitis in cats are infrequent; however, the veterinary clinician should consider this possibility when treating corneal ulcers in cats, especially those which are refractory to the usual treatment.

Specific therapy for herpetic keratitis of the cat should consist of topical idoxuridine* ointment or drops as frequently as every two hours. Idoxuridine is a selective antiviral drug that is widely used in the treatment of viral keratitis of man. Although we have not had the opportunity in our clinic to assess the efficacy of this drug fully, our results agree with the findings of others, and we recommend this drug for the treatment of proven or highly suspected cases of feline herpetic keratitis. An affected cornea should simultaneously be treated with topical antibiotics.

## UVEITIS

Uveitis in the cat usually makes itself manifest to the owner as an accumulation of proteinaceous exudate within the anterior chamber. The findings are usually bilateral, although not necessarily equal in severity. The exudate may fill the anterior chamber, but in most instances the exudate gravitates ventrally and occupies some portion of the inferior anterior chamber. A wide variety of ocular abnormalities usually accompanies this more obvious sign of uveitis. These require closer inspection to be identified, and they most commonly include keratic precipitates, iridal adhesions to the lens (posterior synechiae), lens opacities, vitreous opacities and retinal hemorrhages and detachments. It is important to identify all these findings for a thorough understanding of the severity of the disease, in order to initiate the proper therapy and, perhaps most importantly, because certain signs may provide diagnostic clues to the etiology.

In our clinic, in addition to the physical examination and hemogram, we rely on aqueous humor analysis and serologic tests, including FIP and toxoplasmosis titers, FeLV status, total protein and protein fractionation.

Excellent clinical and pathologic descriptions of some of the ocular manifestations of three major infectious diseases of cats have been previously described (FIP, toxoplasmosis, cryptococcosis). A review of these reports is recommended to supplement the

---

*Herplex®, Allergan Pharmaceuticals, Irvine, California.

discussion of uveitis. In addition to the aforementioned known causes of uveitis in cats, one must consider other viruses, fungi and parasites as well as bacteria, hypersensitivity reactions and trauma.

The etiology of uveitis in most cases cannot be determined solely from the clinical findings and often will remain undiagnosed in spite of exhaustive diagnostic work-ups.

At the Veterinary Medical Teaching Hospital, University of California at Davis, two diseases account for more than 75 per cent of all feline uveitis cases, as proved by serology, hematology and histopathology. These diseases are feline infectious peritonitis (FIP) and the feline lymphosarcoma complex.

To add to the findings of the general physical examination and aid in the positive diagnosis of FIP prior to necropsy, we rely on the characteristic ocular signs and serologic testing. The ocular signs which are considered "typical" are the presence of keratic precipitates on the corneal endothelium which often either are ringed with RBC's or have a center of RBC's surrounded by WBC's. In addition, ophthalmoscopy may reveal an active retinal vasculitis with perivascular exudates and hemorrhages. Both the flame-shaped superficial intraretinal hemorrhages and the keel-shaped preretinal hemorrhages may be present owing to FIP. Analysis of the aqueous humor in cases of FIP does not provide a positive diagnosis; however, the cellular morphology is primarily neutrophilic, which in certain cases allows differentiation between FIP and lymphosarcoma. The serum FIP antibody titer is a new, particularly useful diagnostic test currently being evaluated and standardized by Dr. Niels Pedersen at the Veterinary Medical Teaching Hospital. All the proven cases of either the "dry" or "wet" form of FIP that have been tested to date have serum titers of 1:400 or higher. Additionally, total plasma protein values exceeding 7.8 gm./100 ml., serum globulins exceeding 4.6 gm./100 ml. and serum fibrinogen values of 400 gm./100 ml. or higher are considered diagnostic of FIP.

A presumptive diagnosis of toxoplasmosis can be made in cats with signs of uveitis and a positive serum titer. A positive antibody titer against *Toxoplasma gondii* should be considered suspicious, and the titer should

be compared with a second sample 4 to 5 weeks after the initial sample was tested. Paired serum samples taken during active infection in cats should reflect a fourfold, or greater, rise in titer.

In the cat, the frequently documented lesions of toxoplasmosis consist of "mutton-fat" keratic precipitates on the endothelial surface of the cornea and foci of retinitis and retinochoroiditis. In the posterior portion of the eye, the retina is the primary tissue affected. The retinitis is usually multifocal, the individual areas of inflammation varying in size from pinpoint to larger than the optic disc. Retinal hemorrhages and exudative detachments may also be observed.

In general, the management of uveitis in cats should consist of a careful medical evaluation, with specific therapy if a definite cause is discovered, and nonspecific corticosteroid and cycloplegic treatment to provide comfort and minimize permanent intraocular damage that may make the difference between a seeing eye and a blind one.

Corticosteroid therapy for uveitis may be administered by topical (Maxitrol® ointment, Alcon, or Predforte® suspension, Allergan), subconjunctival (Depo-Medrol®, Upjohn) or systemic routes. Whether all three of these routes are necessary will depend on the severity and response of the uveitis. If signs of an anterior uveitis (keratic precipitates, hypopyon, miosis, photophobia) are evident, topical cycloplegic therapy with atropine sulfate ointment or solutions is necessary.

## RETINAL DISEASES

The retinal disorders encountered most frequently in our clinic are degenerations, which may be focal or diffuse, and inflammatory changes, which are usually multifocal. With the exception of the diffuse retinal degenerations and retinal detachments, retinal diseases of cats do not cause apparent visual problems or pupillary abnormalities and therefore remain unknown unless ophthalmoscopy is performed. Important diagnostic signs of systemic disorders are frequently observed in the cat's fundus, and ophthalmoscopy should be included in every physical examination.

**Focal Retinal Degenerations.** The retinal degenerations observed most frequently in cats are focal. In most instances, these appear as a single, well-demarcated lesion located either centrally near the optic disc or at the superior peripheral margin of the tapetal fundus. Approximately 50 per cent of these are bilaterally symmetrical. These focal areas of degeneration are usually observed to overlie the tapetum and appear as an area of hyperreflectivity with a somewhat darker border, which sets them off from the adjacent normal tapetal reflection. The central focal lesions were first described by Bellhorn and Fischer in 1970. Bellhorn, Aguirre and Bellhorn in 1974 demonstrated by electroretinography and electron microscopy that in addition to the ophthalmoscopically visible focal retinal degeneration, there was also a generalized cone abnormality.

In the general cat population, these central or peripheral focal lesions are inactive, cause no apparent visual loss and may be assumed to be nonprogressive. Periodic reexamination should be performed to substantiate this assumption. We have reexamined a number of affected cats for up to five years and to date none of the lesions has progressed.

**Diffuse Retinal Degenerations.** This particular retinal atrophy is diagnosed with surprising frequency in our clinic. It is usually seen in adult cats that in all other respects are healthy. Sometimes more than one cat in the same household is affected. Despite thorough questioning with particular emphasis on diet and genetics, we have been unable to determine a cause for this retinal disease in the cats we have examined.

The signs at the time of presentation are dilated, poorly responsive pupils and behavioral abnormalities attributable to poor vision. By the time most owners become aware that a visual problem exists, their cats' retinas are severely affected. The clinical findings are bilateral and in addition to the presenting signs, ophthalmoscopy reveals a marked increase in tapetal reflectivity, marked vascular attenuation and pallor of the optic disks.

Diffuse retinal atrophy has been reported to occur in kittens and adults being maintained on synthetic diets that utilized casein as the principal source of protein. A recent investigation utilizing cats maintained with a taurine-free casein diet demonstrated that the critical dietary factor was the amino acid taurine. Taurine appears to be critical for photoreceptor viability in the cat.

A report of diffuse retinal degeneration occurring by 15 weeks of age in 2 of 6 kittens in two successive litters suggests that this disorder may also have, in certain cases, a genetic basis.

While the discovery and subsequent follow-up examinations of the retinal degenerations of cats are rewarding for the veterinary ophthalmologist, it remains a fact that there are no known treatments at this time.

### SUPPLEMENTAL READING

Bellhorn, R. W., and Fischer, C. A.: Feline central retinal degeneration. J. Am. Vet. Med. Assn., *157*:842–849, 1970.

Bellhorn, R. W., Aguirre, G. D., and Bellhorn, M. B.: Feline central retinal degeneration. Invest. Ophthalmol., *13*:608–616, 1974.

Bistner, S. I., *et al.*: Ocular manifestations of feline herpesvirus infection. J. Am. Vet. Med. Assn., *159*:1223–1237, 1971.

Cello, R. M.: Clues to differential diagnosis of feline respiratory infections. J. Am. Vet. Med. Assn., *158*:968–973, 1971.

Doherty, M. J.: Ocular manifestations of feline infectious peritonitis. J. Am. Vet. Med. Assn., *159*:417–424, 1971.

Fischer, C. A.: Intraocular cryptococcosis in two cats. J. Am. Vet. Med. Assn., *158*:191–199, 1971.

Gelatt, K. N., Peiffer, R. L., and Stevens, J.: Chronic ulcerative keratitis and sequestrum in the domestic cat. J.A.A.H.A., *9*:204–213, 1973.

Roberts, S. R., *et al.*: Dendritic keratitis in a cat. J. Am. Vet. Med. Assn., *161*:285–289, 1972.

Rubin, L. F., and Lipton, D. E.: Retinal degeneration in kittens. J. Am. Vet. Med. Assn., *162*:467–469, 1973.

Schmidt, S. Y., Berson, E. L., and Hayes, K. C.: Retinal degeneration in cats fed casein. 1. Taurine deficiency. Invest. Ophthalmol., *15*:47–51, 1976.

Vainisi, S. J., and Campbell, L. H.: Ocular toxoplasmosis in cats. J. Am. Vet. Med. Assn., *154*:141–152, 1969.

# CONGENITAL AND HEREDITARY DISEASES OF THE CANINE AND FELINE EYE

G. A. SEVERIN, D.V.M.,
*and* J. D. LAVACH, D.V.M.
*Fort Collins, Colorado*

Congenital and inherited diseases are being observed more frequently in purebred cats and dogs. Even mixed breed animals can be affected. Early recognition and understanding of the inheritance of these conditions are necessary so that conscientious breeders can eliminate them from among breeding animals.

A congenital lesion is defined as a lesion present at birth. It results from arrested or defective prenatal development and may be the result of genetic factors or extrinsic factors affecting development of the eye. Collie eye syndrome is an example of a congenital inherited disease. The disease is present at birth and can be diagnosed as soon as the animal is old enough to be examined. Noninherited congenital diseases are the result of extrinsic factors that cross the placental barrier and affect ocular development. These factors include infectious agents, especially viral; toxic compounds or drugs; dietary insufficiency; and irradiation. The stage of development of the eye and the nature of the extrinsic factor involved will determine the degree of abnormal ocular development.

Whenever a congenital lesion is observed, it is of vital concern to the breeder to determine whether genetic factors are involved. A thorough history is needed to determine the possibility of inheritance; when questioning the breeder, be sure to ascertain the following:

1. Have there been previous litters from this mating? If so, were any animals affected?

2. How many of this litter are affected?

3. What was the survival rate of this litter?

4. Are the parents normal?

5. Was the bitch (queen) ill during pregnancy?

6. What was her diet?

7. Was she given any drugs?

8. Did she have access to chemicals?

Not all inherited diseases are present at birth; some are acquired as the animal matures, thus requiring reexamination until the patient reaches the age when the lesion will be seen. Unfortunately, owners of animals with lesions that do not become clinically evident until the animal is age 5 years or older will often be breeding them, unaware of the problem and thereby disseminating the condition to large numbers of animals. This can be the case in some animals with retinal atrophy.

Determining the mode of inheritance can be difficult because lesions may be recessive or dominant, autosomal or multisomal, and have variable penetrance. Most of the diseases in which inheritance has been determined are autosomal recessive, resulting in healthy appearing carriers in the heterozygous state. This becomes a major difficulty in selecting breeding stock. The current method used to determine a carrier animal is test mating of the animal in question with an affected one and then examining the offspring. Dominant autosomal lesions are the simplest to determine. Unfortunately there may not be complete penetrance of the trait and, therefore, breeding data may be confusing. Some diseases are the result of, or enhanced by, multiple factors, of which color genetics and physical characteristics desired in the breed are major factors. Color-dilute animals (merles or harlequins) will have more iris and fundus abnormalities, and this may increase the severity of concurrent inherited eye diseases. Brachycephalic animals commonly have prominent eyes and nasal folds, predisposing exposure ketatopathies.

Analysis of pedigrees is of limited value in determining the mode of inheritance, since often the status of some animals in the pedigree cannot be determined because of death or lack of cooperation from individual owners. The best sources of information are well-designed breeding studies, but unfortunately these are expensive and time-consuming, especially if the trait does not show up until the animal is in middle age. Only through combined efforts and cooperation among breeders, pet owners and veterinarians, using well-designed breeding programs, will it be possible to determine whether inheritance plays a part in some of the congenital and spontaneous diseases observed in animals.

A positive immediate step is for breeders to have breeding stock examined and to breed only animals with normal-appearing eyes. This will lead to progressive upgrading of the breeds but will not eliminate recessive diseases or dominant diseases with incomplete penetrance. The Canine Eye Registration Foundation* (CERF) has been formed to act as a registry for normal-eyed dogs. It is cooperating with The American College of Veterinary Ophthalmologists to serve as a center for the accumulation of vital statistics on normal dogs and dogs affected with hereditary eye diseases. These data are being studied according to breed and disease and will increase our knowledge about eye diseases.

In the following discussion the authors will mention the breeds that are most frequently associated with specific conditions. The reader should keep in mind that variations occur within a breed between geographic areas, and that inherited conditions may be observed in breeds in which they have not been previously reported.

---

*Canine Eye Registration Foundation, Inc., P.O. Box 15095, San Francisco, California 94115.

# THE GLOBE

## MICROPHTHALMIA

Microphthalmia is congenital smallness of the eye. It can vary from eyes that appear normal in structure and function, with smallness as the only defect (nanophthalmos), to vestiges that require microscopic examination to differentiate true anophthalmia. Microphthalmia is often complicated with multiple ocular defects such as hypoplasia of the iris, cataract, persistent hyperplastic primary vitreous, retinal dysplasia and coloboma. It may be associated with cyst formation or, rarely, unusual intraocular contents, such as lung or lacrimal gland tissue. Microphthalmia occurs sporadically in all small animals but is most common in small breeds of dogs and collies. It is a very rare condition in the cat. Breeding color-dilute animals, i.e., merles or harlequins, to obtain homozygous offspring will increase the incidence of microphthalmia. Hearing deficiencies may also be detected. A bilateral microphthalmia-microphakia syndrome occurs in beagles as a dominant nonsex-linked trait.

## STRABISMUS

Strabismus is an abnormal deviation of the axis of the eye or eyes from the normal axis. Most cases of congenital strabismus in small animals are bilateral. This is a common condition of the brachycephalic breeds of dogs. The eyes are often slightly exophthalmic and exhibit a divergent strabismus (exotropia). This is not associated with any visual deficit, and surgical correction is not recommended because the corrections usually are only temporary, since the condition recurs in most cases. A convergent strabismus or esotropia (cross eyes) is inherited as a simple autosomal recessive gene in Siamese cats. Convergent strabismus may be associated with microphthalmia and/or horizontal nystagmus in collies.

## NYSTAGMUS

Nystagmus is rapid, repetitive, involuntary movement of the eyes. Animals that are born blind or nearly blind will be noted to have searching eye movements. Both eyes will wander in a nonspecific pattern, unable to fix on any object. These animals will often have obvious ophthalmic lesions such as microphthalmia or congenital cataracts. Nystagmus in young animals with normal-appearing eyes may be due to brainstem disease in which the central control of eye movements is damaged. Horizontal nystagmus is seen in collies and is often associated with convergent strabismus. Nystagmus is observed more frequently in the Siamese than in other breeds of cats. Many cases of congenital nystagmus will improve with age, and treatment is not recommended.

## EXOPHTHALMIA

Congenital exophthalmia is a rare condition. It may be produced by abnormal contents of the orbit forcing the globe out of the orbit. One anomaly that may produce exophthalmia is a choristoma. This is histologically normal-appearing mature tissue that is growing in the wrong site in the body and is represented by dermoid, epidermoid cyst, teratoma and ectopic lacrimal gland. Another congenital condition that may produce exophthalmia is a hamartoma. This is an anomalous formation of tissues that are normally found in the affected site, and examples are congenital hemangioma, lymphangioma or multiple hamartoma (phakomatosis). Other rare conditions include embryonal rhabdomyosarcoma or vascular anomalies including arteriovenous communication and varices.

## OCULAR DERMOIDS

Ocular dermoids are relatively common in dogs but are rare in cats. The eyelids, conjunctiva or cornea may be involved individually or in combination with adjacent tissue. The more common sites are the lateral canthus and the cornea. Lateral canthus lesions can extend over the globe to the cornea. Fortunately, the eyelids are usually completely formed, with the dermoid located in the canthus, thus permitting surgical removal with excellent cosmetic results. Corneal lesions are usually near the temporal canthus and may extend over the sclera. Dermoids are not considered to be inherited.

# EYELIDS AND LACRIMAL APPARATUS

Congenital disease of the eyelids includes palpebral agenesis, coloboma, small palpebral fissure, entropion, ectropion, eyelash abnormalities, nasolacrimal atresia and excessive nasal fold. The lesions involving the nictitating membrane are encircling third eyelid, eversion of the cartilage and prolapse of the gland.

## PALPEBRAL AGENESIS

Inheritance has been proposed for eyelid agenesis in cats in which a segment of the eyelid margin and the tarsal plate are absent. If multiple defects are present (palpebral agenesis, iris and lens abnormalities), extrinsic factors should be considered. Coloboma is a rare disease characterized by a fissure or notch.

## SMALL PALPEBRAL FISSURE

Small palpebral fissure can occur as a congenital lesion with microphthalmia (the size of the palpebral fissure being directly related to the size of the eye); as a breed characteristic (especially in bull terriers and Bedlington terriers); and as a primary eyelid malformation occurring with a normal eye.

## ENTROPION

Entropion in dogs is usually inherited but can result from scarring or can be spastic, secondary to disease with corneal or conjunctival pain. Lesions can develop before weaning, and inheritance should be considered in all dogs that develop entropion before reaching maturity. Carefully examine entropion patients for a primary cause such as distichiasis or keratoconjunctivitis sicca.

The more commonly affected breeds are chow chow, Irish setter, golden retriever, Chesapeake Bay retriever, Great Dane, St. Bernard and bulldog. The lower eyelid is usually affected but the upper may be involved, especially in the chow chow. In the St. Bernard, the typical change is lateral canthus entropion and central ectropion.

Entropion in cats is usually acquired except for some lines of Peke-faced Persians that have a high incidence, suggesting inheritance.

## ECTROPION

Ectropion is common in dogs and nearly nonexistent in cats. Breeds with excessive or loose facial skin, such as spaniels, St. Bernards and some hounds, especially bloodhounds and bassets, are predisposed. Secondary ectropion may occur from scar tissue contraction and eyelid paralysis. A physiologic change is observed in some hunting dogs, owing to fatigue of the facial muscles. These dogs look normal in the morning and by evening have ectropion.

## EYELASH ABNORMALITIES

Congenital eyelash disease is probably the most common congenital eye problem observed in dogs. Poodles, cocker spaniels and Pekingese universally have a high incidence, but any breed may be affected. This is an inherited disease, and clients with affected animals should be advised accordingly.

Distichiasis with cilia coming from meibomian gland openings is the common form of the disease. Cocker spaniels and poodles typically have long, fine lashes that float in the tear film with minimal irritation, but if the cilia are coarse and touch the cornea, irritation and blepharospasm will result. Occasionally cilia originating in meibomian glands penetrate the palpebral conjunctiva and are directed toward the cornea, causing severe discomfort and ulceration.

Congenital trichiasis involving the temporal upper eyelid is occasionally seen in the Pekingese.

Distichiasis is rare in the cat but can be associated with cilia-bearing meibomian glands.

## NASOLACRIMAL ATRESIA

Nasolacrimal atresia is common in the dog and rare in the cat. Any animal with epiphora should be closely examined for nasolacrimal abnormality.

In dogs the palpebral puncta may be small, absent or misplaced. If both puncta are affected, epiphora will result. If one punctum is normal and the other is missing or small, epiphora is usually minimal. Atresia of the puncta is seen in cocker spaniels, schnauzers and in Bedlington and Sealyham terriers. Atresia of the palpebral canaliculi is less common, and the author has not observed atresia of the nasal punctum.

In cats, cicatricial obstruction of puncta following neonatal conjunctivitis is more frequent than congenital malformation. Conjunctivitis also causes adhesions between the palpebral conjunctiva and symblepharon.

## EXCESSIVE NASAL FOLD

Brachycephalic breeds with an excessive nasal fold often develop secondary keratoconjunctivitis and epiphora. The breeds most commonly affected are Pekingese, pug, Japanese spaniel, English toy spaniel and bulldog. Unfortunately, breed standards encourage heavy folds and the problem is perpetuated accordingly. Animals with heavy folds often have prominent eyes with a physiologic lagophthalmia offering additional irritation.

## ENCIRCLING THIRD EYELID

An encircling third eyelid is seldom seen in dogs and is not reported in cats. When present, it may be seen with additional adnexal lesions and microphthalmia. Removing the band that dorsally encircles the eye is satisfactory treatment.

Beagles and cocker spaniels frequently have a pigmented encircling remnant that is easily identified during examination. This remnant does not cause any clinical problem.

## EVERSION OF THE CARTILAGE

Eversion of the cartilage is of clinical significance only in the dog and may be inherited or acquired. The inherited form is seen most frequently in Weimaraners, Newfoundlands, Chesapeake Bay retrievers and St. Bernards and usually occurs before 6 months of age. It may be acquired following third eyelid injury or improper third eyelid suturing.

## PROLAPSE OF THE NICTITANS GLAND

Prolapse of the gland of the third eyelid occurs frequently in dogs and rarely in cats. Congenital lack of connective tissue to fix the gland to periorbital tissue is the common cause, but occasionally prolapse may be secondary to trauma of the orbit or third eyelid. Hypertrophy of the gland is frequently observed, and it is difficult to determine whether this is the initiating cause of prolapse or the result.

Beagles, bulldogs and Boston terriers are most frequently affected. Animals as young as 4 weeks of age may be affected.

## SCLERA

### CONGENITAL MELANOSIS

Melanin deposits or nevi are sometimes seen in the sclera. These can be quite extensive and extend into the stroma of the cornea. They may be stationary or grow slowly and always have the potential of becoming neoplastic.

### COLOBOMA OF THE SCLERA

Congenital fissure (coloboma) of the sclera is seen in collies and related breeds as one of the fundic abnormalities of collie eye syndrome. The lesion is enhanced in animals with color dilution (merle or subalbinotic animals). Coloboma usually occurs in the sclera near the optic disk but can occur as far forward as the equator.

## CORNEA

Congenital corneal lesions are more common in dogs than in cats. They include dermoid, opacity (dystrophy) and anterior staphyloma.

### CORNEAL OPACITY

Primary congenital corneal opacities, some of which are hereditary, are observed in dogs and cats. They are usually bilateral, central, superficial and stationary. Any layer of the cornea may be affected, with lesions occurring as subepithelial plaques, stromal fibroplasia, stromal edema, lipid deposits and abnormalities in Descemet's membrane or endothelium. Opacity may become less severe with time, as seen with most cases of persistent pupillary membrane, or be progressive, leading to loss of sight.

A hereditary corneal dystrophy has been reported in the Manx cat and is charac-terized by stromal edema followed by epithelial edema and blindness.

Opacities observed secondary to other congenital disease will become less severe if the initiating lesions regress. This occurs with absorption of persistent pupillary membrane strands that involve the cornea.

### CONGENITAL ANTERIOR STAPHYLOMA

Congenital anterior staphyloma is rare. If small and near the limbus, it will not affect sight, but if large or central, it can cause blindness.

## IRIS

The majority of iris defects have minimal adverse effect on vision. The most frequently observed defects include heterochromia, coloboma, persistent pupillary membrane, iris hypoplasia, corectopia and congenital cysts. The rare lesions are polycoria, ancoria and aniridia.

### HETEROCHROMIA AND IRIS HYPOPLASIA

Heterochromia is difference in color between the irides or part of one iris having a different color. It does not affect vision. Iris hypoplasia is poor development of the iris, especially the pigment layer. Both conditions are related to color-coat genetics and frequently occur together. The animals most commonly affected are blue merle collies and Shetland sheepdogs, Australian sheepdogs, harlequin Great Danes, Dalmatians, Old English sheepdogs, huskies, malamutes, and Siamese and white cats.

Some white cats and dogs with blue eyes have an associated deafness similar to Waardenburg's syndrome in man. In severe hypoplasia, the circular artery of the iris will be easily visible on the iris surface, and the iris will be so poorly developed that an examiner can see through it when the eye is transilluminated. As the animal ages, these irides are susceptible to atrophy.

### PERSISTENT PUPILLARY MEMBRANE

Clinical signs of persistent pupillary membrane vary, depending on where they are attached and the number involved. There is no clinical problem if the strands attach only to iris, but when attached to the lens or cornea, opacity may result. Most strands disappear before maturity, with the secondary corneal or lens lesion becoming stationary or regressing.

The disease is inherited in basenjis, but inheritance has not been proved in other breeds. If observed with multiple ocular abnormalities, suspect extrinsic factors. Persistent pupillary membrane is occasionally seen in cats.

## COLOBOMA

Iris coloboma may vary in severity from a small notch in the pupil or perforation at the base of the iris to a defect extending from the pupil to the iris base. Dogs are more frequently affected than are cats, and patients with iris hypoplasià are predisposed.

## CORECTOPIA (ECTOPIC PUPIL)

Many dogs have pupils that are not centered but are slightly superior and temporal. Severe corectopia results in diminished vision that will be exaggerated if lens or corneal opacity is also present. When ectopic pupil is seen in cats, it usually occurs with multiple lesions involving the lens, cornea and/or eyelid. It is rarely seen as a single lesion.

## ANTERIOR UVEAL CYSTS

Anterior uveal cysts arising from iris or ciliary pigment epithelium can be congenital or acquired. When attached to the edge of the pupil, they are easily seen as dark-colored masses. If in the posterior chamber or extending from the ciliary body between the lens and vitreous, they will not be seen except during a complete eye examination. They do not interfere with sight until they become large enough to fill the pupillary space.

# LENS AND VITREOUS

The close embryologic relationship between the vitreous and developing lens may result in lesions involving both. The most common lens lesion is cataract; less frequently seen is displacement, and rarely observed are microphakia, aphakia, coloboma and lenticonus. Congenital lens and vitreous diseases are rare in cats, and when seen, they often occur with multiple ocular abnormalities.

## PERSISTENT HYALOID ARTERY AND TUNICA VASCULOSA LENTIS

A persistent hyaloid artery remnant (hyperplastic primary vitreous) may occur as an opaque nonvascular tube or small artery extending from the optic disc to the lens. If there is also persistence of the posterior tunica vasculosa lentis, the lesion is referred to as persistent hyperplastic primary vitreous (PHPV). PHPV may occur as a small hyaloid artery with "crows' foot" vessels on the posterior capsule of a normal lens; as a vascularized lens; or as a vascularized dense white opacity over the posterior lens surface, with overdevelopment of the ciliary processes. The disease is usually bilateral, without hereditary tendencies.

## CATARACT

Congenital cataracts may be inherited or secondary to extrinsic factors. In beagles a dominant gene with incomplete penetrance has been proposed; and in miniature schnauzers simple autosomal inheritance has been proposed. Noninherited congenital cataracts usually will have additional ocular changes such as synechiae or chorioretinal lesions.

Acquired inherited cataracts have been reported in many breeds, and in some, the mode of inheritance has been proposed. These are: Afghan, simple autosomal recessive; golden retriever, dominant with variable penetrance; poodle, recessive; and German shepherd, dominant. In other breeds, such as Labrador, cocker spaniel and Old English sheepdog, the mode of inheritance has not been determined.

## LENS DISPLACEMENT

Lens displacement is a common acquired hereditary disease in terriers. Wire-haired fox terriers and Sealyham terriers are most frequently involved, with occurrence in Welsh terriers and Manchester terriers less frequently reported. Cocker spaniels and Boston terriers are sometimes affected. The disease is associated with poorly developed zonules, leading to lens displacement and secondary glaucoma.

## OPTIC NERVE AND RETINA

Absence of the optic nerve is rare, while micropapilla, a small optic nerve, is seen in several breeds, especially those with microphthalmia. Hereditary coloboma is seen in collie eye anomaly and related breeds. In other breeds of dogs or cats, coloboma is rare and not hereditary.

Congenital disease of the retina includes color abnormality, coloboma, atrophy, hemeralopia, detachment and dysplasia. Collie eye anomaly may have color abnormalities, coloboma and detachment as simple recessive inheritance. Similar changes are observed in Shetland sheepdogs.

### FUNDUS COLOR ABNORMALITIES

Albinism and subalbinism in dogs and cats result in lack of pigment in the retinal pigment epithelium and choroid, allowing visualization of choroidal blood vessels.

Breeds most frequently affected are blue merle collies and Shetland sheepdogs, Australian sheepdogs, Dalmatians, harlequin Great Danes, light-colored breeds of dogs, Siamese cats and some Persian cats.

### PROGRESSIVE RETINAL ATROPHY

Hereditary progressive retinal atrophy may be generalized or central. It has been observed in many breeds of dogs, even mongrels, and has been proposed in cats. The mode of inheritance has been determined to be autosomal recessive in the poodle, Irish setter, Norwegian elkhound and Samoyed. Central retinal atrophy has been proposed to be dominant in golden retrievers and Shetland sheepdogs. Inheritance should be assumed in other breeds as well.

### SUPPLEMENTAL READING

(For supplemental reading, see "A Catalog of Genetic Disorders of the Dog" in Section 1.)

# Section
# 8

# DISEASES OF CAGED BIRDS AND EXOTIC PETS

Fredric L. Frye, D.V.M.
*Consulting Editor*

*(Continued)*

## INTRODUCTION

While I do not encourage or condone the possession of wild
animals as household pets, I acknowledge that it has been part of
man's history to keep lesser species in a state of domestication or
captivity even when these creatures do not serve a utilitarian
purpose. The earth is rapidly being depleted of its animal resources, many of which are not renewable. If we, as veterinarians
responsible for providing health care and advice in the subspe-
cialty of exotic animal medicine, can help preserve and encourage the captive breeding of some of these animals, the pressures
on the native populations will be lessened.

FREDERIC L. FRYE, D.V.M.
*Consulting Editor*

670

# AVIAN RADIOGRAPHIC TECHNIQUE AND INTERPRETATION

SAM SILVERMAN, D.V.M.
*Davis, California*

Radiography is a routine diagnostic procedure performed on approximately 75 per cent of the avian patients in our practice. Radiography often provides information regarding the organ system involved as well as the classification of the pathologic process, i.e., traumatic, infectious, etc. This information is necessary to formulate a diagnosis and treatment regimen. It is not uncommon to base a diagnosis primarily on radiographic changes when the clinical signs are nonspecific. The frequency of nonspecific clinical signs and the limitation imposed on clinicopathologic studies by the small size of the patient increase radiology's importance in the pet bird practice.

## ANATOMY

Birds are rather well suited for radiographic evaluation because the air sacs provide a negative contrast for the abdominal and thoracic structures. The small size of the patient makes whole body surveys practical. The abdominal and thoracic cavities are continuous because of the absence of the diaphragm.

The lungs are located in the dorsal portion of the thoracic cavity. On the lateral projection, the lung parenchyma appears as a honeycombed structure; the majority of the lucent (air-filled) structures are tertiary bronchioles viewed on end. The walls of the bronchioles normally are well defined and distinct. The bronchioles appear as transverse, indistinct, linear structures on the ventrodorsal projection. The lateral projection of the lungs is of most value in evaluating pulmonary pathology; however,

the ventrodorsal projection must be included in the study to evaluate the laterality of the lesions.

The air sacs can normally be identified as lucent areas in the thoracic and abdominal cavities, but can become opacified by pathologic processes. The volume of the air sacs can be altered by changes in the size or position of abdominal and thoracic organs.

The crop, a diverticulum of the esophagus, is located in the region of the thoracic inlet. It is normally distended with ingesta. The size of this structure varies with species. In some species, it is absent.

The proventriculus is the straight tubular portion of the digestive tract located between the esophagus and the ventriculus (gizzard). The size and shape of this structure vary with species. The proventriculus can be identified on the lateral projection in the caudal portion of the thoracic cavity and the anterior portion of the abdominal cavity, traversing toward the ventriculus.

The ventriculus is round or oblong in shape and can easily be identified by the radiodense grit it usually contains. The normal location of this organ is at the level of the acetabula, slightly to the left of the midline, and two thirds to three fourths of the distance from the spine to the sternum. Certain pathologic conditions can characteristically displace the ventriculus.

The intestines occupy the caudal portion of the abdomen. The cloaca can occasionally be identified as an air-filled round structure.

The dorsal portion of the mid and posterior abdominal regions is occupied by the kidneys, adrenals and gonads. The anterior

671

poles of the kidneys protrude ventrally from the pelvic bones and can, therefore, be identified, whereas the major portion of the kidneys is embedded in the pelvic skeleton and is, therefore, not clearly defined radiographically.

## EQUIPMENT

X-ray equipment for avian radiography should be capable of producing at least 80 kvp at 100 ma., with exposure times of 1/60th of a second or faster. A focal spot size of 0.5 mm. or less will help enhance radiographic detail. The focal film distance should be adjustable. The fast exposure times are necessary to compensate for respiratory motion.

Screen film with ultradetail intensifying screens and nonscreen film are used. Selection of the film type depends upon the size of the patient, the detail required to define the lesion, and the capabilities of the x-ray unit.

## RESTRAINT

Most examinations of birds smaller than cockatiel size can be accomplished without sedation. The larger of more fractious psittacine patients can be sedated with ketamine hydrochloride (Vetalar®, Parke, Davis) at a dose of 10 to 20 mg./kg. of body weight intramuscularly. Galliformes (fowl) and Anseriformes (waterfowl) birds usually require higher levels of ketamine hydrochloride; 40 to 80 mg./kg. of body weight are necessary for these birds. No adverse effects have been seen at these dosages. Adequate immobilization of adequate duration is produced and the patient is usually ambulatory within 45 minutes.

The patient is restrained with masking tape on a plastic sheet (Plexiglas®, Rohm & Haas, Philadelphia, Pa.). A sheet ⅛ × 30 × 30 inches is adequate for most birds. The plastic sheet and the masking tape are relatively radiolucent. Masking tape is preferred to other forms of adhesive tape because it is more radiolucent, is less traumatic to the skin and feathers and can be more readily removed.

In most examinations, tape is applied at the distal portion of the wings, tarsometatarsal regions and anterior cervical region. If the patient is not sedated, a piece of tape is also applied across the body. The tape should not be applied so that it will compromise the patient's respiratory movements. Expansion of the thoracic and abdominal walls is necessary for respiration in birds.

## POSITIONING

The lateral radiograph is obtained by placing the patient in lateral recumbency and extending the wings and legs away from the body (Fig. 1). The dependent extremities are positioned anterior to the contralateral extremity. The dependent side and the anteriorly positioned extremities are marked with an appropriate right or left lead marker. Full extension of the extremities will preclude their superimposition on the abdominal and thoracic organs.

The ventrodorsal projection is most informative if the wings and legs are fully and symmetrically extended (Fig. 2). Patient rotation can be minimized by positioning the sternum parallel to the spine.

The x-ray cassette is placed under the plastic sheet after the patient is restrained and positioned. The film can be easily replaced without repositioning the patient. This is advantageous if multiple exposures are required. The patient can be taped directly to the x-ray cassette if the plastic sheet is not used.

The stress associated with the radiographic examination can be minimized by the administration of supportive treatment to the patient before, during and after the examination. A heat lamp is often focused on the patient during the study. Upon completion of the examination, the patient is placed in an incubator, where the temperature, humidity and oxygen can be regulated.

## EXPOSURE TECHNIQUES

Table 1 lists some of the exposure factors for the species of birds commonly encountered in our practice. Standardization of the exposure factors and processing are of the utmost importance in order to obtain comparable follow-up radiographs. Very slight exposure variations can produce marked alterations of the radiographic image when radiographing birds. For this reason, an aluminum step-wedge is often included in the study to allow rapid comparison of the exposure techniques. This is especially important in skeletal surveys for conditions

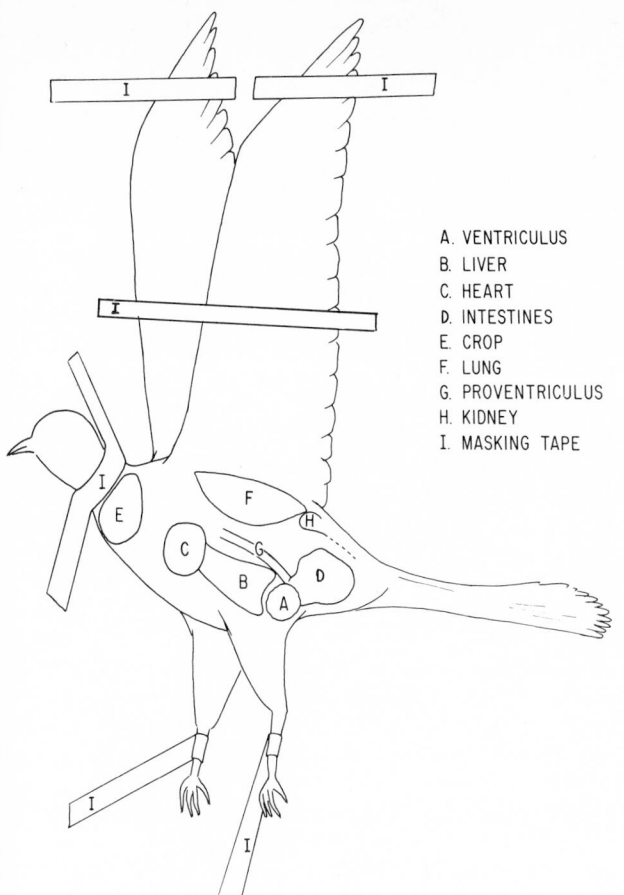

A. VENTRICULUS
B. LIVER
C. HEART
D. INTESTINES
E. CROP
F. LUNG
G. PROVENTRICULUS
H. KIDNEY
I. MASKING TAPE

**Figure 1.** Positioning technique for lateral radiograph. Masking tape is used to restrain the patient. The location of some of the internal organs is indicated.

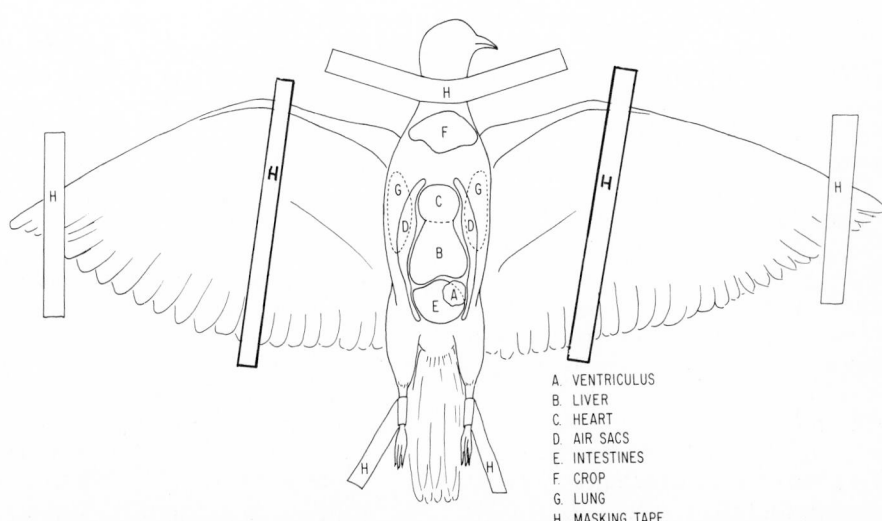

A. VENTRICULUS
B. LIVER
C. HEART
D. AIR SACS
E. INTESTINES
F. CROP
G. LUNG
H. MASKING TAPE

**Figure 2.**   Positioning technique for ventrodorsal body radiograph. The location of some of the internal organs is indicated.

## Table 1. *Avian Radiographic Techniques*

| PATIENT | FILM TYPE | MA. | KVP | EXPOSURE TIME (second) | FOCAL FILM DISTANCE (inches) |
|---|---|---|---|---|---|
| Canary | Nonscreen* | 100 | 70 | $1/60$ | 30 |
| Parakeet | Nonscreen* | 100 | 72 | $1/60$ | 27 |
| Parrot | Nonscreen* | 100 | 70 | $1/60$ | 21 |
| Red tail hawk | Screen† | 100 | 65 | $1/60$ | 40 |
| Pigeon | Screen† | 100 | 60 | $1/60$ | 40 |
| Macaw | Screen† | 100 | 72 | $1/60$ | 40 |
| Macaw | Nonscreen* | 100 | 72 | $1/60$ | 21 |

*Kodak NS54T (Eastman Kodak Co.). Patient restrained on cassette.
†Cronex 6 (E. I. DuPont & Co.) with ultradetail intensifying screens.

## Table 2. *Pathologic Radiographic Changes*

| PATHOLOGIC CONDITION | RADIOGRAPHIC CHANGES |
|---|---|
| Impacted crop | Distention of crop with excessive material. |
| Hepatomegaly | Ventrodorsal projection: liver wider and larger than normal, with possible compression of the air sacs. Possible caudal displacement of the gizzard.<br>Lateral projection: liver enlarged with gizzard displaced caudally and slightly dorsally. Abdomen less lucent than normal. |
| Air sacculitis | Increased density of air sacs, varying from very slight increased opacity to complete consolidation. |
| Pneumonia | Walls of the bronchioles thickened, decreased lucency of bronchioles, possible complete obliteration of the "honeycombing effect." |
| Peritonitis | Increased homogenous density to abdominal and thoracic cavities. Distention of the caudal abdomen. Possible anterior displacement of the gizzard and/or intestines. |
| Gonadal or renal tumor or cyst, etc. | Increased density in the dorsal pelvic region. Ventral displacement of the gizzard and intestines. Possible free abdominal fluid. |
| Calcium, vitamin D deficiency or calcium phosphorus imbalance | Decreased bone density and cortical thickness. Pathologic fractures. |

such as metabolic bone disease. The exposure will be slightly greater when the acrylic sheets are used to restrain the patient.

## INTERPRETATION

Basic radiographic changes such as alteration of density, size, shape and contour are indices of pathology in the avian as well as the mammalian species. The radiologist must be familiar with normal and abnormal radiographic anatomy in order to obtain the maximum amount of information from radiographic studies. The establishment of a cross-referenced filing system keyed to species and pathologic process is also of value. Radiographic changes seen in some of the more common avian diseases are listed in Table 2.

## SUPPLEMENTAL READING

Lafeber, T. J.: Treatment of hepatopathies in budgerigars. Animal Hosp., 3:191–193, 1967.
Lafeber, T. J.: Radiography in the caged bird clinic. Animal Hosp., 4:41–48, 1968.
Morgan, J. P., Silverman, S., and Zontine, W. J.: Techniques of Veterinary Radiography 1975, pp. 255–268. Vet. Rad. Assn., Davis, California.
Silverman, S.: Avian radiographic techniques. *In* Ticer, J. W. (ed.): Radiographic Techniques in Small Animal Practice. Philadelphia, W. B. Saunders Co., 1975.

# FEATHER DISORDERS OF COMMON CAGED BIRDS

T. J. LAFEBER, D.V.M.
*Niles, Illinois*

In any feather disorder, evaluation begins with a physical examination, with special attention to the feathers and feather tracts. The veterinarian should note areas of alopecia; broken, damaged or chewed feathers; evidence of active feather regeneration; and the density of the down. Measurement of a packed cell volume and total protein should be part of every physical examination. In feather problem cases, special procedures can be employed, such as skin scrapings and examination of the quills of chewed feathers for evidence of mites. If an evaluation of feather regeneration is necessary, a tail or flight feather may be plucked.

As a result of this examination and with knowledge of the following basic facts, the veterinarian should be able to solve most feather problems.

## FEATHER FACTS

1. A bird is insulated by its feathers, which are equivalent to an expensive down jacket. Besides protecting it from the cold, its feathers are waterproof and act as an effective "windbreaker." Without protective feathering, the bird's health and even its life are in jeopardy.

2. Feathers grow only in special patches or tracts, with intervening featherless spaces.

3. The density and strength of the contour feathers (surface) protect the bird mechanically and thermally. The thickness of the dead air spaces between the feathers can be regulated to keep the body temperature within the appropriate comfort zone.

4. Water repellency depends upon structure and network and not upon oils on the feathers.

5. Feather coloring is the result of a combination of pigments and light refraction.

6. Lubrication of feathers decreases wear and is the function of the preening gland and powder down.

7. The preening or uropygial gland secretes an oil which the bird spreads with its beak onto its feathers and claws. In the pet bird class, some of the psittacines lack a uropygial gland.

8. Disintegration of the tips of powder down feathers produces a fine powder that helps to waterproof, lubricate and preserve the feathers.

9. A bird's feathers must be replaced before they become worn out. The annual molt, replacing old feathers with new ones, is a dangerous time in the bird's life, since the expenditure of energy to replace its feathers leaves the bird vulnerable to illness.

10. The feather follicle normally begins to grow a new feather as soon as the quill of the old feather is removed. Within two weeks, the feather is one fourth- to one half-inch long.

11. Preening for a bird is more important than is hair grooming for a person, and it should be encouraged. Birds preen their feathers continuously but at irregular intervals. Stress will cause a bird to alter its preening habits.

12. Birds maintain their feathers by means of a number of different types of baths—splashing in a pool of water, showers, dust baths, sun baths, swimming and walking through wet greens.

13. Complete feather care cannot be accomplished unless the bird is healthy both mentally and physically. Mental health demands companionship, a pleasant environment and security from stress. Physical health is related to a balanced diet, good

sanitation and housing and control of diseases.

## FEATHER DISORDERS

### FEATHER PICKING

Feather picking is primarily a disease of confinement and results from stress and poor husbandry. Feather mites may be a cause, but this possibility should be ruled out during the physical examination.

The stress of captivity is based on one factor—insecurity. A bird feels safe only when it can immediately fly away from any disturbance and then hide in a sheltered area. Birds can become very fearful when caged, and unless they can establish a protected area, they are apt to begin to act unnaturally. These birds are described as being somewhat nervous, unfriendly, apprehensive and introverted. Before the feather picking vice is initiated, the bird will lessen its normal preening habits and gradually substitute feather chewing. A common cause of picking is the added tension the bird experiences during a molt. The bird's instincts direct it to increase preening with gentle handling of the feathers, but because of its mental state, it reacts violently—chewing, picking and plucking them.

Other stressful situations that may induce feather picking include isolation from other birds or limited contact with people, since birds are social animals and need companionship; insufficient rest (lack of darkness); malnutrition; fright from many sources, including noise; and close confinement.

Feather picking would not be a problem (1) if bird cages were designed to provide a place for concealment, (2) if birds had an owner or another bird as a companion, and (3) if good basic husbandry practices were followed, which includes providing a balanced diet, 8 to 12 hours of darkness, frequent baths and protection against agitating situations.

**Protective Collars.** Once the feather picking vice has become established, it may be exceedingly difficult to arrest. If success is not achieved after three months of the conservative treatment suggested above, a device can be used to help the bird break the habit (Fig. 1). A combination tube and Elizabethan collar is placed around the bird's neck. The tube collar would be applied first in order to decrease the flexibility of the neck by straightening its normal curve and, thus, extending the head. It

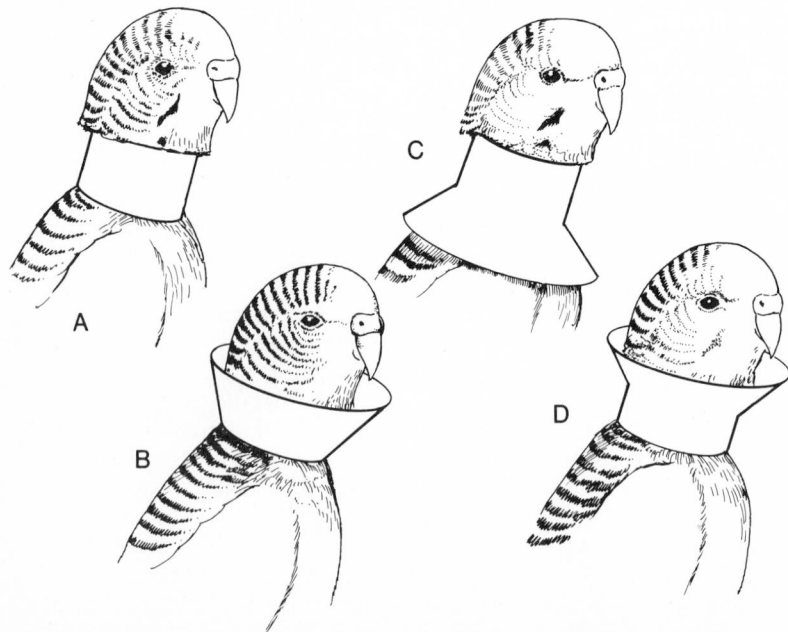

**Figure 1.** A, Tube collar. B, Elizabethan collar. C, Combination tube and reverse Elizabethan collars. This is the type most commonly used. D, Combination tube and Elizabethan collars. This type is also very effective.

likewise serves as a base for attachment of the Elizabethan collar. Since the latter collar will be worn for a considerable length of time, the tube collar protects the skin and feathers of the neck from being damaged by the Elizabethan collar. The tube collar is meant to fit loosely around the neck in both directions. It can be made from any piece of cardboard and wrapped with adhesive tape. The bird should be watched closely for a day or two after placement of the tube collar to be sure that it has adjusted well to the device and is eating and acting normally.

The Elizabethan collar should be cut out of a piece of x-ray film following the pattern shown in Figure 2. The tabs will allow the collar to be taped securely to the tube and coned down over the body or up toward the head. A "pop" rivet, applied with a special tool, holds the collar together. Even parrots

**DISADVANTAGES:**
—Difficult to apply (may require 2 or 3 handlers)
—Does not always prevent feather chewing habit
—Interferes with bathing or preening
—May be destroyed by the bird

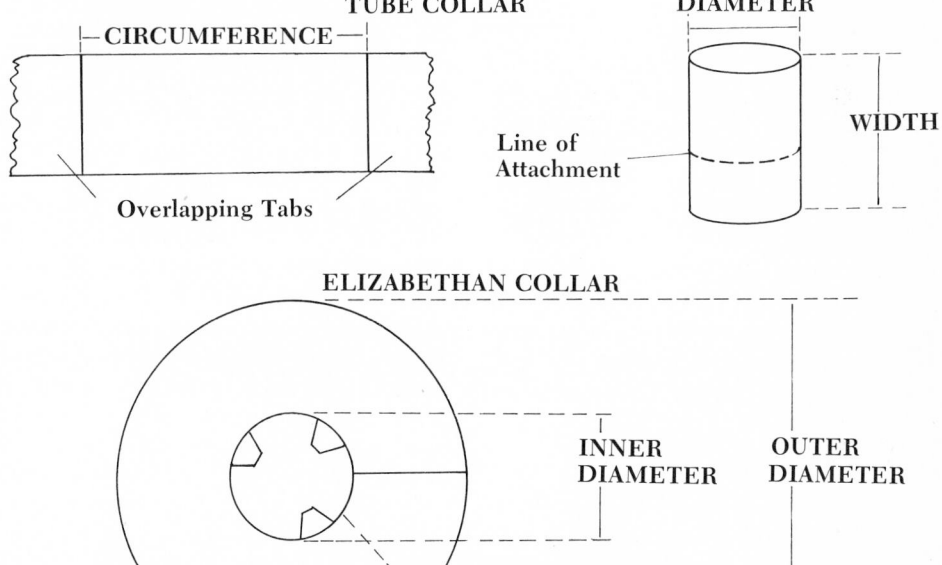

| | TUBE COLLAR | | | ELIZABETHAN COLLAR | |
| | | | | *Inner* | *Outer* |
| | *Circumference* | *Diameter* | *Width* | *Diameter* | *Diameter* |
|---|---|---|---|---|---|
| Parakeets | | | | | |
|   Collar down | 2 to 2¼" | ⅝" | ⅝ to ¾" | ¾" | 2¾" |
|   Collar up | 2" | ⅝" | ⅝" | ⅞" | 2½" |
| Cockatiels | | | | | |
|   Collar down | 2⅜" | ¾" | ¾" | 1" | 3½ to 4¼" |
| Half Moons | Approximately the same as for the cockatiel. | | | | |
| Lovebirds | Approximately the same as for the cockatiel. | | | | |
| Parrots | Birds vary greatly in size, so that the collars should be made proportionately larger. | | | | |

**Figure 2.** Patterns and measurements for Elizabethan collars.

fail to open the rivets. Once the collar is in place, the bird will have to be watched closely for 1 to 2 hours to make sure it has adjusted well to the device and can perch and eat normally. If there seems to be some difficulty in adjustment, the collar should be replaced with a smaller one after a day or two. Some birds will never accept a collar.

The disadvantages of collars are temporary loss of equilibrium, emotional upset, anorexia, sores where the collar touches the wing when it is extended, inability to preen feathers and matting of feathers under the tube portion of the collar if it becomes wet.

### BROKEN FEATHERS

Confinement in cages that are too small will cause damaged feathers. The feathers break as they strike the sides and bottom of the cage. Damaged feathers in no way affect the bird's health—they only mar its appearance.

If a mature feather has been damaged, chewed or in any way destroyed, a replacement feather will not grow until a regular molting cycle occurs or until the damaged feather has been plucked. The only practical therapy is to remove it. Tail and flight feathers may be very difficult to extract, and general anesthesia may be required. The skin may be torn if more than one feather is removed at a time and if the feather is not pulled in the direction of growth.

### HEMORRHAGE FROM FEATHERS

Mysterious bleeding in pet birds is usually caused by a broken or cracked regenerating feather. If a feather is in the process of growing, and the quill is cracked or broken to the depth of the papilla, hemorrhage results. Bleeding should stop immediately when the quill is plucked out of the feather follicle. A broken or cracked feather is painful, and the bird will chew on it until it is removed.

### RUFFLED FEATHERS

Conserving body heat is the most important function of feathers. The greater the thickness of the feathers, the better the insulation around the bird. Ruffled feathers signal that a pet bird is chilled and has a real need for heat. Birds chill under adverse conditions, either when the ambient temperature is very low or when the bird is ill.

A bird that is ill and cold is also hungry. Ruffled feathers in a pet bird are a warning sign and should be attended to; if not, the bird will soon die. Ruffled feathers are not a sign of a feather problem; they function as a body defense mechanism against chilling.

### POOR PLUMAGE

Outward appearance often provides an initial clue to the condition of internal tissues. The relationship between a bird's health and the condition of its plumage has been well documented in both lay and scientific literature. Poor plumage in caged birds usually reflects some nutritional deficiency, but the degree of nutritional abnormality varies. Almost all birds hospitalized for feather disorders have been fed a limited diet of packaged seed only. Rarely, if ever, has a bird on a balanced diet, receiving and eating a variety of foods, developed a feather problem.

It is usually difficult, if not impossible, to evaluate the exact quality of an individual bird's diet, i.e., whether it is well balanced, marginal or deficient. One must consider not only which foods are fed but also how much of each is actually eaten. One bird, when supplied with only a packaged seed of poor variety, may select mainly those seeds of highest nutritional value and will manage to maintain itself on its marginal diet for years. Another bird, given the same brand of seed, may be less selective and may soon develop a critical deficiency. Marginal nutrition is often difficult to detect and in an adult bird may not be obvious for many years.

## MOLTING DISORDERS

Molting disorders include failure to molt, incomplete molt or complications of a complete molt. During molting there is an important relationship between the environment and internal processes, involving nutritional reserves and the endocrine, circulatory and integumentary systems. The environment provides warmth, humidity lengthening photoperiods and a luxurious food supply. The bird must be healthy, with energy reserves and hormonal function adequate to undertake a molt—a balanced process that can be potentially disastrous for the bird when problems arise.

## FAILURE TO MOLT

One of the most common feather irregularities sustained by caged birds is failure to molt. The symptoms of this condition are multifarious, but all stem from the same cause—the feathers that should have been molted and replaced become old and degenerate. Individual feathers are usually dull and dirty and often have ragged, asymmetrical edges. Some feathers may be missing, having been molted but not replaced. Often they become extremely brittle and break easily when in contact with the perch or bars of the cage. In some cases, the old feathers appear to irritate the bird, and many nonmolting birds pull these feathers out or chew on them. Often entire sections of the body may be completely devoid of feathers. Perhaps the most universal symptom is an overall unkempt appearance, which is often not recognized by the owner until it becomes severe.

The diagnosis of this condition is often hypothyroidism of unknown origin. Synthroid®* (1/4 of a 0.1 mg. tablet in the drinking water for birds of all sizes) will cause the bird to begin a molt within 30 days. Alternatively, it will take nine months. Synthroid should be given until the molt is completed. In these cases the other factors of health and feather care are presumed to be normal or to have been corrected.

## INCOMPLETE MOLT

It is not uncommon to find a bird that has started a molt, replaced a number of its old feathers and then stopped molting. Diagnosis is made based on subtle abnormal variations in the bird's appearance. The feathers are generally worn, old and shabby. These birds may be poor preeners—the vanes are split and the new feathers have not been adequately opened and cared for. The feathers of the head are still contained in their keratin sheaths, and small shafts protrude from the head.

The veterinarian should recognize and diagnose this problem and give a guarded

---

*Flint Laboratories, Deerfield, Illinois.

prognosis. The causes of the problem may include disorders discussed earlier (under Molting Disorders) or any avian disease. Laboratory aids should be used in evaluating these birds. "Shotgun" treatment and frequent follow-ups may be necessary.

## COMPLICATIONS OF A COMPLETE MOLT

Ailing birds brought to veterinary hospitals are often in some stage of the molting process. The stress of molting has lowered the birds' resistance to opportunistic bacteria that may cause gastrointestinal or respiratory infections. Following treatment for the secondary infection, improvement and remission result, and the bird may again resume the molting process. Relapse is possible until the molt is completed. One of the most essential factors in treating this type of problem involves keeping the bird at a temperature of 80° to 85° F.

### Recommendations for any Bird in a Molt:

1. *Heat.* In a normal molt, no area of the bird's body ever loses all its feathers. However, the feathering is definitely thin, and this may cause the bird to chill. To avoid this, the room temperature should not be allowed to drop. Should the bird's feathers become ruffled, the room temperature should be raised. If this is not successful, the bird should be placed in an incubator, with the temperature elevated and maintained at about 80° F. A homemade incubator may be prepared by placing a heating pad alongside the cage and wrapping the cage with a plastic wrap. An opening for ventilation is made at the cage door. It is desirable to maintain the heat until the molt is complete. Depending upon the quality of the molt, this could continue longer than eight weeks. Remember, the bird with the abnormal molt will require the longest care and nursing.

2. *Rest.* Eight to 12 hours of total darkness per day will be required during the annual molt.

3. *Security.* Feather picking and other vices are more apt to begin during the molting period. With all the bird's energy being used to grow new feathers, and with the loss of some flight and tail feathers, its instincts render it more susceptible to predatory animals. Confinement in an open cage en-

hances its fears and creates emotional problems, manifested as feather picking and hostility.

4. *Quiet.* In nature, a molting bird resides in a peaceful, safe area. Molting pet birds should be kept in an area free of disturbances.

5. *Preening.* As the molting process begins, the bird becomes increasingly concerned with its plumage. When the quills begin to loosen, the bird removes them and is then ready to care for the new feathers. Each new feather is wrapped in a protective keratin casing. As the feather grows in length, this sheath must be removed before it can open. (The sheath is like a cover on an umbrella—the umbrella cannot be opened until the cover has been removed.) After the bird removes the protective coating, the feather is still curled and the vein (flat part) is narrow. Preening flattens the feather and opens it to its full width.

With hundreds of new feathers regenerating, the bird must preen constantly. A white flaky material resulting from the bird's preening will collect on the cage paper and may alarm the owner, because it resembles heavy dandruff. Coupled with intense preening, it will cause some owners to think that the bird has dry, flaky, itchy skin. A natural but erroneous conclusion would be that oil is needed on the bird's skin and feathers. However, this powder is simply the residue of the keratin sheath, which the bird removes from around the feather—a normal and desirable process.

6. *Luxurious Food Supply.* To supply the bird with a variety of food is relatively easy; to assure that the bird eats a variety of food can be quite difficult. Molting is a test of the adequacy of the bird's nutritional state. Nutritional deficiencies are exposed probably more often during molting than at any other time of the bird's life. A specific molting food does not exist, and if the owner waits until a molt to feed the bird a balanced diet, there will be problems. An owner may add egg to the bird's diet during the molting period. The eggs can be prepared so that they are appetizing to the bird or may be included in other foods, such as egg biscuits, pound cake or cookies with a high egg content.

7. *Bathing.* For many birds, bathing is a refreshing experience that encourages preening. A bath to some birds is splashing in a dish of water; to others, it is being "rained on" or rolling in wet greens.

## FEATHER CYSTS

Subcutaneous cysts containing curled feathers, keratinous flakes and cellular debris are most apparent when they occur on the wings. Surgical excising is the best treatment. Canaries are an exception; once feather cysts begin to erupt, many more follow and may defy complete surgical extirpation.

## HEMORRHAGE FROM FEATHERS

Mysterious bleeding in pet birds is usually caused by a broken or cracked regenerating feather. Finding a bleeding feather with only a small crack in the quill can be difficult, particularly if the feather has stopped bleeding for the moment. Sometimes, two or three new feathers are growing in side by side, and more than one examination may be needed to isolate the feather that is causing the problem. It would be unwise to leave the bird for any length of time without having corrected the problem. If the exact feather cannot be located, it would be acceptable to remove two or three feathers in the area of the bleeding.

Pain occurs as a warning signal to the bird that the new feather has become damaged. The natural response to this is for the bird to investigate the problem. Blood may cover the underside of the wing and the body where the wing was held to the bird's side. Since part of the bird's job is to keep its feathers clean, it will remove the blood from the wing and the body. In the process, the bird may cause the broken feather to bleed even more or may cause other feathers to bleed.

The bird owner must wash off the blood, find the feather that is bleeding and remove it. The bird should be placed in a dark, warm area to recover from the shock. If the bird continues to pick and chew at its feathers, an emergency Elizabethan collar may have to be slipped around its neck.

## OILY FEATHERS

When feathers are coated with oil they lose their primary function—maintenance of a warm body temperature. A sudden reduction of body heat will result in shock and eventual death. A gradual reduction of body heat chills the bird and allows secondary infections to occur, usually of the respiratory system and bowel. Continued chilling, combined with secondary infection, will become critical if proper treatment is not initiated promptly. Removal of the oil from the feathers alone is insufficient treatment. Physiological changes are complex and require intense and proper medical care. Usually the outcome of treatment will be determined within 5 to 7 days, but in many cases birds have died several months after treatment as a result of complications. Depending upon the bird's general condition, a decision must be made as to which of the following steps should be taken.

1. *Incubation.* The bird is placed in an incubator at 90° to 95° F. and allowed to warm up gradually. The temperature and length of incubation will depend upon the individual bird's progress.

2. *Tube Feeding.* Initially, warm 10 per cent dextrose or lactated Ringer's solution may be placed in the bird's crop or subcutaneously, depending upon the degree of dehydration. If the bird's crop is empty, tube feeding with a mixture of warm Neo-Mullsoy® and Geveral® is repeated three times a day until the bird will eat on its own.

3. *Shock.* Intensive care would include heat, oxygen, fluids, antibiotics and cortisone.

4. *Secondary Infection.* Because bacteria are always present, a broad-spectrum antibiotic should be used for 4 to 7 days to prevent infection.

5. *Skin Lesions* A bird is very likely to pick, chew and scratch localized areas of the skin that have reacted to the oil. Self-mutilation will quickly compound the problem and, if allowed to proceed, can cause an astounding degree of damage. Provided that the skin has not become raw and ulcerated, the oil can be removed and a soothing water-soluble antibiotic steroid salve can be applied several times daily. It may be necessary to protect the area by applying an Elizabethan collar or hobbling the bird's feet.

## CONTROLLING FLIGHT

There are a number of reasons why a bird owner would want either to limit the bird's flying ability or to prevent it altogether. To do this, the main feathers used for flight should be removed. The quills of the long flight feathers are firmly anchored in deep follicles that overlie the bones of the wing. The other feathers on the wing are attached only to skin.

Flight feathers may be either plucked or cut out, each method having advantages and disadvantages. In birds smaller than a cockatiel, the flight feathers may be plucked without the need for general anesthesia, and with no harm to the skin as long as the feathers are plucked one at a time. The advantage of plucking feathers rather than cutting them is that the feathers will regenerate in about six weeks. During this time, training can be well advanced.

Clipping flight feathers can be done so that the defect will be practically unnoticeable. To understand this method, note that on both upper and lower surfaces of the wing, there are overlapping feathers that cover the quills of the primary and secondary flight feathers. These are called contour feathers, and they help to complete the flight surface. Do not cut these feathers but lift them up or brush them aside to reveal the underlying quills of the flight feathers. All the secondary flight feathers should be cut at the quill; the primary flight feathers are also cut, except for the outer three or four. This procedure should be performed on only one wing.

The next step is to evaluate the bird's ability to fly. Usually after three or four unsuccessful attempts at flying, the bird will resign itself to the fact that it is incapacitated.

The disadvantage to clipping feathers is that the new feathers will not grow in until the bird goes through a natural molt, which may not take place for a year or two. When cutting the flight feathers, be sure to avoid cutting any growing feathers. Incising the regenerating feather papilla will cause bleeding that will cease only with extraction of the entire quill.

### SUPPLEMENTAL READING

Petrak, M. L. (ed.): Diseases of Cage and Aviary Birds. Philadelphia, Lea & Febiger, 1969.

# PARASITIC DISEASES OF CAGED BIRDS

ROBERT B. ALTMAN, D.V.M.
*Franklin Square, New York*

It would seem that parasitic diseases in birds would be a problem of enormous proportions, since it is estimated that there are approximately 350,000 species of helminths alone that parasitize birds. Yet, with these overwhelming numbers, it is felt that only 2 to 4 per cent of deaths in zoo birds can be attributed to parasites, and the percentage is even considerably smaller in cage and aviary birds.

## ECTOPARASITES

### LICE AND FLEAS

Many species of biting lice (order, Mallophaga) affect domestic and wild birds. They are not particularly significant parasites as far as the pet owner is concerned, but they can be a problem in an aviary and to the breeder.

Most species are large and can be seen crawling on the feathers, particularly on the feathers of the ventral surface of the outstretched wing. The entire life cycle is spent on the host. The eggs (nits) are attached to the primary shaft of the feathers. Adults survive only a few days off the bird, therefore facilitating control. The adults eat the debris of sloughed feathers and skin. Birds are constantly picking and scratching and are very restless. The feathers become ruffled and the skin becomes irritated. Pigeons and wild birds carry the lice and infect pet birds when they are placed near an open window on which the wild birds may perch.

This parasite affects passerines more commonly than it does psittacines. Products to control lice, such as those produced by Geislers and Hartz Mountain, are readily purchased in pet shops and many food and drug stores. They are effective for control and are extremely safe.

Diagnosis is made by identification of eggs, nymphs or adult lice on the feathers.

The head and wing of the bird are the regions most often affected.

Control is relatively simple. Complete fumigation and cleaning of the cage and single, direct application of rotenone or pyrethrin spray or powder to the bird is usually sufficient. One half to 2 per cent pyrethrin extract and talc is an effective topical powder. Malathion is also effective.

Fleas cause few problems and are controlled in the same manner as are lice.

Nesting birds are more likely to be infected with fleas. The eggs are laid in small batches on the host, but the majority drop off in the nest and hatch there.

The use of dichlorvos has been reported; however, this product is toxic to many birds.

## ARACHNIDS

### TICKS

Ticks are relatively unimportant parasites of cage birds with the exception of outdoor aviary birds and captured wild birds. The two most commonly encountered species are *Argas persicus* and *Ixodes ricinus*.

In very small species and young birds, blood loss can result in death. Recognition of larval, nymphal or adult stages confirms the diagnosis. The parasites will be found in the cracks and crevices of the cage and perches.

Organophosphorus is effective for control.

Treatment consists of manual removal of the parasites with forceps. Be sure to include mouth parts. The cage and cage environment should be sprayed with lindane and then thoroughly washed and cleaned.

### PATHOGENIC FEATHER MITES

The red mite *(Dermanyssus gallinae)* and the northern fowl mite *Ornithonyssus sylviarum* are diminishing in importance as common parasites of pet birds. The incidence of these mites, once probably the most common of all external parasites, is greatly reduced because of present-day cage hygiene and effective insecticides. These macroscopic red to gray-brown mites *(D. gallinae)* attack the bird at night and inhabit the crevices and corners of the cage and nest during the daylight hours. They are also under the feed, watering cups and droppings. The mites are blood suckers and cause severe anemia in nestling birds. They produce an intense irritation of the skin.

*D. gallinae* transmits *Lankesterella garnhami* to canaries and sparrows. Evidence also points to the transmission of trypanosomes and the virus of Eastern equine encephalitis.

Warm and humid weather speeds up the reproduction cycle of these mites. The gravid female mite lays its eggs 12 to 24 hours after a blood meal in the cracks and crevices of the cage and nest. The eggs hatch in 48 to 72 hours. Adult birds display symptoms of pruritus and restlessness. Since these mites are nocturnal feeders, diagnosis can be made by placing a white cloth over the cage at night and examining the undersurface of the cloth in the morning. The small mites (about 2/3 mm. in length) can be seen clearly on the undersurface of the cloth as well as at the ends of the perch and beneath the cage.

Control consists of direct spraying of rotenone or pyrethrin on the bird and disinfection of the cage during the day by immersing it in boiling water and then spraying it with one of the previously mentioned compounds. Old perches should be discarded rather than washed or disinfected.

*O. sylviarum* attacks the bird both day and night; therefore the bird must be treated.

Quill mites *Syringophilus bipectinatus* and *Dermoglyphus elongatus)* destroy the feathers early in their development; part or all of the feathers may be lost. These mites enter the feather shaft of the quill during its early development. A powdery mass of eggs, larvae, molted skin, excrement and debris is clearly visible in the feather shaft. The mites are also found in dermal cysts and tumors. They are easily seen because they are large. Though all species are affected, canaries are the most common host. In psittacines, particularly parakeets and

cockatoos, *Pterolichus* is the most common of the Dermoglyphidae found. The life cycles of these species are unknown.

The feather mites Analgesidae and Proctophyllodidae spend all their life cycle on the bird. Eggs are deposited along the shafts of the feathers. These mites are not particularly common and are usually transmitted from swallows, sparrows, robins and other wild birds. *Analges passerinus* is probably the most common species encountered in passerines.

The mites cause skin irritations with scab formation that result in feather picking. Examination of the feathers reveals the mites. Treatment and control are the same as for the previously described mite conditions. Cross and Folger described the use of malathion powder on the floor of the cage, which allows the birds to dust themselves when making contact with the powder.

These treatments are not particularly effective and culling of infected birds to prevent reinfection should be undertaken.

## SCALY LEG OR SCALY FACE MITE

The scaly leg or scaly face mite *(Cnemidocoptes pilae)* is probably the most commonly seen mite in the budgerigar today, and it has been a great problem to the bird owner and breeder. This mite attacks the nonfeathered parts of the bird and is found in the skin surrounding the beak, on the margins of the cere and eyelids, on the legs distal to the tibiotarsal joint and occasionally around the margin of the cloacal opening and wing tips.

The scaly leg mite is seen primarily in budgerigars, but other species of birds are affected. *Procnemidocoptes janssensi* is a similar mite and has been reported in love birds.

*C. pilae* spend their entire life cycle on the host, burrowing into the skin and feather follicles, and feed on connective tissue, forming tunnels that give the characteristic honeycomb appearance. The mite is easily found by microscopic examination of the skin scrapings taken from affected areas. In advanced cases the mite burrows into the germinal part of the upper beak, causing distorted growth that results in malocclusion and various types of beak deformities. In canaries the feet are the primary site of infection. The mite is readily transmitted, and infected birds should be isolated until the full course of treatment has been completed.

Lesions are usually seen in young adult birds. Many birds that have been exposed as nestlings will develop lesions at a later time and others on which live mites have been found will never develop lesions. It is therefore felt that some predisposing factor creating an imbalance in the host-parasite relationship causes clinical signs in some birds and not in others. This is probably the reason why the disease will appear only in a moderate percentage of the birds in an aviary and will not involve the entire flock.

The histopathologic findings consist of marked papillomatous proliferation of the skin with cystic degeneration of the feather follicles, focal hyperkeratosis and parakeratosis.

Early recognition of the disease shortens the duration of treatment and decreases the possibility of beak deformity. A fine, white, crusty coating or film is seen at the margins of the cere in early cases. Scraping and microscopic examination confirm the diagnosis. In very advanced cases a guarded prognosis must be given. The mortality rate is increased possibly because of an increased absorption rate of topical acaricidal medication from surface area involvement. Advanced lesions of the toes frequently cause necrosis, with loss of one or more of the involved digits.

Treatment consists of thorough cleansing of the cage (even though the mite spends its entire life cycle on the bird) and topical application of a 10 to 12.5 per cent solution of benzyl benzoate, crotamiton (Eurax®, Geigy) or rotenone and orthophenylphenol (Goodwinol cream®, Goodwinol). The latter softens the crusts, is easily applied and is relatively nontoxic when applied topically; when used sparingly and according to directions, it is our drug of choice.

*Extreme care should be taken when using Goodwinol cream.* It is essential that when applying to the face and beak, the bird be restrained in such a way as to insure its inability to ingest any medication. When applied to the feet, a very thin film is all that is necessary to prevent ingestion of the ointment, which may produce *severe toxicity*. In advanced cases it is advisable to use light mineral oil for the first 3 to 5 applications to break down encrustations and reduce the amount of Goodwinol needed.

Since the author feels that this product is the best acaricidal product available for this treatment, the results justify the necessary precautions that must be taken. The manufacturer recommends the use of this product for dogs and cats only.

All medication should be vigorously applied directly to the area around the face with an applicator stick swab to break down the crusty material and to penetrate the skin. **The owner should be instructed in the proper method of holding the beak closed to assure that the bird does not ingest any of the ointment, since it is highly toxic orally.**

The legs are treated by massaging well with the fingertips. **A thick layer of the cream should be avoided.** This medication is applied every other day for the first week, twice a week for the second week and weekly for the next four to six weeks. The feet should be treated regardless of whether lesions appear. All exposed birds showing no lesions should be treated once or twice prophylactically.

## DEPLUMING SCABIES

Depluming scabies *(Cnemidocoptes laevis)* is relatively rare in cage birds, but it is seen most commonly in parrots and macaws. This mite is active only during the summer months and disappears in the fall and winter. During the active state, the mite is easily transmitted from one bird to another. The mites embed themselves in the tissues or scales at the base of the quill. Starting in one localized area on the body, the lesions spread to the legs, neck and head.

The symptoms are those of feather pulling, with resultant feather loss, crusting and scab formation of the skin. The feathers shed or break off close to the level of the skin. The resultant habit of feather pulling can be more serious than the mite infection.

Treatment consists of disinfection of the dermis, warm soapy water baths to remove the crusty formation, topical application of nitrofurazone on the scabby areas and application of a rotenone or pyrethrin powder.

## TRACHEA MITE

The trachea mite *(Sternostoma tracheacolum)* has been recorded in South America and North and South America in canaries and some species of finches, and in the United States in canaries, parakeets and some species of dwarf parrots.

Little is known about the life cycle of this mite other than that it spends its entire cycle on the surface of the respiratory tract (paranasal sinuses, trachea, syrinx, bronchi, air sacs, and occasionally encysted on the lungs). Larval, nymphal and adult forms can be found.

Clinically, a characteristic clicking sound accompanies coughing and sneezing. The birds breathe with difficulty and stop singing. A nasal discharge is followed by open-mouth breathing as the result of the granulomatous pneumonia with mucous exudate. Most infections either are mild, causing no problems, or cause death about 3 weeks after the first signs of dyspnea are evident.

Diagnosis is made according to the clinical signs, occasionally accompanied by the discovery of live mites on laryngeal swab. However, for the most part, identification is made from postmortem findings. These very small blackish mites are found in the seromucous exudate in the respiratory tract.

As suggested by Lafeber in 1967, treatment consists of nebulization of a 10 per cent solution of malathion with a mucolytic detergent (Alevaire®, Breon) for one hour at a rate of 40 ml./hr. in an area of 1 cu. ft. Repeat treatment for five weekly doses.

Sulfaquinoxaline (0.05 per cent solution) in the drinking water for six weeks has also been used with success.

This mite is easily transmitted, but the mode of transmission is unknown.

## NEMATODES

### HAIRWORMS OR THREADWORMS

*Capillaria columbae* is occasionally seen in pigeons, and *Capillaria* spp. are common in both canaries and psittacines. The life cycle of the various capillarids is unknown. Most have a direct cycle but a few are indirect. Eggs passed in the feces embryonate in approximately 2 weeks. They can remain infective for many months. The larvae burrow into the mucosa of the small intestine, become adults and mature in about 21 days. Occasionally they can be found in the esophagus and crop. Light infections are of little consequence, but moderate to heavy infections cause greenish diarrhea. The birds develop anorexia and become lethar-

gic and emaciated. Anemia can develop as the result of leakage of plasma protein from the inflamed and sloughing intestinal mucosa. Death is occasionally sudden but in most cases insidious.

Diagnosis is made by the identification of the characteristic thick-shelled bipolar plugged oocysts that measure about 50 $\mu$ × 25 $\mu$ in the droppings or by identification of the hairlike adult worm, which measures approximately 20 mm, in length and is burrowed into the intestinal mucosa. The eggs are readily found by means of standard flotation methods.

Treatment of choice is levamisole used orally or parenterally (intramuscularly) at a dose of 40 mg./kg. Promintic®* (5 per cent methyridine) has also been used at a dose of 200 mg./kg. given subcutaneously or as a 1 per cent solution in the drinking water. Promintic can cause several hours of incoordination and edema at the injection site in some birds. Since eggs are no longer shed in the droppings after 48 hours, the birds should be placed in a new or well cleaned environment 48 hours after treatment.

### ROUNDWORMS

Ascarids are the most common helminth found in avian species. *Ascaris hermaphrodita* is seen in many species of psittacine birds, but canaries are unaffected. *A. ornata* and *A. galli* are also occasionally found. The life cycle is direct. After 2 to 3 weeks, infective larvae develop within the ovum. After being ingested, the larvae migrate into the intestinal mucosa. The adults are in the intestinal lumen and are about 30 to 40 mm. long.

Ascariasis in birds causes few clinical problems. However, heavy infestations can produce retardation of growth, poor condition, diarrhea, and, rarely, intestinal obstruction. Diagnosis is made with standard fecal flotation techniques.

Piperazine citrate (4 gm./ qt. water) is administered daily as the drinking water for three days and repeated in 14 days. Thiabendazole, 1 to 2 gm./kg. in single oral doses or a 0.5 per cent medicated mash, is fed daily for 7 to 14 days for *A. columbae* in pigeons; levamisole, 40 mg./kg., is given 14

---

*Imperial Chemical Industries Ltd., Alderley Park, Macclesfield, Cheshire, England.

days apart. All these treatments are effective.

Good hygiene is necessary to prevent future outbreaks because of the longevity of the eggs.

## GAPEWORM

*Syngamus trachea* has been reported in all species. The adult gapeworm is found in the trachea and bronchi and appears as a red Y-shaped worm attached to the respiratory mucosa.

Young birds of all species are affected, and as maturity is reached, the birds develop resistance to infection. The severity of the disease depends upon the size of the bird and the number of worms involved, because obstruction of the air passage results in dyspnea and asphyxia. Since these nematodes are bloodsuckers, birds can also die of starvation and anemia. The life cycle is direct.

Diagnosis is based upon identification of the parasite ante or post mortem or by demonstration of the ovum in the droppings. The egg is a bipolar operculated ovum with a multilobed nucleus. Necropsy findings vary in severity of congestion and irritation in the trachea, bronchi and lungs.

For treatment, thiabendazole is administered orally at the rate or 40 mg./kg. of body weight for 10 days.

## PROVENTRICULAR AND GIZZARD WORMS

*Habronema incertum* is the most common species affecting cage birds. If affected birds do not die from acute disease, they become emaciated with watery droppings containing mucus.

Necropsy findings reveal the mature worms in the proventriculus. Occasionally, perforation of the proventriculus is seen, with peritonitis and air sac involvement.

Diagnosis can be made by demonstrating eggs in the droppings at necropsy or from postmortem findings.

There is no treatment. Since arthropods such as sow bugs and cockroaches serve as intermediate hosts, good roach control is necessary.

## CESTODES (TAPEWORMS)

Because they all require an intermediate host, tapeworms are less commonly seen in birds that eat predominantly seed and fruit.

Clinical signs are variable, and birds become debilitated, develop diarrhea, become weak and die. Diagnosis is made on observation of proglottids or eggs in the droppings or on postmortem examination. There is no effective treatment. However, niclosamide (Yomesan®, Chemagro) has been used in a single dose of 250 mg./kg.

*Table 1.* *Summary of Nematodes*

| NEMATODE | COMMON NAME | SPECIES AFFECTED | ORGANS CONTAINING ADULT WORMS | OVUM |
|---|---|---|---|---|
| *Capillaria* sp. | Threadworm | Canaries, parakeets, wild passerines | Crop, intestinal mucosa | ×250 Bipolar plugs |
| *Ascaridia* sp. | Roundworm | Psittacines | Duodenum, small intestine | ×240 |
| *Syngamus trachea* | Gapeworm | All species of cage birds | Trachea, bronchi | ×200 Bilateral opercula |

# PROTOZOA

## TRICHOMONAS

*Trichomonas gallinae* has been found in pigeons (causing canker), falcons (causing frounce), canaries, various finches and sparrows and psittacines. Clinically, the birds become lethargic, anorectic and puffed and have diarrhea and, in many cases, dyspnea. Death can occur suddenly in peracute cases, and birds have been known to be carriers, showing no clinical manifestation. Hard, caseous, necrotic foci or plaques are found in the epithelium in the pharynx, esophagus and crop. Diagnosis is generally made by finding characteristic lesions and identifying the organism on wet smears or on postmortem examination. Live flagellates can be found in the lesions as swimming organisms as long as two days after death. Environmental and other forms of stress are thought to be predisposing factors. Contaminated food and water along with direct contact are means of transmission.

Treatment consists of mixing 1 gm. of Enheptin® (2-amino-5-nitrothiazide; American Cyanamid Co.) in 1 liter of water and using the mixture as the only source of water for 6 to 7 days, or adding metronidazole to the ration at 5 mg./100 gm. of body weight for 5 days.

Good hygiene is necessary to prevent reinfection.

The incidence of this condition in the United States is low, and it is seen mostly in pigeons.

## COCCIDIUM

There are several species of coccidia in wild and cage birds, but because of the lack of research, many have not been classified. The genera *Eimeria* and *Isospora* are the most commonly seen, *Eimeria* spp. infecting parakeets and pigeons and *Isospora* spp. infecting passerines, psittacines and raptors.

## PLASMODIUM

A great deal of work has been done on avian malaria; however, because there is little problem clinically in the United States, only very basic material will be presented here.

Malaria is seen primarily in passerines; canaries are highly susceptible. The birds become puffed-up and ataxic. Death usually occurs within 48 hours after symptoms appear. Occasionally, swelling of the eyelids is observed.

Diagnosis is established by identification of intraerythrocytic schizonts and gametocytes in blood smears.

Treatment consists of mosquito control and quinacrine hydrochloride (Atabrine®, Winthrop) given at the rate of 0.24 mg./gram of body weight daily for at least one week.

Necropsy findings include splenic and hepatic enlargement and subcutaneous hemorrhage. Anemia is generally evident.

### SUPPLEMENTAL READING

Lafeber, T. J.: Respiratory diseases. Vet. Clin. N. Amer., 3:224, 1973.

---

# HUSBANDRY OF CAPTIVE WILD BIRDS

JAN F. DETRICK, D.V.M.,
*and* MALCOLM I. RAFF, Ph.D.
*Berkeley, California*

Many publications pertaining to the care and ecologic rehabilitation of displaced wild birds have recently been issued. Unfortunately, the lack of scientific temperance in the approach and recording of findings makes it difficult to recommend much of this material. The fact that each species has its specialized requirements and that trial-and-error methods abound makes it incumbent upon the veterinarian to refer these birds to an organization or particular veterinarian knowledgeable in the field. Also, all native wild birds are protected by federal laws which prohibit captive maintenance. A veterinarian may legally administer emergency treatment, but for anything more, authorization must be sought through the local Bureau of Sport Fisheries and Wildlife and the U.S. Department of the Interior as well as the state wildlife authorities.

## INITIAL HANDLING

In general, birds should be taken from the environment only as a last resort. Birds under one week of age (nestlings) are very difficult to raise, and losses by mishandling are very common. All efforts should be made to return a young bird to the nest. If return to the environment is not feasible, the following steps should be taken.

1. A natural tranquilizing effect can be achieved by placing the bird in a warm, dark, quiet enclosure. The correct temperature is dependent upon the degree of growth and the condition of the bird's feathers. In naked nestlings, the correct temperature is close to 100° F., while it is nearer 85° F. in a fledgling or adult in poor condition. Dehydration is rapid in birds. To protect against further dehydration caused by these high temperatures, three steps should be taken: First, the heat should be applied to the bird and not to the environment. This is accomplished by the use of a heating pad or an electric mantle as used in chemistry laboratories for heating flammable liquids. These are made into a nest and lined with an absorbent material, such as a paper towel, that is frequently changed. Second, a shallow pan of water should be placed in the enclosure where the bird cannot possibly reach it. Third, the enclosure should be large enough to house all the above and yet small enough so that the humidity will cause just a slight condensation. If adequate humidity is difficult to achieve, a sponge may be placed in the water pan to increase the surface area. The competition and body warmth evoked among nestlings by keeping more than one bird per nest is mutually beneficial. This is not recommended for adult birds, however. The birds kept together may be of different age and different species, but they should be of approximately the same size.

2. Dehydration and hypoglycemia are usually coexistent and need to be corrected together. This can be accomplished in small birds and nestlings by the oral administration of an initial solution of dextrose, Karo syrup or honey that is approximately 15 per cent in strength. This solution may then be increased to approximately 20 per cent or replaced with the hummingbird mixture (see below, p. 692). These fluids should be administered every 10 to 15 minutes initially. Care should be exercised so that none of this is spilled onto the feathers. In larger birds the medial tarsal or the wing vein may be used to administer a balanced electrolyte solution containing 10 to 15 per cent dextrose. The established rule is to give 10 ml./kg. over a 5- to 10-minute period; however, experience shows that it is difficult to overhydrate birds, since any excess fluid enters the intestinal lumen and apparently does not cause pulmonary edema.

3. Dexamethasone at a dosage of 4 mg./kg. one or two times IV if possible (otherwise IM) may be helpful. Administration of a broad-spectrum antibiotic is worthwhile, since many bird diseases are opportunistic.

4. Inanition is invariably present to some degree in captive birds. With adaptation to flight, body stores of fat are very scant, and with their very high metabolic rate, birds must constantly eat to survive. Therefore, the bird must eat as soon as possible. If the correct diet is not known, mashed scrambled chicken egg and/or killed soft insects are usually safe until a more adequate diet can be assembled. Force-feeding may be necessary initially, although natural foods may act as a stimulant to self-feeding.

5. When adequately recovered, fully fledged birds and adults can be maintained at room temperature (65 to 75° F.) in an environment commensurate with their normal habitats, essentially free from human exposure. Normal photoperiodicity should be maintained and desires to tame the birds must be avoided, otherwise successful release will be seriously jeopardized.

## IDENTIFICATION AND GENERAL PRINCIPLES

Because of the vast array of environmental niches filled by birds, it is imperative to identify the species as soon and as accurately as possible. However, this may be difficult in fledglings and next to impossible in nestlings. The expertise of local zoologists or qualified Audubon personnel should be sought. Knowledge of habitat, nesting behavior and geographic range of different species is helpful.

Depending on the species, the young hatchling is either altricial or precocial. Precocial chicks frequently have a longer incubation period, are well covered with down and are usually able to feed themselves at hatching. The smaller species of birds usually have a shorter incubation period (commonly 14 days) that results in an altricial chick or "nestling." These birds are generally born blind, helpless and more or less naked. Unless the parents are known, identification may be impossible until the chicks are fledged. However, their state of immaturity dictates their needs better than does an exact species identification. Most of these nestlings possess "lips" that make up the commissures of their beak. These allow the young bird to gape and provide the parent with a target through which it can place food in the nestling's gullet. Pigeons and doves, raptors and many water birds present the exceptions to this observation.

The law of form and function is also expressed in the beak of the adult birds and has led aviculturists to classify the smaller birds on the basis of the beak morphology. "Hard-bills" (the supposed seed-eaters) include the finch-like birds (buntings, grosbeaks, waxbills, cardinals, etc.) and the parrot family. "Soft-bills" (the supposed insectivores and fructivores) include warblers, thrushes, flycatchers, mockingbirds, orioles, starlings, woodpeckers, bushtits, doves, crows, ravens, etc. Although this classification may aid in selecting food preferences, all these birds should be considered omnivores, since they have been shown to eat a varied diet as dictated by their needs and probably by the seasonal availability of food.

The remaining birds, for practical purposes, may be placed in one of the following categories: predatory land birds (vultures, hawks, falcons and owls); predatory water birds (grebes, loons, gulls, shorebirds, etc.); omnivorous water birds (coots, rails, most waterfowl, etc.); and fruit- and nectar-eaters (hummingbirds). The gallinaceous birds will not be included, for their care and feeding is like that of domestic fowl.

## FEEDING TECHNIQUES

Voluntary food intake is necessary if any degree of success is to be realized. Unfortunately, most captive birds, especially the immature, will need either hand-feeding or force-feeding. Before the proper method can be selected, the bird's normal method of feeding must be identified. As pointed out earlier, the nestlings and fledglings of most species rely on "gape." A systematic method of stimulus presentation should be established and would include such gestures as tapping on various parts of the head, wiggling the nest, making squeaking sounds or whistles and alternately shadowing and unshadowing the bird, even if it is too young to have its eyes open. If these gestures fail initially, they should not be abandoned, since later attempts may be successful. However, if the beak must be forced open, it is usually easily and safely accomplished by inserting a fingernail in the commissure of the beak and applying gentle prying pressure.

Most fledglings and occasionally some adults must initially be force-fed or hand-fed, and they must be weaned off to self-feeding with caution. The following methods of force-feeding have proved successful.

1. A soft tube or catheter with the largest diameter that comfortably fits down the esophagus is passed from the left side of the beak well into the esophageal opening to the right of the glottis. The catheters employed range from a No. 5, for fringillids, to a No. 18, for birds 500 gm. and larger. This procedure minimizes the chances of the tube entering the glottis. A catheter-tipped 35-ml. syringe is especially well adapted to deliver food of semi-moist consistency. However, a 3-ml. or tuberculin syringe with the end of the barrel opened will also work.

2. With the aid of a smooth, rounded chopstick or similar tool, semi-moist food molded into pellets may be gently coaxed down the esophagus.

3. Smooth-tipped hemostats may be employed to grip suitable food and deliver it well below the glottis.

In all cases, except for very liquid food, water should be given after each bolus of food. This is most safely accomplished by placing drops of water on the beak, or upper palate if the bird is gaping, and letting capillary action carry it to the pharynx. Birds generally shake the excess water out unless they are very weak.

## TYPES OF FOOD AND SUPPLEMENTS

It is often necessary to institute feeding before the bird is identified and proper ingredients are assembled. In this case the hummingbird mixture (p. 692) may be given, but owing to the high protein requirement in nestlings, it is advisable to supplement it with bits of scrambled egg that have been forced through a strainer. Insectile food is considered safe, since most nestlings are initially fed insects, but it may be important to kill live insects before feeding them to the bird. The basic mixture outlined under omnivorous birds is generally safe and is the best balanced of all the foods. Commerical "nestling" food is available but tends to be very expensive and is of questionable value.

It should be stated that nutritive requirements for all birds are generally the same, in that the need for energy, protein, vitamins and minerals tends to be similar, and the use of complicated mixtures should not be necessary. However, exact nutritive requirements are not well enough established to recommend a general simplified diet. The following is a list of generally used ingredients fed separately or used in mixtures.

1. Insectile foods include any adult insects or their larval forms. Because of the quantities needed, it is best to select a species that can be cultured or purchased in large quantities. Some are too chitinous for nestlings, since chitin is indigestible, much of the calcium is not able to be utilized. The mealworm is a classic example: it should be squeezed to remove its shell and head before it is fed to birds of less than one week of age, or the freshly molted (white) form can be used. Other choices include honeybee larvae, fruit flies, dipteran larvae and earthworms. "Dried flies" are available commercially and may be used to supplement live food.

2. The "meat" foods include high-protein canned dog food such as p/d\*, kibbled dog food (puppy or high-protein may be the best), scrambled or hard-boiled chicken egg, strained beef, baby food, etc.

3. The grain foods include high-protein dry baby cereal, wheat germ, cornmeal, oatmeal, pigeon food and other commercial seed mixtures. Commercial poultry starter mash (28 per cent crude protein) is an excellent food and it should be spun in a blender and sifted to remove the large pieces when used in mixtures. All the above may be offered *ad lib.* to the self-feeders.

4. Carrots and red peppers are often used for their lipochromes to assure adequate formation of the carotenoid pigments.

5. Fruits are good foods for almost any species. Diced apples, grapes strawberries, pears, bananas, etc., make mild nutritional additions to the mixtures. Water-soaked dry fruits and raisins are also good.

6. Powdered gelatin can be employed as a protein supplement in nestlings that have a high protein requirement. This gelatin may be used sparingly in the mixture or fed as a separate ingredient.

7. A vitamin/mineral supplement that contains vitamin $D_3$ (e.g., Vet Nutri®†) should be provided for all birds. Additional calcium in the form of a commercial preparation should be added to mixtures, and a mineral block should be provided to all self-feeders.

8. Grit should be insoluble and may be supplied in small amounts to all self-feeders that do not otherwise have a source of minerals.

## AMOUNT AND FREQUENCY OF FEEDING

There is no replacement for experience in this matter, but here are some general rules that may help. A program of weighing and palpation of the pectoral (breast) muscles is used to gauge if the amount of nutrients is adequate. A finger pressed lightly against the keel-sternum should detect the pectoral musculature on each side. Weighing is more accurate only if adequate records are kept and compared, and it is especially useful during the transition from hand- or force-feeding to self-feeding.

The character of the stool can give valuable information as to the state of hydration and digestion. In order to evaluate this, one must know normal variations of stool for each species. For example, stools tend to be wet in sea birds, moist in carnivores and dry in fringillids.

---

\*Hill Packing Company, Topeka, Kansas.

†Squibb and Sons, Princeton, New Jersey.

It is generally safer to feed too much than too little, and begging birds may be given a little more than they request. In general, each feeding should provide enough food to fill the esophagus, or the crop (in those birds possessing one), and the limit is realized when regurgitation or filling of the pharynx is observed. It is important to note here that insufficient supplemental warmth in nestlings leads to slow digestion and inadequate nutrition. A problem arises in infant birds, who will stuff themselves to the point at which damage to the esophagus may occur. This may happen in a properly stimulated nestling because it will automatically call for more food when the stimulus is presented. Proper evaluation and monitoring of the bird is paramount because behavior may remain spirited and "normal" until death. The nonspirited birds are usually extremely serious problems.

The frequency of feeding is usually every 30 to 60 minutes in nestlings, owing to their high metabolic rate and the limited capacity of their digestive system. Until the nestling is gaping well, the frequency may be as often as every 15 minutes. Other frequencies are listed with the particular species under consideration.

## OMNIVOROUS BIRDS

These include the following Orders:

Passeriformes (perching birds)
Piciformes (woodpeckers, flickers, sapsuckers)
Psittaciformes (parrots)
Apodiformes (swifts)
Caprimulgiformes (nighthawks, whippoorwills)
Cuculiformes (cuckoos, anis, roadrunners)
Columbiformes (pigeons, doves)

The self-feeding adults and immature birds in this group should be offered a variety of foods *ad lib.* Grit and solid seed mixtures such as wild bird seed, parakeet or canary mixes, sunflower seeds, peanuts, pigeon mix, etc., should be selected to parallel most closely their domesticated counterparts. A correlation has been shown between bill size and the size of seed selected, while no correlation has been shown between the size of the bird and seed size. Meat foods, such as dog food (dry or canned), and live foods (mealworms, etc.) should also be available. Fresh or water-soaked dry fruits are welcomed by most species. A mineral block and enough water for drinking and bathing should be offered continuously.

The following mixture is employed in hand-feeding and force-feeding young birds:

2 Hard-boiled eggs with shells
1 Pound high-protein dog food (p/d)
1 Ounce powdered gelatin (Knox)
½ Cup insect food (mealworms, etc.)
2 Tablespoons (heaped) wheat germ
⅓ Cup seedless raisins
1 Tablespoon powdered vitamin supplement (Vet Nutri®)
1 Tablespoon calcium supplement

These ingredients are blended in a food grinder or blender with 2 cups of water (or less). The proper consistency is achieved by adding Gerber's High Protein Baby Cereal® and spun, sifted turkey mash. This makes about 1 quart of mix and may be frozen or refrigerated in small containers and used as needed.

Specific requirements of the most commonly encountered birds are listed below.

**Supposed Meat- and Fruit-eaters: Thrushes (Robins), Jays, Woodpeckers, Crows, Ravens, etc.** These birds will eat dog food, whole mealworms and almost any captured insects. They will accept the widest variety of foods and are therefore fairly easy to maintain. The adults can be force-fed lumps of dog food, berries, etc. The capacity of an adult, robin-sized bird is 8 to 12 ml. every 2 hours, or about 100 to 150 medium-sized mealworms daily. The nestlings require 3 to 4 ml. of solid food, or 4 to 8 ml. of liquid food every 1 to 2 hours.

**Supposed Seed-eaters: Sparrows, Finches, Grosbeaks, Towhees, etc.** The basic mixture is slightly modified by the addition of one more hard-boiled egg and Petamine®*, a commercial, balanced grain food for aviary birds. For birds one week or older, 0.5 to 1.0 ml. is hand-fed or force-fed every 30 to 60 minutes. The crop should be checked before feeding, and if full, the amount fed should be reduced. If the bird begs, more frequent feedings should be instituted. These birds are difficult to raise before one week of age (no pin feathers yet) but have been successfully hatched and reared under artificial conditions. (Lanyon and Lanyon, 1969).

**Heavily Insectivorous Species: Flycatchers, Swallows, Bushtits, Swifts, Whippoor-**

---

*Carnation Co.

wills and Woodpeckers (Supposed Sap-feeders). These birds have been maintained on small pieces of dog food either moistened, or thinned to eyedropper consistency. Freshly killed insects should also be offered, such as mealworms or bee larvae. The sap-feeding woodpeckers can also be given the hummingbird mixture (at right) and fruit bits.

"Milk-feeding" altricial young: Columbiformes (Pigeons and Doves) and Psittaciformes (Parrots). The nestlings of these birds are unique because they are fed a cheeselike secretion produced by the parents for the first 5 to 10 days, a diet which tapers to seed and water. In the Columbiformes, the so-called "pigeon milk" is simply the desquamated epithelial lining of the crop, regurgitated, which the young obtain by thrusting their beaks into the parent's gullet. The secretion of the Psittaciformes seems to be produced in the proventriculus and is also regurgitated and passed directly to the beak of the young.

Birds under 1 week of age can be fed a mixture of egg, baby cereal, Petamine, and spun turkey mash, with the feeding frequency and quantity governed by crop palpation and fecal examination. Feeding is best accomplished with the use of a 3-ml. syringe with the end of the barrel cut off and smoothed. Alternatively, dampened seeds can be gently placed in the esophagus.

Birds over 1 week old can be fed a mixture of grain and seeds soaked with water in a small cup. In the pigeons and doves, the head may be inserted into the tipped cup, and it may be necessary to push the beak into the food almost to the nostrils. The water requirements are high and the crop contents should always feel watery.

In older birds, a commercial pigeon mix of corn, milo and peas is used. In sick birds, the mouth and crop should be checked for the caseous lesions of trichomoniasis. If no evidence is found, and the crop smells sour, a forced drink of bicarbonate of soda, diluted 1 teaspoon per cup of water, may be helpful.

## FRUIT- AND NECTAR-EATERS

These include Trochiliformes (hummingbirds). The adults do well on 4 parts water to 1 part dextrose (or table sugar) with a few drops of vitamins. This mixture is offered to self-feeding birds. However, additional nutrition *must* be provided with protein foods such as fruit flies or squeezed mealworms. Protein can be added to the liquid mixture by mixing Similac® (Ross) or mockingbird food. The following mixture is recommended:

> 1 Cup water
> 4 Drops ABDEC® (Parke, Davis) Baby Vitamins (or Avitron® [Lambert-Kay])
> 10 Mealworms
> 2 Tablespoons Soyalac® (Loma)
> ¼ Cup sugar
> Blend thoroughly and refrigerate.

The food should be administered to adults with a red-tipped eyedropper or hummingbird's feeder. If the bird is weak, it can be forced to eat by placing its beak tip into the eyedropper. If this does not work, a pipette may be carefully inserted into the mouth and a small amount given frequently. Generally, the hummer needs to drink its fill every 20 to 30 minutes. If the baby hummer gapes, it can be fed with a cut-down infant catheter attached to a tuberculin syringe.

Do not allow the mixture to come into contact with the bird's feathers. This very sticky material is impossible for the bird to preen off and thus destroys the insulation and renders it difficult to maintain the normal body temperature (about 110° F.).

## PREDATORY LAND BIRDS

These include the Orders Falconiformes (vultures, hawks, falcons) and Strigiformes (owls). All these birds seem to be obligate carnivores, so all that is needed to assure adequate nutrition is healthy, live, freshly killed, or frozen food. Although vultures will eat carrion in the wild, and the hawks and falcons will take reptiles, it is easiest to feed these birds healthy mice, rats, guinea pigs, chicks, etc. Variety is probably important. Butcher meats are adequate only as occasional meals. The nestlings and young birds can be fed diced chicken, mice or rats. If their eyes are not open, or they otherwise refuse to eat by visual stimulation, the food may be rubbed gently against the sensitive bristle-like feathers on each side of the beak. The young grow alarmingly fast (a young barn owl will double its weight every 10 days), and they need to be fed about 2 to 3 times daily. Dipping the diced pieces of food in water provides a liquid supplement.

At about 4 weeks of age the birds will take the prey in their talons, and whole animals may be given. The adults should receive one or two feedings per day and be given as much as they will eat. An adult red-tailed hawk will eat four to five mice or a whole rat daily, and a healthy kestrel will eat one large mouse or one chick daily.

Barn owls will often not eat for the first two or three days and must be force-fed. This is accomplished by gently pushing a wet baby rat or mouse head-first into the esophagus using water for additional lubrication. Care must be taken to insure that the talons are under control. It is not necessary to add pellet material to the diet of raptors, as is commonly thought. It is also not necessary to "teach" raptors to hunt, for their hunting and survival instincts are very strong, and they revert to their natural habits within a week or two of their release. However, to accomplish this it is very important that they be neither tamed nor imprinted.

## PREDATORY WATER BIRDS

These include both fresh and sea water birds of the following Orders:

Charadriiformes (shorebirds, gulls, auks)
Ciconiiformes (herons, storks, etc.)
Pelicaniformes (pelicans and cormorants)
Procellariiformes (albatrosses and petrels)
Graviiformes (loons)
Coraciiformes (kingfishers)
Podicipediformes (grebes)

A mild fish such as white bait (smelt, 10 to 15 grams each) provides adequate nutrition and is readily available frozen. These fish should be fed to the adults head-first. Unfortunately most of these birds will need force-feeding initially. This is accomplished by placing the fish well back in the pharynx and closing the bill. The fish is then "milked" down by gently squeezing the esophagus so as not to disrupt the neck feathers. The following guide gives the approximate number of fish per day and should be divided into 3 or 4 equal feedings. Thiamine should be supplied every two to three days at a dose of 50 to 200 mg., depending on the size of the bird, to counteract any thiaminase in the fish.

Gulls: Large (over 1 kg.) 30 to 35 fish/day
       Small (0.5 kg.) 12 to 25 fish/day
Auks (murres): 30 fish/day if healthy, 40 to 50 if emaciated
Cormorants: 30 to 50 fish/day

If the bird is unable to handle whole fish, they may be puréed, or very slightly diluted strained baby food meats may be fed by gavage. The amount should be from 60 to 80 ml. every 2 hours. In very young birds, some whole egg may be substituted. In adult birds, dog food can be substituted, and they should be encouraged to self-feed on it.

These birds should be supplied with enough water for bathing and head immersion. However, orphaned young birds may become water-logged and therefore must be prevented from swimming for long periods. These birds should be handled as little as possible to avoid disruption of the plumage, which would retard their waterproofing. The shore birds may be stimulated to self-feed by placing mealworms and fish bits in a container filled with sand and enough water just to cover the sand.

Kingfishers seem to be obligate carnivores of both fresh and salt water, and the adults can be maintained on a diet of small fish, frogs, etc.

## OMNIVOROUS WATER BIRDS

These include both fresh and sea water birds of the Orders Gruiformes (cranes, coots, rails) and Anseriformes (waterfowl). The adult birds will do well if a variety of food is offered. This should include poultry starter mash, dog food, insectile food, fish and possibly some water weeds. Water should be provided as mentioned above, and the same precautions should be taken.

Precocial beak-feeding chicks (cranes, coots, rails) require a considerable amount of care, and the attempt is often discouraging. The parents of these birds offer insects, seeds and weeds by dangling them from their beaks. This can be simulated with forceps, but, as with the gaping chicks, the correct stimulus must be found. These chicks should be fed hourly.

### SUPPLEMENTAL READING

Cucuel, J. P. E.: Husbandry of captive wild birds. See Kirk, R. W. (ed.): Current Veterinary Therapy V. Philadelphia, W. B. Saunders Co., 1974.

Farnar, D. S., and King, J. R. (eds.): Avian Biology. 4 vols. New York, Academic Press, 1972–1974.

Fiennes, R.: Feeding Animals in Captivity. International Zoo Yearbook, 1966, pp. 58–67.

Lanyon, W. E., and Lanyon, V. H.: A technique for rearing passerine birds from the egg. The Living Bird, 8:81–93, 1969.

Petrak, M. I. (ed.): Diseases of Cage and Aviary Birds. Philadelphia, Lea & Febiger, 1969, pp. 143–174.

Welty, J. C.: The Life of Birds. 2nd ed. Philadelphia, W. B. Saunders Co., 1975.

# TREATMENT, HUSBANDRY AND REHABILITATION OF OIL-SOAKED BIRDS

JAMES M. HARRIS, D.V.M.
*Oakland, California*

*and* DAVID C. SMITH, B.S.
*Berkeley, California*

The veterinarian who is interested in caring for wildlife and in the problems involving the environment and who is practicing along the coasts or any major waterways on which petroleum is transported will have to deal with oil-soaked birds.

Oil-soaked birds presented to the clinician must be treated for the following acute conditions: hypothermia, shock and stress, starvation, toxic effects of the oil and acute traumas. Birds that successfully survive the acute stages of exposure to petroleum products then have to face the following chronic problems which the veterinarian must prevent and/or treat: long-term stress, malnutrition, toxicity, aspergillosis, ammonia fume–associated irritation to the mucous membranes, cloacal impaction, bumblefoot-like lesions and sternal bursitis.

## IMMEDIATE TREATMENT

The insulatory ability of oiled feathers is reduced, thus allowing body heat to escape at a greatly increased rate. The bird's metabolic rate increases by up to a factor of three to maintain its normal temperature. Since a 3-cm. diameter spot of oil on the breast of a bird can result in severe heat loss, hypothermia is almost always present in oil-soaked birds presented for evaluation and treatment. In addition, the oiled bird ceases to forage for food, resulting in catabolism of subcutaneous fat stores and pectoral muscles for needed energy.

It is imperative that warmth be provided so that these birds can survive long enough to be treated for the other concurrent problems. Piles of rags in the bottom of boxes used to transport these birds and ventilated boxes of fairly solid structure, such as cardboard, will greatly help in keeping the birds warm. Heaters in clinics and/or treatment centers are also essential to reduce the chilled state of these patients.

Concurrent with hypothermia are shock and stress due to exposure, handling and transport. Following is the recommended precleaning treatment of oil-soaked birds:

1. Loosely wrap the body of the captured bird in cloth (rags, towels or diapers); place it in a covered, ventilated cardboard box (one bird to a box); and immediately transport it to a treatment center. This prevents further ingestion of oil, slows heat loss and minimizes visual stress.

2. Band the bird when it arrives at the center and begin individual records. This allows a biologist to establish differential treatment for purposes of research.

3. Introduce 40 ml./kg. hydrating solution (see Table 1) into the proventriculus (upper stomach) with a No. 14 to 18 French catheter attached to a large disposable syringe. Repeat every hour for the first 3 hours and then 4 times a day thereafter.

4. Administer intravenously or intramuscularly 3 mg./kg. dexamethasone and 1 ml./kg. 50 per cent dextrose. (Intravenous medication can easily be given in the tarsal or wing vein using a 22- to 25-gauge needle.) Place a poncho on the bird and delay further treatment for 30 minutes.

5. Introduce 10 ml./kg. heavy medicinal mineral oil into the proventriculus. Wipe the exterior of the catheter dry before intubation to minimize the possibility of aspiration of the mineral oil. Delay further treatment for 30 minutes.

6. Provide suitable food, deep bedding (except for alcids), and an ambient temperature between 24° and 27° C. (75 to 80° F.).

7. Decide which birds are ready to be cleaned and what cleaning agent is to be used. A decision key is provided in Table 2.

8. Before cleaning, check the bird's record to

694

determine whether it has had an injection of dextrose and dexamethasone within the previous 4 hours. If not, it should receive another dose and be given 40 ml./kg. 5 per cent dextrose *per os*. Then the bird should be cleaned.

Many birds that have been oiled, having been at sea for a number of days, may be in a state of starvation. This can be easily detected by palpating the keel of the bird. Marked reduction in the muscle mass of the pectoral muscles usually indicates starvation and dehydration. It is best not to attempt to clean birds that are in this state until they have been hydrated, given nourishment and allowed to rest for one to four days. Signs of oil toxicity may be readily apparent, especially if oil is ingested, and include respiratory distress, diarrhea mixed with petroleum and cutaneous inflammation. The enteritis associated with oil toxicity can be controlled by giving orally either neomycin with methscopolamine (Biosol-M®, Upjohn) or kaolin and pectin with neomycin.

Traumas associated with capture and wave and sea action should also be treated. Fractures, lacerations, contusions, avulsions and other traumatic injuries should be treated as for any other patient. When antibiotics are needed, those with a broad spectrum seem to be most helpful. Chloramphenicol given intravenously is effective against a wide range of pathogens affecting wildfowl. When possible, culture and sensitivity studies are helpful. Injuries requiring anesthesia can be handled well using Ketaset® (Bristol) or nitrous oxide-fluothane anesthesia. Ketaset has been our anesthetic of choice in almost all cases, at a dose of 0.5 to 1.0 mg./15gm. of body weight.

Since the feet of most water birds are particularly sensitive to drying and heat, bland ointment such as A and D ointment®, (Schering), petrolatum or a lanolin-based ointment should be applied on a regular basis. Accurate medical records should be kept on each patient, for as long as the patient is under medical supervision. Admittance weight, cloacal temperature and observations should be recorded in addition to treatments and other clinical impressions.

## TREATMENT OF CHRONIC PROBLEMS

Birds whose feathers do not regain waterproofing and insulating qualities must be kept a considerable length of time. During this period, many of the chronic problems listed above develop. Long-term stress may be associated with population density, light exposure, temperature, noise and salt. All these factors must be considered in order to reduce stress to its lowest possible level.

Malnutrition is frequently a problem with birds kept for any length of time. An adequate diet is essential. Fresh or frozen fish or substitute foods, such as dog food pellets and commercial duck foods, can be used for some species.

Long-term oil toxicity is difficult to treat. The degree of toxicity depends upon the amount of oil absorbed by the birds upon first exposure to the petroleum product. The liver, kidneys, spleen, intestinal mucosa and heart can be affected by petroleum products. Depending upon the individual bird and which organ or organs are affected, the symptoms of toxicity will vary over a period of time.

Aspergillosis is a common problem encountered in wildfowl kept in captivity for long periods of time. Using bedding material that will not encourage the growth of *Aspergillus* seems to be the most practical way of preventing it. Rags, foam rubber, serval or crushed sugar cane and pine shavings seem to make the best bedding for birds. Straw and hay should not be used. All bedding should be changed regularly and frequently.

Although a number of drugs have been

---

*Table 1.   Medications and Solutions*

Corticosteroid:
  Dexamethasone
    3 mg./kg. intramuscularly or intravenously once or
      twice daily only
Intestinal antispasmodic:
  Biosol-M® (Upjohn)
    3 drops/kg. orally every 6 hours
Gastric demulcent:
  Kaopectate® (Upjohn)
    10 mg./kg. stomach tube every 4 hours
Hydrating solution (hypotonic, for dehydration and
    hypoglycemia):
  Mix: 5 gm. (1 level teaspoon) table salt
    25 ml. 50% dextrose *or* 12 gm. table sugar (3
      level teaspoons)
    1 liter (or 1 quart) fresh water
  Administer 40 ml./kg. by stomach tube
Isotonic sugar solution (approximately 5 %):
  Mix: 100 ml. 50 per cent dextrose *or* 50 gm. table
      sugar (4 level teaspoons)
    1 liter (or 1 quart) fresh water
  Administer 40 ml./kg. by stomach tube

used for the treatment of aspergillosis, none has proved to be practical or effective. If the bedding is not changed regularly, the ammonia fumes produced by decomposing droppings cause serious irritation to the conjunctiva and nictitating membranes. Good sanitation is of primary importance at all times.

Most sea birds are used to defecating in water. Birds kept out of water will frequently develop impactions of the cloaca. Mineral oil inserted through the vent will help to relieve this problem, but often, just making sure the birds enter water periodically will suffice.

Lesions of the joints, very similar to bumblefoot in domestic fowl, are frequently encountered. To date, every conceivable form of treatment for these joint lesions has been tried. Success has been uniformly poor but we believe that prevention through the use of proper bedding and access to water can be accomplished. Sternal bursitis, similar to breast blisters in chickens, is also frequently seen. This is best treated as an open, granulating wound. Topical proteolytic enzymes, chloramphenicol, furacin dressing and powder and hydrogen peroxide are all helpful in treating these open lesions.

## CLEANING AND REHABILITATION

In addition to the above medical care, a veterinarian may also be asked to advise and to help with the capture, preliminary treatment, transportation, cleaning, rehabilitation and release of oil-soaked birds.

Birds should be transported one to a box, preferably in a cardboard box with a top large enough to hold an adequate supply of soft, warm bedding. Birds should not be cleaned until they are adequately hydrated, warm, out of shock and not in a state of starvation. The cleaning method employed should completely eliminate the oil from the feathers but should not produce long-term reduction in waterproofing and insulating effects of the feathers.

The following is an annotated list of current cleaning methods:

*Cleaning with Solvent.* The first requirement is for human safety. Shell Sol-70® has produced fair results and does not ignite easily (flash point 40° C. or 104° F.), but once burning, it burns fiercely. Therefore, it is necessary to ban smoking and provide adequate fire extinguishers. The area should be well-ventilated and everyone should wear a suitable respirator and protective clothing, boots, gloves, masks and hoods.

Warm solvent (35° C. or 95° F.) is placed in 3 to 5 basins, and the bird is given serial baths, taking care not to damage feathers.

Following the baths, the plumage must be rinsed out with flowing solvent. We have built a portable unit that dispenses warm solvent under pressure to 12 nozzles arranged in 6 stations. For lightly oiled birds this rinsing unit is all that is needed for cleaning. When the bird is clean, it is blotted with clean diapers and thoroughly dried with a warm-air dryer such as those used for show dogs.

Final steps in the process involve hydration and rest in a "drunk tank" for 6 to 9 hours until the bird recovers from its intoxicated state caused by the solvent. The bird can then be immediately placed in a pool with easy egress, where it can swim, preen, drink and eat. An audiovisual teaching package is available to train volunteers in the details of this cleaning technique.

*Cleaning with Mineral Oil.* When cleaning with mineral oil, use all the techniques used for cleaning with a solvent except for warm-air drying. Respirators, fire extinguishers and the drunk tank are unnecessary. The bird must be warm and introduced to water gradually, since its plumage will neither be waterproof nor provide effective thermal insulation for some days after cleaning.

*Cleaning with Detergent.* We simply have not been able effectively to clean nor subsequently to release aquatic birds in excellent condition using detergent. Those who have been successful recommend serial baths of a 1 per cent detergent solution warmed to 40° to 45° C. (104° to 113° F.). Thorough rinsing with jets of warm water (40° to 45° C.) is necessary to remove hydrophilic detergent residues.

The reason for our lack of success with this method is probably related to the types of polluting oil we have been encountering. Most of the birds we have received were covered with either very aged heavy oils or lubricating oils, neither of which can be readily emulsified by detergents.

(Please refer to Table 2 for a treatment and cleaning key.)

Following cleaning, good husbandry and rehabilitation is instituted. The plumage of water birds will deteriorate when kept out of water because of contamination, mechanical disruption and diminished care by the bird. Seabirds in the wild depend upon the impeccable condition of their plumage for protection from the cold air and water, and when kept in warm and dry surroundings they neglect their plumage to some extent

*Table 2.* *Treatment and Cleaning Key*

1. Clear the mouth and nostrils of oil. Go to 2.
2. Administer IV: 3 mg./kg. dexamethasone and 1.5 cc./kg. 50 % dextrose. Go to 3.
3. a. Oil is nearly solid and caked on. Go to 4.
   b. Oil is fairly fluid or gooey. Go to 5.
4. Use a catheter to introduce 40 cc./kg. water into the proventriculus. Go to 6.
5. Clearing oil from digestive tract: Rapidly introduce 150 cc. water by catheter into the proventriculus. Follow in 15 minutes with 15 cc. mineral oil. Go to 8.
6. a. Bird is energetic and alert, its cloacal temperature is within 1° C. of normal and it shows no signs of hydrocarbon toxicosis.* Go to 14.
   b. Bird is weak and hypothermic or shows some symptoms of toxicosis. Go to 7.
7. Feed and water for 2 days. Provide considerable warmth. Go to 6.
8. a. Oil is easily emulsified by detergents.** Go to 9.
   b. Oil is *not* easily emulsified by detergents. Go to 10.
9. a. Oil is *not* completely nontoxic.† Go to 6.
   b. Oil is *not* completely nontoxic. Go to 11.
10. a. Bird is showing severe symptoms of hydrocarbon toxicosis.* Go to 12.
    b. Bird is showing mild symptoms of hydrocarbon toxicosis. Go to 13.
    c. Bird is showing minimal/no symptoms of hydrocarbon toxicosis. Go to 14.
11. a. Bird is showing severe symptoms of hydrocarbon toxicosis.* Go to 12.
    b. Bird is showing some symptoms of hydrocarbon toxicosis. Go to 15.
    c. Bird is showing no symptoms of hydrocarbon toxicosis. Go to 14 or 15.
12. Euthanize.‡
13. Clean in warm mineral oil. Go to 6.
14. Clean in warm solvent.
15. Clean in warm detergent solution.

* Symptoms of hydrocarbon toxicosis include anorexia, inability to digest foods, asthenia, ataxia, opisthotonos, blood in stool, convulsions. In wild birds, anorexia is often a result of stress and not of toxicosis.

** To determine: Mix 0.1 cc. of oil with 100 cc. 3% detergent solution.

† Only mineral oil (white oil) and most vegetable oils are nontoxic.

‡ The decision to euthanize might also be dependent upon the scarcity of a particular species or the estimated recuperative capabilities of individual birds.

Putting a weakened bird immediately into a harsh environment is not the answer, because exposure adds to the bird's state of exhaustion and stress. Intermediate steps are needed such as lightly spraying the bird occasionally or placing it into a pool that is somewhat protected from the weather and from which the bird can easily leave. In practice, a properly cleaned bird may be put into a protected artificial pool 8 hours after cleaning and then may be put into an unprotected environment (with plenty of food) within two or three days. One observation is that many aquatic birds refuse to remain in the water of a small pool (1.2 meters square) but will more willingly remain in the water of a larger pool (2 m. x 3 m.). Pools must have constant surface overflow, since bird droppings contain large amounts of fish oils which in still water will form a surface film and will re-oil birds' feathers.

Many questions still remain. Is there a cleaning method that will allow immediate release? What are the species' specific dietary requirements? What specific drugs and antibacterials, if any, would be more effective, and at what levels should they be administered? Are released birds able to survive and breed?

Great progress has been made in the care and treatment of oil-soaked birds as of this writing. Whereas three to four years ago, a 2 per cent survival rate was good, present methods now are producing a 50 per cent return to the wild. Since birds are excellent biologic monitors of the oceans and shore areas, these efforts are worthwhile.

Recently a number of excellent publications have been printed on this subject and are listed below for supplementary reading.

## SUPPLEMENTARY READING

Clark, R. B., and Kennedy, J. R.: Rehabilitation of Oiled Sea Birds. Newcastle-upon-Tyne, England, University of Newcastle-upon-Tyne, 1968.

Naviaux, J. L.: After Care of Oil Covered Birds. Pleasant Hill, California, National Wildlife Health Foundation, 1972.

Recommended Treatment of Oiled Sea Birds. Newcastle-upon-Tyne, England, Department of Zoology, University of Newcastle-upon-Tyne, 1972.

Stanton, P. B.: Operation Rescue. Washington, D.C., The American Petroleum Institute, 1972.

# PSITTACOSIS— ORNITHOSIS*†

R. A. BANKOWSKI, D.V.M.
*Davis, California*

PAUL ARNSTEIN, D.V.M.
*Berkeley, California*

*and* K. F. MEYER, M.D.‡
*San Francisco, California*

It has been known for almost 100 years that certain birds, particularly psittacines, harbor microorganisms that may cause severe pneumonia in man. Conclusive evidence is now available that the microparasite responsible for psittacosis in birds and in man belongs to a unique group of microbes assigned the name *Chlamydia* and classified in the order Rickettsiales. They cannot be considered as typical rickettsiae, viruses or bacteria but rather constitute a distinct category. They are obligate intracellular parasites; in purified suspensions they show the presence of both ribonucleic acid and deoxyribonucleic acid. Their multiplication appears to be by binary fission; characteristic clusters of elementary bodies are formed in cells infected by single infectious particles. Very unlike the true viruses, they are susceptible to some antibiotic compounds, particularly tetracyclines, which act by arresting their multiplication.

When classified by their principal hosts, the *Chlamydia* fall into three groups— human, other mammalian and avian. Psittacosis and ornithosis (avian *Chlamydia* infections) are true zoonoses; they are directly transmissible from the infected animal to man.

Several diseases in addition to psittacosis and ornithosis of household pet birds are important in veterinary medicine; for example, bovine and ovine infectious abortion; lamb polyarthritis; bovine, ovine, caprine and feline pneumonitis; feline follicular conjunctivitis; and turkey and duck ornithosis. In this article, however, we will consider only psittacosis and ornithosis of pet birds. The usual terminology applied to chlamydial diseases in pet birds is psittacosis if the patient is of the family Psittacidae (parrots, parakeets, cockatoos, macaws and so forth) and ornithosis if the patient belongs to any other avian family. In instances in which these agents cause disease in man, the disease is commonly called psittacosis regardless of the reservoir host from which man acquired it.

All birds are susceptible to virulent chlamydial strains originating in avian reservoirs. Numerous strains have been tested to determine their relative infectivity and pathogenicity for various species of birds, and it has been observed that the avian *Chlamydia* constitute a broad spectrum of varying pathogenicity. Of the commonly encountered cage birds, parrots, parakeets and pigeons can be considered potential reservoir species; the other pet cage birds, such as canaries, finches, rice birds and mynahs, although highly susceptible to ornithosis, usually contract it from one of the previously mentioned reservoir species.

## SYMPTOMS AND PATHOLOGIC LESIONS

Chlamydial infections in birds cause systemic disease, with septicemia and fecal excretion of the microorganism common during the acute phases. Outward appearance of the bird is no different from that seen in other febrile systemic illness, ruffled feathers, depression, sleepiness, lack of appetite, watery feces and rapid loss of weight have been observed in acutely diseased birds. Later, there is commonly a temporary reduction in the quantity of feces, which tend to be extremely dark and tenacious. If disease persists beyond the

*This investigation was supported in part by Public Health Service Research Grant No. AI-04406, from the National Institute of Allergy and Infectious Diseases.

†Disclaimer: Trade names are provided as information only, and their inclusion does not imply endorsement by the Public Health Service of the U.S. Department of Health, Education and Welfare.

‡Deceased.

698

twentieth day, stools usually become copious again—very watery and whitish. At this time dry, sticky exudate may appear at the nares. The mortality rate may approach 100 per cent among species having little or no resistance (such as parakeets, conures, Amazons, canaries and finches) if no specific antibiotic medication is given.

In relatively more resistant hosts, such as the cockatoos and the various breeds of pigeons, the mortality rate is lower, varying from 10 to 50 per cent, depending upon the virulence of the infecting *Chlamydia*.

In typical aviary epizootics among the common parakeets (*Melopsittacus undulatus*), psittacosis mortality rates of 20 to 90 per cent have been observed under field conditions and confirmed in the laboratory. The variance is undoubtedly a result of differences in microbial virulence and in genetic susceptibility of the hosts.

If canaries, South American parrot species, lorikeets, rosellas, finches and rice birds infected with ornithosis or psittacosis are untreated, they commonly suffer extremely severe illness, usually terminating in death. The exceptional birds that recover spontaneously do so after prolonged periods of weakness and depression. Such convalescing birds harbor and shed infective *Chlamydia* for many months.

A tentative diagnosis of psittacosis or ornithosis can usually be established following dissection and careful examination of dead birds. The infectious agent, although systemic in its distribution, causes gross lesions that often form a characteristic pattern in the host, especially in advanced acute or severe chronic disease. The lesions to look for are (1) a significant enlargement of the spleen, sometimes accompanied by softening, gray discoloration and pearly foci in this organ; (2) liver abnormality, particularly swelling, fragility, yellowish discoloration, rounded edges and focal necroses; (3) exudate, cloudiness or yellowish clots in the air sacs; (4) purulent, serous or fibrinous pericarditis; and (5) congestion of the intestinal tract, particularly the serosa.

The lungs of most terminal psittacosis or ornithosis cases in birds are remarkably free of gross pathologic lesions.

## DIAGNOSIS

Confirmation of psittacosis or ornithosis is difficult in the live patient because symptoms resemble those of other avian diseases. Only a tenative diagnosis usually is possible, based on association of the bird with an infected or suspected reservoir host and no confirmed diagnosis of other disease. In larger psittacines and in pigeons, acute and convalescent blood specimens can be tested for complement-fixing antibody and for infectious *Chlamydia* by experienced microbiologic laboratories. Satisfactory blood specimens can be obtained by jugular vein or wing vein puncture. Confirmatory isolation of the etiologic agent from blood or feces proves the presence of psittacosis or ornithosis, but this may take three weeks or longer in the laboratory. Specialized laboratory training and facilities are essential for reliable identification of chlamydial isolates. Because these infections may be transmitted to man, it is probably safest to deal with suspects as with confirmed cases.

In fatal avian cases, the typical gross lesions and the demonstrations of typical chlamydial elementary bodies in smears are strong evidence that the bird died of psittacosis (or ornithosis). The best diagnostic smears are made from the air sac membranes or the pericardium, if exudate is present. The smears are stained by Machiavello's method. The *Chlamydia* are seen under high power, oil immersion magnification ($1000\times$) as characteristic clusters of red spherules, approximately 250 to 400 $m\mu$ in size. Additional laboratory work is necessary for final confirmation. Frozen or refrigerated liver and spleen samples can be processed for isolation of the etiologic agent if promptly submitted to specialized microbiologic laboratories.

## TREATMENT

Early chemotherapy with tetracyclines arrests multiplication of the *Chlamydia* and usually completely eliminates the agent. Since the tetracyclines inhibit rather than inactivate the organism, extended therapeutic schedules lasting as long as 45 days are required. Because of the wide choice of formulations in which it is available, chlortetracycline is probably the most practical antimicrobial drug currently available for psittacosis or ornithosis control. It has been extensively tested against chlamydial microorganisms and has shown particularly potent inhibitory activity. Chlortetracycline is readily absorbed from the gastrointestinal tracts of birds. Administration of the antibiotic in feed requires minimal manipulation of infected birds, reducing risk of infection for the therapist. It is also very effective therapy and is the method chosen under usual conditions.

## PROPHYLAXIS

There is no effective vaccine for psittacosis control; since recovery from natural infection results in only partial immunity, it is unlikely that a vaccine would be practical. Prophylactic chemotherapy and subsequent protection from exposure are the recommended control measures. Parakeets, parrots and pigeons are probably the most frequently encountered psittacosis (or ornithosis) suspects in veterinary practice. Management procedures for them are described in further detail.

**Parakeets.** Several cooperating wholesale centers routinely feed the antibiotic (chlortetracycline-impregnated millet, 0.5 mg. chlortetracycline/gm.) for 15 consecutive days to all parakeets just before they are consigned to retail channels.

This voluntary prophylactic disinfection procedure has been practiced for almost 10 years. It is estimated that about 70 per cent of parakeets offered for retail sale in the United States have undergone this treatment. As a result, parakeet psittacosis is not seen nearly as frequently today as it was before the initiation of these programs.

In spite of considerable improvement in the epidemiology, parakeet psittacosis cannot be described as nearing eradication; each year serious cases of psittacosis in humans are traced to parakeets, often bringing to light large numbers of diseased, infective birds. The reason is that there is no easy way to ascertain whether any one specific parakeet or collection is a psittacosis hazard. Treated birds cannot be differentiated from untreated ones; in addition, psittacosis could be contracted by the bird after chemotherapy.

The most beneficial recommendation to the pet owner is to give all his parakeets an effective antichlamydial regimen at least once after purchase. The easiest method is to feed millet seed impregnated with 0.5 mg. chlortetracycline/gm. of seed (Keet Life®). This formulation is readily available and effectively controls psittacosis. It should be fed exclusive of all other feed for 15 consecutive days if the bird is well and for 30 days or longer (depending upon severity of the disease and rate of clinical improvement) if the bird is ill or suspected of having active psittacosis infection. After treatment the bird can be reinfected; treated birds should therefore be kept isolated from potential sources of infection.

Of course, if more than one bird is in a household, all should be treated prophylactically at the same time. If new parakeets are to be added to the household, they should undergo the prophylactic oral regimen before being put in contact with the previously treated birds.

Parakeets that are clinically ill, refuse to eat and are suspected of harboring psittacosis may be administered chlortetracycline injections into the pectoral muscles; 5 to 10 mg. daily, contained in 0.5 ml. of inoculum, can be given for as long as five days. By this time, the bird should be able to eat the medicated millet; at least 15 full days' oral treatment with medicated millet should be given after the bird's daily consumption returns to normal.

When giving injections, the operator must use aseptic procedures and wear a face mask. Intramuscular injection of psittacosis-infected birds poses a risk to the operator; this procedure is not highly recommended and euthanasia is preferable, provided the owner is amenable.

Other small, seed-eating birds, such as canaries, finches and rice birds, may be fed the chlortetracycline-impregnated millet prophylactically or therapeutically if they are exposed to psittacosis or if the infection is diagnosed in an early phase.

**Parrots.** Psittacines larger than parakeets will not subsist on a diet of millet only. In order to obtain satisfactory blood levels of chlortetracycline (at least $2 \mu g./ml$ of blood), the concentration of chlortetracycline in the feed of large psittacines must be approximately 4 to 10 mg./gm. (0.4 to 1 per cent). A satisfactory feed base for incorporating the antibiotic is cooked rice and hen scratch. A convenient source of chlortetracycline is a 22 per cent mixture in soybean meal (chlortetracycline hydrochloride, 220 gm./kg., Aureomycin SF66®, Lederle).

For the preparation of the ration, rice is mixed with hen scratch feed and water in a weight ration of 2:2:3 (for example, 1 lb. rice, 1 lb. hen scratch and 1½ pints water).

This mixture may be cooked in a pressure cooker, autoclave or ordinary cooking utensil until it is soft but not mushy. Ten to 15 minutes in a kitchen or canning pressure cooker is about right. The chlortetracycline must be added after the feed has cooled. If the 22 per cent concentrate is used, a simple procedure is to weigh the needed quantity of cooked and cooled feed first; subsequently, add chlortetracycline concentrate in a quantity equivalent to 2 per cent of this weight. Mixing must be very thorough. A small amount of brown sugar may be added last for greater palatability.

Using this formula, the final concentration of pure chlortetracycline will be 4.4 mg./gm. of cooked feed. As much of the medicated feed should be portioned out as the bird consumes in 24 hours. A bird needs a quantity equivalent to approximately one fifth its weight daily after it has become used to the diet. Consumption differs, and the amount offered should vary accordingly. On this ration, birds tested have within a few days built up blood levels of 2 to 10 $\mu$g. of chlortetracycline/ml. of blood.

Other feed should not be offered during the treatment period. A small supply of coarse sand or fine gravel is given in a separate dish, preferably combined with a vitamin and mineral source, such as chick starter or broiler chow. Fresh water should be available to the bird at all times. It is recommended that medicated mash be fed exclusively for 30 and preferably 45 consecutive days. The ration must be prepared fresh daily.

Dry, stable pellets containing essential daily nutrients and 0.5 per cent chlortetracycline have been developed and tested. They are accepted by all seed-eating parrots and effectively control psittacosis in known infected groups. Administration is the same as described for the cooked mash, but daily preparation is unnecessary because the pellets maintain potency at least six months and probably longer.

In experimental groups of freshly captured normal parrots as well as in groups of known infected birds, a diet consisting exclusively of chlortetracycline-nutrient pellets maintained birds in satisfactory condition for 45 days and longer and resulted in excellent control of psittacosis. Subsequently, these pellets have been used in treatment centers for prophylactic medication of birds prior to importation into the United States. Under these field conditions, they also proved to be practical and effective. The chlortetracycline-nutrient pellets are not sold commercially at this time; information regarding their future availability may be requested from Hartz Mountain Pet Foods, Inc., 700 South Fourth Street, Harrison, New Jersey 07029.

It is strongly recommended that one of the 30- to 45-day oral chlortetracycline treatments be given on a prophylactic basis to all newly acquired pet parrots and parrots intended for exhibit purposes, in order to eliminate latent, inapparent psittacosis.

Parrots may be treated by intramuscular injections of a tetracycline (oxytetracycline, tetracycline or chlortetracycline) at a dosage level of 40 to 50 mg. daily, depending on the size of the bird. This route is recommended only if the animal is too ill to eat the medicated ration. The operator should exercise extreme caution to avoid inhaling infective aerosols during handling; he should wear a mask at all times.

NECTAR-FEEDING BIRDS. The Loriidae (lories and lorikeets), which are becoming more popular as pets among fanciers of the unusual, ordinarily feed on nectar and fruit in nature. In order to obtain satisfactory blood levels of chlortetracycline, an all-liquid diet furnishing moisture and nutrients and the needed concentration of drug is the medicament of choice.

The base ration consists of 4 parts water, 1 part honey and 1 part liquid dietary canned food (Nutrament®, Drackett). To this mixture, chlortetracycline from opened oral capsules is added fresh daily in a quantity of 500 mg./liter (or 0.05 per cent); the bird must be fed in glass or plastic cups. A small amount of kibbled dog food or boiled rice is added to each feed cup as an attractant and a source of additional nutrients. During the 30 to 45 days when this feed is given, no other feed is offered.

**Pigeons.** The same antibiotic concentrate (22 per cent chlortetracycline in soybean meal) used for parrots has proved useful in preparing medicated rations that produce blood levels of chlortetracycline considered adequate for ornithosis control. The basic nutrient is uncooked dry hen scratch feed, processed as follows:

Weigh out the needed amount of scratch feed, and add chlortetracycline concentrate amounting to 4 per cent of the weight of the hen scratch. Moisten with just enough water to make the chlortetracycline concentrate stick to the seeds of hen scratch feed, and mix very thoroughly.

The final concentration of pure chlortetracycline is 0.89 per cent. Pigeons usually eat only 10 to 15 gm. of this mix for the first few days. When the pigeon becomes accustomed to it, consumption averages 50 gm. daily. The level of chlortetracycline in the pigeon's blood is 2 to 4 $\mu$g./ml., which is adequate for ornithosis control if maintained for 30 to 45 days.

In a recent important paper, it has been documented that the inhibitory effect of antibiotics on chlamydial multiplication is reversible. The ability of *Chlamydia psittaci* to resume normal multiplication after its macromolecular syntheses have been brought to a near standstill by chemotherapy agents may, in part, be responsible for the difficulty with which psittacosis infections are eradicated by drug therapy (Tribby *et al.*, 1973).

The chlortetracycline-containing nutrient pellets described for parrot medication have been tested on small numbers of pigeons. Excellent blood levels were produced.

### RESULTS OF CONTROL MEASURES

The utilization of chlortetracycline in bird rations as a method of antichlamydial prophylaxis has become widespread. Desirable changes probably attributable to the practicability of this antimicrobial regimen have occurred. Cases in humans that are traceable to pet birds have declined in the past 10 years from about 150 a year to less than 50 a year for the entire United States. This decline is even more significant when viewed in the light of increased popularity of psittacine pets in United States homes during this time; more than 3 million are sold in retail stores each year, and about 70 per cent of them have probably been prophylactically treated at one of the wholesale centers. The vigor and plumage of the average bird are reportedly superior following completion of the chemotherapy; this may well be because subclinical bacterial or mycoplasmal infections susceptible to chlortetracycline are controlled.

Establishment of antichlamydial effects of chlortetracycline following oral treatment and its mandatory application during quarantine allowed safe and legal importation of psittacines. From 1971 to 1972, it was estimated that over 2 million birds have been imported and there are over 26 million pet birds in homes and in aviaries. Only very rarely have cases of psittacosis in humans been associated with these imported and exotic birds. According to *Morbidity and Mortality*, January 13, 1973, pigeons were the most probable source of infection in nine cases, parrots in six, parakeets in four, canaries in two, chickens in one and turkeys in one. Thus the main source of human and pet bird psittacosis and ornithosis probably remains at the epizootically infected breeding aviaries, particularly those in which parakeets and pigeons are raised.

Additional significant reduction of cases could result from the elimination of these foci by chlortetracycline therapy of entire aviary populations, including all breeding stock and juveniles. Following such flock treatment lasting 30 to 45 days (depending upon whether the flock is a known or suspected chlamydial harbor or the treatment is for prophylaxis only), the birds can return to their usual diets. Of course, all additions to such psittacosis- and ornithosis-free flocks would have to be from other similar flocks or placed in quarantine and treated before integration into the aviary. An added benefit in treated aviaries may be the reduction of nonspecific maladies, chronic enteritides and respiratory problems, many of which are probably of bacterial or mycoplasmal etiology and responsive to chlortetracycline treatment.

### IMPORT AND DISEASE CONTROL REGULATIONS

Prior to 1972, importation of psittacine birds for commercial use was regulated by the Department of Health, Education and Welfare. Regulations required that all birds in the psittacine family be treated prophylactically for psittacosis at one of the Public Health Service approved treatment centers in a foreign country before their arrival in the United States. During 1970 and 1971, evidence was accumulated substantiating the presence of exotic Newcastle disease in psittacine, greater and lesser Indian Hill mynah and other exotic birds which were being imported. This resulted in outbreaks of the exotic form of Newcastle disease in various pet bird and commercial poultry operations. To protect the industries of the United States from exotic Newcastle and other communicable diseases of poultry, importation of all birds into the United

States was placed under the regulations of the Animal and Plant Health Inspection Service of the United States Department of Agriculture.

The following are requirements for commercial birds imported for the purpose of resale, research, breeding or public display: (1) an import permit in advance of shipment; (2) a health certification by a full-time salaried veterinarian in the government in the country from which the birds are shipped; (3) each lot must be quarantined for a minimum period of 30 days in a facility provided by the importer in the immediate vicinity of the port of entry; and (4) during the quarantine period, all exotic birds of the psittacine family must receive treatment with chlortetracycline as a precautionary measure against psittacosis in accordance with guidelines previously set up by the United States Public Health Service. Such guidelines may be obtained from the Director, Center for Disease Control, U.S. Public Health Service, Atlanta, Georgia 30333, or from the Deputy Administrator, Veterinary Services, Animal and Plant Health Inspection Service, U.S. Department of Agriculture, Washington, D.C. 20250.

Special arrangements can be made for two personal pets per family when the Deputy Administrator, Veterinary Services, determines that such importations will not involve the risk of introduction or spread of any communicable disease of poultry. Details concerning importation procedures of these birds may be obtained from Deputy Administrator, Veterinary Services, Animal and Plant Health Inspection Services, U.S. Department of Agriculture, Hyattsville, Maryland 27082.

Most state health departments require prompt notification of confirmed or suspected psittacosis and ornithosis in either humans or animals. This is similar to the regulations dealing with other zoonoses. Some states require identification bands on all parakeets sold locally or transported interstate, for purposes of tracing sources of psittacosis infection.

### SUPPLEMENTAL READING

Crawford, K., et al.: Psittacosis in Maryland. J. Infect. Dis., 121:236–238, 1970.

Meyer, K. F.: The present status of psittacosis-ornithosis. A.M.A. Arch. Env. Hlth., 19:461–466, 1969.

Tribby, I. I. E., Friis, R. R., and Mowlder, J. W.: Effect of Chloramphenicol, Bifampicin and Nalidixic Acid on Chlamydia psittaci growing in L cells. J. Infect. Dis., 127:155–163, 1973.

---

# DISEASES OF THE AVIAN URINARY SYSTEM

ROBERT B. ALTMAN, D.V.M.
*Franklin Square, New York*

It is important to remember a few basic anatomic and physiologic facts that apply to the avian species. These facts are of importance in diagnosis and particularly in interpretation of necropsy findings.

Avian kidneys are metanephric and contain many small glomeruli. The kidneys are buried in the pelvic girdle and are partially trilobed, extending from the ventral surface of the ilium between the sixth and eighth ribs to the sacral region. The right and left kidneys of the budgerigar are often joined posteriorly. The ureter, extending along the ventral surface of the kidneys, enters the cloaca. The urinary bladder is absent.

All the purine nitrogen and most of the amino nitrogen is excreted as uric acid, which is seen in the droppings as the central white material surrounded by a black, green or brown fecal ring. There is reabsorption of water in the cloaca. Tubular excretion accounts for more than 60 per cent of the urinary nitrogen excreted as uric acid. The kidney plays an important role in regulating the acid-base balance and osmosis.

## ACUTE NEPHRITIS

Acute renal disease is almost impossible to diagnosis ante mortem. The course is too rapid and the symptomatology too varied. The only signs may be abnormal droppings, lethargy, rapid breathing and death. The etiology of acute nephritis is infectious (as seen in fowl) in which a purulent nephritis and ureteritis are seen. This form of nephritis is rarely found in caged birds.

Toxic nephritis is seen in disorders such as sodium chloride poisoning. This condition is observed in canaries in which the food is salted or beach sand is fed to the bird. Salt poisoning is noted less frequently in parakeets because this species has the ability to handle hypertonic drinking solutions. Necropsy findings with salt toxicity show only congestion of the kidneys and occasionally enteritis.

With acute nephritis, histopathologic sections may show congestion (nephrosis) and hemorrhage.

## CHRONIC NEPHRITIS

Chronic nephritis is seen with greater frequency than is acute nephritis, but diagnosis is still difficult.

The symptoms of this condition are variable and can apply to many other syndromes. These birds have generally been sick for several weeks and show inappetence, weight loss, depression and puffiness. The character of the droppings varies from a solid fecal ring surrounded by clear watery fluid, with little or no urates evident initially, to a copious amount of watery, nonsolid, green liquid.

The cere, beak and legs may be cyanotic, and the legs may be swollen with engorged vessels. Polydipsia is not consistently evident.

The differential diagnosis of chronic nephritis must be made utilizing the laboratory for clinical blood studies. Blood uric acid levels as determined by micromethods have been reliable. Only 10 lambda (0.01 ml.) of serum are required for this test. Values up to 10 mg./100 ml. in the budgerigar are considered normal, and values of 10 to 15 mg./100 ml. are considered suspicious. Above 15 mg./100 ml. indicates definite renal impairment. High phosphorus levels (normal 1.6 to 9.7 mg./100 ml.; mean 4.3) are also an indication of renal impairment.

Glucose levels should be determined to eliminate the possibility of diabetes. Glucose levels in excess of 550 mg./100 ml. serum must be considered positive. Screening for urine glucose can be done with the use of Clinitest® (Ames) tablets.

Treatment is empirical, and since it is impossible to confirm a diagnosis in a recovered bird, its efficacy is questionable. The bird should be kept warm (85° to 90°F.) and placed on a low-protein diet (millet seed). Vitamin supplements with high levels of vitamins A and B complex should be administered via the drinking water in a water-soluble form or orally. Antibiotics can be given orally or parenterally.

## NEOPLASTIC RENAL DISORDERS

Neoplastic renal problems are seen with increasing frequency. Symptoms are more specific and diagnosis is less difficult than in other renal disorders. These birds show signs of depression, polydipsia and polyphagia, with moderate to severe weight loss. Abdominal distention is often seen with occasional evidence of ascites. A relatively consistent symptom is unilateral or bilateral paresis of the toes and legs. Pressure on the sciatic nerve at the point at which it crosses the enlarged kidney creates this problem.

The droppings are usually less frequent but voluminous or extremely watery as the result of loss of normal urates in the urinary part of the droppings.

The prime diagnostic feature is positive confirmation of a mass by abdominal palpation. Since this technique is of such importance diagnostically, great care should be taken to explore the abdomen thoroughly by deep palpation.

Confirmation of an abdominal mass or renal enlargement, if not made by abdominal palpation, may often be identified radiographically. Normal serum glucose and elevated uric acid levels may also confirm the diganosis.

Treatment is futile and euthanasia should

be advised as early as positive diagnosis can be established.

Most of these tumors are renal adenocarcinomas, particularly in the parakeet. Sarcomas and, rarely, adenomas have been reported.

## RENAL CYSTS

Cysts (solitary or multiple sites) are most often associated with tumors. The abdomen is soft and fluctuating, and aspiration reveals a clear yellow fluid often containing floccular material made up of clumps of white blood cells. In canaries, renal cysts not accompanying tumors are seen on the dorsal aspect of the pelvic girdle through a pelvic foramen.

## GOUT

Gout, a relatively common disease found primarily in the parakeet but affecting all species, has an unknown etiology. In a high percentage of cases, associated renal disease is found. Metabolic dysfunction is considered a possible cause.

Uric acid is deposited at the joints and along tendon sheaths of the extremities (articular gout) or in the visceral organs (visceral gout), including the surface of the serous membranes, the epicardium, pericardium, liver, intestines, and connective tissue. These deposits are extracellular. Articular gout is the form most often seen.

A sign of articular gout is restlessness; the bird shifts its weight from one leg to the other. The toes do not always curl around the perch, and the joints show signs of swelling and blood vessel engorgement. Careful inspection of the legs shows small yellow-white nodules (tophi of uric acid crystals) at the joints. There is much pain associated with this condition.

Surgical curettage of the larger tophi offers some relief, but euthanasia is indicated because treatment is useless and the prognosis hopeless. Microscopic examination of the curetted material reveals needle-shaped or amorphous crystals.

# AVIAN ANESTHESIA

WILBUR B. AMAND, V.M.D.
*Philadelphia, Pennsylvania*

Keeping birds as pets has increased in popularity over the past few years so that the number of caged birds closely rivals the number of cats and dogs. The small animal practitioner is frequently confronted with an avian patient requiring medical or surgical treatment. All too often, veterinarians are reluctant to engage in avian surgery because of the small size of the patient and the surgeon's unfamiliarity with the anesthetic tolerance of birds. In these sensitive animals, it has been found that the anesthetic technique can be more important to the successful outcome of surgery than can the surgical technique. The ability to anesthetize a bird requires, in part, a simple appreciation of the unique avian respiratory system. The avian response to general anesthetics is essentially similar to the mammal's despite the marked anatomic and physiologic differences. Petrak (1969) presents an excellent review of basic avian respiratory anatomy and physiology.

## PRE-ANESTHETIC EVALUATION

A pre-anesthetic examination is a must for each potential surgical or elective anesthetic patient in order that an appropriate anesthetic agent may be selected for each individual case. The choice of an anesthetic agent is likely to be influenced by several factors: age of the patient, general physical condition, coexisting disease, severity of the present surgical disease and the extent and anticipated duration of the surgical procedure. Other factors such as the availability of technical assistance, ease of administration and personal preference will undoubtedly influence the choice of agent. In general, it is advisable to use an agent familiar to the surgeon.

Where a medically treatable disease coexists with a surgical condition, anesthesia should be delayed until such time as the medical condition has been corrected, if such a delay would not needlessly risk the life of the patient. It is especially important to recognize any respiratory disease which would make the risk of general anesthesia prohibitive.

Birds are noted for their poor cutaneous sensation and seem to experience little if any pain upon incising or suturing the skin. However, certain areas such as the head, scaled parts of the legs, limb joints and vent are highly sensitive, and painful stimuli can be readily provoked. Despite the differences in response to pain stimuli, anesthesia should be used for avian patients to the same extent as is considered necessary for mammalian patients. On occasions, when an ultrashort surgical procedure is required, such as lancing an abscess or amputating a toe, the risk of anesthesia may far outweigh its usefulness.

## LOCAL ANESTHESIA

Local injectable anesthetics have been advocated by some individuals, while others claim them to be toxic for birds. These agents have limited use in avian practice because of the need for manual restraint and the associated shock, especially to the smaller birds.

Injectable agents such as procaine or xylocaine can be used to anesthetize the base of a pedunculated cutaneous or adnexal tumor and the surrounding skin. A 0.25 per cent procaine solution has been used successfully in parakeets. At higher concentrations, procaine may be toxic, producing ataxia, seizures and finally death. The dosage must be accurately calculated to avoid the toxic effects. A 1 ml. tuberculin or preferably a microliter syringe with a 25 or 26 gauge needle is essential for the administration of these drugs. One should avoid injecting large amounts of the local anesthetic or injecting into deep or vascular tissues. Local anesthetics containing adrenalin are to be avoided in avian practice.

Topical spray anesthetics such as ethyl chloride or Cetacaine® (benzocaine, Cetylite) are useful in avian practice for lancing an abscess or replacing a prolapsed cloaca or oviduct. These spray agents are generally safe when used in small quantities.

## GENERAL ANESTHESIA

The stages of narcosis and anesthesia in birds have been classified by Arnall (1961). These stages are as follows:

### Narcosis

1. Light narcosis: The bird appears sedated and is lethargic; the eyelids tend to droop.

2. Medium narcosis: The feathers are ruffled and the head hangs low; the bird can be aroused but offers little resistance to handling.

3. Deep narcosis: At this stage, there is little or no response to sounds; fluttering may be provoked by painful stimuli, and shrill cries may be emitted after the stimulus is discontinued (especially with barbiturate narcosis). Respiration is usually fairly rapid, regular and deep but may become irregular following stimulation.

### Anesthesia

1. Light anesthesia: Reflexes (palpebral, corneal, cere, pedal) are present but there is a lack of voluntary movement; the bird exhibits no response to vibration or postural changes.

2. Medium anesthesia: The palpebral reflex is lost and the pedal and corneal reflexes become sluggish. Respiration is slow, deep and regular. This is the anesthetic stage where most operations can be performed.

3. Deep anesthesia: All reflexes are absent and respirations are very slow but may be regular. Any further deepening of anesthesia will further depress respirations until they cease.

### Signs of General Anesthesia

There are two general signs which one may use to assess the stage of anesthesia: (1) reflex responses and (2) respiratory rate.

1. The disappearance of reflex responses (palpebral, corneal, cere or comb and wattle, pedal) has minor variation among species of birds. The most sensitive areas such as the comb or wattle, cere and the interdigital web are usually the last to show absence of response to painful stimuli. The corneal and palpebral response is generally a less reliable indicator of the depth of anesthesia.

2. Once surgical anesthesia has been attained, observation of the depth, rate and

pattern of respiration is frequently the most reliable, if not the only, means by which one can monitor the patient. Sudden changes in any of the respiratory parameters may signal trouble and should indicate a need for further evaluation of the anesthetic state.

General anesthetics are by far the most satisfactory agents for avian anesthesia, as they allow the surgeon more freedom and reduce the danger of shock and trauma to the patient. The general anesthetics may be divided into two groups: inhalation and injectable. The inhalation anesthetics are the agents of choice for avian anesthesia, for they allow the surgeon to control or adjust the concentration of the anesthetic in the inspired air, thereby reducing the chance for toxicity to the patient. This is in contrast to injectable anesthetics which, once injected, are rapidly absorbed, and a small error in dosage may result in acute toxicity and death. A possible exception to the latter statement is the injectable cyclohexamines which will be discussed below under Injectable Anesthesia.

## INHALATION ANESTHESIA

Halothane, methoxyflurane, ether, ethyl chloride and cyclopropane are inhalation anesthetics which may be used with varying degrees of safety in avian patients. Nitrous oxide should be considered only in augmenting the effect of other anesthetic agents. When nitrous oxide-oxygen anesthesia has been used, only slight narcosis was achieved even at levels of 95 per cent nitrous oxide. However, nitrous oxide-oxygen, in combination with other acceptable inhalation anesthetics such as halothane, may be used to induce surgical planes of anesthesia.

Chloroform is an extremely potent anesthetic and quite "toxic" to most avian species. Although some investigators have successfully used chloroform, it cannot be recommended for use an an anesthetic in *any* species of cage or aviary bird. This agent is better regarded as an agent of euthanasia rather than as an anesthetic drug.

Halothane is the safest inhalation anesthetic, permitting very precise control of the inspired concentration, a short induction period and a rapid postanesthetic recovery. Induction can be achieved by placing the bird's head (including the cere-nasal openings) into a mask and delivering a 2.5 to 3.0 per cent concentration of halothane in a 0.5 to 1.0 liter flow of oxygen. A nonrebreathing system such as an Ayers "Y" Piece is convenient for small birds. Anesthesia is normally induced within three to four minutes, after which the concentration of halothane should be reduced to a maintenance concentration of 1.25 to 1.5 per cent. In larger birds (mynah birds, parrots, fowl, etc.), a small endotracheal tube can be inserted and the anesthetic delivered directly into the trachea. Once the bird is anesthetized, it is important to observe the rate, depth and pattern of its respiration, as these are frequently the only objective signs readily available for determining the depth of anesthesia. As a bird approaches surgical anesthesia, it will frequently experience a transient excitement period. The wings will tremble or actually flap and the nictitans will oscillate beneath the closed lids. When the bird relaxes, it can be placed on its back with the mask either taped or held manually in place. Recovery from halothane anesthesia is rapid, usually taking no more than 5 to 10 minutes.

Methoxyflurane has become a very popular anesthetic agent for birds. Doubtless, this popularity has resulted from the low toxicity and wide margin of safety of this agent. The major disadvantage of methoxyflurane is the longer induction period (8 to 10 minutes) and similarly longer recovery period, as compared with halothane. Methoxyflurane, like halothane, is nonexplosive at room temperature and can be used safely with electrocautery. Induction requires a concentration of 3.5 to 4.0 per cent, while a concentration of 2.0 per cent will usually maintain the patient during surgery.

Ether and ethyl chloride have long been used as general anesthetics for birds. These agents are generally administered by the open drop method or by placing a small pledget of cotton, which has been saturated with the anesthetic, over the nares until anesthesia has been induced. Anesthesia can be maintained by intermittent exposure to the agents. Ether has the disadvantage of being very irritating to the mucous membranes. However, the major disadvantage of both ether and ethyl chloride is their explosive properties, a major consideration before employing electrocautery. With the advent of newer and safer anesthetics, ether and ethyl chloride have become less popular as general anesthetics except perhaps for very short procedures.

Cyclopropane (25 to 45 per cent) with oxygen may be used to produce graded planes of anesthesia in birds. This seems to be a simple, easily managed and predictable inhalation anesthetic. A serious drawback is the highly explosive nature of cyclopropane, which limits its safe use. In large birds, anesthesia may be induced with intravenous pentobarbital and then maintained on cyclopropane via an endotracheal tube, or anesthesia may be attained with cyclopropane by mask, thus avoiding the need for barbiturates.

There are two serious complications which may be encountered when anesthetizing small psittacine birds. Because of the small oral cavity and the position of the larynx, it is usually impossible to insert an endotracheal tube. As a bird relaxes under general anesthesia, its large fleshy tongue frequently falls back over the laryngeal opening, causing an obstruction to respiration. This hazard can be corrected by keeping the tongue pulled forward and down. A paper clip molded to the contour of the lower beak works well for this purpose.

Vomiting and aspirating present still another hazard which can be avoided by placing a small diameter polyethylene tube in the esophagus. In the event of vomition, the material will pass through the tube and be directed away from the airway.

Occasionally, it is difficult or unwise to remove a conscious bird from its cage for purposes of examination or therapy. In these instances, the cage may be placed in a clear plastic bag and attached to an anesthetic machine. A high oxygen inflow is used with the vaporizer set at moderate to full position, thereby flooding the cage with the anesthetic. The object is to induce a light plane of anesthesia which will permit one to safely remove the bird from the cage and perform the necessary procedures. If a surgical plane of anesthesia is required, additional anesthetic may be administered by mask or via an endotracheal tube as described above.

## INJECTABLE ANESTHESIA

Injectable anesthetics have been used in birds with varying degrees of success. It is extremely important that the patient be weighed accurately on a gram scale. The importance of this step cannot be overemphasized. A slight error in the calculation of the dose of an injectable anesthetic may be fatal to the small avian patient. Small birds can be placed in a plastic bag or lightweight plastic container to facilitate weighing them. Larger birds can be wrapped in a light cardboard cylinder. The average budgerigar weighs 30 gm.; the average canary weighs 20 gm.

Once injected, the anesthetic is rapidly absorbed. If an overdose has been administered, the patient should be kept warm while oxygen is administered and the other supportive measures deemed necessary are performed.

There are three routes whereby parenteral anesthetic agents may be injected: intramuscular, intravenous and intraperitoneal. The intramuscular route is the most commonly used. Either the pectoral muscles or thigh muscles are acceptable sites of injection. When injecting into the pectoral muscles of small birds, the needle should be inserted at an angle deep into the craniolateral aspect of the muscle mass. Avoid penetrating any air sacs.

The intravenous route may be employed for administering parenteral anesthetics to larger birds such as falcons, hawks and poultry. The most accessible veins are the wing or brachial vein and the jugular vein. However, the poor clotting qualities and thin-walled veins which are a characteristic of birds may cause unsightly hematomas and ruptured vessels following venipuncture. Intravenous anesthesia is difficult to achieve in small birds owing to the small size of the readily accessible veins and the danger of shock to the patient by restraining it in an unnatural position; however, in larger birds (ducks, ornamental fowl, etc.), the intravenous route is acceptable.

Intraperitoneal injection of parenteral anesthetics is often convenient in birds. Injections should be made anterior to the cloacal ring in a cranial direction midway betwen the cloaca and the sternum, on the midline. Extreme care should be exercised when administering anesthetics intraperitoneally because of the danger of accidentally penetrating an abdominal organ or rupturing an air sac.

Of the several injectable anesthetics available, Equi-Thesin®*, a mixture of

---

*Jen-Sal.

chloral hydrate, magnesium sulfate and sodium pentobarbital, is the safest, most reliable and most satisfactory. Administered intramuscularly at a dosage of 2.5 ml./kg. of body weight, Equi-Thesin produces anesthesia in 5 to 15 minutes and lasts for 30 minutes to one hour. Birds that are weak, debilitated or in shock should be given a smaller dose, 2.0 to 2.2 ml./kg. of body weight.

Intramuscular pentobarbital sodium may be used when other anesthetics are unavailable; however, it is somewhat unreliable, having a poor margin of safety. When used, it should be given at the rate of 1.5 mg./30 to 35 gm. of body weight.

The cyclohexamines (phencyclidine, tiletamine, ketamine, etc.) are a group of related drugs which have enjoyed much popularity in recent years. These drugs produce a "dissociative state," are analgesic and, in appropriate dosage, produce a state resembling anesthesia. The specific effects of these drugs seem to vary with the species of animal but, in general, ocular, oral and swallowing reflexes are present, the eyes remain open and muscle tone is increased. Excessive doses may produce tremors and convulsions.

Cyclohexamine anesthesia in birds was first reported in 1964. Phencyclidine was the first drug in the group to be used. However, more recently ketamine has become the favored drug in the group. Numerous reports have advocated its use as a preanesthetic or the sole anesthetic in a variety of avian species requiring general anesthesia. However, the dosages reported have covered a rather wide range.

For parakeets and other small birds, a dose of 1 to 3 mg./30 gm. of body weight (33 to 99 mg./kg.) has been reported. At the higher dosage (2 to 3 mg./30 gm.), complete surgical anesthesia may be evident in three to five minutes and lasts for 5 to 20 minutes. Recovery from anesthesia may be complete in 20 to 30 minutes following the 2-mg. dose but lasts for 40 to 90 minutes at the higher 3-mg. level. Surgical anesthesia was not attained at the lower dosage (1 mg./30 gm.); however, simple procedures such as trimming beaks and splinting broken bones could be easily performed at this lower level.

No signs of toxicity to ketamine appeared in parakeets even at 3 mg./30 gm. (although recovery time was prolonged). A transient excitatory phase (flapping wings) may occur in some birds during the recovery phase. To minimize the possibility of injury during this period, a simple restraining device such as a piece of stockinette or fiberboard cannister may be placed around the bird. This excitation phase in some ways resembles the psycomimetic effect seen in man when given ketamine, in which hallucinations, confusion and agitation occur.

The use of ketamine in larger birds such as fowl and various raptors has likewise been successful. A dosage of 15 to 20 mg./kg. injected intramuscularly produces immobilization and anesthesia in one to five minutes, the effect lasting from 30 minutes to six hours, depending upon the dose. Anesthesia may be maintained in prolonged procedures by additional injections of ketamine (10 mg./kg.) as required or by switching to an inhalation anesthetic.

As with other anesthetics, the *exact* dosage of ketamine must be calculated and the dosage reduced for debilitated birds. Recognizing that ketamine is eliminated via the kidneys, fluid therapy may be indicated in debilitated birds or in those exhibiting a prolonged recovery period. In large birds, fluid may be given intravenously. In small birds, fluid is best given subcutaneously in the wing web or loose skin of the neck.

## ANESTHETIC EMERGENCIES

Evaluating the depth of general anesthesia is relatively difficult in birds. The reflex responses and respiratory rate give the best indication of the stage of anesthesia. (See discussion above under General Anesthesia.) It is advisable to maintain the bird in a light to medium plane of surgical anesthesia, thereby minimizing the chance of respiratory and/or circulatory arrest. This emergency may occur suddenly with little if any warning and may be precipitated by the loss of a large volume of blood, a sudden drop in blood pressure or obstructed respiration.

Apnea may occur during induction or recovery from anesthesia with volatile anesthetics. This usually results from an accumulation of the anesthetic gas in the air sacs. Therefore, it is important to maintain an adequate (but appropriate) oxygen flow during both the period of induction and of recovery. Although the anesthetic gas accumulates in the air sacs, there appears to be no absorption from this site. The air sacs act as a reservoir for the gas. It is recirculated from the air sac to the recurrent bronchi where absorption occurs with each respiration.

If respiratory arrest should occur or if breathing should become slow and/or labored, the inhalation anesthetic must be immediately discontinued and 100 per cent oxygen should be delivered via face mask or endotracheal tube. If apnea exceeds five seconds, artificial respiration should be administered by exerting slight digital pressure on the thorax at the rate of 2/second, using the thumb and forefinger. In larger birds, with an endotracheal tube in place, oxygen can be forced through the lungs and air sacs to flush out any residual anesthetic.

Administration of central nervous system stimulants to aid resuscitation has been reported. The recommended dose for a parakeet is 0.2 ml. of bemegride (3.5 mg./ml.) injected intramuscularly.

If a large amount of blood is lost during surgery, fluids should be administered subcutaneously or intravenously to maintain an adequate intravascular volume and to prevent circulatory colapse. If cardiac arrest occurs, 100 per cent oxygen should be administered while applying closed cardiac massage. Unfortunately, respiratory and cardiac arrest frequently occur simultaneously and are usually fatal.

## PRE- AND POSTANESTHETIC CONSIDERATIONS

Whenever possible, the avian patient which requires anesthesia should be admitted to the hospital for a period of acclimation 12 to 24 hours before the procedure. The bird should be kept in quiet, warm quarters (80° to 85° F. or 27° to 29° C.).

Because of the high metabolic rate of birds, prolonged fasting before anesthesia is undesirable, as the glycogen stores of the liver may be depleted, thereby reducing its detoxifying capacity and generally weakening the bird.

Following anesthesia, the bird should be allowed to recover in warm, quiet surroundings. It should be placed in a small, empty cage which has one or two perches close to the floor of the cage. A source of light may hasten the recovery. Food and water should be offered as soon as the bird is conscious and has regained full control of its balance and locomotion.

### SUPPLEMENTAL READING

Arnall, L.: Anesthesia and surgery in cage and aviary birds (I). Vet. Rec., 73:139–142, 1961.

Beck, C. C.: Chemical restraint of exotic species. J. Zoo Animal Med., 3:45, 1972.

Bennett, R. R.: The use of "metofane" in experimental laboratory birds. Pract. Vet.:184–186, 1961.

Borzio, F.: Ketamine hydrochloride as an anesthetic for wildfowl. Vet. Med./Small Animal Clin., 68:1364, 1973.

Bree, M. M., and Gross, N. B.: Anesthesia of pigeons with CI-581 (ketamine) and pentobarbital. Lab. Animal Care, 19:500–502, 1969.

Friedburg, D. M.: Anesthesia of parakeets and canaries. J. Am. Vet. Med. Assn., 141:1157, 1962.

Gandal, C. P.: Satisfactory general anesthesia in birds. J. Am. Vet. Med. Assn., 128:332–334, 1956.

Graham-Jones, O.: Restraint and anesthesia of small cage birds. J. Small Animal Pract., 6:31–39, 1965.

Jordan, F. T. W., Sanford, J., and Wright, A.: Anesthesia in the fowl. J. Comp. Path., 70:437–448, 1960.

Kittle, E. L.: Ketamine HCl as an anesthetic for birds. Mod. Vet. Pract., 52:40–41, 1971.

Mandelker, L.: Ketamine hydrochloride as an anesthetic for parakeets. Vet. Med./Small Animal Clin., 67:55–56, 1972.

Mattingly, B. E.: Injectable anesthetics for raptors. Raptor Res., 6:51–52, 1972.

Myers, R. E., and Stettner, L. J.: Safe and reliable general anesthesia in birds. Physiol. Behav., 4:277–278, 1969.

Petrak, M. L. (ed.): Diseases of cage and aviary birds. Philadelphia, Lea & Febiger, 1969.

Raises, M. B.: Anesthesia of cage birds. Australian Vet. J., 43:594, 1967.

Seidenstricker, J. C., and Reynolds, H. V.: Preliminary studies on the use of a general anesthetic in falciform birds. J. Am. Vet. Med. Assn., 155:1044–1045, 1969.

Soma, L. R. (ed.): Textbook of Veterinary Anesthesia. Baltimore, The Williams & Wilkins Co., 1971.

Whittow, C. E., and Ossorio, N.: A new technic for anesthetizing birds. Lab. Animal Care, 20:651–656, 1970.

# GENERAL TECHNIQUES FOR AVIAN SURGERY

WILBUR B. AMAND, V.M.D.
*Philadelphia, Pennsylvania*

Surgery is frequently required in the treatment of avian diseases: tumors (testicular, ovarian, lipomas, fibrosarcomas, etc.); abscesses; fractures; retained eggs; amputations; and hernias. The small size of many birds makes the surgical procedure very tedious and requires precise judgment. With a few important exceptions, general surgical principles can be applied to avian surgery.

## SURGICAL PREPARATION

Surgical preparation of the avian patient differs somewhat from that used for mammals. Preoperative medication is not routine. Because of the high metabolic rate and energy requirements of birds, food need not be withheld for any longer than 2 to 3 hours, except for a 4- to 6-hour fast prior to crop surgery. Prolonged fasting may adversely affect the patient's tolerance to the stress of surgery and prevent a satisfactory recovery.

Once the bird is anesthetized, the feathers should be plucked from a liberal area over and around the surgical site. Feathers should not be broken or cut, since the feather shafts thereby left embedded in the skin may cause irritation to the bird and may possibly lead to self-mutilation of the site.

Skin should be washed with a germicidal soap, dried and swabbed with 70 per cent alcohol. Tincture of iodine may be applied, although this is not absolutely necessary. Strict aseptic surgical technique is extremely difficult to achieve when operating on very small birds; however, every attempt should be made to maintain reasonable cleanliness.

Maintaining the bird's body temperature is very important throughout the surgical procedure. The bird should be placed on a hot-water bottle that has been wrapped in a clean towel or laid on a heating pad* with circulating warm water, such as is used in pediatric surgery. The patient may be held in place by an assistant or taped to the surface of the heating unit. If the latter method is used, narrow strips of adhesive or cellophane tape would be placed across the wings and tail only. Tape should not be placed over the body, since this may restrict respiration. The legs of large birds may be taped or tied to the operating table; however, this step is unnecessary in the smaller species.

Cloth drapes are not necessary and are usually undesirable in small birds, since they restrict visual monitoring of respiration and general anesthetic status. An acceptable substitute for cloth drapes is the commercially available transparent polyethylene drape, which will allow complete visualization of the small avian patient. With larger birds, small laparotomy drapes may be used to maintain a clean surgical field.

Sterile eye instruments are most convenient for avian surgical procedures. The instrument set should include iris scissors, strabismus scissors, plain and rat-toothed forceps, several smal hemostats and an orbital speculum. A small needle holder–scissors combination is very handy. An adequate number of sterile cotton-tipped applicators should be available, since they are excellent as sponges and for use in blunt dissection. A small pan of warm sterile saline should be on the set to be used for maintaining tissue moisture. A No. 15 blade is convenient for making the initial skin incision. Suture material may be absorbable or nonabsorbable, depending on preference and location of surgery; small-caliber material, 3-0 to 5-0, is most satisfactory.

*Gorman-Rupp Industries Division, Bellville, Ohio 44813.

711

## HEMOSTASIS

Hemostasis is essential in avian surgery because blood losses from a small bird may be fatal. Since cutaneous vessels are clearly visible through the transparent skin, whenever possible large vessels should be clamped and ligated with 3-0 catgut before transection. If large vessels are accidentally cut, they should be immediately clamped and ligated.

An electrocautery unit is most helpful, but caution is necessary to prevent excessive damage to surrounding tissue. The unit should be set up and properly grounded for immediate use in any extensive procedure in which hemostasis is anticipated to be a serious problem. Note that electrocautery cannot be used with volatile anesthetics such as ether or ethyl chloride. Be sure that all the alcohol has evaporated from the surface of the skin before using electrocautery, since the alcohol may ignite and severely burn the patient.

Silver nitrate, dilute epinephrine (1:10,000) and absorbable Gelfoam®* may be used on an oozing surface to effect hemostasis. A word of caution about the use of absorbable Gelfoam in small birds: the amount of blood absorbed before coagulation may be a fatal volume, although seemingly small. When the volume of blood lost is rather large, it is advisable to use subcutaneous or intraperitoneal saline in small birds and intravenous fluids in larger birds to maintain intravascular volume and prevent circulatory collapse. A 2.5 per cent dextrose in half-strength saline solution has been found to be adequate for this purpose.

## SURGICAL DISORDERS ENCOUNTERED IN THE AVIAN PATIENT

The following discussion of surgical disorders is meant to provide the reader with an appreciation for the scope of conditions that one may encounter when handling avian patients. It is not to be considered encyclopedic. Space does not permit a detailed description of each surgical technique. References listed at the end of this article should be consulted prior to engaging in any surgical procedure with which

---

*Upjohn Company, Kalamazoo, Michigan 49001.

one lacks familiarity. Giving attention to detail will increase one's surgical success rate when dealing with birds of all sizes.

### HEAD AND NECK

**Eyes.** Severe trauma to or infection in the eye may occasionally be encountered in which enucleation will be indicated. A review of the anatomy and an appreciation for the large size of the globe will aid in successful removal of the eye. Most enucleations will be successful unless concurrent ocular disease would either complicate or contraindicate surgical intervention. The small size of some avian patients may make enucleation difficult if not impossible. Lid closure and postsurgical management should follow established practices in mammals. Cataracts are not uncommon in canaries, parakeets, parrots, ducks and others. The disorder is usually bilateral and may be seen at any age but usually occurs in older birds. The techniques for removal are as those described for dogs. Owing to technical problems, cataract surgery has not been recommended in birds smaller than a pigeon or mynah bird.

**Sinuses.** It is not uncommon to encounter a chronic or residual sinusitis following a bout of upper respiratory disease. Signs are generally those of periorbital swelling, closure of the lid(s) and nasal discharge. If caseous material can be identified in the sinuses, removal should be attempted. The area should be surgically prepared, an incision made over the swelling and the material removed with a blunt curette or by flushing. Cultures of the sinus material assist in determination of appropriate medical aftercare. The incision may be left open to facilitate flushing and instillation of antibiotics post operation.

**Nares and Cere.** Rhinoliths have rarely been reported. These appear to be an amalgam of dust and dirt with nasal mucus. They produce a ball-valve effect that may obstruct breathing. Surgical enlargement of the nasal orifice facilitates removal of the obstructing material.

Hypertrophy of the cere has been reported in female parakeets. This condition may on occasion obstruct the nares. Remedial action consists of simply trimming away the keratinized material.

**Beak.** The beak is subject to a variety of insults, such as parasitic infestation with cnemidocoptic mites, trauma with hemorrhage or fracture and neoplasia—all of which may require some degree of surgical intervention. Simple trimming and cosmetic remodeling may be all that is needed to correct the beak distortions seen with the mite infestation.

Laminar hemorrhage following trauma must be differentiated from neoplasms involving the beak, since each has a different prognosis. Laminar hemorrhage needs little care unless the damage affects the vascular nutrition of the beak. Neoplasms of the beak generally have a poor prognosis unless they are detected early and appropriate measures are taken.

Small beak fractures may be stabilized through the use of lateral splints or of small pins that traverse the fracture site and add support until healing is complete.

Major beak fractures that compromise circulation and result in necrosis of the beak distal to the fracture site or traumatic avulsion of a beak carry a poor prognosis. A prosthesis may be considered. Unless the animal can be nutritionally sustained, it is best to consider euthanasia.

**Mouth.** Occasionally small papilloma-like masses are observed at the commissures of the mouth in parakeets. These masses are quite vascular. They rarely cause a problem unless they become too large and interfere with eating or are traumatized and bleed. Not uncommonly these masses spontaneously regress. If necessary they can easily be removed by crushing the base with a small hemostat and excising. Hemostasis should be a major consideration.

Lingual and palatine abscesses are commonly seen in the larger psittacines and some passerines. These are frequently associated with a prior upper respiratory infection. These lesions usually have an ovoid caseous core. The lesion may interfere with prehension of food and/or mastication. Treatment consists of surgically incising over the lesion and removing the inspissated pus. The raw denuded base which remains should be cleaned with antiseptics and dressed with antibiotics. These lesions usually heal rapidly with little obvious discomfort to the bird.

Foreign bodies such as seeds or sharp metallic, glass or plastic objects, etc., will occasionally penetrate the tissues of the mouth. These are handled as in any other species.

Tumors of the mouth or tongue have only rarely been reported and carry a poor prognosis.

**Crop.** Crop fistula, crop impaction and chronic dilatation of the crop are conditions which frequently require surgical intervention.

Crop fistulas are among the more difficult conditions to treat. These usually result from a laceration, penetration or pressure necrosis of the crop. Immediate attention improves the chances of healing. Where possible, the crop should be sutured independently with a second suture line in the overlying skin.

Every attempt should be made to relieve crop impactions asurgically. Oils, gentle external massage and flushing or purging the crop should be tried. Surgery, when required, should be done as aseptically as possible. Again, the incision should be closed in two lines wherever possible.

Where the crop has been chronically dilated and an abundance of redundant tissue exists, it is possible surgically to excise the excess crop tissue and tighten the structure in resuturing the tissue. There can, however, be no guarantee that the condition will not recur.

## BODY

**Cutaneous and Subcutaneous Neoplasia.** Both benign and malignant tumors are among the most common indications for surgery in the avian patient. Neoplasms may be encountered on the skin and in the subcutaneous tissues, abdominal organs and skeletal structures. Tumor surgery demands good surgical anesthesia. The surgical incision should be of ample size to provide adequate visualization of the lesion and assist in good control of hemostasis.

Lipomas or lipogranulomas are the most common subcutaneous tumors. This type of tumor must be differentiated from a pure granuloma, cyst and abscess. Benign subcutaneous tumors occur most frequently over the breast and abdomen and less frequently in the cervical area or over the extremities. Benign tumors usually have a soft consistency, are well-circumscribed and tend to shell-out easily. Fibrosarcomas and adenocarcinomas are frequently encountered malignant tumors. Malignant cutaneous and subcutaneous tumors are commonly found in the cervical area and the upper part of the leg and wing. They tend to have a firmer consistency with a broad invasive base, which makes complete surgical excision very difficult.

The uropygeal gland (preen gland), found at the base of the tail, is the site of a variety of disorders that may require surgical attention. Both benign papillomas and malignant adenocarcinomas are seen at this site. The adenocarcinomas are quite invasive and destructive. The anatomic area makes surgical removal quite difficult unless the tumor is seen very early in its development. Any swelling of the uropygeal gland should be differentiated from ductal obstruction, abscess or neoplasia.

Feather cysts involve one or more feather follicles and contain undeveloped feathers as well as amorphous materials. Although the cysts may be seen on any part of the body that is feathered, they are seen most frequently on the wings and dorsal aspect of the body. The cyst(s) should be incised, the contents removed by gentle curettage and the lining membrane cauterized with silver nitrate. When hemorrhage creates a problem, the cyst can be packed with Gelfoam, and stay sutures can be put in place to assist hemostasis.

**Abdominal Surgery.** Neoplasia, hernias and disorders of the ovary and oviduct are the most common problems requiring abdominal surgery. Disease involving the gastrointestinal system may occasionally require surgical intervention.

When performing abdominal surgery, one should incise the skin and peritoneum separately. A midline, a transverse or a cruciate approach is acceptable. Following the initial skin incision the scalpel should not be used again. Proceed with blunt dissection using a scissors, hemostat and moist cotton-tipped applicator. Frequently abdominal surgery is complicated by numerous adhesions involving the viscera. These adhesions must be carefully broken down by blunt dissection, while vessels are ligated as they are encountered. It is important to identify *all* structures before ligating or cutting, since it is difficult to anastomose structures in the smaller birds. Either 3-0 or 5-0 catgut can be used for vessel ligation and closure of the peritoneum and muscle. In the skin, 4-0 silk has been found to be satisfactory if it is removed in 7 to 10 days postoperatively; otherwise, catgut or other absorbable synthetic suture of appropriate size is acceptable. Either simple continuous

or interrupted skin sutures can be used. In small birds in which the peritoneum cannot be closed separately, the skin and muscle should be adequately closed with simple interrupted sutures.

The kidneys and gonads are the most common sites for abdominal neoplasia. Tumors involving these two organs are usually malignant, though they rarely metastasize. The tumors are usually quite large before signs appear or before the bird is presented for treatment. The anatomic site of the kidneys and large size of the tumors have made management very difficult; nevertheless, in selected cases surgery may be successful.

Neoplastic testes are quite common. Radiography and/or exploratory surgery may be needed to differentiate gonadal from renal neoplasia adequately, since the close anatomic proximity of both organs in an otherwise small abdomen frequently results in similar signs.

Neoplastic testes in a small bird are best removed through an abdominal incision. In larger birds, such as mynah birds, pigeons, parrots, etc., the testes may be removed by using the standard caponizing technique. The incision is made between the 6th and 7th rib on the right side. A rib spreader (ophthalmic speculum) may be used to open the incision and afford a better view into a rather small surgical field. A small pinpoint light source (such as Flexi-lum®*), which can be placed in the abdomen, assists in the visualization of very small organs. Normal testes vary greatly in size, shape and color and are located at the anterior pole of the kidney. Neoplastic testes often are quite vascular. These vessels should be ligated. Not infrequently both testicles will be neoplastic.

Ovarian cysts or neoplasms are indications for surgery in the female bird. A technique similar to that for castration in the male bird is used; however, the approach should be from the left side, since in most female birds the right ovary and oviduct degenerate. The anterior end of the oviduct should be ligated prior to transection.

Abdominal hernias are, for all practical purposes, a disease of female birds. The condition seems to be associated with excessive egg-laying. Obesity is frequently a coexisting disorder, and cholesterol may be

---

*Flexible surgical light, Concept, Inc., Airport Station, St. Petersburg, Florida 33732.

infiltrating the skin. A standard laparotomy is performed through the hernia, excessive muscle and skin are excised and the surgical wound is closed in two layers. It has been recommended that the skin suture line not lie directly over the musculature suture thereby assisting in sealing the abdomen and preventing infection. Hernias may recur.

Female birds may exhibit surgical diseases of the reproductive tract other than ovarian cysts and tumors. In older birds, ova will occasionally accumulate in the abdomen, causing distention. The ova can be removed through a standard surgical laparotomy. When the egg ruptures, a severe yolk peritonitis may develop and requires aspiration, flushing, vigorous antibiotic therapy and good nursing care.

Eggs may on occasion become lodged in the oviduct. The yolk material becomes inspissated and the shell leathery. Following laparotomy, the oviduct may be entered using the technique for a gastrotomy. If the egg has produced pressure necrosis of the oviduct, removal of the oviduct and ovary is advisable. Finally, prolapse of the oviduct in egg-bound birds may require some degree of surgical intervention to effect a successful treatment.

Foreign bodies, tumors, abscesses, impaction and obstruction involving any portion of the gastrointestinal tract may require surgical intervention in order to treat the condition adequately. Whenever any portion of the gastrointestinal tract is surgically entered or transected, extreme care must be taken so as not to compromise the circulation or lumen. Foreign bodies occasionally appear in the gizzard. The gizzard is a very muscular and vascular structure. Use the smallest incision possible to deliver the object and place as few sutures as necessary to seal the organ.

Although tumors, granulomas and abscesses are seen in the lungs of birds, these are usually diagnosed at necropsy. The anatomy of the respiratory system in birds severely limits the ability to perform surgery in this area, even if an antemortem diagnosis can be established.

## EXTREMITIES

**Wings.** Tumors, fractures and techniques to render a bird permanently flightless are the most common indications for surgery in this region of the body.

Tumors involving the wing are fairly common. The ratio of benign to malignant tumors is 2:1. Benign masses are small and well-localized and usually occur on the dorsal surface of the wing and in the region of the humeroradial joint. These are easy to remove; however, malignant masses are usually diffuse, invasive and difficult to dissect free of contiguous tissues. These latter tumors are frequently best managed by amputation of the wing. The amputation technique is similar to that for mammals.

Wing fractures may be managed by either external or internal fixation. In small birds, external immobilization is usually successful if the device is used for 3 to 5 weeks. In larger birds or where external fixation is not the method of choice, internal fixation may be accomplished by either intramedullary pinning or compression plates. Complications to be aware of are infections following compound fractures, development of malunions and nonunions, contraction of tendons and muscles and vascular and neural damage distal to the fracture site.

In zoologic or ornamental birds, it is frequently necessary to render a bird permanently flightless (pinioning). This may be accomplished by neurectomy, tenectomy, wing web resection or amputation. Of these several alternatives, amputation of the distal two thirds of the fused 2nd and 3rd metacarpals, leaving the alula intact, seems to be the most consistently satisfactory and cosmetically acceptable procedure. When done in young birds at 7 to 10 days of age, the procedure is comparable to tail docking. When performed in an older bird, the technique is only slightly more complicated.

**Legs.** Tumors, fractures, "bumblefoot" lesions and gout are among the disorders affecting the lower extremities that may require surgery.

Tumor types seen on the leg are similar to those of the wing. When the tumor is extensive, invasive, malignant or affecting bone, it is advisable to amputate the leg, using techniques described for mammals. Birds are able to adapt quite well with only one leg, using the beak to climb, balance, etc.

Fractures of the leg are handled in a manner similar to those described for the wing. It may be advisable to provide some external support for 1 to 2 weeks after pinning a leg fracture. One should check birds for long or curled toenails, since these may frequently lead to leg fractures in caged birds. In addition, leg bands which become too tight may lead to vascular embarrassment and dry gangrene. Amputation of the limb is indicated in advanced cases of gangrene.

Bumblefoot, a severe infection of the pad of the foot, is seen in larger caged birds, waterfowl, penguins, falcons, etc. The disorder is caused by chronic trauma to the bottom of the foot and secondary bacterial infection. Surgical excision of the lesions is usually required, after which vigorous medical treatment is indicated.

Gout, a crippling metabolic disorder seen in birds, affects the joints of the lower leg and foot and, less commonly, joints in the wing. There is no effective medical treatment. Urate deposits (tophi) may occlude the circulation to the distal extremities, resulting in necrosis and gangrene. In such cases amputation may be indicated. Large urate deposits may be incised and curetted to give some temporary relief. The tissue about the tophi is frequently quite vascular, and hemorrhage may be a problem.

## POSTSURGICAL MANAGEMENT

Prophylactic use of antibiotics postsurgically is not a routine procedure. When an infection exists at the time of surgery or develops postsurgically, antibiotics (potassium penicillin, tetracyclines, chloramphenicol, etc.) should be given orally or intramuscularly.

Some birds may be irritated by the skin sutures. If the bird picks at the surgical site, an Elizabethan collar made from lightweight, sturdy cardboard, oak tag or x-ray film may be secured about the bird's neck. The collar should fit snugly but not impinge on the esophagus or trachea. Some birds will react violently when a collar is first used; however, with time and patience, the bird should accept the device. A common mistake is to attach a collar too loosely, thereby allowing the bird to catch a leg or beak in it and possibly traumatize itself.

Following surgery the bird should be returned to a small cage devoid of toys, mirrors and food and water cups. One or two low perches may be left in the cage, since most birds will prefer to perch upon regaining consciousness. The ambient temperature should be 80° F. A bright light will aid in arousing a bird immediately after surgery, thereby shortening the postanesthetic period. If it is desirable to keep the patient quiet for a period of time after surgery, the cage should be covered or placed in a darkened room. Food and water may be returned as soon as the bird is conscious and has control of its locomotion.

Birds are normally discharged on the second or third postoperative day. The owner should be instructed to keep the bird warm and free from drafts at home, to supply ample food and water, to clean the cage regularly and to keep the bird confined to the cage until the surgical incision has completely healed. The cage should not be cluttered with toys, because they may be a source of trauma to the surgical site. Frequently, bird's feces will exhibit a change in color and consistency for several days postoperatively. This should not be a cause for concern unless attended by other signs of disease. All birds should be reexamined within two weeks postoperatively.

### SUPPLEMENTAL READING

Arnall, L.: Some common surgical entities of the budgerigar. Vet. Rec., 72:888–890, 1960.

Arnall, L.: Anesthesia and surgery in cage and aviary birds. Vet. Rec., 73:139–142, 173–178, 188–192 and 237–241, 1961.

Bush, M.: Avian orthopedics. Proc. Am. Assn. Zoological Veterinarians, Atlanta, Georgia, November, 1974, pp. 111–113.

Gandal, C. P.: Removal of an intra-abdominal tumor in a pigeon by radical incision. Avian Dis., 5:250–252, 1961.

Gandal, C. P., and Saunders, L. Z.: The surgery of subcutaneous tumors in parakeets (*Melopsittacus undulatus*). J. Am. Vet. Med. Assn., 134:212, 1959.

Keymer, I. F.: Cage and aviary bird surgery. Mod. Vet. Pract., 41:28–36, 1960.

Lafeber, T. J.: Infraorbital sinusitis of caged birds. J.A.A.H.A., 5:49–57, 1969.

Petrak, M. L. (ed.): Diseases of Cage and Aviary Birds. Philadelphia, Lea & Febiger, 1969.

Schwarte, L. H.: Poultry surgery. *In* Biester, H. E., and Schwarte, L. H. (eds.): Disease of Poultry, 5th ed. Ames, Iowa, Iowa State University Press, 1965.

Thorson, T. E.: Removal of cysts and cystic tumors from budgerigars. Mod. Vet. Pract., 52:39, 1971.

Wallach, J. D.: Surgical techniques for cage birds. Vet. Clin. N. Amer., 3:229–236, 1973.

# FRACTURES OF THE EXTREMITIES OF BIRDS

ROBERT B. ALTMAN, D.V.M.
*Franklin Square, New York*

For fractures of the pelvic extremities in passerine and small psittacine species, the simplest type of coaptation splintage is employed. This basic flap splint is lightweight and offers adequate support. It is simple to apply, does not require anesthesia, is easily made from adhesive tape and can be contoured to fit any shape leg at any point on the extremity.

For fractures of the pectoral extremities, adhesive tape is used to support and confine the wings to the body. This technique can be used in small and medium-sized birds (parrots, mynahs, macaws) and is simple to apply, rarely requiring anesthesia.

The techniques mentioned above are used in species in which approximation of the fragments can be accomplished, and in birds which can support their own weight without loss of support of the appliance.

In the event that alignment of proximal and distal segments cannot be accomplished, a surgical approach with pinning or plating must be considered.

If, because of the size or weight of the bird, it is felt that adhesive tape splintage would not be adequate to maintain support, plaster or fiberglass is used in a similar manner. With the application of plaster or fiberglass, anesthesia is generally necessary.

Fiberglass has replaced plaster for the most part, since it is much lighter, is more easily applied and dries faster; one or occasionally two layers are all that is required in contrast to at least twice that amount of plaster. Birds can chew through plaster much more easily than through fiberglass.

## FRACTURES OF THE LEGS

When applying a flap splint, the fracture should be reduced manually by digital pressure after the feathers have been plucked from the area to which the tape is to be applied. Prior to the application of the tape, the skin and surrounding feathers should be swabbed with alcohol.

**Midtarsometatarsal Fractures.** The bird is held by an assistant in a ventrodorsal position, with the fractured leg facing the clinician. Tension is applied by holding the leg in a straight upright position by the middle toe. A ¼- to ¾-inch wide piece of adhesive tape, approximately 4 inches long, is flapped around the leg (tarsometatarsal area) (Fig. 1) with three or four layers, leaving a ⅛- to ¼-inch flap on each side of the limb. With the fingers, this flap is pinched together close to the leg to fix the fractured ends. Tightly compress the flaps with a heavy hemostat (Fig. 2A). Total fixation is accomplished, giving rigidity to the splint

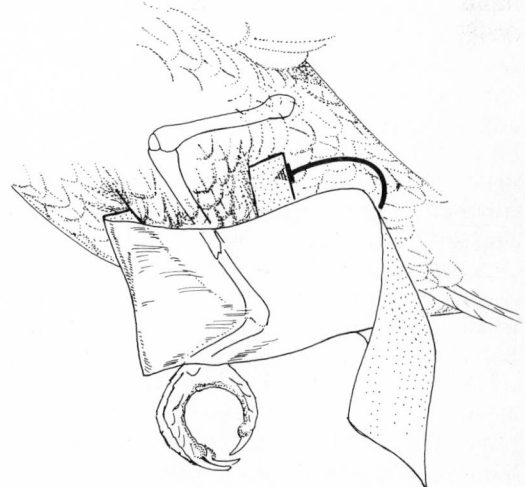

**Figure 1.** Mid tarsometatarsal fracture. First step in application of a "flap splint." The free end of the tape is then carried around for several more layers. Leg is flexed in normal standing position in diagram for illustration purposes only. During actual application, leg is held straight with tension and then flexed in final fixed position.

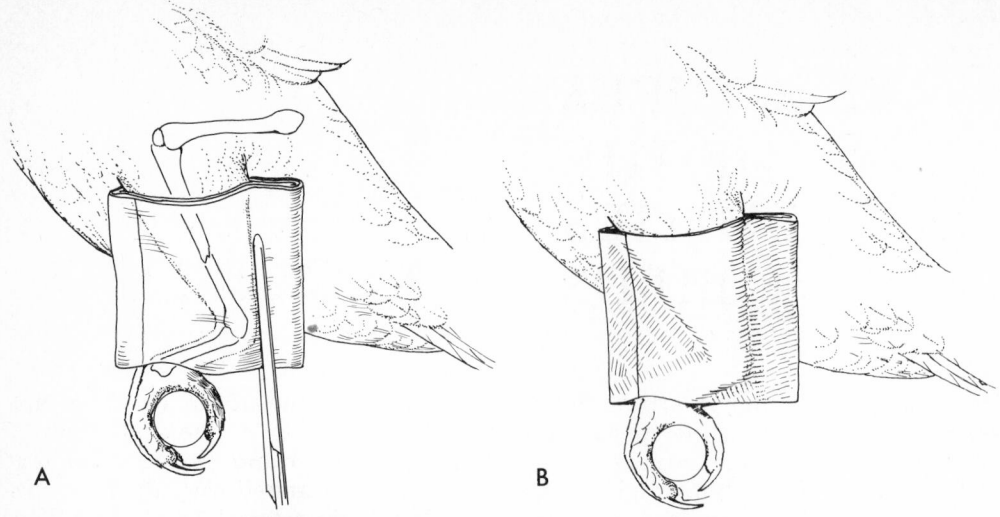

**Figure 2.** *A,* Compressing tape with hemostat to secure tape and increase stability. *B,* Mid tarsometatarsal fracture—completed "flap splint."

(Fig. 2B). Most other techniques are variations of this basic splint.

**Fractures of the Tibiotarsal-metatarsal Joint Area.** A fracture involving the proximal third of the tarsometatarsus or the distal third of the tibiotarsus is set by applying tension and approximating the bones in the extended position. A band of adhesive ¾- to 1-inch wide is placed around the extended leg. It is then clamped only on the posterior and proximal anterior border. The anterior distal border of the flap is cut at the margin with a dental crown scissors through all layers to the point at which the joint flexes and the tarsometatarsus lies fixed in the splint at an angle (Fig. 3). For canaries, the angle should be approximately 45 degrees; for a budgerigar, it should be about 65 degrees. The entire splint is then tightly pinched over the tarsometatarsus and compressed with a hemostat.

A *fracture of the distal third of the tarsometatarsus* close to the metatarsalphalangeal articulation is set without the flap (Fig. 4). A narrow piece of adhesive, cut to fit the part, is laid under the claws and carried up the lateral side of the metatarsal bone. This should be fitted tightly to ensure fixation of the bones. A piece of ½-inch adhesive tape is flapped around the lower portion of the metatarsal bone. This piece of adhesive should be rolled tightly enough to fix the bones and to hold the underlying supporting adhesive in place. Be very careful not to create too much pressure and inhibit circulation.

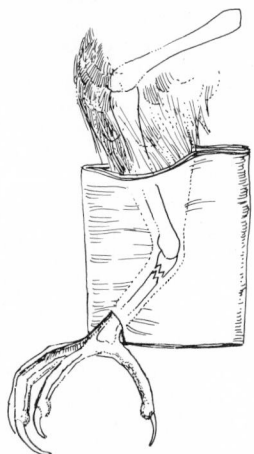

**Figure 3.** Proximal one-third tarsometatarsal fracture. When angulating tibiotarsal-tarsometatarsal joint, care must be taken to insure angulating joint rather than fracture.

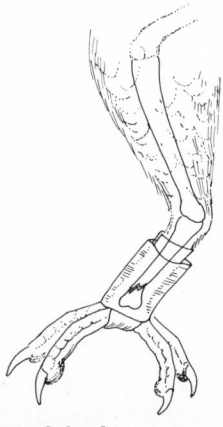

**Figure 4.** Distal third tarsometatarsal fracture.

**Femoral Fractures.** Since the femur lies within the confines of the body contour, a different approach is necessary to set femoral fractures. Unless the fractured femur is pinned, a form of body fixation is necessary. If the leg is completely flexed and held against the body, the broken ends of the bones fall in nearly normal apposition and heal normally.

In a canary, the feathers of the body on each side of the tightly flexed leg are brought together and tied with suture material. This forms a sling, immobilizing the flexed leg. If the feathers are tied too far anteriorly or posteriorly, the leg tends to slip out of the sling.

The feathers of parakeets are not as long or easily manipulated as those of canaries and are more readily plucked from the body. In this case, a body splint of tape must hold the fractured leg flexed against the body. This is accomplished with a ½-inch adhesive strip wrapped around the flexed leg and continued around the body posterior to the wings to fix the leg close to the body.

**Fractured Claws.** These are easily set by approximation next to the adjoining toe and are held in place with flexible collodion or collodion and cotton. If the toe is displaced and difficult to keep in place, use a flap splint in the horizontal plane. This fits nicely around the perch.

Use no gravel on the bottom of the cage and do not remove the perches. The swing should be removed. Keep food and water in their normal places so that birds are forced to perch and to use the splint as a crutch.

**General Care.** All splints should be examined at least once a week for adjustments. In all but very serious cases, the splint may be removed at the end of two weeks. In cases in which severe soft tissue damage has occurred, or in which there is much distraction of the fragments, loss of function is possible from nerve damage and/or severe vascular involvement. Necrosis of the affected limb is a possible sequela and will occur within the first week. If the limb is viable, grasping function of the toes is usually restored to the affected limb 24 to 72 hours after splinting.

General anesthesia may be given when setting fractures but it is usually unnecessary. Ketamine HCl at a dose of 60 to 80 mg./kg. of body weight or halothane can be used. Ketamine anesthesia is prolonged, lasting up to four hours at this dosage rate.

In removing the splint, gradually pry apart the tape with the jaws of a dental crown scissors, and cut from proximal to distal edges of the tape. After two weeks, enough feather growth has occurred under the tape to facilitate this procedure. Ether may be employed to loosen the tape.

## FRACTURES OF THE WINGS

The basic principle for setting wing fractures is the body splint method. The most common fractures are of the humerus and radius and ulna. An assistant should hold the bird in a dorsoventral position, with the fractured wing facing the clinician. One hand supports the anterior part of the body; the other hand holds the legs posteriorly, the posterior part of the body and the base of the tail.

A piece of ½-inch wide adhesive tape, 6 to 8 inches long, is used to fix the wings. After the fragments of the wing are brought into apposition with the wing flexed against the body, the tip of the fractured wing is placed on top of the normal wing. A ½-inch band of adhesive tape is placed under the fractured wing at the anterior margin and is carried over the wing and wound around the body, confining the normal wing too (Fig. 5). Allow the remaining adhesive tape to hang free.

Another piece of adhesive tape of the same width is placed perpendicularly over the anterior margin of the first piece of tape, carried straight back along the top line of the body, over the crossed wing tips, and flapped under the posterior border of the wing tips. The first piece of tape is then continued twice around the body. A small piece of ½-inch wide adhesive tape is placed around the wing tips, parallel to the first strip and perpendicular to the second hori-

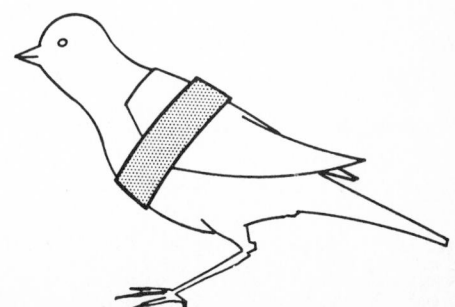

**Figure 5.** Placement of the first strip of adhesive around the body.

zontal strip (Fig. 6). This strip ties the wings together and acts as a counterbalance. Four to 12 hours is usually required for the bird to establish stability and to learn to balance itself with the new splint.

In two weeks, the three strips are cut and the tape is removed with the aid of ether. By holding the base of the feathers with a finger, the strips of adhesive are easily peeled off. Be careful to do this gently. Some feathers are removed with the tape.

After the tape has been removed, the wing may droop slightly, but this usually corrects itself with exercise. Often, however, the bird is unable to fly.

## SURGICAL FIXATION

Most of the extremity fractures that are badly distracted are compound and often comminuted. As a result, contamination is a problem. Osteomyelitis is not a common sequela to compound fractures, but bone cysts at the fracture site are.

When orthopedic surgery of any type is performed, strict asepsis should be accomplished.

Fractures of the humerus and femur do not heal as rapidly as those of other long bones because pneumatic bones have less marrow and vascularization.

When intramedullary pinning is employed, the same principles as applied to mammals should be followed for birds. Avoid invading joints, when possible, and use the largest possible diameter intramedullary pin. The weight of the appliance should be kept as light as possible.

Cross-pinning with Kirschner wires and Rush pinning are techniques frequently used. When Rush pinning is used, it is often

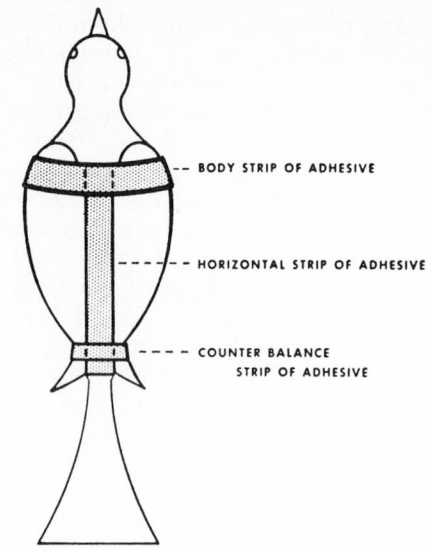

**Figure 6.** The completed splint for fractures of the wings.

necessary to improvise by cutting and bending small intramedullary pins.

In large species, plating is the method of choice, since additional coaptation splinting is not required, and immediate function is restored to the limb. When plating is not employed, coaptation splints frequently must be used in conjunction with the surgical repair. It is preferable, when possible, to remove internal fixation devices.

Mandibular cracks and fractures can be approached in two ways. If the crack is incomplete, an epoxy resin can be used as filler to prevent further fracture. If the mandibular fracture is complete, the fracture fragments must be immobilized by wiring. Drilling holes with a 19- or 20-gauge hypodermic needle and passing the wire through the needle facilitate placement of the wire. Epoxy can be used as an adjunct.

# RESTRAINT AND PHYSICAL EXAMINATION OF MONKEYS AND PRIMATES

JAMES M. HARRIS, D.V.M.
*Oakland, California*

After 18 years of experience as a practicing veterinarian treating primates, I feel I should preface my remarks with the statement that the practitioner should not accept these animals as patients unless proper equipment is at hand in working order, the operator has full knowledge and experience in using the equipment, and the practitioner also has a competently trained assistant or animal handler.

Before any equipment is obtained, it is most important to be sure that one wishes to assume the risks and go through the often exasperating experiences of handling primate patients. If the reader has any common sense, I strongly advise him to stop at this point, ignore primates and go on to the next section of this book. On the other hand, if the reader is a glutton for punishment, it is hoped that the following information will be helpful in working with these patients.

Primate patients can be divided into two groups; those owned by private parties as pets and those residing in academic and research institutions. Every effort should be made to discourage private parties from owning primates as pets, as there are numerous health hazards and great potential physical dangers.

Most primate-owning clients have set attitudes that usually are a handicap to the clinician. They generally have little knowledge of the animal, spend little or no time training them, and often, because their animals are kept as child substitutes, overprotect and undercontrol their pets. All of this makes for a most difficult doctor-client-patient relationship. On the other hand, if the client is knowledgeable and has spent time with his primate pet, he may be a great help to the veterinarian in supplying a good case history and in controlling the animal.

In order to properly physically examine a primate patient, control and restraint are of primary importance. Little can be done unless the patient is adequately restrained.

The following equipment is suggested for restraint and handling of primate patients.

1. Monkey handling gloves*: heavy leather gloves that protect hands and at least a half of the forearm, preferably with a double cuff.
2. A strong net: a salmon fishing net with at least a 4-foot pole and a 2-foot diameter to the hoop.
3. Noose and pole: the pole should be rigid and at least 6 feet in length. (The standard "come-along" used for handling particularly aggressive canine patients is satisfactory.)
4. Examination rooms with securely closing doors—preferably self-closing. All equipment in the rooms must be under cover.
5. Properly constructed escape-proof cages with solid sides, top and back. Double locking doors, food boxes and water bottles that lock on the cage, and excrement pans that lock in the cage. I have found the primate cages made by Abdco Wire and Metal, Hayward, California are quite satisfactory for most smaller primates.
6. Chemical restrainers: phencyclidine hydrochloride and/or ketamine hydrochloride.
7. For primates over 5 kg., a squeeze cage.

"Hand catching" with proper gloves is the preferred way of catching primates. It is also best to have the primate presented in a cage or carrier. One must always attempt to grasp the primate by the upper arm. Never grasp the forearm, as struggling on the part of the patient may produce spiral fractures of the humerus. Once a firm hold is ob-

---

*Simmons Glove Co., Oakland, California.

tained on the upper arm, the patient can be withdrawn from its cage, the other arm grasped and both elbows brought together behind the patient's back. The arms should be grasped above the elbows firmly and pressed together. Both rear legs should then be grasped near the ankles and the animal stretched out on the examination surface. Held in this manner, the patient can also be sat upright on the edge of the examination table, with the arms pinned behind the chest and the legs extended down the side of the table. With an assistant holding the patient in this manner, the clinician can then control and manipulate the head and perform necessary procedures.

Alternate methods for catching primates include pressing the net in front of a cage door and opening the door, allowing the primate to leap into the net. The net is then twisted on itself or quickly pressed on the floor and the primate grasped by the upper forearm with a gloved hand.

Larger primates can be snared with a noose and pole or "come-along" and pushed into a corner of their cage to facilitate manual grasping of the animal or administration of injectable sedation. On occasion, a sheet of plywood, with a firm handle attached that is the size of the cage opening, can be used to press the primate to the rear of the cage. If a number of ports are placed in the barrier, sedating injections can be administered through this structure.

In extremely fractious, intractable patients, administration of phencyclidine hydrochloride in indicated dosages will produce depression and a cataleptoid state in three to five minutes.

Hand carried primates can be difficult to restrain. Clients should be encouraged to bring their pets in a container. If it is not presented in a container, every effort should be made to restrain and examine the animal as soon as possible after admittance to the examination room. The longer one waits, the more set the primate becomes, making capture and restraint that much more difficult.

It is best to have all necessary paper work and owner complaint and, if possible, history recorded before the patient enters the hospital and/or clinic for examination. This cannot be overemphasized. I strongly suggest that those practitioners who wish to practice primate medicine make every effort to *plan ahead.* Clients contacting our hospital for care of primates are asked to come in and fill out medical records for their pets in advance of routine visits, and every effort is made to obtain a case history on the phone prior to their appointment.

In the case of the more tractable species (woolly and spider monkeys; young chimpanzees), a series of orientation visits are sometimes most helpful in establishing good rapport among patient, client and clinician. These cases must be carefully selected, but, when possible, a large degree of trust can be established between the animal and doctor, making the actual physical examination a much easier task requiring little if any restraint.

I must again emphasize that this is the exception and not the rule. Clients who own these animals are usually most willing to pay for service and the extra visits are most worthwhile.

The physical examination, although at times somewhat acrobatic, can and should be as complete as possible. Body weight can be obtained by weighing the animal and its container first, then removing the patient and reweighing the container. The skin, coat and general condition should be noted. The head, including eyes, ears, buccal cavity and throat, should be examined. (In the rhesus macaque, ulcers in the buccal cavity and tongue may be lesions of monkey B virus, which produces a fatal encephalitis in humans. Extreme caution should be taken with animals showing these lesions.) The thorax and abdomen should be thoroughly auscultated, percussed and palpated. When indicated, fecal material should be collected for *Salmonella* and *Shigella* screening and parasitic surveys.

During the course of the physical examination, while the animal is restrained, a tuberculosis test can be administered. This procedure should be done at regular intervals on all primates kept as pets or research animals. Macaques should be tested quarterly. New world species should be tested for tuberculosis at least once a year.

# RESTRAINT MORTALITY IN WILD ANIMALS

MURRAY E. FOWLER, D.V.M.
*Davis, California*

Veterinarians are frequently called upon to care for wild animals. Some refuse, citing the danger of personal injury and the high incidence of mortality of such species during restraint. Why such high restraint mortality in wild animals? Numerous factors are involved (Table 1). An analysis of these may assist the clinician in preventing death.

These factors may also affect domestic species. However, since domestic animals are usually docile and able to be handled by man, the effects are much less intense. The physiological response of wild animals to restraint is intense and normal homeostatic mechanisms may extend to cause bodily harm.

## PERACUTE MORTALITY

**Trauma.** Head and neck injuries are more commonly a hazard during attempts to capture hooved animals, but small mammals and birds may fling themselves against cage walls, causing concussions and fractures. Improper use of nets may result in trauma from the hoop striking the head.

**Hypoxia.** Excitement and increased activity create greater demand for oxygen. Suffocation is not uncommon. The restraint method may interfere with breathing through pressure exerted on the thorax or obstruction of the airway.

It is not uncommon to see a handler twisting the head to one side, or stretching the head and neck in an abnormal position. The nostrils may be obstructed with muzzles, hoods or blinders. The tiny canary or budgerigar that has a "heart attack" may well have died instead from a heavy hand encircling the thorax, preventing respiration.

Heavy gloves decrease tactile sense and may encourage a handler to exert excessive pressure in order to maintain a grip on the animal. Hands should never completely encircle the throat during restraint. Carotid sinus pressure could result in hypotension and cerebral ischemia.

Excessive chasing to capture, especially in unconditioned animals, may result in pulmonary edema and hypoxia.

Regurgitation and obstruction of the trachea more commonly occur during chemical immobilization, but many birds and a few mammals will regurgitate when excited. Manipulation may encourage aspiration.

Hypoxia coupled with acidosis, common with increased muscular exertion, may sensitize the cardiac muscle to the effects of catecholamines (epinephrine and norepinephrine), and ventricular fibrillation may ensue.

**Cholinergic Bradycardia.** Fatal syncope is an extension of the common phenomenon of fainting in man. Cerebral ischemia brought about by rapid carotid hypotension causes unconsciousness. As soon as the person lies flat on the floor, normal pressure is restored, and consciousness returns.

**Table 1.** *Etiology of Restraint Mortality*

*Peracute* (Minutes)
Trauma—concussion
Hypoxia—strangulation, pulmonary edema, regurgitation
Cholinergic bradycardia (fatal syncope)
Ventricular fibrillation
Hemorrhage
Hypoglycemia

*Acute* (Minutes to Hours)
Gastric dilatation—bloat
Hyperthermia
Hypothermia
Acidosis
Hypoglycemia
Fracture of cervical vertebrae
Chemical restraint agent idiosyncrasy

*Delayed* (Hours to Days)
Gastric dilatation—bloat
Gangrenous pneumonia—regurgitation
Hypothermia
Shock—trauma

Another normal cholinergic bradycardia is the diving reflex of marine mammals. Why does this normally protective mechanism cause death during restraint? During restraint, the typical adrenergic alarm response is initiated. There is vasoconstriction and hypertension. Centers in the hypothalamus normally stimulate the sympathetic system. However, similar centers in the hypothalamus can also stimulate the parasympathetic system.

Under intense stimulation, in some animals the cholinergic response overpowers the adrenergic, resulting in a precipitous fall in blood pressure. Unconsciousness may result. In man, this effect is transient. Why do animals die? The answer is not known. It is known that animals can go into irreversible hypovolemic shock at this point. Also, consider the following: fatal syncope can occur in man if the upright position is maintained. Crucifixion caused death through a form of recurrent syncope, brought about in this manner. Some individuals in panic-stricken, wedged crowds experience similar mortality. Perhaps veterinarians might do well to consider this. If we have the animal in hand, and such syncope occurs, we can prevent the animal's death if we permit it to lie out flat, giving it a chance to recover.

**Ventricular Fibrillation.** This is a rapidly fatal condition resulting from catecholamine stimulation of the cardiac myocardium. The alarm response is characterized by excess catecholamine production triggered by stimulation of the sympathetic nervous system and the adrenal medulla. Normally the animal is capable of coping with this excessive catecholamine through the typical alarm reaction. However, if the myocardium has been previously sensitized by either acidosis or hypoxia, it is likely that ventricular fibrillation may occur. During fibrillation, the heart is incapable of serving as a pump. There is failure of blood flow to the brain and to the cardiac muscle. Clinical signs include failure to detect a pulse or viable heart beat. Mucous membranes become darkened and dyspnea due to anoxia occurs. The animal becomes unconscious, with typical anoxic struggling, and dies in moments. In clinical situations, it is unlikely that any successful therapeutic measures, short of electrical defibrillation, can be instituted to correct such an effect.

**Hemorrhage.** Hemorrhage may be an important cause of mortality in tiny animals. The torn claw of a parakeet or canary is life-threatening. Hematomas from venipuncture in birds are also dangerous. Hemostasis should always be given immediate attention.

**Hypoglycemia.** Unfortunately, wild animals, particularly those kept as pets, are frequently malnourished. Glycogen reserves may be depleted. At the time of restraint, when there is a vital demand of the body for energy, it may not be there. Hypoglycemic shock may ensue, characterized by convulsions, muscle tremors, paresis, hypothermia, and death.

## ACUTE MORTALITY

**Gastric Dilatation.** Restrained animals are usually placed in abnormal positions. This may inhibit normal eructative mechanisms. Quickly accomplished procedures rarely cause such problems. It is, however, possible to cause a torsion of the intestine by rapidly rolling an animal. Dilatation under these circumstances may occur much later. The signs are those of an acute abdomen.

Bloat is quite common during chemical immobilization of ruminants. Constant attention must be given until the animal is able to maintain itself in sternal recumbency.

**Thermal Extremes.** Muscular activity produces heat. Many small mammals and birds have no physiologic thermoregulatory mechanism to cope with heat stress. These animals' only defense against excessive heat is behavioral—to avoid the heat source. We frequently abolish all means of heat dissipation, so the body temperature soon elevates to lethal levels. Rectal temperature should be continually monitored. Hypothermia, although less common, must also be given consideration, especially during recuperation from chemical immobilization. Cold cage floors or surgery tables conduct heat rapidly from tiny animals.

**Acidosis.** Acidosis may result from lactic acid production during anaerobic oxidation in active muscles. Acidosis is not likely to cause serious problems in the wild pet brought into the clinic. It could be a factor in the capture of a zoo animal which has been chased.

A syndrome called capture myopathy occurs in animals chased and captured from the wild. A pH change down to 6.8 may occur in a 3-minute chase. Skeletal and cardiac muscle necrosis results.

Slight acidosis may be a contributing factor to ventricular fibrillation by sensitizing the cardiac muscle to epinephrine.

**Chemical Restraint.** Some believe that the answer to all the foregoing problems is the use of chemical restraint agents. Such chemical agents are all potent drugs with diverse pharmacologic effects. None is universally applicable to all species. These agents are indispensable to wild animal restraint but must be used with great care.

Numerous factors modify the expected response of these agents. A discussion of these is a treatise in itself. Suffice it to say here that mortality does result from the use of these agents. A clinician, inexperienced in the use of these agents, would do well to consult a local zoo veterinarian before attempting such immobilization.

## DELAYED MORTALITY

Most wild animals survive handling and restraint procedures without visible scars. Nonetheless, all such manipulations initiate nonspecific responses involving the hypothalamic-hypophyseal-adrenocortical pathway. These effects are cumulative.

The clinical manifestations of chronic stress are more difficult to evaluate than are those of the alarm response. Anorexia, weight loss, weakness and lethargy are common signs. Decreased resistance to infections and parasitic diseases are also common.

Clinicians should be fully aware that malnourishment, inability to develop and exercise behavioral patterns, constant intimidation and temperature extremes can be devastating to the homeostatic mechanisms of wild animals.

An animal presented for restraint may be on the verge of adrenal exhaustion. Handling such an animal may initiate shock, resulting from the animal's inability to adapt further to a stressful situation. The signs of hypoadrenalism in wild species are unknown. In the dog there is progressive weakness, weight loss, vomiting, dehydration, polyuria and polydipsia.

The astute clinician must carefully observe and evaluate the presenting signs of each wild animal before initiating manipulative procedures. Laboratory findings are of little help in diagnosis because of the wide variation from species to species. Furthermore, one must restrain the animal in order to obtain laboratory samples.

## PREVENTION AND THERAPY

The severity of the alarm response is primarily dependent on the intensity and duration of stimulation to the animal. To reduce alarm, minimize stimulation. Decrease sight stimulation by dimming the light when capturing a diurnal bird in a cage. Eliminate extraneous noise and avoid boisterous talking when handling wild animals. Move slowly and steadily when approaching wild animals.

Extremes of heat and cold are very deleterious to wild species. When it is obvious that an animal is either hypo- or hyperthermic, correct the situation before proceeding further. If the animal is cold, immerse it in warm water with a temperature of 112° to 114° F. Warm-water enemas and warm broth given via stomach tube are beneficial. The deep body temperature can be elevated as much as 15° F. in 5 to 10 minutes using these techniques.

Hyperthermia can be corrected by using cold water in place of warm. Monitor the animal for some time to see that it equilibrates.

Avoid painful manipulations without the use of anesthesia or sedation. Be prepared to carry out procedures quickly to minimize prolonged touch or pressure stimulation by grasping the animal.

A factor frequently overlooked by a handler is the position of the head, body or limbs. Maintain as nearly natural positions as is possible. Aside from the nonspecific stress effect, respiration may be inhibited by peculiar positioning.

The clinician has less opportunity to institute preventive therapy in chronic stress states. Use techniques similar to those for acute stress to minimize stimulation. Theoretically, the administration of corticosteroids should prevent hypoadrenal shock; however, the author has had little success with their use.

The treatment of an animal that becomes unconscious during restraint cannot await laboratory confirmation of hypoglycemia or hypoxia. Clear the airway and provide supplemental oxygen to the lungs. Cole* endotracheal tubes of various sizes are ideal for

---

*Air Products, 656 Toland Place, San Francisco, California, (415) 824-3933.

intubation. Artificial respiration may be used in lieu of resuscitation equipment. Once oxygen is supplied, consider the need for glucose, intravenous steroids and perhaps cardiac massage.

Suspected acidosis may be corrected with intravenous infusion of sodium bicarbonate.

---

# INDIVIDUAL CARE AND TREATMENT OF RABBITS, MICE, RATS, GUINEA PIGS, HAMSTERS AND GERBILS

STEPHEN M. SCHUCHMAN, D.V.M.
*Castro Valley, California*

Diagnosis and treatment of diseases of laboratory animals is not unlike those of other, more familiar, species. Their differences and similarities are neither more nor less than those between horses and cows or dogs and cats. Once this mental bridge is spanned from familiar species to laboratory species, cross application of principles of diagnosis, treatment and prevention of disease becomes possible.

## PHYSICAL EXAMINATION

The physical examination is divided into two parts: (1) general information and (2) systematic examination of the animal.

### GENERAL INFORMATION

The questions listed are designed to obtain basic information from the client as to the animal's care, general condition and micro- and macroenvironment.

#### CHECK LIST

1. Species.
2. Sex.
3. Age.
4. Weight in grams, pounds or ounces.
5. What kind of diet is fed and by whom?
6. How is water dispensed and by whom?
7. Room and cage temperature.
8. Humidity.
9. Type of cage.
10. Frequency of cage cleaning.
11. Number and kind of animals owned.
12. What age group is affected?
13. What is major complaint? How long has it been going on?
14. What does client think is the problem?
15. Has the animal had a litter or has it been bred?
16. Has the animal been on medication in the past?

### SYSTEMIC EXAMINATION OF THE ANIMAL

Under each system, specific items are listed. These are guides to help identify clinical signs. It should be remembered that a high percentage of clinical illnesses seen in laboratory species are either primary or secondary to nutritionally deficient diets or poor animal husbandry practices.

#### EXAMINATION

1. Integument and hair coat:
   a. General condition.

b. Signs of scratching or fighting.
c. Alopecia, distribution.
d. Pustules.
e. Fluorescence of hair shafts that are not considered normal (Wood's light examination).
f. Cutaneous swelling, neoplastic/non-neoplastic, or infectious.
g. Skin scraping, cellophane tape test for mites, black paper test for mites.

2. Digits and tail:
   a. Necrosis of digits.
   b. Ulcerated or abscessed foot pads.
   c. Circumscribed lesions or sores around base of tail.
   d. Sores randomly spaced anywhere on tail.
   e. Gray-blue coloration of tail of mice (cyanosis).
   f. Fecal soiling of ventral surface of tail near base.
   g. Congenital absence of tail, or loss of tail.
   h. Presence of ingrown toenails.

3. Ears:
   a. Examination of ear canal.
   b. Scratching around ears.
   c. Sores on ears.
   d. Drooping ears in rabbits (in which this is not a breed characteristic).
   e. Cyanotic appearance of pinna.
   f. Congenital absence of ears or evidence of traumatic loss of part or all of the pinna.

4. Locomotion:
   a. Reluctance to move.
   b. General weakness of all four limbs.
   c. Paraparesis or paraplegia.
   d. Palpate appendicular skeleton.
   e. Lameness.
   f. Favors a particular side when lying down (fractures or soreness on opposite side).
   g. Radiographic examination.

5. Musculature:
   a. Relative amount and condition of muscle mass.
   b. Pain on palpation.

6. Central nervous system:
   a. Cranial nerve deficit.
   b. Spinal reflexes.
   c. Postural reflexes.
   d. Gross CNS disturbance (head tilt, paraplegia, circling, convulsions, flaccid or spastic paralysis).
   e. Ophthalmoscopic examination (in species in which this is practical).

7. Respiratory system:
   a. Labored breathing.
   b. Open-mouth breathing.
   c. Sneezing, epistaxis.
   d. Evidence of nasal discharge, staining of nares, staining of medial surface of forelegs.
   e. Cyanotic coloration of pinna and tail.

f. Auscultation of thorax.
g. Radiographic examination of thorax.

8. Circulatory system:
   a. Auscultation of chest.
   b. Palpate pulse.
   c. Radiographic examination of thorax.
   d. Electrocardiogram.
   e. CBC and necessary blood chemistries.
   f. Color of mucous membranes.

9. Gastrointestinal system:
   a. Check incisors and molars.
   b. Check cheek pouches for impaction or other abnormalities.
   c. Examine tongue and oral mucosa.
   d. Palpate abdomen.
   e. Examine anus and surrounding area for signs of diarrhea or other abnormalities.
   f. Check consistency and number of fecal pellets.
   g. Fecal flotation, sedimentation examination, protozoan examination and fecal culture.
   h. Radiographic examination of abdomen.

10. Lymphatic system:
    a. Examine for lymphadenopathy.
    b. Abscessation of nodes.
    c. Neoplasms.

11. Mammary glands:
    a. Neoplasm.
    b. Mastitis.
    c. Enlargement of glands in milk production.

12. Urogenital system:
    a. Determine sex.
    b. Penis—sores, ulcerations.
    c. Vaginal discharge.
    d. Palpate for fetus.
    e. Urinalysis.

**Sexing Mature and Immature Laboratory Animals.** A standard rule used to determine the sex of any mature laboratory species is that the anogenital distance is longer in the male than in the female. This is easiest to determine when both sexes are present, as is the usual case when a litter is born. To determine the sex of a mature laboratory animal, consult Table 2.

## MANUAL RESTRAINT OF RODENTS AND LAGOMORPHS

Two basic methods are described that allow for secure and safe manual restraint of rodents. The restraining procedure for rabbits differs and is described separately. Familiarity with each species minimizes the necessity of excessive restraint.

Long-tailed rodents may be removed from their cages by gently lifting them near the base of the tail and placing them either

## *Table 1.* *Useful Information*

| | HAMSTER | RABBIT | MOUSE | RAT | GERBIL | GUINEA PIG |
|---|---|---|---|---|---|---|
| Weight at birth | 2 gm. | 100 gm. | 1.5 gm. | 5.5 gm. | 3 gm. | 100 gm. |
| Puberty | (F) 28–31 days (M) 45 days (best to breed 70 days) | 4–9 months | 35 days | 50–60 days | (F) 3–5 months (M) 10–12 weeks | (F) 20–30 days (M) 70 days |
| Duration of estrus cycle° | 4 days | 15–16 days | 4 days | 4 days | 4 days | 16 days |
| Gestation | 16 days | 28–36 days | 19–21 days | 21–23 days | 24 days | 62–72 days |
| Separation of adults during parturition and weaning | Yes | Yes | No | No | No (mates for life) | No |
| Number per litter | 4 to 10 | 7 | 10 | 8–10 | 1–12 | 1–4 |
| Eyes open | 15 days | 10 days | 11–14 days | 14–17 days | 16–20 days | Prior to birth |
| Wean at | 25 days | 42–56 days | 21 days | 21 days | 21 days | 14–21 days or 160 gm. |
| Postpartum estrus | Within 24 hours | 14 days | Within 24–48 hours | Within 24–48 hours | Within 24–72 hours | Within 24 hours |
| Breeding life | 11–18 months | 1–3 years (maximum 6 years) | 12–18 months | 14 months | 15–20 months | 3–4 years |
| Adult weight | (F) 120 gm. (M) 108 gm. | (F) 4 kg. (M) 4.3 kg. | (F) 30 gm. (M) 30 gm. | (F) 300 gm. (M) 500 gm. | (F) 75 gm. (M) 85 gm. | (F) 850 gm. (M) 1000 gm. |
| Life span | 2–3 years | 5–7 years | 3–3½ years | 3 years | 4 years | 4–5 years |
| Body temperature (°F.) | 97–101 | 101–103.2 | 96.4–100 | 99.5–100.6 | 100.8 | 100.4–102.5 |
| Daily adult water consumption | 8–12 ml./day | 80 ml./kg. body weight | 3–3.5 ml./day | 20–30 ml./day | 4 ml./day | 10 ml./100 gm. body weight |
| Daily adult food consumption (varies with age and condition) | 7–12 gm./day | 150–100 gm./day | 2.5–4 gm./day | 20–40 gm./day | 10–15 gm./day | 30–35 gm./day |
| Diet | Commercial rat, mouse or hamster chow supplemented with kale†, cabbage†, apples, milk | Commercial rabbit pellets, greens in moderation | Commercial mouse chow | Commercial rat or mouse chow | Commercial mouse or rat chow (lowest fat possible), sunflower seeds | Commercial guinea pig chow, good quality hay, kale, cabbage, fruits (cannot rely on vitamin C levels of commercial ration) |
| Room temperature (°F.) | 65–75 | 62–68 | 70–80 | 76–78 | 65–80 | 65–75 |
| Humidity (per cent) | 50 | 50 | 50 | 50 | less than 50 | 50 |

°All species listed are seasonal polyestrus.
†Better source of vitamin C than lettuce.

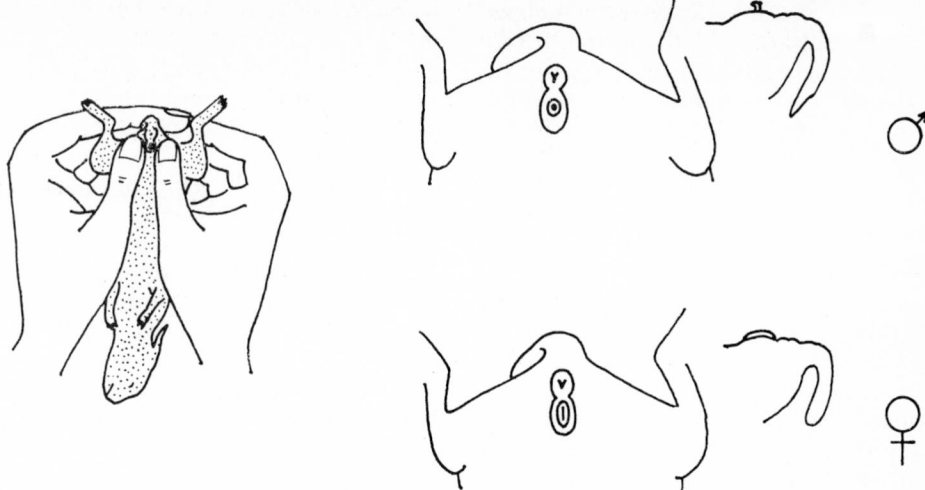

**Figure 1.**   Sexing young rabbits. The penis of the male is a rounded protrusion 1.2 mm dorsal to the anus; a pair of reddish-brown specks occur near the vent. The vulva of the female has a slit-like opening and is less than 1.2 mm from the anus; no specks are apparent. (From Sanford: Reproduction and Breeding of Rabbits. Fur & Feather, Yorkshire, England, 1958.)

**Table 2.**   *How to Determine the Sex of Mature and Immature Laboratory Rodents and Lagomorphs*

| MALE | FEMALE |
|---|---|
| *Mature Hamsters, Mice, Rats, Guinea Pigs and Gerbils* | |
| 1. Anogenital distance longer in the male. | 1. Anogenital distance shorter in the female. |
| 2. Manipulate "genital papilla" (prepuce) to protrude penis. | 2. Have three external openings in the inguinal area: (a) anus (most caudal opening); (b) vaginal orifice (middle opening); |
| 3. Palpate for testicles either in a scrotal sac (if present) or subcutaneous in inguinal region. | (c) urethral orifice at tip of urethral papilla (most anterior opening). |
| 4. Males have only two external openings in the inguinal area: (a) anus; (b) urethral orifice at tip of penis. | In these animals the urethral papilla is located outside the vagina (unlike the dog or cat). |
| In very fat males there may be a depression between the penis and anus. This depression can be obliterated by manipulating the skin in that area. | In very fat females or young females, the vaginal orifice may be either hidden by folds of skin (the former) or sealed (latter). Gentle manipulation of the skin in this area will divulge the orifice. |
| *Mature Rabbits* | |
| 1. Protrude penis by manipulating skin of prepuce. | 1. There is a common orifice for both the vagina and urethra (like the dog and cat). |
| 2. Palpate for testicles. | 2. No structure like a "penis" can be protruded from the urogenital orifice. |
| 3. Anogenital distance is longer. | 3. Anogenital distance is shorter. |

in your hand or on a nonslip surface such as a wire cage top. Short-tailed species, if too aggressive to be picked up by the palm or cupped hands, can be removed by grasping the loose skin over the neck with long-nosed forceps.

Most routine examinations are done without any restraint other than gently holding the animal in the hand. If a procedure requires more than this, the following methods are used.

Small jumpy rodents (hamsters, mice, gerbils) should be examined at ground levels to prevent injuries resulting from falls from the examining table. It is important to assure that all exits from the examining room are closed.

## TOWEL METHOD

This method is used for an aggressive animal or for one that might bite as a result of a required procedure. An opened towel of desired thickness (depending on the size of the animal's teeth) is placed in the hand used to hold the patient. The rodent is allowed to walk on a wired surface while the tail (if present) is held taut. The animal is then gently grasped behind the head, using the toweled hand. Once a secure hold is established, the body can be supported in the palm of the same hand or with the free hand. Routine injections, laboratory collection of specimens, minor surgical procedures, or close examination of the oral cavity can be accomplished using this procedure.

## NO TOWEL METHOD

Small rodents or less aggressive large ones may be securely restrained by placing the animal on a nonslip surface and, while holding the tail or caudal end of the animal, slowly and gently grasping enough loose skin over the neck region so that the animal's head and neck are restricted in movement. The rest of the body is held in the palm or supported with the other hand.

## LIFTING, CARRYING AND MANUALLY RESTRAINING RABBITS

Care should be taken when removing rabbits from their cages. The animal's quick, jerky motions can result in fracture of its back. The animal is removed by grasping the loose skin over the dorsum of the neck and lifting gently while the hind legs are supported with the other hand. The animal can be carried in this manner if held close to your chest.

When ordinary means of restraint are undesirable, the following method can be used. The rabbit is placed on a nonslip surface of a table and positioned on either its back or sternum. Both fore- and hindlimbs are tied individually and gently but firmly stretched in their respective directions. The bindings are secured at the ends of the table. An assistant (standing in front of the animal) places each hand on the respective side of the animal's head and applies gentle but firm traction in an anterior direction. Traction is continued until the desired procedure is completed. It is thought that this procedure places the animal in a cataleptic state. Once traction is released and the animal is untied, it immediately becomes active.

## BLOOD AND SERUM COLLECTING TECHNIQUES

When first using either of the following techniques, the clinician is asked to recall his first experience in collecting blood from a cat and how difficult it was until the technique was perfected. This experience will apply to the collection of blood from laboratory species. (See Tables 3 and 4.) A study was done on our Hospital Colony using the technique from Table 3; the results are reported in Table 4.

Needle-hub venipuncture and orbital bleeding are two methods of blood collecting that are safe, supply adequate amounts of blood and are cosmetically acceptable. Both procedures are carried out with manual restraint only. Sedation or anesthesia is unnecessary and often contraindicated. Routine research blood collecting techniques such as cardiac puncture and cutting digits or tails have a high risk factor or are otherwise unsuitable for use on a client's animal.

Total blood volume for rodents and lagomorphs averages 5 to 7 ml./100 gm. of body weight. This figure is helpful in determining amounts of blood that can be safely collected.

*Text continued on page 735*

*Table 3.  Techniques for Performing Routine Blood Chemistries on Small Laboratory Animals*

| TEST | METHOD | AMOUNT OF SAMPLE (λ)* | | | INSTRUMENT USED | WAVE LENGTH | COMMENTS** |
|---|---|---|---|---|---|---|---|
| | | Regular Plasma | or | Serum | | | |
| Glucose† | Ortho-toluidine (Communicable Dis. Center, U.S.D.H.E.W., P.H.S., 1965) | 20 | or | 20 | Coleman 6/20 | 630 | Plasma or serum must be removed from cells within 40 minutes |
| Glucose‡ | Ortho-toluidine | 25 | or | 25 | Coleman Jr. II | 595 | Use Dow reagent, which uses 100 μl; can use 25 μl. by cutting all solutions by 75% |
| BUN† | Diacetylmunoxime (Crocker, 1967) | 10 | or | 10 | Coleman 6/20 | 520 | Use Pfizer BUN-tel, which uses 20 lambda; can use 10 lambda by cutting all solutions by 50% |
| BUN§ | Eskalab | 2 | or | 2 | Eskalab | | |
| Calcium or Phosphorus | Harleco | — | | 250 | Eskalab | | Standard Harleco procedure requires twice the serum; solutions used are cut by 50% |
| | | — | | 100 | | | |
| Calcium§ | Harleco calcium | — | | 500 | | | Titration with EDTA |
| Calcium‡ | O-cresophthalein complexone | — | | 25 | Perkin-Elmer Coleman 55 | 565 | Use Dow reagent, which uses 50 μl; can use 25 μl. by cutting all solutions by 50% |
| SGPT† | Sigma Frankel | 100 | or | 100 | Coleman 6/20 | 505 | Sigma Frankel uses 200 lambda; use 100 lambda by cutting all solutions by 50% |
| SGPT§ | Eskalab | 50 | or | 50 | Eskalab | | |
| SGPT‡ | Henry et al. (1960) (modified) | 50 | or | 50 | Chemetrics Analyzer Computer | 340 | |
| SGPT§ | Eskalab | 50 | or | 50 | Eskalab | | |

*Continued on next page*

*Table 3.*   *Techniques for Performing Routine Blood Chemistries on Small Laboratory Animals—Continued*

| TEST | METHOD | AMOUNT OF SAMPLE (λ)* | | | INSTRUMENT USED | WAVE LENGTH | COMMENTS** |
|---|---|---|---|---|---|---|---|
| | | Regular Plasma | or | Serum | | | |
| SGOT§ | Henry (1960) Amador and Wacker (1962)(modified) | 50 | or | 50 | Chemetrics Analyzer Computer | 340 | |
| Alkaline phosphatase§ | Eskalab | — | | 25 | Eskalab | | |
| Alkaline phosphatase‡ | Berger and Rudolph (1965)(kinetic PNP) | — | | 25 | Perkin-Elmer Coleman 55 | 405 | Use 1 ml. of substrate |
| Sodium and Potassium‡ | Coleman flame photometer | 50 | or | 50 | Coleman flame photometer | | Add 50 lambda plasma or serum to 5 ml. of working diluent |
| Potassium and Sodium | IL flame photometer | — | | 50 | IL flame photometer | | |
| Bilirubin, total and direct | Evelyn Malloy (diazo technique) | 100 (Add 100 more for direct) | or | 100 | Coleman 6/20 | 550 | Add 100 lambda to volume of 1 ml. water; this is 10% of regular method and must use microcuvettes |
| Bilirubin, total and direct‡ | Jendrassik bilirubin; Nosslin (modified) | 50 (Add 50 more for direct) | or | 50 | Coleman Jr. II | 600 | |
| Amylase‡ | Dy-Amyl-L® (dyed amylopectin) | — | | 50 | Perkin-Elmer Coleman 55 | 540 | For sample, dilute 50μl. with 0.95 ml. saline |
| Amylase† | Caraway | — | | 50 | Coleman 6/20 | 660 | Use dilution of 50 lambda to 0.2 ml. saline; use 1–5 dilution in technique |
| Cholesterol‡ | Lieberman direct | 200 | | — | Coleman 6/20 | 640 | |
| Cholesterol‡ | Lieberman direct (modified) | — | | 25 | Coleman Jr. II | 625 | Use 1.5 ml. color reagent with microcuvettes |

| Analyte | Method | | | Instrument | nm | Comments |
|---|---|---|---|---|---|---|
| Cholinesterase‡ | S-butyrylthiocholine hydrolysis | — | 10 | Perkin-Elmer Coleman 55 | 405 | |
| Chloride‡ | Schales and Schales | — | 50 | | | Titration with mercuric nitrate (0.01 N) |
| $CO_2$‡ | Van Slyke (modified) | 50 (Heparinized only) or | 50 | | | Titration with NaOH (0.50 N) diluted 1:10 for use |
| Triglycerides‡ | Pinter et al. (1967) Garland and Randle (1962) | — | 200 | Gilford 3400 E | 340 | (Worthington Biochemical Corp.) |
| Uric Acid‡ | Urica-Quant | 250 or | 250 | Perkin-Elmer Coleman 55 | 405 | Use BMC, which uses 500 $\mu$l.; can use 250 $\mu$l. by cutting reagents by 50% |
| LDH‡ | Amador et al. (1963) Wacker et al. (1956) (modified) | — | 25 | Chemetrics Analyzer Computer | 340 | |
| Phosphorus‡ | Hycel | — | 100 | Coleman Jr. II | 650 | Use Hycel, which uses 200 $\mu$l.; can use 100 $\mu$l. by cutting reagents by 50% |

*10 lambda = 0.01 ml.
†Techniques of H. Weitzman, Director of Hayward Medical Laboratory, Hayward, California.
‡Techniques of J. Alberti and L. Krusee, Veterinary Disease Laboratory, Campbell, California.
§Technique of A. Ramans, Valley Veterinary Hospital, Ygnacio Valley Road, Walnut Creek, California.
**10 microliters ($\mu$l.) = 0.01 ml.

*Hospital Colony Study\* Using Techniques† from Table 3*

| TEST | SPECIES | NO. OF TESTS RUN | MEAN | UNITS | S.D. | CV (%) |
|------|---------|------------------|------|-------|------|--------|
| BUN | Mouse | 3 | 21.0 | mg. % | 2.64 | 12.50 |
| | Rat | 6 | 15.3 | mg. % | 1.21 | 7.89 |
| | Hamster | 6 | 15.6 | mg. % | 1.14 | 7.30 |
| | Guinea pig | 6 | 22.3 | mg. % | 2.94 | 13.10 |
| | Rabbit | 4 | 15.0 | mg. % | 2.58 | 17.20 |
| SGPT | Mouse | 2 | 26.0 | IU/l. | 1.41 | 5.43 |
| | Rat | 4 | 16.7 | IU/l. | 2.21 | 13.20 |
| | Hamster | 7 | 59.1 | IU/l. | 26.20 | 44.40 |
| | Guinea pig | 6 | 23.0 | IU/l. | 2.09 | 9.12 |
| | Rabbit | 3 | 39.3 | IU/l. | 10.00 | 25.40 |
| Alkaline Phosphatase | Mouse | 3 | 76.0 | IU/l. | 2.51 | 3.29 |
| | Rat | 7 | 125.0 | IU/l. | 20.10 | 16.00 |
| | Hamster | 8 | 54.6 | IU/l. | 9.39 | 17.10 |
| | Guinea pig | 6 | 23.1 | IU/l. | 4.95 | 21.30 |
| | Rabbit | 4 | 60.7 | IU/l. | 8.53 | 14.00 |
| Sodium | Mouse | 2 | 152.0 | mEq./l. | 2.82 | 1.86 |
| | Rat | 6 | 138.0 | mEq./l. | 2.17 | 1.56 |
| | Hamster | 8 | 141.0 | mEq./l. | 3.44 | 2.43 |
| | Guinea pig | 6 | 133.0 | mEq./l. | 0.81 | 0.61 |
| | Rabbit | 3 | 144.6 | mEq./l. | 6.11 | 4.22 |
| Potassium | Mouse | 2 | 7.00 | mEq./l. | 0.14 | 2.02 |
| | Rat | 6 | 5.06 | mEq./l. | 0.51 | 10.10 |
| | Hamster | 8 | 4.72 | mEq./l. | 0.76 | 16.20 |
| | Guinea pig | 6 | 4.76 | mEq./l. | 0.27 | 5.72 |
| | Rabbit | 3 | 4.70 | mEq./l. | 0.45 | 9.75 |
| Total Protein | Mouse | 3 | 5.90 | gm. % | 0.23 | 3.89 |
| | Rat | 6 | 5.88 | gm. % | 0.36 | 6.21 |
| | Hamster | 7 | 5.67 | gm. % | 0.31 | 5.64 |
| | Guinea pig | 6 | 5.01 | gm. % | 0.20 | 4.06 |
| | Rabbit | 3 | 6.10 | gm. % | 0.51 | 5.21 |
| Total Bilirubin | Mouse | QNS | — | — | — | — |
| | Rat | 6 | 0.42 | mg. % | 0.14 | 35.30 |
| | Hamster | 6 | 0.77 | mg. % | 0.28 | 36.50 |
| | Guinea pig | 6 | 0.57 | mg. % | 0.08 | 14.40 |
| | Rabbit | 3 | 0.40 | mg. % | 0.10 | 25.00 |
| Cholesterol | Mouse | 2 | 119.50 | mg. % | 4.94 | 4.14 |
| | Rat | 3 | 40.00 | mg. % | 3.46 | 8.66 |
| | Hamster | 3 | 88.00 | mg. % | 14.70 | 16.70 |
| | Guinea pig | 2 | 60.00 | mg. % | 6.36 | 10.50 |
| | Rabbit | QNS | — | — | — | — |
| Creatinine | Mouse | QNS | — | — | — | — |
| | Rat | 3 | 0.43 | mg. % | 0.15 | 35.20 |
| | Hamster | 3 | 0.20 | mg. % | 0.10 | 50.00 |
| | Guinea pig | 3 | 0.57 | mg. % | 0.05 | 10.10 |
| | Rabbit | QNS | — | — | — | — |
| Lipase | Mouse | 2 | 0.025 | Tietz | 0.01 | 28.20 |
| | Rat | 6 | 0.072 | Tietz | 0.01 | 24.00 |
| | Hamster | 7 | 0.130 | Tietz | 0.02 | 20.30 |
| | Guinea pig | 6 | 0.060 | Tietz | 0.02 | 43.90 |
| | Rabbit | 3 | 0.190 | Tietz | 0.03 | 19.50 |

\*Boulevard Pet Hospital, Castro Valley, California.
†Techniques of J. Alberti and L. Krusee, Veterinary Disease Laboratory, Campbell, California.

*Table 4.   Blood Values and Some Values of Chemical Constituents of Serum**

| | RATS | MICE | HAMSTERS | GUINEA PIGS | RABBITS | MONGOLIAN GERBIL |
|---|---|---|---|---|---|---|
| SGPT (Sigma-Frankel units) | 25–42 | 32–41 | 22–36 | 10–25 | 14–27 | – |
| Alkaline phosphatase (Bodansky units) | 4.1–8.6 | 2.4–4.0 | 2–3.5 | 1.5–8.1 | 2.1–3.2 | – |
| BUN (mg./100 ml.) | 10–20 | 8–30 | 10–40 | 8–20 | 5–30 | 18–24 |
| Sodium (mEq./liter) | 144 | 114–154 | 106–185 | 120–155 | 100–145 | 144–158 |
| Potassium (mEq./liter) | 5.9 | 3.0–9.6 | 2.3–9.8 | 6.5–8.2 | 3.0–7.0 | 3.8–5.2 |
| Bilirubin total (mg./100 ml.) | 0.42 | 0.18–0.54 | 0.3–0.4 | 0.24–0.30 | 0.15–0.20 | – |
| Blood Glucose (mg./100 ml.) | 50–115 | 108–192 | 32.6–118.4 | 60–125 | 50–140 | 69–119 |
| RBC × 10^6 | 7.2–9.6 | 9.3–10.5 | 4–9.3 | 4.5–7 | 3.2–7.5 | 8.3–9.3 |
| Hemoglobin (gm./100 mL) | 14.8 | 12–14.9 | 9.7–16.8 | 11–15 | 10–15 | 10–16 |
| Hematocrit (per cent) | 40–50 | 35–50 | 40–52 | 35–50 | 35–45 | 35–45 |
| WBC × 10^3 | 8–14 | 8–14 | 7–15 | 5–12 | 8–10 | 9–14 |
| Segmented | 30 | 26 | 16–28 | 42 | 30–50 | 10–20 |
| Nonsegmented | 0 | 0 | 8 | 0 | 0 | 0 |
| Lymphocyte | 65–77 | 55–80 | 64–78 | 45–81 | 30–50 | 70–89 |
| Eosinophil | 1 | 3 | 1 | 5 | 1 | 1 |
| Monocyte | 4 | 5 | 2 | 8 | 9 | 0 |
| Basophil | 0 | 0 | 0 | 2 | 0 | 0 |

*These are values found in healthy-appearing animals and can be used as guides but should not be interpreted as physiologic normals for the species listed.

## NEEDLE-HUB VENIPUNCTURE TECHNIQUE

Needle-hub venipuncture method can be used on laboratory species that have veins large enough to be cannulated with a 25-gauge needle. It can be used on rabbits, guinea pigs, mature rats and hamsters. Each species is restrained in an appropriate manner by an assistant. A rubber band tourniquet is placed above the elbow or stifle. Rabbits and guinea pigs can be bled from the cephalic vein, while rats and hamsters are sampled from a large vein on the lateral surface of the thigh. Clipping the hair and extending the limb facilitate visualization of the vein. A 25-gauge ⅝-inch hypodermic needle (without syringe) is inserted into the occluded vessel. Blood will flow into the hub of the needle. Collection is made (*in situ*) directly from the hub of the needle with a micro-hematocrit tube.* If skin contamination will not affect the sample, lancing of the occluded vessel without cannulation can be done. The blood sample is then collected directly from the surface of the skin.

---

*Micro-hematocrit tubes (length, 75 mm.; O. D., 1.47 mm.; I. D., 0.56 mm.; a larger size can be used accordingly), Clay Adams, a division of Becton-Dickinson and Co.

## ORBITAL BLEEDING TECHNIQUE

Orbital bleeding technique (Riley, 1960) is used when venipuncture or lancing a vein is not practical. This is the method of choice for mice but can be used on rats, hamsters and gerbils. An assistant is not required. The animal is placed on a nonslip surface to facilitate handling.

The thumb and forefinger stabilize the head and neck and tighten the loose skin in this area. The index finger is free to lightly bulge the eye outward. With the clinician's free hand, a micro-hematocrit tube is placed just lateral to the medial canthus and gently but firmly slid posteriorly and medially under the globe to the venous plexus that lines the back of the orbit. A controlled thrust is required when collecting samples from rats or hamsters. In the mouse, the vessels of the plexus rupture easily when the tube contacts them. Slight withdrawal of the tube allows blood to fill the capillary tube.

When collecting is completed, direct pressure over the lid expedites hemostasis. Weekly sampling has been done on the same animals without clinically affecting their health. A 40-gm. mouse has a total blood volume of 2 ml. If healthy, 0.1 to 0.2 ml. can be safely collected. The capacity of a micro-hematocrit tube is 0.02 ml.

## CBC, PLASMA AND SERUM COLLECTION

White blood cell pipettes* can be filled and blood smears made directly from the pooling blood.

Specimens for routine serology are obtained by using plain hematocrit tubes. When plasma is needed, heparinized tubes are substituted. After the tube is filled and spun, the clot or red cell layer can be broken off and discarded, leaving a column of plasma or serum for diagnostic testing.

## VIRUS DIAGNOSTIC TESTING†

Table 5 indicates viral infections that can be serologically identified and the species of laboratory animals usually tested. Testing programs such as these are used mainly for commercial colonies but have been modified for clinical application.

## URINE COLLECTION

Collection techniques vary depending upon species. Mice and rats will urinate if picked up quickly. Urine may then be collected from the table surface (if clean) with a micro-hematocrit tube. Animals that will not urinate spontaneously can be placed in modified metabolic cages. These can be made by placing a plastic bag or sheet of plastic on the floor of a cage that has been elevated slightly at one end. Usually within one hour, an adequate sample is obtained. It should be remembered that gerbils produce only 2 to 3 drops of concentrated urine a day (appreciably less than other laboratory species). Rabbits' urine may be collected either by manual expression of the bladder or by centesis. Catheterization is only practicial in the male. A 3½ French urinary catheter is used, although the urethra will accommodate a larger size. Extreme caution should be used when attempting this procedure, since the urethra in this species is easily traumatized and ruptured.

## URINALYSIS

Bili-Labstix®‡ are used to check urine for pH, protein, glucose, ketones, bilirubin and blood. The small volume of urine obtainable in some species necessitates multiple collections to complete an analysis. Specific gravity is measured with a refractometer.§ Centrifuged urine sediment samples can be obtained by filling a micro-hematocrit tube and centrifuging.

Lithuria and basic urine may be found in hamsters, guinea pigs and rabbits. Amorphous calcium carbonate and triple phosphate crystals are the predominant types found. Rat and mouse urine is acid-reacting and comparatively free of crystals. Proteinuria is a consistent finding in these two species.

## ECTOPARASITE MONITORING

Mite and fungal infestations are two of the more common dermatologic problems encountered. Examination of the animal may be expedited by the use of a hand lens or binocular loupe. Scrapings, Wood's light examination and fungal culture are the tests of choice. When mite infestation is suspected but cannot be demonstrated by skin scraping, it may be helpful to place an anesthetized or chemically immobilized animal on black paper. If the test is conducted long enough and infestation is moderate to heavy, the mites will migrate from the skin to the hair shafts where they can be seen. They may also be visible on the black paper.

## FECAL ANALYSIS FOR HELMINTHS, PROTOZOA AND BACTERIA

Analysis of feces is an important part of a laboratory animal's health program,

---

*Unopette®, Becton-Dickinson, Rutherford, N.J.

†Laboratory Animal Virus Testing Service, Microbiological Associates, Inc., 4733 Bethesda Ave., Bethesda, Maryland 20014.

‡Ames Co., Elkhart, Indiana 46514.

§Protometer B5991 or Total Solids Meter B5996, Scientific Products, 1430 Waukegan Road, McGaw Park, Illinois 60085.

**Table 5.** *Serologically Identifiable Viral Infections and Laboratory Animals Used**

| VIRAL INFECTION | HAMSTER | GUINEA PIG | RAT | MOUSE |
|---|:---:|:---:|:---:|:---:|
| Reovirus, type 3 | X | X | X | X |
| Pneumonia virus of mice (PVM) | X | X | X | X |
| K virus (newborn mouse pneumonitis) | | | | X |
| Theiler's encephalomyelitis (GD–VIII) | X | X | X | X |
| Polyoma | | | | X |
| Sendai | X | X | X | X |
| Minute virus of mice (MVM) | | | X | X |
| Mouse adenovirus (MAdV) | | | X | X |
| Mouse hepatitis (MHV) | | | X | X |
| Lymphocytic choriomeningitis (LCM) | X | X | X | X |
| Ectromelia | | | | X |
| Toolan H-1 | | X | X | |
| Simian myxovirus (SV5) | X | X | X | X |
| Kilham rat virus | | | X | |
| Rat coronavirus | | | X | |

*Laboratory Animal Virus Testing Service, Microbiological Associates, Inc., 4733 Bethesda Ave., Bethesda, Maryland 20014.

whether the animal is used for research or as a pet. The examination should consist of (1) fecal sedimentation examination; (2) fecal flotation examination; (3) protozoan smear examination; and (4) bacterial culture of feces on selective media. The analysis should specifically check for (1) ova of *Hymenolepis nana;* (2) ova of *Syphacia, Aspicularis* and other nematodes; (3) overgrowth of protozoa; and (4) *Salmonella* and *Pseudomonas.*

Coprophagy, feces-contaminated food or bedding and contamination of feed during processing all contribute to heavy infestation if the life cycle of the pathogenic organism is direct. Semi-yearly examinations are advised if the animal population remains closed. If new animals enter the household, testing should be more frequent.

## CLINICAL SIGNS AND DISEASES MOST COMMONLY SEEN*

The following information is tabulated (Tables 6 to 10) for each species:
1. The systems most commonly affected by diseases.
2. Clinical signs most commonly seen when that system is affected.
3. Description of disease.
4. Brief approach to treatment.
5. Differential diagnosis in some cases.

The systems and diseases are listed in order of decreasing frequency.*

## DIAGNOSTIC RADIOGRAPHY FOR SMALL RODENTS

Diagnostic radiographs can be obtained by using the technique chart (Table 11).† Individual calibration of the machine to be used is necessary for best results. Rabbits and large rats require the same technique as that for cats. Kodak Blue Brand® or Sakura® medical x-ray film is used in high-speed cassettes.

To facilitate positioning of a small mammal, 4 strips of adhesive tape, ½ x 12 inches long, are wrapped around the individual extremities. Thus, adequate positioning can be obtained even while wearing lead gloves.

## PARENTERAL ROUTES OF MEDICATING

Intramuscular and subcutaneous injections are the preferred routes of parenteral

(*Text continued on page 750*)

---

*Based on the author's experience.

†Radiographic technique of R. P. Barrett, Castro Valley, California.

*Table 6.* Diseases of Rabbits

| CLINICAL SIGNS | AGE GROUP | MORBIDITY | MORTALITY | TESTS | ETIOLOGY | TREATMENT | MISCELLANEOUS |
|---|---|---|---|---|---|---|---|
| *Respiratory System* | | | | | | | |
| Unilateral or bilateral purulent nasal discharge; stained hairs around nostrils; sometimes staining of medial aspect of paws; nasal discharge may be present only on exercise; conjunctivitis; some cases may show marked dyspnea | Usually mature | H(±) | ± | Culture, radiographs of thorax | *Pasteurella multocida* | Antibiotics 1. Pencillin 2. Furazolidone 3. Tetracyclines 4. Sulfonamides | Common name—"snuffles"; primarily a respiratory disease, but same organism can cause septicemia, abscess, urogenital disease in males and females |
| | | | | | | | Other less common diseases that can cause respiratory signs |
| | | | | | *Pasteurella pseudotuberculosis* | | *Pseudotuberculosis* |
| | | | | | *Vaccinia* virus | | *Rabbit pox:* (Usually rash, pock-type lesions on skin and ears) |
| | | | | | *Myxoma* virus | | *Myxomatosis:* Very high morbidity and mortality; may see edema of head resulting in drooping of ears; also, in chronic cases, fibrotic nodules on nose and ears |
| | | | | | | | Nonspecific conjunctivitis, (conjunctivitis only sign) |
| *Integument and Ears* | | | | | | | |
| Crusty accumulation in ear canals; shaking head; scratching at ears | Any | ± | L | Otoscopic and microscopic examination | *Psoroptes cuniculi; Chorioptes cuniculi* | Rotenone in oil; clean cage | Common name—ear canker |

| Clinical Signs | Age/Animal Affected | | Diagnosis | Etiology | | Treatment | Comments |
|---|---|---|---|---|---|---|---|
| Crusty skin; pruritus; alopecia, patchy or generalized; usually head and ears affected but can be any place on body | Any | ± | UV light; KOH preparations; fungal culture | *Microsporum sp.; Trichophyton sp.* | L | Griseofulvin | Communicable disease<br><br>Other pruritic disease; *Sarcoptes* |
| Alopecia on chest area; animal biting out hair | Mature female | 0 | Rule out other dermatologic diseases | Hair pulling for nesting behavior | 0 | Nothing | |

*Digestive System*

| Clinical Signs | Age/Animal Affected | | Diagnosis | Etiology | | Treatment | Comments |
|---|---|---|---|---|---|---|---|
| Large subcutaneous abscess anywhere on body, usually under side of neck | Any (but more in males) | L | Culture | *Pasteurella multocida* (unless proved otherwise) | L | Open drain; appropriate antibiotics (penicillin) | Usually associated with fighting or from a chronically irritated area; staphylococci second most common cause |
| Slobbering; difficulty eating; may get teeth caught on wire cage | Usually mature | L | Examination of oral cavity | Probable congenital malocclusion | L | Routine cutting of overgrown or ingrown incisors or molars | Continuous growing incisors must be continually worn down; if not, this condition may result. Lack of gnawing on hard objects is not a major cause. Malocclusion is. |
| Small warts on tongue and oral mucosa | Any over a month old | ± | Biopsy | Rabbit oral papillomatosis | L | Remove wart or vaccinate | |
| Bloat; profuse mucoid diarrhea; anorexia; borborygmus; huddling | Any | + (young) | Fecal analysis to check for other problems | Unknown; may be:<br>1. Due to deficiency of amylase<br>2. Nutritional<br>3. Bacterial<br>4. Viral | ± (young) | Increase roughage in diet; prevent secondary septicemia and dehydration | Commonly referred to as mucoid enteritis<br><br>Other less common diarrhea-causing diseases<br>1. Salmonellosis<br>2. Coccidiosis |

(*Table 6 continued on the following page.*)

**Table 6.**  *Diseases of Rabbits (Continued)*

| CLINICAL SIGNS | AGE GROUP | MORBIDITY | MORTALITY | TESTS | ETIOLOGY | TREATMENT | MISCELLANEOUS |
|---|---|---|---|---|---|---|---|
| *Mammary Gland* | | | | | | | |
| Anorexia; polydipsia; mastitis | Mature female | L | ± | Culture | *Streptococcus; Staphylococcus; Pasteurella* | Antibiotics; drain; hot pack | Usually associated with nursing |
| *Urogenital System* | | | | | | | |
| Lithuresis; pH urine 8–9; urine dries and leaves large amount of white crystals | Any; usually mature when noticed | 0 | 0 | Urinalysis | Normal rabbit urine | None | When urine dries, it has chemical consistency similar to that of boiler scale |
| Ulceration; scab-covered lesion about genitals, either sex; can have ulcers in other areas; vesicles may be on skin surrounding genitals | Mature | | | Look for organism in exudate using dark field microscopy | *Treponema cuniculi* | Penicillin | Not communicable disease |
| *Miscellaneous* | | | | | | | |
| Hepatomegaly, irregular surface to liver; abdominal enlargement; poor general condition; diarrhea (±); in young, mild hemorrhagic diarrhea (a healthy rabbit usually seen); hepatic lesions may only be seen as an incidental finding) | Any | ± | ± | Microscopic examination of feces; both types have oocysts that appear in stool | *Eimeria* sp.; both intestinal and hepatic types occur in rabbit | Wire floors; sulfaquinoxaline; sulfamethazine | Other less common diseases affecting liver 1. *Pasteurella tularensis* causes small yellow-gray necrotic foci on liver; spleen is covered with miliary necrotic foci 2. Tyzzer's disease; necrotic foci on liver, along with enteritis |
| Subcutaneous swellings | Any | L | L | Biopsy | Pox virus | | Shope fibroma only seen in wild cottontails |

*Table 7.  Diseases of Guinea Pigs*

| CLINICAL SIGNS | AGE GROUP | MORBIDITY | MORTALITY | TESTS | ETIOLOGY | TREATMENT | MISCELLANEOUS |
|---|---|---|---|---|---|---|---|
| *Lymph System; Respiratory System* | | | | | | | |
| 1. Active, healthy looking animal with enlarged lymph nodes; nodes may discharge pus | Usually mature | ± | ± | Culture | β-Hemolytic streptococci, Lancefield type C | Antibiotics; drainage; quarantine | Called "lumps"; other diseases (less common) with same signs; pseudotuberculosis; streptobacillosis |
| 2. Acute; death | Any | ± | H | Culture; necropsy | β-Hemolytic streptococci | | Generalized septicemia; other diseases causing acute death; salmonellosis; pseudotuberculosis |
| 3. Chronic duration: anorexia, ruffled haircoat, huddling, dyspnea, nasal discharge, crusty dried mucus on medial aspect of forelegs, purulent conjunctivitis, lymphadenitis | Usually mature | ± | H | Culture | β-Hemolytic streptococci, Lancefield type C | Antibiotics; supportive care | Other diseases with similar signs |
| | | | | | *Bordetella bronchisepticus* | | *Bordetella*: usually just confined to respiratory tract |
| | | | | | *Salmonella typhimurium* or *Salmonella enteriditis* | | *Salmonella*; respiratory signs usually lacking; may not have diarrhea |
| | | | | | *Pasteurella pseudotuberculosis* | | Pseudotuberculosis: palpate for enlarged mesenteric lymph nodes; chronic emaciation may be only sign |
| | | | | | | | Pneumococci pneumonia |
| | | | | | | | Virus pneumonia |
| | | | | | | | *Pseudomonas* |
| | | | | | | | *Klebsiella* |
| | | | | | | | *Corynebacterium* |

(Table 7 continued on the following page.)

## *Table 7.* Diseases of Guinea Pigs (Continued)

| CLINICAL SIGNS | AGE GROUP | MORBIDITY | MORTALITY | TESTS | ETIOLOGY | TREATMENT | MISCELLANEOUS |
|---|---|---|---|---|---|---|---|
| *Integument and Hair* | | | | | | | |
| Alopecia; can be generalized or patchy; may be symmetrical in distribution; non pruritic | Any age | ± | L | Rule out other dermatologic diseases | Unknown; in weanlings or females, may be due to stress; in males, a similar looking disorder is due to grooming between two animals | Feed hay, cabbage or kale or do nothing | Usually seen only in colony or heavy stress situations |
| Scaly patchy skin lesions; broken hair shafts; can be generalized; pruritic | Any | ± | L | UV light; KOH preparation culture | *Tricophyton Microsporum* | Griseofulvin (use cautiously, since derived from *Penicillium* cultures) | Communicable disease |
| Sores on hocks or plantar surface of foot; abscesses | Mature | ± | L | Culture | *Corynebacterium pyogenes* | Put on softer surface; treat symptomatically (daily medicated dressings) | Problem encountered when animal is usually raised on wire |
| *Diseases of Pregnant Females* | | | | | | | |
| Sow in late pregnancy; lethargy; anorexia; huddling; may die within 24 hours | Mature | ± | + | | Pregnancy toxemia | Steroids; supportive care; calcium gluconate. Cesarean section. | Friable yellow liver on necropsy; normal fetus; may be prevented by feeding good quality diet last part of gestation |
| *Digestive Tract* | | | | | | | |
| Difficulty chewing or moving mouth; slobbering when eat- | Mature | ± | L | Physical examination; | Nutritional (possibly); | Correct diet; file or cut | Diseases of salivary glands may mimic clinical signs; chemical |

| Clinical Signs | Age | | | Diagnosis | Etiology | Treatment | Remarks |
|---|---|---|---|---|---|---|---|
| | | | | | poor quality hay diet; chronic fluorosis | | |
| Blood-tinged diarrhea; acute death sometimes in young; usually asymptomatic | Young | ± | ±(L) | Fecal analysis | *Eimeria caviae* or protozoan overgrowth (*Trichomonas*) | Coccidiostats | Coccidiosis usually not a problem; other internal parasites not usually a problem but should check for them; nematode of cecum (*Paraspidodera*) is reported to be most common |

*Miscellaneous*

| Clinical Signs | Age | | | Diagnosis | Etiology | Treatment | Remarks |
|---|---|---|---|---|---|---|---|
| Poor weight gain; rough coat; greater incidence of disease; increased huddling; hesitancy to move about; enlarged joints (±); subconjunctival hemorrhage (±) | Any | ± | ± | Serum ascorbic acid levels of feed and analysis | Ascorbic acid deficiency | Ascorbic acid in water and feed; kale, cabbage, citrus fruits, orange juice instead of water; ascorbic acid supplement 1–3 mg./100 gm./day | Occurs even on fortified commercial diet<br>1. Poor quality control of commercial ration<br>2. Shelf life of guinea pig feed is short<br><br>Other diseases causing soreness of limbs or inability to move<br>1. Fractures<br>2. Muscular dystrophy (vitamin E deficiency)<br>3. Myositis (viral?)<br>4. Guinea pig paralysis (viral?) |
| Cachexia; generalized loss of condition | Usually mature males | ± | | Possibly radiography and/or electrolyte studies | Thought to be improper Ca:P ratio or its relationship to Mg | Put on balanced diet | Diffuse calcification of internal viscera |

*Table 8. Diseases of Hamsters*

| CLINICAL SIGNS | AGE GROUP | MORBIDITY | MORTALITY | TESTS | ETIOLOGY | TREATMENT | MISCELLANEOUS |
|---|---|---|---|---|---|---|---|
| *Gastrointestinal Tract* | | | | | | | |
| Diarrhea-stained anus; lethargy; anorexia; prolapsed rectum; can die within 48 hours to one week after symptoms start | Any | ± | H | Culture feces; fecal analysis; direct smear | Wet tail; exact etiology unknown; overgrowth of *E. coli* and protozoan organisms (trichomonads); improper caging; overcrowding; lack of fresh water | Supportive care 1. Fluids sq. 2. Antibiotics (Gentocin) 3. Sulfonamides 4. Improve husbandry 5. Fresh food 6. Whole milk or butter milk 7. Surgery | Very common; guarded prognosis; normal bacteria, flora and fauna are gram-negative bacilli resembling *Bacterioides*, *Lactobacilli* (gram-positive type), *Streptococcus bacillus*, *Escherichia*, *Staphylococcus*, spirochetes, large coccus forms, *Giardia* and trichomonads; prolapsed rectum is usually accompanied by an intussusception of the colon |
| Mild diarrhea; animal relatively healthy in appearance | Mature | L | L | Microscopic examination of stool | Overgrowth of *Trichomonas*, *Giardia*, *Chilomastix* | High protein diet fed for 7 days; 45% ground beef liver, 42% lean ground beef, 11% lard, 2% calcium carbonate or carbarsone *per os*; 15.6 mg./100 gm. body weight per day for 21 days | |
| Constipation; diarrhea may be associated with it | Young | ± | ± | Palpate abdomen; x-ray abdomen | Inadequate amount of water to drink | Assure adequate water intake; milk of magnesia | |

| Clinical signs | Age | | | Diagnostic method | Etiology | Treatment | Comments |
|---|---|---|---|---|---|---|---|
| Usually no clinical signs other than mild enteritis | Any | ± | L | Fecal analysis | Hymenolepis nana; Syphacia obvelata and others | Proper anthelmintic; Piperazine | *H. nana*; communicable disease |

*Integument*

| Clinical signs | Age | | | Diagnostic method | Etiology | Treatment | Comments |
|---|---|---|---|---|---|---|---|
| Alopecia about the face, but can be generalized | Usually mature | ± | ± | Skin scrapings | Demodex sp.; Notoedres sp. | Pyrethrum insecticides; Eurax (crotomiton) | Common; although looks like a poor prognosis they respond; pruritus is not a major finding |

*Miscellaneous*

| Clinical signs | Age | | | Diagnostic method | Etiology | Treatment | Comments |
|---|---|---|---|---|---|---|---|
| Paresis; inactivity; inability to lift head; crawls | Mature | ± | ± | Physical examination, radiographs | Nutritional deficiency | Vitamin D | Commonly called cage paralysis; other musculoskeletal diseases: 1. Nutritional muscular dystrophy (vitamin E deficiency) 2. Polymyopathy and myocardial necrosis (congenital and genetically controlled gradual onset) |
| Ocular discharge; chattering; ruffled haircoat; huddling; nasal discharge ± | Young; more susceptible | ± | L | | Possible viral etiology and/or pneumococci, streptococci | Antibiotics: chloramphenicol; tetracyclines | |
| Change in behavior; lethargy; inactivity; sleeping long periods; slow heart rate; respiratory rate slow; all animals in group may not be in this condition; low body temperature | Usually not in very old animals | | ± | Physical examination | Hibernation: large fluctuation in ambient temperatures; precold exposure in history | Raise environmental temperature | Animal will go into hibernation for a few days, then out; may be repeated; heart rate can be as slow as 4–15 beats/minute |

*Table 9.*  *Diseases of Mice and Rats*

| CLINICAL SIGNS | AGE GROUP | MORBIDITY | MORTALITY | TESTS | ETIOLOGY | TREATMENT | MISCELLANEOUS | SPECIES |
|---|---|---|---|---|---|---|---|---|
| *Integument and Appendages* | | | | | | | | |
| Scratching around head and ears; abrasions; scabs; bald spots | Haired animals | ± | L | Skin scraping; blue paper test | *Myobia*; *Mycoptes*; *Radfordia*; *Notoedres* | Dichlorovos strips; ectocide; pyrethrum powder | Common in mice | Mice, rats |
| Sores around ears and on pinna; scabs and wounds randomly positioned on caudal two thirds of tail | Mature males | L | L | Observation | Fighting | Separate males | | Mice |
| Circumscribed necrotic lesion usually at base of tail | Any | ± | L | | Humidity too low | Adjust humidity to 50–55 per cent | Ringtail syndrome | Mice |
| Congenital absence of tail | At birth | O | O | Genetic studies | Hereditary | | | Mice |
| Bluish or pale color of pinna or tail | Any | ± | H | Any that are necessary | Cyanosis, usually associated with severe respiratory illness or septicemia | Antibiotics; fluids; general supportive care | Poor prognostic sign | Mice |
| Bald spots; scaliness; pruritus (±) | Haired | + | L | Wood's light examination; KOH slide culture | *Trichophyton*; *Microsporum* | Griseofulvin; tolnaftate cream 1 per cent | There may be some normal fluorescence of hair shafts | Mice, rats |
| Sloughing and/or necrosis of digits and tail; papules or pustules (±) | Any | H | H | Serology | Pox virus (ectromelia) | Vaccination; supportive care if requested; euthanasia advised | Often a latent infection; vaccination of healthy stock | Mice |

*Respiratory System*

| Clinical Signs | Age | | | Diagnosis | Etiology | Treatment | Remarks | Species |
|---|---|---|---|---|---|---|---|---|
| Sneezing; chattering; labored breathing; nasal discharge; epistaxis; pawing at nose; unkempt coat; arching of back; generalized depression; vestibular disease; conjunctivitis | Usually mature | ± | ± | Culture if possible; serology | Not a specific disease entity but due to one or more of the following: enzootic bronchiectasis (rats) (probable virus); infectious catarrh (*Mycoplasma pulmonis*); disease syndrome referred to as chronic murine pneumonia | Antibiotics; long-term if necessary 1. Tylosin 2. Sulfonamides | Other less common diseases with similar signs; *Pasteurella pneumotropica*; *Bordetella bronchiseptica*; pneumonia virus of mice; adenovirus; K virus; *Diplococcus pneumoniae* (common in rats); streptococcal infections | Mice, rats |

*Gastrointestinal Disease*

| Clinical Signs | Age | | | Diagnosis | Etiology | Treatment | Remarks | Species |
|---|---|---|---|---|---|---|---|---|
| Prolapsed rectum | 3 weeks and older | ± | L | Fecal analysis; cellophane tape test not reliable | *Aspicularis tetraptera*; *Syphacia obvelata* or other heavy parasite infestation | Appropriate anthelmintic therapy: 1. Piperazine compounds 2. Yomesan | Pinworms and *Hymenolepis nana* are common (M) | Mice, rats |
| Mustard color soiling around tail and caudal part of body; watery stools; acute death; fecal impaction | Suckling age | H | H | Fecal cultures if necessary to rule out other diseases | Epizootic diarrhea of infant mice (EDIM); epizootic diarrhea of suckling rats | Filter caps over top of cage prevent transmission; antibiotic therapy sometimes helpful | Filter caps and sanitation are effective in stopping outbreaks | Mice, rats |
| Mild diarrhea; usually healthy looking animal | Any age | ± | L | | *Giardia* or other protozoan overgrowth | Feed apples, cabbage, ground beef; furazolidone, antibiotics | | |
| Acute death; focal necrosis of liver (white spots); may have enteritis; diarrhea may be present | Any age | ± | H | Difficult to culture; histopathology with special staining technique may demonstrate organisms | Tyzzer's disease; *Bacillus piliformes* | Antibiotics | Can be latent; other diseases with similar signs; salmonellosis; *Pseudomonas* septicemia following stress | Mice, rats |

(*Table 9 continued on the following page.*)

*Table 9.*   Diseases of Mice and Rats (Continued)

| CLINICAL SIGNS | AGE GROUP | MORBIDITY | MORTALITY | TESTS | ETIOLOGY | TREATMENT | MISCELLANEOUS | SPECIES |
|---|---|---|---|---|---|---|---|---|
| *Central Nervous System* | | | | | | | | |
| Head tilt; circling | Mature | L | L | Radiography; neurologic examination | *Mycoplasma* or bacterial infection of vestibular apparatus associated with upper respiratory infection | Antibiotics; steroids | | Mice, rats |
| *Mammary Glands* | | | | | | | | |
| Neoplasm | Mature female | L | L | Biopsy | Mammary tumor, adenocarcinoma (M); fibrosarcoma (R) | Surgical excision | Usually recur after removal; located anywhere on body | Mice, rats |
| *Lymph Nodes* | | | | | | | | |
| Lymphadenopathy | Mature | L | ± | Culture or biopsy | *Pasteurella pseudotuberculosis* | Antibiotic if bacterial | | Mice, rats |
| *Miscellaneous* | | | | | | | | |
| Enlargement of salivary glands causing swelling of neck region | Mature | ± | L | Biopsy | Sialodacryadenitis; viral etiology | Steroids; antibiotics | Usually latent | Rats |
| Marked depression; hunched up posture; roughened coat; conjunctivitis; anorexia; lethargy; death; stunting in surviving animals | Any; young more commonly affected | ± | ± | Fecal culture | *Salmonella*; *Pseudomonas* | Antibiotics; hyperchlorination of water (10 ppm); euthanasia advised (if communicable disease) | These are nonspecific signs of septicemia; any latent disease can cause infection if animal is stressed; examples are mouse hepatitis virus, reovirus; heavy parasitism | Mice |

*Table 10.*  *Diseases of Gerbils**

| CLINICAL SIGNS | AGE GROUP | MORBIDITY | MORTALITY | TESTS | ETIOLOGY | TREATMENT | MISCELLANEOUS |
|---|---|---|---|---|---|---|---|
| | | | | *Miscellaneous* | | | |
| Bare spots on base of tail | Mature | ± | L | | Fighting due to overcrowding | Correct overcrowding | |
| Inflammation and ulceration around the nose and jaw | Mature | | | Rule out other dermatologic problems | Thought to be from mechanical abrasion | Remove source of mechanical abrasion | |
| Protrusion of nictitating membrane, conjunctiva and eye itself | Older animals | ? | ? | | Unknown | | Evaluate for glaucoma or retrobulbar pressure |
| Scanty or patchy growth of hair | Young not weaned | ? | ? | | Unknown | None; hair will grow in as animal gets older | Seen in some strains of mice also |
| Seizures when handled: body stiffens; legs stiffen and tremble | More common in young animals | | | | Thought to be a form of catalepsy | Dilantin has been used but may be unnecessary | Seizuring occurs with less frequency as the animal gets older |
| Sneezing; chattering; labored breathing | Any | ± | ± | Physical; culture; radiography | Virus? Bacterial? Mycoplasm? | Penicillin; tetracyclines | Usually follows stress |
| Diarrhea mild | Any | ± | ± | | | | No one enteric disease is prevalent but should consider enteritis due to: 1. *Salmonella* 2. Unwashed vegetables 3. Parasitism, although very few natural parasites; gerbils are very susceptible to most experimental infestation 4. Protozoan overgrowth (*Entamoeba* may be a normal finding) |

*From Schwentker, V.: Tumblebrook Farm, West Brookfield, Mass. Personal communication.

*Table 11.   Technique for Small Mammals**

| THICKNESS (Cm.) | FFD (INCHES) | KVP | Ma | SECONDS | MaS |
|---|---|---|---|---|---|
| | | *Bone†* | | | |
| 0.5 | 36 | 40 | 100 (Fine Focal Spot) | 1/30 | 3.3 |
| 1 | | 42 | | | |
| 2 | | 44 | | | |
| 3 | | 46 | | | |
| 4 | | 48 | | | |
| 5 | | 50 | | | |
| 6 | | 52 | | | |
| 7 | | 54 | | | |
| | | *Soft Tissue* | | | |
| 1 | 36 | 38 | 100 (Fine Focal Spot) | 1/30 | 3.3 |
| 2 | | 40 | | | |
| 3 | | 42 | | | |
| 4 | | 44 | | | |
| 5 | | 46 | | | |
| 6 | | 48 | | | |
| 7 | | 50 | | | |
| 8 | | 52 | | | |
| 9 | | 54 | | | |
| | | *Thoracic* | | | |
| 2 | 36 | 34 | 200 | 1/60 | 3.3 |
| 3 | | 36 | | | |
| 4 | | 38 | | | |
| 5 | | 40 | | | |
| 6 | | 42 | | | |
| 7 | | 44 | | | |
| 8 | | 46 | | | |

*Radiographic technique of R. P. Barrett, Castro Valley, California.
†If animal is immature, it might be better to use 50 ma.

administration of medications. Accurate dosing is accomplished by using a tuberculin or a microliter syringe* equipped with a 25- to 27-gauge needle. Microliter syringes are used when doses are 0.1 ml. or less.

Intravenous injections can be given when necessary. A 25- to 27-gauge needle is chosen according to vein size. The vein of choice for an intravenous injection in each species is listed below.

| SPECIES | VEIN OF CHOICE |
|---|---|
| Rabbit | Marginal ear vein or cephalic vein |
| Guinea pig | Cephalic vein |
| Rat | Vein on the caudolateral aspect of the thigh or the vein on the dorsal surface of the tail.† |
| Hamster | Vein on the caudolateral aspect of the thigh |
| Mouse | Tail vein† (very difficult without practice) |

*Microliter syringe (0.001 to 0.1 ml.), The Hamilton Co., Reno, Nevada.
†Wrap or immerse the tail in warm water prior to venipuncture.

## INTRAGASTRIC INTUBATION AND ARTIFICIAL ALIMENTATION

Intragastric intubation and the use of a liquid replacement diet can help support an anorectic patient's nutritional needs. Liquid diets‡ fortified with baby foods (fruits, vegetables, cereals, meats) have been used satisfactorily. Usually, a volume of 2 to 3 ml./100 gm. of body weight is infused at one time. Karo syrup, honey or vegetable oil can be added if caloric requirements necessitate it. The daily caloric requirement for a healthy mature rodent is roughly 15 to 35 Kcal./100 gm. of body weight. The higher caloric requirement pertains to mice and hamsters, while the lower requirement is for rats, guinea pigs and rabbits. Growth, lactation or a febrile condition can double the daily caloric requirement.

‡Esbilac® (Borden), Initol® (Hill), Neo Mull-Soy® (Borden) and Pet Kalorie® (Haver-Lockhart) made into a slurry.

Intragastric intubation can be accomplished with either a flexible rubber tube* or a rigid metal cannula† with a ball-tipped end. Sharp incisors can easily cut a flexible tube unless the jaws are manually held open. Passage of the tube between the interdental space (between incisors and molars) may help avoid this problem. If this is not possible, a tongue depressor or a small flat stick with a hole drilled in its center can be used as a mouth gag. The gag is placed on edge just behind the incisors. A tube can then be passed through the hole in the mouth gag. Speculums are not needed when using metal cannulas. These are designed specifically for use in laboratory species. With a little practice, they can be passed quickly and atraumatically. With either method of gastric intubation, two points of resistance are usually encountered. The first is just before the tube reaches the esophagus, the second point being just before the tube reaches the cardia. Gentle manipulation of the tube (not pressure) will help it pass atraumatically.

## ENDOTRACHEAL INTUBATION IN THE RABBIT

The rabbit's oral cavity architecture and its extremely posteriorly positioned larynx make endotracheal intubation challenging. Intravenous ketamine HCl (11 mg./kg.) or sodium thiamylal‡ (1 ml./2.25 kg.) and atropine sulfate (0.04 mg./kg.) is used to facilitate intubation. A rabbit or dog mouth speculum is placed in position. The animal is placed upon its sternum and its head and neck are held extended, forming approximately a 45- to 60-degree angle with the table surface. Gentle manual traction is applied on the tongue. A laryngoscope with a No. 1 Miller blade§ is inserted as far back as possible into the oral cavity. Pressure is placed on the laryngoscope handle so as to press the blade against the base of the tongue and the floor of the oral cavity. If the laryngoscope blade and the head of the

animal are held correctly, the glottis can be seen. Once the glottis is visualized, it is helpful to turn the laryngoscope handle a quarter turn to the right (from the 6 o'clock to the 3 o'clock position). This allows better visualization and more room to work. A semi-rigid probe is passed into the oral cavity, starting from the left commissure of the lips. It is placed into the opening of the glottis. A 4-mm. (I.D.) uncuffed endotracheal tube is fed down the probe and manipulated until it enters the trachea. Laryngeal spasm is not a problem in this species.

## DRUG DOSAGES

The following dosages are ones that I have used in my practice (Table 12). They have a fair degree of safety and efficacy. Serum level studies of the chemotherapeutics have not been carried out by the author and will not be discussed here.

## SURGERY AND ANESTHESIA

Surgical and anesthetic procedures are routine, with just a few exceptions. Induction of anesthesia is accomplished by masking with either halothane or methoxyflurane. Endotracheal intubation is practical only in the rabbit. After intubation, the animal is connected directly to the anesthetic machine. In species not intubated, planes of anesthesia can be maintained by intermittent masking. Face masks of varied lengths and diameters can be made by cutting the closed end off disposable syringe containers. Depths of anesthesia are best monitored by observing respiratory rates and the color of the albinotic iris.

Postsurgical care of laboratory animals presents particular problems. Rabbits will invariably chew away sutures unless the incision is bandaged for three to four days postoperatively. Temperature regulation and body heat conservation are paramount problems in very small rodents. Small body size and its relationship to exposed surface area make them more vulnerable to heat loss. Exogenous heat sources, such as hot water bags or a well covered heating pad on a low setting, are indicated. Full recovery from the anesthesia should be accomplished before the animal is returned to its cage.

---

*3 to 12 French rubber stomach tube by Davol.

†Oral Administration Needle, Aloe Scientific, 1831 Olive Street, St. Louis, Missouri 63103; or Biomedical Needles, Animal Feeding Stainless Steel, Popper & Sons, Inc., New York, New York 10010.

‡Surital® (Parke, Davis) (sodium thiamylal for injection, N.F.) veterinary, 5 gm., made into a 2 per cent solution.

§Harris-Lake Inc., Cleveland, Ohio.

*(Text continued on page 756.)*

*Table 12.* Drug Dosages*

| DRUG | MANUFACTURER'S CONCENTRATION/ML. | MG./100 GM. (OR KG. WHEN LISTED) OF BODY WEIGHT | ROUTE | VOLUME OR AMOUNT TO BE GIVEN/100 GM. OF BODY WEIGHT (OR /KG.) | MISCELLANEOUS |
|---|---|---|---|---|---|
| Innovar-Vet | Comes in a standard concentration containing a mixture of Fentanyl, 0.4 mg./ml., and Droperidol, 20.0 mg./ml. | — | Intramuscular | 0.02–0.05 ml./100 gm. | Up to 0.15 ml./100 gm. may be necessary in hamsters; 0.02–0.05 ml. dose works best in rats, guinea pigs and mice; 0.02 ml. for rabbits |
| Nalline | 5 mg./ml. | 0.5 mg./100 gm. | Subcutaneous; intramuscular; intravenous | 0.1 ml./100 gm. | Intravenous route for quickest response; 5 mg. is the largest dosage usually given |
| Ketamine HCL | 100 mg./ml. | 4.4 mg./100 gm. | Intramuscular | 0.05 ml./100 gm. | Produces a mild form of sedation; good for minor surgical procedures and oral examination; short duration; less than 20 minutes |
| Ketamine HCL | 100 mg./ml. | 11 mg./kg. | Intravenous | 0.11 ml./kg. | Used in rabbits; good for endotracheal intubation and minor surgical procedures; very short duration (less than 10 minutes) |
| Surital (5 gm.) stock bottle | 2 per cent solution | — | Intravenous | 1.0 ml./2.27 kg. (1.0 ml./5 lb.) | Used in rabbits for endotracheal intubation; use anesthetic to effect |
| Atropine sulfate | 1/150 gr./ml. or 0.4 mg./ml. | 0.004–0.01 mg./100 gm. | Subcutaneous; intramuscular; intravenous | 0.01–0.025 ml./100 gm. | |
| Dexamethasone | 1 mg./ml. | 0.06 mg./100 gm. | Subcutaneous; intramuscular; intravenous; intraperitoneal | 0.06 ml./100 gm. | |
| Prednisone | 10 mg./ml. | 0.05–0.22 mg./100 gm. | Subcutaneous; intramuscular | 0.005–0.022 ml./100 gm. | |

| | (active ingredients) | | Oral ration or a single dose *per os* | | Instructions |
|---|---|---|---|---|---|
| | | | | | ...thoroughly one pulverized tablet/1 lb. of finely ground feed; small amounts of water are added to ground mixture to facilitate reshaping into a kibble type ration; air dry or feed as mash; we have used it on large numbers of mice (male, female, some pregnant) without problems; have not had opportunity to use on large numbers of other species; medicated feed is fed for 3 days, off for 3 days, on for 3 days; repeat in 2 weeks if necessary; procedure described can be used also in hamsters, although its efficacy has not been documented; I have no personal experience using it in guinea pigs, rabbits or gerbils |
| Piperazine citrate or adipate | 500 mg. tablets or can buy bulk | 50–100 mg./100 gm. | Oral | ½–1 tablet/50 ml. water | Put in drinking water; use the following regimen for pinworms (for mice and rats): 7 days on medication; 7 days off medication; 7 days on medication. Clean cages thoroughly just before putting animal on medication and when taking it off medication; do all animals in same room at same time; pinworm eggs may be air-borne; filter caps may help; 5 per cent sucrose solution may increase palatability of medicated water |
| Sucrose | | | Oral | 25 gm./487 ml. of water | Used to increase palatability of medicated water |
| Griseofulvin | 50 mg./tablet | 2 mg./100 gm. | Oral | Consult chart for amount of feed consumed | Mix one (50 mg.) tablet/lb. of feed; follow mixing instructions for yomesan; use cautiously in guinea pig since griseofulvin is derived from *Penicillium griseofulvin* |
| Shell Pest Strips (DDVP) | — | — | — | — | Place a strip 1 × 2 × 2 inches on top of average size mouse cage; keep it away from animal so it will not chew on it; use for 3 days; take off for 3 days; serum cholinesterase levels will fall with long-term use but will go back to normal when strips are removed; production may be lowered; can be used safely on mature, healthy (not systemically ill) animals |
| Ectocide | — | — | — | 1/16 tsp./100 gm. if nursing; 1/64 tsp./adult | Put desired amount of ectocide into a paper bag (lunch bag size); place animal in bag and shake; this method distributes medication evenly over animal; *only do on mature animals* |

*Long-term antibiotic therapy (greater than five days at therapeutic levels) may result in fatalities due to destruction of symbiotic bacteria in the gastrointestinal tract. This is especially true in guinea pigs and hamsters. Unless otherwise stated, chemotherapeutics may be used on any species.

(*Table 12 continued on the following page.*)

*Table 12. Drug Dosages (Continued)*

| DRUG | MANUFACTURER'S CONCENTRATION/ML. | MG./100 GM. (OR KG. WHEN LISTED) OF BODY WEIGHT | ROUTE | VOLUME OR AMOUNT TO BE GIVEN/100 GM. OF BODY WEIGHT (OR/KG.) | MISCELLANEOUS |
|---|---|---|---|---|---|
| Crotomiton (Eurax) | 10 per cent lotion | – | Topical | – | Apply one to two times a day |
| Chloramphenicol palmitate | 125 mg./4 ml. | 2–5 mg./100 gm. | Oral | 0.07 ml.–0.16 ml./100 gm. | Give two to three times a day† |
| Chloramphenicol succinate | 100 mg./ml. | 0.66 mg./100 gm. | Intramuscular | .0066 ml./100 mg. | Give one to two times a day (dose can be doubled if needed) |
| Tylosin | 50 mg./ml. | 0.2–0.4 mg./100 gm. | Intramuscular | 0.004 ml.–0.008 ml./100 gm. | Give one to two times a day (dose can be doubled if needed) |
| Gentamicin sulfate (Gentocin) | 50 mg./ml. | 0.44 mg./100 gm. | Intramuscular | 0.008–0.016 ml./100 gm. | Give one to two times a day; has been used with good results in hamsters with wet tail |
| Tetracycline (Panmycin) | 100 mg./ml. | 1.5–2 mg./100 gm. | Oral | 0.015–0.02 ml./100 gm. | Give two to three times a day† |
| Oxytetracycline (intravenous terramycin) | 100 mg./ml. | 0.6–1 mg./100 gm. | Intramuscular | 0.006–0.01 ml./100 gm. | Give one to two times a day |
| Chlortetracycline (intravenous) | 100 mg./ml. | 0.6–1.0 mg./100 gm. | Intramuscular | 0.006–0.01 ml./100 gm. | Give one to two times a day |
| Sulfamerazine | | 5–8 mg./100 gm. | Oral | 30–80 mg, added to sufficient quantity of water to make 100 ml. of solution | Put in drinking water or administer proper dosage for weight *per os* |

| | | | | | |
|---|---|---|---|---|---|
| Sulfaquinoxaline | Concentrate stock solution 3.44 gm./100 ml. | — | Oral | 0.25 gm.–1.0 gm./1000 ml. of water (0.025–0.1 per cent solution) or 0.256 gm./500 gm. of feed (0.05 per cent ration) | Medicate for 30 days; improve sanitation and animal husbandry methods |
| Sulfadimethoxine (Bactrovet) | 12.5 per cent oral suspension | 2.0–5.0 mg./100 gm. | Oral | 0.016–0.04 ml./100 gm. | Give once a day† |
| Procaine penicillin G | 300,000 units/ml. | 2000 units/100 gm. | Intramuscular | 0.0066 ml./100 gm. | Has been used in all laboratory species; anaphylaxis can occur in guinea pigs; use other antibiotics if possible |
| Furazolidone (Furoxone) | 100 mg./ml. | 0.5 mg./100 gm. | Oral | 0.005 ml./100 gm. | 0.55 gm./100 ml. of water = 0.055 per cent solution or 5 mg./100 gm. of feed for long-term therapy (30 days); used mainly in rabbits |
| Nitrofurazone (Furacin) | 0.2 per cent solution (0.2 gm./100 ml.) | 8 mg./kg. | Oral | 4 ml./kg., added to daily water | 100 mg./1000 ml. of water or 0.01 per cent solution for long-term therapy in rabbits |
| Vitamin A, U.S.P. | 100,000 units/ml. | 50–500 units/100 gm. | Intramuscular | 0.0005–0.005 ml./100 gm. | |
| Vitamin D, U.S.P. | 100,000 units/ml. (1 ml. of stock solution can be diluted with 10 ml. of saline) | 20–40 units/100 gm. | Intramuscular | 0.002–0.004 ml. of diluted stock solution/100 gm. | |
| Vitamin C, U.S.P. | 100 mg./ml. | 2–20 mg./100 gm. | Intramuscular | 0.02–0.2 ml./100 gm. | |
| B complex (Vitaxin) | $B_1$ 100 mg./ml. $B_2$ 2.0 mg./ml. $B_{12}$ 100 mcg./ml. | — | Intramuscular | 0.002–0.02 ml./100 gm. | |

†This formula can be used to calculate the amount of chemotherapeutic and water that will be placed in the drinking bottle.

$$\frac{\text{Total daily dosage of chemotherapeutic} \times 5\ddagger}{\text{Total amount of daily water consumed for the species being treated (Table 1)} \times 5} = \frac{\text{The amount of chemotherapeutic to be placed in the water per day}}{\text{The amount of water to be placed in the drinking bottle per day}}$$

Example for a 100-gm. hamster on Panmycin:

$$\frac{0.06 \text{ ml. of Panmycin} \times 5}{12 \text{ ml.} \times 5} = \frac{0.30 \text{ ml. of Panmycin}}{60 \text{ ml. of water}} \text{ to be placed in drinking bottle}$$

‡Use this factor (5) if daily volume of water to be consumed is less than 1 oz. (30 ml.); this will give adequate volume to fill water bottle and account for any wastage.

For specific information and particular surgical procedures of either a clinical or experimental nature, the reader should consult:

1. Farris, E. J., and Griffith, J. Q.: The Rat in Laboratory Investigation. Rpt. 1963. Philadelphia, J. B. Lippincott Co., 1967, pp. 168–180, 434–452.

2. Markowitz, J., Archibald, J., and Downie, H. G.: Experimental Surgery. 4th ed. Baltimore, The Williams & Wilkins Co., 1959.

## COMMUNICABLE DISEASES

Dermatomycosis, salmonellosis and *Hymenolepsis* are relatively common in laboratory animals. If diagnosed, the disease's public health significance should be explained to the client. Consultation with a physician familiar with communicable diseases can be helpful.

Leptospirosis, tularemia, sylvatic plague, lymphocytic choriomeningitis and rabies can occur as natural diseases in laboratory species. Although extremely uncommon, their existence and significance should not be forgotten.

Vaccination against rabies and leptospirosis is not routinely performed unless the incidence of the disease in a specific area warrants it, or an owner specifically requests it. Killed vaccines are used if they must be given.

### SUPPLEMENTAL READING

Crocker, C. L.: Rapid determination of urea nitrogen in serum or plasma without deproteinization. Am. J. Med. Techn., *33*:361–365, 1967.

Farris, E. J., and Griffith, J. Q.: The Rat in Laboratory Investigation. Rpt. 1963. Philadelphia, J. B. Lippincott Co., 1967.

Green, E. L., *et al.*: Biology of the Laboratory Mouse. 2nd ed. New York, McGraw-Hill Book Co., 1966.

Hafez, E. S. E.: Reproduction and Breeding Techniques for Laboratory Animals. Philadelphia, Lea & Febiger, 1970.

Hoffman, R. A., Robinson, P. F., and Magalhaes, H.: The Golden Hamster, Its Biology and Use in Medical Research. Ames, Iowa, The Iowa State University Press, 1968.

Laboratory animals. J. Lab. Animal Sci. Assn., Laboratory Animals Ltd., 7 Warwick Court, London, WCIR 5DP.

Laboratory Animal Science. Joliet, Ill., American Association for Laboratory Animal Science.

Riley, V.: Adaptation of orbital bleeding technique to rapid serial blood studies. Proc. Soc. Exp. Biol. Med. *104*:751–754, 1960.

Schwentker, V.: The Gerbil: An Annotated Bibliography. Presented by Tumblebrook Farm, West Brookfield, Mass.

Weisbroth, S. H., Flatt, R. E., and Kraus, A. L.: The Biology of the Laboratory Rabbit. New York, Academic Press, 1974.

Wescott, R. B.: An Outline of Diseases of Laboratory Animals. Columbia, Mo., University of Missouri Press, 1969.

# EXOTIC ANIMAL RADIOLOGY

SAM SILVERMAN, D.V.M.
*Davis, California*

Radiology is often quite useful in the medical and surgical management of small mammals and reptiles maintained as pets or used as laboratory animals. The small size of these animals and the difficulty encountered in restraint are factors which may complicate radiographic procedures. High-capacity x-ray generators (300 ma.) are necessary to produce adequate milliamperes, with fast exposure times (1/60 second or faster). This is especially true in animals with rapid respiratory rates (mice and hamsters). One method that can be utilized to increase the usable output of the x-ray generator is to decrease the focal film distance from the conventional one meter (as was described in the article on "Avian Radiographic Technique and Interpretation"). The intensity of x-rays is inversely proportional to the square of the distance from the x-ray tube to the x-ray film (inverse square law). Therefore, halving the focal film distance will allow a fourfold reduction in the exposure time without altering milliamperes (quantity of x-rays at the x-ray film).

The availability of new immobilization drugs such as the phencyclidine derivatives has greatly simplified patient restraint and positioning for x-ray procedures. If these drugs are not acceptable for the species being examined, one of the gaseous anesthetic agents may be acceptable. The majority of our examinations of small mammals and reptiles are performed with some chemical immobilization. The small size of these animals makes it very difficult to prevent accidental x-ray exposure of the radiographer if manual restraint is used. Paper masking tape and small sandbags are used to position the patient. It is often helpful to have several small pieces of radiolucent sponge available to assist in the precise positioning of these animals.

Nonscreen film can be used for examinations of small mammals, but this type of film requires a higher radiation exposure and thus often a longer exposure time. We therefore use par speed film and high-detail intensifying screens, since these can also be processed through an automatic processor. Nonscreen dental film is not acceptable because of the long exposure time required. Furthermore, it is often difficult to include the entire area of interest on this small format film.

The radiographic examination of the various types of small animals will be discussed according to conformational group (small mammals, rabbits, lizards, turtles and tortoises, and snakes). It is not possible to give exposure radiographic factors that are acceptable for all x-ray units; however, I will give a representative set of factors that have been acceptable with our equipment.

## SMALL MAMMALS

### Mice, Rats, Hamsters, etc.

If the patient is debilitated or otherwise easily accepts restraint, it may be possible to examine these animals without anesthesia. Most of our studies are performed on anesthetized animals; we maintain a bell jar with cotton pledgets impregnated with methoxyfluorane in the bottom of the jar for this purpose. After the animals are anesthetized, they should not be placed in a small cage or a well ventilated area, since their fur absorbs the anesthetic vapors and recovery from the anesthetic can be prolonged.

Dorsoventral radiographs are easier to produce than ventrodorsal studies. The legs should be pulled laterally and taped to the

x-ray cassette with masking tape. The animal's head should be taped to the cassette to provide additional restraint if it is not deeply anesthetized.

Lateral studies are performed similarly to studies in larger animals. The dependent legs (those closest to the x-ray cassette) are positioned cranial to the contralateral legs, and the dependent side is indicated on the x-ray film with a radiopaque marker. In this way it is possible to identify the laterality of abnormalities detected in the appendicular skeleton.

Representative exposure factors for small mammals using par speed film and high-detail intensifying screens include

| PATIENT | MA | TIME (SEC) | KVP. |
|---------|-----|------|------|
| Rat | 100 | 1/60 | 64 |
| Mouse | 100 | 1/60 | 58 |

### Rabbits

These animals present a unique problem to the radiographer. It is possible to injure their spines severely (fracture and/or luxate the caudal lumbar spine) if they are not restrained properly and they extend their legs abruptly in a kicking movement. It is therefore necessary to restrain these animals to prevent free movement of the hindlegs. Anesthesia or manual restraint is required when radiographing rabbits. The lateral projection is easiest to obtain. The legs are extended gently for this study. Ventrodorsal studies are more difficult. Rabbits seem to resist being placed on their back. We find it best to position the rabbit for the lateral study and then rotate it into the ventrodorsal position. The radiographic exposure is made immediately after the animal is in the ventrodorsal position.

Radiographic exposure technique used for rabbit studies is quite similar to that used for cats.

We have performed gastrointestinal contrast studies on rabbits with some success to rule out gastrointestinal foreign bodies, obstruction, etc. Conventional upper gastrointestinal micropulverized barium suspensions (25 to 30 per cent) are acceptable. At least 50 cc. is required for a medium-sized rabbit.

### Reptiles

Lizards are among the easiest animals to radiograph if certain precautions are taken.

The animal's environmental temperature should be gradually reduced to room temperature if its cage is heated. This will decrease the animal's activity to an acceptable level. Extreme hypothermia is not a recommended form of sedation, owing to the possible severe metabolic depression, etc. Phencyclidine derivatives have been successfully used on several types of reptiles, but the prolonged sedation is not necessary for most radiographic procedures. Masking tape is used to restrain lizards to a thin (3 mm.) radiolucent sheet of plastic. The animal is placed in the prone position, and tape is fastened across the neck, body, tail and legs. The plastic sheet with lizard attached is then placed on an x-ray cassette and the exposure is made. If the study must be repeated, e.g., technique is not adequate, the plastic sheet is placed on a second cassette. This precludes repositioning the lizard for supplemental studies. Most lizards readily accept this form of restraint.

Dorsoventral projections are the only routine projections obtained on most lizards. Lizards do not tolerate being placed in lateral recumbency; therefore, lateral projections are obtained with the lizard in the prone position. The x-ray cassette is placed as close to the side of the lizard as possible, and the x-ray beam is directed horizontally.

Exposure factors for a medium-sized *iguana* are 100 ma., 1/60 seconds and 36 to 40 kvp. Par speed film and high-detail intensifying screens are used. The added aluminum filtration can be removed from the collimator to maximize utilization of the lower kvp. x-rays; however, humans should not be in the room when the exposure is made because of the increased radiation hazard.

### Snakes

Snakes are not difficult to radiograph. Small snakes can be coiled in a natural position on an x-ray cassette or taped to the cassette in a straightened position. It is also possible to place the snake in a thin plexiglass tube and radiograph it through the tube. This method is useful for obtaining lateral projections of snakes by taping the tube to a vertically positioned x-ray cassette and using a horizontally directed x-ray beam. Snakes can also be taped to padded boards and then placed in apposition to the x-ray cassette.

Owing to the similarity of skeletal anatomy throughout the majority of a snake's body, it is useful to place lead markers at specific intervals on the snake's skin when performing whole body studies. This will allow more accurate localization of the radiographic abnormalities, etc. Sequential numbers are the most useful marking system.

Acceptable exposure factors for a medium-sized snake are 100 ma., 1/60 seconds and 45 kvp., using par speed film, and high-detail screens.

### Turtles and Tortoises

Turtles and tortoises are among the easiest animals to radiograph. The dorsoventral projection is obtained by placing the animal on the x-ray cassette and restraining it with a piece of masking tape attached to the caudal portion of the carapace and the cassette. The animal will attempt to walk against this restraint. The radiographic exposure is made when the head and legs are fully extended from the shell. The dorsoventral view is ideal for examination of the digestive tract but is not acceptable for the respiratory system, owing to superimposition of the lungs on the other viscera.

The respiratory system is evaluated using a horizontal x-ray beam directed in a cranial to caudal direction. The x-ray cassette is placed in a vertical position, and the animal is placed on a small platform, e.g., cardboard box, etc., directly in front of the x-ray cassette, so that it is looking into the x-ray beam. The lungs occupy the dorsal portion of the body cavity.

Acceptable exposure factors for a medium-sized tortoise (6 cm. dorsoventral dimension) are 300 ma., 1/60 seconds and 52 to 58 kvp., using par speed film and high-detail screen.

### SUPPLEMENTAL READING

Morgan, J. P., Silverman, S., and Zontine, W. J.: Techniques of Veterinary Radiography. Veterinary Radiology Associates, Davis, California, 1975, pp. 269–285.

# HEMATOLOGY OF SOME ZOO ANIMALS AND EXOTIC PETS

FRED K. SOIFER, D.V.M.
*Houston, Texas*

Special consideration must be given these unusual animals when considering their hematology. Very few of them can be restrained for bleeding without considerable stress or the use of chemical restraint. However, because of the owners' inability to detect early signs or symptoms of the disease, laboratory tests become more important in establishing and substantiating the diagnosis.

When the animal can be bled with a minimum of restraint (Fig. 1), chemical agents should not be used. However, any severe stress will produce an altered blood picture. This includes a leukocytosis, neutrophilia and eosinopenia. Several of the chemical restraint medications show no apparent effect on the hematology. Phencyclidine (Sernylan®, Parke, Davis) and ketamine are effective and safe; research has shown that they do not affect the patient's blood picture (Fig. 2). The tranquilizers may be administered later for deeper sedation or longer duration but should not be given before blood is collected.

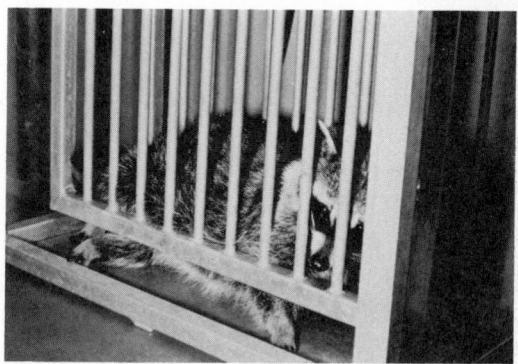

**Figure 2.** Raccoon in squeeze cage to restrain for administration of sedation and subsequent bleeding.

## METHODS OF BLOOD COLLECTION

The exotic cats can be bled from the cephalic, femoral, saphenous or jugular veins. Raccoons, coatis, kinkajous, skunks and ferrets are probably bled most easily from the jugular veins, although the other veins mentioned above may be used on the larger or older animals. The nonhuman primates may all be bled from the femoral vein with ease (Fig. 3). The laboratory ani-

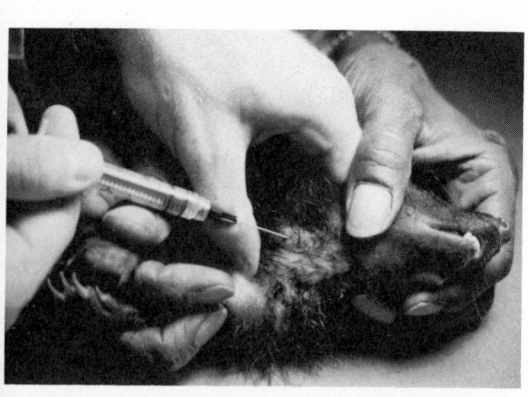

**Figure 1.** Manual restraint to jugular bleed a young raccoon.

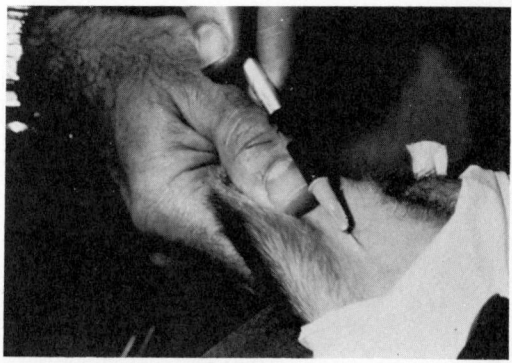

**Figure 3.** Femoral bleeding of monkey.

*Table 1.*   Hematologic Data of Some Exotic Species

| ORDERS | RBC 10⁶ | Hb (mg/100 mL.) | PCV | ESR (mm./hour) | WBC 10³ | Neutrophil | Lymphocyte | Monocyte | Eosinophil | Basophil | NO. OF ANIMALS REPRESENTED |
|---|---|---|---|---|---|---|---|---|---|---|---|
| Monotremata | —† | | | | | | | | | | |
| Marsupialia | | | | | | | | | | | |
| Opossum | 4 | 10 | 32 | — | 12 | 39 | 46 | 10 | 5 | 0 | 20 |
| Tasmanian devil | 6 to 7.3 | — | 35 to 40 | 1 to 3 | 8 to 10 | 70 | 30 | 0 | 0 | 0 | 2 |
| Chiroptera | | | | | | | | | | | |
| Fruit bats | — | — | 45 | 1 to 3 | — | 67 | 29 | 4 | 0 | 0 | 6 |
| Primates | | | | | | | | | | | |
| Gibbon | — | — | 45 to 50 | — | 8 to 11 | 55 | 35 | 5 | 5 | 0 | 8 |
| Chimpanzee | 5.3 | 13 | 40 to 45 | — | 12 | 44 | 50 | 2 | 4 | 0 | 20 |
| Orangutan | — | — | 35 to 40 | — | 10 to 11 | 56 | 35 | 5 | 4 | 0 | 2 |
| Gorilla | — | 12 to 14 | 35 to 45 | — | 8 to 14 | 47 | 45 | 3 | 5 | 0 | 5 |
| Capuchin | — | — | 35 to 40 | 0 to 3 | 10 to 12 | 51 | 40 | 2 | 3 | 0 | 30 |
| Squirrel | 7 | 14 | 35 to 40 | 0 to 3 | 10 to 12 | 45 | 45 | 4 | 6 | 0 | 45 |
| Spider | — | — | 35 to 40 | 0 to 5 | 10 to 12 | 52 | 40 | 3 | 5 | 0 | 23 |
| Wooly | — | — | 35 to 40 | 0 to 3 | 11 to 14 | 63 | 32 | 3 | 2 | 0 | 36 |
| Marmoset | 6 | 14 | 45 to 50 | 0 to 3 | 10 to 12 | 50 | 41 | 2 | 3 | 0 | 260 |
| Macaque | 5 to 7 | 12 | 35 to 45 | 1 to 9 | 12 to 15 | 35 | 60 | 2 | 3 | 0 | 312 |
| Baboon | 5 to 7 | 14 | 43 | 0 to 5 | 6.5 | 30 | 64 | 3 | 3 | 0 | 26 |
| Edentata | | | | | | | | | | | |
| Tamandua | | | — | | | | | | — | | |
| Pholidota | | | | | | | | | | | |
| Pangolin | | — | 33 | 1 to 9 | — | 63 | 36 | 1 | 0 | 0 | 4 |
| Lagomorpha | | | | | | | | | | | |
| Rabbit | 5.5 | 12 | 35 to 45 | 2 to 4 | 8 to 10 | 42 | 38 | 9 | 1 | 0 | 39 |
| Rodentia | | | | | | | | | | | |
| Squirrel | — | — | 35 to 45 | 0 to 1 | 5 to 9 | 67 | 25 | 6 | 10 | 0 | 21 |
| Porcupine | 5.5 | 14.5 | 35 to 45 | 2 to 4 | 9 to 12 | 42 | 45 | 8 | 5 | 0 | 46 |
| Guinea pig | 7 | 16 | 45 to 50 | 0 to 1 | 8 to 10 | 30 | 67 | 2 | 1 | 0 | 62 |
| Hamster | 8 to 9 | 14 | 35 to 50 | 1 to 2 | 12 to 15 | 26 | 65 | 4 | 1 | 0 | 43 |
| Rat | 9 | 15 | 40 to 50 | 1 to 2 | 8 to 14 | 30 | 66 | 5 | 3 | 0 | 24 |
| Gerbil | 7 to 8 | 14 to 16 | 35 to 45 | 0 to 2 | 11 | 22 | 75 | 2 | 3 | 0 | 12 |
| Pinnipedia | | | | | | | | | | | |
| Sea lion | 4 | 13 | 38 | — | 5 to 9 | 60 | 35 | 3 | 2 | 0 | 11 |
| Seals | 4 to 5 | 20 | 35 | — | 7 to 10 | 61 | 22 | 4 | 9 | 2 | 16 |
| Tubulidentata | | | — | | | | — | | | | |
| Proboscidea | | | | | | | | | | | |
| Indian elephant | 2.5 | 10 to 11 | 35 | 61 | 9 to 10 | 33 | 56 | 4 | 7 | 0 | 10 |
| Artiodactyla | | | | | | | | | | | |
| Camel | 8 | 14 | 28 to 30 | — | 18 to 20 | 40 | 45 | 6 | 9 | 0 | 4 |
| Guanaco | 15 | 15 | 40 | 1 | 12 | 64 | 24 | 3 | 5 | 0 | 7 |
| Sheep | 12 | 12 | 35 | 0 | 7.5 | 30 | 62 | 3 | 5 | 0 | 10 |
| Deer° (spotted fallow); aged female | 10.3 | 17.1 | 42 | 4 | 4.3 | 39 | 23 | 1 | 35 | 2 | 4 |
| Deer (white tail) | 18 | 18 | 55 | — | — | 40 | 55 | 3 | 2 | 0 | 8 |
| Poor condition goat | 13 | 11 | 35 | 0 | 9 | 36 | 56 | 3 | 5 | 0 | 29 |
| Bernstein° dik-dik | 16 | 19 | 49 | — | 8.7 | 70 | 25 | 4 | 1 | 0 | 1 |
| Bernstein° Suni antelope | 17 | 20 | 63 | — | 7 | 20 | 80 | 0 | 0 | 0 | 1 |
| Eland (baby) | 8 | 11 to 12 | 35 to 40 | 1 | 7 to 8 | 61 | 38 | 1 | 0 | 0 | 2 |
| Mouse deer | 74 | 14.3 | 65° | 0 | 8.4 | 14 | 70 | 3 | 11 | 2 | 2 |

*Table 1.  Hematologic Data of Some Exotic Species (Continued)*

| ORDERS | RBC $10^6$ | Hb (mg/100 ml.) | PCV | ESR (mm./hour) | WBC $10^3$ | DIFFERENTIAL COUNT (PER CENT) | | | | | NO. OF ANIMALS REPRESENTED |
|---|---|---|---|---|---|---|---|---|---|---|---|
| | | | | | | Neutro- phil | Lympho- cyte | Mono- cyte | Eosino- phil | Baso- phil | |
| Carnivora | | | | | | | | | | | |
| Canidae | | | | | | | | | | | |
| Wolves and foxes | 7 to 8 | 12 to 16 | 35 to 45 | 0 to 2 | 10 to 12 | 60 | 38 | 1 | 1 | 1 | 90 |
| Ursidae | | | | | | | | | | | |
| Black bear | 8 | 16 | 45 to 50 | 0 | 11 to 14 | 70 | 25 | 3 | 2 | 0 | 6 |
| Grizzly | 8 | 22 | 45 to 50 | 1 to 9 | 6 to 8 | 65 | 20 | 7 | 7 | 1 | 2 |
| Polar | 6 | 16 to 18 | 50 to 55 | 0 | 10 to 14 | 75 | 12 | 7 | 6 | 0 | 2 |
| Kodiak° (cubs) | 4 to 6 | 9 to 11 | 30 to 40 | 1 | 8 to 12 | 60 | 35 | 4 | 1 | 0 | 6 |
| Procyonidae | | | | | | | | | | | |
| Raccoon | 11 | 10 to 11 | 35 to 40 | 1 to 3 | 13 to 16 | 45 | 49 | 2 | 3 | 0 | 18 |
| Coatis | 11 | 10 to 11 | 35 to 40 | 1 to 3 | 13 to 16 | 45 | 49 | 2 | 3 | 0 | 23 |
| Kinkajous | 10 to 12 | 11 to 12 | 35 to 45 | 1 to 3 | 14 to 18 | 56 | 38 | 6 | 0 | 0 | 14 |
| Mustelidae | | | | | | | | | | | |
| Skunk | —† | — | 35 to 40 | 1 to 3 | 12 to 15 | 47 | 50 | 1 | 2 | 0 | 23 |
| Ferret | — | — | 35 to 40 | 1 to 3 | 9 to 13 | 65 | 35 | 0 | 0 | 0 | 16 |
| Viverridae | | | | | | | | | | | |
| Binturong | 11.2 | 22.2 | 55 | 1 to 6 | 10 to 14 | 68 | 30 | 0 | 2 | 0 | 7 |
| Genet | — | — | — | — | — | — | — | — | — | — | — |
| Felidae | | | | | | | | | | | |
| Lion | 7 to 8 | 8 to 12 | 35 to 40 | 0 to 5 | 10 to 15 | 63 | 30 | 5 | 2 | 0 | 12 |
| Tiger | 6 to 8 | 9 to 14 | 35 to 45 | 0 to 5 | 10 to 15 | 63 | 30 | 5 | 2 | 0 | 6 |
| Leopard | 6 to 8 | 8 to 13 | 35 to 45 | 0 to 5 | 10 to 14 | 63 | 30 | 5 | 2 | 0 | 4 |
| Jaguar | 6 to 8 | 8 to 13 | 35 to 45 | 0 to 5 | 10 to 14 | 63 | 30 | 5 | 2 | 0 | 3 |
| Cheetah | 6 to 8 | 8 to 13 | 35 to 40 | 0 to 5 | 10 to 12 | 63 | 30 | 5 | 2 | 0 | 4 |
| Cougar | 7 to 8 | 10 to 18 | 35 to 50 | 0 to 4 | 8 to 12 | 63 | 32 | 2 | 3 | 0 | 7 |
| Ocelot | 7 to 8 | 10 to 18 | 35 to 40 | 0 to 8 | 8 to 13 | 65 | 33 | 0 | 2 | 0 | 28 |
| Margay | 7 to 8 | 10 to 18 | 35 to 40 | 0 to 8 | 8 to 13 | 65 | 33 | 0 | 2 | 0 | 16 |
| Jagarundi | 7 to 8 | 10 to 15 | 35 to 40 | 0 to 5 | 8 to 13 | 65 | 33 | 0 | 2 | 0 | 8 |

°Dr. Jon Bernstein provided these figures.
†Dashes indicate that no data were available at time of publication.

mals may be bled from the jugular vein in the larger species (with practice and care) and from the tail tip (by trimming) in the long-tailed species. Birds may be bled from the jugular vein or the axillary or wing vein. Toenails may be trimmed short in any of the above animals when a small amount of blood is all that is required. Snakes, lizards and alligators must be cardiac bled. The author has not bled turtles or tortoises, but it has been suggested that nails may be trimmed short or a hole may be drilled in the plastron and a cardiac puncture performed.

Table 1 gives guidelines for hematologic data of some exotic species.

---

# DISEASES OF EXOTIC FELINES

ROBERT M. MILLER, D.V.M.
*Thousand Oaks, California*

All species of exotic cats are kept as pets and may be presented to the veterinarian for treatment. The ocelot is so popular that conservationists fear for survival of the species, particularly because they breed poorly in captivity. Margays, bobcats, jungle cats and jaguarundi are also popular. Occasionally one will see little leopard cats *(Felis bengalensis)* and golden cats *(Felis temminchi)*. In our practice, pet pumas are seen as often as ocelots, and leopards, cheetahs, jaguars and tigers are not unusual.

Basically, the veterinarian should remember that all the aforementioned animals are cats and, medically speaking, if they are treated like domestic cats, most problems will be avoided.

## NUTRITION

Suckling kittens may be reared on a formula, such as Borden's KMR or Esbilac®. As soon as solid food is taken, it may be added to the diet. Many commercial canned cat foods are excellent. One, Science Diets Zupreme®, has been formulated specifically for exotic cats. Commercial dog foods have also been used successfully. The feeding of baby chicks, whole chickens and mice or rats is nutritionally sound but impractical and unnecessary considering the availability, convenience and excellence of some commercial cat foods.

The diet to avoid, and the one that the owner most often employs, consists of red meat, liver or heart. Such a diet causes nutritional secondary hyperparathyroidism in all species of cats because of its low calcium and relatively high phosphorus content. This bone disease is characterized by loss of bone density, bone deformity and spontaneous pathologic fractures. It is the most common disease of young exotic cats, and it is often improperly called cage paralysis or osteogenesis imperfecta. The bone deformities can cause irreversible abnormalities. Pelvic narrowing may lead to chronic constipation and megacolon. Vertebral deformity may cause lordosis, posterior incoordination and partial or complete paresis. Many of these cats display lens opacities and strabismus.

Of course, red meat, heart and liver may be supplemented with calcium compounds to prevent this disease, but it is more practical and better nutritionally simply to feed one of the previously recommended foods. Also, because of the palatability of red meat, some cats are easily addicted to it and refuse other foods. Some cats enjoy a treat of asparagus, celery, lettuce or chicken necks. These, or an occasional bit of raw fish, are not objectionable. The same vitamin supplements that the practitioner uses for his domestic feline patients are suitable for exotic cats.

## VACCINATIONS

Exotic cats are highly susceptible to feline panleukopenia and must be diligently immunized. Because controlled data on the best method of vaccination are not available, we must rely upon practical experience. Using killed feline distemper vaccine, we give several injections at two-week intervals. Dosages are increased for larger cats.

We have used modified live virus vaccine (Leukogen TC [Fromm]), followed by a killed vaccine (Felocine [Norden]) two weeks later. Both manufacturers recommend their vaccines for exotic cats. In the larger cats, we double the dose. A booster after six months and annually thereafter may be valuable in maintaining immunity.

More recently we have been using modified live vaccine combined with rhinotracheitis and calicivirus vaccines (Pitman-Moore). We do not know if exotic cats are truly susceptible to these viruses but we have seen no adverse reactions to these new vaccines.

## PARASITES

Imported exotic cats are often heavily parasitized. Diagnostic and therapeutic procedures used in domestic cat practice are suitable for exotic cats. For ascarids we have used piperazine, except in the African lion, in which we have noted prolonged ataxia. Similar reactions have been reported in the cheetah. In the latter species, Dizan (Corvel) may be used. Dizan is also excellent for hookworms, although other drugs may be used. Mebendazole has replaced Dizan as our preferred treatment for hookworms and ascarids in exotics. However, this drug has not been officially cleared for use in cats. Yomesan® (niclosamide, Farbenfabriker Bayer) and Scolaban® (bunamidine HCl, Cooper and Nephews) are the best drugs for tapeworms. For coccidiosis we use nitrofurazone or a sulfonamide.

## OTHER DISEASES

In general, the experienced small animal practitioner's knowledge of feline medicine will safely guide him in the treatment of exotic cats. Upper respiratory infections are common. Tylocin (Elanco) has been a useful antibiotic for such infections and need be injected only once daily. The dosage we use is 20 mg./kg. of body weight initially and 10 mg./kg. thereafter.

## ANESTHESIA

Probably the greatest difference in the treatment of domestic and exotic cats is in the field of anesthesiology. Pentobarbital sodium should never be used. The well-known high mortality rate in exotic cats from general anesthesia stems largely from the use of this anesthetic. By using the methods of anesthesia to be discussed, the risk in anesthetizing an exotic cat should be no greater than in a domestic cat.

For short surgical procedures, intravenous thiamylal sodium, given slowly to effect, is satisfactory. A pre-anesthetic tranquilizer is advisable, as are atropinization and endotracheal intubation.

For more prolonged procedures, methoxyflurane administered via gas machine is suitable for maintaining anesthesia.

For difficult to handle patients, we inject phencyclidine (Sernylan®, Park, Davis) intramuscularly, at the rate of 2 to 4 mg./kg. of body weight. This drug produces convulsive muscular movements, which can be suppressed by injecting any phenothiazine tranquilizer such as acepromazine, at the rate of 1.0 mg./kg. (In very large cats, this dosage may be reduced.) It also causes salivation, which should be controlled with atropine. Many surgical procedures, including abdominal surgery, can be satisfactorily performed under this drug alone. If the patient is insufficiently anesthetized, either thiamylal sodium or methoxyflurane may be used to induce a deeper plane. More recently, we have used ketamine hydrocholoride satisfactorily to immobilize the smaller Felidae. The dosage is the same as for domestic cats, and the addition of a low level dose of a phenothiazine tranquilizer smoothes the effect of the ketamine.

For cats of any size, a combination of Rompun (Haver-Lockhart) and ketamine HCl provides very safe and satisfactory general anesthesia. Rompun is administered first intramuscularly, 2 to 3 mg./kg. of body weight. As soon as the animal is adequately sedated, we follow with an intramuscular dose of ketamine HCl at a dosage of 10 to 15 mg./kg. of body weight. Atropine is used to prevent salivation and an ophthalmic ointment is used to prevent drying of the cornea. Recovery from this combination is smooth and uneventful. We find this especially useful for removing claws and "fangs."

## SURGICAL PROCEDURES

### CELIOTOMY

The most common indication for celiotomy in our experience is for the relief of intestinal obstruction due to foreign bodies. Ocelots are prone to swallow fabric and rubber toys. We have noted a tendency for considerable reaction to catgut in this species and think that stainless-steel wire is the best suture material with which to close the abdominal incision.

### CASTRATION AND SPAYING

These operations are performed in the same manner as in the domestic cat.

### DEFANGING

We strongly disapprove of grinding or cutting off the teeth. The pulp cavity extends nearly to the tip of the cat's tooth, and exposure of the pulp is inevitable if enough of the tooth is cut off to blunt it. Removing the four great canine teeth is a better answer to the problem of biting. The cat can and will bite after it is defanged, and it can still inflict damage, but the danger of severe injury to humans is greatly reduced. In immature cats with deciduous teeth, the teeth are simply elevated out with care and patience. In such cats, the embryonic permanent tooth may then be removed through the same opening. It is medial and deep to the deciduous tooth and may be recognized as a pearly, slippery "bud"!

The fangs of mature cats can be very difficult to remove. We make a gum flap, and then remove the lateral overlying bone with a dental surgical burr and carefully elevate the tooth. We then suture the gum closed with simple interrupted sutures of catgut. In such patients, the lower fang root often constitutes the bulk of the thickness of the mandible over the alveolus. Great care must be taken not to fracture the mandible. If the mandible is inadvertently fractured, do not remove the opposite tooth. Instead, wait six or eight weeks for the jaw to heal, and then remove the remaining fang.

### DECLAWING

Basically, the declawing procedure in exotic cats is similar to that in house cats. In exotic cats that are the size of house cats, the technique is identical, using the Resco nail trimming instrument. This instrument, when properly used, neatly disarticulates the second and the third phalanx, but preserves the entire pad and a small portion of the third phalanx, that volar proximal process upon which the deep digital flexor tendon inserts. This tendon unsheathes the claw.

In cats too large for the Resco technique, we try to duplicate the Resco action by using a scalpel and White's nail trimmer. In larger cats we employ bone cutting shears, and in full grown lions or tigers we use a Gigli saw. The paw is routinely prepared for surgery. If the hair is long, it is clipped. An elastic bandage is then wrapped from the paw proximally to the elbow to force as much blood as possible from the leg. A tourniquet is placed above the elbow and the elastic wrap is removed. The surgical field should be relatively bloodless.

A Backhaus towel clamp is used to grasp the claw and it is extended by traction. An incision is made around the base of the nail, including an adequate amount of corium, but not including any pad or the folds of skin on either side of the nail. The articulation of the second and the third phalanx is severed. All that now holds the amputated portion to the rest of the paw is the previously mentioned volar proximal process of the third phalanx. We cut through it with a suitable instrument. On the dewclaw we totally disarticulate the third phalanx. Nitrofurazone powder is applied to each wound. On very large cats and on the dewclaws of medium-sized cats, we often close the incision with interrupted sutures of catgut.

Next, the paw is dressed. A strip of adhesive tape is folded in half longitudinally, sticky side out. It is wrapped around the paw above the level of the dewclaw. Tube-gauze bandage is then applied to the paw, proximally adhering to the tape, and drawn firmly distally to pull the edges of each incision over the exposed tissues. Several thicknesses of gauze are applied and then the entire dressing is covered with Elasticon bandage (Johnson & Johnson), applied not too tightly. Finally, the tourniquets are removed, and penicillin is administered intramuscularly (Bicillin® [Wyeth], 1 to 3 ml., depending upon size). Removal of the tourniquet is frequently followed by hemorrhage which soaks through the dressing. In these cases, the tourniquet should be replaced and left on as long as needed to control serious bleeding. The bandages are removed in two or three days for smaller cats, but for larger cats, such as lions, they should be left in place for a considerably longer period of time (up to one week for lion cubs). To remove the dressings on intractable cats, we give phencyclidine or ketamine, for restraint purposes.

## MISCELLANEOUS INFORMATION

The life span, gestation period, body temperature and normal blood and urine values of small exotic cats are the same as in the domestic cat.

Ocelots average 15 kg. at maturity, but they can exceed 25 kg. Margays show the same size range as the domestic cat. The American bobcat ranges midway in size between the ocelot and the margay but, of course, lacks their striking color pattern.

The litters of exotic cats tend to be small. The ocelot usually has two kittens, and the bobcat about four. Ocelots mature at two years of age and come into heat in midsummer, often becoming quite temperamental at that time.

Cheetahs are unique in that their claws are not retractable, and they should never be declawed. The cheetah is like a dog in other ways and can make a tractable and affectionate pet.

# ANTHELMINTICS FOR EXOTIC AND ZOO ANIMALS

FRED K. SOIFER, D.V.M.
*Houston, Texas*

Diagnosis and treatment of parasitic diseases in exotic animals have some rather unique features. Many of the animals exhibit unfamiliar helminth ova in their feces. In addition, exotic animals (even some of the small mammals) cannot safely be caught and restrained for the administration of anthelmintics. Because of these problems, we must use anthelmintics that are broad-spectrum in activity and palatable enough to be administered in the food or water. When an exotic pet is not eating and parasites are contributing factors to the illness or inappetence, a broad-spectrum injectable anthelmintic becomes necessary.

The author's philosophy concerning exotic animals and parasitism is dogmatic. *If an animal is parasitized, administer an anthelmintic.* Many wildlife management investigators argue that animals live out their lives infested with parasites, but we must remember that a relationship exists in the wild that is absent in captivity. Animals in their natural habitat live in a relatively large area, eat a variety of nutritious foods and are rarely stressed. On the other hand, when we import exotic pets, great numbers may be crammed into small crates, and they are often poorly fed and excessively stressed. In these cases, parasitism contributes to their demise.

### METHODS OF ADMINISTERING ANTHELMINTICS TO EXOTIC ANIMALS (MONOTREMES, EDENTATA, MARSUPIALS AND CHIROPTERA)

Drugs may be mixed with food as in the case of TBZ, piperazine, Task® (Shell), levamisole and other palatable and semipalatable anthelmintics. Unpalatable medications or drugs for animals not feeding regularly can be placed in suspension or

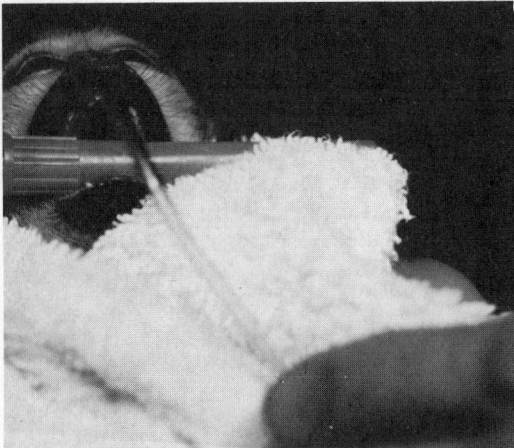

Figure 1. Administration of anthelmintic to monkey via stomach tube.

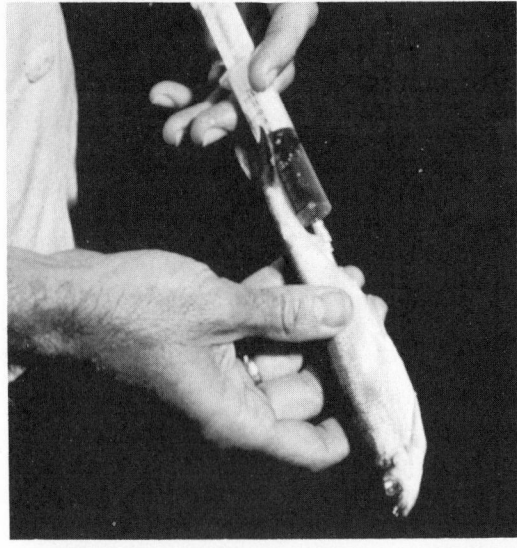

Figure 2. Injection of Tramisole into fish.

solution and given via stomach tube. Products such as D.N.P. or the experimental levamisole solution may be injected.

**Primates.** Thiabendazole (TBZ) as Equizole® and piperazine are palatable. Other medications must be flavored, tubed or injected (Fig. 1).

**Lagomorphs and Rodents.** These may be medicated orally when the drugs are palatable, tubed if desired, injected or fed low levels in the drinking water.

**Pinnipeds.** Most of the medications may be given by injecting them into, or embedding them in, the food given to the animals (fish, squid, etc.) (Fig. 2). Experimental levamisole (Tramisole®) has been injected subcutaneously and intramuscularly with some success.

**Proboscidea.** Drugs are given in sweet foods.

**Hooved Stock.** Low level feeding or oral dosing is used in young or restrainable animals.

**Carnivora.** Drugs are given as in dogs and cats.

**Aves.** These may be medicated via stomach tube or low levels added to the food or water.

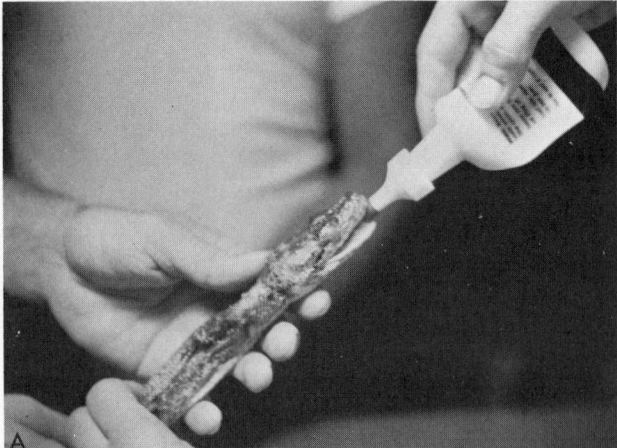

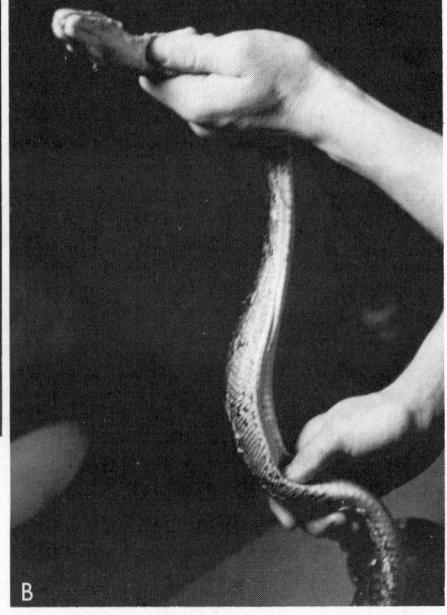

Figure 3. *A,* Tubing snake with oral anthelmintic. *B,* Expressing oral anthelmintic distally in snake to discourage regurgitation.

**Table 1.** *Anthelmintics for Exotic Pets and Zoo Animals (Continued)*

| ANIMAL GROUP | DRUG | SOURCE | DOSAGE |
|---|---|---|---|
| "Hooved Stock" | Thiabendazole (Equizole®) (Omnizole®) | Merck | *Zebra:* 50-100 mg./kg.<br>*Ruminants:* 50-100 mg./kg.<br>All low level feedings: 10 lb. Crumbles/100 lb. of feed for 1 to 3 days, 10 days off, then 1 lb. Crumbles/100 lb. of feed 10 days on, 10 days off, etc. |
| | Dichlorvos (Equigard®) (Atgard® V) | Shell | *Zebra:* 40 mg./kg.<br>*Ruminants:* 8-10 mg./kg. daily for 5 days, or 5 gm./500 kg. (2.5 mg./kg.) in a single dose—repeat in one week |
| | Levamisole | Cyanamid | As directed on package (3-4 mg./kg.) |
| | Mebendazole (Telmin®) | Pitman-Moore | 12 gm./250 kg. |
| Aves | Thiabendazole (Equizole®) | Merck | 250-500 mg./kg. single oral dose for large birds<br>0.125-0.25 mg./gm. for small (or aged) birds; can lower dosage and give low level 5 to 12 days |
| | Piperazine | Many | 200-500 mg./kg. single oral dose or 6-10 gm./gal. drinking water for 1 to 4 days<br>(0.3-0.5 mg./gm. single dose in small caged birds) |
| | Bunamidine hydrochloride (Scoloban®) | Cooper USA, Inc. | 20-40 mg./kg. |
| | Levamisole (Levasole®) | Cyanamid | 20 mg./kg. (or 0.5-1.0 gm./gal. drinking water for 2 days) |
| | Mebendazole (Telmin®) | Pitman-Moore | 20-40 mg./kg. for 3 to 5 days |
| Reptiles* | Thiabendazole (Equizole®) | Merck | 50 mg./kg. (hydroscopic—be sure to mix with enough water) |
| | Piperazine | Many | 50-80 mg./kg. |
| | Dichlorvos (Task®) | Shell | 12-16 mg./kg. for 2 doses<br>Contraindicated with kidney or liver damage or obstipation |
| | Bunamidine hydrochloride (Scoloban®) | Cooper USA, Inc. | 50 mg./kg. |
| | Levamisole (Ripercol®) | Cyanamid | 10-20 mg./kg. injected IM<br>EXPERIMENTAL—do not use in weak or debilitated reptiles |
| | Mebendazole (Telmin®) | Pitman-Moore | 20 mg./kg. daily for 2 to 4 daily doses |

*Vermifuges should be administered to chelonians at half the measured body weight to allow for the weight of the shell.

---

# AMPHIBIAN DISEASES*

G. E. COSGROVE, M.D.
*Oak Ridge, Tennessee*

Veterinarians may be confronted with sick or abnormal amphibians from several sources: Many are kept as pets or curiosities in aquaria or terraria; if they survive for a while, the owners may develop sufficient attachment to them to seek help when prob-

lems arise. Other animals may be noticed in the wild because of some unusual appear-

*By acceptance of this article, the publisher or recipient acknowledges the right of the U.S. Government to retain a nonexclusive, royalty-free license in and to any copyright covering the article.

ance or activity. Such sporadic encounters would be only a minor concern in normal veterinary practice. There are some situations, however, which would call for a veterinarian to practice extensive amphibian medicine. Most zoos have amphibian collections, some of which contain quite valuable specimens. Likewise, schools or laboratories often have colonies large and valuable enough to warrant some attempts at diagnosis or treatment when problems arise. A growing industry in certain parts of the country is "frog farming." Because of the large investment of capital and the intensive culture, and because the product is sold for food or to research institutions, the health of the animals is of prime importance. The amphibians raised usually are either urodeles—tail-bearing amphibians like salamanders, whose young usually resemble miniature adults—or anurans—tailless amphibians like frogs and toads, whose tadpole young do not resemble the adults at all.

Many types of problems occur, varying considerably in importance. The most common is the microbiologic complex called "red leg," which is a septicemic disease with a variety of generalized signs. Probably no other microbial problem is nearly so important. When red leg starts in grouped amphibians, a high mortality can be expected. Alterations in the environment of the captive animals can also be devastating. Heat, dehydration, fouling as a result of improper cleaning or feeding, entrance of toxicants such as chlorine or other chemicals into the water, etc., are causes of deaths. Simple inspection of the environment of the animals is often diagnostic. Starvation often occurs because the animals involved refuse to eat, slower or smaller individuals do not get their share or the diet is deficient in some way. Since amphibians pass through life stages, conditions tolerated in one stage may be suddenly or slowly lethal in another. Knowledge of the biology of the animal is essential when evaluating requirements for successful life. Anuran metamorphosis is an especially stressful time, and if conditions are suboptimal, mortality can be expected.

Of great importance in environmental causation of disease is the shipping of amphibians from supplier to user. If the animals survive this critical process, they should not be too rapidly introduced into the new and different habitat. Once safely in the colony, they are subject to damage if husbandry practices are too vigorous or prophylactic therapies are carried out without adequate pretesting for effects. Since the amphibian skin is always moist and readily crossed by many materials, special problems are created by tank additives.

Of little importance to the health of the colony, but extremely interesting to the observer, are the sporadic conditions encountered in individuals. These include various types of lumps or swellings which may occur in any organ or tissue. Some of these are neoplasms, although they are rare except for frog renal adenocarcinoma, which is virus-initiated and "epidemic" in certain frog populations. Cold-blooded tuberculosis in amphibians is transmissible but usually slowly progressive. Other granulomas are due to fungi or degenerating parasites. Parasites often occur in cysts or nodules in any tissue, and some congenital malformations are also nodular. A great variety of other disease problems occur in sporadic form.

Mild degrees of parasitism are ubiquitous in amphibians, but accompanying lesions are often nonexistent or mild—they are usually more of a curiosity than a colony health problem.

## TREATMENT

A visit to the habitat, with inspection for improper conditions and advice on correction of these, is important. Especially important aspects to observe include environmental temperatures, air humidity, soil substrate and acidity of a terrarium, water pH and oxygen of an aquarium or tank, associated plants and their health, illumination, crowding and food and feeding techniques.

If the amphibians are grouped, diseased individuals should be removed when noted and either quarantined or killed. Pathologic and microbiologic studies may reveal whether there is any danger of an epidemic.

Little information is available about treatment of amphibian disease with the exception of red leg, in which a variety of antibiotic and bacteriostatic regimens have been reported to be successful. These include penicillin, tetracycline* (Achro-

---

*See cautionary note regarding the use of tetracycline hydrochloride on page 776.

mycin®), nitrofurazone, gentamicin or other antibiotics added to the water, given by stomach tube or in food or injected. Increasing the salinity of the tank water up to but not exceeding 0.6 per cent is highly recommended for crowded lab tanks of certain species. Water circulation and filtration may physically remove potential pathogens. No matter what additive treatments are used, a test for toxicity should be made on an isolated individual before the whole tank is treated. Dosage experimentation is often necessary. When a pathogenic agent is isolated, sensitivity to various therapeutic agents should be tested if possible.

Subtoxic tank additives such as fungicides, parasiticides or chemicals successfully reduce surface fungal or ectoparasitic infestations. The principles are very similar to those routinely applied in fish aquaria, and many of the same substances are used, e.g., malachite green, methylene blue, very dilute potassium permanganate, potassium iodide, tincture of iodine, trypaflavine, etc. Visceral lesions of tuberculosis or fungal granulomas apparently have not been successfully treated by tank additives. Treating individual animals by feeding, tubing or injection might be successful, but the effort is often prohibitive. Possibly amphibians could be used as chemotherapeutic models in this way.

Little has been written about transmission of amphibian disease to man. The red leg pathogens are not usually human pathogens. Cold-blooded tuberculosis from fish has rarely occurred in the skin of people, so amphibian tuberculosis might behave likewise. Probably none of the parasites are transferrable except by direct consumption of raw amphibian flesh or use of flesh poultices, as practiced in certain parts of the world. The fungi that infect amphibians have not been incriminated as human pathogens.

More experimentation in the treatment of amphibian disease is certainly needed. Effective drugs should be found and tested to determine the best routes of administration and the tolerance levels of each. The possibility of treating a tankful of animals at once with an agent which can then cross the animals' skin barriers is unique to the care of amphibians. Microbiologic studies for identification of pathogens and necropsies for studying ramifications of the diseases in the tissues should be more widespread.

Amphibians could be used more exten-sively as comparative pathology teaching materials as they already are used in comparative anatomy, zoology-parasitology, etc. As a by-product of veterinary care of amphibians, some valuable specimens should be accumulated for teaching purposes, collections, registries of comparative pathology or tumors in lower animals as well as for use in consultation on amphibian disease. Photographs of lesions and sick amphibians would be useful additional resources for the veterinarian.

At present, consultation on amphibian disease is not easily obtainable. There are a few centers of amphibian research with disease orientation, and some pathology registries have amphibian experts.

## CENTERS FOR AMPHIBIAN DISEASE STUDY

Amphibian Facility
University of Michigan
Ann Arbor, Michigan 48106

Department of Microbiology
Aquatic Microbiology Section
Louisiana State University
Baton Rouge, Louisiana 70803

Ultrascience, Inc.
Skokie, Illinois 60076

Registry of Tumors of Lower Animals
U.S. Museum of Natural History
Smithsonian Institution
Washington, D.C. 20560

Registry of Comparative Pathology
Armed Forces Institute of Pathology
Washington, D.C. 20306

### SUGGESTED READING

Amphibians: Guidelines for the breeding, care, and management of laboratory animals. NRC, NAS-NAE, 1974, 153 pp.

Balls, M., and Clothier, R. M.: Spontaneous tumors in amphibia. A review. Oncology, 29:510-519, 1974.

Cosgrove, G. E., and Jared, D. W.: Diseases and parasites of *Xenopus*, the clawed toad. *In* Amborski, R. L., Hood, M. A., and Miller, R. R. (eds.): Gulf Coast Regional Symposium on Diseases of Aquatic Animals, 1974 Proceedings. Center for Wetlands Resources, Louisiana State University, Baton Rouge, 1974, pp. 225-242.

Dawe, C. J., and Harshbarger, J. C.: A symposium on neoplasia and related disorders of invertebrate and lower vertebrate animals. Natl. Cancer Inst. Monograph, Vol. 31, 1969, 772 pp.

Gibbs, E. L., Gibbs, T. J., and Van Dyck, P. C.: *Rana pipiens*: Health and disease. Lab. Animal Care, *16*:142-160, 1966.

Glorioso, J. C., Amborski, R. L., Amborski, G. F., and Culley, D. D.: Microbiological studies on septicemic bullfrogs (*Rana catesbeiana*). Am. J. Vet. Res., *35*:1241-1245, 1974.

Mizell, M. (ed.): Recent Results in Cancer Research: Biology of Amphibian Tumors. New York, Springer-Verlag, 1968, 484 pp.

Nace, G. W.: The amphibian facility of the University of Michigan. BioScience, *18*:767-775, 1968.

Nace, G. W., Waage, J. K., and Richards, C. M.: Sources of amphibians for research. BioScience, *21*:768-773, 1971.

Priddy, J. M., and Culley, D. D., Jr.: The frog culture industry, past and present. Proc. 25th Ann. Conf. Southeast. Assoc. Game and Fish Commission, 1971, pp. 597-601.

Reichenbach-Klinke, H., and Elkan, E.: The Principal Diseases of Lower Vertebrates. New York, Academic Press, 1965, 600 pp.

# GENERAL CONSIDERATIONS IN THE CARE OF CAPTIVE AMPHIBIANS

FREDRIC L. FRYE, D.V.M.
*Berkeley, California*

## INTRODUCTION

The Class Amphibia encompasses frogs, toads, salamanders (which include hellbenders, sirens, mudpuppies, newts, Congo eels, mole salamanders and lungless salamanders) and the lesser known caecilians, many of which are suited to captive husbandry and study by amateur herpetologists.

Amphibians are usually, but not always, four-legged animals that do not possess a scaly skin. Their skins secrete moist, often mucoid, substances elaborated from glands distributed over most body surfaces to help prevent them from drying out when they are not in contact with their usual watery or damp environment. Some frogs, toads and a few salamanders possess highly specialized skin glands that produce poisonous secretions which function as a defense against predators.

There are approximately 3500 different species of living amphibians known at this time which are assigned to three major orders:

1. Order Apoda (without legs)

These are slender, wormlike creatures called *caecilians*, who live most of the time entirely buried in forest litter. They are rarely encountered in exotic animal dealers' collections. Most are from tropical countries.

2. Order Caudata (with tails)

These are the tailed amphibians, commonly called salamanders. Salamanders usually have well-developed forelimbs and hindlimbs; sirens have only poorly developed forelimbs; and Congo eels have miniscule forelimbs and hindlimbs, which can be easily overlooked.

3. Order Anura (without tails)

This order includes frogs and toads. Both forelimbs and hindlimbs are present in adult animals. Herpetologists prefer to call all anurans "frogs," since the distinction between frogs and toads breaks down completely when they are studied on a worldwide basis. In the United States, however, it is a workable distinction: here, frogs are jumpers and have relatively smooth, moist skin, whereas toads are hoppers and have dry, warty skin.

Another characteristic of amphibians is their preference for far cooler environmental temperatures than those associated with most reptiles. Like reptiles, which they may superficially resemble, amphibians are *poikilothermic*—their body temperatures are largely dictated by the surrounding environmental temperature. In contrast, mammals and birds can and do regulate their body temperatures over a wide range of exterior temperatures.

Perhaps the greatest difference between reptiles and amphibians is that amphibians undergo a major *metamorphosis* during their early life. The eggs of frogs are laid in water, where they are fertilized, develop and hatch out as tadpoles or "pollywogs." As these tadpoles develop and grow larger, most of them grow legs: first the hindlegs and then the forelegs, and gradually the tail is resorbed and disappears. The larvae's gills, which exchange needed oxygen and carbon dioxide in the aquatic environment, disappear and are replaced with air-breathing lungs in most species. The larvae of salamanders are merely referred to as larvae. Lungless salamanders lay their eggs in damp places (under logs, etc.), never in water. Metamorphosis takes place in the egg, and at hatching, a miniature of the adult emerges.

Some species, such as mudpuppies and axolotls, develop lungs but retain gills throughout their lives; other species, such as lungless salamanders, perform their respiratory functions through transpiration and gas exchange across their skin.

During the time that frog and toad larvae live in their aquatic environment, their gastrointestinal system is best suited to digest algae and other plant life, whereas all salamander larvae eat simple water animals and, accidentally, decaying organic material. As metamorphosis progresses, the digestive system changes and matures, so that more complex animal material can be assimilated.

Some frogs and toads, such as the African clawed frog, are entirely aquatic and rarely, if ever, venture from their watery milieu.

## OBTAINING AMPHIBIANS

**Wild-Caught Amphibians.** Often, the woodlands surrounding a major urban center will yield a variety of amphibian species, and a careful search in streams and ponds or under rocks, fallen trees, or loose bark may turn up members of either the Order Anura or Caudata. Be sure to observe the local fish and game conservation regulations and take only one or two amphibians from a particular site—there is no excuse for greed.

When it is their turn to breed, many amphibians return to the exact geographic area where they were hatched and matured through their metamorphosis; if and when a decision is made to release wild-caught pets, an attempt should be made to do so in the exact spot where they were acquired.

Care should be taken to note the natural habitat from which the amphibian is taken, and the artificial habitat should reproduce it as much as possible. Pieces of tree bark, moss, soil, forest litter, etc., greatly enhance the microhabitat. A precaution: some vegetative matter will rot and release acids and other harmful substances in an aquarium.

Many newly caught animals, including amphibians, suffer some degree of shock from the stress imposed by the act and conditions of capture as well as by the immediate captivity. To lessen the untoward effects of this reaction, always try to handle the newly acquired animal as little and as gently as possible and provide some shelter in which it may seek privacy and darkness.

**Purchased or Traded Amphibians.** Exotic or foreign amphibians sometimes are found in pet shops or through trades with other collectors. There are many herpetologic societies whose memberships cooperate in developing husbandry, breeding and morphologic data; there are opportunities to trade with such informed persons.

Many amphibians purchased from commercial souces have been exposed to high population densities in communal cages or tanks, so that the attendant exposure to bacterial, fungal and/or parasitic disease organisms is greater than would be the case in the wild; therefore, strict quarantine for 4 to 6 weeks before introduction into the resident, conditioned population is recommended. These amphibians have been subjected to the multiple stresses of capture, shipment (perhaps several times), dietary changes and disease agents; as for wild-caught amphibians they should be treated very gently and handled only when absolutely necessary.

## HOUSING CONSIDERATIONS

Most amphibians reside in a moist, relatively cool environment and, depending on whether the specimen is terrestrial or aquatic, small terrarium or aquarium tanks can serve well as captive homes.

Amphibians should never be housed with

reptiles, birds or mammals. Large predatory amphibians should not be kept in the same enclosure with smaller, more delicate species. (Bullfrogs and giant salamanders are cannibalistic and will surprise the unwary amateur herpetologist with a steadily diminishing collection if this precaution is not heeded.)

If woodland species such as most toads, terrestrial frogs, tree frogs, salamanders or newts are to be kept satisfactorily as pets or scientific study animals, a well-planned terrarium setting should be set up and prepared *before* the animals are obtained. A suitable tank or cage large enough to allow free movement should be filled partially with slightly moistened sand, fine gravel, potting soil, humus, leaf mold, etc. Rocks, pieces of heavy *nonresinous* tree bark, moss and either natural or artificial plants may be used to create a natural setting pleasing to both the inhabitants and human observers.

Some amphibian species are only semiaquatic or semiterrestrial, and some provision must be made to afford not only bathing facilities but also an opportunity for the animal to "haul out" and leave the water entirely. A small pond or pool that can be removed or drained easily for routine cleaning without disturbing the entire habitat or its lodgers is ideal. A simple rock or float may be provided for the more aquatic setting, so that those specimens which leave their watery medium only occasionally may crawl out at will. When larvae complete their metamorphosis, breathing is accomplished more and more with the new lungs and less with the now-disappearing gills; at this point, a place to climb out becomes essential to survival.

## WATER TREATMENT

With the more aquatic species, a means must be found to help clean and purify the water medium between total volume changes. Aquarium filters often are quite suitable for this purpose if the volume is not too great, and a visit to a well-stocked aquarium shop or pet supply store to discuss the intended project with those familiar with the various pieces of filter equipment is a wise investment in time.

Snails, freshwater clams, crawfish and small catfish may also be employed as biologic filters, but often they end up on the menu of the amphibians housed with them.

Since chemicals have been added to render most municipal water supplies safe for human consumption, it is generally advisable to allow a quantity of this tap water to stand for a day or two in a jug or gallon pickle jar before use to help dissipate the dissolved chlorine. The water may also be brought to a boil to help hasten the removal of chlorine, but then it may take many hours before it will be cool enough to introduce into the tank. Dechlorinating drops and tablets are available from aquarium and pet shops. Distilled water is also quite suitable for immediate use.

Much of the waste material excreted by amphibians is rich in nitrogen-containing compounds, particularly ammonia. Great care must be taken to insure that an adequate rate of flushing or exchange of water is provided to prevent an accumulation of these compounds, many of which may reach levels toxic to captive amphibians. Dangerously large amounts of ammonia may also be produced by bacterial action upon nitrogen-rich wastes. Obviously, great attention must be paid to hygiene if successful husbandry is to be achieved.

Aquatic salamanders and frogs shed their skins frequently, and this shed skin may block a filtering system unless it is removed with small forceps.

When changing the water in the tanks, be sure to dispose of the waste water in a toilet or other waste-water system. Do not use the kitchen sink or any other area where food is prepared, because such waste water is absolutely teeming with bacteria.

Many woodland amphibians imbibe moisture directly through their skins, and unless direct access to a pool or pond is available, a sprinkle or shower once a day is imperative. A spray bottle is ideal for delivering such a shower; this water also must not contain toxic levels of chlorine.

Besides the obvious requirements of clean water, shelter, food, temperature and light, gill-breathing species of amphibians also must have an adequate supply of oxygen-rich water in which to swim in order to thrive. Normally, if there is sufficient oxygen to support living fishes, it should be adequate for a small number of gill-breathing amphibians. A professional aquarist or dealer can help in the selection of suitable aquarium plants and/or air pumps and airstones.

**pH Maintenance.**    A pH range of 6.5 to 8.5 has been found to be ideally suited to most aquatic amphibians. Generally, an attempt to maintain the pH at the lower end of this range should be made.

The acidity or alkalinity of a particular water sample can be ascertained easily with test paper strips, which give a colorimetric value depending upon the hydrogen-ion concentration of the sample. More accurate results may be obtained with an electronic pH meter.

Raising or lowering the pH value of a water sample can be accomplished safely by adding sodium hydroxide or calcium sulfate, respectively. Acetic acid also can be used to lower the pH of particularly alkaline water further and perhaps, in such cases, it would be more prudent to use distilled water as a starting point.

**Temperature Requirements.** Most authorities have recommended a room and water temperature of 65° to 68° F. (18° to 20° C.). For some larvae, a temperature of 68° to 72° F. (20° to 22° C.) is advised. For actively feeding frogs from the more temperate climates, a room and water temperature of 72° to 78° F. (22° to 25° C.) is more appropriate, while tropical species would find 78° to 86° F. (26° to 30° C.) more to their liking. Some of the aquatic salamanders are more comfortable in water which is cooled to 45° to 55° F. (7° to 12° C.).

**Light Requirements.** While specific data on photoperiod or light-dark cycles are not available for all species of amphibians, a general rule can be stated: in those equatorial species from the tropics, an equal day/night cycle of about 12 hours each is desirable; whereas for the more temperate zone-dwelling species, a photoperiod of about 14 to 16 hours of light to 8 to 10 hours of dark may be more appropriate. Since the seasons change, some variation in amount of light to darkness is desirable. At no time, however, should a constantly light environment be provided, since this imposes a severe stress upon captive animals.

## FEEDING

Some examples of correct nutrition follow.

**Most Toad and Frog Larvae.** These may be fed romaine lettuce, ground rabbit or guinea pig pellets, small pieces of kibbled dog food, finely minced hard-boiled egg yolk, brewers' yeast, raw beef and beef liver. Great care must be exercised to pre-vent accumulation of uneaten food which would spoil and quickly foul the water. The ground rabbit or guinea pig pellets as a main food source plus small amounts of kibbled dog food and supplemental feeding of egg yolk or meat once or twice weekly appear both to be nutritionally sound and to allow water quality to be maintained most easily. Larvae should be fed daily to thrice weekly, depending upon age and size (young ones being fed more often).

**Clawed Frog (*Xenopus*) Larvae.** The recommended diet for these interesting creatures is finely ground, dried green peas or unseasoned, dried split-pea soup base, which has the consistency of flour; it should be mixed with water to produce a slurry before being fed to the larvae. Later, as the larvae grow larger, finely ground or crushed rabbit or guinea pig pellets are substituted for the dried peas. As the larvae begin to form rear limbs, finely ground lean beef and powdered milk (mixed together) should be added to their diet. *Tubifex* worms and *Daphnia* may also be fed.

**Axolotls, Mudpuppies and Other Salamander Larvae.** These youngsters can be fed brine shrimp, *Tubifex* worms and *Daphnia*. As growth progresses, earthworms, beef heart and raw beef liver cut into thin strips will be taken. Later, earthworms, corn grubs, etc., can be fed three to four times weekly. Commercial Trout Chow® (Purina), a well-balanced ration containing required vitamins and minerals and rich in protein, also has been used successfully as a feed for these animals.

**Most Adult Frogs and Toads.** With few exceptions, the adults of most anuran species can be fed earthworms, corn grubs, crickets and sow bugs. For tree frogs, which usually are somewhat smaller than most species of terrestrial frogs and toads, genetically wingless fruit flies are very useful and can be obtained from most genetics departments of a university or college; they can be bred easily in small culture bottles and have the decided advantage of being flightless. Baby crickets also are an excellent diet for smaller frog and toad species. It must be remembered that most terrestrial frogs and toads will respond only to *moving* bait.

**Adult Clawed Frogs.** Perhaps the easiest to feed of the anurans, these aquatic frogs commonly are fed earthworms, raw beef, beef heart, trout chow and small live fish. If beef, heart or raw liver is fed exclusively, a powdered vitamin-mineral supplement should be mixed with the above meats to prevent deficiencies. The natural diet of earthworms is recommended because it is the most simple and well balanced and causes the fewest management problems relating to water fouling.

**Adult Salamanders.** Earthworms, corn grubs and crickets provide a stable, well-balanced diet with minimal effort for adult salamanders.

**Caecilians.** These secretive, legless creatures feed well on earthworms and small grubs.

*SPECIAL NOTE:* If commercial trout chow is to be fed, there are some special considerations concerning its use. If any of the pellets remain uneaten, they will disintegrate and produce water fouling. This tendency can be lessened in two ways: (1) feed only enough chow at one time so that surplus material is not left behind and (2) mix a binder, such as unflavored gelatin or agar, in with the pellets. This is best accomplished by mixing the gelatin or agar according to the instructions on the package, stirring in the trout chow and, after the gelatin or agar-chow mix sets thoroughly, cutting it into suitable pieces. The recipe is

2 cups trout chow
1 to 2 packages unflavored gelatin
Mix per instructions on package of
gelatin.

High-protein baby cereal, in varying proportions, may be added. In this form, it may be fed as needed, and the unused portion can be stored for future use in the refrigerator for about two weeks. It may be stored in a frozen state for several months and thawed before feeding.

## DISEASES

While it is beyond the scope of this article to discuss in depth the diagnosis and treatment of all the major diseases affecting captive amphibians, it would be appropriate to cover briefly the most common medical problems encountered in these animals.

### STARVATION AND DEHYDRATION

Unfortunately, all too frequently, starvation and dehydration are the result of ignorance regarding general care and feeding of a particular species. Obviously, the attempted feeding of a totally inappropriate food item to an animal who continually refuses to eat will result in disaster for the animal and disappointment for the owner. The deprivation of an adequate water supply in a suitable delivery system for terrestrial species eventually will cause death from the effects of dehydration and kidney failure.

### VITAMIN-MINERAL IMBALANCES AND DEFICIENCIES

Vitamin-mineral imbalances and deficiencies usually are induced by the feeding of an artificial diet. For instance, the feeding of raw beef or heart without supplemental provision of a calcium-vitamin $D_3$ source will result in developmental bone diseases such as rickets and/or fibrous osteodystrophy. The exclusive feeding of raw liver will produce multiple vitamin and mineral imbalances.

The use of natural food items such as earthworms, corn grubs, crickets, *Tubifex* worms and fruit flies will aid greatly in the *prevention* of such diet-induced problems.

### VIRAL, BACTERIAL, FUNGAL, PROTOZOAN AND METAZOAN PARASITIC INFECTIONS AND INFESTATIONS

Viral, bacterial, fungal, protozoan and metazoan parasitic infections and infestations have been described in captive amphibians. Many can be traced back to overcrowded conditions and poor sanitation. Often a frog, toad or salamander may not appear to be "sick" but rather may exhibit only subtle signs, consisting of appetite loss, sluggishness or abdominal distention or bloating, which could easily be overlooked or mistaken for something else.

**Tetracycline hydrochloride is not a** *"cure-all"!* There is a widely held belief that tetracycline hydrochloride may be added to the water of aquatic amphibians as a means of treating bacterial diseases, especially "red leg." Such injudicious use of this drug is likely to produce more harm than good, since it is now well known that tetracycline will induce severe toxic skin reactions when present in significant concentrations in amphibians' water. Also, the amount that could possibly be absorbed through the intact skin of these animals would be totally inadequate to serve as an effective antibiotic.

The *only* effective means of administering tetracycline to amphibians is by a carefully inserted gastric tube at a dosage of 5 mg. tetracycline/30 gm. body weight of the amphibian. This dosage should be repeated twice daily for about one week. A prepared therapeutic concentration yielding 25 mg. tetracycline/ml. has been suggested to limit the volume required to treat some amphibians properly.

Because of the delicate and highly absorptive nature of amphibian skin, the use of topical antiseptics, antifungal agents, etc., may be of limited usefulness.

## INJURIES

Injuries are seen occasionally, especially in populations in which the more aggressive frog, toad and salamander species are housed with smaller, less aggressive members of their own kind. Overcrowding also may stimulate antisocial behavior, resulting in traumatic injuries. Rivalry over food, shelter or sexual partners may result in fights and/or attempted cannibalism. The appearance of abrasions, lacerations or lost digits or entire limbs is ample evidence that some drastic housing changes must be made.

## THERMAL SHOCK

Thermal shock is seen when an amphibian is allowed to become either overheated or suddenly chilled, and both causes can be eliminated by careful attention to the habitat needs of the animals and *gradual* changes to cooler water. If ice is to be used to help cool the aquatic environment, be certain that it is made from chlorine-free water.

## BREEDING AND REPRODUCTION

Breeding and reproduction of amphibians could fill an entire volume of a textbook. Many amateur herpetologists have been successful not only in rearing amphibians from fertilized eggs found in the wild, but also in bringing about captive mating, ovulation, fertilization and metamorphosis in selected individuals.

Before captive breeding can be accomplished successfully, nutrition and general husbandry must be near optimum. The selected reading list at the end of this article provides specific references for consultation.

## SUGGESTED READING

Bardach, J. E., Ryther, J. H., and McLearney, W. O.: Aquaculture. New York, Wiley-Interscience, 1972, 868 pp.

Bennett, G. W.: Management of Artificial Lakes and Ponds. New York, Reinhold, 1962, 283 pp.

Bishop, S. C.: Handbook of Salamanders. The Salamanders of the United States, of Canada, and of Lower California. Ithaca, New York, Comstock Publishing Co., Inc., 1947, 555 pp.

Branch, H. E.: A Laboratory Manual of *Cryptobranchus alleganiensis* Daudin. New York, Vantage Press, 1959, 79 pp., 5 plates.

Brown, A. L.: The African Clawed Toad. London, Butterworth, 1970, 120 pp.

Buterenbrood, E. L.: Newts and Salamanders (Ch. 52, pp. 867-892). *In* UFAW Handbook on the Care and Management of Laboratory Animals. 3rd ed. London, Livingston, 1966.

Cairns, A. M., Bock, J. W., and Bock, F. G.: Leopard frogs raised in partially controlled conditions. Nature, *213*:191-193, 1967.

Cochran, D. M.: Living Amphibians of the World. Garden City, New York, Doubleday Co., 1961, 199 pp.

Committee on Animal Nutrition, National Research Council: No. 10: Nutrient Requirements of Laboratory Animals. 2nd ed. National Academy of Sciences, Washington, D.C., 1972, 117 pp.

Conant, R.: A Field Guide to Reptiles and Amphibians of Eastern North America. Boston, Houghton-Mifflin Co., 1958, 366 pp.

Cosgrove, G. E.: Amphibian Diseases. *In* Kirk, R. W. (ed.): Current Veterinary Therapy VI. Philadelphia, W. B. Saunders Co., 1977.

Cullum, L., and Justus, J. T.: Housing for aquatic animals. Lab. Anim. Sci., *23*:126-129, 1973.

Frazer, J. F. D.: Frogs and Toads. (Ch. 51, pp. 853-866). *In* UFAW Handbook on the Care and Management of Laboratory Animals. 3rd ed. London, Livingston, 1966.

Frye, F. L.: Husbandry, Medicine and Surgery in Captive Reptiles. Bonner Springs, Kansas, VM Publishing, Inc., 1973, 140 pp.

Gibbs, E. L.: An effective treatment for red-leg disease in *Rana pipiens*. Lab. Anim. Care, *13*:781-783, 1963.

Goin, C. J., and Goin, O. B.: Introduction to Herpetology. 2nd ed. San Francisco, W. H. Freeman, 1971, 356 pp.

Gurdon, J. B.: African clawed frogs. *In* Wilt, F. H., and Wessells, N. K. (eds.): Methods in Developmental Biology. New York, Thomas Y. Crowell Co., 1967, pp. 75-84.

Justus, J. T., and Cullum, L.: A new method of housing axolotls and other aquatic amphibians. Lab. Anim. Sci., *21*:110-111, 1971.

Mertens, R.: The World of Amphibians and Reptiles. New York, McGraw-Hill Book Co., Inc., 1960, 207 pp.

National Academy of Sciences: Amphibians. Guidelines for the Breeding, Care, and Management of Laboratory Animals. Printing and Publishing Office, National Academy of Sciences, Washington, D.C., 1974, 153 pp.

Nickerson, M. A., and Mays, C. E.: The Hellbenders: North American "Giant Salamanders." Publications in Biology and Geology (No. 1), Milwaukee Public Museum, 1973, 106 pp.

Oliver, J. A.: The Natural History of North American Amphibians and Reptiles. Princeton, New Jersey, D. Van Nostrand Co., Inc., 1955, 359 pp.

Porter, K. R.: Herpetology. Philadelphia, W. B. Saunders Co., 1972, 524 pp.

Reichenbach-Klinke, H., and Elkan, E.: The Principal Disease of Lower Vertebrates. New York, Academic Press, 1965, 600 pp.

Salthe, S. N.: The egg capsules in the amphibia. J. Morphology, 113:161-171, 1963.

Savage, R. M.: The Ecology and Life History of the Common Frog. London, Sir Isaac Pitman & Sons, Ltd., 1961, 221 pp.

Stebbins, R. C.: A Field Guide to Western Reptiles and Amphibians. Boston, Houghton-Mifflin Co., 1966, 277 pp.

Witschi, E.: Studies on sex differentiation and sex determination in amphibians. J. Esp. Zool., 56:149-165, 1930.

---

# MANAGEMENT AND NUTRITIONAL PROBLEMS IN CAPTIVE REPTILES

JOEL D. WALLACH, D.V.M.
*Douglasville, Georgia*

The demise and disappearance of the prehistoric terrestrial reptiles can be traced to a single factor—a dramatic change in the earth's environment. Infectious diseases, parasites and predation were tolerated by the great populations of giant poikilotherms until just before the Ice Age, when the universal crisis came. A great chill came over the earth, and although vegetation and prey animals were still found in abundance, only the homeotherms (mammals and birds) could utilize these raw materials and convert them into the basic chemicals of life.

Hypothetical necropsy records of the time would have listed a variety of "descriptive" causes of death, for example:

1. Fatty liver
2. Parasitism—*Entamoeba invadens*
3. Parasitism—oxyuriasis
4. Gastric impaction
5. Exhaustion—mired in tar pit

Although there appears to be a great variety of causes of death for the dinosaur, there was a common denominator—herpatecology, or the change in environmental dynamics. For example, a fatty liver can result from the cessation of cellular metabolism. As for parasitism, a few thousand one-celled animals would hardly seem ambitious enough to tackle healthy 50-ton reptiles with whom they had been living in harmony for millions of years; pinworms have caused a lot of itchy tails but can hardly be blamed for the disappearance of these beasts. Gastric impaction of materials normally ingested would seem unlikely as the cause of death for a healthy adult dinosaur. Lastly, why did the great poikilotherms huddle around the tar pits only to push several of their comrades into the mire to die of exhaustion? The common denominator—lack of environmental heat.

To determine whether or not our modern scientific community has advanced in the field of reptilian management since one million B.C., the data collection of zoos, its interpretation and resulting actions were examined.

In the husbandry section of the *International Zoo Yearbook* (Volume 12) it was reported that "to many zoos the mortality rate is synonymous with the number of animals brought to post-mortem. The remaining zoos answering the survey (56.8%), regardless of animal population, indicated that reptiles dying in the collection were omitted from post-mortem examination." An article in *The American Journal of Veterinary Research* stated that 42 per cent of the snakes lost at a large public institution were not traceable or not necropsied.

A recent article in *The American Journal of Veterinary Research* described an outbreak of entamebiasis in which 51 species of reptiles were affected. The reptiles were housed under a variety of sophisticated caging systems complete with filters and treated water; however, the water reservoir was shared by snakes, turtles and crocodilians. The article stated "that cultures of *Entamoeba invadens* grown at 35° C. can still infect and be pathogenic in snakes, provided that the host is kept at 26° C., but such cultures are not infective if the snakes are kept at 35° C. Environmental temperature of the snake host is, in part, a method of controlling the infection. At high temperatures (35° to 37° C.) the infection dies out and at low temperatures (13° to 14° C.) pathogenicity is absent."

The 1967 records of the U.S. Fish and Wildlife Service show that animal dealers imported 27,759,332 fish, 405,134 reptiles, 203,189 birds, 137,697 amphibians and 74,304 mammals into the United States for the exotic pet trade and laboratory use. The majority of those imports will have died as a result of a lack of understanding of their basic needs. Congressional acts have been conceived and voted into law to protect mammals and birds but only the rarest of reptiles find federal protection. State laws are on the books to protect certain local species but enforcement is difficut.

Despite a potential life span of 10 to 100 years, the captive reptiles' average life as a pet or as a zoologic exhibit is less than 2 years. Although reptiles may survive in captivity for up to 2 years when kept under suboptimal conditions, relying on body stores of energy and essential nutrients, the reptiles eventually succumb to secondary infections or nutritional diseases after such stores are depleted.

Investigation into the causes of early deaths of reptiles shows them to result from a poor understanding of reptilian physiology or gross nutritional abuse. In contrast, reptiles that are well cared for, with husbandry programs designed for their unique physiologic processes, thrive throughout their expected life span and reproduce in captivity.

## TEMPERATURE

Reptiles as a group possess more crude homeostatic mechanisms than do birds or mammals. Because reptiles are less dependent on strict homeostasis than mammals and birds, they are more tolerant of short-term changes in their internal environment. Feral reptiles withstand extended unfavorable environmental conditions by reducing their metabolic rate to almost zero and becoming torpid.

Reptiles have a relatively high ratio of surface area to body volume because of small size and, as a result, absorb or lose internal heat rapidly in response to fluctuations in environmental temperatures. The wide variations in the internal temperatures of reptiles are thought to result from their inability to maintain a high metabolic rate. A comparison of the metabolic rate of two desert rodents and a desert iguana of comparable size at an environmental temperature of 37° C. indicated that the lizard's metabolism was only one seventh that of the mammals.

A monitoring organ thought to be located in the hypothalamus of reptiles registers temperature alterations of the blood. This hypothalamic "system" appears to aid in regulation of body temperature by initiating physiologic changes (variations in skin pigmentation in lizards and changes in cardiovascular circulatory patterns in all reptiles) that help restore the animal's temperature to its original level.

The term "preferred optimal (PO) body temperatures" reflects temperatures to which a particular species is physiologically adapted (Table 1). The PO temperatures for most reptiles fall between 20° and 39.5° C. (68.0° to 103.1° F.). The notable exception is the tuatara from New Zealand, which has a PO requirement of 12.8° to 21.0° C. (55° to 70° F.). Rapid acclimation to captivity will be ensured by placing a freshly captured reptile in the specific PO temperature range required by that species; this will ensure optimal metabolic rates.

Only limited metabolic compensations are made by reptiles maintained at temperatures lower than the PO. The reptile may live for a considerable length of time (1 to 2 years) without readily apparent ill effects.

*Table 1.   Cloacal Temperatures of Reptiles*

| SPECIES | RANGE OF ACTIVE REPTILES | PREFERRED OPTIMAL BODY TEMPERATURE | CRITICAL HIGH |
|---|---|---|---|
| American alligator | 26.0–37.0° C. (78.0–98.0° F.) | 32.0–35.0° C. (89.6–95.0° F.) | 38.0–39.0° C. (100.4–102.2° F.) |
| Boa | — | 26.0–34.0° C. (78.0–93.7° F.) | — |
| Racer | — | 24.8–36.0° C. (76.0–96.8° F.) | 42.4° C. (108.0° F.) |
| Gopher snake | 16.0–34.6° C. (60.8–94.0° F.) | 22.0–31.0° C. (71.6–87.8° F.) | 40.5° C. (104.9° F.) |
| Garter snake | 16.0–35.0° C. (60.8–95.0° F.) | 20.0–35.0° C. (68.0–95.0° F.) | 38.5–41.0° C. (101.3–105.0° F.) |
| American chameleon | — | 22.6–30.4° C. (72.3–86.9° F.) | 41.8° C. (107.0° F.) |
| Green iguana | 26.7–42.4° C. (79.7–108.5° F.) | 29.5–39.5° C. (85.1–103.1° F.) | 46.1° C. (114.8° F.) |
| Five-lined skink | 13.5–37.0° C. (56.3–98.6° F.) | 28.0–36.0° C. (82.4–96.8° F.) | 41.0° C. (105.8° F.) |
| Painted turtle | 8.0–30.2° C. (46.4–86.0° F.) | — | 39.0–41.0° C. (102.2–105.8° F.) |
| Desert tortoise | 19.0–37.8° C. (66.2–100.4° F.) | 26.7–29.4° C. (80.6–85.1° F.) | 39.5–43.0° C. (103.1–109.0° F.) |

Reptiles may be active (Table 1) and even eat at temperatures considerably lower than the PO temperature; however, it is generally agreed that they should be exposed to PO temperatures for at least part of the day, so that physiologic processes such as digestion, defecation and reproduction can be completed. Failure to provide adequate PO temperature permits the decomposition of food in the alimentary canal when there is insufficient normal enzymatic activity. It has been observed that some species of geckos have a higher PO temperature in captivity than can possibly be attained in the natural state. In such cases it is recommended that cage temperatures similar to those reported in the natural habitat be used.

Although the PO temperature is required, it has been dramatically demonstrated that exposure time to such temperatures must be limited, inasmuch as margins of safety regarding excessive heat are narrow. The upper limit of the PO body temperatures may be only a few degrees below the critical high (lethal) temperature (Table 1). In the wild state, reptiles voluntarily limit such exposure.

Experimental groups of *Sceloporus* lizards were subjected to temperatures of 12°, 25° and 35° C. for 2 weeks, after which they were tested for thermal preference in a thermal gradient. Those lizards conditioned to environments of 12° and 25° C. preferred their appropriate temperatures, whereas the group acclimated to 35° C. constantly chose lower temperatures. The mean activity temperature of this species in the wild is 35° C. Such evidence tends to support the belief that a behavioral mechanism is used to limit the period of exposure to PO temperatures.

One investigator subjected *Sceloporus* lizards to PO temperature for 13 weeks. This resulted in the death of many of the lizards and functional thyroid hypertrophy in the survivors. A second experiment demonstrated that lizards exposed to continuous temperatures only 1 to 3 degrees above the PO range developed anorexia and atrophy of skeletal muscle and showed inhibited spermatogenesis. Iguanids that were continuously exposed to the PO temperature developed similar clinical signs; these signs failed to appear in another group for which the temperature was allowed to drop at night.

Earless lizards are capable of maintaining a daytime body temperature of 38.5° C., with fluctuations of only 3 degrees despite radical changes in the surrounding air temperature. Such efficiency is not entirely physiologic in nature but in the main is behavioral. Behavioral mechanisms of temperature regulation are most important for those species that live in environments that have a wide diurnal variation in temperature (e.g., the desert).

Basking (exposing the body to the sun) is the usual method of facilitating absorption of radiant heat. Reptiles are very efficient at basking. They align their bodies perpendicular to the rays of the sun. Lizards and tortoises commonly use sloping surfaces, rocks or other objects to tilt against so as to facilitate such positioning. Some species prefer to climb high onto plants to bask, whereas others press themselves against a warm substrate. By drawing the rib cage forward and outward, snakes and lizards are able to flatten their bodies and increase the surface area exposed to the source of radiant heat. Small species heat up very rapidly, whereas larger forms require some time to increase their body temperatures. Observations on a 5-foot-long (1.5 m.) alligator showed that it required 7.5 minutes of basking time to increase its temperature 2° C.

Reptiles can be positioned in a display that provides hot spots, with incandescent spotlights focused on desired locations. Heat coils in the cage floor should occupy only a portion of a cage and are definitely contraindicated for species that burrow in the substrate to escape the sun's heat or for those that do not manifest heat-avoidance behavior (e.g., rain forest dwellers). When a display contains many species with varying PO temperature requirements, temperature gradients in the environment are essential.

The reptilian skin is thought to be cool to the touch from evaporation of small amounts of water vapor, but the skin is devoid of sweat glands and is, therefore, an inefficient cooling mechanism. Reptiles in general cool themselves by altering body posture, panting, burrowing or entering the water. They can make themselves slimmer and align themselves parallel to the rays of the sun, or they may stand up to lift their ventral surface from any hot substrate. Some species scrape away any hot substrate immediately beneath themselves and lie on relatively cool, freshly exposed sand. Panting occurs in desert iguanas and collared lizards when their body temperatures reach 43° C.

Retreats should be provided if the heat source of an aquarium or cage cannot be controlled readily and if there is likelihood of excessive heat accumulation. Psychologically acceptable cool retreats (e.g., broken pottery, tree bark, rock or box shelters) or thermal gradients are used voluntarily and should be provided for most species. Exceptions are the tropical forest species that do not normally manifest heat-avoidance behavior.

## HUMIDITY

Chelonians (tortoises and turtles) and snakes drink by dipping their snouts in a water source and take in water by suction. By contrast, most lizards do not drink from dishes or bodies of water but drink from water droplets by lapping them with the tongue. In nature, dew makes up their principal water source. *Anolis* lizards (American chameleons) will not drink from a pan, so cages should be sprayed daily to provide water droplets for drinking.

Water makes up 70 per cent of the reptilian body, compared with approximately 60 per cent in man. Fresh-water reptiles contain 73 per cent water and marine forms contain 65 per cent. Reptiles conserve considerable amounts of body water by utilizing the microenvironments of a burrow. Use of metabolic water by reptiles is questionable because increased oxygen requirements resulting from beta oxidation cause heavy loss of water via panting.

Reptilian kidneys are elongated paired organs of up to 15 per cent of body length. They are located in the dorsum of the abdominal cavity, and in snakes the right kidney is usually located slightly more cranial than the left. The kidneys are smooth organs in lizards and are heavily lobulated in chelonians, snakes and alligators. A urinary bladder is present in some species of lizards and is best developed in chelonians.

Terrestrial chelonians, all lizards and snakes excrete uric acid as the greater part of their nitrogenous wastes. Uric acid requires relatively large amounts of water to stay in solution and is carried by the blood from the liver (the site of production) to the glomeruli and the lining of the renal tubules (90 percent by the latter route in iguanids), where it is excreted. Water is resorbed by the renal tubules and cloaca. The concentrated uric acid in the collecting ducts precipitates out of solution as a chalky white, crystalline mass with a low water content.

Captive reptiles do well under conditions of varying relative humidity. Relative humidity within the human comfort range, approximately 33 to 60 per cent, appears to be adequate for most reptiles. Clinical signs resulting from excessively low relative humidity include improper and incomplete ecdysis (shedding of skin). The reptile often will manage to complete ecdysis without assistance if a water dish of sufficient size is provided to allow total immersion. If this does not occur, the reptile may be placed in an appropriate-sized jar or 20-gallon can half-filled with water. The unshed tags of skin may then be gently removed after the snake has been "soaked" for several hours. Reptiles kept in very dry facilities (e.g., heated buildings) should be lightly sprayed daily with a fine water mist to prevent excessive drying.

Desiccation and "renal constipation" are more severe manifestations of dehydration and usually result in death of the specimen. Normal urine contains a large amount of urates and uric acid, which precipitate out of solution in the renal tubules just prior to death of a reptile. This results in a mottled yellow to peach-colored appearance of the kidneys. Microscopic examination of formalin-fixed renal specimens following embedding and staining will reveal little in the way of pathologic changes other than postmortem degeneration. The embedding process places the urates and uric acid back into solution, thus differentiating the lesions from true visceral gout, which produces classic microscopic tophi.

Excessive humidity can also be detrimental. When peat moss or other absorbent substrates are used, they collect moisture and act as an excellent culture medium for bacterial production. Blister disease is a common finding in snakes kept in facilities that are chronically damp, and it may be observed even in aquatic forms. Clinical signs of blister disease include the appearance of large fluid-filled vesicles between the layers of skin. In uncomplicated cases the fluid is clear and viscid. The lesions, however, often become secondarily infected and fill with caseous exudate. Treatment includes drainage of the lesion, after which it is flushed with a surgical disinfectant. Antibiotics should be administered parenterally in secondarily infected cases.

## LIGHT

Light and temperature requirements of reptiles are interrelated. One investigator has found that seasonal gonadal development in the *Anolis* lizard can be stimulated only when long photoperiods are accompanied by PO temperatures. It is generally agreed that the daily photoperiod should vary during the year so as to stimulate endocrine systems (e.g., thyroidal and gonadal activity).

Feeding activity of reptiles is directly affected by light and temperature. If PO temperatures are provided but subminimal light is available, feeding may be delayed in a freshly caught reptile for up to ½ to 2 years. Feeding may never occur if proper light is not provided, and the reptile will eventually die of caloric exhaustion or from a secondary infectious disease.

Placing reluctant feeders previously exposed only to incandescent light under a wide-spectrum artificial light will usually stimulate feeding within a few days. It is recommended that commercially available wide-spectrum light tubes be used as the basic light source. Incandescent spotlights can be used in the cage to provide hot spots for basking sites.

## POPULATION DYNAMICS

Snakes, crocodilians, lizards and chelonians are commonly housed together in displays for purposes of showmanship and convenience of maintenance. In such facilities there are invariably violent interactions that result in severe trauma or the death of individual specimens. Care must be taken, especially when feeding such groups. A feeding frenzy develops, and formerly peaceful cagemates injure each other as a result of their voraciousness. Crocodilians severely lacerate or crush chelonians while snatching away particles of food. Often two snakes will seize the same prey animal with the final result that one snake will ingest the other along with the prey. Both snakes may die of suffocation if they are of equal size. Venomous snakes strike violently at each other, and although they are immune to the venom of their own species, they can inflict deep puncture wounds.

Generalized subcutaneous edema may appear in iguanids and true chameleons kept under conditions of high population densities. Reduction of animal numbers in the cage usually produces a spontaneous regression of the clinical signs.

Hypoglycemic shock has been reported in crocodilians subjected to the stresses of high population densities. Restraint or chronic social pressures produced by high population densities and competition for food result in low liver glycogen content in the affected animal. Repeated adrenergic stimulation has a glycogenolytic effect on the hepatic and skeletal muscle glycogen stores of the alligator.

Hypoglycemic shock is characterized by mydriasis, tremors, loss of the righting reflex and reduction of the metabolic rate. It has been reported in several species of crocodilians, including the American alligator, false gavial and caiman. Animals from 18 inches to 5 feet in length were most often affected. The earliest sign, pupillary mydriasis, usually appears following the addition of a new individual to a group. This subtle sign may last several weeks. The mydriasis may spontaneously disappear if the animal adjusts. Continued agitation will cause the disease to progress to opisthotonos and eventually to a complete state of catatonia, whereupon the animal may drown. Determination of blood glucose content at the advanced stage will reveal concentrations less than 5 mg./100 ml. of plasma.

Alligators normally display a winter physiologic hypoglycemia in both the wild and captive state (the lowest value, 50 mg./100 ml., occurs in October; the high value, 100 mg./100 ml., occurs in July or August). Normally, this fluctuation does not have any adverse effect, however, if there is a concurrent adrenergic response; the resulting epinephrine appears to deplete the already low glycogen stores and precipitates hypoglycemic shock. The clinical signs are reproduced readily in alligators by administering 1000 units/kg. of body weight of regular insulin.

Treatment of hypoglycemic shock includes relief of any population pressures and oral (by means of stomach tube) or parenteral administration of glucose at the rate of 3 gm./kg. body weight.

## CAGE SUBSTRATES

Reptiles feeding on live prey should not be fed on tanbark or other fibrous substrates. Pursuit of the prey by the reptile through the coarse material often results in plant awns or fibers becoming embedded in the soft tissues of the mouth or head. Such injuries initially go unnoticed but eventually result in the production of exuberant foreign body granulomas. It is recommended that such reptiles be housed on pea gravel, artificial grass or brown paper.

If absorbent substrates such as peat moss are used, they should be changed often so as to prevent development of bacterial flora and excessive humidity.

Rocks or branches should be available to all snakes as aids to ecdysis. Arboreal reptiles should have limbs available as perches for their primary substrate. Without such psychologic props, the reptile may fail to adjust to captivity despite the availability of proper temperature, humidity and light spectrum.

## FEEDING AND NUTRITIONAL DISEASES

Most modern reptiles are carnivorous to some extent, with the exception of a few highly specialized herbivores (large tortoises and iguanid lizards). In general, all reptiles are carnivorous in their immature stages, and those that become herbivorous do so only as they become mature (Table 2).

The stomachs of reptiles are, in general, simple structures. In snakes, the stomach is a long fusiform organ; in chelonians and most lizards, the stomach is a saclike dilatation of the anterior alimentary canal. Crocodilians have two distinct chambers: the anterior one (gizzard) is thick-walled and often contains stones thought to aid in physical digestion of food; the posterior chamber (pyloric region) is thin-walled. The gastric glands produce hydrochloric acid and pepsin or its precursors. Both products are thought to be produced by a single cell form in contrast to the more specialized gastric cells found in mammals.

**Table 2.** *Feeding Preferences of Reptiles*

| SPECIES | IMMATURE | ADULT |
|---|---|---|
| Snakes | Worms, arthropods, amphibians | Birds, mammals, eggs, reptiles, fish, amphibians |
| Chelonians | Arthropods, worms | Worms, mollusca, arthropods, fish, tadpoles, birds, mammals, plants |
| Crocodilians | Arthropods, worms, amphibians | Fish, amphibians, mammals, birds |
| Lizards | Arthropods, worms | Arthropods, amphibians, reptiles, birds, mammals worms, eggs, plants |

The small intestine is comparatively longer in herbivorous species of reptiles than in the carnivorous ones. Tortoises, iguanids or agamids have larger small intestines than do carnivorous species of comparable size. The small intestine produces enzymes of digestion and is very efficient in the absorption of amino acids.

The liver produces bile salts for the emulsification and absorption of ingested fats. The gallbladders of snakes are located at the caudal poles of the liver and possess a long bile duct that runs back caudally to the duodenum.

The pancreas produces enzymes for the digestion of protein, carbohydrates and fat. This organ is intimately associated with the spleen in snakes.

A modified cecum is found in chelonians, crocodilians and some species of lizards. The cecum tends to be large and well-developed in the large herbivorous tortoises. Its function is thought to be similar to that of the equine cecum.

The colon's major function is to conserve water by resorbing water from the fecal mass.

Reptiles are intermittent feeders in nature. Captive snakes are usually fed every week or every 2 weeks, whereas crocodilians, chelonians and lizards may be fed daily or on alternating days. Captive reptiles kept under continuous optimal conditions tend to become obese, thus lowering their tolerance to high environmental temperature and often rendering males infertile.

Failure to feed eventually leads to death from caloric exhaustion. An Indian python 2.4 m. (8 feet) long reportedly lost 10 per cent of its body weight following a 140-day fast. A boa 2.7 m. (9 feet) long lost 50 per cent of its body weight following a fast that lasted 506 days. Gila monsters have reportedly fasted for 1 year. Chelonians can survive for 1 year without feeding.

Environmental temperatures directly affect the digestion of reptiles. A python 2.44 m. (8 feet) long was able to digest a rabbit completely after 5 days at a temperature of 28° C. and after 7 days at 22° C. At 18° C., an ingested rabbit was not digested after 15 days. Carnivorous lizards provided with PO temperatures can digest insects in 12 hours.

A boa 2.13 m. (7 feet) long was radiographed periodically following a feeding on a rat. Observations on the rat's skeleton during digestion were as follows:

TIME ELAPSED (HOURS)

27   Decalcification recognizable.
47   Skeleton noticeably less distinct
52   Skull almost completely invisible.
118  Only a faint shadow of one femur remaining

At no time did any part of the rat's skeleton pass through the pylorus while being digested. Normal feces from a python will contain undigested material such as hair, feathers, horns and scales. Teeth of the host or prey animals may also be found in the digestive tract.

Both the arthritic and the visceral forms of gout have been reported in reptiles. The arthritic form is most often recognized clinically, whereas the visceral type is usually discovered at necropsy. Both forms are manifested by the deposition of uric acid crystals in the joint or the periarticular tissue (tophi), which are often surrounded by multinucleated giant cells.

Naturally occurring cases of gout have been observed in all forms of reptiles without evidence of primary renal disease in 13 cases reported by three different investigators. High-protein diets of reptiles and concurrent dehydration are thought to be the etiologic factors. In general, terrestrial reptiles are uricotelic, whereas alligators may be uricotelic or ammonotelic, depending on their state of hydration.

Investigators have artificially reproduced gout in alligators by means of intraperitoneal injections of the amino acid D-serine. An increase in uric acid excretion could be obtained when DL-alanine, D-alanine and L-arginine were administered at the rate of 15 mg./kg. of body weight. Glycine and DL-arginine were ineffective in altering uric acid excretion in the alligator because of rapid renal deaminization to ammonia.

Uric acid is the metabolic end product of both protein and purine metabolism in reptiles. Investigators have demonstrated that the rates of uric acid excretion in the alligator were just as great with purine-free diets (e.g., gelatin) as with high-purine diets (e.g., rabbit tissue).

The normal concentration of uric acid in blood plasma of alligators ranges from 1.0 to 4.1 mg./100 ml. In alligators with gout, the uric acid content increases to 70 mg./100 ml. of serum. A study revealed the normal excretion rate of nitrogenous wastes in alligators to be 20 per cent urea, 10 per cent uric acid and 70 per cent ammonium salts; this ratio is subject to change, depending on the amount of protein in the diet and the animal's state of hydration. In alligator embryos, these values were 4.6, 7.3 and 46.5 per cent, respectively.

Studies have shown the percentage of uric acid wastes to be 93 to 98 per cent in lizards, 89 per cent in a python and 63 per cent "in a snake." The excretion rates for black snake embryos are 60 per cent urea, 20 per cent uric acid and 10 per cent ammonium salts.

Recommended treatment includes rehydration and reduced frequency of high-protein meals. Prognosis is extremely guarded.

Extended fasts in reptiles encourage the development of severe avitaminoses and mineral deficiencies. The rate of nutritional disease is lower in snakes that feed well because whole-animal diets tend to reproduce the natural diet. Deficiency diseases occur frequently in all other forms of reptiles (lizards, chelonians and crocodilians) because of general misconceptions concerning their natural diets. Little basic information is available in reference to specific reptilian requirements of micronutrients; however, it is recommended that reptilian diets be supplemented with 1 mg. of a vitamin-mineral mix/gm. of body weight up to 30 gm. of supplement.

Avitaminosis A is a common malady of chelonians and is characterized by palpebral edema resulting from an occlusion of the ducts draining the harderian glands by keratinized debris. In advanced cases, generalized anasarca appears. Supplementation of the diet with a few drops of cod liver oil daily will reverse early signs in the acute stage and will arrest the more chronic forms. Once the disease is controlled, routine vitamin supplementation is recommended.

Avitaminosis D causes classic rickets in all forms of reptiles. Clinical signs include depression, ataxia, anorexia, enlarged articulations, soft shells and a variety of skeletal and shell deformities. Vitamin D is usually ingested by the carnivorous species in the form of liver stores or yolk sacs of the prey animal. Some reptilian species (iguanas) are thought to utilize ultraviolet light sources for meeting vitamin D requirements. Treatment of clinical disease can be in the form of a few drops of cod liver oil, egg yolk, day-old chicks or vitamin-mineral supplements (1 mg./gm. of body weight).

Hypervitaminosis D occurs in reptiles and has been reported most often in iguanids. Overzealous supplementation with vitamin D preparations and prolonged exposure to ultraviolet light can result in the classic medial calcification of elastic blood vessels. Advanced cases can be diagnosed radiographically.

Avitaminosis E has been reported in crocodilians fed mackerel and in snakes fed obese laboratory rodents. Steatitis and skeletal muscle atrophy are classic findings, although either lesion may be seen alone. Steatitis appears as a generalized induration of adipose tissue. The well-circumscribed lesions are heavily pigmented with a yellow ceroid lipofuscin. This pigment emits a yellowish-orange fluorescence upon exposure to ultraviolet light. Microscopic examination of such lesions reveals an acid-fast, basophilic, amorphous material surrounded by fibroblasts and macrophages. Reticuloendothelial cells and macrophages of the liver are laden with globules of ceroid. Linear ulcerations of the cloacas in crocodilians are filled with a yellow keratinized debris. These ulcerations are thought to correspond to those found in the gastric squamous epithelium of pigs suffering from vitamin E deficiency. Lesions of steatitis involve focal induration of intramuscular, subcutaneous and abdominal fat deposits. The well-circumscribed foci are made up of a yellow or tan, greasy, friable, soaplike material which is well encapsulated by a thin connective tissue wall.

Because anorexia often is the only clinical sign, this disease is usually diagnosed in reptiles at necropsy. It is therefore essential to obtain a detailed dietary history from the owner. Dietary or parenteral administration of vitamin E is recommended for treatment; routine dietary supplementation should be practiced.

Ascorbic acid deficiency has been reported in snakes and lizards. Ascorbic acid deficiency is thought to be the initiating cause of ulcerative stomatitis, with the resultant disruption of the oral mucosa allowing invasion of bacteria normally found in the reptilian mouth. The acute lesion appears as edema and erythema and is characterized in the advanced stages by inflammation of the gingiva of the upper and lower dental arcades. As the disease progresses, it becomes secondarily infected. Copious amounts of caseous yellow to gray exudate accumulate between the dental arcade and the lips and palate. Untreated cases usually progress to secondary osteomyelitis. The exudate is eventually aspirated or swallowed, resulting in terminal pneumonia or gastroenteritis.

Treatment includes local cleansing of the affected areas with thimerosal, hydrogen peroxide or a sulfonamide in the early stages. More advanced cases require careful débridement of injured and necrotic tissue and flushing with previously mentioned products. Local treatment should be supplemented with 10 to 30 mg. of ascorbic acid and a broad-spectrum antibiotic daily for 10 days. This is followed by continuous local treatment and dietary supplementation with ascorbic acid.

One of the most common nutritional diseases encountered in reptiles presented for clinical examination is calcium deficiency. The disease has been reported both in carnivorous and herbivorous forms. Reptiles fed an all fish or all red-meat diet receive respective dietary calcium to phosphorus ratios (Ca:P) of 1:44 and 1:25. Insectivorous reptiles are notoriously susceptible to calcium deficiency, since there is no calcium in the chitinous exoskeleton of insects. The results of calcium deficiency because of improper Ca:P ratios in reptiles are fibrous osteodystrophy, nutritional secondary hyperparathyroidism and urinary calculi. Calcium-deficient diets adequate in vitamin D hasten the more severe signs as a result of the mobilization of skeletal stores of mineral by vitamin D.

The easiest way to supplement calcium to small insectivorous lizards and small chelonians is to provide commercially available lime water as a source of drinking water. The disease is rarely reported in the larger species of snakes fed whole birds or mammalian prey animals. Those that eat ground meat should be fed a nutritionally complete commercial dog food or carnivore sausage rather than horse meat or beef. If horse meat or fish must be fed, calcium carbonate should be supplemented at the respective rates of 400 to 900 mg./100 gm. and 1.5 gm./100 gm. of food.

Next to calcium deficiencies, the most commonly reported mineral deficiency is iodine deficiency. The lack of dietary iodine or the goitrogenic effects of large anionic goitrogens (nitrates) in green forages result in classic goiter. The disease is most often observed in herbivorous lizards or chelonians. Signs include lethargy and a palpebral enlargement at the thoracic inlet.

Goiter may be prevented by supplementing the diet with a complete vitamin-mineral preparation at the rate of 1 mg./gm. of body weight or iodized salt fed at the rate of 0.5 per cent of the total diet.

## DISCUSSION

While we are obligated to treat the vast variety of reptiles in our charge with chemical and machine, it is, in the final analysis, attention to the details of herpatecology that will provide the best preventive medicine in the management of the captive poikilotherm.

### SUPPLEMENTAL READING

Donaldson, M., Heynman, D., Dempster, R., and Garcia, L.: Epizootic of fatal amebiasis among exhibited snakes: Epidemiologic, pathologic, and chemotherapeutic considerations. Am. J. Vet. Res., 36:807–817, 1975.

Frye, F. L.: Bacterial diseases of captive reptiles. In Kirk, R. W. (ed.): Current Veterinary Therapy V. Philadelphia, W. B. Saunders Co., 1974, pp. 626–628.

Kauffeld, C.: Snakes: The Keeper and the Kept. Garden City, New York, Doubleday and Co., Inc., 1969.

Laszlo, J.: Observations on two new artificial lights for reptile displays. Intern. Zoo Yearbook, 9:12–13, 1969.

Licht, P.: Decreases in spermatogenesis in lizards exposed to elevated temperatures. Copeia, 4:428–436, 1965.

Marcus, L. C.: Parasitic Diseases of Captive Reptiles. In Kirk, R. W. (ed.): Current Veterinary Therapy V. Philadelphia, W. B. Saunders Co., 1974, pp. 632–638.

Murphy, J. B.: Notes on iguanids and varanids in a mixed exhibit at Dallas Zoo. Internl. Zoo Yearbook, 9:39–41, 1969.

Pallaske, G.: Hypervitaminosis D in a lizard. Berlin Münch. Tierarztl. Wchnschr., 74:132, 1961.

Pawley, R.: Observations on a prolonged food refusal period of an adult fer-de-lance, Bothrops atrox asper. Internl. Zoo Yearbook, 9:58–59, 1969.

Peaker, M.: Some aspects of the thermal requirements of reptiles in captivity. Internl. Zoo Yearbook, 9:3–8, 1969.

Stebbins, R. C., and Barwick, R. E.: Radiotelemetric study of thermoregulation in a lace monitor. Copeia, pp. 541–547, 1968.

Wallach, J. D.: Medical care of reptiles. J. Am. Vet. Med. Assn., 155:1017–1034, 1969.

Wallach, J. D.: Nutritional diseases of exotic animals. J. Am. Vet. Med. Assn., 157:583–599, 1970.

Wallach, J. D.: Diseases of reptiles and their clinical management. Current Veterinary Therapy IV. Philadelphia, W. B. Saunders Co., 1971, pp. 433–439.

Wallach, J. D.: Environmental and nutritional diseases of captive reptiles. J. Am. Vet. Med. Assn., 159:1632–1643, 1971.

Wallach, J. D., and Hoessle, C.: Hypervitaminosis D in green iguanas. J. Am. Vet. Med. Assn., 149:912–914, 1966.

Wallach, J. D., and Hoessle, C.: Visceral gout in captive reptiles. J. Am. Vet. Med. Assn., 151:897–899, 1967.

Wallach, J. D., Hoessle, C., and Bennett, J.: Hypoglycemic shock in captive alligators. J. Am. Vet. Med. Assn., 151:893–896, 1967.

Wallach, J. D., and Hoessle, C.: Fibrous osteodystrophy in green iguanas. J. Am. Vet. Med. Assn., 153:863–865, 1968.

Wallach, J. D., and Hoessle, C.: Steatitis in captive crocodilians. J. Am. Vet. Med. Assn., 153:845, 1968.

# BACTERIAL AND FUNGAL DISEASES OF CAPTIVE REPTILES

FREDRIC L. FRYE, D.V.M.
*Berkeley, California*

## INTRODUCTION

When dealing with suspected bacterial diseases, an attempt should be made to identify the causative agent whenever possible. Standard microbiologic techniques are employed as with other species. Often, what at first may appear as a "typical" infection with ubiquitous reptilian pathogens eventually may be found to be something entirely different and may, therefore, require a different antimicrobial agent.

The following disease entities represent the most frequently encountered bacterial and fungal conditions in captive reptiles.

## ABSCESSES

Subcutaneous abscess formation is common in all captive reptiles but especially in turtles, tortoises, lizards and snakes. It may be initiated by external wounds, bites from arthropod parasites, and hematogenous spread from distant sites.

A number of microorganisms have been isolated from reptilian abscesses. Both pure and mixed cultures have been found. *Aeromonas hydrophila, Aeromonas aerophila, Aeromonas aerogenes, Citrobacter* spp., *Enterobacter* spp., *Escherichia coli, Mycobacterium* spp., *Pasteurella* spp., *Peptostreptococcus, Proteus morgani, Proteus rettgeri, Pseudomonas* spp., *Salmonella marina* and *Serratia* spp. have been reported.

It is obvious that some protection should be afforded the clinician handling patients capable of transmitting such potentially zoonotic disease organisms as enumerated above. Disposable examination gloves are an inexpensive and effective barrier to contamination.

Massive internal abscesses are encountered occasionally. These may be suspected when firm swellings are palpated within the body cavity of snakes, lizards or crocodilians. Radiography should be employed to help confirm the diagnosis. A stained blood film from the patient usually reveals a marked leukocytosis with eosinophilia. Snakes and lizards affected with such large abscesses frequently are found with metastatic pulmonary lesions and purulent pericarditis.

Quarantine of infected animals always must be strictly observed. A "clean to dirty" routine should be established and maintained, i.e., the healthy animals are always handled first and no cross contamination is allowed. Thorough attention to hygiene is mandatory in this, as well as other, subspecialities of veterinary medicine.

Superficial abscesses are treated by incision and evacuation of the usually inspissated contents. If practicable, the interior periphery of the abscess cavity should be thoroughly curetted, or at least debrided, to be sure that no residuum remains. The defect should be flushed with hydrogen peroxide (3 per cent by volume) and Betadine® solution (Purdue Frederick). An antibiotic pack may be employed using a debriding agent such as Kymar® ointment (Armour-Baldwin), Elase® (Parke, Davis), etc. Furacin® ointment (Eaton) also is of value as a packing agent.

In the case of some maxillary abscesses in turtles and tortoises, a defect may remain following treatment. This defect leaves an open communication to the oropharynx. It can be repaired easily with a prosthesis made from rapid polymerizing epoxy resin (Devco 5-Minute Epoxy Cement®) and an appropriate fabric patch. (This technique has been described previously [Frye, 1973a].)

## INFECTIOUS STOMATITIS ("MOUTH ROT")

Infectious stomatitis is one of the most frequently encountered lesions in captive snakes. Stress, poor hygiene, malnutrition and oral wounds all contribute to the progression of the disease. The etiologic agent most often cultured from these lesions is *Aeromonas hydrophila*. If the condition is left untreated for a sufficiently long time, osteomyelitis will result. Hypovitaminosis C may be implicated.

Treatment consists of thorough, but gentle, cleansing of all oral tissues. The mouth can be kept open with a tape-padded tongue depressor held at a right angle to the mandibles. Any loose teeth are removed gently, and the resultant open alveoli and gingival tissues are flushed or swabbed with 3 per cent hydrogen peroxide followed by full-strength Betadine solution. Systemic antibiotics, particularly Chloromycetin®, sodium succinate (chloramphenicol sodium succinate; Parke, Davis) and Gentocin® (gentamicin sulfate; Schering), are injected. Multi-B vitamin complex and injectable ascorbic acid are used as adjunctive therapy. In the past, sulfamethazine and sulfaquinoxyline also have been used both locally and in the drinking water. The injectable antibiotics appear to be most effective.

## SEPTICEMIC CUTANEOUS ULCERATIVE DISEASE (SCUD)

Septicemic cutaneous ulcerative disease is characterized in aquatic turtles by cutaneous ulceration, anorexia, lethargy and paralysis. In advanced cases, areas of necrosis are seen in the visceral organs, particularly the liver. The etiologic agent has been reported to be *Citrobacter freundii*.

Treatment consists of daily injections of Chloromycetin sodium succinate in appropriate dosages. Local treatment of the cutaneous ulcers with Betadine promotes more rapid healing after these lesions have been debrided.

## RESPIRATORY INFECTIONS

Respiratory infections are common to all captive reptiles, but they are of particular importance in snakes, turtles and tortoises. The most frequently identified microorganisms associated with reptilian respiratory infections are *Aeromonas* spp., *Proteus* spp. and *Pseudomonas* spp., although many others have been implicated.

The clinical signs are nasal discharge, open-mouth breathing, wheezing, inappetence and torpor. Occasionally, the presenting sign or complaint (as described by the owner or keeper) is the loss of normal swimming equilibrium in turtles. This is seen as a longitudinally slanted appearance of the turtle in the tank, with one side lower than the other. Since the pulmonary system of the aquatic chelonians also functions as an efficient hydrostatic organ for maintaining various states of buoyancy, a unilateral loss of the functional pulmonary bed will cause the turtle to swim with a marked list, and the affected, nonaerated side will be lowermost.

The inspiratory effort in the chelonians is largely an active process, and expiration is mostly passive; therefore, the clearance of exudates from distal respiratory spaces is very inefficient. The high incidence of respiratory infection in captive reptiles of all families attests to the jeopardy in which these animals are placed once they are stressed sufficiently to become clinically diseased.

Treatment with gentamicin sulfate and ampicillin or Chloromycetin sodium succinate plus sodium ascorbate has been most effective. Injection sites are the posterior aspect of the rear legs and the thigh area. Intraperitoneal injections may be used for some agents but generally are not as desirable as intramuscular injections. (See Table 1 for dosages.)

Husbandry practices also should be improved; most new arrivals or newly acquired reptiles have been severely stressed from the moment of capture until they reach their ultimate destination.

An effort should be made to increase the environmental temperature of reptiles that have been shown to have bacterial infections. Many of the aeromonads will prove lethal to reptiles kept at lower than optimal temperature but will lose much of their pathogenicity when the host animals are maintained at higher ambient temperatures.

## CEPHALIC, INTERMANDIBULAR AND PHARYNGEAL CELLULITIS IN SNAKES

A specific syndrome that seems to occur in snakes is characterized by massive edema and cellulitis involving the head and neck, particularly the intermandibular and pharyngeal areas. The onset is usually sudden, often within 24 hours. The most frequently encountered pathogenic organisms found in microbiologic cultures from these lesions have been *Aeromonas* spp. and *Pseudomonas* spp.

The treatment that has proved most effective has been the daily administration of an experimental antibiotic, Butirosin sulfate, a relatively new member of the deoxystreptamine family of antibiotics (which includes neomycin, kanamycin, paromomycin and gentamicin). It is administered in a dosage of 40 to 60 mg./kg. subcutaneously daily for six days. Parenteral fluid therapy must be provided to prevent nephrotoxicity and other manifestations common to this class of antimicrobial agents. At this writing, the antibiotic is under clinical investigation and is not available for general use.

## BLISTER DISEASE

Blister disease is a condition seen in reptiles, especially snakes and lizards kept in a captive environment that is too damp and also contaminated with feces-borne bacteria. It is characterized by multiple dermal vesicles that at first are filled with fluid but soon become filled with caseous debris.

Treatment consists of thorough washing of the patient with a mild germicidal soap or solution. The animal should be moved to dry quarters. Appropriate antibiotic therapy with parenteral Chloromycetin or ampicillin should be initiated.

## SALMONELLOSIS

While salmonellosis usually does not produce signs of overt disease in the reptilian host, it has received much publicity recently because of the potential public health hazard associated with contact exposure to some chelonians. The genesis of this problem stems from the practice of rearing and collecting turtles for the pet trade in sewage-contaminated ponds and marshes. Another source of infection in these turtles has been the practice of feeding the feral breeding population slaughterhouse offal, condemned carcasses and other waste materials. These items frequently are heavily contaminated by organisms of the *Salmonella* spp. and *Arizona* spp.

Late in 1972, federal and several state statutes severely curtailed the interstate shipment of these animals.

The exclusion of turtles and tortoises from the menageries of young children would seem desirable from two standpoints: first, the incidence of turtle-associated salmonellosis in children would be greatly reduced;

*Table 1.* *Parenteral Antibiotics for Use in Reptiles*

| DRUG | MANUFACTURER | ROUTE OF ADMINISTRATION | FREQUENCY OF ADMINISTRATION | RECOMMENDED DOSAGE |
|---|---|---|---|---|
| Ampicillin trihydrate (Polyflex) | Bristol | Intramuscular; subcutaneous | Once daily | 3–6 mg./kg. every 24 hours |
| Benzathine penicillin with procaine penicillin (Flocillin) | Bristol | Intramuscular | Varies with species and ambient temperature | 10,000 units total penicillin activity/ kg. every 24–72 hours |
| Chloramphenicol (Chloromycetin succinate)* | Parke-Davis | Intravenous; intramuscular; subcutaneous | Once daily | 10–15 mg./kg. in divided doses |
| Gentamicin sulfate (Gentocin)* | Schering | Intramuscular; subcutaneous | Once daily | 3 mg./kg., 6 days |
| Kanamycin sulfate (Kantrex)* | Bristol | Intravenous; intramuscular; also as a wound-flushing agent | Once daily | 10 mg./kg. in divided doses |
| Lincomycin (Lincocin)* | Upjohn | Intramuscular | Once daily | 6 mg./kg. |
| Neomycin sulfate with methscopolamine (Biosol-M)* | Upjohn | Oral | Once daily; twice daily | 2.5 mg./kg. |
| Neomycin sulfate with polymyxin sulfate (Daribiotic)* | Beecham-Massengill | Intramuscular; intravenous; also as a wound-flushing agent | Once daily | 10 mg./kg. |
| Oxytetracycline hydrochloride (Liquamycin injectable and intramuscular)† | Pfizer | Intravenous (Liquamycin injectable); intramuscular (Liquamycin intramuscular) | Once daily | 6–10 mg./kg. |
| Polymyxin B* | Pfizer | Intramuscular | Once daily | 1–2 mg./kg. |
| Potassium penicillin G, buffered, U.S.P.‡ | Squibb | Intramuscular; intraperitoneal; also as a wound-flushing agent | Varies widely | 20,000 – 80,000 units/kg. |
| Streptomycin sulfate, buffered U.S.P.* | Squibb | Intramuscular | Twice daily | 6 mg./kg. |
| Sulfadimethoxine (Symbio)* | Affiliated Lab. | Intravenous; intramuscular | Once daily | 30 mg./kg. first day; 15 mg./kg. second to fourth day |

*Should not be used in presence of impaired renal or hepatic function or dehydration. Parenteral fluids should be employed.
†May produce some local inflammation at injection site (Liquamycin intramuscular).
‡May cause cardiac arrest at high and rapid uptake dosages owing to K+ ion.

and second, the high morbidity and mortality of these turtles would be ameliorated.

## NECROTIC ENTERITIS OR ENTEROGASTRITIS

A variety of pathogenic organisms have been associated with enteritides in reptiles. Whether a specific organism is actually the etiologic agent or merely an opportunist or casual contaminant may be academic.

The signs of enteritis in a reptile are identical to those exhibited by mammalian and avian species, namely, diarrhea that usually contains mucus, blood and cellular debris. Since amebic enterohepatitis associated with *Endamoeba invadens* may produce identical signs, the feces should be examined for the presence of amebic cysts and/or trophozoites.

A number of antibiotics have been employed with success. Oral neomycin sulfate, with or without methscopolamine, has proved quite effective. If *Pseudomonas* organisms are identified, polymyxin B may be of benefit.

## SHELL "FUNGUS" OR SHELL "ROT"

Shell "fungus" or "rot" is a common disorder of aquatic chelonians. While not necessarily caused by mycotic agents, it should be included with any discussion of the principal bacterial and/or mycotic diseases of captive reptiles. Often a wide variety of bacteria may be isolated, while fungal cultures may be negative. Wallach (1975) reported a specific pathogen, *Beneckea chitinovora*, an organism common to crustaceans, to be implicated in an outbreak of shell rot in turtles.

Typically, the lesions of shell rot involve punctate to diffuse ulcers of the shell plate tissues that may progress to a pesudomembrane. The more common shell "fungus" is manifested as pitted, excoriated, pale areas of lifted shell substrate. It is highly infectious; therefore, isolate all affected individuals.

Treatment consists of local débridement and painting of the lesions with Betadine solution. While undergoing treatment, affected turtles should be kept dry, except to feed.

## MYCOTIC GRANULOMAS

A number of mycotic granulomatous lesions have been described in reptiles. Upon routine histopathologic sectioning and staining with periodic acid–Schiff, fungal elements are demonstrated easily. The gross lesions may be either soft and fluctuant or dry and gangrenous. *Aspergillus* spp. and *Paecilomyces* spp. are the most commonly identified pathogens associated with these lesions.

Treatment is confined to wide excision or amputation if the area involved will permit it. At this time there is no effective medical treatment that can be substituted for surgical excision.

### SUPPLEMENTAL READING

Aronson, J. D.: Spontaneous tuberculosis in snakes. J. Infect. Dis., *44*:215–223, 1929.
Boever, W. J., and Williams, J.: *Arizona* septicemia in three boa constrictors. Vet. Med./Small Animal Clin., *70*:1357–1359, 1975.
Frye, F. L.: Clinical evaluation of a rapid polymerizing epoxy resin for repair of shell defects in tortoises. Vet. Med. Small Animal Clin., *68*:51–53, 1973a.
Frye, F. L.: Husbandry, Medicine and Surgery in Captive Reptiles. Bonner Springs, Kansas, VM Publishing, Inc., 1973b.
Frye, F. L., and Dutra, F. R.: Mycotic granulomata involving the forefeet of a turtle. Vet. Med./Small Animal Clin., *69*:1554–1556, 1974.
Kluger, M. J., Ringler, D. H., and Anver, M. R.: Fever and survival. Science, *188*:166–168, 1975.
Marcus, L. C.: Infectious diseases of reptiles. J. Am. Vet. Med. Assn., *159*:1626–1631, 1971.
Murphy, J. B.: A review of diseases and treatment of captive chelonians—bacterial and viral infections. H.I.S.S. News-Journal, *1*:77–81, 1973.
Murphy, J. B.: A brief outline of suggested treatments for diseases of captive reptiles. Society for Study of Amphibians and Reptiles, 1975, pp. 1–13.
Page, L. A.: Diseases and infections of snakes: A review. Bull. Wildlife Dis. Assn., *2*:111–126, 1966.
Reichenbach-Klinke, H., and Elkan, E.: The Principal Diseases of Lower Vertebrates. New York, Academic Press, 1965.
Wallach, J. D.: The pathogenesis and etiology of ulcerative shell diseases in turtles. J. Zoo Animal Med., *6*:11–13, 1975.

# HEMATOLOGY OF CAPTIVE REPTILES (WITH EMPHASIS ON NORMAL MORPHOLOGY)

FREDRIC L. FRYE, D.V.M.
*Berkeley, California*

## INTRODUCTION

The title has included the adjective "normal" with full knowledge that, even under the most enlightened captive husbandry conditions, a certain bias of stress resulting from captivity must be imposed upon the subject. In addition, the stress of recent capture may also introduce artifacts into the data obtained.

## OBTAINING THE SPECIMEN

Depending on the volume of whole blood required, several techniques may be employed without endangering the subject's life in the process.

In very small lizards, turtles, tortoises or snakes, it is obvious that only a limited volume blood sample (a few drops to perhaps 0.5 ml.) may be obtained. In such instances, the hematologic examination may, of necessity, consist of a stained blood film, microhematocrit, total protein determination and perhaps—depending upon micro methods available—hemoglobin, plasma proteins, etc. Even in small fence lizards (for example, *Sceloporus occidentalis*), several drops of blood may be gathered easily by clipping a *rear* toe just at the junction of terminal phalanx and claw. A sharp fingernail or toenail clipper works very well to produce a clean clip from which a small quantity of blood will flow, and the blood flow usually will cease spontaneously or may be stanched with an appropriate styptic. The loss of a rear toenail will not unduly hamper the locomotion of these animals.

In larger specimens, cardiocentesis may be performed using a thin-walled, small-gauge needle. The desirability of employing anticoagulants is determined by the circumstances (field or laboratory) and by which laboratory tests are to be done.

The sites for cardiac puncture vary widely with the species and overall physical condition. In lizards and snakes, the preferred site is approached ventrally and anteriorly.

In snakes, a location ventrally, near the midline, usually will place the large single ventricle within the path of the directed needle. In most small to medium-sized snakes, the beating heart, which is usually situated about one fifth to one third of the total body length posterior to the head, may be located by visual means if the snake is restrained gently on its back. Often, the location of the heart in smaller snakes may be found by using a transilluminator. In boas, for example, the heart is conveniently located at almost exactly one fourth the snake's length posterior to the snout.

In larger snakes, the heart usually can be palpated and, infrequently, auscultated with a delicate stethoscope. In the giant snakes, the external jugular veins, which are located on either side of the snake's neck in shallow furrows, may be employed to yield blood samples; approach as in mammals.

The crocodilians may be bled in a number of ways. In juveniles, cardiocentesis is the most practical method. As these animals increase in size, jugular and lateral caudal veins can be used for whole blood sampling.

The bony skeletal plates of the chelonians (turtles, tortoises, terrapins) pose access problems, except in soft-shelled turtles of the genus *Trionyx* and a few other species. Again, small volumes of blood may be obtained from toe-clipping. Cardiocentesis is most practical except in the giant Galapagos and aldabra tortoises and marine turtles, which may weigh several hundred kilograms; in these reptiles, other sites, such as jugular, flipper or ventral sinus veins, may have to be utilized. An alternative in these chelonians is to cut a claw transversally so that the nail bed is exposed. A styptic such as ferric subsulfate must be used to insure hemostasis—which may be more easily discussed than accomplished!

In the smaller chelonians, cardiocentesis may be performed using hypodermic needles or biopsy needles bearing stylets, or by actually drilling a small hole that can be sealed with epoxy resin. The site is approximately midway and posterior to the axillary fossae (Fig. 1).

Obviously, when either venipuncture or cardiocentesis is performed, the site(s) should be prepared appropriately to achieve asepsis.

A new technique for collecting blood from lizards entails needle aspiration from the ventral caudal spinal vessels (Esra *et al.*, 1975).

Depending upon the specific reptile,

bone marrow is present in several sites. In normal snakes, for instance, the major location for erythropoietic activity is the vertebral bodies. Between spicules of bone are typical colonies of myeloid and erythroid stem cells and their progeny in various stages of maturation (Figs. 2 A and B). Similar cell masses of marrow are found in the medullary cavities of those species which possess limbs (Fig. 1 B) and within the cancellous shell spaces of turtles and tortoises.

For all practical purposes, a bone marrow biopsy is possible in most reptilian species, provided that the size of the animal will permit the procedure. Excellent bone marrow specimens can be gathered from most of the larger lizards, crocodilians and turtles by aspirating from an appropriate long bone site after routine restraint and aseptic preparation functions have been accomplished. In snakes, the biopsy needle is directed into the ventral portion of the spinal vertebral centra. If necessary, radiography may be employed to aid in directing the path of the needle to help prevent injury to the overlying spinal cord.

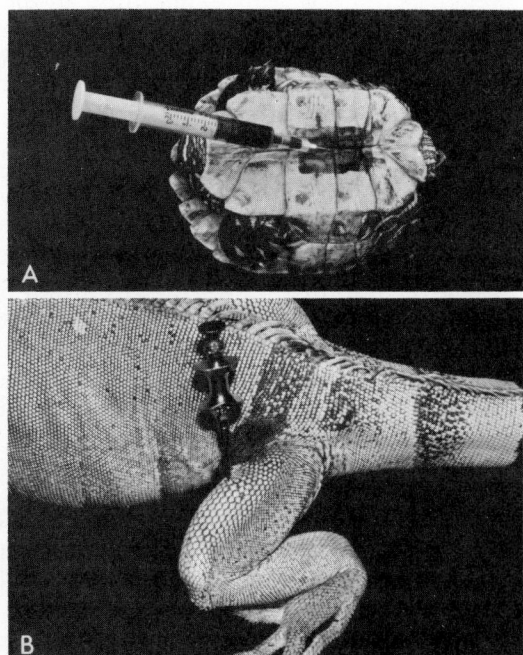

**Figure 1.** *A*, Correct location for collecting a blood sample from a chelonian via cardiocentesis. *B*, Correct placement of bone marrow needle for obtaining bone marrow from iguana femur.

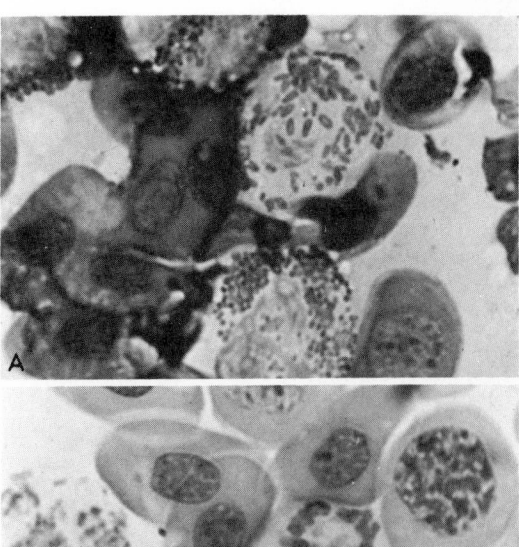

**Figure 2.** *A* and *B*, Typical appearance of myeloid and erythroid cell populations seen in reptile bone marrow.

## STAINING TECHNIQUES

Most Romanowsky-type stains will give satisfactory results. I prefer Gugol's Wright's stain, Kleineberger-Noble or Jenner-Giemsa for permanent mounts, and methylene blue for nonpermanent, quick screening examination of blood films. Considering the small volumes of blood obtainable from the smaller reptiles, the traditional, permanent stains are more appropriate.

Blood films should be made as thinly as practice allows and air-dried very quickly to preserve not only blood cell morphology but also morphology of any hemoparasites that may be present. If a permanent stain preparation is to be made, prior fixation with absolute methanol is advised, because it will help preserve the quality of the smears during transit from the field.

## MORPHOLOGY

*Note:* All reptiles possess nucleated erythrocytes, leukocytes and thrombocytes. For this reason, the use of automated white cell counters will give spurious results. The red cell number can be approximated with automated counters, but accuracy can be obtained easily with the hemocytometer and standard methodology.

**Erythrocyte.** The erythrocyte is an oval hemoglobin-containing cell bearing a more or less centrally placed nucleus, the outline of which may be markedly irregular. When viewed partially from the side or edge, these cells appear "flapjack"-shaped rather than truly biconcave disk–shaped, as in most mammals (Fig. 3). While seemingly contradictory by definition, true reticulocytes as well as polychromatic juvenile reptilian erythrocytes can be demonstrated easily with new methylene blue and similar stains. Similarly, Howell-Jolly bodies are sometimes encountered in reptilian erythrocytes. Spindle-shaped, pyriform and other anomalous forms of erythrocytes are seen occasionally in blood films. Some of these are artifactual but, in some individual animals, the frequency of finding these abnormal cells is sufficiently high to preclude any explanation except atypical erythrogenesis. Sometimes, erythrocytes are found either with multiple nuclei or lacking nuclei altogether, and so far, the clinical significance of such anomalous cells is in question.

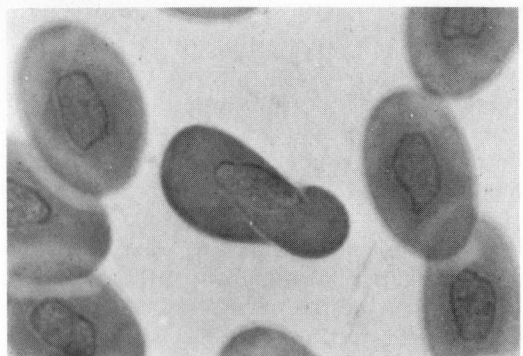

**Figure 3.** Reptilian erythrocytes exhibiting typical "flap-jack" configuration.

**Lymphocyte.** In reptiles, as in mammals, the lymphocyte is quite variable in size, with both large and small mononuclear cells being represented. The cytoplasm is finely granular and, as in mammals, stains light blue with Romanowsky stains and may contain azurophilic and/or hyaline inclusions. Juvenile lymphocytes or prolymphocytes usually contain a single well-defined nucleolus (Fig. 4).

**Monocyte.** The monocyte is reminiscent of that seen in mammals. A single, indented nucleus helps identify this mononuclear leukocyte. This cell is usually, but not invariably, larger than a large lymphocyte. The finely granular cytoplasm also stains light blue to blue-gray. The nuclear chromatin is fine in appearance (Fig. 5).

**Neutrophil.** Until recently, the neutrophil was not recognized in reptiles; however, specialized staining in my laboratory has proved conclusively that this cell does exist. This leukocyte is characterized by its usually nonsegmented nucleus—similar to the Pelger-Huët anomaly in mammals—

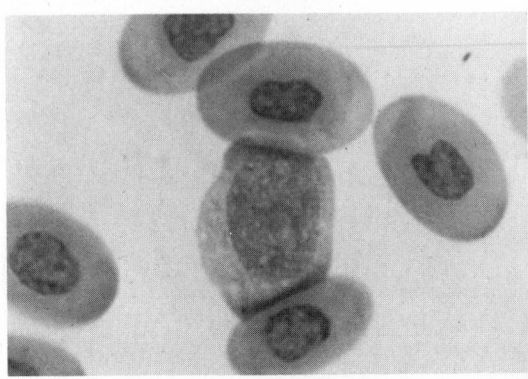

**Figure 4.** Reptilian lymphocyte.

*Table 1.* Some Blood Values

| | ALLIGATOR MISSISSIPIENSIS (ALLIGATOR)* | PSEUDEMYS SCRIPTA ELEGANS (RED-EARED SLIDER TURTLE) | NATRIX SIPEDON (WATER SNAKE) | TERRAPENE CAROLINA (BOX TURTLE)* | THAMNOPHIS SIRTALIS (GARTER SNAKE) | (BOA CONSTRICTOR)† |
|---|---|---|---|---|---|---|
| Plasma volume (ml./kg.) | 60.1 | 74.0 | — | — | — | — |
| RBC volume (ml./kg.) | 12.6 | — | — | — | — | — |
| Venous hematocrit (% cells) | 22.7 | 12–25.4 | — | — | — | — |
| Whole blood volume (ml./kg.) | 72.7 | 72.5–110.2 / 90.8 | — | — | — | — |
| RBC count ($\times 10^5$/cu. mm.) | 0.67 | 0.53–0.78 / 0.69 | 0.77 | 0.41–0.83 / 0.65 | 0.71–1.39 / 1.05 | 1.71 |
| PCV (%) | 30 | 15–21 / 17.5 | 35.5 | 20–38 / 28.6 | 19–37 / 28 | 18.5 |
| MCV (cu. $\mu$) | 450 | 211–296 / 255 | 465 | 309–587 / 442 | 266–268 / 267 | 108.2 |
| Hgb (gm./100 ml.) | 8.2 | 5.9–8.9 / 7.3 | 10 | 5.0–8.5 / 5.9 | 5.8–11.3 / 8.5 | 5.1 |
| MCHC (%) | 123 | 96–118 / 106 | 131 | 79–131 / 91 | 82 | — |
| RBC size, dry film ($\mu$) | 12.1 × 23.2 | — | 11 × 19.6 | 9 × 19 | 10.3 × 18.1 | — |
| WBC, total (per cu. mm.) | — | 9,700 | — | 7,500 | — | 6,700 |
| Neutrophils (%) | — | 12 | — | 0.3 | — | 9 |
| Eosinophils/ heterophils (%) | — | 34:12 | — | 10:8 | — | 4:32 |
| Basophils (%) | — | 1.5 | — | 8.0 | — | 2 |
| Lymphocytes (%) | — | 39.5 | — | 56.1 | — | 51 |
| Monocytes (%) | — | 1 | — | 9.4 | — | 2 |

*Data from Altman and Dittmer, 1964.
†Data from Frye, 1973.

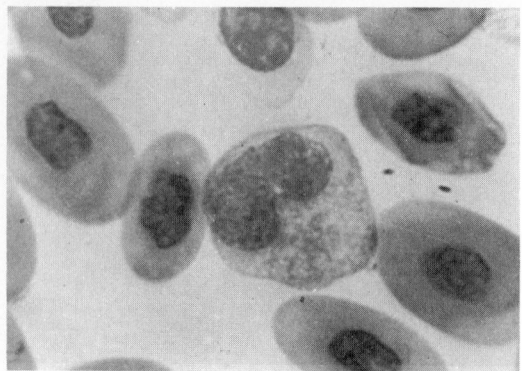

**Figure 5.** Reptilian monocyte.

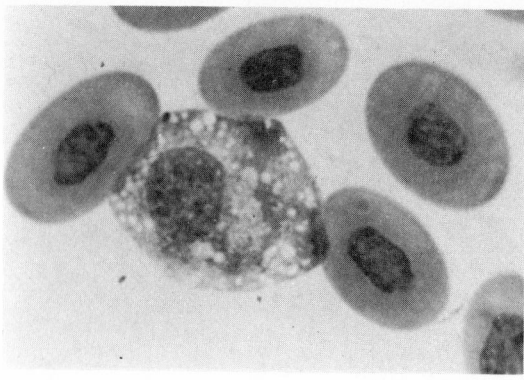

**Figure 7.** The so-called "toxic" neutrophil seen in systemic disease.

whose edges may be somewhat scalloped, and by its cytoplasm, which usually contains basophilic, eosinophilic and azurophilic granules and fibrillar strands. The nuclear chromatin is coarse, with significant clumping interspersed between a fine ground substance (Fig. 6).

As is the case in mammals, the neutrophil is sometimes seen with a "foamy" cytoplasm or containing "toxic granules." These granulocytes are found most frequently in reptiles exhibiting generalized infectious diseases such as severe respiratory infections and widespread abscess formation with signs of septicemia. An example of such a cell is illustrated in Figure 7.

**Heterophil.** The heterophil is a granulocyte whose fusiform, rod- or fibril-shaped intracytoplasmic inclusions or granules may stain intermediately between

those of the eosinophil and basophil. In those instances in which both heterophils and eosinophils accept the red eosin equally, the identification rests upon the shape of the intracytoplasmic inclusions. The nucleus usually is situated somewhat eccentrically (Fig. 8).

**Eosinophil.** The eosinophil is identified easily by its spherical, beadlike granules, which accept the eosin dye in the conventional blood stains. The nucleus stains pale blue and usually, but not always, is centrally located (Fig. 9). In response to a systemic disease process, the reptilian eosinophil may degranulate without actually lysing. These eosinophils do not exhibit the intense red-staining cytoplasmic granules but can be identified readily by examination under a microscope whose substage condenser has been lowered to increase the light contrast (Fig. 10).

**Basophil.** The basophil is encountered frequently in reptiles. Its cytoplasmic gran-

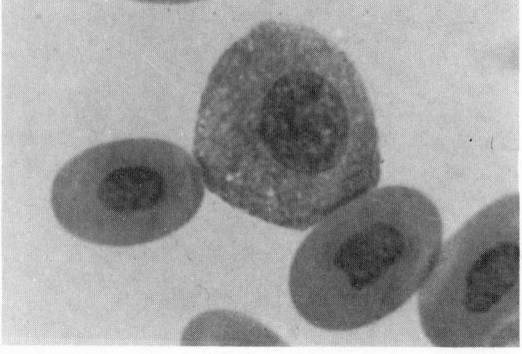

**Figure 6.** Neutrophil. These cells have demonstrated marked alkaline phosphatase and peroxidase activity similar to that seen in mammalian neutrophils. Note the dense nuclear chromatin and finely granular cytoplasm. The nucleus is not lobed as in the mammals.

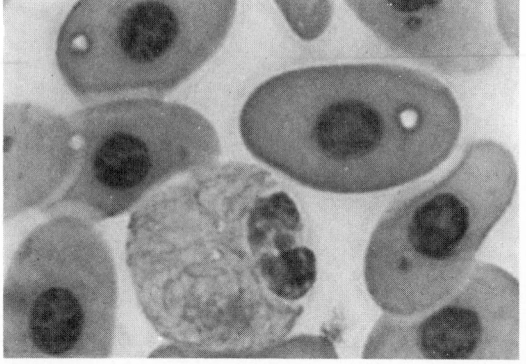

**Figure 8.** Typical reptilian heterophil. Note the rod-shaped cytoplasmic granules.

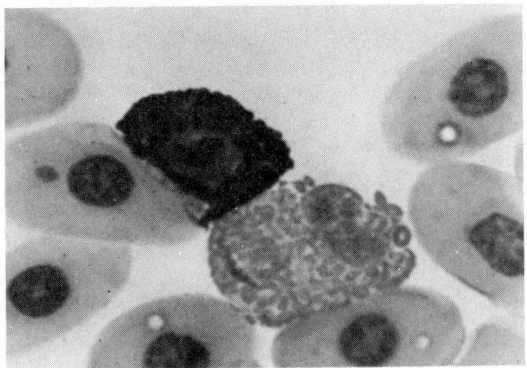

Figure 9. Eosinophil in central portion of field. The darker-staining cell to the left is a basophil.

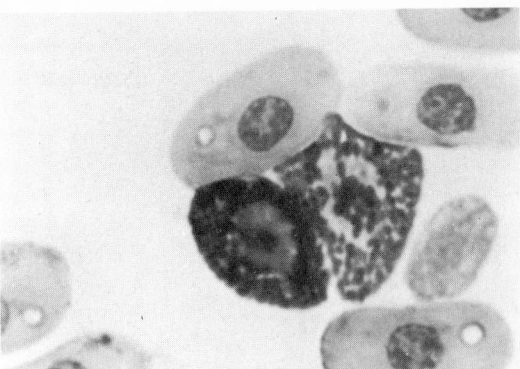

Figure 11. Two reptilian basophils.

ules may be spherical or rod-shaped and stain intensely dark blue (Fig. 11).

**Thrombocyte.** The reptilian thrombocyte is an elliptical cell which is usually smaller but sometimes approaches the dimensions of reptilian erythrocytes. Because it does not contain hemoglobin, the finely granular cytoplasm stains pale blue. The centrally located nucleus tends to be relatively large and smooth-edged and stains dark blue, with a dense chromatin pattern (Fig. 12). This cell apparently is capable of active phagocytosis; heme pigment, bacteria and amorphous cellular debris have all been found to be engulfed.

## COMMONLY ENCOUNTERED ABNORMAL FINDINGS

Some of the more commonly encountered abnormal findings seen during routine examination of stained reptilian blood films

are hemoprotozoa, particularly *Hemogregarines*, *Hemoproteus*, *Leucocytozoon* and trypanosomes. These parasites are demonstrated readily by conventional stains. Their mere presence in the blood of reptiles may or may not be *clinically* significant, because some, particularly the hemogregarines, appear to produce minimal signs of disease unless they are present in a large percentage of the cells (Figs. 13, 14, 15 and 16).

There appears to be a degree of periodicity. While not seen in many samples obtained in the morning or afternoon, these hemoparasites may be seen with higher frequency in evening samples; logically, this would follow the feeding habits of many arthropod vectors for these hemoparasites.

Erythrophagocytosis, bacteriophago-

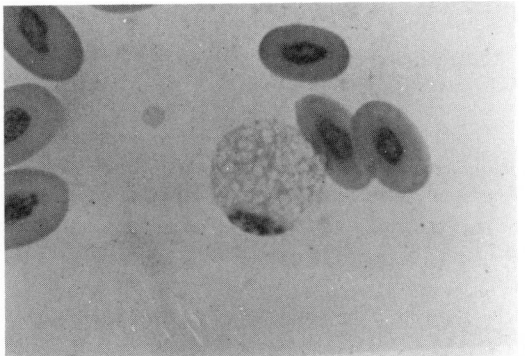

Figure 10. An eosinophil which has been degranulated. These cells are frequently seen in systemic disease or in animals subjected to significant stress.

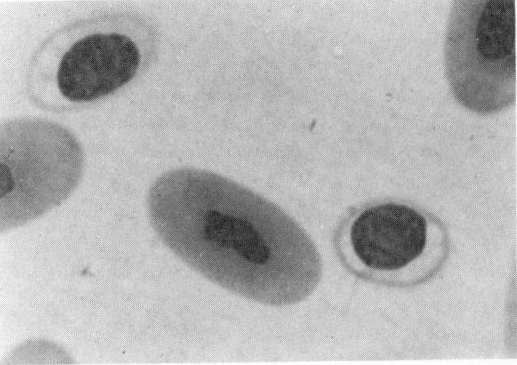

Figure 12. Thrombocytes. Note that the shape is similar to that of the reptilian erythrocyte, but the thrombocytes have almost clear blue cytoplasm, do not contain hemoglobin except when involved in erythrophagocytosis, and possess a slightly larger and more dense nucleus than that of the erythrocyte.

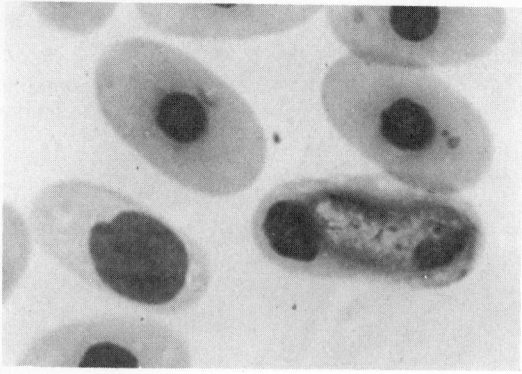

**Figure 13.** A hemogregarine hemoprotozoon parasite within a reptilian erythrocyte.

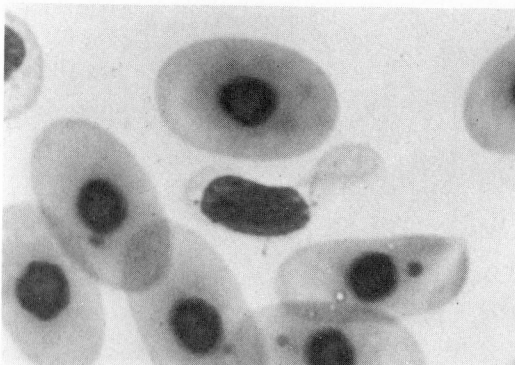

**Figure 15.** A *Haemoproteus* parasite. These are usually extracellular.

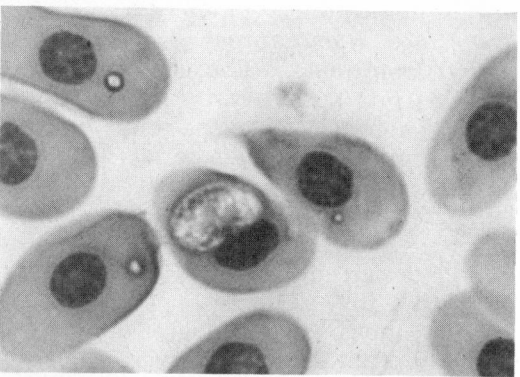

**Figure 14.** Another form of a hemogregarine parasite. These organisms are capable of entering and exiting from intact cells without creating lysis.

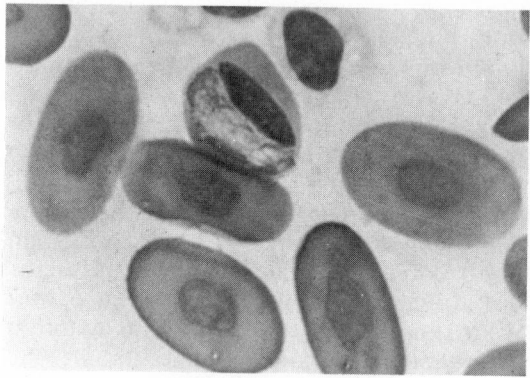

**Figure 16.** A *Leucocytozoon* parasite. These organisms, as their name implies, inhabit white cells rather than erythrocytes of their host species.

cytosis and other signs of cellular activity also are seen in some stained blood films. Obviously, such findings should be correlated with clinical signs exhibited by a particular patient.

Lupus erythematosus-like cells, lymphoblasts and erythroblasts also have been found in the blood of captive reptiles.

### SUPPLEMENTAL READING

Altman, P. L., and Dittmer, D. S.: Biology Data Book. Washington, D.C., Federation of American Societies for Experimental Biology, 1964.

Esra, G. N., Benirschke, K., and Griner, L. A.: Blood collecting technique in lizards. J. Am. Vet. Med. Assn., *167*:555–556, 1975.

Frye, F. L.: Husbandry, Medicine and Surgery in Captive Reptiles. Bonner Springs, Kansas, VM Publishing, Inc., 1973.

Gans, C., Bellairs, A. d'A., and Parsons, T. S.: Biology of the Reptilia. Vols. 1 to 4. Morphology A through D. New York, Academic Press, 1969–1973.

U.S. Armed Forces Institute of Pathology: Manual of Histologic and Special Staining Techniques. 2nd ed. New York, McGraw-Hill Book Co., 1960.

# SALMONEL-
# LOSIS IN
# REPTILES

LEONARD C. MARCUS, V.M.D.
*Boston, Massachusetts*

Salmonellosis is the major zoonosis associated with reptiles. More than 200 serotypes of *Salmonella* and the *Arizona* group of Enterobacteriaceae have been isolated from their intestinal flora (Kaufman and Morrison, 1966). Aquatic turtles, land tortoises, snakes, lizards and crocodilians from various parts of the world have been found to be infected with these bacteria. Although turtles have been incriminated more often than other herpetofauna as a source of human salmonellosis, for all practical purposes, all reptiles should be considered possible reservoirs.

Most of the turtles kept as pets in the United States (the most common species being the red-eared turtle, *Pseudemys scripta elegans*) are raised on farms in the South (Baker *et al.*, 1972; Kaufmann *et al.*, 1972). Original stock animals, caught in the wild, may be naturally infected with *Salmonella*. They are then raised in crowded conditions in ponds where the water is often stagnant. The turtles on many of these farms are fed uncooked meat scraps and offal from local abattoirs, feed which is often heavily contaminated with enteric pathogens. Soil in the banks of the ponds, where the turtles nest, is often heavily contaminated. Since *Salmonella* can penetrate turtle eggs (Feeley and Treger, 1969), baby turtles emerge from the egg already infected (Kaufmann *et al.*, 1972). The combination of crowding, stagnant water and contaminated feed is conducive to dissemination of *Salmonella* and the problem is compounded when the animals are packed together for shipment and later kept in a common display case in a pet shop. It is not unusual for 25 to 50 per cent of turtles in a pet shop to harbor *Salmonella* and *Arizona*.

Salmonellosis is usually asymptomatic in reptiles, the animal acting as a carrier. Turtles may carry the infection asymptomatically for at least 12 months (Kaufmann *et al.*, 1967). Rarely, reptiles suffer enteritis or septicemia with necrotic foci in the liver and other viscera. Sick animals might have diarrhea, anorexia and listlessness. Differential diagnosis would include amebiasis, gastrointestinal helminthiasis, chemical intoxication and septicemia by *Aeromonas hydrophila* (Marcus, 1971). Specific diagnosis of salmonellosis in the individual live animal is only possible on the basis of positive cultures from stool, cloacal swab or blood. On postmortem examination, cultures should be taken of lesions, blood, bile, intestinal contents and the female reproductive tract. To determine the presence of *Salmonella* in a group of animals kept together, water from their enclosure should be sampled.

Because the organisms are so common and the public health hazard so great, it would seem prudent to culture the stool of any reptilian pet to determine if it is a *Salmonella* carrier. For various technical reasons a single culture may fail to reveal the organisms, the most important being that *Salmonella* excretion rate is variable, and a turtle that is a heavy shedder one time may have a negative stool culture the next (Kaufmann *et al.*, 1967). Therefore the sanitary precautions outlined below must be maintained in caring for reptiles. Although there is considerable variation in pathogenicity of different serotypes for different host species, any *Salmonella* or *Arizona* serotype found should be considered a potential human pathogen.

Definitive, controlled studies on the efficacy of antibiotic treatment of *Salmonella* infections in reptiles have not been published. In a limited study, 200 mg. of neomycin sulfate per 5 gallons of tank water kept at 29.5° C. (85° F.) for four days seemingly eliminated enteric *Salmonella* in three asymptomatic turtles. Two other turtles whose water temperature was not controlled required four more days with twice the above concentration of neomycin to eliminate the infection (Thorson, 1974). In another study, apparent elimination of *Sal-*

*monella* from the gut (on the basis of three successive negative stool cultures) was achieved in tortoises by treating them with 50 mg. of oxytetracycline orally daily for six days (Weber, 1973).

In man it is often difficult to eliminate the carrier state, especially with *S. typhi*, which may require cholecystectomy, since typhoid organisms residing in the gallbladder may not be susceptible to chemotherapy. *Salmonella* have been isolated from the biliary tract of turtles (Kaufmann and Morrison, 1966) but it is self-evident that cholecystectomy in these animals is not a practical approach to the problem. Unless one were prepared to do very carefully controlled studies with adequate precautions guarding human health, it would seem more advisable to kill rather than treat infected reptiles. If any attempt is made to treat salmonellosis in pet reptiles, the veterinarian is obligated to warn the owner of the hazard to human health and to give advice on proper isolation of the animal and the hygienic precautions to be taken, including sanitary disposal of feces, disinfecting potential fomites and thorough washing of hands after handling the animal or its cage. Small children should not be permitted to handle reptiles, their cages or items contaminated with their stool unless their hands can be washed by an adult immediately afterward. Herpetofauna and their containers should neither be held nor washed in the kitchen sink or otherwise brought into contact with areas where human food is kept.

Based on data available on other species, chloramphenicol or ampicillin is the drug of choice for systemic (extraintestinal) salmonellosis. In man, antibiotic treatment for enteric salmonellosis prolongs the period of shedding organisms in the stool. Therefore, human *Salmonella* enteritis is usually treated symptomatically, e.g., with fluid therapy. If reptile carriers are treated with antibiotics, several stool cultures should be taken, at least up to several weeks after cessation of treatment, to be sure that the infection is eliminated. As explained above, one negative stool culture cannot be considered definitive.

Reinfection can occur via food items such as rats and mice fed to snakes. Packaged turtle foods, commonly found in pet stores, have not been found to contain *Salmonella* and, if nutritionally balanced (many are not), are a suitable diet for pet turtles.

Numerous case reports and epi-demiologic studies have proved that reptiles, especially baby fresh-water turtles, are a major source of human salmonellosis, especially in children (Altman *et al.*, 1972). It was estimated that 14 per cent, or 280,000, of the approximately 2 million human cases of salmonellosis occurring yearly (1970, 1971) in the United States were contracted from turtles (Lamm *et al.*, 1972). Attempts to control the problem by testing turtles for *Salmonella* failed, and numerous human infections were traced to turtles certified as "*Salmonella*-free." Therefore, the Food and Drug Administration has ruled that it is illegal to sell viable turtle eggs or live turtles with a carapace length less than four inches in the United States (Federal Register, 1975). (Marine turtles are excepted from this law, because they have not been demonstrated to be a significant reservoir of *Salmonella*. Sale of these sea animals should be restricted, however, because they are endangered species which do not reproduce in captivity. Viable turtle eggs and baby turtles sold for "bona fide scientific, educational, or exhibitional purposes" are also exempted from this federal law.)

## SUPPLEMENTAL READING

Altman, R., Gorman, J. C., Bernhardt, L. L., and Goldfield, M.: Turtle-associated salmonellosis. II. The relationship of pet turtles to salmonellosis in children in New Jersey. Am. J. Epidemiol., 95:518–520, 1972.

Anonymous: Ban on sale and distribution of small turtles, Federal Register, 40:22543–22546, 1975.

Baker, E. F., Anderson, H. W., and Allard, J.: Epidemiological aspects of turtle-associated salmonellosis. Arch. Environ. Health, 24:1–9, 1972.

Feeley, J. C., and Treger, M. D.: Penetration of turtle eggs by *Salmonella braenderup*. Pub. Health Rep., 84:156–158, 1969.

Kaufmann, A. F., and Morrison, Z. L.: An epidemiologic study of salmonellosis in turtles. Am. J. Epidemiol., 84:364–370, 1966.

Kaufmann, A. F., Feeley, J. C., and DeWitt, W. E.: *Salmonella* excretion by turtles. Pub. Health Rep., 82:840–842, 1967.

Kaufmann, A. F., Fox, M. D., Morris, G. K., Wood, B. T., Feeley, J. C., and Frix, M. K.: Turtle-associated salmonellosis. III. The effects of environmental Salmonellae in commercial turtle breeding ponds. Am. J. Epidemiol. 95:521–528, 1972.

Lamm, S. H., Taylor, A., Gangarosa, E. J., Anderson, H. W., Young, W., Clark, M. H., and Bruce, A. R.: Turtle-associated salmonellosis. I. An estimation of the magnitude of the problem in the United States, 1970–1971. Am. J. Epidemiol., 95:511–517, 1972.

Marcus, L. C.: Infectious diseases of reptiles. J. Am. Vet. Med. Assn., 159:1626–1631, 1971.

Thorson, T. E.: Salmonellosis in pet turtles. Modern Vet. Pract., 55:31–32, 1974.

Weber, A.: Therapeutic trial in tortoises with latent *Salmonella* infections. Kleintier-Praxis, 18:48–50, 1973.

# PARASITIC DISEASES OF CAPTIVE REPTILES

LEONARD C. MARCUS, V.M.D.

*Boston, Massachusetts*

Reptiles are host to a great variety of protozoan and metazoan parasites. If the enteric protozoa are included, virtually 100 per cent of reptiles in the wild harbor some kind of parasite. The parasitic population is often very dense and every body surface and tissue can be invaded by a parasite of some kind. Many of these parasites, e.g., most of the intestinal ciliates and flagellates, are commensal or, at least, not obviously pathogenic. It is often problematic to relate the presence of given parasites to specific disease problems. This discussion will emphasize those parasites that have been proved pathogenic in reptiles but will also deal briefly with some common parasites of little pathogenic significance. Further information on reptilian parasites can be gathered from the text of Reichenbach-Klinke and Elkan (1965), from the chapter by Kaplan (1973), from references cited below and from bibliographies in these sources.

Stresses of captivity such as inadequate space, heat or light, inappropriate or inadequate diet and concurrent illness can disrupt usual host-parasite relationships and result in disease. In general, it is those parasites with a direct life cycle that can increase disproportionately and produce the greatest morbidity and mortality in captive specimens. If reptiles are fed exclusively on laboratory or homebred feed items (rats, mice, mealworms, etc.), it is not likely that they will contract parasites with indirect life cycles because of the nonavailability of suitable intermediate hosts.

A specific diagnosis of a particular parasite can only be made by identifying the parasite or its egg. There are very few reptilian parasites that cause pathognomonic signs or lesions that would permit definitive diagnosis on clinical or pathologic grounds alone. In general, a severely parasitized reptile shows decreased activity, progressive weight loss and anorexia. These are nonspecific signs that can be seen in other disease entities (Marcus, 1968).

## PROTOZOAN DISEASES

**Amebiasis.** Several species of amebae are found in reptiles, but the only one recognized as a common and significant pathogen is *Entamoeba invadens*. This organism can cause explosive epizootics or smouldering enzootic disease in a reptile collection, with high mortality in snakes and, to a lesser extent, in lizards.

Amebiasis may be characterized by the nonspecific signs of parasitism referred to above, or may present with rapidly progressive dehydration due to severe enteritis and diarrhea. With amebic infection of the stomach, there may also be fluid loss through vomiting. The vomitus and stools usually contain blood which is often grossly visible, though in early or mild cases it may only be detectable chemically (guaiac test). The case fatality rate in susceptible animals usually approaches 100 per cent.

Snakes and lizards become infected by ingestion of amebic cysts which are passed in the stools of other infected reptiles. The mature cyst of *E. invadens* is tetranucleate and gives rise to four trophozoites by excystation in the gut. The trophozoites, which move by extension of pseudopodia, invade the gastrointestinal mucosa and multiply by binary fission. Together with enteric bacteria they cause progressive ulceration of the gut. The amebae commonly invade the blood stream and metastasize to distant organs where they may be found on histopathologic examination, with or without accompanying necrosis and inflammation. As in human amebiasis, the most common extraintestinal lesions are found in the liver, where there may be diffuse inflammation (amebic hepatitis) or, more commonly, focal necrosis (amebic abscess).

The life cycle is completed when trophozoites in the gut encyst, and the cysts, which are the infective form, are passed in the stool. Trophozoites, which are the invasive form, may also be passed in the stool, but do not survive very long in the external environment. Definitive diagnosis depends on finding cysts or trophozoites in the stool.

As in human amebiasis, disease in reptiles is associated with the presence of massive numbers of trophozoites. A patient, human or reptile, passing cysts, but having few or no trophozoites in the stool, is likely to be a chronic carrier without overt disease, unless something happens to upset the balance and trophozoites become predominant. It has been suggested that the cyst form is favored by the presence of starch and, therefore, turtles whose diet consists of vegetable matter are likely to be chronic carriers and act as a source of infection for other reptiles (Meerovitch, 1958). It has also been suggested that there may be different strains of amebae from different geographic areas and, when snakes from different parts of the country or world are put together in a collection, they are exposed to virulent strains (Telford, 1971).

Prevention of amebiasis depends on adequate quarantine procedures before introducing new animals to a collection, appropriate separation of host species and adequate sanitation or disinfection of cages and cleaning utensils to prevent fecal contamination between cages.

I am not aware of any rigorous, well controlled studies to determine the efficacy or hazards of various forms of treatment of amebiasis in reptiles. Diloxanide (Entamide®) at a daily dosage of 500 mg./kg. of body weight, given orally, is reported to be effective. Paromomycin (Humatin®, Parke, Davis), 25 to 100 mg./kg. per day for 4 weeks is also effective, but it is expensive. Oral tetracyclines, iodochlorhydroxyquin (Entero-Vioform®, Ciba), diiodohydroxyquin (Diodoquin®, Searle) and emetine hydrochloride have also been recommended. Emetine hydrochloride is a parenteral drug and is especially effective against extraintestinal lesions; the other agents are given orally and their effectiveness is limited to enteric lesions. Metronidazole (Flagyl®, Searle), given orally, is now the drug of choice for both enteric and extraintestinal amebiasis in man and has been proved effective at 200 mg./kg. body weight in reptiles. Since so little is known about drug dosages or effects in reptiles, I can only suggest that dosage rates recommended for man be used and then altered by empiric adjustments for proper therapeutic effects. *Entamoeba invadens* is not known to be infective for man.

**Coccidiosis.** Numerous species of coccidia have been found in the gut and gallbladder of various reptiles, and one coccidian species (*Klossiella boae*) has been found in the kidney of a boa constrictor. Most of these infections are not thought to be clinically significant, although this question may not have been adequately studied. Histologically, there is evidence of epithelial destruction in the gut and gallbladder associated with at least some coccidian infections in reptiles. Coccidiosis in reptiles responds to sulfa drugs and to some coccidiostats used in poultry.

**Blood-Borne Protozoa.** Routine examination of reptilian blood films commonly reveals the presence of trypanosomes in the plasma or malarial organisms (*Plasmodium* spp.) in the red blood cells. Other common intraerythrocytic sporozoa include *Hemoproteus* and *Schellackia* spp. and the hemogregarines (*Hemogregarina, Hepatozoon* and *Karyolysus* spp.). All of these hematozoa have no known clinical significance and, at least in North America, no known public health or agricultural significance.

All of these blood-borne protozoa are transmitted by certain insects, mites or leeches. In the absence of these intermediate hosts, transmission cannot occur in captivity.

## CESTODES

Adult tapeworms are commonly found in the gut of many reptiles, and larval forms are not unusual in reptilian muscles and viscera. The adult cestodes compete with the host for absorption of nutrients but, if the diet is adequate, there is food enough for both and the host does not suffer overtly. Certain larval cestodes, particularly the larvae of Pseudophyllidean tapeworms (spargana), can cause tissue damage in their migration, the nature and severity of clinical signs depending on their numbers, location and host resistance.

The presence of adult tapeworms in the gut can be diagnosed by finding segments or eggs in the stool. Sparganosis may be suspected when subcutaneous or intramuscular lumps are palpated. If the larvae are actively migrating, the location of these lesions will change with movement of the worm. The most common cause of subcutaneous nodules in reptiles is abscesses (Marcus, 1971), and differential diagnosis also includes tumors, geotrichosis, myiasis, mycobacterial infections and filariasis. Visceral sparganosis is unlikely to be diagnosed ante mortem.

Adult tapeworms in reptiles can be treated with dichlorophen (Anthophen®) (Jackson, 1972). Spargana and other larval cestodes can be surgically excised.

## TREMATODES

It is very common to find adult flukes in the alimentary tract and larval trematodes in various tissues of reptiles. Renifers are a group of flukes often found in the mouth of certain snakes, e.g., indigo snakes (*Drymarchon corais cooperi*) and king snakes (*Lampropeltis* spp.). These flatworms often move down the esophagus when they are exposed to light when the snake's mouth is opened. Diagnosis of other flukes residing in the gastrointestinal tract, biliary system or lungs depends on finding operculate eggs in the stool. The eggs of certain flukes which live in the urinary tract may be found in the urinary component of the droppings. Larval trematodes are usually incidental postmortem findings.

Unless they are present in unusually large numbers or have migrated out of their usual site, adult flukes generally cause no obvious problems in reptiles. The same is true of most larval forms, but some larval flukes, e.g., *Alaria* spp., can cause severe necrosis and inflammation in their migratory path through tissues and can probably cause some debility.

Most drugs effective against flukes are fairly toxic. Since most trematode infections of reptiles are asymptomatic, they are best left untreated.

All digenetic flukes, which include all the trematodes of man, domestic birds and mammals, and a great majority of reptilian flukes have complex life cycles with at least one and usually two or more intermediate hosts; thus, transmission in captivity is unlikely unless the reptiles are being fed wild caught prey, e.g., frogs (including frogs bought from dealers, since these are originally caught in the wild).

## ACANTHOCEPHALA

The larvae of thorny-headed worms are occasionally found in the abdomen or subcutis of terrestrial reptiles. No specific signs have been associated with such infections; they are not likely to be diagnosed clinically and no specific treatment is known. The larvae are acquired by ingestion of arthropod intermediate hosts.

Adult thorny-headed worms are found in the small intestine of certain aquatic turtles which have become infected by eating specific snail intermediate hosts. These adult worms can cause nodular granulomas of the intestinal wall at the site of attachment and can also cause intestinal perforation. Diagnosis of infection can be made by finding the characteristic thick-shelled oval eggs containing rostellar hooklets (these eggs can be differentiated from Cyclophyllidean tapeworm eggs which also contain hooklets, but are round). Chemotherapy for acanthocephaliasis in turtles has not been studied, but therapeutic agents used for the analogous condition in swine could be tried.

## NEMATODES

Reptiles are host to a huge variety and number of nematodes, most of which inhabit the alimentary tract or lung. Only a few of the more common or clinically significant nematodes of reptiles can be mentioned here.

Ascarids are found in many reptiles, the best known being *Ophidascaris* spp. in snakes (Sprent, 1970). These are large, stout-bodied worms which are transmitted via intermediate hosts such as frogs or rodents. The fourth stage larvae of some *Ophidascaris* species congregate in the stomach where a mass of these worms may be found with their heads imbedded in a focal area of the gastric mucosa, the bodies of the tightly grouped worms extending into the lumen like Medusa's head. The adult worms are usually found in the small intestine. It is likely that heavy infection with these ascarids can cause some debility in the host.

Diagnosis of ascariasis depends on identification of the characteristic round, thick-shelled eggs, which bear close enough resemblance to ascarid eggs commonly passed by dogs, cats or pigs that they are readily identified. Occasionally, an intact ascarid may be vomited or defecated.

Ascarids in reptiles can be treated with 2,2 dichlorvinyl dimethyl phosphate (DDVP) (Atgard V®), using one oral dose of 24 mg./kg. of body weight (Dobbs, personal communication). Treatment can be repeated in a week, if necessary. An alternative treatment is thiabendazole, 100 mg./kg., *per os*.

*Kalicephalus* is a genus of hookworm-like nematodes parasitic in snakes. Depending on the species, these worms can be found anywhere in the alimentary tract from the esophagus to the rectum. Their presence has been associated with hemorrhagic ulcers of the gastrointestinal tract, so it is probable that in some cases, at least, these worms can be significant pathogens.

*Kalicephalus* infections can be diagnosed by demonstrating the thin-walled, transparent oval eggs in the stool or in swabs of the esophagus. The eggs are in the morula stage when laid, but may contain the first stage larva, or the larva may have hatched by the time the egg has been defecated.

The life cycle of *Kalicephalus* apparently is direct, infection occuring by ingestion of infective larvae. Percutaneous penetration by the larvae, as in mammalian hookworm infection, is also thought to be possible. This is a parasite that can increase in captive reptiles. Prevention depends on adequate removal of stools from cages and prevention of fecal contamination in the cages. Treatment for *Kalicephalus* is thiabendazole, 100 mg./kg., *per os* (Cooper, 1971).

Lungworms (*Rhabdias fuscovenosa*) have been reported in certain water snakes (*Natrix natrix, N. tessellata*) and garter snakes (*Thamnophis sirtalis*), and infection apparently can cause respiratory distress in these animals. A major differential diagnosis would be bacterial pneumonia. Diagnosis of lungworm is based on finding the larvae in the stool. Recommended treatment is tetramisole (Ripercol®), 10 mg./kg., given in-trapleuroperitoneally (since snakes have no diaphragm, there is one body cavity) (Zwart, 1969).

Oxyurids are among the most common and numerous intestinal helminths of lizards and turtles. Like their counterparts, *Enterobius vermicularis* in man, *Passaleuris ambiguus* in the rabbit and *Oxyuris equi* in the horse, these pinworms usually live in the lower gastrointestinal tract and usually produce no obvious disease. They are occasionally passed as intact adults in the stool and they can also be diagnosed by finding their eggs in the stool. In some species, the eggs are oval with one flattened side, as is the situation with the mammalian pinworms referred to above. Oxyurid life cycles are direct. No treatment is indicated for reptilian pinworms.

Filarial worms are found in snakes, lizards and crocodilians. Depending on the species, adult worms may be in major vessels or connective tissue, e.g., the subcutis. In large numbers, especially in abnormal hosts, blood and lymphatic vessels may be occluded, resulting in edema and necrosis of the area supplied by the thrombosed vessel. Severe, necrotic dermal lesions due to the filaria *Macdonaldius oschei* have been described in captive pythons.

As in mammalian filariasis, diagnosis is made by finding the microfilariae in the blood or finding adult filariae or microfilariae in lesions. Prevention of filariasis depends on elimination of blood-sucking arthropods, e.g., ticks and mosquitoes. Chemotherapy for reptilian filariasis has not been reported, to our knowledge, but agents used for analogous veterinary and medical conditions could be tried, e.g., diethylcarbamazine. It has been reported that adult *M. oschei* in boa constrictors (*Constrictor constrictor mexicanus*) can be killed by keeping the snakes at a constant ambient temperature of 35° to 37° C. for 24 to 48 hours (Telford, 1965).

## PENTASTOMES

Pentastomes are a phylum of parasites which show some of the characteristics of arthropods and annelid worms. The great majority of pentastome species are found in reptiles at some stage of their life cycle, the adult form being the stage most commonly seen in dissection of reptilian hosts.

For those pentastomes which we will deal with here, the life cycle pattern is as follows: The adult worm, which often has a characteristic series of annular thickenings around its body, resides in the respiratory tract (usually the lungs) of snakes, lizards or crocodilians (a few species are found in turtles). Eggs are deposited containing the primary larva which may have four leg-like appendages, giving it a superficial resemblance to a mite. The eggs are brought up in the sputum, passed in the stool, develop to an infective stage and are swallowed by a suitable intermediate host, e.g., rodent, primate or ungulate. Man may accidentally enter the cycle at this stage (see below). The larvae develop into infective nymphs in the mesentery, liver and other tissues of the intermediate host and develop into adults in the reptilian respiratory tract after the intermediate host is swallowed by the definitive reptilian host.

Pentastomes have a great capacity to bore through tissue and, on occasion, adult worms may bore through the lung and body wall and protrude from the skin. They have also been seen to emerge from the mouth of snakes. Pentastomes often occur in great numbers, both as adults in the definitive host and as larvae and nymphs in intermediate hosts, yet, despite their numbers and their capacity to migrate through tissue, most pentastome infections (larval and adult) are asymptomatic. In some cases, however, there may be significant damage to the reptilian host, e.g., by direct destruction of tissue or by occlusion of the trachea.

Examples of common adult pentastomes in reptiles include *Armillifer armillatus* in African pythons and vipers, *Porocephalus crotali* in the cottonmouth moccasin *(Agkistrodon piscivorus)* and North American rattlesnakes *(Crotalus* spp.) and *Kiricephalus* spp. in colubrid snakes (including many of the nonpoisonous snakes of the United States) and *Sebakia* spp. in crocodilians. *Armillifer armillatus* commonly uses primates, rodents and small antelopes as intermediate hosts, and man is commonly an accidental host in Africa. Despite the fact that the great majority of human infections are asymptomatic, appropriate sanitary precautions should be taken to prevent ingestion of eggs in the event someone has an infected snake.

There is no known effective treatment for pentastomiasis in reptiles. An extensive review and bibliography of the Pentastomida has been published (Self, 1969).

## LEECHES

Leeches are common ectoparasites on aquatic reptiles, and, in our experience, are especially common in turtles. After these blood suckers feed to repletion, they drop off the host, so they are not commonly seen in captive reptiles. Adequate quarantine procedures before introducing new specimens in a collection should effectively prevent these worms from becoming established in such potentially suitable environments as a turtle pond in a zoo.

Leeches should not simply be pulled off, as this may traumatize the host's skin or leave the mouthparts imbedded in the host. Topical application of concentrated salt solutions, alcohol or vinegar can encourage the leech to release its hold. Many of the leeches that attack reptiles are not very host-specific and may attack man and other animals, and the same treatment to remove the leeches can be used on these hosts.

Leeches can act as intermediate hosts for hemogregarines in turtles (see p. 802).

## DIPTERA

In the wild, reptiles are commonly attacked by mosquitoes and biting flies. This may have agricultural and public health significance, since reptiles may be a significant reservoir for such arthropod-borne diseases as eastern and western encephalitis and Japanese B encephalitis. Some of the flies and mosquitoes that attack reptiles will also bite birds and mammals, including man.

Myiasis is a common problem of tortoises in the wild, and it is not unusual for someone to present a box turtle *(Terrapene carolina)* with maggots under its skin. These can be surgically excised.

## MITES

A number of mites commonly infect reptiles, the best known being the snake mite, *Ophionyssus natricis (serpentium)*. This mite, which can be seen as a tiny gray dot moving between and under the scales of snakes (and, less commonly, lizards), especially in the areas of the chin, eye and cloaca, is a serious pathogen. Under unsanitary conditions in captivity, the mite population can increase enormously and heavily infested reptiles become debilitated through blood loss. In addition, these mites transmit *Aeromonas hydrophila*, a gram-negative rod that causes pneumonia and hemorrhagic septicemia in reptiles.

Infestation with mites can be treated topically with 4% ammonium fluorosilicate powder (Dri-Die SG67, Davidson, National Biocide), which dehydrates the mites. This powder should be used with caution on very small reptiles, because it can also have a dehydrating effect on them. Hanging DDVP-impregnated fly strips (Vapona®, Shell) reportedly eliminates the mites in time, but in my experience such compounds can be toxic to small reptiles. When we placed a 3-inch piece of a cat flea collar, which contains the same organic phosphate as the fly strip, in a cage with some anole lizards (*Anolis carolinensis*), the lizards rapidly developed a progressive, generalized flaccid paralysis which could be reversed by removing the insecticide strips. Two agents which reportedly are highly effective and safe are Ortho Dibrom 8-E (California Chemical) using 2 to 4 ml./gallon of water, and Diazinon 25E (Geigy) diluted at least 1:480 in water; both agents are used as sprays and can be reapplied, if needed, in two to four weeks (Camin *et al.*, 1964).

Reptiles can be treated with one of the above agents before they are introduced into a collection to prevent infestation of the other specimens. Sanitary measures that will help reduce mite populations include removing shed skins, pieces of bark and other items in the cage where the mites can hide.

Chiggers are six-legged larvae of Trombiculid mites which rather indiscriminately parasitize the skin of reptiles, birds and mammals, including man. The eight-legged nymphs and adults are free-living, feeding on other small arthropods and their eggs. Chiggers have been given the colloquial name "red bugs" and in heavy infestations, which can be debilitating, clumps of these larval mites are grossly apparent as red spots on the host's skin. They often prefer to attach at skin folds, e.g., axilla and hip. Because the free-living nymphs and adults do not readily survive indoors, infestation with chiggers is usually limited to newly arrived specimens. In light infestations, chiggers can be individually picked off with very fine forceps, taking care to remove the imbed-

ded mouthparts and swabbing the site of attachment with an antiseptic. In heavy infestations, one of the treatments for mites, described above, can be used.

Ticks are commonly found on terrestrial reptiles. Like chiggers, these ectoparasites most often attach to body folds, although in one instance we saw a tick with its mouthparts imbedded in the carapace of an African tortoise. Ticks are blood suckers but are rarely present in sufficient numbers to cause significant blood loss. Ticks may be vectors of certain blood parasites. More important, however, is the fact that some ticks which parasitize reptiles will also feed on mammals. Therefore, all exotic reptiles should be examined and treated for ticks because of the potential hazard of importing foreign diseases of man or domestic animals with these vectors. Ticks can be removed manually, taking care not to leave the mouthparts imbedded in the skin.

## SUPPLEMENTAL READING

Camin, J. H., Clarke, G. K., Goodson, L. H., and Shuyler, H. R.: Control of the snake mite, *Ophionyssus natricis* (Gervais), in captive reptile collections. Zoologica, 49:65–79, 1964.

Cooper, J. E.: Disease in East African snakes associated with Kalicephalus worms (Nematoda: Diaphanocephalidae). Vet. Rec., 89:385–388, 1971.

Dobbs, J. S., and Vandeford, A. D.: Personal communication.

Jackson, O. F.: Helminth infestation in snakes. Vet. Rec., 90:51, 1972.

Kaplan, H. M.: Parasites of laboratory reptiles and amphibians. *In* Flynn, R. J.: Parasites of Laboratory Animals. Iowa State University Press (Ames), 1973, pp. 507–644.

Marcus, L. C.: Diseases of snakes and turtles. *In* Kirk, R. W. (ed.): Current Veterinary Therapy III. Philadelphia, W. B. Saunders Co., 1968, pp. 435–442.

Marcus, L. C.: Infectious diseases of reptiles. J. Am. Vet. Med. Assn., 159:1626–1631, 1971.

Meerovitch, E.: Some biological requirements and host-parasite relations of *Entameba invadens*. Canad. J. Zool., 36:513–523, 1958.

Reichenbach-Klinke, H., and Elkan, E.: The Principal Diseases of Lower Vertebrates. New York, Academic Press, 1965.

Self, J. T.: Parasitological reviews. Biological relationships of the Pentastomida: a bibliography on the Pentastomida. Exper. Parasitol., 24:63–119, 1969.

Sprent, J. F. A.: Studies on ascaridoid nematodes in pythons: the life history and development of *Ophidascaris moreliae* in Australian pythons. Parasitology, 60:97–122, 1970.

Telford, S. F., Jr.: Some observations on the effects of varying ambient temperature in vivo on filarial worms of snakes. Jap. J. Exper. Med., 35:291–300, 1965.

Telford, S. R., Jr.: Parasitic diseases of reptiles. J. Am. Vet. Med. Assn., 159:1644–1652, 1971.

Zwart, P., and Jensen, J.: Treatment of lungworm in snakes with tetramisole. Vet. Rec., 84:374, 1969.

# ANESTHESIA OF REPTILES

JOEL D. WALLACH, D.V.M.
*Douglasville, Georgia*

There are a variety of anesthetic alternatives available to the clinician restraining or performing surgery on reptiles. A basic consideration that the clinician must appreciate is the primitive homeostatic mechanism possessed by reptiles. Because of the varied metabolic pathways, reptiles are more tolerant of short-term changes in their internal environment than mammals and birds. Reptiles have also developed a variety of respiratory adaptations associated with their physical shape and their environmental niches. Reptiles lack a functional diaphragm; most snakes have only one lung; the primary muscles of respiration in the turtle are those of the limbs. Some species of turtle can change from aerobic to anaerobic metabolic pathways and survive atmospheres of 100 per cent nitrogen for periods over 24 hours long. Diving reptiles can breath-hold for over four hours. Such respiratory adaptations directly affect the induction and recovery rates of reptiles anesthetized with inhalant anesthetic agents.

Manual restraint supplemented with local infiltration of 2 per cent xylocaine hydrochloride (Xylocaine®, Astra) around the surgical site is perhaps the least complicated method of making analgesia available to the reptilian patient. This technique is satisfactory for removing neoplasms and bacterial and foreign-body granulomas, suturing lacerations and for other minor surgical procedures.

Hypothermia has been used extensively for restraining reptiles during surgery. It is thought that hypothermia also imparts some degree of anesthesia. Hypothermic restraint and anesthesia is induced by placing the reptile patient in a refrigerator set for 5° C. for two hours. The effective level of hypothermic restraint is maintained during surgery by placing the animal in a tray of ice water. The reptile's unique metabolic pattern allows rapid recovery from hypothermic immobilization following rewarming to room temperatures.

The use of electroanesthesia has been reported in the green iguana. Both low and high frequency sine waves were used simultaneously. Bitemporal electrode placement was employed. The anesthetic period lasts for 35 to 75 minutes. Rapid induction and recovery are assets for use of this technique in reptiles.

**Injectable Agents.** Succinylcholine chloride (Anectine®, Burroughs Wellcome) will produce complete skeletal relaxation in four minutes when given to alligators at the rate of 1.35 to 2.25 mg./lb. (0.45 kg.) of body weight. Recovery will take place in seven to nine hours. Nicotine alkaloid (Cap-Chur-Sol®, Palmer Chemical and Equipment Co.) used at the rate of 0.23 to 1.35 mg./lb. (0.45 kg.) of body weight produces tonic-clonic convulsions in alligators; consequently, it does not provide satisfactory immobilization.

The immobilizing and analgesic qualities of the opium derivative, M-99 (Etorphine®, D-M Pharmaceuticals), have been used to advantage for crocodilians, turtles, tortoises and snakes for clinical and surgical procedures, including thyroidectomy and surgical removal of neoplasms. Crocodilians ranging in body weight from 0.5 to 129 lb. (9.23 to 58.56 kg.) received 0.05 to 20 mg. M-99. Turtles averaging about 4 lb. (1.82 kg.) body weight received 0.5 to 5.0 mg. M-99. Galapagos tortoises ranging in weight from 100 to 138 lb. (45.40 to 62.65 kg.) were given 10.0 to 15.0 mg. M-99. A variety of snakes received from 2.0 to 15.0 mg.

Intramuscular administration of M-99 was used for the crocodilians. Intraperitoneal administration shortened the induction time, but did not alter the total effect. For snakes, the agent was administered via the pleuroperitoneal cavity in the posterior third of the body on the ventral midline. For turtles and tortoises, the intramuscular route gives satisfactory immobilization and analgesia. The induction periods ranged from two minutes to 20 minutes, resulting in 30 to 180 minutes of effect. Recovery was apparent in a few hours.

Injectable anesthesia has been in use for some time for reptiles. Thiopental sodium (Pentothal sodium®, Abbott) administered at the rate of 0.016 to 0.025 mg./gm. of body weight of snake in the pleuroperitoneal cavity results in the loss of the righting reflex and a light plane of anesthesia lasting from 25 to 45 minutes. Pentobarbital sodium (Nembutal sodium®, Abbott) administered at the rate of 0.015 to 0.050 mg./gm. of body weight of snake had results similar to that obtained with the thiopental sodium. Pentobarbital sodium administered to tortoises at the rate of 18.2 mg./kg. of body weight reportedly produces reliable deep anesthesia for two to four hours. This is the drug of choice for tortoises that are cachectic. Sodium pentobarbital (Cap-Chur-Barb®, Palmer Chemical and Equipment Co.) tranquilizes American alligators when administered intramuscularly at the rate of 3.5 to 4.0 mg./lb. (0.45 kg.) of body weight; recovery takes place in two to three hours.

Tricaine methanesulfonate (Finguel®) administered to snakes at the rate of 0.178 to 0.272 mg./gm. of body weight gives a light plane of anesthesia similar to the two aforementioned agents. This product produces complete muscular relaxation in American alligators in 10 minutes after intramuscular administration at the rate of 40.0 to 45.0 mg./lb. (0.45 kg.) of body weight; recovery occurs in 9 to 10 hours.

Phencyclidine hydrochloride (Sernylan®, Parke, Davis) produces immobilization in the American alligator after a 50- to 60-minute induction period when given at the rate of 5.0 to 10.0 mg./lb. (0.45 kg.). Its effects last for six to seven hours.

A sister compound to phencyclidine is ketamine HCL-CI 581 (Ketalar®, Parke, Davis). When administered intramuscularly to reptiles at the rate of 10 to 40 mg./lb. (0.45 kg.), this compound will produce a series of effects ranging from tranquilization to deep anesthesia. Induction occurs in approximately 30 minutes; drug effects at standard doses last from 6 to 10 hours with total recovery in 24 hours. Ketamine HCL-CI 581 produces excessively long recovery rate and may produce respiratory arrest at doses of 45 to 60 mg./lb.

Tribromoethanol (TBE) (Avertin®) is another anesthetic drug of choice in debilitated tortoises. This may be administered intraperitoneally at the rate of 250 mg./kg. of body weight together with 125 mg. amylene hydrate (AH)/kg. of body weight. The induction period ranges from 40 to 70 minutes. Deep anesthesia persists for one to two hours, followed by postanesthetic depression for an additional 12 to 16 hours. This anesthetic may also be administered per rectum at the rate of 400 mg. TBE and 200 mg. AH/kg. of body weight. The induction period to deep anesthesia is one to two hours. Deep planes of anesthesia are maintained for 1.0 to 1.5 hours, followed by depression for 6.0 to 9.0 hours.

## INHALANT ANESTHESIA

Inhalant anesthesia is currently being used with success in reptiles. Probably the agent most universally employed is halothane, which has the advantage of rapid induction and recovery. Induction periods of less than 10 minues are average, and surgical anesthesia lasting up to 20 minutes can be induced by a single exposure to the vapors.

Halothane is administered by absorbing 5 ml. of the liquid into a gauze sponge and then placing it in a shallow box with a sliding transparent lid. Two or three respiratory exchanges at room temperature are sufficient to induce anesthesia. Turtles' response to inhalant anesthesia is variable, since they may hold their breath for a considerable length of time. Turtles are more resistant to anoxia than are snakes and crocodilians. Induction periods with ether may last up to three hours.

More sophisticated techniques for inhalation anesthesia include the use of endotracheal tubes and gas machines. Semi-open (Ayer's "Y" Piece) and nonrebreathing systems are suggested for reptiles weighing less than 5 kg. The flow of gas must be high enough to flush out the reservoir tube during the exhalation pause; this flow is at least two times greater than that for mammals, and for most reptiles ranges between 300 and 500 ml./minute.

Reptiles present an anesthetic picture sufficiently different from that of mammals to warrant some voluntary practice on animals procured for that purpose.

### SUPPLEMENTAL READING

Calderwood, H. W.: Anesthesia for reptiles. J. Am. Vet. Med. Assn., *159*:1618–1625, 1972.

Glenn, J. C., Straight, R., and Snyder, C. C.: The clinical use of dl 2-(o-chlorophenyl)-2-(methylamino) cyclohexanone hydrochloride (Ketamine HCL-CI 581) as an anesthetic agent for snakes. Am. J. Vet. Res., 33:1901–1903, 1972.

Wallach, J. D.: Medical care of reptiles. J. Am. Vet. Med. Assn., *155*:1017–1034, 1969.

# SURGERY IN CAPTIVE REPTILES

FREDRIC L. FRYE, D.V.M.
*Berkeley, California*

*"The most useful equipment for a successful surgeon is a pessimistic pathologist."*
JOHN ROWAN WILSON
(1919– )

## INTRODUCTION

With the quantum increase in the interest and expertise in clinical exotic animal practice has come the concomitant development of operative techniques applicable to poikilothermic animals, especially reptiles.

This discussion will cover the more frequently encountered surgical conditions and how they may be resolved practically using familiar current veterinary surgical methods. The only special item required to accomplish these aims is the surgeon's interest.

In order to be successful in reptile surgery, as in any other surgical endeavor, strict attention must be paid to sterile technique. **There is absolutely no excuse for nonsterile surgery.** There are those clinicians who think nothing of breaking sterile protocol because their particular patients are considered to be immune to asepsis. Pre- and postsurgical antibiotic therapy is no substitute for sterile technique. This applies to all types of surgery, except of course abscess incision and drainage.

## INSTRUMENTS

The instruments employed in reptilian surgery are sterilized in routine fashion. The patients are prepared as for any other surgical procedure with appropriate scrubbing and disinfecting methods. The actual surgical sites are draped as usual before surgery commences.

Specialized equipment *per se* usually is not required. We prefer to use small dental curettes and spatulas for the enucleation of the commonly inspissated abscess contents. Small cerumen loops are also useful, especially in removing the contents of infraorbital and periorbital abscesses; these loops are smooth and less likely to produce corneal or blepharic trauma. Five-inch, angled wire suture scissors with serrated jaws have many applications; they are particularly suited for the trimming of chelonians' overgrown external mouth parts. The Dremel Moto Tool®, with a variety of bits, wheels and circular saw blades, is very useful for a wide range of conditions, especially for trimming overgrown beaks of the larger turtles and tortoises. These devices can be purchased from most hardware and hobby stores for a relatively modest cost, and they are sterilized easily by appropriate ethylene oxide gas methods. The high-speed nitrogen Hall drill is employed for most actual hard-tissue surgery.

## SUTURE MATERIALS

Suture materials used are the same as those employed in other species. Chromic gut, Dexon® (polyglycolic acid), polyester Dacron (Mersilene® [Ethicon], Polydek®, Tycron®, etc.) and Vetefil® have all been used with success. In the very heavy crocodilians, the preferred suture material is monofilament stainless-steel wire carried on a very stout reverse-cutting needle, because it will withstand abrasion better than any other material. This is particularly important in the case of ventral incisions and those made in the palmar and plantar regions, which are subject to contact with rough surfaces.

## SUTURE PATTERN

The suture pattern employed in most reptilian surgery is at the discretion of the surgeon, but we prefer to use a simple interrupted pattern. Continuous sutures are used sometimes when inversion of the incised skin edges is less likely to occur—especially in chelonians and crocodilians. In snakes and lizards, however, great care must be exercised to produce a slightly *everting* skin closure; there is a natural tendency for the skin of snakes and lizards to roll inward at the edge. When suturing the skin of snakes and lizards, the suture needle is directed inward and outward, so as to create a slightly outward-facing skin closure.

In general, we prefer to start suturing in the middle of the incision and to work toward the two outer ends to help prevent puckering and therefore promote primary healing.

Upon the first ecdysis following suture removal, the surgical incision scar usually disappears with the old epidermis.

## SOME SURGICAL PROCEDURES

**Shell Repair.** Fractured chelonian shells are repaired by debriding and elevating the depressed and devascularized bone and shell fragments. Single or multiple patches of previously sterilized fiberglass cloth and Devco 5-Minute Epoxy Cement® are applied (see Frye, 1973a, for description of technique). Clear epoxy is preferred because it has a very rapid polymerization time, does not evolve a harmful amount of exothermic heat and is cosmetically acceptable. Other materials which have been used are the more slowly polymerizing expoxies and dental acrylics. Occasionally, interfragmentary wiring or plating may be necessary. The tensile strength of these fiberglass–epoxy resin prostheses and splints is excellent, and resistance to abrasion as the animal crawls is superior to the natural shell.

In the juvenile or still-growing individual, the patched areas overlying growth interfaces must be removed as soon as healing is complete to allow unimpeded growth. This healing can be ascertained by radiography. A rotary burr or similar instrument is used to remove the overlying fiberglass and epoxy resin. [A word of caution: there is every reason to believe that, like asbestos and gypsum particles, fiberglass-epoxy dusts may be carcinogenic when inhaled, ingested or left in contact with mucosa for prolonged periods. Therefore, the operator should be protected with an appropriate respiratory filtration mask and goggles or face mask.]

**Celiotomy.** When the coelomic cavity of a hard-shelled chelonian must be invaded surgically, a Hall drill with a cutting drill-burr fitted to the chuck is preferred. The actual surgical site is located just anterior to the ventral pelvic girdle; this can be visualized easily with radiography. A square portion of plastron is excised entirely; usually, a 6- to 10-cm. quadrilateral incision is adequate. Once excised, the piece is held in lactated Ringer's solution until replacement at the initiation of shell repair. (This technique is described elsewhere.)

A layer of epoxy resin is applied to the outside surface of the excised bone fragment in such a way that contact of the epoxy with the freshly incised edge surfaces is precluded. Temporary support of the fragment within the celiotomy void is afforded with two disposable needles placed into the cancellous bone at opposite ends of the flap or fragment. The round or oval piece of trimmed fiberglass cloth is now laid upon the freshly mixed epoxy resin; digital or mechanical "working in" of the resin into the interstices of the cloth is done to insure a thorough bond of the two materials.

Once polymerization has taken place, the bone flap is removed temporarily, the two disposable needles are withdrawn and the flap is set aside while the outer periphery of the incision site is dressed with freshly prepared resin. After resin has been applied carefully to the outer periphery of the incision site, the bone flap is replaced, and the skirt of raw fiberglass cloth is embedded in the epoxy resin just applied. The fiberglass is now treated (as described above) and additional resin is supplemented, as necessary, to complete the repair.

**Beak Trimming.** Occasionally, the mandibular, premaxillary or maxillary horny beak parts will split or be avulsed. A very suitable repair can be made with epoxy cement alone after thorough cleansing of the surrounding area with ether and alcohol before applying the cement. After a hard cure is achieved, the repair is dressed to match the natural mouth parts.

**Amputations.** When individual phalanges or entire digits require surgical removal, these amputations are best done at the appropriate palmar or plantar junctions, respectively. The patient is left with a stumpless and highly functional limb, and the cosmetic results are satisfactory.

When an entire limb must be sacrificed owing to irreparable tissue loss or neoplasia, it is preferable to remove the affected arm or leg at its respective scapulohumeral or coxofemoral articulation; this results in a totally stumpless postoperative effect. Again, the result is maximally comfortable and free from additional trauma.

If a tail must be shortened surgically, some judgment must be exercised as to whether the stump is to be sutured. In those lizards whose tails will regenerate, it is best *not* to suture the stump, since this will interfere greatly with caudal regeneration. In snakes, crocodilians, chelonians and those lizards whose tails do not regenerate, a ventral-dorsal flap incision is created and sutured in routine fashion.

**Soft Tissue.** Internal soft tissue structures are operated upon as in other species. When a hollow viscus is invaded, the recommended closure is one in which two layers of sutures are placed.

## SUPPLEMENTAL READING

Frye, F. L.: Surgical removal of a cystic calculus from a desert tortoise. J. Am. Vet. Med. Assn., *161*:600–602, 1972.

Frye, F. L.: Clinical evaluation of a rapid polymerizing epoxy resin for repair of shell defects in tortoises. Vet. Med./Small Animal Clin., *68*:51–53, 1973a.

Frye, F. L.: Husbandry, Medicine and Surgery in Captive Reptiles. Bonner Springs, Kansas, VM Publishing, Inc., 1973b.

Frye, F. L., and Schuchman, S. M.: Salpingotomy and caesarian delivery of impacted ova in a tortoise. Vet. Med./Small Animal Clin., *69*:454–457, 1974.

Frye, F. L.: Clinical obstetric and gynecologic disorders in reptiles. Proc. A.A.H.A., 1974, pp. 497–499.

# Section
# 9

# NEUROMUSCULAR DISORDERS

ALEXANDER DE LAHUNTA, D.V.M.

*Consulting Editor*

# EXAMINATION OF THE CEREBROSPINAL FLUID

DAMON R. AVERILL, JR., D.V.M.
*Boston, Massachusetts*

Examination of the cerebrospinal fluid (CSF) is an essentially ancillary procedure in the evaluation of patients with neurologic disorders. The techniques required for cerebellomedullary cistern puncture (cisternal puncture) and measurement of spinal fluid pressure, cell count, cytology and total protein content are simple and should be available to every practicing veterinarian. The spinal tap should be planned carefully and carried out when it is clear that the risk of the procedure is outweighed by the value of the data to be obtained. CSF findings will not be sufficient for definitive diagnosis and must be interpreted with respect to careful physical and neurologic examinations. The CSF analysis is about as useful in differential diagnosis of neurologic disorders as the complete blood count is for the diagnosis of systemic diseases.

## INDICATIONS FOR CISTERNAL PUNCTURE

Rare clinical problems such as neck pain and fever (suggesting meningitis) or progressive clouding of consciousness with no obvious cause require immediate sampling of CSF. Either of these syndromes can represent life-threatening disorders and the spinal fluid tap should be done so that proper treatment can be started as soon as possible.

Animals with seizure disorders are candidates for CSF examination. In general, cisternal taps should be done on the older age groups (over five years) as part of the preliminary examination, since they are at risk for brain tumors. Very young animals (less than two to three months) should also have CSF examinations because of the high association between pediatric-onset seizure disorders and structural abnormalities of the brain. Mature animals with benign seizure

disorders should have their CSF studied as soon as they become refractory to anticonvulsant medication to make sure there is no progressive intracranial lesion.

A neurologic finding suggestive of a structural brain lesion such as personality change, hemiparesis, cortical blindness or multiple cranial nerve deficits necessitates cisternal puncture for differential diagnosis.

Normal cerebrospinal fluid in a patient with a structural brain lesion is unusual and may be interpreted as suggestive of toxic, metabolic or functional disorders. It must be remembered, however, that patients with small neoplasms or focal encephalitis may have normal spinal fluid findings.

## CONTRAINDICATIONS FOR CISTERNAL PUNCTURE

The major contraindication for cisternal puncture is the danger of general anesthesia. Animals with brain lesions which involve or compress the pontomedullary respiratory centers are more vulnerable to anesthetic accident. Care must be taken to estimate this risk as in any surgical procedure, and careful monitoring of respiratory rate and depth is of extreme importance.

Increased intracranial pressure due to tumor or other cause of brain swelling may result in the brain shifting towards the site of CSF removal if excessive or rapid withdrawal of CSF occurs. Subsequently, the needle may damage the cerebellum and/or medulla as they herniate through the foramen magnum. Any indication of increased intracranial pressure, e.g., papilledema or radiographic implication of space-taking lesion, gives cause for reevaluation of the necessity for cisternal tap. If pressures over 250 mm. CSF are found at the beginning of the procedure, then the amount of CSF removed should be only that necessary for the most important laboratory studies (usually 0.5 ml.) and it should be aspirated *slowly*.

Skin infection at the site of cisternal puncture excludes this site for needle placement into the cerebellomedullary cistern as meningeal contamination is possible.

## COMPLICATIONS OF CISTERNAL TAP

At the time of dural perforation, bleeding may occur from transverse venous plexuses or from subarachnoid capillaries if the aspiration of CSF is too rapid. Aliquots of CSF can be removed safely over a one- to two-minute period of time with very gentle aspiration. In careful hands, serious bleeding occurs in about 0.5 per cent of cases. Bleeding around the cerebellum and medulla results in vestibulocerebellar signs which resolve in several weeks if brain swelling is controlled with corticosteroids. Meningitis can be prevented if aseptic technique is strictly followed.

## PROCEDURE

The cerebellomedullary cistern is the space between the caudal surface of the cerebellum and the medullary roof just rostral to the foramen magnum. This space is best entered with the dog in lateral recumbency and with the head flexed 90 degrees to the midline of the back. The muzzle should be lifted from the table so that the midline of the skull parallels the table top. Attention must be given to avoid excessive flexion of the neck, because endotracheal tubes kink when flexed and may obstruct the tracheal airway. Care must be taken to avoid any thoracic or abdominal pressure by leaning on the animal, as this will raise the intracranial pressure.

A 3-inch, 20-gauge needle with short bevel and stylet is used so that the gloved operator can manipulate the needle with both hands. The needle is inserted at the point where a line drawn caudally from the external occipital protuberance along the median plane crosses a line drawn between the cranial tips of the wings of the atlas. The needle may be inserted perpendicular to the back line or directed cranially and "walked" down the occipital bone to the atlanto-occipital joint space. The needle is advanced slowly with the bevel in horizontal plane, so that the longitudinal fibers of the dura are separated rather than split. The dura mater may be felt as a mild pressure which quickly disappears on perforation. The needle is advanced 1 to 2 mm. further and then the stylet is removed to see if fluid flows. If so, a three-way stopcock with vertical calibrated manometer and small syringe already attached is placed on the needle and the opening pressure can be measured before the 1- or 2-ml. sample is taken. If no fluid is obtained, the stylet should be replaced and the needle withdrawn for another try. It is not wise to advance the needle without beginning the entire insertion, as medullary puncture may result. If excessive bleeding occurs in CSF, the tap should be repeated in 24 to 48 hours so that the erythrocytes will be cleared.

## ANALYSIS OF CSF

The opening pressure and the appearance of the spinal fluid should be recorded at the time of the procedure. The cell count and cytologic examination must be done within 30 minutes after the tap, or the cell morphology will be badly damaged. Total protein remains constant during weeks of refrigeration, providing no evaporation takes place.

1. *Opening pressure:* The normal pressure recorded is less than 180 mm. of CSF. Small pulsatile fluctuations of the meniscus will correspond to arterial pulse, and larger ones, to respiratory excursions. A simple method of determining the rate of CSF production is by removing a known volume of CSF (e.g., 1 ml.) and then measuring the time required for the manometer to fill to the opening pressure level. This time corresponds to that required to produce 1 ml. of CSF. Normal value for CSF production in the dog is about 0.040 ± 0.005 ml./minute. The rate of CSF absorption may be determined if a constant infusion pump is available (Davson, 1967) and this varies directly with the intracranial pressure. The cisternal pressure subsequent to withdrawal of the sample is of no clinical value.

2. *Appearance of CSF:* CSF is normally crystal clear. If there is any doubt about a particular sample, it can be compared to tap water in an identical container. A hazy pink color results from erythrocytes in suspension and, if bleeding occurred more than 48 hours prior to the tap, the supernate following centrifugation will be yellow (xantho-

chromic). Xanthochromia may also result from a very high CSF total protein (>400 mg./100 ml.). When it is apparent that red blood cells are present in the spinal fluid, as it is withdrawn, several samples should be collected and erythrocyte counts done on the first and third sample. If subarachnoid hemorrhage antedates the tap, the third tube will have the same erythrocyte count as the first tube; if bleeding occurs at the time of the tap, there will be fewer erythrocytes in the third tube than in the first tube.

3. *Cells:* CFS is transferred immediately to one chamber of a hemocytometer and the cells in all nine squares counted. This number multiplied by 1.1 gives the total cell count. A second sample drawn into a capillary tube wet with glacial acetic acid and counted similarly will give the white cell count, and the difference between the two counts equals the red cell count. The normal CSF has no erythrocytes but, since fragile subarachnoid vessels are commonly damaged during aspiration, fresh erythrocytes are common until some expertise is gained. The differential cell count is done by centrifuging the sample, pouring off the supernate, adding a few drops of canine serum, smearing and staining as in a blood film. Cytologic details are nicely preserved with this method.

Polymorphonuclear leukocytes are never found in normal CSF. The total of small and large mononuclear cells should not exceed 10/cu. mm. An occasional polygonal ependymal cell or arachnoidal cell may be found; they are much larger than the large mononuclear cells. Malignant cells are typically extremely large and arranged in clumps and rafts. Millipore filter techniques are available (Rozel, 1972) and have the advantage of allowing study of every cell present in the sample filtered.

4. *Total protein:* Normal total protein of CSF does not exceed 35 mg./100 ml. in our laboratory determined by a modification of the Folin-Wu method. Methods using sulfosalicylic acid precipitation methods give values consistently lower than this, and several normal samples should be sent to the clinicians' laboratory to determine normal levels for that laboratory. Most infections of the nervous system cause an elevated gamma globulin fraction of the total protein. This may be determined by indirect tests (colloidal gold test) (Shafer, 1966) or immunoelectrophoresis (Cutler, 1969), if available. In general, the total protein becomes elevated because of the production of antibodies in the subarachnoid space or leakage of serum protein from damaged blood vessels.

## CHARACTER OF CSF IN BRAIN DISEASES

Most dogs and cats with recurrent generalized seizures which have no other neurologic abnormalities (idiopathic epileptics) have normal spinal fluid. Normal CSF, therefore, from an animal with a recurrent seizure disorder supports the diagnosis of idiopathic epilepsy.

Contrary to widely held opinion, the cisternal and ventricular CSF pressure in canine hydrocephalics is usually well within normal limits. This is probably due to the fact that most cases are presented to the hospital in a compensated state, i.e., enough ventricular enlargement has occurred to compensate for decreased CSF absorption via transependymal resorption of CSF. Many hydrocephalics have xanthochromic spinal fluid and it is common to find hemosiderin-laden macrophages in the cell population. These findings result from leaking capillaries at the ventricular surface. The total protein is normal in clear samples and elevated to 50 to 100 mg./100 ml. in xanthochromic specimens.

Canine distemper encephalitis produces an increase in CSF protein, but the content may be as low as 40 to 50 mg./100 ml. or as high as 500 mg./100 ml. The globulin fraction of this protein is almost invariably elevated (Cutler, 1969). The cell count is usually normal although small mononuclear cells may be increased to 25 to 50/cu. mm.

Both cryptococcal meningitis and *Toxoplasma* encephalitis result in large increases in CSF protein and usually an increased cell count. Cryptococci may be easily seen in wet India ink preparations of CSF and *Toxoplasma* organisms are sometimes found in the stained smear.

Intracranial tumors, if larger than 2 to 3 cm. in diameter, cause an elevated CSF pressure which may range from 200 to 550 mm. CSF. Tumors usually leak protein as well, and typical levels are 50 to 100 mg./100 ml.

The CSF in lead poisoning is usually within normal limits.

SUPPLEMENTAL READING

Cutler, R. W. P., and Averill, D. R., Jr.: Cerebrospinal
fluid gamma globulins in canine distemper encephalitis. Neurology, 19:1111, 1969.
Davson, H.: Physiology of the Cerebrospinal Fluid.
London, J. A. Churchill Ltd. 1967.

Rozel, J. F.: Membrane filtration of canine and feline
cerebrospinal fluid for cytologic evaluation. J. Am.
Vet. Med. Assn., 160:720, 1972.
Shafer, H., et al.: Extravascular fluids: the colloidal
gold test for CSF proteins. In Page, L. B. and Culver,
P. J. (eds.): A Syllabus of Laboratory Examination in
Clinical Diagnosis. Cambridge, Harvard University
Press, 1966.

# EPISODIC WEAKNESS IN THE DOG

MICHAEL D. LORENZ, D.V.M.
*Athens, Georgia*

## EPISODIC WEAKNESS— THE PROBLEM

Episodic weakness in the dog is a sign of disease in different systems of the body that tends to wax and wane in intensity. Affected animals are lethargic and may stagger and fall while walking. Most patients tire easily with exercise and prefer to lie down or sleep. The pet may seem depressed. Diseases in which episodic weakness is the outstanding sign are perplexing because different systems may be involved. In order to reach a definitive diagnosis, a thorough diagnostic evaluation of the patient is necessary. The purpose of this chapter is to discuss the diagnostic evaluation of a case presented with the problem of waxing-waning (episodic) weakness. A detailed discussion of many of these diseases can be found in other sections of this book and will not be covered in this article.

Diseases which produce episodic weakness as an outstanding clinical sign can be classified as follows:

1. Metabolic causes:
   a. Hypoglycemia
   b. Adrenal insufficiency
   c. Hypokalemia
2. Cardiovascular causes:
   a. Arrhythmias (ventricular tachycardia, atrial fibrillation)
   b. Heart block
   c. Canine dirofilariasis and congestive heart failure
3. Neuromuscular causes:
   a. Myasthenia gravis
   b. Polymyositis

## PATHOPHYSIOLOGY

Hypoglycemia may be caused by the increased utilization of glucose as occurs in functional beta cell tumors, insulin overdose or poisoning with sulfonyl-urea compounds. Hypoglycemia is also caused by failure of glucose secretion as occurs in glycogen storage diseases, adrenal insufficiency, hepatic insufficiency and starvation. Whatever the cause, a rapid decrease in the blood glucose concentration is likely to cause seizures and severe weakness. A slow decline in the blood glucose level results in weakness, depression and, at times, peculiar behavior. The signs of hypoglycemia are more pronounced with exercise because of the increased utilization of glucose by muscle tissue. These signs improve with rest or with the ingestion of food. Thus, waxing-waning episodes of weakness are characteristic of hypoglycemic patients. All the effects of hypoglycemia depend on the fact that the nervous system requires glucose as its main substrate for energy. If the blood glucose decreases, a decrease in cerebral oxidation occurs, producing the signs of hypoglycemia.

Adrenal cortical atrophy, usually of unknown cause, occurs in the dog. Destruction of the adrenal cortex creates a deficiency of both mineralocorticoids and glucocorticoids. A deficiency of aldosterone, the primary mineralocorticoid in the dog, is responsible for the hyponatremia and hyperkalemia present in patients with adrenal cortical insufficiency. The production of nerve impulses and cardiac and skeletal muscle contractions are dependent upon the proper gradients of sodium and potassium ions in the body. Hyperkalemia results in muscle weakness or paralysis, bradycardia and depressed reflexes. These effects are more severe when the sodium concentration is simultaneously low. In addition, hypoglycemia is occasionally encountered in patients suffering from adrenal insufficiency. If present, hypoglycemia will compound the weakness created by the electrolyte disturbances outlined above. In many cases of adrenal insufficiency, a history of periodic weakness is present. Terminally, most cases show severe weakness and circulatory collapse.

Other causes of hyperkalemia, which may be manifested in affected patients as weakness, include diabetes mellitus, chronic renal failure and severe acidosis. Signs of episodic weakness may accompany the more classic signs of these diseases.

Hypokalemia may be caused by many diseases involving different systems of the body. Hypokalemia causes severe weakness and paralysis of skeletal muscle. Hyporeflexia and apathy are common manifestations of hypokalemia. Intercompartmental shifting of potassium, excessive loss or decreased intake of potassium are causes of hypokalemia. In diabetic acidemia, potassium levels in the blood may be elevated prior to therapy. With insulin therapy, potassium is driven back into the intracellular compartment and extracellular hypokalemia results. Hypokalemia can also be caused by severe vomiting and diarrhea. In the former, losses occur by the gastric and renal routes, while in the latter the losses are in the feces.

Cardiovascular diseases which result in decreased cardiac output and, therefore, decreased blood supply to nervous tissue and muscle will result in severe weakness. Many of these diseases intermittently affect the patient, and signs of episodic weakness occur. The patient at rest or with minimal exercise may appear normal. However, episodes of severe weakness may follow more prolonged periods of exercise. Cardiac arrhythmias, such as ventricular tachycardia and atrial fibrillation, produce a decreased cardiac output because of poor cardiac filling during an abbreviated period of diastole. Decreased oxygenation of tissue occurs and severe weakness results.

First- and second-degree heart blocks occur commonly in brachiocephalic breeds of dogs and usually do not produce any clinical signs. Third-degree heart block produces dramatic signs of severe weakness, lethargy and syncope. In complete third-degree block, the beat arising in the ventricle occurs at a slow rate. Cardiac output per unit time is markedly decreased and poor tissue perfusion occurs. Weakness secondary to tissue hypoxia occurs. In certain cases, the heart block is intermittent and episodes of weakness are created.

Canine dirofilariasis commonly produces signs of exercise intolerance, coughing and weakness. The presence of adult *Dirofilaria immitis* in the right ventricle, pulmonary arteries, and right atrium creates an obstruction in the pulmonary vascular bed, resulting in pulmonary hypertension and subsequent right heart failure. Exertional fatigue develops because the circulatory and respiratory systems cannot supply increased amounts of oxygen necessary for muscle activity during exercise.

Myasthenia gravis is the outstanding cause of episodic weakness due to a neuromuscular etiology. Although commonly reported to occur in humans, the disease has been reported infrequently in the veterinary literature. The cause of myasthenia gravis in man is unknown, but dysfunction of neuromuscular transmission is suspected. The action of acetylcholine may be altered at the neuromuscular synapse by excessive cholinesterase activity or by inadequate release of acetylcholine. An immunologic disorder has recently been advocated as the basic cause of myasthenia gravis. Circulating antibodies may interfere with the activity of the motor end-plate. Whatever the cause, the failure of acetylcholine to function at the neuromuscular synapse results in severe muscle weakness which is more severe with exercise.

Polymyositis has rarely been reported in dogs. It occurs infrequently in man. The etiology in man is obscure, but much evidence has been presented that supports an autoimmune mechanism which involves many muscles of the body. Inflammation and necrosis of muscle result in severe pain, weakness and atrophy of affected muscles. The disease is usually progressive with a waxing-waning course. It may occur as one manifestation of other diffuse connective tissue diseases.

## HISTORY—THE SUBJECTIVE DATA BASE

Episodic weakness is one problem which can easily be identified as a sign of many diseases. It may be the primary complaint of the owner or one of many signs present in the patient. The duty of the clinician is to develop a history which may identify other problems or progression of signs more characteristic of the diseases outlined above.

As stated before, hypoglycemia may be caused by several diseases. Functional hypoglycemia has been reported in hunting dogs after exercise and is manifested as seizures and weakness. Glycogen storage diseases have been reported primarily in puppies of the toy breeds. Signs include weakness and seizure. In some cases, signs of hepatic insufficiency develop. Functional beta cell tumor has been reported in most breeds of middle-aged to older dogs. The boxer breed is over-represented in numbers in most reports of this disease. Weakness and convulsions may occur one to two hours after feeding or after exercise. In all cases of hypoglycemia, feeding may improve the signs. Improvement after feeding is not characteristic of the other diseases causing episodic weakness.

Adrenal cortical insufficiency also has a nonspecific history. In the classic disease, episodes of vomiting and diarrhea may precede the signs of weakness as shock. There is no breed or sex predisposition for this disease. Diarrhea may be the outstanding problem of the patient with hypokalemia. Polyuria, polydipsia and increased appetite are classic signs in diabetes mellitus.

A history of cough, syncope and weakness may be present in patients with cardiovascular diseases. Other signs such as ascites or cyanosis may also be present. A history of having lived in an endemic heartworm area may be offered by the client.

A history of weakness made more severe with exercise characterizes myasthenia gravis. In addition, sialosis, dysphagia, urinary incontinence and depresssion may be present. There is no breed or age predisposition for this disease. Polymyositis causes severe muscle pain during the acute phase of the disease. The owner may complain about lameness, stiffness or pain when the patient is handled. Severe muscle atrophy and weakness may be the initial complaint

of the owner in the chronic phase of the disease.

## PHYSICAL AND ANCILLARY EXAMINATIONS—THE OBJECTIVE DATA BASE

Physical examination of the patient with episodic weakness may reveal findings which are suggestive of one particular disease. Patients with hypoglycemia are often normal on physical examination or show the nonspecific signs of weakness, coma or convulsions. Dogs with adrenal insufficiency are often presented in adrenal crisis. Severe pallor of the mucous membranes, dehydration and a slow weak pulse are present. The temperature is usually subnormal and the patient may be comatose. Chronic adrenal insufficiency usually presents a course of weakness and depression. Patients with cardiac arrhythmias also may have pale mucous membranes and poor capillary profusion. Simultaneous palpation of the femoral pulse and auscultation of the heart may reveal a pulse deficit. Careful auscultation of the chest is necessary to detect ventricular premature contractions or atrial fibrillation. In third-degree heart block, a slow heart rate is found. Auscultation of the heart may reveal normal atrial rhythm and a very slow idioventricular rhythm. A split second heart sound may be auscultated in patients with heartworm disease. The patient should be examined for other signs of right heart failure. Ascites, peripheral edema or a jugular pulse may be present.

Physical findings in patients with myasthenia gravis include urinary incontinence, sialosis,dyspnea, a weak voice and dehydration. Neurologic examination may reveal depressed peripheral reflexes, ataxia and weakness with exercise. The pharyngeal muscles may have poor tone as determined by the gag reflex. An inability to swallow food or water produces severe dehydration and moderate weight loss. The patient may gag in an effort to swallow saliva or water. The eyelids may droop and poor tone may be present in muscles of the eyelids and lips. Vomiting can be associated with esophageal dilatation in certain cases.

The outstanding physical findings of polymyositis are asymmetrical muscle atrophy in chronic cases and asymmetrical muscular pain in acute cases. A thorough palpation of all muscles should be performed on every case affected with episodic weakness.

## ANCILLARY EXAMINATIONS— THE DIAGNOSTIC PLAN

Diagnostic tests or procedures are necessary to differentiate the many diseases causing episodic weakness. A minimal data base should be collected on each case. Laboratory analysis should include a complete blood count, microfilaria check, urine analysis, fasting blood glucose prior to and after 15 minutes of exercise, and blood electrolytes. Electrocardiographic examination of the patient should always be performed. ECG findings of spiked T waves, widening of the QRS complex, atrial standstill and bradycardia are characteristic of hyperkalemia. Hypokalemia is manifested as a prolonged QT interval on the ECG. Third-degree heart block and cardiac arrhythmias can be definitively diagnosed only with an ECG. Signs of right ventricular enlargement in the ECG tracing would support a diagnosis of suspected heartworm disease.

If the information collected from the minimal data base does not yield a confirmed diagnosis, more definitive tests are indicated. Pharmacologic testing with neostigmine should be performed in patients suspected of having myasthenia gravis. Neostigmine methyl sulfate, 0.04 to 0.06 mg./kg., is given by intramuscular injection. If no improvement in the clinical signs occurs within 15 minutes, the dose of neostigmine should be repeated. To prevent abdominal cramping, vomiting or diarrhea, atropine sulfate, 0.04 mg./kg., should be administered 15 minutes prior to testing with neostigmine. Electromyographic testing may also be utilized to confirm a diagnosis of myasthenia gravis. This procedure is limited to institutions that have the necessary equipment to perform the test.

Evaluation of certain serum enzymes may be of help in documenting a diagnosis of polymyositis. Lactic acid dehydrogenase (LDH), glutamic oxaloacetic transaminase (GOT) and creatine phosphokinase (CPK) are released during active necrosis of muscle cells, and elevations of these enzymes can be detected in the blood during acute episodes of polymyositis. Muscle enzyme levels are usually normal during the chronic phase of polymyositis. Muscle biopsy is another method of documenting a diagnosis of polymyositis. Histologic changes are characteristic for this disease.

Radiographic examination of the thorax may reveal changes characteristic of heartworm disease even though a normal ECG or negative microfilaria examination is present. A dilated esophagus may be present in cases of myasthenia gravis and can be detected in thoracic radiographs.

## TREATMENT—THE THERAPEUTIC PLAN

Definitive therapy can be offered once a diagnosis has been established. The reader is referred to other sections of this book where an in-depth discussion of each disease is offered. Since myasthenia gravis is not discussed elsewhere, the management of this disease will be discussed here. Definitive therapy for myasthenia gravis includes drugs that enhance the effect of acetylcholine at the neuromuscular junction. Drugs of the anticholinesterase group, such as neostigmine, are used. The exact dose of neostigmine is not known but probably varies with individual need. A dosage of 0.5 mg./kg. of neostigmine bromide orally three times a day should be given initially. The dosage is then individualized to each patient's needs. Underdosing results in poor clinical response or transitory improvement. Overdosing can cause weakness by a depolarizing block at the neuromuscular junction. Therapy in many cases can be discontinued without relapse after a few weeks of treatment.

## SUMMARY

The initial diseases that produce periodic (episodic) weakness may be difficult to distinguish from neurologic diseases that also cause severe weakness. Polyneuropathies such as coonhound paralysis, tick paralysis and brachial neuritis may present severe weakness, but the course is progressive and signs do not wax and wane. However, in their initial phase, each of these diseases may be remarkably similar. Table 1 summarizes the diagnostic plan one should follow in evaluating a case presented with episodic weakness. Through a logical elimination process utilizing diagnostic tests or procedures, a confirmed diagnosis can be documented. Rational therapy based on a documented diagnosis can resolve the initial problem of episodic weakness.

**Table 1.**  *A Diagnostic Plan for Patients with Episodic Weakness*

| DISEASE | DIAGNOSTIC TEST | POSITIVE RESULT |
|---|---|---|
| Hypoglycemia | Fasting blood glucose | 50 mg./100 ml. or less |
| Adrenal insufficiency | Serum electrolytes | Potassium >5.2 mEq.<br>Sodium <135 mEq.<br>Na:K ratio <25:1 |
|  | ECG | Tall spiked T waves<br>Wide QRS; absence of P waves<br>Bradycardia |
| Hypokalemia | Electrolytes | Potassium <2.4 mEq. |
|  | ECG | Prolonged QT interval |
| Cardiac arrhythmias<br>  Ventricular tachycardia<br>  Atrial fibrillation | <br>ECG<br>ECG | <br>Series of PVC's<br>No P waves; presence of "f" waves; rapid<br>  irregular rates |
| Heart block<br>  Third degree | ECG | P waves unassociated with QRS complexes;<br>  atrial rate normal; ventricular rate very slow |
| Heartworm | Modified Knott's<br>ECG<br>Thoracic radiograph | Microfilaria of *D. immitis*<br>Right heart enlargement; enlarged pulmonary<br>  arteries; enlarged pulmonary outflow tract;<br>  right ventricular enlargement |
| Myasthenia gravis | Response to neo-<br>  stigmine testing | Improvement in weakness and greater<br>  exercise tolerance |
| Polymyositis | Muscle enzymes<br>Muscle biopsy | Increase in LDH, GOT and CPK; inflamma-<br>  tion and necrosis of muscle |

### SUPPLEMENTAL READING

Ettinger, S. J., and Suter, P. F.: Canine Cardiology. Philadelphia, W. B. Saunders Co., 1970.
Fraser, D. C., Palmer, A. C., and Senior, J. E. B.: Myas-thenia gravis in the dog. J. Neurol. Neurosurg. Psychiat., 33:431–437, 1970.
Sodeman, W. A., and Sodeman, W. A., Jr.,: Pathologic Physiology: Mechanisms of Disease. 5th ed. Philadelphia, W. B. Saunders Co., 1974.

# POLYMYOSITIS IN THE DOG

DAMON R. AVERILL, JR., D.V.M.
*Boston, Massachusetts*

Polymyositis is an inflammatory disease of many skeletal muscles. It occurs with sufficient frequency at our hospital to warrant consideration in any patient with appendicular, esophageal or brachial muscle weakness.

Dogs with histopathologically documented polymyositis have represented many breeds, but the German shepherd dog is the most commonly affected. Mature dogs are affected more often than very old or very young ones. Females outnumber males slightly.

The usual presentation is a mild progressive weakness of all limbs which is frequently much worse following exercise, although episodes of severe weakness may occur without obvious exertion. Some dogs appear entirely normal until physically stressed on a leash or while climbing stairs.

About half of the dogs have postprandial vomiting, a hoarse bark or difficulty chewing and swallowing. Some cases have swollen or atrophic temporalis muscles or a mechanical limitation of jaw abduction. Rare cases have exertional muscle trembling and contraction which is interpreted as cramping.

On physical examination, there is a slightly stiff but symmetrically coordinated gait. The dog becomes weak during exercise and may collapse and recover sufficiently in a few minutes to regain its feet and walk a shorter distance before collapsing again. The temporal fossae may be concave or excessively convex owing to temporalis muscle atrophy or swelling, respectively. There may be painful proximal muscles but the palpable peripheral nerves (e.g., radial and ulnar) are not painful. The neurologic examination demonstrates normal affect and cranial nerve function. Prehension of food and water may be poor and repeated swallowing efforts without success may be seen while the dog tries to drink water. Dogs with swallowing difficulty may have a very sensitive gag response. The postural reactions (hopping, placing, etc.) and pain perception are normal. The segmental reflexes may be decreased but are most often normal. The rectal temperature is normal.

Several conditions may cause a very similar clinical syndrome. Among these are polyneuritis and myasthenia gravis–like weakness which may also cause weakness of swallowing muscles. Other disorders such as cervical spinal cord damage, hypoadrenocorticism and nutritional bone disease are similar to polymyositis only in respect to the appendicular weakness.

Except for myasthenia gravis–like weakness, the differential diagnosis may be clear on physical examination. Cervical spinal cord signs are only rarely intermittent and cause increased segmental reflexes which result in the limbs having increased resistance to passive manipulation. There is usually some degree of position-sense loss in all four limbs not found in polymyositis.

Dogs with hypoadrenocorticism often have bradycardia and a small heart which may be determined by thoracic auscultation or percussion. Their femoral pulses are usually weak as well.

Dogs with polyneuritis (see "Canine Polyneuritis") usually have a rapidly progressive course without exertional episodes and have severely diminished or absent segmental reflexes. Polyneuritis may cause muscle pain and the peripheral nerves may also be painful.

Nutritional bone disease (nutritional secondary hyperparathyroidism) may present with apparent tetraplegia, actually reluctance to walk, and bone pain may be misinterpreted as muscle pain. On further examination the discomfort can be localized to the epiphyseal regions of the long bones. This disorder occurs in young, rapidly growing dogs and can be confirmed by laboratory tests and radiographic study. (See article on "Parathyroid Glands and Calcium Metabolism.")

Myasthenia gravis–like weakness occurs rarely in the dog and cannot be differentiated from polymyositis on physical examination. None of the reported cases of myasthenia gravis–like weakness in the dog has had muscle pain, but difficulty in swallowing and esophageal dilatation are common enough to make the presentation nearly identical to polymyositis. Dogs with myasthenia gravis–like weakness have circulatory muscle enzyme concentrations within normal limits as well as normal muscle biopsies. Transient abolition of weakness may result from the administration of neostigmine to myasthenic dogs but, since this drug may increase the strength of the patient with polymyositis, the value of this test is limited to those who can quantitate the improvement by measuring a decreased latency of neuromuscular transmission.

The laboratory findings in polymyositis may include a slightly increased white blood cell count with mild eosinophilia. Most helpful is the elevation of any one of the following enzymes: serum glutamic-oxaloacetic transaminase (SGOT), lactic dehydrogenase (LDH), creatine phosphokinase (CPK) or aldolase. (See Appendix for "A Roster of Normal Values.") In some cases, all these enzymes are elevated; in others, only one is above normal.

The CPK and aldolase are enzymes found only in skeletal muscles and are the most reliable. The others are found in other organs and should be interpreted with respect to known normal functions in those other organs. For example, we interpret an elevated SGOT as a significant documentation of myositis only when there is no physical suggestion of liver disease and when the serum glutamic-pyruvate transaminase (another enzyme released by the liver) is within normal limits. It must be remembered that all these circulating enzymes are excreted by the kidney so that renal failure may severely alter their serum concentrations. Theoretically, a sudden loss of many muscle fibers during exercise will turn the urine brown with the muscle pigment myoglobin. This has not been observed in our cases.

Radiographic examination of the thorax of some dogs with polymyositis demonstrates esophageal dilatation, and fluoroscopic examination during barium swallow has shown decreased esophageal contraction in two examples. We have seen restriction of deglutition of barium resulting from a swollen inflamed thyropharyngeus muscle in one dog.

It is important to confirm the diagnosis of polymyositis by histopathologic examination once the physical diagnosis has been supported by ancillary studies because the cause of the myositis will determine the appropriate treatment. Tissue must be selected from muscles which are clearly affected clinically and, since the inflammatory foci may be widely disseminated, several blocks should be fixed from the same muscle.

The most commonly reported cause of polymyositis in the dog is *Toxoplasma gondii* infection which usually produces a severe necrotizing myositis. The treatment for this disease is described elsewhere in this text. More common in our practice is a mononuclear interstitial myositis with muscle fiber necrosis and occasional necrosis of small arterioles. To date, it is suspected that this lesion has an immunologic basis, since the inflammatory cells are lymphocytes and plasma cells, no organisms can be demonstrated in the lesion and, in a few cases, we have found hypergammaglobulinemia or serum antinuclear antibody activity.

A third histologic type especially found in German shepherd dogs from which temporalis muscle biopsies have been taken is also interstitial, but the predominant inflammatory cell is the eosinophil. It is not known if this is a separate entity or an early phase of mononuclear myositis.

Since the most effective treatment of idiopathic inflammatory polymyositis is the early and vigorous use of corticosteroids, and the use of these drugs in the presence of infection is injudicious, it is essential to rule out toxoplasmosis and bacterial myositis before applying this therapy.

The prognosis for noninfectious polymyositis is generally good, providing the esophageal and laryngeal muscles have not been badly damaged. The oral administration of prednisolone at a dose of 0.25 to 0.5 mg./kg. every eight hours results in relatively rapid amelioration of muscle pain, and most dogs show great improvement in strength and exercise tolerance within 48 hours. If no improvement is shown by this time, the dose of prednisolone should be doubled for another 48 hours and this plan followed until clinical remission begins. A broad-spectrum antibiotic such as penicillin or tetracycline may be given to avoid bacterial infection, but this is not usually done unless the dog is treated at home away from daily examination in the hospital. The prednisolone should be continued until all signs of illness are gone. If the temporalis muscles have undergone fibrosis, jaw contracture will not resolve with this medication and mechanical force may have to be applied to relieve this restriction. In some cases the esophageal dilatation will disappear within three to seven days. A decrease to normal of the muscle enzymes found elevated during the illness can be a good indicator of the efficacy of treatment (Table 1).

Once the signs are gone and the serum enzymes are normal, the corticosteroid should be withdrawn gradually over a 7- to 10-day period. During this time, the dose should be cut in half for each succeeding day.

An insufficient number of cases has been studied to give an estimation of long-term prognosis. Several cases, however, have had clinical recurrences as long as eight months following a clinical attack. It is well known that eosinophilic myositis of the masticatory muscles of German shepherd dog types

*Table 1.  Serum Enzyme Concentrations Considered Within Normal Limits at Angell Memorial Animal Hospital*

| ENZYMES | NORMAL VALUES |
|---|---|
| Aldolase | <6 mg./ml. |
| CPK | 0 to 12 units |
| SGOT | 20 to 77 mg./ml. |
| SGPT | 4 to 40 S.F. units |
| LDH | 62 to 430 g./ml. |

commonly relapses and may smoulder subclinically for many months. These observations suggest that periodic serum enzymes, measured at regular intervals, may predict the onset of a recurrence of polymyositis and give support for corticosteroid treatment before clinical weakness begins.

The treatment of polymyositis in the dog is satisfying, but the diagnosis cannot be made without reasonable clinical suspicion, availability of laboratory determinations of serum enzymes and histopathologic confirmation of the cause of the disease.

### SUPPLEMENTAL READING

Adams, R. D., Denny-Brown, D., and Pearson, J.: Diseases of Muscle. New York, Harper & Row, 1967.

Innes, J. R. M.: Myopathies in animals. Brit. Vet. J., *107*:131, 1951.

Meier, H.: Myopathies in the dog. Cornell Vet., *48*:313–330, 1958.

# CANINE POLYNEURITIS

JOHN F. CUMMINGS, D.V.M., *and* ALEXANDER DE LAHUNTA, D.V.M.
*Ithaca, New York*

Polyneuritis, i.e., simultaneous inflammatory involvement of multiple spinal and cranial nerves, is a form of lower motor neuron disease. The general signs of peripheral nerve disease include muscle weakness, hypotonia, hyporeflexia, muscle wasting and sensory impairment.

Canine polyneuritides have been recognized only recently. Both acute and chronic forms are now identified but complete nosologic characterization is lacking in the chronic forms.

## ACUTE POLYNEURITIS

### COONHOUND PARALYSIS

In our experience, the most frequently occurring acute polyneuritis is that of coonhound paralysis. This is primarily an occupational hazard for coonhounds although it occurs in suburban dogs that encounter raccoons. A raccoon bite or scratch precedes the onset of signs by 7 to 14 days. The onset is marked by weakness in the pelvic limbs and, in the incipient stage, this syndrome can be confused with musculoskeletal disorders. Paralysis usually progresses rapidly, and most often the veterinarian is presented with a symmetrically tetraparetic animal. Recumbent animals remain alert and afebrile. Spinal reflexes are reduced or absent. Hypotonia of the limb musculature is manifested by reduced resistance to passive manipulation. In severe cases, the neck and tail are paretic. Frequently, the voice is feeble and facial weakness also may be evident. Although motor impairment is invariably more striking than sensory change, there is often evidence of hyperalgesia in the extremities. Paralysis usually reaches a peak within 10 days of onset. The animal's condition then remains stable for a variable period before paralysis abates.

The pathologic changes are concentrated in the ventral spinal roots and spinal and peripheral nerves. Lesions consist of segmental demyelination with axon preservation, wallerian degeneration of axons and myelin, and perivenular leukocytic infiltration. In its clinical and pathologic features, this canine affliction closely resembles the idiopathic polyneuritis of Guillain-Barré in man. Onset of this human paralytic syndrome is often preceded by an infection which involves the upper respiratory tract, and it has been postulated that autoimmune processes may be involved in the etiology. A similar etiology may be suggested for coonhound paralysis, but the raccoon's role in initiating this demyelinating neuritis remains enigmatic.

Treatment must first be directed at supporting the patient through the early critical phase of paralysis, and subsequently the dystrophic effects of denervation must be minimized.

Shortly after the onset, i.e., in the progressive phase of paralysis, the animals require constant monitoring. Formerly, this syndrome was considered benign, but recently we have observed with increased frequency a very rapidly advancing paralysis that leads to respiratory failure unless a respirator is employed.

Affected dogs maintain a normal appetite, but those with cervical paresis require assistance in order to eat and drink. Fecal and urinary retention may occur transiently. Soap and water enemas relieve constipation, and catheterization and urinalysis are used to guard against cystitis. Whirlpool baths at 100° F. for 20 minutes twice daily are advocated to stimulate appendicular musculature and prevent contractures. Following cleansing in the bath, decubital ulcers are treated with 3 per cent hydrogen peroxide. The animals are best maintained on a straw bed and turned hourly in an effort to minimize these ulcers which otherwise develop rapidly in the tetraplegic phase.

While corticosteroid therapy (dexamethasone, 1 to 2 mg./kg./day) has been suggested, there is little indication that it influences the course of the illness. Should corticoids be employed, concurrent broad-spectrum antibiotic therapy is advisable especially in patients with deep, infected bed sores.

Occasionally, recovery is rapid and virtually complete in three to four weeks, thus suggesting extensive neuropraxic involvement in these animals. More often, abatement of paralysis is slower, and sometimes is incomplete. Paralysis regresses in the reverse sequence in which it developed. In severely paralyzed patients, recovery of motor activity in the thoracic limbs is accompanied by reduction in hyperalgesia and initial healing of decubital ulcers. When the animal is capable of bearing weight, it should be exercised for short periods four or five times daily. Animals are usually discharged when they are capable of walking several hundred feet unaided.

The prognosis in the progressive phase of paralysis should be guarded and, with passage of this critical stage, a good prognosis for recovery may be given. However, intercurrent processes (infections, gastric torsion, etc.) have been fatal in the stabilized or regressing phases of paralysis. Animals with protracted paralysis and marked muscle wasting may fail to recover completely.

Examination of a large number of cases has strengthened our conviction that animals, once afflicted with coonhound paralysis, are prone to redevelop the syndrome on subsequent encounters with raccoons. For this reason, we adivse clients to prevent such encounters. This advice goes unheeded by most raccoon hunters.

### BRACHIAL PLEXUS NEURITIS

Recently, we observed an acute bilateral brachial paresis that developed about 48 hours after an episode of generalized urticaria, facial edema and vomiting. Immunologic testing suggested that the antecedent allergic manifestations were related to ingestion of a horsemeat diet. The onset, distribution and course of this paresis closely resembled those found in severe forms of serum neuritis and neuralgic amyotrophy in man.

In contrast to the coonhound syndrome, this paresis developed more rapidly and in fact appeared to be maximal at the onset. Moreover, the weakness was asymmetrical and confined to the thoracic limbs. The animal could advance the limbs at the shoulder, but there was marked weakness distal to the elbow. The biceps reflex was absent on the left as was the triceps reflex on the right. Flexor reflexes were depressed bilaterally. Antebrachial pain perception was blunted and sensory nerve biopsy specimens revealed extensive axonal destruction.

In further contrast to coonhound paralysis, the pathologic changes consisted of wallerian degeneration exclusively. This degeneration appeared to be initiated in the ventral branches of the spinal nerves that form the brachial plexus. In the comparable human syndromes, it has been suggested that paralysis results from compressive perineural edema. However, it is most difficult to reconcile this pathogenesis with the asymmetrical, all-or-none type of muscle involvement observed in the thoracic limbs.

Treatment in this one case was supportive and essentially the same as that employed in coonhound paralysis. Both electrodiagnostic and biopsy findings indicated extensive axonal disruption, and for this reason a poor prognosis was given for rapid restoration of thoracic limb function. This prognosis proved accurate as the animal remained markedly incapacitated with severe muscle atrophy seven weeks after the onset of signs.

# CHRONIC POLYNEURITIS

Chronic polyneuritis denotes a rather characteristic assemblage of clinical findings rather than a discrete disease entity. Studies of tissue from several affected animals reveal varying pathologic changes which suggest diverse and, as yet unknown, pathogenetic mechanisms.

Affected dogs have been mature, i.e., 6 to 12 years old. Signs develop gradually over a period of months, and while there may be temporary remission, neurologic impairment becomes progressively more severe and more generalized. Initial weakness is usually mistaken for a skeletal disorder. Thus, it is only after elimination of diagnosis such as cruciate ligament rupture, osteoarthritis, or hip dysplasia that one considers lower motor neuron disease. Weakness is asymmetrical and initially it may be obvious in only one extremity. Because of progression with partial remission, one may be presented with a history of shifting lameness. Later, in the course, tetraparesis may be noted.

On neurologic examination, weakness in the extremities may be demonstrated as reduced ability to perform postural reactions. Cranial nerve deficits may be evidenced as unilateral or bilateral facial weakness and altered voice. Findings on spinal reflex examination vary with the stage and distribution of paresis. Tendon reflexes are often reduced or absent. Flexor reflexes may be impaired also. Hypalgesia in the dog becomes clinically evident only with extensive damage to sensory nerves; thus pain perception will seem intact despite moderate involvement of such nerves. Reduced muscle tone is obvious in severely affected extremities and muscle wasting becomes more pronounced with time.

Sensory nerve and muscle biopsy, electromyography and determination of nerve conduction times are most useful in establishing a diagnosis of polyneuritis, especially in the early stages. As diverse pathogenetic processes are involved, cerebrospinal fluid findings vary in chronic polyneuritis. In one animal, there was a persisting albuminocytologic dissociation, i.e., elevated protein without concomitant leukocytosis. Cerebrospinal fluid findings were unremarkable in other animals.

Pathologic changes in one individual included segmental myelin loss as well as wallerian degeneration of moderate intensity in spinal roots and peripheral nerves. Axonal destruction in the proximal portions of the dorsal roots resulted in degeneration in the dorsal columns of the spinal cord. In the dog with the albuminocytologic dissociation, there were heavy perivenular leukocytic infiltrations in the spinal roots and cranial and peripheral nerves. Both segmental demyelination and wallerian degeneration were prominent in the infiltrated areas. Spinal changes secondary to peripheral axon disruption included central chromatolysis in the ventral gray columns and degeneration in the dorsal columns. Regeneration in some nerves and roots was signaled by the presence of thin clusters and onion bulb formations. Another animal suffered from a severe interstitial inflammation of the spinal roots and cranial and peripheral nerves. The epi-, peri-, and endoneurial sheaths were heavily infiltrated by lymphocytes, plasma cells and large mononuclear cells. Myelin loss of both segmental and wallerian types was marked. Similar inflammatory changes occurred in the leptomeninges, brain and spinal cord and, in these locations, they were reminiscent of those found in granulomatous reticulosis of the central nervous system.

To date, all forms of therapy, including treatment with corticosteroids and cytotoxic agents, have proved ineffective in halting the insidious progress of these neuritides. Admittedly the incidence is low, but it is important to distinguish this type of neuritic involvement from those musculoskeletal disorders which are amenable to therapy.

## SUPPLEMENTAL READING

Cummings, J. F., and Haas, D. C.: Coonhound paralysis: an acute idiopathic polyradiculoneuritis in dogs resembling the Landry-Guillain-Barré syndrome. J. Neurol. Sci., 4:51–81, 1967.

Cummings, J. F., et al.: Canine brachial plexus neuritis: a syndrome resembling serum neuritis in man. Cornell Vet., 63:589–617, 1973.

Cummings, J. F., and de Lahunta, A.: Chronic relapsing polyradiculoneuritis in a dog. A clinical, light- and electron-microscopic study. Acta Neuropath. (Berlin), 28:191–204, 1974.

Kingma, F. J., and Catcott, E. J.: A paralytic syndrome in coonhounds. N. Amer. Vet., 35:115–177, 1954.

# AVULSION OF THE BRACHIAL PLEXUS IN THE DOG

I. R. GRIFFITHS, F.R.C.V.S.
*Glasgow, Scotland*

Brachial plexus avulsion, which has also been called the radial paralysis syndrome, is the commonest neurologic condition of the canine forelimb. The onset of clinical signs is sudden and invariably associated with trauma, usually a car accident. To understand the diagnostic and prognostic aspects of the problem fully, the anatomy and pathology must be appreciated.

## ANATOMY AND PATHOLOGY

The brachial plexus originates from the ventral branches of the spinal nerves C6 to T1. Occasionally, either C5 or T2 also contributes to the plexus. The spinal nerves are formed in the usual manner from the junction of the dorsal and ventral nerve roots. The named peripheral nerves arise from the brachial plexus. The more important nerves are suprascapular, musculocutaneous, axillary, pectoral, radial, median and ulnar and the lateral thoracic nerves. For full details of the anatomy, the reader should refer to Miller *et al.* (1964).

The pathology of plexus avulsions is complex and can vary from case to case. The commonest finding is avulsion of the dorsal and/or ventral nerve roots from the spinal cord, with resultant neuroma formation in the leptomeninges. Axonal ruptures also occur in the ventral branches and into the plexus itself, but loss of continuity of the nerve in the ventral branches plexus or peripheral nerves is uncommon. The damage is therefore not a single focal lesion but a diffuse one. The nerve root avulsion may involve all roots from C6 and T1 or may involve either the cranial part of the plexus (i.e., C6 and C7) or the caudal part of the plexus (i.e., C8 to T1). Often the loss of fibers is not complete and a varying proportion of motor fibers may survive intact. These surviving fibers are important in the process of reinnervation of the muscles. Fuller details of the neuropathology have been presented by Griffiths (1974).

## CLINICAL DIAGNOSIS OF THE CONDITION

The clinical signs will vary depending upon the number of nerve roots and branches involved and the degree to which they are affected. Nevertheless, the motor disability can be divided into three types.

**Involvement of the Complete Plexus C6 to T1.** This causes the most severe disability and results in complete lack of function in the limb. The leg hangs limp and useless, and the characteristic position is one of "dropped elbow" with carpal flexion, so that the affected limb may appear longer than the normal limb. Occasionally the brachium may be advanced when the dog is walking. This movement results from the action of the brachiocephalicus muscle, which receives its innervation from the plexus. After approximately three weeks post injury, muscle atrophy becomes obvious, especially in the triceps muscle, and eventually involves the whole limb, including the supra- and infra-spinatus muscles. No reflexes (triceps or biceps jerks or pedal reflexes) are obtained in the limb. The dorsum of the paw is often dragged along the ground, resulting in severe excoriation of the skin. There is usually complete sensory loss in the distal part of the limb. Two patterns of desensitization are seen, as depicted in Figure 1. Occasionally, immediately after the accident, the area of sensory loss is greater than that shown in the figure, but within one to two weeks, the desensitized area reduces to that shown.

The ipsilateral panniculus reflex is absent owing to damage to the nerve roots and branches of C8 and T1, which together with

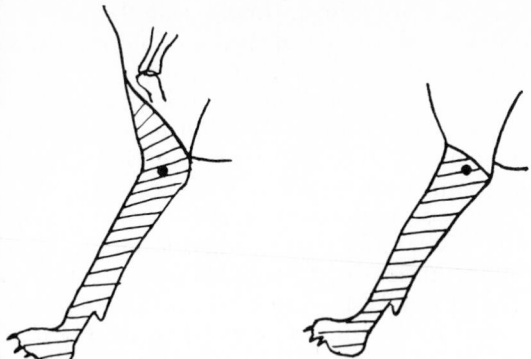

**Figure 1.** Lateral view of two patterns of desensitization (hatched areas) in total plexal avulsion. (From Bennett and Vaughan: J. Small Animal Pract., 15:177–182, 1974.

the lateral thoracic nerve form the efferent pathway for the reflex. Stimulation of the ipsilateral flank causes a consensual reflex muscle twitch seen on the contralateral side. The presence of the consensual response indicates that the afferent fibers from the site of stimulation to the cord and the interneurons to the contralateral C8 and T1 motor neurons are intact.

Approximately 55 per cent of cases show miosis of the ipsilateral pupil, and very occasionally, a slight ptosis is seen. The pupil dilates in shade and constricts in light, but in both situations it remains smaller than the normal pupil. The pupillary abnormality and occasional ptosis are due to interruption of the preganglionic sympathetic fibers in the ventral nerve root of T1. The sympathetic supply to the pupil arises mainly from the intermediolateral gray matter of T1 and passes up the neck in the vagosympathetic trunk. The synapse occurs in the cranial cervical ganglion. The clinical signs therefore constitute a partial Horner's syndrome and are unequivocal evidence of a nerve root lesion.

**Avulsion of the Caudal Part of the Plexus.** This is a fairly common form of brachial plexus lesion and accounts for 33 per cent of the cases. The injury involves predominantly the nerve roots and ventral branches of C8 and T1. Any damage to C6 and C7 tends to be minor. The C8 and T1 roots and branches supply the majority of the innervation to the triceps muscle and the muscles below the elbow joint. The dog cannot bear weight on the limb, owing to the paralysis of the extensor muscles, and may adopt the "dropped-elbow position." It

is more common, however, for the leg to be carried with the elbow and shoulder flexed because the flexor muscles of these two joints receive an adequate innervation from segments C6 and C7. It is possible to demonstrate elbow flexion ability by inducing the dog to jump up at a person or on a table or by testing for an ocular placing reflex with the normal leg held. There is also loss of the ipsilateral panniculus reflex, with a consensual response on the contralateral side. There is often ipsilateral miosis due to sympathetic dysfunction. The sensory level can vary considerably, and four patterns of loss are shown in Figure 1 and 2.

**Damage to the Cranial Part of the Plexus.** This implies damage to primarily the C6 and C7 nerve roots and branches with relative sparing of C8 and T1. This is a relatively uncommon form of brachial plexus injury. The extensor muscles still retain the majority of their innervation, and the dog can bear weight on the limb. The main disability involves lack of elbow flexion, a decreased protraction of the limb and atrophy of the supra- and infraspinatus muscles. The panniculus reflex is intact, and sympathetic dysfunction does not occur.

The patterns of skin desensitization in brachial plexus avulsion have been illustrated in Figures 1 and 2, but these can vary from case to case. This is because the patterns of dorsal nerve root avulsion do not necessarily match the patterns of ventral nerve root avulsion. It is also possible in rare cases for pain sensation to remain intact despite severe motor dysfunction. With in-

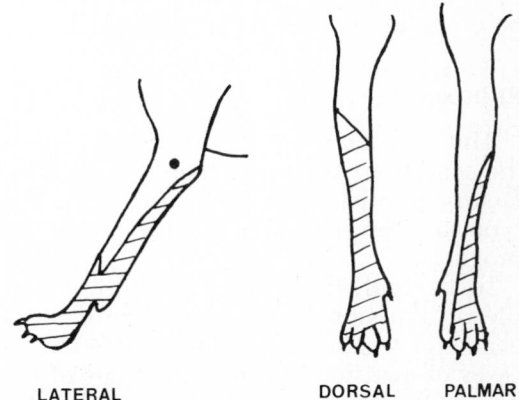

LATERAL                DORSAL      PALMAR

**Figure 2.** Two patterns of sensory loss seen in incomplete plexal lesions. The lateral view depicts one pattern; the dorsal and palmar views depict the other pattern. (From Bennett and Vaughan: J. Small Animal Pract., 15:177–182, 1974.

creasing duration from the time of injury the area of desensitization will decrease as nerve fibers sprout into the desensitized skin from the contiguous innervated area.

## OTHER AIDS TO DIAGNOSIS

Radiography may sometimes reveal concurrent injuries such as fractured ribs or fractures of the long bones in the ipsilateral limb. Such fractures should be regarded as coexistent with the nervous lesion but not the cause of it.

One of the more useful investigations that can be performed in special centers is electromyographic (EMG) and nerve conduction studies. These can reveal the state of innervation or denervation of a muscle and are especially useful in detecting minor degrees of denervation that are not clinically appreciable. Such a situation can occur in the biceps and brachialis muscles following damage to the caudal part of the plexus. These muscles, while retaining the majority of their innervation, are often partially denervated owing to damage to the C8 nerve root. Provided that the case is seen immediately after injury, the percentage of nerve fiber loss in a peripheral nerve can be estimated by serially recording the amplitude of the evoked muscle action potential (Griffiths and Duncan, 1974). A combination of EMG and nerve conduction studies will usually reveal whether the muscle is completely or partially denervated. Electromyography can also demonstrate the early stages of reinnervation before it is clinically detectable. It is, however, a specialized procedure and will not be discussed further in this article.

## PROGNOSIS

This is often the most difficult aspect of the condition. At present there are no satisfactory published reports correlating the type and severity of the injury with the prognosis.

In general, those animals with a total plexal avulsion have an extremely poor chance of regaining useful limb function. In cases of avulsion of the caudal part of the plexus, the prognosis depends on the severity of the denervation. The denervation of the triceps and lower limb muscles is usually partial, and the outlook depends upon the number of surviving nerve fibers and

their potential for reinnervating the muscle with collateral axonal sprouts. In some cases it is evident initially that there is some triceps function, although not sufficient to allow weight-bearing. These dogs often have a good prognosis, and function returns as reinnervation proceeds. Dogs with a clinically complete denervation of the triceps and distal limb muscles at one month after injury generally have a bad prognosis. Although on EMG some remaining innervation can be demonstrated, it is seldom enough to provide adequate functional innervation. For dogs with the rarer cranial plexal avulsion, the prognosis is reasonably good.

The above statements are generalities based on clinical experience. Better assessments of the prognosis will be available when we understand more fully the exact mechanisms by which function is regained and also which aspects of the electrophysiologic examination are the best indicators of prognosis.

## MANAGEMENT OF THE CONDITION

At present there is no "direct" treatment of the condition. The diffuseness of the nerve fiber damage precludes surgical intervention and nerve suture. There are three courses of management that can be adopted:

1. Amputation of the limb.
2. No treatment other than dressing of any excoriations that occur and prevention of contractures.
3. Various tendon translocations, particularly biceps translocation to the olecranon and a carpal flexor to the extensor position.

Amputation is indicated when the limb becomes badly ulcerated and self-mutilated. This is particularly the case in total plexal avulsion. It is also indicated if contractures develop in other forms of plexal avulsion. Previously, amputation was also employed in cases of caudal plexal avulsion, but current policy is to leave the limb if at all possible.

No direct intervention is indicated in avulsion of the cranial plexus and in certain cases of caudal plexal involvement, particularly when this is partial and the triceps retains some function. Temporization is probably the best course to adopt initially in all cases of plexal avulsion, so that the full extent of the lesion can be revealed.

If the limb can be left for a longer time (several months), it is easier to gauge the degree of reinnervation and returning function. If tendon translocations are required, they can be performed at this stage (see Hussain and Pettit (1967) and Bennett and Vaughan (1976) for details of tendon translocations.)

### SUGGESTED READING

Bennett, D., and Vaughan, L.: The use of muscle relocation techniques in the treatment of peripheral nerve injuries in the dog and cat. J. Small Animal Pract., 17:99–108, 1976.

Griffiths, I. R.: Avulsion of the brachial plexus. I. Neuropathology of the spinal cord and peripheral nerves. J. Small Animal Pract., 15:165–176, 1974.

Griffiths, I. R., and Duncan, I. D.: Some studies of the clinical neurophysiology of denervation in the dog. Res. Vet. Sci., 17:377–383, 1974.

Hussain, S., and Pettit, G. D.: Tendon transplantation to compensate for radial nerve paralysis. Am. J. Vet. Res., 28:335–344, 1967.

Miller, M. E., Christensen, G. C., and Evans, H. E.: Anatomy of the Dog. Philadelphia, W. B. Saunders Co., 1964, p. 578.

# INTRACRANIAL INJURY

J. E. OLIVER, JR., D.V.M.
*Athens, Georgia*

Trauma cases accounted for 12.8 per cent of admissions at one metropolitan teaching hospital (Kolata et al., 1974), the distribution between dogs and cats being about the same as that for the total hospital population. Motor vehicle accidents accounted for over half the injuries in dogs but for only 16.3 per cent in cats, and head injuries from these accidents occurred in about 25 per cent of dogs and in almost 40 per cent of the cats. In a survey of 600 dogs involved in motor vehicle accidents, 30 had skull injuries and 12 had brain injuries (Kolata and Johnston, 1975). Seventy-five dogs died or were euthanatized as a result of their injuries. None of the dogs with brain injuries died, but two were euthanatized. Similar data on human motor vehicle accidents indicate that 50,000 deaths occur each year in the United States and that more than two thirds of these include head injuries (Javid, 1974).

These data suggest that the dog is relatively resistant to intracranial injury as compared to man. Considering the heavy temporal muscle and relatively thick skull of most dogs, this is probably true. However, many injured dogs die and are not accounted for in hospital statistics.

Management of acute intracranial injury must be instituted at the earliest possible moment if brain function is to be preserved. In man, 60 per cent of deaths from brain injury occur in the first 24 hours (Javid, 1974). Animals with acute intracranial injury frequently are in shock and have incurred injuries to other body systems. Emergency treatment, as outlined in the section on treatment, may be necessary to preserve life before a complete evaluation can be made.

## DIAGNOSIS

A rapid, but thorough, physical examination should be made. Open chest wounds or gross hemorrhage may require immediate attention. A general assessment of the patient's injuries provides a more accurate prognosis, an estimate of the therapy required and the probable duration and cost of hospitalization. A neurologic evaluation is then made to determine the location and extent of brain injury.

## NEUROLOGIC EXAMINATION

Clinical evaluation of the levels of consciousness, motor function and neurophthalmologic signs (pupils, eye movements) provide sufficient information to localize the level of the brain injury and to make a reasonably accurate prognosis (Oliver, 1972; Ommaya and Gennarelli, 1974; Overgaard *et al.*, 1973).

Consciousness is maintained by pathways from the rostral reticular formation in the brain stem (reticular activating system) to the cerebral cortex. Decreasing levels of consciousness indicate increasing disconnection of this system. Loss of consciousness indicates complete disconnection.

Consciousness may be graded as awake and alert, lethargic, stuporous or comatose. The patient that is lethargic will tend to sleep when undisturbed but is easily aroused with mild stimulation. The stuporous patient can only be aroused with strong, usually painful, stimulation. Strong, painful stimulation does not arouse the patient in coma, although some motor activity can be elicited.

Motor function includes voluntary and involuntary (reflex) activity. An awake animal will usually have intact voluntary motor activity, although some degree of paresis may be present. Severe paresis or paralysis in an awake, alert animal is likely to indicate spinal cord damage. A lethargic animal may have some paresis but usually will still have voluntary motor function. A stuporous animal will often exhibit a hemiparesis or tetraparesis. Some voluntary activity is usually preserved. Myotatic reflexes may be exaggerated. Voluntary motor activity is lost in coma. Coma may be further graded as (1) normal spinal reflex responses; (2) decerebrate rigidity, including extension of all four limbs, "clasp-knife response" and possibly opisthotonos; or (3) hypotonia of the muscles and depression of spinal reflexes.

Pupillary light reflexes and oculocephalic responses are also useful indications of the extent of intracranial injury. Constricted pupils are usually seen with lesions in the diencephalon (hypothalamus). Lesions of the oculomotor nucleus (midbrain) or nerves produce pupillary dilation that is unresponsive to light. Brain-stem lesions encompassing the oculomotor nuclei and descending sympathetic pathways will result in a pupil in midposition that is unresponsive to light.

A summary of the clinical findings with lesions at various levels of the brain stem is presented in Table 1. It is important to realize that the level of the lesion indicated by clinical signs is the lowest level of significant injury. Areas rostral to that level have generally suffered serious damage also (Ommaya and Gennarelli, 1974).

The time course of the clinical signs and the presence of lateralizing signs are also of importance in establishing a diagnosis and prognosis. Brain-stem hemorrhage, the most frequently encountered lesion in severe head injury, is characterized by loss of con-

sciousness immediately after injury. Herniation of the cerebrum under the tentorium cerebelli, compressing the brain stem, occurs more slowly and may be accompanied by unilateral clinical signs (see Table 2 and Figure 1).

## PROGNOSIS

Clinical evaluation of levels of consciousness, neurophthalmologic signs and motor signs provides an accurate prognosis (Oliver, 1972, Ommaya and Gennarelli, 1974, Overgaard *et al.*, 1973). Animals that are unconscious from the time of injury and remain unconscious for 48 hours rarely recover. Those that do recover usually have severe motor deficits.

Slowly progressive signs of loss of consciousness, decreasing voluntary motor activity and pupillary dilation indicate increasing intracranial pressure from an expanding hematoma or from brain swelling. These cases can be saved if adequate treatment is instituted early (Table 3).

## PATHOLOGY

Because the brain is encased in an inelastic compartment, virtually all the pathologic sequelae to head injury result in increased intracranial pressure. Depressed skull fractures, intracranial hemorrhage or brain swelling all increase the volume of material within the calvaria. Brain tissue is compressed or displaced, creating focal or generalized dysfunction. Increased pressure causes displacement of the cerebral hemispheres under the tentorium cerebelli caudally, causing compression of the brain stem. Further increases in pressure will produce herniation of the cerebellum through the foramen magnum compressing the medulla oblongata. Death rapidly ensues from respiratory arrest.

Brain swelling or cerebral edema is an increase in fluid, primarily extracellular in white matter and intracellular in gray matter. Edema may be a sequela to any insult to nervous tissue, including trauma, hypoxia, hypercarbia, cold, heat, toxins, etc. It is safe to assume that any significant head trauma will produce some degree of cerebral edema.

Hemorrhage may be extradural, subdural, subarachnoid or intracerebral. Subarachnoid hemorrhage is probably the most

*Table 1.* *Signs Characteristic of Severe Damage to the Brain Stem at Various Levels*

| LEVEL | CONSCIOUSNESS | PUPILS | EYE MOVEMENTS | MOTOR FUNCTION | AUTONOMIC RESPONSES |
|---|---|---|---|---|---|
| Early Diencephalic | Apathy | Small but reactive | Normal | Hemiparesis | Normal to irregular respirations |
| Late Diencephalic | Stupor | Small but reactive | Normal | Hemiparesis to tetraparesis | Cheyne-Stokes respiration |
| Midbrain | Coma | Bilateral dilation | Poor oculocephalic response | Decerebrate rigidity | Hyperventilation |
| Pons | Coma | Midposition, unresponsive | Oculocephalic response absent | Flaccid paralysis | Rapid shallow respirations |
| Medulla | Coma | Misposition, dilated terminally | Absent | Flaccid paralysis | Irregular to apnea, pulse slowing |

Modified from Plum and Posner: The Diagnosis of Stupor and Coma, 1966, and Oliver, J. E., Jr.: Vet. Clin. N. Am., 2:341, 1972.

*Table 2.* *Signs Characteristic of Progressive Unilateral Tentorial Herniation*

| LEVEL | CONSCIOUSNESS | PUPILS | EYE MOVEMENTS | MOTOR FUNCTION | AUTONOMIC RESPONSES |
|---|---|---|---|---|---|
| III N. | Normal to stupor | Ipsilateral dilation | Normal to slight lateral strabismus | Normal to hemiparesis | Normal |
| Early midbrain | Stupor | Ipsilateral to bilateral dilation | Ipsilateral ventrolateral strabismus | Hemiparesis ipsi- or contralateral | Normal |
| Late midbrain to pons | Coma | Dilated bilateral to fixed midposition | Ventrolateral strabismus to fixed midposition | Decerebrate rigidity | Hyperventilation |
| Pons | Coma | Midposition, unresponsive | Oculocephalic response absent | Flaccid paralysis | Rapid, shallow respirations |
| Medulla | Coma | Midposition, dilated terminally | Absent | Flaccid paralysis | Irregular to apnea, pulse slowing |

Modified from Plum and Posner: The Diagnosis of Stupor and Coma. 1966, and Oliver, J. E., Jr.: Vet. Clin. N. Am., 2:341, 1972.

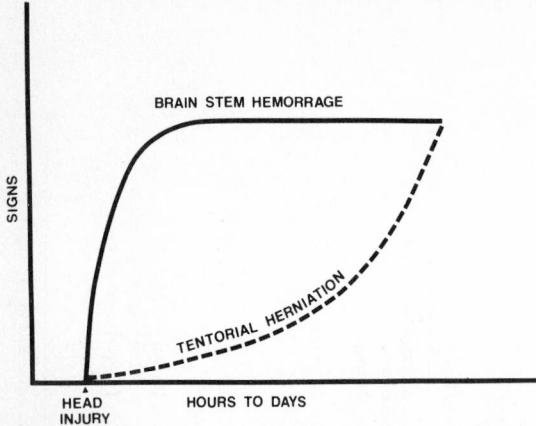

**Figure 1.** Sign time graph of head injury. Tentorial herniation and brain stem hemmorrhage may be differentiated by the clinical course. (From Oliver: Vet. Clin. N. Am., 2:341, 1972.)

frequent, with intracerebral hemorrhage the most severe.

Fractures may be linear or depressed, simple or comminuted, and closed or compound. Fractures may be significant if they are depressed into the brain, if they lacerate a blood vessel or if they are compound with the possibility of introducing infection into the brain. Basilar fractures may lacerate the cavernous sinus, dorsal calvarial fractures may lacerate the dorsal sagittal sinus and lateral calvarial fractures may lacerate the middle meningeal artery.

## MANAGEMENT

Acute head injury requires treatment as early as possible and careful monitoring for changes in the condition of the animal. Stuporous or comatose animals should be monitored continuously if treatment is to be successful. Figure 2 provides a guide to management based on the clinical signs of the animal.

Unconscious animals may need attention before they reach the veterinary clinic. Owners can be instructed on the telephone to maintain a patent airway by extending the animal's head and neck and pulling the tongue forward. If possible, the animal should be carried on a piece of plywood or some similar rigid support to avoid displacement of the spinal column.

When the animal is presented for treatment, maintenance of a patent airway is still the most important consideration. An endotracheal catheter or tracheostomy tube should be used if any difficulties in respiration are encountered. Hypoxia and hypercarbia are primary causes of brain swelling.

Treatment of shock, gross hemorrhage and penetrating chest wounds must be instituted to maintain life. (Details of management are described in other articles.) Adrenal corticoids are ususaly given for shock and are also beneficial in the treatment of cerebral edema. Dexamethasone at a dose of 2 mg./kg. body weight intravenously or a comparable dose of other steroids is recommended. If intravenous fluids are administered for hypovolemic shock, the volume should be monitored carefully to avoid overhydration, which aggravates cerebral edema. Central venous pressure measurements may be useful for evaluation of fluid therapy.

A stuporous or comatose animal should receive an osmotic diuretic. Mannitol (20 per cent solution) at a dose of 2 gm./Kg. IV is preferred, although urea may be used. Mannitol should be given in a slow drip at a rate of approximately 30 drops a minute.

*Table 3.* *Comparison of Acute Brain-Stem Hemorrhage with Tentorial Herniation Following Head Injury*

| | BRAIN-STEM HEMORRHAGE | TENTORIAL HERNIATION |
|---|---|---|
| Onset | Early | Delayed |
| Course | Static to progressive | Progressive |
| Pupils | Constricted early, dilated late | Unilateral dilation progressing to bilateral dilation |
| Consciousness | Stuporous to comatose | Alert of apathetic, progressing to coma |
| Muscle Tone | Decerebrate rigidity or flaccid paralysis | Normal or weak progressing to decerebrate rigidity to flaccid paralysis |
| Reflexes | Usually symmetrical | Often unilateral asymmetry |

From Oliver, J. E., Jr.: Vet. Clin. N. Am., 2:341, 1972.

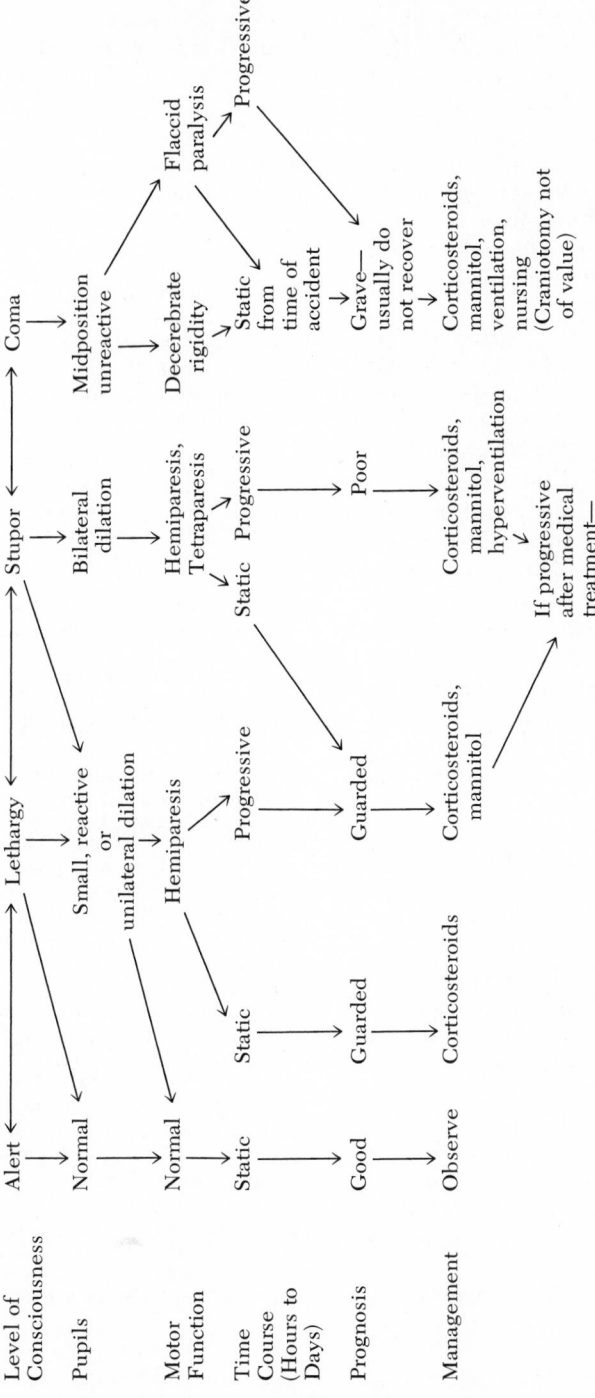

**Figure 2.** Management of intracranial injury.

Renal output should be monitored by means of an indwelling urethral catheter. Mannitol should be repeated at 4- to 6-hour intervals for 3 to 4 doses. At that time the corticosteroids should be exerting maximal effect and mannitol can be discontinued. It is very easy severely to dehydrate an animal with mannitol. General dehydration is not necessary to achieve reduction of brain swelling, therefore adequate fluids should be administered simultaneously to maintain hydration. Mannitol may be dangerous in animals with severe blood loss (Parker, 1973). Maintenance of an adequate blood volume should precede the administration of osmotic diuretics.

Several experimental studies have suggested that dimethyl sulfoxide (DMSO) is effective in treating cerebral edema. Adequate data are not available to make a final judgment, so use of DMSO should be considered experimental at this time.

Coma from the time of injury and persisting for 48 hours in spite of medical treatment is evidence of brain-stem hemorrhage (Tables 3 and 4). Prognosis for recovery is grave, and treatment is limited to nursing care. The animal should be turned frequently to prevent hypostatic congestion, the bladder should be emptied at least three times daily, body temperature should be maintained in the normal range and fluid balance should be maintained.

Progressive deterioration indicates an expanding mass or uncontrolled cerebral edema. Hematomas will usually produce signs of unilateral compression (see Table 2). Progressive signs constitute an emergency and indicate the need for craniotomy. Bur holes may be placed and the hematoma evacuated or a lateral craniotomy performed for complete decompression (Oliver, 1966, 1968).

Surgery is warranted in the first 24 to 48 hours in the absence of progressive signs if there is a skull fracture depressed more than the thickness of the calvaria, if the fracture is compound or if there are bone fragments in the brain.

Postoperative and medical treatment include good nursing care as previously described. Antibiotics are usually indicated, especially if shock or open wounds are present.

Post-traumatic epilepsy is a possible sequela to head injury. Prophylactic anticonvulsants have been recommended, but their efficacy is not clearly established. Phenobarbital (2 mg./kg./day) and diphenylhydantoin (2 to 10 mg./kg./day) are given to all animals with open head injury or following craniotomy.

## SUPPLEMENTAL READING

de la Torre, J. C., Kawanaga, H. M., Rowed, D. W., Johnson, C. M., Goode, O. J., Kajihara, K., and Mullan, S.: Dimethyl sulfoxide in central nervous system trauma. Ann. N.Y. Acad. Sci., *243*:362, 1975.

Hoerlein, B. F.: Canine Neurology. 2nd ed. Philadelphia, W. B. Saunders Co., 1971.

Javid, M.: Current Concepts—Head Injuries. New Engl. J. Med., *291*:890, 1974.

Kolata, R. J., and Johnston, O. E.: Motor vehicle accidents in urban dogs: a study of 600 cases. J. Am. Vet. Med. Assn., *167*:938, 1975.

Kolata, R. J., Krant, N. H., and Johnston, O. E.: Patterns of trauma in urban dogs and cats: a study of 1000 cases. J. Am. Vet. Med. Assn., *164*:499, 1974.

Oliver, J. E., Jr.: Principles of canine brain surgery. Animal Hosp., *2*:73, 1966.

Oliver, J. E., Jr.: Surgical approaches to the canine brain. Am. J. Vet. Res., *29*:353, 1968.

Oliver, J. E., Jr.: Management of the patient with acute head injury. Proc. Gaines Veterinary Symposium, Purdue University, Lafayette, Indiana, 1969.

Oliver, J. E., Jr.: Neurologic emergencies in small animals. Vet. Clin. N. Am. *2*:341, 1972.

Oliver, J. E., Jr.: Craniotomy, Craniectomy and Skull Fractures. *In* Bojrab, M. E. (ed.): Current Techniques in Small Animal Surgery. Philadelphia, Lea & Febiger, 1975.

Ommaya, A. K., and Gennarelli, T. A.: Cerebral concussion and traumatic unconsciousness. Brain, *97*:633, 1974.

Overgaard, J., Christensen, S., Hvid-Hansen, O., Haase, J., Land, A., Hein, O., Pedersen, K., and Tweed, W. A.: Prognosis after head injury based on early clinical examination. Lancet, *2*:631, 1973.

Parker, A. J.: Blood pressure changes and lethality of mannitol infusions in dogs. Am. J. Vet. Res., *34*:1523, 1973.

Plum, E., and Posner, J. B.: The Diagnosis of Stupor and Coma. Philadelphia, F. A. Davis Co.,1966.

Sabin, T. O.: The differential diagnosis of coma. New Engl. J. Med., *290*:1062, 1974.

# EVALUATION AND THERAPY OF SPINAL CORD TRAUMA

T. H. BRASMER, D.V.M.
*St. Paul, Minnesota*

In the owner's mind, all spinal cord disease is related to trauma. Dogs with spinal cord neoplasia, congenital anomalies, infectious diseases, degenerative diseases, canine disk disease and some nonspinal systemic conditions are often presented with apparently valid histories which indicate that some external trauma was the direct cause. Certain key questions help to separate the traumatic conditions from the nontraumatic.

1. Was there a direct witness of the trauma?
2. Did the clinical signs begin *immediately* following the trauma?
3. Was the trauma truly violent, i.e., was the animal struck by automobile, kicked by horse?
4. Is there other clinical evidence of trauma?
5. Have the clinical neurologic signs changed since the trauma?

If, after careful questioning, it is apparent that the neurologic deficit began at the time of trauma and has remained stable or has improved, then trauma is the probable cause. If the history indicates a vague relationship to trauma with a progressive worsening of the deficit, trauma is unlikely to be the cause.

Once trauma has been established as a probable cause, obvious neurologic signs should be temporarily ignored. Injury of sufficient force to produce spinal cord trauma frequently produces other life-threatening injury. As always, a careful complete physical examination is the rule. We must be extremely careful not to narrow our vision too rapidly. The beautifully repaired spinal fracture patient who dies from intestinal rupture does little to satisfy our ego. Abdominal or thoracic trauma may be difficult to appreciate immediately after injury, therefore the visceral evaluation should continue for several days. But since

spinal cord trauma should be surgically or medically treated without delay, procrastination or "waiting for developments" must be avoided. Shock, major abdominal or thoracic hemorrhage, visceral rupture or ventilation abnormalities are treated first and then the spinal cord trauma is reevaluated.

The length of the vertebral column, from occiput to tail, is carefully palpated. Visible or palpable distortion may be present. Such distortion should be verified initially by neurologic examination and finally by radiographic examination.

Clinically, the canine spinal cord can be divided into four segments. These are cranial cervical; caudal cervical–cranial thoracic; thoracolumbar junction; and lumbosacral. Trauma to each of these segments produces rather specific neurologic deficits. A few simple neurologic tests will concentrate our x-ray beam so that more definitive examinations are possible. Multiple lesions may occur, but a single site of injury is the rule.

Since the patient is rarely ambulatory and should not be extensively manipulated, the neurologic examinations are best conducted with the animal in lateral recumbency and prior to any sedation or analgesia.

The reflexes selected and their method of evaluation ignore the subtleties of a definitive neurologic examination. We observe only the crudest (grossest) of responses in order to help localize the lesion.

Table 1, although confusing at first glance, is extremely simple in use and can be helpful in pinpointing the source of trouble. For example, we examine a patient, just struck by a car, who exhibits hindlimb paralysis, intact patellar and withdrawal reflexes, good anal sphincter tone, Schiff-Sherrington syndrome, poor pain response in hindlimbs, and normal motor function and segmental reflex in the forelimbs. Im-

**Table 1.**   *Outline of Important Reflex Abnormalities in Spinal Cord Trauma*

| TOPOGRAPHIC AREA | | | |
|---|---|---|---|
| I | II | III | IV |
| $C_1$–$C_4$ * | $C_5$–$T_2$ | $T_3$–$L_3$ | $L_4$–$S_3$ |

*Vertebral column segments.

Loss of anal sphincter reflex—IV
Loss of hindlimb segmental reflexes (patellar and withdrawal)—IV
Loss of hindlimb voluntary motor function (paresis or paralysis)—I, II, III, or IV
Loss of hindlimb pain response—I, II, III or IV
Loss of forelimb segmental reflex (withdrawal)—II

Schiff-Sherrington syndrome (foreleg hyperextension)—III
Loss of forelimb voluntary motor function (paresis or paralysis)—I or II
Loss of forelimb pain response—I or II
Horner's syndrome—II
Paresis of respiratory muscles—I or II

mediately, our examination can be narrowed down to the area between $T_3$ and $L_3$. Experience tells us further that the most likely area is the T-L junction. Palpable distortion of the spinous process may or may not be present. But we know the general area of the lesion for a more definitive examination. In a similar manner, if the dog lacks anal sphincter tone, lacks patellar and withdrawal reflexes in the hindlimbs, and exhibits analgesia of the rear quarters, we can feel reasonably certain that the lesion is below the level of $L_3$.

These reflexes may be accurately evaluated within minutes after injury. Spinal shock (total areflexia caudal to the lesion) lasts a very short time in the dog or cat. By the time the traumatized patient is presented for examination, the veterinarian may safely assume that spinal shock will not confuse his examination.

Following complete physical and neurologic evaluation, the affected topographic area should be radiographed. As always, both lateral and ventrodorsal views are necessary. Usually the animal is anesthetized prior to x-ray examination. Any trauma patient must be considered a questionable anesthetic risk; atropinization, induction with an ultrashort-acting barbiturate, tracheal intubation and maintenance on a volatile or gas anesthetic with assisted ventilation are all important steps in a safe procedure. Light-plane anesthesia is maintained until the films have been read. Frequently, the animal should be taken to surgery immediately.

Obvious fracture-luxations are easily recognized. Compression fractures may be more difficult to diagnose and radiographic changes can be very subtle even with severe neurologic signs. Do not overlook a narrow intervertebral disk space from which disk material has extruded into the vertebral canal. We should *not* assume that the displacement seen radiographically is a faithful reflection of the actual displacement which occurred at the moment of trauma. From a prognostic viewpoint, a complete fracture luxation with marked displacement is an unfavorable sign; however, minimal displacement is *not* necessarily a favorable sign. The radiographs are used to pinpoint the lesion. The neurologic signs are used to assist in giving the owner a reliable prognosis.

Prognosis must be based on past experience. It is now becoming more obvious that we have erred in the past by being too conservative. Newer therapeutic and surgical techniques seem to be broadening the possibility of functional recovery. All spinal cord trauma must be viewed as serious. Many patients are beyond repair. But recent experience has shown that rapid rational medical and/or surgical therapy offers far greater hopes than had previously been thought possible.

Dyspnea, associated with cervical trauma, is an emergency situation of highest priority. Cranial cervical cord trauma (area I) may reduce thoracic respiratory drive, leaving only the phrenic nerve and diaphragm functional. The animal exhibits a gasping respiratory motion of the mouth and head, with little or no chest movement. When blood gases are examined, the arterial oxygen tension may be as low as 40 mm. Hg. Carbon dioxide tensions may be either high, low or normal, depending on the minute respiratory volume. If the $PO_2$ is low and the $PCO_2$ low or normal, only additional oxygen is required. This can be supplied by face mask, nasal catheter, oxygen cage or a catheter introduced directly into the trachea between tracheal rings. If the arterial carbon dioxide is high, then the animal should be immediately placed on a mechanical respirator.

This complication, which can occur following either accidental or iatrogenic trauma, is exceedingly serious. Few veterinary hospitals are prepared to maintain an animal on a respirator for extended periods. The use of the respiratory itself can produce severe respiratory and circulatory complications. The owner must be made aware of the grave prognosis. Despite the gravity of the situation, the occasional animal who completely recovers will make all of the efforts seem very worthwhile.

Two criteria are helpful in separating those patients which can be managed conservatively from those which require surgery. These are vertebral column stability and degree of spinal cord damage. If the animal is ambulatory, even with some paresis and deficits in proprioception, he may be temporarily placed in the conservative category. Radiographs should then be carefully reviewed. The key question then becomes one of fracture-luxation stability. Where the fractures involve only spinous or transverse processes, surgery is unnecessary. But if the lamina are distorted, the vertebral body fractured, several articular facets fractured, or there is luxation distortion, reduction and immobilization are necessary. Conversely, patients who exhibit paralysis usually require immobilization and almost always require decompression and reduction.

Medical therapy, in addition to that directed at traumatic lesions elsewhere in the body, should be instituted immediately and continued while radiographs are taken and surgical decisions are made. Both dexamethasone and mannitol reduce edema of the central nervous system. Dexamethasone alcohol (Azium® Solution [Schering Corp.]) is one of the readily available products; the usual dose in neurologic trauma is 2 to 4 mg./kg. This corticosteroid is diluted with any isotonic solution (such as lactated Ringer's solution) and given intravenously as a rapid drip. The mode of action of dexamethasone is controversal, but it appears to be most effective in reducing intracellular edema, which most seriously affects the gray matter. On the other hand, a direct bolus injection with a syringe has produced cardiac arrest in a few cases, and some authorities have expressed concern over the speed of activity of this compound. Although no firm data are available, our clinical impressions indicate that there is marked activity within 30 minutes after administration.

Mannitol, usually given as a 20 per cent solution, acts as a hypertonic agent to reduce brain and spinal cord edema. Two grams (10 ml. of 20 per cent solution) per kg. is given in the same rapid intravenous drip. Since mannitol produces marked diuresis, a urinary catheter should be introduced into the bladder. Both of these drugs may be repeated every six hours if necessary.

External support (plaster casts, splints, etc.) may be useful in some fractures of the cervical and cranial thoracic areas. They should not be considered as a substitute for adequate surgical decompression. A variety of internal fixation methods have been described. All these methods will provide rigid support when properly used. Flexible plastic plates, vertebral body plates and vertebral body pinning have proved superior to any method of external support. Body casts are used only when there is good fracture-luxation stability, minimal vertebral canal distortion and minimal neurologic deficit.

There is no simple answer to the question: Is this animal operable or is the situation hopeless? The dog and the owner stubbornly refuse to be simply a statistic. Each patient must be individually evaluated in the light of neurologic signs, radiographic findings, time since injury and, unfortunately, the enthusiasm and financial cooperation of the owner. The following outline, although far from precise, may help to categorize the prognosis.

1. Fair to good prognosis.
   a. Paresis only.
   b. Intact pain sensation.
   c. Minimal distortion of vertebral canal.
   d. Injury less than four hours.
2. Guarded to fair prognosis.
   a. Paraplegia-tetraplegia.
   b. Intact pain.
   c. Intact segmental reflexes.
   d. Minimal distortion of vertebral canal.

   e. Injury less than eight hours.
3. Guarded prognosis.
   a. Paraplegia-tetraplegia.
   b. Analgesia.
   c. Moderate distortion of vertebral canal (over 40 per cent of canal diameter).
   d. Schiff-Sherrington syndrome.
   e. Injury over eight hours.
4. Poor prognosis.
   a. Paraplegia-tetraplegia.
   b. Analgesia.
   c. Marked distortion of vertebral canal.
   d. Injury over 24 hours.
5. Unfavorable prognosis.
   a. Severe distortion of vertebral canal.
   b. Impatient, uncooperative owner.

Recently, we have begun to offer the owner an alternative to simple treatment or euthanasia. Even animals who are in the poor prognosis category deserve an immediate exploration, decompression and direct examination of the spinal cord. This technique has added a new and often surprising dimension to our evaluation of spinal trauma. There is no real substitute for direct observation of the lesion. If the spinal cord is severed, crushed or severely malacic, the decision is obvious and the owner and patient are spared a long hospitalization period. If, on the other hand, the cord is firm and intact, and we decompress the bony lesion, open the dura mater, reduce the distortion and stablize the vertebral column, the results are often gratifying. Time is critical, but it appears that some patients previously considered hopeless can be salvaged if an all-out effort is immediately instituted. Specific surgical techniques have been discussed in the veterinary literature, but this rapid evaluation and repair should include:

1. Dexamethasone and mannitol.
2. Rapid wide dorsal decompression.
2. Fracture-luxation reduction and stabilization by any acceptable method (dorsal plating, cross pinning, vertebral body plating).
4. Local spinal cord hypothermia by the slushing technique.
5. Dorsal incision of the dura mater.

6. Careful evaluation of the spinal cord.
7. Broad-spectrum antibiotics.

Corticosteroids, usually dexamethasone, are normally continued for three to four days. Two mg./5 kg. twice daily seems to be sufficient after spinal surgery. Patients managed conservatively are also given this dosage. The antibiotic umbrella is continued for several days after the corticosteroids are discontinued.

After severe trauma, a few animals rapidly become ambulatory. The majority remain severely paretic or paralyzed for long periods. Patience and excellent nursing care are often rewarded. A simple, but effective, routine includes:

1. Bedding deeply (12 to 18 inches) in shavings or sawdust.
2. Manually expressing bladder at least twice daily.
3. Swimming or whirlpool exercise twice daily.

Even the large breeds, who cannot easily be given whirlpool exercise, will tolerate long periods of tetraplegia if they are bedded in deep shavings. Decubital ulcers are rarely a problem with this routine.

We hope to see some sign of neurologic improvement every day or at least every other day. In general, pain responses are the first to return, followed by motor function and, lastly, proprioceptive function. But the client must be warned that the improvement can be agonizingly slow. Most patients who are going to make a functional recovery do so within six weeks. If after 45 days there is little or no improvement, the client should be cautioned against further optimism. Occasionally, however, dogs will become functionally sound months after injury. That is, they will regain sufficient walking ability to do well in a protected environment. Some of these may be true "spinal" walkers with no functional spinal cord tracts.

## SUPPLEMENTAL READING

de Lahunta, A.: Small animal neurologic examination. Vet. Clin. N. Am., 1:191–206, 1971.
Oliver, J. E., Jr.: Neurologic emergencies in small animals. Vet. Clin. N. Am., 2:341–359, 1972.

# CANINE INTER-VERTEBRAL DISK DISEASE

ERIC J. TROTTER, D.V.M.
*Ithaca, New York*

The pathophysiology of the intervertebral disk would probably be only a matter of academic interest were it not for the central nervous system (CNS) lesions which often result subsequent to disk degeneration. Degenerative disk disease itself is an asymptomatic, systemic disease process which affects all breeds of dogs. The various degenerative processes within the disk are important only as they affect the predisposition of the disk to dorsal protrusion or extrusion, with resultant spinal cord compression. A basic understanding of the pathophysiology of the intervertebral disks is essential to the rational prophylaxis and treatment of the intervertebral disk syndrome.

## PATHOPHYSIOLOGY OF THE INTERVERTEBRAL DISK

The distinction between disk degeneration in chondrodystrophoid and nonchondrodystrophoid breeds has been reported in detail by various authors. In all breeds, it is a continuous process concomitant with aging. In the chondrodystrophoid breeds, the degeneration begins at an earlier age (two to nine months) than in the nonchondrodystrophoid breeds (one to seven years), and progresses at a more rapid rate. The neurologic manifestations of disk degeneration are seen in the former breeds at an earlier age, usually three to six years, whereas clinical signs of disk protrusion are most often seen in the latter breeds at a later age, most often from 5 to 12 years. The disk syndrome in the nonchondrodystrophoid breeds is thus often termed geriatric disk disease.

In the chondrodystrophoid breeds, the disk degeneration is essentially a chondroid metaplasia with, or leading to, dehydration, necrosis and dystrophic calcification. Degeneration of the annulus fibrosis occurs simultaneously with degeneration of the nucleus pulposus. With degeneration, the nucleus loses its normal shock-absorbing function and becomes predisposed to protrusion or extrusion. The weakened, degenerate annulus is no longer able to restrain the equally degenerate nucleus and to properly distribute the loads applied to this shock-absorbing system. Even minimal stresses, such as normal movement of the vertebral column, are sufficient, at this stage, for the initiation of disk prolapse.

Severe, acute vertebral column trauma, even in the presence of diffuse intervertebral disk degeneration, is more apt to result in vertebral fractures and luxations than in disk protrusion. Although ventral and lateral disk protrusions or extrusions may occur, with or without nerve root compression, the majority are dorsal extrusions, through the thinner dorsal laminations of the annulus. These extrusions of nuclear material have been previously classified as Hansen type I protrusions, and result commonly in a compressive myelopathy.

In the nonchondrodystrophoid breeds, fibroid metaplasia, with dehydration, necrosis, fibrosis and, occasionally, calcification, predominates. These changes begin at an older age, and progress more slowly. The majority of the subsequent protrusions are dorsal bulgings of the intact, degenerate annulus, without true extrusion of nuclear material into the epidural space. These protrusions have been previously classified as Hansen type II protrusions. Again, a compressive myelopathy is the usual result.

## SPINAL CORD PATHOLOGY

Except for the fortunately small percentage of thoracolumbar disk extrusions which result in myelomalacia, the basic lesion in the intervertebral disk syndrome is a compressive myelopathy, usually involving from one to four segments of the spinal cord. The spinal cord lesion has been attributed to a number of factors. These included: mechanical distortion or derangement of the nervous elements, hemorrhage, edema, venous stasis, ischemia and anoxia, with resultant demyelination, gliosis, focal malacia and cavitation. The severity of the spinal cord lesions is influenced not only by the magnitude of the protrusion, but also by its rate of development. A small, rapidly occurring protrusion will usually result in a much more severe neurologic dysfunction than will a large slowly progressive protrusion. The "dynamic force" with which the disk extrudes, the inflammatory reaction in the epidural space and the specific location of the extrusion with respect to the diameter of the vertebral canal are also important factors which determine the severity of the spinal cord lesion. A "vicious cycle," beginning with the extrusion, and including many of the above factors, is probably responsible for the compressive myelopathy.

In contrast to this focal compressive myelopathy, thoracolumbar disk extrusion may result in a diffuse, necrotic myelopathy. This has previously been referred to as hematomyelia, ascending syndrome, hemorrhagic myelomalacia and ascending cord necrosis. Owing to the progressive nature of the lesion and the predominance of hemorrhage and necrosis, it may be better designated ascending-descending myelomalacia.

The pathogenesis of myelomalacia is also unknown, although numerous mechanisms have been proposed. These include vasospasm, thrombosis, venous occlusion and rupture of medullary vessels, with resultant ischemia anoxia. The onset is typical of that of a compressive focal myelopathy subsequent to thoracolumbar disk extrusion. However, usually within 24 hours of the onset of clinical signs, the spinal cord lesion begins to progress. The extension of the lesion may consist of both ascension and descension, or either component may predominate. Analgesia and areflexia become more extensive as the multisegmental hemorrhagic necrosis continues. The neck is often held in extension, contributing to the general impression of extreme apprehension and exquisite pain. Extensor rigidity of the forelimbs (Schiff-Sherrington phenomenon) due to the destruction of ascending inhibitory neurons precedes thoracic limb motor deficits. The necrotic phenomenon may spontaneously arrest but, in most cases, death due to respiratory failure ensues within four days of onset.

At postmortem examination, extradural and intradural hemorrhage are often extensive. Examination of transverse sections of involved segments of the spinal cord reveals varying degrees of hemorrhage, necrosis and cavitation. The ascending or descending lesion may "skip over" some segments, or involve all segments of the spinal cord from cauda equina to medulla.

When these signs become apparent, early euthanasia is recommended because of the extensive, irreparable nature of the spinal cord lesion, the animal's acute suffering and the hopeless prognosis.

## BREED AND SITE INCIDENCE OF DISK PROTRUSION

The incidence of the intervertebral disk syndrome has been investigated by various authors. The chondrodystrophoid breeds predominate. Although obviously influenced by geographic distribution and changing breed popularity, dachshunds, Pekingese, cocker spaniels, poodles and beagles seem most commonly affected. Of the nonchondrodystrophoid breeds, German shepherds and Labrador retrievers predominate.

Hoerlein (1971) and others have published extensively on the breed incidence and anatomic sites of disk protrusion in the dog. The thoracolumbar region is most commonly affected. In this region, the intervertebral disk at $T_{12-13}$ and $T_{13}$–$L_1$ account for the greatest percentage of protrusions. In the cervical region, protrusions occur most commonly at $C_{2-3}$ and $C_{3-4}$.

## NEUROLOGIC EXAMINATION IN THORACOLUMBAR DISK PROTRUSION

Protrusions of the thoracolumbar disks most often result in an upper motor neuron (UMN) and general proprioceptive (GP) lesion, with varying degrees of pain and bilaterally symmetrical pelvic limb paresis and ataxia. Hind leg segmental spinal reflexes are usually normal or hyperreflexic. Muscle tone may be normal, hypotonic or hypertonic. The crossed-extensor reflex may be present. The Schiff-Sherrington phenomenon is not commonly associated with thoracolumbar disk protrusion unless myelomalacia ensues. Conscious perception of pain, not to be confused with the flexor, or withdrawal reflex, may be normal, decreased or absent, thus classifying the patient as eugesic, hypalgesic or analgesic. Postural reactions of the pelvic limbs may be absent or poorly performed. Bladder function may be normal or "spinal": retention or retention-reflex. Defecation is rarely affected. The approximate site of the lesion may often be localized by the panniculus reflex, or by the animal's hyperesthetic response to pressure applied to the spinous processes. In severe cases, a line of analgesia to noxious stimuli may be traced on the abdominal wall.

Further classification of the degree of paresis or paralysis has proved useful. The grading system utilized is as follows:

Grade 5: Normal strength.
Grade 4: Supports,* minimal paresis-ataxia.
Grade 3: Supports, frequently stumbles, moderate paresis-ataxia.
Grade 2: Supports with assistance, stumbles, and falls.
Grade 1: No support, slight movement when supported by tail.
Grade 0: Absence of purposeful movements.

In some cases, the lesion may be a mixed UMN and lower motor neuron (LMN) type. These lesions result from a compressive myelopathy involving the spinal cord segments containing the cell bodies of the lower motor neurons to the perineum, tail or pelvic limbs. The previously described neurologic signs of the pure UMN lesion are complicated by LMN signs such as hyporeflexia or areflexia. Disk protrusions or extrusions at $L_{3-4}$, $L_{4-5}$, and $L_{5-6}$ may result in varying degrees of dysfunction of the spinal cord segments or roots of the femoral, sciatic, perineal and caudal neurons which are evidenced by altered muscle tone and segmental spinal reflexes. The prognosis in these cases is not as favorable as in pure UMN lesions because of the involvement of the cell bodies themselves, rather than the axons. Differentiation of these LMN lesions from myelomalacia is essential because of the radical differences in prognosis and treatment. The tone of the abdominal musculature, the cranial extent of the line of analgesia, and the character of the respirations may be utilized in the differential diagnosis.

Exact recording of the neurologic status of the patient at the time of admission and during the preoperative and postoperative periods is essential for optimum patient care and objective evaluation of therapeutic techniques.

## NEUROLOGIC EXAMINATION IN CERVICAL DISK PROTRUSION

Cervical disk protrusions most often result in extreme cervical pain. This may be due to direct spinal cord compression or to radicular involvement. The typical dog with a protruded cervical disk is apprehensive, reluctant to move and appears stiff because of contraction of the cervical musculature. Any manipulation of the head or neck results in severe pain. Occasionally, cervical disk extrusion results in an UMN and GP lesion in the pelvic and thoracic limbs. With caudal cervical lesions, there may be an associated LMN lesion in the thoracic limbs. The lesion may result in varying degrees of ataxia and tetraparesis. The pelvic limb deficit is usually more obvious than that of the thoracic limbs.

## RADIOGRAPHIC EXAMINATION

The area of the lesion must be approximated as exactly as possible to allow for efficient radiographic examination. Proper radiographic technique is essential for the production of high quality diagnostic films. General anesthesia is necessary for the elimination of motion and for precise positioning of the patient which will allow for adequate visualization of the intervertebral disk spaces. Accurate placement of the central x-ray beam over the suspected area of involvement aids in the prevention of false interpretation of narrowed disk spaces.

In most cases, conventional radiographs are adequate if the approximate location of the lesion has been determined by neurologic examination. However, if any uncertainty regarding interpretation of the plain radiographs exists, a myelogram should be performed.

## THERAPY OF THORACOLUMBAR DISK PROTRUSION

The veterinary medical literature contains many conflicting claims for the relative safety and efficacy of a wide variety of treatments for thoracolumbar disk protrusion. The very nature of the disk disease

---

*Support implies voluntary motor activity to achieve standing position.

process has been responsible for much of the controversy. The lesion is difficult, if not impossible, to reproduce experimentally for a controlled evaluation of therapeutic techniques. Because of the high incidence of spontaneous recoveries, particularly in mild cases, and the absence of a standard neurologic classification, evaluation of various therapeutic regimens approaches the impossible. The superiority of surgical over nonsurgical therapy for those cases in which disk protrusion has resulted in severe paresis or paralysis has, however, been well documented.

The formulation of a protocol for the treatment of TL intervertebral disk protrusion, although somewhat arbitrary, does provide for a systematic approach to a controversial problem. The protocol presently in use at this clinic is shown in Table 1.

As related previously, high quality diagnostic films may be utilized as a decisive factor in the determination of the treatment regimen of a specific patient. In cases of grade 3 paresis and ataxia, the choice of surgical technique is often based on the radiographic findings. An extremely narrowed intervertebral disk space, suggesting complete extrusion of disk material, is an indication for laminectomy rather than fenestration, as is the presence of radiographically observable disk material in the epidural space. Chronic, progressive lesions with grade 3 neurologic signs would seem to suggest the feasibility of fenestration.

### Table 1. Protocol for Treatment of Thoracolumbar Disk Protrusion

| CATEGORIES, AS DETERMINED BY HISTORY AND NEUROLOGIC EXAMINATION | THERAPY |
| --- | --- |
| Pain only, first attack | Medical |
| Pain only, recurrent attacks | Fenestration |
| Mild paresis and ataxia (grade 4), first attack | Medical |
| Mild paresis and ataxia (grade 4), recurrent attacks | Fenestration |
| Moderate paresis and ataxia (grade 3) | Fenestration *or* decompression |
| Severe paresis (grades 2 and 1) and paraplegia (grade 0) | Decompression |

## MEDICAL THERAPY OF INTERVERTEBRAL DISK PROTRUSION

Resorption of extruded disk material, the formation of a stable fibrosis in the offending disk, and the impressive compensatory ability of the canine spinal cord may account for the relatively high incidence of spontaneous improvements in cases with mild to moderate neurologic dysfunction. Medical therapy is utilized in mild cases mainly as supportive therapy for these reparative mechanisms. Analgesics,* muscle relaxants,** antiarthritic preparations† and corticosteroids‡ must be used with caution during the healing stages of the disk protrusion. Overzealous administration of these medications may lead to complete relief of the beneficial self-limiting pain. Resultant overactivity at this stage may result in the extrusion of further disk material and a worsening of the neurologic dysfunction. Excessive pain should be lessened with medication, but not completely relieved. Enforced cage rest, preferably under the supervision of a veterinarian, is essential during the administration of these preparations.

Various authors have alluded to the greater incidence of recurrence of cervical and thoracolumbar disk protrusions following medical rather than surgical therapy. Firm recommendations regarding the advisability of medical therapy and of prophylactic disk fenestration await more extensive, long-term comparison survey.

## SURGICAL THERAPY OF THORACOLUMBAR DISK PROTRUSION

Recurrent cases of thoracolumbar pain, or pain and minimal paresis and ataxia, have responded well to fenestration of the offending and adjacent disks. The mechanism of action, according to Olsson (1951a), is the production of an acute inflammatory reaction which stimulates phagocytosis, resorption of necrosis and the formation of a stable

---

*Aspirin, Bufferin® (Bristol-Myers), Demerol® (Winthrop).
**Robaxin® (methocarbamol, Robins), Maolate® (chlorphenesin carbamate, Upjohn).
†Cordex®, Cordex-Forte® (Upjohn), Butazolidin® (phenylbutazone, Geigy), indomethacin.
‡Azium® (Schering), prednisolone, prednisone.

fibrosis in the disk. There is little, if any, immediate decompressive effect. However, further protrusion of disk material is probably prevented. The technique may thus be both therapeutic and prophylactic in cases of mild to moderate paresis and ataxia. With minimal operative trauma, all of the "high incidence" disks may be fenestrated by the ventral approach, as described by Leonard (1960).

In cases of moderate to severe paresis and ataxia, or paraplegia, a more aggressive approach is indicated. Adequate decompression of the spinal cord, with removal of the extruded disk material, has proved successful in a high percentage of cases. Hemilaminectomy has been well described, and practiced with excellent results. However, dorsal laminectomy appears to have several advantages.

The laminectomy presently in use at this clinic is a modification of the Funkquist type B dorsal laminectomy (Figs. 1 and 2). It results in excellent exposure and decompression with no hazard of secondary spinal cord compression due to constrictive fibrosis. Complete removal of the caudal articular processes and undercutting of the laminectomy edges allow the removal of extruded or protruded disk material. "Sling" sutures of 5-0 swaged, cardiovascular silk

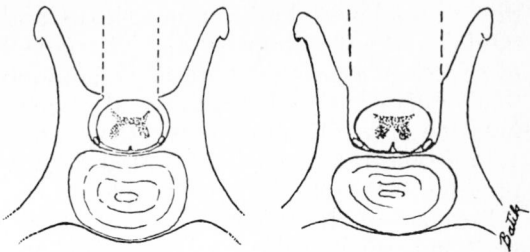

**Figure 2.** Transverse sections through areas of dorsal laminectomies according to Funkquist B (*left*) and modified dorsal laminectomy (*right*) techniques.

may be placed in the dura mater to facilitate atraumatic spinal cord manipulation during removal of disk material from the epidural space. By means of dura scissors,* or bent, disposable 20-gauge hypodermic needle, the dura mater is incised on the dorsal midline for the full length of the laminectomy. Incision of the inelastic dural sheath is thought to result in greater decompression of the spinal cord. It also permits the formulation of a more accurate prognosis, since focal malacia and thrombosis or rupture of the spinal cord vasculature, if present, are readily observable.

## SURGICAL THERAPY OF CERVICAL DISK PROTRUSION

The superiority of surgical over nonsurgical therapy, both in terms of results and recurrence rate, has been previously reported.

With pain as the only predominant clinical sign, ventral fenestration is employed. Routinely, the offending disk and all other safely accessible cervical disks are fenestrated with a claw-type tarter scraper. This usually includes the first four cervical intervertebral disks, which comprise the majority of commonly protruding or extruding disks. Medical therapy alone is utilized only if financial consideration or serious systemic disease is a major deterrent to surgery.

As in the case of thoracolumbar disk protrusion, significant degrees of paresis and ataxia necessitate a more aggressive approach. A wide, dorsal laminectomy, continued cranially and caudally until normal amounts of epidural fat are visualized, may be performed. The exposure of the cervical spinal cord is superior to that achieved with a ventral decompression. Hemorrhage from

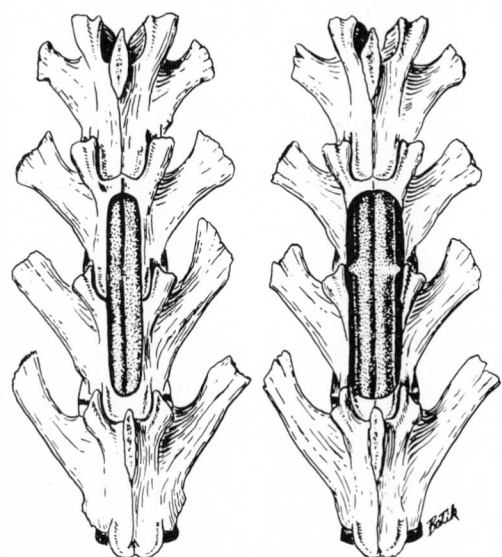

**Figure 1.** Dorsal view of decompressive laminectomies to illustrate the increased exposure and decompression of the spinal cord with the modified dorsal laminectomy (MDL) technique. Narrow dorsal laminectomy (*after* Funkquist type B) (*left*)- modified dorsal laminectomy (MDL) (*right*).

---

*Schmieden-Taylor dura scissors.

the internal vertebral venous plexus and trauma to the vertebral vessels have proved to be less of a problem with this technique than with either ventral cervical decompression or hemilaminectomy. However, in ventral midline extrusions, ventral decompression is the preferred technique.

Because of the greater diameter of the vertebral canal in the cervical region, undercutting of the laminectomy edges and the placement of dural "sling" sutures are usually unnecessary for the removal of the extruded disk material. The dura mater is routinely incised to achieve increased spinal cord decompression and to allow for a more accurate prognosis.

Enforced cage rest in the hospital is recommended for one week postoperatively in all cases of cervical disk protrusion. Restricted exercise and the avoidance of collars or lead ropes for at least six weeks are recommended at discharge to prevent postoperative exacerbations. Postoperative care in those cases requiring dorsal laminectomy is essentially identical to that of thoracolumbar laminectomy.

## SUPPORTIVE THERAPY IN CERVICAL AND THORACOLUMBAR DISK SURGERY

"Improvement in neurosurgical results has been achieved not only with perfection of operative techniques, however, but also because of increased ability to protect the central nervous system during and after surgical procedures" (Matson, 1965).

A 20 per cent solution of mannitol (Osmitrol®, Travenol) in water may be administered intravenously through a filtered fluid administration apparatus at a dosage of 2 gm./kg. of body weight. The calculated amount is given over a 10- to 20-minute period to achieve maximum osmotic effect. This is often repeated in three to four hours, especially in acute, severe cases in which edema of the spinal cord is believed to be a prominent factor in the production of the spinal cord lesion. The administration of mannitol is usually begun after all soft tissue dissection has been completed because of its tendency to increase hemorrhage markedly. The hypertonic solution of inert, nontoxic mannitol effectively lowers cerebrospinal fluid pressure and brain and probably spinal cord mass with little, if any, rebound effect.

Large doses of corticosteroids (Azium) are administered intravenously at the time of surgery, or in the early preoperative period if immediate decompressive surgery is not possible. Dexamethasone is utilized at a one-time dosage of 2 mg./kg. of body weight. The calculated dosage of dexamethasone is mixed into a balanced electrolyte solution (lactated Ringer's solution) which is administered during the operative procedure. The beneficial effects of corticosteroids in neurosurgical patients have been reported by various authors. They result primarily from the reduction of inflammation and edema of the nervous tissues.

Broad-spectrum antibiotics are administered preoperatively and are mixed into the balanced electrolyte solution which is administered during surgery.

Balanced electrolyte solutions are administered in the intraoperative period to maintain normovolemia and to offset the dehydrating effect of the potent osmotic diuretic, mannitol.

Hyperventilation is achieved by means of mechanically assisted respiration (Bird Mark 7 respirator) in order to produce a mild respiratory alkalosis. This technique has proved to be an effective means of preventing CNS edema due to acidosis and a safeguard against inadvertent laceration of the internal vertebral venous plexus. The undercutting procedure of the laminectomy is continued only during the expiration phases of the ventilator when the sinuses are collapsed because of decreased intrathoracic pressure and subsequent increased venous return to the right heart.

Proper positioning of the patient is essential for the prevention of venous engorgement and possible CNS edema due to stasis. It has been shown that occlusion of the external jugular veins or caudal vena cava results in markedly increased flow through the internal vertebral venous plexuses.

The implementation of selective regional spinal cord hypothermia in all laminectomy cases has appeared to be one of the major factors in the improvement of neurosurgical results. Although utilized mainly for its beneficial effects in reducing iatrogenic spinal cord trauma, it has been previously proved to be of great benefit in the early treatment of impact injuries of the spinal cord. Although the mechanism of action of spinal cord hypothermia is as yet unknown, it does appear to "allow doing extensive dissection, manipulating, and unavoidably caused surgical trauma heretofore prohibitively dangerous" (Brasmer, 1972).

Experimental and clinical data have indicated the efficacy of a relatively simple and practical technique for the production of selective regional spinal cord hypothermia. Wide mouth, autoclavable, 250-ml. centrifuge bottles* are filled with lactated Ringer's solution and placed in a deep freeze ($-80°$ C). After remaining at this temperature for 40 minutes, the bottles are removed and shaken vigorously to produce fine ice crystal "slush" similar to commercial soft drink "Sno-Cones." The laminectomy defect is then gently filled with the slush, which is allowed to remain in position for 20 minutes. Internal spinal cord temperatures of $6°$ C. have been realized with this technique. The slush is then melted with room temperature lactated Ringer's solution and removed with suction prior to a secure closure of the dorsal lumbar fascia. Absorbable gelatin sponge† is "tented" over the laminectomy defect prior to closure.

## POSTOPERATIVE CARE OF THE NEUROSURGICAL PATIENT

Hypertonic solution and corticosteroid administration are often continued into the postoperative period to aid in alleviation or prevention of spinal cord edema. Catastrophic gastrointestinal complications have been seen infrequently in patients treated with massive doses of corticosteroids following neurosurgery. However, because of the low incidence of these complications and the overwhelming experimental and clinical evidence supporting the beneficial effects of steroids, their administration is still recommended. Since clinical studies in man have shown that the decrease in mucous viscosity and the increase in gastric acidity and pepsin do not develop before the seventh day of ACTH administration, steroid therapy should not be used for more than six days. In the postoperative care of laminectomy cases, the dosages of corticosteroids are gradually decreased during the first four to five postoperative days to prevent suppression of adrenal function due to the exogenous steroid administration.

---

*Nalge screw-cap centrifuge bottles.
†Gelfoam (Upjohn).

Broad-spectrum antibiotic therapy is continued for at least three days after the discontinuation of steroid therapy.

Utilization of foam rubber cage pads, air mattresses, small water beds or cedar shavings has markedly reduced the incidence of decubitus in paralyzed patients.

Whirlpool baths reduce muscle spasticity, improve circulation, promote paddling movements of the pelvic limbs, aid in the prevention of muscle atrophy and add to the general sense of well being of the patient. The addition of a whirlpool concentrate of povidone-iodine (Betadine®, Purdue Frederick) is beneficial for the prevention of urine scald, superficial pyodermas and infection of decubital sores.

Well lubricated, aseptically maintained indwelling urinary catheters seem to decrease the bladder trauma associated with repeated manual expressions, and aid in the prevention of retention cystitis and urine scald. Broad-spectrum antibiotic solutions (Furacin®, nitrofurazone [Eaton]) may be flushed into the bladder after evacuation.

Maintenance of a high plane of nutrition to overcome negative nitrogen balance, enthusiastic nursing care and generous amounts of affection cannot be overemphasized.

Exercise carts, easily constructed from inexpensive aluminum rod and lawn mower wheels, aid in the prevention of pressure sores and the stimulation of early postoperative pelvic limb activity. Tailing exercises are substituted in the occasional animal which develops total dependence on the exercise cart.

Paralyzed patients are discharged from the hospital as soon as conscious control of micturition is regained. Most owners are delighted to participate in the rehabilitation program. Early return to familiar surroundings promotes patient enthusiasm and early return to normal function.

Continued communication with the owner in the form of both short- and long-term progress reports is essential for the objective evaluation of the therapeutic regimen in use.

## RESULTS

Although there is much individual variation, the guidelines for anticipated postoperative improvement in cases of severe paresis or paralysis are given in Table 2.

**Table 2.** *Guidelines for Anticipated Postoperative Improvement in Severe Paresis or Paralysis*

| NEUROLOGIC STATUS | POSTOPERATIVE DAY |
|---|---|
| Return of normal urination | 10 to 21 |
| Return of normal pain sensation to pelvic limbs | 10 to 21 |
| Onset of voluntary paddling movements in pelvic limbs | 14 to 35 |
| Return of support (voluntary activity initiated to achieve standing posture) | 14 to 42 |
| Ambulation | 14 to 90 |
| Return of normal proprioception | 21 to 180 |

The attitude of the majority of veterinary surgeons toward laminectomy has remained conservative, probably because of the fear of transforming, with surgery, a reversible to an irreversible lesion. With the advent of effective ancillary neurosurgical techniques for the prevention of spinal cord trauma during surgery, and the refinement of neurosurgical techniques, the risks have been minimized. The neurologic status of the patient has been only rarely worsened by laminectomy according to the previously described technique. Not only is the recovery period shortened, but the recovery rate is greatly enhanced by neurosurgery.

**SUPPLEMENTAL READING**

Brasmer, T. H., and Lumb, W. V.: Lumbar vertebral prosthesis in the dog. Am. J. Vet. Res., 33:499, 1972.
Funkquist, B.: Thoracolumbar disc protrusion with severe cord compression in the dog. I, II, III. Acta. Vet. Scand. 3, 1962.
Funkquist, B.: Decompressive laminectomy in thoracolumbar disc protrusion with paraplegia in the dog. J. Small Animal Pract., 11:445–451, 1970.
Griffiths, I. R.: The extensive myelopathy of intervertebral disc protrusions in dogs (the ascending syndrome). J. Small Animal Pract., 13:425–437, 1972.
Hansen, H. J.: A pathologic-anatomical study on disc degeneration in dog. Acta Orthop. Scand., Suppl. 11: 1952.
Hoerlein, B. F.: Canine Neurology. 2nd ed. Philadelphia, W. B. Saunders Co., 1971.
Knecht, C. D.: The effects of delayed hemilaminectomy in the treatment of intervertebral disc protrusions in dogs. J. Am. Animal Hospit. Assn., 6: 1970.
Leonard, E. P.: Orthopedic Surgery of the Dog and Cat. 2nd ed. Philadelphia, W. B. Saunders Co., 1971.
Martin, J. G.: The feasibility of delayed surgery in intervertebral disc protrusion causing paraplegia or paresis. Proc. Am. Animal Hosp. Assn., 423, 1969.
Matson, D. V.: Treatment of cerebral swelling. New England J. Med., 272:626, 1965.
Olsson, S. E.: Observations concerning disc fenestration in dogs. Acta Orthop. Scand., 20:349, 1951a.
Olsson, S. E.: On disc protrusion in dog. Acta Orthop. Scand., Suppl. 8:1951b.
Olsson, S. E.: The dynamic factor in spinal cord compression. A study on dogs with special reference to cervical disc protrusions. J. Neurosurg., 15:308, 1958.
Russell, S. W., and Griffiths, R. C.: Recurrence of cervical disc syndrome in surgically and conservatively treated dogs. J. Am. Vet. Med. Assn., 153, 1968.
Swaim, S. F.: Ventral decompression of the cervical spinal cord in the dog. J. Am. Vet. Med. Assn., 162, 1973.
Valergakis, F. E. G., Critides, S., and Winokur, G. L.: Gastrointestinal complications in neurosurgical patients treated with steroids. Am. J. Gastroent., 1972.

# OTITIS EXTERNA AND MEDIA

R. E. HOFFER, D.V.M.
*Ithaca, New York*

Otitis externa is an inflammation of the auditory canal. Otitis media is an inflammation of the middle ear and is generally an extension of otitis externa. Otitis interna is generally secondary to otitis media.

## ANATOMY OF THE EAR

The pinna of the ear is a platelike extension of the auricular cartilage, covered by skin on both sides. In dogs, its shape is often characteristic of the particular breed. The pinnas of cats are usually the same shape, regardless of the breed. The auricular cartilage is attached to the external acoustic meatus by the tubular-shaped annular cartilage (Fig. 1). The vertical ear canal is formed at the base of the pinna where the thin cartilage plate is rolled into a tube. At the rostral border of the opening into the

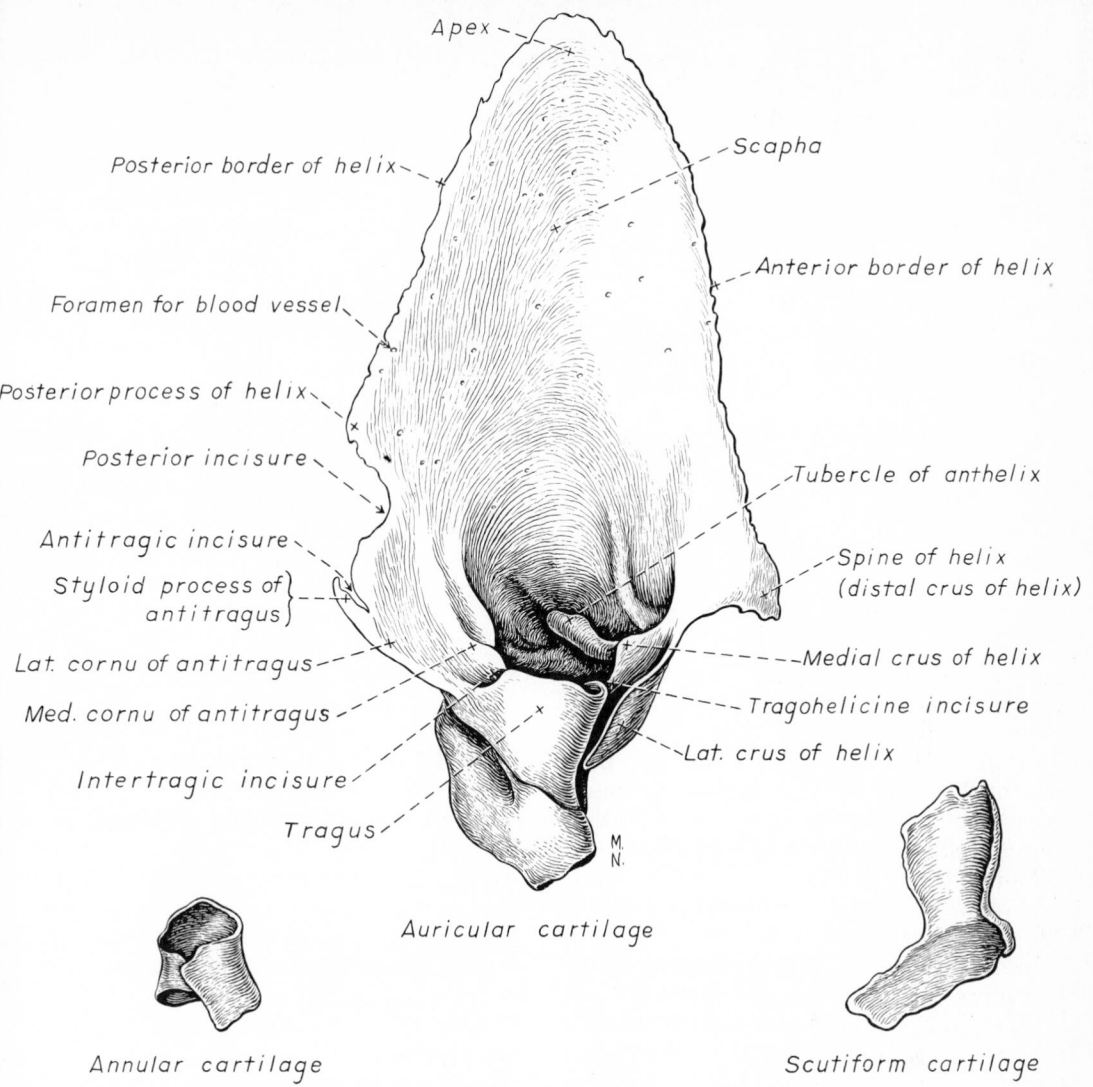

Apex

Posterior border of helix

Scapha

Anterior border of helix

Foramen for blood vessel

Posterior process of helix

Posterior incisure

Tubercle of anthelix

Antitragic incisure

Spine of helix
(distal crus of helix)

Styloid process of
antitragus

Lat. cornu of antitragus

Medial crus of helix

Med. cornu of antitragus

Tragohelicine incisure

Lat. crus of helix

Intertragic incisure

Tragus

M.
N.

Auricular cartilage

Annular cartilage

Scutiform cartilage

**Figure 1.** Pinna and auricular cartilages. (From Getty *et al.*, 1956.)

vertical ear canal is the tragus, the thick, irregularly quadrangular plate of the auricular cartilage. The intertragic notch between the tragus and the antitragus is located at the lateral boundary of the opening into the ear canal, and the tragohelicine notch is located at the medial aspect of this opening.

The horizontal ear canal is formed by the auricular cartilage laterally and the annular cartilage medially. In the modified Lacroix-Zepp's operation it is important to include in the excision a portion of the horizontal canal so that the junction of auricular and annular cartilages can be visualized. The annular cartilage attaches by ligaments around the osseous external acoustic meatus.

The oval-shaped tympanic membrane separates the horizontal external ear canal from the middle ear. The external portion of this membrane is concave. The middle ear cavity of the dog has two portions: (1) a larger, ventral portion and (2) a narrow, dorsal portion, which contains the auditory ossicles. The vestibular and cochlear windows communicate with the inner ear. The auditory tube, which communicates with the nasopharynx, is located at the level of the external acoustic meatus and rostral to the cochlear window (Fig. 2).

## INCIDENCE

Otitis externa is one of the most common disease problems in the dog and cat and is particularly prevalent in dogs. The reported

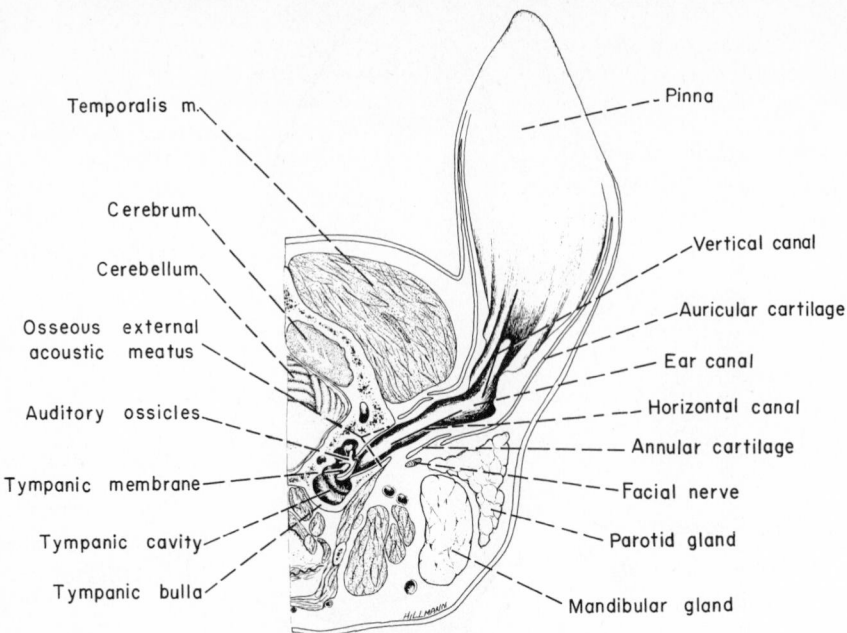

**Figure 2.**   Transverse section through head showing ear canal. (Modified after Sis.)

incidence varies from 7.5 per cent to 20.4 per cent. The incidence in the cat has been reported as 2 per cent, but many feel that the incidence is higher.

The incidence of otitis media in dogs has been reported as 16 per cent for patients with acute otitis externa and 50 per cent in chronic otitis cases. The incidence of primary otitis media is low and has not been observed by Spruell, Fraser or the author. It is generally accepted that the accumulation of debris, hair and foreign bodies results in extension through or rupture of the tympanic membrane, with subsequent extension of the inflammation into the middle ear.

Certain breeds have been reported to be more prone to otitis than have others. Dogs with pendulous ears have the highest incidence of the disease, and it appears to be more frequent in older animals. The breeds with the highest incidence are the cocker spaniel and the miniature poodle. In the cat and dog, incidence of bilateral disease is higher than unilateral.

## ETIOLOGY

The cause of otitis externa is complex. Many factors have been incriminated but the exact etiology has not been determined. It has been suggested that by the time the animal presents for treatment the initial cause may not be apparent.

Factors associated with otitis are foreign bodies, matted hair, dried wax, trauma to the ear from cleaning and examination, ectoparasites, allergic response (generally associated with other allergic skin problems), bacterial and fungal flora in the ear and excessive moisture.

Probably the cause of otitis externa is a combination of these factors. Two factors that seem to be frequently involved and may predispose to otitis externa are ear mites and trauma. Ear mites in dogs and even more so in cats may be a major factor in the development of otitis externa. Even if the mites are not found during the physical examination, it has been suggested that they initiate the problem and subsequently are driven out by the inflammation.

All the factors listed, including mites, trauma and excessive moisture, produce irritation to the ear, which predisposes to the development of otitis externa. This irritation can be aggravated by the conformation of the ear.

The most frequent isolates from the ears of dogs and cats were yeasts of the *Pityrosporon* spp. and bacteria of the *Pseudomonas* spp., *Proteus* spp. and *Staphylococcus* spp. It is felt that *Proteus* spp. and *Pseudomonas* spp. can be primary pathogens in the disease. However, *Staphylococcus* spp. may be found in normal ears and may grow only in response to inflammation initiated by some other factor.

*Pityrosporon* is considered by some to be a primary pathogen and by others to be similar to *Staphylococcus*. If a pure culture of *Pityrosporon* is isolated, it may be considered to be the causative factor but could also be a secondary pathogen. Often there will be mixed cultures from the ears, especially in chronic cases.

Otitis media is usually the result of the extension of otitis externa and therefore the same organisms are identified in most cases.

## PHYSICAL FINDINGS

In the acute phase of otitis externa, the dog or cat may show a black or tan odoriferous discharge from the ears. They may scratch their ears and shake their heads. As the infection becomes worse, they will show pain on palpation of the ear. On otoscopic examination the ear will be full of debris, and often the tympanic membrane cannot be visualized.

The epithelium of the ear canal will be reddened and may be swollen in the acute phase of otitis externa. As the disease progresses, ulceration will appear, and the ear canal will become more stenotic, with excessive proliferation of the epidermis. This may even progress to small tumor-like masses within the ear canal.

The disease, when chronic, shows a thickening of the skin of the auditory canal, and often ulceration will occur. The cartilage of the auditory canal will feel hard and in severe chronic cases may become ossified.

Otitis media generally shows only the symptoms of otitis externa. However, if severe inflammation of the middle ear occurs, the patient may show a head tilt with other signs of vestibular system disturbance. Occasionally a facial palsy can occur as a result of extensive inflammation affecting the facial nerve as it passes by the bulla. Occasionally the animal will be reluctant to open its mouth.

If the tympanic membrane is ruptured, the diagnosis of otitis media is confirmed. Occasionally in the acute states the tympanic membrane will be intact, but instead of being concave, pearly gray in color and glistening, it may show changes that indicate extension of inflammation. If the membrane bulges and is dull in appearance, it indicates a severe middle-ear problem. Occasionally the middle ear will be full of debris or granulation tissue. In this case, the tympanic bulla usually will show increased density upon radiographic examination.

## TREATMENT

When an animal presents with suspected otitis externa (with or without otitis media), the most important procedure is to clean the ears thoroughly. To do this properly, it is almost always necessary to anesthetize the patient or use heavy sedation. This will permit complete examination of the auditory canal and tympanic membrane. Prior to cleaning the ears, a sterile swab for culture and sensitivity should be obtained. A slide made from the debris in the ear should be examined by microscopy to identify mites if present. After thorough examination, the decision should be made to treat the ears medically or surgically.

After anesthesia, the ear is cleaned by filling it with a ceruminolytic agent and allowing it to set. The ear canal is then filled with Betadine® scrub (Purdue Frederick, Yonkers, New York 10701) and massaged. The canal is flushed using a 2-oz. rubber bulb syringe, and this process is repeated until the ear is perfectly clean. An alternate method is to use a Water-Pik® to clean the canal. When the bulb syringe is used, care should be taken not to occlude the canal completely; otherwise, excessive pressure could cause the tympanic membrane to rupture.

After a thorough cleaning, the ear canal is dried with cotton-tipped applicators, and the canal and tympanic membrane are examined with an otoscope. If debris or excessive hair is still present, it may be removed by use of an alligator forceps under direct visualization through the otoscope. An antifungal-antibiotic action ointment can then be instilled in the ear until results of the culture are obtained. If the tympanic membrane is ruptured, only water-soluble ointments should be utilized to prevent their buildup in the ventral portion of the middle ear.

Once instituted, medical therapy should be continued for three to four weeks. The ears should be examined and cleaned once each week if necessary. *Pityrosporon* spp.

may be treated with nystatin or by changing the pH of the ear canal with vinegar.

If ear mites are present, these should be treated for a period of four weeks with Canex® (Pitman-Moore) and mineral oil applied once every three days in the ear canal. The entire animal has to be treated with a good flea powder and flea collar if mites complicate the otitis externa.

Acute otitis externa should respond to proper treatment and result in a cure. If the condition recurs, check to see if there is something in the environment or handling of the dog, such as bathing, swimming or excessive plucking of the ears, that predisposes the dog to flare-ups. Then eliminate the problem or compensate for it with medication. Proper treatment of most acute otitis cases will prevent the development of chronic otitis and otitis media.

Surgical intervention is necessary if (1) chronic otitis is present with physical changes in the ear canal, (2) there are repeated acute flare-ups of chronic otitis, (3) there is no response to treatment and (4) there are symptoms of otitis media.

There are four procedures that may be utilized for treating otitis externa and/or otitis media. The procedures are well described in the standard small animal surgical textbooks and are

1. Modified Lacroix-Zepp's procedure
2. Resection of the vertical ear canal
3. Ablation of the ear
4. Bulla osteotomy

These procedures may be utilized in a stepwise manner:

A modified Lacroix-Zepp's is the initial procedure. It removes the lateral aspect of the vertical ear canal. The most important aim of this procedure is to obtain complete drainage of the horizontal ear canal. If there is extensive physical change of the vertical ear canal, it may be removed completely. This is especially indicated if there is excessive proliferation of tissue of the vertical canal.

After performing either a modified Lacroix-Zepp or a vertical canal resection, it is important to clean all debris and granulation tissue thoroughly from the middle ear.

If the horizontal ear canal is stenotic, owing to scarring or excessive proliferation, complete ear ablation may be necessary. If this is done, the bulla must be drained. This can be done by placing a tube that has an external diameter as large as the osseous

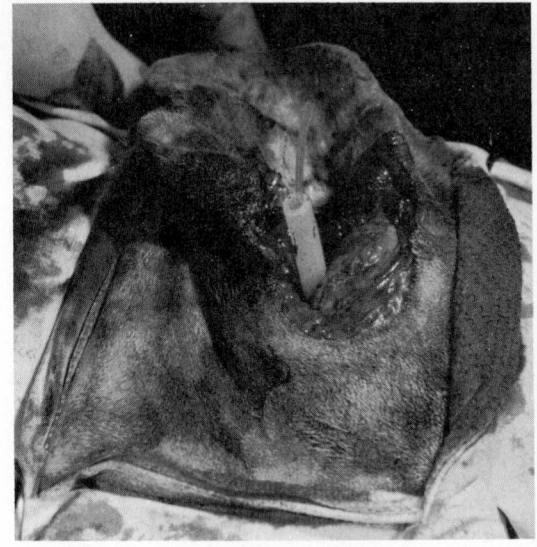

Figure 3.

meatus into the bulla and then placing a smaller tube within the larger tube (Fig. 3). Following surgery, the outer tube is fixed to the ear and then bandaged. The bulla is flushed with appropriate antibiotics or antiseptics through the smaller inner tube; the larger tube acts to drain the bulla.

If tubes cannot be placed into the bulla or there is evidence of severe middle-ear inflammation, a bulla osteotomy should be performed. Generally this is done in conjunction with ear ablation, but it may also be done with a Lacroix-Zepp's procedure.

If otitis media extends to otitis interna, the prognosis is more guarded.

Generally, if a modified Lacroix-Zepp's procedure is properly performed before progression of the otitis externa, results will be good.

### SUPPLEMENTAL READING

Barter, M., and Lawler, D. C.: The incidence and microbiology of otitis externa of dogs and cats in New Zealand. N. Zeal. Vet. J., 20:29–32, 1972.

Fraser, G., Gregor, W. W., MacKenzie, C. P., Spruell, J. S. A., and Withers, A. R.: Canine ear disease. J. Small Animal Pract. 10:725–754, 1970.

Getty, R.: The ear, *In* Miller, M. E., Christian, G. C., and Evans, H. E. (eds.): Anatomy of the Dog. Philadelphia, W. B. Saunders Co., 1964, pp. 847–853.

Grono, L. R.: Observation on the incidence of otitis externa in the dog. Aust. Vet. J., 45:417–419, 1969.

Grono, L. R.: Studies of the ear mite, *Otodectes cynotis.* Vet. Rec., 85:6–8, 1969.

Grono, L. R., and Frost, A. J.: Otitis externa in the dog. Aust. Vet. J., 45:420–422, 1969.

Hoffer, R. E., and H. E. Jensen: Stereoscopic Atlas of Small Animal Surgery. St. Louis, The C. V. Mosby Co., 1973.

Pugh, K. E., Evans, J. M., and Hendy, P. G.: Otitis externa in the dog and cat—An evaluation of a new treatment. J. Small Animal Pract., 15:387–400, 1974.

Spruell, J. S. H.: Otitis media of the dog. In Kirk, R. W. (ed.): Current Veterinary Therapy V. Philadelphia, W. B. Saunders Co., 1974, pp. 657–683.

Trotter, E. J.: Drainage of the bullae. Personal communication, 1976.

# EPILEPSY

WILLIAM J. KAY, D.V.M.
*and* WILLIAM R. FENNER, D.V.M.
*New York, New York*

Epilepsy is one of the most common symptoms of disturbance of the central nervous system in cats and dogs and is the most gratifying to treat. An epileptic is any animal who suffers from recurring cerebral seizures, regardless of etiology. The bizarre clinical manifestations of many epileptics are often overinterpreted, and structural disease is assumed to be present. For this reason, care must be taken to determine the true nature of an animal's seizure disorder because true epilepsy, which can mimic the most serious neurologic lesions, can be treated. The severity of the animal's clinical signs may not be a true reflection of the condition of the animal's brain if epilepsy is present; in this instance, diligent therapy often yields gratifying results.

In order to establish any paroxysmal disorder as being a cerebral seizure or epileptic event, the events must be repetitive and generally similar. Other organ systems can demonstrate paroxysmal manifestation of disease as well, but there is usually no repetitive, similar pattern.

While we are concerned with seizures of a cerebral nature, syncopal attacks of a cardiovascular nature, cervical and lumbar radicular pain (spinal root pain), hypoglycemia and paroxysmal labyrinthine disorders (vestibular in nature) can mimic epileptic seizures and can make the establishment of the nature of the disorder difficult. Intermittent or mild forms of vestibulitis can be quite difficult to distinguish from seizures, especially if the neurologic examination is normal. Short periods of head tilt or head tremors not accompanied by other manifestations of an epileptic attack, such as autonomic hyperactivity, unconsciousness, thrashing and tonic and clonic movements, indicate vestibular, labyrinthine or inner ear lesions until proved otherwise.

Epilepsy is only a symptom of an underlying neurologic (neuronal) dysfunction occurring primarily within the brain or, secondarily, caused by toxic substances or metabolic or electrolyte abnormalities; however, it is often the only treatable symptom or the only symptom of clinical significance. Thus, controlling the seizures becomes the clinical and therapeutic objective of the veterinarian. This discussion will deal primarily with the diagnosis of seizure disorders and their management with oral or parenteral medication, depending on their severity.

## INCIDENCE

In most cases, the inherited nature of seizures has not been established, but there are certain breeds that often present with this problem. Among the breeds that appear to have a high incidence of convulsions are the German shepherd, St. Bernard, Irish setter, poodle and beagle. Statistics are not available concerning the incidence in particular breeds. In our institution, epileptic attacks are at least one of the clinical signs in over 1000 of the 80,000 cases seen annually.

## THE COMPONENTS OF AN EPILEPTIC ATTACK

All epileptic events are characterized by paroxysms that are preceded by an aura. The series of clinical signs heralding the event may include restlessness, nervousness, whining, shaking, salivation, affection, wandering and hiding. The duration of the aura may be a few seconds to several days, and it may be unnoticed by the owner. Careful historical evaluation and a request that the client observe the animal carefully for such phenomena usually lead to establishment of the aura. The aura is often so apparent to the client that anticonvulsant therapy exceeding maintenance levels can be instituted during the aura, thus preventing or lessening the severity of the actual ictus or epileptic attack.

Following the aura, the animal manifests the ictus. (See Classification of Seizures.) Although the attack can be so brief that it is barely discernible, it is usually noticed. The ictus can last from a few seconds to several minutes unless the animal is in status epilepticus (see page 865) or approaching that state. Clients often report that ictal events last for several minutes. It has been our experience that most attacks last from one to three minutes. Longer duration is often reported because the owner misinterprets the postictal phase immediately following the attack, during which some motor movements may occur.

The phenomena immediately following the ictus represent the postictal phase. This may be the only phase actually observed by the client and the veterinarian, as many seizure disorders occur only at night. In this period, confusion, disorientation, salivation, pacing, wandering, restlessness, unresponsiveness and/or transient blindness may present clinical problems, and the postictal phenomena are often of far greater concern than the actual seizure. To control, shorten and change the postictal phase are important therapeutic goals, as many clients will tolerate the ictus itself, and proper therapy can minimize the manifestations of the postictal period.

There does not seem to be a direct correlation between the severity of the individual seizures and the severity and duration of the postictal phase. Mild seizures may be followed by very severe postictal phenomena, and severe seizures may have mild postictal phenomena. The confusion, disorientation and other signs are thought to occur because the neuronal cells are exhausted and cannot utilize required metabolites. The ictal event creates electrical energy which is transmitted in a grossly abnormal manner through brain circuits not normally used, and the brain is temporaily exhausted as a result. Following multiple, serious seizures, the postictal phase can last for days. Again, one should be cautious about interpreting a serious and complex postictal phase as indicating a structural lesion of serious consequence.

## CLASSIFICATION OF SEIZURES

The presence of seizures, without regard to etiology, may be determined quite easily in animals with generalized major motor seizures (grand mal seizures), tonic or tonic-clonic seizures or seizures characterized by gross movements of the head, face, body or extremities. Seizures of a milder, shorter or relatively infrequent nature (such as focal motor seizures involving one small part of the body, generalized minor motor seizures, hysterical seizures and so-called psychomotor or behavorial seizures which have a variety of clinical manifestations) are more difficult to classify as being epileptic.

**Psychomotor or Behavioral Seizures.** Special mention should be made of a common disorder affecting dogs, in which the outward manifestations of the paroxysmal events are behavioral. Patients with this particular form of epilepsy can have what appears to be taste sensation (visceral or autonomic sensations, with manifestations such as salivation, vomiting and retching), auditory sensation or hallucination sensation (when the patient seems to see something). Animals with the latter manifestation have been called "fly chasers." Another form of behavioral epilepsy is the paroxysmal rage reaction. Animals with this form of epilepsy often attack their owners and are seemingly unaware of their actions.

It must be cautioned that only if the events are paroxysmal and are preceded by an aura and followed by a postictal phase can the behavioral features of the event be regarded as having epileptic significance. To diagnose psychomotor or behavioral epilepsy without evidence of repeated events is to base that diagnosis on insufficient evidence. In our experience, animals with abnormal personality manifestations—those with so-called "personality problems"—are usually not epileptics. The areas of the cerebrum in which seizures with this manifestation originate have not been identified accurately; the discharges may originate in the temporal lobe and the limbic system.

**Petit Mal Epilepsy.** Petit mal in animals

has not truly been established. Animals exhibiting short motor seizures, akinetic seizures (so-called drop attacks) or brief spells could have petit mal epilepsy or a variant of petit mal. True petit mal is an electroencephalographic diagnosis, and the disease has not been diagnosed accordingly in animals.

**Hysterical Seizures.** Epileptic attacks characterized by hysterical behavior are common. These events are paroxysmal and similar, thus allowing them to be considered epileptic, but the outward manifestations of body movement, autonomic hyperactivity and uncontrolled thrashing are usually absent. Patients with this disorder generally run wildly during the seizure, bumping carelessly into objects. They often act confused and dazed following the seizure and will then sleep.

Although running attacks are not unusual manifestations of epilepsy, such a diagnosis should be withheld unless the events are repetitive. Lead poisoning (plumbism) should be ruled out when the attacks are hysterical. When gastrointestinal signs are associated with such events, the possibility of lead poisoning is increased. Because of the serious nature of lead poisoning, we routinely screen any animal exhibiting running attacks for lead poisoning; in addition to obtaining a careful history to determine the possibility of lead ingestion, tests include radiographs of the abdomen, hematologic examination for basophilic stippling and determination of blood and urine lead levels.

## OBJECTIVES OF THE NEUROLOGIC EXAMINATION

The purpose of any neurologic examination is to determine whether all the clinical signs exhibited by the patient are referrable to one small focal site within the central nervous system. Etiologies should not be considered until the clinician has satisfactorily determined the anatomic substrata or site relating to the animal's problem. If the clinical signs exhibited by the animal are truly epileptic, then the attacks in and of themselves are of localizing value because the discharges originate in the cerebrum. Epilepsy is an active irritating neuronal discharge within the cerebrum, distinguishing it from nearly all other cerebral lesions, which destroy the neurons.

There are two major types of epilepsy: so-called idiopathic (functional) epilepsy and symptomatic epilepsy. When a careful history, a complete neurologic examination and a diagnostic evaluation which may include cerebrospinal fluid analysis yield no evidence of an actual structural or organic lesion, the disease is considered idiopathic.

When the seizures are accompanied by a structural or organic lesion of a focal, multifocal or diffuse nature, the disease is considered symptomatic. Even when structural diseases, especially structural lesions of a nonprogressive nature (such as postdistemper, encephalitis or a healed infarct), produce the clinical signs of epilepsy, it is important to realize that the seizures can often be controlled successfully with anticonvulsants. Seizures due to progressive lesions, such as brain tumors, can sometimes be controlled for a period of time.

Animals may have epilepsy as a symptom of a functional disease with few or no other signs of central nervous system dysfunction. However, in symptomatic epilepsy, the epileptic attacks reflect an underlying structural lesion. In many animals with symptomatic epilepsy, the neurologic examination reveals one or more neurologic deficits. Deficits in motor strength, vision or sensation are common; not only can they indicate the localization within the cerebrum but, when the neurologic examination is done in a serial manner (i.e., several successive examinations), their progression or regression is used as a guide to evaluate the relative improvement or deterioration of the nervous system. The presence of a progressive focal motor, focal sensory or focal visual deficit is usually indicative of a space-occupying lesion. More subtle changes such as personality alteration, dementia or unresponsiveness are indications of a more diffuse disturbance in neurologic function, either from a focal, multifocal or diffuse disease process. Animals exhibiting signs of either focal deficit or diffuse hemispheric dysfunction, apart from the actual seizure, must be treated more aggressively if long-term success is to be expected.

The actual content and visible manifestation of the aura, the seizure and the postictal phase can sometimes suggest more precise localization to a particular aspect of the cerebrum. The manifestations of the seizure indicate the site and rate of discharge of the neurons and the neuronal pathway affected by the electrical energy but do not lead to identification of etiology. So-called chewing-gum seizures (masticator seizures), for example, may be due to brain tumors, bacterial or viral infections or hypoglycemia, or may follow trauma. Animals with idiopathic epilepsy often have chewing-gum seizures, reflecting discharges from certain areas of the brain only. Chewing-gum seizures do *not* imply canine distemper in many cases.

When the epilepsy is secondary, other clinical or diagnostic signs may allow a positive etiologic diagnosis. Seizures arising secondarily are usually transient and may not require chronic oral medication after the incitive condition has been controlled.

## CAUSES OF EPILEPSY

The causes of epilepsy are numerous, since nearly every pathologic process can and does result in epileptic attacks in dogs and cats. There are no significant studies to determine the percentage of cases that, with a particular etiology, will have epileptic attacks. It is important to understand that epilepsy can be a functional disorder with no underlying pathologic condition.

Included among the causes of epilepsy are viral diseases (canine distemper); fungal diseases (toxoplasmosis and cryptococcosis); bacterial infections (either direct or systemic); intracranial neoplasms (primary or metastatic); vascular diseases (including emboli, thrombi and vasculitis); and a variety of systemic hematologic disorders (including thrombocytopenia and autoimmune hemolytic anemia). Trauma and congenital disorders such as globoid cell leukodystrophy have all resulted in seizure disorders, hydrocephalus, and many of the inherited metabolic disorders of the nervous system. The nature, severity and frequency of epileptic attacks are not dependent on or related to the etiology. Serious organic progressive disorders such as brain tumors can have a mild or short epileptic attack, while serious episodes of status epilepticus can be functional.

"Chewing-gum" or mastication seizures are quite common in dogs but are not caused by any specific etiology. Certainly, "chewing-gum" seizures are not pathognomonic for canine distemper and therefore should not imply a serious or guarded prognosis.

The onset of seizures in relationship to the etiology is not a factor of time in most instances. Seizures can develop at the time of onset of the disease or months to years later. In summary, it is difficult to determine the etiology of any seizure disorder from observing the actual seizure or by its description. The outlook for the control of seizures and for the prognosis of the animal should be based on a complete evaluation.

## IMPORTANCE OF THE HISTORY TO THE CLINICAL EVALUATION

The history (anamnesis) is often critical to the diagnosis of either epilepsy or a more serious, "less treatable" disease. In order to establish a pattern for the treatment of chronic epilepsy, the importance of a careful history cannot be overemphasized. The client should be questioned to determine whether the animal has been circling, wandering, bumping into objects or restless; whether there is dysfunction of the extremities, indicated by stumbling or knuckling; whether the animal has undergone a recent or longstanding personality change; and whether endocrine dysfunction is present, as indicated by polydipsia, polyuria or polyphagia. Changes in sleeping and excretory habits are all potentially important, as they increase the likelihood of a structural lesion.

Historical evidence of a neurologic deficit is often sufficient to establish the presence of a cerebral lesion. If a focal neurologic deficit coexists with the seizures, the suspicion of a potentially serious disease of the cerebrum is increased. However, it should be emphasized that *historical information suggesting signs of a focal, multifocal or diffuse neurologic deficit is truly significant only when such findings occur apart from the actual epileptic event or events.* Many of the above signs which seemingly suggest serious brain lesions are really, in fact, components of the epilepsy itself.

The presence of a focal neurologic deficit or a history of neurologic signs other than the seizures does not necessarily lead to a guarded or grave prognosis. Although a single ictus seldom lasts longer than a few minutes (30 seconds to five minutes), the entire event, from the aura to the postictal phenomena, can last hours or even days. Indeed, multiple seizures can visibly alter the animal's behavior for several days. If the neurologic examination is performed during the aura, the ictus or the postictal phase, conclusions concerning the nature and severity of the disorder will generally be overstated.

When sudden unconsciousness is accompanied by unilateral or bilateral postural abnormalities of the head and extremities and by any focal or diffuse motor movements, the clinician is forced to consider epilepsy as a cause of the unconsciousness. However, if the animal does not begin to regain consciousness within 10 to 15 minutes, with nearly full recovery in about an hour, epilepsy can be ruled out unless the patient has experienced several violent generalized seizures or has been in status epilepticus, since a true epileptic attack is characterized by returning function within a few minutes. If a patient fails to respond after a short time or if the neurologic examination suggests a serious structural lesion within one cerebral hemisphere or both or within the brain stem, then the original assumption of epilepsy is incorrect. Neurologic disorders causing unconsciousness that are often misdiagnosed as epileptic include intracranial hemorrhage, intracranial infarction, acute encephalitis, brain trauma and occasionally intracranial tumors.

As a practical principle, we attempt to give the animal a "good disease." In this manner, signs generally interpreted as grave are normally considered as aspects of the seizure disorder rather than indications of serious parenchymal damage to the brain unless there is specific evidence to the contrary. An example of this is the animal with significant hemiparesis following serious seizures. The hemiparesis can, of course, be the result of a serious intracranial lesion within the contralateral cerebral hemisphere, but it can also be a transient phenomenon resulting from electrical exhaustion of the hemisphere which may persist for a few minutes to a few hours. This phenomenon, called postictal hemiparesis, indicates a contralateral cerebral focus of seizure activity, but it does not necessarily reflect a serious underlying lesion.

When an epileptic is refractory to treatment or when the seizure disorder is progressive, progressive disease of the substance of its brain is not necessarily indicated. In other words, the epilepsy can become more severe or can change without reflecting a serious organic disease, because repeated epileptic attacks tend to create neuronal pathways which the electrical discharges "learn" to follow with relative ease. Thus, the disorder is still considered "treatable." Again it is useful to remove from the evaluation those signs associated only with the epileptic seizure.

As is true for the seizure events themselves, the severity of the postictal phase also does not reflect the true nature of the underlying neurologic dysfunction. In addition, we have found no correlation between the quality and content of the seizure and the length and consequence of the postictal phase. Animals having generalized major motor attacks of brief duration, which do not seem excessively devastating, can have long, rather serious postictal phases. The reverse is also true in that animals having violent, repetitive seizures may have mild postictal phenomena of very short duration. The postictal phase is often the most lengthy, most serious aspect of the entire epileptic sequence and the one causing greatest concern to both client and veterinarian.

At our hospital, an animal is considered to have idiopathic epilepsy alone until proved otherwise. Treatment begins with both the veterinarian and the client hopeful of success. It should be kept in mind that the older the animal, the greater the possibility of a serious, progressive, organic disease of the brain. In addition, the first historical and physical signs of a serious underlying neurologic disease are often epileptic attacks, and neurologic evaluation during or just after an attack is not contributory. In such cases, the history is not germane to the establishment of structural disease, and the diagnosis must be based on serial neurologic examinations and laboratory data, including cerebrospinal fluid analysis.

## DIAGNOSTIC EVALUATION

In making the differential diagnosis, all forms of treatable disease of the central nervous system should be ruled out before instituting chronic anticonvulsant therapy. Epilepsy may have various structural causes, including neoplasms, infections, intracranial hemorrhage, trauma and congenital disorders. These diseases are generally progressive, and the animal may be presented with many neurologic signs other than epileptic seizures. In these diseases, the epileptic attacks may occur at any point in the disease process, or epilepsy may never be a component. In addition, several systemic and metabolic diseases may lead to epilepsy; these include uremia, hepatic dysfunctions, insulin-secreting tumors of the pancreas, lead poisoning, electrolyte imbalances and various toxic substances. If these diseases are treated appropriately, epilepsy usually does not remain as a problem. The presence of epileptic attacks, especially severe, violent or repetitive epileptic attacks, makes the neurologic evaluation of the patient quite difficult, and the animal that is presented during or immediately following a series of epileptic events is a difficult diagnostic and prognostic problem. The reason for this is that the epileptic attacks "cloud" the cerebrum, making a truly fastidious examination quite difficult.

It is especially important that extracranial causes of epileptic seizures be evaluated and treated either primarily or concurrently with the seizures. Because seizures are often a reflection of an active disease or dysfunction of the central nervous system, a complete evaluation of the animal is essential. When an active infection of the nervous system is suspected, the evaluation should include cerebrospinal fluid analysis and culture. Ophthalmic examination should be done routinely.

In any or all animals exhibiting nonprogressive or progressive disturbance in neurologic function, it is essential to perform diagnostic tests. The animal should first have a complete medical evaluation to determine the function of all organ systems. A complete hematologic evaluation, a liver and kidney function, a urinalysis and a complete cardiac evaluation are part of our routine work-up. A complete ophthalmic examination including funduscopy is also performed. Skull x-rays and an examination of the cerebrospinal fluid (CSF) are usually performed after the above medical and ophthalmic evaluations are made. Other tests can be done but require more sophisticated equipment, including cerebral angiography, radioactive isotope scanning and electroencephalography.

*Cerebrospinal fluid analysis* is performed whenever there is historical or physical evidence of organic neurologic disease or when an animal has proved refractory to all methods of treatment. The fluid is collected, with the animal under general anesthesia and in lateral recumbency, by passing a 20-gauge 1.5- or 3-inch spinal needle into the subarachnoid space at the medullospinal junction while the neck is flexed, after the skin has been clipped and prepared aseptically. The needle is directed carefully between the occipital bone and the atlas directly on the midline until it penetrates the dura mater and the arachnoid. Fluid pressure is then measured with either a vertical or horizontal manometer.

Following the measuring of CSF pressure, the fluid is collected either by allowing it to drip into a sterile container or by attaching a syringe and withdrawing the fluid very gently. Depending upon the size of the animal, 1 to 3 ml. are collected and submitted for laboratory analysis. The laboratory analysis consists of a total and differential white blood cell count, an analysis of the total protein, glucose determination and bacterial culture; exfoliative cytology should be performed when the method is available. Electrophoresis can also be performed.

It is not within the scope of this article to describe in detail the findings of CSF analysis, but the presence of increased CSF pressure and elevated protein levels indicate a space-occupying lesion, usually a neoplasm. Increased cellularity is usually compatible with an infectious process, either viral or bacterial, or, rarely, a fungal disease. The presence of red blood cells can be indicative of an intracranial hemorrhage from a variety of etiologies. The presence of blood in the CSF can, however, be iatrogenic—the result of a bloody cisternal puncture. Xanthochromia, which is the result of red blood cell breakdown from a previous hemorrhage, results in a yellowish or slightly brownish discoloration in the CSF.

Again it is important to remember that many serious disturbances of neurologic function, even with significant deficits or evidence of widespread dysfunction of the cerebrum, are either treatable, as in bacterial infection, or reversible, as in intracranial hemorrhage, if the basic cause of the hemorrhage can be determined and treated. In any event, when recurring epileptic seizures are present, anticonvulsant therapy should be instituted.

## USE OF ELECTROENCEPHALOGRAPHY

Electroencephalography can offer valuable information to the clinician to whom i is available. At the present time, no standard method for recording electroencephalograms exists; a representative method may be found in Klemm (1969).

Epilepsy may be diagnosed when it was not previously suspected. We have seen two animals presented in a coma with no history of motor signs. Electroencephalographically, however, both were in status epilepticus and responded to anticonvulsant therapy.

The electroencephalogram may diagnose a disease other than epilepsy. When a patient is presented with a history of seizures and its electroencephalogram exhibits patterns differing from the usual abnormalities of an epileptic, an etiology other than "idiopathic epilepsy" should be entertained.

Electroencephalographic findings in epilepsy may include spiking or sharp waves, which may be focal or diffuse. Some epileptics set up mirror foci, and so the discharges may be seen in similar locations in each hemisphere. Among the more common abnormalities suggesting etiologies other than epilepsy are focal areas of slow wave activity, suggesting a space-occupying mass; diffuse slowing, suggesting metabolic encephalopathy or diffuse encephalopathies; the high voltage slowing of the hydrocephalic; and fast, low voltage activity with spiking, suggesting encephalitis. All artifacts should be noted and should not be misinterpreted as "pathology."

When used appropriately, electroencephalography may contribute greatly to your handling of an epileptic patient. It is a tool and does not replace a complete history and neurologic examination. It should be remembered that the electroencephalogram suggests etiologies and does not diagnose with certainty. Most importantly, a normal electroencephalogram does not exclude any condition.

## ESTABLISHING A THERAPEUTIC REGIMEN

There is no absolute rule regarding the time or conditions necessary for the initiation of medication for the chronic control of epilepsy. Several guidelines are commonly used in determining whether anticonvulsant therapy should be instituted:

### Indications Suggesting Therapy

1. The intolerance of clients to seizure phenomena of any severity or frequency.

2. Individual seizures becoming more complex or longer in duration.

3. If the postictal phase increases in severity and length and is accompanied by viciousness or incontinence, restlessness, pacing, wandering and transient blindness.

4. When the first attack is very violent or involves multiple seizures.

5. When the diagnosis of certain paroxysmal events remains in question and anticonvulsant therapy is used to attempt a therapeutic diagnosis.

### Indications Suggesting that Therapy may be Delayed or Contraindicated

1. When the seizures are short, not violent, and infrequent.

2. When the paroxysms or events witnessed are not definitely epileptic and further events must be observed before a diagnosis is made.

3. When the cost or difficulty of medicating the patient exceeds the value of the medication in the control of the patient, e.g., when the seizures are infrequent or when the animal refuses to accept medication.

## CHOOSING AN ANTICONVULSANT

The ideal anticonvulsant should completely suppress seizures, regardless of the type, at a low dosage level. The drug should be low in cost, widely available in different dosages for different sized patients, easily administered and without undesirable side effects. Such an ideal anticonvulsant is not yet available. Only those that have proved effective over the years for a large number of animals will be considered (Table 1).

**Diphenylhydantoin (DPH).** Diphenylhydantoin (Dilantin®, Parke, Davis) is thought to exert its anticonvulsant activity at the neuronal dendritic level, thus preventing the spread of the spontaneous electrical discharge. It does not prevent the initial ictal discharge but suppresses its potentiation. It is useful in controlling generalized major motor seizures, focal motor seizures, hysterical seizures and psychomotor or behavioral seizures.

The advantages of diphenylhydantoin include the absence of sedative effects, its effectiveness, low toxicity, few side effects, low cost, worldwide availability and availability in combination with phenobarbital. Diphenylhydantoin in combination with phenobarbital is not, at this time, a substance controlled by the Bureau of Narcot-

*Table 1.*   *Drugs, Dosages, Advantages and Disadvantages of the Most Commonly Used Anticonvulsant Drugs*

| DRUG | INDICATION USES | DOSE AVAILABILITY | DOSE RANGE | ADVANTAGES | DISADVANTAGES |
|---|---|---|---|---|---|
| Diphenyl-hydantoin (Dilantin) | Generalized major motor seizures, minor motor seizures and behavioral seizures | Capsules: 30 mg. 100 mg. 100 mg. with 0.25 gr. pheno-barbital | 4 mg./kg/day 100 mg./kg/day | Absence of sedation<br><br>Effectiveness in a high per cent of cases<br><br>Low toxicity and absence of many side effects noted in humans<br><br>Low cost<br><br>Not a controlled substance (BNDD)<br><br>Worldwide availability<br><br>In combination with phenobarbital, is not a controlled substance | Transient ataxia<br><br>Rapid metabolism, difficulty in maintaining adequate blood levels; possibly is poorly absorbed in dogs<br><br>Some polyphagia, polydipsia, polyuria<br><br>Relatively toxic in cats; generally not desirable as an anticonvulsant in cats<br><br>Does not stop initial ictal discharge |
| Phenobarbital | Generalized major motor seizures, minor motor seizures and behavioral seizures | Tablets: 0.125 gr. 0.25 gr. 0.5 gr.<br><br>Liquid<br><br>Injectable: 0.5 to 1 gr./ml. | 0.125 gr. twice daily to 2 gr. four times daily | High efficacy<br><br>Rapid action, few hours<br><br>Low toxicity in animals<br><br>Can be administered by several routes (intravenously, intramuscularly and orally)<br><br>Generally the most effective drug in status epilepticus<br><br>Low cost<br><br>Worldwide availability<br><br>Drug of choice in cats | Sedative effects<br><br>Restricted drug<br><br>Long-term prescription not honored<br><br>Polyphagia, polydipsia, polyuria<br><br>Reverse effects, irritability and restlessness<br><br>Length of sedation precluding a neurologic examination, following intravenous, intramuscular and oral administration, is often several hours |

| Drug | Indications | Dose Form | Dose | Advantages | Disadvantages |
|---|---|---|---|---|---|
| Primidone (Mysoline), (Mylepsin) | Generalized major motor seizure, minor motor seizure | Tablets: 50 mg. scored, 250 mg. scored | 8 mg./kg./day 40 mg./kg./day  May vary both up and down | High level of efficacy  Rapid action  Useful in most clinical seizure disorders  Not controlled by BNDD  Widely available | Sedation dramatic and severe in many animals; sedation may be transient as the patient becomes accustomed to the medication  Great variability in dose tolerances  Only one form available; no parenteral form  Only two size tablets available (50 mg. and 250 mg.) |
| Diazepam (Valium) | Control of the exacerbation of seizures  Control of status epilepticus  Feline seizure epilepticus | Tablets: 2.5 mg. 5 mg. 10 mg.  Injectable: 5 mg./ml. in 2-ml. vials | 2.5 to 100 mg. intravenously or intramuscularly to effect | Effectiveness in stopping status epilepticus and other generalized seizure disorders  Rapid action  Safety  Relative brevity of action; neurologic evaluation can be done shortly afterwards; few hours if further seizures do not occur  Useful in cats, parenterally or orally  Can be used as a tranquilizer | Relatively short action; often needs to be repeated several times in status epilepticus management  Cannot control violent status epilepticus  Relatively expensive  Controlled by BNDD  Seldom used for oral prevention and control  Reverse effects sometimes seen, restlessness, viciousness |

ics and Dangerous Drugs (BNDD). Diphenylhydantoin is well tolerated in dogs. Disadvantages are that the drug causes transient ataxia in high dosages; it has a lag in initial effectiveness of several days in some cases; and it is rapidly metabolized and seems to be poorly absorbed from the gastrointestinal tract in dogs, as indicated by the fact that large dosages can be administered without side effects. Diphenylhydantoin is ineffective when administered parenterally. It is not effective in treating an acute exacerbation of seizures or status epilepticus but is, rather, used prophylactically. There is some mild but persistent polyphagia, polydipsia and polyuria associated with the use of diphenylhydantoin.

**Phenobarbital.** Phenobarbital is an extremely effective anticonvulsant, having been in use for this purpose for nearly 60 years in man. Its mode of action is believed to be at the nerve cell body, and it prevents the initial ictal discharge.

Phenobarbital is effective in all forms of epilepsy seen in dogs and cats—generalized seizure disorder, minor motor and focal motor seizures, hysterical seizures and psychomotor seizures. It is the drug of choice in the cat.

Phenobarbital is highly effective, and there is little time lag involved. There is low toxicity in animals. It can be administered by several routes, so that medication may be continued during exacerbation of seizures, status epilepticus or during diagnostic studies under anesthesia in an epileptic animal whose seizures are under control. Phenobarbital is the drug of choice for treating an animal presented while having an epileptic attack or one in status epilepticus. The cost is low, and the drug is widely available.

Some of the disadvantages of phenobarbital for the control of seizure disorders include its sedative effects and its restriction by the BNDD. Polyphagia, polydipsia and polyuria are encountered routinely, and patients treated with phenobarbital often become restless and irritable. Following parenteral administration of phenobarbital, several hours to several days may pass before a meaningful neurologic evaluation can be performed.

**Primidone.** Primidone (Mysoline®, Ayerst) has been used as an anticonvulsant for nearly 20 years and has a respected place in the treatment of epilepsy in the dog. Although its action at the nerve cell body is similar to that of phenobarbital (approximately 25 per cent of the drug is converted to phenobarbital by the liver), the specific action of the drug is unique. Primidone has proved effective in controlling generalized seizures, focal motor seizures, sensory seizures and behavioral seizures. The advantages of primidone include its high efficacy rate, its rapid action when administered orally, its wide availability and lack of restriction by the BNDD. Disadvantages include heavy sedation which, in many cases, is transient; the wide variation in dosage ranges; the lack of a parenteral form; and polyphagia, polydipsia and polyuria in nearly all cases. The drug also causes irritability, restlessness and personality changes in many animals. Animals maintained on high doses of primidone must be evaluated periodically for signs of liver disease.

**Diazepam.** Diazepam (Valium®, Roche), usually administered parenterally, has proved effective in control of exacerbated seizure disorders and status epilepticus. Although diazepam is a tranquilizer whose mode of action is considered to be at the presynaptic level, the drug has definite anticonvulsant properties. Generally speaking, diazepam is the only tranquilizer that is used in the treatment of epilepsy. The drug can be used as a premedication for epileptic animals requiring anesthesia, surgery or diagnostic procedures. The oral form is seldom used to control seizure disorders in dogs but is sometimes employed in generalized seizure disorders in cats, either alone or in combination with phenobarbital.

The advantages of diazepam include its effectiveness in stopping status epilepticus and exacerbated seizure disorders; its rapid action; and its brevity of action, which allows the neurologic examination to be performed within hours of administration of the drug. Its relatively short action is also a disadvantage, however, in the sense that repeated injections are necessary to control status epilepticus. In addition, it is expensive, and adverse effects including irritability are occasionally seen.

## GENERAL ANESTHESIA

General anesthesia should be employed with extreme caution for the control of an exacerbated seizure disorder or for status epilepticus. In our institution, general anesthesia is administered only after large doses of diazepam and phenobarbital have failed to prevent further generalized attacks.

**Dosages.** There is no single drug or combination of drugs which has proved useful for all patients. It is certainly desirable to initiate treatment with a single drug alone, but this guideline is not always adhered to strictly; combinations of drugs are often employed. The therapeutic goal is to stop the seizure even at the risk of inducing sedation, at least initially. However, the client often prefers that his animal be given a lower dosage of anticonvulsant, risking the recurrence of seizures because he does not wish the animal to be sedated.

Diphenylhydantoin is the drug of choice initially. The dosage of this drug is seldom calculated on a per kg. body weight basis. It ranges from 8 mg./kg./day to 120 mg./kg./day, depending upon the severity of the seizure and the animal's previous response to the drug if it has been treated previously. The clinician should revise the dosage according to the degree of control achieved and the presence of side effects. We find that if diphenylhydantoin is going to cause side effects, they will occur early in the course of therapy. Clients should be informed of the side effects and should be aware that control of the seizures may take time and require trials of various dosages and medications.

If the seizures are violent or serious, diphenylhydantoin can be supplemented with phenobarbital. Because of the rapid action of phenobarbital, anticonvulsant therapy begins almost immediately, and the lag period before effectiveness is shortened considerably. We routinely use diphenylhydantoin and phenobarbital in combination, but the clinician can elect to dispense the drugs separately to obtain precise control of dosage rates.

In refractory epileptics, we often administer much higher dosages of anticonvulsants than those listed in Table 1. We have found that effective control of seizures is very difficult in some breeds, such as the German shepherd, Irish setter, Great Dane, St. Bernard and Shetland sheepdog. Large dogs, in particular, often require very high dosage rates. We have often treated such animals with dosage combinations as high as 1500 mg. of diphenylhydantoin and 7½ gr. of phenobarbital per day without significant sedation.

We routinely add primidone to the therapeutic regimen when diphenylhydantoin and diphenylhydantoin with phenobarbital have not adequately controlled the seizures. The client must be clearly aware that seizure control is a partial phenomenon and that decreases in the frequency, duration and severity of the seizures, as well as altering the postictal phase, are all considered therapeutic gains. Therefore, in making a decision to employ a different drug or to add a drug to therapeutic regimen, the hoped for gain is weighed against the side effects.

We find that many animals are adequately controlled with one drug but not with another. For example, when seizures are not controlled with diphenylhydantoin or diphenylhydantoin with phenobarbital, but when significant improvement is achieved with primidone, we reduce the dosages of diphenylhydantoin and phenobarbital. The dosage of primidone required to achieve chronic oral control of seizures must be determined on an individual basis. Effective dosages have been as low as 10 mg. twice daily in dogs of toy breeds, and as high as 500 mg. three times daily in dogs of giant breeds.

Diazepam is seldom used in the oral prophylactic control of seizure disorders. Occasionally, the drug is administered to animals which have been refractory at high levels of the other anticonvulsants. It is used routinely in the parenteral control of status epilepticus.

It is important not to change medication too quickly, instead allowing enough time for full evaluation of the effectiveness of the anticonvulsant chosen (up to two months in some cases). One drug should not be discontinued immediately in favor of another, but rather both should be administered for several weeks. Failure to do this can lead to a serious exacerbation of the seizure disorder because of the possible lag in effectiveness of the added drug.

If an epileptic previously controlled under a therapeutic regimen suddenly becomes refractory, updated historical information and serial neurologic examinations become particularly important, as an animal formerly considered to have idiopathic epilepsy may actually have a structural disorder of greater consequence.

We know of no sure way to determine anticonvulsant medication that will prove immediately effective in a given animal, either singly or in combination, and dosage levels are similarly not absolute. We have found that the most satisfactory regimen begins with increasing levels of diphenylhydantoin and is followed by the addition of phenobarbital if necessary and, finally, the addition of primidone. It should also be noted that, while primidone is an extremely effective anticonvulsant, its numerous side effects have limited its usefulness in many animals.

## SOME REASONS FOR FAILURE IN THE MANAGEMENT OF EPILEPSY

Any of the circumstances listed below can result in exacerbation of a seizure disorder or make control difficult.

1. Failure of the client to give the anticonvulsant as directed.
2. Dosages that are too low.
3. Changing anticonvulsants without adequate drug overlap.
4. Progressive structural disease.
5. The presence of other diseases or situations stressful to the animal, causing a higher-than-normal level of electrical discharges.
6. Serious systemic disease.

## EPILEPSY IN THE CAT

Although epilepsy is generally similar in the dog and cat, there are several special considerations in feline epilepsy.

## THE MANIFESTATIONS OF EPILEPSY IN CATS

All forms of epilepsy known to occur in dogs also occur in cats, and all the components of a seizure are present—the aura, the ictus and the postictal phase. Cats experiencing seizures frequently demonstrate what seems to be a rage reaction or hysteria. They may hiss and growl and yet remain unresponsive to verbal or visual stimuli. Motor movements, including twitching, may or may not be associated manifestations. Events such as those described above should be repetitive in nature, as in dogs, in order to be considered epileptic.

Although idiopathic epilepsy has not been documented in the cat, the assumption that all seizure disorders are of a structural and progressive nature has not been borne out by our clinical experience. However, when a cat is presented with a history of epilepsy or with spells that are confusing to both the client and the veterinarian, it should be examined carefully for an organic lesion.

## CAUSES OF FELINE EPILEPSY

The most common causes of epilepsy in the cat include infectious feline peritonitis (IFP), toxoplasmosis, cryptococcosis, lymphosarcoma, meningioma, toxic and metabolic disorders such as thiamine deficiency, and congenital disorders such as hydrocephalus and lipid storage diseases.

Special mention should be made of thiamine deficiency, which represents a neurologic emergency in the cat. The neurologic signs are of a diffuse nature, including dilated pupils, gait ataxia, cerebellar tremor, an abnormal "doll's head" or oculovestibular reflex, and epileptic seizures often characterized by ventral flexion of the head on the sternum. Thiamine deficiency can be treated effectively early in its course, before irreversible neurologic damage has occured, with injectable thiamine hydrochloride intravenously or intramuscularly. Doses of 50 mg./day for two to three days have proved effective. Thiamine deficiency can result from the debilitating effects of a number of other systemic disorders, including diseases characterized by anorexia. Because of the frequency with which the condition leads to epileptic seizures, we routinely treat seizures in the cat with thiamine hydrochloride in addition to the usual anticonvulsant medication. The consequences to the cat are grave if a seizure disorder induced by thiamine deficiency is not treated. Cats not properly treated usually die.

## DIAGNOSIS AND TREATMENT

To determine the etiology of epileptic seizures in the cat, a complete history, neurologic examination and diagnostic tests including cerebrospinal fluid analysis should be completed. Funduscopy has proved useful in diagnosing a number of the more serious diseases of the feline nervous system, such as toxoplasmosis. The presence of active or inactive fundic lesions, including chorioretinitis, should raise the clinician's suspicion of organic disease.

In treating epilepsy in the cat, we use first

phenobarbital and then diazepam (Valium). We have found diphenylhydantoin to be of little value in the cat. The dosages in the cat require constant monitoring, as there is a very fine line between therapeutic and sedative levels. On an outpatient basis, treatment may begin with a dosage of 0.25 gr. (16 mg.) of phenobarbital twice daily, with instructions to the client to increase or decrease the level by 0.25 or 0.125 gr. until an effective level is reached. Diazepam has proved of value in the chronic oral control of feline epilepsy in dosages of 2.5 to 5 mg. two or three times daily.

Status epilepticus is uncommon in cats, but management is similar to that in dogs except for significantly decreased dosage levels. Valium can be used in dosages of 2 to 10 mg. intravenously or intramuscularly, and phenobarbital, in dosages of 5 to 100 mg. either intravenously or intramuscularly. Occasionally, general anesthesia is necessary to stop very serious status epilepticus in the cat.

## STATUS EPILEPTICUS

"Status" is defined as "a fixed or enduring state." In the context of neurology, status epilepticus means that seizures or epileptic attacks are continuous. Seizures of either a focal or a generalized nature occur either repetitively or follow each other so closely that the animal fails to recover between attacks. Status epilepticus is one of the most serious of the neurologic disorders. It is a neurologic emergency that can lead to irreversible coma and death unless it is quickly and effectively controlled.

Any epileptic can experience one or more episodes of status epilepticus and, in some animals, the first manifestation of epilepsy is a serious attack of status epilepticus. An animal with a history of prior status epilepticus or one presented in status must be treated aggressively: *the seizure must be stopped.*

Animals in status epilepticus are generally presented in a state of altered consciousness, either mild or serious in nature. There is no correlation between the seriousness of the status epilepticus and the underlying etiology; for example, many cases of violent status are considered as idiopathic epilepticus. As is true of any seizure, no conclusion should be drawn during the attack concerning the localization, etiology or prognosis.

The following therapeutic regimen is suggested:

1. To stop the seizure, give diazepam and/or phenobarbital to effect: diazepam (Valium), 10 to 35 mg. intravenously or intramuscularly; phenobarbital, 60 to 120 mg. intravenously or intramuscularly. If the seizures have not stopped or subsided materially within a few minutes after the administration of diazepam, phenobarbital should be administered without hesitation.

2. If the above measures fail to control the status epilepticus, anesthetize the patient with either an intravenous barbiturate, volatile anesthetic, or other anesthetic of choice. Anesthetize only to effect.

3. Place an indwelling catheter as soon as possible into the cephalic, saphenous or jugular vein.

4. Draw blood for routine laboratory tests.

5. Determine the blood glucose level as soon as possible in the event that hypoglycemia was the causative factor.

6. If necessary, administer 50 per cent dextrose intravenously in adequate amounts to raise the blood glucose at least to fasting levels; for example, we administer 2 ml. in a Yorkshire terrier and 50 ml. in a Great Dane.

7. Calcium gluconate should also be administered intravenously if there is a question of hypocalcemia.

After these measures have been taken, the animal should be examined carefully and a detailed history obtained.

Caution must be observed in administering any anticonvulsant (intravenously or intramuscularly) to an animal which has had a serious attack of status epilepticus and which later exhibits an occasional focal seizure, a minor motor seizure or diffuse twitchings and jerkings. Overtreatment of an already depressed animal can result in its death. We usually allow the animal to undergo brief seizure activity after an attack of status epilepticus, but additional anticonvulsant medication must be administered if the seizures again become generalized.

Animals seen following several severe, generalized seizures but which are not in status epilepticus must also be considered as having serious problems. Such animals are given diazepam and phenobarbital and are either hospitalized or observed closely for further seizure activity.

The neurologic examination of an animal either in status epilepticus or recently treated for status epilepticus yields little valuable information. The clinician should always approach the examination as if the animal has an uncontrolled form of epilepsy without serious structural disease unless the history, neurologic examination and laboratory data suggest a different conclusion.

There are three distinct possible causes for the altered state of consciousness exhibited by the animal:

1. Seizures themselves can alter the state of consciousness.

2. When parenteral anticonvulsants have been administered, the neurologic situation becomes more complex in that two distinct influences are altering the animal's nervous system.

3. Seizures, parenteral anticonvulsants and underlying structural disease may all contribute to the animal's comatose or unconscious condition.

Determining the relative roles of each of the above factors is a true diagnostic challenge. A careful history, thorough medical examination and laboratory studies including cerebrospinal fluid analysis will do much to suggest the proper conclusion. Again, attempts to evaluate an animal which has undergone several serious seizures while it is under the influence of anticonvulsants can be discouraging.

Animals that are unconscious following an attack of status epilepticus should be maintained on intravenous fluid therapy. The "piggy back" technique of administering a constant, slow intravenous infusion of anticonvulsant is an effective means of maintaining blood levels of necessary anticonvulsant which avoid the depressing effect of a large bolus of medication.

It is imperative that oral medication be instituted as soon as possible. The animal should be given large amounts of diphenylhydantoin with phenobarbital as soon as it can swallow. Sedative levels of diphenylhydantoin and phenobarbital or diphenylhydantoin, phenobarbital and primidone should be given until it is certain that the animal will not relapse. An altered state of consciousness can persist for several days, and relapses are common. This is especially true of epileptics previously under control with oral anticonvulsants which, because of the acute onset of status epilepticus, cannot be maintained on their routine oral medication.

Any animal that is in or has recently undergone an attack of status epilepticus should be hospitalized.

## APPENDIX I

### RULES OF THUMB IN SEIZURE MANAGEMENT

1. Careful discussion with the client must always precede therapy.

2. Except in status epilepticus, animals will seldom die from a seizure.

3. Most seizure disorders, regardless of etiology, will worsen if not controlled or treated.

4. In almost every seizure disorder (even those well controlled), relapses will occur.

5. The exacerbation of a seizure disorder after successful management may mean that a more rigorous course of therapy is needed. It probably does not mean that the animal has a serious structural lesion.

6. The discontinuation of anticonvulsants in seizure patients will often precipitate a series of seizures or status epilepticus.

7. In general, the younger the animal, the more successful will be the treatment of seizures if no serious or progressive structural lesion exists.

8. The evaluation of the animal immediately following a seizure is difficult, and a prognosis usually cannot be made at that time.

9. Clients must be told that successful management of seizures often requires several medications. A trial with one or more is often needed before a successful combination or dosage level is found.

10. Oral medication usually takes several days to have a therapeutic effect, and clients must be told this because seizures will often occur shortly after medication is instituted.

11. The prognosis in even serious seizure disorders, including status epilepticus, is not necessarily grave without a history or physical findings of structural disease.

12. There is no correlation between the severity of the seizure and the underlying disease (idiopathic seizures can be as serious as, or more so than, those associated with large intracranial neoplasms).

13. Changing patterns of seizures may indicate uncontrolled or improperly medicated seizures, rather than progressive brain disease.

14. There does not seem to be a correlation between the severity of the seizure and the duration, nature and severity of the postictal phase. Short focal seizures can have more complex postictal phenomena than many generalized seizure disorders.

15. Most seizures have a prodrome or aura which should be looked for by the veterinarian or the client.

16. Generally speaking, the longer the animal has had the seizure disorder, the better the prognosis.

17. Most seizure patients without progressive structural disease can be at least partially controlled.

## APPENDIX II

1. *The Aura*—The clinical signs beginning a few seconds to several hours before the actual epileptic event, including restlessness, nervousness, whining, shaking, salivation, affection, wandering and hiding.

2. *Epilepsy*—The occasional sudden, excessive, rapid and local electrical discharges of cerebral neurons.

3. *Ictus*—A fit or convulsion: the actual epileptic attack.

4. *Focal Seizure (Focal Motor Seizure)*—A seizure involving one part of the body such as the lips, ears, leg or even one side of the body.

5. *Generalized Seizure*—An epileptic event characterized by unconsciousness, motor movements and tonic or tonic-clonic movements.

6. *Paroxysm*—A sudden onset of a disease or of its symptoms, especially if they are recurrent.

7. *Postictal Phase*—The clinical signs seen following the epileptic attack, including bumping, restlessness, autonomic discharge and transient blindness.

8. *Seizure Disorder*—A clinical condition in which epileptic attacks or seizures are a clinical problem (usually seizures of a repetitive or recurring nature).

9. *Status Epilepticus*—Unremitting seizures.

## SUPPLEMENTAL READING

Cammermeyer, J.: Frequency of meningoencephalitis and hydrocephalus in dogs. J. Neuropath. Exp. Neurol., *20*:386–398, 1961.

Cunningham, J. G.: Canine seizure disorders. J. Am. Vet. Med. Assn., *158*:589–597, 1971.

DeMyer, W.: Technique of the Neurologic Examination. 2nd ed. New York, McGraw-Hill Book Co., 1974.

Holliday, T. A., Cunningham, J. G., and Gutnick, M. J.: Comparative clinical and electroencephalographic studies of canine epilepsy. Epilepsia, *11*:281–292, 1970.

Jasper, H. H., Ward, A. A., and Pope, A.: The Basic Mechanism of the Epilepsies. Boston, Little, Brown & Co., 1969.

Kiloh, L. G., McComas, A. J., and Osselton, J. W.: Clinical Electroencephalography. 3rd ed. London, Butterworths, 1972.

Klemm, W. R.: Animal Electroencephalography. New York, Academic Press, 1969.

Penfield, W., and Jasper, H. H.: Epilepsy and the Functional Anatomy of the Human Brain. Boston, Little, Brown & Co., 1954.

Schmidt, R., and Wilder, B. J.: Epilepsy: A Clinical Textbook. Philadelphia, F. A. Davis Co., 1968.

Woodbury, D. M., Penny, K. J., and Schmidt, R. P.: Anti-Epileptic Drugs. New York, Raven Press, 1972.

# INHERITED METABOLIC DISORDERS OF THE NERVOUS SYSTEM IN DOGS AND CATS

HENRY J. BAKER, D.V.M.
*Birmingham, Alabama*

At the turn of this century a practicing physician, Sir Archibald Garrod, proposed an entirely new concept of disease—*inborn errors of metabolism*. In its present-day context, this idea asserts that certain diseases result from the mutation of a single gene which effects production of a defective enzyme. As a result, cells lose their ability to carry out the specific metabolic reaction governed by the altered enzyme. Since the advancement of this revolutionary concept, several hundred inherited metabolic diseases of man have been reported. While relatively few corresponding animal diseases have been recognized to date, those described here represent some of the best examples of clinically significant inherited metabolic diseases of dogs and cats.

## CLINICAL SIGNS

The eight diseases summarized in Table 1 are remarkably similar in many aspects of their clinical manifestations. All are *progressive*, degenerative disorders of the nervous system. Clinical signs usually begin as discrete tremors or dysmetria and advance at varying rates to generalized locomotor disease. Pelvic limb disability frequently appears first and becomes most severe. The age at which clinical signs first appear varies considerably and is characteristic of each entity. However, the initiation of neurologic signs in all except one of these diseases (feline metachromatic leukodystrophy) occurs at the time of or following weaning. This hallmark, coupled with the progressive nature of these diseases, helps to differentiate them from congenital defects such as viral induced cerebellar hypoplasia of kittens. Advanced signs include paraplegia, blindness and grand mal seizures. In some instances, involvement of visceral organs also contributes to the total clinical syndrome (e.g., feline sphingomyelin lipidosis).

## ETIOLOGY

The specific underlying biochemical defect is unique for each of these clinical entities. However, all are characterized by absence or severe deficiency of a specific degradative enzyme, which leads to an abnormal accumulation of the biochemical substrate normally hydrolyzed by that enzyme. Identification of the accumulated material provides a biochemical basis for differentiating some of these diseases which have similar clinical signs and histologic lesions. Furthermore, the clinical designation for these diseases is often derived from the nature of the chemical which accumulates (e.g., $GM_1$ gangliosidosis).

## INHERITANCE

All these diseases, for which a mode of inheritance has been established, are transmitted as recessive traits. In each instance, only homozygous recessive individuals (i.e., both alleles of a gene pair are mutant) develop clinical signs of disease. Heterozygotes (i.e., one mutant and one normal allele) are entirely normal in physical appearance, although they carry the disease trait and have enzyme levels approximately half that of homozygous normal animals (Table 2). Therefore, heterozygote carriers are key to the perpetuation and exten-

*Table 1.  Inherited Metabolic Disorders of the Nervous System in Dogs and Cats*

| DISEASES* | BREEDS AFFECTED | LESIONS | AGE OF ONSET | SIGNS | BIOCHEMICAL LESION |
|---|---|---|---|---|---|
| Canine globoid cell leukodystrophy (Krabbe's disease) | Cairn terriers; West Highland white terriers; beagles; mixed breeds | Demyelination; globoid cells | 4 to 5 months | Progressive motor disability | Cerebroside accumulates; β-galactosidase deficiency |
| Feline globoid cell leukodystrophy | Domestic cat | Same as canine GLD | 5 to 6 weeks | Same | Unknown |
| Feline sphingomyelin lipidosis (Niemann-Pick disease) | Siamese cat | Vacuolation of neurons and macrophages in liver, spleen, etc. | 2 to 4 months | Same | Sphingomyelin accumulates; sphingomyelinase deficiency? |
| Feline metachromatic leukodystrophy | Domestic cat | Demyelination; gliosis | 2 weeks | Same; rapidly progressing to convulsions; opisthotonos | Sulfatid accumulates; arylsulfatase deficiency? |
| Feline CNS glycogenosis (Pompe's disease) | Domestic cat | Neuronal accumulation of glycogen | Young adult | Unknown | Glycogen accumulates; α-glucosidase deficiency? |
| Canine GM₂ gangliosidosis (Tay-Sachs disease) | German shorthair pointers | Vacuolation of neurons | 9 to 12 months | Ataxia; blindness; seizures | Gm₂ ganglioside accumulates; hexosaminidase deficiency? |
| Feline GM₂ gangliosidosis (Sandhoff's disease) | Domestic cat | Vacuolation of neurons and hepatocytes | 8 to 10 weeks | Tremors; incoordination; paraplegia | GM₂ ganglioside accumulates; hexosaminidase deficiency |
| Feline GM₁ gangliosidosis | Siamese cat, domestic cat | Vacuolation of neurons and hepatocytes | 10 to 16 weeks | Tremors; incoordination; paraplegia | GM₁ ganglioside accumulates; β-galactosidase deficiency |

*Terms in parentheses refer to eponyms used for analogous human disorders.

**Table 2.** *β-Galactosidase Activity in Skin from Cats of Feline GM₁ Gangliosidosis Family*

| PHENOTYPE | GENOTYPE | ENZYME ACTIVITY |
|---|---|---|
| Normal | Homozygous normal | 77.2 ± 16.4* |
| Normal | Heterozygous (carrier) | 29.7 ± 8.1 |
| Diseased | Homozygous recessive | 5.4 ± 2.7 |

*Activities expressed as mean ± 1 SD nanomoles of substrate cleaved per milligram protein per hour.

sion of these traits. For example, 50 per cent of the progeny of matings between carrier and normal individuals will be inapparent carriers of the defect. Thus, unless the existence of these traits is recognized by the occurrence of clinical disease in the progeny of carrier parents, the genetic defect can readily become widespread in a family or breed. Although most of these diseases occur in specific breeds, some have also been observed in mongrels. In both instances, consanguinity is a key element in the expression of disease, because it increases the probability of mating between heterozygous carriers.

## DIAGNOSIS

The pattern of histologic lesions in tissues of diseased animals is sufficiently unique to establish a tentative diagnosis. However, specific diagnosis depends upon identification of the material which accumulates in brain and other organs. Two major types of histologic lesions are associated with these diseases, including (1) vacuolation of cells resulting from the accumulation of complex lipids in the cytoplasm, and (2) extensive loss of myelin. Those disorders characterized by the latter lesion are often referred to as leukodystrophies (e.g., metachromatic leukodystrophy). Diagnostic histologic lesions are not present in the tissues of heterozygous carriers. In those instances where the specific enzyme deficiency has been established, it is possible to detect carriers by finding reduced enzyme activity in their tissues, such as biopsied skin (Table 2).

## PREVENTION

These diseases are inherited disorders of purebred animals and consequently have the same devastating potential of other, better known, inherited diseases such as progressive retinal atrophy. Furthermore, the recessive mode of inheritance precludes recognition of these traits until a specific diagnosis is made on a homozygous diseased animal. Therefore, the crucial first step in the prevention of these disorders depends upon the alert clinician who is aware that these entities exist and maintains a high level of suspicion for unusual, progressive neurologic diseases. Assistance in the specific identity of a disease thought to be of this type can be secured from laboratories specializing in the study of these conditions. Once the trait is known to be present in a family or breed, carriers can be identified by enzyme testing or breeding trials, and appropriate steps can be taken to eliminate the trait.

## COMPARATIVE STUDY

All of the diseases being considered here were first recognized in man, followed by discovery of the animal counterparts. In the few instances where breeding stock has been available to permit extensive investigation of the animal diseases, their pathologic processes have been found to be remarkably similar to the analogous human disorder. The ultimate benefit, for both animals and man, to be derived from such comparative studies is obvious. Practicing veterinarians have an unprecedented opportunity to make major contributions to the advancement of biomedical science through continued recognition of the established entities and in the discovery of additional examples of inborn errors of metabolism.

### SUPPLEMENTAL READING

Baker, H. J., et al.: Animal model of human disease.: Feline GM₁ gangliosidosis. Am. J. Path., 74:649–652, 1974.

Crisp, C. E., et al.: Lipid storage disease in a Siamese cat. J. Am. Vet. Med. Assn., 156:616–622, 1970.

Fletcher, T. F., Kurtz, H. J., and Low, D. G.: Globoid cell leukodystrophy (Krabbe type) in the dog. J. Am. Vet. Med. Assn., 149:165–172, 1966.

Hegreberg, G. A.: Morphologic changes in feline leukodystrophy. Fed. Proc., 30:341, 1971.

Johnson, K. H.: Globoid cell leukodystrophy in the cat. J. Am. Vet. Med. Assn., 157:2057–2064, 1970.

Karbe, E., and Schiefer, B.: Familial amaurotic idiocy in male German shorthair pointers. Path. Vet., 4:223–232, 1967.

Sandstrom, B.: Glycogenosis of the central nervous system in the cat. Acta Neuropath., 14:194–200, 1969.

# CLINICAL BEHAVIORAL PROBLEMS: AGGRESSION

KATHERINE A. HOUPT, V.M.D.
*Ithaca, New York*

The three most common behavioral problems presented to small animal practitioners are: house-soiling with urine or feces due to a failure to learn or to retain bladder or bowel control; destructiveness in the owner's absence; and aggression. House-soiling may be primarily a medical problem if due to enteritis, cystitis or diabetes, but more commonly it is entirely a behavioral problem which must be dealt with psychologically. Destructiveness in the home has a simple but often impractical solution: do not leave a dog alone in a house for long periods of time. Fortunately, there are also behavioral means to cope with this problem when a dog must be left alone. Aggression is the most serious of these common behavioral problems and can be treated medically, surgically or behaviorally.

Aggression can take several forms, and it is important to determine the type of aggression because the treatments differ. Aggression can be intraspecific or interspecific. If interspecific, it may be directed at other animals or at people. A good behavioral history will reveal whether the major behavioral problem is interspecific or intraspecific aggression. The character of the onset of the aggressiveness is also worth noting. Aggression of sudden onset is more likely to be the result of organic disease or a drastic change in the animal's environment. Such changes in the environment need not be limited to physical or geographic changes. An alteration of the social environment by the addition or subtraction of an animal or person may influence aggressive behavior. Dogs often show aggression toward a new pet and, not uncommonly, toward a new infant or new spouse.

Intraspecific aggression occurs among strange dogs. A group of dogs will normally form a dominance hierarchy, that is, a social order that determines which animal has first access to food, shelter and sexual partners. Overt violence is often evident at first, but as the hierarchy is established, subtle threats replace such violence. Nearly all social species form hierarchies in order to reduce aggression and to insure that the fittest will survive when supplies of food are limited. Cats are not a social species and form dominance hierarchies with difficulty. As a result, aggression may persist for prolonged periods, especially when adult cats are mixed.

There are several factors which may contribute to the development of intraspecies aggression. Scarcity of any necessity, in particular, food, increases aggression. Crowding also increases the incidence of aggressive behavior. If possible, animals should be fed individually, or, if that is not possible, individual dishes and an abundant amount of food should be provided. A less palatable, more bulky diet, such as meal, rather than a highly palatable diet of meat should be used in group feeding situations. Crowded conditions not only increase the level of aggression but also prevent the loser of a battle from fleeing to a safe distance.

Intraspecies aggression can usually be avoided by housing dogs individually and by using proper restraint. The most serious problems arise in dogs that must work together as a team. Prefrontal lobotomy, although still in the experimental stage in veterinary medicine, has been shown successfully to attenuate intraspecific aggression in malamutes and to permit formerly aggressive dogs to work together in harness with other dogs (Allen *et al.*, 1974).

Interspecies aggression can be directed at other animals (predatory behavior) or toward humans. Predatory behavior or hunting is probably not innate but rather is learned behavior. Cats may chase small, fast-moving objects like mice but usually will not kill them unless they have seen adult cats, usually their mother, do so. Kittens raised in an environment in which they did not observe adult cats killing rats seldom kill rodents, and kittens raised with rats never kill rats. In general, of course, predatory behavior in cats is not considered misbehavior unless it is directed against songbirds, but predatory behavior by dogs is often a clinical problem. Dogs that kill chickens, deer, lambs or cats are frequently presented for treatment. The easiest approach is proper restraint of the dog. A dog on a leash or in a pen not only is prevented from killing other animals but is also no longer at risk of automobile-induced trauma. A more drastic treatment may also be used. Many mammals, including canids, are able to learn to avoid a food that they associate with illness. If the dog not only kills but also eats its prey, this phenomenon of taste aversion can be used to eliminate predatory behavior. For example, if the dog kills and eats chickens, it can be allowed to do so and shortly afterward can be injected intraperitoneally with lithium chloride (10 ml. 0.3 M LiCl/kg. body weight), or a dead chicken (0.1 gm./kg.) can be baited with an equivalent amount of LiCl in a capsule. Two or three exposures to the nausea associated with lithium should suffice to teach the dog to avoid attacking chickens. Similar treatment taught coyotes, which formerly killed lambs, to avoid both live and dead lambs (Gustafson *et al.*, 1974).

The most common type of aggression presented to veterinarians is aggression directed toward humans. The practitioner is particularly concerned with aggression toward the veterinarian and he soon learns to recognize the two potentially difficult types of aggressive dogs: the dominant and threatening dog, with erect ears and slowly wagging tail but whose teeth are bared; and the fear-biter, the submissive dog with ears flattened against it head and tail between its legs but which also bares its teeth. The fear-biter will bite when its critical distance is invaded by the veterinarian in order to examine it and it cannot escape. Small dogs can be restrained manually and larger dogs can be chemically restrained. The introduction of tranquilizers and sedatives that can be administered intramuscularly or orally has greatly facilitated handling of large intractable dogs. Xylazine (Rompun®,

Chemagro) 2 ml./kg. IM or piperacetazine (Psymod®, Pitman-Moore) 0.5 mg./20 kg. orally have proved particularly useful. One drawback is the masking of clinical signs by tranquilization. Another is that powerful sedative drugs should not be used on dogs with serious liver or kidney disease because the drugs will not be excreted or metabolized at the normal rate.

Aggression toward humans is by far the most serious veterinary behavior problem. One million dog bites are reported in the United States per year, and many biting episodes that occur within the dog's home probably go unreported. Since most of the victims of dog bites are children, the problem can not be dismissed as affecting only the dog and its owner. The clinician should develop a therapeutic approach to aggression which first uses a purely behavioral approach and then escalates to medical and finally surgical treatments (Fig. 1). Of course, if the patient is a large dog that has already inflicted serious wounds and there are small children in the household, the most efficacious treatments should be used.

The behavioral approach involves counseling owners of dogs that are genetically predisposed to aggressive problems, e.g., German shepherds and malamutes. When large breed dogs are puppies, the owner should make every effort to establish dominance over the animal because many behavioral problems develop when there is a question of dominance or when a dog is dominant over the owner. Picking up a dog

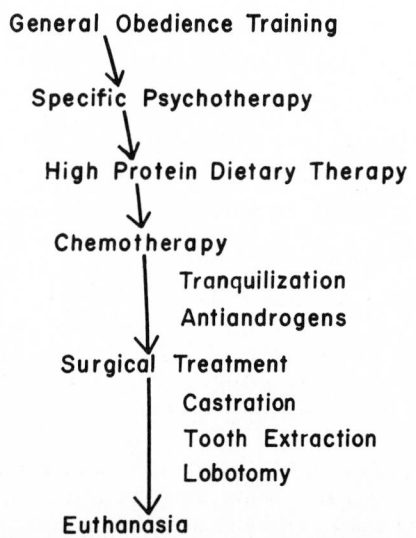

**Figure 1.** Progressive therapies for aggression.

is a good and nonpainful way to establish dominance. Play-fighting should be discouraged as well as the slightest indication of threats toward strangers. Good obedience training will at least insure that the dog is controllable in the owner's presence. Once an aggressive behavior problem has developed, there are ways in which the dog's aggression can be attenuated behaviorally. The success rate of these methods has not been evaluated objectively, but they have reduced aggression in some cases (Campbell, 1974).

High-protein diets (24 per cent) have also been recommended to reduce aggression' and hyperactivity in dogs. High-protein diets may alter behavior by increasing the level of the brain neurotransmitter serotonin, which would tend to sedate the animal.

Tranquilization is the next level of treatment. The major tranquilizers like promazine are commonly used in veterinary practice for this purpose, but some clinicians have seen increases rather than decreases of aggression after such tranquilizers have been given. When this occurs, the dog is probably a fundamentally dominant and aggressive animal that has developed inhibitions against attacking. These inhibitions are removed by the central nervous system depressant effect of the tranquilizers. Tranquilizers will be most effective in dogs that are fundamentally fear-biters. Diazepam (0.5 mg./kg.) (Valium®, Roche) is particularly effective in reducing anxiety in humans and animals. It may be more useful than the major tranquilizers in reducing aggressive behavior.

Testosterone not only organizes those cells in the fetal brain which are involved in emotional behavior so that the male has a lower threshold for aggression but also stimulates aggression in the adult. The effect of castration on aggressive behavior has been known for centuries, although many dog owners are unwilling to consider it. Castration is particularly effective in young dogs and in middle-aged terrier-type dogs (6 to 7 years old) that are becoming increasingly aggressive with age. Removing the source of testosterone will probably not be effective in a mature dog that either has been aggressive for much of its life or has shown a sudden onset of marked aggression rather than a gradual increase in grouchiness. Owners should be convinced that it is not cruel to castrate male dogs and

that it is as irresponsible to allow a dog with aggressive traits to breed as it is to allow a dog with any other inheritable physical defect to do so. If owners still object to surgical castration, temporary chemical castration may be achieved with 2.2 mg./kg. megestrol acetate (Ovaban®, Schering) orally per day. Castration is of particular value in reducing intraspecies aggression. The American public has long accepted castration as a means of preventing fighting among male cats but seems unwilling to recognize its value in dogs. The female hormones do not, as a rule, stimulate aggression, so that ovariectomy seldom attenuates aggression in female dogs or cats. The exception is bitches that are prone to pseudopregnancy with accompanying aggression. Ovariohysterectomy will usually eliminate the aggression.

Aggression of sudden onset may be caused by tumors or abscesses in the brain. Lesions of the hypothalamus or other limbic system structures that inhibit aggression may cause aggression. Conversely, removing those areas of the brain which facilitate aggressive behavior has been advocated in both human and veterinary medicine. As discussed above, prefrontal lobotomy does appear useful for eliminating intraspecific aggression but does not appear to reduce interspecific aggression. Those dogs and cats which were returned to their home environment gradually increased in aggressiveness postoperatively. Obviously, further studies should be undertaken to refine the surgical techniques and to determine which areas should be abolished in order to reduce aggression most effectively. The ethical problems troubling the human psychosurgeon need not be a concern as long as the animal can function as a healthy pet.

If the more moderate forms of therapy for aggression do not attenuate the problem, or if the dog has already inflicted serious injury, a more drastic surgical approach can be used. The incisor and canine teeth can be extracted, thus rendering the dog relatively harmless. Interestingly, dogs so treated appear to decrease in aggressive behavior as if aggressiveness without the pleasure of an ounce of human flesh or at least a marked human fear reaction is not rewarding. Dogs can still prehend and masticate commercial foods, so there is no nutritional disadvantage to the procedure. However, there is eventually an unfortunate cosmetic result, because the muzzle conformation will change as the gums atrophy. Nevertheless, tooth extraction is the most certain way to prevent further harm to the dog's victims. The only other alternative with a more certain outcome is euthanasia. In a situation in which the owners are reluctant to consent to the death of a beloved pet but are concerned about the safety of their children, of their friends and of themselves, dental extraction has much to recommend it.

None of the suggested treatments for aggression—behavioral, medical or surgical—is guaranteed to eliminate aggression, although all may attenuate it. The owner of an aggressive dog must be made aware that aggression is of a complicated genetic and environmental etiology and is no more easily eliminated than is any chronic disease, such as arthritis or valvular heart disease. In particular, the client should be made to feel that euthanasia of a large aggressive dog is often wise. If the household consists of adults who are willing to take the risks of serious bites, behavioral techniques, tranquilization and castration should be utilized. If there are small children in the household, no risks should be taken.

### SUPPLEMENTAL READING

Allen, B. D., Cummings, J. F., and de Lahunta, A.: The effects of prefrontal lobotomy on aggressive behavior in dogs. Cornell Vet., 64:201, 1974.

Campbell, W. E.: Behavior Problems in Dogs. American Veterinary Publications, Santa Barbara, California, 1975.

Fox, M. W.: Abnormal Behavior in Animals. Philadelphia, W. B. Saunders Co., 1968.

Gustafson, C. R., Garcia, J., Hankins, W. G., and Rusiniak, K. W.: Coyote predation control by aversive conditioning. Science, 184:581, 1974.

Hart, B.: Drug choice in feline psychopharmacology. Feline Practice. 3:8, 1973.

# OSTEOCHON-DROSIS DISSECANS, ENOSTOSIS (EOSINOPHILIC PANOSTEITIS) AND HYPERTROPHIC OSTEODYS-TROPHY (LAMENESS)

JEFFREY A. LA CROIX, D.V.M.
*Ithaca, New York*

Lameness, when it occurs in growing dogs of the large and giant breeds, presents a diagnostic challenge to the clinician. The etiology in the majority of such cases will be trauma in one form or another to bones, joints or their supporting soft tissues. Yet, a significant number of these cases of lameness will be caused by specific diseases of bone.

Among the causes of lameness in young

dogs of the large and giant breeds, the following conditions will be found:

Hematogenous osteomyelitis
Septic arthritis or polyarthritis
Overnutrition
Vitamin A poisoning
Vitamin D poisoning
Rickets
Hyperparathyroidism
Elbow dysplasia
Hip dysplasia
Genu valgum
Radius curvus
Osteochondrosis dissecans
Enostosis (eosinophilic panosteitis)
Hypertrophic osteodystrophy

This article will deal with the last three conditions listed. While the exact etiology of osteochondrosis dissecans (OD), enostosis and hypertrophic osteodystrophy (HOD) remains in doubt, recent experiments with overnutrition have produced "hypertrophic" bone diseases, the histopathologic changes of which closely resemble those seen in clinical cases of OD, enostosis and HOD.

## OSTEOCHONDROSIS DISSECANS (OD)

Reports of OD appear in the veterinary literature of the early 1960's. Although widely recognized as appearing at the shoulder joint (humeral head), it is also observed at the stifle (usually lateral femoral condyle) and, more rarely, at the elbow and hock joints.

### CLINICAL SIGNS AND RADIOGRAPHIC APPEARANCE

Osteochondrosis dissecans produces a persistent lameness in the involved limb. The age at onset is from 4 to 12 months. When the shoulder is affected, pain can usually be elicited by extension of the limb with pressure applied either to the point of the shoulder or at the caudal aspect of the joint. A similar manipulation at the stifle will usually cause pain if this joint is the site of the lesion.

When the disease involves the humeral head, a lateral radiograph of the affected limb with the leg in extension will show the lesion as a lytic defect or flattening at the centrocaudal aspect of the humeral head. In more severe cases, a saucer-shaped lesion is produced by rarefaction of subchondral bone at this point. A separated fragment (slab) of subchondral bone and its overlying cartilage may be seen within the saucer-shaped defect, or this fragment may become displaced, resulting in a free-body or joint mouse.

While clinically the lameness is usually unilateral, a radiograph of the opposite shoulder will in many cases show a less severe but similar lesion.

### HISTOPATHOLOGY

Histopathologically, the defect is the result of a delay in enchondral osteogenesis. The articular cartilage cells have failed to produce epiphyseal trabeculae, causing a loss of continuity between the articular cartilage and the epiphysis. The result is a collapse or fracture of the articular cartilage and subchondral bone, producing the typical radiographic lesion described previously. Biomechanical considerations may explain the site predilections for the disease.

The separated or collapsed fragment of articular cartilage and subchondral bone remains viable, and the bone marrow of the defect produces granulation tissue at the interface.

### THERAPY

Therapy may be conservative or surgical. Proper case selection is often difficult.

Visualization of an extensive or deep lesion, appearance of a completely separated slab fracture at the articular surface and a free-body within the joint are all indications for surgery. Surgical treatment consists of exposure of the joint as described by Piermattei and Greeley or by Dingwall and Flipo. The procedure of the latter authors does not require ostectomy of the acromion. Free-bodies are removed manually or by flushing the joint with a sterile physiologic solution. The fractured cartilage is separated from its bed, and the lesion is gently curetted so as to remove all granulation tissue, leaving a cavity, the surface of which bleeds freely. The edges of the articular defect should be rounded before final flushing and closure.

Postoperative care consists of 4 to 5 days' confinement followed by restricted exercise for 2 weeks. Full function can be expected by 4 to 6 weeks.

Conservative therapy involves *complete* rest. The patient should, under no circumstances, be allowed to run free, and rough play must be discouraged. If necessary, tranquilizers may be administered to reduce the animal's level of activity.

In the author's opinion, long periods of confinement in a cage or crate have not proved to be more beneficial than more moderate restriction of activity. Furthermore, such confinement may have a negative effect on the patient's general emotional and physical development.

Analgesics and corticosteroids are contraindicated, since the lessening of pain and discomfort is likely to encourage a greater degree of movement and consequently more trauma to the lesion.

Conservative therapy is most likely to be successful if the patient is a placid individual. Vigorous active dogs are likely to traumatize the diseased bone continuously, making the defect more severe or causing an intraarticular fracture.

If conservative therapy (rest) has not resulted in significant improvement in 6 to 8 weeks, the affected joints should be radiographed again. If the lesion is static, rest may be continued. However, if the lesion is more severe, surgery is recommended.

## ENOSTOSIS

Enostosis (eosinophilic panosteitis) was first described in Europe in 1951. It was initially thought to be an infectious process (possibly streptococcal), but experimental work and clinical observations seem to contradict this early opinion.

### CLINICAL SIGNS AND RADIOGRAPHIC APPEARANCE

Enostosis produces an intermittent, often shifting, limb lameness that lasts for a few days to several weeks. Signs first appear at from 4 to 16 months of age. More rarely, cases have been reported to occur initially in dogs up to 20 months of age. Males are affected more frequently than females. The lameness is unaffected by either rest or exercise. Concurrent signs of systemic illness are not seen. Eosinophilia is, at best, an inconsistent sign and, when present, is probably due to other causes. Upon physi-

cal examination, pain can usually be elicited by deep palpation of the affected bone along its diaphysis.

Radiographically, the lesions are seen in the long bones, especially the tibia, femur and humerus, and can be visualized within 3 to 5 days of the onset of clinical signs. An oval area of increased density appears within the medullary canal, often located adjacent to a nutrient foramen. These areas represent an increase in trabecular bone— "hypertrophic bone." Less commonly, and later in the course of the disease, a linear, homogeneous thickening of the cortex along the diaphyseal shaft may become apparent.

Remission of clinical signs is not necessarily correlated with a resolution of the radiographic changes. Radiographic changes within the bone may persist for 2 to 3 months following the acute episode of lameness.

Since the radiographic changes may be subtle, it is often helpful to take identical views of the opposite limb.

### HISTOPATHOLOGY

Histopathologically, ectopic medullary bone resulting from failure of resorption accounts for the increased medullary density seen radiographically. Excessive subperiosteal bone formation is responsible for the cortical thickening seen later in the course of the disease.

### THERAPY

Although the course is somewhat variable, the disease is self-limiting, and signs usually disappear by the time the patient is 18 to 24 months of age. Treatment is therefore probably unnecessary and extremely difficult to evaluate.

Corticosteriods, phenylbutazone and salicylates have been used without noticeably influencing the course or outcome of the disease.

## HYPERTROPHIC OSTEODYSTROPHY (HOD)

Hypertrophic osteodystrophy has been diagnosed in the dog since the 1950's. Recently the term has been given a broader meaning to include the so-called "hypertrophic osteodystrophies" induced by overnutrition, especially overnutrition with calcium, which results in hypercalcitoninism. This discussion will be limited to the classic form of HOD.

## CLINICAL AND RADIOGRAPHIC APPEARANCE

The age at the onset of signs is usually from 3 to 6 months. Signs include lameness and evidence of a more generalized soreness, fever, depression, inappetence and reluctance to move. Tonsillitis or another focus of infection such as pyoderma or pneumonia may be noted. Albuminuria and leukocytosis occur during fever episodes. Firm, warm, swollen metaphyseal regions (most prominent at the distal ends of the radius, ulna, femur and proximal tibia) are nearly pathognomonic of the disease.

While a diagnosis can be based on clinical signs, radiographs will confirm the diagnosis by showing changes at the metaphyses of the affected bones.

The metaphysis, usually seen as a region of fairly dense trabecular bone blending smoothly into the diaphysis, loses its normal architecture. A transverse zone of rarefaction (called the scorbutic zone) can be seen in the metaphysis on the diaphyseal side of the epiphyseal plate. The affected metaphyses are usually wide (flared), and mineralized deposits can be seen along the surface of the cortex in this region.

The exact cause of HOD is unknown. The disease is, however, most likely to occur in the fastest growing individuals in which growth has been encouraged further by oversupplementation of the diet, especially with minerals and fat-soluble vitamins.

The clinical picture of a dog suffering from overnutrition or more specifically hypercalcitoninism (from a diet high in calcium) is quite similar to HOD. Dogs with induced hypercalcitoninism show lameness and have swollen metaphyses and generalized skeletal pain. Fever is absent, and unlike HOD, dietary correction alone will result in improvement in the condition.

## HISTOPATHOLOGY

Histopathologically, the causes of the visible radiographic changes are seen to be fibrous periosteal thickening, subperiosteal hemorrhage and extraperiosteal new bone growth. Normal metaphyseal architecture is disrupted as mineralization of cartilage and replacement with osteoid fails to take place (scorbutic zone).

## THERAPY

The radiographic and histopathologic changes of HOD resemble those seen in human scurvy (vitamin C deficiency). In addition, dogs with HOD have been shown to have lowered serum vitamin C levels, with the levels rising along with induced or spontaneous recovery from the disease.

Treatment consists of correction of any dietary imbalance. Special attention should be given to correcting the amounts of calcium and phosphorus and to lowering the caloric intake. This can be accomplished by feeding a high-quality commercial dry dog food along with a small amount of meat to improve palatability. All nutritional supplements should be discontinued.

While response to treatment is variable, this clinician recommends the administration of 1000 mg. vitamin C intravenously b.i.d. for 5 days. If improvement occurs, treatment is continued orally with 500 mg. vitamin C b.i.d. for one month.

Antibiotics are indicated if any infection is present. Disagreement exists concerning the use of corticosteroids. Corticosteroids have been shown to decrease the population of osteoblasts. This effect may not be unwanted during the acute stage of a "hypertrophic" bone disease. It is the clinical opinion of the author that the use of corticosteroids lessens subperiosteal pain, contributes to the general well-being of the patient and exerts no demonstrable effect on the bone that can be interpreted as delaying resolution of the disease. The prognosis in all cases of HOD should be guarded, since response to therapy is not consistent.

## SUPPLEMENTAL READING

Cotter, S. M.: Enostosis of young Dogs. J. Am. Vet. Med. Assn., 153:401–410, 1968.

Dingwall, J. S., and Flipo, J.: Joints of the forelimb. *In* Canine Surgery. Santa Barbara, California, 1974, pp. 1056–1057.

Hedhammar, A., Krook, L., Whalen, J. P., *et al.*: Overnutrition and skeletal disease: an experimental study in growing Great Dane dogs. Cornell Vet., 64 (Suppl. 5), 1974.

La Croix, J. A.: Diagnosis of orthopedic problems peculiar to the growing dog. Vet. Med./Small Animal Clin., 65:229–239, 1970.

Meir, H. *et al.*: Hypertrophic osteodystrophy associated with disturbance of vitamin C synthesis in dogs. J. Am. Vet. Med. Assn., 130:483–491, 1957.

Piermattei, D. L., and Greeley, R. G.: An Atlas of Surgical Approaches to the Bones of the Dog and Cat. Philadelphia, W. B. Saunders Co., 1966, pp. 38–41.

Van Sickle, D. C.: Selected orthopedic problems in the growing dog. Am. Anim. Hosp. Assoc., 1975, pp. 20–35.

---

# CANINE HIP DYSPLASIA

STEN-ERIK OLSSON
*Stockholm, Sweden*

## DEFINITION

In the dog, hip dysplasia is a developmental condition and not a congenital anomaly. Subluxation of the femoral head leads to abnormal wear, with erosion of the joint cartilage, inflammatory changes in the synovia and synovial membrane, thickening of the joint capsule and formation of osteophytes. These changes may start comparatively early but are not severe until in late adolescence or early adulthood. The end result is an acetabulum more shallow than normal and a flattened femoral head. The trigger mechanism may be either slight joint laxity or poor support in weight-bearing by a slanting roof of the acetabulum. Either way, a vicious circle of increased luxation, increased remodeling with more flattening and more shallow acetabulum is started. Osteoarthrosis, increasing in severity over the years, is always seen.

## ETIOLOGY AND PATHOGENESIS

The etiology of hip dysplasia is multifactorial. Anything that causes abnormal weight-bearing by the hip joint in a growing dog can lead to the morphologic changes characteristic of hip dysplasia. The cause of hip dysplasia can be local, as for example a fracture of the femoral shaft healed in malalignment, or it can be a unilateral sacralization of the seventh lumbar vertebra, giving rise to an asymmetrical pelvis. In these cases hip dysplasia is usually unilateral. Most cases of hip dysplasia are, however, caused by generalized constitutional factors governing the growth and development of the skeleton. The reason why only the hip joints react to these generalized stimuli in the way they do is their anatomic shape—the hip joints are unique in that they are the only joints with no horizontal support in weight-bearing.

Some of the pathologic findings in the cartilage of dysplastic hip joints are consistent with findings in osteochondrosis, which is a generalized condition in fast-growing dogs. The possible relationship between osteochondrosis and hip dysplasia is under investigation.

## DIAGNOSIS

At present the only reliable diagnosis of hip dysplasia in the dog is the one made on radiographs taken when the animal is over 18 months of age but not older than 5 or 6 years. The reason for the upper age limit is the fact that primary osteoarthrosis of old age may be impossible to differentiate from slight hip dysplasia. Below the age of one year it is sometimes difficult to draw the line between what is normal and abnormal. Palpation at an early age, i.e., estimation of the amount of laxity of the hip joints, has little prognostic value except in puppies in which the hip joints are very tight. There is a great chance that these hip joints are going to develop into sound joints.

## GENETICS AND PREVENTION

Hip dysplasia as it is seen in most breeds of large dogs is an inherited defect with a polygenic mode of inheritance. This means that many genes are responsible for its development. It is also quantitative in nature, i.e., its phenotypic expression can vary from only very minute changes to complete luxation with almost no acetabulum. As any other inherited defect with a polygenic mode of inheritance, the expression of hip dysplasia is subject to modification by a variety of environmental factors. The amount of influence by environmental factors can be calculated and expressed as a heritability index. (A condition that is completely controlled genetically has a heritability index of 1. If there is no hereditary influence, the heritability index is 0.

The most recent heritability index, calculated on unbiased data from one kennel with more than 2500 German shepherd puppies, was found to be 0.33. In previous studies heritability figures have varied from 0.25 to 0.50, but the latest figure is probably the most reliable. A heritability index of 0.33 means that heritability is moderate, indicating that it is possible to lower incidence and severity of hip dysplasia considerably by genetic selection. One could expect relatively rapid results if good hip joints were the only factor considered in dog breeding. Since this is not the case, breeders must understand that simultaneous genetic selection for many desirable characteristics, for example, a certain conformation, good disposition, good working ability and good hip joints, makes it difficult to obtain immediate results.

Selection for better hip joints is usually based only on the breeding of phenotypically normal individuals, i.e., dogs with radiographically normal hip joints. This is of course better than no selection at all, but the limitation of the method is obvious, when one knows that male dogs with excellent hip joints may have offspring in which the incidence of hip dysplasia varies from 21 per cent to 68 per cent. Rather than using individual selection (mass selection) it is recommended that individual performance (progeny testing) and family performance (sibling evaluation and pedigree depth) be used. This is, however, difficult to accomplish, since most dog breeding occurs on a small scale.

It was shown recently that incidence and severity of hip dysplasia can be influenced by nutrition during growth in offspring of dogs with hip dysplasia. A high-calorie diet increases incidence and makes dysplasia more severe, while a low-calorie diet decreases incidence and makes hip dysplasia less severe. This finding and the observation that overfeeding (feeding *ad libitum*) of puppies causes many other skeleton problems in fast-growing dogs clearly demonstrate that restricted feeding of growing dogs is important for normal development. On the other hand, puppies that develop normal hip joints despite overfeeding probably have a better genetic constitution (genotype).

It is imperative for all breeders to decide what kind of dog they want. If good function and working ability is high on the priority list, special attention should be paid to good hip joints in breeding. If more irrational characteristics such as conformation and color have top priority, hip dysplasia may be of less concern. It should always be remembered that the radiographic diagnosis of hip dysplasia is one thing, the clinical problem of hip dysplasia another. Many times there is poor correlation between the degree of hip dysplasia as diagnosed on radiographs and the clinical signs. Many dogs with hip dysplasia have no noticeable clinical sgns. One must understand that the radiographic diagnosis of hip dysplasia in a clinically healthy dog is nothing but a memo to the owner, saying that the owner must put the status of the dog's hip joints on the negative side of the balance sheet when he sums up what makes the animal suitable or unsuitable for breeding.

## CLINICAL SIGNS

The clinical signs of hip dysplasia vary widely from very slight discomfort to severe crippling disease. There are great differences in individual temperament, which will influence the signs of hip dysplasia. Young dogs may walk with a swaying gait and may "bunny hop" on the hind limbs when running. One should not forget that improvement or even disappearance of signs is not uncommon, and adult dogs may not show any evidence of hip dysplasia until old age, when severe osteoarthrosis complicates the picture.

Dogs with clinical signs of hip dysplasia should be allowed to choose their own level of exercise but if necessary may be encouraged to a moderate level of activity. Forced sudden activity such as playing ball or jumping should be discouraged. Older dogs can be given the usual medication for pain caused by osteoarthrosis.

At the present time, there are four surgical procedures available for cases in which for various reasons surgery is indicated. The simplest and most "innocuous" method is pectineomyotomy, for which there is wide indication. Following this type of surgery, improvement has been seen both in young dogs with unstable hips and in old dogs with severe osteoarthritis. Pectineomyotomy changes the gait pattern of the hind legs somewhat, allowing for more abduction in weight-bearing. This is probably the reason why it seems to alleviate pain. However, the effectiveness of pectineomyotomy has been seriously questioned.

Another sugical procedure is pelvic osteotomy. It is aimed at improving the support by the acetabular roof. The acetabulum is rotated over the femoral head and in this way further subluxation is prevented. This procedure is technically difficult and requires long-term postsurgical care. The long-term result is questionable.

Resection arthroplasty, i.e., removal of the femoral head, is a salvage procedure for dogs with severe hip dysplasia. This operation is comparatively easy to perform, but postoperative care and rehabilitation are time-consuming. Intensive physical training and exercise such as swimming and running are imperative during the first 4 to 6 months after surgery in order to get good functional nearthrosis. Resection arthroplasty should be reserved for young, active dogs and preferably should be done on both sides in one and the same operation.

In recent years the total hip prosthesis has been used successfully in dogs with severe hip dysplasia but nothing is known about the long-term result. One should remember, however, that fitting and insertion of a well-functioning total hip prosthesis is a technically difficult and expensive procedure.

# OSTEO-CHONDROSIS IN THE DOG

STEN-ERIK OLSSON
*Stockholm, Sweden*

It has long been known that there are certain skeletal problems characteristic of growing dogs of the large breeds. Several conditions were described in the 1950's and 1960's, such as osteochondritis dissecans of the shoulder, ununited anconeal process of the elbow and retained cartilage of the distal ulna. Lesions of this nature in the hind limbs have also been known for a long time, such as hip dysplasia and *genu valgum*. More recently lesions such as osteochondritis dissecans of the medial condyle of the humerus and fragmentation of the coronoid process (ununited coronoid process) of the ulna were described. In the hind limbs interest is now focused on epiphysiolysis of the femoral head and osteochondritis dissecans of the knee and of the hock. A few cases of osteochondritis dissecans of the cervical intervertebral joints have also been described.

The various lesions have been looked upon as separate entities and not until 1975 was there an understanding of the morphologic similarities and the generalized background of these lesions. Similar lesions in horses, cattle, pigs, turkeys and poultry have been studied, and this has contributed to an even better understanding of the generalized nature of the condition now called osteochondrosis.

Of all the lesions described, hip dysplasia seems to be the only one which does not entirely fit into the picture of osteochondrosis, but there is little question that some of the features of hip dysplasia are consistent with osteochondrosis.

The basic mechanism behind osteochondrosis is a disturbance of endochondral ossification. The various lesions considered to be manifestations of osteochondrosis occur at sites where cartilage with an abnormal growth rate is exposed to pressure or tension. It should be pointed out that all cartilage in the growing skeleton may be affected, i.e., both the growth plates and the joint cartilage. While it has been recognized that certain lesions in the growth plates, such as retained cartilage of the distal ulna, are the result of overgrowth and a failure of calcification and ossification, the nature of the lesion in the joint cartilage (osteochondritis dissecans) was not understood. The reason for this is obviously that one has not reckoned with joint cartilage as a growth cartilage. It should therefore be emphasized that the joint cartilage is in fact the *growth cartilage* of the epiphysis in the same manner as the cartilage of the growth plates of the long bones is the growth cartilage of the metaphysis.

Normal growth of the epiphysis takes place by proliferation of chondrocytes near the joint surface. As cartilage continues to grow, vesiculation, degeneration and calcification of the cells take place. The calcified layer of the cartilage is invaded by vessels from the bone marrow. Some of the calcified cartilage is resorbed, but remnants of cartilage are used as a framework for bone, which is laid down by osteoblasts. The process is called *endochondral ossification*.

In osteochondrosis the normal differentiation process of the chondrocytes is disturbed (vesiculation, degeneration and calcification do not take place in a normal way), and the cartilage gets thicker than normal. At certain sites of pressure or tension, vessels from the bone marrow do not penetrate the cartilage and formation of bone ceases. If this process is localized to only a part of a joint cartilage, this will lead to a defect in the bone as bone formation continues in the calcified layer of the surrounding cartilage. Cracks and fissures often occur in the thickened cartilage that fills the defect, and once this has happened, the condition is called osteochondritis dissecans. If similar changes take place in a metaphyseal growth plate, epiphysiolysis may occur or the normal shape of the bone may be changed, because growth is interfered with. It should be emphasized, however, that many lesions do not advance that far. Some lesions are seen only on radiographs. They heal spontaneously and never cause any clinical problems.

Radiographic and pathologic investigations have demonstrated that osteochondrosis is truly generalized, since pathologic lesions are often found at several sites in the same animal. Osteochondritis dissecans, for example, is often bilateral and symmetrical and frequently occurs in more than one pair of joints.

In the pig, an animal which is bred and fed to grow fast, osteochondrosis occurs with a frequency of about 80 per cent, and osteochondritis dissecans is common in almost all joints. If growth is slowed down by nutritional or genetic means, osteochondrosis does not occur. Also, in the dog, osteochondrosis is related to rapid growth. Retained cartilage of various growth plates and osteochondritis dissecans of various joints are found only in dogs of medium or large size. Male dogs that grow faster than females are affected twice as often as are females.

## OSTEOCHONDRITIS DISSECANS OF THE SHOULDER JOINT

For a long time osteochondritis dissecans was known to exist in the dog only in the shoulder joint. It was first recognized in the 1950's, and a large number of papers have appeared on the subject. Osteochondritis dissecans of the shoulder joint is seen in all large and medium size dogs, predominantly in males. The first clinical signs are usually noticed between the ages of 4 and 7 months. Lameness of one or both forelimbs that is insidious in onset and gets worse after exercise is the most prominent sign. Stiffness after rest is another important sign. Pain can usually be elicited by palpation, flexion and extension of the shoulder. The clinical signs may vary in severity over periods of weeks or months.

The definite diagnosis is made by means of radiographic examination. A mediolateral radiograph of the extended shoulder joint usually reveals a defect in the subchondral bone of the humeral head. In mild or early cases only a flattening of the dorsocaudal contour of the humeral head is seen. It is imperative that radiographs be of good quality. Sedation or anesthesia is, as a rule, necessary. The dog is placed on the cassette with the side to be radiographed toward the table. The affected limb is pulled in a cranioventral direction and the opposite limb is pulled caudally, out of reach of the well collimated x-ray beams.

In dogs with advanced lesions there is usually sclerosis of the subchondral bone and sometimes calcification of the cartilage flap, which covers the defect. In many cases the defect is sometimes located to the caudolateral instead of the caudal side of the humeral head. Hence, a radiograph made in lateral projection does not visualize the lesion as a defect in the contour of the bone, but rather as an area of decreased density in the caudal part of the head. It should be remembered that the lesion in most cases is bilateral and for this reason both shoulders should always be radiographed, ever if there is no history or sign of bilateral lameness.

It is usually easier to make the diagnosis of osteochondritis dissecans of the shoulder joint than to decide what kind of therapy to use. The simple reason for this is that many cases of osteochondritis dissecans of the shoulder heal spontaneously. The pedicle of the cartilage flap may rupture and the flap may become dislodged. Eventually this flap, now turned into a joint mouse, is resorbed by the joint fluid through enzyme activity. Sometimes the natural course is entirely different. The flap remains intact and as long as it covers the floor of the defect no outgrowth of scar tissue will take place. It is not unusual to find that a lesion in the humeral head on one side heals spontaneously, while the one in the humeral head of the other limb continues to cause problems.

Because the animals show pain and lameness, restriction of exercise has been recommended as part of the treatment by many investigators. In contrast, the present author is of the opinion that a dog with osteochondritis dissecans of the shoulder should be allowed to move around as much as possible, because in this way the chance is greater that the flap will be dislodged. If necessary the dog can be given analgesics. If there is no obvious improvement after 4 to 6 weeks, surgery should be contemplated seriously. If one can prove the presence of a calcified flap or piece of cartilage in the defect, surgery should be performed with no further delay. Even in cases in which the signs are not severe or may have subsided, it is safe to do a repeat radiographic examination. If the radiographs reveal that bone has not filled the defect, an arthrogram should be made to demonstrate whether or not there is a flap or loose piece of cartilage in the defect. If the arthrogram is positive, surgery is indicated, but surgery is not necessary if there is no loose piece or flap *in the defect*, as healing in this case will take place spontaneously. If there is a joint mouse, it is usually lodged in the ventrocaudal pouch of the joint where in most cases it does not cause any clinical signs.

Eventually it will be digested, but it can also remain viable and grow in size. If a joint mouse is lodged in the sheath of the biceps tendon, it may give rise to pain and lameness and necessitate surgery.

Arthrography of the shoulder joint is easy to perform. The anesthetized dog is placed on the table with the side to be examined facing upward. A needle is inserted into the shoulder joint slightly caudal to the tip of the acromion. Depending on the dog's size, 4 to 6 ml. of a 20 per cent solution of Skiodan® (methiodal sodium [Winthrop]) or a similar compound is injected. The dog is turned over on the other side, and the limb is passively moved for about one minute in order to distribute the contrast medium evenly in the joint. Two films are then taken at an interval of about 2 to 3 minutes. If it is seen on previous plain films that the defect is located to the caudolateral part of the humeral head, the limb should be held in 5- to 10-degree supination during the second exposure to make the central beam hit the floor of the defect as tangentially as possible.

Surgery consists of removal of the cartilage flap or piece of cartilage that is lying in the defect and trimming of the edges of the defect. The postsurgical care includes restricted exercise for about 4 weeks.

## MANIFESTATIONS OF OSTEOCHONDROSIS IN THE ELBOW JOINT

In the very young dog it is sometimes not easy to differentiate between lameness caused by pain in the elbow and pain in the shoulder. It is therefore to be recommended that in doubtful cases both the elbow and the shoulder be radiographed. The radiographic examination is of great importance for early diagnosis of lesions in the elbow joint, provided that proper technique is used. Two projections are necessary, one mediolateral with the elbow *fully flexed*, the other anteroposterior with about 30- to 40-degree flexion of the elbow. It is sometimes useful also to have a mediolateral view of the elbow in only a few degrees of flexion.

There are three lesions in the elbow joint, all of which are manifestations of osteochondrosis: osteochondritis dissecans of the medial condyle of the humerus, fragmentation of the coronoid process (ununited coronoid process) and ununited anconeal process. They are all very important, not only because they give rise to lameness in the young dog, but because they lead to severe osteoarthrosis.

The three lesions have a similar clinical appearance, at least in the early stages. The owner of a dog with any of these elbow lesions usually complains that the dog has a stiff gait during the first few minutes after a period of rest. This sign is usually seen when the dog is about 4 to 5 months old. Front limb lameness is rarely noticed until the dog gets a little older. The lesions are often bilateral. For this reason the dog gets lame on both front limbs and this is difficult for the owner to observe. The bilateral lameness is usually seen as a slightly stiff, stilted gait of the forelimbs. The front limbs are usually held slightly laterally rotated, with elbows close to the chest. Careful clinical examination reveals some pain in the elbows on extension and sometimes on flexion.

Radiographic examination of the elbows at the age of 4 to 5 months is essential for the diagnosis of one of the three lesions, i.e., the one which seems to be the least common, the ununited anconeal process. The other two lesions do not give rise to radiographic signs at that age.

## UNUNITED ANCONEAL PROCESS (ELBOW DYSPLASIA)

This lesion has long been recognized and was recently considered to be the most common cause of osteoarthrosis of the elbow joint. It is found in many breeds of dogs of large size but seems to be a problem mainly in the German shepherd. There are indications that the condition has a genetic trait because the lesion is frequently found in littermates. Hence, it is not advisable to use a dog with ununited anconeal process for breeding.

In the German shepherd, the anconeal process ossifies at about age 10 to 13 weeks and unites with the rest of the ulna about 2 to 4 weeks later. Hence, in a normal dog the anconeal process should be united with the ulna at the latest at an age of 18 to 20 weeks. If not united at that time, there is little question that the anconeal process will remain ununited. In such a case, changes typical of osteochondrosis with cracks and fissures

can be seen histologically in the cartilage between the separate ossification center and the ulna. The end result is usually a large piece of bone, which is connected with the ulna by only a bridge of fibrocartilage or connective tissue.

Treatment of ununited anconeal process is surgical. The most common procedure is to remove the ununited process via a lateral incision between the lateral epicondyle and the olecranon. It has also been suggested that osteosynthesis should be done, i.e., to screw the process to the ulna in order to avoid the instability which is said to occur when the anconeal process is loose or removed. More research seems to be needed in order to evaluate the result of this kind to treatment. There seems to be a time factor to consider when one decides to do surgery. There are indications that surgery should not be done until the dog has reached an age of 9 to 12 months. If it is done earlier, i.e., during the period of very fast growth (4 to 8 months), secondary changes (remodeling and osteoarthrosis) seem to develop more easily after surgery than if the ununited anconeal process is left in place until a time when growth is almost completed.

## FRAGMENTATION OF THE CORONOID PROCESS OF THE ULNA (UNUNITED CORONOID PROCESS) AND OSTEOCHONDRITIS DISSECANS OF THE MEDIAL CONDYLE OF THE HUMERUS

These two lesions were recently described as causes of osteoarthrosis of the elbow joint and were found to be more common than the ununited anconeal process, at least in certain breeds. The two lesions are particularly a problem in golden and Labrador retrievers, but they occur separately or together in most breeds of large dogs. As a separate lesion, it is most common to find fragmentation of the coronoid process, except in the golden retriever, in which osteochondritis dissecans of the medial condyle of the humerus is the most common.

While the clinical signs of the two lesions are very similar to those of the ununited anconeal process in the early stages, the radiographic picture is entirely different. As a rule, nothing abnormal can be seen on radiographs before the dog is about 7 months of age, although clinical signs may have been present since an age of 4 or 5 months. It is therefore imperative to advise the owner of a young dog with slight clinical signs from the elbow joint to return the dog for a repeat radiographic examination 4 to 8 weeks after the first examination. Too many cases have hitherto been missed by veterinarians who have fallen back on the erroneous and diffuse diagnosis of "growing pain." There is no justification for making this diagnosis or, what is even worse, injecting corticosteroids intraarticularly, even if the clinical signs are vague and the radiographic picture is normal in a young dog.

The fragmentation of the coronoid process can usually not be visualized on radiographs. The first radiographic signs are instead small osteophytes on the dorsal aspect of the anconeal process and medially on the coronoid process. The osteophytes on the anconeal process can be seen only if the radiograph is made with the elbow joint in full flexion. If there is a lesion only on one side, the diagnosis is usually comparatively easy to make, since the difference between the normal and diseased side is obvious, provided that one knows what to look for. The differential diagnosis between a case of fragmentation of the coronoid process and a case of osteochondritis dissecans of the medial condyle of the humerus is more difficult. In typical cases of the latter lesion, a small triangular defect can be seen in the weight-bearing surface of the medial condyle. This defect is often surrounded by a sclerotic zone.

It is obvious that the two lesions have gone unrecognized until recently, mainly because the early radiographic changes have been overlooked. Once the dog is over a year of age, the radiographic signs are obvious and the diagnosis of osteoarthrosis is made. This often means a negative attitude by the veterinarian toward a search for rational treatment, since osteoarthrosis (if no obvious cause is found) is considered to be caused by wear and tear.

In the case of fragmentation of the coronoid process and osteochondritis dissecans of the medial condyle of the humerus, surgery should preferably be done at the age of 8 to 11 months. Only the medial approach to the elbow joint can be used. A slightly bowed incision in the skin and underlying fascia is made from over the distal part of the humeral shaft, over the pro-

tuberance of the medial condyle and down over the forearm. The pronator teres muscle and the flexor carpi radialis muscle are then dissected and cut as close as possible to their origins at the medial condyle of the humerus. This will give free access to the joint capsule and allow the median nerve to be seen and the position of the underlying artery and vein to be known. The joint capsule and the medial collateral ligament can thereafter be incised along the joint space without risk of damaging any of these structures. The incision must be long enough to allow some luxation of the joint to make it possible to inspect the joint surface of the medial condyle of the humerus and of the coronoid process of the ulna.

In early cases of osteochondritis dissecans of the medial condyle of the humerus, there is a defect in the weight-bearing surface, covered by a flap of cartilage. The flap should be removed and the edges of the defect trimmed. In later cases, there is usually no flap. Instead it may have been turned into a large cartilaginous body that may be found adhering to the joint capsule. It may even have been resorbed. In a joint with only a defect and no flap, only the edges of the defect should be trimmed. Whatever the findings, the coronoid process should be carefully inspected, since osteochondritis dissecans of the medial condyle is frequently combined with fragmentation of the coronoid process. The most common finding in fragmentation of the coronoid process is an elongated ossicle, covered with cartilage, which lies between the coronoid process and the head of the radius. Sometimes, the coronoid process is fragmented in several small pieces. On the opposing joint surface, there is always considerable erosion caused by the loose fragments. All fragments should be removed. The joint capsule, the muscles and the skin are then closed. The dog is caged for about 10 days and kept on restricted exercise for a period of 4 to 6 weeks. If the only finding at early surgery is fragmentation of the coronoid process and the fragments can be completely removed, prognosis is good. If surgery is done late (after the appearance of large osteophytes), prognosis is guarded. The joint will usually become pain-free, but range of motion will remain limited. In cases of osteochondritis dissecans of the humeral condyle or in cases with a combination of the two lesions, prognosis is always guarded, even if surgery is done early. However, surgery should always be tried, since an untreated case of either of the two lesions or a case with the two lesions combined usually develops into very severe osteoarthrosis. It should be remembered, however, that in many dogs with fragmentation of the coronoid process, the lesion can remain undetected for years. This usually happens in dogs with bilateral lesions and whose owners who are not very observant. These dogs are often not brought to a veterinarian until there is acute lameness due to trauma to one of the severely osteoarthrotic elbow joints.

## OSTEOCHONDRITIS DISSECANS OF THE KNEE (STIFLE)

This is a much more common lesion in dogs of large size than was previously assumed. Diagnosis is often difficult, since the clinical signs in most cases are diffuse in the young dog. The hip joints are apt to be suspected as the cause of the lameness rather than the knees. There is no obvious lameness, rather a disturbed gait pattern of the hind limbs somewhat similar to the "slinky gait" of hip dysplasia. Radiographs are essential for early diagnosis, but only technically good radiographs made in the right projections will reveal a flattening or defect of the lateral or medial condyle, particularly if the lesion is small. A mediolateral radiograph should be made on a cassette with low-speed, high-resolution screens. Two posteroanterior views with the knee in different angulations should be used.

The most common site of a defect is the lateral femoral condyle, particularly its weight-bearing surface. The lesion can easily be missed if the central beam from the x-ray tube does not hit the lesion tangentially.

Many cases of osteochondritis dissecans of the knee remain undetected and heal, sometimes leaving only a scar in the condyle. In other cases severe osteoarthrosis develops. Roughly 10 to 15 per cent of all cases of osteoarthrosis seen in the larger breeds are caused by osteochondritis dissecans. Once osteoarthrosis has developed there seems to be little one can do to improve the situation other than the conventional medical and physical therapy. If it is a young dog with acute lameness and a large

lesion in either the lateral or medial condyle, an exploratory arthrotomy should be contemplated and a flap or joint mouse removed.

More research has to be done before any definite conclusions can be drawn about why some cases of osteochondritis dissecans of the knee heal without any secondary changes, while others give rise to very severe osteoarthrosis. There seems to be no straightforward indication for surgery at the present time other than in cases of acute lameness, in which a large flap or a joint mouse can be seen.

## OSTEOCHONDRITIS DISSECANS OF THE HOCK JOINT

Osteochondritis dissecans of this joint is not as common as the one in the shoulder, elbow or knee but is common enough to warrant special attention in cases of slight lameness in the hindlimbs of young dogs. The lesion seems to be particularly common in Labrador and golden retrievers, but it does occur in other breeds. The clinical signs usually begin at 4 to 5 months of age and are usually very vague. The lesion is more often unilateral than osteochondritis dissecans in other joints. The most typical findings are a slightly shorter step than normal for the affected limb and pain on extension and flexion of the hock. Rather early the range of flexion is decreased considerably. In some dogs there is obvious joint effusion. As in osteochondritis dissecans of other joints, the radiographic examination provides the diagnosis. The lesion is located to the medial ridge of the talus, and it is best demonstrated as a defect in the ridge on an anteroposterior film. Sometimes a fragment can be seen because it is calcified or ossified. In old cases the fragments can be very large in size. Sometimes a lateral radiograph with the hock joint in as much flexion as possible is useful.

A rather high percentage of loose bodies removed from hock joints contain bone. This is in contrast to osteochondritis dissecans in other joints of the dog, where ossicles are extremely rare.

Surgery is the treatment of choice. The hock joint can be reached by a longitudinal incision caudally to the medial malleolus. With the leg in flexion, the loose bodies can easily be removed. Prognosis is good if surgery is performed early.

## OSTEOCHONDROSIS OF THE CERVICAL INTERVERTEBRAL JOINTS

Compression of the cervical cord caused by instability of the cervical vertebrae (so-called spondylolisthesis) has been described. It is mostly seen in Great Danes and in dogs of breeds of similar size. The reason for instability has remained obscure. The present author has encountered a few cases in growing Great Dane dogs in which the cause of instability was a lesion in the cranial part of the ventral facets of one or two pairs of intervertebral joints. The lesion had all the criteria of osteochondrosis and it was very similar to the lesion seen at the same location in pigs. It was obvious in these cases of osteochondrosis of the intervertebral joints that treatment should aim at stabilizing the cervical spine by plating rather than trying to restore normal function of the diseased joints.

## OTHER MANIFESTATIONS OF OSTEOCHONDROSIS

Retained cartilage of various growth plates is seen. In most cases clinical signs are not caused by these changes, and they usually heal spontaneously. Only advanced lesions in the growth plates of the distal ulna and of the distal femur or proximal tibia seem to give rise to serious deformation. In cases of ulnar involvement, decrease in growth rate of the ulna leads to asymmetry of growth of the forelimb between ulna and radius. The distal part of the radius is bowed around the distal metaphysis and epiphysis of the slower-growing ulna. This leads to lateral deviation of the distal part of the forelimb. When the distal femur and proximal tibia are involved, it usually leads to *genu valgum*. Once there is deformation, surgical correction has to be done, but it is safe to wait until growth is complete. If a dog is seen at an early stage of osteochondrosis with only slight deformation, it should be put on a restricted but well-balanced diet, and exercise should also be restricted.

Slipped femoral capital epiphysis is a common lesion in osteochondrosis in pigs, and there is good reason to suspect that even in the dog slipped epiphysis can be caused by osteochondrosis. This is again an example of a lesion that should be treated surgically once it has developed but that one should be able to prevent by not pushing growth by overfeeding.

Finally, a few words about osteochondrosis and hip dysplasia: Recent findings have indicated that one of the reasons why hip dysplasia gets worse in dogs that are overfed during the most active growth period is the appearance of osteochondritis dissecans at the acetabular rim. Degeneration and fissures occur and lead to the formation of small cartilage flaps. The normal growth of this part of the acetabulum is in this way interfered with, and hip dysplasia gets worse. More research is needed, however, to clarify the role of osteochondrosis in the development of hip dysplasia.

# MULTIPLE CARTILAGINOUS EXOSTOSES IN DOGS

PAUL C. GAMBARDELLA, V.M.D.
*Boston, Massachusetts*

### INTRODUCTION

Multiple cartilaginous exostoses (MCE) is a benign proliferative disease of cartilage and bone. Common synonyms of MCE include hereditary multiple exostoses, diaphyseal aclasis, osteochondromatosis, and deforming chondrodysplasia. It may affect any bone formed by endochondral ossification. The disease is common in man and has been reported in the dog, horse and cat.

## PATHOGENESIS

In man, multiple cartilaginous exostoses is a hereditary disease, characterized by autosomal dominance with full penetrance, and most often referred to as hereditary multiple exostoses. In the dog, a familial tendency is probable, but the exact mode of inheritance is not known. There is apparently no breed predilection.

The pathogenesis of MCE has not been conclusively established, but there is general agreement that it is related to abnormal differentiation of cartilage cells. It has been postulated that pluripotential cells are forced from the center of the epiphyseal plate during normal growth and expansion of the plate. Instead of differentiating into osteoblasts as they meet the osteogenic groove (the transition zone between the epiphyseal plate and the osteogenic layer of the periosteum), the cells remain chondrogenic in nature and give rise to a cartilaginous layer that produces new bone by endochrondral ossification. Although cartilaginous exostoses originate near active growth plates, they may become associated with the diaphysis as the bone grows. The degree to which the latter occurs apparently depends on the extent and duration of the lesion. Ordinarily the lesions stop growing when the normal growth plates close, and they may range in size from a few millimeters to several centimeters in diameter when growth ceases. In man, individual lesions that have been dormant for years may undergo a spurt of growth. This phenomenon is rare in man and has not been reported in the dog.

## CLINICAL FINDINGS

Clinical signs of MCE usually become manifest during the period of active bone growth. If the lesions do not cause clinically evident abnormalities, the disease may remain undetected. The disease has never been detected in the newborn.

Exostoses may appear on any bone that develops from endochondral ossification. In man, the lesions are often bilaterally symmetrical and may be as few as 1 or as many as 1000 per patient. Forty-seven exostoses were recognized in one canine patient. The axial and appendicular skeletons are affected with equal frequency in dogs; however, the tarsal and carpal bones are rarely affected. The lesions themselves are nonpainful when palpated. Pain or loss of function develops when tendons, nerves, vessels or other soft tissues are compressed and distorted by the exostoses. When the vertebrae are affected, spinal cord compression and resultant neurologic deficits may occur.

Chondrosarcomas have been reported to develop in the lesions of 5 to 20 per cent of affected human beings. This malignant transformation may occur spontaneously in lesions that have been inactive for many years. Malignant neoplasms (chondrosarcoma and osteosarcoma) developed in the lesions of two reported cases of MCE in dogs. Both dogs were over 8 years of age.

## RADIOGRAPHIC FINDINGS

Exostotic bony lesions may protrude from any bone except the skull and are characterized as radiopaque osseus densities of variable size interspersed with large radiolucent areas. The radiolucent areas represent hyaline cartilage. The cortex of an affected bone may or may not be incorporated within the lesion. When the lesions originate from long bones, the metaphyses are generally involved and the lesions are variable in shape. Lesions originating from vertebrae and ribs tend to be more circular in shape. The smooth, sclerotic borders of the lesions suggest a slow growth rate.

## LABORATORY FINDINGS

Evaluation of laboratory data from those cases encountered by the author plus data from other reported cases has revealed no abnormalities. In particular, the concentrations of serum calcium, phosphorus and alkaline phosphatase activity were within normal limits. This is also the finding in species other than the dog with MCE.

## HISTOPATHOLOGIC FINDINGS

The microscopic appearance of MCE is characterized by normal cortical and cancellous bone capped with hyaline cartilage. Because the exostoses grow by endochondral ossification, the microscopic appearance of the cartilage cap resembles a normal physis. Although the appearance of the cartilage varies with the age of the lesion, an outer zone of proliferation, a middle zone of hypertrophy and an inner zone of provi-

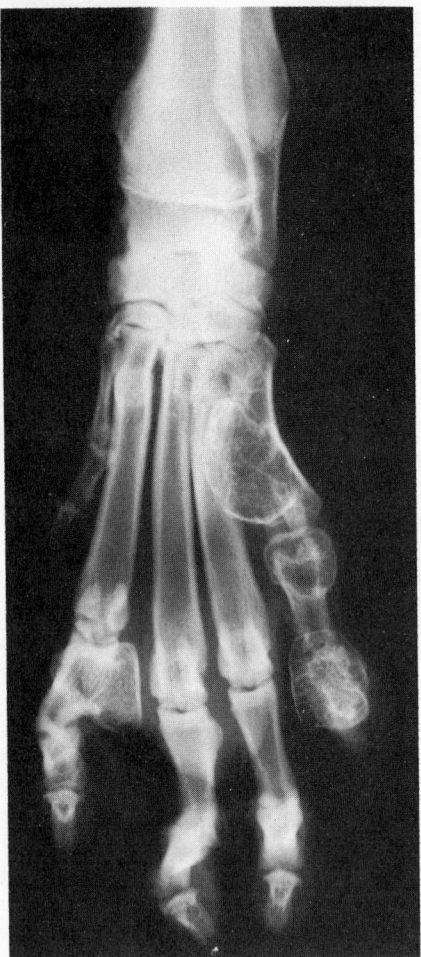

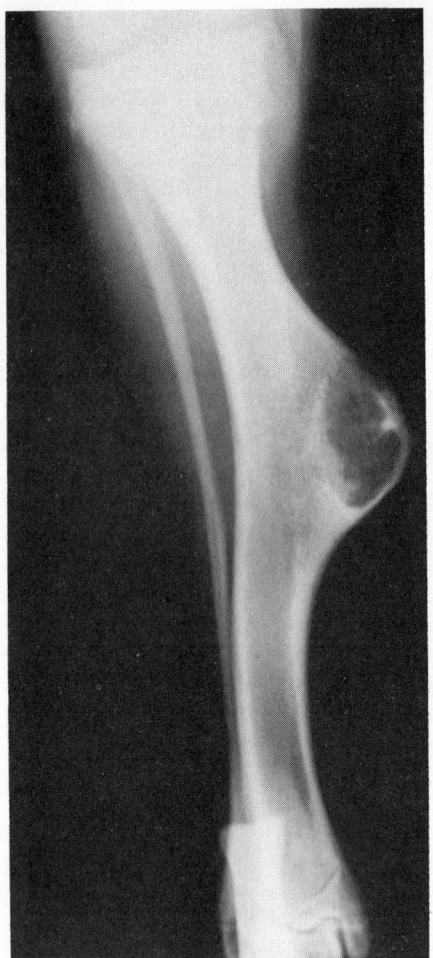

**Figure 1.** Anteroposterior radiograph of the left forepaw of a dog with multiple cartilaginous exostoses. (From Gambardella *et al.*: J. Am. Vet. Med. Assn., *166*:762, 1975.)

**Figure 2.** Anteroposterior radiograph of the right tibia of a dog with multiple cartilaginous exostoses. This exostosis has distorted the normal cortex. (From Gambardella *et al.*: J. Am. Vet. Med. Assn., *166*:762, 1975.)

sional calcification may be observed. During the active growth phase of a young patient, these zones are quite distinct. However, as the lesion matures and the growth phase slows and finally stops, the zones of hypertrophy and provisional calcification may no longer be distinguished. In such lesions, normal subchondral cancellous trabeculae separate the cartliage cap from the remaining exostosis.

## DIAGNOSIS

Abnormal findings obtained from the history and physical examination help to localize the disease process in the body. Inasmuch as exostoses may arise from many bone sites, signs referrable to any body sys-tem may develop. Lameness due to pain or mechanical interference with the musculoskeletal system and neurologic deficits due to spinal cord compression are common sequelae of multiple cartilaginous exostoses in the dog. Hard nonpainful masses in multiple areas of the skeleton may be found incidentally when a new puppy is presented for vaccination.

Radiography may provide strong supportive evidence of MCE, but a definitive diagnosis must be based on microscopic examinations of biopsy specimens.

## PROGNOSIS

The prognosis depends on the location of the lesions, the age of the patient at the time

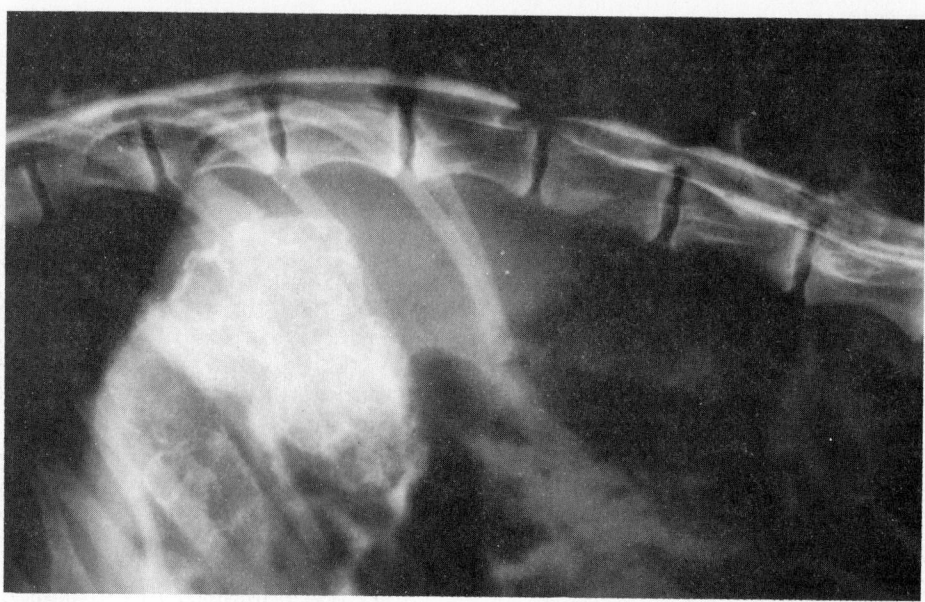

**Figure 3.** Myelogram of a dog with multiple cartilaginous exostoses. Exostoses are causing spinal cord compression at the level of $L_2$—$L_3$. Exostoses are also present on the ribs. (From Gambardella *et al.*: J. Am. Vet. Med. Assn., *166*:762, 1975.)

of diagnosis and the presence or absence of clinical complications. If a patient with multiple cartilaginous exostoses is physically mature and there are no associated clinical abnormalities, a good prognosis should be given. The possibility of malignant transformation in later years should be mentioned to the owners. They should be instructed to have the patient reevaluated in the event of any change in the size, shape or sensitivity of the lesions. If a patient with MCE is growing, a guarded prognosis should be given, because the development of complications is uncertain. If a patient with MCE has developed clinical complications, the prognosis depends on the system(s) involved, the severity of the complications and the surgical accessibility of the lesion(s).

## TREATMENT

Because most exostoses stop growing after closure of the physes, treatment is unnecessary unless the growth of exostoses results in clinical sequelae. Surgical removal of the lesions should be considered if dysfunction of the skeletal, muscular or neurologic systems develops. Regrowth of an exostosis after partial removal does not normally occur if normal bone growth has stopped. Because the disease appears to be familial, breeding should be discouraged.

### SUPPLEMENTAL READING

Aegerter, E. E., and Kirkpatrick, J. A., Jr.: Orthopedic Diseases: Physiology, Pathology, Radiology. 4th ed. Philadelphia, W. B. Saunders Company, 1975.

Gambardella, P. C., Osborne, C. A., and Stevens, J. B.: Multiple cartilaginous exostoses in the dog. J. Am. Vet. Med. Assn., *166*:761–768, 1975.

Langenskiold, A.: The development of multiple cartilaginous exostoses. Acta Ortho. Scand., *38*:259–266, 1967.

Prata, R. G., Stall, S. G., and Zaki, F. A.: Spinal cord compression caused by osteocartilaginous exostoses of the spine in two dogs. J. Am. Vet. Med. Assn., *166*:371–375, 1975.

Solomon, L.: Hereditary multiple exostoses. Am. J. Hum. Genet., *16*:351–363, 1964.

# CANINE POLYARTHRITIS

RALPH E. BARRETT, D.V.M.
*Pullman, Washington*

## INTRODUCTION

*Polyarthritis* is defined as the simultaneous inflammation of several joints. There are numerous causes of polyarthritis. It may present as a specific disease entity (e.g., rheumatoid arthritis) but more commonly it is a manifestation of, or is present concurrently with, another polysystemic disease (e.g., systemic lupus erythematosus, chronic infection, septicemia, neoplasia, etc.). Table 1 presents the conditions that should be considered in a differential diagnosis of polyarthritis. Included in the table are conditions that may be confused with polyarthritis prior to localization of the lesion to

**Table 1.** *Differential Diagnosis of Polyarthritis*

---

A. Noninflammatory
  1. Degenerative joint disease (Osteoarthritis)
    a. Primary
    b. Secondary
B. Inflammatory
  1. Infectious
    a. Bacterial
    b. Fungal
    c. Mycoplasma
    d. Protozoal (e.g., leishmania)
  2. Noninfectious
    a. Immune-mediated
      (1) Erosive
        (a) Rheumatoid arthritis
      (2) Nonerosive
        (a) Systemic lupus erythematosus
        (b) Polyarthritis occurring secondary
          to primary infectious or
          neoplastic processes
    b. Nonimmunologic
      (1) Crystal-induced arthritis (gout,
        pseudogout)
      (2) Hemarthrosis
        (a) Hemophilia
        (b) Multiple myeloma with
          hyperviscosity syndrome
        (c) Many bleeding diatheses
C. Nonarticular conditions that may mimic
  polyarthritis
  1. Hypertrophic osteodystrophy
  2. Pulmonary hypertrophic osteoarthropathy
  3. Eosinophilic panosteitis
  4. Polymyositis
  5. Peripheral neuropathy
  6. Spinal cord dysfunction

---

the joints. In addition to the causes of polyarthritis, there are many conditions that may affect single joints. These include synovial neoplasia, neoplastic extension from surrounding soft tissues and bacterial infection from penetrating trauma or extension from surrounding soft tissues. Also, the causes of polyarthritis may occasionally present as monarthric disease initially or when one joint is disproportionately affected.

Since the etiology, clinical course, prognosis and therapy vary widely in polyarthritis, a thorough diagnostic work-up is emphasized. Clinical pathology, radiography, special serology, joint fluid analysis and synovial biopsy are usually necessary for a definitive diagnosis. Several of the more common causes of polyarthritis, including degenerative joint disease, bacterial polyarthritis, systemic lupus erythematosus (SLE) (and other inflammatory nonerosive polyarthritides) and rheumatoid arthritis (RA), will be discussed.

## DEGENERATIVE JOINT DISEASE

### DEFINITION

Degenerative joint disease (osteoarthrosis, osteoarthritis) is a chronic joint disease characterized by degenerative and proliferative joint changes. Degenerative joint disease is not usually classified as a form of polyarthritis because the lesions are not inflammatory, and it usually does not involve multiple joints. It is included in this discussion because it is the most common cause of canine joint disease and must be considered in the differential diagnosis. It is classified as primary or secondary. Primary degenerative joint disease, which is common in man, is the result of the wear and tear of aging and pathologically is considered a "normal" response to aging. Few cases of possible primary canine degenerative joint disease have been seen. Secondary degenerative joint disease occurs when abnormal stresses are placed on the joints that hasten the rate of cartilage loss.

## ETIOPATHOGENESIS

The etiopathogenesis is not known. Secondary stress may arise from acquired and congenital postural and orthopedic abnormalities, dysplastic joints, trauma, inflammatory joint diseases, damage to supporting structure of the joints and obesity.

## CLINICAL MANIFESTATIONS.

Clinical signs may be absent early in the disease. Later signs may include mild joint pain on palpation, stiffness, limitation of movement and disuse muscle atrophy. If only one joint is involved, differentiation from other polyarthritic conditions is not difficult. However, hip dysplasia, osteochondritis dissecans and ununited anconeal process, which precede degenerative joint disease, can be bilateral, or multiple conditions may be present in some dogs.

## DIAGNOSIS

Age and breed of dog should be considered for genetic predisposition. Joint swellings are due to bone changes rather than soft tissue changes such as in infectious or immune-mediated nonerosive arthritic diseases.

Degenerative joint disease is characterized radiographically by periarticular new bone proliferation, a decreased joint space (articular degeneration), deformation of subchondral bone and increased density of subchondral bone. Vary rarely, bone cyst formation occurs. There is poor correlation between severity of radiographic changes and clinical signs.

Joint fluid is usually normal (see Table 3). There is a small volume of clear, nonclotting fluid with a normal or slightly elevated total WBC count (<3,000 WBC/cu. mm.). Mononuclear cells predominate. Viscosity is normal.

## THERAPY

There is no specific treatment of degenerative joint disease. The goals of therapy are to allow continued joint function and to slow the progression of degeneration.

1. *Restricted exercise.* Abnormal weight-bearing activities and strenuous exercise are harmful, but normal exercise may be helpful.

2. *Analgesics.* Salicylates (buffered aspirin) at a dosage of 30 mg./kg. t.i.d. is often beneficial. Arquel® [Parke, Davis]), at a dosage of 2 mg./kg. p.o. once daily indefinitely has been used successfully to control the pain in chronic, severe degenerative joint disease. Toxic gastroenteritis can be observed as an uncommon side effect. Phenylbutazone (Butazolidin®, Geigy) may be used as a short-term analgesic and anti-inflammatory. Long-term usage is contraindicated because of potential ulcerogenic effects and hematopoietic toxicities. Dosage is 50 to 200 mg. p.o. every 8 hours.

3. *Anti-inflammatory drugs.* Use of systemic and intraarticular corticosteroids is controversial. Their usage may make the animal more comfortable and decrease secondary inflammation and pain; however, this may allow for increased traumatization and may speed up the degenerative process.

4. *Diet.* Reduce body weight.

5. *Surgery.* Several orthopedic techniques may slow down or eliminate the degenerative process by reestabilizing the joint, reestablishing alignment or eliminating pain. Examples include anterior cruciate repair, patellar luxation and stifle deformity repair, femoral head excision, curettage of osteochondritis lesions, ununited anconeal process removal or repair and arthrodesis.

Prognosis for total remission in degenerative joint disease is poor. These animals usually experience a slow, progressive clinical deterioration. However, properly treated cases can be maintained satisfactorily for years.

## BACTERIAL POLYARTHRITIS

Although viral, *mycoplasma*, protozoal and mycotic infections are possible, the most common type of infectious polyarthritis in the dog is bacterial. Monarthric bacterial arthritis due to localized joint damage or extension from surrounding soft tissue infection is more common than polyarthritis associated with septicemia. The polyarthritis of subacute bacterial endocarditis may be caused by hematogenously spread bacteria or by the deposition of antigen-antibody complexes in the synovial membrane (see inflammatory nonerosive joint diseases). Septic polyarthritis will be discussed here.

When true septicemia is present, involvement of other organ systems may also occur. Pneumonia, endocarditis and pyelonephritis are often present concurrently. Bacterial polyarthritis associated with sepsis is an uncommon disease and accounts for only a small percentage of polyarthritis cases.

## ETIOLOGY

The most common organisms involved are *Streptococcus* spp. and *Staphylococcus* spp., but *E. coli, Pseudomonas* spp. and other enterics are less commonly involved.

## CLINICAL MANIFESTATIONS

Signs of septic arthritis include lethargy, weakness, anorexia, lameness or reluctance to walk. Pyrexia is present in acute cases, while recurrent fever may be seen in chronic cases. The joints affected by the polyarthritis are inflamed. Pain, swelling, heat and erythema are often present. A previous systemic disease or infection may be of historical significance. A local infection of the skin, bone, teeth, pharynx, prostate, anal glands, uterus or umbilicus of neonates may be concurrent. Bacterial endocarditis with a systolic or rarely a diastolic (aortic valve) murmur may be present. Mitral valve involvement is most common. Cardiac arrhythmias are uncommon but may occur if myocarditis has occurred. Evidence of pyelonephritis with lumbar pain, hematuria, pyuria, proteinuria and bacteriuria may also be present. Petechial hemorrhages of mucous membranes due to endotoxemia and vasculitis are rarely seen.

## DIAGNOSIS

Diagnosis can be made only after identification of the microorganism. Routine aerobic and anaerobic cultures of joint fluid are employed as well as direct Gram stains of synovial fluid. In addition, two or three serial blood cultures prior to antibiotic therapy are recommended. Bacteriologic studies of other organ systems (e.g., urinary) may be helpful in identifying the source and type of organism.

The joint fluid has a decreased viscosity and will clot on exposure to air. Total synovial fluid WBC counts are typically over 110,000 WBC/cu. mm. (see Table 3). More than 90 per cent are neutrophils, and floccules of mucopurulent material may be present. Phagocytized or free bacteria may be observed in the fluid. An elevated RBC count due to severe inflammation is common.

Radiographic signs are uncommon during the first week. Later radiographic abnormalities include destruction of periarticular bone, articular erosion and massive bone proliferation around the joint margins.

## THERAPY

Identification of the organism and use of the appropriate systemic antibiotics are imperative. Symptomatic therapy should be instituted after cultures have been acquired if the dog is critically ill. Parenteral sodium penicillin in dosages of 40,000 to 100,000 units/kg. IV every 6 hours or procaine penicillin IM b.i.d., with streptomycin at 10 to 20 mg./kg. IM b.i.d., is usually effective. In resistant cases, penicillin and kanamycin at 6 mg./kg. IM b.i.d. is more effective. *Pseudomonas* infections may only be sensitive to gentamicin at 2 mg./kg. IM b.i.d. When possible, the antibiotics should be changed to the oral route and administration continued for 4 to 6 weeks. Response to therapy should be monitored with blood and joint fluid cultures as indicated. Rarely, one or two severely affected joints may require needle aspiration or surgical drainage for decompression and to facilitate response to systemic therapy. Intraarticular therapy is rarely required, owing to the excellent vascular supply of the joint. With vigorous, appropriate antibiotic therapy, the prognosis for complete elimination of the organism is good.

# SYSTEMIC LUPUS ERYTHEMATOSUS (SLE) POLYARTHRITIS

## DEFINITION

SLE is a chronic multisystem inflammatory disease. It is characterized by autoimmune phenomena. Many organ systems can be affected and clinical signs including autoimmune hemolytic anemia, thrombocytopenia, glomerulonephritis, skin lesions, polymyositis, meningitis, myelopathy and polyarthritis have been observed in the dog. The most common clinical sign in the dog is polyarthritis.

## ETIOPATHOGENESIS

Many factors have been shown to be associated with exacerbations of SLE. Exposure to sunlight, certain drugs, infectious agents, endocrine factors and genetic factors have all been incriminated. Virus participation is highly suspected. Cell-free filtrates have been prepared from dog spleens. When injected into normal dogs and mice, antinuclear antibodies are formed. Also, positive LE clot tests and autoimmune hemolytic anemia have been seen in cats infected with feline leukemia virus. SLE in the NZB strain of mice is possibly related to an underlying leukemia virus infection. Present information suggests that an abnormal immune response in genetically predisposed SLE patients may result in the development of cell-mediated immunity and autoantibodies to cellular contents released during chronic viral infection or to new cell antigens which result from the viral infection. Although autoantibodies may affect numerous tissues they have not been shown to be cytotoxic, but they will cause formation of antigen-antibody complexes. Many of the clinical manifestations of SLE are due to deposition of these immune complexes in the tissues. Activation of complement and noncomplement systems has been incriminated as producing the lesions seen, particularly those occurring in the glomerulus of the kidney.

## CLINICAL MANIFESTATIONS

The polyarthritis form of the disease often presents with a history of a shifting leg lameness and chronic relapsing pyrexia, which is not responsive to antibiotics. The lameness often undergoes periods of exacerbation and remission. Enlargements of the joints are seen in about half the cases. In acute cases, local redness, swelling and heat or only arthralgia may be seen. Joint enlargements in the chronic cases are usually due to fibrosis of the joint capsule. Lymphadenopathy may be seen during periods of exacerbation. Cachexia and generalized muscle atrophy are proportional to the severity and chronicity of the disease.

## DIAGNOSIS

Definitive diagnosis of the nonerosive polyarthritis of canine SLE can only be reached by positive serologic tests and elimination of other causes of polyarthritis. Radiographs are usually negative for joint abnormalities other than periarticular soft tissue swelling. The hematologic examination may show a leukocytosis, neutrophilia and moderate anemia. A mild increase in serum globulins may be seen.

The joint fluid in SLE often has a reduced viscosity and will form a clot on exposure to air. The fluid is turbid and the color is occasionally yellow owing to presence of hemosiderin. The total WBC count is over 3,000 WBC/cu. mm., and may be as high as 400,000/cu. mm. The percentage of neutrophils is increased to 20 to 85 per cent of the cells (normally 10 per cent) (see Table 3). Bacterial, *Mycoplasma, Chlamydia* and virus cultures are negative. Rarely, LE cells may be seen in direct smears of joint fluid; however, LE cells may be seen nonspecifically in inflamed joints regardless of the cause and are therefore not specific for SLE.

Serologic diagnosis is based on the finding of a positive LE cell test and a positive fluorescent antinuclear antibody (FANA) test. However, at present, available commercial tests may often be inaccurate. The LE clot test is subject to human error, and is a more indirect test than the FANA test. The LE cell can rarely be seen in chronic infectious diseases of the dog, but is still the most specific for SLE. False positives can occur with the FANA test. Other evidence of autoimmune disease, including autoimmune hemolytic anemia with a positive Coombs' test, thrombocytopenia, immune complex glomerulonephritis, polymyositis, meningitis and myelopathy, would add further support to a diagnosis of SLE. Rheumatoid factor test is usually negative but may be positive in SLE.

Histologically the synovial membrane may be swollen and a primarily neutrophilic infiltrate is present. The largest numbers of these cells are found within and adjacent to the synovial cell layer. There are usually a few small aggregates of plasma cells near small blood vessels beneath the synovium. Joint destruction, deformity and narrowing are rare. If these are present, a diagnosis of an overlap syndrome (rheumatoid arthritis–lupus) should be suspected.

## THERAPY

The goals of therapy are symptomatically to control the arthralgia and to slow or stop progression of the arthritis. The immune-mediated polyarthritis of SLE is responsive to corticosteroids in over half the cases. Prednisolone is recommended at a dosage of 2 to 4 mg./kg. p.o. divided b.i.d. for 2 to 4 weeks; it is then reduced to 1 mg./kg. divided b.i.d. for 2 weeks, reduced again to 0.5 mg./kg. divided b.i.d. for 2 weeks and then stopped. If exacerbation of clinical signs occurs, maintenance for life at the lowest effective dosage is indicated. Often periods of months may lapse before relapse occurs. Alternate-day prednisolone therapy with the total dosage given every other morning is occasionally satisfactory. Alternate-day prednisolone therapy may lapse before relapse occurs. This will reduce the side effects of long-term corticosteroid therapy, allow the hypothalamic-pituitary-adrenal axis to recover and prevent prolonged immunosuppression.

In cases resistant to corticosteroid therapy Pedersen *et al.* (1976*b*) have produced remissions using more potent immunosuppressive drugs. Cyclophosphamide (Cytoxan®, Mead Johnson) is given at a dose of 1.5 to 2.5 mg./kg. p.o. daily for 4 consecutive days of each week. Dogs 10 kg. and less receive 2.5 mg./kg. daily, dogs 10 to 20 kg. receive 2.0 mg./kg. daily, and dogs over 20 kg. receive 1.5 mg./kg. daily for 4 consecutive days of each week. Azathioprine (Imuran®, Burroughs Wellcome) is given at a dose of 2 mg./kg. p.o. daily.

After two weeks on combination drug therapy the prednisolone dose is reduced to half the initial dose, and after the arthritis is in complete remission, half the initial dose is given every other morning if possible. Complete blood counts are done weekly for the first month, every two weeks for the second month and monthly thereafter on all dogs receiving cyclophosphamide and azathioprine. If the white blood cell counts remain above 7,000/cu. mm., the doses of these two drugs are not changed. If the white blood cell count falls to between 5,000 and 7,000/cu. mm., the doses of these two drugs are reduced by one-fourth. If the white blood cell count falls below 5,000/cu. mm., cyclophosphamide and azathioprine are discontinued until the count increases, and then they are reinstituted at half the initial doses. Remission usually occurs within 2 to 12 weeks. Only a small percentage of dogs fail to respond completely. Dogs with residual joint damage may show pronounced improvement but may retain some minimal lameness.

After the arthritis is in remission for at least 2 months, the dose of azathioprine is reduced to 2 mg./kg. every other morning. When the disease is in complete remission for at least 4 months, an attempt is made to withdraw all cytotoxic drugs. If this is successful, corticosteroids are eventually discontinued. If the joint disease recurs, the disease is maintained in remission with the lowest possible dose of these drugs.

Side effects from chronic use of these drugs are not a problem in most cases. Delayed hair growth, or hair loss, may occur as an effect of the cytotoxic drugs. Sterile hemorrhagic cystitis can be a side effect of prolonged cyclophosphamide usage. Bone marrow depression due to cytotoxic drugs is occasionally seen, but the dosages can usually be readjusted before it becomes a problem. Liver disease resulting from chronic use of azathioprine is not a problem at this dosage, although dogs with preexisting liver problems should not be given this drug.

## OTHER CAUSES OF NONEROSIVE POLYARTHRITIS

A polyarthritis clinically and pathologically similar to canine nonerosive SLE polyarthritis has been observed in dogs with chronic bacterial infections, chronic fungal infections, bacterial endocarditis, dirofilariasis and neoplastic diseases. In some of these cases the joint disease may be the main manifestation of the underlying infectious disease process. As in SLE, the pathogenesis of the joint disease in these animals probably involves the deposition of immune complexes in the synovial membrane. The joint disease usually subsides with correction of the primary infectious process. However, corticosteroids may be needed to hasten resolution of the lameness if it is severe. Concurrent use of cyclophosphamide, azathioprine and prednisolone as described above may be necessary.

# RHEUMATOID ARTHRITIS

## DEFINITION

Rheumatoid arthritis (RA) is a severe, erosive, often progressive polyarthritis associated with immunologic mechanisms. Numerous cases of RA have been reported in the dog but not in the cat. RA is not a common disease, but reported incidence is increasing as diagnostic techniques improve and awareness of the disease increases. RA is a specific disease entity in the dog, and the term RA should not be used unless diagnosis has been confirmed.

## ETIOPATHOGENESIS

Exact etiology and pathogenesis of RA are unknown. Most present theories on etiology propose that an unknown infectious organism initiates RA, and this agent directly or indirectly results in immune-complex disease, hypersensitivity and autoimmunity. Numerous agents including bacteria, viruses, phages, *Mycoplasma*, protozoa and physical agents have been suspected as initiators. Pathogenesis of the joint destruction in RA has been postulated to involve several immune-mediated steps: (1) An altered immunoglobulin G (IgG), possibly as a result of reaction with antigen, is produced; (2) rheumatoid factor (RF), produced by B lymphocytes and plasma cells in the synovial membrane, reacts with the altered IgG; (3) RF-IgG complexes are formed, near the joint capsule, and fix complement (C); (4) chemotactic factors are released and attract neutrophils to the joint; (5) RF-IgG-C complexes are phagocytized in the joint space by neutrophils; (6) lysosomal enzymes are released by the neutrophils and cause the tissue damage. Evidence for presence of T cell–mediated destruction has also been suggested.

## CLINICAL MANIFESTATIONS

History of a chronic, relapsing and progressively worsening lameness involving several limbs or generalized stiffness is common. Initially there is a shifting lameness, with soft tissue swelling around involved joints. There is pain on palpation and movement of the joints. Depression, fatigue, anorexia and weight loss are often present. Advanced cases may have crepitus or may present with nonfunctioning joints due to destruction and ankylosis. Pyrexia, lymphadenopathy and splenomegaly occur uncommonly. Joint involvement is most severe in the carpal and tarsal joints, but in some cases elbows and stifles may show severe changes. Other joints usually do not become as severely involved. Evidence of concurrent SLE occasionally is present. Subcutaneous nodules, fibrinous pericarditis and pleuritis, interstitial pneumonia, ocular lesions and vasculitis reported in man have not been seen in the dog.

## DIAGNOSIS

Nine criteria should be evaluated in the diagnosis of RA in the dog (Table 2). Six of the nine criteria should be satisfied for a diagnosis of classic canine RA. Diagnostic emphasis should be placed on the radiographic appearance of RA and the presence of characteristic histologic changes in the synovium.

Several nonspecific clinical pathologic abnormalities may be present. A normochromic, normocytic anemia not responsive to hematinics is occasionally seen. Mild leukocytosis and neutrophilia may be present. Serum protein determinations and electrophoresis are variable but often reveal hypoalbuminemia, hyperglobulinemia and elevations of the alpha$^2$- and beta-globulin fractions. Proteinuria associated with renal amyloidosis may be present.

Rheumatoid factors (RF) are autoantibodies to altered IgG (see article on "Laboratory Diagnosis of Immunologic Disorders"). RF is mainly immunoglobulin M (IgM), and immunoglobulin A (IgA) may be involved as RF in certain cases. IgM is

**Table 2.** *Diagnostic Guidelines in Canine Rheumatoid Arthritis*

1. Morning stiffness.
2. Pain or tenderness in one or more joints.
3. Soft tissue swelling or effusion in one or more joints.
4. Swelling of any other joint.
5. Symmetrical onset of joint symptoms and swelling.
6. Roentgenographic evidence of RA.
7. Positive RF.
8. Poor mucin precipitate of synovial fluid.
9. Characteristic histologic changes in the synovium.

*Table 3.*   *Synovial Fluid Changes in Various Types of Canine Arthritis*

| CONDITION | NUCLEATED CELLS/CU. MM. | DIFFERENTIAL (% TOTAL) | | MUCIN CLOT | MICRO-ORGANISMS | IgG AND C'3 INCLUSIONS |
|---|---|---|---|---|---|---|
| | | Mononuclear Cells | Neutrophils | | | |
| Normal* | 0–2,900 (430)† | 88–100 (99) | 0–12 (1) | Good to fair | Absent | Absent |
| Degenerative* joint disease | 0–3,470 (990) | 88–100 (96) | 0–12 (4) | Good to poor | Absent | Absent |
| Rheumatoid-like arthritis (6 cases) | 3,000–38,000 (13,600) | 20–80 (45) | 20–80 (55) | Fair to poor | Absent | Present |
| Nonerosive, non-infectious arthritis (51 cases) | 4,400–371,000 (66,300) | 5–85 (27) | 15–95 (73) | Good to poor | Absent | Absent to rare |
| Septic arthritis (9 cases) | 110,000–267,000 (173,560) | 1–10 (4) | 90–99 (96) | Poor | Present** in 90% cases | Not tested |

From Pedersen, N. C.: Proc. A.A.H.A. Convention, May, 1976.
*Cell count and differential values reconstructed from Sawyer, D. C.
**Culture and stained smears.
†Numbers in parens are means.

the predominant RF detected by standard agglutination tests. RF titer is determined by the sensitized sheep red blood cell (Rose-Waaler) method or by the latex particle agglutination (LPA) method. Human rheumatoid latex reagent is unsatisfactory in the dog. A specific latex reagent must be prepared for dogs. Positive RF titers in dogs by the Rose-Waaler method range from 1:16 to 1:128. RF may be positive in dogs with other autoimmune (e.g., SLE) or chronic infectious diseases. Also, serologic abnormalities such as LE cell factor and antibodies can be seen in dogs with RA but less frequently than in SLE. Because there is some degree of overlap of these factors, it seems unwise to separate SLE and RA based on serologic tests alone. Separation should be based on the type of joint disease associated with each. RA is usually erosive in nature; SLE and other hypersensitivity arthritides are usually nonerosive.

Characteristic radiographic changes develop within weeks to months as the condition progresses. Signs include soft tissue swelling or joint capsule distention, subchondral bone rarefaction, marginal erosions at the site of attachment of the joint capsule, joint space widening or narrowing, periarticular soft tissue or joint capsule calcification, irregular articular surfaces and disuse muscle atrophy and osteoporosis. Severe joint deformity and ankylosis may be present in advanced cases. These changes are symmetrical, involving several joints.

An exudative joint fluid similar to SLE is characteristeric (Table 3). Total WBC count is usually not as high.

Histologic evaluation of synovial membrane biopsies are characterized by a diffuse, proliferative synovitis, with infiltration of lymphocytes and plasma cells. Increased collagenous connective tissue and hyperplastic synoviocytes are present. Villous hypertorophy occurs and may protrude into the articular space and attach to a fibrous pannus that has replaced an eroded articular cartilage.

## THERAPY

The goals of therapy are to control pain and slow the progressive, erosive joint damage. Quinacrine, gold salts and D-penicillamine have been shown to be beneficial in human RA but have not been evaluated in the dog. Buffered aspirin will occasionally control symptoms and pain associated with RA, but the disease usually progresses in spite of therapy. A dosage of 30 mg./kg. t.i.d. is recommended, but higher dosages may be necessary. Corticosteroids have a temporary beneficial effect on canine RA, but progressively higher dosages become necessary with time, and they do not change the progressive course of the joint destruction. Short-term benefits may be seen with prednisolone at a dosage of 2 mg./kg./day divided b.i.d. Immunosuppressive drug therapy with cyclophosphamide, azathioprine and prednisolone has arrested the progression of the disease in several cases in which it has been tried (Pedersen *et al.*, 1976*a*) (regimen described under SLE discussion). It is important that therapy be instituted before advanced joint destruction occurs. In cases of advanced joint destruction with only a few joints involved, arthrodesis may allow the return of some function.

## SUPPLEMENTAL READING

Biery, D. N., and Newton, C. D.: Radiographic appearance of rheumatoid arthritis in the dog. J. Am. Anim. Hosp. Assn., *11*:607–612, 1975.

Hardy, R. M., and Wallace, L. J.: Arthrocentesis and synovial membrane biopsy. Vet. Clin. N. Am., *4*:499–462, 1974.

Miller, J. B., Perman, U., Osborne, C. A., Hammer, R. F., and Gambardella, P. C.: Synovial fluid analysis in canine arthritis. J. Am. Anim. Hosp. Assn., *10*:293–398, 1974.

Newton, C. D., Lipowitz, A. J., Halliwell, R. E., Allen, H. L., Biery, D. N., and Schumacher, H. R.: Rheumatoid arthritis in dogs. J. Am. Vet. Med. Assn., *168*:113–121, 1976.

Pedersen, N. C., Pool, R. C., Castles, J. J., and Weisner, K.: Non-infectious canine arthritis. II. Rheumatoid-like arthritis. J. Am. Vet. Med. Assn., *169*:295–303, 1976*a*.

Pedersen, N. C., Weisner, K., Castles, J. J., Ling, G. V., and Weiser, G.: Non-infectious canine arthritis. I. The inflammatory, non-erosive arthritides. J. Am. Vet. Med. Assn., *169*:304–310, 1976*b*.

Sawyer, D. C.: Synovial fluid analysis of canine joints. J.A.V.M.A., *143*:609, 1963.

Schultz, R. D.: Immunologic disorders in the dog and cat. Vet. Clin. N. Am., *4*:153–173, 1974.

# CANINE HEPATIC ENCEPHALOPATHY

RALPH E. BARRETT, D.V.M.
*Pullman, Washington*

## INTRODUCTION

Hepatic encephalopathy (HE) is defined as a disturbance in cerebral and brain-stem function caused by severe liver disease that has sensitized the brain to the deleterious effect of various toxins and metabolic derangements. This condition is being diagnosed with an increased frequency in dogs as veterinarians become more aware of the variable clinical syndromes of HE.

Neurologic signs of HE have been seen in dogs with three types of liver diseases: (1) congenital portal vein anomalies, (2) urea cycle enzyme deficiencies and (3) advanced liver disease (Table 1). Signs of HE are not seen in the common canine liver conditions of fatty infiltration, chronic or acute obstructive jaundice and chronic passive congestion. Also, HE is extremely uncommon in infectious canine hepatitis.

**Table 1.** *Differential Diagnosis of Hepatic Encephalopathy in the Dog*

| |
|---|
| I. Hepatic Diseases |
|   A. Congenital portal vein anomalies |
|   B. Acquired portal vein anomalies |
|   C. Urea cycle enzyme deficiencies |
|   D. Advanced liver failure |
|     1. Cirrhosis |
|     2. Neoplastic infiltration |
|     3. Toxicosis |
| II. Nonhepatic Diseases |
|   A. Metabolic |
|     1. Hypoglycemia |
|     2. Uremia |
|     3. Barbiturate toxicity |
|     4. Lead toxicity |
|   B. Central nervous system diseases |
|     1. Neoplasia |
|     2. Trauma |
|     3. Abscess |
|     4. Encephalitis |
|     5. Thrombosis |
|     6. Idiopathic epilepsy |
|     7. Hydrocephalus |

## PATHOGENESIS

The exact pathogenesis of hepatic encephalopathy is unknown, but present theories revolve around the interrelated factors of increased cerebral sensitivity, metabolic derangements and cerebral toxins. It is no longer valid to consider the simplistic view that hyperammonemia is the sole agent producing HE.

*Increased cerebral sensitivity* relates to the fact that the brains of patients with severe liver disease exhibit increased sensitivity to factors that depress the level of consciousness (e.g., sedatives, infection, electrolyte disturbances, hypoxia, etc.). Patients without liver disease are more tolerant of these factors. This increased sensitivity suggests that the liver produces substances that are important to brain function.

Several *metabolic derangements* may precipitate hepatic encephalopathy in susceptible patients (Table 2). These factors summate with the effects of cerebral toxins and may precipitate an episode of HE.

*Cerebral toxins* have received the most attention in the search for the pathogenesis of HE. Many substances have been incriminated in the induction of HE. Ammonia, methionine (and methanethiol derived from methionine), phenylalanine, tryptophan (and indoles and skatoles from tryptophan), glutamine, alpha-ketoglutaramate, short-chain fatty acids, serotonin and false neurotransmitters (octopamine and beta-phenylethanolamines) have all been suspected.

Although the pathogenesis of HE is a complex phenomenon, probably caused by a multiplicity of factors, most believe that ammonia still represents the key cerebral toxin. This is based on the findings that (1) increased blood and cerebrospinal fluid (CSF) ammonia concentrations are usually found in patients with HE, (2) elevated

**Table 2.** *Conditions that May Precipitate Hepatic Encephalopathy*

| CONDITION | MECHANISM(S) |
|---|---|
| Increased Protein Intake | Increased substrate for production of nitrogenous substances. |
| Gastrointestinal Hemorrhage | Increases protein substrate<br>Hypovolemia compromises hepatic, cerebral and renal function.<br>Hepatic hypoxia. |
| Alkalosis | Increases intracellular transport of ammonia and amines. Shifts $NH_3 + H^+ \leftrightarrows NH_4^+$ to the left. $NH_3$ is more diffusible across cell membranes and is "trapped" intracellularly. |
| Hypokalemia | Reduced conversion of $NH_3$ to glutamine by liver mitrochondria.<br>Causes extracellular fluid alkalosis.<br>Increased production of $NH_3$ by renal tubular cells. |
| Uremia | Increased enterohepatic circulation of urea nitrogen with increased ammonia production.<br>Direct cerebral effect of uremia. |
| Hypovolemia | Compromises hepatic, cerebral and renal function.<br>Compromise of renal function increases enterohepatic urea nitrogen cycle and increases ammonia production. |
| Infections | Increased tissue catabolism leads to increased endogenous nitrogen load and increased ammonia production.<br>Dehydration and decreased renal function.<br>Hypoxia and hyperthermia potentiate ammonia toxicity. |
| Constipation | Increased production and absorption of nitrogenous substances. |
| Methionine | Metabolic products (e.g., methanethiol) are neurotoxic. |
| Increased Fatty Acids in Diet | Synergistic toxicity with methanethiol and ammonia. |
| Stored Blood for Transfusion | Contributes ammonia. |
| Commercial Protein Hydrolysates | Amino acid imbalances contribute to HE. |
| Diuretics | Induce hypokalemic alkalosis.<br>Increased renal vein ammonia output.<br>Overvigorous→hypovolemia and prerenal azotemia. |
| Tranquilizers and Anesthetics* | Direct depressive effect on brain.<br>Hypoxia.<br>Prolonged metabolism in liver disease. |

*Chlordiazepoxide (Librium®, Roche), barbiturates, chlorpromazine, diazepam (Valium®, Roche), morphine, meperidine.

glutamine (the end product of cerebral ammonia detoxication) is usually found in the CSF of patients with HE, (3) patients with congenital urea cycle enzyme deficiencies often have hyperammonemia and (4) ammonia will precipitate HE in experimental animals. Evidence against the sole role of hyperammonemia as a cause of HE includes the observations that (1) some patients with HE have normal or only slightly elevated blood ammonia and (2) massive dosages of ammonia are necessary to produce HE in experimental animals.

The basic cerebral mechanisms for ammonia toxicity are not known. Suggested causes include (1) interference with brain energy metabolism; (2) an accumulation of an inhibitory neurotransmitter, gamma-aminobutyric acid; (3) a decrease in the neurotransmitter acetylcholine; and (4) a direct inhibitory effect on the neuronal membrane. Interference with brain energy metabolism has the most support at present.

## PATHOLOGY

Since both acute HE and HE seen in chronic liver injury are potentially clinically reversible, it is assumed that HE is not associated with permanent morphologic abnormalities of the brain. Thus, HE is considered to be a metabolic abnormality in which there is some biochemical alteration of cerebral function.

In acute HE, no morphologic abnormalities in the brain are seen, although cerebral edema may rarely be present. In dogs with chronic congenital portosystemic shunting, a spongy degeneration, called polymicrocavitation, and hyperplasia and nuclear enlargement of astrocytes, which are referred to as Alzheimer type II astrocytes, may be seen. Alzheimer type II astrocytosis may reflect increased metabolic activity in the detoxification of ammonia. The exact nature and pathogenesis of the polymicrocavitation is not understood. Most assume these cavities to be dilated interstitial spaces or myelin sheaths without axonal degeneration and with no cellular response.

## DIAGNOSIS

The clinical features of hepatic encephalopathy in the dog are extremely variable. Thus the clinician must have a high index of suspicion. In addition to the primary liver diseases that cause HE, several metabolic and central nervous system diseases must be considered and eliminated from the differential diagnosis (Table 1). Numerous neurologic signs have been observed in dogs with HE (Table 3). Clinical signs often follow a large meal, especially if it is high in protein.

The syndrome most often associated with canine HE is *congenital portal vein anomaly*. In this syndrome variable amounts of portal venous blood are shunted away from the liver. Seven types of anomalies have been identified: (1) persistent ductus venosus, (2) portal vein atresia, (3) portal vein to caudal vena cava shunt caudal to the liver, (4) anomalous connection of the portal vein to the azygos vein, (5) shunting of the portal vein and caudal vena cava into the azygos vein, (6) splenic vein to caudal vena cava shunt and (7) mesenteric veins to caudal vena cava shunts.

The history usually consists of a variable combination of neurologic (Table 3), urinary tract and gastrointestinal signs. Clinical signs other than neurologic signs that may be observed include (1) polyuria and polydipsia, (2) stunted growth, (3) ascites, (4) anorexia, (5) weight loss, (6) vomiting, (7) diarrhea, (8) cystic calculi (urate or ammonium biurate), (9) hypersalivation, (10) bloating after eating, (11) anesthetic or tranquilizer intolerance and (12) enlarged kidneys. It must be emphasized that animals with congenital portal vein anomalies may present with any one or several of the neurologic or non-neurologic signs. Thus, this syndrome should be included in the differential diagnosis of polyuria and polydipsia, ascites, cystic calculi, CNS disease, poor growth and weight loss.

**Table 3.**  *Neurologic Signs Observed in Canine Hepatic Encephalopathy*

Listlessness and depression
Compulsive pacing or circling
Head pressing
Ataxia
Grand mal seizures
Sudden viciousness
Disorientation and staring
Blindness
Craving attention
Tremors
Walking along walls
Climbing walls
Hypermetria
Coma or stupor

Ancillary diagnostic aids include routine and special clinical pathology and radiography. The two consistent biochemical abnormalities in this syndrome are an increased retention of plasma sulfobromophthalein (BSP) and an elevated fasting and postprandial blood ammonia. Since values and techniques for blood ammonia determination vary between laboratories, it is not possible to establish normal values. Results should be compared to controls for each laboratory. The increased BSP retention (>5 per cent at 30 minutes) may be moderate (5 to 10 per cent) but is usually quite high (15 to 20 per cent).

There are variable abnormalities in several other blood biochemistry determinations. There may be hypoproteinemia, hypoalbuminemia, slightly elevated serum glutamic pyruvic transaminase (SGPT), slightly elevated serum alkaline phosphatase (SAP) and a below normal blood urea nitrogen (BUN). In a significant number of these cases, urate or ammonium biurate crystals or calculi are found in the urine. Repeated urinalyses may be necessary before these crystals are detected. The pathophysiology of these abnormalities has been described elsewhere (Barrett *et al.*, 1976; Cornelius *et al.*, 1975; Ewing *et al.*, 1974).

Plain and contrast abdominal radiography are beneficial in diagnosing congenital portal vein anomalies. Plain radiographs often demonstrate a small liver. If ascites is present, fluid drainage and a pneumoperitoneogram may be necessary to evaluate the liver silhouette. Differentiation from other causes of reduced liver size must be made by means of liver biopsy and contrast radiographic techniques.

Selective arteriography of the cranial mesenteric or celiac artery, percutaneous splenoportography and portal or splenic venography have been utilized to diagnose portal vein anomalies. Fluoroscopic monitoring is necessary for positioning the catheter in selective arteriography. Splenoportography has three disadvantages: (1) it is often difficult to isolate the spleen percutaneously, (2) the contrast agents may damage the spleen and (3) the density of the contrast agent as it passes through the portal circulation is less than with other techniques. Portal venography performed following laparotomy and placement of a Silastic® intravenous catheter (Dow Corning) into the portal vein via a jejunal vein offers excellent visualization of the shunts following contrast agent injection. Sodium iothalamate (80 per cent) (Angio-Conray®, Mallinckrodt Pharmaceuticals, St. Louis, Missouri) at a dosage of 1 cc./kg. can be used as the contrast medium. Hand pressure injection followed by immediate exposure of the radiographs is usually adequate for diagnosis. A single study by only one of these techniques may occasionally be inadequate for diagnosis. Multiple contrast studies should be considered if there is a high index of suspicion for this syndrome. It must be emphasized that contrast radiography is the most reliable diagnostic aid in this syndrome. Abnormal shunting is often difficult to detect on exploratory laparotomy or gross necropsy.

Hepatic encephalopathy may rarely be seen in end-stage hepatic disease. Dogs with *chronic cirrhosis, diffuse hepatic neoplastic infiltration* and advanced *hepatic toxicosis* may have hyperammonemia and show signs of ataxia, stupor and coma shortly before death. HE is not the dominant clinical syndrome. Signs of chronic, advanced liver failure such as emaciation, anorexia, vomiting, diarrhea, polyuria and polydipsia, jaundice and ascites are more prevalent. Hematologic examination, clinical biochemistries, radiography and liver biopsies will establish the diagnosis of these conditions.

Two cases of *urea cycle enzyme deficiency* in the dog associated with hyperammonemia have been reported (Strombeck *et al.*, 1975a). One dog showed signs of anorexia, listlessness, depression, vomiting, emaciation and chronic diarrhea. The other dog had signs of stunted growth, occasional vomiting and seizures characterized by shaking, muscle stiffness and disorientation. Routine laboratory tests for liver function including SGPT, SAP and BSP retention were normal. The hyperammonemia was associated with a deficiency of arginosuccinate synthetase, one of the urea cycle enzymes.

Since the diagnosis of HE may be difficult to differentiate from other causes of encephalopathy, other diagnostic tests may be done prior to evaluation of liver function or blood ammonia. The cerebrospinal fluid in HE is clear, normocellular and under normal pressure, except when cerebral edema is present. The electroencephalogram

(EEG) may be of diagnostic value. The EEG shows various degrees of changes from the regular alpha rhythm to a delta-wave pattern. As coma progresses, the EEG loses all high-frequency waves, appearing at 7 to 8 cycles per second. This EEG pattern will help differentiate the causes of metabolic CNS diseases from organic CNS diseases but is not specific for HE. These EEG changes can also be seen in canine hypoglycemia and uremia.

In summary, the diagnosis of HE depends on the presence of hepatic failure, neurologic signs and eliminating other potential causes of encephalopathy. Laboratory tests including a BSP retention, SGPT, SAP, total protein, albumin, globulin, BUN, urinalysis, fasting and two-hour postprandial blood ammonia should be done if HE is suspected. Additional diagnostic aids such as plain and contrast liver radiographs, liver biopsy, urea cycle enzyme analysis and EEG may be necessary. To eliminate other causes of encephalopathy, electrolytes, fasting blood glucose, blood lead, lupus erythematosus cell test and CSF tap should be normal.

## THERAPY

There are two primary goals in the treatment of hepatic encephalopathy: (1) reversal of the presenting HE crisis and (2) long-term prophylactic and supportive management of the precipitating factors of HE (Table 4).

**Treatment of the HE Crisis.** Severe encephalopathy can be precipitated by numerous factors (Table 2). It must be considered to be a life-threatening metabolic emergency that requires immediate correction. Total *withdrawal of dietary protein* is mandatory. This removes the substrate for production of further nitrogenous toxins. *Cessation of drugs* such as diuretics, tranquilizers and methionine that may have precipitated HE is necessary. Barbiturates can be removed by peritoneal dialysis. *Gastrointestinal bleeding* that increases protein substrate and worsens hypovolemia should be corrected. *Blood transfusions* or *parenteral hyperalimentation* that may have initiated the HE crisis should be stopped. *Intravenous fluid therapy* for correction of dehydration, alkalosis and hypokalemia is beneficial in several ways. Correction of hypovolemia enhances renal elimination of

**Table 4.** *Current Established and Experimental Therapeutic Measures for Hepatic Encephalopathy*

I.  General Supportive Care
   *A.  Replace fluid and electrolyte imbalances
   B.  Reverse precipitating causes (see Table 2)
II.  Prevention of Ammonia and Other Nitrogenous Substances from Entering Circulation from Gastrointestinal Tract
   A.  Protein restriction
      *1. Homemade low-protein diet[1]
      *2. Commercial "low-protein" diets (k/d[a], Nephro Diet[b], Diet N[c], Clinicare N[d])
   B.  Sterilization of intestinal tract
      *1. Neomycin (and other antibiotics)
   C.  Gastrointestinal cleansing
      *1. Cathartics
      *2. Enemas
   D.  Altered gastrointestinal environment
      1. *Lactobacillus* administration[2,3]
      2. Lactulose therapy[4]
      3. Colonic bypass surgery[5]
      4. Induction of antibodies to urease[6]
      5. Acetohydroxamic acid (inhibitor of urease) therapy[7]
III.  Anti-CNS Toxin Therapy
   A.  L-dopa (L-dihydroxyphenylalanine)[8,9,10]
   B.  Exchange transfusions[11]
   C.  Plasmapheresis[12]
   D.  Hemodialysis[13]
   E.  Isolated liver perfusion[14]
   F.  Cross-circulation[15]
   G.  Charcoal hemoperfusion[16]

---

*Used successfully in the dog.
[a]Hill Packing Company, Topeka, Kansas.
[b]Atlas Canine Products, Inc., Glendale, L.I., New York.
[c]C. P. Bernard Packing Company, Camden, New Jersey.
[d]Chas. Pfizer & Company, New York, New York.

[1]Bovee, K. C.: What constitutes a low protein diet for dogs with chronic renal failure? J. Am. Animal Hosp. Assn., 8:246–253, 1972.
[2]Read, A. E., McCarthy, C. F., Heaton, K. W., and Laidlow, J.: *Lactobacillus acidophilus* (Enpac) in the treatment of hepatic encephalopathy. Brit. Med. J., 1:1267–1269, 1966.
[3]Van der Zwan, J. C., Gips, C. H., Qué, G. S., and Boonstra, S.: Milk protein in the treatment of chronic portosystemic encephalopathy. Neth. J. Med., 17:42–49, 1974.
[4]Fessel, J. M., and Conn, H. O.: Lactulose in the treatment of acute hepatic encephalopathy. Am. J. Med. Sci., 266:103–110, 1973.
[5]Resnick, R. H., Ishihara, A., Chalmers, T. C., and Schimmel, E. M.: A controlled trial of colon bypass in chronic hepatic encephalopathy. Gastroenterology, 54:1057–1069, 1968.
[6]Thomson, A., and Holmes, A. W.: Immune inhibition of urea breakdown in patients with cirrhosis. Gastroenterology, 52:14–17, 1967.
[7]Summerskill, W. H. J., Thorsell, F., Feinberg, J., and Aldrete, J. S.: Effect of urease inhibition in hyperammonemia: Clinical and experimental studies with acetohydroxemic acid. Gastroenterology, 54:20–26, 1968.

[8]Abramsky, O., and Goldschmidt, Z.: Treatment and prevention of acute hepatic encephalopathy by intravenous levodopa. Surgery, 75:188–193, 1974.

[9]Fischer, J. E.: False neurotransmitters and hepatic coma. Res. Publ. Assn. Nerv. Ment. Dis., 53:53–73, 1974.

[10]Weiss, A., and Pitman, E. R.: Arousal response in hepatic encephalopathy with L-dopa. Am. J. Gastroenterol., 62:497–503, 1974.

[11]Gelfand, M. L.: Successful treatment of hepatic coma by exchange transfusion. Proc. Rudolf Virchow Med. Soc., 28:1–10, 1970.

[12]Lepore, M. J., and Martel, A. J.: Plasmapheresis with plasma exchange in hepatic coma. Ann. Intern. Med., 72:165–174, 1970.

[13]Weg, J. G., Harris, R. E., Miller, N. B., Wiltsie, D. S., McPhaul, J. J., and Finkel, M.: Treatment of hepatic coma by hemodialysis. Texas Med., 60:736–740, 1964.

[14]Ranek, L., Hansen, R. E., Hilden, M., Ramsoe, K., Schmidt, A., and Tygstrup, N.: Pig liver perfusion in the treatment of acute hepatic failure. Scand. J. Gastroent., 6 *(Suppl. 9)*:161–169, 1971.

[15]Burnell, J. M., Dawborn, J. K., Epstein, R. B., Gutman, R. A., Leinbach, G. E., Thomas, E. D., and Volwiler, W.: Acute hepatic coma treated by cross-circulation or exchange transfusion. New Engl. J. Med., 276:935–943, 1967.

[16]Gazzard, B. G., *et al.*: Charcoal hemoperfusion in the treatment of fulminant hepatic failure. Lancet, 1:1301–1307, 1974.

$NH_3$, corrects prerenal azotemia and decreases enterohepatic urea nitrogen cycling. Correction of alkalosis and hypokalemia will reduce the intracellular transfer of ammonia and amines. *Cleansing enemas* with warm water will help reduce the colonic content of bacteria and nitrogenous products. Instillation of neomycin in the colon after the enemas may help reduce bacterial production of $NH_3$. *Intravenous antibiotic* therapy is indicated if concurrent infection is thought to be a precipitating factor. Chloramphenicol at a dosage of 40 mg./kg. IV t.i.d., or high dosages of sodium penicillin (100,000 μ/kg.) IV q.i.d. with kanamycin at 6 mg./kg. IM b.i.d. are often beneficial in septicemias. *Oxygen therapy* may be helpful in correcting renal and hepatic hypoxia. Resultant increased renal and hepatic function will decrease the enterohepatic circulation of urea nitrogen. There is no evidence that *corticosteroid therapy* is beneficial in HE. Corticosteroids have been shown to be of value only in chronic active hepatitis in man and the dog.

**Long-Term Prophylactic Therapy.** Therapy in chronic HE is aimed at preventing entrance of ammonia and other nitrogenous toxins from the gastrointestinal tract into the circulation. Three techniques are utilized to manage HE in patients with no precipitating cause: (1) protein restriction, (2) "sterilization" of the intestinal tract and (3) gastrointestinal cleansing. *Dietary protein restriction* reduces intraluminal nitrogenous substances responsible for ammonia formation and may reduce the total body urea pool. Urea plays an important role in the control of ammonia production. Enterohepatic circulation of urea is present in animals. Circulating urea diffuses into the small intestine and is hydrolyzed to ammonia by urea-splitting bacteria and mucosal urease in the colon. The ammonia is absorbed back into the circulation and reconverted to urea by the liver. Whenever hepatocellular disease or portosystemic shunting is present, the ammonia is not converted to urea and enters the circulation.

Dietary protein restriction can be accomplished by feeding commercially prepared low-protein diets or, more efficiently, by homemade low-protein diets. Dogs with congenital and experimentally produced portacaval shunts have been maintained for years with minimal clinical signs of HE with protein restriction as the only means of therapy.

The recommended diet for chronic HE is a high-carbohydrate, low-fat, low-quantity and high–biologic value protein diet. Certain short-chain fatty acids have been shown experimentally to potentiate the signs of HE. Thus, high-fat diets should be avoided.

*Oral broad-spectrum antibiotics* have also been used to interrupt the enterohepatic urea cycle by reducing the colonic bacterial flora. Controlled therapeutic trials have not been conducted in the dog. However, oral antibiotics have been of little value in dogs with severe portosystemic shunting, and protein restriction alone has been sufficient in some dogs with less severe shunting.

Neomycin is the most commonly used antibiotic. An initial dosage of 20 mg./kg. b.i.d. is recommended. The dosage is gradually reduced until the drug is stopped or until the minimal dosage that prevents the signs of HE is found. Other antibiotics (e.g., tetracycline, kanamycin and sulfonamides) may also be effective. Animals with renal disease should be monitored closely while receiving neomycin, since a small amount of neomycin is absorbed from the gastrointestinal tract, and it is potentially ototoxic and nephrotoxic.

If ascites is present it should be controlled symptomatically. A low-sodium diet (Prescription diet h/d, Hills Division, Riviana Foods, Topeka, Kansas) and diuretics are recommended. Since diuretics (e.g., thiazides and furosemide) may cause potassium depletion, they should be used cautiously or with oral potassium supplementation.

## EXPERIMENTAL AND THEORETICAL THERAPEUTIC MEASURES

Many methods of therapy for human HE are currently under investigation. Some are expensive and require elaborate technical facilities. These procedures have been listed in Table 4 with selected references for further discussion of the rationale and techniques involved (Table 4, III—B through G).

Many procedures utilized in humans have not been particularly successful. Administration of *Lactobacillus acidophilus* will replace the normal colonic flora with these nonurease-producing organisms, but very large amounts of bacterial culture are needed and clinical effects are variable. *Antibodies to urease* can be induced by parenteral administration of jack bean urease. In clinical trials, severe reactions to the jack bean extract occurred, and clinical benefits in patients with HE were not apparent. Administration of *acetohydroxamic acid*, an inhibitor of urease, will lower blood ammonia levels, but little clinical improvement occurred in a small number of human cases. *Colonic bypass* surgery is a radical technique that appears to have little justification in veterinary patients.

Two procedures that have not been used in canine HE appear to be economically feasible and practical for veterinary patients. These are lactulose therapy and L-dopa therapy.

*Lactulose* is a nonabsorbable synthetic disaccharide (beta-1, 4-galactoside fructose). Several studies in man have shown it to be an effective alternative to neomycin therapy in treating and preventing recurrent HE. Two mechanisms are suggested for the mechanisms of action of lactulose: (1) colonic acidification and (2) catharsis. Lactulose is not hydrolyzed in the small intestine, owing to a lack of appropriate intestinal disaccharidases. It is hydrolyzed by colonic bacteria to acetic, lactic and formic acids. This acidifies the colonic contents, favoring the formation of $NH_4^+$, which is less diffusible through the intestinal mucosa than $NH_3$. These acids also produce an osmotic and fermentative diarrhea. An increased acid environment in the colon also favors growth of lactobacilli, which have no urease and, in contrast to the usual colonic bacteria, cannot convert urea to ammonia. The dosage of lactulose is adjusted until 2 to 3 semiformed stools are produced daily, or stool pH decreases to 5.5 or less. The human dosage is approximately 15 to 30 ml. q.i.d. following loading dosages of 50 to 700 ml. Lactulose therapy would be indicated in patients with HE that are nonresponsive to protein restriction and neomycin therapy. This drug is not licensed for use in the United States but has recently become available in Canada (Wm. S. Merrell Company).

Administration of L-dopa to human patients with unresponsive HE has recently received much attention. Its use is based in part on the false neurotransmitter hypothesis. This theory states that in HE the toxic amines or their precursors accumulate in the CNS in adrenergic neurons and displace the putative transmitters norepinephrine and dopamine. However, the effects of L-dopa in HE may be secondary to a variety of actions. In experimental animals with HE secondary to end-to-side portacaval shunt, L-dopa administration may lower blood ammonia levels and protect against HE. Since gastrointestinal upset is a problem with orally administered L-dopa, intravenous therapy appears to be the treatment of choice. The human dosage is given as 0.1 per cent L-dopa in a 0.9 per cent saline solution for a total of 600 to 1200 mg. daily. The use of L-dopa would be limited to the short-term treatment of the acute HE crisis.

## SUPPLEMENTAL READING

Barrett, R. E., de Lahunta, A., Roenigk, W. J., Hoffer, R. E., and Coons, F. H.: Four cases of congenital portacaval shunt in the dog. J. Small Animal Pract., *17*:71–85, 1976.

Breen, K. J., and Schenker, S.: Hepatic coma: Present concepts of pathogenesis and therapy. *In* Pepper, H., and Schaffner, F. (eds.): Progress in Liver Disease. Vol. 4. New York, Grune and Stratton, 1972, pp. 301–331.

Cornelius, L. M., Thrall, D. E., Halliwell, W. H., Frank, G. M., Kern, A. J., and Woods, C. B.: Anomalous portosystemic anastomoses associated with chronic hepatic insufficiency in six young dogs. J. Am. Vet. Med. Assn., *167*:220–228, 1975.

Ewing, G. O., Suter, P. F., and Bailey, C. S.: Hepatic insufficiency associated with congenital anomalies of the portal vein in dogs. J. Am. Animal Hosp. Assn., *10*:463–475, 1974.

Fischer, J. E.: Hepatic coma in cirrhosis, portal hypertension, and following portacaval shunt. Arch. Surg., *108*:325–336, 1974.

Schenker, S., Breen, K. J., and Hoyumpa, A. M.: Hepatic encephalopathy: Current status. Gastroenterology, *66*:121–151, 1974.

Strombeck, D. R., Meyer, D. J., and Freedland, R. A.: Hyperammonemia due to a urea cycle enzyme deficiency in two dogs. J. Am. Vet. Med. Assn., *166*:1109–1111, 1975*a*.

Strombeck, D. R., Weiser, M. G., and Kaneko, J. J.: Hyperammonemia and hepatic encephalopathy in the dog. J. Am. Vet. Med. Assn., *166*:1105–1108, 1975*b*.

# THE "SWIMMING PUPPY" SYNDROME

MICHAEL D. LORENZ, D.V.M.
*Athens, Georgia*

The swimming puppy syndrome is an uncommon developmental abnormality observed primarily in certain chondrodystrophoid breeds of dogs. Occasionally the abnormality is observed in cats and other breeds of dogs; however, the syndrome appears to be most common in those breeds of dogs that have short legs and wide thoracic cavities. The English bulldog, basset hound and Scottish terrier are especially predisposed to this syndrome.

The cause of the syndrome is unknown, although various undocumented theories have been formulated. These include altered neuromuscular synapse function, improper or delayed myelination of peripheral nerves, slow muscular development and ventral horn dysfunction (neuronopathy).

## CLINICAL SIGNS

Regardless of the cause, signs of the syndrome may be seen as early as the second week of life and are usually pronounced by the fifth to sixth week after birth. Early in the syndrome, affected animals appear to be weak and unable to stand or move about. Progressive movements are made by the animal pushing itself along in sternal recumbency. Affected neonates usually nurse well and continue to grow well despite the locomotor dysfunction. Apparently, failure of the trunk to be supported by the appendicular skeleton results in dorsoventral compression of the thorax, abdomen and pelvis. This compression causes malpositioning of the limbs in a lateral manner, so that support of the body is impossible. At this stage of the disease, affected animals make characteristic "swimming movements" with the limbs in an attempt to move about. Joint deformities commonly develop because of the altered limb angulation. Neurologic examination usually reveals no detectable signs of neurologic deficit. Clinical signs of dyspnea may occur in cases with severe thoracic compression. Aspiration pneumonia is a common finding, and constipation, as a sequela to abdominal and pelvic compression, is also observed. Decubital ulcers and urine scalds are associated problems. Necropsy studies have not revealed a pathogenesis for this syndrome.

## MANAGEMENT

Both environmental and genetic factors may play an important role in the development of this syndrome, and *prevention is the best management*. Slick, hard surfaces in the kennel or whelping box provide little or no traction for the rapidly developing puppy or kitten. Difficulty in standing or walking is greatly accentuated. Breeders of chondrodystrophoid dogs should be advised to place soft mats in the whelping area for the puppies to walk on. A satisfactory mattress can be made by covering clean straw with a bed sheet or blanket. The thick straw mattress supports the clumsy puppy or kitten and decreases the mechanical forces on the body that tend to produce dorsoventral compression. This bed is inexpensive and easy to change if it becomes soiled. Balls of wadded newspaper can also be covered with inexpensive cloth if straw is not available. In one case, a breeder of bulldogs utilized a blanket-covered air mattress with great success. Breeders should be encouraged to take the puppies outside twice a day on grass for exercise beginning at 2½ to 3 weeks of age. This encourages the puppies to walk and develop muscular strength. If the weather prohibits outside exercise, puppies should be exercised on a large piece of patio carpet.

Slow development of muscular or ligamentous strength in relationship to the size or weight of the body may also be important in the development of this syndrome. Passive manipulation or massage of the appendicular skeleton may strengthen muscle tone. Hobbles that prevent the legs from splaying laterally can also be used to help the limbs support the body. The hobbles are made with half-inch adhesive tape and are changed weekly or sooner if the tape becomes too tight. The owner is instructed to inspect the feet daily for evidence of swelling or edema. Tape irritation may occur, and the owner should also be advised to watch for this problem.

Affected animals that have severe dorsoventral compression of the trunk respond poorly to hobbles, casts or other means of support. Euthanasia should be considered in these cases. Breeders should be advised that genetic factors *may* influence this syndrome and the breeding of affected ambulatory animals should be discouraged.

---

# FELINE ISCHEMIC ENCEPHA-LOPATHY—A CEREBRAL INFARCTION SYNDROME

ALEXANDER DE LAHUNTA, D.V.M.
*Ithaca, New York*

A neurologic syndrome has been recognized in cats that consists of a peracute onset of signs of a cerebral disturbance, most often unilateral. These signs are caused by an extensive ischemic necrosis of cerebral tissue. Since 1966, 27 cases have been recognized, 17 in 1974 and 1975. Twelve of the 17 were presented only for pathologic examination.

The disease affects adult cats of any age and both sexes. Although it tends to occur more commonly in the summer months, a few cases have occurred in the fall and winter.

The onset is sudden and the signs are variable. Some animals show only severe depression with mild paresis and ataxia. They may pace or circle continuously in one direction. Others may begin by exhibiting seizure activity that may be unilateral and may consist of tonic or clonic activity of the muscles on one side of the head, trunk and limbs. Changes in attitude and behavior are common and may involve severe aggression. Pupils are often dilated, and blindness may be apparent. For the first 1 to 2 days there may be an observable mild hemiparesis. Fever may accompany the onset of this disease.

These acute signs usually resolve in a few days to residual signs of a nonprogressive unilateral cerebral lesion. Destruction of the sensorimotor cortex or its cerebral pathway causes an obvious deficit in the contralateral postural reactions, but there is no interference with gait. The loss of the visual cerebral cortex or optic radiation causes a contralateral failure to respond to a menace gesture, but pupillary responses to light are normal. Unilateral cerebral lesions often cause an animal to pace slowly in a circle toward the side of the abnormal cerebrum. Lesions in the frontal lobe or rostral thalamus may cause head-turning and circling toward the diseased side. This is referred to as the adversive syndrome. Occasionally the eyes also deviate in the same direction. Although their specific cause is not known, these are fairly reliable signs.

Occasionally a cat will continue to have seizures. These may be generalized or partial motor seizures in which the seizure activity is observed in the muscles on the side of the head and body opposite the diseased cerebrum. The latter shows the influence of the cerebral upper motor neuron on the lower motor neuron to the opposite side of the head and body. Involvement of limbic system structures such as the amygdala and hippocampus may be the cause of the behavioral change, which is often paramount and permanent.

Occasionally bilateral blindness has persisted with dilated unresponsive pupils because of ischemic necrosis of the optic chiasm. Careful examination early in the disease may reveal a unilateral facial hypalgesia contralateral to the cerebral lesion. This results from the lesion in the somesthetic cortex or its thalamocortical projection. Nevertheless, a contralateral limb and trunk hypalgesia has not been detected. No other cranial nerve deficits have been observed. Spinal flexor reflexes are normal, as is pain perception from the limbs. There may be mild hypertonia and hyperreflexia of tendon reflexes, which may be more pronounced on the side where the postural reactions are deficient.

## DIFFERENTIAL DIAGNOSIS

If the acute onset of signs, lack of progression and signs referable to a cerebral disturbance are recognized, the differential diagnosis is limited. Only intracranial injury would produce a similar syndrome. If the disease is initiated with seizures, thiamine deficiency should be considered. A history of fish diet or prolonged anorexia and preictal signs of ataxia would suggest this diagnosis. Treatment with 1 to 2 mg. of thiamine should produce an immediate response. Intoxication with lead, organophosphates, chlorinated hydrocarbons or ethylene glycol could all produce signs of an acute encephalopathy. Without a history of exposure, antemortem differentiation may be difficult. However, these all produce a diffuse abnormality. No localizing signs would be apparent. If the onset and course are unknown, the various causes of feline encephalitis must be considered. These include *Toxoplasma gondii, Cryptococcus neoformans* and the agent of feline infectious peritonitis. These inflammations usually produce a more insidious onset and show evidence of a progressive disturbance. Signs are usually more diffuse. Cerebral neoplasms must be considered in the older cat, especially if the onset is not clearly documented and seizures occur.

Hematology and urinalyses have been normal. CSF often has a mildly elevated protein content with normal leukocytes or a mild mononuclear pleocytosis. Scintigraphy in the chronic stage and electroencephalography have sometimes indicated the location of the lesion.

## PATHOLOGY

The lesion consists of a variable degree of ischemic necrosis of the cerebral hemisphere, usually unilateral but occasionally bilateral. Most of the necrosis is entirely ischemic. Occasionally hemorrhages occur in the parenchyma or in the leptomeninges. The necrosis may be multifocal in the cortex, or the infarction may involve up to two thirds of one entire cerebrum. Usually the major infarction lesion has been in the distribution of the middle cerebral artery. In chronic cases, gross atrophy is most marked in the vicinity of this vessel on the lateral side of the infarcted cerebrum. However, the lesion also involves areas supplied by other cerebral vessels. In a few cases ischemic lesions have been found in the brain stem.

Vascular lesions have been found in only a few cases. These have consisted of a large thrombus in the middle cerebral artery, venous thrombosis and vasculitis, consisting of mononuclear cells in old cases and neutrophils in early cases. The patient with the thrombosed middle cerebral artery had an extensive associated vasculitis with neutrophils and eosinophils. In one case, autopsied 3 months after the onset, a dead nematode was found in the thalamus. Its significance remains to be proved.

Neutrophils are abundant in the degenerate tissue of an acute ischemic lesion if the blood supply remains. These are soon replaced by mononuclear cells that phagocytize the dead debris. In most cases there is no evidence of a primary inflammatory lesion associated with blood vessels. No lesions have been found in other organs, including the heart. To date, tissue culture viral isolation studies have been unrewarding.

## PROGNOSIS

The prognosis for life is good, for it is not a progressive disorder. Only one patient has died and that was an acute death 12 hours after the onset of clinical signs. All others have lived; however, their behavioral change has often interfered with their previous relationship to the owner. In a few instances persistent circling and uncontrollable seizures have been a problem.

## TREATMENT

Without knowledge of the specific cause of this disease, rational therapy cannot be offered. The acute onset of tissue destruction, which may be accompanied by hemorrhage and edema, should be treated as one would treat an intracranial injury. This would include high levels of corticosteroids such as dexamethasone at 2 to 4 mg./kg. every 8 hours for 2 days and at a decreasing dosage schedule for the next few days and a hypertonic solution such as 20 per cent mannitol at 2 gm./kg. intravenously given at the onset and repeated 3 hours later.

The only residual sign that may be amenable to therapy is seizure. Phenobarbital is the drug of choice in cats and should be administered at the rate of 2 mg./kg. orally two to three times daily. No treatment has been tried for the persistent alteration of behavior that is often seen. Tranquilizers should be considered for this.

# FIBRO-CARTILAGINOUS EMBOLIC ISCHEMIC MYELOPATHY

ALEXANDER DE LAHUNTA, D.V.M.
*Ithaca, New York*

Fibrocartilaginous embolic ischemic myelopathy has been observed in adult dogs (2 to 9 years of age) of many breeds and both sexes and at all levels of the spinal cord. The location and extent of the ischemic myelopathy will determine the nature of the clinical signs.

For example, complete infarction of the right lateral funiculus and adjacent dorsal and ventral gray columns from C6 through C8 will produce a total spastic upper motor neuron (UMN) paralysis of the right pelvic limb and flaccid lower motor neuron (LMN) paralysis of the right thoracic limb. Pain perception and reflexes will be absent from the thoracic limb. Reflexes will be normal to hyperactive in the pelvic limb, and pain perception will be intact. Horner's syndrome will occur in the ipsilateral eye.

Bilateral infarction of gray and white matter in the caudal thoracic or cranial lumbar segments will produce a spastic paraplegia with hypertonia and hyperreflexia. Caudal to the lesion there will be analgesia or hypalgesia, depending on whether any tracts are spared in the white matter at the lesion site.

If the infarction is bilateral through the gray and white matter of the L4 through caudal segments of the spinal cord, there will be complete flaccid paralysis of the tail, anus and pelvic limbs. All tone, reflexes and pain perception will be absent.

This lesion has been observed unilaterally and bilaterally in the lumbosacral intumescence, the caudal thoracic and cranial lumbar spinal cord segments and the cervical intumescence. Clinical cases of a unilateral or bilateral cervical spinal cord lesion cranial to C6 have been observed. Those cases with more of a unilateral lesion and one that spares the gray matter of either intumescence have shown a remarkable degree of recovery or compensation. Signs of improvement have usually been observed within 7 days of the onset. Of 15 cases diagnosed with this disease, 7 have made some significant degree of recovery.

Except for one case the signs have been peracute in onset and have peaked within 12 to 24 hours of the first observation of an abnormality. In one case it took between 48 and 72 hours for the signs to develop fully. The signs are nonprogressive, and pain is not associated with the lesion.

CSF usually contains an elevated protein content. Leukocytes may be normal or slightly increased. No xanthochromia has been observed.

## DIFFERENTIAL DIAGNOSIS

If the acute onset and lack of a progressive course are recognized, the differential diagnosis is mostly limited to external injuries (automobile, gunshot) or internal injuries from sudden intervertebral disk extrusions. History, associated pain and radiographic studies should confirm these diagnoses. In the absence of these, a myelogram will distinguish the extradural disk lesion from a mild intramedullary swelling that often occurs in this ischemic myelopathy.

Inflammatory lesions and neoplasia produce less evidence of an acute onset and signs of a progressive course.

## PATHOLOGY

The lesion consists of an ischemic and sometimes hemorrhagic infarction of gray and/or white matter, usually limited to a few adjacent segments of the spinal cord. Occasionally they have been multifocal in a number of adjacent spinal cord segments. The pattern of infarction cannot be explained by the compromise of any single parenchymal blood vessel. Multiple vessel involvement in the leptomeninges or parenchyma must occur. Emboli can be found in the small arteries and veins of the leptomeninges and the parenchyma at the site of the lesion. These are pale blue in color with hematoxylin and eosin, blue with azocarmine, and tan with phosphotungstic acid hematoxylin, which is typical of fibrocartilage and not the fibrin of thrombotic material.

The source of this material is unknown. In the cases necropsied, no evidence of concurrent intervertebral disk degeneration was found. There is no justification yet in these dogs to assume that this is intervertebral disk material that has extruded into the marrow of a vertebral body to reach the venous circulation.

## TREATMENT

The only rational therapy to offer is treatment for an intraspinal injury. Edema and hemorrhage are components of the lesion and should be somewhat amenable to high-level corticosteroid therapy. Dexamethasone should be administered intravenously immediately at the rate of 2 to 4 mg./kg. and repeated at 8-hour intervals for 2 days. The dose should then be progressively reduced over the next few days. An initial intravenous administration of 20 per cent mannitol at the rate of 2 gm./kg. and repeated in 3 hours may also be efficacious.

There are insufficient clinical data as of yet to substantiate the value of this therapy.

### SUPPLEMENTAL READING

de Lahunta, A., and Alexander, J. W.: Ischemic myelopathy secondary to presumed fibrocartilaginous embolism in nine dogs. J. Am. Animal Hosp. Assn., *12*:37–48, 1976.

Zaki, F., Prata, R. C., and Kay, W. J.: Necrotizing myelopathy in five great danes. J. Am. Vet. Med. Assn., *165*:1080–1084, 1974.

# Section
# 10

# DISEASES OF THE GASTROINTESTINAL SYSTEM

### PETER THERAN, V.M.D.
*Consulting Editor*

# THE ORAL CAVITY

DONALD L. ROSS, D.V.M.
*Houston, Texas*

The tissues of the oral cavity have evolved to exist in a state of continual stress and destruction. Microorganisms, trauma and developmental and genetic defects are the primary causes of altered structure or function of the oral tissues. The microorganisms are the major factor in oral pathology, and oral health is dependent on the day-to-day process of repairing tissue damage. The mouth provides an excellent medium for growth of microorganisms and, therefore, oral hygiene becomes an important part of therapy for both hard and soft tissues in the mouth.

The relationship between oral infections and the function of other body systems has not been completely defined. The products of oral infections must be removed on a daily basis by the body's defense mechanisms, and the malfunction of other body systems reduces the repair capability of the oral tissues. Any factor affecting oral function to such an extent that nutrient intake is reduced obviously affects the health of the individual. Trauma is the most important factor in this category. The interaction of the nasopharynx, sinuses, salivary glands and other structures in the head and neck region often complicates oral pathology and function.

In understanding oral function and dysfunction, the normal occlusal pattern should be studied carefully. The occlusion of the carnivore is anatomically designed to function in a pattern similar to that of the German shepherd dog, and it is referred to as a "scissor bite." The maxillary incisors overlap the facial surfaces of the mandibular central and intermediate incisors, contacting the cingulum of the upper teeth. The lower lateral incisor rests on the small distal cusp of the upper intermediate and on the medial cusp of the upper lateral incisor. The lower canine should interdigitate in the interproximal space between the maxillary lateral incisor and canine teeth. There should be no contact between the lower canine and either upper tooth. The large cones of the mandibular premolars close into the interproximal space anterior to their maxillary counterparts. The large cusp of the mandibular first molar must go in front of the maxillary first molar. The mandibular second molar occludes with the maxillary first and second molars. The mandibular third molar may or may not occlude with the maxillary second molar.

With this occlusal pattern, 95 per cent of all defects that severely affect oral function involve either the anterior teeth or the comparative lengths of the two opposing jaws. Most breed standards are based on the position of the incisors; however, these teeth are so susceptible to trauma that they are a poor choice for this purpose.

## GENETIC AND DEVELOPMENTAL DEFECTS

### THE CLEFT PALATE COMPLEX

This group of oral abnormalities is the result of incomplete mesoderm development during the separation of the oral and nasal cavities. In the primary palate (cleft lip), the defect is produced by the separation of epithelial tissues when the supporting connective tissue stroma fails to develop. In the secondary palate (cleft palate), the lateral palatine processes fail to develop and to unite along the midline of the palate. The clinical picture seen with these defects will vary markedly among affected individuals. The origin of these traits is generally considered to be a recessive genetic factor. Other factors such as excessive corticosteroid therapy, abnormal levels of vitamin A and severe stress conditions have produced these abnormalities in several species of animals. On a clinical basis, the nongenetic causes of cleft defects are rare in the dog and cat; however, judicious steroid use during pregnancy is advisable.

The cleft lip usually presents as a unilateral defect in the lip, floor of the nostril or dental arch, extending into the incisive foramen. Much less frequently, it exists as a

913

bilateral nasal defect or in combination with a cleft palate. The majority of these animals are capable of sustaining life, and the defect becomes primarily a cosmetic consideration. Since there is usually no absence of tissue, correction consists of adjusting the position of the soft tissues to close the defect. The cleft palate usually presents as a defect of varying widths that extends from the incisive foramen posteriorly through the hard and soft palates. In this form, the cleft palate is incompatible with life. The inability to form a vacuum between the tongue and palate prohibits effective nursing, and supplemental nourishment must be provided. Milder forms of cleft palate range from soft palate defects to a mere displacement of the palatal rugae as they meet along the midline of the roof of the mouth (Fig. 1). When soft palate defects alone are present, chronic irritation and inflammation of the nasopharynx are the major clinical findings.

Euthanasia or neutering of affected individuals is to be recommended to reduce the genetic pool of these defects. If salvage of these animals is to be attempted, surgical correction must be postponed until the animal is at least 6 to 8 weeks of age. This delay reduces the surgical risk in the very young and gives the affected tissues time to mature and develop. It is not uncommon for two or more surgical procedures to be required to complete the restoration of the normal oral anatomy. There must be at least a 4- to 6-month interval between surgical procedures to allow complete revascularization of the tissues.

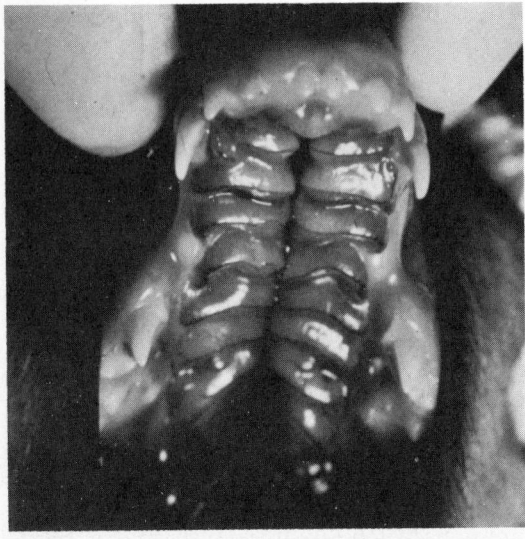

**Figure 1.**   Cleft palate. Note the mismatched rugae.

## MICROGNATHISM

Micrognathism is the term applied to the defect that results from extreme variance in size between the maxilla and the mandible. This defect is usually quite noticeable within the first few weeks of life. The exact genetic mechanism is difficult to evaluate, because many of the factors controlling jaw size, position and forms are inherited independently. Man has selectively bred for a micrognathic maxilla in several breeds (bulldogs, pug, Boston terriers, etc.). This change in jaw size is often accompanied by a posterior shift of the soft palate in relation to associated nasopharyngeal structures and results in chronic respiratory distress. The soft palate extends too far into the pharynx, the lateral nasal cartilages collapse, the tonsils protrude into the pharynx, the lateral laryngeal ventricles evert into the lumen of the trachea and the tracheal rings collapse—all these are common problems in these animals. Surgical correction of these problems early in life is recommended to prevent the cardiopulmonary changes that follow chronic respiratory embarrassment.

Micrognathism of the mandible is recognized as a severe genetic defect in all breeds. Prehension difficulties and palatal trauma from the lower canines are the only common problems associated with this defect. Tongue size usually corresponds closely to mandible size, and pharyngeal problems are not seen. The length of the mandible can be increased with a bilateral mandibular body osteotomy, but the decreased width in the canine area makes correct occlusion difficult to achieve. A more practical approach would be the amputation of a portion of the lower canines to relieve palatal trauma. This must be accompanied by a root canal or pulp capping procedure to preserve pulp tissue health and insure tooth longevity.

## PROGNATHISM

Strictly defined, the term prognathism refers to the abnormal protrusion of either jaw. However, in clinical usage, the term has come to be associated with mandibular protrusion and corresponds with the lay term "Undershot." Excessive length of the maxilla is described as "brachygnathic" or "overshot." Either condition may be observed in the young animal as the result of either a genetic defect or a developmental problem. The developmental and genetic forms present similar clinical pictures and usually cannot be differentiated by means of occlusal examination. Eruption of deciduous teeth at a time when jaw lengths are unequal will result in a dental interlock capable of blocking normal jaw growth. Genetic factors strong enough to alter bite patterns after the eruption of the deciduous or permanent teeth must be considered very strong traits and likely to reproduce themselves in succeeding generations.

To differentiate the mechanical defect from the genetic defect, the teeth involved in the dental interlock should be removed at 8 to 10 weeks of age. If correction of jaw relationships occurs by the time the permanent dentition erupts, the condition may be considered mechanical in origin; if it does not, it must be placed in the genetic category. The extraction of teeth does not stimulate jaw growth; it only allows unimpeded development of jaw structures. Based on clinical observation, this procedure results in significant improvement or total correction in about 50 per cent of jaw length discrepancies seen in the young dog. Care must be taken during the extractions to avoid injury to the epithelial membrane of the permanent-tooth bud. Areas of enamel hypoplasia may be produced on the permanent tooth if the elevator damages this membrane prior to completion of enamel formation. Teeth from the short jaw that would interfere with its forward growth should be selected for extraction. Extractions are generally limited to the canine and incisor teeth.

There are forms of prognathism that are not expressed until the permanent dentition is in place and the animal is 7 to 10 months of age. During this growth phase, the mandible tends to lengthen more than the maxilla, and shifts in the occlusal pattern occur. These are of genetic origin and will take one of two forms: (1) the lower jaw may suddenly develop a reverse scissor pattern in the incisal area, with corresponding shifts in position of the posterior teeth; or (2) the incisal pattern may remain stable and the lengthening of the jaw may be accommodated by a ventral bowing of the mandible.

There are two forms of prognathism that are not usually associated with prognathism. The first of these types of abnormal occlusion is referred to in lay terms as "wry bite" or "wry mouth," in which the halves of either jaw do not develop equally. Severe cases appear to have a prognathic occlusion on one side and a normal pattern of occlusion on the other side. In some individuals, the unequal growth of the lower jaw, with a strong dental interlock between the two arches, produces a deviation of the maxilla toward the same side. This can be detected by tracing the midline of the head from the occipital crest through the midpoint between the eyes and down across the nose pad. If these three points do not lie along the same line, close examination of the occlusion should reveal the extent of the defect. The second type of abnormal occlusion is termed "level bite" and is just a degree of prognathism. Unfortunately, it has been accepted in some breed standards as a normal bite pattern. This pattern is anatomically inefficient, does not tend to breed true, often shifts during life and usually results in excessive wearing in the incisal area.

## ANTERIOR CROSSBITE

Individual animals may have correct occlusion of the canines and premolars and yet one or more maxillary incisors may occlude on the lingual of the lowers. The causes of this type of occlusal pattern include crowding of the maxillary incisors, incorrect angulation of the mandibular incisors and traumatic displacement of the incisors. Genetic involvement has been hard to prove or disprove, but the likelihood that the condition will be passed on to succeeding generations is much less than with prognathism.

The condition is characterized by a flat or blunt maxillary incisal arch. This is best seen by looking up into the open mouth to view the arch. Correction is usually easy if there is adequate space to move the lower incisors posteriorly without overcrowding or rotation of the teeth. It is much easier to pull the lowers in than to push the uppers out. The lower incisors are fitted with orthodontic brackets, which are connected with an archwire. Elastics are placed along the wire and attached to some form of stable base, usually an acrylic base, in the posterior of the mouth. Therapy usually requires 6 to 8 weeks.

## RETENTION OF DECIDUOUS TEETH

The retention of deciduous teeth past the time of eruption of the permanent teeth is a common problem in many breeds and perhaps one of the most important in terms of long-term oral health. The resulting malocclusions frequently produce soft tissue trauma or abnormal and accelerated attrition of teeth. The retention of these teeth for as short a period as two weeks can produce occlusal defects in the permanent dentition. The mechanism governing resorption of the root structure of the deciduous teeth is not fully understood. The presence of the developing permanent-tooth bud does stimulate the resorption process but is not the sole governing factor. When deciduous teeth are retained, it is the permanent tooth that deviates from its normal eruptive pathway and comes into the arch in an unnatural position.

Changes are produced in the soft tissue when the permanent tooth erupts alongside the deciduous tooth that can be as harmful as those caused by the malocclusion. The permanent-tooth surface in contact with the deciduous tooth is often deprived of normal periodontal tissues, and a slight periodontal defect persists after loss of the deciduous tooth. Once a periodontal lesion is established, gradual progression over a period of years is likely.

The permanent teeth have a characteristic eruption pathway when the deciduous teeth are retained. The incisors, lower canines and premolars erupt lingual to the deciduous teeth. The lower canines tend to damage the soft tissues of the palate as they erupt to their full length. The maxillary canines erupt mesial to the deciduous canines, and the resulting occlusal defect is seen in the lower jaw. The lower canines are forced forward to maintain their position anterior to the maxillary canines. They move the lower incisors forward and produce an abnormal occlusion resembling prognathism.

The presence of a deciduous tooth in the arch long past the normal period of eruption indicates a lack of its permanent replacement. These deciduous teeth will often remain in the mouth for 3 to 5 years. While not capable of full oral function, the deciduous teeth will persist until their root structure is eventually resorbed. It is usually recommended that intraoral radiographs be taken prior to the extraction of deciduous teeth unless there is visual evidence of a permanent tooth near the gingival surface.

## OVERCROWDING OF TEETH

The rotation of teeth in the dental arch occurs when the teeth are not proportional to jaw structure. Head and jaw size is much easier to change by selective breeding than is tooth size. Consequently, in many of the smaller breeds tooth development resembles that of their larger ancestors. Rotations in the incisal area due to minor variations in tooth size can be relieved by reducing the width of each incisor slightly. This is best accomplished using a safe-side diamond disk, under water irrigation, at about 8 months of age. In the premolar region, extractions are indicated to preserve gingival health and longevity of adjacent teeth.

## ABNORMAL FORM AND NUMBER OF TEETH

Anodontia (absence of teeth) is rare in the dog, but oligodontia (reduced number of teeth) is a commonly seen entity. The most commonly affected areas are the premolars, incisors and the last molars. The absence of a single tooth is a condition less likely to be passed on to succeeding generations than is that of the absence of the same tooth on both sides of the arch or the absence of several adjacent teeth. If a tooth or a pair of teeth is absent and the adjacent teeth enlarge to fill the dental arch, the defect is almost certain to be passed on to a high percentage of the offspring. Enlargement of teeth occurs when there is a total lack of tooth buds in the adjacent spaces to inhibit its development. Absence of teeth must be differentiated from impacted teeth by means of intraoral radiographs.

Supernumerary teeth are seen in most breeds and rarely present severe health problems. Extra teeth are frequently seen in association with other oral defects and occur in such abnormal positions as the floor of the mouth and the hard palate. When they are present in the dental arch, they generally result in crowding and rotation of teeth. This crowding results in abnormal gingival contours, entrapment of food debris, early onset of periodontal disease and loss of teeth. The obvious solution to extra teeth in the mouth is extraction. Determination of the correct tooth for extraction generally involves selection of the tooth most likely to cause gingival alterations and removal of which would allow adjacent teeth to shift into the most desired occlusal form. This defect is considered to be low on the hereditability scale, and little emphasis is placed on it in a breeding program.

Impaction of teeth as seen in the dog and

cat is generally a result of the tooth's inability to penetrate the alveolar bone and gingival tissues. Usually, the simple removal of the soft tissue and bone covering a tooth will allow it to complete its eruptive pattern and assume its normal position in the mouth. Occasionally, a tooth will be lodged behind an adjacent tooth and form a true impaction. When this occurs, orthodontics and/or oral surgery is usually required to bring the impacted tooth into the mouth and move it into an acceptable occlusal position.

The term "fusion" denotes a joining of two tooth buds into a single tooth unit. This generally presents little or no health problem in the mouth and is of general academic interest only. The enamel covering is usually complete, and the teeth are capable of remaining healthy and functional for an indefinite period of time. The term "gemination" indicates an attempt on the part of a tooth to split into two teeth. This generally results in an excessively large tooth crowded into the dental arch and an altered gingival anatomy. Overcrowding of the teeth produces early periodontal disease and loss of teeth.

Dens in dente (translated as "tooth within a tooth") is a developmental defect involving the infolding of the enamel-forming epithelium and mesoderm of the permanent-tooth bud. This results in the formation of additional layers of enamel, dentin and pulp within the shell of the primary tooth. At the time of eruption, the area of involution usually leaks bacterial contamination into the pulp chamber and initiates an acute pulpal infection and periapical abscess. Therapy consists of removal of areas of gnarled enamel that protrude from the crown and performing endodontic therapy. An apicoectomy–retrograde amalgam filling is usually required. The most difficult part of treatment often is the long-term antibiotic therapy required to control apical infection until the root apex matures enough for endodontic treatment.

Enamel pearl is a developmental defect in which a small amount of enamel is displaced out onto the root. The periodontal tissues are incapable of attachment to the displaced enamel, and a food trap forms in the subgingival area. The result is early periodontal disease and tooth loss. This is only one of several conditions that produce localized gingivitis. These areas should be carefully explored, especially in the young dog, and eliminated or controlled if at all possible prior to development of severe periodontal disease.

## CARTILAGINOUS MANDIBULAR SYMPHYSIS

The mandibular symphysis begins as a very soft cartilaginous area in the neonate and matures into a stable fibrocartilaginous union of the mandibles in the adult. If this maturation fails to occur, the mandibular symphysis cartilage partially surrounds the root structure of the central incisors and affects the alveolar bone structure in the area. The incisors increase their anterior angulation because of the force of tongue thrust and the lack of bone support. Repositioning of these teeth affords only temporary relief. The early onset of periodontal disease frequently results in loss of these teeth.

Invasion of the mandibular symphysis by oral bacteria may destroy the symphysis, resulting in complete separation of the jaws. When the condition is known to exist, the lower central incisors should be removed to halt bacterial invasion of these tissues. The condition is seen primarily in the toy breeds but has been noted in the giant breeds. Comparison of intraoral films of the symphysis area of a few animals will quickly demonstrate the affected individuals. If the symphysis is lost, lag-bone screws or circum-mandibular wires in the area of the first premolar will usually provide adequate stabilization of the jaws for oral function if infection can be eliminated from the area.

## MYOFASCITIS

A condition has been noted in several young adult dogs in which extreme pain is evidenced upon opening of the mouth. These animals are incapable of opening their mouths more than an inch wide and are usually anorectic. The first attacks occur in the 8- to 12-month-old individual and last for 3 days to 2 weeks. The attacks recur with irregular frequency until the animals are 15 months to 2 years old. The symptoms of the condition can be relieved with steroid therapy. With growth and maturity, the attacks subside in intensity and duration until the animal becomes symptom-free.

The condition is probably best compared with a condition seen in humans when an asymmetrical development of the two halves of the body produces a myofascitis of the muscles of mastication. The unequal stresses initiate the inflammatory response. Although the presenting symptoms are similar to those of a retrobulbar abscess and eosinophilic myositis, a differential diagnosis can be made on the basis of the relatively normal blood counts and the immediate relief provided by steroid therapy.

## INFECTIONS OF THE ORAL CAVITY

### PERIODONTAL DISEASE

The term periodontics refers to the diagnosis and treatment of the diseases of the supporting tissues of teeth. This group of tissues includes the gingiva, the periodontal ligament, the cementum and the alveolar bone. Periodontal diseases are the most common infections in the oral cavity and result in greater destruction of soft tissue and teeth than occurs with any other disease process. Periodontal disease is basically the result of the bacterial population in the mouth and its destruction of soft tissue as compared to the body's immune response and ability to repair the damage as it occurs. Factors affecting the onset and progress of periodontal disease would include diet, chewing exercise, oral hygiene programs, dental prophylactic care, other disease or body defects, the immunologic defense mechanism and oral trauma.

The symptoms of periodontal disease, commonly termed pyorrhea, in its advanced stages include halitosis, gingival recession, calculus accumulation, purulent discharge from the root bifurcations, loosened teeth, alveolar infection and eventual loss of teeth. The theory that periodontal disease is initiated by the mechanical irritation of calculus has been overemphasized for many years. In many animals large calculus deposits may accumulate while the periodontal tissues remain healthy. Periodontal disease, in all forms, can exist in the absence of calculus. By viewing periodontal disease as the daily interaction of the periodontal tissues and the oral microflora, one can better evaluate the disease in animals, and meaningful therapy can be chosen.

The normal gingival crevice (formed by the gingival margin overlying the enamel surface of the tooth) is 1 to 3 millimeters deep. This crevice is lined by a one-cell thick epithelial layer of tissue and is continually inhabited by microorganisms. The disease process begins with the invasion of the gingiva by oral microorganisms through small ulcerations of the soft tissue wall of the gingival crevice. A destructive cycle follows in which each change in the periodontal structure facilitates entrapment of food debris in the gingival pocket, thereby increasing the number of bacteria that accelerate periodontal tissue destruction. In most cases, calculus formation follows rather than initiates the development of periodontal disease. The importance of calculus on the surface of teeth is in its medium-like properties supporting extremely large bacterial populations in and around the area of the gingival crevice.

Four separate steps should be considered in developing a therapeutic and prophylactic program for periodontal disease:

The first step in any program is scaling of the teeth to remove calculus, plaque, microorganisms and food debris from the teeth surfaces. The objective of this procedure is to give the periodontium the opportunity to repair itself before large numbers of bacteria again rebuild on the surface of the teeth and in the gingival crevice. Incorrectly accomplished scaling procedures, especially in the subgingival area, can be harmful to the soft tissues and diminish the beneficial effects of scaling. The ultrasonic scaling instruments are the most efficient and effective means of removing calculus and plaque from the surfaces of the teeth. However, these instruments do have limitations, and incorrect usage may damage the soft tissue or the tooth surfaces. The working tips of these instruments generate heat and must be continually cooled with a water spray to prevent excessive heat build-up. Ultrasonic instruments should not be used in the subgingival scaling procedures because the coolant spray is ineffective in the periodontal pocket, and burning of soft tissue may result. In using the instrument on the surface of teeth, the working tip should be directed at the calculus-enamel interface and should be moved lightly and rapidly in a continuous motion over the surface of the teeth. Excessive pressure applied to the working tip of the instrument will cause microetching of the enamel surface and will enhance the reattachment of microorganisms and food debris to the tooth surface. Care should also be exercised in the use of veterinary hand scaling instruments. These instruments are frequently too large to fit correctly into the subgingival crevice or the periodontal pocket. The excess bulk of metal will cause tearing of additional periodontal ligament fibers during the scaling process. Therefore, subgingival scaling should be done with fine, sharp, human dental instruments (Fig. 2).

The second phase of a dental prophylactic program should include root planing and subgingival curettage, accomplished at the same time as the scaling. Root planing is the smoothing of dentinal irregularities on exposed root surfaces by repeatedly passing the scaling instrument over the surface of the exposed root structure. Subgingival curettage is the removal of necrotic cellular debris from the soft tissue wall of the periodontal pocket. This allows maximal opportunity for reattachment of periodontal structures to the roots of the tooth and the reestablishment of the epithelial covering of the soft tissue wall of the periodontal pocket. Scaling instruments used in human dentistry have a double cutting edge so that both surgical steps are performed simultaneously. The instrument is inserted to the depth of the periodontal pocket and, on the cutting stroke, one surface acts against the root structure and the other against the soft tissue of the periodontal pocket. Correctly accomplished subgingival curettage will usually draw blood from the depth of the periodontal pocket.

The third step in the dental prophylactic program is the polishing of the exposed surfaces of the tooth. This step is aimed at re-

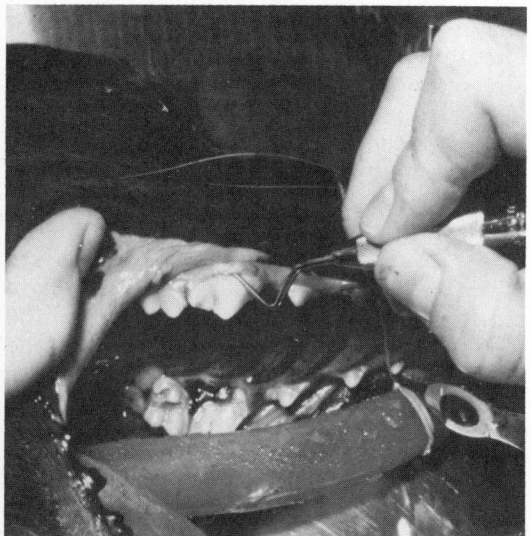

**Figure 2.** Subgingival scaling should be accomplished with fine, sharp instruments.

tarding the rate of bacterial repopulation by removing irregularities of the enamel and exposed dentinal structures. It has secondary benefits of making home cleaning of teeth easier to accomplish and future dental prophylactic procedures less difficult and time-consuming. Polishing of tooth structures is accomplished with a rubber "prophy" cup and polishing paste used with a dental hand instrument of low torque and high rpm. Polishing can create tremendous heat build-up and damage both pulp and periodontal tissues when accomplished with insufficient paste or high-torque electric motors.

The fourth step in a dental prophylactic program is an oral hygiene program at home. Severe periodontal disease cannot be controlled in a veterinary office. Without a home care program, the periodontal tissues receive only a slight break in the destructive forces of the disease process. The home care program can be divided into three areas: diet, chewing exercises and cleaning of the teeth. In the area of diet, dry animal food provides significant gingival stimulation and tends to scrape plaque and food debris from the surfaces of the teeth. It has been shown that animals on a dry diet tend to build less tartar and plaque on their teeth. Chewing exercise would include such things as Milk Bone®, rawhide chew strips and vinyl rubber chew toys. All these materially reduce the accumulations on the surface of the teeth and provide gingival stimulation to enhance oral health. The susceptibility of some individuals to periodontal disease is so great that a program of teeth cleaning must be introduced to control the disease process totally. The most effective method of cleaning teeth is a soft infant toothbrush used with baking soda or hydrogen peroxide as a dentifrice. The brushing program, using only water initially, should be introduced to the dog over a period of several weeks. If an individual animal totally refuses to accept the toothbrush, then a soft rag wrapped around the end of the finger may be substituted in the oral hygiene program. The root bifurcation areas and deep periodontal pockets are difficult to clean with a brush, and a water flush is needed to remove debris from these areas. This water flush may come from an electric Water-Pik®, a dental irrigator, an injection syringe, a water pistol or a water hose.

Commercial toothpastes are not recommended for animal use because of the detergent content of these dentifrices. The detergent produces a sudsing, foaming action that tends to increase anxiety and nervousness in the dog. If swallowed on a daily basis, the detergent may provide enough irritation to set off periodic gastrointestinal problems. In general, animals' teeth should be cleaned and polished professionally at least once a year, beginning at about age 18 months. The frequency of home care should be once a week in the healthy animal and increased, as needed, in those individuals with periodontal disease problems. The accumulation of plaque on the surface of the teeth must be avoided if control of periodontal disease is to be achieved.

There has been no conclusive evidence establishing a relationship between periodontal disease and other organ malfunction. On a clinical basis, improvement in total health and vitality of the animal has been noted when oral infections are eliminated. As a rule of thumb, if as much as one third of the root structure remains in healthy alveolar bone, teeth can be returned to a healthy, functional state in most individuals (Fig. 3). However, if a home oral hygiene program cannot be provided, body health is better served by extracting teeth severely affected by periodontal disease. Extraction is to be preferred to prolonged periods of gingival infection and gradual loss of teeth over a period of years. Extractions are also indicated when gingival recession destroys gingival tissue beyond the mucogingival junction at any point around the tooth. The mucosal tissue is incapable of attaching to root structure and of withstanding occlusal trauma.

Acute gingival infections are rarely seen in animals. This type of infection converts rapidly to chronic periodontal disease in most instances. Occasionally, subgingival caries will keep acute gingival infection active over a prolonged period of time. There are several other forms of periodontal disease. In response to periodontal infection, gingival hyperplasia may result instead of gingival resorption. The hyperplastic reaction leads to a gradual increase in pocket depth and loss of periodontal attachment, and the teeth are lost from the mouth as rapidly as if there had been gingival recession. Careful exploration of a gingival crevice is needed to detect presence of this type of pocket. A familial gingival hyperplasia exists as a genetic trait in some breeds. The breeds most often affected are Boxers, Great Danes, Collies, Doberman pinschers and Dalmatians. Gingivectomy is the preferred treatment for all gingival hyperplastic reactions (Fig. 4).

The oronasal fistula is also a form of periodontal disease. The destruction begins on the lingual surface of the maxillary canine, gradually working up the root structure, destroying the periodontium and hard palate and establishing a tract between the mouth and the nasal passage. Over a period of years, the process continues destroying maxillary alveolar bone, until the tooth is finally lost from the mouth. During this period of oral tissue destruction, the animal may exhibit sneezing, purulent nasal discharge and symptoms of sinusitis or nasal foreign bodies. Three to five years is generally required to complete avulsion of the maxillary canine following the establish-

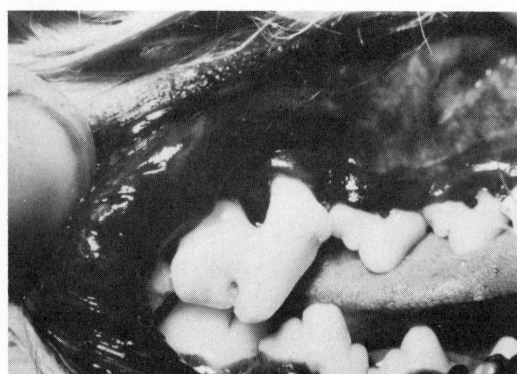

**Figure 3.** Proper oral hygiene can return severely damaged teeth to a healthy condition. (From Ross, D. L.: Veterinary dentistry. *In* Ettinger, S. J.: Veterinary Internal Medicine. Philadelphia, W. B. Saunders Co., 1975.)

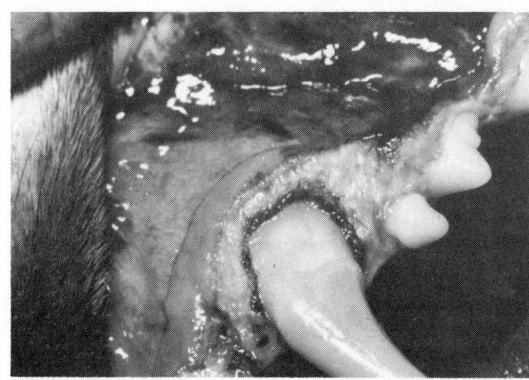

**Figure 4.** Gingivectomies eliminate periodontal pockets and allow proper cleansing of the area.

ment of a periodontal pocket along its lingual root surface. If the condition is noted early, a program of oral hygiene at home will retard bone destruction and allow careful monitoring of the developing fistula, so that extraction may be accomplished prior to the loss of massive amounts of maxillary bone.

The mandibular canines are also frequently involved in periodontal disease. A severe infection and loss of bone structure occurs on the buccal surface of the mandibular canine. The process becomes so severe that the lip area, in effect, becomes a periodontal pocket and food trap. If detected early, this problem may be brought under control by means of a mandibular frenectomy and gingival surgery. This combined surgery eliminates the periodontal pocket and allows the waste products to pass to the posterior part of the mouth. The animal and client are then able to keep the area clean and healthy.

## ENDODONTICS

Endodontics is the diagnosis and treatment of the diseases of the pulp tissues of teeth. Therapy for these conditions is commonly termed root canal therapy. The pulp consists of nerves, vessels and connective tissue that support the odontoblastic cells throughout life and provide internal sensory and metabolic function to the interior of the teeth. Pulp therapy is indicated when pulp tissue is exposed to oral flora either by breakage, by wearing away or via the apex of a root with severe periodontal disease. Any factor that devitalizes the pulp, such as pulpal hemorrhage or trauma, is also an indication for pulp therapy. The vitality of the pulp tissue can be evaluated based on the color of the dentine over the end of the pulp chamber or the translucent characteristics of the tooth. If the pulp tissue is black, the pulp has been exposed for an extended period of time and is necrotic. If the tissue is red or pink, exposure occurred recently and pulpal death will usually occur in the next 6 to 18 months. Any exposure of over 12 hours should be considered sufficient indication for endodontic therapy. If the end of the pulp chamber is tan or brown in color, the tooth has been able to protect the pulp tissue by secondary dentine deposition, and the tooth will remain vital. Pulpal hemorrhage is indicated by a pinkish translucent

hue to the enamel of the crown. Pulpal devitalization from other causes will give a dull gray character to the tooth.

The typical pathologic progression of an exposed pulp chamber is as follows: bacterial invasion of the pulp chamber, death and necrosis of the pulp tissue, spreading of the bacterial infection through the apex of the root into the surrounding alveolar bone and establishment of a chronic periapical abscess. The abscess then progresses to destroy the periodontal ligament and alveolar bone over a period of years until sufficient supporting structure has been removed to cause the avulsion of the tooth. A draining fistula below the eye is usually associated with an abscessing maxillary fourth premolar. Any tooth in the mouth is capable of producing such a fistula, and once established, it is difficult to treat without endodontic therapy or extraction of the tooth. In reality, less than 10 per cent of teeth with periapical abscesses progress to the point of fistula formation and draining to the external surface.

Swelling below the eye is commonly associated with the fourth premolar, but this syndrome can be produced by a variety of causes. When either of the buccal roots of this tooth is involved, the condition is usually alveolar osteitis with drainage through the thin buccal cortical plate. When the lingual root of the fourth premolar, the distal root of the third premolar or the mesial root of the first molar is involved, the drainage is frequently via the maxillary sinus and may produce external swelling but rarely actual fistulization. The maxillary sinus may become infected from a variety of nondental causes. The zygomatic salivary gland may produce a swelling in the same general area when it becomes inflamed or obstructed. A careful examination is required of the teeth, periodontal tissue and glands in the area to make a precise diagnosis. If the swelling is of sinal, but nondental, origin, ventral drainage may be established by directing a Steinmann pin into the sinus from between the buccal roots of the fourth premolar. The area should be thoroughly irrigated with an antibiotic solution, and a drain or packing may be placed in the area if desired. If the infection is of pulpal origin, the tooth can be salvaged by performing endodontic therapy to eliminate the source of the exposure, establishing ventral drainage and instituting antibiotic therapy.

Other pathologic conditions occasionally seen following pulpal exposure include internal dentinal resorption, in which the infection and destruction of the pulp tissue sets off a removal of the dentinal matrix similar to that seen in resorption of the roots of deciduous teeth. This process may continue until nothing is left except the enamel shell of the tooth, at which point any minor blow is sufficient to fracture the tooth. This condition is commonly seen following subgingival bacterial decay activity in the cat. The body may also institute a root resorptive process, beginning at the apex of the root and working gradually toward the crown structure. When sufficient root structure has been lost, the tooth is avulsed from the mouth, much as a deciduous tooth is lost.

The objectives of endodontic therapy are removal of cellular debris from the pulp chamber, filling the pulp chamber so as to establish a seal on the apical end of the root chamber and sealing the crown of the tooth. This is accomplished by using root canal files of gradually increasing sizes to extract the pulp tissue and to file the walls of the pulp chamber until they are smooth. The canal preparation is continued until clean dentinal shavings are withdrawn from the entire length of the pulp chamber. During this filing procedure, the canal is flushed with solutions of sodium hypochlorite (Chlorox®), hydrogen peroxide and saline. The flushing action removes debris from the chamber and lubricates the chamber walls, making canal preparation much easier.

After the canals have been cleaned and prepared, filling of the pulp chamber can be accomplished in any of several ways. With the exception of the canine teeth, the easiest method is to use silver cones of the same size as the last file used in preparing the canals. The canal is coated with a paste of zinc oxide and eugenol to act as a cement for the silver cone. Then the silver cone is fitted into place and cut off just below the opening in the crown structure of the tooth. A seal or restoration is placed in the crown to complete the restorative process. In the canine teeth, it is necessary to achieve an apical seal via an apicoectomy (the surgical exposure of the apex of the root structure). This surgical procedure is necessary because of the length and curvature of the canal of the canine teeth. It is impossible to establish a hermetic seal with standard

human endodontic techniques in the canine teeth. On the maxillary canine, the apicoectomy procedure is begun by making an incision 2 millimeters above the mucogingival junction from the mesial border of the maxillary third premolar forward to the posterior border of the maxillary lateral incisor. A periosteal flap is raised over the root structure of the maxillary canine, and the apex of the root structure is exposed with a dental bur. A hole approximately the size of the end of a pencil eraser is usually sufficient to establish adequate visualization and allow sealing of the root canal apex. The site for the apicoectomy can be more precisely determined by introducing a root canal file into the pulp chamber, measuring its length of insertion, and withdrawing and laying the root canal file alongside the canine to indicate the apical end of the root canal. A small amalgam restoration is placed in the apical end of the canal. The canal is then filled with a paste of zinc oxide and eugenol. The periosteal flap is repositioned and sutured with absorbable sutures. The crown surface of the tooth is restored with an appropriate material to complete the sealing of the pulp chamber. In most canine teeth, coronal access to the pulp chamber is best accomplished from the anterior surface of the tooth just above the gingival margin, with the bur directed toward the apex of the root structure. On the mandibular canine, the apicoectomy is accomplished via an incision through the skin on the ventral surface of the mandible. The apex of the mandibular canine lies just lateral and slightly anterior to the posterior border of the mandibular symphysis. Endodontically treated teeth have a potential life span equal to that of the normal tooth. A tooth should be considered worthy of endodontic treatment if as little as 6 millimeters of tooth structure shows above the gingival line and there are no fractures running under the edge of the gingival tissue that would interfere with periodontal health.

An endodontic technique that is of value in many instances is amputation of the canine teeth (Fig. 5). Unwarranted use of the canine teeth as weapons is an undesirable trait in some animals. By eliminating the crown portion of the tooth, the base can be preserved for its function in holding and grasping objects, yet the offensive weapon portion of the tooth is eliminated. This technique seems to have marked psycholog-

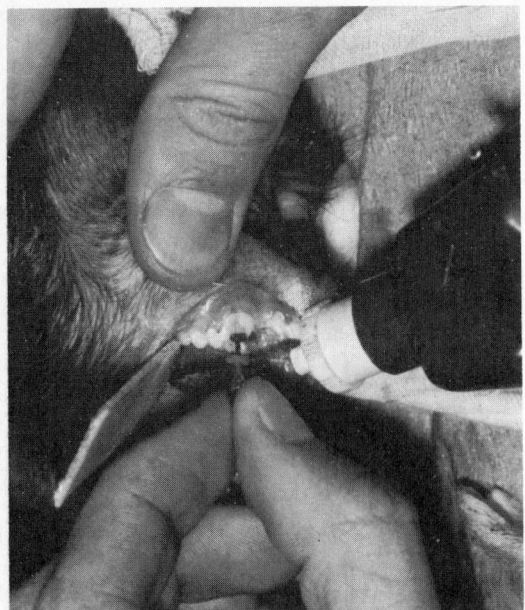

**Figure 5.** The canine teeth can be eliminated as weapons by amputation and endodontic therapy.

ical effects on the individual animal and frequently converts the very aggressive animal into one that is easily managed and suitable as a domesticated pet. The procedure is begun by using a diamond disk under water irrigation to amputate the crowns of the canine teeth until they are level with the adjacent teeth. This leaves a flat, blunt canine tooth protruding into the mouth approximately 6 to 12 millimeters. The procedure should be accomplished under conditions as aseptic as possible. The pulp tissue is extracted with root canal files and the canal is cleaned and enlarged in a normal manner. Filling of the canal can be accomplished with a paste consisting of iodoform and glycerine injected into the canal, and the crown of the tooth is then sealed with a restoration of choice. Teeth treated in this manner are capable of establishing a fibrous biologic seal across the apex of the root structure of the tooth. The technique is successful because there have been no oral microorganisms introduced into the canal and no periapical disease is present. In the very young animal, the technique may be modified slightly by amputating the tooth, drilling down 3 millimeters into the pulp chamber with a sterile dental bur and placing a layer of calcium hydroxide (Dycal®) across the exposed pulp tissue to provide a bacteriostatic, thermal insulating layer over the pulp tissues. A restoration of choice may then be placed on the crown of the teeth. This modification should not be attempted in animals over 3 years of age.

## BACTERIAL DECAY

For many years, the process of bacterial decay has been considered to be rare in the dog and cat and of very little consequence in the overall oral health of these animals. However, on a clinical basis, an increased frequency of this process has been noted. In man, the bacterial decay process affects primarily the enamel-covered crown of the tooth. In the dog and cat, the lesions on the enamel surface are infrequent, but any exposed root surface seems to be as susceptible to bacterial decay as it is in man. These lesions begin in the periodontal crevice or pocket, destroying the dentin of the root structure and progressing rapidly into the pulp chamber. Once the infection reaches the pulp tissue, internal dentinal resorption occurs at a rapid rate. The tooth is reduced to a hollow shell that succumbs to any trauma and fractures at or below the gingival surface. If these lesions are detected early, small restorations may be used to stop the progress of the decay.

The cat appears to be particularly susceptible to the bacterial decay process. Clinically, the syndrome begins as a marginal gingivitis overlying the early carious lesion. It is not uncommon to see 3 to 10 teeth affected at the same time in the susceptible animal. Restoration of these lesions is possible early in the process by surgical removal of the overlying gingival tissue in order to place the filling in the root structure. The feasibility of this procedure is dependent upon the amount of tooth structure affected and the amount of gingival tissue that must be removed for access to the bacterial decay area. Frequently, the combination of tooth and gingival destruction makes restoration impractical by the time the lesions are detected on clinical examination. Extractions are indicated if restorations cannot be accomplished. Individual animals that have one or more carious lesions in the mouth are very likely to develop additional lesions as time goes by. It is estimated that 20 per cent of total teeth lost in the cat can be traced to bacterial decay problems; in the dog, the figure is probably 10 per cent or slightly less. In susceptible animals, oral hygiene efforts are particularly necessary to reduce the daily bacterial populations in and around the gingival crevice and hopefully reduce the number of carious lesions that would have developed in the mouth.

## INFECTIONS OF OTHER SOFT TISSUES IN THE MOUTH

**The Oral Cavity.** All the soft tissues in the mouth are subject to infection by the various microorganisms in and around the oral cavity. In general, most of these infections respond to cleaning and systemic antibiotics or antifungal therapy. However, there are a few specific diseases that deserve brief mention. *Cheilitis* is often associated with infections involving the other soft tissues of the mouth and usually responds to gentle cleaning with bactericidal soaps. Occasionally, a steroid cream may be required to bring the localized reaction under control. Chronic lip-fold dermatitis is seen in some breeds, and management may require surgical resection of the lip fold in the most stubborn and recurring cases. Careful attention to culture and sensitivity testing is indicated in all recurring oral infections. Before culture samples are taken, oral lesions should be cleaned on the surface; samples should be taken from the depths of the lesion. Any oral culture and sensitivity should involve a fungal culture. The most common fungal agent involved in soft tissues of the mouth is *Candida albicans*. This agent responds to topical application of nystatin two to four times daily.

*Oral papillomatosis* is generally considered to be a viral disease in puppies and young dogs. The wartlike developments are generally self-limited, and intervention is generally necessary only when the warts are traumatized during the chewing process. Surgical removal is reported to stimulate the immune response and hasten regression of these lesions. A lasting immunity is conferred upon the animal once the oral papilloma viral agent has been brought under control by the normal body immune response. Mycotic infections of the mouth are generally a complicating factor in other infections but occasionally are seen as a separate clinical entity. Ulceration of the mucosal surface is characteristic. Lesions are usually painful, and anorexia is a major complaint. Thickened salivary excretions,

halitosis and a whitish film or strings of tissue around the lesions are commonly noted.

*Vincent's stomatitis*, or trench mouth, is a disease of the gingival tissues produced by a combination of spirochete and fusiform bacilli. The onset of the oral infection is usually rapid, starting with the gingival tissue and proceeding rapidly toward the apex of the root, denuding bone in its path. Halitosis and ropy salivation accompany the necrotic process in the mouth, and pain may be so severe as to limit intake of food. Therapy is directed toward maintaining blood levels of penicillin for one to three weeks. Good oral hygiene and other supportive therapy, such as high-protein diets and vitamin supplementation to maintain body condition until the repair process is complete, should be provided in all severe oral infections.

Little is known of the effect of many viral agents in the mouth. Many diseases are thought to be viral in origin, triggered by viruses or complicated by viral agents. With these types of lesions, therapy must be directed toward maintaining adequate intake of food and water, relieving oral pain and suppressing secondary bacterial and fungal contaminants until the autoimmune system has eliminated the viral agent from the body.

*Recurring necrotizing stomatitis* is an ulcerative disease seen on the mucosal surfaces of the oral cavity, most commonly noted on those surfaces that contact the enamel surface of the teeth. The disease is characterized by a diffuse inflammation with deep mucosal ulceration at tooth contact points. Halitosis and pain are pronounced. Cultures of the lesions usually yield *Staphylococcus* and *Candida*, and the lesions respond to therapy directed at these agents. The relationship between mucosal contact ulceration and healthy gingiva and teeth is unexplained. Recurrence of the attacks are frequent. Repeated applications of the antibiotic and antifungal agents are needed to bring the process under control and to reduce the number and severity of the attacks until a point is reached at which the animal and owner can coexist in reasonable comfort. Occasionally, steroids or analgesics are needed to reduce the inflammation and pain during an attack, to permit adequate food ingestion and for the application of medications.

*Systemic stomatitis* is known to occur in

he dog and the cat. In general, a wide range of systemic malfunctions may result in a secondary oral inflammatory reaction. Reported cases of systemic stomatitis are usually due to advanced systemic disorders with other signs of the primary dysfunction being easily observed in any individual animal. Among the particular dysfunctions reported are advanced renal disease, vitamin deficiency, diabetes, canine pemphigus and some heavy-metal poisonings. It is unlikely that oral lesions are caused by early systemic problems, but is is probable that borderline systemic problems prevent normal response to oral therapy. Conversely, severe periodontal infections can alter response to therapy for systemic problems.

In the cat, both *feline rhinotracheitis* and *feline leukemia virus* are capable of producing ulcerative lesions in the mouth. Feline ulcerative lesions may produce such extensive pain that a pharyngostomy tube for feeding may be necessary to provide the necessary nutrients until the body can overcome the infection. Pemphigus and lupus erythematosus are also commonly associated with oral ulcerative complications.

Many ulcerative and inflammatory lesions in the mouth may be associated with early *tumor formation*, and any lesion that does not respond to selected antibiotics and antifungal therapy should be biopsied. In the cat, eosinophilic granuloma or labial granuloma is commonly seen in the upper lips in the region of the maxillary canine teeth. Continued licking of the area aggravates the condition and may cause the spread of the lesion to other areas of the mouth. Currently, one successful method of treatment is steroids administered as a combination of local injection and suppository. Surgery to remove these lesions is usually unrewarding, and reconstructive surgery may be necessary to eliminate the unsightly scar tissue resulting from the initial surgical attempts.

**Other Oral Structures.** Infections of the soft tissues in other areas of the oral cavity are usually of a general nature, and variance in clinical signs is related to tissue function and location. This group includes glossitis, pharyngitis, tonsillitis, infections of the palate and sialadenitis. The origin of these infections includes trauma, foreign bodies, chemical and mechanical factors and often secondary involvement from other oral problems. A differential diagnosis is rarely difficult, but therapy response may be slower than desired. Utilization of aids such as radiology, sensitivity tests and biopsy is encouraged in these areas if immediate diagnosis and healing are not realized. Use of cautery is to be discouraged in the mouth.

A majority of tongue problems are secondary to other oral problems. *Primary glossitis* is frequently of traumatic origin (embedded foreign objects, strangulation, lacerations, chemicals). Some dogs have one or two rows of hair follicles along the tongue midline, and these may become irritated and inflamed. The area should be cleansed, the hairs removed and antibiotic coverage instituted. Blocked venous drainage may create sublingual swelling that resembles a ranula. Severe lacerations may be debrided and sutured. Removal of too much tissue can result in deviation of the tongue after healing. The organisms involved in glossitis are almost always those seen in the normal oral flora.

*Pharyngitis* is common in the dog and cat. It is almost always associated with an upper respiratory disease. Involvement of the retropharyngeal lymph node may complicate pharyngitis. Pain, swelling and/or drainage may interfere with respiration and eating. Surgical intervention may be required for drainage or node removal.

*Tonsillitis* is usually thought of as any condition that elevates the node out of the crypt. However, in the cat, the inflamed node may not protrude. The character of the tissue is a more reliable diagnostic sign than is node size. In severely affected tonsils small abscesses may form across the surface of the tonsil. A second form of tonsillitis is produced with chronic dysfunction of associated organ systems (vomition, coughing and respiratory distress). In the first form, the animal is "sick," and treatment involves antibiotics, analgesics, small doses of steroids and a soft diet. With therapy, most animals overcome or outgrow this type of tonsillar problem. Mechanical obstruction of the pharynx is the most common reason for tonsil removal. In this surgery, the cutting and ligating technique is preferred to cautery because of the reduced postoperative swelling and discomfort and the faster healing of the tissues.

*Infections of the soft palate* are rarely primary. More often, mechanical dysfunction of the soft palate with either excessive or inadequate length creates problems for the associated tissues. Again, electrosurgery and cautery are best avoided in surgery of the soft palate. A lack of adequate soft palate length is one form of the cleft palate syndrome.

*Sialadenitis* is not a common problem in the dog or cat. When it does occur, it is usually seen in the parotid gland. Rarely, it will occur in the mandibular gland. Swelling of the gland and a purulent discharge from the affected duct are diagnostic. Sensitivity tests, antibiotics and moist hot packs generally reduce swelling and bring the process under control. If the zygomatic gland is affected, a syndrome similar to a retrobulbar abscess ensues. Fortunately, the same drainage technique is effective for both problems.

More frequent occurrences in animals are problems related to saliva flow. Ranula, cervical salivary mucocele, pharyngeal mucocele and sialoliths are the entities in this group. Surgical intervention may be an elective or emergency procedure, depending on the degree of oral or pharyngeal obstruction. It is often possible to handle these situations with periodic drainage of the affected area, but recurrence and pet esthetics generally make surgery the technique of choice. Sialograms are of great diagnostic value. Traumatic incidents may open the salivary ducts, but these seldom cause permanent defects. Blockage of the parotid duct may be produced by a maxillary oronasal abscess, and severance is possible during extraction of maxillary molars.

## ORAL RESTORATIVE THERAPY

### ORTHODONTICS

Orthodontics is the phase of dentistry that deals with the prevention and correction of malocclusion. Perhaps no other area of dentistry is as controversial as the repositioning of teeth with the dental arch. According to ethical guidelines, all animals are entitled to a healthy bite, but not all animals are entitled to a perfect bite. The alleviation of genetic defects for cosmetic purposes in breeding and show animals is clearly unethical and to be avoided. The classification of an orthodontic defect should be made only after careful observation and analysis of the tooth structure, location, dental arch form and upper and lower jaw relationship. Malocclusions will produce early wearing

of the teeth; rotation and crowding of the teeth, resulting in periodontal diseases; soft tissue trauma in many mouths; and occasionally, complete inability of the mouth to function as a prehensile organ.

The orthodontic movement of teeth is based on the biomechanics of pressure on the periodontal ligament. The body attempts to equalize pressure in all directions on the periodontal ligament of a tooth. Thus, it will remove alveolar bone in areas of reduced periodontal ligament force and add alveolar bone in areas of periodontal ligament stress. The movement of teeth must be at a speed consistent with the biologic ability of the bone to remodel and re-form itself. Excessive pressure or excessive speed in moving teeth will result in the avulsion of the tooth. During movement of teeth in the dental arch, the principle that for every force there is an equal but opposite force must be kept in mind. Thus, for any tooth being moved in one direction, there is a force applied on other teeth to move in the opposite direction. The resistance of teeth to movement is directly proportional to the surface area of the root structure. The teeth composing the force base must have a larger total root surface area than the tooth or teeth to be moved.

Some minor tooth movements may be accomplished with rather simple orthodontic appliances. Posterior movement of a lower incisor may be accomplished with a wire twisted around the neck of the tooth, a hook bent in the wire on the posterior surface of the tooth, and an elastic stretched over the lower canine and attached to the hook on the incisor. Elastics used in orthodontic appliances must be closely observed at all times. An elastic may slip below the surface of the gingival tissue and become hidden from view. It will continue to work its way toward the apex of the roots of the tooth, destroying alveolar bone in the process, until the tooth is avulsed or the segment of bone is amputated by the elastic band.

Other forms of more sophisticated orthodontic appliances are quite applicable to veterinary dentistry. The biteplate is an excellent device to use in spreading the lower canine teeth to permit a correct relationship with the upper arch. The biteplate consists of an acrylic splint made to fit on the palate of the mouth, with a build-up of acrylic in the area contacted by the lower canines when the mouth is closed. The bite pressure exerted during closing will force the lower canines to move along an inclined plane into correct occlusal position. This same type of appliance is effective in moving incisor teeth in humans but has proved to be ineffective in animals. Because of the difficulty in banding canine teeth, the acrylic appliance has become a major tool in veterinary orthodontics. It can be adapted to a wide range of situations, incorporating an assortment of force-applying mechanisms in its action. Hooks for attachment of elastics, finger springs for direct force application, screw-type appliances and direct occlusal pressures are methods by which the acrylic appliance may provide force to move malpositioned teeth into a desired occlusal pattern. Because of the canine occlusion, brackets and arch wires are generally limited in their application to incisor teeth. The direct bonding cements allow direct attachment of the orthodontic bracket to the enamel surface of the tooth. The orthodontic bracket may then be used for the stabilization of an elastic attachment on a tooth, the attachment of a finger spring to a tooth, the joining of several teeth into a single unit with an arch wire and as a point of attachment to hold removable appliances in the mouth. Orthodontic brackets must be carefully positioned on teeth to avoid occlusal interference from other teeth and soft tissue trauma and to provide correct force application to the tooth being moved. In designing an orthodontic appliance, all force vectors must be carefully analyzed to insure the desired end result. Orthodontic appliances for the animal populations must be designed on an individual basis to accomplish individual needs.

Growth patterns may allow the correction of minor tooth displacements. The crowding of incisal teeth in the young adult can usually be eliminated by the reduction in width of the incisors and allowing shifting of the incisors during the growth processes. As a rule of thumb, no more than 20 per cent of a tooth should be removed during this form of therapy. It is desirable to remove lesser amounts from all teeth in contact with each other in the anterior arch rather than to remove a large amount of tooth structure from any single tooth. Tooth movement must be accomplished fairly rapidly in veterinary dentistry as compared to human orthodontic techniques. Oral hygiene levels are hard to maintain during orthodontic treatment. Accumulations of food debris around orthodontic appliances lead to soft tissue infection and loss of periodontal tissues. Most tooth movement procedures should be accomplished in 8 weeks or less, and the retainer phase of therapy should be limited to 4 weeks if possible. Orthodontic techniques designed around removable appliances are desirable if at all possible, since the appliances can be removed on a daily basis for cleaning of the appliance and the oral structures. Frequently, it is desirable for force applications and in-mouth time for appliances to be limited to 12 to 14 hours per day. Oral hygiene should be stressed with any form of intraoral appliance.

## ORAL SURGERY

Oral surgery encompasses a wide range of techniques in veterinary dentistry, but perhaps the most common area of surgical problems is fracture fixation. The most common fracture is the split mandibular symphysis. Figure-eight wiring techniques of various designs are adequate for symphysial fracture fixation if the mandibular canines flair to the outside at an adequate angle. Vertically positioned mandibular canines result in unequal compression along the symphysis and frequently allow movement between the two mandibles. In these instances, it is desirable to make a skin incision on the ventral surface of the mandible over the posterior border of the mandibular symphysis and to wire the mandibular symphysis together at that point. Application of the figure-eight wire around the canine can then achieve mandibular stabilization and correct occlusal positioning. Fractures of the body of the mandible present a problem not seen in fixation of long bones. The mandibular canal is not a medullary cavity. It is filled with large blood vessels, lymphatics and nerve bundles. The introduction of intramedullary pins and/or bone screws into the mandibular canal results in the destruction of the vascular supply and the innervation to the teeth and anterior part of the lower jaw. The preferred technique for fixation of mandibular fractures anterior to the fourth premolar is the intraoral acrylic splint (Fig. 6). The procedure consists of establishing a correct occlusion, usually by wiring the segments together. An impression

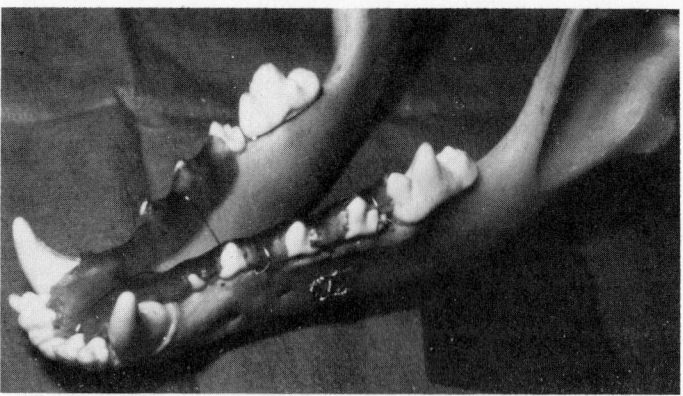

**Figure 6.** The intraoral acrylic splint is a versatile technique for fracture fixation.

and oral cast is made of the area. An orthodontic acrylic is used to form an intraoral splint that rests on the surface of the lower teeth and around the floor of the mouth. Circum-mandibular wires are then used to attach the intraoral splint to the jaw. The advantage of this type of appliance lies in the bearing of pressure of stabilization by the surfaces of the teeth and the ventral surface of the mandible in the area of wire placement. The vascular supply through the mandibular canal and through the soft tissues on the exterior of the mandible is not compromised, and healing may proceed at its maximal rate. The circum-mandibular wires are placed by attaching a surgical needle to a 24- or 26-gauge wire, penetrating the skin on the ventral surface of the mandible and pushing the needle through the periosteum, walking the needle off one edge of the mandible along the periosteum of the mandible and into the mouth. The needle is removed and attached to the opposite end of the wire and is taken back through the same skin hole and up the opposite side of the mandible into the mouth. The two free ends of the wire extending into the mouth are then brought across the acrylic splint and twisted together until the desired tension is achieved and stabilization is accomplished. In general, it is preferred that two wires be placed posterior to the fracture site and at least one wire anterior to the fracture. In most fractures the splint should be extended around the arch, and an additional wire should be placed on the other mandible. This type of fracture fixation is effective in simple, compound and multiple fracture situations in the anterior part of the mandible.

For fractures posterior to the mesial surface of the lower fourth premolar, wiring techniques are generally preferred. Adequate planning must be given to take into consideration all force vectors produced by occlusion and muscular pull. It is essential that wire of the largest gauge possible be used for each fracture situation. Cerclage and figure-X wiring of fracture sites are the most common patterns of wire placement. Fractures in the angle of the mandible and in the vertical ramus are also best stabilized by wiring techniques. Bone plates on the mandible have the disadvantage of placement of one or more bone screws into the mandibular canal or into tooth roots. These leave lasting scars on the tooth roots and may result in impaired vascular supply via the mandibular canal. Fractures of the temporomandibular joint usually result in partial joint dysfunction and eventual arthritic changes within the joint. Occasionally, complete jaw immobility results from temporomandibular joint fractures or trauma. The condyle of the mandible may be surgically removed and a false joint formed in the area, as is possible in the coxal femoral joint area. The surgical exposure of the temporomandibular joint is via a skin incision on the anterior border of the ear and careful dissection of the soft tissue away from the cartilage of the ear canal down to the temporomandibular joint.

Fractures of the maxilla most commonly involve a multiple fracture line situation. Fractures generally extend across the hard palate and dorsally in a variety of patterns to involve the bridge of the nose and the inferior orbit of the eye. Wiring of the maxillary bone at the point of the bridge of the nose, at the inferior orbit of the eye and at the dental arch is generally sufficient to achieve stabilization of maxillary fractures. Fractures of the incisive or premaxilla bone are best stabilized with an acrylic splint in the roof of the mouth, held in place by a circum-maxillary wire placed across the bridge of the nose. These splints may also be used to stabilize avulsed teeth and to cover oronasal tissue defects until healing is completed. Unless fractures of the hard palate are badly fragmented, it is rarely necessary to wire the hard palate itself. A simple fracture of the midline of the hard palate is usually adequately stabilized by a circum-maxillary wire applying compressive forces across the hard palate. Fractures of the zygomatic arch are usually angular and may be adequately stabilized with cerclage wiring.

Surgical repositioning of teeth is a technique that may allow rapid correction of orthodontic problems in the young animal. This technique should be reserved for those animals under 10 months of age in which open apical root structures still exist. The procedure consists of elevating the affected tooth free of its attachment to the alveolar bone, making an incision through the soft tissue to the point of desired positioning, swinging the tooth through an arc about the apex of the root into the correct position and splinting the tooth in the new position for two to three weeks. If apical blood supply remains undisturbed during the surgical movement of the tooth, the procedure has an excellent chance of achieving the desired occlusal pattern and maintaining a healthy, vital tooth. It may be necessary to create an alveolar pocket or socket in the site of the new tooth position. Attempting this procedure in older animals with closed apical root structures or the avulsion of the tooth during the procedure generally results in the loss of the tooth from the mouth.

The oronasal fistula following the loss of the maxillary canine tooth from severe periodontal disease is best closed by a periosteal flap technique. The procedure is begun by preparing a tissue bed around the circumference of the fistula site. An incision is made on the mesial and distal sides of the fistula, extending upward toward the bridge of the nose. The incision extends down through the periosteum, so that a tissue flap containing a normal periosteal membrane may be elevated free of the maxillary bone. It is necessary that the periosteal flap be of sufficient length to cover the oronasal fistula without tension. The periosteum is incised at the apex of the flap and the soft tissue incisions are extended dorsally until a flap may be positioned over the fistula without tension on the soft tissues. The flap is sutured in place with nonabsorbable sutures or Dexon® in a retention suture pattern. These sutures are removed in two weeks and healing is evaluated at that time. Generally, closure of 75 per cent or more of the oronasal fistula will be adequate to allow normal function with a minimal amount of nasal tissue irritation from food impaction. If repeat surgical procedures are required to close the fistula, they should be postponed for 4 to 6 months to allow the establishment of completely normal vascular patterns in the tissue area. Repeated attempts at surgical repair will certainly result in repeated failure if this revascularization process is not complete prior to surgical intervention.

Extraction of teeth is indicated if the teeth are incapable of being retained in a healthy state in the mouth. This may be due to an inability on the part of the owner to provide correct oral hygiene or to a lack of adequate healthy tissue to support the teeth. In general, a tooth may be maintained in the mouth if as much as one third of its root structure remains in healthy alveolar bone, if fracture lines do not extend under the gingival margin and if endodontic diseases are eliminated with the root canal therapy. On multirooted teeth, lack of attachment to healthy bone on a single root is adequate reason for extraction, regardless of the health of the tissue surrounding the other root structures of that tooth. Extraction techniques are a matter of gradual stretching and breaking of periodontal ligament fibers and not of brute force application to a tooth. In general, all multirooted teeth should be sectioned into their component parts prior to extraction procedures. Extraction should be begun by severing the gingival attachments down to the crest of the alveolar bone. The gingival tissue is incised around the surface of adjacent teeth so that the gingival tissue may be laid back as a flap technique to reveal the crest of the alveolar bone. A dental bur is used to remove 3 to 5 millimeters of the alveolar bone crest. The elevator is then inserted between the root segments perpendicular to the long axis of the root. A gentle rocking action is instituted with the elevator gradually to stretch and break the periodontal fibers of the tooth. No more than the thumb and the first two fingers should be used in this procedure. The rocking of the tooth elevator should be continued for a period of 2 or 3 minutes, and moving the elevator gradually around the circumference of the root structure will result in its loosening and easy removal. Because of the lack of manual force applications to the tooth structure, this procedure tends to become tedious. However, a period of gentle rocking action of the tooth elevator over a period of 3 to 5 minutes generally results in removal of the tooth without fracture of either the root tip or the alveolar bone. The dental elevator is an instrument that gains its mechanical advantage because of the difference in the diameter of the working tip of the instrument as opposed to the handle of the instrument. It was not designed as a gouging or probing instrument. Attempts to dislodge root structure by pushing the dental elevator into the alveolar socket result in alveolar bone fracture or breakage of the root structure or the tooth. Extraction forceps are also designed to apply gradual or limited pressure to the periodontal ligament. Extraction forceps should be applied as close to the alveolar crest as possible and used in a buccolingual, rocking motion. When dealing with single root segments, a slight torquing action may be applied to enhance the stretching and breaking of the periodontal ligament fibers. The most common instruments used in dental extractions are the No. 301 elevator and the Nos. 150-S and 151-S pediatric extraction forceps. The removal of the alveolar crest is desired following the extraction of the tooth to facilitate soft tissue repair over the alveolar socket and, in the absence of infection, to allow suturing of the soft tissue over the alveolar socket. Broken root tips are most easily removed by using a dental bur to drill down into the alveolar socket, reducing the root tip to dentinal shavings. The alveolar socket is then irrigated with a sterile saline solution. With experience, it is easy to differentiate between the feel of the drill cutting dentin and feel of the drill in alveolar bone. This allows the complete removal of the root tip without fracture of alveolar bone or unnecessary damage to surrounding soft tissues. The procedure is accomplished quickly and easily.

## SUPPLEMENTAL READING

Bojrab, M. J.: Current Techniques in Small Animal Surgery. Philadelphia, Lea & Febiger, 1975.

Burkett, L. W.: Oral Medicine. 6th ed. Philadelphia, J. B. Lippincott Company, 1971.

Egelberg, J.: Local effect of diet on plaque formation and development of gingivitis in dogs. Odontol. Rev., *16*:31, 1965.

Grossman, L. T.: Endodontic Practice. 7th ed. Philadelphia, Lea & Febiger, 1970.

Hammer, D. L., and Sachs, M.: Clefts of the primary and secondary palate. *In* Bojrab, M. J. (ed.): Current Techniques in Small Animal Surgery. Philadelphia, Lea & Febiger, 1975.

Harvey, C. E., and O'Brien, J. A.: Disorders of the oro-pharynx and salivary glands. *In* Ettinger, S. J. (ed.): Textbook of Veterinary Medicine. Philadelphia, W. B. Saunders Co., 1975.

McCall, J. D., and Wald, S. S.: Clinical Dental Roentgenology. 4th ed. Philadelphia, W. B. Saunders Co., 1957.

O'Brien, J. A., and Harvey, C. E.: Diseases of the upper airway. *In* Ettinger, S. J. (ed.): Textbook of Veterinary Internal Medicine. Philadelphia, W. B. Saunders Co., 1975.

Orban, B. J.: Oral Embryology and Histology. 6th ed. St. Louis, The C. V. Mosby Co., 1966.

Prichard, J. F.: Advanced Periodontal Disease. Philadelphia, W. B. Saunders Co., 1972.

Reitan, K.: Biomechanical principles and reactions. *In* Graber, T. M., and Swain, B. F. (eds.): Current Orthodontic Concepts and Techniques. 2nd ed. Philadelphia, W. B. Saunders Co., 1975.

Ross, D. L.: Comparison of Single Appointment Endodontic Therapy Using Absorbable and Nonabsorbable Filling Techniques. Thesis. Houston, The University of Texas Graduate School of Biomedical Science, 1972.

Ross, D. L.: Anterior mandibular fracture fixation. *In* Bojrab, M. J. (ed.): Current Techniques in Small Animal Surgery. Philadelphia, Lea & Febiger, 1975.

Ross, D. L.: Occlusion in the dog. Southwest. Vet., *28*:247, 1975.

Ross, D. L.: The teeth. *In* Bojrab, M. J. (ed.): Current Techniques in Small Animal Surgery. Philadelphia, Lea & Febiger, 1975.

Ross, D. L.: Veterinary dentistry. *In* Ettinger, S. J. (ed.): Textbook of Veterinary Internal Medicine. Philadelphia, W. B. Saunders Co., 1975.

Ross, D. L., and Heller, R. A.: Endodontics in a Capuchin monkey: Reduction of the length of the canine crown. Vet. Med./Small Animal Clin. 68:255, 1973.

Ross, D. L., and Myers, J. W.: Endodontic therapy for canine teeth in the dog. J. Am. Vet. Med. Assn., *157*:1713, 1970.

Rudy, R. L.: Fractures of the maxilla and mandible. *In* Bojrab, M. J. (ed.): Current Techniques in Small Animal Surgery. Philadelphia, Lea & Febiger, 1975.

Seltzer, S.: Endodontology—Biologic Considerations in Endodontic Procedures. New York, McGraw-Hill Book Co., 1971.

Shulze, C.: Developmental abnormalities of the teeth and jaws. *In* Gorlin and Goldman (eds.): Thoma's Oral Pathology. 6th ed. St. Louis, The C. V. Mosby Co., 1970.

Socransky, S. S.: Relationship of bacteria to the etiology of periodontal disease. J. Dent. Res., *49*:203, 1970.

Stockard, C. F.: The Genetic and Endocrine Basis for Differences in Form and Behavior. American Anatomical Memoirs. Philadelphia, Wistar Institute of Anatomy and Biology, 1941.

Wallace, L. J.: An alternate procedure of cleft hard and soft palate in the dog. *In* Bojrab, M. J. (ed.): Current Techniques in Small Animal Surgery. Philadelphia, Lea & Febiger, 1975.

# DISEASES OF THE ESOPHAGUS

RICHARD E. HOFFER, D.V.M.
*Ithaca, New York*

Diseases of the esophagus have become more significant in veterinary medicine since the advent of better methods of diagnosis and treatment. Most esophageal diseases are surgical problems, although some may respond to medical therapy. Esophageal disease may be divided into four categories: (1) traumatic, (2) parasitic-neoplastic, (3) congenital and (4) neuromuscular.

## TRAUMATIC DISEASES

The most common cause of esophageal trauma is foreign bodies. Foreign bodies may be smooth or sharp. Generally, a sharp foreign body produces more trauma more rapidly than a smooth one. Changes secondary to esophageal foreign bodies may result from pressure on the esophageal wall. This pressure usually involves only the esophageal mucosa. However, lesions can extend through the esophageal muscularis, predisposing to esophageal perforation.

Sharp objects such as plastic or metal materials may produce mucosal lacerations or full-thickness esophageal lacerations. Pointed objects, such as fishhooks, may perforate the esophagus and involve other adjacent structures, such as the aorta.

Esophageal foreign bodies usually lodge in four areas: (1) high cervical esophagus, (2) thoracic inlet, (3) base of the heart and (4) esophageal hiatus. These represent areas where the esophagus is normally compressed.

Wounds of the cervical esophagus may result from fights or other traumatic injuries. Traumatic stricture and diverticulum of the esophagus can result from foreign bodies, wounds or ingestion of caustic material. A stricture usually occurs and, if it persists, results in esophageal dilatation anterior to the narrowed area. A stricture can be caused by improper or traumatic removal of a foreign body, with subsequent damage to the esophageal wall.

## PARASITIC-NEOPLASTIC DISEASES

Primary neoplasms of the esophagus are rare. Leiomyoma, squamous cell carcinoma and sarcomas have been reported. *Spirocerca lupi* granulomas are uncommon except in endemic areas, but the lesion produced by the parasite has the same effect as a neoplasm and may become neoplastic.

## CONGENITAL DISEASES

A congenital esophageal diverticulum may be seen. This resembles a traumatic diverticulum but is seen in young dogs with no history of trauma and no evidence of strictures.

A vascular ring produces stenosis of the esophagus, with esophageal dilatation. This condition presents as an esophageal problem (see article on "Persistent Right Aortic Arch").

## NEUROMUSCULAR DISEASES

Cricopharyngeal achalasia is seen in young dogs. The condition is characterized by dysphagia resulting from failure of the cricopharyngeal sphincter to relax, thus preventing passage of food from the pharynx into the esophagus. The exact etiology of this condition is unknown, but abnormal innervation of the cricopharyngeal muscles may be suspected.

Neuromuscular diseases of the esophagus affect the normal peristaltic activity of the esophagus and are manifested by failure of progressive peristalsis and asynchronous function of the intrinsic gastroesophageal sphincter. There are two disease entities in the dog that produce this effect. The first is *achalasia*, found in the mature dog without previous esophageal disease. Dogs do not recover from this condition, since it is a permanent neuromuscular defect. The second condition is *idiopathic megaesophagus*, which is seen in the young or immature dog.

Some puppies with this neuromuscular deficit will outgrow it and develop normal esophageal function by the time they reach maturity. However, not all dogs will outgrow the condition, and consequently some dogs never improve at all.

When a normal dog swallows a bolus of food, a progressive peristaltic contraction begins in the cervical esophagus and carries the bolus down the esophagus. Just before the bolus reaches the intrinsic gastro-esophageal sphincter, the sphincter relaxes so that the food can enter the stomach. This sequence can be demonstrated by measuring pressure changes within the esophagus and by the use of fluoroscopy with barium swallows.

A dog affected with either of the above diseases shows abnormalities in the normal esophageal motility pattern. A dog with achalasia does not have any progressive peristaltic contractions or local peristaltic contractions. The bolus will advance through the lumen only as the result of gravity. In addition, the intrinsic gastroesophageal sphincter does not relax in response to a swallow. However, the sphincter will relax and allow emptying of the esophagus in response to an intraluminal pressure increase.

A dog with idiopathic megaesophagus may show various types of esophageal peristalsis and intrinsic esophageal sphincter function, depending upon the stage of the disease. In the early stages of the disease, the esophageal body motility and sphincter function are the same as that seen with achalasia. However, as the dog matures, and if the dog is one that is going to respond, local peristaltic contractions progressing to normal peristaltic contractions are visualized. In the early stages the sphincter is completely asynchronous, but as the disease responds, relaxation and contraction of the sphincter become more normal and synchronize with the primary peristaltic contractions.

The etiology of these two diseases has not been demonstrated. It has been suggested that achalasia is the result of a defect in the nucleus ambiguus, resulting in a lack of innervation of the esophagus. With achalasia this is a permanent defect. It has been suggested that idiopathic megaesophagus is a developmental immaturity of the esophageal innervation and/or musculature. Since the condition may be seen in litter mates, it has been suggested that this is a congenital defect and may be hereditary. Studies utilizing manometric measurements of esophageal contraction and simultaneous fluoroscopic evaluation should help to clarify and define further these very confusing disease entities.

Polymyositis, myasthenia gravis and systemic lupus erythematosus are disease entities that can present as acquired achalasia. The presence of these conditions should be ruled out before initiation of therapy.

## DIAGNOSIS

The diagnosis of esophageal diseases depends mainly upon radiographic techniques; however, a complete history and physical examination and the use of esophagoscopy are necessary for a valid diagnosis and prognosis.

Most animals have a history of vomiting and dysphagia, regardless of the cause of the esophageal disease. A careful history aids in establishing the probability of the disease. Information as to whether the dog is fed bones or chews up various objects may help to indicate a condition involving a foreign body.

The age of onset is valuable in the diagnosis. Congenital conditions may be suspected in the young animal and neoplasms in the older ones. Foreign bodies may occur at any age.

A detailed history of previous illness is necessary. If the dog has been treated for a foreign body, ingestion of caustic material or a cervical wound, the possibility of a stricture is increased. If the dog has had distemper, the possibility of acquired achalasia may be considered. The area of the country in which the dog is located could suggest S. *lupi*.

The character and frequency of vomiting and the time between feeding and vomiting are useful in the diagnosis. Persistent dysphagia and attempts to swallow solid food with simultaneous expulsion of the food from the mouth indicate cricopharyngeal achalasia or a high esophageal foreign body. Vomiting of solid, undigested food shortly after eating would indicate an obstruction without dilatation, i.e., foreign body or early stricture. Vomiting of liquid, foul-smelling vomitus with a large quantity of mucus occurring at varied intervals after eating would indicate esophageal dilatation, i.e., achalasia, diverticulum or vascular ring. If the frequency of vomiting has increased but smaller amounts of material are vomited, or if the animal appears to regurgitate rather than vomit, an esophageal dilatation should be suspected.

The diet may also aid in differentiating the main type of esophageal disease. The more liquid the diet, the narrower the stricture. However, if the diet has no effect on the pattern of vomiting, esophageal dilatation should be suspected.

A thorough physical examination of the animal should be performed. In most cases, an animal with a chronic esophageal problem is emaciated. Evidence of trauma should be sought, especially in the cervical region. A specific abnormality that may be seen with achalasia or a vascular ring is a ballooning of the cervical region of the esophagus at the thoracic inlet. This may be seen and palpated after the animal has been fed. It may also be demonstrated by occluding the nares, closing the mouth and sharply compressing the thorax.

Auscultation is helpful in establishing a prognosis, because many esophageal dilatations are accompanied by secondary aspiration pneumonia. Also, a patent ductus may be detected that would influence one's approach to a vascular ring.

In a *S. lupi* endemic area, a fecal specimen should be examined for possible ova of the parasite.

Esophagoscopy is valuable in diagnosing neoplasms, strictures or foreign bodies. Esophagoscopy enables one to examine the mucosa, to visualize a mass that penetrates the esophageal mucosa or to see some foreign bodies.

There are various types of esophagoscopes available. The most recent are the flexible fiberoptic types of endoscopes. These permit excellent visualization of the esophageal lumen but are not very effective for removing a foreign body. Some fiberoptic scopes may be utilized to obtain a biopsy. The major disadvantage of this type of equipment is that at present it is very expensive. There is some indication that fiberoptic scopes may become available to the veterinarian at a much reduced price in the near future.

Rigid tube types of lighted endoscopes of different sizes are at present the most adaptable as well as affordable instruments for esophagoscopy in the canine.

The dog should be placed in dorsal recumbency under a short-acting anesthetic. The lubricated esophagoscope is passed into the esophagus and then slowly down the esophagus into the stomach. When passing the esophagoscope, it is important that the lumen of the esophagus be followed. If the lumen cannot be seen, the esophageal wall in an involved area could become perforated by pushing the esophagoscope blindly. A more detailed description of the technique of esophagoscopy may be obtained from the supplemental reading and on page 988.

The use of a stomach tube to check blindly for a foreign body can result in a misleading diagnosis or even a perforation.

## RADIOGRAPHY

Radiography with the use of fluoroscopy is the most necessary diagnostic aid for esophageal conditions. Routine lateral and ventrodorsal views of the cervical and thoracic regions of the esophagus demonstrate esophageal dilatation and opaque foreign bodies. The use of barium demonstrates a nonopaque foreign body, a stricture, dilatation, diverticulum and other conditions that compress the esophagus, such as neoplasm and vascular ring. If there is any indication of esophageal perforation, barium should not be utilized for esophageal evaluation; instead, injectable contrast materials should be utilized. Barium motility studies of the esophagus should always be done in an animal that is not under the effects of tranquilization or anesthesia. These drugs may interfere with normal esophageal motility and could give a misleading radiograph.

A useful technique in demonstrating diverticula or esophageal dilatation is to hold the animal upright (spine vertical) when administering barium and taking the radiograph. This outlines the dilatation, and when there is lack of function of the gastroesophageal sphincter, it demonstrates this narrowed area of the esophagus.

A fluoroscopic examination while administering barium is necessary for a positive diagnosis of esophageal neuromuscular disease. In achalasia this examination demonstrates the lack of progressive peristalsis and the failure of the narrowed segment (the gastroesophageal sphincter) to relax and allow esophageal emptying. With idiopathic megaesophagus it will show the abnormal peristalsis and asynchronous function of the gastroesophageal sphincter. The amount of abnormality visualized will depend upon the stage of the disease. In the late stages of idiopathic megaesophagus the only abnormality seen will be retention of a small amount of barium in the most distal esophagus, an indication of minor motility dysfunction at this point.

Barium administration is useful in differentiating a diverticulum from generalized esophageal dilatation. Fluoroscopy may also be used to demonstrate the failure of a barium meal to pass from the pharynx to the esophagus, denoting cricopharyngeal achalasia.

## TREATMENT

**Foreign Bodies.** Foreign bodies may be removed by esophagotomy or by the use of forceps and an endoscope. When an endoscope is used, the foreign body may be removed through the oral cavity or pushed into the stomach, where it can be subsequently removed if necessary. Utilizing esophagoscopy, Ryan and Greene have reported a recovery rate of 98.4 per cent in 51 cases of esophageal foreign bodies removed by esophagoscope. They have successfully utilized this technique even when there was esophageal perforation and suggested the use of a pharyngostomy tube when there was evidence of a small perforation or mucosal laceration.

Esophagoscopy, to be done successfully in cases with foreign bodies that have perforated or have the potential to lacerate, requires good equipment and an operator that is totally familiar with the equipment and techniques.

Esophagotomy is utilized for the removal of esophageal foreign bodies. Esophagotomy allows direct visualization of the esophagus, and the degree of damage to the esophagus can be assessed and repaired at the time of removal. When large esophageal tears occur or when a large amount of esophageal necrosis is suspected, the esophagotomy approach should be utilized. The esophageal incision for an esophagotomy should be made in viable tissue, and the foreign body is removed through this site.

The closure of an esophagotomy is best accomplished with a two-layer suture pattern. The first layer is closed with a simple continuous suture pattern of 5-0 silk through the esophageal mucosa and submucosa. Care is taken to close the ends of the incision. The second layer is closed with a simple interrupted suture pattern of 3-0 chromic gut through the muscularis of the esophagus.

If the esophagus is severely damaged, resection and anastomosis are necessary. Anastomosis is performed in an end-to-end manner using the same suture pattern as for an esophagotomy, provided that there is no tension on the anastomosis. If an extensive resection is necessary, resulting in tension on the suture line, two rows of simple interrupted sutures should be used to complete the anastomosis. The mucosa and submucosa are sutured with a simple interrupted suture pattern of 3-0 silk with the knots tied in the lumen. The muscularis is sutured with 3-0 chromic gut with the knots tied on the outside of the lumen. The anastomosis should be checked for leaks after the mucosal layer is closed.

**Strictures.** Strictures usually do not respond to dilatation, but this method of treatment may be attempted. A second method that may help is a myotomy of the strictured area. This technique is also usually unsuccessful. A third method of enlarging the lumen is insertion of a patch graft from an adjacent muscle such as the sternocephalicus in the cervical region. This technique was recently described by Howard *et al.* (1975). Resection and anastomosis is a most effective treatment and is accomplished with a two-layer simple interrupted pattern, depending upon the amount of tension.

**Diverticulum or Local Dilatation.** Local dilatation should be treated by attempting to correct the cause. If the dilatation is anterior to a stricture, repair of the stricture may cause the diverticulum to decrease and result in a normal esophageal lumen. If a true diverticulum is present, it must be resected. It should be sutured with the two-layer suture pattern, and the resulting lumen should have the same diameter as the normal esophagus. The sac should be resected in stages and sutured after each small incision. Occasionally, the diverticulum and the involved esophagus may have to be completely resected.

When a long section of the esophagus must be resected, the tension can be relieved by dissecting the esophageal hiatus and mobilizing a portion of the stomach into the thorax through the hiatus. The hiatus must then be fixed to the stomach to prevent diaphragmatic hernia.

**Cricopharyngeal Achalasia.** Immediate relief of dysphagia is produced by performing a cricopharyngeal myotomy. All the fibers of the cricopharyngeus muscle must be severed in order to insure recovery.

**Neuromuscular Disease.** Idiopathic megaesophagus may respond to medical management. Not all cases will respond, but some do. Some animals will improve but will never become normal, while others will return completely to normal esophageal motility patterns. The recommended treatment is feeding the dog in an elevated position and training the dog to remain elevated for at least 10 minutes after eating. A slurry of the consistency of pea soup has been very successful. The total dietary requirement should be divided into 2 or 3 feedings. The animals are given water *ad lib*. We have placed the bowl on a table or stepstool and trained the patients to remain elevated following feeding. Some of these patients will periodically develop inhalation pneumonia and will require intermittent therapy for this condition if they are going to respond. It has been our experience that dogs with idiopathic megaesophagus have demonstrated improvement by the time they are one year of age, at the latest.

Acquired achalasia, achalasia of cats and possibly nonresponsive idiopathic megaesophagus should be treated by a modified Heller myotomy (esophagomyotomy). The results of this procedure in acquired achalasia have been good. However, with congenital achalasia, surgical therapy has not been overly successful. The object of the surgery is to produce relaxation of the gastroesophageal sphincter. This produces better emptying of the esophagus by eliminating the functional obstruction.

Following surgery, the esophageal dilatation will generally persist, with consequent intermittent regurgitation. Regurgitation may be controlled by feeding the animal in an elevated position. Some dogs will respond to a diet of dry kibbled dog food fed *ad lib*. Others will do better on a scheduled feeding plan with moist dog food or slurry. The diet must be adjusted by trial and error to fit the particular dog.

## POSTOPERATIVE CARE

Postoperative care following esophageal surgery should include antibiotics and the following diet regimen: no food orally during the first 24 hours, a liquid diet during the next 24 hours, a semisolid diet for the next 48 hours and a gradual return to a regular diet by the seventh postoperative day.

If resection and anastomosis is performed, oral intake of food and water should not be permitted for 72 hours, and the animal should be supported with parenteral fluids. After 72 hours, the oral intake of fluid should start, and the previously discussed diet schedule should be followed carefully.

A pharyngostomy tube may be utilized following esophagoscopic removal of a foreign body. Also when the animal is in poor nutritional condition as the result of acquired achalasia, pharyngostomy may be utilized initially to build the dog up.

## COMPLICATIONS

The primary complication of surgery for cricopharyngeal achalasia or esophageal achalasia is perforation of the esophageal mucosa, resulting in cervical cellulitis or pleuritis. This can be avoided by injecting the occluded esophageal lumen with sterile saline following completion of the myotomy and observing it for leaks.

Complications of esophageal surgery are leakage of the suture line and breakdown of the anastomosis with pleuritis. Usually this is evident by the fifth postoperative day. A stricture may occur following an esophageal anastomosis; however, it can usually be avoided with the use of proper surgical technique.

Complications of foreign body removal may be stricture and perforation. It is necessary to use good judgment in deciding which approach to use in the removal of foreign objects.

### SUPPLEMENTAL READING

Clifford, D. H., Pirsch, J. G., and Maudlin, M. L.: Comparison of motor nuclei of the vagus nerve in dogs with and without esophageal achalasia. Proc. Soc. Exper. Biol. Med., *142*:878, 1973.

Diamant, N., Szczepanski, M., and Mui, H.: Manometric characteristics of idiopathic megaesophagus in the dog: An unsuitable animal model for achalasia in man. Gastroenterology, *65*:216–223, 1973.

Hoffer, R. E.: Diseases of the esophagus. *In* Kirk, R. W. (ed.): Current Veterinary Therapy V. Philadelphia, W. B. Saunders Co., 1974.

Howard, D. R., Lammerding, J. J., and Dewevre, P. B.: Esophageal reinforcement with sternothyroideus muscle in the dog. Canine Pract., July/Aug., 1975, pp. 30–35.

Reed, J. H.: Esophagus. *In* Archibald, J. S. (ed.): Canine Surgery. Santa Barbara, California, American Veterinary Publishing Company, 1974, pp. 482–483.

Rosin, E.: Surgery of the canine esophagus. Vet. Clin. N. Am., 2:17, 1972.

Ryan, W. W., and Greene, R. W.: The conservative management of esophageal foreign bodies and their complications: A review of 66 cases in dogs and cats. J. Am. Animal Hosp. Assn., 11:243, 1975.

---

# TREATMENT OF GASTRIC DILATATION AND TORSION IN THE DOG

DUDLEY E. JOHNSTON, M.V.Sc.
*Philadelphia, Pennsylvania*

Acute gastric dilatation in the dog causes marked pathophysiologic changes. Posterior vena caval pressure rises together with a fall in cardiac output and arterial blood pressure. Compression of the posterior vena cava by the dilated stomach is probably the underlying cause of the increased caval pressure and of the reduced venous return to the heart. Venous return from the stomach is reduced, and respiratory embarrassment occurs, owing to the increased size and pressure of the stomach.

Rapid and complete decompression of the stomach should be the immediate aim when treating cases of gastric dilatation and torsion. Immediate laparotomy to decompress and reposition the stomach has been advocated; however, it is necessary to anesthetize and operate on an animal that is in severe cardiac and respiratory distress. A method has been devised to decompress the stomach rapidly and without the need for general anesthesia; this decompression is followed by a period during which the animal is stabilized before definitive surgical procedures are carried out.

## PROCEDURES ON PRESENTATION

Once the diagnosis of gastric dilatation is made, attempts at gastric decompression are instituted immediately. Initially, in acutely distressed dogs, 18-gauge hypodermic needles are inserted into the stomach to evacuate some of the gas to relieve the dog's critical condition. Then, if the dog's condition and temperament allow, and if it can be accomplished without undue stress, a large-bore stomach tube is passed in an attempt to decompress the stomach. This can be done successfully in most cases of gastric dilatation and in some cases of gastric dilatation with torsion. If the stomach tube can be passed easily, the stomach is emptied and gastric lavage is performed.

If the dog is in a critical condition or passage of the stomach tube is unsuccessful or causes additional stress, immediate gastrostomy is performed.

In the few minutes while the dog is being prepared for gastrostomy, or immediately following gastric decompression by stomach tube, supportive therapy is instituted to stabilize the patient. An 18-gauge indwelling catheter is placed in either the jugular or the cephalic vein. If the jugular vein is used, central venous pressure is monitored during therapy. A multiple electrolyte solution of the replacement type is given at an initial rate of up to 80 ml./kg./hour. If clinical signs or blood pH studies indicate acidosis, sodium bicarbonate is administered intravenously at a rate of 2 to 5 mEq./kg. body weight over 4 to 8 hours. Antibiotics and corticosteroid drugs are administered systemically.

## Gastrostomy

Immediate gastrostomy is done in those dogs that will not tolerate passage of the stomach tube or in which passage of the stomach tube is unsuccessful. The procedure takes only a few minutes, does not appear to add to the stress of the dog and effectively decompresses the stomach. The administration of sedatives for this procedure is usually unnecessary; however, if the animal cannot be physically restrained without stress, meperidine hydrochloride, 1 mg./kg., is administered intramuscularly. The dog is restrained in left lateral recumbency, or the procedure is performed with the dog standing. The incision is made in the most prominent point of distention of the stomach in the right paracostal region. Local anesthetic solution is injected in the form of an L-block. A 5-cm. incision is made in the skin approximately 2 cm. behind and parallel to the costal margin. The external and internal abdominal oblique muscles and the transverse abdominal muscle and peritoneum are split in the direction of the muscle fibers. This exposes the wall of the dilated stomach (Fig. 1). If omentum is covering the stomach, a hole is made in it to gain access to the stomach wall; however,

care should be exercised to avoid damaging blood vessels. The stomach is attached to each end of the skin incision by two stay sutures of 2-0 silk (Fig. 2). The long ends of the stay sutures are used to suture the stomach to the margins of the skin incision with a simple continuous suture, thus isolating an area of stomach wall from the peritoneal cavity. The stomach wall is incised, and the gastric contents are allowed to escape, thus decompressing the stomach (Fig. 3). The cut edges of the stomach are oversewn with 3-0 chromic surgical gut to control bleeding, if this is found necessary. Following evacuation of stomach contents, the interior of the stomach is lavaged through the gastrostomy with saline, and the stomach wall is inspected for signs of ischemia.

## Stabilization of the Animal

Following gastric decompression (either by passage of a stomach tube or gastrostomy), hydration, renal function and electrolyte balance are assessed, and corrections are made to stabilize the animal completely.

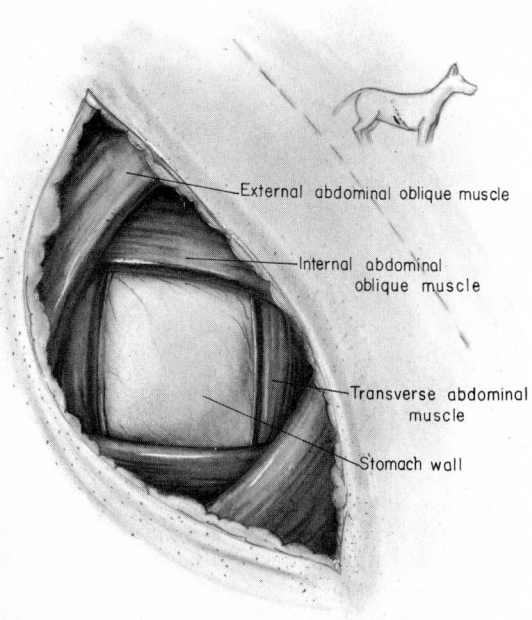

External abdominal oblique muscle

Internal abdominal oblique muscle

Transverse abdominal muscle

Stomach wall

**Figure 1.**  The dilated stomach is exposed through a 5-cm. paracostal skin incision and blunt dissection of the abdominal muscles. (Courtesy of The Journal of Small Animal Practice, *14*:131, 1973.)

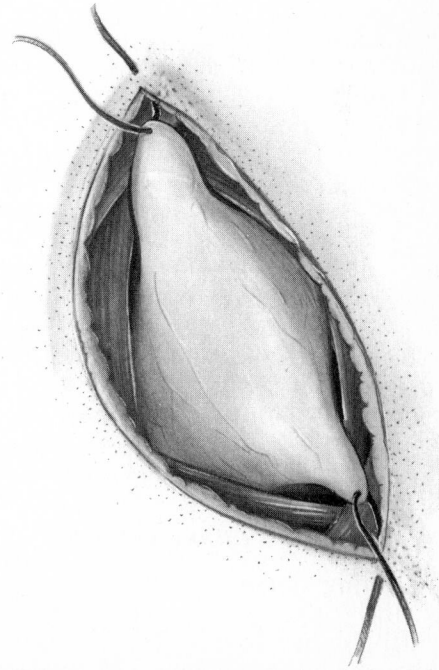

**Figure 2.**  Stay sutures of 2-0 silk are used to attach the stomach wall to each end of the skin incision. (Courtesy of The Journal of Small Animal Practice, *14*:131, 1973.)

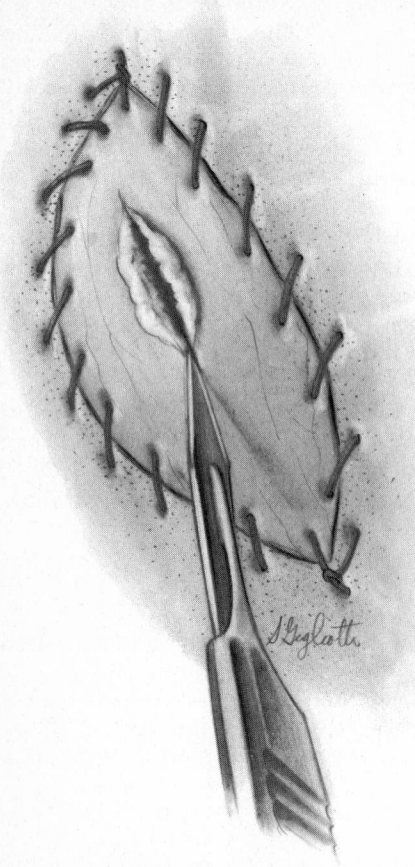

**Figure 3.** The stomach wall is sutured to the skin with 2-0 silk suture and the stomach wall is then incised. (Courtesy of The Journal of Small Animal Practice, *14*:131, 1973.)

**Table 1.** *Feeding Regimen for a Large Dog (e.g., German Shepherd) Following Treatment of Gastric Dilatation and Torsion*

| | |
|---|---|
| First 24 hours after surgery: | No oral food or water |
| | Intravenous fluid (60 ml./kg.) |
| Second day after surgery: | 08.00 1/3 can moist dog food |
| | 09.00 500 ml. water |
| | 11.00 1/3 can moist dog food |
| | 12.00 500 ml. water |
| | 13.00 1/2 can moist dog food |
| | 14.00 water *ad lib* |
| | 16.00 1/2 can moist dog food |
| | 20.00 1/2 can moist dog food |
| Third day and thereafter until discharge: | 1/2 can moist dog food 4 times per day. Water *ad lib*. |
| After discharge from hospital: | The owner is advised to divide the dog's normal diet into several portions and feed the dog three or four times per day. The dog should not be exercised for at least one hour after eating. |

From Pass, M. A., and Johnston, Dudley E.: J. Small Animal Pract., *14*:131, 1973.

## PROCEDURE FOLLOWING DECOMPRESSION BY STOMACH TUBE

If subsequent dilatation does not occur, exploratory laparotomy is usually not necessary. Food and water are restricted as outlined in Table 1. Recurrence of gastric dilatation may indicate the presence of a gastric torsion or a continuing problem, and exploratory laparotomy should be performed.

## PROCEDURE FOLLOWING DECOMPRESSION BY GASTROSTOMY

Following decompression by gastrostomy, the patient is completely stabilized, as outlined previously. In general, this stabilization occurs over a period ranging from 2 to 24 hours. The animal is then anesthetized, and a definitive surgical procedure is performed.

The first, and sometimes the only, procedure is closure of the gastric fistula. The incision in the stomach wall is closed temporarily with a simple continuous suture. The previously clipped area of skin is cleaned and draped. The stomach wall at both ends of the incision is grasped with Babcock forceps, the silk sutures between the stomach and skin are removed and the stomach wall is lifted from the abdomen. Dry towels are placed on the skin, and warm, saline-soaked towels are packed around the abdominal incision to prevent contamination of the peritoneal cavity. The area of stomach wall containing the sutured gastrostomy incision is excised. The gastric mucosa is closed with simple interrupted sutures of 3-0 surgical gut, and the muscular and serosal layers are closed with a Cushing suture of 3-0 surgical gut. The stomach wall is cleansed with warm saline and returned to the abdomen.

At this time, one can determine by observation and palpation whether gastric torsion or splenic torsion is present and whether other complications, such as necrosis of the stomach wall, have occurred. If no complications exist, the muscular layers of the abdominal wall are closed in layers, and the skin incision is sutured.

If complications are found, a midline exploratory laparotomy is done following closure of the gastrostomy incision, and definitive surgical correction is instituted.

## EXPLORATORY LAPAROTOMY

The abdomen is entered through a midline incision that extends from the xyphoid process of the sternum to a point caudal to the umbilicus. The stomach is located, the direction of torsion is determined and the stomach is untwisted. If an associated spenic torsion is present, the spleen is removed. The stomach wall is examined for any areas of ischemic necrosis, and such areas are carefully excised.

Finally, in order to prevent postoperative accumulation of gas in the stomach, a tube gastrostomy is performed. A soft rubber tube, approximately No. 22 French, or a Foley catheter is inserted into the stomach, using one of two accepted methods. A simple method is to insert the tube into the lumen through a small stab incision. The incision and 2 to 3 cm. of tube length are covered by a series of inverting Lembert or Cushing sutures. A second method is to insert the tube into the lumen through a small stab incision that has first been surrounded by a purse-string suture. This suture is tightened and tied, inverting an area of gastric wall. A second purse-string suture is inserted to invert still more gastric wall around the tube. The gastrostomy tube is brought out through a stab incision in the abdominal wall. The area of stomach surrounding the tube is sutured to the abdominal wall with simple interrupted sutures of 2-0 surgical gut to prevent leakage of gastric contents into the peritoneal cavity and to form a gastropexy.

## POSTOPERATIVE CARE AFTER LAPAROTOMY

No oral food or water is permitted during the first 24 hours following surgery. The dog is maintained by intravenous administration of a replacement and a maintenance type of multiple electrolyte solution at a total dose rate of 60 ml./kg. in 24 hours. Oral feeding is begun on the second postoperative day. The feeding and watering regimen for a large dog is outlined in Table 1. The gastrostomy tube is removed 2 or 3 days after surgery by simply pulling it out. It should be left in place for longer periods if postoperative accumulation of gas is occurring. The tube should be clamped between aspirations of gas to avoid loss of acid gastric fluids.

### SUPPLEMENTAL READING

Pass, M. A., and Johnston, D. E.: Treatment of gastric dilatation and torsion in the dog. Gastric decompression by gastrostomy under local analgesia. J. Small Animal Pract., 14:131, 1973.
Walshaw, R., and Johnston, D. E.: Treatment of gastric dilatation/volvulus by gastric decompression and patient stabilization before major surgery. J.A.A.H.A., 12:162, 1976.

# NEOPLASMS OF THE DIGESTIVE TRACT IN THE DOG

AMIYA K. PATNAIK, D.V.M.,
and ARTHUR I. HURVITZ, D.V.M.
New York, New York

Neoplasms of the gastrointestinal tract are not uncommon in animals and form a significant part of the neoplastic process in the dog. The oral cavity has the highest incidence of tumors in comparison with any other segment of this tract. Adenocarcinomas of the stomach and intestines are more common than benign epithelial

**Table 1.** *Distribution of Tumors of the Intestinal Tract of the Dog\**

|  | ADENO-CARCINOMA | CARCINOID | LEIOMYO-SARCOMA |
|---|---|---|---|
| Duodenum | 7 | 2 | 3 |
| Jejunum | 4 | 0 | 6 |
| Ileum | 1 | 0 | 1 |
| Cecum | 0 | 0 | 4 |
| Colon | 9 | 2 | 3 |
| Rectum | 10 | 0 | 0 |
| Unknown | 3 | 0 | 2 |
| TOTAL | 34 | 4 | 19 |

\*From a survey of necropsies at The Animal Medical Center.

tumors and benign or malignant connective tissue tumors. Cancers of the colon, rectum and duodenum are more common than those of other segments of the bowel. The average age of animals with adenocarcinomas of the stomach (10 years) and the bowel (9 years) is lower than that of animals with connective tissue tumors (15.8 and 11.4 years). Incidence in males was predominant for all gastric tumors and adenocarcinomas of the bowel. Leiomyosarcomas of the intestines occurred more frequently in females than in males. Although no obvious breed predisposition was seen in cases of gastrointestinal tract tumors, it was significant that none of the intestinal adenocarcinomas occurred in the boxer breed of dogs, which has often been considered to be more predisposed to various neoplastic processes.

## TUMORS OF THE MOUTH

Melanoma is the most common tumor that occurs in the oral cavity. Of 68 oral melanomas, more than half occurred in the gum. The next most common sites, which represented only 7 to 10 per cent of the tumors, were the tongue, lip and palate. The average age of these animals was 11.4 years, and 59 per cent of the tumors occurred in males. A predisposition of cocker spaniel dogs to oral melanomas has been documented. Obvious local invasion occurred in 81 per cent of these animals, and 50 per cent were presented with ulceration at the tumor site. Melanomas occurring in the oral cavity were less melanotic and more malignant in comparison to melanomas of other sites.

Among the other common tumors seen in the oral cavity, including the tongue, are fibrosarcoma, squamous cell carcinoma and adenocarcinoma. The rarer tumors seen are lymphosarcoma, mast cell tumors of the lips and ameloblastoma involving the gum. Soft tissue tumors sometimes infiltrate the maxilla and mandible and on rare occasions metastasize to these bones from other sites. Chondrosarcoma rather than osteosarcoma is the more common primary tumor of the bones in the oral cavity. Melanomas, carcinomas and squamous cell carcinomas readily metastasize to the regional lymph nodes and other sites. Fibrosarcomas and primary bone tumors, on the other hand, rarely metastasize, but often form massive destructive lesions in the oral cavity.

A highly malignant tumor of a primitive cell is seen in young animals (6 months to one year of age) that may initially be considered non-neoplastic because of the young age. This tumor is presented as a primary lesion of the oral cavity, especially of the palate and gum. Diagnosis of cancer can be positively made from biopsy, but these tumors are not distinguishable as carcinoma or sarcoma with light microscopy. The maximal survival time of these animals after the tumor diagnosis is less than 6 months.

Common clinical signs associated with neoplasms of the oral cavity are increased salivation, difficulty in eating and anorexia. Sarcomas are often ulcerating mass lesions in the oral cavity, whereas mass lesions are less obvious in cases of epithelial tumors. Biopsy of the tumor serves as the best aid to diagnosis. Neoplasms arising from the major salivary glands are rare but are highly malignant and often show local invasion as well as distant metastasis. Malignant mixed tumors, mucoepidermoid adenocarcinomas and adenocarcinomas are the common types of tumors seen in these glands. The differential diagnoses to be considered in this region are salivary gland cysts, chronic lymphadenitis, lymphoma, carotid body tumor, thyroid neoplasms and metastatic oral tumors.

## TUMORS OF THE ESOPHAGUS

Primary tumors of the esophagus are very rare, except for fibrosarcomas and extraskeletal osteosarcomas occurring in the endemic areas of *Spirocerca lupi* infection, where the parasites are responsible for these tumors. Leiomyomas are more common than carcinomas. Thyroid adenocarcinomas, mammary adenocarcinomas and lymphosarcomas are among the most common primary tumors that metastasize to the esophagus. Clinical signs result from esophageal constriction, and diagnosis can be made by contrast radiography, endoscopic examination and pathologic examination of biopsy specimens.

## TUMORS OF THE STOMACH

In a survey of 10,270 canine necropsies done at The Animal Medical Center, 26 cases of adenocarcinomas of the stomach were diagnosed with a frequency rate of 0.25 per cent. The pyloric area was the most common site. The leiomyomas were the second most common type of tumor seen, followed by leiomyosarcoma, lymphosarcoma and benign epithelial tumors. The average age of dogs with adenocarcinoma was 10 years, much lower than the average age of dogs with leiomyomas, which was 15.8 years in this series. The adenocarcinomas (61 per cent) as well as the leiomyomas (71 per cent) were seen predominantly in the males. Obvious breed predispositions were not seen in either of the tumors.

The most common presenting clinical signs of dogs with adenocarcinomas are persistent vomiting, weight loss, anorexia and depression. Ascites, jaundice, diarrhea, coughing and dyspnea are less common signs. Although most of the leiomyomas were small and were detected only at necropsy, the presenting signs were similar to those for adenocarcinoma. Most adenocarcinomas and all lymphosarcomas have various sized gastric ulcers, and both these tumors are seen as diffuse lesions with thickened walls, but the lesions are very firm in cases of adenocarcinoma. All the lymphosarcomas occurring in the stomach were reticulum cell sarcomas. Both the benign and malignant tumors of the muscles were usually seen as extramucosal localized mass lesions. On examination, abdominal masses are sometimes palpated in all types of tumors. Plain and contrast radiography, gastroscopy and biopsy aid in diagnosis.

On rare occasions, metastatic tumors are seen in the gastric wall. These include adenocarcinomas of the mammary gland, intestines and pancreas; lymphosarcomas; hemangiosarcomas; and undifferentiated sarcomas. Eosinophilic gastroenteritis is a rare condition in dogs but should be considered as a differential diagnosis, since the clinical and radiographic signs may be similar.

## TUMORS OF THE INTESTINES

Table 1 shows the frequency of the two most common tumors seen in the intestinal tract of the dog, as reviewed in a survey of 10,270 necropsies at The Animal Medical Center. A total of 34 adenocarcinomas and 4 carcinoids were seen with an incidence rate of 0.37 per cent, which is higher than that of the gastric carcinomas. The duodenum, colon and rectum were almost equally involved. This distribution is close to that in man and contrasts with the incidence in cats, in which more than 50 per cent of the adenocarcinomas are seen in the ileum, and the colon and rectum are rarely involved. Leiomyosarcomas seem to occur more frequently in those sites where adenocarcinomas do not occur. For example, adenocarcinomas are not seen in the cecum, which is a common site of leiomyosarcomas.

The average age of the dogs with adenocarcinoma of the intestinal tract was 9 years, and the incidence in males was greater than that in females. The leiomyosarcomas occurred in a slightly higher age group (11.4 years), and sex distribution was the reverse of that of adenocarcinoma, with 66 per cent occurring in females. No obvious breed predispositions were noted. The boxer breed, with its recognized predisposition for various tumors and specific enteropathies such as boxer colitis, was conspicuously absent in this review of adenocarcinomas of the small and large bowel.

Lymphosarcoma of the intestines is rare and usually involves multiple segments of the bowel and the adjoining lymph nodes. These are usually ulcerating mass lesions, and malabsorption is an important clinical feature in addition to other clinical signs. Other rare tumors of the bowel are the carcinoids, mast cell tumors and neurofibromas. Bowel walls are not uncommon sites of metastasis. Besides direct infiltration from the pancreas, bile ducts and generalized neoplastic process of the peritoneal cavity, distant metastases are seen in both the muscular wall and the mucosa from a number of tumors (e.g., hemangiosarcoma, intestinal adenocarcinoma, mammary adenocarcinoma, lymphosarcoma and plasma cell tumors). One case was seen in which the clinical, endoscopic and histologic examination revealed a condition similar to human juvenile polyposis in a 1-year-old dog.

As in the stomach, eosinophilic enteritis should be remembered when considering the diagnosis of neoplasm of the bowel, especially lymphosarcoma. In eosinophilic enteritis the bowel wall may be greatly thickened and the draining lymph nodes are often enlarged. These cases may resemble intestinal lymphoma, except for the presence of eosinophilia.

Animals with tumors of the small bowel may be presented because of weight loss, anorexia, vomiting, diarrhea (sometimes with blood) and ascites. Palpation sometimes reveals an abdominal mass. Radiographic contrast studies and exploratory surgery aid in diagnosis. Dogs with tumors of the colon and rectum are usually presented with straining, rectal bleeding, diarrhea, anorexia, depression, rectal prolapse and ascites. Rectal examination demonstrates stenosis or palpable mass lesions. Proctoscopy usually shows ulcerating lesions, and proctoscopic biopsies are helpful in diagnosis. In both cases of duodenal carcinoid in our series, the animals presented with diarrhea in addition to other nonspecific clinical signs.

## TUMORS OF THE ANUS

Apart from perianal gland tumors, which are usually benign and seen mostly in aged male dogs, adenocarcinomas and melanomas are only occasionally seen in the anal area. Anal melanomas are as malignant as those of the oral cavity.

## THERAPY

Oral tumors are treated with chemotherapy, immunotherapy, conventional surgery, cryosurgery and different combinations of these. Malignant tumors have only temporarily responded to treatment, but these procedures have prolonged the survival time of the animals.

Tumors of the remainder of the gastrointestinal tract, except the rectum, hardly respond to treatment, and most animals die or are euthanatized. In cases of rectal carcinomas, cryosurgery seems to have prolonged the life of the animal, although complete elimination of the tumor is rarely achieved.

The reader is referred to the articles on the management of cancer patients for a more complete discussion (see pages 479 to 490).

# THE MAL-ABSORPTION SYNDROMES

NEIL V. ANDERSON, D.V.M.
*Manhattan, Kansas*

The malabsorption syndromes are chronic diarrheal diseases characterized by weight loss and constant or recurrent large-volume diarrhea (Ewing, 1971; Schall, 1974; Van Kruiningen, 1968). Defecation occurs 4 to 6 times daily, usually without tenesmus. Mucus-entrapped gas may impart a foamy consistency to the feces. Steatorrhea is the hallmark of the malabsorption syndromes and is noted by the rancid odor or as liquid or congealed fat in the feces.

The client may describe weakness or reduced vigor, dull hair coat, steatorrhea, borborygmus and flatulence. Voracious appetite is a common sign, but some dogs reduce their food intake. Hyperphagic dogs may have abdominal distention. Vomiting occurs but is not a prominent complaint. Edema is noted in some cases. Lack of sustained response to symptomatic treatments is usual for all malabsorption syndromes.

The physical findings confirm the client's observations. The degree of debilitation is related to duration of illness and severity of the lesion. Abdominal distention may occasionally be due to hypoproteinemic ascites, but increased volume of intestinal content is the usual cause. Thickened or distended loops of small intestine may be palpable. Fever and abdominal pain are not common.

The clinician uses "malabsorption syndrome" as a working hypothesis based on observation. It is not a diagnosis unless qualified as to etiologic agent, or anatomic or biochemical defect. If steatorrhea is not present, digestion and absorption of nutrients may in fact not be greatly impaired, and one should rule out common causes of chronic diarrhea as described below. When maldigestion or malabsorption is suspected on the basis of history and physical examination, a hematologic data base should be gathered and reviewed. Anemia, leukocytosis, lymphocytosis, lymphopenia or eosinophilia is present in certain of these syndromes. Further testing may reveal hypoproteinemia, hypoalbuminemia, hyperglobulinemia, hypocholesterolemia, hyperglycemia or hypoglycemia. Review of all abnormalities in the data base will usually give a strong sense of diagnostic perspective toward the probability of malabsorption.

## DIAGNOSTIC WORK-UP

The clinical work-up of the malabsorption syndromes is time-consuming for the veterinarian and expensive for the client. Recognizing that these constraints exist, certain common causes of chronic diarrhea should be ruled out before the malabsorption syndromes are given further serious consideration.

The problem-oriented approach to diagnosis (POVMR) (Welser, 1975) is particularly helpful in the work-up of the malabsorption syndromes. The rule-out designator (R/O) as used below means that the disease is probably present, based on history, signs and findings, or is a common disease that should be ruled out before proceeding with the work-up. When the initial data base (history, physical findings and initial laboratory data) does not permit diagnosis nor guide therapy, the most probable diagnoses may be ranked in decreasing order of probability and ruled out by an appropriate diagnostic plan. Alternatively, one may rank the rule-outs on the basis of least cost, deferring the more expensive diagnostic procedures until later. Several excellent algorithms, each compatible with the problem-oriented method, have been devised for guiding the diagnostic work-up (Lorenz *et al.*, 1975; Van Kruiningen and Hayden, 1972). The stepwise work-up described below has been useful to the author, when the case at hand lacks distinguishing features that would lead more directly to the diagnosis.

The initial rule-outs (R/O) are made by review of the history and by fecal examinations.

(a) *R/O Endoparasitism*: Direct microscopic and fecal flotation examinations should both be done. Unless the condition of the animal requires immediate treatment, a triad of fecal examinations at 48-hour intervals can be done before the animal is hospitalized for more extensive work-up. The latter approach is particularly indicated for the kennel-dwelling dog. If endoparasitism is confirmed, treatment is given and the dog is observed for 14 to 28 days. If no improvement occurs, the malabsorption work-up is continued. *Coccidia* and *Giardia* parasitize mucosal cells and thus may produce a malabsorption syndrome. Repeated direct microscopic examination of feces in warm saline and flotation examinations are quite reliable for demonstrating these protozoan parasites. Rarely, giardiasis is diagnosed by means of intestinal intubation or mucosal biopsy.

(b) *R/O Microbial Infection*: Persistent diarrhea of less than 14 days' duration will often resolve spontaneously after immunity to microbial agents has developed. Alternatively, extended antibiotic therapy may result in cure.

(c) *R/O Dietary Cause*: A trial change of ration supervised by the veterinarian should precede the work-up, unless it has already been properly done by the client or by another veterinarian. Habitual scavenging can cause recurrent diarrhea. Confinement at home for at least a week with feeding of a standard complete ration is an inexpensive alternative to hospitalization. Exclusion of milk from the test diet may control the diarrhea (Hill, 1972). If reintroduction of milk is followed by diarrhea, a tentative diagnosis of milk intolerance is made. Further resolution of the problem requires intestinal biopsy and assay of lactose activity on the mucosal surface.

(d) *R/O Emotional Factors*: Some dogs respond to emotional stress with recurrent or persistent diarrhea. General health usually remains excellent, and debilitation does not occur. The carefully taken history should adequately rule out this possibility.

## MALDIGESTION

The next diagnostic effort, the above diagnoses having been ruled out, is to identify whether maldigestion exists. Three causes of maldigestion are summarized in Table 1.

Pancreatic maldigestion is characterized by weight loss, hyperphagia, diarrhea and steatorrhea. Large-volume fecal passage occurs five or more times daily. Feces are pungent and have a greasy texture. Coprophagia may be noted. Rarely, edema due to hypoalbuminemia exists in cases of long duration.

Fasting hyperlipidemia and hyperglycemia (100 to 180 mg./dl.) occur in end-stage chronic pancreatitis. Dogs with JPA often have fasting plasma glucose values of 100 to 130 mg./dl. but are not hyperlipidemic. Differentiation between juvenile pancreatic atrophy and end-stage chronic pancreatitis is based on age of onset (<2 years vs. 5 to 8 years) and breed (JPA is predominantly but not exclusively a disease of the German shepherd breed). Past history of painful anterior abdominal disease or of a severe vomiting syndrome is often given for chronic pancreatitis. Abdominal exploration and biopsy will differentiate the two forms of pancreatic disease but are seldom indicated if response to replacement therapy is obtained. The use of pancreatic extract as a combined diagnostic and therapeutic tool is frequently the first step in office practice. If it is successful, much time and effort have been conserved; if it fails, one proceeds with the laboratory phase of the clinical work-up.

Approximately 75 per cent of all the malabsorption syndromes in dogs are caused by pancreatic exocrine insufficiency (Schall, 1974). The severity of steatorrhea in this disorder sets it in a class apart from gastric and biliary disease, in which mild steatorrhea occurs. Vomiting, anorexia, hematemesis and anterior abdominal pain and mass are likely to predominate in gastric disease, while icterus usually accompanies biliary obstruction. Prospectively, one might investigate for fat malabsorption in long-standing cases of nonicteric liver disease, e.g., in congenital vascular anomalies causing liver atrophy and in hepatic fibrosis.

**Tests of Maldigestion.** Steatorrhea is demonstrated by applying Sudan III or IV or oil red O stain to fresh feces on a glass slide (Van Kruiningen and Hayden, 1972). The number of orange-stained globules of undigested lipid per high-power field is compared to that of a healthy dog fed a standard commercial ration. As many as three globules per high-power field may be seen in normal feces. Larger numbers of

*Table 1.   Maldigestion in Dogs*

| DISEASE | FUNCTIONAL ABNORMALITY | DIAGNOSTIC PROCEDURE |
|---|---|---|
| Pancreatic Exocrine Insufficiency | Incomplete digestion | Sudan or oil red O stain |
|   Juvenile pancreatic atrophy (JPA) | Steatorrhea | Fecal trypsin test ↓ |
|   Chronic pancreatitis | Creatorrhea | Fat absorption test ↓ |
| | Amylorrhea | Glucose tolerance test ↓ |
| | | Fecal fat analysis ↑ |
| | | Exploratory laparotomy |
| Gastric Disease | Rapid emptying and | Radiocontrast studies |
|   Surgical resection |   incomplete chymification | Gastroscopy |
|   Chronic gastritis | Steatorrhea | |
| Biliary Obstruction | Hepatic atrophy | |
| | Bile-salt deficiency | Sudan or oil red O stain |
| |   and incomplete lipolysis | Observe for icterus |
| | Steatorrhea | Van den Bergh test ↑ |

stained globules occur in pancreatic mal-digestion, as well as when excessive dietary fat has been consumed. Dietary-fat overload is ruled out by history or by repeating the test after the dog has been on a standard commercial ration for several days. If the feces are grossly fatty, criteria being odor, appearance and tactile impressions, but lack stained globules, digestion has proceeded normally and malabsorption is suspected. In these instances, one should inspect the slide for unstained, needle-like fatty-acid crystals.

The clinician should also search for mal-digestion of other nutrients. Undigested meat fibers are found by Lugol's iodine stain, preferably after fresh, raw chunks of meat are fed. Commercial canned meat foods usually do not contain intact fibers. Fecal starch content is variable in normal dogs. Persistent gross amylorrhea, also de-tected by iodine stain, suggests that mal-digestion is of pancreatic origin.

Pancreatic maldigestion is ruled out by demonstration of tryptic activity of feces on a gelatin substrate (tube test is preferred) at 1:100 dilution. Feces from dogs with pan-creatic maldigestion may liquefy gelatin at a lesser dilution, e.g., 1:10, perhaps because bacterial proteases are present, but such false positive results are avoided by concur-rent use of a 1:100 dilution. The test may be performed daily for 3 to 5 days if results are equivocal.

Plasma turbidity after a fat meal is reli-able evidence of normal pancreatic lipolytic activity. Vegetable oil (3 ml./kg. body weight) is fed after a 16-hour fast. Most dogs will readily lap the oil from a feeding pan, obviating the need for passing a stomach tube. Anticoagulated blood samples are drawn initially and at 2 and 3 hours after feeding. Readily visible turbidity of the plasma constitutes a positive test result and is interpreted as adequate digestive and ab-sorptive capacity for lipid. The zero-time sample is taken to rule out fasting hyper-lipidemia, which may occur in end-stage chronic pancreatitis, diabetes mellitus, hypothyroidism, renal amyloidosis and the nephrotic syndrome.

Both fecal trypsin and fat absorption tests are subject to false negative results. Fecal trypsin activity varies greatly from day to day as a result of variations in daily secre-tion and in rate of degradation of enzyme during transit through the gut. Plasma tur-bidity may not be achieved during the test period because of delayed or erratic gastric emptying or because of enteritis or other in-testinal lesion. However, false positive re-sults do not occur with the fat absorption test if a fasting plasma sample is always used as a control. These two tests share the advantage of being inexpensive and easy to perform and are within the capabilities of every veterinarian.

Glucose tolerance is usually reduced in pancreatic maldigestion. Both the oral and high-dose intravenous glucose tolerance tests (OGTT and H-IVGTT) have been used to demonstrate that most dogs with JPA are prediabetic according to glucose tolerance criteria (Greve and Anderson, 1973; Hill and Kidder, 1972). A critical comparison of the two tests has not been reported. If other data are equivocal, and quantitative fecal fat analysis or exploratory laparotomy is not a viable option, one might do a glucose toler-ance test. The OGTT has the added advan-tage of testing the absorptive capacity of the intestinal mucosa but is more time-consuming to perform.

The dose for the OGTT is 2 gm. glucose/ kg. body weight as a 12.5 per cent solution. One gm. glucose/kg. body weight is the dose for the H-IVGTT. A 50 per cent solu-tion is given IV as a bolus in 30 to 45 sec-onds. Samples are drawn at 0, 30, 60, 90, 120, 150 and 180 minutes for OGTT, and data are plotted on conventional graph paper. The curve should not exceed 160 mg./dl. and should return to the fasting value by 180 minutes or before. The H-IVGTT data are plotted on semilogarithm paper and the k-value, or steepness of slope of the curve, should exceed 2.0. The curve should return to the fasting value by 60 minutes.

Quantitative fecal fat analysis is done by determining total and split (digested) fats on an aliquot of a total 72-hour quantitatively collected fecal specimen. Fecal fat excre-tion in excess of 5 gm./24 hr. in a large dog and a predominance of unsplit fats (neutral triglyceride) confirms the diagnosis of pan-creatic exocrine insufficiency (Hayden and Van Kruiningen, 1976) but does not rule out concurrent malabsorption of fat. If lipid is predominantly digested and fecal trypsin is normal, pancreatic exocrine insufficiency is ruled out and malabsorption is suspected.

## MALABSORPTION

When maldigestion has been ruled out, the work-up of intestinal malabsorption begins. The data base should be expanded to include not only hematologic data but serum electrophoresis and chemical tests as well. The malabsorptive diseases are grouped in Table 2 in the approximate order of complexity of diagnostic effort.

The protozoal diseases will probably have been ruled out earlier in the work-up. Warm 0.85 per cent saline solution is recommended for direct microscopic examinations for trophozoites. Tap water will lyse or distort these parasites. Lugol's solution is useful for identifying protozoan cysts. Always examine under high-dry and oil-immersion objectives. PAF fixative is help-

ful in preserving and concentrating protozoa in feces (Buckner and Ewing, 1974). Thionin or azure A stain is recommended for improved visualization of the protozoa.

*Lactase deficiency* may have been ruled out during the outpatient phase of the work-up. If not, careful exclusion of dietary lactose by use of an all-meat or a hamburger and rice ration should be done in the hospital. Rarely, mucosal biopsy and lactase assay may be necessary for diagnosis.

*The stagnant loop syndrome* is a debilitating diarrheal disease resulting from stasis of ingesta anterior to partial obstruction of the small bowel. The lesion site is usually quite distal in the small bowel, and vomiting is infrequent or may not occur. Congenital or acquired stenoses, foreign bodies, tumors, intussusception and cecal

*Table 2.* *Intestinal Malabsorption in Dogs*

| DISEASE | FUNCTIONAL ABNORMALITY | DIAGNOSTIC PROCEDURE | CHANGE FROM NORMAL |
|---|---|---|---|
| Protozoal Enteritis Coccidiosis Giardiasis | Hypermotility Osmotic diarrhea due to intraluminal retention of water by unabsorbed particles | Flotation and direct fecal examinations | |
| Lactase Deficiency | Osmotic diarrhea due to colonic bacterial production of volatile fatty acids from lactose | Milk-free ration Lactase assay of mucosal biopsy | ↓ |
| Stagnant Loop Syndrome (partial obstruction of small bowel) | Putrefaction, osmotic diarrhea Deconjugation and dehydroxylation of bile acids, reducing fat absorption | Abdominal palpation Radiocontrast studies Exploratory laparotomy | |
| Eosinophilic Gastroenteritis Visceral larva migrans Other causes | Hypermotility Osmotic diarrhea | Eosinophil count Full-thickness biopsy | ↑ |
| Lymphangiectasia | Fat malabsorption, steatorrhea Fatty-acid hydroxylated by bacteria → "castor-oil" effect | Lymphocyte count Serum albumin Serum globulin Serum cholesterol $^{51}$Cr-albumin in feces Augmented fat absorption test Vitamin A absorption Fecal fat excretion D-Xylose absorption Full-thickness biopsy | ↓ ↓ ↓ ↓ ↑ ↓ ↓ ↑ ± |
| Other Diseases Villus atrophy Lymphocytic-plasmacytic enteritis Histoplasmosis Chronic "bacterial" enteritis Malignant lymphoma Amyloidosis | Fat malabsorption, steatorrhea Fatty-acid hydroxylated by bacteria → "castor-oil" effect Osmotic diarrhea | Leukocytosis Serum albumin Augmented fat absorption test $^{51}$Cr-albumin in feces Fecal fat excretion Full-thickness biopsy | ↓ ↓ ↑± ↑ |

inversion are some of the causes. The stagnant loop tends to dilate with the passage of time, and the dilated loop and the site of obstruction may be palpable.

Putrefaction of nutrients in the stagnant loop interferes with normal digestion and promotes osmotic retention of water in the static loop of bowel. Intermittent, often explosive diarrhea alternating with passage of partially formed feces is a distinguishing feature of the stagnant loop syndrome. Bacterial colonies attach to the mucosal surface and not only interfere with nutrient absorption but may induce net secretion of water into the lumen. Bacterial deconjugation and dehydroxylation of bile acids occurs and may be a cause of steatorrhea (Wilson and Dietschy, 1971). Decreased absorption of vitamin $B_{12}$ and iron has been postulated as a cause of anemia in dogs with stagnant loop syndrome.

Short-term clinical and hematologic improvement may be obtained with broad-spectrum antibiotic therapy. Suppression of bacterial numbers in the stagnant bowel often proves deceiving to patient, clinician and client. Relapse invariably occurs after antibiotic therapy is discontinued and serves as a strong clue to the diagnosis. Radiocontrast studies are most helpful in confirming the diagnosis.

*Eosinophilic gastroenteritis* is an allergic disease occurring in dogs of all ages past the neonatal period. Soft to fluid diarrhea, often with blood, is usually observed, as are low-grade fever, partial anorexia, depression and weight loss. Thickened, tender loops of small intestine may be palpated. An absolute eosinophilia of 2000/cu. mm. or more is commonly, but not invariably, detected. Radiocontrast studies may reveal thickening of small bowel but do not further refine the diagnosis.

Some cases of eosinophilic gastroenteritis are caused by visceral larva migrans of *Toxocara* spp., particularly in dogs under 3 years of age. The lesions tend to be focal and very thick and are not limited to the gastrointestinal tract. Other cases have diffuse infiltration of eosinophils into the lamina propria, including the villus core, or deeper into the submucosa and muscularis. The latter do not have histopathologic evidence of larval migration. Food allergy has not been proved to be a cause of eosinophilic gastroenteritis in dogs. Food allergy and food intolerance have presented as vomiting or vomiting-diarrhea syndromes, in the author's experience, rather than as malabsorption syndromes.

The remaining diseases constitute the "hard core" of intestinal malabsorption syndromes because of insidious onset, inconstancy of signs, slowly debilitating course and usual absence of pain. The clinical signs and many of the laboratory test results are related to the location and severity of the lesion rather than to the etiologic agent. Thus, intestinal biopsy is essential to the diagnosis in many cases.

*Lymphangiectasia* is a severe protein-losing enteropathy with obstructed, dilated lacteals in one or more layers of the small bowel. Diarrhea is usual but inconstant. Weight loss, lassitude, variable appetite, vomiting, ascites and peripheral edema are characteristic, particularly in the advanced case.

Absorption of long-chain fatty acids into lymph is impaired. Bulk loss of lymph into the intestinal lumen results in lymphopenia, hypoproteinemia, hypoalbuminemia and hypoglobulinemia. The serum cholesterol value is often below 140 mg./dl. Low total serum calcium (7.0 to 8.5 mg./dl.) is associated with hypoalbuminemia, as it is in a number of diseases in which serum albumin is decreased. Hypocalcemia and calcium gluconate–responsive "seizures" have been reported in a dog with lymphangiectasia (Finco *et al.*, 1973). Moderate anemia may exist.

Fecal excretion of digested fat is increased. Alternatively, the augmented fat absorption test may be used to assess fat malabsorption. Pancreatic enzyme–treated lipid (one teaspoonful per 10 ml. of vegetable oil) is incubated for 20 minutes at room temperature before feeding as a fat meal. Positive plasma turbidity at 2 and 3 hours rules out severe fat malabsorption. The use of $^{131}$I-triolein, $^{131}$I-oleic acid and vitamin A absorption to assess fat absorptive ability is limited to referral centers for the former and to commercial laboratories for vitamin A determinations. Proteinuria as a cause of protein loss must be ruled out by serial urinalysis. Liver disease must also be ruled out as a cause of hypoalbuminemia.

D-Xylose absorption may be decreased in severe lymphangiectasia. Xylose is a pentose sugar that is absorbed passively and by facilitated diffusion from the small intestine. Both false positive and false negative results are obtained. A peak absorption value of 45 mg./dl. or greater is evidence for adequate absorption but does not rule out intestinal disease in the dog. Values below 45 mg./dl. suggest but do not prove that intestinal malabsorption exists. False negative results may occur. As with other function tests, the nature of the intestinal lesion is not revealed.

Other intestinal function tests include oral glucose, lactose and starch tolerance tests. A "flat" glucose curve for each indicates malabsorption. Lymphangiectasia is suspected on the basis of hypoproteinemia, lymphopenia, hypocholesterolemia and one or more abnormal absorption tests; biopsy confirms the diagnosis.

*Villus atrophy* occurs when intestinal mucosal cells are depleted in numbers and villi become atrophic, blunted or fused. Epitheliotropic viral infections cause acute, reversible villus atrophy in piglets, kittens and calves, but the cause of persistent villus atrophy in dogs is not known. The failure of absorption predisposes to diarrhea, as bacteria in the ileum and colon metabolize the undigested food and cause an increase in osmolality of colon contents. Villus atrophy can be suspected by intestinal function tests but is ruled out with assurance only by means of intestinal biopsy.

*Lymphocytic-plasmacytic enteritis* may be a persistent immunologic reaction to chronic bacterial infection or to other ingested or inhaled antigen(s). Diagnosis is made by means of biopsy.

*Histoplasmosis* can involve the small intestine as well as other gastrointestinal organs and causes weight loss, fever and bloody diarrhea. Diagnosis is made by demonstration of *Histoplasma* bodies in circulating neutrophils or buffy-coat culture, by fecal culture or by biopsy of lymph node, colon or small intestine. A rising titer to *Histoplasma* antigen is helpful in diagnosis, primarily in retrospect because of the time factor. Punch biopsy of colon via a colonoscope is a valuable technique in the diagnosis of histoplasmosis.

*Chronic "bacterial" enteritis* is a hypothesis rather than a proven diagnosis. Quantitative bacterial culture methods are only now approaching the degree of specificity needed to make them useful in diagnosis of the chronic enteritides. When judged by favorable response to treatment with certain antibiotics, a persuasive case may be made for a bacterial cause in many cases. Hypergammaglobulinemia has been reported in chronic enteritis in dogs. (Hayden and Van Kruininger, 1976.)

*Malignant lymphoma* of the small bowel may be suspected when diarrhea is associated with thickened intestine and enlarged mesenteric nodes. A mature neutrophilia and leukocytosis are consistent with but not diagnostic of malignant lymphoma. Lymphocytosis and abnormal lymphocyte morphology may be observed in some cases.

*Amyloid deposition* in kidney, liver and spleen is more common than in bowel, but persistent proteinuria and malabsorption syndrome might be resolved to amyloidosis if intestinal and renal biopsies are positive.

## INTESTINAL BIOPSY

Biopsy may be, and frequently is, the diagnostic procedure of choice after the initial work-up of routine hematologic tests, urinalysis, fecal examinations and observations in the hospital. The decision as to when to biopsy is influenced by several factors. Palpable thickening or firmness of the small intestine, mesenteric lymphadenopathy, tenderness or pain on palpation, one or more abnormal tests of function and rapidly declining condition favor the use of biopsy early in the work-up. Conversely, negative physical examination of the abdomen, slowly changing or stable physical condition and absence of fluid accumulations serve as cautions. Further observations, review of history with the client and several tests of intestinal absorption are in order before surgical biopsy is elected in the latter instance. Pre- and postsurgical transfusions of plasma (albumin) may be essential for effective healing. After surgery, oral protein intake is maximized to the limit of the patient's ability to digest and absorb it.

A standard laparotomy is done. Transverse elliptical biopsies of duodenum, jejunum and ileum are made and mounted, mucosal surface up on a rigid surface before fixation in buffered neutral formalin. A mesenteric node, wedge of liver and lobule of pancreas are also removed. These six specimens should always be taken even if no gross abnormalities are observed. Additional biopsies are taken as indicated by findings at laparotomy. Biopsy for suspected malabsorption syndrome should be regarded as a standardized sampling procedure. If hypoalbuminemia exists, the client must understand that the prognosis for post-surgical healing is less than favorable. In many cases, debilitation is severe, and the prognosis is already less than favorable before laparotomy and biopsy.

When biopsy specimens of intestine do not contain evidence to account for the malabsorption syndrome, and when other tests do not yield a diagnosis, one must proceed with empirical treatment and observe for improvement. The cost-benefit ratio for work-up of the malabsorption syndromes is low when the diagnostic effort serves as a guide to successful therapy, but one must acknowledge that the ratio may be very high if all results are negative or equivocal. The client must be counseled carefully as to what may be expected from function testing, laparotomy and biopsy before the work-up begins.

## TREATMENT OF THE MALABSORPTION SYNDROMES

### MALDIGESTION

Replacement therapy for pancreatic exocrine insufficiency begins with a low-residue, high-carbohydrate, moderate-protein and moderate-fat ration of high biologic value. This ration is appropriate for all the syndromes described here. Food is given twice daily. Powdered or granular pancreatin*, thoroughly mixed with moistened food and held at room temperature for 20 minutes, seems to enhance weight gain better than pancreatin tablets do. The benefits of exogenous bile salts to promote micellar digestion of fat and of sodium bicarbonate to raise the pH of chyme are difficult to assess. Suppression of bacteria in the colon by chronic administration of broad-spectrum antibiotic tends to reduce the severity of diarrhea.

Maldigestion of gastric origin, if associated with decreased hydrochloric acid secretion, may respond to glutamic acid HCl (Acidulin® [Lilly]). One-half to 2 capsules per meal is suggested. Salting the food with NaCl may be helpful. If the primary

gastric disease is progressively worsening, treatments will be of little avail.

Bile-salt deficiency requires supplementation with commercial bile salts. The nature of underlying hepatic disease will determine the response and the prognosis.

### MALABSORPTION

Coccidiosis is treated with sulfa-dimethoxine (60 mg./kg./day in divided doses for 7 to 10 days or longer). Low-residue commercial food is fed twice daily. Alternative treatments are amprolium (Amprol® [Merck], 110 to 220 mg./kg./day) and nitrofurazone (Furadex® [Eaton], 5.9 mg./kg. t.i.d.). Supportive treatments with fluids, electrolytes, vitamins and anticholinergics are given as needed.

Giardiasis is treated with metronidazole (Flagyl® [Searle], 66 mg./kg./day) or glycobiarsol (Milibis-V® [Winthrop], 220 mg./kg./day) for 5 days. A high-protein ration is recommended.

Lactase deficiency is managed by exclusion of milk products from the food ration. Stagnant loop syndrome is treated by removal of foreign bodies or excision of stenotic lesions. Functional stagnant loops in the absence of a local organic lesion have not been observed by the author.

Eosinophilic gastroenteritis is treated with prednisone (2.2 mg./kg./day orally in divided doses). The dose is tapered over a 2- to 3-week period, and intermittent (every other day) therapy is given at 10 to 20 per cent of initial dosage if necessary. In the author's experience, the visceral larva migrans variety of eosinophilic gastroenteritis does not respond as well or as completely as that apparently due to other types of antigenic stimulation.

Lymphangiectasia does not respond well to treatment. A regimen of canine albumin (150 to 300 mg./kg. IV) weekly for several months, accompanied by intermittent diuresis to relieve edema, and a low-fat diet (rice and defatted boiled chicken) brought about symptomatic relief in a 7-year-old male dog. Oral protein supplementation and fat- and water-soluble vitamin injections were used. After several months, a commercial diet (i/d® [Riviana Foods]) was gradually introduced. The dog has been clinically well for over one year with the commercial ration and protein supplementation as total therapy. Serum albumin

---

*For example, Viokase® powder, Vio Bin Corp., Monticello, Illinois 61856.

is sustained above 2.0 gm./dl. Follow-up biopsy has not been done. Limited use of medium-chain triglyceride (MCT [Mead Johnson]) in dogs has not been helpful in the experience of others. MCT was not used in this case.

Villus atrophy is treated with injections of cyanocobalamin ($B_{12}$, 20 mcg./kg. once weekly) and folic acid (0.5 mg./kg./day). Additionally, oral antibiotic (tetracycline, ampicillin, tylosin [Tylocine®, Lilly]), multiple vitamin–mineral supplements and anticholinergic therapy may be included. Prednisone (2.2 mg./kg./day orally in divided doses) may be helpful. Tapering of dosage and discontinuation of drugs should be done singly so as to reduce drug treatment to the minimum required for maintenance and to determine which drugs are needed for maintenance.

Chronic enteritis is treated on the basis of biopsy results. Identification of an etiologic agent (e.g., *Histoplasma capsulatum*) provides a basis for specific therapy. If the etiology is not found or if biopsy is not done, the presumption is made that chronic bacterial infection or imbalance of gut flora exists. Long-term antibiotic therapy and other supportive treatment are given, as described for villus atrophy. Tylocine® (Lilly) has proved beneficial in many cases and does not cause recognizable complications. Some cases of chronic enteritis do not respond to therapy.

Lymphocytic-plasmacytic enteritis is treated with the same regimen as is villus atrophy.

Malignant lymphoma is treated with a battery of chemotherapeutic agents initially, followed by regular maintenance therapy. Supportive treatment is given as needed. Intestinal function will improve as the malignant cells are decreased in number.

Amyloidosis is not generally regarded as a treatable disease at present but may be treated with immunosuppressant drugs, as is malignant lymphoma. The residual function of the amyloid-infiltrated intestine may sustain life longer if therapy is given as for villus atrophy.

### SUPPLEMENTAL READING

Buckner, R. G., and Ewing, S. A.: Trichomoniasis. *In* Kirk, R. W. (ed.): Current Veterinary Therapy V. Philadelphia, W. B. Saunders Co., 1974.

Ewing, G. O.: Intestinal malabsorption. *In* Kirk, R. W. (ed.): Current Veterinary Therapy IV. Philadelphia, W. B. Saunders Co., 1971.

Finco, D. R., Duncan, J. R., Schall, W. D., Hooper, B. E., Chandler, F. W., and Keating, K. A.: Chronic enteric disease and hypoproteinemia in 9 dogs. J. Am. Vet. Med. Assn., 163:261–271, 1973.

Greve, T., and Anderson, N. V.: The high-dose intravenous glucose tolerance test (H-IVGTT) in dogs. Nord. Vet.-Med., 25:436–445, 1973.

Hayden, D. W., and Van Kruiningen, H. J.: Control values for evaluating gastrointestinal function in the dog. J.A.A.H.A., 12:31–36, 1976.

Hill, F. W. G.: Malabsorption syndrome in the dog: A study of thirty-eight cases. J. Small Animal Pract., 13:575–594, 1972.

Hill, F. W. G., and Kidder, D. E.: The oral glucose tolerance test in canine pancreatic malabsorption. Brit. Vet. J., 128:207–214, 1972.

Lorenz, M., Schall, W., Finco, D., and Lewis, R.: Problem oriented veterinary gastroenterology. Proc. J.A.A.H.A., 2:15–52, 1975.

Schall, W. D.: Malabsorption syndromes (malassimilation). *In* Kirk, R. W. (ed.): Current Veterinary Therapy V. Philadelphia, W. B. Saunders Co., 1974.

Van Kruiningen, H. J., and Hayden, D. W.: Interpreting problem diarrheas of dogs. Vet. Clin. N. Am., 2:29–47, 1972.

Van Kruiningen, H. J.: The malabsorption syndrome. *In* Kirk, R. W. (ed.): Current Veterinary Therapy III. Philadelphia, W. B. Saunders Co., 1968.

Welser, J. R.: Problem-oriented veterinary medical record. *In* Ettinger, S. J. (ed.): Textbook of Veterinary Internal Medicine. Diseases of the Dog and Cat. Philadelphia, W. B. Saunders Co., 1975.

Wilson, F. A., and Dietschy, J. M.: Differential diagnostic approach to clinical problems of malabsorption. Gastroenterology, 61:911–931, 1971.

# HEMORRHAGIC GASTRO-ENTERITIS

MICHAEL BERNSTEIN, D.V.M.
*Boston, Massachusetts*

Hemorrhagic gastroenteritis (HGE) is an acute, usually nonfatal, gastrointestinal upset seen in all breeds of dogs. It is a problem that is easily treated, especially if recognized early. Although mild cases of this disease may respond well to symptomatic treatment in spite of the clinician's failure to recognize the full extent of the problem, awareness of possible complicating factors is essential if all cases are to be properly cared for.

The cause of hemorrhagic gastroenteritis is unknown, and there does not seem to be a breed, age or individual predilection. Sixty-two cases which were hospitalized in the Intensive Care Unit at Angell Memorial Animal Hospital between 1970 and 1974 were surveyed. Of these, 30 were males, 18 were intact females and 14 were spayed females. The age range was 1 year to 13 years, but 75 per cent of the cases were 5 years old or younger. Most dogs had never had the syndrome before. The breed distribution was consistent with the breed popularity in the pet dog population as a whole.

The typical history in a case of HGE includes vomiting several times (often only white froth or phlegm), followed by episodes of bloody, almost jam- or jelly-like diarrhea. The onset of this syndrome is acute, and dogs are often presented to the hospital after being ill for as short a time as 8 to 16 hours. The most significant findings on physical examination of the dog are simply lethargy and depression and a high and rapidly rising hematocrit. Fevers and significant abdominal pain are *not* characteristic. The stools are not formed but are usually jelly-like and dark red-brown in color.

The most important parameter to monitor in this syndrome is the patient's hematocrit. On presentation the packed cell volume (PCV) may range from the low 50's to the high 70's; without proper fluid therapy, however, it can rise 5 to 10 percentage points within a several-hour period. Other than the elevated PCV, laboratory data are usually not particularly helpful. Although there may be an elevated white blood cell count with a left shift, this is not seen in all cases. Serum protein levels are usually either normal or lower than normal, indicating that these dogs are suffering from a shocklike syndrome rather than true dehydration. Serum amylase levels, when they have been determined, have been normal. Characteristically, the BUN is also normal. The stool should always be checked for parasites.

Treatment of these cases is based on intensive fluid therapy. All dogs with hematocrits of 60 or above are given intravenous fluids, usually via an indwelling cephalic vein catheter. A continuous rapid drip of lactated Ringer's solution is started and is continued until the hematocrit drops to between 45 and 50; the hematocrit is monitored every 2 to 3 hours. After the PCV has been lowered, the dog is maintained on IV fluids at the rate of 65 to 90 cc./kg. divided q.i.d. for the next 2 to 3 days; a continuous drip is reinstituted only if the hematocrit begins to rise again. The dog is allowed no food or water during this time.

If a dog with HGE is presented with a hematocrit between 50 and 55, he may be treated with subcutaneous fluids alone; these are given at the rate of 65 to 90 cc./kg. divided t.i.d. or q.i.d. However, the PCV must be monitored closely, because it can rise rapidly in a short period of time, and subcutaneous fluids may not be absorbed fast enough to counter this rise.

If the patient's hematocrit is between 55 and 60 on presentation, a butterfly IV infusion set may be used to administer an initial cardiovascular volume of IV fluids (90 cc./ kg.) before maintaining the dog on subcutaneous fluids.

In the average case, the patient can be started on small amounts of water and baby food on the third or fourth hospital day, and IV fluids are discontinued if the patient tolerates this well. We often maintain the dog on subcutaneous fluids until discharge on the fourth or fifth hospital day.

Most dogs do not have any vomition or diarrhea after the first hospital day, and it does not appear that atropine or intestinal protectants alter the course of the disease. Broad-spectrum antibiotics are always used in conjunction with an indwelling intravenous catheter, but how large a part these drugs play in the outcome of the case is unknown. Some clinicians advocate the use of steroids in the treatment of HGE, but they are not routinely used at our hospital, and good response to treatment is still obtained.

Of the 62 dogs studied in this survey, 58 recovered without complications. One case, a silky terrier that was presented to our clinic with a hematocrit of 80, suffered brain damage secondary to hemoconcentration. He was left permanently blind and was also ataxic for several weeks following the illness.

Three of the animals in this survey died; one was a 13-year-old spitz that was presented with a PCV of 73; the second case was a 13-year-old poodle with a PCV of 65. The third case was a 2-year-old Chihuahua that was presented hypothermic and with a PCV of 79; this was the only case that was necropsied. The necropsy revealed hemorrhagic ileitis; congestion of the stomach, colon and jejunum; congestion of the liver and spleen; and hemorrhage and congestion of the mesenteric lymph nodes.

In conclusion, the syndrome of hemorrhagic gastroenteritis must be considered whenever a dog is presented with an acute onset of vomiting, bloody diarrhea and collapse. Included in the differential diagnosis must be acute pancreatitis, intestinal obstruction, Addison's disease and septic or endotoxic shock; these syndromes must all be ruled out before the diagnosis of HGE can be made. Treatment of HGE is relatively simple and is usually successful; it is completely dependent on the adequate and intelligent use of fluid therapy.

# OBSTRUCTION OF THE SMALL INTESTINE

WILLIAM E. HORNBUCKLE, D.V.M., and LAWRENCE J. KLEINE, D.V.M. Boston, Massachusetts

Surgery is almost always the final solution to intestinal obstruction and will be discussed briefly at the conclusion of this section. Diagnosis and supportive treatment will receive principal emphasis.

## HISTORY AND PHYSICAL SIGNS

When small bowel obstruction is suspected, history taking should attempt to determine the possibility of a foreign body and previous injury, surgery or illness. Incarceration of a segment of small bowel in a mesenteric tear is not uncommon in trauma victims. Intussusceptions and strictures may complicate intestinal surgery. Repeated episodes of vomiting beginning at an early age might be a clue to a congenital cause of obstruction. It is always wise to inquire about an animal's chewing habits (e.g., bones, toys, string, nursing bottle nipples, clothing, etc.).

Vomiting is reported in the majority of animals with intestinal obstruction. However, this sign occurs with many other disorders (e.g., nonspecific gastroenteritis, acute pancreatitis). The point at which vomiting begins in the course of an illness will help localize the level of obstruction. Early onset is likely with higher obstruction and late onset or absence of vomiting correlates with lower obstruction; slow-moving foreign bodies may manifest characteristics of both. Bilious content of vomitus suggests that the lesion is posterior to the luminal entry of the bile duct; feculent vomitus and/or fecal odor to the animal's breath is associated with lower bowel obstruction (i.e., intestinal adhesions or strictures). If vomiting occurs within several minutes to a few hours after eating, a high obstruction should be suspected.

Diarrhea and/or scanty amounts of blood-stained mucus may indicate an intussusception. Blood in the stool can occur with bowel infarction, ulceration, neoplasia, parasitism or inflammation.

Weight loss may be the result of chronic disease or fluid loss of an acute vomiting episode. Abdominal discomfort is suggested by restlessness, panting or abnormal body posture.

## PHYSICAL EXAMINATION

Physical diagnosis of small bowel obstruction by simple palpation will shorten the diagnostic process and hasten the surgical remedy. However, factors such as body conformation, obesity, pain, shock and the animal's cooperativeness will influence the clinician's ability to palpate the abdomen, so that other diagnostic procedures may be required. Injury can result from abusive or repeated palpation of an abdominal abnormality (e.g., rupture of an infarcted segment of bowel).

A systematic inspection of the abdomen should be preceded by an assessment of the animal's general condition. Supportive treatment needs will be formulated from these findings. A subjective evaluation of the animal's acid-base status by physical examination is not reliable as the sole basis of acid-base correction.

Examination of the abdomen should begin with the animal standing. The often neglected ventral aspect of the body is inspected for hernias, scars and wounds. Abdominal enlargement could be the result of peritoneal effusion or the distention of bowel loops by gas or fluid. Abdominal rigidity might suggest pain or displacement of viscera.

A disciplined, systematic attempt to palpate abdominal organs is important (i.e., bladder, colon, uterus or prostate, left kidney, occasionally right kidney, liver, spleen, mesenteric lymph nodes, ileocecal junction, small intestine and occasionally stomach). This routine establishes the sites where masses, segmental bowel distention or areas of pain are localized; an abnormality should not distract the clinician from completing the examination unless further palpation would complicate the disease process or cause undue pain.

Skillful technique in examination may be crucial in detecting free fluid or an elusive foreign body. Gentle ballottement can create fluid waves and in conjunction with fingertip palpation will localize foreign bodies (e.g., rock) that would otherwise be displaced to areas out of reach by deep deliberate palpation.

Placing the animal in different body positions is helpful when palpating abdominal content that is otherwise out of reach. Elevation of the forelegs and thorax will aid in examining anterior abdominal viscera. When obese animals are placed on their backs, they lack the muscle tone to resist the rolling of abdominal viscera under the examiner's fingers.

Tranquilization and sedation are aids in abdominal palpation but should be used with discretion, since many animals with intestinal obstruction are already in some degree of cardiovascular collapse.

Pendulous kidneys, ileocecal junction, mesenteric lymph nodes, stool, retained testicles and folded spleen represent a few physical findings which may be mistaken for an intestinal mass.

Peritonitis can be a late event in simple obstructions but occurs early in obstructions with vascular interference. A presumptive diagnosis of peritonitis can be made on physical examination in the presence of abdominal pain, fluid and fever. Radiography and paracentesis will be helpful in confirming the presence of this complication.

## RADIOLOGY

When integrated with physical findings, radiology is an important diagnostic aid in the evaluation of the animal with suspected obstruction of the small intestine.

Causes of intestinal obstruction include foreign body, adhesion, intussusception, volvulus, incarcerated hernia, abscess, intramural hemorrhage and stricture. Many times one cannot determine the cause of obstruction but can determine only that complete or partial, proximal or distal small intestinal obstruction is present.

Plain radiography should always precede contrast examination; often, enough information is derived from the plain radiographs to obviate further study. If further radiography is necessary, one will know whether radiographic technique and patient preparation are satisfactory.

In order to provide maximal accuracy in interpretation, one must be able to ascribe the proper significance to the various clinical and radiographic signs that may occur with obstruction. One must be aware that there is no single sign which is diagnostic of either presence or absence of obstruction. For instance, while vomiting is usually an important sign, partial obstruction can be present in the absence of vomiting.

Gaseous distention of the small intestine is usually present shortly after complete obstruction, the amount of gas depending on the degree and duration of obstruction. It may be present in early obstruction and disappear when strangulation follows. Dilatation of the small intestine is a significant finding in obstruction, but there are other causes of distention secondary to altered motility that must be differentiated from intestinal obstruction, including aerophagia due to dyspnea or pain, uremia, shock, anticholinergic drugs, enemas, malabsorption, postoperative abdomen, hypokalemia and peritonitis.

Fluid accumulation in the small intestine must also be considered a possible indication of obstruction. In cases of chronic partial obstruction, fluid accumulation may be more prominent than gas. A similar appearance may occur, however, with excessive water intake or inflammatory lesions of the small intestine.

Plain radiographic findings that indicate the possibility of obstruction include distention of the small intestine with either gas or fluid, an intraluminal filling defect or abnormal location of an organ.

Some clinical findings that may indicate a need for a contrast examination (UGI) include unexplained vomiting, palpable abdominal mass, unexplained anorexia, scanty or tarry stools and unexplained abdominal pain or distention.

If clinical or plain radiographic findings indicate intestinal perforation, no further contrast study should be performed; instead, exploratory surgery is indicated. If contrast examination must be carried out in a case of suspected perforation, an organic iodide should be substituted for barium.

The contrast examination should not be performed on an animal that is under the influence of anticholinergic drugs, since it may be impossible to evaluate the transit time of the contrast medium or intestinal diameter.

If chemical restraint is desirable, acetylpromazine and triflupromazine hydrochloride maleate are effective and have no significant effect on gastrointestinal transit time (Zontine, 1973).

Commercial barium sulfate should be administered to dogs or cats by stomach tube, in a dose of 5 to 8 cc. liquid barium/kg. body weight. Exposures are then made in the ventrodorsal and lateral planes immediately, 30 minutes, 60 minutes, 3 hours, 6 hours and 24 hours following oral administration of contrast medium. The timing of the exposures may be varied depending on the results of the examination.

Several organic iodinated products are available for oral use, but none provides the uniformity of coating, density and transit time of barium suspensions. The iodides suffer from dilution and loss of density at the point where they are needed most, since fluid is often present proximal to an obstruction. These compounds are then absorbed through the intestine, further reducing the density of the contrast medium. For these reasons we seldom use iodides to evaluate patients with suspected obstruction. If an iodinated compound is used, the usual dose is 3 to 5 cc./kg. body weight, with the maximal total dose of 20 cc. in cats and 75 cc. in dogs. Exposures are made immediately, 15 minutes, 30 minutes, 60 minutes and 3 hours following administration. Organic iodides should not be administered to animals that are debilitated or that are just beyond weaning age, for these compounds are hyperosmotic and may cause serious dehydration.

Abnormalities in the UGI study that indicate obstruction are delayed transit time; dilated intestinal lumen; dilution of contrast medium; narrowed lumen, which may be due to an intraluminal filling defect or external pressure; fixed and displaced loops of intestine; opaque foreign body; or ascites. In general, any of the above signs should be seen in more than one film and should be compatible with the clinical findings before it can be considered diagnostic. Careful study of all the films along with knowledge of the clinical findings is essential for accurate diagnosis.

Recognition of intestinal ischemia is difficult in many cases but always of critical importance. Vascular compromise must be recognized as a surgical emergency because infarction and perforation may follow rapidly. When any of the following radiographic signs are present, one must seriously consider the possibility of strangulation:

1. Fixation of dilated loop of intestine in multiple radiographic projections.
2. Thickening of the intestinal wall by edema or hemorrhage.
3. Isolated segment of intestine dilated by fluid.

Signs that may be seen in contrast radiographs include delayed transit, dilution of medium and eccentric indentations of medium ("thumbprinting"). If any of these signs are present along with fever and tachycardia in an animal with obstruction, the diagnosis of strangulation is certain enough to warrant emergency laparotomy.

## LABORATORY AIDS

In cases in which a diagnosis of intestinal obstruction is made at the initial examination, laboratory tests are often limited to rapid screening procedures, i.e., hematocrit, total solids, BUN (Azostix® [Ames]), which help assess and monitor the animal's fluid requirements. In cases of complicated obstruction or in situations in which the diagnosis is obscure and the signs of illness overlap with other disease processes, more specific tests or procedures will be required.

Blood and urine samples should be collected prior to the initiation of fluid and drug infusions to protect the differential features of laboratory data. For example, prerenal azotemia is not uncommon in animals with small bowel obstruction. However, disorders such as acute pancreatitis, hypoadrenocorticism and primary renal disease may also present with azotemia as well as similar historical and physical manifestations. The pretreatment urinalysis and serum levels of amylase, electrolytes, etc., will aid in differential diagnosis.

Monitoring of bicarbonate and blood pH is needed to evaluate acid-base status, to assess the need and effect of bicarbonate replacement and occasionally to provide an early indication of electrolyte alterations (chloride, potassium, calcium). Interpretation of acid-base data, as well as electrolyte balance, requires an understanding of the effects of dilution or dehydration of the extracellular fluid compartment. Acid-base status can be normal in animals with intestinal obstruction, or initial alterations often spontaneously improve when the underlying cause of imbalance is corrected. Therefore, only severe or persistent alterations of acid-base balance require treatment.

Electrolyte studies should at least include sodium, potassium and chloride to assist in differential diagnosis; to evaluate refractory states of ileus, diarrhea or acid-base alterations; and to monitor massive or chronic fluid therapy or potassium supplementation.

The clinician must be prepared to handle biopsy material and effusions for diagnostic examinations. Sterile vials of thioglycolate broth and blood agar plates are recommended for culture of these samples, and 10 per cent buffered formalin is suggested for tissue fixation. Tissue imprints and smears of fluid on glass slides (air-dried) may be stained with Wright's-Giemsa or Gram stain for examination. An effusion should be collected in a sterile tube for culture, a second tube containing a preservative (one drop of 10 per cent buffered formalin per milliliter of effusion) and a third tube containing an anticoagulant (EDTA) for cell counts.

## TREATMENT

**Supportive Medical Treatment.** Some animals with small bowel obstruction are seriously ill when first examined, so that supportive treatment must precede diagnostic studies, drug-specific therapy and surgery. Physical evaluation of the animal and some simple tests (hematocrit, total solids, BUN [Azostix]) will help formulate initial fluid replacement. If bicarbonate and pH meters are available, the clinician can discriminate more specifically with regard to the selection of fluids and acid-base correction.

The indwelling polyethylene vascular catheter is both practical and advantageous for intravenous fluid administration. Subcutaneous fluid support will be sufficient in cases in which symptoms are mild; however, once a diagnosis of obstruction is confirmed and surgery is scheduled, an intravenous catheter should be inserted and intravenous infusions started. If the venipuncture site is properly prepared and maintained, the catheter can be left in the vein for 3 to 5 days with no significant complications. Usually this covers the time necessary for postoperative fluid support; if the animal is not self-supporting at this point, fluid administration should be changed to another vein or to the subcutis. There are a number of indwelling vascular catheters available; the 12-inch 17-gauge Bardic Intracath®* is preferred. One to 2 cc. of heparin-physiological saline solution (1000 units heparin per 100 cc. saline) is used to flush the catheter before and after infusion of fluids or drugs. If the catheter is installed in the jugular vein, the tip should lie within the anterior vena cava.

Urine output is an important monitor of fluid therapy. The volume of urine in the bladder prior to fluid therapy should be approximated by means of abdominal palpation; in more seriously affected animals, the volume of urine should be measured and an indwelling urinary catheter inserted until adequate urine production is recorded.

In general, a balanced electrolyte solution equivalent to Ringer's lactate is an adequate replacement and maintenance fluid. Two clinical situations, however, would indicate the use of physiological saline instead of Ringer's lactate during the initial replacement program.:

1. Early intestinal obstruction with vomiting. Extracellular bicarbonate levels are increased to compensate for chloride loss. Additional bicarbonate is contraindicated; lactate is metabolized by the liver to bicarbonate.

2. In the azotemic animal prior to the diagnosis of intestinal obstruction. Primary renal disease and hypoadrenocorticism are still among the differential diagnoses at this point, and there must be clinical concern for possible increased potassium levels.

In very dehydrated animals, a volume approximating the content of the cardiovascular space (65 to 90 cc./kg. body weight) is given intravenously within the first 2 to 4 hours; half this fluid volume is usually adequate replacement in less affected animals. This same volume of fluid would then be divided into 3 to 4 administrations for daily maintenance. Adjustment in the rate and/or volume of fluid would require periodic appraisal of hydration, urine output, control of vomiting and diarrhea, and monitoring of simple tests (hematocrit, total solids, BUN [Azostix]). The clinician is often guilty of giving too little fluid in the beginning and too much in the end; as the

animal becomes self-supporting, the amount of injectable fluid should be reduced.

In critically ill animals when replacement volumes exceed a single cardiovascular fluid volume, or when volumes of fluid are delivered rapidly, or in animals fragile to fluid administration (e.g., preexisting heart disease), the central venous pressure should be monitored. A single random reading of 0 to 5 cm. of water is considered normal; however, a change of 2 to 3 cm. in a series of readings is an indication of overhydration. Measurements are made in the anterior vena cava via a catheter inserted into the jugular vein and are recorded on a manometer with the animal on its right side.

In most cases of intestinal obstruction, there is time to administer the initial fluid volume (65 to 90 cc./kg.) intravenously prior to surgery. Even if immediate surgery appears to be indicated, it will often take 30 to 90 minutes to get the animal to the operating table; during this time a substantial amount of intravenous fluids can be administered to improve the cardiovascular status of the animal significantly. Surgical correction of less severe forms of obstruction can often be delayed in order to derive the benefit of both replacement and maintenance fluid therapy. During surgery, fluid is administered intravenously at a volume of 11 cc./kg. body weight per hour.

The concept of supplying maintenance needs (e.g., energy sources, amino acids, vitamins, etc.) is discussed elsewhere. If oral alimentation can be started within 3 to 5 days postoperatively, a balanced electrolyte solution is adequate supplementation. Though total caloric needs cannot be supplied, an adequate compromise for fasting periods approaching 7 to 10 days is obtained by adding 50 cc. of 50 per cent dextrose to 500 cc. of Ringer's lactate.

Postoperatively, initiation of oral alimentation depends on the complexity of the surgery, the existence of potential for complications, the control of vomiting and diarrhea and the daily physical assessment of the animal. Most cases (e.g., simple enterotomy) can tolerate oral fluid and broth within the first 2 to 3 days; the consistency of food is gradually increased over the next several days (baby food and/or blended dog food). Other cases (e.g., resection and anastomosis) will require fasting periods of 3 to 7 days before feeding.

---

*C. R. Bard, Inc., Murray Hill, New Jersey.

Empirical supplementation of bicarbonate is rarely harmful but is not recommended in routine treatment of intestinal obstruction. Increased bicarbonate levels associated with high normal to elevated blood pH have been documented in two specific clinical situations that contraindicate additional bicarbonate supplementation:

1. Obstruction associated with the primary chloride loss through vomiting.

2. Hypokalemic metabolic alkalosis. In this circumstance persistent elevations of bicarbonate will be found in spite of surgical correction and in spite of change from Ringer's lactate to physiological saline.

Additional potassium supplementation is seldom necessary in the majority of animals with intestinal obstruction. Most are eating potassium-rich food within a week after surgery; the fasting dog, in contrast to fasting people, is remarkable in its ability to conserve potassium. However, in cases of potassium depletion, as alluded to in the previous paragraph and in situations of extended fasting periods and long-term or massive fluid administration, potassium replacement is appropriate. Potassium deficiency should also be suspected in animals with persistent distention of loops of intestine by gas and fluid (i.e., adynamic or inhibition ileus), but electrolyte studies should be performed to justify supplementation. Addition of potassium is indicated only in the presence of normal renal perfusion and good urine production; periodic electrocardiographic and/or electrolyte monitoring will augment the efficacy and safety of potassium administration. If the oral route is possible, a 10 per cent elixir of potassium chloride is given at a dosage of ¼ to ½ mEq. per kg. body weight divided b.i.d. Intravenous infusions of 10 to 20 mEq. potassium chloride per 500 cc. of 5 per cent dextrose and water or Ringer's lactate can be included in daily maintenance fluid volumes. Tapering of daily fluid volumes will automatically reduce the dosage of potassium chloride; however, daily monitoring of electrocardiograms and serum electrolytes is essential to prevent potassium overload and to make adjustments in dosage.

Judicious use of atropine sulfate is advised in the treatment of intestinal obstruction. Indications for its use are intestinal hypermotility, increase in digestive secretions and preanesthetic support. It is presumed that anticholinergic drugs will protect the obstructed or surgical segment of intestine from the hypermotile consequences of further ischemic injury or intussusception; if this is correct, administration beyond the third postoperative day is seldom necessary. As discussed earlier, atropine sulfate should not be administered prior to or during contrast radiography. A wide parenteral dosage range of 0.02 to 0.11 mg./kg. body weight (2 to 4 times daily) is recorded in veterinary literature.

Tranquilizers and combination compounds of tranquilizers and cholinergic blockers are *not* routinely used in the treatment of intestinal obstruction. These drugs can suppress gastrointestinal signs to the point of delaying detection and timely surgical treatment of obstruction. Fluid therapy is required to protect animals with significant dehydration from the hypotensive properties of tranquilizers. These drugs are useful for restraint of intractable animals, preanesthetic preparation and control of persistent vomiting that has not responded to restriction of oral alimentation and administration of atropine sulfate. In the latter instance, the intramuscular administration of 0.2 to 0.5 gm./kg. of chlorpromazine, after dehydration has been corrected, will occasionally control vomiting for several hours without imposing significant tranquilization or sedation.

The major complication, septic or endotoxic shock, is attributed to the effects of varied intestinal flora. Broad antibiotic coverage is important; a combination of penicillin and kanamycin or ampicillin, chloramphenicol, gentamicin and the cephalosporins has been used with satisfactory results. Culture and sensitivity studies should be done for those animals with significant contamination or reaction of the peritoneal cavity; if irrigation and infusion of antibiotics are required, use the same antibiotic that is being given systemically.

Adrenocorticosteroids are almost never used in animals with intestinal obstruction because of delayed healing and predisposition to sepsis. Fulminating or refractory states of shock and endotoxemia are rare indications for steroid administration in combination with aggressive fluid therapy. Hydrocortisone (minimal dosage of 25 to 30 mg. per kg. body weight) is the drug of choice. Dexamethasone (1 to 2 mg. per kg. body weight) is an economical alternative.

Either drug is administered every 4 to 6 hours until clinical stability is secure.

Blood transfusions will occasionally be necessary in the supportive treatment of animals with intestinal obstruction. This is particularly true in obstructions characterized by vascular interference. Blood loss may not be conspicuous in initial hematocrit readings until sufficient exogenous fluid replacement and/or endogenous fluid compartment shifts occur to reflect decreases in repeated hematocrit readings.

Adynamic ileus, secondary peritonitis and aspiration pneumonia represent special management problems. Experience within this clinic suggests that postoperative ileus seldom reaches the clinical importance of peritonitis and aspiration pneumonia and is apparently not as serious a problem in the dog and cat as it is in man. In fact, profuse diarrhea for several days has been a more common management problem postoperatively; patience and good supportive therapy will usually prevail over this complication. Pneumonia can result either from aspiration of vomitus or from accidental inhalation during barium administration.

**Surgical Treatment.** The abdominal incision should be long enough to assure optimal exposure and accessibility to the area of obstruction. A systematic inspection of the entire abdomen should be routinely made. If the site of obstruction is friable or ruptured, it should be dealt with immediately. However, failure to examine the entire abdomen could result in overlooking an equally significant lesion.

Sterile physiological saline solution (warmed to body temperature) and suction apparatus will be needed for peritoneal lavage. Decompression of distended loops of bowel may be beneficial in selected cases, and a peritoneal drainage system may be indicated if peritonitis is a significant complication (Johnston, 1974).

A nonabsorbable monofilament suture such as nylon or stainless steel is recommended for primary closure of the peritoneal cavity.

### SUPPLEMENTAL READING

Johnston, D. E.: Pathogenesis and management of peritonitis and ileus. Archives, J. Am. Coll. Vet. Surg., 3(3):52–58, 1974.
Zontine, W. J.: Effect of chemical restraint on the passage of barium sulfate through the stomach and duodenum of dogs. J. Am. Vet. Med. Assn., 162:878–884, 1973.

# INTESTINAL PARASITISM

FRED K. SOIFER, D.V.M.
*Houston, Texas*

## INTRODUCTION

**Cestodes.** Until the advent of new anthelmintics, tapeworms had traditionally been considered the least harmful of the intestinal parasites but one of the most difficult to remove from the host.

Tapeworm infestations of cats and dogs are commonly diagnosed by the owner, who observes tapeworm segments in the perianal area, on bedding or on fresh feces. Although tapeworm infestation is often asymptomatic, there can be perianal itching ("scooting"), abdominal cramping, vomiting, diarrhea and excessive gas production.

The tapeworms most often seen in dogs and cats in this country are *Dipylidium caninum, Taenia pisiformis, T. hydatigena, T. multiceps, T. serialis, T. ovis, T. taeniaeformis* and *Echinococcus granulosus.* Several other less common tapeworms of cats requiring intermediate hosts, including frogs, toads, lizards and raw fish, will not be discussed. It is important to keep in mind that an intermediate host is required in the tapeworm disease. The intermediate host is the one that harbors the asexual or larval form of the parasite. The dog or cat is usually the definitive host, that is, the animal in which the adult or sexual stage of the parasite is found.

Man is the intermediate host for *Echinococcus*, hydatid cysts of which may exist in many locations in the body. Infection in man with the coenurus, or intermediate stage, of the *Taenia* parasites is also seen on occasion. Fortunately, these infections are relatively rare in the United States. This is especially true of *Echinococcus*. This parasite is being reported with increased frequency. *Dipylidium caninum* has been reported with some frequency in children who also are definitive hosts and consequently segments of the worm are passed.

Prevention of tapeworm infection can be readily accomplished by the control of the intermediate host. In the case of *Dipylidium*, a strict course of flea control must be instituted. This control must include the dog or cat, the house and the yard. It is important to explain all this to the client, or the reinfection of the pet from the premises will cause owner dissatisfaction. It is recommended that a competent exterminator be consulted to exterminate fleas from the premises. After the pet has been treated for the tapeworm infection, the segments should be washed from the animal and the bedding should be cleaned as part of the control program. Control of *Taenia* spp. infection requires that the pet be prevented from eating small wild mammals containing the larval stages of the parasite. Prevention of *Echinococcus* infection is based on confining the pet so that it is not free to consume the hydatid cysts harbored in the viscera of the intermediate host.

**Nematodes.** Life cycles will again be discussed, because the veterinarian must understand them well in order to treat properly. The prepatent period is between the time of ingestion of the infective stage of the parasite and the time when a stage of the parasite may be recovered from the host. Prepatent periods vary considerably because of the influence of temperature, humidity and the type of surface on which maturation of the infective stage occurs.

Furthermore, in most nematode infections in the dog and cat, two stages of the parasite are within the host concurrently. The adult parasite may be within the lumen of the digestive tract, while the migrating larvae may be present in the host's tissues (liver, lung, etc.). With this in mind, the practitioner must adopt one of several procedures: One, following initial treatment, routine reexamination of the stool for ova at the end of the prepatent period is suggested to determine whether a second treatment is needed. (A fecal examination 1 to 2 weeks following the administration of the anthelmintic may be desirable first to be sure of the efficacy of the vermifuge on adult parasites.) Two, since in mixed infections the prepatent periods vary markedly, a routine "re-worming" may be recommended at a compromise time decided upon by the practitioner (4 weeks is often suggested). Finally, a low level of anthelmintics may be administered repeatedly. The last method is frequently used when decontamination of the premises is not possible. Greyhounds are commonly treated in this manner. Brood bitches are also treated by this method in many areas of the country. The advent of some of the newer anthelmintics that have greater safety and efficacy may influence the selection of a suitable method.

*Ascaris* infections are contracted by the ingestion of infective eggs. The eggs become infective in about 2 to 3 weeks, and the prepatent period is 6 to 10 weeks. This period may vary considerably. Routine fecal examination of bitches prior to breeding may be consistently negative for ascarid eggs. However, stools become positive after the stress of whelping. Hookworm infection takes place either by ingestion or by skin penetration by the infective larvae. Larvae become infective in 5 to 7 days after ingestion, and the prepatent period is about 2 to 3 weeks. In the case of whipworms, ingestion of the infective egg is required for transmission to occur. Eggs become infective in about 2 weeks, and the prepatent period is 10 to 12 weeks. *Strongyloides* infect the host by skin penetration or by ingestion of the infective larvae. The prepatent period is about 1½ weeks. *Strongyloides* infection is diagnosed by the demonstration of free larvae in the stool rather than by embryonated eggs.

As in control of tapeworms, parasite transmission should be discussed with the owner. Pets that run loose in the neighborhood cannot be expected to remain free of intestinal parasites. On the other hand, pets confined to yards that have become contaminated with infective eggs or larvae also present a real problem. The old methods used to kill infective larvae (salt and Borax) have little effect on some of the hardier eggs (especially ascarids), and they also kill grass. Concrete runs (slick concrete instead of rough) can easily be washed free of eggs and larvae if a careful program of sanitation is maintained. Some of the newer insecticides are reputedly larvicidal for hookworms.

Symptoms of nematode infections vary with the parasite in question and often with the number of parasites infecting the host. Ascarids commonly produce a characteristic "pot-bellied" appearance, general unthriftiness, emaciation and digestive disturbances (diarrhea, constipation, flatulence and emesis). Icterus may be caused by the mechanical blockage of the bile duct. Hookworms commonly produce a blood-tinged diarrhea. The anemia produced is not only from the actual blood-sucking of the worm, but as the female worms move from area to area in the gut "looking" for males with which to mate, the areas of buccal detachment continue to bleed. The anemia produced is a typical blood loss anemia. Respiratory symptoms may be present as a result of migrating larvae. Whipworms cause an intermittent diarrhea, usually with excess mucus. Typhlitis may produce the characteristic "side biting" described in the literature. *Strongyloides* usually cause watery, mucoid diarrhea. Bronchopneumonia may also be manifested. (See treatment discussion at end of article.)

**Coccidia.** The pathogenicity of coccidia in small animals is a controversial subject. Coccidiosis is most frequently described as a self-limiting disease of little importance (Conroy, 1964). Others feel that the disease can be self-limiting but may also cause severe illness and may produce a carrier state. Coccidiosis is certainly influenced by regional problems. Coccidiosis is a serious problem in the southern United States, undoubtedly contributed to by the mild weather and higher humidity. On the other hand, coccidiosis is rarely a problem in the northern states except in crowded, poorly kept kennels and some dog pounds.

A five-year study of this parasite in the Houston area produced some interesting statistics. Of the 143 cases in the study, 123 were found in animals under one year of age. Only 11 cases were asymptomatic and were found on routine fecal examination. Species statistics were as follows:

| | |
|---|---|
| Isospora felis | 41 cases |
| I. rivolta | 25 cases |
| I. bigemina (cati) | 15 cases |
| Eimeria canis | 2 cases |
| Mixed infections | 13 cases |
| Species unidentified | 47 cases |

All the above species were observed, measured, identified and in some cases sporulated for further study (Conroy, 1964; Hoskins *et al.*, 1962; Morgan and Hawkins, 1952). Incidental parasitism with rabbit coccidia was observed in several dogs. Passage of these oocysts by the dogs ceased 36 to 48 hours after the pet rabbits and their feces were removed from the premises.

A review of the size and shape of coccidial parasites is necessary before diagnosis, life cycle, pathology, treatment and prevention can be discussed (Kudo, 1939):

1. *I. bigemina (cati)*—8 to 10 $\mu$ × 10 to 15 $\mu$ and slightly elliptical.

2. *I. rivolta*—15 to 20 $\mu$ × 20 to 25 $\mu$ and oval.

3. *I. felis*—26 to 37 $\mu$ × 36 to 48 $\mu$ and egg-shaped.

4. *E. canis*—11 to 28 $\mu$ × 18 to 45 $\mu$ and long oval with a polar micropyle. When sporulated, it has four sporocysts, each with two sporozoites, instead of two sporocysts, each with 4 sporozoites, as in *Isospora* spp.

*I. bigemina (cati)* is reportedly the most pathogenic and *I. felis* the least pathogenic (Galvin and Turk, 1964).

Oocysts can be demonstrated in microscopic examination of a fresh stool specimen (100 to 400 × magnification). Size, shape and the characteristic pinkish cast make these protozoa easy to recognize. While they are easily floated using standard flotation solution, heavily infected animals commonly exhibit oocysts on direct smears. A negative fecal examination does not always mean that there are no coccidia, since signs (diarrhea, etc.) often precede the shedding of oocysts by several days.

The life cycle of this protozoan is described as follows: Unsporulated oocysts are passed in the feces. Sporulation time is approximately 96 hours. Ingestion of the sporulated oocyst produces infection in the susceptible animal. Further development takes place in the subepithelial and epithelial tissues. *I. bigemina (cati)* is most pathogenic, probably because of its more intense subepithelial activity. The prepatent period, or time from ingestion of the infective oocyst until the time when a stage of the parasite can be demonstrated from the stool of the host animal, is between 5 and 7 days (Morgan and Hawkins, 1952). Thus, the puppy or kitten from infected premises may show symptoms as early as 5 days postexposure.

Lesions from coccidiosis are confined to the epithelial and subepithelial tissues of the small intestine and cecum where hemorrhagic enteritis with ulceration and desquamation is produced. A thickening of the mucosa may be seen in animals that have recovered from severe infection. Connective tissue may replace the normal mucosa, which may explain the chronic colitis that may be present in these animals as they mature.

Treatment and prevention must be initiated in any case of coccidiosis. Any animal harboring coccidia may be a potential clinical problem when the resistance of the host is lowered to allow a "take-over" by the parasite and the onset of clinical disease. The carrier animal is continually passing oocysts potentially dangerous to other dogs and cats. Any preventive program must include the immediate and constant removal of fecal material from the premises followed by a thorough clean-up. We have found careful scrubbing with a detergent solution and adequate flushing with lots of water to be effective in mechanically removing oocysts from the premises. Puppies or kittens also may be raised on wire to prevent fecal contamination. Treatment consists of coccidostatic drugs and good supportive therapy as described below:

1. Fluids (Multisol-R® [Abbott] or lactated Ringer's [bicarbonate and electrolyte replacement] as needed).

2. Dietary correction (i/d is useful).

3. Coccidiostatic drugs are probably effective in controlling secondary bacterial infections (intestinal sulfas, and 24-hour systemic sulfas such as sulfadimethoxine).

4. Anticholinergics such as prochlorperazine and isopropamide (Darbazine® [Norden]).

5. Adsorbents and demulcents.

Coccidiostatic drugs are effective against schizontic stages (asexual) only. It is therefore necessary to continue medication long enough to assure "cure." "Spiramycin," produced by the French drug company Rhone-Pulene, has shown decidedly coccidiocidal action clinically and is apparently effective against all stages of the parasite. (Dr. R. D. Turk and Dr. T. J. Galvin). Unfortunately, the drug is not available in the United States at this time. It is used in human medicine under various trade names in Europe and Canada. "Spiramycin" is the most encouraging new therapeutic agent for use on coccidiosis that I have had the opportunity to test. Amprolium (Corid® [Merck]) has been used in cattle and experimentally with some success in birds and rabbits and may have some promise for use in dogs and cats (see page 58 in *Current Veterinary Therapy V*).

A controversy has arisen over whether the shedding of coccidia in cats is in fact coccidia or toxoplasma. *Isospora bigemina (cati)* is 8 to 10 $\mu$ × 10 to 15 $\mu$. *Toxoplasma gondii* is about 10 × 12 $\mu$. Since both organisms have been recovered from cat feces, the question is whether these similar organisms can in fact be differentiated. Dubey (1973) suggests that *I. cati* is usually passed sporulated (the other coccidial oocysts are shed unsporulated), while *Toxoplasma gondii* is passed unsporulated and, at room temperature, takes 1 to 5 days to sporulate and become infectious. If oocysts in the 10 to 15 $\mu$ range are discovered in the examination of cat feces, feline toxoplasmosis cannot be ruled out by the veterinarian, and the necessary precautions should be observed when handling the feces of these animals. Further work is needed to clarify this controversy.

## EXAMINATION OF FECES

A routine fecal examination should include a direct smear, especially if the patient has persistent diarrhea and if flotation examinations have been negative. This method has its merits and its disadvantages. The smear requires only a minute amount of feces and is a simple and rapid test. The smear should be made transparent enough to read through. Too dense a direct smear is almost worthless as a diagnostic tool. The direct smear may disclose the presence of motile bacteria and encysted and trophozoite forms of protozoan parasites. It may reveal fragile, operculated trematode eggs, although the sedimentation method is probably more efficient for detection of this parasite. The thin-walled eggs of *Spirocerca lupi* are often seen on direct smears. These fragile eggs also could be destroyed by the plasmolytic action of some flotation solutions.

It must be emphasized that the direct smear is a qualitative test. An animal may appear negative for intestinal parasites on examination of the direct smear yet harbor many pathogenic parasites. The number of mature female worms producing eggs, the number of eggs reaching the suitable premises for development, the egg-laying capacity of the type of parasite present, the amount and consistency of the feces examined, the age of the specimen and finally the efficiency of the method of examination influence the interpretation of the *degree* of parasitism. We can markedly increase the number or percentage of eggs recovered by examining a sufficient, but not excessive, amount of fresh fecal material. Careful mixing of the feces in a 1:10 ratio with an acceptable flotation solution, waiting the optimal period of time and then *careful* microscopic examination of the specimen for the eggs floated are all required for best results. A methodical search rather than a careless scanning is also important.

The number of parasite eggs found in a given stool sample is not necessarily indicative of the degree of parasitism or the damage being inflicted by the adult parasites upon the host animal. Significant damage can be caused by immature worms and larvae in the intestinal tract; yet neither may produce any ova. We are also aware that some parasites produce more eggs than others. Diarrhea can be deceiving, since it will dilute the number of eggs recovered for fecal examination.

## FLOTATION SOLUTIONS

Studies have shown that the efficiency of the flotation solution varies with the specific gravity (see Figure 1) and the type of eggs being floated (Bello, 1961; Farr and Luttermoser, 1941; Koutz, 1941; Otto *et al.*, 1941). The importance of allowing the eggs sufficient time to rise, using a centrifuge and mixing of the feces thoroughly with the

flotation solution has been reported previously. The proper amount of time for all eggs to rise is 10 minutes for the salt solutions and 15 minutes for the sugar solution.

Using zinc sulfate initially, solutions with eight different specific gravities were prepared (1.00, 1.10, 1.15, 1.20, 1.25, 1.30, 1.35 and 1.40). An egg suspension was prepared by mixing a gram of feces from a dog heavily infected with hookworms with 10 ml. of 0.85 per cent NaCl solution. The suspension was filtered through a single layer of gauze, and enough NaCl solution was added to make 10 ml. of the resultant suspension. A count of eggs indicated that there were 17,500 eggs per gram of feces in the sample being tested. Therefore, 0.1 ml. of this suspension should average approximately 175 eggs. Subsequent tests proved this to be true. Replicate tubes were placed in the test tube racks for each of the eight solutions being tested. Using a calibrated serologic pipette, 0.1 ml. of the agitated egg suspension was introduced into each of the previously prepared tubes (13 × 100 mm., 10 ml.) whose rims had been ground evenly flat. Each test solution was carefully poured on top of the egg suspension to a meniscus. Each replicate tube was thus prepared, and a 22 × 22 mm. coverslip was placed over each meniscus. After 10 minutes, the coverslips were carefully inverted and placed on glass microslides, and the floated eggs were counted. The replicate counts were averaged for each of the eight test solutions. This same procedure was repeated five times, and the averages were recorded (Table 1). Approximately 95 per cent of the floated eggs reportedly are removed on the first coverslip inverted (Bello, 1966). In order to reduce the results to percentages,

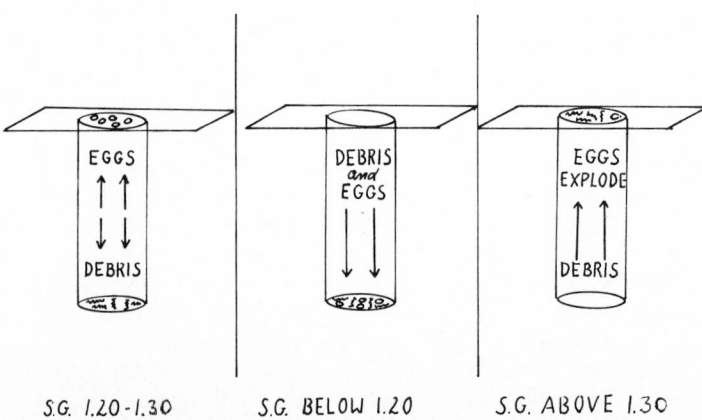

S.G. 1.20-1.30          S.G. BELOW 1.20          S.G. ABOVE 1.30

**Figure 1.** Optimum specific gravity of flotation solutions.

**Table 1.** *Optimum Specific Gravity of Eight Flotation Solutions Using Zinc Sulfate*

| S.G. | % EGGS RECOVERED |
|------|------------------|
| 1.00 | 0 |
| 1.10 | 52 |
| 1.15 | 68 |
| 1.20 | 80 |
| 1.25 | 87 |
| 1.30 | 83 |
| 1.35 | 29 |
| 1.40 | 22 |

95 per cent of the known eggs per 0.1 ml. was calculated to be 166 eggs. Neither the distortion of the eggs nor the amount of debris floated with each solution was recorded. Tests with other flotation solutions showed the same approximate optimum specific gravity of 1.25. Although sodium nitrate was as efficient at higher gravities, the increase in debris floated made these more concentrated solutions unacceptable.

Sodium nitrate proved to be the most efficient flotation solution tested (Table 2). In order to reach an overall "best" solution, the efficiency of each type of solution of each type of eggs was listed. The solutions were rated from 1 through 5, from most effective to least effective; the ratings for each solution were then totaled (Table 3). While NaCl and MgSO⁴ both totaled 11, NaCl was probably better, since it raised a slightly greater total number of eggs than the MgSO⁴.

**Table 2.** *Flotation Solution Rating (All S. G. 1.25 Except NaCl at 1.20)*

| Hookworms | % |
|-----------|---|
| NaNO₃ | 81 |
| NaCl | 59 |
| Sugar | 46 |
| ZnSO₄ | 44 |
| MgSO₄ | 36 |

| Whipworms | % |
|-----------|---|
| NaNO₃ | 88 |
| Sugar | 44 |
| ZnSO₄ | 40 |
| NaCl | 37 |
| MgSO₄ | 19 |

| Roundworms | % |
|------------|---|
| MgSO₄ | 72 |
| NaNO₃ | 48 |
| ZnSO₄ | 45 |
| Sugar | 38 |
| NaCl | 35 |

**Table 3.** *Overall Flotation Solution Ratings*

| | SOLUTION | HOOK-WORMS | ROUND-WORMS | WHIP-WORMS | TOTAL |
|--|----------|------------|-------------|------------|-------|
| Most Efficient ↑ | NaNO₃ | 1 | 2 | 1 | 4 |
| | Sugar | 3 | 4 | 2 | 9 |
| | ZnSO₄ | 4 | 3 | 3 | 10 |
| | NaCl | 2 | 5 | 4 | 11 |
| ↓ Least Efficient | MgSO₄ | 5 | 1 | 5 | 11 |

In determining the "best" flotation solution, one should consider efficiency, ease of preparation and possibly expense. With the exception of common salt (NaCl) solution, which is a saturated solution, all other reagents require scales in their preparation (Small Animal Parasitism, M.V.P., 1965; Turk, 1966) (Table 4). The use of heat facilitates the speed of preparation of all solutions. However, sodium nitrate went into solution with relative ease, while sodium chloride required the most time and heating. With a saturated salt (NaCl) solution, the maximum specific gravity attainable was 1.20. This was attained with rock salt or ice cream salt. (I was not able to reach 1.20 with the table salt probably because of the additives to assure easy pouring.) All solutions required a hydrometer (approximate cost, $4.50) to adjust the S. G. after preparation.

## PUBLIC HEALTH ASPECTS

Although many intestinal parasites are transmissible from animals to man, this rarely occurs. Nevertheless, veterinarians should be aware of the problem in order to inform clients, without alarming them. One should also be aware that a malpractice suit could arise from the casual omission of zoonotic information to the client.

**Table 4.** *Preparation and Cost of Flotation Solutions*

| REAGENT | AMOUNT TO FIX 1 GALLON | COST* |
|---------|------------------------|-------|
| NaNO₃ | 5 lb. | $1.75 |
| Sugar | 10 lb. | $2.80 |
| ZnSO₄ | 5 lb. | $2.10 |
| NaCl | 2 lb. | $ .50 |
| MgSO₄ | 2 lb. | $1.00 |

Adjust S. G. with hydrometer.
*Subject to change.

## Table 5. Anthelmintics

| DRUGS | MODE OF ACTION | EFFICACY Hookworms | Roundworms | Whipworms | Tapeworms | Strongyloides | DOSAGE | COMMENTS |
|---|---|---|---|---|---|---|---|---|
| Carbon tetrachloride Tetrachlorethylene | Protoplasmic poison | + 25% | + 60% | ± 30% | − | − | Not recommended | Hepatotoxic. Requires enema |
| N-Butyl chloride | | | | | | | 1 mg/kg. after 12 hr. fast | |
| Caricide® (Diethylcarbamazine) (Cyanamid) | Narcotic effect | − | + 80% | − | − | − | 3 mg/kg/day orally | Effective on third stage or infective larvae until they reach the heart. Contraindicated if microfilaria present. |
| Piperazine (Many manufacturers) | Narcotic effect | − | + 85% | − | − | − | 100-200 mg/kg. orally, repeat 24 hr. | Caution against overdose, especially with piperazine citrate. |
| Canopar® (Thenium closylate) (Cooper) | Disintegration of mouth parts | + 95% | ± ? | − | − | − | ½ tablet b.i.d. up to 5 kg. to 1 tablet o.d. over 5 kg. | Not absorbed from digestive tract. Some emesis. Cannot use on nursing animals. |
| Dizan® (Dithiazanine iodide) (Elanco) | Interferes with glucose transport | + 80% | + 80% | + 80% | − | + 85% | 4-6 mg/kg. o.d. oral 5-10 days | Requires multiple dosage. Absorbed products may be nephrotoxic. Effective microfilaricide. |
| Task® (Dichlorvos) (Shell) | Cholinesterase inhibitor | + 95% | + 95% | + 90% | − | − | 25-30 mg/kg. as directed | Contraindications include heartworm disease and liver or kidney damage. Do not use in conjunction with other cholinesterase inhibitors. Split dosage to b.i.d. |
| D.N.P. (Disophenol) (Cyanamid) | Unknown | + 95% | − | − | − | − | 7 mg/kg. SC | Overdoses fatal. Do not administer to overheated animals or those with respiratory problems. |
| Milibis-V® (Glycobiarsol) (Winthrop) | Paralysis and death from arsenic and bismuth | − | − | + 75% | − | − | 200 mg/kg. o.d. for 5 days | Developed for treatment of amebiasis. |

| Drug (source) | Mode of action | | | | | | Dosage | Side effects |
|---|---|---|---|---|---|---|---|---|
| Whipcide® (Phthalofyne) (Pitman-Moore) | Unknown—suspect narcotic effect | — | — | + 15 to 30% | — | — | 180 mg./kg. orally after 24 hr. fast | Side effects. Foul odor of by-products. |
| Nemural® (Drocarbil) (Winthrop) | Relaxation of mouth parts of worm and cathartic effect on host | — | — | — | + 50% | — | 4-6 mg./kg. orally after light feeding; repeat 3 wk. | Severe vomiting and diarrhea that may be difficult to control. |
| Yomesan® (Niclosamide) (Farbenfabriken) | Destroys neck and scolex | — | — | — | + 75% | — | 150 mg./kg. orally | Heavy mucus blocks action. |
| Scolaban® (Bunamidine) (Cooper) | Destroys all parts of parasite | — | — | — | + 90% | — | 20-40 mg./kg. on empty stomach; feed lightly in 3 hr. | Best on empty stomach. |
| Thiabendazole (Merck Sharp & Dohme) | Unknown | ± | — | — | — | + 95% | 50-60 mg./kg. o.d. orally | Some emesis. |
| Vermiplex® (2-2 methylenebis, methylbenzene) (Pitman-Moore) | Protoplasmic poison? Irritant | + 95% | + 90% | + 90% | ± 70% | — | Size capsule as directed by manufacturer | Incoordination, emesis, toxicity in excess. |
| Levamisole (L-Tetramisole) (Cyanamid) | Acts like cholinesterase inhibitor | + 60% | + 60% | + 40% | — | ? | 4-8 mg./kg. b.i.d. for 7-10 days | Short life in the body, so b.i.d. dosage essential. High dosage toxicity. Good microfilaricide at dosage shown. |
| *Experimental* Telmin® (Mebendazole) (Pitman-Moore) | Interferes with glucose metabolism of parasite | + 95% | + 95% | + 95% | + 85% | + ? | 20 mg./kg. b.i.d. orally for 3 days or 20 mg./kg. o.d. for 5 days | Excellent in 2½ years testing. No contraindications. |
| Strongid-T® (Pyrantel pamoate) (Pfizer) | Effect on neuromuscular activity of parasite that produces a rigidity and asphyxiation | + 95% | + 95% | — | — | — | 0.8 mg./kg. b.i.d. for one day | Excellent in early testing. |

The larval forms of the dog and cat hookworm produce a cutaneous migration in man known as "creeping eruption" or "plumber's itch." *Toxocara* larvae produce visceral larva migrans and peripheral retinitis in man. The transmission of these parasites to man is an important consideration and is another reason why pets should be kept parasite-free.

## TREATMENT

The facts describing the damage to puppies and kittens by intestinal parasites is documented elsewhere. Nonetheless, we often ignore the adult or geriatric patients, perhaps believing that their resistance to parasites is good and that administering a vermifuge is unnecessary. If a brood bitch is allowed to maintain a constant parasite population, the pups will most certainly pick up the infection either prenatally or shortly after birth. Dogs or cats kept in confined yards and not wormed will build an incredibly large parasite population in a relatively short time. The geriatric patient, although considered relatively resistant to parasitism, can become acutely infected if its resistance is lowered for any reason.

With new and safer anthelmintics, any animal with intestinal parasites should be treated. This is true even of sick and debilitated animals, provided that the complications discussed in this section are considered.

The properties of an ideal anthelmintic are as follows:

1. Low toxicity to the host.
2. High parasiticidal activity.
3. Broad spectrum of activity.
4. Ease of administration.
5. Minimal contraindications and side effects.
6. Low cost.

Drugs injurious to parasites may also be toxic to the host, particularly if administered in sufficient dosage.

[*Editor's Note*: Acute deaths have been reported following the use of bunamidine HCl in normal doses in dogs. If the drug is used, exertion and excitement should be avoided for more than 24 hours after dosage. (See Williams, J. F., and Keahy, K. K.: Sudden death associated with treatment of three dogs with bunamidine HCl. JAVMA *168*:689–690, 1976.)

The anthelmintics listed in Table 5 have been tested by the author over a period of 10 years, in most cases on a clinical basis, and results are based on the cessation of appearance of parasite eggs or segments after the administration of the anthelmintic. Less than 8 per cent of the animals were autopsied to determine absence or presence of parasites. Therefore, the results are strictly the author's opinion.]

## SUPPLEMENTAL READING

Bello, T. R.: Comparison of the flotation of *Metastrongylus* and *Ascaris* eggs in three different levitation solutions. Am. J. Vet. Res., *22*:597–600, 1961.

Bello, T. R.: Personal communication, 1966.

Conroy, J. D.: Feline Medicine and Surgery. American Veterinary Publications, Santa Barbara, California, 1964, p. 130.

Dubey, J. P.: Feline toxoplasmosis and coccidiosis: A survey of domiciled and stray cats. J. Am. Vet. Med. Assn., *162*:873–876, 1973.

Farr, M. M., and Luttermoser, G. W.: Comparative efficiency of zinc sulfate and sugar solutions for the simultaneous flotation of coccidial oocysts and helminth eggs. J. Parasitol., 27:417, 1941.

Galvin, T. J., and Turk, R. D.: Intestinal parasitism. *In* Kirk, R. W. (ed.): Current Veterinary Therapy I. Philadelphia, W. B. Saunders Co., 1964, p. 160.

Georgi, J. R.: Parasitology for Veterinarians. 2nd ed. Philadelphia, W. B. Saunders Co., 1974.

Hoskins, H. P., Lacroix, J. V., and Mayer, K.: Canine Medicine. 2nd ed. American Veterinary Publications, Santa Barbara, California, 1962, pp. 107–108.

Koutz, F. R.: A comparison of flotation solutions in the detection of parasite ova in the feces. Am. J. Vet. Res., 2:95, 1941.

Kudo, R. R.: Protozoology. Springfield, Illinois, Charles C Thomas, 1939.

Morgan, B. B., and Hawkins, P. A.: Veterinary Protozoology. Burgess Publishing Co., Minneapolis, Minnesota, 1952, pp. 85–88.

Otto, G. F., Hewitt, R., and Strahan, D. E.: A simplified zinc sulfate levitation method of fecal examination for protozoan cysts and hookworm eggs. Am. J. Hygiene, *33*:32, 1941.

Small Animal Parasitism. M. V. P., *46*:7–70, 1965.

Turk, R. D.: Class notes. School of Veterinary Medicine. Texas A & M University, 1966.

# TRICHINOSIS

JEAN HOLZWORTH, D.V.M.
*Boston, Massachusetts*

Although sanitary control measures are gradually reducing the incidence of trichinosis, this parasitism of humans and carnivorous animals still occurs virtually worldwide. Autopsy studies indicate that the rate of infection in animals in a given area roughly reflects that in man, yet all but the most serious clinical infections of man go unrecognized, while clinical diagnoses in cats and dogs are almost unheard of. This record would probably be far different if trichinae were routinely looked for in all cases of hemorrhagic gastroenteritis.

Cats, especially young ones, are said, on the basis of experimental studies, to be among the species most susceptible to infection with *Trichinella spiralis*. Dogs are among the more resistant. Carnivores become infected either by scavenging where uncooked pork scrap is available or by preying on other infected animals, notably rodents. In certain areas, bear meat is a serious source of infection for both man and animals.

## CLINICAL SIGNS

Clinical signs may develop within a few hours after infected meat is eaten, for the digestive enzymes of the host act swiftly to release the encysted larvae, which develop rapidly into adults. As observed in three naturally infected cats and in experimental feline infections, signs include inappetence, vomiting and passage of bloody feces containing much mucus and shreds and casts of intestinal epithelium—results of the burrowing activities of the adult trichinae and their first-stage larval offspring. Also described are weakness, wasting, stiffness of the limbs and generalized tenderness on handling. As in man, the effects may range from minimal to death, depending on how many larvae are eaten.

In man, the variety of signs, symptoms and complications are legion. Edema about the eyes and intense myalgia are considered virtually pathognomonic. Myocarditis and pneumonia are often the actual causes of death. The eyes and central nervous system are now and then affected.

## DIAGNOSIS

Trichinosis can be diagnosed definitively by recovery of the parasite at any one of three stages in the cycle of infection. Although the initial intestinal phase is often asymptomatic, the presence of hemorrhagic enteritis, if it occurs, should prompt examination of the stool. Whether or not fecal flotation discloses ova of other parasites, sediment of centrifuged material should also be examined, for it is here that adult trichinae will be found—worms varying in length from about 1.5 to 4 mm. Seeing them for the first time under the microscope, one is startled by their relatively large size and husky appearance. Also, one tends to assume at first glance that, as in many nematodes, the blunt anterior end is the head and the tapered structure the tail; however, just the opposite is the case. The tapered end consists largely of esophagus, with its single column of conspicuous "stichosome" cells, while the thicker posterior is notable for the genital structures. The majority of the worms are female. Just behind the esophagus is the vulva, from which large numbers of first-stage larvae emerge, and behind that is the uterus, in which developing larvae may sometimes be distinguished as fine linear structures. At the posterior rounded end is the ovary. The blunt posterior of the much smaller male is equipped with two copulatory prongs or lobes.

Because of their relatively large size and characteristic form, these worms should not easily be confused with the much smaller, slimmer larvae (all measuring about an average of 300 microns) of several other parasites that might be encountered in cat or dog feces—those of *Strongyloides stercoralis, Aelurostrongylus abstrusus, Crenosoma vulpis, Filaroides osleri, Angiostrongylus vasorum,* or (in stale samples) hookworm species.

Within several days of infection, first-stage larvae, the offspring of the copulating adults, penetrate the intestinal wall to migrate by various routes throughout the body. With luck, they may be detected in circulating blood by a modified Knott's test. One milliliter of EDTA-treated blood is mixed with 9 ml. of 2 per cent formalin, and the centrifuged sediment is stained with methylene blue. The rather rigid cylindrical trichina larvae are just over 100 microns long, in no way to be confused with the much longer, slender, threadlike and wavy microfilariae of *Dirofilaria immitis* or *Dipetalonema reconditum.*

The third method of diagnosis, used most frequently in man, is muscle biopsy. Chances of demonstrating migrating or unencysted larvae in skeletal muscle are best if the procedure is delayed until the fifth week of infection. About a gram of muscle is taken, usually from a limb. A third of the specimen is fixed in formalin for microscopic study; the rest is refrigerated in physiological saline solution to be examined, if need be, by means of digestion or maceration.

For autopsy diagnosis, tongue and diaphragm are generally considered the sites of the most numerous cysts. Calcified larval cysts are evidence of old rather than recent infection.

Important corroborative evidence of clinical trichinosis is eosinphilia, which may appear as early as 10 days after infection, reach a peak in the third or fourth week and subside gradually over weeks or months. In one cat, eosinophils constituted 22 per cent of the total WBC at three weeks from onset of illness and were still moderately elevated several months after recovery (Holzworth and Georgi, 1974).

## TREATMENT

In addition to symptomatic and supportive measures, trichinosis in man, if severe, is usually treated with thiabendazole, which is believed to be effective against the parasite in both the intestinal and migratory phases. Supplementation with corticosteroids is considered advisable to prevent the side effects of thiabendazole and also seems to provide relief from inflammation and pain.

Studies with experimental infections in animals, however, provide inconclusive evidence as to the parasiticidal efficacy of a great variety of drugs, including thiabendazole, and suggest that natural body defenses are lowered in animals treated with corticosteroids, so that adult trichinae remain longer in the intestine, larvae are more numerous, susceptibility to secondary infection is increased and mortality is higher (Gould, 1970).

In one clinical infection in a cat, signs of hemorrhagic enteritis and discharge of adult parasites ceased promptly concurrently with three days' treatment with a preparation containing neomycin, sulfonamides and kaolin (Kaobiotic®[Upjohn] ½ tablet q.i.d.) (Holzworth and Georgi, 1974). Whether this treatment was truly effective or the infection was abating in its natural course cannot be known. Because the cat never showed signs of severe systemic illness, specific parasiticides were not considered.

In man, treatment with thiabendazole is recommended only for severe infection, at a dose of 25 mg./kg. twice a day, until improvement occurs or signs of toxicity develop (vomiting, diarrhea, fatigue and unsteadiness). This dosage is within the range used for other parasitisms of dogs.

Thiabendazole is not generally recommended for cats; however, it has been used to treat *Strongyloides* infection in that species without ill effect at the same dose as in man and dogs (personal communication, William Jackson, D.V.M., Lakeland, Fla.).

### SUPPLEMENTAL READING

Conn, H. F.: Current Therapy 1975. Philadelphia, W. B. Saunders Co.
Gould, S. E.: Trichinosis in Man and Animals. Springfield, Illinois, Charles C Thomas, 1970.
Holzworth, J., and Georgi, J. R.: Trichinosis in a cat. J. Am. Vet. Med. Assn., 165:186–191, 1974.

# GIARDIASIS

GERALD JOHNSON, D.V.M.
*New York, New York*

*Giardia* sp. has received little recognition as a pathogen in the dog, although its pathogenicity has been established in man. In spite of its ubiquity, the organism is seldom detected, perhaps because it has not been considered a pathogen. There have been no detectable differences in the organism found in various hosts, i.e., *G. lamblia* vs. *G. canis*; therefore, it will be referred to here simply as *Giardia* sp. Burrows and Lillis (1967) reported that one third of 660 stray dogs from New Jersey with abnormal stools harbored *Giardia* organisms. Epidemics have been reported in man.

Although dogs may have giardiasis and be asymptomatic, or the infestation may be self-limiting, in the dogs showing signs, treatment is indicated. In our experience, it is seen most often in young dogs. Signs may include soft, light-colored stools—occasionally mixed with mucus and blood—increased frequency of defecation, and tenesmus.

The organism normally inhabits the upper small intestine and does not invade tissue. Morphologic changes in the mucosa associated with *Giardia* sp. have been described in man but not in the dog. Morphologic changes are not always present despite functional changes.

The organisms are found on the mucosal surface and in the intervillous spaces, aligning themselves on the microvillous border of the epithelial cells. Varying degrees of malabsorption have been reported in man. Carbohydrate malabsorption can be demonstrated in infected dogs by means of the oral glucose and D-xylose tolerance tests. In man, there is an association between *Giardia* infestation and immunodeficiency, particularly IgA deficiency. This association has not been documented in the dog.

Detection of trophozoites in the dog is most easily done through saline smears of the stool. It is important that the stool be recently passed or obtained digitally.

Smears made from swabs inserted into the rectum or colon are also satisfactory. To eliminate confusion with other motile protozoa, a wet Lugol's iodine slide or Wright's stain applied to a dried smear may be used to elucidate the characteristic morphology of *Giardia* sp. Methods are also available for detecting cysts, including concentration techniques. Cysts are irregularly passed in man. Difficulty in diagnosis occurs in individual dogs in whom trophozoites or cysts are not detected in stool specimens. The most definite means of diagnosis is biopsy of the small bowel or examination of mucus from the duodenum or upper jejunum, either by aspiration of the duodenum or at celiotomy. Superinfestation should be ruled out.

Response to treatment is usually dramatic and occurs in a few days. Recommended drugs are metronidazole (Flagyl® [Searle]), administered at 25 mg./kg. every 12 hours orally for 5 days, or quinacrine (Atabrine® [Winthrop]), 50 to 100 mg. every 12 hours orally for 3 days, repeated in 3 days.

## SUPPLEMENTAL READING

Alp, M. H., and Hislop, I. G.: The effect of *Giardia lamblia* infestation of the gastrointestinal tract. Australasian Ann. Med., *18*:232–237, 1969.

Ament, M.E., and Rubin, C. E.: Relation of giardiasis to abnormal intestinal structure and function in gastrointestinal immunodeficiency syndromes. Gastroenterology, *62*:216–226, 1972.

Burrows, R. B., and Lillis, W. G.: Intestinal protozoan infections in dogs. J. Am. Vet. Med. Assn., *150*:880–883, 1967.

Soulsby, E. J. L.: Helminths, Arthropods and Protozoa of Domesticated Animals. 6th ed. of Mönnig's Veterinary Helminthology and Entomology. Baltimore, The Williams & Wilkins Co., 1968, pp. 594–596.

Takano, J., and Yardley, J. H.: Jejunal lesions in patients with giardiasis and malabsorption. An electron microscopic study. Bull. Hopkins Hosp., *116*:413–429, 1965.

Zinneman, H. H., and Kaplan, A. P.: The association of giardiasis with reduced intestinal secretory immunoglobulin A. Am. J. Dig. Dis., *17*:793–797, 1972.

# TRICHOMONIASIS

R. G. BUCKNER, D.V.M.
*Stillwater, Oklahoma*

*and* S. A. EWING, D.V.M.
*St. Paul, Minnesota*

*Pentatrichomonas* spp. frequently are associated with mucoid and occasionally hemorrhagic diarrhea in puppies. Clinical symptoms, including diarrhea, lethargy, anorexia, retarded growth and rough hair coat, commonly appear between 6 and 8 weeks of age. The infection has been observed asymptomatically in mature dogs, implying that a carrier state may exist. Puppies born to infected dams may be expected to exhibit symptoms at 3 or 4 weeks of age. The infection has been observed in association with unsanitary kennel conditions and has been reported in dogs eating feed contaminated with mouse droppings. The prepatent period has not been determined accurately.

## DIAGNOSIS

Diagnosis may be made by one of three methods: (1) observation of direct saline (0.85 per cent) smears prepared either with freshly passed feces or from rectal swab, (2) similar study of fresh feces in preserved PAF fixative (Burroughs, 1967) and stained with either thionin or azure A and (3) culture of fresh feces employing egg slant overlaid with either Locke's solution or Locke's solution and inactivated serum. Light infections may be missed by the direct microscopic methods, but culture requires laboratory assistance. The second technique has advantages to the practitioner, because concentration is possible and examination may be delayed.

In the second technique, the fixative and stains are prepared as follows:

PAF FIXATIVE

| | |
|---|---|
| Phenol crystals (white) | 20.0 gm. |
| Normal saline (0.85 per cent) | 825.0 ml. |
| Ethanol (95 per cent) | 125.0 ml. |
| Formaldehyde solution | 50.0 ml. |
| Liquefied phenol (23.0 ml. may be substituted for crystals) | |

STAINS

| | |
|---|---|
| Thionin powder | 10.0 mg. |
| Distilled water | 100.0 ml. |
| Azure A powder | 10.0 mg. |
| Distilled water | 80.0 ml. |

The feces are covered with fixative and permitted to stand at room temperature for one hour or longer. Excess fixative is then decanted, and 1 to 2 drops of the remaining sediment is mixed well, removed and stained. If concentration is desired, the following procedure is useful: (1) strain the fixed sample through gauze, (2) centrifuge the fluid collected at 1000 rpm for two to three minutes and decant the excess fixative, (3) wash and centrifuge the sediment repeatedly (two to four times) with normal saline (0.85 per cent) and (4) stain one to several drops of the washed sediment with thionin or azure A to facilitate recognition. Samples should be examined at 430× for differential diagnosis.

Identification of the organism suspended in a saline (0.85 per cent) smear is made by observing characteristic movement, i.e., undulating, frequently changing shapes and moving with moderate speed. The flagella are not usually visible, but the oval nucleus in the anterior half of the body may be observed. When stained, it is most frequently pear-shaped; however, it may be oval and vary in size from $5\mu$ to $20\mu$ by $3\mu$ to $14\mu$.

## TREATMENT

Treatment of canine trichomoniasis has been most effective using metronidazole (Flagyl® [Searle]) at the rate of 66 mg./kg. of body weight daily, administered orally for five consecutive days. Dogs fed as much as 99 mg./kg. of body weight daily for 30 days have not exhibited toxicity.

An alternative treatment is glycobiarsol (Milibis® [Winthrop]). This has been used

970

in limited trials but its efficacy needs further documentation.

## SUPPLEMENTAL READING

Buckner, R. G., and Besch, E. D.: Transmission studies and control of canine trichomoniasis. Abstracts of the 20th Annual Meeting of the American Association for Laboratory Animal Science, 1969, p. 118.

Burroughs, R. B.: A new fixative and techniques for the diagnosis of intestinal parasites. Techn. Bull. Reg. Med. Techn., 37:208–212, 1967.

Levine, N. D.: Protozoan Parasites of Domestic Animals and of Man. Minneapolis, Burgess Publishing Co., 1969, p. 103.

Soulsby, E. J. L.: Helminths, Arthropods and Protozoa of Domesticated Animals. 6th ed. of Mönnig's Veterinary Helminthology and Entomology. Baltimore, The Williams & Wilkins Co., 1968.

# A DIAGNOSTIC APPROACH TO CHRONIC DIARRHEA

MICHAEL D. LORENZ, D.V.M.
*Athens, Georgia*

## INTRODUCTION

This article describes a logical diagnostic approach to chronic diarrhea. This system is not new; it has been used by clinicians for several years and its usefulness has stood the test of time. The intent here is not to describe the various tests or gastrointestinal disorders, but rather it is to present to the veterinary practitioner a concise and useful plan to follow when pursuing the cause of chronic diarrhea.

## SMALL BOWEL VERSUS LARGE BOWEL

The initial step in the diagnosis of chronic diarrhea is to localize the clinical signs and physical findings to either the small or the large intestine. Animals with small bowel diseases produce stools characterized by a watery or mushy consistency. The volume of stool passed may be normal or increased, and the frequency of defecation may be normal or modestly increased. Mucus and fresh blood are absent except in puppies or kittens, in which small bowel disease may result in some fresh blood in the stool. Blood, when present, is digested and melena results. The patient may experience severe weight loss. Gross steatorrhea is pathognomonic of small bowel disease or pancreatic exocrine insufficiency.

Dogs and cats with chronic large bowel diarrhea produce stools that are soft or semiformed. Stools are passed frequently and in scant amounts. Tenesmus is a classic clinical sign. Fresh blood and mucus are almost always present in the stool. Weight loss is not remarkable except in very chronic cases. From the above discussion, it should be clear that gross examination of the patient's feces and observation of the act of defecation are important initial steps in evaluating the patient with chronic diarrhea.

## SMALL BOWEL DIARRHEA

Small bowel disorders can be classified by means of the presence or absence of fat in the stool. Thus, the clinician should try to document the presence or absence of fat in the stool before proceeding within other in-depth studies. Diseases that tend to cause little or no steatorrhea include chronic endoparasitism, eosinophilic gastroenteritis, neoplasia and dietary allergy. Diseases characterized by the presence of steatorrhea include maldigestion disorders (biliary obstruction, hepatic insufficiency, pancreatic exocrine insufficiency) and malabsorption syndromes (lymphangiectasia, infiltrative neoplasia, other chronic enteropathies). Neutral fat in the stool may be observed grossly or demonstrated microscopically with Sudan IV stain. Sudan IV stains neutral fat droplets reddish-orange; however, fatty acids are not stained. A 24-hour fecal fat excretion study can quantitate the degree of steatorrhea present. This is the preferred method for documenting the steatorrhea resulting from malabsorption inasmuch as the Sudan IV test may be negative. Unlike maldigestion disorders, malabsorption syndromes result in the fecal loss of free fatty acids and monoglycerides. Determining the presence or absence of steatorrhea is the second step in the diagnostic plan for cases of chronic diarrhea of small bowel origin. Once the presence or absence of fat has been established, the clinician should pursue more in-depth studies.

## Steatorrhea Absent

1. *Chronic endoparasitism.* Direct fecal smears, duodenal fluid aspiration or intestinal mucosal biopsy are procedures necessary to rule out *Giardia* infection. Fecal flotations on at least three random stool samples may be necessary to document hookworms. Fecal flotations and direct fecal smears are often diagnostic if numerous stool samples are examined.

2. *Eosinophilic gastroenteritis.* In many cases, this disease is suspected when the fecal flotation is negative and a circulating eosinophilia is found in the hemogram. However, definitive diagnosis of this disease is based upon characteristic morphologic changes in an intestinal biopsy. However, intestinal biopsy is seldom done, because this disorder responds very well to oral glucocorticoid therapy.

3. *Neoplasia.* Intestinal neoplasia usually causes obstruction of the intestinal tract, and vomiting as well as diarrhea occurs. A barium series may demonstrate this obstruction. Unless needed to document obstruction or linear foreign body, a barium series is seldom diagnostic in cases of chronic diarrhea unaccompanied by vomiting. In most cases, the therapeutic benefit of the barium is superior to its diagnostic benefit.

4. *Dietary allergy.* No tests exist that are absolutely specific for this disorder. Dietary elimination studies are the usual methods available to the veterinary practitioner for documenting dietary allergy. A favorable response to the elimination of certain dietary substances is indirect evidence of dietary allergy. Simply changing dog foods should not be the method employed for conducting the test. Instead, careful exclusion of basic nutrients must be performed.

5. *Salmonellosis.* This condition is best documented with fecal cultures. The presence of a positive salmonella culture is not absolute proof that the bacteria is the cause of the animal's illness, since salmonella organisms can be isolated from clinically normal dogs and cats. In most cases, it is wise to treat with the appropriate antibiotic; however, the clinician should be aware that the salmonella organism might be an incidental finding.

## Steatorrhea Present

1. *Maldigestion* (biliary obstruction, hepatic insufficiency, pancreatic exocrine insufficiency). Icterus, ascites or acholic stools may incriminate liver dysfunction. Pancreatic exocrine insufficiency can be documented by fecal trypsin analysis (gelatin tube digestion, x-ray film digestion) and microscopic exam of the stool for starch (Lugol's stain) and muscle fibers.

2. *Malabsorption* (lymphangiectasia, diffuse infiltrative neoplasia, nonspecific chronic enteropathies). Inasmuch as these conditions may result in enteric loss of protein, determinations of total protein and A/G ratio are indicated as well as specific tests for absorption of nutrients. Hypoproteinemia, if present, is characterized by a decrease in both albumin and globulin, since both proteins are lost via the intestinal tract. Specific absorption tests include urine and blood D-xylose, glucose, vitamin $B_{12}$ and radioactive triolein and oleic acid. The oral fat absorption test, before and after enzyme hydrolysis, is an inexpensive test that can be performed in any practice situation without special equipment. A negative fat absorption test after enzyme hydrolysis provides presumptive evidence of malabsorption.

## MINIMUM DATA BASE SUMMARY—SMALL BOWEL

In summary, the *minimum* data base for a case of chronic small bowel diarrhea should include

1. Direct fecal smears and fecal flotations on at least three random fecal samples.

2. Microscopic stool exam with Sudan IV and Lugol's stains.

3. Fecal trypsin (three determinations on random stool specimens).
4. Oral fat absorption test.
5. CBC, urine analysis, total protein and A/G ratio.

## LARGE BOWEL DIARRHEA

Diseases that produce chronic large bowel diarrhea include
1. Histiocytic ulcerative colitis.
2. Eosinophilic ulcerative colitis.
3. Idiopathic ulcerative colitis.
4. Histoplasma colitis.
5. Colonic neoplasia.
6. Cecal inversion.
7. Spastic colon syndrome.
8. Allergic colitis.
9. Protothecal colitis.

The diagnostic plan for these disorders should include routine procedures such as rectal exams, gross stool exams, microscopic stool exams and fecal flotations. In addition, proctoscopic examination with mucosal biopsy is of great diagnostic importance. This procedure can establish a morphologic diagnosis, reveal the etiologic agent and establish prognosis. Examination of colonic mucus and exudates may detect the etiologic agent. Cytologic examination of this material may provide clues to the cause (neoplasia versus inflammation) of the colonic disorder. Barium enema is reserved for cases in which the proctoscopic exam is negative. This procedure can establish the location and nature of disease in the proximal or transverse colon. It is the procedure of choice for confirming a diagnosis of cecal inversion. Fecal cultures are of little diagnostic benefit, but mycotic infections can be diagnosed with this technique. A hemogram and urine analysis screen many body systems and should be considered an extension of the physical examination. Both are included as part of the diagnostic plan.

## MINIMUM DATA BASE
## SUMMARY—LARGE BOWEL

1. Proctoscopic exam with biopsy.
2. Barium enema.
3. Cytology of colonic exudates.
4. Fecal culture.
5. CBC, urine analysis.

## CONCLUSION

This article attempts to give the reader a sound diagnostic plan for evaluating patients with chronic diarrhea. In most cases, a definitive diagnosis can be made following the plans outlined above. The procedures utilized are not time-consuming inasmuch as several procedures may be performed on the same fecal specimen or at the same time in the patient. The reader is referred to other articles in this section for more in-depth discussions of each disorder.

# ACUTE PANCREATITIS

JOHN L. PARKS, D.V.M.
*New York, New York*

## INTRODUCTION

By definition, pancreatitis denotes inflammation of the pancreas. In a broader sense, it is a disease process that presents to the clinician not only signs involving the pancreas but also those associated with biliary, hepatic and gastrointestinal disturbances.

There are two classic forms of acute pancreatitis: the interstitial, edematous form and the fulminating, hemorrhagic, necrotizing form. With the proper management, the former usually affords a favorable prognosis, while the latter can be highly lethal.

Recognition and treatment of pancreatitis are difficult in that there are many intermediate types between these two forms. In addition, the clinical course can be very unpredictable, and recurrent attacks of acute pancreatitis with abscess formation and fibrosis often follow.

There is no age, sex or breed predisposition; however, the disease is usually seen in

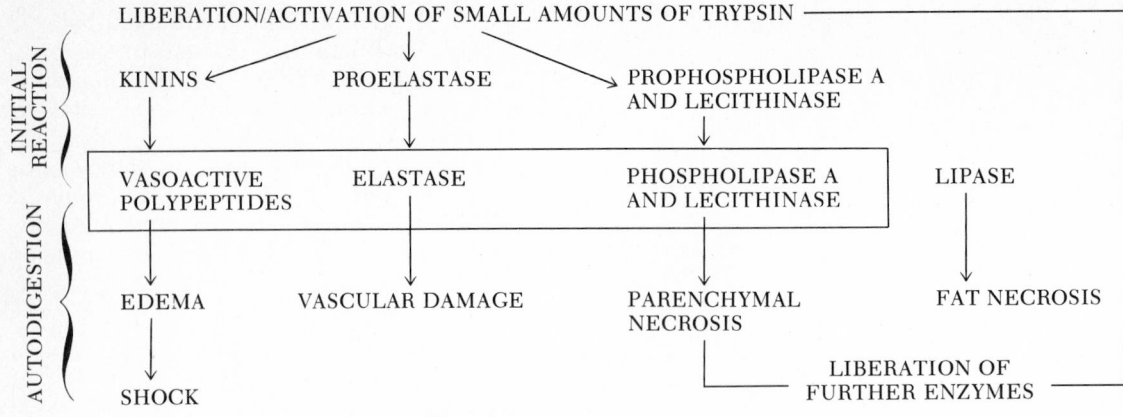

**Figure 1.** Acute pancreatitis.

the middle-aged female dog of the medium to small breeds. Obesity seems to be a common finding among those affected (Anderson, 1968).

The etiology of naturally occurring pancreatitis is unknown. It can be seen following pancreatic surgery and abdominal trauma. Corticosteroids have been found to induce pancreatitis in rabbits in experimental situations (Stumpf *et al.*, 1956).

Pancreatitis is an autodigestive disease process. Enzymes released from the injured tissue not only attack the organ itself but have systemic effects on cardiovascular function (Fig. 1). Pancreatic hemorrhage and necrosis lead to peritonitis, often with fat saponification. Systemically, vasoactive polypeptides released from the pancreas cause peripheral vascular collapse and shock.

## HISTORY

The typical historical findings in patients with pancreatitis include vomition, diarrhea, anorexia, lethargy and depression. These symptoms may come on acutely as with most gastrointestinal disorders, or the disease may take a more chronic course, with periodic bouts of acute illness. Occasionally, an animal is presented in shock with peracute symptoms.

These symptoms are very general and can be attributed to any number of gastrointestinal diseases and metabolic disorders. A thorough clinical examination and appropriate laboratory and radiographic work-ups are necessary to assure a proper diagnosis.

## PHYSICAL EXAMINATION

The physical examination can often be as noncontributory as the historical data. Anterior abdominal pain and shock should alert the clinician to the possibility of pancreatitis. Occasionally, jaundice and an abdominal mass in the area of the pancreas are found. The state of hydration and urine production are important considerations in proper patient management.

## LABORATORY DATA

The laboratory work-up on a suspected pancreatitis patient should include a complete blood count (CBC), broad-based blood screen (SMA-12/60)*, electrolytes, serum amylase and lipase and urinalysis.

Leukocytosis and a shift to the left are variable findings in pancreatitis, depending on the duration and severity of the disease. Patients with chronic pancreatitis often have local abscessation, which favors a more dramatic neutrophilic response (up to 50,000 WBC).

The results of a broad-based blood screen will reflect the secondary effects of pancreatitis on liver and kidney function. Elevations of serum glutamic pyruvic transaminase (SGPT), alkaline phosphatase and total bilirubin are common.

Prerenal elevations of blood urea nitrogen (BUN) and serum creatinine are often found in patients that present in shock.

---

*SMA-12/60 Autoanalyzer,® Technicon Industrial Systems, Technicon Instruments Corp., Tarrytown, New York 10591.

These values should be assessed in conjunction with the results of urinalysis to detect primary renal disease (low specific gravity, 1.008 to 1.012).

Hyperglycemia can be observed in acute pancreatitis. It can be a transient or persistent finding when diabetes mellitus is present. If the blood glucose remains above 180 mg./100 ml., diabetes mellitus should be suspected and treated accordingly.

Hyperlipemia, milky or cream-colored plasma, a nonspecific laboratory finding in pancreatitis, can also be seen with diabetes mellitus, hypothyroidism and hyperadrenalism and following ingestion of a large fatty meal.

The serum electrolyte disturbances again reflect changes secondary to pancreatitis. Serum sodium and, more importantly, serum potassium can be elevated in patients that are significantly dehydrated and in shock with oliguria.

Low serum calcium levels (below 6.2 mg./100 ml.) occur when sufficient fat necrosis has trapped calcium ions in the saponification process. Glucagon released from pancreatic islet cells has also been incriminated as a hypocalcemic factor (Anderson, 1971). Clinically, a marked, rapid fall in serum calcium can cause tetany.

Elevation of serum amylase (2 to 3 times normal value) and lipase (greater than 1 sigma unit) in the absence of poor renal function is the laboratory finding most helpful in diagnosing pancreatitis. The presence of increased enzyme activity in the blood is dependent on the severity of the inflammatory process and the duration of the disease process. Experimentally, serum amylase increases rapidly and remains elevated for a variable period, while lipase activity tends to rise slowly and persist longer. Clinically, this difference may not be valid. Both enzymes are excreted by the kidney and are subject to false elevations in the presence of primary renal disease.

## RADIOGRAPHY

Abnormal radiographic findings are variable and most often localized to the area of the pancreas and adjacent structures. Duodenal ileus is a common finding often associated with an ill-defined fluid density in the pancreatic bed. Localized and generalized peritonitis show up radiographically as hazy fluid densities. Occasionally a mass lesion may be found that displaces both gastric and colonic shadows.

## MANAGEMENT

Management of the pancreatitis patient requires coordination of medical and surgical skills and repeated assessment of the clinical course progression to reverse a potentially lethal disease (Fig. 2). In general, the disease in the mild state can be managed by resting the pancreas from its digestive role while maintaining proper hydration and electrolyte balance. However, the presence of shock, persistence of clinical symptomatology and a progressive failing clinical course indicate the need for surgical intervention to aid the healing process.

**Shock.** The presence of shock is a grave sign and requires prompt and vigorous therapy. A large-bore intravenous catheter (16- to 18-gauge) should be placed in the jugular vein for rapid administration of fluids and central venous pressure (CVP) monitoring. The urinary bladder should also be catheterized to allow for continuous monitoring of urinary output (normally 1 to 2 cc./kg./hr.) as an indirect assessment of blood pressure. Lactated Ringer's solution should be rapidly administered to effect to expand the collapsed circulatory volume while CVP and urine output are monitored. Sodium bicarbonate is administered empirically at a rate of 2 to 4 mEq. per kg. of body weight for each half-hour the patient is in shock. Hydrocortisone sodium succinate (4 to 20 mg./kg./hr.) or dexamethasone (2 to 10 mg./kg./4 to 6 hr.) should be given intravenously. A broad-spectrum parenterally administered antibiotic (chloramphenicol, cephalothin, ampicillin, kanamycin) should be given at recommended dosages and continued for at least 10 days after shock has been reversed.

**Medical Therapy.** Once the shock state has been reversed, the patient should be maintained with medical therapy. These patients in which shock cannot be reversed are candidates for surgical intervention with the realization that they are very poor surgical risks.

As previously stated, the medical management of acute pancreatitis involves resting the pancreas from its digestive functions while restoring and maintaining adequate

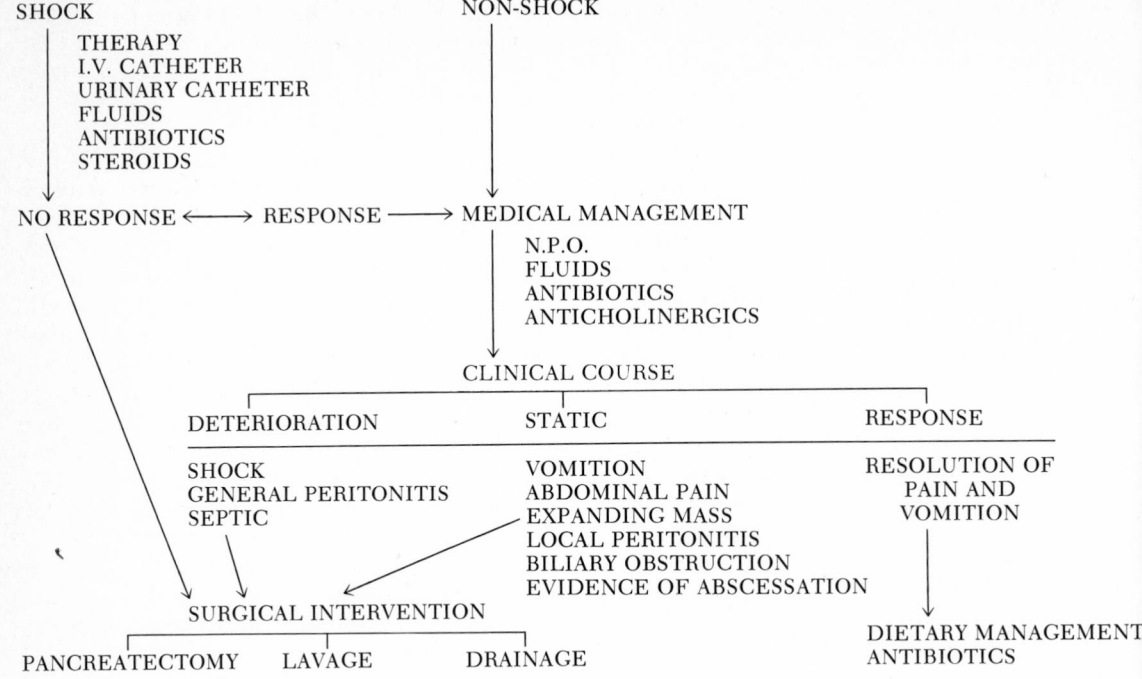

**Figure 2.** Injury to the acinar cell.

fluid and electrolyte balance. Food, water and medicaments should not be given orally until the inflammation has subsided and vomiting has ceased. A balanced electrolyte solution, i.e., lactated Ringer's, should be administered intravenously in the dehydrated or vomiting patient or subcutaneously in those with lesser clinical involvement. Pancreatitis patients should receive a minimum of 40 cc./kg./day divided b.i.d. or t.i.d.

Broad-spectrum antibiotics should be given to combat secondary infection of inflamed pancreatic tissue. Anticholinergic drugs (atropine sulfate, Darbazine® [Norden], Probanthine® [Searle]) are indicated in the vomiting patient and to reduce pancreatic secretion. Overuse of these drugs can lead to patient discomfort from paralytic ileus, thus delaying recovery. Meperidine hydrochloride (5 to 10 mg./kg.) is the analgesic drug of choice if its use is warranted; it is not recommended in the presence of shock or failing clinical course (Anderson, 1969).

Calcium gluconate should be given if hypocalcemia occurs. The dosage of 10 to 30 ml. of a 10 per cent solution should be added to daily fluid volume based on repeated serum calcium determinations.

Diabetes mellitus concurrent with acute pancreatitis should be attacked as vigorously as is the acute pancreatitis; its treatment is described elsewhere in this text.

Once clinical improvement has been achieved (cessation of vomiting, absence of pain, etc.), small amounts of water can be given orally. If fluids are not vomited, small feedings can then be given, beginning with broth and gradually changing to a low-fat, good-quality protein diet. If vomiting resumes, peroral feeding should be stopped and the animal should be thoroughly reassessed.

**Surgery.** The patient that is unresponsive to medical management, continues to vomit, deteriorates or lapses into shock warrants surgical intervention in addition to rigorous medical therapy.

Pancreatic abscessation, biliary obstruction and localized and generalized peritonitis are not uncommon sequelae to acute pancreatitis. Their management can only be achieved by surgical means. Surgical intervention in acute pancreatitis is of high risk but offers an alternative approach to those patients unresponsive to medical therapy alone. Good patient monitoring and sound surgical judgment are important to successful surgery. The surgical procedures indicated include peritoneal drainage, peritoneal lavage and pancreatectomy.

*Peritoneal drainage* is indicated for the treatment of localized pancreatic necrosis and pancreatic abscessation and following pancreatectomy (Parks, 1974). The purpose of drainage is to allow a pathway for exteriorization of the inflammatory process and pancreatic enzymes. Multiple Penrose drains (¼- to ½-inch) should be placed along the involved area of the pancreas. Loosely wrapping the omentum around the drains and involved pancreas will help aid the exteriorization process. The drains should exit through the ventral abdominal wall just off the midline away from the celiotomy incision. Drains must be secured to the skin with sutures or safety-pinned to prevent their excursion or dislodgment by the patient. A sterile bulky dressing should be applied and changed daily. Drains should remain in place until flow ceases and clinical improvement is noted, generally for 3 to 5 days. Drain tract wounds should be kept open by daily gentle probing for several days after the drains have been removed.

*Peritoneal lavage* therapy is advocated for acute hemorrhagic necrotic pancreatitis with resultant generalized peritonitis (Parks *et al.*, 1973). Peritoneal lavage combines the techniques of lavage and drainage in its application. The dilution and spread of the peritoneal fluid allow for greater contact with the body's defense mechanisms in the peritoneum. The flushing and draining action accomplishes the mechanical removal of bacteria, enzymes, cellular debris and toxins. The resultant reduction of inflammation normalizes peritoneal surfaces and allows the pancreas to heal while reducing pain and eliminating ileus.

The lavage system consists of one inflow drain (Nos. 14 to 18 French rubber tube) placed high in the flank area and one or more outflow drains, either Penrose drains or sump, exiting from the ventral abdominal wall. The drains should be placed by an operative approach directly in the pancreatic bed. Drains should be fixed to the skin, and no dressings should be applied to allow unrestricted gravitational drainage of the lavage fluid.

The lavage solution consists of lactated Ringer's to which is added 2500 units of heparin, ½ gram ampicillin and ½ gram kanamycin per liter. The solution is warmed to body temperature and administered by a slow, continuous drip on a b.i.d. to t.i.d. schedule. Patients should receive 40 cc. of lavage solution per kg. of body weight.

The duration of lavage therapy is based on the clinical response and the presence of complications. Daily patient monitoring includes serum sodium and potassium, hematocrit and serum protein. Complications relating to lavage therapy include anemia, hypoproteinemia and hypokalemia. Once lavage therapy is discontinued, drains should remain in place for 24 to 48 hours to allow for collection of any residual fluid.

*Pancreatectomy*, partial or total, involves the excision of pancreatic tissue, a radical procedure requiring considerable surgical expertise. The surgical risks are high, and the difficulty of the procedure is further complicated by the altered anatomy of the diseased state. Endocrine and exocrine deficiency can be expected in total excision, which would require considerable replacement therapy postoperatively.

## SUPPLEMENTAL READING

Anderson, M. C.: Review of pancreatic disease. Surgery, 66:434, 1969.
Anderson, N.: Acute pancreatitis. *In* Kirk, R. W. (ed.): Current Veterinary Therapy III. Philadelphia, W. B. Saunders Co., 1968, pp. 526–531.
Anderson, W.: Boyd's Pathology for the Surgeon. 8th ed. Philadelphia, W. B. Saunders Co., 1971.
Parks, J. L.: Peritoneal drainage. J.A.A.H.A., 10:289, 1974.
Parks, J. L., Gahring, D., and Greene, R. W.: Peritoneal lavage for peritonitis and pancreatitis in 22 dogs. J.A.A.H.A., 9:442, 1973.
Stumpf, H. H., Wilens, S. L., and Somoza, C.: Pancreatic lesions and pancreatic fat necrosis in cortisone treated rabbits. Lab. Invest., 5:224, 1956.

# DISEASES OF THE LIVER

STEPHEN I. BISTNER, D.V.M.
*St. Paul, Minnesota*

The liver, the largest gland in the body, has many complex functions, including formation of bile, ketone bodies, plasma proteins and urea, storage of carbohydrates, control of carbohydrate metabolism, detoxification of many drugs and toxins, inactivation of polypeptides, and metabolism of fats. Because of the wide diversity of function and tremendous regenerative and reserve capacity of the liver, detection of specific hepatic disease is difficult before there is serious impairment of hepatic function.

The onset of hepatic disease can be insidious and the signs vague. Some of the signs frequently seen with hepatic disease (namely, anorexia, emesis, diarrhea, depression, jaundice, ascites, anemia and hemorrhagic tendencies) may also occur as a result of disease processes in other body organs. Hepatomegaly and acholic feces alone may be specific for hepatic disease. Thus, the astute clinician must be observant in order to diagnose and treat disorders of the liver.

In the initial physical examination, the clinician must pay special attention to the history with respect to the onset of illness and the possible ingestion of toxic agents or drugs that could influence hepatic function. The presence of an elevated temperature may indicate an inflammatory or infectious process. The history may reveal the presence of a darker than normal urine, indicating excess bilirubin. The stool may be light in color (acholic) or it may be darker than normal, indicating elevated levels of bile pigments. There may be bleeding tendencies evidenced by bleeding into body cavities. Bleeding tendencies may also be manifested by petechiation of the mucous membranes. The liver may be palpably enlarged behind the costal arch and may be painful. Ascites and edema may be present. In these cases, a complete examination of the heart and lungs is essential to evaluate the possibility of congestive heart disease.

## BILE METABOLISM

Jaundice, or icterus, is the condition recognized clinically by a yellowish discoloration of the plasma, the skin and the mucous membranes caused by staining with bile pigments. It is often the first and sometimes the only manifestation of hepatic disease. Consequently, it is important to understand the mechanisms of the secretory and excretory functions of the liver and the basic metabolism of bile pigments.

Bile is a complex aqueous solution of the organic and inorganic compounds. The major organic solutes of bile are the bile salts (white crystalline, steroid compounds derived from cholesterol), phospholipids, cholesterol and bile pigments.

Bilirubin derived from hemoglobin of senescent erythrocytes and various hepatic hemoproteins constitute the major bile pigments. Hemoglobin is transported in the plasma by haptoglobin to the reticuloendothelial cells where heme is degraded to biliverdin and then to bilirubin. Bilirubin is transported in the plasma as an albumin-bilirubin complex. Bilirubin enters the hepatic cell and is conjugated to become water soluble.

The serum bilirubin level represents a balance between input from the production of bile and hepatic removal of the pigment. Hyperbilirubinemia, therefore, may result from overproduction of bile pigment, which is too great for proper metabolism by the liver; from impaired uptake, conjugation or excretion of bilirubin; and from leakage back of conjugated pigment from damaged cells or bile ducts. In hepatic disease, icterus may be a result of both impaired uptake and metabolism of bile pigments as well as leakage of bile from damaged biliary ducts.

Unconjugated bilirubin is almost insoluble at a physiologic pH and is transported in the blood tightly bound to albumin. Conjugated bilirubin is water soluble and is excreted in the bile in combination with cholesterol, phospholipids and bile salts to form a mixed micelle. Some conjugated bile is excreted by the kidneys and is found in the urine. Bile excreted in the intestinal tract undergoes deconjugation and hydrogenation, forming urobilinoids (urobilinogen). Some of this is absorbed by the intestinal tract and passes to the hepatic portal system, thus giving rise to the enterohepatic circulation of bile pigments.

Bilirubin levels in serum are measured by the diazo (van den Bergh) reaction. Unconjugated bilirubin demonstrates an indirect van den Bergh reaction (requiring the solubilizing effect of alcohol for the coupling reaction), whereas conjugated bilirubin reacts directly (without alcohol). Total serum bilirubin values greater than 1.0 mg./100 ml. offer clear-cut evidence of hyperbilirubinemia. When the major fraction of serum bilirubin is direct reacting, it is interpreted as indicating that some form of regurgitation jaundice is present. When the direct reacting bilirubin constitutes 50 to 80 per cent of the total bilirubin, the cause is most likely to be a primary hepatic lesion. When the direct reacting bilirubin is greater than 80 per cent of the total bilirubin, an extraheptic obstructive process probably exists.

The laboratory report of the van den Bergh test indicates the total bilirubin concentration and the concentration of the direct reacting or conjugated bilirubin. The difference between these is the unconjugated or indirect reacting bilirubin. Elevations in the level of indirect reacting bilirubin in excess of the level of direct reacting bilirubin usually is indicative of a hemolytic process. Other evidence of hemolysis should be looked for, including a low packed cell volume, immature red blood cells and reticulocytes, petechiation of mucous membranes, hemoglobinuria and other clinical signs referable to anemia. It is not unusual for animals with severe hepatic disease to also have decreased red blood cell survival rates. Therefore, increased levels of both conjugated and unconjugated bilirubin may be present in these patients.

Small amounts of direct reacting conjugated bilirubin are normally present in the urine of dogs and cats. Increased levels of bilirubin in the urine imply the presence of hepatobiliary disease. The presence of bilirubin in the urine may antedate overt icterus or an increase in direct acting serum bilirubin and may serve as an early indication of the presence of hepatobiliary dysfunction. The absence of bilirubin in the urine in the presence of jaundice suggests the presence of unconjugated hyperbilirubinemia because only conjugated bilirubin is excreted into the urine.

It is also significant that, in hemolytic states where hemoglobin is saturated onto available protein binding sites, most dogs will show increased amounts of bilirubin in the urine without significant increases in the plasma conjugated bilirubin level. There is an indication that the canine kidney can degrade increased levels of hemoglobin to bilirubin.

Approximately 10 to 15 per cent of the urobilinogens formed in the intestinal tract are absorbed into the portal circulation. Increased levels of urinary urobilinogen may be present when excessive bile pigment forms, as in hemolysis; when intestinal transit time is prolonged, as in constipation; when bacteria invade the small intestine, allowing increased formation and reabsorption of urobilinogen; and when hepatic dysfunction interferes with normal enterohepatic disposition of urobilinogen. Urobilinogen excretion is decreased when entry of bilirubin into the intestinal tract diminishes, as in intra- or extrahepatic obstruction, when the intestinal bacterial flora is reduced, when bilirubin production decreases and when renal insufficiency is present.

Marked decreases in fecal bile pigments result in the presence of acholic stools, which are very white or light colored and greasy in appearance. This occurrence is added evidence of an obstructive phenomenon. Overproduction of bile pigments results in an increase in urobilinogen concentration in the stools, causing the stools to appear darker.

Kernicterus refers to the encephalopathy that may be present in human and animal neonates from unconjugated hyperbilirubinemia. This condition, although uncommon in animals, has recently been reported in dogs and cats. Evidence indicates tha bilirubin uncouples phosphorylative oxidation in neurons, and the condition is more prone to develop in states of acidosis.

## LABORATORY EVALUATION

Laboratory tests in hepatic disease are helpful in many different ways: (1) They are of value in detecting hepatic abnormalities (this is very helpful in the nonjaundiced animal); (2) these tests may suggest the underlying lesions behind the hepatobiliary dysfunction; (3) the tests may provide an index of the extent of hepatic damage and hence a way of giving a prognosis in the condition; and (4) these tests serve as a means of following the course of hepatic disease.

Many tests have been proposed to study hepatic disease; however, no single laboratory procedure fulfills all the objectives just outlined. Therefore, a carefully selected combination of liver function tests (liver profile) is very helpful in carefully examining the status of this organ.

## THE LIVER PROFILE

The liver profile includes tests based on bile pigment metabolism, which have already been discussed, tests based on excretion of foreign dyes via the bile and tests based on evaluation of enzyme activity and of synthesis in the liver.

**Tests Based on Excretion of Foreign Dyes Via the Bile.** Sulfobromophthalein sodium is used extensively in the detection of hepatic dysfunction. Following intravenous administration, the dye is rapidly removed from the blood, primarily by the liver, and is then excreted slowly in the bile. In the tests used most frequently, the concentration of the dye in the plasma is determined at a specific time after a standard dose of dye per unit of body weight (5 mg./kg.) has been administered intravenously.

Impairment of sulfobromophthalein removal from the blood may be due to interference in a number of liver functions: (1) decreased hepatic blood flow as seen in heart failure, hemorrhage and cirrhosis; (2) acquired liver disease that may result from toxins, drug toxicity, hepatic inflammation and tumors; (3) competition for carrier by bilirubin, bile salts or other anionic dyes. In this regard, a sulfobromophthalein test is seldom justified in jaundice; the results may be misleading because of competition for excretion by bilirubin and because an indication of hepatic disease is already present and not much new, useful information can be learned. Retention of more than 10 per cent of the dye in the serum after 30 minutes is considered abnormal. Indocyanine green can also be used to measure dye excretion by the liver.

**Tests Based on Evaluation of Enzyme Activity.** Serum transaminases are a group of enzymes that catalyze the transfer of an amino group to an $\alpha$-keto acid. Measurement of the activity of the two enzymes glutamic oxaloacetic transaminase and glutamic pyruvic transaminase has been used extensively in hepatic disease. In the dog, the serum glutamic pyruvic transaminase (SGPT) levels are more specific for hepatic disease than are the serum glutamic oxaloacetic transaminase (SGOT) levels. Elevated transaminase levels are a sensitive indicator of hepatic cell damage. In the jaundiced animal, SGPT levels in excess of 400 units usually indicate acute hepatocellular disease. When SGPT values are between 50 and 400 units, mild to moderate hepatocellular damage is present.

Serum alkaline phosphatase catalyzes the hydrolysis of a number of organic phosphate esters. The enzyme can be identified in many tissues, including red blood cells and bone; however, its exact function is unknown. There is good evidence that serum alkaline phosphatase is obtained principally from three sources: the skeleton, the hepatobiliary system and the intestinal tract. It is estimated that bone alkaline phosphatase accounts for 40 to 75 per cent of serum activity. The mechanism by which hepatobiliary disease leads to an increase in serum alkaline phosphatase is controversial. In dogs, extrahepatic obstructive jaundice is rare and elevated levels of serum alkaline phosphatase are often associated with hepatocellular jaundice (intrahepatic obstruction). Most evidence suggests that this occurs mainly because of regurgitation of enzymes, formed in the liver, from the intrahepatic biliary tree into the circulation.

Recent evidence indicates that elevations of serum alkaline phosphatase in biliary obstructions may not be associated with excretory blockage but rather with an overproduction of SAP by the liver.

The kidney of the cat is able to excrete alkaline phosphatase; consequently, this test is invalid in obstructive disease in this animal. Normal serum alkaline phosphatase levels in adult dogs are usually less than 8

King-Armstrong units; however, young puppies with rapid bone metabolism may have significantly elevated levels. Values of 9 to 20 King-Armstrong units indicate mild hepatic damage and values exceeding 20 King-Armstrong units are suggestive of severe damage. It is important to note that serum alkaline phosphatase levels can be reported in a number of different units and that values in controls and patients should be expressed in the same units.

Approximate conversion factors for alkaline phosphatase are as follows:

| UNITS | CONVERSION FACTOR |
|---|---|
| Bodansky → King-Armstrong | ×2.80 |
| King-Armstrong → Bodansky | ×0.34 |

**Evaluation of Synthesis in the Liver.** A large portion of the plasma proteins, including all the plasma fibrinogen, the albumin fraction and probably more than 80 per cent of the total globulin fraction, is synthesized by the liver. The remainder of the major plasma proteins, including gamma globulins, are produced by extrahepatic tissue. Normal values in the dog for total serum proteins are 5.3 to 7.5 gm./100 ml. In fibrosis or other chronic diseases of the liver, the albumin levels in the blood may be decreased, thus changing the albumin:globulin ratio (normal is 1.5 to 2.3).

With the salting out technique to determine albumin:globulin ratios, the globulin fraction contains all the gamma globulins, three-fourths of the beta globulins and one-fourth of the alpha globulins. The albumin fraction contains all of the albumins plus most of the alpha globulins and part of the beta globulins. Therefore, the serum electrophoretic method of plasma protein analysis is more valuable (although more complicated) in assessing changes in levels of plasma proteins. Changes in serum protein levels in animals with chronic hepatobiliary disease are quite common. However, alterations in plasma proteins may result from many other causes, such as severe proteinuria, chronic infection and malnutrition.

Cholesterol is the precursor of the steroid hormones and the bile acids. Cholesterol is both ingested as food and synthesized by the liver. The normal total serum cholesterol concentration is between 125 and 250 mg./100 ml., of which 70 per cent is normally esterified. Although total cholesterol levels may be elevated in hepatic disease, the ratio of esterified to nonesterified cholesterol levels may be more valuable in assessing the presence of hepatobiliary disease. Esterified cholesterol levels may be decreased in hepatic disease, altering the ratio of cholesterol ester to total cholesterol (normal is 60:100).

Serum uric acid also has been used as a liver function test. The rationale is that uric acid normally is converted to allantoin, which is then excreted in the urine. If the liver fails to perform this function, the serum concentration of uric acid increases. This test offers little information about liver function; however, when coupled with other tests in the liver profile, it may be of benefit in determining the extent of hepatic damage.

The use of clinical laboratory tests in the liver profile may permit the clinician to gain insight into the type of liver problem that exists. A more conclusive diagnosis based upon histopathologic examination of the liver can be performed via a hepatic biopsy. Hepatic biopsy can be performed by an exploratory laparotomy or by a needle biopsy. The Franklin modified Vim-Silverman biopsy needle is very effective for punch biopsies of the canine and the feline liver. Blind insertion of the biopsy needle through a percutaneous approach can be fraught with difficulty and may result in serious postoperative complications. A more satisfactory method of needle biopsy is the modified keyhole percutaneous liver biopsy technique.

The position of the liver is outlined by palpation behind the last rib. With the dog in dorsal recumbency, an area on the ventral midline is clipped and surgically prepared and an incision site 2 inches long is infiltrated with local anesthesia. A small incision (just large enough to accommodate the gloved index finger) is made in the abdomen. The border of the left hepatic lobe is fixed against the diaphragm or other abdominal organs. A separate skin incision adjacent to the abdominal incision is made to accommodate the biopsy needle. From this position, the needle is guided to the surface of the liver.

Once biopsy material is obtained, impression smears can be made, a portion fixed in buffered 10 per cent formalin and a small piece submitted for culture, if indicated. Liver biopsy techniques are most advantageous when disseminated hepatobiliary disease exists and when focal lesions in the liver can be adequately located and biopsied. Complications of liver biopsy may include excessive hemorrhage, bile-induced peritonitis, and injury to other abdominal organs. Proper evaluation of the patient prior to biopsy is extremely important in avoiding postoperative complications. Any hemorrhagic abnormalities should be controlled prior to biopsy.

## TREATMENT

The treatment of hepatic disease should emphasize four aims: to eliminate or remove if possible the injurious agent, to minimize the harmful effects of the agent on the liver, to encourage healing and regeneration, and to maintain the life of the animal until adequate liver function can be restored.

The animal with acute hepatic disease needs extensive nursing care and frequent evaluation of vital signs. For the animal with ascites, it is important to record body weight daily along with fluid consumption and urine volume. This can best be done by placing the animal in a metabolism cage.

The level of protein in the diet of an animal with hepatic disease can be extremely critical. Too little protein may not provide the animal with adequate nutrients for reparative processes. Too much protein may lead to ammonia retention because of the liver's inability to convert ammonia to urea. The retained ammonia with other nitrogenous products can produce nervous signs and lead to hepatic coma.

The gastrointestinal tract is the most important site of production of ammonia, which is formed from ingested ammonium salts and from the action of bacterial ureases on protein. At the outset, it is best to provide small amounts of proteins of high biologic value. The types of prescription diets used in renal disease can also be used in hepatic disease. Additional calories can be made available by feeding corn syrup orally or by giving glucose solutions parenterally. Glucose decreases tissue protein breakdown, thus helping to prevent an increase in nitrogenous material in the blood. Also, glucose may stimulate the combination of ammonia with glutamic acid to form glutamine, which acts as a storehouse for ammonia and helps to remove it from the blood where it may be toxic.

The use of antibiotics in the treatment of hepatic coma and nervous disorders due to the retention of ammonia has been well founded. Orally administered, poorly absorbed antibiotics, such as neomycin (20 mg./kg. of body weight every six hours) and kanamycin (10 mg./kg. of body weight every six hours), reduce the bacterial content of the gastrointestinal tract and decrease the organisms that form ammonia. Prolonged administration of neomycin may be complicated by development of a malabsorption syndrome or staphylococcal enteritis. Although only small amounts of neomycin are absorbed systemically, toxic blood levels may develop if renal impairment exists. Many types of antibiotics can be used for the treatment of specific hepatic infections. They are used in the same manner as in treating other infections in the body.

All the common hypnotics, sedatives and analgesics may be tolerated poorly by the patient with hepatic disease. Morphine is conjugated in the liver before it is excreted, and in hepatic disease the rate of conjugation may be greatly decreased, thus prolonging its action. Hepatic involvement is not required in meperidine (Demerol) excretion, and because of causing depression of the patient, the drug may be administered in one-half the normal dose. The rapid-acting, long chain barbiturates are detoxified mainly by the liver. Therefore, if barbiturates must be used, one should choose a barbiturate with the greatest renal excretion, such as barbital or phenobarbital. About 60 per cent of the phenothiazine derivative drugs are detoxified by the liver. Thus, the use of analgesics, hypnotics and sedatives in severe hepatic disease may be hazardous and should be avoided if possible. If these drugs are absolutely needed, the dosage should be decreased and the animal carefully observed.

Fluid and electrolyte balance are extremely important in the patient with hepatic disease. In the anorectic animal, fluids and medication can be given via stomach tube if vomiting is not present. If ascites and edema are present, sodium must be restricted. Body weight, fluid intake and urine output, hematocrit and electrolyte balance should be followed to prevent dehydration and hyponatremia.

The administration of corticosteroids may increase appetite and sense of well-being, diminish the bilirubin value and decrease the periportal inflammatory reaction in inflammatory hepatic diseases. There are, however, no good, controlled studies that indicate that steroid therapy alters the degree of hepatic necrosis or increases the rate of healing. Thus, steroids should be used very selectively and seem to be indicated in rare cases of acute hepatic necrosis with a deteriorating course and in hepatic lesions that may be associated with an allergic or autoimmune phenomenon.

Adequate nutrition is extremely important in treating the patient with hepatic disease. Adequate calories must be provided so that body proteins are not broken down and a negative nitrogen balance created. Proteins with a biologic value of 75 or greater should be fed at a rate of 2 to 3 gm./ kg. of body weight daily. Foods containing purine and uric acid precursors, such as fish meal, shellfish and glandular products (spleen, thymus, liver and other meat by-products), should not be fed. Fats should not be fed in excess quantities (not more than 4 per cent of the diet). Fats should be severely restricted if steatorrhea is present .

The term fatty liver usually is synonymous with the hepatic accumulation of triglycerides. The major hepatic lipids include phospholipids, triglycerides, fatty acids, cholesterol and cholesterol esters. Increased amounts of fat in the liver result from increased fatty acid supply to the liver, increased triglyceride formation and decreased synthesis or release of lipoproteins. Substances that decrease the fat content of the liver are known as lipotropic agents. Choline can be manufactured in the body in limited quantities and therefore is not considered a true vitamin. Methionine stimulates the formation of choline. Choline, in turn, is a constituent of the phospholipid lecithin and is required for normal fat transport. Therefore, supplementation of the diet with choline and methionine (Methischol® capsules [USV Pharm.]) may help to reduce fatty infiltration of the liver.

In addition, multivitamins should be administered to malnourished and severely anorectic animals. In severe cirrhosis of the liver, the absorption of the fat-soluble vitamins A, D, E and K may be severely impaired. These may be supplemented by parenteral administration.

Serious hepatobiliary disease may result in abnormal bleeding tendencies. The pathogenesis of the bleeding in hepatic disease is often complex and may be due to several factors: (1) The plasma may be deficient in clotting factors; (2) the blood platelets may be qualitatively and quantitatively defective; (3) endogenous anticoagulant factors may be present; (4) plasma fibrinolytic systems may behave abnormally. The one stage prothrombin time may reflect deficiencies of factor VII, Stuart factor, proaccelerin, prothrombin or fibrinogen. Abnormally long one stage prothrombin time may reflect severe hepatocellular damage or vitamin K deficiency. Four clotting factors in mammalian plasma, namely Christmas factor, Stuart factor, factor VII and prothrombin, are synthesized only if vitamin K is available. In animals with severe hepatocellular damage and prolonged one stage prothrombin times, large amounts of vitamin K may be without obvious benefit because hepatocellular damage prevents the synthesis of normal clotting factors. When vitamin K (AquaMephyton® [Merck Sharp and Dohme]) has to be administered, 5 to 10 mg. total dose can be given every 12 hours. If there is a prolonged clotting time, deep intramuscular injections should be avoided and the intravenous route used with a pressure bandage over the venipuncture site.

Ascites refers to the accumulation of free fluid within the peritoneal cavity. Although it is liable to occur in any hepatic disease, ascites is most commonly associated with cirrhosis of the liver and implies a poor prognosis. The mechanisms leading to the formation of ascites may be classified as primary and secondary. Primary ascites refers to the formation of transudates from the liver and perihilar lymphatics because of increased hepatic intravascular pressure or low plasma protein levels. Intra-abdominal tumors, especially involving the mesentery, may severely interfere with lymphatic drainage and produce ascites. Secondary mechanisms producing ascites are related to impaired renal excretion of salt and water.

Medical treatment of ascites due to hepatic disease does not attack the primary problem; however, it can be very effective in reducing the amount of ascitic fluid present and in making the animal more comfortable. Large amounts of ascitic fluid should not be removed by paracentesis unless the fluid interferes with respiration and other normal physiologic functions to such an extent that removal is mandatory. The rapid withdrawal of large amounts of ascitic fluid can lead to hypovolemic shock, renal failure and the loss of large amounts of protein.

An effective way to remove ascitic fluid is by the use of diuretic therapy, which brings about a slow diuresis during which excess body sodium and water are excreted while essential substances are retained. The diuretic of choice in most animals with ascites is hydrochlorothiazide (2 mg./kg. of body weight orally three times daily). Overzealous use of diuretics may lead to the development of electrolyte abnormalities, renal failure and hepatic coma. Coupled with the use of diuretics should be a low-sodium diet (77 mg./100 gm. diet on dry weight basis or about 100 mg./kg. of canned food) and enforced rest. More potent diuretics, such as ethacrynic acid (0.4 to 1.0 mg./kg. of body weight) are available but must be used with caution.

In patients with sodium retention that is unresponsive to diuretic therapy, microcrystalline spironolactone (25 mg./15 kg. of body weight) may be added to the treatment regimen. When all measures have failed in trying to remove ascitic fluid medically, the administration of prednisolone (10 to 20 mg. daily) may help to promote diuresis. Intravenous mannitol (1 gm./kg. of body weight intravenously) or plasma protein expanders may also help to initiate diuresis in animals with low extracellular fluid volume and plasma protein levels.

## SUPPLEMENTAL READING

Cornelius, C. E.: Liver function. *In* Kaneko, J. J., and Cornelius, C. E. (eds.): Clinical Biochemistry of Domestic Animals. Vol 1. 2nd ed. New York, Academic Press, 1970, pp. 161–230.
Cornelius, C. E.: New concepts in canine hepatic function. J. Am. Animal Hosp. Assn., 9:147–150, 1973.
Medway, W., Prier, J. E., and Wilkinson, J. S.: Textbook of Veterinary Clinical Pathology. Baltimore, The Williams & Wilkins Co., 1969.
Osborne, C. A., Stevens, J. B., and Perman, V.: Needle biopsy of the liver. J. Am. Vet. Med. Assn., 155:1605–1620, 1969.
Schiff, L.: Diseases of the Liver. 3rd ed. Philadelphia, J. B. Lippincott Co., 1969.

# CHOLE-LITHIASIS

WILLIAM D. SCHALL, D.V.M.
*East Lansing, Michigan*

Cholelithiasis is rare in cats and dogs. The prevalence is less than 1 per cent in both species, and about 75 per cent of the reported cases represent incidental postmortem findings. Obstructive icterus can occur, however, if a gallstone obstructs the common bile duct (choledocholithiasis).

## DIAGNOSIS

Because gallstones are rare and seldom cause overt clinical signs when present, the diagnosis of cholelithiasis is rare. Emesis and abdominal pain are clinical signs considered to be compatible with the presence of gallstones, but proof of this association is lacking. Regardless, either emesis or abdominal pain may prompt abdominal radiography, which may result in the discovery of radiodense gallstones. Less than one third of canine and feline choleliths are radiodense, however. Cholecystography or cholangiography may demonstrate radiolucent choleliths, but these contrast procedures are seldom performed. Hematologic and clinical chemistry determinations are noncontributory for the diagnosis of choleliths.

Choleliths may pass into the common bile duct (choledocholithiasis) and cause obstructive icterus. The hyperbilirubinemia is characterized by conjugated bilirubin concentration in excess of 50 per cent of the total. Urine analysis findings include bilirubinuria and a lack of urobilinogen if the obstruction is complete. Acholic feces are also characteristic of dogs and cats with choledocholithiasis if the obstruction is complete.

Obstructive icterus due to choledocholithiasis is also accompanied by increased serum activity of alkaline phosphatase, 5'-nucleotidase and leucine aminopeptidase. These enzymes are produced in greater quantity in response to cholestasis. Depending on the duration of the obstruction, secondary hepatic necrosis may occur and result in increased serum activity of transaminases and other leakage enzymes.

## THERAPY

There is no known specific medical therapy for cholelithiasis or choledocholithiasis. Chenodeoxycholic acid has been used to dissolve human gallstones that are primarily composed of cholesterol, but evidence accumulated to date suggests that cholesterol is not a major constituent of canine and feline choleliths.

Specific therapy of cholelithiasis and choledocholithiasis is restricted to surgery. Cholecystectomy is usually preferred. Presurgical evaluation of patients with choledocholithiasis should include activated clotting time determination. If the clotting time is increased, 5 to 10 mg. of vitamin $K_1$ should be administered intramuscularly prior to surgery.

Since bacterial infection, especially in dogs, may complicate partial or complete cholestasis, antibiotics are probably indicated. In the absence of *in-vitro* antibiotic sensitivity testing, those antibiotics known to be excreted in bile (ampicillin, cephalothin or tetracycline) should be administered.

# URETHRO-RECTAL FISTULAS

CARL A. OSBORNE, D.V.M.
*St. Paul, Minnesota*

Fistulas that connect the lumina of the urogenital tract and the intestines may be congenital or acquired. Although relatively uncommon, they may be associated with signs related to the urinary, reproductive or gastrointestinal systems.

## CONGENITAL URETHRORECTAL FISTULAS

A congenital fistula connecting the urethra and vagina with the ventral floor of the rectum has been reported in a 2-year-old female miniature poodle (Goulden *et al.*, 1973). The anomaly was characterized clinically by the passage of urine from both the anus and the vulva. An asymptomatic rectovaginal fistula was reported in a 1-year-old female Irish setter with urinary incontinence caused by anomalous development of the urogenital system (Knecht and Westerfield, 1971). At the University of Minnesota, an asymptomatic rectovaginal fistula was observed in an incontinent 5-month-old female German shepherd with an ectopic right ureter that connected with the vagina.

Congenital urethrorectal fistulas have recently been observed in three male English bulldogs (Goulden *et al.*, 1973; Osborne *et al.*, 1975). All three dogs had patent fistulas that connected the pelvic urethra with the rectum and voided urine from the anus and through the penis at the same time. This abnormal pattern of micturition was observed by the owners during the first few months of life. The fact that urine was voided through the anus only during micturition was consistent with the finding that there were no abnormal communications between the rectum and the urinary bladder or ureters. One dog had severe perineal dermatitis as a result of urine scald, and another had intermittent diarrhea. Unlike human beings with congenital urethrorectal fistulas, these dogs did not pass fecal material through the urethra. All three dogs had secondary bacterial cystitis caused by *Escherichia coli* and *Proteus* spp.

In man, congenital urethrorectal fistulas are frequently associated with an imperforate anus and anomalies of other body systems (Campbell, 1970). In one of the English bulldogs with a urethrorectal fistula, both ureters entered the mid-dorsal region of the urinary bladder rather than the trigone (Osborne *et al.*, 1975).

In one bulldog, an abnormal orifice located in the ventral wall of the rectum was detected with the aid of a speculum inserted through the anus (Goulden *et al.*, 1973). Urine was aspirated from a urethral catheter inserted into the rectal orifice. Contrast radiography was required to establish a specific diagnosis in all three bulldogs. Communication of the urethral lumen with the rectal lumen was demonstrated by positive contrast retrograde urethrography in two cases and by micturating cystourethrography in one case. Injection of contrast material under pressure during retrograde urethrography was required to force a sufficient quantity into the fistulas to be radiographically visible.

Surgical extirpation of the anomalous fistulas was performed following splitting of the pubic symphysis with an osteotome in two dogs. In the other dog, the lumen of the fistula was obliterated by ligation. A normal pattern of micturition was observed following fistulectomy and ligation. The secondary bacterial cystitis was eliminated by the use of antimicrobial agents selected on the basis of bacterial culture of urine and antibiotic sensitivity tests.

It has been hypothesized that congenital urethrorectal fistulas in man develop as a result of failure of the urorectal septum to separate the cloaca completely into an anterior urethrovesical segment and a posterior rectal segment. The cause of congenital urethrorectal fistulas in dogs is unknown. Although analysis of the pedigrees of the three bulldogs did not reveal any common ancestry, it is tempting to hypothesize that a hereditary predisposition to urethrorectal fistulas exists in this breed. The incidence of urethral prolapse is apparently higher in male English bulldogs than in other breeds; however, there is no evidence that they are related to the occurrence of urethrorectal fistulas.

## ACQUIRED URETHRORECTAL FISTULAS

Acquired fistulas between the urinary tract and the intestinal tract have been reported on several occasions in human beings as a result of inflammatory, traumatic or neoplastic lesions. The paucity with which they have been reported in the veterinary literature indicates that they are uncommon in domestic animals.

### SUPPLEMENTAL READING

Campbell, M. F.: Anomalies of the genital tract. *In* Campbell, M. F., and Harrison, J. H. (eds.): Urology. 3rd ed. Vol. 2. Philadelphia, W. B. Saunders Co., 1970.

Christie, B. A.: Incidence and etiology of vesicoureteral reflux in apparently healthy dogs (voiding cystourethrography described). Invest. Urol., *9*:184–194, 1971.

Goulden, B. E.: Diagnosis of vesico-ureteral reflux. New Zealand Vet. J., *16*:167–175, 1968.

Goulden, B., Bergman, M. M., and Wyburn, R. S.: Canine urethro-rectal fistulae. J. Small Animal Pract., *14*:143–150, 1973.

Knecht, C. D., and Westerfield, C.: Anorectourogenital anomalies in a dog. J. Am. Vet. Med. Assn., *159*:91–92, 1971.

Osborne, C. A., Engen, M. H., Yano, B. L., Brasmer, T. H., Jessen, C. R., and Blevins, W. E.: Congenital urethrorectal fistula in two dogs. J. Am. Vet. Med. Assn., *166*:999–1002, 1975.

# GASTRO-INTESTINAL FIBEROPTIC ENDOSCOPY

JAMES F. ZIMMER, D.V.M.
*Ithaca, New York*

Gastrointestinal endoscopy consists of examination of the mucosal aspect of the alimentary canal *in vivo* using any one of a variety of instruments. Although endoscopic examination of the alimentary canal with associated diagnostic procedures represents a major advance in the field of gastroenterology, it must be regarded as only a supplementary procedure in the diagnostic evaluation of cases of gastrointestinal disease. Endoscopy does not reduce the need for a complete history, a thorough physical examination, or laboratory and radiographic evaluations.

## INSTRUMENTATION

Gastrointestinal endoscopy cannot be considered a recent development. The history of gastric endoscopy dates back to 1868, when Kussmaul successfully inserted a straight metal-tube gastroscope into the stomach of a professional sword-swallower. It is reported that a seventeenth century veterinarian devised a hollow tube for the diagnosis and treatment of a bovine fecalith, thus predating the recorded use of endoscopy in man. During the past few decades, technical developments and enthusiasm for clinical application have resulted in the development of sophisticated endoscopic instruments.

The principle of fiberoptic endoscopy is based on the total internal reflection of light in tiny flexible glass fibers. A spot of light entering one end of a fiber is transmitted by "bouncing" along the walls of that fiber until it emerges at the opposite end. The spot of light that emerges is about 95 per cent as bright as that entering the fiber. To minimize the light loss and to prevent light from one fiber from scattering into adjacent fibers, each fiber is wrapped with insulation, usually a glass coating of a different refractive index. Approximately 200,000 of these insulated fibers are combined to form a bundle approximately ¼ inch in diameter. The fibers of each bundle are joined together only at the proximal and distal ends to provide greater flexibility of the fiber bundles.

In those endoscopes designed for clinical use there are two separate fiber bundles, one for viewing and one for light transmission. The fibers in the visual bundle are spatially oriented, so that the top of the object viewed at one end is in the same spatial orientation at the other end. A lens system at the distal or mucosal end focuses the image on that end of the bundle, and a lens system at the proximal or observer's end magnifies the image emerging from the bundle. The direct internal transmission of light through this flexible glass bundle enables the projection of a visual image from one end of the bundle to the other through curves, coils and even knots in the bundle. Light for illumination at the mucosal end of the endoscope is carried from an external light source through a nonspatially oriented bundle. The intensity of this light is sufficient for visualization and photography, but there is no heat because the light source is outside the patient. Still photography is easily accomplished by the addition of a standard 35-mm. camera with an appropriate adapter.

In addition to the fiberoptic light bundle and the fiberoptic viewing bundle, most endoscopes contain a suction channel that can be used to evacuate mucus, fluid and blood from the viscus being examined. Suction is controlled by a button or valve at the head of the instrument. A similar mechanism allows control of the flow of air from an external air pump into the viscus. This insufflation of air distends the viscus and enables visualization of its mucosa and lumen. Without this distention the walls of the viscus would collapse around the tip of the endoscope and obstruct the examination. Another proximally located mechanism provides control of a fine spray of water over the distal objective lens to rinse away mucus, blood or other material coating the lens.

Most modern endoscopes also have a channel for the passage of biopsy forceps, cytology brushes and catheters for the irrigation of lesions and collection of cytologic specimens. This channel usually is the same as that used for suction. The standard biopsy instruments consist of two small opposing cups mounted on the end of a long flexible shaft. The biopsy forceps are passed through the biopsy-suction channel, and mucosal biopsy specimens are taken under direct visualization. The biopsy specimens are small, often only 2 mm.$^2$ in area and 1 to 2 mm. thick, and must be oriented properly for accurate histologic interpretation. The brush cytology technique consists of the introduction of a small brush through the biopsy-suction channel, rubbing or brushing the area under direct visualization and then spreading the resulting material on slides for staining and examination. The spray cytology technique involves the introduction of a plastic tube with a narrow nozzle through the biopsy-suction channel. Irrigation of the selected lesion is carried out under pressure. The washings are then aspirated, centrifuged and examined. These latter two procedures require the cooperation of a pathologist experienced in exfoliative cytology.

Perhaps the most significant technologic achievement in the field of endoscopy has been the development of a mechanical system by which the distal (mucosal) end of the endoscope can be moved and controlled by manipulation of a deflection control knob or arm on the observer's end of the endoscope. The tip control systems of the more sophisticated (i.e., more expensive) endoscopes enable movement of the distal tip in two planes and various combinations thereof. The relative limitation of movement in one plane is easily overcome by rotation of the entire endoscope on its long axis. This controlled deflection of the distal end of the endoscope allows thorough examination of the mucosal aspect of the alimentary canal and reduces the danger to the patient. The area of mucosa for biopsy, cytology or photography can be selected on the basis of appearance rather than accessibility. Controlled selective visualization and "target biopsy" increase the accuracy and effectiveness of gastrointestinal endoscopy.

## PROCEDURES

To minimize the risk of injury to the animal and to reduce the possibility of damage to the instrument, veterinary patients undergoing fiberoptic endoscopy are placed under general anesthesia following routine preanesthetic preparation. A fast of 12 to 24 hours is recommended for most patients undergoing upper gastrointestinal endoscopy. However, for those cases with indications of delayed gastric emptying, a longer fast (24 to 48 hours) may be necessary to evacuate the stomach completely. In preparation for colonoscopy, a 24- to 48-hour fast is recommended, and a high, warm-water enema is given the evening before and again 2 to 4 hours before the procedure. Such an enema should be administered until the return is completely clear.

One basic principle of endoscopy that cannot be overemphasized is that one should never attempt to advance an endoscope by force. If resistance is met, one must withdraw the instrument and attempt to determine the source of the resistance and how it can best be circumvented. The procedures described are those which the author has found to be successful with the instruments available to him.

### ESOPHAGOSCOPY

**Indications and Technique.** Signs indicating esophageal disease include repeated "regurgitation"* of undigested food and/or

---

*In the veterinary literature, the term regurgitation has been equated with esophageal disease. Specifically, the relatively passive act of emptying the dilated esophagus by animals with megaesophagus has been dubbed regurgitation. Thus, it has been stated that regurgitated material does not contain gastric juice and has a basic pH. By strict definition, however, regurgitation is the expulsion of the contents of the stomach in small amounts without the abdominal retching usually associated with vomiting. To be consistent with the other veterinary literature, the term is used here with the former connotation, but this difference in meaning is denoted by the addition of the quotation marks.

saliva, ballooning of the cervical esophagus, excessive drooling, anorexia or dysphagia and recurrent pneumonia (due to aspiration). In addition to a thorough history and a complete physical examination, it is important to evaluate the esophagus radiographically before endoscopic examination is performed. Interpretation of plain radiographs in conjunction with the clinical findings will indicate whether further plain radiographs or contrast studies are needed. Esophagograms are usually performed using a suspension of barium sulfate as the contrast material. However, if there is a possibility of esophageal perforation, a sterile, readily absorbed contrast medium (Hypaque® [Winthrop]) should be used in place of the barium suspension. This radiographic evaluation will help locate radiopaque and radiolucent foreign bodies or suggest the nature of other abnormalities.

Esophagoscopy allows visualization of the mucosal lining of the esophagus, making it possible to detect inflammation, ulcerations, dilations, diverticula, strictures, foreign bodies, tumors and parasitic infestations. The animal is placed under general anesthesia, intubated with a cuffed endotracheal tube and placed in lateral recumbency. An oral speculum is placed in the mouth. The animal's head and neck are extended and the tongue is pulled forward. The lubricated endoscope is passed dorsal to the larynx and into the esophagus. The esophagus offers little resistance to passage of the endoscope. Insufflation of the esophagus facilitates passage of the endoscope and improves visualization of the mucosa and any pathologic changes. Accumulations of saliva are easily aspirated through the suction channel. Once the instrument is in the lumen of the esophagus, it is advanced slowly to observe the walls of the esophagus. The esophagus extends from the cricopharyngeal sphincter to the cardia of the stomach and is about 30 cm. long in medium-sized dogs. The normal esophageal mucosa is pale pink to pink-gray in color, smooth and glistening. Pulsations of the heart and aorta are transmitted through the wall of the esophagus and are visible at the base of the heart. At this same area, there is a normal slight narrowing of the dilated esophageal lumen. At the gastroesophageal junction, the esophagus normally forms a small closed rosette.

**Abnormal Endoscopic Findings.** In acute esophagitis, the mucosa is hyperemic and unusually friable, as manifested by bleeding and denudation of the epithelium upon contact with the endoscope. Secretions are increased and may be profuse and blood-tinged. Cases of acute esophagitis in dogs have been reported recently. The esophagitis apparently was induced by reflux of gastric fluid into the esophagus as a result of improper positioning during abdominal surgery. Regurgitation of a small amount of grayish fluid during surgery was associated with postoperative anorexia or dysphagia. Spontaneous reflux peptic esophagitis in the dog has also been reported. It was postulated that reflux of gastric contents into the esophagus was related to a defect in the lower esophageal sphincter.

With chronic obstructions of the esophagus, there is usually dilation of the esophagus cranial to the obstruction, with loss of tone of that section. Dilation will be limited to the esophagus cranial to the base of the heart in animals with vascular ring anomalies. Mucosal changes at these sites may be minimal. This is in marked contrast to acquired strictures, in which the normal mucosa is replaced by scar tissue that appears as white ringlike structures or webs.

Endoscopic examination of the esophagus in cases of suspected or diagnosed esophageal foreign bodies is of value in locating the object, identifying any exposed sharp edges and evaluating the degree of damage to the esophageal wall. In those cases in which there is no evidence of pressure necrosis of the esophageal wall (producing mediastinal involvement) and when the object has no apparent sharp edges, removal of the foreign body can be directed by endoscopic visualization. Long alligator grasping forceps or a probang is carefully guided along the endoscope to the foreign body and used to grasp and extract the object under constant visualization. After removal of the foreign body, endoscopic reexamination of the esophagus is performed to evaluate the severity of damage to the esophageal wall and to determine whether further treatment is necessary.

Generalized megaesophagus is a neuromuscular disease of the esophagus occurring in less than 1 per cent of the canine population but producing a high mortality rate. The condition occurs most frequently in young dogs, particularly German shepherds and Great Danes. It is characterized by persistent "regurgitation," dilation of all or part of the body of the esophagus and respiratory tract disease. Radiography is the most practical method of establishing a definitive diagnosis of this condition. The radiographic hallmark of the disease is a greatly dilated esophagus with narrowing of the lumen at the diaphragm. The entire thoracic and, often, the cervical esophagus is dilated. Since the condition results in a functional abnormality, endoscopic examination of the esophagus is generally unrewarding. With the animal under general anesthesia and with insufflation of the esophagus, the judgment that the esophagus is dilated may be difficult unless there is marked dilation. Occasionally, a mild esophagitis will be present as a result of retention of ingesta in the esophagus. A rare condition usually associated with preexisting megaesophagus is gastroesophageal intussusception, also referred to as eversion of the stomach. The clinical signs change from persistent "regurgitation" and vomiting to abrupt depression and the appearance of dark blood in the vomitus. Radiographically, an area of increased density within the thoracic esophagus is evident, and the gas pattern of the fundic portion of the stomach is distorted or absent. Endoscopically, one finds the rugose gastric mucosa filling the lumen of the thoracic esophagus. Immediate surgical intervention is the necessary treatment.

## GASTROSCOPY

**Indications and Technique.** Endoscopic examination of the mucosal aspect of the stomach is indicated when the clinical signs or physical findings suggest the presence of gastric disease and/or when there is a need for confirmation or clarification of radiographic findings. In most cases of gastric disease or dysfunction, persistent vomiting is the chief complaint. To establish clearly what actually is occurring, a detailed description of the act of vomiting should be obtained from the client. The clinician should observe the vomiting act if at all possible. An accurate description of the vomitus itself often provides additional valuable information. Its color and consistency and any changes in these characteristics during the course of the disease should be described. These and other specific details

may indicate the seriousness of the disorder and whether symptomatic treatment or an extensive diagnostic evaluation is warranted. Other clinical signs suggestive of potentially serious gastric disease include hematemesis (vomition of blood), melena, weight loss, anemia and abdominal pain.

Radiographic examination of the abdomen and upper gastrointestinal tract is an important aid in evaluating patients suspected of having gastric dysfunction or disease. Following adequate preparation of the patient, survey radiographs should be taken before other diagnostic procedures are performed, since some radiopaque foreign bodies will be obscured by contrast media. These plain films may reveal the size, shape, position and contents of the stomach. Upper gastrointestinal contrast studies, using either negative or positive contrast media (air or barium sulfate suspensions, respectively), provide some assessment of the function and structure of the stomach. All oral medications and any drugs affecting gastrointestinal motility should be discontinued for an appropriate period prior to such studies.

Gastroscopy allows visualization of the mucosal lining of the stomach, making it possible to detect inflammation, foreign bodies, tumors and ulcerations. The preparation of the animal and passage of the endoscope are the same as for esophagoscopy. Careful examination of the esophageal mucosa and lumen should be conducted as the endoscope is passed through the esophagus. The stomach lies mainly in a transverse position, more to the left of the median plane than to the right of it. There are four major divisions of the stomach: the cardiac portion, fundus, body and pyloric portion. The cardiac portion blends with the esophagus and includes the functional gastroesophageal sphincter. The fundus of the stomach is a rather large, blind outpocketing located to the left of and dorsal to the cardia. The body is the large middle portion of the stomach that extends from the fundus on the left to the pyloric portion on the right. The pyloric portion comprises approximately the distal third of the stomach and is irregularly funnel-shaped. The thin-walled, conical part is referred to as the pyloric antrum and funnels down to the pyloric canal, which is directed cranially. Since the stomach is an asymmetrical organ, positioning of the animal for gastroscopy will influence which portion of the stomach is best visualized. With the patient in right lateral recumbency, any material in the stomach gravitates into the pyloric portion of the stomach. The lumen of the pyloric antrum is occluded, and the antrum is at least partially collapsed. With the patient in left lateral recumbency, the material settles in the fundus and body, and the lumen of the pyloric antrum distends with trapped gas.

Gastroscopy is usually begun with the patient in left lateral recumbency. After the mucosal end of the endoscope passes through the cardia, the stomach is partly inflated. The mucosa of the stomach is normally thrown into folds, the gastric rugae, which persist even in a moderately distended organ. These folds are mainly longitudinal in direction and are very tortuous. They are most prominent on the greater curvature and persist there longest with increasing distention. The normal color of the mucosa in the body and fundus is pink to grayish-red. In the pyloric region it is lighter in color. Following insufflation, the body of the stomach is carefully examined. The linear rugae on the greater curvature are followed upward into the pyloric antrum. Because of the sharp angulation of the lesser curvature in the dog, it may be necessary to flex the endoscope maximally upward toward the pyloric antrum and to push the endoscope gently into the stomach. This causes the flexed end of the endoscope to "slide by" into the pyloric antrum. From this position, the peristaltic activity in the antrum and the function and conformation of the pylorus can be visualized. Normally there should be active peristalsis, with the waves moving down the antrum to the pylorus. Alternatively, the antrum may be static with the pylorus closed. Further retroflexion in this position enables one to examine the shelflike structure representing the mucosal aspect of the lesser curvature, commonly referred to as the gastric angle. Even greater retroflexion brings into view the body, cardia, and fundus of the stomach as viewed from the pyloric antrum. With the animal in left lateral recumbency, any saliva or ingesta present will gravitate to the dependent fundus, forming a "mucus lake." In order to examine the fundus and cardia adequately, it may be necessary to place the animal in right lateral recumbency. Then with the tip of the endoscope just inside the

cardia, the stomach is moderately distended. The tip is then flexed upward toward the fundus along the greater curvature. The endoscope is slowly advanced into the stomach as the flexed tip slides along the greater curvature into the gastric fundus. One can usually see the cardia with the body of the endoscope emerging from it. The combination of these procedures enables the examination of all mucosal aspects of the stomach.

**Abnormal Endoscopic Findings.** Endoscopic examination of the stomach in cases of suspected or diagnosed gastric foreign bodies provides the same advantages and uses as described for esophagoscopy. By definition, acute gastritis is an acute inflammation of the gastric wall, usually limited to the mucosa. Since this condition is commonly characterized by an abrupt onset and a relatively brief course, gastroscopy would be of limited value unless there were indications of more severe involvement, i.e., persistent hematemesis or marked abdominal pain. Chronic gastritis is generally characterized by vague signs, including sporadic vomition unrelated to the time of eating, poor growth rate, dull hair coat, etc. It has been postulated that the causes of chronic gastritis are the same as, but of greater duration than, those of acute gastritis. Pathologically chronic gastritis is virtually always of the hypertrophic type, characterized by thickening of the mucosa. Therefore, endoscopically one would expect to find the gastric mucosa thickened, velvety and covered with a tenacious glassy mucus; the gastric rugae may be exaggerated. Careful endoscopic examination, thorough radiographic evaluation and a clinical laboratory data base are warranted in such cases.

When an older dog is presented with a history of persistent vomition, anorexia and weight loss, one must strongly consider the possibility of gastric neoplasia. Other clinical signs include hematemesis, melena, diarrhea and anemia. Radiographic features supporting a diagnosis of gastric neoplasia include distortion of the lumen, thickening of the gastric wall, filling defects, derangement of the rugal pattern, delayed gastric emptying and rigidity of the gastric wall as seen on multiple radiographs. Endoscopic findings in cases of gastric neoplasia are quite variable. Based on gross pathologic findings and the author's endoscopic experience, approximately half the gastric neoplasms diagnosed have mucosal ulcerations. Other endoscopic findings correlate well with the radiographic features. These include adenomatous polyps or masses producing filling defects; diffusely infiltrating nonulcerating tumors that alter the rugal pattern and affect motility; and raised thickened plaquelike tumors (with or without central ulceration), resulting in a thickened gastric wall. It must be recognized that some gastric tumors will produce no endoscopic abnormalities. Gastric biopsy is necessary to establish the diagnosis of gastric neoplasia. Endoscopic biopsy samples should be taken from the edge of the lesion, rather than from the center, since the center may contain chiefly necrotic tissue and debris. It is important to take as many samples as possible, since some tumors are difficult to document, and one must try to obtain as deep a bite as possible. In some cases, it is necessary to perform an exploratory laparotomy and full-thickness biopsy or excision of the gastric lesion in order to substantiate the diagnosis.

Gastric peptic ulcers are erosive lesions of the gastric mucosa caused by the action of the acid gastric juice. Documented cases in the dog and cat are rare. Clinical signs vary but include chronic vomiting, abdominal pain, anemia, variable appetite, weight loss and sudden collapse and death due to perforation. Vomiting may be associated with eating. Melena and hematemesis may also be observed and may produce anemia. Survey radiographs and contrast studies may be of little value in outlining an ulcer. Based on reported cases and limited endoscopic experience, gastroscopy should reveal round or oval lesions, 1 to 2 cm. in diameter, with a sharply punched-out appearance. The walls of the ulcer should be relatively straight, either perpendicular to or slightly overhanging the ulcer base. The principal sites affected are the nonacid-producing areas of the stomach, i.e., the pyloric antrum and the lesser curvature. Peptic ulceration in the dog has usually been associated with other disorders such as liver disease, malignant mastocytosis and chronic uremia. Some cases of benign gastric ulcers have been drug-induced, aspirin and indomethacin being particularly damaging.

Obstruction of the pylorus in the dog is frequently associated with postprandial projectile vomiting caused by delayed gastric emptying. Hypertrophic pyloric stenosis, either congenital or acquired, produces narrowing of the pyloric canal as a result of thickening of the pyloric musculature. Pyloric stenosis may also be caused by chronic gastritis, gastric ulcers and neoplasms. Radiographic features of pyloric obstruction include gastric distention, delayed gastric emptying and intestinal hypermotility. In a limited number of canine patients with pyloric stenosis due to muscular hypertrophy, gastroscopy revealed the pyloric orifice to be fixed and markedly narrowed. Peristaltic waves passing down the antrum in a normal fashion resulted in some degree of contraction, but complete closure of the orifice did not occur. In the normal animal, the pylorus should remain closed until the antral peristaltic waves are very close to the pylorus, when it should open briefly. In cases suspected of pyloric stenosis, careful gastroscopic examination may reveal other abnormalities in the stomach such as chronic gastritis or ulcers.

## COLONOSCOPY

**Indications and Technique.** The primary indication for colonoscopy is the presence of any colonic symptom, sign or abnormality that is unexplained or needs further clarification. The classic sign of colonic disease is tenesmus. The animal strains and makes frequent attempts to defecate but passes only small amounts of feces. The feces are usually liquid or semisolid and often contain visible amounts of fresh blood and excess mucus. Vomiting may occur occasionally with colonic disease. Weight loss is usually not a problem in animals with colonic disease unless it is chronic and severe. A thorough physical examination may reveal other indications of colonic abnormalities. A careful visual examination of the perineum and circumanal area is recommended. Since many diseases involving the colon also produce lesions in the rectum, a digital rectal examination should be done on every patient with signs of colonic disease unless it would endanger the animal or cause severe discomfort. Following a low, warm-water enema, visual examination of the anal canal and rectum can usually be performed on a conscious animal in the standing position. Simple inexpensive equipment is available for this purpose. Routine laboratory examination of the feces should be done to determine the presence of parasites, protozoa and abnormal cells. In addition, fecal cultures for pathogenic bacteria, fungi and algae should be performed. When combined with mucosal biopsy, colonoscopy is a very effective aid in evaluating animals with signs of colonic disease.

The large intestine of the dog and cat is short and relatively unspecialized. In general, it is a simple tube that extends from the ileocolic sphincter to the anus. The large intestine is anatomically divided into cecum, colon, rectum and anal canal. The colon begins at the ileocolic orifice and ends at the rectum. The colon has three divisions: the ascending colon, the transverse colon, and the descending colon. The short ascending colon courses in a cranial direction from its origin at the ileocolic orifice in the right side of the abdomen. The transverse colon begins at the right colic flexure and forms an arc, which runs from right to left across the abdomen. The descending colon is the longest segment of the colon. It extends from the left colic flexure to the pelvic inlet, where it becomes the rectum without demarcation. The rectum then extends from the pelvic inlet to the anal canal.

Colonoscopy is begun with the animal in right lateral recumbency in order to pool any liquid contents in the transverse and ascending colon. The well-lubricated distal end of the endoscope is inserted into the anal canal and gently advanced into the colon. Insufflation of air dilates the lumen and facilitates insertion. The colonic mucosa is visualized during both insertion and withdrawal of the endoscope. The normal canine colonic mucosa is pale pink, smooth and glistening and distends evenly with insufflation. The lumen of the colon should always be visible. Passage through the left and right colic flexures is accomplished by the "slide by" technique, as described for gastroscopy. The instrument is cautiously advanced as long as the mucosa can be seen to slide smoothly and easily past the tip. In most dogs, it is possible to reach the ileocolic and cecocolic junctions. Care must be taken to avoid calling the ileocolic junction a sessile polyp. To identify the junction, one should recognize a depression or dimple on the top of the "polyp" and see the cecocolic orifice in the background.

**Abnormal Endoscopic Findings.** Colonic mucosal diseases produce superficial ulceration and a granularity of the mucosa. The mucosa becomes friable and bleeds easily upon contact with the endoscope, but the colon distends evenly with insufflation, and no strictures are apparent. The colon maintains its normal length and configuration. On the other hand, transmural diseases of the colon produce deep ulcers with rough, irregular edges. The mucosa is firm, friable and grossly corrugated. The colon tends to distend poorly, and strictures may be apparent. In severe cases, the colon is shortened and contorted.

Colonic polyps may appear as grapelike clusters with pedunculated bases. They are reddish-purple, and the surface may bleed easily. The adjacent colonic mucosa is usually normal. Malignant colonic tumors may appear as grossly ulcerated areas of mucosa. They may bleed easily if traumatized. In other cases of colonic neoplasia, the lumen may be stenotic with the mucosa intact and appearing normal.

To confirm the diagnosis of colonic disease, biopsy of lesions may be accomplished with endoscopic biopsy forceps, a suction biopsy instrument or standard human uterine biopsy forceps.

## CONCLUSIONS

Following recent advances in the design and manufacture of low-cost, simple endoscopes, flexible fiberoptic endoscopy will soon be within the financial reach of many practicing veterinarians. These technical advances combined with increasingly strict regulation of the use of radiography in veterinary medicine have set the stage for the rapid adoption and utilization of fiberoptic endoscopy by the practitioner. Understanding the basic principles of these instruments and recognizing the indications for and limitations of various basic procedures provides a starting point from which further experience can be gained. With such experience, one can then apply endoscopy to a wider variety of cases, conditions and species.

Although flexible fiberoptic gastrointestinal endoscopy has been cited as the single most important advance in the diagnosis of diseases of the gastrointestinal tract, it must be regarded as only an adjunctive diagnostic procedure of value in many, but not all, patients with manifestations of gastrointestinal disease.

## SUPPLEMENTAL READING

### General

Antelyes, J.: Endoscopy and endopalpation. Vet. Med./Small Animal Clin., *60*:391–397, 1965.

Bockus, H. L. (sr. ed.): Gastroenterology. Vol. 1. 3rd ed. Philadelphia, W. B. Saunders Co., 1974.

Bonneau, N. H., and Reed, J. H.: Use of the gastrocamera in the dog. J. Am. Vet. Med. Assn., *161*:185–189, 1972.

Waye, J. D.: Colonoscopy. Surg. Clin. N. Am., *52*:1013–1024, 1972.

### Esophagoscopy

Grier, R. L.: Esophageal disease as a result of improper patient positioning. Arch. Coll. Vet. Surg., *IV*:4–6, Spring, 1975.

Guffy, M. M.: Esophageal disorders. *In* Ettinger, S. J. (ed.): Textbook of Veterinary Internal Medicine. Philadelphia, W. B. Saunders Co., 1975, pp. 1098–1124.

Kleine, L. J.: Radiologic examination of the esophagus in dogs and cats. Vet. Clin. N. Am., *4*:663–686, 1974.

O'Brien, J. A.: Esophagoscopy. Vet. Clin. N. Amer., *2*:99–103, 1972.

Rogers, W. A., and Donovan, E. F.: Peptic esophagitis in a dog. J. Am. Vet. Med. Assn., *163*:462–464, 1973.

Ryan, W. W., and Greene, R. W.: The conservative management of esophageal foreign bodies and their complications: A review of 66 cases in dogs and cats. J.A.A.H.A., *11*:243–249, 1975.

### Gastroscopy

Bonneau, N. H., Reed, J. H., Pennock, P. W., and Little, P.B.: Comparison of gastrophotography and contrast radiography for diagnosis of aspirin-induced gastritis in the dog. J. Am. Vet. Med. Assn., *161*:190–198, 1972.

Cornelius, L. M., and Wingfield, W. E.: Diseases of the stomach. *In* Ettinger, S. J. (ed.): Textbook of Veterinary Internal Medicine. Philadelphia, W. B. Saunders Co., 1975, pp. 1125–1149.

Demling, L., Ottenjann, R., and Elster, K.: Endoscopy and Biopsy of the Esophagus and Stomach. Translated by K. H. Soergel. Philadelphia, W. B. Saunders Co., 1972.

Ewing, G. O.: Indomethacin-associated gastrointestinal hemorrhage in a dog. J. Am. Vet. Med. Assn., *161*:1665–1668, 1972.

Murray, M., McKeating, F. J., and Lauder, I. M.: Peptic ulceration in the dog: A clinico-pathological study. Vet. Rec., *91*:441–447, 1972.

Murray, M., McKeating, F. J., and Lauder, I. M.: Primary gastric neoplasia in the dog: A clinico-pathological study. Vet. Rec., *91*:474–479, 1972.

Sautter, J. H., and Hanlon, G. F.: Gastric neoplasms in the dog: A report of 20 cases. J. Am. Vet. Med. Assn., *166*:691–696, 1975.

### Colonoscopy

Amand, W. B.: Nonneurogenic disorders of the anus and rectum. Vet. Clin. N. Am., *4*:535–550, 1974.

Ewing, G. O., and Gomez, J. A.: Canine ulcerative colitis. J.A.A.H.A., *9*:395–406, 1973.

Lorenz, M. D.: Disorders of the large bowel. *In* Ettinger, S. J. (ed.): Textbook of Veterinary Internal Medicine. Philadelphia, W. B. Saunders Co., 1975, pp. 1192–1218.

Overholt, B. F.: Colonoscopy. Gastroenterology, *68*:1308–1320, 1975.

Van Kruiningen, H. J.: Granulomatous colitis of boxer dogs: Comparative aspects. Gastroenterology, *53*:114–122, 1967.

# CHRONIC PROGRESSIVE HEPATITIS IN BEDLINGTON TERRIERS (BEDLINGTON LIVER DISEASE)

ROBERT M. HARDY, D.V.M.
*and* JERRY B. STEVENS, D.V.M.
*St. Paul, Minnesota*

## INTRODUCTION

In January of 1975, work was begun at the University of Minnesota to define the cause(s) of an apparently familial hepatic disease in Bedlington terriers. We received information from numerous sources throughout the country that many dogs of this breed had been dying from hepatic failure, and that the frequency of such losses appeared to be increasing alarmingly.

Through the cooperation of many local breeders and veterinarians throughout the United States, we have been able to accumulate data on 57 Bedlington terriers from which serum for biochemical tests was obtained. For 35 of these 57 dogs biochemical evidence showed that active hepatocellular disease was present when initally evaluated.

The combined clinical, biochemical and histologic characteristics of this canine disease bear a marked similarity to the hepatic form of Wilson's disease (hepatolenticular degeneration) of man. This inherited human disease is associated with the pathologic accumulation of copper in the liver and other tissues.

## HISTORY AND PHYSICAL FINDINGS

The clinical signs and physical findings in this disease are quite variable. In general, affected animals fall into three groups: (1) the first group, including young adults of either sex whose illness runs a relatively short clinical course, in which the clinical signs often follow or are precipitated by some stressful event (whelping, showing); (2) a chronic form, characterized by a slowly progressing, debilitating type of illness; and (3) a clinically asymptomatic group, in which persistent biochemical evidence of active hepatocellular inflammation or necrosis, i.e., elevated serum glutamic pyruvic transaminase concentrations (SGPT), is the only indication of hepatic disease.

The first group is composed of relatively young dogs (2 to 6 years of age) that, until the onset of signs, tend to have unremarkable medical histories. Their immediate past histories usually include vigorous campaigning in dog shows or, in the case of females, recent whelping. Such physically stressful activities appear to precipitate hepatic failure in susceptible animals. The clinical signs necessitating veterinary care include depression, lethargy, anorexia and vomiting, all of abrupt onset. Jaundice may appear within one to two days following the onset of clinical signs.

A significant number of dogs in this group have such fulminant hepatic failure that death occurs within 48 to 72 hours. Therapeutic efforts in such dogs have been unrewarding. Animals surviving this acute attack may remain clinically asymptomatic for years or be prone to recurrent attacks of a similar but less severe nature later in life.

Physical findings are usually nonspecific. Occasional dogs present with jaundice and hepatomegaly, making localization of the site of disease relatively uncomplicated. For the majority of animals, however, biochemical tests are required for definitive evidence that hepatic disease exists.

The second clinical group is composed of middle-aged to aged dogs whose signs are similar to those in group 1. In general, signs have been present for long periods of time (weeks to months) and are less severe. Appropriately, chronic weight loss and ascites may be noted, in addition to the signs mentioned previously. Evidence of previous attacks of acute hepatitis is generally lacking. The physical examination tends not to contribute to the diagnosis. The liver is non-palpable in most dogs, owing to chronic hepatic necrosis and scar tissue contraction. Ascites, when present, appears late in the disease course and may not be evident when the animal is first evaluated. Anemia may be evident clinically and is due in some cases to an acute hemolytic crisis associated with elevated serum copper concentrations.

The third group is composed of clinically asymptomatic animals. This group is detected only by evaluating biochemical tests used to assess hepatic enzyme activity in serum. This segment of the Bedlington terrier population represents younger dogs that have not experienced an acute crisis or are in the preclinical stages of the chronic progressive group. Some dogs have abnormal SGPT concentrations as early as 12 weeks of age. However, a normal SGPT does not exclude the possibility of the dog having the disease. Three of four adult animals found to have normal SGPT values on initial evaluation later developed elevated SGPT values.

## Diagnosis

In our initial evaluation of these dogs, numerous biochemical and histopathologic studies were carried out. The only consistent serum abnormality of localizing value was a persistent elevation in the serum glutamic pyruvic transaminase concentration SGPT. Values ranged from 43 sigma frankel units to over 2000 SFU (normal = 10 to 40 SFU). Fifty-seven dogs have been evaluated biochemically to date, and 35 have had abnormal SGPT concentrations. Of the 22 dogs with normal SGPT values, 18 were less than one year of age when tested. Of the 4 adult animals with normal SGPT values when first tested, 3 have since developed significant elevations.

In order to characterize the disease and hopefully provide a definitive diagnosis, hepatic biopsies were evaluated in several dogs with abnormal SGPT determinations. Although the liver appeared normal or finely nodular in younger animals, the livers of adult animals were often small when observed at laparotomy. They either had swollen, rounded borders, or presented a coarsely nodular picture characteristic of postnecrotic cirrhosis (Fig. 1). Microscopically, varying degrees of hepatic cell necrosis and associated inflammatory cell reaction and fibrous connective tissue proliferation were noted. Necrotic cells tended to be observed primarily in peripheral lobular areas. Bile duct proliferation was inconsistently present and not dramatic. The hepatocyte cytoplasm contained numerous brownish eosinophilic granules. Affected hepatocytes were generally located at the lobule periphery. However, they have been observed to be distributed throughout the lobules. The granules are characteristic but not specific for this disease. By utilizing a variety of histochemical techniques, it was possible to determine that these granules reacted strongly to two stains used to detect copper in tissues (rubeanic acid and Timms' stains).

On the basis of the strongly positive reaction to copper-specific stains (rubeanic acid), a sample of frozen liver from one of

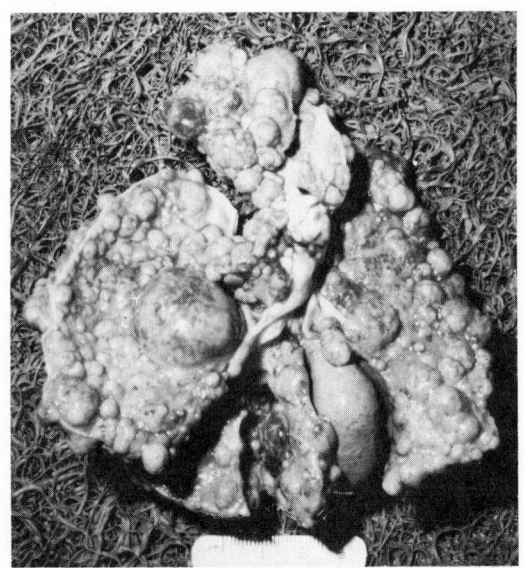

**Figure 1.** Photograph of the liver from a 9-year-old male Bedlington terrier. Gross appearance is characteristic of severe postnecrotic cirrhosis.

the affected dogs was evaluated for its copper content. A value of 226 micrograms per gram of wet weight (PPM) was obtained. Similar analyses on livers from normal dogs have produced values that ranged from 10 to 40 micrograms per gram of wet weight. Since this first detection of abnormally elevated liver copper concentrations, the livers of 17 similarly affected dogs have been biopsied. Eight samples were adequate for tissue copper concentrations, and all eight were massively elevated. In addition, the other nine animals reacted positively to specific copper stains.

Based on the combined data obtained from the clinical histories, biochemical profiles and histologic evaluations of these dogs, a presumptive diagnosis of chronic progressive hepatitis resembling the hepatic form of Wilson's disease was made.

Additional clinical support for the similarity of the canine and human syndrome came from the observation of an acute hemolytic crisis in two of the animals. Hemolysis has been noted frequently in humans suffering from Wilson's disease and is caused by a rapid rise in serum copper concentration, which alters red cell membrane stability and leads to hemolysis. Serum copper concentration increased dramatically in the dogs in which hemolysis was noted. This rapid rise in copper concentration is presumed to be a result of massive hepatocellular necrosis and the rapid release of intracellular copper into the peripheral circulation.

A number of other diagnostic findings in Wilson's disease of man have not been detected in the Bedlingtons. These include a low serum copper concentration, hypoceruloplasminemia (a circulating copper-binding protein) and Kayser-Fleischer rings at the corneoscleral junction. The first two of these abnormalities are nearly always present in the human syndrome. The relative significance of the similarities and dissimilarities between the canine and human syndromes has yet to be resolved.

## THERAPY

Reversal of the disease process by conventional therapeutic measures has been uniformly unsuccessful. Supportive care for hepatic failure (bordering on heroics) has enabled some dogs to survive acute attacks, but a gradual relentless progression of the disease (symptomatic or asymptomatic) is the rule.

A specific copper-chelating drug (d-penicillamine*) has had remarkable success in controlling and reversing the hepatic manifestations in human patients with Wilson's disease. This drug binds copper within the circulation and promotes a marked cupriuresis and negative copper balance. The effectiveness of this drug depends on its being used in conjunction with low copper diets. The therapy is also much more likely to cause a return to normal hepatic function when begun before advanced cirrhotic changes in the liver have occurred. Even when begun in asymptomatic children, many months of therapy are sometimes necessary before laboratory evidence for cessation of inflammation is detected.

Preliminary results of the effectiveness of d-penicillamine in affected dogs have been variable. We currently are evaluating this agent in several dogs, and although SGPT concentrations are decreasing significantly, some activity is still evident after 5 months of continuous therapy. Reports from practitioners working with us on therapeutic trials have not been as encouraging. The prognosis may depend on the severity of the hepatic lesion when therapy and a low-copper diet are instituted. Ideally, the total copper intake should be less than 1 mg. A survey of the copper content of various commercially available canine diets is in progress. A list of foods with low and high copper content is available from the manufacturer of Cuprimine.*

Our current dosage recommendations for this drug are one 250-mg. capsule given once daily. The drug should be given at least 30 minutes prior to any food intake. Giving food along with the medication will reduce the effectiveness of the drug. Many dogs will vomit this drug when it is administered on an empty stomach. If vomiting occurs, the capsule may be divided into approximately two equal portions and administered at 12-hour intervals. This has reduced the incidence of vomiting significantly in many dogs.

---

*Cuprimine®, available from Merck Sharp and Dohme, West Point, Pennsylvania.

Obviously, a great deal remains to be learned about this problem in Bedlington terriers. The mode of inheritance is unknown. Will Cuprimine be effective in diseased dogs? Is there a carrier state? Is the high level of copper really the cause of the problem or an associated abnormality? Hopefully, the answers to these and other questions will be forthcoming in the not too distant future.

## SUPPLEMENTAL READING

Hardy, R. M., Stevens, J. B., and Stowe, C. M.: Chronic progressive hepatitis in Bedlington terriers associated with elevated liver copper concentrations. Minn. Vet., 15:13–24, June, 1975.

Sternlieb, I., and Scheinberg, I. H.: Wilson's disease. *In* Schaffner, F., Sherlock, S., and Leevy, C. M. (eds.): The Liver and Its Diseases. New York, Intercontinental Medical Book Corp., 1974.

Walshe, J. M.: The liver in hepatolenticular degeneration. *In* Schiff, L. (ed.): Diseases of the Liver. 4th ed. Philadelphia, J. B. Lippincott Co., 1975.

# Section

# 11

# METABOLIC
# DISORDERS

AD RIJNBERK, D.V.M.
*Consulting Editor*

# DIABETES MELLITUS

EDWARD CHARLES FELDMAN,
D.V.M.
*Berkeley, California*

## UNCOMPLICATED DIABETES MELLITUS

Diabetes mellitus is a disease process classically characterized by a decreased tolerance to carbohydrate, resulting from a relative or absolute lack of insulin at the cellular level. The generalized chronic metabolic disturbances that develop are ultimately life-threatening.

### PATHOPHYSIOLOGY

In the absence of insulin at the cellular level, glucose obtained from the diet or by hepatic gluconeogenesis is not efficiently utilized by muscle, adipose tissue or the liver itself. Consequently, glucose accumulates in the blood (hyperglycemia), and as its concentration exceeds the renal tubular maximum transport threshold, glucose spills into the urine (glycosuria). The renal threshold for glucose in the dog is between 175 and 220 mg./100 ml. Glycosuria causes an osmotic diuresis, leading to polyuria and thus obligatory polydipsia. The calories lost through glycosuria can represent a large portion of the normal caloric maintenance requirement. Polyphagia thus occurs because the body is literally starving in spite of hyperglycemia. In response to caloric starvation, fat and protein are metabolized to fatty acids and glucose, respectively. As the polydipsia, polyuria, polyphagia and weight loss become evident to the owner, the animal is presented to the veterinarian. Its condition may or may not be complicated by ketosis, which results from the breakdown of large amounts of fatty acids. The present discussion is concerned with the nonketoacidotic form of diabetes mellitus.

Although the exact cause of the diabetes mellitus often cannot be ascertained, several factors are known to interfere with the delicate balance between glucose and insulin. Genetic factors have been implicated in this disease, as have high chronic caloric intake and obesity. Glucocorticoids, ACTH, estrogens, progesterones and numerous other drugs can cause diabetes mellitus; Dilantin® (diphenylhydantoin [Parke, Davis]) and certain diuretics may cause a reversible form by inhibiting insulin secretion. Diabetes mellitus may also be caused by hyperadrenocorticism (Cushing's syndrome) or by destruction of the beta cells of the pancreas (via pancreatitis, neoplasms, trauma or surgery). In patients with a "borderline" state of insulin secretion, acute stress (injury or illness) or pregnancy may precipitate clinical diabetes.

### DIAGNOSIS

The diagnosis of diabetes mellitus is suspected whenever there is a history of polydipsia, polyuria, polyphagia and weight loss. The diagnosis is confirmed by the finding of persistent fasting hyperglycemia. The normal fasting blood glucose concentration in the dog is 60 to 100 mg./100 ml., and the repeated finding of values above 150 mg./100 ml. is usually considered diagnostic of overt diabetes, in the absence of complicating factors. The latter include hyperadrenocorticism, postprandial hyperglycemia and hyperglycemia induced by stress (which can be quite dramatic in the feline).

When blood glucose concentration exceeds the renal threshold, there is concurrent glycosuria, which is easily detected with Diastix® paper strips* or Clinitest® tablets.* Glycosuria without hyperglycemia can be caused by primary renal disease.

Oral glucose tolerance tests (OGTT) should be used only when the diagnosis is in doubt. The most common indications for OGTT are (1) glycosuria with normal blood glucose, (2) borderline hyperglycemia (120 to 175 mg./100 ml.) without glycosuria, (3) borderline postprandial hyperglycemia and (4) a family history of diabetes. In the dog or cat with symptomatic diabetes, an OGTT

---

*Ames Company, Division of Miles Laboratory, Elkhart, Indiana 46514.

1001

may precipitate ketoacidosis and is therefore contraindicated.

Laboratory evaluation in any candidate for long-term insulin therapy should include a complete blood count (CBC), a renal function test (BUN or creatinine), total serum protein, serum glutamic pyruvic transaminase (SGPT), alkaline phosphatase and blood glucose. The thorax and abdomen should be examined radiographically.

As glucose utilization diminishes in the diabetic, fat mobilization becomes excessive and frank lipemia may occur. SGPT and alkaline phosphatase levels are usually elevated in association with the resulting fatty metamorphosis of the liver. The latter leads to hepatomegaly, which may be marked and which is the most common radiographic abnormality.

## TREATMENT

**Oral Hypoglycemics.** These drugs are seldom used in veterinary medicine and should be reserved for the exceptional patient in which glucose tolerance tests are required to confirm the diagnosis of diabetes mellitus. Although tolbutamide is widely used in man, it has severe hepatotoxic effects in the dog and hence should not be used in this animal. Other sulfonylureas, such as chlorpropamide and acetohexamide, have been used successfully in a few cases in dogs.

**Insulin.** By the time diabetes mellitus is diagnosed in the dog or cat, daily injections of insulin are usually required to control the disease. The following discussion is concerned with the use of U40 NPH insulin (40 units/ml.), which is probably the insulin preparation most widely used in veterinary medicine.

NPH insulin, like all insulins, must be refrigerated, and the contents of the vial should be thoroughly mixed before each dose is withdrawn. Following subcutaneous administration, the onset of action is in approximately 3 hours, peak blood levels occur in 8 to 10 hours and the total duration of effect is 18 to 24 hours. As the effect of insulin reaches its maximum, blood glucose concentration is greatly reduced. To avoid the induction of severe hypoglycemia, *feeding must be timed to correspond to the period of greatest insulin activity*.

**Client Instruction.** Diabetes mellitus is a serious disease, and its treatment requires

the assistance of capable and willing owners. Over- or underdosage of insulin for several consecutive days can have serious consequences. Acute overdosage is likely to result in a hypoglycemic episode. Recurrent severe hypoglycemia will result in loss of normal mentation and response. Chronic underdosage can result in the cascade of metabolic changes leading to ketoacidosis. For these reasons, daily monitoring of urine sugar and ketone levels is imperative, a point which should be emphasized repeatedly to the owner. Day-to-day caloric intake and exercise are unavoidably variable and will affect the daily insulin requirement. Hence the owner must understand that adjustments in insulin dosage will be based on the results of daily urine monitoring.

The owner is instructed to maintain a daily diary. This should include the results of morning urine glucose and ketone measurements, the dose of insulin, whether the patient ate in the morning and evening, and the site of insulin injection (which should vary).

**Method of Treatment.** Each diabetic should be hospitalized until its metabolic condition is stabilized. The initial dose of insulin in the dog is approximately ½ unit (U.) per kilogram of body weight, subcutaneously. In the cat, which is more sensitive to exogenous insulin, the initial dose is ¼ U./kg., subcutaneously. It is preferable to begin therapy at a low dose because it is easier to correct for hyperglycemia than to deal with an acute hypoglycemic crisis. In the hospital and at home, a simple schedule is followed for monitoring and treating the diabetic (Table 1).

Early each morning, the urine is tested for sugar and ketone levels by use of Ketodiastix®.* The *corrected* dose of insulin (see below) is then administered subcutaneously, and the patient is given 10 to 25 per cent of its daily food intake. The main meal is given approximately 10 hours later, to coincide with the peak in insulin action. No snacks are allowed. If the animal frequently appears to be weak prior to the evening meal (suggesting hypoglycemia), the meal should be given earlier in the day.

The basic objective of insulin therapy is to maintain the patient at 1/8 to 1/4 per cent

---

*Ames Company, Division of Miles Laboratory, Elkhart, Indiana 46514.

glycosuria in the morning, thereby avoiding the precipitation of a severe hypoglycemic episode prior to the evening meal.

The dosage adjustments each morning are quite simple (Table 2). The adjustments shown in Table 2 are appropriate for a 10-kg. dog; they should be reduced somewhat for smaller dogs and increased for larger ones. When a urine specimen cannot be obtained, the previous day's dose should be repeated. During initial hospitalization, blood glucose concentration should also be measured in the afternoon in order to determine individual patient sensitivity to insulin.

The owner must be instructed to call the veterinarian whenever ketonuria occurs, since this may signal the need for immediate treatment of ketoacidosis.

Rarely, marked glycosuria is observed each morning, even with increasing doses of insulin. When the dose of insulin approaches 1.7 U./kg., there is an increased risk of significant hypoglycemia later in the day. Hence the veterinarian must be consulted whenever high doses appear to be needed. The most common causes for an apparent increase in the dose requirement are improper administration of the dose subcutaneously, inadequate mixing of the insulin prior to its withdrawal from the vial and use of insulin that is outdated or has been inactivated by improper storage. If these possibilities are eliminated, it can be assumed that the administered dose is completely metabolized in 18 to 20 hours. In the hours of inadequate or absent insulin levels in the blood, the blood sugar then rises and glycosuria occurs, resulting in the finding of large amounts of glucose in the morning urine specimen. This problem can usually be resolved by the use of lente insulin, which has a slightly longer duration of effect (Table 3). Thus, the early morning absence of insulin in the blood is eliminated, and improved control can be achieved. It is not recommended that the NPH insulin be

**Table 1.** *Recommended Treatment Schedule*

| |
|---|
| 8:00 A.M.: Collect urine sample and determine amount glycosuria |
| 8:15 A.M.: Administer corrected insulin dose |
| 8:30 A.M.: Feed ⅛ to ¼ total daily food requirement |
| 6:00 P.M.: Feed ¾ the total daily food requirement |

**Table 2.** *Insulin Daily Dosage Adjustment (10-Kilogram Dog)*

| |
|---|
| If urine is 2% glycosuria, increase 2 units. |
| If urine is 1% glycosuria, increase 1 unit. |
| If urine is ½% glycosuria, increase ½ unit. |
| If urine is ¼ to $^{1}/_{10}$% glycosuria, repeat previous day's dosage. |
| If urine is negative, decrease 2 units. |

administered twice daily, since monitoring such a patient becomes quite difficult. The effect of PZI insulin overlaps from day to day and therefore it should not be used.

A phenomenon of severe hypoglycemia followed by rebound hyperglycemia and marked glycosuria can occur. This is known as the "Somogyi effect" and can be misinterpreted as indicating the need for increases in insulin dosage when the dose should actually be decreased. Only close monitoring by the owner and the veterinarian will avoid such complications.

The owner should be instructed to have a glucose-containing syrup, such as Karo Syrup®,* available at all times. If the animal appears to be weak or unusually tired, the syrup should be administered orally immediately. If a convulsion occurs, the syrup should be rubbed on the buccal mucosa. The owner should be instructed to do this *immediately,* even before contacting the veterinarian. Hypoglycemia can produce coma as well as a seizure. For any known diabetic presented to the veterinarian because of an acute generalized central nervous system disturbance, a blood sample should be withdrawn for blood glucose determination and then a minimum of 5 to 10 cc. of 50 per cent dextrose IV (unless ketoacidosis is obvious) should be given immediately.

**Diet.** Once diabetes mellitus has been diagnosed, the patient's diet must be *constant.* The amount of food ingested will directly affect the amount of insulin required to maintain stability. Ideally, a commercial canned food should be found that not only is palatable but also has a constant caloric value.

The patient should be fed according to what the veterinarian believes to be its ideal body weight. A small dog should receive approximately 75 calories per kilo-

---

*Best Foods, Englewood Cliffs, New Jersey 07632.

**Table 3.** *Commonly Used Insulin Preparations*

| TYPE OF INSULIN | SUSPENSION | HOURS AFTER SUBCUTANEOUS INJECTION | | |
| | | *Effects Begin* | *Maximum Action* | *Duration of Effects* |
| --- | --- | --- | --- | --- |
| Regular | Solution | ¼ | 2–4 | 6–8 |
| NPH | Crystalline | 3 | 8–10 | 18–24 |
| Lente | 30% Amorphous and 20% Crystalline | 3 | 10–12 | 18–28 |
| PZI | Amorphous | 3–4 | 14–20 | 24–36 |

gram of body weight, while large dogs should receive approximately 55 calories per kilogram. If weight loss is deemed necessary to reach ideal body weight, total daily caloric intake should be reduced. The reducing diabetic must be monitored closely at home, since the daily insulin requirement will decrease as body weight decreases. Rarely, insulin is no longer required once ideal body weight is achieved.

**Exercise.** The amount of daily exercise will greatly affect the daily insulin requirement and should therefore be as unvaried as possible. Working dogs will require *less* insulin on working days. Although the cause is not well understood, the entry of glucose into skeletal muscle is increased during exercise in the absence of insulin. Hence diabetes is more difficult to manage in the working dog and requires close communication between the owner and the veterinarian. In our experience, dogs exercise much more at home than in the hospital but they also consume more food at home, and the insulin dose requirement usually increases after the animal is released from the hospital.

**Nonspayed Bitches.** Estrus, pseudopregnancy and pregnancy complicate the management of diabetes, since they make the effect of insulin highly erratic. The hormones produced during pregnancy and pseudopregnancy antagonize the effects of insulin, and insulin is destroyed by an insulinase produced by the placenta. The increased energy needs associated with heat cycles, pseudopregnancy and pregnancy often result in the onset of ketosis secondary to the bitch's chronic hyperglycemia, which stimulates fetal growth hormone. Fetuses tend to be large. In the neonate there is an increased risk of a hypoglycemic crisis due to beta-cell hyperplasia, which results again from chronic stimulation by high blood glucose concentrations in utero.

Thus for female diabetic patients, ovariohysterectomy should be performed as soon as possible after their condition is stabilized.

**Elective Surgery.** A simple protocol should be followed when any surgery is performed on the diabetic dog or cat. Ketosis and hyperglycemia must be prevented during and immediately after surgery. Elective major operations should be delayed until the patient's clinical condition is stable.

The day prior to surgery the patient receives the normal dose of insulin and is fed as usual. No food is given after midnight. On the morning of surgery, one half of the calculated dose of insulin for that day is given. During surgery the patient is maintained on an IV drip of 5 per cent dextrose in water or 5 per cent dextrose in saline until oral intake is reestablished. Because the diabetic patient needs carbohydrate to respond to the stress of surgery, the IV dextrose drip is important. Obviously, insulin must also be administered so that the diabetic animal can utilize the dextrose. Since the normal amount of food will not be consumed that day, a lower insulin dosage is administered. It is easier to adjust hyperglycemia than to treat a hypoglycemic crisis.

During and after surgery, total urine output, urine ketones and urine glucose must be monitored at frequent intervals. Measurements of blood glucose may also be required postoperatively. If hyperglycemia and glycosuria occur, small amounts of regular insulin can be given at 4- to 6-hour intervals. The dose of regular insulin in this situation is approximately 20 per cent of the total daily dose of NPH insulin for 4+ glycosuria. The dose is reduced further for smaller degrees of glycosuria or if the long-acting insulin is expected to peak during the given time period.

On the day after surgery the diabetic can

usually be returned to the routine schedule of insulin administration and feeding. If the patient is not eating, it can be maintained on IV dextrose and saline. Since the carbohydrate load in this situation is continuous, it is desirable to maintain a continuous supply of insulin. This is accomplished by giving one half the usual dose subcutaneously at 12-hour intervals until the animal is eating regularly and can be returned to the normal schedule.

## KETOACIDOSIS

Ketoacidosis is a state of deranged metabolism in the terminal phases of untreated diabetes mellitus. It constitutes a medical emergency which requires immediate and intensive care. If intensive care facilities and laboratory services are not available, the veterinarian should refer the patient to a hospital that can provide them. There is no one precise formula for the management of ketoacidosis. The patient does need close observation, so that changes in therapy can be made on the basis of its response. Frequent evaluation of both clinical and laboratory status is the key to success.

### PATHOPHYSIOLOGY

In the absence of adequate insulin, there are abnormalities in the metabolism of carbohydrate, fat and protein. These changes can lead to life-threatening metabolic acidosis and dehydration. Owing to its inability to utilize glucose, the body attempts to meet its energy demands by means of gluconeogenesis and mobilization of free fatty acids. The production of fatty acids may exceed the capacity of the normal hepatic metabolic pathways, resulting in the production of large amounts of the organic ketoacids, namely, betahydroxybutyrate, acetoacetate and acetone. Acidosis is caused by betahydroxybutyric acid and acetoacetic acid in a ratio of approximately 4:1. Ketoacids are excreted in the urine (ketonuria) in the form of sodium ketone salts.

In the absence of insulin, glucose accumulation in the extracellular (hyperglycemia) fluid occurs as a consequence of underutilization of glucose by the tissues and overproduction of glucose by the liver.

This hyperglycemia causes an obligatory osmotic diuresis, resulting in the loss of both water and electrolytes (sodium, potassium and chloride). Further losses of water and electrolytes occur as a result of repeated vomiting.

### DIAGNOSIS

The relevant past history usually includes the typical features of diabetes mellitus: polydipsia, polyuria, polyphagia and weight loss. The recent history is usually one of polydipsia, polyuria (although patients in critical condition may be oliguric or anuric), vomiting, anorexia, depression and hyperventilation. The owner usually reports that the pet has been exhibiting signs of severe illness for only 1 to 4 days. The physical examination reveals a dehydrated, depressed, tachypneic, obtunded patient, often with a strong odor of acetone on the breath.

If diabetic ketoacidosis is suspected, semiquantitative determination for plasma, serum or whole blood ketones should be done immediately by use of nitroprusside (Acetest®*) tablets. Urine should be checked simultaneously for ketones and glucose, using reagent strips (Keto-diastix®*). A strongly positive reaction for ketones in undiluted plasma, "4+" glycosuria and "large" reaction for ketonuria is sufficient cause to initiate therapy for ketoacidosis. However, these findings *must* be followed by additional laboratory tests for adequate initial treatment and for continued monitoring of the ketoacidosis. The additional measurements should include the serum electrolytes (sodium, potassium and chloride); the degree of acidosis, utilizing the venous $CO_2$ level; blood glucose; and BUN and a complete urinalysis. In addition, a CBC should be done, radiographs should be taken of the thorax and abdomen and a complete-lead electrocardiogram should be recorded. The patient is often azotemic (of renal or prerenal origin) and the *serum* potassium is often normal or elevated, although *total body* potassium is usually low. Both serum sodium and serum chloride are usually low. The sodium and chloride levels are of value in determining the amount of electrolyte

---

*Ames Company, Division of Miles Laboratory, Elkhart, Indiana 46514.

depletion that has occurred secondary to ketosis and vomiting. Treatment should commence while the results of these tests are being awaited.

The initial examination should focus not only on the state of hydration and central nervous system depression, but also on possible causes of the ketoacidosis, such as acute infection, trauma, estrus or pregnancy. Additional laboratory studies may be indicated, such as tests of liver and renal function and protein electrophoresis. The measurement of serum lipase can be used to assess pancreatic acinar destruction, but measurement of serum amylase is not reliable in the presence of ketoacidosis.

## TREATMENT

All pertinent treatment data must be recorded. A flow sheet should be maintained until the patient is no longer in critical condition. All administered drugs, including fluids, insulin, alkali and electrolytes, must be charted. Body temperature, pulse rate, respiratory rate, central venous pressure, urine output, the degree of glycosuria and ketonuria and specific gravity of the urine should be recorded regularly. The treatment protocol in ketoacidosis is summarized in Table 4.

**Table 4.** *Treatment of Diabetic Ketoacidosis*

A. Initial Therapy
  1. *Fluids:* 0.45% NaCl.
  2. *Insulin:* "Regular" only—1 U. per kilogram body weight divided (25% IV and 75% IM).
  3. *Bicarbonate:* 25% of calculated dose by intravenous infusion over first 6 hours.
B. Guidelines
  1. Repeat plasma electrolytes, $CO_2$ and blood glucose at 4-hour intervals until normal levels are approached.
  2. Drain *all* urine from bladder every 30 minutes and note amount recovered as well as levels of glycosuria and ketonuria.
  3. Monitor central venous pressure and EKG.
C. Subsequent Therapy
  1. *Fluids:* Change intravenous infusion to 5% dextrose in water (0.45% NaCl and 5% dextrose in water can be combined for long-term maintenance).
  2. *Insulin:* "Regular" insulin every 4 hours at adjusted doses until NPH insulin is instituted.
  3. *Bicarbonate:* Adjust dose depending on subsequent blood $CO_2$ levels.
  4. *Potassium:* If animal is not anuric, add potassium to intravenous infusion after 3 to 4 hours of therapy.

**Fluid Therapy.** Replacement of fluids is accomplished via an indwelling catheter in the jugular or cephalic vein. Since very large amounts of fluids may be administered, assessment of the cardiovascular system is mandatory. Acute congestive heart failure is a potential complication.

The volume of fluid to be administered during the initial 6 to 12 hours is determined by calculating the dehydration deficit and adding this to the maintenance requirements, i.e., urine output and insensible fluid loss. Both central venous pressure determinations and the monitoring of urine output via an indwelling urinary catheter are valuable aids in determining fluid replacement. Fluid administration should be rapid during the first hour and then slowed to a maintenance rate of approximately 2 cc./kg./hr.

The ketoacidotic patient is invariably dehydrated as a result of the osmotic diuresis. The loss of water is relatively greater than that of salt, which leads to hyperosmosis. Thus, hypotonic saline (0.45 per cent NaCl) is the optimal replacement fluid.

The intravenous fluid is subsequently changed to 5 per cent dextrose in water (D5W). Timing of this change is critical. The glucose is provided to prevent a hypoglycemic crisis, to supply a substrate for the insulin and to avoid a precipitous fall in blood glucose concentration, which may induce cerebral edema. The change from hypotonic saline to 5 per cent dextrose in water is made when blood glucose concentration falls below 250 mg./100 ml. Blood glucose concentration should be measured every 30 minutes and for this purpose, Dextrostix®* are excellent.

Alternatively, the change may be made when the urine glucose level falls below ½ per cent (++) on Keto-diastix®*. In order to utilize this method of regulating fluid therapy, frequent measurements of urine glucose are necessary. During the course of insulin therapy, the urine glucose level will fall from its original 2 to 6 per cent (on dilution) to much lower levels. If, for example, the initial value is 2 per cent and with each 60 minutes of treatment there is a decrease of 50 per cent, the urine glucose level after four hours will be 1/10 per cent ("trace" on Keto-diastix). If all the urine produced dur-

---

*Ames Company, Division of Miles Laboratory, Elkhart, Indiana 46514.

ing this period is allowed to mix in the bladder, the resulting glucose value will obviously be higher and hence misleading. With a urinary catheter in place, the bladder can be emptied every 30 minutes, thereby avoiding the dilutional artifact. Urine glucose values above 2 per cent can be measured by the new "2 drop" method using Clinitest tablets.

In animals with severe volume depletion, normal saline (0.9 per cent) should be administered at a rate of 20 to 30 ml./kg./hr. for the first hour, following which 0.45 per cent saline should be used. In patients with persistent vomiting, a 1:1 mixture of 0.45 per cent saline and 5 per cent dextrose in water is preferred.

**Insulin Therapy.** The ketoacidotic diabetic needs insulin immediately. Only regular insulin should be used initially, because its prompt onset of action and short half-life permit rapid evaluation of the response and appropriate adjustments in dosage. The initial dose is 1 U./kg., 25 per cent of the total dose being given as an intravenous bolus and the remainder being given intramuscularly. In cats, the dose should be reduced to 1/2 U./kg.

The half-life of intravenously injected insulin is only 3 to 5 minutes and the concentration falls to less than 1 per cent of the initial value within 25 minutes. After intramuscular injection, the onset of action is within 5 to 15 minutes, the peak effect is within 2 to 3 hours and the total duration of effect is 4 to 6 hours. Intramuscular administration is preferred to subcutaneous in this situation because absorption via the former route is less affected by dehydration and shock. The combination of IV and IM administration provides insulin immediately as well as an adequate level in the blood for approximately 4 hours.

At 4-hour intervals the patient will require additional insulin, with possible adjustments in the dose. The adjustments are based on urine glucose and ketone levels, as shown in Table 5. The change from 0.45 per cent saline to 5 per cent dextrose in water, also noted in the table, is often made at times other than the 4-hour mark.

The change from regular to NPH insulin is usually made between 7 and 9 A.M., once the patient's condition is stabilized and there is no ketosis, acidosis or hyperglycemia. In this way the animal can be monitored during the day and can be fed at a convenient time late in the afternoon. If the animal is due for an injection of regular insulin at the time when the change to NPH insulin is to be made, both preparations can be administered together. The dose of regular insulin should be reduced, however, because there is some regular insulin in the NPH preparation. The NPH insulin will take effect just as the blood level of regular insulin begins to decline.

**Bicarbonate Therapy.** There is a great deal of controversy concerning the use of bicarbonate in ketoacidosis. Since acetoacetate and betahydroxybutyrate can be utilized by the body, serum bicarbonate concentrations begin to return toward normal with fluid and insulin therapy alone. Often, however, the ketoacidotic animal is presented with serum $CO_2$ concentrations as low as 4 to 6 mEq./l. ($CO_2$ concentration = bicarbonate concentration), with the normal level being approximately 24 mEq./l. Measurement of the initial venous $CO_2$ level is thus imperative if one is to determine the correct amount of bicarbonate to be administered. Available bicarbonate preparations are at a concentration of approximately 1 mEq./l.

If the initial serum bicarbonate level is

*Table 5.* Insulin Adjustments in a 10-Kilogram Dog

| URINE GLUCOSE* | URINE KETONES* | INSULIN ADJUSTMENT (add or subtract from previous dose) | ROUTE | IV FLUIDS |
|---|---|---|---|---|
| 2%, 1%, ½% | Large, moderate | Increase 2 U. | IM | 0.45% saline |
| ¼%, 1/10%, Neg | Large, moderate | Increase 2 U. | IM | 5% dextrose in water |
| 2%, 1%, ½% | Small | Increase 1 U. | SC | 0.45% saline |
| ¼%, 1/10%, Neg | Small | No change | SC | 5% dextrose in water |
| 2% | Negative | Increase 1 U. | SC | 0.45% saline |
| 1%, ½% | Negative | Increase ½ U. | SC | 0.45% saline |
| ¼%, 1/10% | Negative | No change | SC | 5% dextrose in water |
| Negative | Negative | Decrease 2 U. | SC | 5% dextrose in water |

*Keto-diastix® determinations, Ames Company, Division of Miles Laboratory, Elkhart, Indiana 46514.

less than 12 mEq./l., approximately 25 per cent of the dose of bicarbonate, determined by the equation below, should be administered in the intravenous infusion during the initial six hours of therapy. The bicarbonate deficit, i.e., the milliequivalents of bicarbonate needed to correct acidosis, is calculated as follows:

$$\text{mEq. bicarbonate} =$$
$$\text{body weight (kg.)} \times 0.4 \times \text{base deficit.}$$

The base deficit is the difference between the patient's serum bicarbonate concentration and the normal value of 24 mEq./l., and the factor 0.4 corrects for the bicarbonate distribution volume (40 per cent of body weight).

There are three main objections to the use of bicarbonate: First, it may result in metabolic alkalosis, as the ketones are metabolized. Second, a rapid elevation of arterial pH may be accompanied by a paradoxical and exaggerated fall in cerebral spinal fluid pH, resulting in deterioration of central nervous system function. Third, alkalinization causes a shift to the left in the dissociation curve for oxygen, thereby limiting delivery of oxygen to the tissues. In addition, administration of sodium (as sodium bicarbonate) in the presence of incipient congestive heart failure must be monitored closely in order to prevent cardiovascular overloading. Conversely, severely acidotic animals (serum $CO_2$ less than 12 mEq./l.) need alkali because severe acidosis can depress consciousness and result in coma. If serum $CO_2$ is measured every 4 to 6 hours and the bicarbonate is administered conservatively, the ketoacidotic animal can be treated without unnecessary risk.

To avoid aggravating cellular dehydration by infusing a hypertonic solution, bicarbonate must be added only to *hypotonic* solutions. If bicarbonate is added to an isotonic solution, a hypertonic solution, which is detrimental to the patient, would be created. Lactate solutions should not be used to correct ketoacidosis because blood lactate concentration tends to be elevated in this condition and there is a danger of creating a mixed keto-lactic acidosis.

**Potassium Therapy.** In the ketoacidotic diabetic, total body potassium is invariably reduced by 5 to 10 mEq./kg. of body weight. The depletion is initiated by the flux of potassium from the cell to the extracellular fluid, which accompanies the depletion of

glycogen stores in ketoacidosis. In addition, lack of insulin causes irregularities in the normal cellular exchange of ions, resulting in intracellular depletion of potassium. As a consequence, potassium accumulates in the extracellular fluid and blood. Although potassium is lost in great amounts in the urine, owing to the diuresis associated with ketosis, and persistent vomiting may further exaggerate the depletion, the initial serum potassium concentration is usually within or above the normal range. As the acidosis is corrected and as potassium accompanies glucose into the cells following the administration of insulin, serum potassium concentration declines. The finding of low or low normal serum potassium levels in ketoacidosis may indicate severe potassium depletion and imminent danger of fatal cardiac arrhythmias. Accordingly, potassium chloride should be administered when serum potassium reaches low normal values (usually within 3 to 4 hours after therapy is begun). If the animal is anuric, potassium is contraindicated, and measures should be taken to induce diuresis.

A dose of 7 mEq. of potassium chloride *added to* each 250 cc. of intravenous fluid, after the initial 3 to 4 hours of therapy, meets the usual requirement of the ketoacidotic diabetic. The animal's size, fluid requirements, urine production rate and general condition determine the actual amount of potassium required. It is safer to add 7 mEq. of potassium chloride to each 250 cc. of fluid than to calculate the dose on the basis of body weight. This regimen of therapy is monitored every four hours with serum potassium levels and electrocardiograms. Potassium must be diluted in the infusion fluid to avoid myocardial irregularities associated with rapid alterations in extracellular potassium concentration. Generally, potassium is administered until the animal begins to eat. If serum potassium concentration rises above normal, the amount of intravenously administered potassium must obviously be reduced.

The electrocardiogram is extremely useful in monitoring the response of the ketoacidotic diabetic, in that it indicates the development of both hypo- and hyperkalemia. Hypokalemia should be suspected when there is a prolonged Q-T interval (merging of T and U waves), depression of the ST segment and depression of T waves. Hyperkalemia is indicated by "peaked" T waves, prolonged P-R intervals and, with increasing severity, disappearance of P waves. If allowed to go unchecked, hyperkalemia will result in ventricular asystole or ventricular fibrillation. Appreciation of the subtle electrocardiographic changes depends upon careful comparison of frequent tracings.

**Complications.** Despite all efforts to revive ketoacidotic animals, deaths still occur. The mortality rate for ketoacidosis in man is about 3 to 10 per cent. Failure to respond to intensive care can usually be attributed to the coexistence of irreversible shock, cerebral edema, overwhelming sepsis, acute pancreatitis or renal failure.

## HYPEROSMOLAR NONKETOTIC COMA

Hyperosmolar nonketotic coma is a disorder characterized by severe hyperglycemia, hyperosmolarity and dehydration. It should be suspected in any severely dehydrated, nonacidotic and lethargic or comatose animal. Accompanying signs in noncomatose animals include weakness, polyuria, polydipsia and anorexia. Clinical signs develop more slowly than in ketoacidosis, and the patient may have appeared to be ill for as long as 1 to 2 weeks.

The diagnosis is suggested by the finding of glycosuria without ketonuria and is confirmed when significant hyperglycemia is demonstrated. The patient usually has an elevated BUN and is never acidotic (venous $CO_2$ analysis). If serum osmolarity cannot be measured directly, it may be calculated by the following formula:

$$\text{mOsm./l.} = 2\,(\text{serum Na} + \text{serum K}) + \frac{\text{blood glucose}}{18} + \frac{\text{BUN}}{2.8},$$

where serum Na and K are in mEq./l. and blood glucose and BUN are in mg./dl. The normal serum osmolarity is approximately 300 mOsm./l. and values above 320 mOsm./l. are considered to be significantly elevated. Serum sodium concentration may be low, normal or high, and serum potassium is usually normal or low.

The aim of therapy is steadily (not precipitously) to correct the hyperosmolarity, hyperglycemia and dehydration, while stimulating diuresis to lower the BUN. Rehydration is accomplished with 0.45 per cent saline for the initial 2 to 3 hours, following which the infusion is changed to normal saline. Regular insulin is utilized at lower doses than in ketoacidosis because there is greater sensitivity to insulin. Serum electrolytes and blood glucose levels must be monitored closely and changes in therapy must be made as required. Urine output, central venous pressure and the electrocardiogram must also be monitored closely. The prognosis for recovery is guarded.

### ACKNOWLEDGMENTS

This paper was supported in part by the Berkeley Veterinary Research Association.

The author wishes to thank Nancy V. Bohannon, M.D., of the Metabolic Research Unit, University of California Medical School, San Francisco, for her assistance.

### SUPPLEMENTAL READING

Diabetes Mellitus. *In* Boedeker, E. C., and Dauber, J. H. (eds.): Manual of Medical Therapeutics. 21st ed. Boston, Little, Brown and Co., 1975.

Felig, P.: Diabetic ketoacidosis. New Engl. J. Med., *290*:1360–1362, 1974.

Gerich, J. E., Martin, M. M., and Recant, L.: Clinical and metabolic characteristics of hyperosmolar nonketotic coma. Diabetes, *20*:228–238, 1971.

# HYPOGLYCEMIA IN THE DOG

ROGER K. JOHNSON, D.V.M.,
*and* CLARKE E. ATKINS, D.V.M.
*Walnut Creek, California*

Hypoglycemia is not a specific diagnosis but rather the manifestation of a more specific disease or physiologic process. Extensive research in human medicine has resulted in the classification of hypoglycemia based on (1) age of onset—neonatal, juvenile or mature onset; (2) occurrence—transient or persistent/recurrent; and (3) hypoglycemic stimulus—reactive or fasting. Furthermore, in man, a list of specific diagnoses has been defined for each classification. Relatively few disease processes characterized by hypoglycemia have been documented in the dog.

The regulation of normal blood glucose concentration is a complex process involving intestinal absorption, hepatic production and peripheral utilization of glucose. In the fasted state, glycogen and glucose are formed in the liver from amino acids (gluconeogenesis), from glycerol derived from lipolysis and from lactate. Normal function of liver enzyme pathways is essential to the hepatic regulation of the blood glucose concentration. In addition, profound influences on both hepatic production of glucose and peripheral glucose utilization are exerted by hormones such as insulin, glucagon, epinephrine, norepinephrine, cortisol, ACTH and growth hormone.

## CLINICAL MANIFESTATIONS

For the most part, the clinical manifestations of hypoglycemia are similar regardless of the etiology. The brain is largely dependent on glucose oxidation for energy and does not have readily available glycogen stores; in addition, glucose enters the neuron predominately by diffusion rather than as an insulin-dependent process. Therefore the blood glucose concentration is of prime importance to the brain, and the signs of hypoglycemia are understandably those of central nervous system dysfunction. The severity of clinical manifestations is related to the rate at which the blood glucose concentration declines and, to a lesser extent, to the degree of hypoglycemia.

We have observed nearly normal behavior in a dog with a decrease in blood glucose concentration to 6 mg./100 ml. over a 36-hour period. Conversely, we have observed a generalized seizure in a dog whose blood glucose concentration dropped from the normal range to 40 mg./100 ml. over a 30-minute period.

Generalized or focal neurologic signs may be observed in dogs with hypoglycemia and include weakness of the rear legs or generalized weakness, muscular twitching, incoordination, amaurotic blindness, generalized seizures or other bizarre neurologic aberrations. Pulmonary edema has recently been described as a possible sequel to hypoglycemia.

When hypoglycemia evolves rapidly, there is a prompt increase in concentrations of growth hormone, cortisol, pancreatic glucagon, epinephrine and norepinephrine. The effect of these hormones is complex, but in general they serve to stabilize or elevate blood glucose concentrations and thus counteract hypoglycemia by increasing hepatic glucose release, inhibiting endogenous insulin release or decreasing peripheral glucose utilization.

When the onset of hypoglycemia is slow, the counter-regulatory mechanism may not be triggered. Likewise, when acute hypoglycemia recurs frequently over a long period of time, the response mechanisms may be exhausted. Consequently, through either mechanism, these recurrent episodes of hypoglycemia are marked by a lessened ability of the dog to restore blood glucose values to normal and may result in severe cerebral damage or so-called "irreversible hypoglycemic brain damage."

## JUVENILE ONSET HYPOGLYCEMIAS

### TRANSIENT JUVENILE HYPOGLYCEMIA

This form of hypoglycemia, seen predominantly in puppies of the toy and miniature breeds that are less than 3 months of age, is usually precipitated by cold, starvation or gastrointestinal disturbances. The signs of transient juvenile hypoglycemia are not dissimilar to those of other forms of hypoglycemia. In our experience, however, the puppies are more commonly presented comatose or severely depressed, with accompanying facial muscle twitching. The blood glucose concentration may be extremely low and is rarely above 30 mg./100 ml.

To prevent irreversible neuronal damage, prompt therapy is imperative. Initially, it should include a total of 1 to 2 cc. of 50 per cent glucose per kg. body weight, administered intravenously as a bolus, diluted in equal parts of sterile water to avoid the possibility of hyperosmolarity.

In the event that clinical signs are not ameliorated by repeated glucose administration, it can be assumed that cerebral edema is present. If the unresponsive signs include generalized seizures, sedation with diazepam is indicated prior to specific therapy for cerebral edema (mannitol and dexamethasone). Ten to 15 per cent glucose should then be administered in a balanced electrolyte solution at a rate sufficient to maintain normoglycemia until oral alimentation is possible. Pups should then be fed frequently, and oral sugar should be administered at regular intervals until normoglycemia is maintained. If the precipitating factors are adequately treated, recurrence of signs is uncommon.

## PERSISTENT OR RECURRENT JUVENILE HYPOGLYCEMIA

In some puppies, hypoglycemia may continue or recur despite therapy, and these puppies should be evaluated for other causes of hypoglycemia. Hereditary defects in carbohydrate metabolism (most commonly the glycogen storage diseases); defects in amino acid metabolism; hormone deficiencies (growth hormone, cortisol and ACTH); and hyperinsulinism (beta cell hyperplasia, leucine sensitivity, islet cell adenoma, etc.) are known causes of persistent or recurrent hypoglycemia in children. Similar reports in the dog are limited to the glycogen storage diseases, and even these are incompletely documented.

Type I glycogen storage disease (von Gierke's disease) is caused by a deficiency of glucose-6-phosphatase, an enzyme necessary for the conversion of glucose-6-phosphate to free glucose. The end result of this enzyme deficiency is a visceral accumulation of glycogen and ensuing hypoglycemia. Children affected with type I glycogen storage disease are characterized by fasting hypoglycemia that responds poorly to glycogen, growth retardation, hepatomegaly, renomegaly, ketosis and acidosis due to lactate accumulation, hyperlipidemia and a bleeding diathesis.

Bardens described type I glycogen storage disease in 6- to 12-week old puppies characterized by symptomatic hypoglycemia with hepatomegaly and less than normal response to glucagon administration. Puppies that responded to initial therapy relapsed and eventually died, and autopsies were reported to reveal glycogen deposition in the liver, kidneys and myocardium. A tentative diagnosis of glycogen storage disease may be made if recurrent or persistent hypoglycemia is found in a puppy that also has hepatomegaly, acidosis and ketosis. To establish a definitive diagnosis, histologic evidence of glycogen accumulation should be provided and specific enzyme analysis performed. The prognosis of glycogen storage disease in the dog is grave; however, if treatment is attempted, it should consist of frequent carbohydrate feedings, glucose supplementation and avoidance of lactose, which may contribute to glycogen accumulation. Diazoxide, an experimental benzothiazide derivative that causes elevations of blood glucose, may prove efficacious in the long-term treatment of type I glycogen storage disease in the dog.

## MATURE ONSET HYPOGLYCEMIA

### BETA CELL TUMOR IN THE DOG

Beta cell tumor or "insulinoma" is used here to describe a "functional" tumor of the beta cells of the pancreatic islets of Langerhans, i.e., one which produces excessive quantities of insulin. *The increased transfer of blood glucose into cells, mediated by excessive insulin, causes periods of hypoglycemia and the resulting neurologic dysfunction.* The infrequent occurrence of insulinoma is suggested by the fact that functional tumors have been reported in only 45 dogs. However, when a high index of suspicion is maintained, this condition, like any other, is recognized more frequently.

Unlike the analogous condition in man, in which 90 per cent of the tumors are benign, 69 per cent of the reported canine "insulinomas" have been malignant and, in our experience with 16 cases, 82 per cent have been malignant. Death may be the result of the so-called "irreversible hypoglycemic brain damage" or euthanasia after unsuccessful management of a vague neurologic disorder or may follow the discovery of a malignancy. Thus, early diagnosis is essential.

"Insulinomas" occur most frequently in older dogs, the average age at the time of diagnosis being about 9 years, but we have documented signs of the disease in a 3½-year-old dog. Signs of hypoglycemia are occasionally overt, and the diagnosis may be ascertained almost immediately; however, it is not uncommon for the disease to persist for as long as two, and occasionally as long as six, years before it is correctly diagnosed.

There is no apparent predilection according to sex or breed except for a slightly higher incidence in boxers, as is the case for several other neoplasms.

## CLINICAL SIGNS

An "insulinoma" is usually very small and does not cause malignant cachexia, nor does it usually cause significant mechanical damage to any organ. We have, however, recently observed two dogs with mild signs of acute pancreatitis associated with islet cell tumors. The clinical signs of "insulinoma" are purely those of hypoglycemia. Stimuli such as fasting, exercise, excitement and eating will frequently drive blood glucose concentrations to subnormal levels in the patient with a functioning beta cell tumor. The ensuing neurologic abnormalities are directly related to the rate at which the blood sugar falls rather than to the degree of hypoglycemia. Therefore, the neurologic signs are characteristically intermittent, except late in the course of the disease, when hypoglycemia may be constant. It may seem paradoxical that eating can cause hypoglycemia, but postprandial hyperglycemia is a potent stimulus for insulin production in the normal patient and is usually exaggerated in the presence of an "insulinoma". In addition, L-leucine, an amino acid found in most proteins, is known to stimulate insulin production in some beta cell tumors in both man and the dog.

Generalized seizures (grand mal) may occur after a hypoglycemic stimulus but are not consistent. With about equal frequency, there may be no history of generalized seizures, seizures throughout the course of disease or seizures only late in the course of the disease. On the other hand, virtually all dogs with "insulinoma" exhibit some signs other than seizures, and it is important to note that these also occur intermittently. Generalized asthenia (weakness); apparent weakness of the rear legs (paraparesis); generalized muscle twitching; and a syndrome of disorientation, incoordination and apparent blindness are among the most common signs in this group. In addition, bizarre signs observed infrequently are irascibility, running and barking, hysteria accompanied by loss of bowel and bladder control, apparent anxiety manifested by incessant barking and twitching of only the facial muscles or periods of persistent yelping as if in extreme pain. One dog exhibited episodes of consistent lowering of the right shoulder accompanied by generalized muscular twitching. The hypoglycemic episodes characteristically become more frequent and more severe during the course of the disease. Nearly any set of neurologic signs, whether focal or generalized, can be caused by hypoglycemia. Based on these signs, the differential diagnosis should include idiopathic epilepsy, brain tumor, lead poisoning, canine distemper, other organic brain diseases, hypoparathyroidism and spinal conditions.

## DIAGNOSIS

Unless the patient is in a hypoglycemic crisis, there may be no relevant physical findings. Similarly, radiographs, hemograms and most blood chemistry analyses are unremarkable. Fasting (12-hour) blood glucose concentrations (ortho-toluidine method) are usually below normal ($< 70$ mg./100 ml.) and are often profoundly low ($< 50$ mg./100 ml.), but repeated testing may be necessary to document hypoglycemia. One normal blood glucose concentration, even after a 24-hour fast, is not sufficient evidence to discount the diagnosis of "insulinoma"; a 48-hour fast may be necessary.

A patient with fasting hypoglycemia and signs that are ameliorated by glucose administration is said to have met the criteria for "Whipple's triad." This triad of signs merely confirms that the neurologic abnormalities are caused by hypoglycemia but does not indicate the etiology of that condition. It is paramount that a definite diagnosis be made before a dog with hypoglycemia, usually aged, is subjected to a laparotomy for removal of an alleged beta cell tumor.

Plasma insulin levels can now be determined by many commercial and research laboratories and should be used to make a positive diagnosis rather than making a diagnosis by exclusion. In our experience, the average fasting immunoreactive insulin (IRI) concentration in normal dogs is about $20\mu$U./ml.; values above 54 $\mu$U./ml. are abnormal. In fasting hypoglycemia due to other causes, plasma IRI concentration is usually normal or below normal, whereas it is usually elevated in dogs with "insulinoma". This concept of cause and effect is best expressed by a ratio between IRI and glucose concentrations (I/G ratio) in samples drawn simultaneously. The average fasting I/G ratio in normal dogs is about 21.5 $\mu$U./mg. $\times$ 100; values above 52 $\mu$U./mg. $\times$ 100 are abnormal.

In the unusual event that the above procedures fail to confirm the diagnosis, or if use of insulin is not feasible, the provocative test of choice is the glucagon tolerance test. Glucagon is a hormone produced by the alpha cells of the islets of Langerhans. When injected intravenously, it causes rapid glycogenolysis and hyperglycemia. Glucagon stimulates insulin production both directly, within three minutes after injection, and indirectly, through its hyperglycemic effect, 15 to 30 minutes after injection. These insulinogenic effects are usually exaggerated in the presence of an insulinoma, and the excessive insulin concentrations are reflected in subnormal blood glucose concentrations (Fig. 1). The glucagon tolerance test is performed after a 12-hour fast, if possible, and 0.03 mg./kg. of glucagon U.S.P. is injected intravenously. Samples for analysis of blood glucose, and preferably IRI, concentrations are drawn optimally at 0, 1, 3, 5, 15, 30, 45, 60, 90, 120 and 180 minutes. As a minimum, samples should be collected at 0, 15, 30, 60 and 120 minutes.

Diagnostic criteria for the glucagon tolerance test are (1) a decrease in blood glucose concentration one or two minutes after injection (caused by rapid release of insulin from the tumor); (2) in the absence of severe liver disease, peak blood glucose concentration <135 mg./100 ml.; (3) hypoglycemia (<50 mg./100 ml.) by 60 or 120 minutes (highly diagnostic); (4) one minute after injection, plasma IRI values >50 $\mu$U./ml. or an average increase from fasting to one minute of > 18 $\mu$U./ml. (highly diagnostic); (5) probably the most diagnostic clinical pathological data that can be obtained, an insulin/glucose ratio one minute after injection of glucagon in which values are > 75 $\mu$U./ml. should be considered clearly diagnostic.

Other tests of less value for the diagnosis of "insulinoma" are the oral glucose tolerance test, intravenous glucose tolerance test, leucine tolerance test and tolbutamide tolerance test.

## COMPLICATIONS

Prolonged, severe hypoglycemia may cause so-called "irreversible brain damage." This is essentially hypoxic damage, because the end result of decreased metabolism is decreased oxygenation of the neuron. Dogs having recurrent single seizures or other transient neurologic signs undergo minimal neuronal damage. However, if glucose is given to a dog in hypoglycemic coma or status epilepticus and amelioration of signs does not occur, some degree of cerebral hypoxia and edema has occurred.

This condition should be treated with (1) 0.5 to 1.0 gm. of dextrose/kg. injected as a 50 per cent solution through a large vein to avoid thrombophlebitis and a rapid continuous infusion of dextrose solution, 10 per cent to small dogs and 20 per cent to large dogs; (2) soluble glucocorticoids administered at the recommended dosage for treatment of shock; (3) 2 mg. of prednisolone/kg. injected intramuscularly; (4) diazepam administered intravenously to effect; (5) oral or intravenous diphenylhydantoin when long-term anticonvulsant therapy is needed; (6) mannitol 1 to 3 gm./kg., repeated at one half the dose in six hours; and (7) local hypothermia (ice pack on the head of the dog).

Continuous dextrose infusion is frequently required to abate hypoglycemia in dogs with insulinoma. During its long-term administration, special attention must be paid to control of sepsis. In addition,

# GLUCAGON TOLERANCE TEST

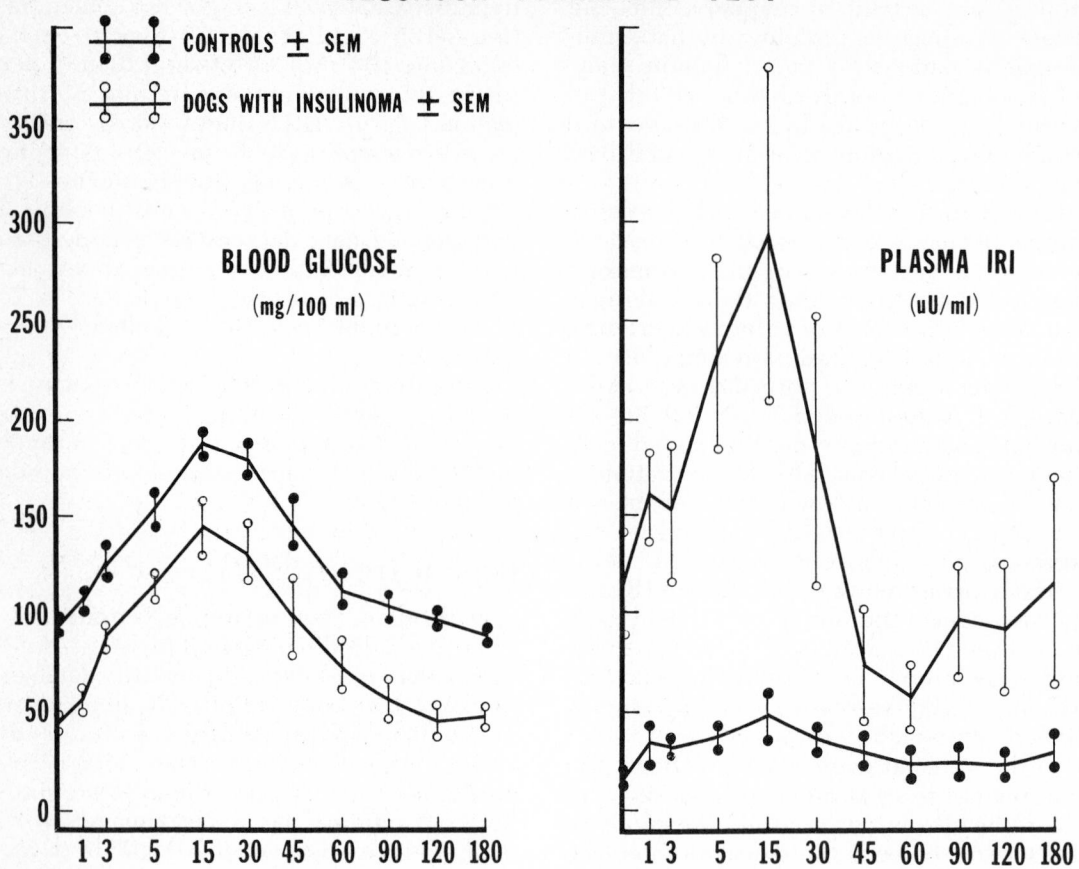

**Figure 1.** Blood glucose and plasma and immunoreactive insulin (IRI) response to intravenous glucagon in normal dogs and in dogs with insulinoma.

hypokalemia is frequently observed during glucose administration to dogs with insulinoma and is caused by the transfer of potassium from extracellular to intracellular fluids. Potassium supplementation is therefore needed.

**SURGICAL THERAPY**

Surgical removal of a functioning beta cell tumor is the obvious therapy of choice but is fraught with problems. The incidence of malignancy among these tumors is very high and, even if the diagnosis is made early in the course of the disease, there is often metastasis to the regional lymph nodes, liver or spleen prior to surgery.

To our knowledge, a histologically malignant, nonmetastasizing tumor has not been surgically removed without hypoglycemia recurring at a later date. Surgery is therefore curative only for the rare adenoma and is only palliative for carcinomas.

Although the majority of insulinomas are grossly visible, the surgeon may occasionally be unable to locate a tumor for the following reasons: (1) a solitary primary tumor may be too small to be seen or palpated; (2) multiple microscopic tumors distributed uniformly throughout the pancreas are equally elusive; and (3) an ectopic pancreatic tumor may be present. We have had one patient with tumorous pancreatic tissue that was located at the hilus of the mesoduodenum and was not found in the pancreas upon careful histologic examination. In the event that no distinct tumor mass is detectable, the surgeon must either do a complete pancreatectomy, remove a biopsy specimen blindly or do nothing, since neither lobe of the canine pancreas has had a greater occurrence of tumors. The majority of dogs with "insulinoma" experience age changes that make them poor surgical risks. In addition, postoperative pancreatitis is a frequent complication even with proper surgical technique.

Preoperative therapy should include the withholding of all food, water and oral medication, i.e., nothing *per os* (NPO), for one day and the parenteral administration of glucocorticoids for two days before surgery. Normoglycemia and hydration should be maintained by administration of parenteral dextrose and balanced electrolyte solutions. The actual technique for removal of pancreatic tumors is discussed elsewhere.

Postoperatively, the patient should be monitored intensively and treated as though pancreatitis were present. Our preferred therapy includes (1) NPO for three to five days; (2) atropine sulfate injectable, U.S.P., 0.2 mg./kg. hourly in intravenous fluids; (3) cephaloridine, 10 mg./kg. every 12 hours; (4) continuous administration of lactated Ringer's solution containing potassium (potassium chloride, U.S.P.) in a concentration of 10 to 20 mEq./500 ml. and dextrose sufficient to cause a mild glycosuria; (5) if necessary, dexamethasone (Azium® [Schering]), 2 mg./kg. every 6 hours, decreasing over a 3- to 5-day period.

Laboratory studies should include daily measurements of blood glucose, sodium, potassium, amylase, lipase and BUN.

Dogs with metastatic disease will usually remain hypoglycemic after surgery, whereas temporary or permanent diabetes may result from the complete excision of the tumor.

Our recommendations for surgery are (1) if a definitive diagnosis of insulinoma has been made and the patient is a good surgical risk, a laparotomy should be performed; (2) if at surgery one finds metastatic disease or a primary tumor that is difficult to remove, especially in the left lobe or the angle of the pancreas, only a biopsy specimen of that tumor should be removed; (3) if an operable primary tumor is found and there are no metastatic lesions, the tumor should be removed.

## MEDICAL THERAPY

Medical treatment is only palliative but can permit a reasonably normal life for some time. Diazoxide (Schering) is an experimental benzothiazide derivative with hyperglycemic effects. We have used it effectively for as long as six months to control hypoglycemia in dogs with insulinoma. The initial dose should be 10 mg./kg. and should be increased as required up to 40 mg./kg. daily. Apparently, however, either a tolerance for diazoxide develops or the tumor's insulin production becomes so great that diazoxide is not solely effective. Diazoxide's hyperglycemic effect may be potentiated by administering hydrochlorothiazide at 2 to 4 mg./kg. daily. To supplement the above therapy, or if diazoxide is unavailable, glucocorticoids, a high-protein diet and frequent feedings may be used to control hypoglycemia.

Propranolol, a beta-adrenergic blocking agent, has recently been effectively used to elevate the blood glucose in a human subject with insulinoma; the method of action remains unclear. If effective in the dog, propranolol, which is readily available at any pharmacy, could be extremely useful in management of canine islet cell tumors, because most are malignant and require medical management.

A new antitumor drug called streptozotocin has been shown to cause regression of beta cell adenocarcinomas in man and is currently under investigation for use in dogs.

## OTHER HYPOGLYCEMIAS

### TUMOR HYPOGLYCEMIA

Some extrapancreatic tumors have been shown to cause hypoglycemia in man, and we have observed this phenomenon in one dog with metastatic mammary carcinoma and another with primary pulmonary adenocarcinoma. Multiple theories have been proposed to explain the cause of hypoglycemia in extrapancreatic tumors; briefly, they include (1) rapid unregulated glucose uptake by massive tumors at a rate faster than production of glucose by gluconeogenesis, and (2) production of insulin or an insulin-like substance (refer to later article in this section, "Ectopic Hormone Production by Nonendocrine Neoplasms.")

### HEPATOGENOUS HYPOGLYCEMIA

Certain liver diseases, when severe, may result in hypoglycemia due to destruction of hepatic enzyme systems responsible for storage or lysis of glycogen. Cirrhosis, fatty degeneration, the glycogenoses (GSD's), neoplasia, portal vein anomalies and acute necrotic and other forms of hepatitis are notable examples.

Occasionally, dogs with severe liver disease are presented because of hypoglycemic signs, but more commonly the signs are those related to liver disease.

## HYPOADRENOCORTICISM

The presenting signs of hypoadrenocorticism are usually those of hypovolemia, hyperkalemia and hyponatremia (refer to article later in this section on "Primary Adrenocortical Insufficiency"). Hypoglycemia occurs not uncommonly in severely ill dogs with hypoadrenocorticism, but what portion of the weakness associated with that disease is from hypoglycemia is debatable. We have observed generalized seizures associated with blood glucose concentrations of 45 mg./100 ml. and 22 mg./100 ml., resulting from a lack of glucocorticoid production in two proven addisonian dogs.

## HUNTING DOG HYPOGLYCEMIA

A hypoglycemia of hunting breeds has been described, usually affecting highly nervous dogs 1 to 2 hours after beginning a hunt. When afflicted, these dogs appear dazed, then stagger and exhibit grand mal type seizures. Recovery generally occurs within minutes, but the dogs remain exhausted for the remainder of the day. Frequent feedings with a protein-rich meal at least one hour prior to the hunt and several smaller carbohydrate-rich meals throughout the hunt have been recommended and found to be successful. Twice daily feedings appear to be adequate on days when the dog is not worked. Adrenocorticosteroids and tranquilizers have also been advocated. Bardens feels that this syndrome may represent a type III glycogen storage disease, but no evidence for this has been provided.

## MISCELLANEOUS CAUSES OF HYPOGLYCEMIA

One of the most common causes of a low blood glucose report from the laboratory is simply the failure to remove the serum from the cells or the failure to utilize an agent such as sodium fluoride to preserve the sample. Whole blood at room temperature is said to oxidize glucose at the rate of 10 mg./100 ml./hour.

It is not uncommon to find a mild to severe hypoglycemia in a patient with a severely debilitating disease. If the underlying disease is adequately treated, blood glucose concentration usually returns to normal.

During routine screening of mature dogs, it is not uncommon in our experience to find blood glucose concentrations below normal. There is often no apparent cause for this finding, and normoglycemia is often found on retesting. The cause for this incidental finding of hypoglycemia is unclear.

Primary renal glycosuria, resulting from an enzymatic defect in the renal tubules, is known to occur in the dog. However, an associated hypoglycemia, which is found in this hereditary disease in man, has not been described in the dog.

Other causes of hypoglycemia may include intestinal malassimilation, insulin overdosage and ingestion of oral hypoglycemic drugs.

## SUPPLEMENTAL READING

Bardens, J. W.: Glycogen storage disease in puppies. Vet. Med./Small Animal Clin., *61*:1174, 1966.

Bardens, J. W., Bardens, G. W., and Bardens, B.: Clinical observations of a von Gierke-like syndrome in puppies. Allied Vet., *32*:4, 1961.

Bleicher, S. J.: Hypoglycemia. *In* Ellenberg, M., and Rifkin, H. (eds.): Diabetes: Theory and Practice. New York, McGraw-Hill Book Co., 1970.

Capen, C. C., Belshaw, B. E., and Martin, S. L.: Endocrine disorders. *In* Ettinger, S. J. (ed.): Textbook of Veterinary Internal Medicine. Vol. II. Philadelphia, W. B. Saunders Co., 1975.

Kogut, M. D.: Hypoglycemia: Pathogenesis, diagnosis, and treatment. Curr. Probl. Pediatr., *4*:1–59, 1974.

# HYPO-THYROIDISM

BRUCE E. BELSHAW, D.V.M.,
*and* AD RIJNBERK, D.V.M.
*Utrecht, The Netherlands*

Hypothyroidism is the state of lowered metabolism resulting from inadequate quantities of circulating thyroid hormone. By far the most frequent form of the disease in the dog is primary hypothyroidism resulting from atrophy of the thyroid gland. Only very rarely does the disease occur in dogs as a result of congenital defects in thyroid hormone synthesis or severe iodine deficiency. Secondary hypothyroidism, *i.e.*, resulting from insufficient secretion of thyroid-stimulating hormone (TSH) by the pituitary, has been recognized in the dog but is also very infrequent. The following discussion is therefore concerned with the usual form of canine hypothyroidism encountered in clinical practice. For a discussion of the less frequent forms of the disease, the reader is referred to the preceding edition of this book.

## PATHOLOGY

Biopsy of the thyroid in dogs with acquired primary hypothyroidism almost always reveals gross atrophy of the gland due to disappearance of the follicular epithelium. The calcitonin-secreting parafollicular cells are unaffected but are usually gathered into clusters as a result of the disappearance of follicles and the collapse of the stroma. There are usually a few follicles, in which degenerating and necrotic follicular cells can be seen, mixed with foci of mononuclear cells and occasional neutrophils, but exudative inflammation does not dominate the histologic picture. The etiology of this lesion remains unknown.

Although chronic lymphocytic thyroiditis is a well-known entity in experimental beagle colonies, it is seldom found to be the cause of clinical hypothyroidism in pets. The histologic picture is that of diffuse and progressive lymphocytic infiltration and replacement of the follicles, and it appears that hypothyroidism occurs only after 75 per cent or more of the follicles have been lost.

## CLINICAL FEATURES

Hypothyroidism is most often observed in dogs of the larger breeds, between the ages of 2 and 5 years. The disease develops insidiously and the animals are usually presented at three to nine months after the onset of the first signs, with a history of slowing of mental and physical activities.

Many of the signs and symptoms (Table 1) can be directly related to a decrease in metabolic rate. The hypothyroid animal apparently has difficulty in sustaining body heat, and rectal temperature may be subnormal. At home, the animal looks for warm places to lie down and tolerates high temperatures very well, without panting. In nearly all cases, an increase in body weight is noted, but severe obesity seldom develops. A reduced appetite is to be expected from the decreased metabolic rate, but this is noted only in a minority of the histories.

Most hypothyroid dogs show signs that suggest some impairment of cerebral function. In particular, there is a delay in reaction to such stimuli as the offering of a favor-

**Table 1.** *Incidence of Signs and Symptoms in 13 Dogs with Acquired Primary Hypothyroidism*

| SIGNS AND SYMPTOMS | NUMBER OF DOGS |
|---|---|
| Lethargy | 13 |
| Sensation of cold | 12 |
| Coarse and scanty hair coat | 12 |
| Thickened skin | 11 |
| Pigmentation | 10 |
| Low body temperature | 9 |
| Puffy appearance | 9 |
| Weak apex beat | 9 |
| Increased body weight | 8 |
| Alopecia | 7 |
| Low pulse rate | 5 |
| Absence of estrus (5♀) | 5 |
| Small testes (7♂) | 4 |
| Reduced appetite | 3 |
| Diarrhea | 2 |
| Hoarseness | 2 |

ite food, the announcement of a walk or a loud noise. The dog does not want to play as much as previously and is remarkably quiet and good-natured.

The main functional change in the cardiovascular system is a decreased cardiac output, which is made clinically apparent by a weak apex beat and a weak and usually slow pulse. The electrocardiogram in hypothyroidism shows a general reduction in voltage, with flattening of the T waves. In some cases, the ear flaps, the extremities and especially the areas of alopecia are cool to the touch, suggesting some impairment of the peripheral circulation.

Changes in hair and skin may be more or less pronounced, depending on the duration of the disease. In long-standing cases, the hair coat on the trunk is coarse and scanty, and the skin is slightly pigmented. In general, the hair on the head and the lower parts of the limbs is less sparse. Alopecia may occur bilaterally on the chest and flanks and on the posterior parts of the thighs; the affected areas are often darkly pigmented and have the texture of emery paper. In some short-haired dogs such as the boxer, the retarded growth and shedding of hair result in a very thick coat resembling a carpet. The skin becomes inelastic and markedly thickened. This thickening is most noticeable on the lower parts of the forelegs and above the eyes. The latter results in a typical puffy appearance, comparable to the myxedematous face in man. In most cases, some blepharoptosis contributes to this tragic facial appearance.

The most common symptom in the gastrointestinal tract of man is constipation. This is not a consistent sign in the dog, and occasionally dogs with severe hypothyroidism are presented with diarrhea as the main complaint.

Most hypothyroid bitches have abnormalities of the estrous cycle. In some, the behavioral changes of estrus are less intense and proestral hemorrhage is replaced by discharge of mucus for a few day. In others, anestrus persists for as long as the hypothyroidism is untreated. In males, testicular atrophy occurs only in very long-standing cases.

Routine laboratory examination may reveal slight anemia, the hemoglobin level being decreased to about 12 mg./100 ml. Occasionally, elevated erythrocyte sedimentation rates and hyponatremia have also

been observed. If the latter is noted, the coexistence of adrenocortical insufficiency should be considered.

## DIAGNOSIS

Hypothyroidism should be suspected in a dog presented with a history of slowing of mental and physical activity, sensitivity to cold and some weight gain and, when the clinical examination shows blepharoptosis, a low pulse rate and a coarse and scanty hair coat with a thick and inelastic skin. However, in some cases, the disease is less advanced or less classic and must be distinguished from "simple" obesity (see p. 1068) or Cushing's disease (see p. 1027).

However obvious the diagnosis of hypothyroidism may seem to be in any given patient, we believe objective laboratory confirmation to be essential. While diagnostic confirmation can be provided by the measurement of thyroid uptake of radioiodine and by thyroid biopsy, neither of these procedures is practical in private veterinary practice, and the obvious method of choice is the measurement of circulating thyroid hormone concentration.

Several direct and indirect methods for measuring circulating thyroid hormone concentration have been evaluated in the dog. Only two are sufficiently sensitive and accurate for use in diagnosing hypothyroidism in this species. These two methods are the measurement of thyroxine iodine (T4I, also called hormone iodine, or HI) by column chromatography, and the measurement of thyroxine (T4) and/or triiodothyronine (T3) by radioimmunoassay. Modifications are required in both procedures for accuracy at the low hormone concentrations that distinguish hypothyroid dogs from normal dogs. The modifications are such that the routine performance of either procedure is only practical in laboratories dealing with large numbers of canine specimens. The correlations between T4 values determined by the two methods is excellent. The advantages of radioimmunoassay are that a much smaller sample of plasma is required, the assay can be completed in a single working day and the special problems of iodine analysis (the final step in the column chromatography procedure) are avoided. Nevertheless, there are also technical problems in radioimmunoassay and, in laboratories with experience in iodine analysis, the column chromatography procedure may well be preferred.

Excellent separation of hypothyroid from euthyroid dogs is achieved by a single measurement of plasma T4*, by either of the above methods, or by the radioimmunoassay of plasma T3.

## TREATMENT

Once treatment for hypothyroidism has been started, it is continued for the remainder of the patient's life. It is therefore of great importance that the diagnosis be firmly established before treatment is begun.

In our experience, the most satisfactory treatment is the oral administration of *l*-thyroxine, once daily, preferably in the morning. The maintenance dose of T4 is 20 μg./kg. of normal body weight. Usually, desiccated thyroid is equally effective, at a dose of 20 mg./kg. In a small proportion of our patients, complete restoration of euthyroidism has not been achieved with desiccated thyroid, even at higher dose levels, although the initial response was quite satisfactory. In such patients, full recovery has ensued when treatment was changed to *l*-thyroxine, but the cause for the limitation of response to desiccated thyroid is not yet known.

The disease has usually been present for several months, and in some cases for two years or more, before the dog is presented for examination and treatment. One may hesitate to reverse the resulting metabolic changes too rapidly and may thus prefer to begin treatment at one fourth or one half the dose. One or two increases can be made to reach the full dose in about four weeks. However, we have never observed an undesirable reaction in dogs in which treatment was begun at the full replacement dose.

After about one week of treatment the hypothyroid dog becomes much more lively and alert and may begin to lose some weight. Subsequently the atrophied skin and hair starts to regenerate, this being manifested initially by extensive shedding and scaling. This may be associated with some irritation and erythema, which may even temporarily require bathing and local treatment until the regrowth of the coat is complete.

Once euthyroidism is restored, the animal need only be reexamined once or twice a year to ascertain that the maintenance dose is correct. An excessive replacement dose usually induces polyuria and restlessness, while inadequate treatment results in the return of signs of hypothyroidism. Recognition of the latter will be aided by review of the original clinical record. Measurement of plasma T4 concentration can also be used to resolve any doubts about the correctness of the replacement dose. The plasma specimen should be collected 24 hours after the preceding daily dose, at which time plasma T4 concentration should still be maintained well within the range of values observed in normal dogs.

In the event that laboratory confirmation of the diagnosis cannot be carried out, the therapeutic trial may be of value. The usual full maintenance dose of *l*-thyroxine or desiccated thyroid is used, and acceptance or rejection of the diagnosis is decided upon the basis of the patient's response after no more than one month of trial therapy.

### SUPPLEMENTAL READING

Belshaw, B. E., *et al.*: The iodine requirement and influence of iodine intake on iodine metabolism and thyroid function in the adult Beagle. Endocrinology, 96:1280–1291, 1975.

Mizejewski, G. J., *et al.*: Immunologic investigations of naturally occurring canine thyroiditis. J. Immunol., 107:1152–1160, 1971.

Rijnberk, A.: Iodine metabolism and thyroid disease in the dog. Thesis, University of Utrecht, 1971.

---

*Radioimmunoassay of T4 in canine plasma is available at Comparative Pathology Laboratory, Inc., 391 Atlantic Avenue, Brooklyn, New York 11217. Diagnostic interpretation of the result is provided on the report.

# THYROID TUMORS

A. RIJNBERK, D.V.M.
*Utrecht, Netherlands*

*and* I. LEAV, D.V.M.
*Boston, Massachusetts*

The term goiter means enlargement of the thyroid gland, regardless of the cause. It should be noted that under normal circumstances the thyroid of the dog is not palpable. The veterinary practitioner will very seldom see dogs with goiter due to diffuse thyroid hyperplasia, the cause of which may be either iodine deficiency or an inborn error in thyroid hormone synthesis (see also article on "Hypothyroidism" in *Current Veterinary Therapy V*). The great majority of goiters seen in veterinary practice are unilateral neoplasms, which have a high incidence of malignancy. These tumors occur in dogs of both sexes, from 4 to 13 years of age (average approximately 9 years), with a predilection for the boxer. The animal is usually presented for veterinary examination because the owner has detected a lump in its neck. However, about 20 per cent of these tumors develop autonomous hyperfunction leading to signs of hyperthyroidism, and in such cases the hyperthyroid state is usually the reason for presentation.

## TOXIC THYROID TUMORS

Thyrotoxicosis can be defined as the clinical and metabolic abnormalities which are the consequence of an excess of circulating thyroid hormone. The terms "thyrotoxicosis" and "hyperthyroidism" are used interchangeably. A disease entity comparable to Graves' disease in man has not yet been observed in the dog. The only type of hyperthyroidism known to occur in the dog is that due to an autonomous hypersecreting tumor.

Radioiodine studies have demonstrated that these tumors are not under TSH control. If the tumor causes frank hyperthyroidism, endogenous TSH secretion is entirely suppressed and the nonaffected thyroid tissue does not take up radioiodine and hence is not visualized by scintillation scanning (so-called "decompensated" toxic thyroid tumor). Injection of TSH (bovine) for three days will activate the remaining thyroid tissue, which then becomes visible on the second scintiscan. When the thyroid hormone production of the tumor causes only a borderline hyperthyroid state, TSH secretion may not be entirely suppressed, and the nonaffected thyroid tissue may still be faintly visible on the first scintiscan (so-called "compensated" toxic thyroid tumor). In dogs with "compensated" tumors, the clinical signs are often unobtrusive and the plasma thyroid hormone levels may be normal. Evolution from the compensated into the decompensated stage has been observed in a few cases, as depicted in the schematic drawing (Fig. 1).

## CLINICAL MANIFESTATIONS

The clinical manifestations of hyperthyroidism may be divided into two categories: (1) changes in the thyroid itself and (2) consequences of an excess of circulating thyroid hormone.

**The Thyroid.** Since the thyroid tumor is

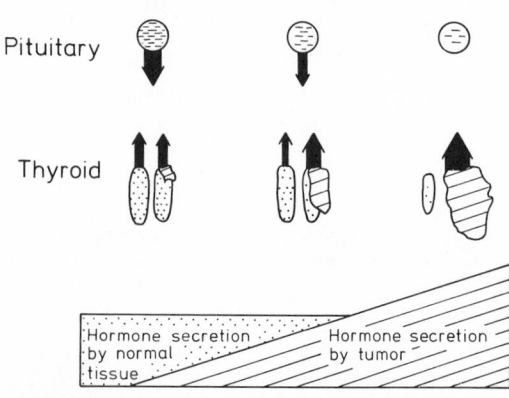

**Figure 1.** Development of a functional tumor into a toxic thyroid tumor of increasing size and with increasing thyroid hormone output. As hypersecretion of thyroid hormone progresses, the TSH release successively declines, and the remaining thyroid tissue becomes inactive.

the underlying cause, a thyroid tumor (usually unilateral) should be found on careful palpation of the neck. The tumors are usually rather small (2 to 5 cm. in diameter) as compared to some of the nonfunctional tumors (see below). Characteristically, a thyroid tumor is easily movable along the trachea.

**Excess of Thyroid Hormone.** The signs of hyperthyroidism vary greatly in severity. Sometimes the onset is abrupt, and the animal is admitted a few weeks later in a clear-cut hyperthyroid state. In other cases, the symptoms develop insidiously, so that the owners may be uncertain as to when they first occurred. The abnormalities may even develop so gradually that the owners believe them to be part of the normal behavior of the animal and are only convinced that the animal had been exhibiting signs of hyperthyroidism by its response to therapy.

Polydipsia is one of the most frequent signs leading to veterinary examination. In some cases, the demand for water increases only slightly, whereas in others the daily intake may amount to many liters. As can be seen from Table 1, the animals show weight loss despite an increased intake of food. Weakness and fatigue become manifest in reduced exercise tolerance. Muscle atrophy along the back and thighs may be observed in severe cases. Intolerance to a hot environment is demonstrated by the dog's habitual search for cool places in which to lie down. Continuous panting may also be observed. Some animals show nervousness mainly characterized by a restless behavior. Tremor is not a common symptom. In a small number of cases, defecation is more frequent than normal, the consistency of the feces being softer but not semiliquid. In most bitches, the hyperthyroid state does not exist long enough to produce an observable effect on estrus. The coat is sometimes reported to have become slightly coarser, but there are usually no striking abnormalities in the hair and skin. Tachycardia has not been listed in Table 1 because pulse rates seldom or never exceed the normal range. On palpation, the femoral pulse and heart beats are usually quite forceful. Electrocardiograms show high voltage in all leads.

## NONTOXIC THYROID TUMORS

In the great majority of cases, patients are presented because the owner has noticed an enlargement in the neck. The tumor may also be an incidental finding during a physical examination performed for an unrelated disease. Apart from functional tumors not leading to a hyperthyroid state, tumors with very little or no functional activity are also encountered in this category. The latter may arise from the follicular epithelium as well as from parafollicular (C-cell) elements (discussed below). These tumors may destroy the affected thyroid lobe entirely. The contralateral lobe can easily compensate for this loss of functional thyroid tissue (see also Figure 2) without a clinically noticeable enlargement.

### CLINICAL MANIFESTATIONS

The physical signs found in 45 dogs with nontoxic thyroid tumors are listed in Table

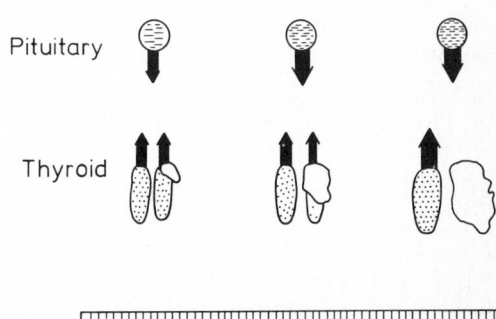

**Figure 2.** During the development of a nonfunctional thyroid tumor destroying the affected lobe, thyroid hormone secretion is sustained via the feedback-controlled increased secretion from the contralateral lobe.

**Table 1.** *Incidence of Signs and Symptoms in 13 Dogs with Hyperthyroidism*

| SIGNS AND SYMPTOMS | NUMBER OF DAYS |
|---|---|
| Goiter | 13 |
| Polydipsia | 13 |
| Weight loss | 10 |
| Polyphagia | 8 |
| Weakness and fatigue | 8 |
| Intolerance to hot environment | 7 |
| Nervousness | 6 |
| Hyperdefecation | 3 |
| Tremor | 3 |
| Absence of estrus (8 ♀) | 2 |

**Table 2.** *Incidence of Signs and Symptoms in 45 Dogs with Nontoxic Thyroid Tumors*

| SIGNS AND SYMPTOMS | NUMBER OF DAYS |
|---|---|
| Unilateral goiter | 39 |
| Bilateral goiter | 6 |
| Consistency: | |
|   Soft | 4 |
|   Firm | 26 |
|   Hard | 15 |
| Irregular shape | 13 |
| Tracheal deviation | 12 |
| Palpable regional lymph nodes | 6 |
| Dysphagia | 6 |
| Local pain | 4 |
| Respiratory distress | 3 |
| Weight loss | 3 |

2. Most of the tumors have a firm or hard consistency. The bigger ones are not freely movable along the trachea. Irregular shapes are found not only in cases with highly malignant growths, but also in some cases of cyst formation. Primary lymphatic drainage of the canine thyroid is in the cranial direction, and hence lymph node enlargement may be detected above and medial to the tumor. Occasionally, both ipsilateral and contralateral cervical lymph nodes may be involved.

The time between the first detection of the tumor by the owner and referral of the dog for veterinary advice may vary from a few days to several years. Slow enlargement does not cause any concern to some owners nor, in fact, to some veterinarians. In long-standing cases, pressure symptoms manifested by dysphagia, hoarseness or tracheal obstruction may be observed at admission.

## DIAGNOSIS

Diagnosis is made by clinical examination. For palpation, the animal should sit in a relaxed position with the head tilted backward. The larynx is first palpated with the thumb and index finger, this being followed by careful bilateral palpation along the trachea using the same fingers. Since the thyroid lobes in the dog are only loosely attached to the trachea and the overlying musculature, neoplastic enlargement causes descent along the trachea. Only in severe cases with metastases and cachexia may routine blood examination reveal abnormalities (e.g., increased erythrocyte sedimentation rate and anemia).

Radiographic examination of the thorax should be performed whenever a thyroid tumor is found, in order to check for the presence of metastases. *In-vivo* radioiodine studies are most helpful in characterizing the thyroid tumor. Suppression of the unaffected thyroid tissue, as demonstrated by scintiscanning, provides evidence for autonomous hyperfunction of the tumor. Hyperthyroid dogs will also show increased thyroidal iodine turnover. However, these techniques are not essential for proper treatment of these neoplasms, since, regardless of their functional status, all operable tumors should be removed.

## TREATMENT

As the great majority of the clinically detected thyroid tumors are malignant, they should be removed in the earliest stage. Very small tumors can easily be removed via a ventral midline approach. With larger tumors, the incision can be made over the tumor, allowing a more lateral approach, which facilitates the ligation of the cranial thyroid artery at its emergence from the carotid artery. The inferior thyroid artery is usually very small and can be ligated with the venous return at the caudal pole of the tumor. When the cervical lymph nodes are found to be enlarged, they should be removed together with the tumor. Severely malignant tumors may invade the surrounding tissues such as muscles, trachea and esophagus. Growth into the thyroid veins and internal jugular vein may also be observed. In such cases, complete removal may be impossible. In our experience, however, a few animals have survived resection that included the carotid artery.

The most threatened structures during this surgery are the recurrent laryngeal nerves and the parathyroid glands. The parathyroid glands and their vessels can only very occasionally be recognized and saved. Unilateral removal of thyroid and parathyroid tissue does not require any replacement therapy, since the contralateral glandular tissue will compensate for the loss. In cases of bilateral thyroid tumor, however, radical surgery will result in hypothyroidism and hypoparathyroidism. In these cases, parathyroid replacement is necessary in addition to full thyroid replacement (20 to 30 $\mu$g./kg. *l*-thyroxine). With the use of plasma calcium and phosphorus levels as a guide, the maintenance dose of dihydrotachysterol and calcium lactate can be determined.

Removal of a toxic thyroid tumor is followed by an increase in body weight and the disappearance of polyuria, restlessness and other clinical signs associated with the hyperthyroid state. In those dogs in which the tumor does not cause thyrotoxicosis, the results of surgery are adversely influenced by the delay in referral for treatment. Rapid regrowth of incompletely removed tumors and rapidly developing metastases may require euthanasia within a few months following surgery.

## PATHOLOGY

The preceding discussion dealt with thyroid tumors in general and was written from the point of view that all tumors observed by the clinician should be regarded as malignant. They may turn out to be benign, but since this is unpredictable, they should be handled from the outset as malignant tumors. A short description of some histopathologic aspects of thyroid tumors is presented below.

The majority of benign canine thyroid tumors (adenomas) are small solid, focal lesions, not commonly detected during life. In some instances, however, these neoplasms are cystic and large enough to be noted in the living animal. Grossly solid adenomas are round or ovoid and a few millimeters to several centimeters in diameter. Although a well-delineated capsule is seldom noted, adenomas are frequently solitary and distinct from the compressed adjacent thyroid. They are usually soft and cream- to red-brown. The large cystic adenomas are turgid and, when cut, exude a clear amber or blood-tinged fluid. The cut surface contains a central cavity that has a smooth or rugose lining. Microscopically most small solid adenomas are characterized by either small or large irregular follicles. Cystic tumors are lined by a dense fibrous capsule from which project fronds of uniform cells arranged in follicular and/or compact cellular patterns. Since cysts are seen in small adenomas, it is likely that cycles of continued growth accompanied by degenerative changes are responsible for the eventual appearance of the tumors.

Carcinomas of the canine thyroid are generally large, solid masses. Their malignant nature may be evident grossly, since large neoplasms will often extend into thyroidal veins or adjacent structures. Metastases are most often to the lungs and/or retropharyngeal lymph nodes.

In all instances, however, the diagnosis of carcinoma can be confirmed only microscopically, which is particularly important, since many small neoplasms are not associated with gross evidence of their malignancy and thus may resemble adenomas. While cellular pleomorphism may suggest a malignant potential, the diagnosis of carcinoma rests solely on finding histologic evidence of capsular and/or vascular invasion. The demonstration of these features is frequently subtle and therefore at least six sections of a neoplasm should be studied before its true nature can be ascertained.

Microscopically, carcinomas of the canine thyroid usually have two patterns contained within a single tumor—follicular and compact cellular—and are therefore referred to as mixed follicular compact cellular carcinomas. Some, however, are largely composed of either pattern and are termed follicular or compact cellular carcinomas. Although these classifications are arbitrary, they may be of clinical importance, since in our experience the follicular neoplasms appear to behave more aggressively than do the other types.

Recently, we have described two cases of medullary carcinoma arising in the canine thyroid. These neoplasms originate from parafollicular cells, which are responsible for the secretion of calcitonin and probably other physiologically active hormones. Microscopically, these tumors have a compact cellular pattern and may therefore be difficult to distinguish from similarly arranged follicular neoplasms. Immunohistochemistry and electron microscopy should be used to identify tumors of parafollicular cell origin accurately. Anaplastic carcinomas of the canine thyroid are rare, highly aggressive neoplasms that have a variety of histologic appearances. For a more in-depth discussion of the morphology of these and other canine thyroid tumors, the reader is referred to our recent publication (Leav *et al.*, 1976).

## MISCELLANEOUS THYROID TUMORS

### ECTOPIC THYROID TUMORS

The frequent occurrence of aberrant thyroid tissue in the dog has been known for a long time. This tissue consists of remnants of the thyroglossal duct and occasionally lies anterior to the thyroid. Usually, however, it descends with the heart into the thorax during fetal development. Neoplasms may arise from these ectopic sites. Intrathoracic neoplasms are seldom detected in the living animal and quite frequently occur in association with carcinoma of the primary gland. Tumors arising from thyroglossal duct remnants usually appear as a midline swelling at the junction of the larynx and hyoid. A few of these tumors have been reported to cause hyperthyroidism.

### MEDULLARY CARCINOMAS

Two of these tumors have now been convincingly documented in the dog by electron microscopy and immunohistochemistry. These tumors arise from the thyroidal parafollicular (C) cells and, in humans, are generally associated with excess secretion of calcitonin. They do not lead to a significant reduction of the serum calcium level. Severe diarrhea is the most striking clinical sign and is currently believed to be due to the elaboration of serotonin and/or prostaglandins by the neoplasm; diarrhea ceases following removal of the tumor.

### THYROID TUMORS IN CATS

Most information on thyroid tumors in domestic cats comes from surveys of pathology collections or scattered case reports. It appears that benign tumors of the feline thyroid are not uncommon, carcinomas are rare and both occur almost exclusively in old cats. The tumors are usually small, and this probably explains why they are rarely detected in the living animal.

### SUPPLEMENTAL READING

Leav, I., *et al.*: Adenomas and carcinomas of the canine and feline thyroid. Am. J. Pathol., 83:61–122, 1976.
Rijnberk, A.: Iodine metabolism and thyroid disease in the dog. Utrecht Drukkerij Elinkwijk, 1971.

---

# PRIMARY ADRENO-CORTICAL INSUFFICIENCY

JOHN A. MULNIX, D.V.M.
*Fort Collins, Colorado*

The term "adrenocortical insufficiency" includes all conditions in which corticosteroid production is inadequate. *Primary* adrenocortical insufficiency is caused by damage to the adrenal cortex itself. In *secondary* insufficiency, the secretion of ACTH by the pituitary gland is insufficient; the adrenal cortex itself is intact but may be atrophic. There is no apparent breed predilection for primary adrenocortical insufficiency, but this disorder appears to be more common in females and in dogs under 5 years of age. The overall incidence appears to be low, and the increasing frequency of diagnosis is most likely due to improved diagnostic methods and wider use of laboratory screening procedures.

### PATHOPHYSIOLOGY

The principal pathophysiologic changes are related to the lack of mineralocorticoids. There is diminished ability to retain sodium and to excrete potassium, leading to a reduction in the total amount of extracellular sodium chloride and hence in intravascular volume. Although the serum potassium levels are consistently elevated in primary adrenocortical insufficiency, the severity of the disease is not related to the degree of elevation of serum potassium. Potassium ions are lost when there is vomiting and diarrhea, and intracellular potassium may actually be depleted. Elevated serum potassium levels cause multiple cardiac conduction defects. The accompanying lack of glucocorticoids results in reductions in cardiac output, renal perfusion and smooth muscle tone, and, in association with a reduced intravascular volume, total vascular collapse can result. Other manifestations of loss of glucocorticoids include muscle weakness, anorexia and gastrointestinal changes.

## CLINICAL SIGNS

The patient may be presented in an acute addisonian crisis or with vague chronic signs. In chronic insufficiency there may only be occasional vomiting, which can rapidly progress to a full crisis. In dogs having undergone adrenalectomy and without maintenance therapy, muscular weakness and anorexia are usually the first signs observed, but coma, ataxia, depression, anorexia and muscular weakness are constantly observed immediately prior to death. In naturally occurring adrenocortical insufficiency, depression, anorexia and a weak femoral pulse are consistently seen. Other signs include vomiting or diarrhea, weakness, dehydration and occasionally bradycardia. Complete collapse and an inability to walk are also observed.

## LABORATORY DATA

Slight to moderate elevation of blood urea nitrogen concentration is a consistent finding and, in the presence of the above clinical findings, should prompt additional laboratory studies. Serum sodium and chloride concentrations are below normal, owing to excess loss in the urine. Serum potassium levels may be only slightly or moderately elevated (usually between 5.5 and 7.0 mEq./l.), although elevations above 7.0 mEq. are sometimes observed. The electrocardiogram can be used to determine immediately whether there is hyperkalemia. The degree of change in the ECG is related to the severity of elevation of serum potassium. The most characteristic change is spiking of the T wave and flatten-

ing of the P wave. With severe hyperkalemia, prolongation of the Q-T interval, complete sinoatrial arrest and bradycardia may also be present. The sodium:potassium (Na:K) ratio is occasionally useful in the diagnosis of marginal cases. Normal Na:K ratios range from 27:1 to 32:1. In primary adrenocortical insufficiency, the Na:K ratio is usually 24:1 or lower. This pattern of laboratory data (elevated blood urea, hyperkalemia and hyponatremia) is fairly specific for primary adrenocortical insufficiency in the dog.

Hypoglycemia does not appear to be common in dogs with adrenocortical insufficiency. Hypercalcemia has been reported but is also uncommon. The total leukocyte count can vary widely but is usually within normal limits. Although eosinophilia and an absolute lymphocytosis are not consistent changes, their occurrence is a further indication of possible adrenocortical insufficiency. The hematocrit of patients in an acute crisis with dehydration may be within the normal range, but once the dog is rehydrated, a normochromic normocytic anemia may be observed. Occasional elevation of the plasma protein concentration reflects the effect of dehydration.

The most specific method of diagnosis is the measurement of plasma corticosteroid concentration. Normal resting plasma cortisol or $11\beta$-hydroxycorticosteroid ($11\beta$-OHCS) levels vary widely, partly depending on the laboratory and the method. Cortisol levels determined by competitive protein binding or radioimmunoassay are always lower than $11\beta$-OHCS levels determined by the fluorometric method.

Once treatment for primary hypoadrenocorticism has been started, it must be continued for the rest of the patient's life. It is therefore of prime importance that the diagnosis be firmly established before tceatment is started. Consequently, an ACTH stimulation test should be performed once the acute crisis has been controlled.

## TREATMENT

In a dog with an addisonian crisis, it is not safe to await laboratory results before beginning therapy. A sterile intravenous catheter should be placed immediately in the jugular or cephalic vein, and appropriate samples collected. A sterile urinary catheter should be inserted in the bladder. Intravenous isotonic saline solution is the fluid of choice, and the total volume to be administered is based on estimation of the degree of dehydration. The rate of administration should be controlled according to the central venous pressure and urine flow rate. Hypertonic saline solution should not be used because it may cause intracellular dehydration. Soluble intravenous glucocorticoids, such as hydrocortisone (50 to 100 mg.), are added to the intravenous drip. Hydrocortisone also provides some immediate mineralocorticoid activity before mineralocorticoids (which are administered IM or SC) are absorbed. Large doses of glucocorticoids are indicated when the crisis is severe.

Mineralocorticoid activity is provided initially in the form of desoxycorticosterone acetate (DOCA) only if the patient is in an acute crisis. Approximately 1 mg. per 12.5 kg. of body weight is given intramuscularly. Large doses of mineralocorticoids do not appear to be necessary to control an addisonian crisis in the dog. Even with marked elevation of serum potassium, the above therapy will result in marked clinical improvement within 30 to 60 minutes.

Intramuscular DOCA is administered once every 24 hours until the acute crisis is controlled, the dosage being adjusted according to serum potassium levels. Daily injections of 1 to 3 mg. DOCA will keep the serum potassium below 5 mEq./l. The intravenous isotonic saline is continued until the volume deficit has been replaced and the patient has remained stable for at least 24 hours. Oral administration of medication is avoided for the first 24 hours to prevent further vomiting. Once the blood urea and electrolyte levels have returned to normal, a routine maintenance program is followed.

For chronic replacement therapy, parenteral administration of mineralocorticoids is preferred. A microcrystalline suspension of trimethylacetate esters of DOCA (Percorten M® [Ciba]) is effective for about three weeks. An injection of 25 mg. provides an absorbed dose of approximately 1 mg. of DOCA per day, which will maintain electrolyte balance. An alternative form of therapy is with desoxycorticosterone acetate pellets. One desoxycorticosterone acetate pellet is implanted subcutaneously on the dorsal midline by sterile surgical technique under local anesthesia. Each pellet contains approximately 125 mg. DOCA and will release 0.5 mg. of desoxycorticosterone per day. This will provide adequate control for an average of six to eight months per implant. Oral glucocorticoids in the form of prednisolone and sodium chloride are also administered daily. A dose of 2.5 to 5 mg. of prednisolone, administered once daily in the morning, is adequate. The owner should be instructed to increase this dosage two- to fourfold in the event of any stress. Sodium chloride is provided daily in the form of tablets (1 g.) or table salt on the animal's food.

Patients should be rechecked every six months for routine clinical and laboratory evaluation and implantation of a new DOCA pellet. This procedure is less risky than waiting until the previous pellet implant has been completely absorbed and the patient is beginning to show signs of mineralocorticoid deficiency.

Oral fludrocortisone acetate (Florinef® [Squibb]) tablets (0.1 mg.) can also be used. This steroid contains both mineralo- and glucocorticoid activity. The usual dosage is 0.1 mg./day. The dose should be adjusted according to the serum potassium level. Treatment with oral fludrocortisone is less satisfactory in the dog, because missing several days of therapy or failure to administer the tablet properly can lead to recurrence of an addisonian crisis.

## SUPPLEMENTAL READING

Anderson, J. G., and Clark, D. R.: Pattern of physiologic effects of adrenalectomy in the dog. Am. J. Vet. Res., 36:1036–1040, 1975.
Halliwell, R. E. W., Schwartzman, R. M., Hopkins, L., and McEvoy, D.: The value of plasma corticosteroid assays in the diagnosis of Cushing's disease in the dog. J. Small Animal Pract., 12:453–462, 1971.
Keeton, K. S., Schechter, R. D., and Schalm, O. W.: Adrenocortical insufficiency in dogs. Mod. Vet. Pract., 53:25–29, 1972.
Mulnix, J. A.: Hypoadrenocorticism in the dog. J. Am. Animal Hosp. Assn., 7:220–241, 1971.
Mulnix, J. A.: Adrenal cortical disease in dogs. Vet. Scope, 19:12–20, 1975.
Rijnberk, A., der Kinderen, P. J., and Thijssen, J. H. H.: Investigations on the Adrenocortical Function of Normal Dogs. J. Endocrinol., 41:387–395, 1968.

# HYPERADRENO-CORTICISM

RONALD D. SCHECHTER, V.M.D.
*San Diego, California*

Hyperadrenocorticism, or Cushing's syndrome, is the clinicopathologic manifestation of excess glucocorticoid production or administration. In the dog, naturally occurring Cushing's syndrome has been associated with either bilateral adrenocortical hyperplasia or, less commonly, neoplasia of the adrenal cortex. Functioning pituitary tumors were present at necropsy in over 80 per cent of the cases of bilateral adrenocortical hyperplasia in one review, although most of these pituitary tumors were quite small and slow-growing. There have also been reports of no pituitary lesions in many dogs with bilateral adrenocortical hyperplasia. It has been suggested that bilateral adrenocortical hyperplasia in man (and probably the dog) is associated with a central nervous system origin and the effect of neurotransmitters, often referred to as adrenocorticotropic releasing factors. This mechanism might increase ACTH production without causing tumor growth in the anterior pituitary gland in some cases or delay tumor appearance until later in the course of the disease in others. Approximately 10 to 15 per cent of dogs with Cushing's syndrome have a primary neoplasm of one adrenal gland.

Excessive or prolonged administration of corticosteroids can also produce Cushing's syndrome in the dog, although the clinical manifestations can be quite variable in appearance and intensity.

## CLINICAL EVALUATION

Findings common to all dogs with hyperadrenocorticism are polydipsia, polyuria, nonpruritic alopecia and an enlarged, pendulous or flaccid abdomen. However, these manifestations vary considerably among individual dogs. Larger dogs tend to develop alopecia more slowly and less extensively, but any breed of dog in the early stages of Cushing's syndrome may lack significant hair loss. It should be stressed, in fact, that the only clinical findings that are invariably found in the early stages of the disease are polydipsia and polyuria. Other frequent signs are lethargy, myasthenia, polyphagia, hyperpigmentation of skin and hair, calcinosis cutis, keratin plugging of hair follicles (especially on the abdomen and around nipples) and testicular atrophy. The absence of estrus in the bitch has also been reported as an early sign. Although some dogs gain weight and appear obese, most merely have an enlarged abdomen and the remainder of the body is quite thin.

Signs relating to progressive central nervous system involvement, such as dumbness, severe lethargy and anorexia, aimless wandering, head pressing and ataxia, may be associated with pressure necrosis or invasion of overlying brain tissue by a pituitary tumor. Horner's syndrome (uni- or bilateral miosis, ptosis and enophthalmos) may also be associated with hypothalamic damage by pituitary tumor growth.

Hepatomegaly and calcification of various tissues (especially the skin, bronchial walls and renal parenchyma) can occasionally be seen radiographically. Erosion of the sella turcica does not occur in the dog with pituitary tumors, as it does in man, due to anatomic differences. Osteoporosis, although present, is not usually recognized radiographically.

## LABORATORY EVALUATION

Lymphopenia (less than 1500/cu. mm.) and eosinopenia (less than 200/cu. mm.) are consistent findings in dogs with Cushing's syndrome. Serum alkaline phosphatase levels are usually elevated, often to very high values, and appear to be partially or entirely due to the induction of a new isoenzyme in the liver by corticosteroids. Serum glutamic pyruvic transaminase (SGPT) values are also frequently elevated because of fatty infiltration and degeneration of the liver. Similarly, the amount of

Bromsulphalein® (BSP) (Hynson) retention is occasionally elevated.

Plasma sodium and potassium concentrations are, with rare exceptions, within normal limits.

Plasma glucose concentrations are usually normal but may be slightly elevated. Occasionally, however, marked elevations are seen in association with diabetes mellitus. Dogs that are not frankly diabetic but are hyperglycemic should be carefully watched for the later development of diabetes.

Plasma cholesterol values are usually elevated in hyperadrenocorticism. Increased cholesterol levels may also be associated with hypothyroidism. Although Cushing's syndrome is often misdiagnosed as hypothyroidism, the two conditions can, in fact, be present simultaneously. Occasionally secondary hypothyroidism may be associated with pituitary tumors that are causing Cushing's syndrome.

The blood urea nitrogen (BUN) concentration should be determined to evaluate renal function, especially in older dogs. In general, however, dogs with Cushing's syndrome are not more susceptible to kidney disease (except for infection) than normal dogs and often have BUN levels below normal because of excessive urinary excretion of urea.

Most dogs with Cushing's syndrome excrete large volumes of urine with a specific gravity often less than 1.012 and sometimes less than 1.005, the latter being suggestive of diabetes insipidus. In our experience, however, neurohypophyseal diabetes insipidus rarely occurs in dogs with hyperadrenocorticism. They are, in fact, capable of concentrating their urine (either before or after therapy) to a degree that precludes the lack of antidiuretic hormone. The widespread belief that diabetes insipidus is frequently associated with functioning pituitary tumors is erroneous.

Special efforts should be made to detect urinary tract infection, utilizing urine analysis, culture and sensitivity, since many dogs with Cushing's syndrome become infected. It must be remembered that the absence of clinical signs usually associated with urinary tract infection does not exclude it as a diagnostic possibility. Catheterization of the urinary bladder should be avoided, since dogs with Cushing's syndrome have little resistance to induced infections. Urine should be collected by either aseptic percutaneous bladder tap or clean midstream catch.

## Endocrinologic evaluation

The most reliable means of confirming the diagnosis of hyperadrenocorticism is by plasma corticosteroid determination utilizing the competitive protein-binding (CPB) technique of Bassett and Hinks.

Plasma should be separated as soon as possible from an anticoagulated (heparin or EDTA) blood sample, placed in a clean glass vial and refrigerated or frozen prior to mailing. The procedure requires 0.1 to 0.2 ml. of plasma, but at least 1 ml. should be sent to the laboratory. If the specimen must be mailed, it should be sent by air mail in a rigid container with adequate protection against breakage; it should be kept cold if possible. Indicate that the sample is from a dog and request plasma corticosteroid (cortisol) assay. The cost is about $15 to $20 per sample.

The CPB method measures cortisol and corticosterone, which are normally secreted in a ratio of about 3:1 in the dog. Resting plasma corticosteroid values (CPB) in normal, caged, unstressed dogs range from 1 to 2.5 $\mu$g./100 ml. However, when evaluating sick dogs, it is more realistic to consider resting plasma corticosteroid values both in normal dogs and in dogs with disease conditions that do not directly involve the pituitary or adrenal glands. In these dogs, resting values range from 1 to 12.5 $\mu$g./100 ml. Resting plasma corticosteroid values in dogs with Cushing's syndrome usually range from 2.5 to 12.5 $\mu$g./100 ml., but occasionally are much higher. Although the mean resting plasma corticosteroid concentration is significantly higher in dogs with Cushing's syndrome (6 $\mu$g./100 ml.) than in dogs without Cushing's syndrome (3.5 $\mu$g./100 ml.), the two ranges overlap considerably. The more measurements, the greater the degree of accuracy, but cost usually limits the number to two or three.

Production of adrenal corticosteroids is markedly increased in dogs with Cushing's syndrome following the administration of adrenocorticotropin (ACTH). However, minimal or no response to ACTH stimulation in a dog that otherwise appears to have

Cushing's syndrome could indicate the presence of an autonomously functioning adrenocortical tumor.

To test the response of the adrenal cortex to exogenous ACTH, 3 to 5 ml. of heparinized blood is collected immediately prior to the intramuscular administration of 2.2 IU of ACTH gel/kg. of body weight. Plasma is again collected two hours after ACTH injection.

The post-ACTH stimulation plasma corticosteroid values in normal dogs with conditions other than Cushing's syndrome range from 9.5 to 22 $\mu$g./100 ml. In dogs with Cushing's syndrome, the post-ACTH plasma corticosteroid response is usually quite exaggerated and values range from 20 to 60 $\mu$g./100 ml. There is very little overlap of values between the two groups of dogs, but when ACTH stimulation produces equivocal results, the test should be repeated.

Plasma corticosteroids can also be satisfactorily determined by a fluorometric method, and this may be the only method available in some areas. However, while as little as 0.1 ml. of plasma is required for the CPB method, 2 to 5 ml. are required for the fluorometric method. In the dog, higher values are generally obtained by fluorometric analysis than by the CPB procedure, and the fluorometric procedure appears to be less specific and precise.

Determination of canine plasma corticosteroids by a radioimmunoassay (RIA) technique has been offered by various laboratories and appears to be quite accurate and reliable. However, values in both normal dogs and dogs with Cushing's syndrome need to be adequately evaluated, ideally for each individual laboratory.

The measurement of urinary 17-ketogenic steroids (17-KGS) has also been used to diagnose hyperadrenocorticism in the dog. However, the necessity for accurate 24-hour total urine collections alone makes this approach cumbersome in private veterinary practice.

Resting plasma corticosteroid values in dogs with iatrogenic Cushing's syndrome will usually be very low (less than 2 $\mu$g./100 ml.) if synthetic steroids were administered recently. Plasma corticosteroid levels can be expected to be elevated, however, if hydrocortisone was administered. Moreover, dogs with iatrogenic Cushing's syndrome can be expected to have lower than anticipated post-ACTH plasma cortisol levels, depending on the degree of adrenocortical atrophy that has been induced. In short, dogs with iatrogenic Cushing's syndrome, despite the clinical findings of hyperadrenocorticism, will usually have paradoxical plasma cortisol values compatible with adrenal insufficiency. Treatment of these patients should include repeated ACTH gel administration until cortisol levels return to normal. Signs of adrenal insufficiency should be treated as required (see article on "Systemic Glucocorticoid Therapy").

## CHEMOTHERAPHY

O,p'-DDD*† (ortho, para prime-DDD) is a specific adrenocorticolytic drug that has been used successfully to treat Cushing's syndrome in dogs since 1969. O,p'-DDD causes necrosis of the zona reticularis and zona fasciculata of the adrenal cortex, thereby decreasing the production of corticosteroids. The zona glomerulosa, which produces aldosterone, tends to be spared at the dose level recommended below; thus, hypoadrenocorticism (Addison's disease) is rarely produced. Overdosage, however, can result in transient and possible permanent adrenal insufficiency requiring replacement therapy. Despite earlier reports that o,p'-DDD was highly toxic, especially to the liver, only the adrenal cortex is significantly affected in the dog. Liver toxicity is so negligible that SGPT and BSP levels do not become elevated and, in fact, return to normal in dogs that have elevated values prior to o,p'-DDD treatment. A few deaths that have occurred either during or shortly after treatment with o,p'-DDD have been attributable to pituitary tumor growth with compression or invasion of overlying brain tissue. Progressive neurologic abnormalities, including Horner's syndrome, have frequently accompanied this tumor growth.

Although no deaths have been directly re-

---

*Lysodren® (Calbio Pharmaceuticals, San Diego, California), supplied as 500-mg. scored tablets; the cost is $30.00 per 100 tablets.

†*Author's Note:* O,p'-DDD has been approved for use in man for the relief of intractable pain. It has not been approved for veterinary use, and its use in man varies substantially from the usage advocated here. Thus o,p'-DDD should be used with appropriate discretion and precaution.

lated to o,p'-DDD toxicity, a very few dogs have died suddenly while receiving the drug. It is conceivable that o,p'-DDD played a contributory role, although the number of such deaths has been too small to permit valid conclusions.

Prior to treatment, it is extremely important that the patient be carefully evaluated in order to confirm the presence of hyperadrenocorticism, to differentiate bilateral adrenocortical hyperplasia from adrenal neoplasia and to recognize concurrent or secondary conditions, such as hypothyroidism, diabetes mellitus, infection, CNS abnormalities and degenerative tissue changes from the excess corticosteroids. If an adrenal neoplasm is suspected (i.e., no response to ACTH stimulation), exploratory laparotomy should be performed after radiographic evaluation of the lungs for metastatic lesions.

It is also very important to determine whether or not corticosteroids have been administered recently in order to rule out the possibility of iatrogenic Cushing's syndrome.

O,p'-DDD is given orally in a dose of 50 mg./kg. of body weight once daily to effect. Most dogs require initial treatment for 5 to 10 consecutive days. In some dogs treatment for 20 days or more may be necessary. The daily dose is not critical, except perhaps in very small dogs, but probably should be calculated to within 50 mg. An occasional dog may develop resistance to o,p'-DDD either during the initial treatment period or after a few months of maintenance therapy. This resistance can be overcome by increasing the amount of o,p'-DDD (up to 75 mg./kg.) and administering this in divided doses.

Initial treatment is best carried out in the hospital. However, if the owners are conscientious and cooperative, administration of o,p'-DDD at home is often feasible and may be preferable. Water consumption should be monitored daily before and during o,p'-DDD therapy. This does not require a metabolism cage and thus can be done in most circumstances, even at home. After five days of treatment, the dog's lymphocyte and eosinophil counts should also be determined. These three indices usually return to normal as plasma corticosteroid levels return to normal, although individual variations in response should be expected. Occasionally lymphocyte counts remain decreased for a number of days despite effective therapy. Treatment should be continued in most cases until water intake and eosinophil counts are normal, but if doubt exists, treatment should be discontinued and a plasma corticosteroid measurement obtained. In any case, the plasma corticosteroid level should be determined after the initial treatment period and should be 3 $\mu$g./100 ml. or less. Ideally, an ACTH stimulation test should be performed in order to prove that the adrenal glands can no longer respond excessively. This test, although not essential, is very helpful in establishing the end point of o,p'-DDD therapy. Post-ACTH corticosteroid levels after a successful therapeutic regimen of o,p'-DDD should be approximately twice those of resting values.

Near the end of or shortly after the initial treatment period, serum sodium and potassium concentrations should be measured. This is especially important if there are signs of adrenal insufficiency, such as lethargy, tremors, abdominal pain, vomiting, diarrhea, collapse and shock (see p. 1025). This development is unlikely with the o,p'-DDD regimen described here, because aldosterone production is preserved.

Side effects from o,p'-DDD have been uncommon and have usually consisted of transient depression, weakness and diarrhea. If these or other side effects occur and are severe, administration of the drug should be discontinued. If further o,p'-DDD therapy is required, treatment can be reinstituted after the side effects have disappeared, using a lower, less frequent or divided dosage regimen. Occasionally neurologic abnormalities occur and may be mistakenly attributed to brain damage from a pituitary tumor. Withdrawal of o,p'-DDD for a few days should result in the remission of toxic signs but will have no effect on tumor-related signs. Recurrence of these abnormalities can often be avoided by dividing the daily dose, administering one half in the morning and one half at night.

During the initial treatment period, methionine, choline and B-complex vitamin preparations should be given, as well as appropriate antibiotic therapy, when indicated.

Coexisting diabetes mellitus should be treated, usually prior to o,p'-DDD therapy. However, until the plasma cortisol levels are reduced, blood glucose levels will be very unstable and difficult to regulate. As plasma corticosteroid levels are decreased during o,p'-DDD treatment, the elevated blood glucose levels will decrease. This will necessitate a corresponding decrease in insulin dosage in order to avoid hypoglycemia.

## LONG-TERM MAINTENANCE THERAPY

When the hyperadrenocorticism is under control, a weekly treatment schedule is begun. The dog is given 50 mg. of o,p'-DDD/kg. of body weight once weekly for the rest of its life. The owners administer the drug at home but are instructed to return the dog for examination every two to three months (or sooner, if necessary) during the first six months. On these visits, lymphocyte and eosinophil counts and serum sodium and potassium levels should be evaluated. The owner should keep a record of the dog's water consumption because polyuria and the resultant polydipsia are often the first indications of the recurrence of hyperadrenocorticism. Regression of all clinical manifestations of Cushing's syndrome is usually complete in six to eight weeks.

Resting and post-ACTH plasma corticosteroid levels should be measured at the time of the first progress visit in order to evaluate adrenal function. If Cushing's syndrome does recur, the daily course of o,p'-DDD should be repeated to effect, followed by the weekly dosage schedule with the interval decreased or the dose increased to 60 mg./kg. or more if tolerated. If post-ACTH cortisol levels decrease to less than 1.5 times the resting values, the dosage interval should be increased so as to avoid the eventual development of adrenal insufficiency.

While the animal is receiving the recommended dose of 50 mg. of o,p'-DDD/kg. of body weight once weekly, a few dogs have developed varying degrees of ataxia or depression that may develop and last for as long as 24 hours after each dose. These side effects have been eliminated by giving one half the dose twice weekly.

Progress examinations and laboratory evaluations should probably be repeated every three to six months.

Owners should also have on hand a supply of a glucocorticoid, such as prednisolone or hydrocortisone, for use if signs of hypoglycemia or adrenal insufficiency occur and immediate veterinary aid cannot be obtained.

O,p'-DDD can also be used in the treatment of inoperable adrenal neoplasms, but the efficacy of this treatment has not been adequately evaluated in the dog.

## SURGERY

Unilateral adrenalectomy is the treatment of choice for localized adrenocortical tumors. Because the nontumorous contralateral adrenal gland is usually atrophied, ACTH gel should be administered for a few days before and after surgery to restore its functional capacity. Careful monitoring for adrenal insufficiency is necessary during and after surgery, and appropriate supportive therapy must be instituted if needed (see p. 1025).

Total surgical adrenalectomy can be used in cases of bilateral adrenocortical hyperplasia. The major disadvantages of this approach are the difficult surgery and postsurgical management, the necessity for lifelong supportive therapy for the resultant hypoadrenocorticism and the cost of both surgery and replacement therapy.

Finally, hypophysectomy may be employed in selected cases of Cushing's syndrome. The indications and technique are described in *Current Veterinary Therapy V*, p. 787.

## PROGNOSIS

The course of Cushing's syndrome in the dog is highly unpredictable, and growth of a pituitary tumor may occur either during the initial treatment or later while the animal is on maintenance levels of o,p'-DDD. Nonetheless, most dogs with Cushing's syndrome can be expected to respond well to o,p'-DDD treatment and, barring problems from other disease conditions, can be expected to live a reasonably healthy and happy life.

It must be emphasized that the evaluation and treatment of dogs with Cushing's syndrome can be quite difficult and demanding, especially in complicated cases. We therefore urge practitioners with limited experience to consult with or refer these cases to their more experienced colleagues either in private practice or at veterinary medical centers.

SUPPLEMENTAL READING

Bassett, J. M., and Hinks, N. T.: Micro-determination of corticosteroids in ovine peripheral plasma: effects of venipuncture, corticotrophin, insulin and glucose. J. Endocrinol., 44:387–403, 1969.
Halliwell, R. E. W., et al.: The value of plasma corticosteroid assays in the diagnosis of Cushing's disease in the dog. J. Small Animal Pract., 12:453–462, 1971.
Rijnberk, A., der Kinderen, P. J., and Thyssen, J. H. H.:
Spontaneous hyperadrenocorticism in the dog. J. Endocrinol., 41:397–406, 1968.
Schechter, R. D., et al.: Treatment of Cushing's syndrome in the dog with an adrenocorticolytic agent (o,p'-DDD). J. Am. Vet. Med. Assn., 162:629–639, 1973.
Siegel, E. T., Kelly, D. F., and Berg, P.: Cushing's syndrome in the dog. J. Am. Vet. Med. Assn., 157:2081–2090, 1970.

# SYSTEMIC GLUCOCORTICOID THERAPY

DANNY W. SCOTT, D.V.M.
*Ithaca, New York*

Glucocorticoids are probably the most used and abused drugs in veterinary medicine. The reasons for frequent use are readily understood. There probably is not a single organ system in the body that does not suffer from one or multiple disease entities that require glucocorticoids for their proper management. On the other hand, their abuse is usually attributable to ignorance and neglect.

## EFFECTS OF GLUCOCORTICOIDS

### ANTI-INFLAMMATORY AND ANTI-ALLERGIC ACTIONS

Glucocorticoids nonspecifically inhibit the inflammatory effects of many noxious agents, including microorganisms, chemical or thermal irritants, trauma and allergens. The anti-inflammatory actions of glucocorticoids include (1) maintenance of cellular membrane integrity and (2) stabilization of the membranes of the intracellular lysosomes, which contain hydrolytic enzymes capable of cell digestion and extension of inflammatory tissue damage. The fibroblastic proliferation, which follows inflammation as part of the reparative process and tends to localize infection, is greatly reduced, and this may potentiate the spread of an infection. However, this action is beneficial in preventing the adverse consequences of excessive fibrosis and scarring.

### IMMUNOSUPPRESSIVE ACTIONS

Various facets of the immune system are affected as follows: (1) macrophages and monocytes (depression of phagocytosis, chemotactic responses, processing of antigens and influx from peripheral blood to sites of inflammation): (2) lymphocytes (lymphocytolytic); (3) neutrophils (depression of phagocytosis, intracellular killing, chemotactic responses and influx from peripheral blood to sites of inflammation); (4) humoral antibodies (decreased synthesis); and (5) complement (inhibition of several major subfractions of the complement system).

It is apparent that glucocorticoids suppress the specific and nonspecific immune response. It is not surprising, then, to find that animals with hyperadrenocorticism (naturally occurring or iatrogenic) have a high incidence of secondary bacterial infections (especially urinary tract, respiratory tract and skin). The critical consideration here is that these infections can be present without any significant physical or laboratory abnormalities (no pyrexia, pain or leukocytosis, etc.), owing to the potent nonspecific anti-inflammatory properties of the glucocorticoids.

Another important consideration concerning immunosuppressive side effects of glucocorticoids (in addition to the increased susceptibility to infection) is the possibility of increased incidence of neoplasia. People on long-term glucocorticoid therapy have a higher incidence of various types of cancer.

## CARBOHYDRATE, PROTEIN AND LIPID METABOLISM

Glucocorticoids promote gluconeogenesis through peripheral and hepatic actions. Physical and laboratory abnormalities that might be expected to arise from these actions include the following:

1. Skeletal muscle wasting and weakness (protein catabolism).
2. Hepatomegaly (fatty liver).
3. Fat redistribution (peripheral pads, liver, omentum).
4. Thin, hypotonic, alopecic skin, with poor wound healing and easy bruising (protein catabolism, inhibition of fibroblast proliferation and collagen deposition; increased vascular fragility).
5. Lameness, bone pain and pathologic fractures (osteoporosis and osteomalacia due to protein catabolism; decreased intestinal absorption of calcium; inhibition of vitamin D activity; increased calcium resorption from bone).
6. Lipemia, hypercholesterolemia (fat mobilization).
7. Hyperglycemia (rarely, overt diabetes mellitus, which usually develops in patients with preexisting latent diabetes).

## WATER AND ELECTROLYTE BALANCE

In man, practically all glucocorticoids tend to cause hypokalemia by increasing urinary losses of potassium. The author has not seen hypokalemia in dogs with naturally occurring or iatrogenic hyperadrenocorticism, nor in any dog treated with long-term glucocorticoid therapy.

Also, in man, sodium retention is potentiated slightly or moderately by natural glucocorticoids (hydrocortisone, corticosterone) and, negligibly, by most synthetic glucocorticoids (prednisone, prednisolone, dexamethasone), while a few glucocorticoids actually enhance sodium excretion (triamcinolone, betamethasone, methylprednisolone). The author has not observed changes in serum sodium in dogs with endogenous or exogenous hyperadrenocorticism.

Glucocorticoids increase free water clearance and promote water excretion in man, dog and cat. This is recognized clinically as polyuria and polydipsia. Although the exact mechanisms for these events are not completely understood, current knowledge suggests (1) increased glomerular filtration rate, (2) inhibition of antidiuretic hormone (ADH) release and/or action and (3) direct action on the renal tubules.

## GASTROINTESTINAL SIGNS

Glucocorticoids (except for triamcinolone) enhance the appetite, which is manifested clinically as polyphagia and weight gain. The author has occasionally seen anorexia in association with glucocorticoid therapy. Glucocorticoids also increase gastric acid and pepsin secretion, while decreasing the rate of gastric mucosal cell proliferation. This may predispose to gastric ulcers. The author has also seen a few dogs and cats that developed diarrhea (often bloody, with large bowel signs predominating) while on prednisolone therapy. The diarrheas disappeared within 48 to 72 hours after prednisolone therapy was withdrawn.

## NEUROLOGIC SIGNS

Glucocorticoids are thought to promote normal psyche. Psychologic abnormalities are common in people on glucocorticoid therapy (behavioral and mood changes, psychoses, depression, mania, etc.). The author has witnessed similar reactions in dogs and cats only rarely (cats become depressed and/or prefer seclusion; dogs become irritable and sometimes vicious). In man, glucocorticoids also increase cerebral cortical irritability, especially in patients with underlying tendencies to a seizure disorder.

## HEMATOLOGIC SIGNS

Glucocorticoids classically produce leukocytosis (neutrophilia), eosinopenia, lymphopenia and lesser degrees of erythrocytosis and thrombocytosis. These findings are inconsistent clinically in man, dogs and cats.

## IATROGENIC HYPERADRENOCORTICISM (CUSHING'S SYNDROME)

*Iatrogenic hyperadrenocorticism* has been described frequently in both man and the dog. The incidence of this unfortunate entity is definitely increasing. The marked increase in incidence may be related to the emergence of the newer, more potent glucocorticoids, especially the repositol injectable form. The findings are essentially identical to those of naturally occurring hyperadrenocorticism (see preceding article). Apparently there is individual variation in susceptibility to the adverse effects of glucocorticoid therapy and in the clinical signs manifested. The author has seen all combinations of clinical signs, from classic hyperadrenocorticism to calcinosis cutis alone.

Laboratory findings in iatrogenic hyperadrenocorticism are usually normal. In our experience the classic findings of naturally occurring hyperadrenocorticism (eosinopenia; lymphopenia; elevations in SGPT, serum alkaline phosphatase, cholesterol, blood glucose, etc.) are rarely seen in the iatrogenic case.

Diagnosis is based on history and clinical findings and results of adrenocorticotropic hormone (ACTH) response tests. The ACTH response test will differentiate between naturally occurring hyperadrenocorticism due to adrenocortical hyperplasia (normal or elevated resting plasma cortisol, with exaggerated response) or adrenocortical neoplasia (high normal to elevated resting plasma cortisol, with little or no response) and iatrogenic hyperadrenocorticism (low or normal resting plasma cortisol, with no response). Occasionally adrenocortical tumors will give normal or high normal ACTH responses. Table 1 summarizes findings in seven cases of iatrogenic hyperadrenocorticism seen by the author in one year. The disease has been caused by various glucocorticoids, given in varying doses, by various routes and for varying periods. This emphasizes the individual variation that exists among dogs with adverse reactions to glucocorticoids.

Treatment requires cessation of excessive exogenous glucocorticoids, while continuing maintenance and stress therapy for the concomitant secondary adrenocortical insufficiency (see below).

## IATROGENIC SECONDARY ADRENOCORTICAL INSUFFICIENCY

The most occult, yet most critical and life-threatening, side effect of glucocorticoid therapy is *iatrogenic secondary adrenocortical insufficiency*. The primary abnormality is a lack of endogenous ACTH. The function of the zona glomerulosa of the adrenal cortex, which is dependent on the renin-angiotensin-aldosterone system and not on ACTH, is preserved. Thus, the electrolyte disturbances associated with mineralocorticoid deficiency and classic hypoadrenocorticism (Addison's disease) are not seen. But, while glucocorticoid secretory capacity is suppressed, the patient is extremely vulnerable to acute glucocorticoid insufficiency and circulatory collapse.

Patients receiving therapeutic doses of glucocorticoids develop ACTH insufficiency with secondary adrenocortical insufficiency as a result of two conditions: (1) sudden withdrawal of long-term exogenous glucocorticoids and (2) acute stress from infection, trauma, surgery, pregnancy, etc., in patients on long-term (low- or high-dose) glucocorticoids. Under normal conditions these patients usually do well, but under stress they cannot respond with adequate endogenous glucocorticoids.

Glucocorticoids may suppress the release of corticotropin-releasing factor (CRF, from the hypothalamus) and/or ACTH (from the pituitary). Suppression of the hypothalamic-pituitary-adrenal (HPA) axis is related to (1) the glucocorticoid being used, (2) the dose, (3) the duration of therapy and (4) the route of administration (the parenteral route causing the greatest suppression, followed in order of decreasing action by the oral route and topical application).

Prolonged exposure to exogenous or endogenous glucocorticoids in quantities sufficient to cause signs of hyperadrenocorticism consistently causes suppression of CRF-ACTH release and consequent adrenocortical atrophy. So, ironically, an individual may be presented with simultaneous evidence of hyper- and hypoadrenocorticism (see Table 1). The crucial factor to remember is that if the dog has received enough glucocorticoids to show signs of hyperadrenocorticism, it also, automatically, must have secondary adrenocortical insufficiency.

Diagnosis is based on history and clinical

**Table 1.** *Findings in 7 Dogs with Iatrogenic Hyperadrenocorticism and Secondary Adrenocortical Insufficiency*

| BREED | AGE (YEARS) | SEX | STEROID THERAPY RECEIVED | HISTORY AND CLINICAL FINDINGS | LABORATORY ABNORMALITIES | ACTH RESPONSE TEST* Plasma Cortisol (µg./100 ml.) | |
|---|---|---|---|---|---|---|---|
| | | | | | | Pre | Post |
| Boxer | 8 | M | 40 mg. repositol methylprednisolone IM, monthly for 7.5 years | Iatrogenic hyperadrenocorticism; acute collapse and shock | Eosinopenia and lymphopenia | 4 | 6 |
| Boston terrier | 2 | Fs | mg. prednisolone PO, b.i.d. for 4 months | Polyuria, polydipsia, polyphagia, acute collapse and shock | — | 0 | 2 |
| Pug | 6 | Fs | 2.5 mg. prednisolone PO, s.i.d. for 3.5 years | Calcinosis cutis | — | 2 | 4 |
| Irish setter | 3 | F | 5 mg. prednisolone PO, s.i.d. for 1 year | Iatrogenic hyperadrenocorticism; episodic weakness and lethargy | — | 2 | 2 |
| German shepherd | 9 | Fs | 40 mg. repositol methylprednisolone IM, every 1 to 2 months for 6 years | Iatrogenic hyperadrenocorticism; calcinosis cutis | — | 4 | 5 |
| Basset hound | 8 | Fs | 10 mg. hydrocortisone PO, t.i.d. for 2 months | Calcinosis cutis | — | 2 | 1 |
| Pug | 3 | M | 0.9 mg. betamethasone IM, monthly for 3 months | Calcinosis cutis; iatrogenic hyperadrenocorticism; episodic weakness and anorexia | — | 6 | 6 |

*ACTH response test: pre-ACTH blood sample, 40 units ACTH gel IM, and post-ACTH blood sample in 2 hours.
Plasma cortisols by fluorometric assay: Normal dog = 5 to 10 µg./100 ml. resting and 10 to 20 µg./100 ml. post-ACTH.

findings, ACTH response test, plasma cortisol response to insulin-induced hypoglycemia and radioimmunoassay for plasma ACTH (the last two are not being used at present in the dog). It should be emphasized that the characteristic serum electrolyte and resultant electrocardiographic abnormalities seen with naturally occurring hypoadrenocorticism are not found, because the mineralocorticoid secretion is intact.

When glucocorticoid therapy is withdrawn, patients will be susceptible to HPF insufficiency for several months. In man, it is advisable to administer appropriate doses of glucocorticoids for daily maintenance and stress for at least *one year* after any course of glucocorticoid therapy that has lasted longer than three months.

From studies on carbohydrate metabolism in dogs after adrenalectomy, it can be recommended that a daily maintenance dose of 0.2 to 0.5 mg./kg. hydrocortisone be administered orally, every morning, between 7 and 10 A.M. Hydrocortisone is the glucocorticoid of choice for replacement therapy. For glucocorticoid replacement, it is necessary to mimic the normal diurnal or circadian cortisol secretory pattern (see below).

During periods of stress it is necessary to increase the dose of hydrocortisone in order to mimic the response of the normal HPA axis. Thus, for minor stresses, cortisol production may increase 2- tm 4-fold, while with major stresses cortisol production may increase 10- to 25-fold.

In the treatment of secondary adrenocortical insufficiency due to exogenous glucocorticoids, one can anticipate the eventual return of normal HPA function. Only rarely is the adrenocortical atrophy irreversible. However, the HPA insufficiency may persist for over a year. In man, the return of HPA function is detected by radioimmunoassay of plasma ACTH or plasma cortisol response to insulin-induced hypoglycemia. However, these procedures are not available at present for animals. Thus, it is safest to follow the previously mentioned rule of thumb used in human medicine (continue maintenance and stress therapy with hydrocortisone for one year). However, future studies may show that the biologically "faster-living" dog may not need such a long period of time to recover.

The usefulness of ACTH therapy, aimed at restoring the mass and functional capacity of the adrenal glands, has been widely debated because the most obstinate block after prolonged glucocorticoid therapy is *not* at the level of the adrenocortical responses to ACTH but in the ability of the HP unit to resume release of adequate amounts of CRF-ACTH. This block cannot be corrected and, in fact, is probably worsened by the use of ACTH. Therefore, ACTH should *not* be used in secondary adrenocortical insufficiency.

## ALTERNATE-DAY STEROID THERAPY

Many attempts have been made to decrease the side effects of glucocorticoid therapy. Changes in molecular structure, concomitant ACTH administration, use of shorter-acting glucocorticoids, reduction in total daily dose regimens and modification of therapy to an intermittent basis have all been tried. These mechanisms have been unsuccessful. For instance, if oral prednisolone is given for three consecutive days of a week and omitted for the remaining four days, the HPA axis is still not protected.

The critical factor in long-term glucocorticoid therapy is the maintenance of the normal diurnal or circadian cortisol secretory pattern. This diurnal rhythm has been described for man and the dog and appears to be determined by the hypothalamus. Plasma cortisol levels are highest in the morning (7 to 10 A.M.) and lowest at night (10 to 12 P.M.). Plasma ACTH levels vary inversely with plasma cortisol.

The alternate-day steroid (ADS) regimen has been developed to preserve the normal diurnal cortisol rhythm and thus to avoid HPA suppression. It has been shown that certain oral glucocorticoids can be administered once, every other morning, when plasma cortisol is normally highest, and ACTH release is already inhibited by natural negative feedback. This still affords control of symptoms on the off days but allows the HPA axis to function normally. The only oral glucocorticoids that can be used in this manner are prednisone, prednisolone and methylprednisolone. Hydrocortisone and cortisone allow HPA function on the off days but often do not control symptoms.

If long-term glucocorticoid therapy is indicated, the ADS regimen should be used whenever possible, since it is the only safe

*Table 2.* Characteristics of Pharmaceutical Derivatives of Adrenocorticosteroids for Oral Administration

| DRUG | GLUCOCORTICOID POTENCY* | MINERALOCORTICOID POTENCY | HPA† SUPPRESSIVE ACTIVITY | SUITABLE FOR ADS‡ | EQUIVALENT DOSE IN MG. |
|---|---|---|---|---|---|
| *Short-Acting* | | | | | |
| Hydrocortisone | 1.0 | ++ | + | No | 20 |
| Cortisone | 0.8 | ++ | + | No | 25 |
| Prednisolone | 4.0 | + | + | Yes | 5 |
| Prednisone | 4.0 | + | + | Yes | 5 |
| Methylprednisolone | 5.0 | 0 | + | Yes | 4 |
| *Intermediate-Acting* | | | | | |
| Triamcinolone | 5.0 | 0 | ++ | No | 4 |
| Paramethasone | 10.0 | 0 | ++ | No | 2 |
| Fluprednisolone | 10.0 | 0 | ++ | No | 2 |
| *Long-Acting* | | | | | |
| Dexamethasone | 30.0 | 0 | +++ | No | 0.75 |
| Betamethasone | 30.0 | 0 | +++ | No | 0.60 |
| Fludrocortisone | 15.0 | ++++ | +++ | No | — |

*Compared with hydrocortisone on a mg.-for-mg. basis.
†HPA = Hypothalamic-pituitary-adrenal.
‡ADS = Alternate-day steroid therapy.

regimen available at present. The author currently has some 200 dogs on ADS. Some have been medicated for periods of up to three years with no untoward side effects. These dogs have not developed clinical signs or biochemical changes suggestive of either iatrogenic hyperadrenocorticism or secondary adrenocortical insufficiency. The only side effects noted by the owners have been occasional polyphagia and/or polydipsia on the day of glucocorticoid administration. Extreme polydipsia, polyuria, polyphagia and weight gain have not been reported. The author's present ADS regimen is as follows:

1. Five to seven days of induction therapy (½ to 1 mg./kg. prednisolone orally, twice daily).

2. Then, 2 mg./kg. prednisolone orally, every other morning between 7 and 10 A.M.

3. Then the ADS dosage is reduced by 50 per cent, at weekly intervals, until the lowest maintenance dose is determined. This maintenance dose varies considerably from dog to dog but usually averages ½ mg./kg. every other morning.

ADS is intended for maintenance therapy. Its purpose is to lessen side effects, especially HPA suppression. It is *not* intended to permit or encourage indiscriminate use of glucocorticoids. The following general principles of glucocorticoid therapy must *always* be enforced:

1. Use glucocorticoid therapy only when a diagnosis has been established, and when less harmful forms of therapy have failed.

2. Use the smallest therapeutically effective dose.

3. Use ADS therapy whenever possible.

Parenteral sustained-release glucocorticoid preparations are unphysiologic, unnecessary, undesirable and in most instances contraindicated in clinical medicine. These preparations are absolutely contraindicated when long-term symptomatic therapy is needed.

### SUPPLEMENTAL READING

Berlinger, F. G.: Use and misuse of steroids. Postgrad. Med., 55:153–157, 1974.

Bondy, P. K.: The adrenal cortex. *In* Bondy, P. K., and Rosenberg, L. E. (eds.): Duncan's Diseases of Metabolism. 7th ed. Philadelphia, W. B. Saunders Co., 1974, pp. 1105–1180.

Fine, R. M.: Physiologic effects of systemic corticosteroids in dermatology. Cutis, 11:217–226, 1973.

Frawley, T. F.: Corticosteroid therapy: Updating of principles. Postgrad. Med., 56:123–129, 1974.

Liddle, G. W.: The adrenal steroids and their functions. In Beeson, P. B., and McDermott, W. (eds.): Textbook of Medicine. 14th ed. Philadelphia, W. B. Saunders Co., 1975, pp. 1733–1752.

Sayers, G., and Travis, R. H.: Adrenocorticotropic hormone; adrenocortical steroids and their synthetic analogs. *In* Goodman, L. S., and Gilman, A. (eds.): The Pharmacologic Basis of Therapeutics. 4th ed. New York, The Macmillan Co., 1970, pp. 1604–1642.

Scott, D. W., and Greene, C. E.: Iatrogenic secondary adrenocortical insufficiency in dogs. J. Am. Anim. Hosp. Assn., 10:555–564, 1974.

Streeten, D. H. P.: Corticosteroid therapy. I. Pharmacological properties and principles of corticosteroid use. J.A.M.A., 232:944–947, 1975.

Streeten, D. H. P.: Corticosteroid therapy. II. Complications and therapeutic indications. J.A.M.A., 232:1046–1049, 1975.

# PARATHYROID GLANDS AND CALCIUM METABOLISM

CHARLES C. CAPEN, D.V.M.,
*and* SHARRON L. MARTIN, D.V.M.
*Columbus, Ohio*

## INTRODUCTION

Parathyroids in animals consist of one or two pairs of glands situated in the anterior cervical region, often in close proximity to the thyroid gland. They are present in all air-breathing vertebrates, first appearing in amphibians coincidentally with the transition from an aquatic to a terrestrial life. Parathyroid glands are composed of a single type of secretory cell, termed a chief cell, that is responsible for the synthesis and secretion of parathyroid hormone (PTH) (Capen, 1975*a*). Recent evidence suggests that a larger biosynthetic precursor ("proparathyroid hormone") is first synthesized on the rough endoplasmic reticulum from which active PTH is cleaved enzymatically during transport through the Golgi apparatus prior to storage in secretion granules and secretion from chief cells (Fig. 1).

In contrast to most endocrine organs, which are under complex controls involving both long and short feedback loops, the parathyroids have a unique feedback control by the concentration of calcium (and to a lesser degree magnesium) ions in serum. PTH is the principal hormone involved in the minute-to-minute fine regulation of blood calcium in mammals. It exerts its biologic actions by directly influencing the function of target cells primarily in bone and kidney (Capen, 1975*b*).

Calcium plays a key role in many fundamental biologic processes, including neuromuscular excitability, membrane permeability and blood coagulation, in addition to being an essential structural component of the skeleton. The precise control of calcium ions in extracellular fluids is vital to the health of animals and man. To maintain a constant concentration of calcium, despite marked variations in intake and excretion, endocrine control mechanisms have evolved that primarily consist of the interactions of three major hormones. Although the direct roles of PTH, calcitonin and vitamin D frequently are emphasized in the control of blood calcium, other hormones such as adrenal corticosteroids, estrogens, thyroxine, somatotropin and glucagon may contribute to the maintenance of calcium metabolism and skeletal homeostasis under certain conditions.

## PRIMARY HYPERPARATHYROIDISM

In primary hyperparathyroidism, parathyroid hormone is produced in excess of normal by a functional lesion in the parathyroid gland. This disease is encountered infrequently in older dogs. Primary hyperparathyroidism does not appear to be a sequela of long-standing secondary hyperparathyroidism in animals.

## PATHOPHYSIOLOGIC MECHANISMS

The normal control mechanisms for PTH secretion by the concentration of blood calcium are lost in primary hyperparathyroidism. Hormone secretion is autonomous, and the parathyroid produces excessive hormone in spite of the increased blood calcium. Cells of the renal tubules are most sensitive to alterations in the amount of circulating PTH. The hormone acts on these cells initially to promote the excretion of phosphate and retention of calcium. A prolonged increased secretion of PTH results in accelerated osteocytic and osteoclastic bone resorption. Mineral is removed from the skeleton and replaced by immature fibrous connective tissue. The bone lesion of fibrous osteodystrophy is generalized throughout the skeleton but is accentuated in local areas, such as in the cancellous bone of the skull.

The lesion in the parathyroid gland responsible for the excessive secretion of PTH in dogs is usually an adenoma composed of active chief cells. Adenomas are usually single and may be located either in the cervical region near the thyroid gland or within the anterior mediastinum near the base of the heart. Parathyroid neoplasms in the precardial mediastinum are derived from ectopic parathyroid anlage displaced into the thorax with the expanding thymus during embryonic development. Histopathologic demonstration of a rim of normal tissue and fibrous capsule in an enlarged parathyroid suggests a diagnosis of adenoma rather than primary hyperplasia.

## CLINICAL FEATURES

Hypercalcemia results in anorexia, vomiting, constipation and generalized muscular weakness due to decreased neuromuscular excitability. Other functional disturbances observed are the result of weakening of bones by excessive resorption. Lameness due to fractures of long bones may occur after relatively minor physical trauma. Compression fractures of weakened vertebral bodies may exert pressure on the spinal cord and nerves, resulting in motor and/or sensory dysfunction. Facial hyperostosis, with partial obliteration of the nasal cavity by poorly mineralized woven bone and fibrous connective tissue, and loosening or

**Table 1.  *Differential Diagnosis of Hypercalcemia***

|  | SERUM CALCIUM | SERUM PHOSPHORUS | SERUM ALKALINE PHOSPHATASE | SOFT BONE LESION | MINERALI-ZATION | PARATHYROID LESION |
|---|---|---|---|---|---|---|
| Primary Hyperparathyroidism | High | Low | Elevated | Severe, generalized | Moderate | Adenoma, Hyperplasia |
| Vitamin D Intoxication | High | High | Normal | Mild or Absent | Severe | Atrophy |
| Malignant Neoplasm with Bone Metastases | High | Normal or Elevated | Moderately Elevated | Multifocal | Moderate | Inactive, Atrophy |
| Pseudohyperparathyroidism (ectopic PTH) | High | Low | Normal or Elevated Slightly | Mild | Moderate | Inactive, Atrophy |

loss of teeth in alveolar sockets have been observed in dogs with primary hyper-parathyroidism.

## DIAGNOSIS

Primary hyperparathyroidism should be included in the differential diagnosis of older dogs with a clinical history of multiple fractures associated with severe generalized skeletal disease and normal renal function. Radiographic evaluation reveals areas of subperiosteal cortical resorption, loss of lamina dura, soft tissue mineralization, bone cysts and a generalized decrease in bone density and fractures in advanced cases.

The most important and practical laboratory test to aid in establishing the diagnosis of primary hyperparathyroidism is quantitation of total blood calcium (Table 1). Although other laboratory findings may be variable, hypercalcemia is a consistent finding and results from accelerated release of calcium from bone. The blood calcium of normal animals is near 10 mg./100 ml., with some variation depending upon the analytic method employed as well as the age and diet of the animal. Calcium values consistently above 11.5 to 12.0 mg./100 ml. should be considered to be in the hypercalcemic range. Dogs with primary hyperparathyroidism usually have a greatly elevated (12 to 20 mg./100 ml. or above) blood calcium. The blood phosphorus is low (4 mg./100 ml. or less) or in the low normal range because of inhibition of renal tubular reabsorption of phosphorus by excess PTH.

The activity of alkaline phosphatase, an enzyme involved in both apposition and resorption of bone, may be elevated in the serum of animals with overt bone disease. The increased activity of this enzyme is thought to result from a compensatory increase in osteoblasts along trabeculae as a response to mechanical stress in bones weakened by excessive resorption. The urinary excretion of phosphorus and often calcium is increased and may result in nephrocalcinosis and urolithiasis. Accelerated bone matrix catabolism is reflected by an increased excretion of hydroxyproline in the urine. The detection of elevated circulating levels of PTH by radioimmunoassay in man has greatly facilitated the early diagnosis of hyperparathyroidism. At present, this laboratory procedure is not readily available for routine use in the diagnosis of parathyroid disease in dogs.

## DIFFERENTIAL DIAGNOSIS

Other causes of hypercalcemia which must be considered in differential diagnosis of primary hyperparathyroidism are vitamin D intoxication, malignant neoplasms with osseous metastases and parathyroid hormone–like activity produced by malignant neoplasms of nonparathyroid origin without metastases to bone (Table 1). The hypercalcemia of hypervitaminosis D may be of a magnitude similar to that in hyperparathyroidism but is usually accompanied by hyperphosphatemia and normal serum alkaline phosphatase activity. Skeletal disease is usually not present, since the increased concentrations of blood calcium and phosphorus are derived principally from augmented intestinal absorption rather than bone resorption.

Malignant neoplasms with osseous metastases may cause moderate hypercalcemia and hypercalciuria, but the alkaline phosphatase activity and serum phosphorus are usually normal or slightly elevated. These changes are believed to be due to release of calcium and phosphorus into the blood from areas of bone destruction at rates greater than those at which they can be cleared by the kidney and intestine. Bone involvement is sharply demarcated and localized to the area of metastasis. Osteolysis associated with tumor metastases has been shown to be the result not only of a physical disruption of bone by neoplastic cells but also of the local production of humoral substances that stimulate bone resorption, such as prostaglandins and osteoclast-activating factor. Hypercalcemia and hypophosphatemia also have been reported in animals and man with several different types of malignant neoplasms in the absence of bone metastases and functional lesions in the parathyroid glands. (Refer to the section on paraneoplastic syndromes on page 1061.) Other sporadic causes of hypercalcemia include multifocal osteolytic lesions associated with septic emboli, complete immobilization and chronic renal disease.

## TREATMENT

The aim of treatment is to eliminate the source of excessive PTH production. An attempt should be made to identify all four parathyroid glands before excising any tissue. Parathyroid adenomas appear as light brown-red, encapsulated nodules usually many times the size of normal glands. A correlation often exists in man between tumor size and the severity of hypercalcemia and bone disease. Parathyroid carcinomas are larger than adenomas, invade adjacent structures (e.g., thyroid glands, cervical muscles) and metastasize to regional lymph nodes and lung.

Single or multiple adenomas should be removed *in toto*. If all four glands are enlarged considerably (e.g., primary chief or water-clear cell hyperplasia) in a patient with severe bone disease and hypercalcemia, three parathyroids should be excised *in toto* and the fourth gland left intact with a good blood supply, provided that secondary hyperparathyroidism has been eliminated. In case all identifiable glands appear to be of normal size and a diagnosis has been established with reasonable certainty, surgical exploration of the thorax near the base of the heart may be necessary to localize the neoplasm.

Successful removal of the functional parathyroid lesion results in a rapid decrease in circulating PTH levels, because the half-life of PTH in plasma is approximately 20 minutes. It should be emphasized that plasma calcium levels in patients with overt bone disease may decrease rapidly and be subnormal within 12 to 24 hours postsurgery, resulting in severe hypocalcemic tetany. Serum calcium levels should be monitored frequently following surgical removal of a parathyroid neoplasm. Postoperative hypocalcemia (5 mg./100 ml. and lower) can be the result of (1) depressed secretory activity of chief cells due to long-term suppression by the chronic hypercalcemia or injury to the remaining parathyroid tissue during surgery, (2) decreased bone resorption and (3) accelerated mineralization of osteoid matrix formed by the hyperplastic osteoblasts but previously prevented from undergoing mineralization by the elevated PTH levels. Infusions of calcium gluconate to maintain the serum calcium between 7.5 and 9.0 mg./100 ml. plus the feeding of high-calcium diets and supplemental vitamin D therapy will correct this serious postoperative complication.

If hypercalcemia persists for a week or more after surgery or recurs after initial improvement, the presence of a second adenoma or metastases from a carcinoma should be suspected. Rapidly developing hypercalcemia of significant magnitude should be considered a medical emergency that, if not promptly corrected, can lead to death of the patient. The extracellular concentration of calcium can be reduced by several means, including (1) drugs that increase urinary calcium excretion, (2) peritoneal dialysis and (3) phosphate preparations that promote calcium deposition in bone and soft tissues.

## SECONDARY HYPERPARATHYROIDISM— RENAL ORIGIN

Secondary hyperparathyroidism as a complication of chronic renal failure is a metabolic state characterized by an excessive, but not autonomous, rate of PTH secretion. This disorder is encountered more frequently in dogs but also occurs in cats. The secretion of hormone by the hyperplastic parathyroid glands usually remains responsive to fluctuations in blood calcium.

## PATHOPHYSIOLOGIC MECHANISMS

The primary etiologic mechanism in this disorder is long-standing, progressive renal disease resulting in severely impaired function. Chronic renal insufficiency in older dogs results from interstitial nephritis, glomerulonephritis, nephrosclerosis or amyloidosis. Several congenital anomalies such as cortical hypoplasia, polycystic kidneys and bilateral hydronephrosis may result in renal insufficiency in younger dogs.

When the renal disease progresses to the point at which there is significant reduction in glomerular filtration rate, phosphorus is retained and progressive hyperphosphatemia develops. Although the concentration of blood phosphate has no direct regulatory influence on the synthesis and secretion of PTH, it may, if elevated, contribute to parathyroid stimulation by virtue of its ability to lower blood calcium.

The calcium ion concentration in the blood is known to be the important factor controlling secretory activity of the parathyroid gland. In normal animals, there is a linear, inversely proportional relationship between the rate of PTH secretion and the concentration of blood calcium over a range of 4 to 12 mg./100 ml. Parathyroid stimulation in patients with chronic renal disease can be attributed directly to the hypocalcemia. Several mechanisms contribute to the development of hypocalcemia in chronic renal failure. As mentioned, when the phosphate concentration increases, blood calcium decreases reciprocally according to the mass-law equation when the serum is saturated with respect to these two ions.

Recent evidence suggests that impaired intestinal absorption of calcium due to an acquired defect in vitamin D metabolism plays a significant role in the development of hypocalcemia in chronic renal insufficiency and uremia. Vitamin $D_3$, prior to acting on target cells in the intestine and bone, is first converted to 25-hydroxycholecalciferol by liver enzymes and is subsequently metabolized to 1,25-dihydroxycholecalciferol by a mitochondrial enzyme ("25-hydroxycholecalciferol-l-hydroxylase") in the kidney cortex. The metabolically active or "hormonal" form of vitamin D is 1,25-dihydroxycholecalciferol. The concentrations of circulating PTH, ionized calcium and phosphate appear to regulate the rate of formation of this active metabolite. Chronic renal disease appears to impair the production of 1,25-dihydroxycholecalciferol by the kidney, thereby diminishing intestinal calcium transport and leading to the development of hypocalcemia.

Parathyroid chief cells initially undergo organellar hypertrophy and subsequently cellular hyperplasia as compensatory mechanisms to increase hormonal synthesis and secretion in response to the hypocalcemic stimulus. Since the parathyroid gland stores comparatively little pre-formed hormone, the rate of polypeptide biosynthesis appears to be rate-limiting for hormonal secretion. Although the parathyroids are not autonomous, the concentration of PTH in the peripheral blood in human patients with chronic renal failure may exceed that of primary hyperparathyroidism. Parathyroid hormone accelerates osteocytic and osteoclastic resorption, resulting in release of stored calcium from bone. The long-standing increase in bone resorption that attempts to return serum calcium to normal eventually results in the metabolic bone disease associated with chronic renal insufficiency. Progressive glomerular and tubular dysfunction with loss of target cells interferes with an expression of the phosphaturic response by the increased circulating PTH in renal disease. Phosphate is retained and the blood concentration continues to rise in spite of the secondary hyperparathyroidism.

## CLINICAL FEATURES

The predominant clinical signs of vomiting, dehydration, polydipsia, depression and ammoniacal breath odor are related to progressive renal insufficiency and uremia. A spectrum of skeletal lesions of secondary hyperparathyroidism may be present, ranging from very minor changes with early (or mild) renal disease to the severe fibrous osteodystrophy of advanced renal failure. Histologic evaluation of the skeleton in dogs with chronic renal disease reveals that a high percentage have generalized fibrous osteodystrophy (Krook, 1957). The volume of affected bones is usually normal (isostotic fibrous osteodystrophy), particularly in older dogs because of the slow onset of renal failure and lower metabolic activity of bones. Hyperostotic bone lesions (e.g., facial swellings) may be seen in younger dogs in which repair by proliferation of fibrous connective tissue and deposition of osteoid exceeds the rate of resorption, resulting in a greater than normal volume.

Although skeletal involvement is generalized with hyperparathyroidism, it does not affect all parts uniformly. Lesions become apparent earlier and reach a more advanced stage in certain areas. Resorption of alveolar socket bone and loss of lamina dura dentes occur early and result in loose teeth which may be dislodged easily and interfere with mastication. Cancellous bone of the maxilla and mandible also is a site of predilection in hyperparathyroidism. Owing to the accelerated resorption, the bones become softened and readily pliable (i.e., "rubber jaw disease"), and the jaws fail to close properly. Long bones of the abaxial skeleton are less dramatically affected. Lameness, stiff gait and the occurrence of fractures after relatively minor trauma may result from the increased bone resorption.

## DIAGNOSIS

Skeletal lesions of varying severity should be suspected in all patients with chronic renal insufficiency and secondary hyperparathyroidism. Roentgenographically, there is evidence of generalized skeletal demineralization in advanced cases with localized areas of accentuation and loss of lamina dura dentes. Several laboratory procedures are particularly useful to establish and assess the extent of renal disease. The blood urea nitrogen (BUN) and creatinine levels are elevated consistently, whereas the glomerular filtration rate and effective renal blood flow are decreased. Specific details of methods for evaluation of kidney function can be found in the section on renal disease.

Serum should be analyzed for calcium, phosphorus and alkaline phosphatase. Results of a single determination of these parameters must be interpreted with an appreciation that considerable variation exists, depending upon the stage of the disease, because of the body's compensatory mechanisms. The blood calcium is variable but is usually near normal (10 mg./100 ml.) because of mobilization of skeletal reserves.

Although the serum calcium in most dogs will be in the low normal range, an occasional dog with long-standing renal failure will have signs of mild hypocalcemic tetany. A small percentage of dogs with chronic kidney disease will have a moderate hypercalcemia. Although the exact mechanism for the development of hypercalcemia with renal disease is uncertain, it may be the result of diminished PTH degradation by the damaged kidney, decreased urinary calcium excretion or hypercitricemia. Hyperphosphatemia of 6 mg./100 ml. and above in older dogs, with slightly higher values in younger animals, is a consistent finding and results from the retention of phosphate by the damaged kidney. Alkaline phosphatase activity may be elevated in animals with overt bone disease. Urinary excretion of calcium and phosphorus is decreased.

## TREATMENT

The aim of treatment with this disorder ideally would be to interrupt the progression of kidney disease and restore or replace renal function to a semblance of normal. Owing to the stage and progressive nature of the disease when the diagnosis is established in animals, treatment is directed realistically toward reducing the excretory load and providing substances (e.g., sodium as chloride or bicarbonate, water, etc.) that the failing kidney is unable to conserve (see article on "Conservative Management of Chronic Renal Disease" in *Current Veterinary Therapy* V, p. 894). A k/d® prescription diet with supplemental calcium (gluconate or lactate) and vitamin D may diminish the severity of hyperparathyroidism and accompanying bone lesions. Recent evidence suggests that 1,25-dihydroxycholecalciferol and other active vitamin D metabolites have considerable potential in the therapy of impaired intestinal absorption of calcium, hypocalcemia and osteomalacia associated with chronic renal disease in humans.

## SECONDARY HYPERPARATHYROIDISM— NUTRITIONAL ORIGIN

The increased secretion of parathyroid hormone in this metabolic disorder is a compensatory mechanism directed against a disturbance in mineral homeostasis induced by nutritional imbalances. The disease occurs commonly in cats, dogs, certain primates and laboratory animals, as well as in many farm animal species.

## PATHOPHYSIOLOGIC MECHANISMS

Dietary mineral imbalances of etiologic importance in the pathogenesis of nutritional secondary hyperparathyroidism are (1) a low content of calcium, (2) excessive phosphorus with normal or low calcium and (3) inadequate amounts of vitamin $D_3$. The significant end result is hypocalcemia which results in the parathyroid stimulation. A diet low in calcium fails to supply the daily requirement, even though a greater proportion of ingested calcium is absorbed, and hypocalcemia develops. Ingestion of excessive phosphorus results in increased intestinal absorption and elevation of blood phosphorus. Hyperphosphatemia does not stimulate the parathyroid gland directly but does so indirectly by virtue of its ability to lower blood calcium. Diets containing inadequate amounts of vitamin $D_3$ (even with normal vitamin $D_2$) cause diminished intestinal calcium absorption and hypocalcemia in certain New World monkeys housed indoors under laboratory conditions.

In response to the nutritionally induced hypocalcemia, all parathyroid glands undergo cellular hypertrophy and hyperplasia. Since kidney function is normal, the increased levels of PTH result in diminished renal tubular reabsorption of phosphate and increased reabsorption of calcium, returning blood levels toward normal. In addition, bone resorption is accelerated and release of calcium elevates blood calcium levels to the low normal range. Continued ingestion of the imbalanced diet sustains the state of compensatory hyperparathyroidism, leading to progressive development of the metabolic bone disease.

## CLINICAL FEATURES

The disease develops in young cats fed a predominantly meat diet (Scott, 1968). For example, beef heart or liver contains minimal amounts of calcium (7 to 9 mg./100 gm.) and has a markedly imbalanced calcium:phosphorus ratio (1:20 to 1:50).

Kittens exclusively fed beef heart develop functional disturbances within four weeks. Clinical signs are dominated by disturbances in locomotion manifested by a reluctance to move, posterior lameness and an uncoordinated gait. The kittens often assume a standing position with characteristic medial deviation of the paws. The skeletal disease becomes progressively more severe after 5 to 14 weeks. The kittens become quiet and reluctant to play. They assume a sitting position or are in sternal recumbency with the hind legs abducted at the pelvis. Normal activities may result in sudden onset of severe lameness due to incomplete or folding fractures of one or more bones. The high content of digestible protein (more than 50 per cent on a wet basis) and fat promotes rapid growth in kittens fed beef heart. They appear well-nourished and their hair coat maintains a good luster.

The disease has been reported more frequently in Siamese and Burmese kittens, but skeletal lesions can be induced readily in other breeds. The indulgence of fussy eating habits with undesirable diets by their owners, rather than a genetic predisposition, probably accounts for the higher incidence in these breeds. A wide variety of synonyms have been used to describe this metabolic disorder in cats, including osteogenesis imperfecta, juvenile osteoporosis and paper-bone or Siamese cat disease. In general, kittens are more susceptible and develop more severe skeletal lesions than adult cats fed a similar diet. Adult cats fed a beef heart diet develop osteoporosis slowly after a period of months in response to increased PTH secretion, whereas the skeleton of kittens develops severe generalized osteitis fibrosa within a few weeks. The disease develops rapidly because the dietary imbalance is wide and the skeletal metabolic rate of kittens is high. Resorption proceeds at a faster rate than repair by fibrous connective tissue proliferation, resulting in a decreased bone volume (hypostotic fibrous osteodystrophy) (Rowland *et al.*, 1968). Vertebral fractures with compression of the spinal cord and paralysis are common in kittens but infrequent in adult cats.

The feeding of a monotonous meat diet to dogs of any age results in secondary hyperparathyroidism, with the development of skeletal disease by mechanisms similar to those described previously in cats. The low calcium content and unfavorable calcium:phosphorus ratio of nonsupplemented all-meat diets are unable to fulfill the daily requirements for either growing pups (528 mg. of calcium and 440 mg. of phosphorus/kg. of body weight daily) or adult dogs (264 mg. of calcium and 220 mg. of phosphorus/kg. of body weight daily).

Lameness is the initial functional disturbance in growing dogs and may vary from a slight limp to complete inability to walk. The bones are painful on palpation, and folding fractures of long bones and vertebrae are not uncommon. Clinical signs are usually related to resorption of jaw bones in adult dogs. Parathyroid hormone–stimulated resorption of alveolar socket bone results in loss of lamina dura dentes, loosening and subsequent loss of teeth from their sockets and recession of gingivae, with partial root exposure in advanced cases.

Secondary hyperparathyroidism of nutritional origin also occurs in collections of aviculturists (domestic and captive birds), zoologic parks (caged lions and tigers, green iguanas, crocodiles, etc.) and laboratory animals (ground squirrels, nonhuman primates, etc.) housed indoors in research laboratories without exposure to sunlight. The metabolic disorder has been recognized in New World monkeys for many years and has received numerous synonyms including cage paralysis, simian bone disease and osteomalacia. Hypocalcemia resulting from either inadequate vitamin $D_3$ or extensive phosphorus in the diet of pet monkeys stimulates the parathyroid gland. The monkeys become inactive, offer less resistance to handling and have difficulty masticating their food. In pet monkeys, maxillary hyperostosis, joint pain and distortion of limbs by palpable fractures without mineralized calluses in advanced stages of the disease often occur.

## DIAGNOSIS

The diet should be evaluated for calcium, phosphorus and vitamin D content in all patients (particularly young and rapidly growing animals) with skeletal disease. In nutritional hyperparathyroidism, there is radiographic evidence of generalized skeletal demineralization, loss of lamina dura dentes, subperiosteal cortical bone resorption, bowing deformities and multiple folding fractures of long bones. Laboratory parameters used to assess renal function should be within normal limits in patients with nutritional hyperparathyroidism.

Analysis of the serum for calcium, phosphorus and alkaline phosphatase should be undertaken with an appreciation that one determination may be of limited diagnostic value. Since the body's compensatory mechanisms with this disease are complex and usually operational when the animal is seen for the first time, serum calcium and phosphorus levels usually are in a low normal range. Alkaline phosphatase activity often is elevated in animals with overt bone disease. The increased secretion of PTH acts on the normal kidneys to increase phosphate and decrease calcium excretion in the urine.

## TREATMENT

The aim of treatment is to decrease PTH secretion by correcting the dietary mineral imbalance or deficiency. Kittens with the disease should be fed a diet that fulfills their high demand for animal protein and meets the daily requirements for calcium (200 to 400 mg.) and phosphorus (150 to 200 mg.). Calcium gluconate, lactate or carbonate alone or in combination should be used as dietary supplements to achieve a 2:1 calcium:phosphorus ratio during the healing phase in cats with severe bone disease. Additional vitamin D is usually not necessary, since the requirements of cats are low (50 to 100 IU of vitamin $D_3$ daily), but may be indicated in severely affected cats to increase intestinal absorption of calcium. Calcium gluconate should be given parenterally if the appetite is depressed. A similar therapeutic regimen should be used for dogs. The feeding of excessive amounts of calcium for prolonged periods should be avoided both therapeutically and under normal conditions, because it may retard growth and alter remodeling of bone in young dogs (Hedhammar *et al.*, 1974; also refer to article on "Nutritional Hypercalcitoninism").

It is essential to keep affected animals closely confined in flat-bottomed cages for at least three weeks after initiation of the supplemental diet. The response to therapy is rapid, and within a week the kittens become more active and their attitude improves. Jumping or climbing must be prevented, because the skeleton is still susceptible to fractures. The restrictions need be less rigid after three weeks, but confinement with limited movement is indicated until the skeleton returns to normal. Improvement of the skeleton during dietary supplementation can be followed radiographically. Fracture calluses become radiodense and the overall mineral density and cortical bone thickness increase progressively with treatment. The skeleton is usually healed after feeding the supplemental diet (calcium:phosphorus ratio of 2:1) for eight to nine weeks. Subsequently, the diet should supply the total daily requirements of calcium and phosphorus and be balanced at about 1.2:1.0. The prognosis for recovery is good unless vertebral fractures have resulted in injury to the spinal cord and posterior paralysis. Even advanced cases respond favorably to dietary supplementation. Good nursing care is essential to prevent complications such as decubital ulcers, constipation and additional fractures. Healed pelvic fractures may predispose to dystocia and obstipation.

New World monkeys kept as pets may develop hyperparathyroidism when fed diets imbalanced with excess phosphorus and often low in calcium. Correction of the dietary imbalance and substitution of vitamin $D_3$ (2000 IU/kg. of diet) for vitamin $D_2$ results in increased intestinal calcium absorption and reversal of the skeletal disease within several months.

## HYPOPARATHYROIDISM

In hypoparathyroidism either subnormal amounts of PTH are secreted by pathologic parathyroid glands or the hormone secreted in unable to interact normally with target cells. Hypoparathyroidism has been recognized sporadically in dogs, particularly in smaller breeds such as schnauzers and terriers. The incidence of hypoparathyroidism in small animal medicine is much lower than that of hyperparathyroidism.

Several pathogenic mechanisms can result in an inadequate secretion of PTH (Table 2). The parathyroid glands may be damaged or inadvertently removed during the course of thyroid surgery. If the parathyroids or their vascular supply has been damaged, there often is regeneration of adequate functional parenchyma and subsequent disappearance of clinical signs. Agenesis of both pairs of parathyroids is a

**Table 2.** *Possible Pathogenic Mechanisms of Hypoparathyroidism*

| |
|---|
| Congenital |
|   (Agenesis, Hypoplasia) |
| Idiopathic |
|   (Degeneration, Lymphocytic Parathyroiditis) |
| Iatrogenic |
|   (Neck Surgery, Irradiation) |
| Metastatic Neoplasms |
| Trophic Atrophy Caused by Hypercalcemia |
|   (Vitamin D Excess, Ectopic PTH Secretion, |
|    Bone Metastases) |
| Failure to Convert Pro-PTH to PTH |
| Inability of Target Cells to Respond to PTH |

rare cause of congenital hypoparathyroidism in pups. Idiopathic hypoparathyroidism in adult dogs may be associated with extensive degeneration of chief cells with partial replacement by adipose connective tissue or diffuse lymphocytic parathyroiditis (Burk and Schaubhut, 1975). The latter may develop by means of an autoimmune mechanism, since a similar destruction of secretory parenchyma and lymphocytic infiltration has been produced experimentally in dogs by repeated injections of parathyroid tissue emulsions. Other possible causes of hypoparathyroidism include invasion and destruction of parathyroids by primary or metastatic neoplasms in the anterior cervical area and trophic atrophy of parathyroids associated with long-term hypercalcemia. Certain cases of idiopathic hypoparathyroidism with histologically normal parathyroids in both animals and man may be due to a lack of the specific "enzyme" in chief cells which converts the proparathyroid hormone molecule to the biologically active PTH secreted by the gland (Fig. 1).

The functional disturbances and clinical manifestations of hypoparathyroidism are primarily the result of increased neuromuscular excitability and tetany. Because of the lack of PTH, bone resorption is decreased and blood calcium levels diminish progressively (4 to 6 mg./100 ml.). Affected dogs are restless, nervous and ataxic with weakness and intermittent tremors of individual muscle groups that progress to generalized tetany and convulsive seizures. Concurrently, blood phosphorus levels are substantially elevated owing to increased renal tubular reabsorption.

Limited experience in the treatment of hypoparathyroidism suggests that initially the tetany should be stopped by returning

CHIEF CELL                    ECF

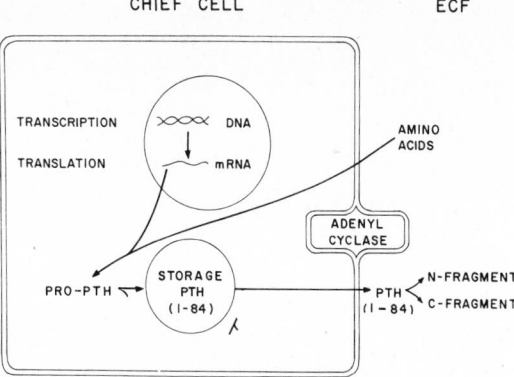

**Figure 1.** Biosynthesis of parathyroid hormone by chief cells. Parathyroid hormone is synthesized as part of a larger biosynthetic precursor molecule (Pro-PTH) that is converted to the active form prior to storage and secretion from the cell.

blood calcium levels to near normal through the intravenous administration of organic calcium solutions. Long-term maintenance of blood calcium in the absence of normal PTH secretion should be attempted by feeding diets that are high in calcium and low in phosphorus and that are supplemented with large amounts of vitamin $D_3$ (25,000 to 50,000 or more units per day). Large doses of vitamin D are often required to elevate the blood calcium in hypoparathyroid patients, because the lack of PTH diminishes the rate of formation of the biologically active vitamin D metabolite by the 1-hydroxylase system in the kidney. In order to prevent the development of hypercalcemia and extensive soft tissue mineralization, the clinician should adjust the dosage of vitamin D by frequently determining the serum calcium levels. Replacement therapy with either parathyroid extract or PTH derived from heterologous species (e.g., bovine) is expensive and ineffective on a long-term basis because of the development of antibodies. Synthetic PTH, especially the biologically active amino terminal (1-34) end of the molecule, and the potent active metabolites of vitamin D (1,25-dihydroxycholecalciferol) may be useful in the treatment of hypoparathyroidism in the near future.

There is little evidence to suggest that puerperal tetany (eclampsia) in heavily lactating bitches is the result of an interference in PTH secretion. Severe hypocalcemia and often hypophosphatemia develop near the time of peak lactation (approximately one to three weeks post partum), probably as the result of an imbalance between the rates of inflow and outflow from the extracellular fluid calcium pool. The administration of intravenous calcium to stop the tetany, combined with temporarily decreasing the lactational drain of calcium by removing the nursing puppies, usually corrects the disruption of calcium homeostasis in the majority of bitches. Supplemental dietary calcium and vitamin D, plus corticosteroids in certain cases, have proved useful in preventing relapses in bitches with puerperal tetany.

Corticosteroids have no logical basis for use in the above treatment regimen, but many clinicians are firmly convinced that they are beneficial. Since these drugs may lower serum calcium by interfering with intestinal calcium transport, their real value in eclampsia is uncertain.

### SUPPLEMENTAL READING

Burk, R. L., and Schaubhut, C. W., Jr.: Spontaneous primary hypoparathyroidism in a dog. J. Am. Anim. Hosp. Assn., 11:784–785, 1975.

Capen, C. C.: Functional and fine structural relationships of parathyroid glands. *In* Brandly, C. A., and Cornelius, C. E. (eds.): Advances in Veterinary Science and Comparative Medicine. New York, Academic Press, Inc., 19:249–286, 1975a.

Capen, C. C.: Parathyroid hormone, calcitonin, and cholecalciferol: The calcium regulating hormones. *In* McDonald, L. E. (ed.): Veterinary Endocrinology and Reproduction. 2nd ed. Philadelphia, Lea & Febiger, pp. 62–114, 1975b.

Hedhammar, A., Wu, F., Krook, L., et al.: Overnutrition and skeletal disease. An experimental study in growing Great Dane dogs. Cornell Vet., 64(Suppl. 5):1–160, 1974.

Krook, L.: Spontaneous hyperparathyroidism in the dog. A pathologic-anatomical Study. Acta Path. Microbiol. Scand., 41:(Suppl. 122):1–88, 1957.

Osborne, C. A., and Stevens, J. B.: Pseudohyperparathyroidism in the dog. J. Am. Vet. Med. Assn., 162:125–135, 1973.

Roth, S. I., and Capen, C. C.: Ultrastructural and functional correlations of the parathyroid glands. *In* Richter, G. W., and Epstein, M. A. (eds.): International Review of Experimental Pathology. New York, Academic Press, Inc., 13:162–221, 1974.

Rowland, G. N., Capen, C. C., and Nagode, L. A.: Experimental hyperparathyroidism in young cats. Path. Vet., 5:504–519, 1968.

Scott, P. P.: Special features of nutrition of cats, with observations on wild Felidae nutrition in the London Zoo. Symp. Soc. London, pp. 21–36, 1968.

# NUTRITIONAL HYPER-CALCITONINISM

LENNART KROOK, D.V.M.
*Ithaca, New York*

## CALCITONIN

Calcitonin is a peptide hormone manufactured by the thyroid C cells (C for calcitonin), also called parafollicular or light cells. Its function is to retard resorption of bone and thus decrease plasma calcium. Calcitonin also decreases the growth activity in articular and epiphyseal cartilage.

Calcitonin secretion is stimulated by hypercalcemia. It is further stimulated, and more powerfully so, by gastrin, a hormone produced by the G cells (G for gastrin) in the gastrointestinal mucosa—hence the term "the G.I.-thyroid axis." Gastrin secretion, in turn, is stimulated by high calcium concentration in the G.I. tract.

## NUTRITIONAL HYPERCALCITONINISM

A diet high in calcium—only twice the recommended levels will qualify—induces hypercalcemia. This stimulates calcitonin production and hence retardation of bone resorption, with the resulting decrease in plasma calcium. One stimulus for increased calcitonin production has thus been controlled but not the other. A high concentration of calcium in the G.I. tract stimulates gastrin production, so that hypercalcitoninism is maintained and thus retards bone resorption. Plasma calcium continues to decrease. High dietary calcium will thus eventually result in hypocalcemia.

## HYPERCALCITONINISM AND THE SKELETON

During growth of bones as organs, the cellular activity in articular cartilage and epiphyseal plates is great. The growth activity depends on proper protein and energy supply and on balance among growth hormone, thyroxine and calcitonin. Growth of bone as a tissue depends on proper balance between apposition and resorption. Apposition is, obviously, required for increase and renewal of bone mass, and resorption is of great importance in modeling of bones. The renewal, or turnover, rate of bone tissue is about 2 per cent *per day* in the growing dog.

Calcitonin acts on both cartilage cells and the resorbing osteocytes. Since the growth potential and the length of the growth period are greater in dogs of large-size breeds, such dogs are especially sensitive to dietary excesses of calcium, protein and energy.

### Calcitonin and Cartilage

OSTEOCHONDROSIS DISSECANS. Experimental exogenous hypercalcitoninism has been shown to cause retardation of the growth activity in articular and epiphyseal cartilage, the same events as occur in nutritional hypercalcitoninism.

In the epiphyseal plate, the resting cartilage, which grows by mitotic division under the influence of growth hormone, is converted into columnar and vesicular cartilage; this maturation is controlled by thyroxine. Vascular penetration of the distal row of vesicular cartilage cells occurs at a regular line, and osteoblasts lay down bone matrix along the chondroid core between the cartilage cells. The morphogenesis is similar in the articular cartilage but growth is slower.

Calcitonin prevents normal maturation of growth cartilage. Columnar cartilage is not transformed into vesicular cartilage. The cartilage cells remain small, and penetration by epiphyseal vessels does not occur. Unopened cartilage cells protrude into the epiphysis, and since there is no formation of epiphyseal trabeculae from such cartilage, a discontinuity between the articular cartilage and the osseous epiphysis results. Loose connective tissue and traumatic hemorrhages replace the trabeculae, and the thickened cartilage is usually elevated above the surrounding intact cartilage. This is the anatomic basis for the radiographic lucency typical of osteochondrosis dissecans.

The site of predilection is the humerus, where the lesions regularly occur in the central part of the caudal one third of the proximal epiphysis. This is by no means the exclusive site. Anatomically similar changes occur elsewhere, notably in the articular processes of vertebrae.

OTHER MANIFESTATIONS OF RETARDED CARTILAGE MATURATION. Normally, the costochondral junction is slightly wider than the cartilage or osseous parts of the rib. The epiphysis rapidly tapers off to the normal contour of the rib. In hypercalcitoninism, the costochondral junction is enlarged for two reasons. First, unopened cartilage grows down, and normal tapering is prevented. Second, there is failure of bone resorption in the perichondral ring (an extension of the cortical bone that embraces the growth cartilage like a cuff). The perichondral ring may be up to 1 cm. wide. The net result is a considerable widening of the costochondral area, the clinical appearance of which is very similar to that of rickets. The etiology and pathogenesis in the two conditions are, obviously, quite the opposite.

Downgrowth of cartilage and failure of formation of primary spongiosa can also occur at the epiphyseal plates of long bones. The discontinuity between cartilage and metaphyseal trabeculae results in epiphysiolysis, which is usually restricted and rarely results in complete detachment of the epiphysis.

### Calcitonin and Bone

HYPERTROPHIC OSTEODYSTROPHY. Bone resorption is retarded and apposition is normal (or enhanced because of the high amounts of protein and energy in many dog foods, especially if meat and meat by-products are the main ingredients). The net result is too much bone tissue. Sites of predilection are areas of rapid growth, i.e., the epiphyseo-metaphyseal regions. The distal radius-ulna usually shows the most pronounced signs. The periosteum is pushed peripherally by the enhanced apposition, and modeling into osteons is delayed. The periosteum is not firmly attached to bone and yields to pressure and tension, with resulting lameness.

ENOSTOSIS ("EOSINOPHILIC PANOSTEITIS"). The morphologic basis for this entity is excessive subperiosteal bone formation, especially in the diaphysis, and ectopic medullary bone formation. The lesions may occur in any long bone; the radius-ulna is the site of predilection.

HIP DYSPLASIA. During growth, modeling and remodeling of the femoral neck and head require very active resorption of bone, especially at the medial aspect of the neck. With retarded bone resorption, the angle between the shaft and the neck of the femur remains too obtuse (coxa valga) and, finally, the head does not reach into the acetabulum but rides on its lateral margin.

THE WOBBLER SYNDROME. The wobbler syndrome is characterized by incoordination of the pelvic and, more rarely, of the thoracic limbs; it is a rather frequent clinical sign in rapidly growing dogs of large-size breeds. The main anatomic feature is a pinching of the cervical spinal cord.

Expansion of the cervical spinal canal must be perfectly synchronized with growth of the spinal cord. Expansion is achieved by resorption of bone inside the border of the spinal canal, with the smooth surfaces receding toward areas of osteocytic osteolysis; surface osteoclasia is not involved.

In hypercalcitoninism, the retarded rate of bone resorption prevents proper expansion of the canal; the site of predilection is the cranial one third in cervical vertebrae II to VI. The dorsoventral diameter of the spinal canal is much decreased, and the contour is irregular. The spinal cord grows independently of the surrounding osseous structures and is therefore pinched by the retained bone. Demyelination of the cord is the foremost change in response to the pinching.

### SPECIFICITY OF THE CLINICAL MANIFESTATIONS

The various clinical entities summarized above have been induced experimentally by feeding high dietary calcium with high protein and energy. This does not imply that the signs are pathognomonic of hypercalcitoninism. Some of the entities do have multifactorial etiology. For example, hip dysplasia, enostosis and osteochondrosis dissecans can be induced experimentally by injection of sex hormones into the pregnant bitch or into neonatal puppies.

## DIAGNOSIS

The clinical diagnosis of the various expressions of hypercalcitoninism offers little difficulty. The clinical signs, radiographic appearance and dietary history are typical. The limitations of clinicopathologic tests should be pointed out. The changes in plasma calcium and alkaline phosphatase over long periods of time in experimental situations depict the pathogenesis of the lesions in bone and bones. The changes are subtle, however, and there are great variations between dogs. Single determinations of calcium and alkaline phosphatase in blood plasma are therefore of limited or no value in the diagnosis, or exclusion, of any of the skeletal manifestations of nutritional hypercalcitoninism.

## TREATMENT

Treatment of clinically manifest nutritional hypercalcitoninism obviously is directed toward removal of excessive dietary calcium (and excessive vitamin D as well as excessive protein and energy). The prognosis is guarded, at best. The enlargement of the epiphyseo-metaphyseal regions does regress somewhat, but restitution cannot be expected. If hip dysplasia has been induced as a result of retarded modeling during growth, remodeling cannot be expected after growth. Diseases caused by defects in cartilage growth are not likely to be corrected after cessation of growth.

Vitamin C has been implicated in the etiology of hypertrophic osteodystrophy. The function of vitamin C is to maintain the integrity of connective tissue cells. In vitamin C deficiency (scurvy) the mesenchymal cells do not mature, and thus there is an osteoblastic insufficiency, i.e., osteoporosis. This means *too little* bone tissue. Hypertrophic osteodystrophy, on the other hand, means *too much* bone tissue. No one will deny that, for unknown reasons, large doses of vitamin C may, in some instances, relieve the pain in hypertrophic osteodystrophy. However, this in no way implicates vitamin C in the etiology of hypertrophic osteodystrophy, no more than the relief of the clinical signs of hangover by consumption of aspirin establishes that condition as an aspirin deficiency.

In any nutritional disease, prophylaxis is of greatest importance. A dog should be fed according to his needs—not too little, not too much. Most pellet dog foods are well balanced. To "reward" a dog with an extra allowance of meat or to supplement the diet with vitamin and mineral pills can do nothing but cause an imbalance in the diet.

---

# POLYURIA AND POLYDIPSIA

J. A. JOLES
*Utrecht, The Netherlands*

*and* J. A. MULNIX, D.V.M.
*Fort Collins, Colorado*

## INTRODUCTION

Polydipsia (pd) and polyuria (pu) refer respectively to excessive fluid intake and urine production. Urine production in the cat and the dog should not exceed 50 ml./kg. body weight/day.

Although urine concentration varies considerably in the course of 24 hours in some dogs, it should not decrease to less than plasma osmolality. Fluid intake varies even more than urine production, being related not only to urine production but also to evaporative loss, water content of the diet, water content of the feces, lactation and other factors. Water consumption of 100 ml./kg. body weight/day may be considered as the upper limit of normal in the dog and the cat.

## REGULATION OF EXTRACELLULAR FLUID

Extracellular fluid (ECF) osmoconcentration is regulated largely by means of two complementary systems: fluid intake and urine production. Fluid intake is controlled by the thirst centers located in the hypothalamus. Urine volume is determined largely by the action of antidiuretic hormone (ADH), which is arginine vasopressin in all mammals except the Suidae (such as the domestic swine), in which it is lysine vasopressin (LVP). ADH is produced in the supraoptic nucleus (SON) and paraventricular nucleus (PVN) in the hypothalamus and is transported via the hypothalamic-pituitary tract to the posterior pituitary (neurohypophysis).

The two major physiologic influences affecting the hypothalamic nuclei and the thirst centers are blood osmotic pressure and blood volume.

Changes in the osmolality of the plasma are detected by osmoreceptors in the hypothalamus. Osmoreceptors are cells or clusters of cells that are neurally connected to the SON and PVN and that regulate the production of ADH in the nuclei as well as the release of ADH from the posterior pituitary. Osmoreceptors also influence the thirst centers which, in turn, induce drinking via cerebral stimulation.

Variations in blood volume are registered by the left atrial volume receptors as well as by baroreceptors in the carotid sinus and aortic arch. Impulses are transmitted via the vagus to the CNS, where they influence the release of ADH.

Little is known of the relative importance of the osmoreceptor and volume receptor systems. Under normal physiologic conditions, they work in concert to influence ADH secretion. In a state of overhydration, blood volume is raised and plasma osmolality is decreased, which depresses the secretion of ADH. When the organism is dehydrated, ADH secretion increases. The influence on the thirst centers is complementary.

Sodium (Na) concentration, which determines ECF volume, is regulated primarily by the mineralocorticoid aldosterone and falls outside the limits of this discussion. Although the two systems are linked, little is known of this coordination.

ADH causes the cells of the renal collecting tubules to become permeable to water, so that water passes from the collecting tubules into the medullary interstitium, from which it is transported to the cortex by the vasa recta. The passage of water through the tubular cells is probably not diffusion but "bulk flow" through aqueous "pores" in the cells. Vasopressin appears to increase the flow by enlarging the radius of individual pores.

The concentration gradient between tubular lumen, interstitium and blood vessel is only slight at any one level. However, the concentration gradient between the cortico-medullary junction, which is the boundary of the isotonic cortex, and the hypertonic medullary papilla is normally very large.

Severely dehydrated subjects produce a more concentrated urine than would be expected from the direct action of ADH alone and, similarly, chronically overhydrated patients, when deprived of water, achieve only a low maximal urinary concentration. These phenomena are due to changes in renal blood flow. In the polyuric state an increased flow in the juxtamedullary (deep) vasa recta "washes out" the solute concentration gradient, while in the oliguric state the flow is decreased and the "trapped" solute increases the concentration gradient.

## CONDITIONS ASSOCIATED WITH POLYURIA

The differential diagnoses of pd/pu include renal disease, diabetes mellitus, liver disease, hyperthyroidism, hypercalcemia associated with (pseudo)hyperparathyroidism, hyperadrenocorticism, insufficient ADH release (diabetes insipidus), nephrogenic diabetes insipidus, excessive water consumption (primary or psychogenic polydipsia) and the pyometra-endometritis complex.

Most of these diseases can be identified by evaluation of the clinical history, physical examination, blood and urine analyses and other routine diagnostic procedures. However, the differentiation of the different forms of diabetes insipidus, primary (psychogenic) polydipsia and, occasionally, hyperadrenocorticism usually requires the Pitressin response test or the water deprivation test.

Diabetes insipidus is a disease state in which there is an inability to concentrate urine, despite the absence of an osmotic diuresis. It is due to

1. The absence of antidiuretic hormone (ADH), as in the hereditary ADH-synthesis disorder in the Brattleboro strain of rats;

2. Unidentified etiology (the so-called idiopathic diabetes insipidus), which is the most frequently occurring category;

3. Traumatic, inflammatory or neoplastic insult to the hypothalamic nuclei or the hypothalamic-pituitary tracts, which results in partial or complete ADH deficiency;

4. Inability of the renal collecting tubules to respond to ADH, i.e., either congenital nephrogenic diabetes insipidus or, more often, an acquired disorder such as results from fibrosis of the renal medulla.

In all forms of diabetes insipidus, plasma osmolality tends to be raised because of the inability to concentrate urine. Polydipsia occurs in response to the hypertonicity of plasma caused by dehydration.

In primary or psychogenic polydipsia, the primary defect is excessive water consumption, and polyuria is the physiologic response to dilution of the extracellular fluid. The distinctive feature of primary polydipsia is that plasma osmolality tends to be decreased to the lower limit of normal or even below. Primary polydipsia can be caused by lesions in the thirst centers or in central cerebral structures. Psychogenic polydipsia is occasionally seen as a manifestation of abnormal behavior.

Polyuria is one of the leading symptoms of hyperadrenocorticism in the dog, and it may be the only clinical sign in the early stages of this disease. The polyuria appears to be directly related to corticosteroid excess, since it can be induced in the normal dog by the administration of corticosteroids, but the mechanism of action is not yet clear. There are two hypotheses: corticosteroids may block the release of ADH from the neurohypophysis, or corticosteroids may oppose the renal action of ADH.

## DIAGNOSTIC PROCEDURES

Since the patient suffering from diabetes insipidus must be treated for the remainder of his life, the decision to impose this treatment on both patient and owner must be based on a confirmed diagnosis.

Two diagnostic tests have proved useful:

**Pitressin Reponse Test.** The least laborious diagnostic approach is to

1. Measure urine flow during a control period of several hours (e.g., 24-hour collection in a metabolism cage).

2. Administer vasopressin (3 to 5 pressor units of Pitressin Tannate in Oil*, SC or IM).

---

*Pitressin® Tannate in Oil, Parke, Davis and Co., Detroit, Michigan 48232.

3. Repeat the measurement of urine production during a similar period of time.

Alternatively, the owner can be instructed to record the animal's water consumption during three consecutive days, before and after the injection of Pitressin. A dramatic reduction (75 per cent or more) in urine flow and water consumption indicates a defect in ADH production or release. Owing to the low medullary tonicity, a patient suffering from diabetes insipidus may fail to form highly concentrated urine in response to this first diagnostic injection, but the effect on diuresis and water intake should be dramatic. If not, a different underlying condition is suspected.

In the water-loaded patient there may be some reduction in urine flow because endogenous ADH production has previously been inhibited by the low plasma osmolality.

In the dog with hyperadrenocorticism there may be a slight decrease in urine volume, and urine concentration will be minimally affected.

When the reduction in urine volume is not impressive, an additional test is required. However, these procedures, as described below, necessitate measurements of plasma and urine osmolality (Uosm). Osmolality is preferable to specific gravity as an index of renal concentrating ability because the change in osmotic concentration is the response of interest and is only reflected approximately by change in specific gravity.

**Modified Water Deprivation Test.** The principle of this test is to determine whether endogenous ADH is released in response to dehydration and whether the kidneys respond to this stimulus.

The modified water deprivation test facilitates differentiation of central diabetes insipidus, nephrogenic diabetes insipidus, primary (psychogenic) polydipsia and hyperadrenocorticism (Fig. 1).

The test should not be performed in patients with severe renal disease or in renal failure.

The patient is deprived of food for 12 hours prior to, and water is withheld at, the start of the test. Urine is collected by spontaneous micturition if the patient is cooperative; otherwise, a urethral catheter is introduced (with a terminal cap or valve) so that the bladder can be emptied each hour. The bladder is emptied at the start of the test. The urine sample should be collected in a clean, dry receptacle to exclude possible

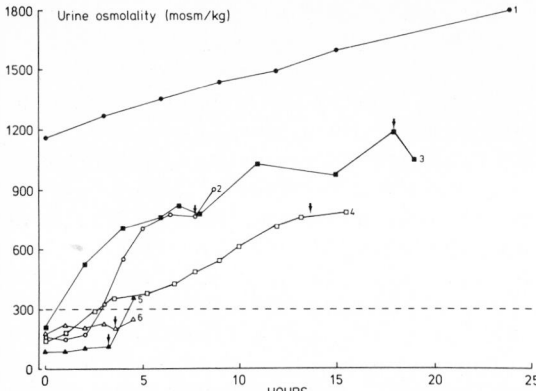

**Figure 1.** Modified water deprivation test. Urine osmolality (mosm./kg.) vs. time (hours). Plasma osmolality (300 mosm./kg.) is indicated by the solid horizontal line. The vertical arrows indicate the time of SC injection of synthetic LVP (3 to 5 pressor units). (*1*) Normal dog; (*2*) partial ADH deficiency diabetes insipidus; (*3*) primary polydipsia; (*4*) hyperadrenocorticism; (*5*) central diabetes insipidus; and (*6*) nephrogenic diabetes insipidus.

contamination that could influence the urine concentration. The patient is weighed hourly and the test is always terminated when the patient has lost 5 per cent of its original body weight, to avoid severe dehydration. Urine osmolality is determined immediately after each hourly collection. When there is a less than 5 per cent increase in urine osmolality between two consecutive samples, maximal urinary concentration by means of endogenous ADH has been achieved. (When the weight loss caused by dehydration is less than 2 to 3 per cent, the stimulus for endogenous ADH release is usually not maximal, and "false" Uosm plateaus may be observed [see curve 3, primary polydipsia, in Figure 1].) When there is less than a 5 per cent increase in urine osmolality between two consecutive samples, a urine sample is collected and, immediately thereafter, 2 to 3 pressor units of aqueous vasopressin (synthetic LVP*) are injected SC. This exceeds the dosage necessary for a maximal concentrating response but is less than the minimal dosage needed to induce a pressor response. The final urine sample is collected 45 to 60 minutes later, and the test is terminated.

In the normal dog, when Uosm reaches a plateau in response to dehydration, endogenous ADH production equals or exceeds the ADH tonicity needed to achieve a maximal renal response. Exogenous ADH causes little or no additional increase in Uosm (less than 10 per cent). The maximal urinary concentration achieved in the normal dog varies from 1100 to 2100 mosm./kg., depending largely on renal medullary tonicity.

Similar results are obtained in dogs with primary polydipsia, although maximal urinary concentration will be somewhat less. Several days of restricted water consumption will result in an increase in maximal urinary concentration in these patients. When the Uosm plateau is reached, the weight loss caused by dehydration in the normal or primary polydipsic dog rarely exceeds 3 per cent. Often, at the termination of the test, in cases of primary polydipsia (or normal dogs), the subjects first start eating *before* drinking, indicating that the sensation of thirst is less than that of hunger.

The patient with severe central diabetes insipidus or nephrogenic diabetes insipidus will not be able to concentrate urine to a level greater than plasma osmolality (300 mosm./kg.). However, after exogenous ADH there is a 50 to 500 per cent increase in Uosm in patients with central diabetes insipidus, while there is essentially no change in those with nephrogenic diabetes insipidus. The subject with partial diabetes insipidus will be able to concentrate urine to levels varying between 300 and 1000 mosm./kg. after water deprivation, and there will be a further increase of 10 to 50 per cent after exogenous ADH.

The patient with hyperadrenocorticism has a Uosm plateau which is similar to that of the patient with partial diabetes insipidus, but exogenous ADH causes little or no additional increase in Uosm. The weight loss due to dehydration in partial hypothalamic-neurohypophyseal diabetes insipidus or hyperadrenocorticism is not as rapid as is the case with severe hypothalamic-neurohypophyseal or nephrogenic diabetes insipidus.

The duration of the test varies considerably. In patients with severe diabetes insipidus the test must usually be terminated after 4 hours, while in normal dogs and those with primary polydipsia a period of 12 to 18 hours of dehydration may be required to achieve maximal ADH release. This entails a weight loss of 3 to 5 per cent.

---

*Vasopressin synthetic, Sandoz Pharmaceuticals, E. Hanover, New Jersey 07936.

## THERAPY

ADH *per se* is the most appropriate therapy in cases of insufficient ADH release (diabetes insipidus). The preparation used most frequently is Pitressin® Tannate in Oil (Parke, Davis), a suspension of ADH in peanut oil, which is administered subcutaneously or intramuscularly. It should be used only in cases of diabetes insipidus with a proven hypothalamic-neurohypophyseal–dependent etiology. Two to three units should be administered once every 36 to 48 hours, depending on the urine production.

*It is essential to warm and shake the ampule thoroughly so that the brown deposit, which is the active substance, is uniformly distributed in the suspension.*

Excessive dosage may cause water retention, intoxication and hyponatremia, as in the Schwartz-Bartter syndrome (inappropriate secretion of antidiuretic hormone, recognized in man). Immunologic reactions against exogenous ADH have not been reported in veterinary medicine.

A different form of therapy is Minrin (DDVP)*, which is used as a nasal spray in human patients. In veterinary practice, it can be administered as eye drops, but this poses difficulties which are often insurmountable to the owner in the case of exophthalmic dogs or poorly manageable cats. In addition, it is expensive.

Primary polydipsia, especially in a young patient, should be approached with a change in the owner-pet relation. Frequent exercise and play, possibly supplemented by a light sedative (e.g., chlorpromazine), may be sufficient to break what has become a habit out of boredom or isolation.

The excess urine production in the patient with nephrogenic diabetes insipidus is not easily reduced. A diet with a low salt and protein content may have some beneficial effect. In our limited experience, chlorothiazide† did not have the marked antidiuretic effect described in medical literature when administered to patients with nephrogenic diabetes insipidus.

### SUPPLEMENTAL READING

Kleeman, C. R., and Vorherr, H.: Water metabolism and the neurohypophyseal hormones. *In* Bondy, P. K., and Rosenberg, L. E. (eds.): Duncan's Diseases of Metabolism. 7th ed. Philadelphia, W. B. Saunders Co., 1974.

---

*Desamino-(D-Arg⁸)-vasopressin, Ferring A. B., Malmö, Sweden.

†Diuril®, Merck & Co., Inc., West Point, Pennsylvania 19486.

---

# TUMORS OF THE TESTES

DANIËL R. G. MATTHEEUWS, D.V.M.,
*and* FRANK H. COMHAIRE, M.D.
*Ghent, Belgium*

## INTRODUCTION

Testicular tumors are remarkably common in the dog; more than 90 per cent of the testicular tumors reported in all domestic animals occur in the dog. In systematic autopsies, their frequency was reported to be 16 per cent in unselected adult dogs and 57 per cent in aged animals; they affect predominantly dogs that have passed midlife, more than 80 per cent occurring beyond the age of 7 years. Neoplasms of cryptorchid testicles, however, tend to occur at younger ages. Some breed predisposition is presumed, since the boxer, the poodle and the wire-haired fox terrier appeared to be overrepresented in some reports; however, this could be due to the higher incidence of these breeds in the population of dogs investigated. An association exists between testicular neoplasia and cryptorchidism but this varies greatly with the tumor type. More tumors are found in the right than in the left testicle, and more than one third occur bilaterally. The coexistence of two or more tumors of different types in one animal is common and amounts to 35% according to some reports.

Changes sufficiently striking to be recognized by the owners can be either local, owing to the presence of a mass in the scrotum, inguinal canal or abdomen, or general, appearing as the so-called "feminization syndrome."

The following is a histologic classification of tumors of animal testes (Nielsen and Lein, 1974):

I.  Germ cell tumors
    A.  Seminoma
        1.  Intratubular, with or without invasion
        2.  Diffuse type
    B.  Embryonal carcinoma
    C.  Teratoma
II.  Sex cord–stromal (gonadostromal) tumors
    A.  Sertoli (sustentacular) cell tumors
        1.  Intratubular, with or without invasion
        2.  Diffuse type
    B.  Leydig (interstitial) cell tumors
        1.  Solid diffuse type
        2.  Cystic-vascular (angiomatoid)
        3.  Pseudoadenomatous
    C.  Tumors with intermediate Sertoli-cell and Leydig-cell differentiation
III.  Multiple primary tumors
IV.  Mesotheliomas
V.  Stromal and vascular tumors
VI.  Unclassified tumors

In the dog, testicular tumors generally originate from either Sertoli cells, cells of the germinative layer, or Leydig cells. Tumorous growths of embryonal tissue, such as embryonal carcinoma and teratoma, have not yet been reported. Mesotheliomas and stromal and vascular tumors are extremely rare, and metastatic localization in the testicle is exceptional. Whereas certain tumors cannot be classified histologically, others are composed of mixed cell types, either combined within the same tumorous mass or appearing as multiple separate tumors within one or both testicles.

Although most testicular tumors in the dog are benign, some are malignant, and metastases of all histologic types have been reported. Malignancy occurs in about 10 per cent of Sertoli cell tumors; it is rare in seminomas and exceptional in Leydig cell tumors.

## CLINICAL FINDINGS

**Sertoli Cell Tumors.** The incidence of Sertoli cell tumors is similar to that of the seminomas and somewhat lower than that of the Leydig cell tumors. Sertoli cell tumors are relatively slow growing, noninvasive and painless, and they may become very large. About half the tumors have a diameter of less than 1 cm.; others may be 10 cm. or more. Normal testicular tissue persists as a compressed peripheral rim in the neoplastic testicle. The tumor is larger than the normal testis and generally similar in shape, although intra-abdominal tumors tend to be more irregular. Slicing of the typical gross specimen reveals a small, pale, brownish-yellow to white, firm or hard mass, irregularly lobulated by rather dense white fibrous bands. Tiny cysts filled with clear fluid are often conspicuous, and the neoplastic tissue commonly has a greasy cut surface. Generally, Sertoli cell tumors occur in testes with tubular atrophy due to either cryptorchidism or senility. Indeed, more than 50 per cent of these tumors are found in undescended testicles, of which three fifths are located in the abdomen and two fifths in the inguinal ring.

Cryptorchidism occurs in about 10 per cent of all adult animals, and the abdominal location is more common than the inguinal one. Whereas in the scrotal testis tumorous degeneration occurs with equal frequency in the right and left testicles, right-side involvement predominates in dogs with cryptorchid Sertoli cell tumors. In the latter, the right-to-left ratio is 1.8:1.0, being similar to the ratio for cryptorchidism. Sertoli cell tumors, although usually unilateral, occur bilaterally in about 10 per cent of cases.

In about one third of the cases, the tumor gives rise to the so-called "feminization syndrome." The first manifestation of this syndrome is usually an alteration of the coat, owing to failure of normal growth, shedding and replacement of hair. Symmetrical hairless areas appear at the sites of maximal abrasion or wear, i.e., the posterior and lateral aspects of the thighs, the ventral thorax and abdomen and occasionally the neck and shoulders, if the animal wears a collar or harness. The dry and brittle hair can be pulled out readily and painlessly. The skin of the hairless sites is often abnormally thin and presents, in some cases, a diffuse dusky-purple pigmentation. In several instances, failure of normal hair growth after clipping first called attention to the disease. Elongation of the nipples, with or without thickening of the mammary tissue, occurs particularly in the two caudal sets of glands. The glands resemble those of recently lactating females and in a few there is secretion of a serous or milky fluid. About one fourth of the dogs with feminization have a definite history of attracting other male dogs but the affected dog usually attempts to fight off the other dog. Affected dogs usually display pendulous swelling of the prepuce, varying degrees of penile atrophy, depressed libido, female posture of micturition, lethargy and premature aging.

Both the size and the location of the tumor appear to be related to the development of this syndrome. The average size of the neoplastic testicle is about two to three times greater in dogs with the syndrome than in those without it, and feminization is more frequent when the tumor is localized in a cryptorchid testis. The incidence of feminization increases from about 15 per cent with scrotally located tumors to 50 per cent in cases of inguinal and 70 per cent in cases of abdominal localization.

Whereas dogs with Sertoli cell tumors without feminization do not show important changes in the prostate for their age, those with feminization can present either atrophy or enlargement of the gland. The latter is usually due to squamous metaplasia of the epithelial elements with formation of large epidermoid cysts or suppurative inflammation. When the Sertoli cell tumor is unilateral, the opposite testis is atrophied, particularly if feminization is present.

**Seminoma.** Seminomas are derived from cells of the germinative layer in atrophic tubules. The tumor passes through an *"in-situ"* or intratubular phase before it invades the interstitial tissue to form a diffuse neoplasm. The diameter of the diffuse tumor ranges from 0.1 to 10 cm., being greater than 3 cm. in more than half the cases. The tumor usually conforms to the shape of the testis and is lobulated by delicate fibrous septa into firm, bulging masses. They have a friable yellowish-white cut surface, frequently mottled by areas of necrosis and hemorrhage. This neoplasm can coexist with either Leydig cell or Sertoli cell tumors in the same or opposite testis.

As for the Sertoli cell tumors, cryptorchidism is a predisposing factor, nearly one third of seminomas being found in cryptorchid testicles. Again, right-side involvement predominates in dogs with cryptorchid seminomas. Though seminomas are usually unilateral and solitary, 10 to 18 per cent are reported to be bilateral and a few are multiple.

Clinical changes are exceptional in dogs with a seminoma; a pendulous penile sheath was reported in one dog and alopecia in two. Skin changes typical of feminization are frequently seen in dogs with the combination of a seminoma and a Leydig cell tumor; feminization has been reported in dogs with both a seminoma and a Sertoli cell tumor, as well as in dogs with all three tumors.

Prostatic disease, including benign hyperplasia, abscesses and cysts, was found in one third of the patients and occurred more frequently in association with scrotal seminomas. Perineal hernias and perianal adenomas are frequently associated with seminomas.

Generally, there are few obvious changes in the other testis, except for slight atrophy if the tumor is relatively large.

**Leydig Cell Tumors.** This is the most common variety of canine testicular tumors. Most of these tumors are found by chance at postmortem examination; they have diameters of 1 to 2 cm. and lie within the substance of the testis. They are well-circumscribed and have a reddish-yellow, bulging, homogeneous cut surface. The larger, clinically apparent tumors are often cystic and may measure up to 9 cm. in diameter. Each consists of a single cyst, which is filled with a colorless fluid, lined by a yellowish heterogeneous tissue and surrounded by a dense fibrous capsule. Frequently, there is a remnant of the testis at one edge of the tumor. Leydig cell tumors can be either solitary or multiple in the same or in the opposite testis, bilateral involvement occurring in some 40 per cent of the cases.

In contrast to the other testicular tumors, Leydig cell tumors occur rarely in cryptorchid testes. No predilection exists for the right or the left side.

Owing to their small size, 75 per cent of Leydig cell tumors are clinically undetectable; in the remaining 25 per cent an enlargement of the testis is noticed. Leydig cell tumors only exceptionally induce feminization, whereas alopecia and other skin changes, without signs of feminization, are more common. Prostatic diseases and/or perianal gland adenomas occur in about one third of the patients.

The contralateral testis shows no characteristic change.

## ENDOCRINOLOGY

It is generally accepted that the so-called "feminization syndrome" is produced by hyperestrogenism. This hypothesis is sustained by several arguments:

1. The clinical syndrome and the pathologic changes are similar to those produced by injections of estrogens.

2. Estrogens were recovered in high concentrations from both the tumor tissue and the urine of some affected animals.

3. Animals return to normal following surgical removal of the tumor, and recurrence of symptoms occurs concomitantly with the appearance of metastases.

Normal testes of adult dogs produce both testosterone and estradiol, the concentration of these steroids in peripheral and spermatic venous blood varying widely among unselected animals. We found a strong correlation between the testosterone and the estradiol concentrations in spermatic venous blood. An abnormal steroid composition was found in 8 out of 15 samples of spermatic venous blood draining tumorous testes, the estradiol concentration being more elevated than would be expected in light of the corresponding testosterone level. Such abnormal steroid composition was found in 2 out of 3 Sertoli cell tumors, 3 out of 8 seminomas and 3 out of 4 Leydig cell tumors. These data suggest that the abnormal steroid secretion is dependent on the tumorous growth itself, the type of testicular cell of which the tumorous proliferation consists being of less importance.

We could not detect differences in the concentration of either testosterone or estradiol between tumor-bearing dogs with and those without feminization.

## DIAGNOSIS

Little difficulty arises in the diagnosis if the dog presents signs of feminization and a testicular tumor can be palpated. One should suspect an ectopic (nonpalpable) testicular tumor when a dog is presented with signs of feminization and one atrophic testis is found on palpation of the scrotum. The enlarged testicle may be found in the scrotum, the inguinal region or the abdominal cavity. However, the number of such cases is small in comparison with those not presenting feminization. In the latter, the disease is frequently overlooked, because of the small size of the testicular tumor. Very careful palpation of the testes should be performed as a rule in all middle-aged and old dogs, especially if they are cryptorchid. A definite diagnosis can be made only by histologic examination.

## TREATMENT AND PROPHYLAXIS

Since cryptorchidism is often hereditary and predisposes to tumorous degeneration, all cryptorchid dogs should be castrated prophylactically. Castration is equally indicated for all types of testicular tumors, if the neoplasm has not metastasized. The signs of feminization and alopecia disappear spontaneously within about four months.

In patients with metastases, palliative surgery, irradiation or chemotherapy may be considered.

## PROGNOSIS

The prognosis is related to the type, the location and the extent of neoplastic involvement, as well as to the presence or absence of metastases. Regardless of the tumor type, metastases can be found in the sublumbar, iliac, mesenteric and inguinal lymph nodes and in the liver, spleen, lungs, pancreas and kidneys.

Histologic examination of the deep inguinal lymph nodes and a cross-section of the spermatic cord adjacent to the site of incision should be carried out whenever possible in order to aid in the prognosis. Whereas the prognosis is usually favorable for the scrotal tumors, it is less so for dogs with intra-abdominal tumors, because the primary tumor tends to be larger when diagnosed, and transabdominal spread is common.

## COMMENT

Alopecia and feminization have been described in dogs without testicular tumors, seborrheic disorders and a ceruminous otitis externa being part of the clinical syndrome in these dogs.

Although this syndrome is usually ascribed to hyperestrogenism, no differences could be detected between affected animals and normal controls in the concentrations of estradiol and testosterone, in either the peripheral or the spermatic venous blood. Moreover, there was no difference in the concentration ratio of these steroids. The cause of alopecia and feminization in some male dogs without testicular neoplasia is still obscure.

## SUPPLEMENTAL READING

Bostock, D. E., and Owen, L. N.: Neoplasia in the Cat, Dog and Horse. London, Wolfe Medical Publications, Ltd., 1975, pp. 72–76.

Brodey, R. S., and Martin, J. E.: Sertoli cell neoplasm in the dog. J. Am. Vet. Med. Assn., 133:249–257, 1958.

Comhaire, F., and Mattheeuws, D.: Testosterone and oestradiol in dogs with testicular tumours. Acta Endocrinol., 77:408–416, 1974.

Comhaire, F., and Mattheeuws, D.: Testosterone and oestradiol in spermatic venous blood in normal dogs and in dogs with testicular tumours. Proc. Voorjaarsdagen, 1975, pp. 34–35.

Dow, C.: Testicular tumours in the dog. J. Comp. Pathol., 72:247–265, 1962.

Kasbohm, C.: Hodenneoplasien des Hundes aus klinischer Sicht. Tierärztl. Prax., 2:435–444, 1974.

Lipowitz, A. J., Schwartz, A., Wilson, G. P., and Ebert, J. W.: Testicular neoplasm and concomitant clinical changes in the dog. J. Am. Vet. Med. Assn., 163:1364–1368, 1973.

Mattheeuws, D., and Comhaire, F.: Oestradiol and testosterone in male dogs with alopecia and feminization without testicular neoplasia. Brit. Vet. J., 131:65–69, 1975.

Moulton, J. E.: Tumors in Domestic Animals. Berkeley, California, University of California Press, 1961, pp. 153–159.

Nielsen, S. W., and Lein, D. H.: Histological classification and nomenclature of tumours of animal testes. Bull. WHO, 50:71–78, 1974.

Reif, J. S., and Brodey, R. S.: The relationship between cryptorchidism and canine testicular neoplasia. J. Am. Vet. Med. Assn., 155:2005–2010, 1969.

Scully, R. E., and Coffin, D. L.: Canine testicular tumors. Cancer, 5:592–605, 1972.

---

# OVARY, OVARIAN HORMONES AND CONTRA-CEPTIVES

F. N. THOMPSON, D.V.M.,
and L. E. McDONALD, D.V.M.
Athens, Georgia

## PROESTRUS AND ESTRUS

The appearance of a sanguineous discharge from the vulva signals the beginning of an estrous cycle. Puberty in the bitch generally occurs between ages 8 and 14 months, occurring earlier in the small breeds. Rapid follicular growth transpires during proestrus, with follicles reaching a mature size of 3.0 to 5.0 mm. in diameter. The duration of proestrus varies from 5 to 12 days, with plasma estrogen peaking late in proestrus.

The onset of estrus is dated from the time when the bitch will first accept the male, a practical event for dating the cycle. Additionally, the onset of estrus coincides with or follows closely a surge in luteinizing hormone. Spontaneous ovulation usually occurs within 5 days after the onset of estrus; 40 per cent of the bitches ovulate within 2 days and 70 per cent within 3 days. The pubertal bitch tends to ovulate on the

first day of estrus; in older bitches ovulation occurs within 5 days of onset of estrus. An individual bitch completes her multiple ovulations within 24 hours following the first ovulation. The duration of estrus varies from only 1 to 3 days to two weeks but averages 7 to 9 days. Follicular cysts from atretic follicles have been associated with prolonged estrus. Symptoms disappeared without treatment.

The best time to breed for maximal fertility appears to be on the first day of estrus and again approximately 3 days later. Maturation of ova occurs in the oviducts, since ova are released prior to the extrusion of the first polar body. Fertility has been reported to be high following a single mating on the first day of estrus; therefore sperm cells have a long viability in the female reproductive tract. Conception rates of 80 per cent to greater than 95 per cent have been reported in some colonies of bitches.

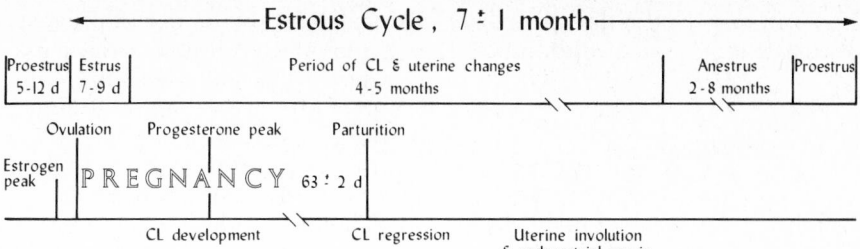

**Figure 1.**   The estrous cycle of the bitch.

## CORPUS LUTEUM AND UTERINE CHANGES

Plasma progesterone levels rise even before ovulation; then, with development of corpora lutea, progesterone levels rise rapidly before the end of estrus and reach a zenith approximately 20 to 25 days post ovulation, gradually waning before their decline at parturition. The ovary is necessary for pregnancy maintenance. In nonpregnant bitches progesterone levels tend to trail off slowly for several weeks longer than in pregnant bitches. The clinical condition of pseudopregnancy, while not understood endocrinologically, is not characterized by abnormal progesterone levels. Likewise, its occurrence is not related to pyometra. The formed corpora lutea bulge slightly above the surface of the ovary. At first they are bright pink, changing to blanched yellow by 50 days post ovulation.

Involution of the uterus requires a period of approximately 120 to 150 days post ovulation. The reason for this lengthy interval is the fact that the endometrium of the canine is particularly sensitive to estrogens and progestins. Administration of either hormone during the time of endometrial hypertrophy predisposes the animal to cystic hyperplastic endometritis, which appears to be related to pyometra. Therefore, use of these hormones is best reserved for the anestrous period.

## ANESTRUS

A variable period (2 to 8 months) of anestrus follows uterine involution. The duration of anestrus determines the interestrous interval, since the life span of the corpora lutea is relatively constant. This interval is generally 7 to 8 months in dogs up to 5 years of age. Longer periods of anestrus are com-

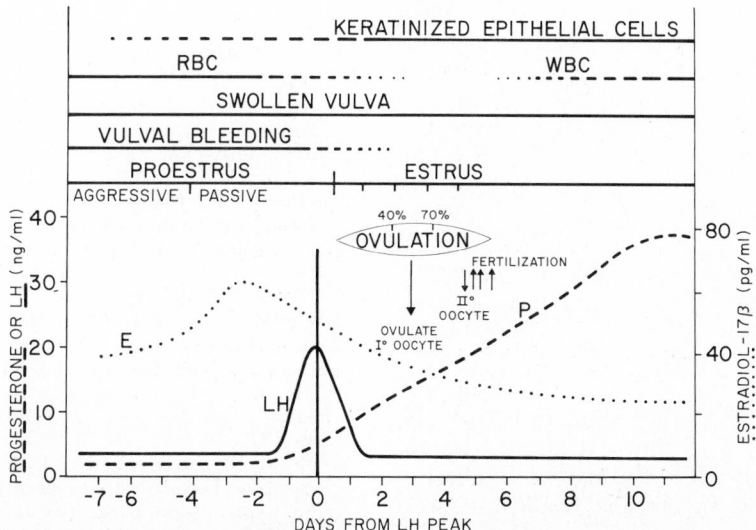

**Figure 2.**   Changes in hormone levels and other events associated with proestrus and estrus in the bitch.

mon in older bitches. Follicular growth is minimal during this period of endometrial quiescence.

*(handwritten: ECP 2mg/ml = 4/10 to 1/20 cc, One 6/10 cc 6.66)*

## ESTRUS INDUCTION

Induction of estrus in the persistently anestrous bitch has been previously disappointing; therefore the work of Arbeiter and Dreier is encouraging. First, to initiate the estrus cycle, 0.1 to 0.5 mg. of estradiol benzoate (IM or SC) was given every second or third day. These injections were given 2 to 4 times or until the vaginal smear revealed that proestrus had begun. The treatment was discontinued if proestrus had not been initiated. However, if the estrogen treatment resulted in proestrus, FSH injections were begun 4 to 8 days after proestrus began. The FSH injections were given every other day until the vaginal smear revealed that estrus had been initiated. Dosage for the FSH was 25 to 50 IU (IM or SC) in the form of PMS (pregnant mare serum). Fifteen of 19 such treated bitches conceived.

## CONTRACEPTIVES

Hormone treatments for the prevention of estrus, the suppression of estrus or the prevention of nidation are efficacious; however, the risk of resultant uterine disease may exist. Oral and injectable progestins are marketed. These function by blocking gonadotropin secretion, thereby inhibiting folliculogenesis and ovulation. Oral progestins, megestrol acetate (Ovaban® [Schering] and Ovarid® [Glaxo]) and medroxyprogesterone (Perlutex® tablets [Leo]) are available for administration to prevent estrus during a specific period. These drugs are contraindicated in the presence of uterine or mammary disease. The manufacturer of Ovaban recommends that 0.55 mg./kg. be given daily for 32 days if therapy is begun during anestrus. Administration should begin at least one week prior to proestrus. Ovaban, 2.2 mg./kg. daily for 8 days, is used to suppress estrus if administration is begun during the *first 3 days* of proestrus. In general, male attraction was found to disappear in 3 to 4 days and other signs of estrus disappeared in 6 to 8 days. It should be remembered that while the use of Ovaban to suppress estrus in clinical trials appeared safe, a much greater risk of causing uterine

damage following use of progestin has been shown to exist during proestrus or estrus as compared to anestrus. Following the cessation of either Ovaban treatment, animals returned to estrus in a range of 1 to 7 months. Most returned to estrus 4 to 6 months later. Fertility was not altered.

The injectable progestin, medroxyprogesterone acetate (Perlutex and Anovulin® [Berk]) in aqueous form, is marketed in Europe. This drug results in the long-term prevention of estrus. The recommended dosage is 50 mg. for dogs that weigh less than 40 kg. and 50 to 75 mg. for dogs that weigh more than 40 kg. An average delay in return to estrus of 12.5 months (range 6 to 26.5 months) has been reported. The drug should be administered only during anestrus after the animal has experienced one estrus. Therefore, to avoid the unwanted interaction with endogenous estrogens and progestins, the drug should not be given until 5 months post estrus. Treatments must be repeated every six months for continued postponement of estrus, but anestrus should not be extended beyond 2 years. Because hair loss has been reported to occur over the injection site, an inconspicuous site is recommended.

Preliminary studies concerning the use of an intravaginal pessary have given mixed responses. Likewise, the use of androgens to block gonadotropin output is being investigated but has not been completely acceptable.

### SUPPLEMENTAL READING

Arbeiter, K., and Dreier, H. K.: Pathognostik und Behandlungsmöglichkeiten der Sub-, Anöstrie und Anaphrodisie bei Zuchthündinnen. Berlin Münch. Tierärztl. Wschr., 85:341–344, 1972.

Edquist, L. E., Johansson, E. D. B., Kasström, H., Olsson, S. E., and Richkind, M.: Blood plasma levels of progesterone and oestradiol in the dog during the oestrous cycle and pregnancy. Acta Endocrinol. (Copenh.) 78:554–654, 1975.

Nett, F. M., Akbar, A. M., Phemister, R. D., Holst, P. A., Reichert, L. E., and Niswender, G. D.: Levels of luteinizing hormone, estradiol and progesterone in serum during the estrous cycle and pregnancy in the beagle bitch. Proc. Soc. Exp. Biol. Med., 148:134–139, 1975.

Smith, M. S., and McDonald, L. E.: Serum levels of luteinizing hormone and progesterone during the estrous cycle, pseudopregnancy and pregnancy in the dog. Endocrinology, 94:404–412, 1974.

# ECTOPIC HORMONE PRODUCTION BY NONENDOCRINE NEOPLASMS

CARL A. OSBORNE, D.V.M.,
*and* SHIRLEY D. JOHNSTON,
D.V.M.
*St. Paul, Minnesota*

## PARANEOPLASTIC SYNDROMES

Neoplasms are often associated with polysystemic signs that cannot be explained by direct invasion of host tissues. In the past, these signs have been lumped under the category of cachexia of malignancy, assumed to be an atypical manifestation of the neoplasm, or attributed to the presence of a concomitant but unrelated disease. In recent years, however, it has become apparent that many clinical signs, biochemical disorders and morphologic abnormalities associated with malignancy are the direct result of immunologic (immune-complex glomerulonephritis, amyloidosis, etc.) and endocrine disorders initiated by the neoplasm.

It has been reported that 15 per cent of human patients with cancer suffer from "paraneoplastic" effects of neoplasms as opposed to the disorders that cancer causes by direct invasion of host tissues (Hall, 1974). Furthermore, the incidence and severity of paraneoplastic manifestations increase with the severity of the neoplastic process. It has been estimated that approximately 75 per cent of all uncured human cancer patients will develop paraneoplastic disorders during the course of their illness (Hall, 1974). Although the incidence of paraneoplastic syndromes in animals is unknown, improved understanding of the biologic behavior of neoplasms and improved laboratory, radiographic and biopsy evaluation of animals with cancer have revealed that they do occur. Continued use of automation for routine biochemical screening may provide a better indication of the frequency of paraneoplastic syndromes in the future.

## ECTOPIC ENDOCRINOPATHIES

### INTRODUCTION

Some systemic derangements associated with neoplasms may be mediated by circulating hormones. It is well known that primary tumors arising from pituitary, parathyroid, thyroid, adrenal, gonadal or pancreatic tissue may produce excessive amounts of the hormone usually produced by that tissue. It is becoming increasingly evident that nonendocrine neoplasms may also produce hormones that in turn induce paraneoplastic syndromes (Table 1). Development of sensitive methods for identification and quantitative measurement of hormones and their biologic effects in man have resulted in widespread recognition of these once rarely recognized phenomena. Because hormone production originates in cells not ordinarily involved in hormone synthesis, these syndromes are commonly called "ectopic endocrinopathies." They include the production of hormones by neoplasms of nonendocrine origin, and the production of the "wrong" hormones by neoplastic endocrine glands. Hormones reported to be produced by nonendocrine neoplasms in man include adrenocorticotropic hormone, alpha- and beta-melanocyte–stimulating hormone, antidiuretic hormone (vasopressin), corticotropin-releasing factor, erythropoietin, gastrin, glucagon, gonadotropins, growth hormone, hypoglycemia-producing factor, parathormone, prolactin, prostaglandins and thyroid-stimulating factor (Odell, 1974).

The mechanism(s) by which nonendocrine neoplastic tissue synthesizes molecules with hormonal activity is not com-

**Table 1.** *Ectopic Endocrinopathies*

| SYNDROME | HORMONE | TUMOR SITE AND TYPE | | |
|---|---|---|---|---|
| | | *Human* | *Canine* | *Feline* |
| Cushing's syndrome | ACTH; MSH | Carcinomas of lung, pancreas, thymus, thyroid, etc. | NR | NR |
| Galactorrhea | Prolactin | Renal cell carcinoma | NR | NR |
| Gynecomastia | Chorionic gonadotropin | Carcinomas of liver, esophagus, etc. | NR | NR |
| Hypercalcemia | PTH; sterols; prostaglandins | Carcinomas of lung, kidney, ovary, etc. | Lymphoma, perianal gland carcinoma, mammary adenocarcinoma | Lymphoma |
| Hypoglycemia | Insulin-like | Retroperitoneal fibromas and sarcomas, etc. | Lymphoma | NR |
| Inappropriate antidiuresis | ADH | Carcinomas of lung, pancreas, prostate, etc. | NR | NR |
| Polycythemia | Erythropoietin-like | Renal cell carcinomas,* cerebellar hemangioblastomas, etc. | Renal cell carcinoma* | NR |

NR=not reported.
*By definition, renal carcinomas are not the source of ectopic erythropoietin; see text.

pletely understood; however, activation (so-called derepression) of genetic structural information has been hypothesized. This genetic information is present in the DNA of all cells but is normally active only in those endocrine tissues that synthesize the hormone. During neoplasia it is proposed that tumor cells undergo dedifferentiation, lose certain genetic repressor mechanisms (i.e., they are derepressed) and express previously inhibited genetic information. The fact that ectopic endocrinopathies in man are manifestations of "simple" polypeptide hormone production rather than "complex" steroid hormone production supports this hypothesis. Polypeptide production is a capability of every cell, whereas steroid hormone synthesis requires an orderly sequence of several enzymatic steps presumably not present in dedifferentiated neoplastic tissue. Derepression is probably not a random event, as demonstrated by the frequent association of specific histologic tumor types in man with specific hormone excesses (Smith, 1975).

The production of hormones by neoplasms of nonendocrine tissues is of great clinical significance. Recognition of these syndromes may aid in the detection of un- suspected neoplasms and may prevent the formulation of therapy directed at nonexistent causes. The therapeutic implications are especially important, since the clinical and biochemical characteristics of ectopic endocrinopathies are often similar to those associated with classic hyperfunctional states of endocrine glands. In addition, correction of the metabolic effects of hormone excess in a patient known to have a neoplasm may produce dramatic clinical improvement and may favor resection of a tumor, the systemic effects of which otherwise suggest metastasis. Detection of significant concentrations of an ectopic hormone in serum or plasma or detection of the biologic effect of the hormone (hypercalcemia, erythrocytosis, hypokalemia, hyponatremia, etc.) may precede recognition of the neoplasm. Several cases have been reported in man in which discovery of an ectopic endocrine syndrome provided the initial clue to the presence of an occult neoplasm in early stages of development. Early recognition of the tumor facilitated resection or treatment of the neoplasm before it could develop further. Ectopic hormones may also serve as a biologic marker (or tag) of a neoplasm. Serial measurement of the ectopic hormone, or its biologic effects, may serve as a useful index of therapeutic response and may signal recurrence of the neoplasm following therapy.

To prove the neoplastic origin of ectopic hormones, several criteria have been suggested, including (a) coexistence of a neoplasm and an endocrine syndrome; (b) detection of nonsuppressible concentrations of the causative hormone in blood or urine; (c) detection of large quantities of the hormone in the neoplasm, and demonstration of an arteriovenous gradient in the hormone concentration across the tumor vascular bed; (d) proof that the hormone did not originate from its usual glandular site; (e) disappearance of, or significant reduction in, the endocrine syndrome following removal or destruction of the tumor; and (f) recurrence of the endocrine syndrome in those patients in whom the tumor recurs. Although many of these criteria have been fulfilled in human patients with several types of neoplastic endocrinopathies, to date most studies in veterinary medicine have been limited to items a, d, e and f. Although the analogy between ectopic endocrinopathies in dogs and cats and in man is far from complete, there have been enough observations made in dogs to support the view that many forms of canine ectopic endocrinopathy can be more completely understood by studying the human analog. With the exception of pseudohyperparathyroidism, the following discussions of ectopic endocrinopathies are based primarily on studies performed in man. This information should provide a basis for more complete evaluation of ectopic endocrinopathies encountered in animals in the future.

## PSEUDOHYPERPARATHYROIDISM

### ETIOPATHOGENESIS

A variety of diseases have the potential to cause hypercalcemia (refer to article on "Hypercalcemic Nephropathy" for details). Hypercalcemia caused by primary parathyroid neoplasms is caused by release of excessive quantities of parathormone. The result is increased mobilization of calcium and phosphorus from bone, increased calcium reabsorption from the renal tubules and intestinal tract and decreased renal tubular reabsorption of phosphorus. The concentration of serum calcium rises, while the serum concentration of phosphorus (in nonuremic patients) falls.

Hypercalcemia associated with malignancy of nonparathyroid tissue usually occurs in man in association with disseminated metastases to bone. The prevalence of hypercalcemia caused by bony metastases of nonparathyroid neoplasms in dogs and cats is not known, but our experience suggests that it is relatively low.

Hypercalcemia has been detected in human beings, dogs and cats with malignant nonparathyroid neoplasms in which bone metastases were not detected by radiographic or necropsy studies. The serum concentration of phosphorus in nonuremic patients with this syndrome was often decreased (but occasionally it was normal). The hypercalcemia and hypophosphatemia are thought to occur as a result of production of parathormone-like substances (or other osteolytic substances, including prostaglandins, vitamin-D–like sterols or osteoclast activating factor) by neoplastic tissue. Unlike parathormone secreted from normal parathyroid glands, however, the secretion of parathormone-like substances from neoplasms is not inhibited by increased concentrations of plasma calcium. The combination of hypercalcemia and hypophosphatemia caused by nonendocrine malignant tumors that have not metastasized to bone is called ectopic hyperparathyroidism or pseudohyperparathyroidism. This name reflects the observation that many of the clinical and laboratory abnormalities associated with pseudohyperparathyroidism are similar to those associated with primary hyperparathyroidism.

Although pseudohyperparathyroidism has been associated with a variety of neoplasms in man (lymphomas, hepatomas, melanosarcomas and carcinomas of the lung, kidney, ovary, urinary bladder, uterus, esophagus, intestines, etc.), it has been almost exclusively observed in association with malignant lymphomas in dogs. The serum calcium concentration was evaluated in 60 adult dogs with malignant lymphoma at the University of Minnesota. Twenty-four (40 per cent) were hypercalcemic (minimum = 11.3 mg./dl.; maximum = 22.3 mg./dl.; mean = 15.8 mg./dl.). Five dogs had a serum concentration of calcium between 11 and 12 mg./dl. One case of leukemia associated with hypercalcemia has been reported in a cat (Chew *et al.*, 1975). Pseudohyperparathyroidism has also been reported in 3 dogs with malignant perianal gland neoplasms (Rijnberk, 1970). We observed hypercalcemia (complicated by calcium nephropathy) in a 5-year-old female St. Bernard with a mixed mammary gland adenocarcinoma.

## CLINICAL FINDINGS

Clinical signs observed in patients with pseudohyperparathyroidism are related to hypercalcemia and the site(s) of neoplasia. Signs caused by hypercalcemia tend to be similar, regardless of underlying cause. Although hypercalcemia may be associated with signs referable to many body systems, signs referable to the urinary tract, gastrointestinal tract and central nervous system are most commonly observed (refer to the section on calcium nephropathy for specific details). Clinical signs specifically related to the growth and metastases of neoplasms in patients with pseudohyperparathyroidism are variable, being dependent on the site(s) of neoplasia, the extent to which normal structures have been altered or destroyed and the duration and severity of the disease process. We have encountered several cases of pseudohyperparathyroidism in which there were no overt clinical signs of neoplasia (lymphoma).

## LABORATORY FINDINGS

Laboratory findings associated with pseudohyperparathyroidism mimic those associated with primary hyperparathyroidism. Nonuremic patients with either disease characteristically develop hypercalcemia, hypercalciuria, hypophosphatemia and hyperphosphaturia. Either disease may be associated with normal or increased alkaline phosphatase activity. Abnormal secretion of parathormone (primary hyperparathyroidism) or parathormone-like substances (pseudohyperparathyroidism) induce hypercalcemia by mobilizing calcium from bones and increasing renal and intestinal absorption of calcium. Hypercalciuria occurs as a result of increased renal clearance of calcium from plasma. Hypophosphatemia and hyperphosphaturia occur as a result of a parathormone-mediated decrease in the renal tubular reabsorption of phosphorus.

In our experience, pseudohyperparathyroidism associated with canine malignant lymphoma has been a far more common cause of hypercalcemia than primary hyperparathyroidism. In both diseases, however, patients are often admitted with signs indicative of renal failure (consult the article on "Hypercalcemic Nephropathy"). Of 24 hypercalcemic lymphoma dogs evaluated at the University of Minnesota, 15 had primary renal failure induced by hypercalcemia at the time of admission to the hospital. Lack of evaluation of the serum concentration of calcium and phosphorus in patients with primary renal failure has undoubtedly contributed to the infrequency with which pseudo- and primary hyperparathyroidism have been recognized in animals in the past. It is probable that many cases of pseudo- and primary hyperparathyroidism in dogs (and cats?) have been erroneously diagnosed as primary renal failure with secondary renal hyperparathyroidism.

Hypercalcemia can also cause significant functional and structural alterations of the kidneys, resulting in renal failure (refer to the article on "Hypercalcemic Nephropathy" for details). As the severity of hypercalcemic renal damage progresses, glomerular filtration decreases to a point where increased serum urea nitrogen and creatinine concentrations may be detected. Progressive reduction in glomerular filtration rate is associated with a progressive increase in serum phosphorus concentration and a progressive decrease in urine calcium concentration. In contrast to secondary renal hyperparathyroidism, which is characterized by varying degrees of hyperphosphatemia and hypocalcemia, renal failure associated with pseudohyperparathyroidism and primary hyperparathyroidism is characterized by varying degrees of hypercalcemia and normo- to hyperphosphatemia. In our experience, the degree of hyperphosphatemia has usually been much greater in dogs with chronic secondary renal hyperparathyroidism than in dogs with renal failure caused by pseudo- or primary hyperparathyroidism.

## RADIOGRAPHIC FINDINGS

Absence of radiographically demonstrable osteolytic lesions characteristic of disseminated neoplastic metastases is a prerequisite to establishment of a diagnosis of pseudo- and primary hyperparathyroidism. Generalized skeletal demineralization has not been a prominent feature in our series of dogs with pseudohyperparathyroidism, presumably because of the relatively short duration of the disease process prior to its correction or because of the rapid demise of the patient. Although extensive demineralization and pathologic fractures of bones have been reported in association with primary hyperparathyroidism in dogs, the latter undoubtedly represents an advanced stage of the untreated disease. We have encountered two cases of primary hyperparathyroidism in dogs in which the owner's complaint was related to signs of renal failure. Although both dogs had some skeletal demineralization, pathologic fractures were not detected.

## TREATMENT

Once hypercalcemia is recognized, it may assume an important role in formulation of therapy for a patient with neoplasia (consult the article on "Hypercalcemic Nephropathy" for specific details concerning symptomatic therapy of hypercalcemia). Treatment of neoplasms associated with hypercalcemia is dependent on their biologic behavior and location and may consist of surgical removal, irradiation, chemotherapy and/or immunotherapy. (Consult other articles for specific recommendations about therapy of neoplasms.) Successful therapy of neoplasms that produce parathormone-like substances is typically associated with a reduction of serum calcium concentrations to normal values within a few days. We have encountered several dogs with hypercalcemia due to lymphoma in which the serum calcium concentration became subnormal (6 to 8 mg./dl.) two to three days following therapy. Post-treatment hypocalcemia may occur as a result of depressed secretory activity of the parathyroid glands due to long-term suppression by hypercalcemia and accelerated mineralization of bones. In our experience, it has usually been unnecessary to treat the hypocalcemia unless it drops below 6 to 7 mg./dl. Oral calcium gluconate and vitamin D supplements may be considered, however. Oral calcium lactate should be avoided, since alkalinization may decrease the plasma concentration of ionized calcium. Signs of hypocalcemic tetany should be controlled with intravenous calcium gluconate.

## POLYCYTHEMIA

Renal erythropoietic factor (REF) is elaborated primarily by as yet unidentified cells in the kidney in response to anemia, hypoxia or impaired circulation. REF is rapidly activated to erythropoietin by combining with an alpha-globulin produced by the liver. Erythropoietin stimulates committed stem cells in bone marrow to differentiate and mature to erythroblasts and results in increased release of immature erythrocytes into the peripheral blood. Increased production of red cells increases the total body red cell mass and provides an appropriate compensatory response to the initial stimulus of tissue hypoxia.

Inappropriate production of erythropoietin has been reported in human beings with a variety of neoplastic (adenomas, adenocarcinomas, nephroblastomas) and non-neoplastic (hydronephrosis, cysts) renal diseases and was suspected in two dogs with renal adenocarcinomas associated with erythrocytosis. The mechanism(s) by which renal neoplasms stimulate increased production of REF is not clear, but there is evidence that the neoplastic cells produce REF or an erythropoietin-like substance (Hammond and Winnick, 1974). In many human cases, and in one case in a dog, removal of the renal neoplasm was followed by correction of the erythrocytosis. In addition, erythropoietin activity has been detected in tumor extracts obtained from human beings. It is also possible that neoplastic and non-neoplastic renal diseases compromise the renal microcirculation, or constrict the renal artery or vein, and induce local renal hypoxia. Renal hypoxia in turn would be expected to stimulate the production and release of additional REF.

Since the kidney is the normal site of production of REF, the production of excessive REF by renal neoplasms is not an ectopic endocrinopathy. However, inappropriate erythrocytosis has been observed in human beings with cerebellar hemangioblastomas, hepatomas, uterine fibromas and pheochromocytomas. Increased erythropoietin activity was detected in serum and/or tumor extracts obtained from these patients.

Clinical signs of erythrocytosis (injected mucous membranes, vertigo, headache, dyspnea, etc.) are common, regardless of underlying cause. With the exception of laboratory evidence of erythrocytosis (increased hematocrit, hemoglobin, RBC count, etc.), there may be no other laboratory evidence of excessive REF production. There may be, however, a conspicuous lack of clinical dehydration, cardiopulmonary disease and other common causes of erythrocytosis. Unlike polycythemia vera (a neoplastic condition of uncommitted bone marrow stem cells), in which patients may have erythrocytosis, leukocytosis and thrombocytosis, inappropriate elaboration of REF from neoplasms is characterized only by erythrocytosis.

## ECTOPIC ACTH PRODUCTION

Numerous cases of hyperadrenocorticism have been reported in human patients with nonadrenocortical nonpituitary tumors (primarily oat cell carcinomas of the lung; also, thymomas and noninsulin-producing islet cell tumors of the pancreas; infrequently, neoplasms of the thyroid, ovary, prostate, liver, parotid gland and neural tissue). Neoplastic production of ACTH by nonendocrine tumors has not been reported in the dog or cat. Tumors of many human patients have been found to contain an ACTH-like substance (by radioimmunoassay and bioassay) that behaves like pituitary ACTH. The adrenal glands of such patients are typically hyperplastic, but the ACTH content of their pituitary glands is depressed.

The clinical and metabolic manifestations of this ectopic endocrinopathy are highly variable, being dependent upon the level of cortisol stimulation by the ectopic ACTH and upon the duration and severity of the neoplastic disease. Although the serum concentrations of ACTH and cortisol are extremely high, less than one half the patients with ectopic ACTH production develop the typical features of Cushing's syndrome. This may be related to the relatively short duration of the disease. With few exceptions, the production of ACTH by tumors is autonomous and cannot be suppressed by dexamethasone.

Treatment of the syndrome should be directed toward eradication of the neoplasm.

If the latter is unfeasible, production of cortisol from the hyperplastic adrenal glands may be suppressed with metyrapone, o,p'-DDD (Lysodren® [Calbio]) and/or aminoglutethimide (Smith, 1975).

## INAPPROPRIATE ANTIDIURESIS

The physiologic regulation of antidiuretic hormone (vasopressin) is controlled primarily by plasma osmolality (high osmolality stimulates ADH release) and blood volume (low blood volume stimulates ADH release).

Secretion of ADH becomes inappropriate when it continues to be elaborated despite normal or low plasma osmolality and normal or elevated intravascular volume. The syndrome of inappropriate secretion of antidiuretic hormone (SIADH) has been observed in human beings with carcinomas of the lungs, duodenum and pancreas and with thymomas and lymphomas. It has not been reported in animals. These neoplasms have been found to release vasopressin that appears to be identical to the arginine vasopressin released by the pituitary gland.

Antidiuretic hormone released by either the pituitary gland or neoplasms increases the permeability of the distal nephrons and collecting ducts to water. The result of excessive ADH production is water retention characterized by increase in body weight, expansion of extracellular fluid volume, reduction in plasma osmolality and hyponatremia. Hyponatremia is caused by reabsorption of water by the kidneys and natriuresis and is aggravated by a shift of extracellular sodium into cellular fluid, which has become hypotonic as a result of water intoxication. Increased renal excretion of sodium and decreased renal excretion of water result in the formation of urine that is hypertonic to plasma. Cardiac, renal and adrenal function is typically normal (except for secondary suppression of aldosterone by the adrenal glands).

The clinical signs of SIADH are related to the rate of decrease in plasma sodium and osmolality rather than to their absolute values. When serum sodium and osmolality decline slowly, the only indications of SIADH may be fatigue, lethargy and disorientation. In these patients, hyponatremia is often a chance finding during routine evaluation of patients with malignancy.

When there is a rapid decline in serum sodium and osmolality, the signs may be more profound but equally nonspecific. They usually include anorexia, vomiting, confusion and occasionally convulsions and coma.

A diagnosis of SIADH may be established in patients with hyponatremia, low plasma osmolality, hypernatriuresis and hypertonic urine. In contrast to the hyponatremia associated with adrenocortical insufficiency, there is a conspicuous lack of clinical and laboratory evidence of dehydration in patients with SIADH.

Sustained hypersecretion of vasopressin is not associated with clinical signs unless unlimited access to water is permitted. Rigid restriction of water intake to match insensible losses typically is associated with an increase in serum sodium concentration and osmolality and remission of signs produced by water intoxication. Long-term therapy should be directed toward eradication of the tumor.

## OTHER ECTOPIC ENDOCRINOPATHIES

### GONADOTROPINS

Neoplasms of nonpituitary and nonplacental origin (carcinomas of the lung, esophagus, liver, ovary, etc.) may produce gonadotropins, which in turn cause sexual precocity in children and gynecomastia in men.

### INSULIN-LIKE SUBSTANCES

Severe fasting hypoglycemia and its associated clinical signs have been observed in human patients with extrapancreatic tumors. Large retroperitoneal and intrathoracic sarcomas have been incriminated most frequently, but hypoglycemia has also been observed in patients with hepatomas, adrenocortical carcinomas, bronchogenic carcinomas and undifferentiated adenocarcinomas of the stomach and colon. Hypoglycemia has also been re-

ported in a dog with leukemia and pseudohyperparathyroidism (DeSchepper *et al.*, 1974).

Although the underlying cause of neoplastic hypoglycemia has not been determined, a noninsulin hypoglycemia-producing substance is suspected in most cases. A few investigators have reported the presence of insulin or an antigenically similar substance in an occasional patient with extrapancreatic neoplasia and hypoglycemia.

### OTHERS

Neoplastic production of thyroid-stimulating hormone, prolactin and growth hormone are less common causes of ectopic endocrinopathies in man.

## SUPPLEMENTAL READING

Chew, D. J., Schaer, M., Liu, S., and Owens, J.: Pseudohyperparathyroidism in a cat. J. Am. Anim. Hosp. Assn., *11*:46–52, 1975.

Christy, N. P.: Endocrine syndromes associated with cancer. *In* Beeson, P. B., and McDermott, W. (eds.): Textbook of Medicine. 14th ed. Philadelphia, W. B. Saunders Co., 1975.

DeSchepper, J., *et al.*: Hypercalcemia and hypoglycemia in a case of lymphatic leukemia in the dog. Vet. Rec., *94*:602–603, 1974.

Gomez-Uria, A., and Pazianos, A. G.: Syndromes resulting from ectopic hormone-producing tumors. Med. Clin. N. Am., *59*:431–440, 1975.

Hall, T. C.: Ectopic synthesis and paraneoplastic syndromes. Cancer Res., *34*:2088–2091, 1974.

Hammond, D., and Winnick, S.: Paraneoplastic erythrocytosis and ectopic erythropoietins. Ann. N.Y. Acad. Sci., *230*:219–227, 1974.

Odell, W. D.: Humoral manifestations of nonendocrine neoplasms—ectopic hormone production. *In* Williams, R. H. (ed.): Textbook of Endocrinology. 5th ed. Philadelphia, W. B. Saunders Co., 1974.

Osborne, C. A., and Stevens, J. B.: Pseudohyperparathyroidism in the dog. J. Am. Vet. Med. Assn., *162*:125–135, 1973.

Rijnberk, A.: Pseudohyperparathyroidism in the dog. Tijdschr. Diergeneesk, *95*:515, 1970.

Scott, R. C., and Patnaik, A. K.: Renal carcinoma with secondary polycythemia in the dog. J. Am. Anim. Hosp. Assn., *8*:275–283, 1972.

Smith, L. H.: Ectopic hormone production. Surg. Gynec. Obstet., *141*:443–453, 1975.

# OBESITY

JAN J. de BRUIJNE, M.S.,
*and* ALEID A. M. E. LUBBERINK,
D.V.M.
*Utrecht, The Netherlands*

Although obesity is rarely of endocrine origin, it is often presented to the veterinarian as a "metabolic problem." Frequently, owners of animals affected with this disease are convinced that "there is something wrong with the glands." This illusion must be dispelled. Nevertheless, reference to the endocrine system is inevitable in any discussion of obesity, if only to exclude metabolic abnormalities as a significant causative factor in the vast majority of cases.

The function of the adipose tissue is to store, in the form of triglycerides, the surplus calories not metabolized immediately after ingestion and, when necessary, to liberate free fatty acids for oxidation in the peripheral tissues to provide energy. This storage and releasing function is essential, because the supply of calories is intermittent, while cellular metabolism requires "fuel" 24 hours a day. It is particularly important for wild animals because it provides energy during periods when food is not available.

Dogs closely follow human behavior in their way of life. An abundance of food of high quality and severe restrictions of daily exercise are two consequences of our modern urban society. The obvious effect is an increase in the frequency of obesity.

## DEFINITION

Obesity can be defined as an excessive accumulation of fat in the adipose tissue. All available evidence indicates that this accumulation of body fat arises because caloric intake exceeds requirements. There is no simple technique to measure the mass of adipose tissue in the dog. In practice, it is usually necessary to rely on subjective evaluation of body configuration in association with body weight. We suggest that an increase of 15 per cent above the desired or ideal weight be regarded as obesity.

## ETIOLOGY

Although the pathogenesis of obesity is relatively easy to understand, we still lack knowledge about many of the factors normally concerned with the regulation of energy balance and appetite. Studies in animals have demonstrated the presence of medial satiety and lateral appetite centers in the hypothalamus. The responsiveness of these centers might be altered in some obese dogs, but obesity that is proved to be due to organic hypothalamic disease is very rare.

As is the case in man, environmental factors appear to be of some importance. For example, obesity is more frequent among dogs owned by obese people than among dogs owned by people of normal physique (Mason, 1970). Most probably this refers mainly to the slightly overweight, middle-aged dog that is fundamentally normal but eats a little too much and exercises too little. However, the grossly overweight dog that has had this problem throughout life suffers from a disorder that we do not yet understand and are unable to cure.

## CLINICAL FEATURES

Some dogs are admitted for obesity as such, but usually there are additional complaints, such as the inability to take long walks and locomotor disturbances. Some animals are described by their owners as having a ravenous appetite, but the complaint that an animal gets fat in spite of being a "small eater" is also heard. Of course, the latter statement overlooks the question of energy expenditure. It has been observed repeatedly in human medicine that obese patients expend more energy than lean ones in the performance of a physical act. However, the more energy is needed to perform a physical act, the less likely it is to be carried out.

Unlike animals in which the obesity is due to endocrine abnormalities, dogs that are "simply overweight" are usually quite alert and are not dermatologically affected. The fat is usually distributed diffusely over the trunk, but in some obese animals a striking bilateral accumulation of fat is seen in the lumbar area. The genital functions are unaffected.

## DIAGNOSIS

The diagnosis of obesity can be made in dogs in which the history and physical examination are in agreement with the above-mentioned findings, after the two main differential diagnoses have been excluded: hyperadrenocorticism and hypothyroidism (Table 1).

An ACTH-stimulation test and thyroid function studies should be performed in addition to routine blood and urine analyses when the diagnosis of "simple" obesity is not entirely supported by the clinical findings alone. This is particularly important when hair coat abnormalities, absence of estrus or striking lethargy accompany the weight gain.

## TREATMENT

Interest and enthusiasm on the part of both veterinarian and owner are required for successful treatment of obesity. A feeling of mutual confidence should be established. This is particularly true when simple caloric restriction is chosen as treatment.

**Diet.** The following guidelines may be helpful when this mode of therapy is chosen. The dog should be weighed, and a realistic target weight should be established. The prescribed caloric intake should be 50 to 60 per cent of that required by the dog at its desired target weight. The dog's food should be different from what it has been up to the beginning of the diet and a not very palatable commercial dog food is a good choice, since it is simple to give instructions to the owner when such a diet is used.

The dog should be seen every two weeks for control examination and weighing. The weight should be recorded and a graph showing the progress of weight reduction is sometimes helpful in encouraging the owner's cooperation.

We have not found that expensive prescription diets are more effective than the weight reduction program described above. In cases of continued failure, total starvation is employed.

**Total Starvation.** Starvation is a simple and very reliable method of treatment. During the past few years, we have gathered some information on the effects of therapeutic starvation. No severe clinical or chemical changes have been observed in the patients, some of which underwent this treatment for as long as six to eight weeks (Fig. 1). The only disadvantage is the need for prolonged hospitalization, which is indispensable because owners cannot be expected to accomplish such a strict regimen themselves.

The main purposes of starvation are

—to demonstrate to the owner that considerable weight loss, resulting in a livelier dog, is possible;

—to reach a point beyond which the animal will increase its energy expenditure, so that less severe dietary restrictions can be used successfully when the dog returns home.

Slight diarrhea may occur during the first two weeks of total starvation. Urine production decreases to about 10 ml./kg./day. No severe metabolic changes have been ob-

*Table 1.* *Symptoms and Signs that Aid Differentiation of Obesity from Hyperadrenocorticism and Hypothyroidism\**

| | OBESITY | HYPER-ADRENOCORTICISM | HYPO-THYROIDISM |
|---|---|---|---|
| Age at occurrence | All ages | Middle-age | <5 years |
| Overweight | ++ | ± | ± |
| Location of fat | Trunk | Belly | Trunk |
| Polydipsia/polyuria | − | ++ | − |
| Polyphagia | ± | ++ | − |
| Absence of estrus | − | + | + |
| Lethargy | ± | + | ++ |
| Decreased exercise tolerance | ± | +± | ++ |
| Alopecia | − | + | ± |
| Heat intolerance | − | + | − |
| Sensation of cold | − | − | + |

\*It should be noted that the classic picture of each disease has been used for the composition of this table.

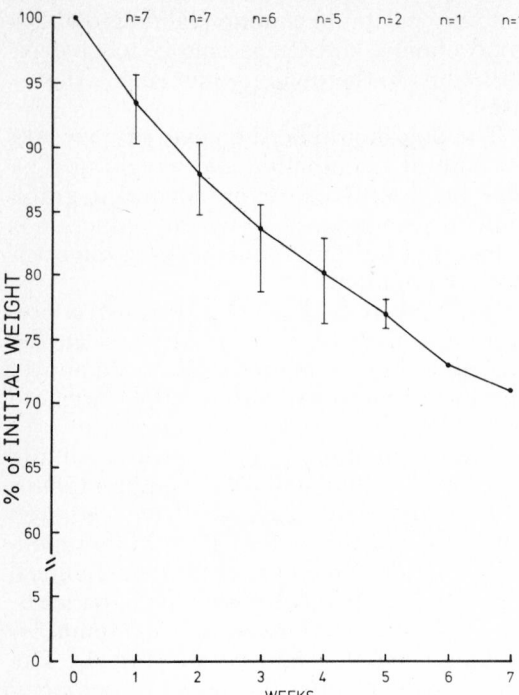

**Figure 1.** Weight loss related to initial weight during total starvation. *Note:* The vertical bars represent the highest and lowest values found.

served. As can be expected, BUN values decrease drastically, owing to a decreased protein metabolism. Circulating ketone bodies rise only moderately, indicating that obese dogs utilize them more efficiently than do other animals, including man. Metabolic acidosis, a frequent problem in fasting human patients, does not occur. On the contrary, by the end of a few weeks of starvation, a slight alkalosis may occur. The results of liver function tests usually remain within normal limits; serum alkaline phosphatase values increased in only one of our dogs, but this dog was subsequently found to have hyperadrenocorticism. Within a few days, sodium excretion decreases to very low values (about 1 mg./kg./day), whereas daily potassium excretion remains at about 10 mg./kg. The serum sodium and potassium values remain within normal range, as do those of calcium.

We conclude that canine "simple" obesity can be safely treated by total starvation. This is not astonishing if one remembers that the dog used to be an animal of prey and had to overcome rather long fasting periods without losing its ability to capture another prey. Apparently, domesticated dogs still behave metabolically, as do animals of prey. This explanation might prove helpful when one must convince a reluctant owner of the fact that total starvation is not as cruel as it may seem.

**Drugs.** Appetite suppressants have no role in the treatment of obesity. Fenfluramine was recently used without result in the treatment of six overweight spayed bitches (Bronson and Parker, 1975). Thyroid hormones should never be used unless the patient has proven thyroid deficiency.

### SUPPLEMENTAL READING

Bronson, L., and Parker, C. H. L.: Effect of fenfluramine on overweight spayed bitches. Vet. Rec., 96:202–203, 1975.

Edney, A. T. B.: Management of obesity in the dog. Vet. Med./Small Animal Clin., pp. 46–49, January, 1974.

Lemieux, G., and Plante, G. E.: The effect of starvation in the normal dog including the Dalmatian Coach Hound. Metabolism, 17:620–630, 1960.

Mason, E.: Obesity in pet dogs. Vet. Rec., 86:612–616, 1970.

# Section
# 12

# GENITOURINARY DISORDERS

CARL A. OSBORNE, D.V.M.
*Consulting Editor*

# The Kidneys

# URINARY TRACT EMERGENCIES

RICHARD C. SCOTT, D.V.M.,
*and* RICHARD W. GREENE,
D.V.M.
*New York, New York*

Most urinary tract emergencies are associated with imbalances of body fluid composition and quantity, and collectively these are called the acute uremic syndrome. Clinical signs are caused by these imbalances, and therapy must be designed to correct them so as to prevent death prior to recovery from the initial insult that caused acute renal failure.

## BODY FLUID ABNORMALITIES

### DEHYDRATION

Dehydration is a common abnormality resulting from acute renal failure. It is caused by loss of body fluid as a result of vomiting and diarrhea and/or by diminished water intake by the patient. Diuresis following oliguria from acute renal failure or from preexisting chronic renal failure may also contribute to dehydration if the patient is unable to drink enough water to replace the deficits that occur. Clinical signs include lethargy and loss of skin elasticity, which varies with the severity of dehydration (see article on "Fluid Therapy").

Therapy is aimed at replacing body fluid deficits together with insensible body fluid losses and urine output, the latter being measured by attaching an empty parenteral fluid bottle to a urinary catheter with a fluid administration set. The catheter is sutured to the prepuce in the male or attached to a Foley catheter in the female. The bottle must be vented by passing a hypodermic needle through the stopper in the top, and appropriate antibiotics should be administered to prevent urinary tract infection (see article on "Adverse Drug Reactions in the Uremic Patient").

Initially, the type of fluid should be balanced and isotonic. Lactated Ringer's solution is usually the fluid of choice for this reason. Additional body fluid and electrolyte abnormalities will determine which drugs are to be added to this fluid; this will be discussed later in this article. Rehydration fluid volumes should be replaced rapidly (in 6 to 8 hours), unless congestive heart failure is also present. When urine output is monitored, daily volumes can be replaced more accurately, and overzealous fluid administration during initial therapy will be prevented.

### OVERHYDRATION

Overhydration resulting from anuria or oliguria is rare, since most patients lose or fail to take in fluid volumes in excess of the body water that is produced during metabolism and not subsequently excreted by the damaged kidneys. If overhydration occurs, it is usually caused by overzealous fluid therapy. Clinical symptoms include dyspnea and coughing, which result from pulmonary edema, dependent edema and depression from cerebral edema.

Therapy includes tapering fluids to very low volumes or discontinuing their administration completely. Oxygen should also be given if dyspnea is severe. An attempt should be made to promote diuresis with an intravenous diuretic such as furosemide (Lasix® [Hoechst]) at a dosage of 10 to 20 mg./kg. of body weight. If diuresis does not occur after 30 minutes, the initial dose of diuretic is doubled and again administered intravenously. If this fails to promote diuresis within 30 minutes, excess body water should be removed by means of peritoneal dialysis. If dyspnea is very severe, dialysis should be started earlier. The concentration of dextrose in the dialysate should be as high as 7 per cent for the first 2 to 3 exchanges if life-threatening pulmonary edema is present. Most states of overhydration can be controlled by using 4.25 per cent and 1.5 per cent dextrose on alternate exchanges until dyspnea is diminished (see article on "Peritoneal Dialysis"). After this, 1.5 per cent dextrose is usually sufficient.

## EDEMA

Edema usually results from hypoalbuminemia associated with the nephrotic syndrome. Clinical symptoms and therapy are discussed in the article on "Glomerulonephropathy and the Nephrotic Syndrome."

# BODY FLUID COMPOSITION ABNORMALITIES

## ACID-BASE DISTURBANCES

Metabolic acidosis usually occurs in acute uremia as a consequence of organic acids retained by the damaged kidneys. This acidotic state may be partially or completely compensated by respiratory mechanisms (see article on "Fluid Therapy"). Although rare, metabolic alkalosis may occur and surpass acidosis when excessive vomition (of hydrogen ions) occurs.

Clinical symptoms of acidosis include variable lethargy and deep, rapid (Kussmaul) respirations. If metabolic alkalosis occurs, symptoms include apprehension, restlessness, ataxia and weakness, in addition to severe vomiting.

Sodium bicarbonate added to parenteral fluids is indicated if symptoms are severe or if there is laboratory evidence of severe acidosis. If metabolic alkalosis is present (pH below 7.3), intravenous chloride (in normal saline) is indicated, together with bowel-coating agents and antiemetics (Darbazine® [Norden]) to prevent vomition (see article on "Fluid Therapy").

## ABNORMALITIES IN POTASSIUM LEVELS

Hyperkalemia during anuric or oliguric primary renal failure is caused by retention of potassium by the damaged kidneys. Infection and tissue damage, excessive alimentation of foods rich in potassium and acidosis, which shifts intracellular potassium to the extracellular fluid during buffering of hydrogen ions each accounts for potassium-loading that can overwhelm the damaged kidney's ability to excrete potassium. Emergency therapy is indicated *only* if hyperkalemia is life-threatening, as indicated by *severe* lethargy or coma, severe bradycardia (heart rate below 40 beats per minute) and electrocardiographic evidence of severe hyperkalemia (severe bradycardia, tall peaked T waves, diminished P waves, or atrial standstill, and occasionally ventricular arrhythmias such as idioventricular beats). It should *never* be assumed that emergency therapy for hyperkalemia is always indicated in acute uremia of any cause. Only if death is imminent is such therapy advisable. Laboratory findings will usually show serum potassium levels above 9.0 mEq./l. in this setting.

If indicated, sodium bicarbonate therapy should be administered to correct acidosis. In addition, if hyperkalemia is life-threatening, intravenous dextrose and regular insulin will usually avert hyperkalemia. Insulin is administered intravenously at 0.7 unit/kg. of body weight. Immediately after this, dextrose is administered at the rate of 2 gm./unit of insulin in order to prevent hypoglycemia. Half this dose is given intravenously, and half is given in parenteral fluids as a 2.5 per cent dextrose solution. It is usually necessary to administer insulin and dextrose only once to treat life-threatening hyperkalemia. If oliguria or anuria persists, peritoneal dialysis should be performed to treat hyperkalemia (see article on "Peritoneal Dialysis").

Hypokalemia can be caused by excessive loss of potassium as a consequence of diuresis after renal function improves. Clinical symptoms are lethargy, weakness, restlessness and ataxia with serum potassium levels below 3.0 mEq./l. Therapy is aimed at cautiously replacing losses with potassium chloride in parenteral fluids, avoiding administration of more than 0.5 mEq./kg./hr. (Greene and Scott, 1975) (see article on "Fluid Therapy"). Potassium-containing elixirs can also be given if oral therapy is tolerated by the patient. Initial doses are 2.5 to 5.0 cc. t.i.d., and therapy is adjusted by monitoring serum potassium (see article on "Fluid Therapy"). The dosage is raised or lowered by 2.5 to 5.0 cc. per day until the appropriate dosage is attained.

## ABNORMALITIES IN SODIUM LEVELS

Hyponatremia can be caused by diuresis of sodium with water, in combination with replacement of this fluid loss with water via alimentation or administration of fluids not containing sodium (e.g., dextrose in water). Clinical symptoms include lethargy, ataxia, vomition and weakness. Laboratory findings will disclose serum sodium concentration below 130 mEq./l. in most cases that are symptomatic. Therapy includes adjustments in fluid therapy until serum sodium is normal. Hyponatremia can be treated with intravenous administration of normal saline (0.9 per cent NaCl) until serum sodium is normal. Such therapy should be given cautiously to prevent overhydration when oliguria or anuria is present. Water restriction is indicated only when dilutional hyponatremia is suspected on the basis of serum osmolality determinations (less than 240 mOsm. water).

## OBSTRUCTIVE NEPHROPATHY

Acute obstruction can be caused by stones that prevent passage of urine at any level in the outflow tract; usually they obstruct the urethra. In the male cat, urethral plugs containing struvite crystals and mucus are most common. Acute obstruction can also be caused by trauma that causes swelling and hemorrhage, by neoplasia associated with hemorrhage or swelling from edema and by incarceration of the bladder into perineal or traumatic hernias.

Gradual obstruction caused by neoplasia, congenital anomalies of the urinary tract and posttraumatic strictures usually result in hydronephrosis. Ureteral obstruction causes an acute uremic syndrome if it is bilateral, or if it is unilateral, with the opposite kidney involved in some other generalized disease.

Clinical symptoms are the same as those of acute uremia of any cause and include vomition, depression, anorexia and dehydration associated with fluid losses. Obstruction of the bladder neck or urethra is associated with strangury; hematuria and pyuria may occur with obstruction at any level. Laboratory data will reveal elevation of the serum concentration of BUN and creatinine, together with other electrolyte imbalances discussed earlier.

Relief of obstruction must be the aim of initial therapy. Catheterization of the bladder, together with back-flushing with sterile solutions, will relieve most obstructions of the urethra and bladder neck caused by uroliths in dogs and cats. If obstruction cannot be relieved in this way, cystocentesis with fine needles can be performed until surgery is feasible (Scott and Wilkins, 1974). Other therapeutic measures are the same as those described earlier for acute uremia and include fluid therapy and correction of acid-base and electrolyte disturbances (see article on "Fluid Therapy").

Obstruction of the ureters or the ureteropelvic junction must be treated surgically after the patient has been stabilized (DeHoff *et al.*, 1972).

Following relief of obstruction, a profound postobstructive diuresis may develop. During this time, daily parenteral fluid volumes must be estimated carefully by monitoring urine output. If this is not done, severe dehydration and decreased renal perfusion may complicate renal failure. If hypokalemia and/or hyponatremia develops during this time, it should be corrected (see article on "Fluid Therapy").

## RENAL TRAUMA

Severe abdominal trauma, especially if applied ventrally, can cause damage to one or both kidneys as a result of direct compression of renal parenchyma and/or from hemorrhage into the renal parenchyma. If hemorrhage occurs through the renal capsule into the retroperitoneal space or peritoneal cavity, severe anemia from blood loss can occur. Avulsion of the kidney from the aorta may result in exsanguination and death.

Clinical symptoms reflect blood loss in most cases. Depression, pale mucous membranes, slow capillary refill and shock (in severe blood loss) will be present. The abdomen is frequently tucked up and painful, especially in the area of the kidneys. Hematuria will be present if the damaged kidney(s) continues to function following trauma. A progressive reduction in PCV may be observed if hemorrhage is gradual. Severe, acute hemorrhage will not be followed by a reduction of PCV until inter- and intracellular fluid enter the vascular compartment.

Bilateral renal trauma may be associated with elevation in the serum concentration of BUN or creatinine. Shock that decreases renal perfusion will cause prerenal uremia. Urinalysis will reveal a specific gravity above 1.025 if prerenal uremia occurs. However, if bilateral trauma causes primary renal uremia, impaired ability to concentrate or dilute urine will develop. Microscopic and gross hematuria frequently occur. If urine sediment examination is performed immediately after collection, red blood cell casts may be observed, hallmarking involvement of the kidney. Abnormalities of other laboratory data are dependent on the extent of damage to other organs in the abdominal cavity (i.e., liver, intestines, spleen, etc.). Whole blood may be obtained by means of abdominal paracentesis if severe hemorrhage from the kidney and/or other organs has occurred.

Radiographs of the abdomen may show an irregular, hazy density throughout the abdomen if a large amount of blood is present in the peritoneal cavity. If blood does not enter the peritoneal cavity, there will be increased density and expansion of the retroperitoneal space, which causes loss of the renal outlines and psoas shadows (lateral projection). Intravenous pyelography using the high-dose, rapid-infusion technique will reveal a blotchy irregular nephrogram phase and variable excretion of dye by the damaged kidney(s), depending on the severity of renal damage.

Emergency treatment to correct severe hemorrhage may be required. Evidence of severe abdominal hemorrhage causing hypovolemic shock should be treated with intravenous corticosteroids, whole blood and antibiotics, followed by intravenous fluids. As soon as the patient is stable, exploratory laparotomy should be performed to locate and control the source of hemorrhage. Mild hemorrhage can be treated medically by stabilizing the patient with fluids in most cases, although whole blood tranfusions may be needed.

If surgery must be performed and severe renal trauma with hemorrhage is found, a complete nephrectomy should be performed, provided that the other kidney is capable of maintaining adequate function, as determined by renal function tests prior to surgery (Archibald and Owen, 1974; De-

Hoff *et al.*, 1972). When 50 per cent or less of the renal parenchyma is injured, partial nephrectomy using a guillotine technique (Archibald and Owen, 1974) is the recommended treatment. With only mild renal damage, minor surgery, as described elsewhere, may suffice (DeHoff *et al.*, 1972).

Postoperatively, the patient should receive antibiotics, fluids and other supportive therapy.

## URETERAL TRAUMA

In addition to causing damage to the kidney(s), severe abdominal trauma can also cause rupture of the ureter at any point along its course to the bladder. Most ruptures either occur near the renal pelvis or involve the renal pelvis.

Clinical signs are similar to those of renal trauma, the major difference being that hemorrhage is usually not as severe unless the kidney or other organs are also involved. The abdomen is frequently painful and tucked up. If sufficient time has elapsed after trauma, urine will be extravasated into the retroperitoneal space or peritoneal cavity. If sufficient urine escapes into the peritoneal cavity, abdominal distention may occur.

Radiographs may reveal irregular blotchy density of the abdomen and widening of the retroperitoneal space by a fluid density caused by urine that has entered this area. Intravenous pyelograms will show extravasation of dye around the kidney if the renal pelvis is ruptured, or into the retroperitoneal space if the ureter is damaged. Occasionally urine is seen in the peritoneal cavity. Laboratory data will reveal a decreased PCV if severe hemorrhage has occurred. If sufficient time has passed after trauma, abnormal renal function tests due to reabsorption of metabolic products from extravasated urine may be detected. Other laboratory data will vary with the severity of damage to other abdominal organs, including the kidneys. Urinalysis frequently reveals microscopic or gross hematuria.

Surgery is indicated after the patient has been stabilized with fluids, antibiotics and steroids (if indicated because of shock). At surgery, rupture of the ureter can be managed by stenting alone or stenting and suturing. A No. 4 French catheter is passed retrograde from the bladder to the kidney and then *distally* from the bladder through the urethra, where it is sutured in place. Complete rupture of the ureter in the upper and middle segments may be repaired by anastomosis with fine chromic catgut, using an interrupted pattern about the entire circumference of the ureter. Small tears in the ureter can be treated by stenting alone, but larger rents should be stented and sutured with an interrupted pattern. If the ureter is severely damaged near the bladder, it can be reimplanted into the bladder (Archibald and Owen, 1974; DeHoff *et al.*, 1972).

Postoperative care includes fluid and electrolyte management, as discussed earlier (see article on "Fluid Therapy"). Broad-spectrum antibiotics that are excreted by the kidney should be used. The catheter should be left in place for 5 to 10 days to allow healing of the ureter.

The surgical procedures for managing ureteral trauma are discussed further elsewhere (Archibald and Owen, 1974; DeHoff *et al.*, 1972).

## TRAUMA TO THE BLADDER AND RUPTURED BLADDER

Acute urethral obstruction that causes severe bladder distention and that is subsequently manipulated by catheterization to relieve obstruction is a cause of ruptured bladder. Severe trauma to the abdomen or bony pelvis can also cause bladder rupture if the bladder is distended at the time of trauma. Severe cystitis, which erodes and weakens the bladder wall, may also cause rupture.

Trauma to the abdomen will be associated with abdominal pain and, if associated with a ruptured bladder, hematuria that is variable in severity. If no urine is passed, hematuria may not be present. Abdominal distention will occur if sufficient urine extravasation has taken place. This latter symptom varies with the size of the bladder tear. Clinical signs may include depression, vomition and fever if peritonitis has developed, although most bladder ruptures remain asymptomatic for up to 24 hours (Burrows and Bovee, 1974). Laboratory data will show an elevation in the serum concentration of BUN and creatinine and other abnormalities, including hyponatremia and hypochloremia. Paracentesis will usually show serosanguineous fluid with signs of inflammation on cytologic examination. The concentration of creatinine rather than BUN in this fluid will more reliably demonstrate that it is urine, if there remains a question as to its character (Burrows and Bovee, 1974).

When bladder rupture is suspected, a urinary catheter should be passed into the bladder, and a positive contrast cystogram should be performed to demonstrate extravasation of dye into the peritoneal cavity and/or around the bladder neck and urethra. An intravenous pyelogram should also be performed if renal or ureteral trauma is suspected.

Treatment of bladder rupture initially is aimed at stabilizing the patient with intravenous fluids and antibiotics. During this time, a urinary catheter is left in place to allow for drainage of the bladder (Burrows and Bovee, 1974). Shock after trauma may also require treatment, as discussed earlier. Following this, surgery is indicated to repair the bladder tear, followed by antibiotics and other supportive therapy postoperatively.

## SUPPLEMENTAL READING

Archibald, J., and Owen, R.: Urinary system. *In* Archibald, J. (ed.): Canine Surgery. 2nd Archibald ed. Santa Barbara, California, American Veterinary Publications, Inc., 1974, pp. 673–701.

Burrows, C. F., and Bovee, K. C.: Metabolic changes due to experimentally induced rupture of the canine urinary bladder. Am. J. Vet. Res., 35:1083–1088, 1974.

DeHoff, W. D., Greene, R. W., and Greiner, T. P.: Surgical management of abdominal emergencies. Vet. Clin. N. Am., 2(2):301–330, 1972.

Greene, R. W., and Scott, R. C.: Lower urinary tract disease. *In* Ettinger, S. J. (ed.): Textbook of Veterinary Internal Medicine. Philadelphia, W. B. Saunders Co., 1975, pp. 1541–1577.

Pullman, T. N., and Coe, F. L.: Chronic renal failure. CIBA Clin. Symp., 25:2, 1973.

Scott, R. C., Wilkins, R. J., and Greene, R. W.: Abdominal paracentesis and cystocentesis. Vet. Clin. N. Am., 4(2):413–417, 1974.

# NEPHRO-TOXICITY

DONALD G. LOW, D.V.M.
*and* GAYLORD M. CONZELMAN, JR., Ph.D.
*Davis, California*

## PATHOPHYSIOLOGY

Nephrotoxicity includes any adverse structural or functional change in the kidneys caused by a chemical or biologic product. The kidney is unusually susceptible to toxicities for at least two reasons:

1. The unusually large blood supply to the kidneys predisposes them to exposure to toxins and poisons.

2. The kidneys have the capacity to extract substances from the blood and concentrate them within the renal parenchyma or in the tubular lumen.

Not all potentially nephrotoxic agents (Table 1) are known to cause nephrotoxicity in domestic animals, but all have been reported to produce renal lesions in one or more animals, including man. Kidney abnormalities can be caused by the unchanged drug, a metabolite or an excretory product. In addition to injury to the kidneys, which may result in clinical signs, many of the agents are harmful to other organs and systems as well. For example, ingestion of glycol-type antifreeze often results in severe depression, ataxia and coma; signs of uremia develop only if the patient survives for a sufficient period of time. Likewise, thiacetarsamide sodium produces hepatic injury as well as renal damage. The clinician must be cognizant of both in order fully to appreciate the problem with which he is confronted.

Excretion of various drugs and chemicals is thought to produce renal lesions by several different mechanisms:

1. Because of reabsorption of salt and water, nonabsorbable substances may be concentrated along the luminal border of the tubular cells and produce their most severe injury there.

2. Some drugs such as the penicillins and iodinated contrast agents are secreted by cells of the proximal convoluted tubules and actually occupy an intracellular position for a brief time.

3. The countercurrent mechanism may cause certain drugs to become concentrated to a marked degree in the interstitial fluid of the medulla. This occurs in man following excessive and prolonged ingestion of phenacetin.

**Table 1.** *Types of Nephrotoxins*

I. *Heavy Metals and Their Compounds*

| | | |
|---|---|---|
| Antimony | Cadmium | Mercury |
| Arsenic | Copper | Silver |
| Beryllium | Gold | Thallium |
| Bismuth | Iron | Uranium |
| | Lead | |

II. *Organic Solvents*
   Carbon tetrachloride
   Methanol
   Tetrachlorethylene

III. *Glycols*
   Diethylene glycol
   Ethylene dichloride
   Ethylene glycol
   Ethylene glycol dinitrate

IV. *Therapeutic Agents*
   A. Antibacterial
      Amphotericin B
      Bacitracin
      Cephaloridine
      Gentamicin
      Kanamycin
      Neomycin
      Penicillin
      Streptomycin
      Sulfonamides
      Tetracycline
   B. Analgesics
      Phenacetin
      Phenylbutazone
      Salicylates
   C. Anticonvulsants
      Phenurone
      Trimethadione
   D. Pesticides
      Chlorinated hydrocarbons
      Phosphorus
   E. Physiologic substances at abnormal concentration
      Hypercalcemia
      Hypokalemia
   F. Miscellaneous
      Cantharides
      Cyclophosphamide
      Hemolysins
      Penicillamine
      Snake venom
      Thiacetarsamide sodium

Drug-induced nephrotoxicity may occur because of dose-related inherent toxicity, as is encountered in the use of amphotericin B, or the injury may be caused by drug allergy that is unpredictable and follows a period of sensitization. On rare occasions, penicillin induces this type of renal injury.

Contact with nephrotoxic agents comes most often through use of nephrotoxic drugs or through accidental ingestion or inhalation of nephrotoxic chemicals. Unless the owner is an unusually astute observer, however, if may be difficult to establish whether exposure to nephrotoxic agents has occurred. When the clinician is using a potentially nephrotoxic drug, he should be most attentive to functional performance of the patient's kidneys.

The onset of signs is usually sudden and often consists of depression, anorexia, vomiting, diarrhea or constipation, and oliguria or anuria, in addition to signs caused by damage to other body organs or systems (see article on"Medical Management of Oliguric and Anuric Primary Renal Failure"). If urinalysis is performed shortly after the kidneys have been damaged by nephrotoxic drugs or chemicals, one often finds proteinuria, numerous casts, red blood cells, white blood cells and renal epithelial cells. If the patient survives and further exposure to the nephrotoxin is prevented, these abnormalities often disappear in a few days. A renal biopsy is often useful in helping to establish the reversibility of the underlying lesions.

## PREVENTION OF NEPHROTOXICITY

Whenever a clinician is utilizing a potentially nephrotoxic drug, he must carefully monitor the kidneys for deleterious effects. This may be accomplished by frequent examination of the patient, by noting approximate water consumption and urine output and by determining serum BUN or creatinine levels at appropriate intervals before and during therapy. Careful evaluation of the patient for signs of nephrotoxicity is obviously more important when using a drug like amphotericin B than when using penicillin, with which nephrotoxicity is rarely encountered. Marked reduction of urine output accompanied by depression, anorexia and gastrointestinal upset often heralds the onset of acute generalized renal injury. The clinician may be able to prevent or minimize renal injury by taking steps to insure adequate urine flow. If oral medication is tolerated, urine flow may be augmented by administering sodium chloride tablets at a dosage of 1 to 2 gm./5 kg. of body weight/day in divided doses. If the patient is unable to tolerate oral medication, urine flow may be supported by the parenteral administration of lactated Ringer's solution. Of the drugs in common use, thiacetarsamide sodium and amphotericin B require careful observation on the part of the clinician. In most instances, if renal injury is recognized early, no treatment is needed other than to withdraw the nephrotoxic drug and to continue the sodium diuresis. If damage is more severe and if the patient develops oliguria or anuria, a more intensive therapeutic approach may be required (see articles on "Medical Management of Oliguric and Anuric Renal Failure," "Peritoneal Dialysis" and "Intensive Diuresis in Polyuric Renal Failure").

The danger of nephrotoxicity is substantially greater when a potentially nephrotoxic drug is administered to a patient with extensive preexisting renal disease; this danger is intensified even further when the drug is excreted through the kidneys. Under such circumstances, extremely high blood and renal tissue concentrations may be attained even though the recommended dosage is used, because the kidneys are unable to excrete the drug at the usual rate. Reduction of dose or increased maintenance dosage intervals are necessary under these conditions if serious toxicity is to be avoided (see article on "Adverse Drug Reactions in the Uremic Patient").

### SUPPLEMENTAL READING

Czerwinski, A. W., and Pederson, J. A.: Drug induced renal disease. Kidney, 8:20–23, 1975.

Faulkes, E. C., and Hammond, P. B.: Toxicology of the kidney. *In* Casarett, L. J., and Doull, J. (eds.): Toxicology: The Basic Science of Poisons. New York, Macmillan Publishing Co., Inc., 1975.

# HYPER-CALCEMIC NEPHROPATHY

CARL A. OSBORNE, D.V.M.,
*and* JERRY B. STEVENS, D.V.M.
*St. Paul, Minnesota*

During the past few years, more consistent evaluations of electrolyte abnormalities in patients with primary renal failure have revealed that hypercalcemia is a far more common cause of renal disease and renal failure in the dog than is generally recognized. Most cases have been caused by pseudohyperparathyroidism, but calcium nephropathy caused by primary hyperparathyroidism and hypervitaminosis D has been encountered as well. Since the renal lesions induced by hypercalcemia are reversible during early stages, early recognition of this problem is of great clinical significance.

## CAUSES OF HYPERCALCEMIA

Although a variety of diseases have been reported to cause hypercalcemia in man, the occurrence of hypercalcemia in dogs and other species has not been critically evaluated (Table 1).

**Osteolytic Neoplasia.** Hypercalcemia associated with malignancy of nonparathyroid tissue usually occurs in man in association with disseminated metastases to bone. The hypercalcemia is thought to occur in association with neoplastic osteolysis, which causes release of calcium and phosphorus at rates that exceed bone repair and the capacity of the kidneys and intestines to remove excessive quantities of these electrolytes from the blood. As a result, the serum concentrations of calcium and phosphorus in these patients are elevated.

Recent studies in man have revealed that many patients with hypercalcemia and disseminated metastases of neoplasms to bone also have elevated plasma concentrations of parathormone (Benson *et al.*, 1974). These results were interpreted to indicate that parathormone-like polypeptides released from tumors may play an important role in the genesis of hypercalcemia in patients with neoplastic osteolysis.

The prevalence of hypercalcemia caused by bony metastases of nonparathyroid neoplasms in dogs and cats has not been determined, although in our experience it appears to be uncommon.

**Hypervitaminosis D.** Animals receiving excessive amounts of vitamin D and calcium in the form of dietary supplements may develop hypercalcemia. The severity of hypercalcemia associated with hypervitaminosis D may be similar to that which occurs in patients with primary and pseudohyperparathyroidism, but it is usually accompanied by hyperphosphatemia (Capen, 1975). Skeletal demineralization is not a consistent feature of hypervitaminosis D, since the increased concentrations of blood, calcium and phosphorus are derived primarily from increased intestinal absorption rather than from bone resorption.

**Primary Hyperparathyroidism.** Hypercalcemia associated with primary hyperparathyroidism is caused by release of excessive quantities of parathormone from hyperplastic or neoplastic parathyroid glands. The result is increased mobilization of calcium and phosphorus from bone, increased calcium reabsorption from the renal tubules and intestinal tract, and decreased renal tubular reabsorption of phosphorus. The serum concentration of calcium rises, while the serum concentration of phosphorus falls (in nonuremic patients).

**Pseudohyperparathyroidism.** Hypercalcemia has been detected in human beings, dogs and cats with malignant nonparathyroid neoplasms in which radiographic and necropsy evidence of bone metastases was not detected. The serum concentration of phosphorus in nonuremic patients with this syndrome was often decreased. Hypercalcemia and hypophosphatemia are thought to occur as a result of production of parathormone-like substances by neoplastic tissue. Unlike normal parathormone secreted from parathyroid glands, however, the secretion of

**Table 1.** *Causes of Hypercalcemia*

| CAUSE | SPECIES | | |
| --- | --- | --- | --- |
| | *Human* | *Canine* | *Feline* |
| Primary hyperparathyroidism | Yes | Yes | Unknown |
| Tertiary hyperparathyroidism | Yes | Unknown | Unknown |
| Pseudohyperparathyroidism | Yes | Yes | Yes |
| Hyperthyroidism | Yes | Unknown | Unknown |
| Hyperadrenocorticism | Yes | Unknown | Unknown |
| Myxedema | Yes | Unknown | Unknown |
| Disuse osteoporosis | Yes | Unknown | Unknown |
| Osteolytic neoplasia | Yes | Yes | Unknown |
| Hypervitaminosis D | Yes | Yes | Unknown |

parathormone-like polypeptides from neoplasms is not inhibited by increased concentrations of plasma calcium. The combination of hypercalcemia and hypophosphatemia caused by nonendocrine malignant tumors that have not metastasized to bone is called ectopic or pseudohyperparathyroidism. This name reflects the observation that many of the clinical and laboratory abnormalities associated with pseudohyperparathyroidism are similar to those associated with primary hyperparathyroidism. Although pseudohyperparathyroidism has been associated with a variety of neoplasms in man, it has almost exclusively been observed in association with malignant lymphomas in dogs (refer to the article on "Ectopic Hormone Production by Nonendocrine Neoplasms" for specific details). It has also been observed in a cat with leukemia.

Recently, metabolites other than tumor-derived parathormone-like polypeptides have been incriminated in the pathogenesis of hypercalcemia of some malignancies in man and laboratory animals. They include vitamin D and its metabolites, nonvitamin D sterols, prostaglandins and a class of osteoclast-activating factors found in the medium of cultured human leukocytes. The significance of prostaglandin $E_2$ as a mediator of hypercalcemia of malignancy is of great clinical interest, since the hypercalcemia may be corrected with indomethacin, a potent inhibitor of prostaglandin synthesis (Brereton *et al.*, 1974; Seyberth, 1975; Tashjian *et al.*, 1974).

## RENAL PATHOLOGY

The microscopic changes associated with early or mild cases of hypercalcemic nephropathy are characterized by varying degrees of calcification, degeneration, necrosis and sloughing of the epithelium of the ascending Henle's loop, distal tubules and collecting ducts. A significant amount of tubular damage may occur without histologically demonstrable precipitates of calcium. The morphologic appearance of the glomerular tufts is usually normal.

More severe states of hypercalcemia are usually associated with calcification of tubular epithelium and basement membranes. Calcium deposits are not commonly associated with an influx of inflammatory cells. Obstruction of tubular lumina with casts causes dilation of portions of nephrons located above the casts.

With severe or prolonged hypercalcemia, calcium deposits may be distributed throughout the renal parenchyma, including the interstitial tissue, basement membranes of glomerular capillaries, Bowman's capsules and walls of vessels, in addition to tubular epithelium and basement membranes.

## CLINICAL SIGNS

Hypercalcemia may be associated with a variety of clinical manifestations, depending on the nature of the underlying cause and the duration and severity of hypercalcemia. Clinical signs caused by hypercalcemia tend to be similar, regardless of underlying cause. Although hypercalcemia may be associated with signs referable to many body systems, signs referable to the urinary tract, gastrointestinal tract and central nervous system are most commonly observed.

Increased serum calcium concentration depresses the excitability of nervous tissue and the contraction of smooth, skeletal and cardiac muscle. Generalized muscular weakness occurs as a result of decreased tonus of skeletal muscle. Loss of tonus of smooth muscle of the gastrointestinal tract results in gastric atony associated with anorexia and vomiting, and intestinal atony associated with constipation. Hypercalcemia may also cause bradycardia, cardiac arrhythmias and, in some patients, ventricular fibrillation. Signs referable to the central nervous system include depression and coma.

During early stages, hypercalcemia is usually associated with polyuria and compensatory polydipsia. Marked dehydration may develop as a result of vomiting and polyuria. If the degree of calcium nephropathy is severe enough to cause renal failure, signs of uremia may be observed. Unfortunately, clinical signs caused by hypercalcemia mimic many of the signs associated with uremia caused by renal diseases other than calcium nephropathy.

Clinical signs specifically related to growth and metastases of neoplasms in patients with pseudohyperparathyroidism and neoplastic osteolysis are variable, being dependent on the site(s) of neoplasia, the extent to which normal structures have been destroyed and the duration and severity of the disease process. We have encountered several cases of pseudohyperparathyroidism associated with malignant lymphoma in which there were no overt clinical signs of neoplasia.

## LABORATORY FINDINGS

Laboratory findings associated with hypercalcemic nephropathy are dependent on the nature of the underlying cause. The common denominator of all these diseases, however, is hypercalcemia. Therefore, accurate determination of serum calcium is extremely important. The serum calcium concentration of normal adult dogs is approximately 9.5 to 11 mg./dl.; that of immature dogs is approximately 10 to 12 mg./dl. Since calcium values vary with the analytical method employed, normal values should be determined for each laboratory. Calcium values consistently above 11 mg./dl. but below 12 mg./dl. in adult dogs should be considered to be suspect, whereas calcium values consistently above 12 mg./dl. should be considered abnormal.

The significance of serum calcium concentration should be considered in association with the serum protein concentration, since approximately 50 per cent of the serum calcium is bound to protein. It follows that hypoproteinemia (especially hypoalbuminemia) may be associated with a decrease in total serum calcium concentration but a normal ionized calcium concentration. If hypoalbuminemia accompanies malignant disease, it may obscure an abnormal rise in ionized calcium concentration.

Laboratory findings associated with pseudohyperparathyroidism mimic those associated with primary hyperparathyroidism. Nonuremic patients with either disease characteristically develop hypercalcemia, hypercalciuria, hypophosphatemia and hyperphosphaturia. Abnormal secretions of parathormone (primary hyperparathyroidism) or parathormone-like substances (pseudohyperparathyroidism) induce hypercalcemia by mobilizing calcium from bones and increasing renal and intestinal absorption of calcium. Hypercalciuria occurs as a result of increased renal clearance of calcium from plasma. Hypophosphatemia and hyperphosphaturia occur as a result of a parathormone-mediated decrease in the renal tubular reabsorption of phosphorus.

In man, hypercalcemia associated with neoplastic osteolysis is often associated with hyperphosphatemia as well as hypercalcemia. This occurs because calcium and phosphorus are released at rates that exceed both bone repair and the capacity of the kidneys and intestines to remove excessive quantities of these electrolytes from the blood. Although not documented, a similar situation in dogs and cats might be expected to occur.

Whether increased serum concentrations of alkaline phosphatase occur depends in part on the severity of bone disease and the presence or absence of concomitant hepatic disease (Table 2).

One of the earliest clinical manifestations of calcium-induced nephropathy is impaired ability to concentrate urine. During early stages of naturally occurring hypercalcemia in man and experimentally induced hypercalcemia in dogs, glomerulotubular imbalance may occur as evidenced by the severity of hyposthenuria, which is often much greater than would be predicted by evaluation of the serum concentration of

**Table 2.** *Differential Diagnosis of Primary Hyperparathyroidism, Renal Secondary Hyperparathyroidism, Pseudohyperparathyroidism and Hypercalcemia Due to Neoplastic Osteolysis*

| FACTORS | PRIMARY HYPERPARATHYROIDISM | RENAL SECONDARY HYPERPARATHYROIDISM | PSEUDOHYPER-PARATHYROIDISM | NEOPLASTIC OSTEOLYSIS* |
|---|---|---|---|---|
| Serum calcium | Elevated | Normal to decreased | Elevated | Elevated |
| Serum phosphorus | Decreased unless uremic; then normal to increased | Increased | Decreased unless uremic; then normal to increased | Frequently increased |
| Serum alkaline phosphatase | Normal to increased | Normal to increased | Normal to increased | Normal to increased |
| Blood urea nitrogen; creatinine | Normal unless uremic; then increased | Increased | Normal unless uremic; then increased | Normal unless uremic; then increased |
| Bone radiographs | Varying degrees of demineralization | Varying degrees of demineralization | Varying degrees of demineralization | Disseminated osteolytic lesions |

*Findings reported in human beings.

urea or creatinine. Inability to concentrate urine following administration of antidiuretic hormone indicates that the hyposthenuria is renal in origin. In some patients, prerenal azotemia may be superimposed on this state of renal hyposthenuria as a consequence of fluid loss from vomiting and impaired renal conservation of water. Unlike primary renal azotemia, which occurs in association with more severe states of hypercalcemic nephropathy, correction of hypovolemia by fluid therapy will result in restoration of glomerular filtration rate and a rapid reduction in the serum concentration of creatinine and urea nitrogen. Impaired ability to concentrate urine will persist, however.

Although examination of the urine sediment usually does not reveal any abnormalities, variable numbers of casts, RBC and WBC may be detected.

As the severity of hypercalcemic renal damage progresses, glomerular filtration decreases to a point at which increased serum urea nitrogen and creatinine concentrations may be detected. Progressive reduction in glomerular filtration rate is associated with a progressively increasing serum phosphorus concentration and a progressively decreasing urine calcium concentration. In contrast to secondary renal hyperparathyroidism, which is characterized by varying degrees of hyperphosphatemia and hypocalcemia, renal failure associated with pseudohyperparathyroidism and primary hyperparathyroidism is characterized by varying degrees of hypercalcemia and normo- to hyperphosphatemia (Table 2). In our experience, the degree of hyperphosphatemia is usually much greater in dogs with secondary renal hyperparathyroidism than in dogs with renal failure caused by pseudo- or primary hyperparathyroidism.

## RADIOGRAPHIC FINDINGS

Calcium nephropathy associated with radiographic evidence of renal calcification has not been observed in our series of dogs with primary hyperparathyroidism (2 cases) and pseudohyperparathyroidism (24 cases).

Absence of radiographically demonstrable osteolytic lesions characteristic of disseminated neoplastic osteolysis is considered to be a prerequisite to establishment of a diagnosis of primary or pseudohyperparathyroidism. Generalized skeletal demineralization has not been a prominent feature in our series of dogs with pseudohyperparathyroidism, presumably because of the relatively short duration of the disease process prior to its correction, or the rapid demise of the patient.

Although extensive demineralization and pathologic fractures of bone have been reported in dogs with primary hyperparathyroidism, the latter undoubtedly represents an advanced stage of the untreated disease. We have encountered two cases of primary hyperparathyroidism in dogs in which the owner's complaint was related to renal failure. Although both dogs had some skeletal demineralization, pathologic fractures were not detected.

## DIAGNOSIS

Evaluation of the concentration of serum calcium is essential to help distinguish primary renal failure due to hypercalcemia from primary renal failure associated with renal secondary hyperparathyroidism. Lack of evaluation of serum concentrations of calcium and phosphorus in patients with primary renal failure has undoubtedly contributed to the infrequency with which calcium nephropathy has been recognized in the past. It is probable that many cases of pseudo- and primary hyperparathyroidism in dogs (and cats?) have been erroneously diagnosed as primary renal failure with renal secondary hyperparathyroidism.

The findings of hypercalcemia in a patient with renal failure strongly suggest, but do not prove, that hypercalcemia is the underlying cause of the nephropathy. In dogs and cats, secondary renal hyperparathyroidism is rarely associated with hypercalcemia. Long-standing renal failure associated with hypercalcemia suggests the development of tertiary hyperparathyroidism, especially if the renal failure is known to have been preceded by hypocalcemia. Although tertiary hyperparathyroidism has not been well documented in dogs (we have encountered one probable case), it has been well documented in human beings (Table 1). It occurs when hyperplastic parathyroid glands caused by the hypocalcemia of very long-standing renal failure become autonomous.

Renal failure associated with congenital or familial renal diseases in immature dogs may be misdiagnosed as calcium nephropathy if one neglects to consider the fact that the normal serum calcium concentration of young dogs is higher than that of mature dogs.

In our experience, pseudohyperparathyroidism associated with canine malignant lymphoma has been a far more common cause of hypercalcemic nephropathy than primary hyperparathyroidism. In both diseases, however, patients are often admitted with signs indicative of renal failure. Of 24 hypercalcemic lymphoma dogs evaluated at the University of Minnesota, 15 had primary renal failure at the time of admission to the hospital. As mentioned previously, both our patients with primary hyperparathyroidism were admitted with signs of renal failure.

Clinical findings which indicate that calcium nephropathy is due to pseudohyperparathyroidism include (1) hypercalcemia; (2) absence of radiographic or postmortem evidence of disseminated neoplastic osteolysis; (3) absence of hyperplastic or neoplastic parathyroid glands (the parathyroid glands are normal or atrophic); (4) presence of a malignant nonparathyroid neoplasm; (5) remission of hypercalcemia after successful treatment of the neoplasm; and (6) exacerbation of hypercalcemia in those patients in whom the neoplasm recurs after therapy.

Clinical findings which indicate that calcium nephropathy is due to primary hyperparathyroidism include (1) hypercalcemia; (2) absence of malignant nonparathyroid neoplasms; (3) absence of radiographic or postmortem evidence of disseminated neoplastic osteolysis; (4) presence of hyperplastic or neoplastic parathyroid glands; and (5) remission of hypercalcemia following surgical extirpation of the abnormal parathyroid gland(s).

Antemortem differentiation between pseudo- and primary hyperparathyroidism may be difficult if there are no overt signs of neoplasia. We have established a diagnosis of malignant lymphoma in several hypercalcemic dogs without peripheral lymphadenopathy by performing aspiration biopsies of normal-sized peripheral lymph nodes. In other instances of extranodal canine lymphoma, the diagnosis was established by obtaining a liver biopsy sample at the same time that a renal biopsy sample was obtained.

Clinical findings which indicate that calcium nephropathy is due to neoplastic osteolysis include (1) hypercalcemia; (2) presence of radiographic or postmortem evidence of disseminated neoplastic osteolysis; (3) presence of malignant nonparathyroid neoplasms; and (4) absence of hyperplastic or neoplastic parathyroid glands.

Clinical findings which indicate that calcium nephropathy is due to hypervitaminosis D include (1) hypercalcemia; (2) evidence of increased consumption or injection of abnormally large quantities of vitamin D; (3) absence of radiographic or postmortem evidence of neoplastic osteolysis; (4) absence of malignant nonparathyroid neoplasia; (5) absence of hyperplastic or neoplastic parathyroid glands; and (6) remission of hypercalcemia following correction of vitamin D intake.

## TREATMENT

**Symptomatic Treatment of Hypercalcemia.** Once hypercalcemia is recognized, it may assume an important role in the formulation of therapy for a patient with neoplasia (parathyroid or nonparathyroid) or hypervitaminosis D. The urgency and regimen of therapy for hypercalcemia are dependent on its duration and severity. Regardless of the severity of hypercalcemia, however, dehydration should be corrected by vigorous replacement therapy with polyionic, isotonic solutions such as lactated Ringer's solution. In addition to replacing fluid and electrolyte deficits, hydration with solutions that contain significant quantities of sodium enhances renal excretion of calcium.

Mild cases of hypercalcemia (12 to 14 mg./dl.) may be treated by eliminating the underlying cause (see below, Specific Treatment of Cause). Restriction of calcium in the diet is of little value in correcting excesses of calcium derived primarily from bone. In the event that the patient has concomitant heart failure, caution must be used when administering cardiac glycosides, since hypercalcemia potentiates the cardiotoxic effects of those drugs.

Since prolonged or severe (>15 mg./dl.) hypercalcemia may result in severe debilitation and even death, symptomatic therapy should be used to reduce the extracellular concentration of calcium until more definitive measures can be instituted to control the underlying cause. Several therapeutic agents have been reported to have anti-hypercalcemic activity in man and dogs. These agents may be classified as drugs that (1) promote urinary excretion of calcium, (2) promote calcium loss from the body by extrarenal routes and (3) remove calcium from extracellular fluid by promoting its deposition in soft tissues or bone. Calci-uretic agents include sodium sulfate, furosemide and ethacrynic acid (Walser, 1961, 1970; Fulmer, 1972; Ong, 1974; Osborne and Stevens, 1973). Although furosemide does not alter the ratio of calcium and phosphorus excreted in urine, it markedly increases renal excretion of both ions. In contrast, thiazide diuretics decrease the renal excretion of calcium and are therefore contraindicated. Intravenous administration of furosemide to dogs at a dosage of 5 mg./kg. has been effective in reducing the severity of hypercalcemia, provided that concomitant fluid therapy was used to prevent depletion of extracellular fluid volume during the course of diuresis (Ong, 1974). Peritoneal dialysis may also be used temporarily to remove calcium from the body and may be of benefit in the treatment of severe uremia as well. Although oral and intravenous administration of phosphate preparations has been recommended to alleviate hypercalcemia by promoting calcium deposition in bone and soft tissue (Spaulding, 1970; Fulmer, 1972), we have had no experience with these agents. The severity of neoplastic hypercalcemia may also be temporarily relieved by the administration of corticosteroids. The pharmacologic mechanism(s) by which corticosteroids lower high serum calcium concentrations is unknown, but in some situations it may be related to their destruction of the tumor (e.g., lymphoma). The value of corticosteroids in treating hypercalcemia should be weighed against their gluconeogenic effect in patients with severe renal failure (consult the article on "Glomerulonephropathy and the Nephrotic Syndrome"). Other agents being considered for use in human patients include mithramycin and calcitonin (Chopra *et al.*, 1975; Vaughn and Vaitkevicius, 1974).

**Treatment of Renal Failure.** Once uremia caused by calcium nephropathy has developed, no regimen of therapy will eliminate the renal lesions. The renal damage that has occurred, however, may heal spontaneously over a period of weeks if the hypercalcemic state is controlled or eliminated. The objective for patients with renal failure should be to keep the patient alive until the body processes of regeneration, repair and compensatory adaptation allow the nephrons to regain sufficient function to reestablish and maintain an adequate degree of biochemical homeostasis. This may be accomplished by minimizing deficits and excesses in fluid, electrolyte and acid-base balance with various combinations of conservative medical management, intensive diuresis and peritoneal dialysis.

**Specific Treatment of Cause.** In patients with mild hypercalcemia, or following treatment of patients with severe hypercalcemia, every effort should be made to reduce the extracellular concentration of calcium by eliminating or controlling the underlying cause. Primary hyperparathyroidism should be treated by surgical removal of the affected parathyroid gland(s). We obtained good results by removing a parathyroid adenocarcinoma from an 11-year-old female cocker spaniel with calcium nephropathy. Treatment of neoplasms associated with hypercalcemia is dependent on their biologic behavior and location and may consist of combinations of surgical removal, irradiation, chemotherapy and immunotherapy. Hypercalcemia and calcium nephropathy underwent remission following surgical extirpation of a mammary gland adenocarcinoma from a 5-year-old female St. Bernard under care at the University of Minnesota.

Successful therapy of neoplasms that produce parathormone-like substances is typically associated with a reduction of serum calcium concentrations to normal values within a few days. We have encountered several dogs with malignant lymphoma and two dogs with primary hyperparathyroidism in which the serum calcium concentration became subnormal (5 to 8 mg./dl.) two to three days following surgery or chemotherapy. Posttreatment hypocalcemia may occur as a result of depressed secretory activity of the parathyroid glands due to long-term suppression of hypercalcemia and accelerated mineralization of bones. In our experience, it has usually been unnecessary to treat the hypocalcemia unless calcium concentration drops below 6 to 7 mg./dl. Oral calcium gluconate and vitamin D supplements may be considered, however. Oral calcium lactate should be avoided, since alkalinization may decrease the plasma concentration of ionized calcium. Signs of hypocalcemic tetany should be symptomatically controlled with intravenous calcium gluconate therapy.

## PROGNOSIS

If patients with hypercalcemic nephropathy are in need of extensive supportive and symptomatic therapy, every effort should be made to determine the reversibility of the underlying renal lesion and the reversibility of the underlying cause of hypercalcemia.

The degree of reversibility of renal lesions caused by metastatic calcification depends on the nature and severity of damage to nephrons. Lesions confined to tubular epithelium may heal by regeneration of viable epithelial cells. Nephrons with more severe and generalized lesions, however, are often irreversibly damaged.

Consult other sections for details concerning the prognosis associated with various types of neoplasms.

### SUPPLEMENTAL READING

Benson, R. C., et al.: Radioimmunoassay of parathyroid hormone in hypercalcemic patients with malignant disease. Am. J. Med., 56:821–826, 1974.
Brereton, H. D., et al.: Indomethacin-responsive hypercalcemia in a patient with renal cell adenocarcinoma. New Engl. J. Med., 291:83–86, 1974.
Brewer, H. B.: Osteoclastic bone resorption and the hypercalcemia of cancer. 291:1081–1082, 1974.
Capen, C. C., et al.: Endocrine disorders. In Ettinger, S. J. (ed.): Textbook of Veterinary Internal Medicine: Diseases of the Dog and Cat. Vol. 2. Philadelphia, W. B. Saunders Co., 1975.
Chopra, D., and Clerkin, E. P.: Hypercalcemia and malignant disease. Med. Clin. N. Am., 59:441–447, 1975.
Epstein, F. H.: Nephropathy of hypercalcemia. In Strauss, M. B., and Welt, L. G. (eds.): Diseases of the Kidney. Vol 2. 2nd ed. Boston, Little, Brown & Co., 1971.
Fulmer, D. H., et al.: Treatment of hypercalcemia. Comparison of intravenously administered phosphate, sulfate, and hydrocortisone. Arch. Int. Med., 129:923–930, 1972.
Mundy, G. R., et al.: Bone-resorbing activity in supernatants from lymphoid cell lines. New Engl. J. Med., 290:867–871, 1974.
Ong, S. C., et al.: Effect of furosemide on experimental hypercalcemia in dogs. Proc. Soc. Exp. Biol. Med., 145:227–233, 1974.
Osborne, C. A., and Stevens, J. B.: Pseudohyperparathyroidism in the dog. J. Am. Vet. Med. Assn., 162:125–135, 1973.
Seyberth, H. W., et al.: Prostaglandins as mediators of hypercalcemia associated with certain types of cancer. New Engl. J. Med., 293:1278–1283, 1975.
Spaulding, S. W.: Treatment of experimental hypercalcemia with oral phosphate. J. Clin. Endocrinol., 31:531–538, 1970.
Tashjian, A. H., et al.: Prostaglandins, calcium metabolism and cancer. Fed. Proc., 33:81–86, 1974.
Vaughn, C. B., and Vaitkevicius, V. K.: The effects of calcitonin in hypercalcemia in patients with malignancy. Cancer, 34:1268–1271, 1974.
Walser, M.: Calcium clearance as a function of sodium clearance in the dog. Am. J. Physiol., 200:1099–1104, 1961.
Walser, M.: Treatment of hypercalcemias. Mod. Treat., 7:662–674, 1970.

# RENAL TUBULAR ACIDOSIS

JERRY A. THORNHILL, D.V.M.
*Berwyn, Illinois*

Two types of functional renal tubular abnormalities predispose patients to metabolic acidosis: proximal renal tubular acidosis (proximal RTA) and distal renal tubular acidosis (distal RTA). These disorders are associated with positive hydrogen ion balance caused by impaired urinary acid excretion. They are characterized by an inability to acidify the urine normally (distal RTA) or by a defect in bicarbonate reabsorption in the presence of normal urinary acidification (proximal RTA). In pure form these disturbances occur with normal glomerular filtration rates. The term renal tubular acidosis has been used to distinguish these disorders from the acidosis that develops owing to renal failure caused by a reduction of functional nephron mass. Renal tubular acidosis may eventually promote kidney damage resulting in nephron failure. When this occurs, acidosis due to renal failure is superimposed on renal tubular acidosis, producing severe metabolic acidosis.

Renal tubular acidosis is well recognized in human medicine and has been the subject of extensive reviews. Owing to the paucity of veterinary literature concerning this disorder, the ensuing discussion is intended to improve recognition of RTA in animals. An understanding of the normal renal acidification process is prerequisite for comprehension of the pathophysiology of distal and proximal RTA.

## NORMAL RENAL REGULATION OF ACID-BASE BALANCE

In mammals the kidney regulates acid-base balance by regulating the concentration of plasma bicarbonate. The renal acidification process maintains plasma bicarbonate at physiologic concentrations by reabsorbing all filtered bicarbonate and excreting an amount of acid equal to the amount of fixed nonvolatile acid (i.e., acid which is not in equilibrium with $CO_2$). These acids (primarily sulfuric and phosphoric derived from dietary sulfoproteins and phosphoproteins) are produced endogenously as end-products of metabolism.

**Bicarbonate Reabsorption in the Proximal Tubule.** Approximately 85 per cent of filtered bicarbonate is reabsorbed in the proximal tubule (Fig. 1). Sodium and bicarbonate ions enter the proximal tubule as a result of glomerular filtration. Sodium ions passively diffuse into the tubular cells down a concentration and electrical gradient and are actively pumped into the peritubular interstitial fluid for uptake into plasma. Hydrogen ions are actively pumped from the interior of the cell to the tubular lumen in exchange for sodium ions. In the tubular lumen hydrogen ions combine with bicarbonate ions to form carbonic acid. A high concentration of carbonic anhydrase in the brush border of the proximal tubule catalyzes the dehydration of carbonic acid to carbon dioxide and water. The carbon dioxide formed diffuses into the tubular cells where, in the presence of intracellular carbonic anhydrase, it combines with water to form carbonic acid. Carbonic acid ionizes into bicarbonate and hydrogen ions. The hydrogen ions generated are actively secreted into the lumen in exchange for sodium ions. The bicarbonate ions gener-

ated diffuse down an electrical gradient into the peritubular plasma accompanying reabsorbed sodium, thus helping to preserve the normal basic pH of blood.

**Bicarbonate Reabsorption in the Distal Tubule.** In the distal nephron, the remaining bicarbonate is reabsorbed. Final acidification of the urine takes place by secretion of hydrogen ions against a large H ion gradient. Bicarbonate reabsorption is again dependent on hydrogen ion secretion in exchange for sodium ion. However, owing to lack of brush border carbonic anhydrase in the distal tubules and collecting ducts, dehydration of carbonic acid formed in the lumen is sluggish.

Approximately 98 per cent of the hydrogen ion secreted into the lumen is utilized in reclaiming filtered bicarbonate (85 per cent reclaimed in the proximal tubule, 15 per cent in the distal tubule). The remaining 2 per cent of secreted $H^+$ is utilized in providing for the delivery of additional bicarbonate to the blood at a rate equal to that of endogenous nonvolatile acid production. In new-bicarbonate addition to peritubular plasma, the fate of secreted hydrogen ion generated by intracellular ionization of carbonic acid is to combine with other buffers in the lumen, mainly phosphate and ammonia.

Sulfuric acid (produced by metabolism of dietary sulfoproteins) and phosphoric acid (produced by metabolism of dietary phosphoproteins and the catabolism of phospholipids) are buffered by sodium bicarbonate to form two salts, disodium sulfate ($Na_2SO_4$) and sodium monohydrogen phosphate ($Na_2HPO_4$), which are filtered into Bowman's space. Loss of these salts in excreted urine would deplete the body of sodium bicarbonate, the main extracellular buffer that neutralizes fixed acids. The kidneys prevent this depletion of sodium bicarbonate by two means: (a) the excretion of titratable acid (T.A.), which applies mainly to filtered $Na_2HPO_4$; and (b) the excretion of ammonium ($NH_4^+$), which applies to the handling of filtered $Na_2SO_4$. In both situations, bicarbonate is newly formed within the tubular cells and returned to the peritubular plasma along with sodium that was filtered.

**Excretion of Titratable Acid (T.A.).** In this process (Fig. 2) the buffer salt sodium monohydrogen phosphate ($Na_2HPO_4$) in the tubular urine is converted to sodium dihy-

## PROXIMAL TUBULE

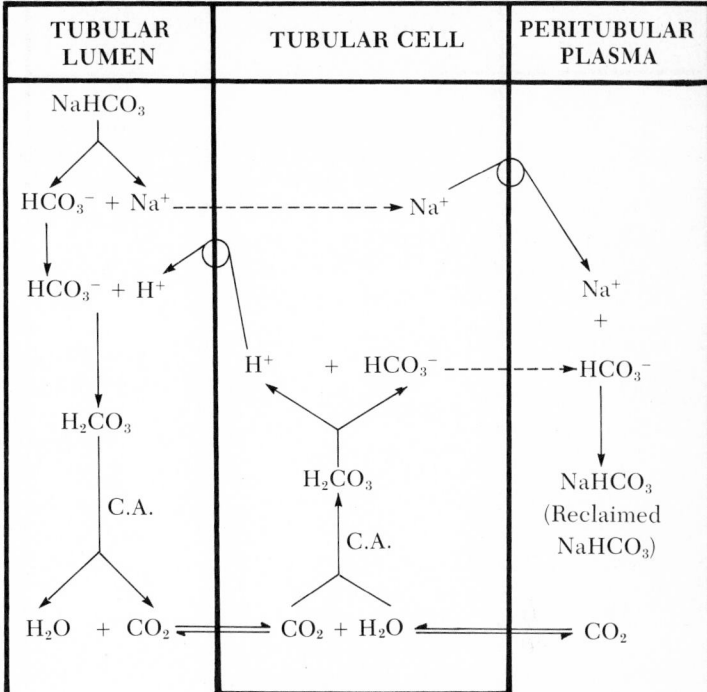

**Figure 1.** Mechanism for reabsorption of filtered bicarbonate ($HCO_3^-$) in the proximal tubular cell. Tubular fluid is exposed to carbonic anhydrase in the brush border of the proximal tubule but not in the distal tubule. Virtually all of the filtered $HCO_3^-$ is reclaimed (85 per cent in the proximal nephron, 15 per cent in the distal) through reabsorption.

C.A. = carbonic anhydrase

– – ▸ = passive diffusion down an electrical-chemical gradient

⟋○▸ = active transport

drogen phosphate ($NaH_2PO_4$) by exchanging one hydrogen ion from the tubular cell for one sodium ion of sodium monohydrogen phosphate. Sodium dihydrogen phosphate is then eliminated in the urine. Formation of such acid salts reduces the pH of the urine. The amount of strong base required to titrate the acid urine back to a pH of the glomerular filtrate (pH=7.4) is equal to the amount of titratable acid that was excreted in the urine.

The pKa of a weak acid is the pH at which the weak acid and its conjugate base exist in equal concentrations in solution. At a pH of 7.4, phosphate (pKa 6.8) exists mainly as $Na_2HPO_4$; as the urine becomes more acid, it is progressively converted to $NaH_2PO_4$. The phosphate buffer pair is the main constituent of the urinary titratable acid pool. Although many organic acids (lactic, acetic, acetoacetic and $\beta$-hydroxybutyric) contribute to the buffer pool, they all have very low pKa values and therefore are poor buffers (poor $H^+$ acceptors) at the pH of urine.

Since about 75 per cent of filtered phosphate is reabsorbed, the availability of the most important T.A. buffer is limited. Accordingly, a second buffer, ammonia, must usually carry the major burden of accepting the additional hydrogen ions in acidosis.

**Excretion of Ammonium.** About 60 per cent of the metabolic $H^+$ produced each day is excreted as ammonium ions formed in the kidney by the reactions of ammonia ($NH_3$) with free $H^+$ secreted by the tubule cell. The remaining 40 per cent of metabolic $H^+$ is excreted as titratable acid.

Unlike phosphate, $NH_3$ gains entry to the tubular lumen by tubular synthesis and diffusion into the lumen. In the dog, the most significant precursor of ammonia is the amide nitrogen of circulating plasma glutamine. Though other amino acids are involved (alanine, glycine and glutamic acid), ammonia is formed within tubular cells mainly as a result of the action of glutaminase on glutamine (Fig. 3). At the glomerular filtrate pH of 7.4 (or less, as the

## DISTAL TUBULE

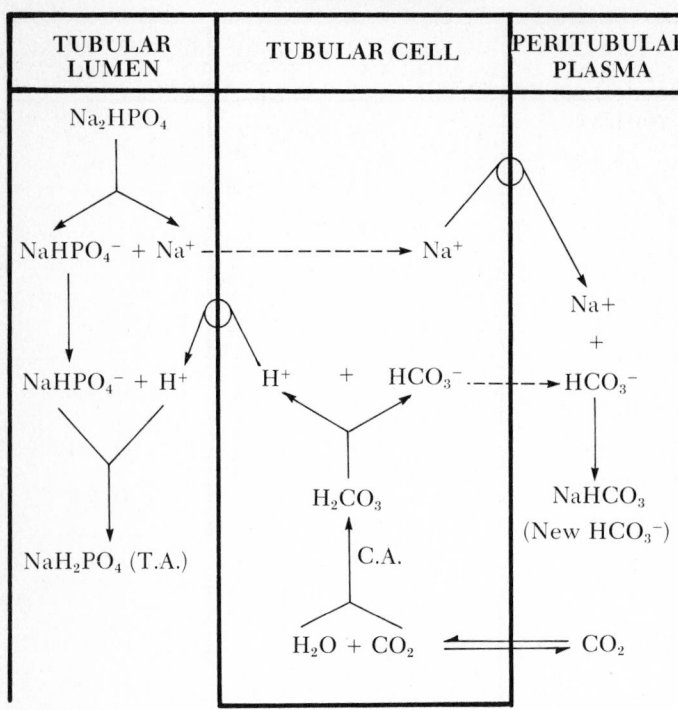

**Figure 2.** Mechanism for formation of titratable acid in the tubular lumen and the generation of new bicarbonate to replenish that which is utilized in neutralizing fixed acids.

C.A. = carbonic anhydrase

T.A. = titratable acid

– – ► = passive diffusion down an electrical-chemical gradient

⟋◯► = active transport

ultrafiltrate courses down the nephron), virtually all $NH_3$ gaining entrance to the tubular lumen will immediately pick up hydrogen ions to form $NH_4^+$. Ammonia is nonionized and highly lipid-soluble; thus, it readily diffuses across the tubular cell membrane. In contrast, ammonium ion is charged and is highly lipid-insoluble. Thus, it is trapped in the tubular lumen and excreted in the final urine.

The process by which the nonionized member of a buffer pair ($NH_3$) can readily diffuse across a cell membrane while the ionized member ($NH_4^+$) cannot results in ion trapping. The formation of ammonium in the tubular lumen diminishes the intraluminal concentration of ammonia, so that the diffusion of ammonia from the cell to the tubular lumen continues in accord with its concentration gradient. Since the ammonia is converted to ammonium almost as fast as it enters, the concentration of ammonia in the lumen is low, and the concen-

tration gradient from cell to lumen is maintained. Free ammonia synthesized within the cell diffuses into both the peritubular plasma and the tubular lumen. As the pH of the tubular fluid decreases because of increased acid secretion, more ammonia in the tubular fluid will be converted to ammonium ion by $H^+$ trapping, thus favoring greater diffusion of ammonia into the tubular lumen than into the plasma.

Urinary ammonium secretion is inversely related to the pH of the urine. As the urine pH falls, there is an increase in ammonium excretion. Depletion of intracellular ammonia due to nonionic diffusion into the tubular lumen results in increased synthesis of ammonia in the tubular cell. As the urine becomes more alkaline, urinary ammonium excretion almost ceases.

The ammonium trapped within the tubular lumen is excreted in the form of neutral salts, such as $NH_4Cl$ or $(NH_4)_2SO_4$. In the process, the bicarbonate (which is newly

## DISTAL TUBULE

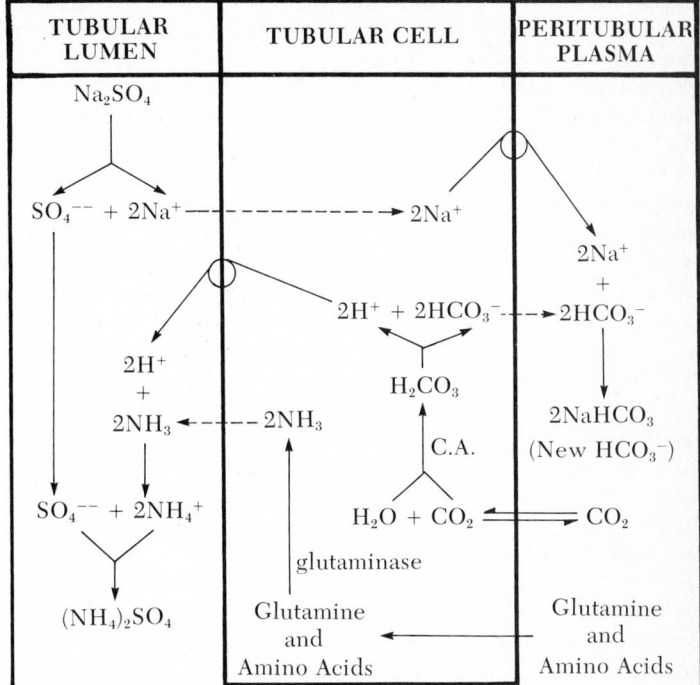

| TUBULAR LUMEN | TUBULAR CELL | PERITUBULAR PLASMA |
|---|---|---|

**Figure 3.** Mechanism for formation of ammonia from amino acid precursors, mainly glutamine, and the subsequent excretion of ammonium. There is generation of new bicarbonate to replenish that which is utilized in neutralizing fixed acids.

C.A. = carbonic anhydrase

$-\!-\!\rightarrow$ = passive diffusion down an electrical-chemical gradient

$\sim\!\!O^{\!\!-\!\!\rightarrow}$ = active transport

formed within the tubular cell) is added to the blood along with the filtered sodium that is reabsorbed. Just as in the excretion of T.A., the result of the $NH_4^+$ mechanism is the excretion of $H^+$, the replenishment of the body $HCO_3^-$ stores and the reabsorption of filtered $Na^+$.

### PATHOPHYSIOLOGY

**Distal Renal Tubular Acidosis.** Distal RTA represents a functional impairment of the distal tubule and collecting duct to lower urine pH below 6.0 (Simpson, 1971). This implies that the distal nephron is unable to generate high intraluminal hydrogen ion concentrations because it is unable to excrete hydrogen ions against a high concentration gradient. The failure of $H^+$ to be secreted into the lumen is probably due to error in membrane transport, whereby there is a defect in active transport of $H^+$ across the epithelial cell membrane.

Distal RTA is characterized by normal reabsorption of bicarbonate in the proximal tubule and by normal glomerular filtration rate in early stages. Bicarbonate reabsorption in the distal segment, however, may not be complete. Owing to the decrease in hydrogen ion secretion in this region, less than the normal 15 per cent may be reabsorbed, resulting in slight urinary bicarbonate loss. Failure to generate high luminal $H^+$ concentration also affects the rates of excretion of titratable acid and ammonium, which are inversely related to urinary pH. Although urinary pH may vary greatly (from 5.0 to 7.0) during the day in the normal dog, the capacity to attain a pH of less than 6.0 seems necessary for elimination of appropriate amounts of $H^+$ via T.A. and $NH_4^+$ to balance daily $H^+$ production.

With reduction in appropriate excretion of metabolic $H^+$, T.A. and $NH_4^+$, and with slight reduction in $HCO_3^-$ delivery to the blood, metabolic acidosis develops. Acidosis stimulates bone buffering of $H^+$ and increased $NH_3$ production by the renal tubule cell. Urine pH, however, remains high, and most of the free ammonia synthesized is lost by diffusion into the peritubular plasma. As acidosis increases, ammonia production further increases. Eventually the concentration may become high enough that the fraction of $NH_3$ accepting $H^+$ in the lumen is sufficient, together with bone buffering and a small amount of titratable acid excretion, to remove $H^+$ at a rate equaling $H^+$ production, thus stabilizing the acidosis. Stabilization, however, probably does not occur clinically and the animal remains in positive hydrogen ion balance, inducing serious biochemical consequences.

The skeletal system plays a role in the body buffering mechanism in metabolic acidosis. In man, dissolution of bone salt as a compensatory mechanism to buffer excess hydrogen ions leads to bone changes, hypercalciuria, secondary renal calculi and medullary nephrocalcinosis. Bone dissolution and excessive urinary calcium loss in human patients with renal acidosis may result in a state of negative calcium balance. This has been confirmed by evidence of a mild reversible hyperparathyroidism stimulated by the hypocalcemia (Coe, 1975). The modest secondary hyperparathyroidism represents an "appropriate" secretion of parathormone (i.e., parathyroid hormone production is sensitive to plasma ionized calcium and is necessary to restore ionized calcium levels to normal). The condition can be reversed if proper alkali therapy for the acidosis reverses the hypercalciuria. Reduced plasma phosphate with a normal or high urinary output of phosphate may be due to increased phosphate clearance seen with secondary hyperparathyroidism, although chronic acidosis may have a minor influence in increasing phosphate output.

High urinary pH, hypercalciuria and decreased excretion of citrate contribute to nephrocalcinosis and urolithiasis in distal RTA of human beings. Calcium salts are known to be relatively insoluble in an alkaline media. Citrate, which forms a soluble and undissociated complex with calcium, is excreted in increased amounts in an alkaline urine and therefore plays a role in preventing the precipitation of calcium salts which might otherwise occur. Citrate excretion, however, is dependent on intracellular pH. Despite an alkaline urine, excretion of citrate is characteristically low in cases of distal RTA. The hypocitraturia is probably due to increased tubular reabsorption of

citrate caused by the intracellular acidosis. Pyelonephritis can occur in any renal disease complicated by nephrocalcinosis. Secondary fibrosis around the calcium deposits predisposes the renal parenchyma to infection.

Hyperchloremic acidosis is commonplace in distal RTA as a consequence of distal tubular insufficiency predisposing to impaired hydrogen-sodium exchange. Sodium exchange for hydrogen ion in the distal tubule is reduced, so that sodium is excreted together with anions entering the distal tubule which normally are excreted with hydrogen ion. Urinary loss of sodium, however, is without concomitant loss of chloride, since chloride ion is reabsorbed normally by the proximal tubule. The fall in extracellular fluid volume (ECFV) accompanying sodium loss stimulates a mild secondary hyperaldosteronism. The resulting retention of sodium and chloride tends to reexpand the ECFV. However, reabsorption of sodium, chloride and water aggravates the hyperchloremia and the acidemia by diluting the already low plasma bicarbonate and increasing the concentration of chloride relative to that of sodium.

In addition to sodium-wasting in distal RTA, potassium-wasting is also a common complication. Reduction in the net rate of $Na^+$–$H^+$ exchange in the distal nephron, imposed by failure of $H^+$ to be secreted against a concentration gradient from tubular cell to lumen, obligates an increase in renal $Na^+$–$K^+$ exchange (Schultze, 1973). This initiates hyperkaluria, with resulting hypokalemia. Even with this exchange, large amounts of sodium are lost in the urine, resulting in sodium depletion and decreased ECFV. The secondary hyperaldosteronism stimulated necessitates $Na^+$–$K^+$ exchange, since $H^+$ is not available, and further adds to the renal wasting of potassium (Morris, 1969). Most patients with distal RTA do not require potassium supplements to maintain normokalemia, provided that correction of their acidosis and decreased ECFV is sustained.

Patients with distal RTA pass large volumes of urine of low specific gravity (1.010). The defect in urinary concentrating ability may result from both hypercalciuria and potassium deficiency. Hypercalciuria produces a diuresis of salt and water by interfering with the tubular reabsorption of sodium. This affects the countercurrent mechanism by decreasing the concentration of sodium in the medullary interstitial fluid. Hypercalciuria may also interfere with renal concentration by interfering with the action of ADH on the permeability of collecting ducts to water. The ability to develop a maximally hypertonic urine is markedly impaired in potassium deficiency in man and animals. This may be due to either a decrease in free water (i.e., water that is free of solutes) absorption or decreased accumulation of solute in the medullary interstitium. In early stages of the disease, hyposthenuria may be corrected by adequate control of acidosis and potassium deficiency. Following nephrocalcinosis and tubular damage, however, the specific gravity becomes fixed.

**Proximal Renal Tubular Acidosis.** Proximal RTA existing as only a defect in bicarbonate reabsorption is rare in man and primarily occurs in children. RTA usually exists as a multiple functional disturbance of the proximal tubule. In proximal RTA, the Tm (transport maxima) for bicarbonate reabsorption is reduced, probably as a result of an error in membrane transport. The basic deficiency is reduction in hydrogen ion secretion from tubular cell to lumen, with subsequent reduction in bicarbonate reabsorption. At physiologic concentrations of plasma bicarbonate (24 to 26 mEq./l.), the proximal tubule in this disorder is unable to reabsorb the 85 per cent of filtered bicarbonate as it normally does and characteristically "wastes" approximately 15 to 20 per cent. The distal nephron, which is responsible for reabsorbing 15 per cent of the filtered bicarbonate, is flooded with the bicarbonate excess, and its reabsorptive ability is overwhelmed. Bicarbonate is lost in the urine, and plasma bicarbonate concentration falls. Owing to the initial bicarbonaturia and distal swamping of $H^+$ secretion, urine pH is high, and titratable acid and ammonium excretion are low. As the plasma concentration of $HCO_3^-$ steadily falls, eventually a level is reached (approximately 12 to 14 mEq./l.) at which the Tm is not surpassed, and, again, 85 per cent of the bicarbonate present in glomerular filtrate is reabsorbed by the proximal tubule, even in the presence of reduced hydrogen ion secretion. The distal tubule (normal hydrogen ion secretion) reabsorbs its 15 per cent and bicarbonaturia ceases. Urinary pH falls into the acid range (i.e., there is no disturbance in distal urinary acidification in proximal RTA), and titratable acid and ammonia are secreted appropriately.

In patients with proximal RTA, there is a limit to the degree of acidosis that can develop. Once the Tm for bicarbonate reabsorption in the proximal tubule is not exceeded, the acidosis stabilizes. Stabilization here implies that $H^+$ ion is in a steady state, with input equaling output. However, the total amount of free $H^+$ ion in the body is greatly increased because of defluent buffering by bicarbonate. The degree of acidosis imposed on a patient with a plasma bicarbonate concentration of 12 to 14 mEq./l. has biochemical consequences, especially in bone buffering.

Unlike distal RTA, gradual leaching of bone, leading to osteomalacia and hypercalciuria stimulated by the metabolic acidosis in proximal RTA, does not usually cause nephrocalcinosis. The reason is that the distal nephron can acidify the urine after stabilization. In addition, citrate excretion is not impaired before stabilization, when urine pH is high.

Potassium- and sodium-wasting with secondary hyperaldosteronism are common complications of both distal and proximal RTA. Although the mechanism is not completely understood, aldosterone secretion and excretion may remain increased in proximal RTA even after acidosis has been corrected. In contrast with distal RTA, patients with proximal RTA frequently show an increased severity in renal potassium-wasting when acidosis is corrected with alkali therapy. This can be attributed in part to excessive sodium bicarbonate delivery to the distal nephron. Raising the plasma bicarbonate concentration with sodium bicarbonate therapy exceeds the Tm for bicarbonate reabsorption, and both sodium and bicarbonate flood the distal system. Delivery to the distal nephron of supernormal amounts of sodium and bicarbonate leads again to saturation of the $H^+$-ion–secreting mechanism and resultant bicarbonaturia plus, in the presence of hyperaldosteronism, an increased exchange of sodium with potassium. Bicarbonaturia also increases intraluminal negativity, which augments net potassium secretion in the distal nephron and promotes renal potassium-wasting.

Hyperchloremic acidosis is also characteristic of proximal RTA for the same mechanism as outlined in distal RTA. In addition, a fall in plasma bicarbonate with retention of hydrogen ions in both disorders is accompanied by a compensatory increase in plasma chloride concentration.

**Proximal RTA—The Fanconi Syndrome.** The Fanconi syndrome is a disorder involving multiple proximal tubular defects due to errors in membrane transport. Characteristically, these are defects of bicarbonate, phosphate, glucose and amino acid reabsorption. Proteinuria (primarily globulins) is usually present. This presumably reflects tubular cell damage, in contrast to albuminuria resulting from glomerular leakage.

Plasma amino acid concentration is normal, but increased amino acid clearance and reduction in tubular reabsorption lead to gross aminoaciduria. In man, glutamine, asparagine, alanine, proline, glycine, valine and cystine are mainly lost. The urinary chromatogram, however, may resemble that of a plasma ultrafiltrate with all amino acids represented.

High phosphate clearance due to decreased reabsorption in the proximal tubule leads to hypophosphatemia. This complicates and possibly hastens the potential osteomalacia predisposed by bone-buffering excessive hydrogen ions in metabolic acidosis. Bicarbonaturia is the initiating cause of the metabolic acidosis.

Patients with Fanconi syndrome usually have some degree of hypercalciuria. This, coupled with heavy phosphaturia, could lead to calculi formation. Nephrocalcinosis and nephrolithiasis are rare, however, owing to protective mechanisms of citrate excretion and urinary acidification once acidosis has developed.

Renal glycosuria is due to reduction of the total tubular reabsorptive capacity for glucose.

Potassium-wasting is also present and is increased with alkali therapy via the same mechanisms described for proximal RTA.

## CLASSIFICATION AND ETIOLOGY

Tables 1 and 2 outline the classification and clinical spectrum (possibly etiologies) of distal RTA (Type I) and proximal RTA (Type II). Although these tables have been adopted and modified from human medicine, much of the contents are applicable to veterinary medicine. Because of the paucity of information about genetically transmitted

**Table 1.** *Clinical Spectrum of Renal Tubular Acidosis—Type I (Distal RTA, Classic RTA, Gradient RTA)*

| |
|---|
| Metabolic disorders causing nephrocalcinosis |
|   Hyperparathyroidism |
|   Hyperthyroidism |
|   Vitamin D intoxication |
| Autoimmune disorders |
|   Idiopathic hypergammaglobulinemia (nonmyelomatous) |
|   Hyperglobulinemic purpura |
|   Cryoglobulinemia |
|   Lupus erythematosus |
| Primary renal disease |
|   Medullary sponge kidney |
|   Pyelonephritis(?) |
| Amphotericin B nephropathy |
| Hepatic cirrhosis |

disorders of proximal and distal RTA in the dog, however, hereditary forms described in man have been omitted.

## CLINICAL SIGNS

Clinical signs depend on the causal disease, the electrolytes and other substances which are lost in the urine, and the degree of acidosis present.

**Distal RTA.** Most of the clinical manifestations of this disorder in man are consequences of prolonged metabolic acidosis and dehydration. Polyuria, polydipsia, anorexia, weight loss, constipation and weakness due to potassium loss may occur.

**Table 2.** *Clinical Spectrum of Renal Tubular Acidosis—Type II (Proximal RTA, Bicarbonate-Wasting RTA, Rate RTA) Associated with Single or Multiple Dysfunctions of the Proximal Tubule*

| |
|---|
| Metabolic disorders associated with chronic hypocalcemia and/or secondary hyperparathyroidism |
|   Vitamin D deficiency |
|   Chronic renal insufficiency |
| Disorders of protein metabolism |
|   Multiple myeloma |
|   Amyloidosis |
|   Nephrotic syndrome |
| Primary renal disease |
|   Medullary cystic disease |
| Heavy metal poisoning |
|   Lead |
|   Cadmium |
|   Mercury |
| Drugs |
|   Acetazolamide |
|   Sulfanilamide |
|   Outdated tetracycline |

Disturbances in gait and bone pain on palpation of back and extremities due to osteomalacia may also be detected. Radiographic evidence of osteomalacia may occur without bone pain. Owing to a high incidence of nephrocalcinosis and nephrolithiasis in distal RTA, dogs may present with an acute abdomen due to renal colic pain when passing a calculus.

**Proximal RTA.** Human patients with this disorder do not have a defect in urinary concentrating ability and do not form renal calculi. However, all other manifestations of acidosis, dehydration and potassium loss may be present.

**Proximal RTA—The Fanconi Syndrome.** Owing to renal glycosuria, pronounced polyuria and polydipsia are common. Weight loss is attributed to longstanding acidosis and dehydration rather than to aminoaciduria. These patients have

a predilection for osteomalacia and bone pain. Hypercalciuria and renal loss of phosphate with resultant hypophosphatemia seem to be the primary causes of bone disease in this syndrome. Nephrocalcinosis and nephrolithiasis, however, are rare in man and animals. Weakness from hypokalemia may be present.

## LABORATORY FINDINGS

Table 3 outlines expected biochemical findings in dogs with RTA. Hyperchloremic acidosis is consistent in the three disorders listed. In all, a base deficit, low plasma $CO_2$ capacity and low plasma bicarbonate concentration indicate the presence of metabolic acidosis. The $PCO_2$ is normal, indicating respiratory balance. However, there is a mild compensatory respiratory alkalosis, for the $CO_2$ content is usually lower than the

***Table 3.*** *Biochemical Findings Expected in Dogs with RTA*

| BLOOD AND URINE | | DISTAL RTA | PROXIMAL RTA | FANCONI SYNDROME |
|---|---|---|---|---|
| **Blood** | | | | |
| Electrolytes | | | | |
| Calcium | mg./dl. | L 8.0–8.5 | L 8.0–8.5 | L 8.0–8.5 |
| Phosphorus | mg./dl. | L to N 2.5–4.5 | L to N 2.5–4.5 | L to N 2.5–4.5 |
| Sodium | mEq./l. | N to H 135–155 | N to H 135–155 | N to H 135–155 |
| Potassium | mEq./l. | L to N 3.5–4.0 | L to N 3.5–4.0 | L to N 3.5–4.0 |
| *Chloride | mEq./l. | H 113–120 | H 113–120 | H 113–120 |
| Chemistries | | | | |
| BUN | mg./dl. | N 10–20 | N 10–20 | N 10–20 |
| Creatinine | mg./dl. | N 0.8–1.2 | N 0.8–1.2 | N 0.8–1.2 |
| Alk. p'tase | IU | N to H 50–150 | N to H 50–150 | N to H 50–150 |
| Total protein | gm./dl. | N to L 4.0–7.5 | N to L 4.0–7.5 | N to L 4.0–7.5 |
| Albumin | gm./dl. | N to L 2.5–4.5 | N to L 2.5–4.5 | N to L 2.5–4.5 |
| Globulin | gm./dl. | N to H 1.5–5.0 | N to H 1.5–5.0 | N to H 1.5–5.0 |
| Glucose | mg./dl. | N 70–110 | N 70–110 | N 70–110 |
| Gases | | | | |
| *pH | | L 7.20 | L 7.18 | L 7.18 |
| $PCO_2$ | mm. Hg | N to L 37 | N to L 35 | N to L 35 |
| *$CO_2$ content | mEq./l. | L 20.0 | L 14.0 | L 14.0 |
| $CO_2$ capacity | mEq./l. | L 21.0 | L 14.5 | L 14.5 |
| Standard $HCO_3^-$ | mEq./l. | L 20.0 | L 20.0 | L 14.0 |
| *Actual $HCO_3^-$ | mEq./l. | L 19.0 | L 13.0 | L 13.0 |
| *Base deficit | mEq./l. | H 7.0 (26−19) | H 13.0 (26−13) | H 13.0 (26−13) |
| *Urine* | | | | |
| Analysis | | | | |
| *Specific gravity | | 1.001–1.012 | > 1.018 | > 1.018 |
| *pH | | > 6.0 | < 6.0 | < 6.0 |
| Protein | | Trace | Trace | Trace |
| *Glucose | | Negative | Negative | Strong positive |
| Ketone | | Variable | Variable | Variable |
| Electrolytes | | | | |
| Calcium | mg./kg./day | > 3.0 | > 3.0 | > 3.0 |
| Phosphorus | mg./kg./day | >30.0 | >30.0 | >30.0 |
| Sodium | mEq./kg./day | > 8.0 | > 8.0 | > 8.0 |
| Potassium | mEq./kg./day | >10.0 | >10.0 | >10.0 |
| Chloride | mEq./kg./day | 2.0–10.0 | 2.0–10.0 | 2.0–10.0 |

*Key laboratory work.
L=low; N=normal; H=high.

$CO_2$ capacity and the actual bicarbonate is lower than the standard bicarbonate.

Because these patients show an increased serum chloride concentration, the "anion gap" is normal. Anion gap is the difference between the sum of the measured cations (Na + K) and the sum of the measured anions ($HCO_3$ + Cl). The concentration of anions such as phosphate, sulfate, organic acid and protein is not ordinarily measured. The concentration of the cation calcium is also not used, for changes in its value in mEq./l. are minimal and do not significantly affect the anion gap value. The normal anion gap is approximately 16 mEq./l. An abnormally high anion gap is associated with diabetic ketoacidosis and azotemia. The following formula is used to determine the presence of an abnormal gap:

$$Anion\ gap = (Na + K) - (HCO_3 + Cl)$$

*Example 1 (Normal dog)*
    Na=142,  K=4,  $HCO_3$=27,  Cl=103 mEq./l.
Anion gap = (142 + 4) − (27 + 103)
         = 16

*Example 2 (Proximal RTA)*
    Na=140,  K=3.5,  $HCO_3$=13.5,  Cl=114 mEq./l.
Anion gap = (140 + 3.5) − (13.5 + 114)
         = 16

*Example 3 (Diabetic ketoacidosis)*
    Na=155,  K=4.5,  $HCO_3$=15,  Cl=100 mEq./l.
Anion gap = (155 + 4.5) − (15 + 100)
         = 44.5

The urinary sediment may not reflect infection in early stages of renal tubular acidosis, but bacterial culture and antibiotic sensitivity tests should be performed on all suspect patients.

## RADIOGRAPHIC FINDINGS

Osteomalacia is softening of bone due to loss of calcium salts. Osteomalacic lesions may be seen in long bones, vertebral bodies or bones of the skull. Pseudofractures may be present.

In distal RTA, renal calculi may occur as well as striations of nephrocalcinosis. However, in early stages of the disease, the degree of mineralization may be insufficient to be detected radiographically. An intravenous pyelogram (IVP) should be performed on all distal RTA patients. The technique gives a good anatomic survey of the urinary tract including pelves, ureters and bladder.

## DIAGNOSIS

Coupled with the symptoms and signs, renal tubular acidosis should be suspected if a patient shows hyperchloremic metabolic acidosis.

**Distal RTA.** Diagnosis is confirmed by failure of the kidneys to secrete a known ingested acid load. The ammonium chloride loading test is commonly employed. Ammonium ion ($NH_4^+$) is acidic because it can dissociate to ammonia (which is removed by conversion to urea in the liver) and $H^+$. When this compound is ingested, the kidneys should normally secrete the excess of hydrogen ion (Wrong, 1959).

Procedure:
—No food is taken after midnight.
—8:00 A.M. ammonium chloride is administered orally at 0.1 gm./kg. body weight.
—Hourly specimens of urine are collected between 10:00 A.M. and 4:00 P.M., and the pH of each specimen is measured immediately with pH paper (pH meter is best).
—If the pH of any specimen falls below 6.0, the test may be stopped.
Interpretation:
—In normal dogs, the urinary pH falls below 6.0 between 2 and 8 hours after the dose.
—In renal tubular acidosis, this degree of acidification fails to occur.

Author's opinions differ concerning the pH to which human patients with distal RTA can acidify urine (6.0 [Simpson, 1971]; 6.6 to 7.0 [Pitts, 1974]; 5.4 [Rodriguez-Soriano, 1969]). This variation emphasizes that renal tubular acidosis is not an entity that can be strictly defined in relation to urinary pH, just as obesity cannot be defined in relation to variation in body weight. What the urine pH does tell is that under the strong stimulus of spontaneous systemic acidosis or ammonium chloride ingestion, the patient cannot secrete the excess hydrogen and correct the acidosis.

**Proximal RTA.** Bicarbonate titration tests are needed to establish the diagnosis of this disorder. Since this test is not readily available in most clinical settings, a diagnosis can frequently be made by using a therapeutic trial of bicarbonate. Patients with proximal RTA may require up to 10 mEq. of sodium bicarbonate/kg. of body weight/day to maintain plasma bicarbonate levels near normal.

THE FANCONI SYNDROME. Diagnosis is confirmed by the presence of glycosuria with a normal glucose tolerance test, therapeutic trial of bicarbonate ranging up to 10 mEq./kg./day to correct the acidosis and hyperphosphaturia with hypophosphatemia. Urinary chromatography to analyze amino acids lost in the urine is valuable but the cost is prohibitive for most clinical settings.

## TREATMENT

The aims of treatment are to correct the acidosis by restoring the bicarbonate which has been lost, to correct the hypokalemia and to arrest the progression of osteomalacia. If a particular disorder predisposing to renal tubular acidosis has been diagnosed, specific therapy should also be initiated.

In renal tubular acidosis with normal glomerular function, treatment for osteomalacia with sodium bicarbonate alone has been very successful in man (Richards *et al.*, 1972). Owing to vitamin D resistance in uremia, osteomalacia in patients with chronic renal failure does not improve with sodium bicarbonate therapy alone.

**Distal RTA.** Acidosis, hypercalciuria and potassium-wasting are usually corrected by the oral administration of 1.0 to 1.5 mEq. of sodium bicarbonate/kg./day in divided doses. Vitamin D and calcium administration for osteomalacia are discouraged in distal RTA because of the predisposition to nephrocalcinosis and calculi formation. The amount of sodium bicarbonate given should be sufficient to return pH and serum bicarbonate to a normal range. Several months may be required before radiographic osteomalacic lesions are resolved.

**Proximal RTA and The Fanconi Syndrome.** Large doses of sodium bicarbonate are required to treat the base deficit associated with these disorders. From 2 to over 10 mEq./kg. of $NaHCO_3$ daily in divided doses may be required to return pH and serum bicarbonate concentrations to within a normal range. Because treatment aggravates the existing hypokalemia, potassium supplementation is also required. Potassium gluconate rather than potassium chloride should be given because of the hyperchloremic metabolic acidosis. Potassium gluconate elixir* provides 20 mEq. of elemental potassium per tablespoonful. Even if the plasma concentration of potassium is known, the quantity required to replace a deficit is not easily calculated because plasma concentration may not reveal the intracellular deficit. A dosage of 1 mEq./kg./day in divided doses can be given safely, but potassium and all other electrolytes should be monitored carefully during the correction of metabolic acidosis. If patients are developing renal failure, potassium therapy should not be initiated.

In all forms of renal tubular acidosis, specific long-term antibiotic therapy should be introduced if urinary infection is present. Sulfanilamide, being a carbonic anhydrase inhibitor, is contraindicated.

## PROGNOSIS

The exact prognosis is unknown. Renal tubular acidosis is slowly progressive, with renal function remaining apparently unchanged over long periods of time. In well-controlled patients, especially in distal RTA, progressive renal damage from fibrosis secondary to nephrocalcinosis and resistant pyelonephritis may occur. Although the prognosis might be more favorable in proximal RTA, since nephrocalcinosis does not tend to develop, a case has been reported in which a dog with the Fanconi syndrome developed resistant pyelonephritis and died from uremia (Thornhill, 1977).

### SUPPLEMENTAL READING

Coe, F. L., and Firpo, J. J.: Evidence for mild reversible hyperparathyroidism in distal renal tubular acidosis. Arch. Intern. Med., *135*:1485, 1975.

Morris, R. C., Jr.: Renal tubular acidosis. New Engl. J. Med., *281*:1405, 1969.

Pitts, R. F.: Physiology of the Kidney and Body Fluids. 3rd ed. Chicago, Year Book Medical Publishers, 1974.

Richards, P., Chamberlain, M. J., and Wrong, O. M.: Treatment of osteomalacia of renal tubular acidosis by sodium bicarbonate alone. Lancet, 2:994, 1972.

Rodriguez-Soriano, J., and Edelman, C. M., Jr.: Renal tubular acidosis. Ann. Rev. Med., *20*:363, 1969.

Schultze, R. G.: Recent advances in the physiology and pathophysiology of potassium excretion. Arch. Intern. Med., *131*:885, 1973.

Simpson, D. P.: Control of hydrogen ion homeostasis and renal acidosis. Medicine, *50*:503, 1971.

Thornhill, J. A.: A case report of the Fanconi syndrome in a basenji. (In preparation, 1977.)

Wrong, O. M., and Davies, H. E. F.: The excretion of acid in renal disease. Quart. J. Med., (N.S.)28:259, 1959.

*Kanon® elixir, Warren-Teed Pharmaceuticals, Inc., Columbus, Ohio 43210.

# APPARENT PSYCHOGENIC POLYDIPSIA

ARTHUR L. LAGE, D.V.M.
*South Weymouth, Massachusetts*

## INTRODUCTION

Psychogenic polydipsia (PP) or compulsive water drinking is frequently considered in the differential diagnosis of polydipsia, although in veterinary medicine there is a paucity of documented cases of PP. Because psychiatric analysis of animals is not feasible, and because the diagnosis of PP is often based on indirect diagnostic analyses or exclusion of other diagnoses, the term apparent psychogenic polydipsia (APP) is preferred for animals.

In man, psychogenic polydipsia is generally considered to be a mental (psychotic or neurotic) disorder—at least when the initial problem begins. The patient often has other psychoses or neuroses such as anxiety, compulsive eating, phobias or schizoid behavior. The etiology of APP in animals is unknown. In two canine cases, physiologic environmental thirst induction was the probable cause. Although some dogs are nervous, none have been neurotic. Regardless of the mental illness initiating the polydipsia, the countercurrent mechanism of urine concentration may be altered by medullary washout of ions secondary to prolonged or severe polydipsia and resultant polyuria. Loss of renal medullary hypertonicity may make it difficult to distinguish APP from pituitary diabetes insipidus or renal diabetes insipidus.

There is an area of the brain called the "drinking center" localized on each side of the hypothalamus. In those animals in which the site of the drinking center has been studied, it was located lateral and caudal to the supraotic nuclei. Its close proximity to the supraotic nucleus (the site of hormone synthesis) may explain why factors causing increased intake of water are sometimes associated with increased renal conservation of water. Physiologically, the four most important causes of thirst are extracellular dehydration, low cardiac output, intracellular dehydration and dryness of the mouth. These stimuli probably excite the thirst center directly and are thought to be mediated through one stimulus—intracellular dehydration. The act of drinking and fullness of the gastrointestinal tract seem to inhibit thirst. These two acts probably excite peripheral sensory receptors that transmit inhibitory impulses into the thirst center. Both extracellular dehydration and circulatory failure can produce intracellular dehydration.

When an animal is maintained on a low or limited salt intake for long periods of time, the osmolar concentration of the extracellular fluid may fall. The extracellular fluid volume may also decrease. When extracellular volume drops, the animal begins to drink large volumes of water. Unless sodium chloride is available, however, the normal extracellular fluid volume may not be restored, and excessive drinking may continue. Continued drinking, excessive urination and low sodium intake will eventually result in loss of ions from the renal medulla. If an adequate amount of sodium chloride is added to the water or fed to the animal, the extracellular volume will usually return to normal.

Many nephrophysiologists and clinical nephrologists believe that prolonged polyuria, even without decreased sodium intake, will cause medullary ionic washout.

## DIAGNOSTIC PROCEDURES

Causes of polyuria and polydipsia include apparent psychogenic polydipsia, pituitary diabetes insipidus (DI), nephrogenic diabetes (NDI), primary polyuric renal failure, pyometra, hyperadrenocorticism, diabetes mellitus, liver failure and hypothyroidism. Confusion may arise in differentiating APP, DI and NDI. Most of the latter diseases are associated with profound polydipsia and polyuria (4 to 6 times normal urine volume).

The most useful test used to establish a diagnosis of APP is the water deprivation–urine concentration test. The second most useful test is the Hickey-Hare test (refer to the article on "Nephrogenic Diabetes Insipidus" for technique and interpretation). Other tests employed and parameters measured in cases of suspected APP include water balance studies, urinalysis and urine and plasma osmolalities.

The Hickey-Hare test is used to detect the ability of the kidneys to reduce urine flow as a result of release of ADH in response to increasing plasma osmolality. In man, it is an important test used to establish a diagnosis of psychogenic polydipsia. It is best used in veterinary medicine after a water deprivation–urine concentration test has first been performed.

The recommended method of clinical evaluation is to admit the patient into the hospital after the physical exam and to perform a hemogram, urinalysis and water balance study on the first day. A presumptive diagnosis of APP, DI or NDI may be made in those cases with a water diuresis associated with a urine specific gravity of 1.001 to approximately 1.006. It has been suggested by many nephrologists in human medicine that when urine specific gravity is maximally dilute (1.001) the diagnosis will usually be APP and *not* NDI or DI. Experience has shown this to be true in about half the cases involving dogs. In cases of APP that I have evaluated, urine osmolalities were quite low (102 to 112 mOsm./kg.). The serum osmolalities were slightly low (285 to 295 mOsm./kg.) and serum sodium concentration was normal to low (131 to 140 mEq./l.).

The next procedure is to perform a water deprivation–urine concentration test. If the patient concentrates urine, the diagnosis is APP; if the patient does not concentrate urine, APP, DI and NDI must still be considered. Three of the cases presented herein did not concentrate urine following water deprivation. Concentration of urine following Hickey-Hare tests, however, revealed the presence of APP. Urine concentration was also observed after limiting the water intake and administering oral sodium in the form of sodium bicarbonate and sodium chloride. A patient that becomes dehydrated following the concentration test, but who still cannot concentrate urine, should be rehydrated and evaluated by an exogenous ADH response test. Inability to concentrate urine following an ADH response test should be followed by the Hickey-Hare test. An abnormal Hickey-Hare (i.e., increased urine flow) indicates the presence of pituitary or nephrogenic diabetes insipidus.

The cases listed in Table 1 are given in the order of increasing clinical complexity. Reference to Table 1 may help the reader better understand the relatively wide spectrum of clinical findings in cases of APP.

Half the cases of canine APP have been encountered in German Shepherd dogs. About 75 per cent of the cases have been in dogs over 30 kg. and about 25 per cent in dogs approximately 15 kg. in weight. APP was not diagnosed in toy breeds of dogs or in cats. The sex distribution has been essentially equal. The age distribution has been 2 to 9 years, with a mean of 5 years. The chief presenting complaint in all cases is PUPD. In about half of all cases, the owners stated that they observed polydipsia prior to the development of polyuria. About two thirds of the cases had intermittent nocturia, while one third had no nocturia. The duration of signs observed before the patient was presented to the hospital ranged from one week to six months. The longer the duration of PUPD before therapy, the more difficult it was to obtain successful treatment. Urine output ranged from 4 to 6 times normal, with a mean of about 4 times normal. Urine specific gravity ranged from 1.001 to 1.003, with about 75 per cent in the 1.000 to 1.002 area. Urine osmolality ranged from 102 to 110 mOsm./kg. water and plasma osmolality from 285 to 295 mOsm./kg. The water deprivation–urine concentration test resulted in urine concentration in about two thirds of the cases, and eventually was normal in most cases. The Hickey-Hare test resulted in decreased urine volume in all cases in which it was used. The BUN concentration was normal in every case.

## THERAPY

After the diagnosis has been substantiated, limiting water intake or administering sodium (sodium chloride and sodium bicarbonate) along with limiting water intake is recommended. As mentioned before, the diagnostic tests of water deprivation–

### Table 1. *Apparent Psychogenic Polydipsia*

| CASE | SEX | WEIGHT (LB.) | AGE (YR.) | PRESENTING COMPLAINT* | DURATION | DURATION AFTER AND WITH Rx** | WATER BALANCE $H_2O$ Intake (ml.) | Urine Output (ml.) |
|---|---|---|---|---|---|---|---|---|
| German shepherd † | M | 74 | 4 | PUPD No nocturia Precede PU? | 2 weeks | Immediate response | 6010 | 5920 (4x normal) |
| Labrador retriever | M | 82 | 3 | PUPD No nocturia Precede PU-yes | 1 week | Immediate response | 5750 | 5570 (4x normal) |
| Terrier † | SF | 32 | 3½ | PUPD Nocturia ± Precede PU? | 2 weeks | Immediate response | 3720 | 3650 (6x normal) |
| German shepherd | M | 85 | 8 | PUPD Nocturia ± Precede PU-yes | 3 weeks | 3 weeks | 6310 | 6120 (4x normal) |
| Collie | F | 63 | 2 | PUPD Nocturia ± Precede PU-yes | Increasing over 3 months | 1 month | 6300 | 6100 (5x normal) |
| Standard poodle | M | 63 | 3 | PUPD No nocturia Precede PU-yes | 3 months | 6 weeks | 6020 | 5670 (5.5x normal) |
| German shepherd † | SF | 90 | 8 | PUPD Nocturia ± Precede PU-yes | 2 months | 2½ months: Limited $H_2O$ and gave Na; HH | 8700 | 8400 (5x normal) |
| White shepherd † | SF | 96 | 7 | PUPD Nocturia ± Precede PU? | 2 months | 4 months: Reasonably, then always, had to limit $H_2O$ | 11,100 | 10,950 (6x normal) |
| Beagle | SF | 31 | 9 | PUPD Nocturia ± Precede PU-yes | 6 months | Never normal unless $H_2O$ limited | 3610 | 3535 (5.5x normal) |
| Stump-tail monkey | M | 25 | 3 | PUPD Psychotic | 3 weeks | Never normal unless Librium® and limited $H_2O$ | 3140 | 2990 (6x normal) |

*Key to Table 1:*
    * Presenting complaint = three items are listed in this column: (1) the presence or absence of PUPD; (2) the presence or absence of nocturia; (3) whether or not polydipsia preceded polyuria. Question mark indicates client did not know. Plus and minus before question indicates not reliable information from the client.
    ** Duration after and with therapy = the duration of clinical signs following diagnosis and therapy.
    † Urine concentration test = water deprivation–urine concentration test.
    ‡ Behavior = the possible causes of APP are listed in addition to behavior patterns of the patient.
    PUPD = polyuria polydipsia.
    HH = Hickey-Hare test.

**Table 1.** *Apparent Psychogenic Polydipsia (Continued)*

| URINE S.G. | OSMOLALITY (mOsm./kg.) Urine | OSMOLALITY (mOsm./kg.) Plasma | URINE CONCENTRATION TEST† | HICKEY-HARE TEST | SERUM Na (mEq./l.) | BEHAVIOR‡ |
|---|---|---|---|---|---|---|
| 1.003 | N.D. | N.D. | 1.040 | N.D. | N.D. | Normal, not nervous |
| 1.001 | 102 | 286 | 1.042 | N.D. | 140 | Hunting on hot day and continued to drink large volumes; normal behavior, not nervous |
| 1.001 | N.D. | N.D. | 1.036 | N.D. | N.D. | Nervous |
| 1.002 | N.D. | N.D. | 1.030 | N.D. | N.D. | Hot spell in Boston area and dog was taken bicycling; not nervous |
| 1.003 | 112 | 295 | 1.031 | Normal response | 137 | In a kennel; started drinking and was very nervous |
| 1.002 | 105 | 290 | 1.018 After HH, 1.026; after 4 days restricted H₂O, 1.040 | Normal response | 134 | Not nervous |
| 1.002 | 103 | 294 | 1.035 | Normal response | 135 | Nervous |
| 1.001 | 110 | 285 | 1.008 After HH, 1.018; after 3 days limited H₂O, 1.036 | Normal response | 135 | Only abnormal change was a new child in the house; nervous |
| 1.001 | N.D. | N.D. | 1.009 After HH and 1 day on oral Na, 1.021; after 3 days limited water and Na, 1.036 | Normal response | 131  135  139 | Not nervous |
| 1.001 | N.D. | N.D. | 1.040+ | N.D. | N.D. | Psychotic |

urine concentration and/or Hickey-Hare may provide the initial boost for beginning effective therapy (i.e., there may be repletion of renal medullary ionic balance).

Therapy consists of giving calculated normal water volume to the patient after the water deprivation test and/or Hickey-Hare test. In those cases where this method is successful (about one third of the patients), the animal is usually content, does not drink from outside sources and does not constantly bark for water.

In those cases in which the animal does not act normal, drinks from any source, constantly barks, drinks his own urine, acts weak or becomes dehydrated, nearly unlimited water volume should be allowed for one day. Water intake should then be reduced by segmental increments (i.e., reduce by 25 per cent of the calculated amount that is above normal intake each week). This is continued until a nearly normal urine output and water consumption have been established. In cases in which this procedure is used, oral sodium chloride and sodium bicarbonate are administered to the patient for 3 to 5 days. Recommended dosage is 0.6 gm. of sodium bicarbonate and 1 gram of sodium chloride per 30 kg. body weight twice daily. Three to 10 weeks may lapse before an animal will be able to handle free-choice water without developing polydipsia. In specific cases, two dogs and one monkey could not be given free-choice water, or be allowed contact with extra liquid sources, without developing high-volume polydipsia. The monkey was treated with 5 mg. of chlordiazepoxide (Librium® [Roche]), given twice daily, and was allowed limited water intake. Chlordiazepoxide was used because of the true psychotic state of the monkey.

## LOW-VOLUME PSYCHOGENIC POLYDIPSIA

Low-volume APP (water intake only 1½ to 2 times normal) also exists in animals. Most of these patients are presented for something else (such as routine vaccinations), and the client volunteers the information that the animal has been drinking slightly more water than usual. Evaluation of water balance studies in these cases have indicated PUPD. Water deprivation–urine concentration tests were normal. These cases may represent early or mild forms of APP. Control of water consumption will eliminate the problem. It is unknown whether these patients will develop high-volume polydipsia. In human medicine these patients are called polydipsics; no therapy is recommended, provided that the polydipsia remains at a low level (1½ to 2 times normal).

### SUPPLEMENTAL READING

Schrier, R. W., and Berl, T.: Nonosmolar factors affecting renal water excretion (Part I). New Engl. J. Med., 292:81–88, 1974.
Schrier, R. W., and Berl, T.: Nonosmolar factors affecting renal water excretion (Part II). New Engl. J. Med., 292:141–145, 1974.

# NEPHROGENIC DIABETES INSIPIDUS

ARTHUR L. LAGE, D.V.M.
South Weymouth, Massachusetts

Nephrogenic diabetes insipidus (NDI) is a chronic disorder characterized by polyuria, urine of low specific gravity or osmolality, polydipsia and lack of response to either exogenous antidiuretic hormone (ADH) or the release of endogenous ADH via the Hickey-Hare test. Use of the term nephrogenic diabetes insipidus should be reserved for cases in which water diuresis results from impaired ability of the distal tubules and collecting ducts to respond properly to ADH, regardless of whether the defect is hereditary, acquired, functional or anatomic. This disorder is primarily a disturbance of water metabolism and must be differentiated from other diseases (apparent psychogenic polydipsia and diabetes insipidus) and physiologic states causing a water diuresis (Table 1). Although there are many diseases that cause polyuria and polydipsia (PUPD), the magnitude of PUPD is usually much greater in patients with NDI, apparent psychogenic polydipsia (APP) and diabetes insipidus (DI).

The basic defect in the nephrogenic type of diabetes insipidus is failure of distal tubules and collecting ducts to respond to ADH, whereas the basic defect in the pituitary type of diabetes insipidus is lack of formation and/or release of endogenous ADH. In APP there are no basic or initiating renal or pituitary defects, because water diuresis is a normal response to polydipsia. If there is a defect initially, it may be related to sodium metabolism and renal medullary ionic concentration (refer to the article on "Apparent Psychogenic Polydipsia"). Figure 1 depicts the diagnostic flow in the form of a modified algorithm. Difficulty in establishing a diagnosis often occurs as a result of renal medullary washout of ions causing a disturbance of the countercurrent mechanism of urine concentration. If this defect exists in a patient with any of the three diseases associated with water diuresis, it must be corrected in order to establish a specific diagnosis and to provide effective therapy.

In order to illustrate medullary solute washout, the following example, which was investigated according to the algorithm in Figure 1, is presented. A 13-week-old female German shepherd dog is presented with a history of PUPD. Physical examination reveals that the dog is thin and small for its age. In order to verify the presence of polyuria and polydipsia, a fluid balance study is done after obtaining the minimum data base (MDB) for a PUPD patient. The MDB suggested is a complete blood count, urinalysis and determination of BUN. The MDB is normal and the urine specific gravity is 1.003, supporting the presence of polyuria. A fluid balance study performed with the aid of a metabolism cage reveals that the urine volume is 6 times normal (the dog weighs 5.5 kg. and the total urine output is 1457 ml./day). These findings indicate that the underlying disorder is associated with one of the diseases in the upper portion of the flow sheet, because the patient has severe polyuria characterized by a urine specific gravity which is significantly below that of glomerular filtrate. The age of the dog, normal findings on abdominal palpation and the absence of neutrophilic leukocytosis eliminate pyometra as a diagnostic probability.

A water deprivation test is then performed. If the patient responds by concentrating urine, the diagnosis is APP. A water diuresis state can be shown to exist by determining the ratio between urine osmolality and plasma osmolality (U/P ratio). During water diuresis a U/P ratio less than 1 indicates that solute is being reabsorbed in excess of water. In pituitary and nephrogenic diabetes insipidus, the U/P ratio following water deprivation is still less than 1. In this case, it is 0.35 before and 0.35 after the water deprivation test, because the urine specific gravity changed only from 1.003 to 1.004 in 12 hours, despite the development of marked dehydration. Since the patient is unable to concentrate urine following water deprivation, the three causes of water diuresis must still be considered. Diabetes insipidus is not always easily distinguished from APP, because persistent polydipsia and compensatory polyuria reduce the maximal urinary concentrations that may be achieved following dehydration or infusion of hypertonic saline solutions. If a patient with APP cannot concentrate urine following a water deprivation test, or responds poorly to the test (i.e., partial response), medullary washout of ions must be complicating the syndrome. Since the great majority of patients with APP concentrate urine following water deprivation, inability to concentrate urine should be followed by an exogenous ADH response test. A positive response to this test indicates the presence of pituitary diabetes insipidus. A near-normal response indicates the presence of pituitary diabetes insipidus associated with renal medullary washout of ions. The latter should be substantiated by repeating the exogenous ADH response test following ionic replacement (using any of the methods described). A negative or very poor response (as exists in the example) indicates that either NDI or APP with advanced medullary washout of ions is the cause of PUPD.

***Table 1.*** *Overview of Clinical Water Diuresis States*

| DIABETES INSIPIDUS SYNDROME* | CLINICAL WATER DIURESIS STATES** | BASIC PRIMARY DEFECT | SOME CAUSES OF PRIMARY DEFECT |
|---|---|---|---|
| Primary diabetes insipidus (compulsive water drinking) | Apparent psychogenic polydipsia | Abnormal thirst causing polydipsia and secondary polyuria | 1. Habit or psychotic state<br>2. A vicious cycle response to original polydipsia which was caused as a normal physiologic response to thirst, i.e., excessive exercise<br>3. Possible functional lesion of thirst center<br>4. Possible anatomic lesion in or around thirst center |
| Pituitary diabetes insipidus or hypothalamoneuro-hypophyseal diabetes insipidus | Pituitary diabetes insipidus | Inadequate secretion of ADH | 1. Injury to secretory neurons<br>  a. Neoplasia<br>  b. Inflammation<br>  c. Trauma<br>  d. Ischemia<br>2. Idiopathic<br>3. Functional defect of secretory cells (not proven) |
| Nephrogenic diabetes insipidus | Nephrogenic diabetes insipidus | Distal tubules and collecting ducts insensitive to ADH | 1. Functional defect<br>  a. Congenital and/or hereditary renal tubular defect<br>  b. Acquired defect<br>    (1) Drug toxicity<br>    (2) Prolonged severe diuresis causing renal medullary depletion of ions<br>2. Anatomic defect<br>  a. Inflammation of the renal medulla<br>  b. Fibrosis of renal medulla<br>  c. Hypercalcemic nephropathy<br>  d. Hypokalemic nephropathy |

*Nomenclature established by use in the literature.
**Nomenclature useful to the clinician.

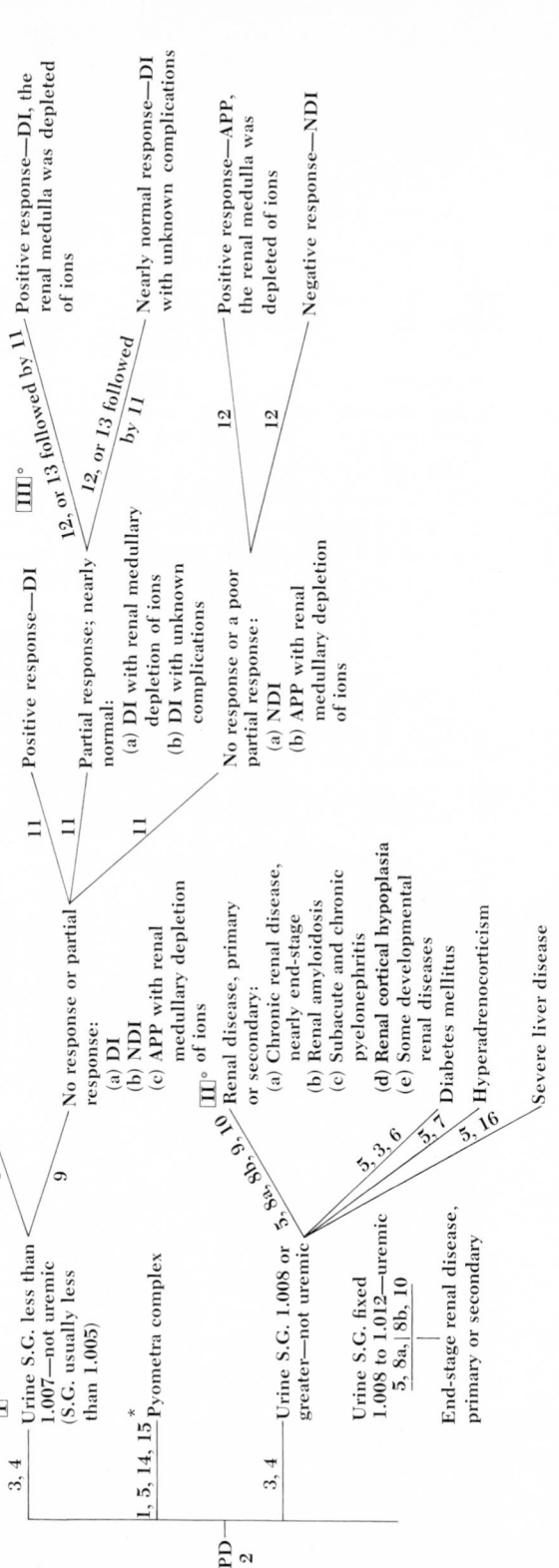

**Figure 1.**

*Key to Figure 1*

This algorithm is to be used as a general guide to assist the clinician. It is not meant as a substitute for in-depth text material, and it in no way covers every aspect of diagnosis. The suggested tests used to achieve a diagnosis are not in every instance chronologic (e.g., #5, physical examination, is used to help diagnose the pyometra complex and would certainly be performed before a fluid balance study). One should use the supplemental reading list to review each test, with the exception of the Hickey-Hare test.

1. History.
2. Fluid balance study; measurement of fluid intake and fluid output using a metabolism cage.
3. Urinalysis; multiple tests will be needed to determine if the specific gravity is truly fixed.
4. BUN or serum creatinine.
5. Physical examination.
6. Fasting blood glucose; may need a glucose tolerance test.
7. Plasma cortisol.
8. Renal function tests.
   a. Endogenous creatinine clearance.
   b. Phenolsulfonphthalein excretion.
9. Water deprivation–urine concentration test; may use either urine specific gravity or osmolality. If osmolality is used, check the plasma osmolality so that a U/P ratio of osmolalities can be determined.
10. Renal biopsy.
11. Exogenous antidiuretic hormone response test.
12. Hickey-Hare test; this procedure may be used both as a diagnostic test and as a therapeutic procedure to help replete the renal medulla of apparently washed-out ions.
13. Oral sodium chloride and sodium bicarbonate loading for two days.
14. CBC.
15. Radiography.
16. Liver function tests.
* If renal disease exists as a result of the pyometra complex, the urine specific gravity will usually be 1.003 to 1.006. There is usually no response to ADH; therefore, pyometra complex should be an early rule-out in the diagnostic plan.
I A urine to plasma osmolality ratio should be performed at this point to evaluate and substantiate the severity of the water diuresis.
II The urine specific gravity may or may not be fixed (1.008 to 1.012) initially.
III These tests (12 and 13) are now used both diagnostically and therapeutically.

The Hickey-Hare test is performed next. A positive response is diagnostic of APP, while a negative response is diagnostic of NDI. (All the tests used in this discussion except the Hickey-Hare test are clearly described in *Canine and Feline Urology* [Osborne *et al.*, 1972]). The Hickey-Hare test is another means of inducing a decrease in urine flow as a result of release of ADH in response to increasing plasma osmolality. It has been used in man to diagnose psychogenic polydipsia. The test is performed in the dog by first administering water (20 ml./kg. of body weight) via stomach tube. An indwelling catheter is placed in the urinary bladder, and a collection vessel or apparatus is used to collect all urine. Urine flow per minute is determined. Sodium chloride solution (2.5 per cent) is infused for 45 minutes at the rate of 0.25 ml./kg. of body weight/minute. Urine volume is recorded every 15 minutes during and 15 minutes after infusion. In man, a normal (or positive) response to the Hickey-Hare test is characterized by a progressive reduction in the rate of urine flow throughout the test period. In patients with NDI or DI, the rate of urine flow will not decrease; in fact, it may increase. In the case described here, the initial urine flow was approximately 1 ml./minute, and the urine volume was 30 to 32 ml. at the end of each of the first three collection periods. The urine volume dropped to 22 ml. 15 minutes after infusion.

The Hickey-Hare test could be performed before the exogenous ADH response test (some physicians do perform this test first);

however, in veterinary medicine, it is better to perform this test after the exogenous ADH response test in most cases for two reasons: First, the Hickey-Hare test is much easier to perform in humans (except in babies and children) than in animals. Second, the great majority of clinical cases associated with water diuresis have been diagnosed as either pituitary diabetes insipidus without severe renal medullary washout or apparent psychogenic polydipsia without severe renal medullary washout. These diagnoses can be readily established by use of the water deprivation–urine concentration test and the exogenous ADH response test.

The mode of therapy for NDI in both human and veterinary medicine is to administer therapeutic dosages of hydrochlorothiazide. Human patients tend to respond to this form of therapy better than do veterinary patients; however, we have had very little experience with documented cases of NDI in veterinary medicine. If a specific cause of NDI, such as drug toxicity, is diagnosed, therapy should be directed toward correction of the potentially reversible cause.

### SUPPLEMENTAL READING

Lage, A. L.: Nephrogenic Diabetes Insipidus in a Dog. J. Am. Vet. Med. Assn., *163*:251–253, 1973.
Osborne, C. A., Low, D. G., and Finco, D. R.: Canine and Feline Urology. Philadelphia, W. B. Saunders Co., 1972.
Weyner, M. J.: Thirst—Proceedings of the First International Symposium on Thirst in the Regulation of Body Water. Pergamon Press, 1964.

# PYELO-NEPHRITIS

DELMAR R. FINCO, D.V.M.
*and* ANATOLE KERN, D.V.M.
*Athens, Georgia*

The term pyelonephritis has been used or abused in a variety of ways in medical literature. The lack of agreement on the meaning of the term reflects the lack of knowledge, in both human and veterinary medicine, regarding urinary tract infection and its possible relationship to chronic nephritis.

In this discussion, the term pyelonephritis will refer to bacterial infection of the kidney, renal pelvis and cranial ureters. For reasons subsequently discussed, the renal medulla and juxtamedullary area are more vulnerable than the cortex to bacterial infection. Excluded from the definition are polysystemic diseases that affect the kidney (leptospirosis, etc.) and cases of chronic nephritis from which bacteria cannot be isolated at the time of examination of the patient.

The prevalence of pyelonephritis in the dog and cat is unknown because clinical tools for proving upper urinary tract (kidney, pelvis, ureter) infection are inadequate, and because bacterial culture of kidneys is not performed by pathologists as a routine autopsy procedure.

## CONFIRMATION OF URINARY TRACT INFECTION

Although urinary tract infection (UTI) may be suspected on the basis of history and physical examination, further examinations are necessary for its confirmation. Demonstration of WBC and bacteria in a urine specimen may be either highly significant or meaningless, depending on the technique used to obtain and store the specimen.

Infection is indicated by the presence of any bacteria in urine obtained by cystocentesis if sterile technique is used to obtain, store and process the specimen. This interpretation is valid because bladder urine is sterile in the normal dog and cat, and therefore bacteria in any number must be considered abnormal. However the presence of bacteria in midstream urine obtained during voiding or by catheterization may not indicate infection because of contamination of sterile bladder urine by urethral or genital debris. Quantitative urine culture is used in an attempt to differentiate infection from contamination, on the assumption that large numbers of organisms indicate UTI, and small numbers indicate contamination. Our study of 32 normal dogs that had sterile urine when sampled by cystocentesis revealed that 11 had $10^2$, 3 had $10^3$, 9 had $10^4$ and 2 had $10^5$ or greater organisms per ml. of midstream-voided urine. Thus, 25 of 32 gave positive cultures on midstream-voided specimens. On catheterized specimens from the same 32 dogs, 28 had no growth, 3 had $10^2$ and 1 had $10^4$ organisms per ml. of urine. We concluded that on samples obtained by catheterization, $10^5$ or more organisms per ml. would not be expected unless infection were present. Unfortunately, large numbers of organisms (most of which are potential pathogens) present in midstream urine obtained from normal dogs make quantitative culture unreliable for differentiation of infection and contamination in these specimens. Culture of midstream urine is more reliable in the cat, because less contamination occurs in this species, but errors in interpretation may also occur.

Overall, our recommendations for urine culture in the dog and cat are as follows:

1. Obtain culture samples by cystocentesis if possible. As a rule, cystocentesis can be performed easily if the urinary bladder can be localized by abdominal palpation. A 5-cm. diameter area of the caudal ventral abdomen is surgically prepared, and while the bladder is localized with one hand, the bladder is punctured with a 22-gauge needle and attached syringe. No anesthetic is required.

2. Obtain a midstream urine specimen from the dog by catheterization as a second choice. The dog's genitalia should be thoroughly cleaned with soap and water, and sterile technique and equipment should be used for catheterization.

3. Obtain urine from the cat by manually expressing the bladder as an alternative to cystocentesis. Catheterization of the female cat is difficult, and routine catheterization of the male is to be avoided because of potential urethral trauma.

4. Routinely use quantitative urine culture procedures. Although any growth on cystocentesis samples is indicative of an abnormality, large numbers of organisms usually present with infection remove doubt concerning the possibility of contamination of sterile urine during procurement or handling. Quantitative urine culture is essential for midstream specimens obtained by catheterization.

5. Interpret $10^5$ or greater organisms per ml. as infection on either cystocentesis or midstream catheter specimens in dogs or on either cystocentesis or midstream expressed samples in cats. Interpret $10^3$ or fewer organisms on midstream catheter or expressed specimens as contamination. Intermediate values require reevaluation of the patient. Urine for quantitative culture should be used for enumeration studies soon after procurement, so that numbers reflect *in-vivo* conditions rather than bacterial growth subsequent to urine collection. Dipstick methods for estimating the quantity of bacteria in urine are available for use in prac-

tice. These methods use direct visualization of bacteria for estimation of numbers or indirect methods based on visualization of chemical reactions caused by products of bacterial metabolism (see article on "Bacterial Infections of the Urinary Tract").

Abnormal numbers of WBC in the urine (greater than 5 per high-power field) may be detected with inflammation due to any cause. The genitalia must be ruled out as the source of WBC when they are found in urine. This can be done by cystocentesis or by meticulous cleaning of the genitalia prior to catheterizing the patient. Obviously WBC found in the urine are from the patient, unless the receptacle is grossly contaminated. The time between sampling and observation is not critical, except that with prolonged standing, WBC may be more difficult to identify because of autolysis. Absence of WBC in urine does not rule out UTI in man. Studies regarding absence of WBC in proved cases of infection have not been reported in the dog and cat, but it is likely that the same situation exists in these species as in man.

It is important to remember that UTI usually represents a transient or persistent defect in the patient's normal innate defense mechanisms against infection. The clinician should always consider factors known to predispose to infection including trauma to the urothelium, urine retention, glucosuria and presence of calculi.

## DIFFERENTIATING PYELONEPHRITIS FROM LOWER TRACT INFECTION

The lower urinary tract (bladder, urethra) serves as a storage receptacle and conduit for excretion of urine. Infection of the lower tract may result in physical discomfort for the patient but infection confined to this anatomic site is rarely life-threatening. By contrast, upper urinary tract infection involves an organ the dysfunction of which can lead to death from azotemia. This distinct difference provides the incentive for differentiating upper from lower urinary tract infection.

Current evidence favors the theory that UTI is most commonly a consequence of ascent of infection via the urethra. The role of vesicoureteral reflux in ascent of infection from the bladder to the ureters and kidneys in the dog and cat has not been adequately studied. The clinical differentiation of upper and lower tract infection may be complicated in some cases because infections in the two sites are not mutually exclusive, and thus positive criteria for identification of infection at one site does not eliminate the possibility of infection at the other site.

## CHARACTERISTICS—LOWER TRACT INFECTION

Lower urinary tract infection is usually noticed because of dysuria. Dysuria is not pathognomonic for lower tract infection; other causes include calculi, soft tissue masses or any cause of epithelial damage, including trauma. Observing dysuria focuses attention on the lower urinary tract but does not eliminate the possibility of concomitant upper tract disease.

Hematuria may occur with several abnormalities, including infection. Confirmation of hematuria is not always helpful in differentiating upper and lower urinary tract disease. Dysuria associated with the passage of bright red blood at the end of urination is indicative of lower tract disease. Blood mixed throughout urine may be of either upper or lower tract origin. Blood in the urine of male dogs may occur as a result of urethral reflux of blood from the prostate gland.

Fever and leukocytosis are uncommon in infection of the urinary bladder, but both may be observed in acute bacterial prostatitis. A urinary sediment devoid of casts is suggestive but not confirmatory for lower tract infection.

## CHARACTERISTICS—UPPER URINARY TRACT INFECTION

In man, acute pyelonephritis is characterized by lumbar pain, fever, leukocytosis, bacteriuria, pyuria and possibly urinary casts. Radiographic alterations are usually absent. As previously indicated, comprehensive studies that document the prevalence of pyelonephritis in the dog and cat do not exist. Our clinical impression is that acute pyelonephritis is uncommon in both species. When observed, it is usually associated with renolithiasis and ureterolithiasis. Clinical signs observed in dogs are the same as those described in man.

Chronic pyelonephritis is more common in the dog and cat. Fever and pain are absent in these patients; the diagnosis is supported by proving urinary tract infection and by demonstrating coexistent renal abnormalities. The latter may be numerous casts on urinalysis or radiologic evidence of abnormalities of the kidneys, renal pelvis or ureter. Renoliths are frequently associated with chronic pyelonephritis, but a cause-effect relationship is not apparent. The affected kidneys may be normal or decreased in size. With chronic pyelonephritis the renal pelves seem to retain contrast media, and moderate dilatation of pelves and ureters may be present.

The finding of UTI and radiographic evidence of renal abnormalities are highly suggestive but not confirmatory for upper tract infection. This fact has been acknowledged in man, and more precise methods of establishing renal infection have been sought. Ureteral catheterization via a cystoscope has been performed to obtain urine prior to its entrance into the bladder. This technique is reliable but not applicable to most patients in veterinary medicine.

A bladder washout technique used in man apparently gives results that correlate well with ureteral catheterization techniques. This procedure entails instillation of enzymes into the bladder to remove mucus and nucleoprotein, followed by antibiotics to kill bladder microorganisms. Subsequently, the bladder is rinsed several times, and quantitative bacterial culture is performed on the final rinse and on serial urine samples subsequently collected. If infection is restricted to the bladder, nearly all the bacteria and subsequent cultures will be sterile or have low bacterial numbers. If renal infection is present, bacteria-laden urine continues to enter the bladder after antibiotic is removed by rinsing; thus, serial cultures reveal a rapid increase in numbers of bacteria. Unfortunately, the time and expense required for the procedure does not lend itself to routine use in veterinary practice. Our limited use of the technique has revealed that prostate infection as well as renal infection can result in a rapid increase in numbers of bacteria. This is apparently due to reflux from the prostate to the bladder around the urinary catheter.

Recent studies in man suggest that upper and lower UTI can be differentiated on the basis of antibody-coating of bacteria. Bacteria originating from the kidney are apparently coated with antibody, but bacteria from the bladder are not. Fluorescent antibody techniques provide a quick and relatively easy method of determining whether antibody-coating exists. Studies in rabbits indicate that local production of antibody (IgG) occurs in the bladder as well as in the kidney. This observation suggests that the reliability of the antibody-coating test must be validated for the species in question, since species variation in immune mechanisms may occur.

Enzyme activity in urine may vary, depending on whether upper or lower tract infection is present. Urinary lactic dehydrogenase isoenzyme 5 levels were significantly higher in upper UTI than in lower UTI in children. Studies are needed to determine whether similar differences exist in dogs and cats.

It can be concluded that certain common clinical tools aid in differentiating upper and lower urinary tract infection but that differentiation is not invariably possible without more elaborate techniques.

## TREATMENT OF PYELONEPHRITIS

A basic principle of treatment of urinary tract infection is the removal of primary causes that are identified. If renoliths are present and functional renal parenchyma remains, nephrolithotomy is indicated. If urine retention is present, efforts should be directed toward solving this problem.

An ancillary form of therapy for treatment of pyelonephritis is induction of polyuria. The medulla of the kidney has been referred to as an immunologic desert because the normal hypertonicity depresses migration of leukocytes, abolishes phagocytosis and inhibits complement activity. Vigorous diuresis may reduce medullary hyperosmolality and may facilitate action of normal immune mechanisms. Furosemide has been used to induce diuresis in man. However, there is some question about enhancement of nephrotoxicity when cephaloridine, cephalothin, colistin and kanamycin are used coincidentally with furosemide. For this reason these antibiotics should be avoided if furosemide is used. A more economical approach than furosemide would be to induce medullary washout by oral administration of salt.

Antibiotics should be the main therapeutic tool for treatment of pyelonephritis. Urine culture and sensitivity testing should be used as a general guide for choice of antibiotic, but unfortunately several factors other than *in-vitro* sensitivity may affect *in-vivo* effectiveness of an antibiotic in pyelonephritis. Sensitivity disks contain quantities of antibiotic that are roughly comparable to serum levels of drug rather than urine levels. Most antibiotics excreted by the kidney may have a urine concentration that is 10- to 100-fold greater than that of serum. The higher concentration in urine results in some instances in which *in-vitro* resistance is accompanied by *in-vivo* sensitivity. Sensitivity testing with disks having antibiotic concentration of urine rather than serum has been advocated to rectify this problem, but the situation is complicated when consideration is given to the intrarenal distribution of antibiotics. Since pyelonephritis is predominantly a disease of the renal medulla, the concentration of antibiotic in the medullary interstitium is probably the most important factor in successful therapy. Several factors have been identified that influence renal distribution of antibiotic, including serum protein binding of the antibiotic, pH-dependent diffusion of the antibiotic, renal tissue binding of the antibiotic, state of hydration of the patient (i.e., urine concentration) and degree of disease in the kidneys. At present, specific data are not available for all antibacterial agents with regard to the role of all these factors at different gradations of renal dysfunction. From data available, it appears that in the normal kidney, urine pH has the following effects.

1. Acid urine enhances interstitial medullary diffusion of the following drugs: sulfisoxazole, tetracycline, cephalothin, nitrofurantoin, and sulfamethoxazole.
2. Alkaline urine enhances interstitial medullary diffusion of gentamicin and trimethoprim.
3. Urine pH is immaterial with regard to interstitial medullary diffusion of ampicillin, cephaloridine and cephalexin.

For most antibiotics, water restriction increases the concentration of antibiotics in the renal medulla. An exception is ampicillin; its medullary concentration is not altered by urine specific gravity. However, the levels of antibiotics achieved during diuresis are usually adequate, and the advantages previously described for diuresis cannot be ignored. Consequently, water diuresis is the preferable type of therapy.

Studies measuring the effect of severe renal disease in man on renal content and distribution of antibiotic revealed very low antibiotic concentrations in all parts of the kidney. This suggests that in the azotemic patient, serum antibiotic levels are probably more meaningful than are urine levels.

Of the antibacterial agents previously listed, some have not had extensive veterinary use. A sulfamethoxazole-trimethoprim combination (Bactrim®, Hoffman-La Roche) is rapidly absorbed from the gut and excreted by means of both glomerular filtration and tubular secretion. Both drugs act by interfering with bacterial folate metabolism and together are synergistic in their activity. In man, the combination has been reported to be highly effective in the treatment of urinary tract infection sensitive to sulfonamides.

Antibiotics with known nephrotoxic properties are less desirable in the treatment of pyelonephritis, since further renal parenchymal destruction is not in the best interest of the patient. Kanamycin, neomycin, gentamicin and cephaloridine should not be used for treatment of pyelonephritis unless organisms are resistant to other drugs. When they are used, renal function should be carefully monitored by urinalysis and BUN for detection of nephrotoxicity.

Empirically, chloramphenicol appears to be a good choice for treatment of pyelonephritis in the dog and cat. A high urine level is achieved after systemic therapy, and sensitivity of a high percentage of urinary pathogens exists.

Antibiotic therapy of pyelonephritis should be conducted for at least 3 weeks, regardless of apparent response during this time. Response to therapy must be judged by urine cultures performed 5 days or more after cessation of therapy. At least two cultures taken at monthly intervals should be sterile before it is concluded that infection has been eradicated.

Urease inhibitors are at present under investigation as adjuvants in the therapy of pyelonephritis. These drugs inhibit the conversion of urea to ammonia by bacterial urease. As a consequence, urine pH is not increased as it usually is with infection caused by urea splitters. Proof of effectiveness and mechanism of efficacy (if it exists) are still speculative. Urease inhibitors are not commercially available for therapeutic use at present.

Urinary acidifiers and alkalinizers may be of use in adjusting urine pH to achieve optimal renal medullary concentration of antibiotic. With regard to direct antibacterial activity, acidifiers are impotent therapeutic agents and should not be relied upon as the sole mechanism of treatment of bacterial infection.

Urine antiseptics such as methenamine are likewise not the preferred mode of therapy, but may have application in cases in which organisms are resistant to all antibiotics available. A urine pH of 5.5 or less is necessary for the antiseptic action of methenamine.

## SUPPLEMENTAL READING

Braude, A. I.: Current concepts of pyelonephritis. Medicine, 52:257–264, 1973.
Carvajal, H. F., Passey, R. B., Berger, M., Travis, L. B., and Lorentz, W. B.: Urinary lactic dehydrogenase isoenzyme 5 in the differential diagnosis of kidney and bladder infections. Kidney Int., 8:176–184, 1975.
Griffith, D. P., Musher, D. M., and Campbell, J. W.: Inhibition of bacterial urease. Invest. Urol., 11:234–238, 1973.
Jones, S. R., Smith, J. W., and Sanford, J. P.: Localization of urinary tract infections by detection of antibody-coated bacteria in urine sediment. New Engl. J. Med., 290:591–593, 1974.
Romankiewicz, J. A.: Factors influencing renal distribution of antibiotics—A key to therapy of pyelonephritis. Drug Intell. Clin. Pharm., 8:512–519, 1974.
Stamey, T. A.: Urinary Infection. Baltimore, Williams & Wilkins Co., 1972.
Whelton, A., and Walker, W. G.: Intrarenal antibiotic distribution in health and disease. Kidney Int., 6:257–264, 1974.

# RENAL AMYLOIDOSIS

KARIM JERAJ, B.V.Sc.,
and CARL A. OSBORNE, D.V.M.
St. Paul, Minnesota

## DEFINITION

Amyloidosis is an idiopathic disease process characterized by the extracellular accumulation of an amorphous, homogeneous substance in close association with basement membranes, vessel walls and stromal connective tissue of various organs and body tissues, especially the kidneys. The term amyloid was coined by Virchow in the mid-1800's because he believed that the substance was composed primarily of carbohydrates. It is now known that amyloid is composed primarily of protein. Purified amyloid contains only small quantities of carbohydrates, which may accumulate following amyloid deposition. Electron microscopic examination of amyloid reveals that it is composed primarily of nonbranching fibrils, typically arranged in a random fashion. Amyloid fibrils are responsible for the characteristic apple-green birefringence that is observed when sections of tissue stained with Congo red are examined by means of polarization microscopy.

## ETIOLOGY

Chemical and immunologic analyses of purified amyloid deposits have revealed that there are at least two types of amyloid fibrils. One type is composed primarily of proteins the amino acid sequences of which are similar to those of light chains and fragments of light chains of immunoglobulins. The other type is composed primarily of nonimmunoglobulin protein (protein A). This chemical difference in amyloid composition presumably represents different causes of amyloid production.

In man, a correlation between the chemical type of amyloid and its pattern of deposition within the body has been observed. Amyloid containing a large quantity of immunoglobin light chains has been found primarily in the tongue, gastrointestinal tract, heart, skeletal and smooth muscle, nerves, skin and carpal ligaments of patients with multiple myeloma or plasma cell dyscrasias. This type of amyloid is commonly referred to as primary or pattern I type.

Protein type-A amyloid has been observed primarily in the kidneys, liver, spleen and adrenal glands of patients with chronic suppuration, necrosis or neoplasia. It is commonly referred to as secondary or pattern II type.

Manifestations of both types of amyloid may be observed in the same patient. In a small percentage of patients, amyloid may be localized to one tissue or organ and is often surrounded by numerous plasma cells. This type is called localized amyloidosis.

Although the etiology of amyloidosis is still unknown, it appears to be related to an immunologic disturbance. The hypothesis that amyloid forms as a result of deposition of circulating antigen-antibody complexes has been rejected, since no evidence has been generated to support this theory (refer to the article on "Glomerulonephropathy and the Nephrotic Syndrome").

Observations in cats, dogs, laboratory animals and man have been interpreted to suggest that the genesis of amyloid is related to local production of this insoluble substance by dystrophic protein-synthesizing cells. It has been theorized that cells altered in some fashion by prolonged antigenic stimulation produce an insoluble glycoprotein that accumulates in nearby extracellular spaces rather than producing soluble proteins that can circulate throughout the body. A variety of cell types have been implicated, including reticuloendothelial cells, plasma cells, glomerular mesangial cells, glomerular epithelial cells, endothelial cells, pancreatic acinar cells and thyroid carcinoma cells.

Following the identification of immunoglobin light chains in some patients with amyloidosis, it was suggested that an increased concentration of circulating free immunoglobin light chains (as in multiple myeloma) may be the precursor of amyloid fibrils in the vascular system. An alternative hypothesis has incriminated proteolytic degradation of antigen-antibody complexes by phagocytes and the production of insoluble amyloid fibrils that accumulate in juxtaposition to the cells.

## PATHOGENESIS

Amyloidosis may alter many body functions. Its potential for widespread distribution is responsible for the polysystemic manifestations of this disease.

Because amyloid is poorly immunogenic, it is not associated with a marked inflammatory response. It is insoluble in physiologic solutions and resists proteolytic digestion. The deleterious effect of amyloid in the body is thought to be related to the depression of body functions by its physical presence. As perivascular amyloid deposits increase in quantity, they encroach on vascular lumina. As a consequence, blood flow becomes compromised, and surrounding cells undergo ischemic atrophy and necrosis. Amyloid may also depress cellular function by restricting metabolic fluid and gaseous exchange across vessel walls.

**Canine Renal Amyloidosis.** In dogs, the glomeruli are sites where amyloid deposition is of major clinical significance. This fact is probably related to the reticuloendothelial activity of glomerular mesangial cells (refer to discussion of applied anatomy in the article on "Glomerulonephropathy and the Nephrotic Syndrome"). In man, the mesangium is the earliest and primary site of amyloid deposition.

Renal amyloidosis in dogs is a chronic irreversible renal disease characterized by generalized and progressive glomerular destruction. It is classified as a primary glomerular disease, because in most cases signs referable to renal destruction are related to amyloid deposition in the glomeruli. Characteristically all the glomeruli are affected by amyloid deposition in a similar fashion. Because of the functional interdependence of glomeruli, renal tubules and interstitial tissue, progressive irreversible destruction of glomeruli invariably results in progressive loss of function in remaining portions of affected nephrons. Amyloid may also be deposited in blood vessels, interstitial tissue and tubular walls, but when involved, they are usually not as severely affected as are glomeruli.

Renal amyloidosis may also be associated with variable degrees of amyloid deposition in other tissues and organs of the body. As a generality, however, these areas are not as severely affected as are the kidneys and uncommonly are associated with the development of clinical signs.

The appearance of the renal lesion is dependent on the rate of amyloid deposition, the quantity of amyloid present, the duration of its existence and the presence or absence of concomitant renal diseases. Depending on the state of the disease, the kidneys may be grossly normal, enlarged or reduced in size.

Renal size is not significantly altered during early stages of the disease when relatively small quantities of amyloid have accumulated in the kidneys. With the exception of persistent proteinuria, this stage of the disease is usually not associated with clinical findings indicative of renal dysfunction.

Increased renal size occurs in association with rapid and massive accumulations of amyloid but prior to the occurrence of a significant degree of ischemic atrophy, necrosis and connective tissue replacement of involved nephrons. Amyloid-enlarged kidneys are usually pale and have a firm, rubbery texture. If the condition is uncomplicated by other renal diseases, the renal capsule usually strips with ease to reveal a relatively smooth or slightly roughened external surface. The cut surfaces of the kidneys often have a waxy appearance. Microscopically, the glomeruli become large, bloodless, homogeneous hyaline structures. Clinically this stage of the disease is characterized by persistent and severe proteinuria. Progressive obliteration of glomerular circulation by amyloid manifests itself functionally as renal insufficiency. Evaluation of tubular function early during this stage of the disease may reveal that it is normal or not as severely affected as is glomerular function (so-called glomerulotubular imbalance).

If the progress of the disease is sufficiently slow to allow the dog to adapt to progressive renal insufficiency, and if the patient does not die from a predisposing disease, the kidneys may become small and scarred (end-stage amyloid-contracted kidneys). Generalized and severe ischemic atrophy and necrosis of renal tubules occurs secondary to progressive reduction of glomerular and peritubular capillary blood flow. Because effective regeneration of nephrons that have been destroyed as a result of progressive depositions of amyloid does not occur, damaged nephrons are replaced with fibrous connective tissue. As a result of progressive contraction of connective tissue elements, these changes are manifested macroscopically as contracted end-stage kidneys. Amyloid-contracted

kidneys have a finely pitted capsular surface and grossly resemble those of chronic generalized glomerulonephritis. A portion of the glomerular capillary circulation must persist in such advanced cases in order for the patient to survive long enough for these chronic changes to occur. For this reason, heavy proteinuria continues, although it may become less severe as glomerular circulation progressively diminishes. Abnormalities related to tubular insufficiency may be detected and are superimposed on those related to progressive destruction of the glomeruli.

The patient may die of renal failure at any time during the course of renal amyloidosis. The rate of progression of renal insufficiency is variable and is dependent on the rate of amyloid deposition in the kidneys, on the distribution and severity of amyloid deposition in other organs and tissues of the patient and on the presence or absence of predisposing diseases or concomitant renal disease. Although the progression of renal amyloidosis in most dogs is such that they develop chronic progressive renal failure associated with small kidneys, we have encountered three dogs with severe oliguric renal failure caused by almost complete obliteration of the glomeruli and amyloid-enlarged kidneys. The mechanisms that precipitate rapid accumulation of amyloid and cause death from renal failure in patients with amyloid-enlarged kidneys, but that allow other patients to survive until amyloid-contracted kidneys have developed, are obscure. The rate of progression of renal failure may be related to the pattern of distribution of amyloid within glomeruli.

**Feline Renal Amyloidosis.** Unlike the disease in dogs, renal amyloidosis in cats is not consistently associated with glomerular disease. Although the glomeruli may be affected, the greatest accumulation of amyloid has been observed in the renal medulla. A similar pattern of renal distribution has been observed in the bovine. Progressive destruction of medullary vessels and tubules would be expected to result in atrophy and fibrosis of affected nephrons. It has been suggested that occlusion of medullary vessels secondary to progressive accumulation of amyloid may also result in papillary necrosis.

The paucity of reported cases of renal amyloidosis in cats may be associated with the unusual location of amyloid in the kidneys of this species. Proteinuria may not be a significant clinical finding in cats in which glomerular involvement is not an important lesion. Because of the common occurrence of amyloid in glomeruli of most other species, cat kidneys may have been erroneously assumed to be free of amyloid on the basis of unaffected glomeruli. If this hypothesis is valid, the clinical nature of renal amyloidosis in cats would be similar to that associated with other types of nonglomerular renal disease (pyelonephritis, etc.).

## CLINICAL HISTORY

The following discussion applies to renal amyloidosis in dogs. Evaluation of the clinical and laboratory findings of renal amyloidosis in cats has been too meager to establish any meaningful generalizations.

The owner's complaint may be related to a predisposing cause. With improvement and widespread use of antimicrobial agents, there has been a decrease in the number of cases of renal amyloidosis associated with chronic suppuration. In contrast, increased use of diagnostic laboratory procedures has resulted in an increase in the recognition of renal amyloidosis with malignant neoplasia. We have also observed renal amyloidosis in dogs with *Dirofilaria immitis* infection. Signs related to amyloid deposition in other organs and tissues of the body may occur, but they are encountered infrequently. When present, they usually are not as severe as the clinical signs associated with renal amyloidosis.

The most striking clinical signs usually occur when renal function is seriously impaired by amyloid deposition. They may provide the first and sometimes the only clinical clue to the presence of amyloidosis. The owner may indicate that his pet has progressive polyuria, polydipsia and nocturia. Less commonly, oliguric renal failure may occur. The animal may show weakness, depression, anorexia and weight loss. If the patient is uremic, vomiting, diarrhea or constipation may develop.

## PHYSICAL EXAMINATION

If the patient is uremic, signs of chronic renal insufficiency, including stomatitis, brick-red discoloration of the tongue, pallor of the mucous membranes, scleral injection,

dehydration, weight loss, depression and weakness, may be detected by physical examination. These findings are similar to clinical manifestations of renal failure caused by other generalized, chronic, progressive, irreversible renal diseases.

If amyloidosis is generalized, enlargement of organs such as the spleen and liver may be detected by means of abdominal palpation. In our experience, these findings occur infrequently in association with renal amyloidosis in dogs.

A high incidence of thrombosis has been observed at necropsy in dogs with renal amyloidosis. Pulmonary thrombosis was most commonly encountered, although thrombi were also observed in the coronary, splenic, renal, mesenteric, iliac and/or brachial arteries. Retrospective evaluation of the cases revealed clinical signs (sudden dyspnea, sudden death, progressive limb dysfunction, etc.) referable to the affected system in some patients. We have encountered several dogs with immune-complex glomerulopathy that died suddenly following thrombosis of major pulmonary arteries, indicating that disorders of blood coagulation are not limited to patients with amyloid glomerular disease.

## LABORATORY FINDINGS

No laboratory tests are specific for the detection of renal amyloidosis. The results of laboratory procedures are dependent on the organs and tissues involved with amyloidosis, the duration and extent of amyloid deposition and the presence or absence of predisposing disease. Although marked and persistent proteinuria is a consistent finding, it is only an indication of generalized glomerular disease (refer to article on "Glomerulonephropathy and the Nephrotic Syndrome"). Proteinuria may persist for months in the absence of clinical signs of renal disease. The quantity of protein excreted in the urine may vary from less than 1 to more than 30 gm. in 24 hours. It is composed predominantly of albumin, but globulins are present in variable quantities.

The results of renal function tests are related to the amount of amyloid deposited in the kidneys. If only a minimal amount of amyloid is present in the renal parenchyma, abnormalities in renal function are not usually detectable by conventional laboratory tests. The only finding suggestive of the glomerular abnormality caused by amyloid deposition is persistent proteinuria.

As the quantity of amyloid in the glomerular capillaries increases, abnormalities referable to decreased glomerular perfusion become evident and are characterized by a progressive increase in blood urea nitrogen and creatinine, and a progressive decrease in glomerular filtration rate. In spite of the decrease in glomerular filtration, a disproportionately large degree of tubular function may persist during early stages of the disease. This usually is manifested by retention of some ability of the kidneys to concentrate urine (maximum urine S.G. of approximately 1.017 to 1.024; refer to discussion of prerenal azotemia and glomerulotubular imbalance in the article on "Glomerulonephropathy and the Nephrotic Syndrome").

If the patient survives for a sufficient period of time to allow development of amyloid-contracted kidneys, abnormalities related to renal tubular insufficiency may become obvious. Impaired ability to concentrate or dilute urine and impaired response to a vasopressin concentration test occur. These findings become superimposed on abnormal findings related to glomerular disease and are similar to those seen in dogs with renal failure caused by generalized glomerulonephritis, generalized pyelonephritis and other types of generalized renal disease. The severity of proteinuria, however, is usually much greater in patients with generalized glomerular disease. Patients with chronic progressive renal amyloidosis also develop varying degrees of nonregenerative anemia and renal osteodystrophy.

Hyaline, granular or waxy casts may be present, but they are not a consistent finding. Amyloid fibrils have been detected by electron microscopy in the urine sediment of human patients with renal amyloidosis.

Evaluation of serum proteins in patients with renal amyloidosis associated with severe albuminuria often reveals hypoalbuminemia. Serum globulins may be normal, decreased or increased in quantity. Evaluation of the concentration of total serum protein without regard to albumin and globulin concentrations may mask hypoalbuminemia in patients with elevated globulin concentrations. If the hypoalbuminemia is severe (i.e., serum concentra-

tion of albumin below approximately 1 gm./100 ml.), the associated decrease in plasma colloidal osmotic pressure may initiate edema and a nephrotic syndrome. Compensatory release of antidiuretic hormone and aldosterone enhances and perpetuates the edema (consult the article on "Glomerulonephropathy and Nephrotic Syndrome").

Hyperlipemia and hypercholesterolemia are frequent findings in dogs with renal amyloidosis. The percentage of cholesterol esters in the serum is usually normal. The mechanisms responsible for hypercholesterolemia are unknown but are related to the hypoalbuminemia.

## DIAGNOSIS

The detection of persistent proteinuria in the absence of hematuria and pyuria should arouse a high index of suspicion of glomerular disease. Although persistent proteinuria is a consistent finding in dogs with renal amyloidosis, it also occurs in association with other generalized glomerular diseases and may be associated with nonrenal disorders. (For further details, consult the article on "Glomerulonephropathy and the Nephrotic Syndrome.")

Persistent proteinuria of renal origin that occurs in association with chronic suppuration, tissue destruction and neoplasia, or enlargement of parenchymatous organs such as the spleen and liver, suggests amyloidosis as a diagnostic probability. Our experience has revealed that renal amyloidosis occurs in association with neoplasia and chronic inflammatory disease more frequently than has been generally recognized.

One must employ renal biopsies in order to confirm an antemortem diagnosis of renal amyloidosis because the clinical findings are not sufficiently specific to allow establishment of a diagnosis other than glomerular disease. Since glomerular amyloid deposits may resemble the lesions of membranous glomerulonephropathy (so-called spicular glomerular amyloidosis), and since biopsy specimens may contain only small deposits of amyloid, formalin-fixed biopsy samples should be routinely stained with Congo red or thioflavin-T and examined for green birefringence by polarization microscopy, in addition to routine examination with hematoxylin and eosin. When possible, demonstration of the characteristic fibrillar structure of amyloid by electron microscopy is also desirable.

Rectal biopsy has become a useful diagnostic aid for the detection of amyloidosis in human beings with renal involvement because amyloid frequently accumulates in the arterioles of the rectal submucosa. We have had no experience in evaluating rectal biopsies obtained from dogs and cats for the presence of amyloid.

## TREATMENT

Effective methods for prevention and treatment of amyloid have not been established because the etiopathogenesis of amyloidosis remains unsolved. No known regimen of therapy consistently results in control or cure; most patients ultimately succumb to renal failure or a predisposing disease, when this is present.

Elimination of predisposing diseases (neoplasms and chronic suppuration) has been reported to halt or reverse amyloid deposition in the kidneys of a few human beings. For this reason, each patient with renal amyloidosis should be evaluated for the presence of endogenous or exogenous stimuli with the goal of eradicating them. Active control or elimination of neoplastic or chronic inflammatory disease may be effective in minimizing or preventing progressive renal damage, provided that renal function is not too severely impaired. If renal amyloidosis has progressed to the stage where it induces primary renal failure, it may be too far advanced for treatment of the predisposing cause to have a significant effect on the course of the renal disease.

Although corticosteroid therapy has not been critically evaluated in dogs or cats with renal amyloidosis, we do not recommend it. Our basis for this recommendation is related to the following:

(1) Corticosteroids enhance experimental production of amyloidosis in laboratory animals.

(2) Corticosteroids may aggravate the severity of clinical signs associated with renal failure because they induce gluconeogenesis. Deamination of amino acids during conversion to carbohydrates increases the quantity of protein metabolic waste products that must be excreted by failing kidneys.

(3) Corticosteroids have been of no benefit to human patients with renal amyloidosis.

Immunosuppressant drugs (e.g., cyclophosphamide [Cytoxan®, Mead Johnson]; melphalan [Burroughs Wellcome]) have been used in the treatment of human beings with amyloid containing the light chains of immunoglobulins (primary amyloidosis or pattern I type) with varying degrees of success. The drugs are given with the expectation that they will inhibit or impair the production of amyloid precursors by decreasing plasma cell proliferation. D-penicillamine has also been reported as a useful agent to mobilize *in-situ* amyloid deposits. Available information is insufficient to permit establishment of meaningful recommendations concerning the use of these drugs for the treatment of amyloidosis in dogs and cats.

Although renal amyloidosis in dogs and cats is a progressive and irreversible disease, symptomatic and supportive treatment of progressive renal failure is often of benefit. Many dogs receiving such treatment at the University of Minnesota have lived for more than a year after the diagnosis of renal amyloidosis was established by means of biopsy. We have been successful in controlling the nephrotic syndrome in several dogs with renal amyloidosis by oral administration of furosemide. Drug-induced hypokalemia was not observed in our series. (Consult the article on "Glomerulonephropathy and the Nephrotic Syndrome" for further information regarding symptomatic and supportive treatment of generalized glomerular disease.)

## PROGNOSIS

The long-term prognosis for patients with renal amyloidosis is poor, because specific treatment that will eliminate the primary abnormality is not available. As a generality, renal amyloidosis in dogs is progressive and irreversible. If amyloidosis occurs secondary to an underlying disease that is amenable to therapy, there is a chance that the progressive nature of amyloid deposition may be halted or reversed. If the underlying disease is not curable, it may become the limiting factor with respect to survival.

The short-term prognosis for patients who respond satisfactorily to symptomatic and supportive therapy of the nephrotic syndrome and/or renal failure is guarded to fair.

## SUPPLEMENTAL READING

Andsell, I. D., and Joekes, A. M.: Spicular arrangement of amyloid in renal biopsy. J. Clin. Path., 25:1056–1062, 1972.

Cohen, A. S., and Cathcart, E. S.: Amyloidosis and immunoglobulins. In Stollerman, G. H. (ed): Advances in Internal Medicine. Vol. 19. Chicago, Year Book Medical Publishers, 1974.

Cohen, H. J., et al.: Resolution of primary amyloidosis during chemotherapy. Ann. Int. Med., 82:466–473, 1975.

Crowell, W. A., et al.: Generalized amyloidosis in a cat. J. Am. Vet. Med. Assn., 161:1127–1133, 1972.

Derosena, R., et al.: Demonstration of amyloid fibrils in urinary sediment. New Engl. J. Med., 293:1131–1133, 1975.

Franklin, E. C.: The complexity of amyloid. New Engl. J. Med., 290:512–513, 1974.

Glenner, G. C., and Terry, W. D.: Characterization of amyloid. Ann. Rev. Med., 25:131–135, 1974.

Gruys, E.: Ultrastructural and enzyme histochemical aspects of amyloidosis in the bovine renal medulla. Vet. Pathol., 12:94–110, 1975.

Hobbs, J. R.: An ABC of amyloid. Proc. Roy. Soc. Med., 66:705–710, 1973.

Jao, W., and Pirani, C. L.: Renal amyloidosis: Electron microscopic observations. Acta Path. Microbiol. Scand., 80A:217–227(Suppl. 233), 1972.

Lender, M.: Amyloidosis associated with neoplastic diseases. South African Med. J., 48:1944–1946, 1974.

Osborne, C. A., Low, D. G., and Finco, D. R.: Canine and Feline Urology. Philadelphia, W. B. Saunders Co., 1972.

Osserman, E. F.: Plasma cell dyscrasias. In Beeson, P. B., and McDermott, W. (eds.): Textbook of Medicine. 14th ed. Philadelphia, W. B. Saunders Co., 1975.

Slauson, D. O., and Gribble, D. H.: Thrombosis complicating renal amyloidosis in dogs. Vet. Path., 8:352–363, 1971.

# GLOMERULO-NEPHROPATHY AND THE NEPHROTIC SYNDROME

CARL A. OSBORNE, D.V.M.
St. Paul, Minnesota

Clinical investigation of renal disease in veterinary medicine has undergone major change in the past decade. Widespread use of percutaneous renal biopsy techniques, increased knowledge about the pathogenesis of kidney diseases and the use of immunofluorescent and electron microscopy have revealed that clinically significant "primary" glomerulonephropathy is relatively common in dogs and cats. Glomerulonephropathy has also been observed in association with polysystemic diseases such as canine lupus erythematosus, canine pyometra, canine adenovirus–infectious hepatitis infection, a variety of canine and feline malignancies and Dirofilaria immitis infection. In some cases, the severity of glomerular disease has been sufficient to cause the nephrotic syndrome, renal failure or both. Renal amyloidosis is also a common cause of generalized glomerular injury that may induce the nephrotic syndrome or renal failure (or both) in dogs. (Refer to the article on "Renal Amyloidosis" for further details.)

## DEFINITION

Glomerulonephropathy is a disease characterized by morphologic abnormalities in glomeruli, which, if progressive, may induce changes in the renal tubules, blood vessels and interstitial tissue. Primary glomerulonephropathy is distinguished from other types of primary renal disease (i.e., tubular disease, pyelonephritis, interstitial nephritis) by changes that initially and predominantly affect glomeruli.

The terms glomerulonephropathy and glomerulonephritis with various qualifying prefixes (proliferative, membranous, membranoproliferative, etc.) are commonly used to describe the variable response of different cells and structures within glomeruli to injury. These terms are analogous to the terms enteritis and dermatitis in that lesions of a specific anatomic area are implied without reference to a specific cause or pathogenic mechanism. Since the etiopathogenesis as well as the clinicopathologic and immunologic manifestations of this disorder are highly variable, a diagnosis of glomerulonephritis (-opathy) does not imply a specific diagnosis.

The nephrotic syndrome is characterized by proteinuria, hypoproteinemia, hypoalbuminemia, hypercholesterolemia and, frequently, edema. These abnormalities occur as a result of increased permeability of glomerular capillaries to plasma protein, especially albumin. It is commonly observed in dogs and cats with membranous or membranoproliferative glomerulonephropathy and in dogs with renal amyloidosis (see Nephrotic Syndrome, page 1122).

## APPLIED ANATOMY

Familiarity with glomerular anatomy is a prerequisite to understanding the pathophysiology of glomerulonephropathy. The renal corpuscles are composed of a tuft of highly branched capillaries (glomeruli) surrounded by a capsule (Bowman's capsule). Glomeruli contain capillary endothelial cells, visceral and parietal epithelial cells, mesangial cells and mesangial matrix and capillary basement membranes (Fig. 1).

Glomerular capillary endothelial cells are similar to endothelial cells lining capillaries in other parts of the body, except that the

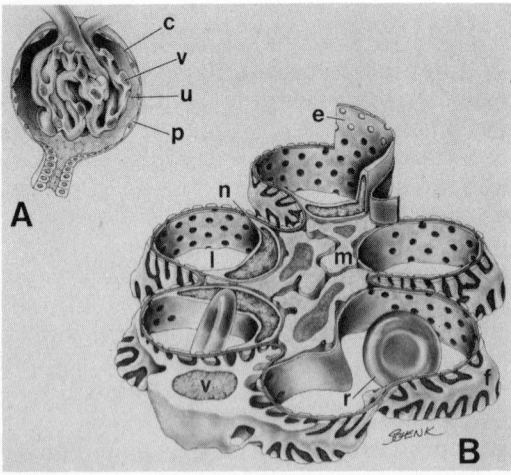

**Figure 1.** *A*, Renal corpuscle with glomerular tuft, urinary space and Bowman's capsule. *B*, Cross section of a portion of a glomerulus: *c*, Bowman's capsule; *u*, urinary space; *p*, parietal epithelial cell; *v*, nucleus of visceral epithelial cell; *f*, foot processes of visceral epithelial cell; *n*, nucleus of capillary endothelial cell; *e*, cytoplasm of capillary endothelial cell containing large pores; *m*, mesangial cells; *l*, capillary lumen; *r*, red blood cell.

former contain large pores (or fenestrae). They offer no significant barrier to filtration.

The glomerular basement membrane (GBM) is located between endothelial cells and visceral epithelial cells in peripheral portions of capillaries, and between mesangial cells and visceral epithelial cells in other portions of the glomerular tuft (Fig. 1). The GBM does not surround the entire capillary lumen, as is the case with other capillaries in the body, but covers the glomerular tuft in a fashion somewhat analogous to the serosa of the abdominal cavity. It is not located between endothelial cells and mesangial cells. Although the GBM serves as the main filtration barrier to large, high molecular weight proteins present in plasma, it does not prevent filtration of smaller molecules. Special structures (called slit-pore membranes) associated with the cytoplasm of visceral epithelial cells are thought to act as the filtration barrier for smaller substances but are permeable to molecules the size of hemoglobin or smaller.

Glomerular capillaries are covered with epithelial cells (commonly called podocytes) characterized by an elaborate layer of primary, secondary and tertiary cytoplasmic processes which extend to the GBM. The spaces between the epithelial foot processes are called filtration slits or slit pores. Ultrastructural studies have revealed the presence of thin membranes (slit-pore membranes) that close the spaces between the foot processes. As mentioned previously, it is presumed that filtration occurs at these sites. Visceral epithelium is thought to produce one or more components of the GBM.

Mesangial cells occupy a space between capillaries and are separated from capillary lumina by endothelial cytoplasm and mesangial matrix rather than by GBM. Mesangial cells are separated from visceral epithelial cells by GBM. These cells are able to phagocytose material in a fashion similar to that of reticuloendothelial cells. The cells extend cytoplasmic processes between capillary endothelial cells and the GBM, where they remove filtration residues that might otherwise interfere with filtration or damage the GBM (Fig. 1). Mesangial cells also help to anchor (or support) the GBM, which does not completely surround glomerular capillary lumina. Mesangial cells are separated from each other by a variable quantity of dense basement membrane–like material called mesangial matrix. It has been suggested that mesangial matrix is formed in part from deposition of "old" GBM following turnover and renewal of the GBM. Changes in mesangial cells and mesangial matrix reflect much of the injury to glomeruli associated with inflammation, and these areas appear to be the sites where hyaline material accumulates in patients with diabetes mellitus and amyloidosis.

The various components of the glomerulus are thought to function as a unit. The basement membrane acts as the main filter of plasma. The endothelium acts as a valve that controls access to the filter by the number and size of its pores. The visceral epithelium may also play a role as a filtration barrier and may act as a monitor which partially recovers proteins that leak through the filters. The mesangium reconditions and unclogs the filter by incorporating and disposing of filtration residues that accumulate on the endothelial side of the GBM.

## APPLIED PHYSIOLOGY

A conceptual understanding of the physiology of glomerular function is a prerequisite to diagnosis, prognosis and treatment of glomerular disease. Formation of urine by the kidneys results from three basic processes: glomerular filtration, tubular reabsorption and tubular secretion. It is well established that the formation of glomerular filtrate from plasma is a major function of glomeruli. Factors that influence the quantity and quality of glomerular filtrate include hydrostatic pressure, volume, colloidal osmotic pressure of blood in glomerular capillaries, permeability of glomerular capillaries and renal intratubular and interstitial pressure. The ability of substances to filter through glomerular capillary walls is primarily related to their size. Since cells, most proteins and most lipoproteins are too large to pass through glomerular capillary walls, they are retained within the vascular system and are not present in glomerular filtrate in significant quantities. In terms of homeostasis, the retention of these vital substances by the body would be expected.

The glomerulus functions as a sieve that increasingly restricts the passage of macromolecules with increasing diameter and molecular weight. Most substances in glomeruli have a molecular weight of less than 70,000. Thus, the common denominator of substances which appear in the glomerular filtrate is not their potential value to the body but rather their size. In order for the kidneys to regulate body fluid and electrolyte balance, it is essential that both beneficial and worthless metabolites of similar size be subjected to potential loss in urine. Some filtered substances (creatinine, phenols, etc.) cannot be reutilized by the body and therefore are not reabsorbed by the tubules. Other filtered substances (amino acids, vitamins, glucose, etc.) are essential for body homeostasis. Since they are too small to be retained by glomerular capillaries, however, they are dependent on tubular reabsorption for retention in the body. The body's requirement for water, electrolytes and other filtered substances is variable, being dependent upon intake metabolism and loss by other routes. The kidneys regulate conservation or excretion of these substances by selective partial or total tubular reabsorption. Some filtered substances such as potassium may be reabsorbed and secreted. The overall effect of these tubular functions is vital to homeostasis.

## MORPHOLOGIC RESPONSE TO INJURY

Although the canine glomerulus has good capacity to repair acute inflammatory lesions, repair of persistent, severe or chronic lesions seldom results in a normal glomerulus. The fact that new glomeruli and tubules cannot be formed following maturation in order to replace irreversibly damaged nephrons is an important event related to the evolution of progressive glomerular disease. Progressive irreversible glomerular damage is usually associated with healing by replacement fibrosis and scarring.

These generalities should not be interpreted as indicating that all glomerular diseases are clinically irreversible. Several types of glomerulonephropathy, as exemplified by human acute poststreptococcal proliferative glomerulonephritis and canine pyometra nephritis, may be associated with complete functional recovery. Others may be associated with irreversible but nonprogressive lesions. We observed one case of membanous glomerulonephropathy in a 4-year-old male Great Dane that was characterized by complete functional recovery, despite persistent nonprogressive glomerular lesions. Functional recovery may be complete even when considerable nephron destruction has occurred, since remaining viable nephrons may increase their functional capacity by compensatory hypertrophy. Progressive renal failure results only if continued nephron destruction exceeds the capacity of viable nephrons to compensate.

Morphologic changes reflecting injury to various components of glomeruli may be distributed in either focal or generalized fashion throughout the kidneys and in local or diffuse fashion within individual glomeruli. Although the components of glomeruli may be altered by a large number of disease processes (infection, toxic agents, ischemia, metabolic defects, immune disorders, etc.), the morphologic characteristics of the alterations, and the body's compensatory and reparative responses to them, are limited. For this reason, the morphologic response and functional consequences of etiologically unrelated kidney diseases are often similar. Even though each component of the glomerulus has a limited response to injury and disease, clinical and experimental observations in several mammalian species have revealed that certain morphologic reactions, either alone or in combination, are characteristic of specific clinical entities (e.g., acute proliferative glomerulonephritis, membranous glomerulonephritis, embolic glomerulonephritis, etc.).

Exudation of PMN's may accompany activation of the complement system following interaction of complement-binding antibodies (IgM or IgG) with various antigens or may occur by activation of the alternate complement pathway.

Endothelial and mesangial cell swelling and proliferation (hyperplasia) often occur in association with acute glomerular injury. Mesangial cell proliferation is associated with many types of glomerular injury and is thought to be related to the phagocytic function of these cells. Although endothelial and mesangial cell proliferation may interfere with glomerular filtration by narrowing capillary lumina and decreasing capillary perfusion, they are potentially reversible alterations.

A consistent reaction of visceral epithelial cells to glomerular injury associated with proteinuria is swelling (formerly thought to be fusion) of their cytoplasmic foot processes and reduction of slit-pore width. Experimental studies in dogs and rats have revealed that foot-process swelling is a result rather than a cause of proteinuria.

Proliferation of parietal epithelial cells lining Bowman's capsule may result in the formation of multiple layers of cells (called epithelial crescents) that protrude into Bowman's space. This reaction is observed in severe acute and subacute glomerulonephropathy and is thought to occur as a result of exudation of fibrin into Bowman's space. Epithelial crescents usually indicate the presence of severe injury that is often irreversible.

Thickening of the GBM is a common manifestation of glomerular injury. A common sequela to GBM thickening is increased permeability to larger molecules normally retained in the vascular compartment. It may seem paradoxical that an increase in the thickness of the GBM is associated with increased permeability to larger molecules. The fact that the thickening may be caused in part by abnormal substances such as amyloid or immune complexes, or by an increased quantity of mesangial matrix, in addition to membranous material, may be a partial explanation of this discrepancy. The fact that splitting or fraying of the GBM imparts an appearance of increased thickness may be another factor. Proteinuria may also be associated (at least in part) with changes in the slit-pore membranes connecting the foot processes of visceral epithelial cells as well as with lesions in the GBM.

## FUNCTIONAL RESPONSE TO INJURY

Damage to various components of glomeruli may alter glomerular filtration by interfering with glomerular blood flow and/or altering the selective permeability of the GBM. Depending on the nature, location and severity of the damage, several different clinical symdromes may be recognized.

**Prerenal Azotemia.** Inadequate perfusion of normal glomeruli with blood, regardless of cause (e.g., dehydration, cardiac disease, shock, hypoadrenocorticism, etc.), may cause prerenal azotemia. Prerenal azotemia is associated with structurally normal kidneys that are capable of quantitatively normal renal function, provided that compromised renal perfusion is corrected.

If the prerenal cause of reduced renal perfusion is allowed to persist, varying degrees of ischemic tubular disease may develop. Development of primary renal failure due to ischemia reduces the likelihood of complete recovery. A diagnosis of prerenal azotemia should be considered if abnormal elevation in the serum or plasma concentration of BUN or creatinine is associated with a high urine specific gravity (greater than 1.025) in patients with no specific evidence of generalized glomerular disease. Detection of a urine specific gravity greater than approximately 1.025 in association with azotemia indicates that a sufficient quantity of functional nephrons is present to concentrate urine (i.e., at least one third of the total nephron population). Significant elevations in the serum or plasma concentration of BUN or creatinine due to primary renal failure cannot be detected until approximately 75 per cent of the nephron population is nonfunctional. The elevation in urine specific gravity associated with prerenal azotemia probably reflects a compensatory response by the body to combat low perfusion pressure and blood volume by secreting antidiuretic hormone (and possibly other substances) to conserve water filtered through glomeruli.

Another form of potentially reversible prerenal azotemia may develop in glomerulonephritic patients with severe hypoproteinemia. Decreased renal blood flow and glomerular filtration occurring in association with marked reduction in vascular volume secondary to a reduction in colloidal osmotic pressure may result in a proportionate degree of retention of substances normally cleared by the kidneys (i.e., urea, creatinine). Therefore the significance of an abnormal increase in the serum concentration of creatinine or urea nitrogen must be carefully defined in hypoproteinemic nephrotic patients. Azotemia cannot be accepted as irrefutable evidence of severe primary glomerular lesions, since it may be associated with a potentially reversible decrease in renal perfusion caused by hypoalbuminemia.

**Glomerulotubular Imbalance.** An abnormal elevation in the serum concentration of BUN or creatinine may also occur in association with an elevated urine specific gravity in *some* patients with primary renal failure caused by generalized glomerular disease. The renal lesion in such patients must be characterized by glomerular damage that is sufficiently severe to impair renal clearance of urea and creatinine but that has not yet induced a sufficient degree of ischemic atrophy and necrosis of renal tubular cells to prevent urine concentration. This group of patients may be differentiated from patients with prerenal azotemia by failure in a search for one of the causes of poor renal perfusion, by the presence of persistent proteinuria and by lack of response to restoration of vascular volume and perfusion with the appropriate therapy.

**Proliferative Glomerulonephritis.** If glomerulonephritis is associated with swelling and proliferation of endothelial and mesangial cells, and/or influx of inflammatory cells, narrowing of glomerular capillary lumina will compromise renal blood flow. As a result, substances normally cleared by the glomeruli (urea, creatinine, phosphorus, etc.) are retained in the body. Evidence of an inflammatory process may be detected in urine (hematuria, pyuria, proteinuria, casts). If reduction in glomerular filtration is severe or progressive, clinical signs characteristic of uremia will develop.

**Membranous Glomerulonephropathy.** Most forms of glomerulonephropathy are associated with a variable degree of increased permeability of the GBM to protein molecules. Since the quantity of various proteins excreted in the urine correlates inversely with their molecular weight, albumin (molecular weight = 68,000) is the principal protein found in urine. Lesser quantities of plasma globulins may also be found. Morphologic changes in the GBM occurring in the absence of significant cellular influx or proliferation are often associated with persistent and ultimately severe proteinuria.

The characteristic, and occasionally the only, indication of membranous glomerular disease is persistent proteinuria, which is usually not associated with significant hematuria or pyuria. If enough plasma protein is lost, a nephrotic syndrome may develop. Hyaline, granular or waxy casts may be observed in urine sediment but are not a constant finding. Except in the later stages of progressive membranous glomerulonephropathy, renal clearance of substances normally present in glomerular filtrate is not significantly impaired, and signs of renal failure are usually absent.

**Membranoproliferative Glomerulone-**

**phropathy.** Glomerular diseases are often characterized by proliferation of cellular components of the glomeruli (especially the mesangium) in addition to thickening of the basement membrane. The functional result of these changes is variable, being dependent on the severity and extent of damage to each of the glomerular components. Affected patients may develop proteinuria, renal failure, and/or the nephrotic syndrome.

**Chronic Glomerulonephropathy.** Proliferative, membranous and membranoproliferative glomerulonephropathy may progress to chronic generalized glomerulonephropathy. Progressive reduction of blood flow through the glomeruli, and thus through the postglomerular peritubular capillaries, ultimately results in progressive ischemic atrophy and fibrosis of the renal tubules. Although the morphologic alterations of glomeruli may be characteristic of a particular disease syndrome during earlier phases of the abnormality, progressive destruction of nephrons results in end-stage kidneys with similar gross and microscopic alterations, regardless of the underlying cause. Not only may the precipitating glomerular lesion be difficult or impossible to identify, but difficulty may be encountered in differentiating end-stage kidneys caused by glomerulonephropathy from end-stage kidneys caused by other diseases (pyelonephritis, interstitial nephritis, etc.).

During early stages of glomerulonephropathy, laboratory evaluation of renal function may reveal abnormal glomerular function but normal or only slightly impaired tubular function (i.e., glomerulotubular imbalance). During more advanced stages of the disease process, changes related to abnormal tubular function become superimposed on changes related to abnormal glomerular function.

The ultimate functional result of chronic generalized glomerulonephropathy is chronic renal failure. Progressive reduction in the number of functioning nephrons results in renal failure characterized by impaired ability to concentrate or dilute urine and by varying degrees of abnormal retention (urea, creatinine, phosphorus, etc.) and loss (bicarbonate, chloride, sodium, etc.) of metabolites normally regulated by the kidneys. Varying degrees of nonregenerative anemia and renal osteodystrophy may also develop.

**Nephrotic Syndrome.** Prolonged severe proteinuria and the resultant hypoproteinemia that occur secondary to damage to the glomerular capillary wall initiate physiologic, metabolic and nutritional defects associated with the nephrotic syndrome.

If the proteinuria that occurs secondary to damage to the filtration barrier(s) in the capillary walls is persistent and severe, urine protein (especially albumin) loss may exceed the capacity of the liver to maintain normal plasma protein concentration. In uremic patients, increase in the rate of endogenous catabolism of albumin and decreased dietary intake of protein may also contribute to hypoalbuminemia. Since albumin molecules account for approximately 77 per cent of plasma colloidal osmotic pressure, progressive hypoalbuminemia is associated with a proportionate decrease in plasma colloidal osmotic pressure. According to the Starling-Landis cycle of capillary-interstitial fluid exchange, a marked decrease in colloidal osmotic pressure will initiate an abnormal shift of fluid from the vascular compartment to the extravascular compartment, resulting in hypovolemia and edema. The edema is usually most severe in dependent portions of the body (ventral midline, limbs), because venous hydrostatic pressure is greatest in these locations. In severe cases, ascites and hydrothorax may develop.

In addition to the reduction in colloidal osmotic pressure that occurs as a result of glomerular loss of plasma protein, body compensatory mechanisms play a role in the development and maintenance of edema. As a result of loss of vascular fluid into the extravascular tissue spaces, vascular volume is reduced. Reduction of renal blood flow associated with decreased vascular volume initiates the compensatory release of aldosterone through the renin-angiotensin system (Fig. 2). Reduction in vascular volume may also stimulate the release of antidiuretic hormone. These hormones promote the resorption of sodium and water from glomerular filtrate by the renal tubules. Because the resorbed sodium and water molecules are not large enough to be retained selectively in the vascular compartment by the capillary walls, they rapidly equilibrate with extravascular fluid compartments. The pharmacologic effects of these hormones tend to perpetuate and ag-

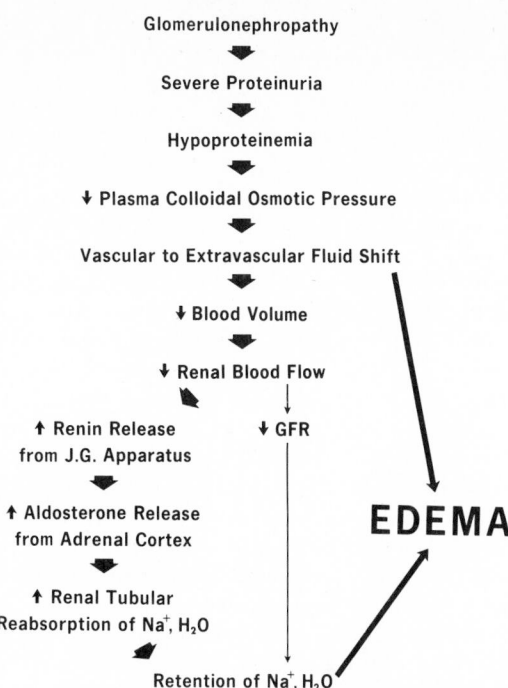

Glomerulonephropathy

Severe Proteinuria

Hypoproteinemia

↓ Plasma Colloidal Osmotic Pressure

Vascular to Extravascular Fluid Shift

↓ Blood Volume

↓ Renal Blood Flow

↑ Renin Release from J.G. Apparatus    ↓ GFR

↑ Aldosterone Release from Adrenal Cortex

**EDEMA**

↑ Renal Tubular Reabsorption of $Na^+$, $H_2O$

Retention of $Na^+$, $H_2O$

**Figure 2.** Pathophysiology of nephrotic edema.

gravate the edema in addition to expanding vascular volume.

Although the nephrotic syndrome is a well-established complication of generalized glomerular disease in dogs and cats, not all patients with generalized glomerular disease develop a nephrotic syndrome. A specific glomerular disease in its mildest form may result in mild proteinuria that is insufficient to cause severe hypoalbuminemia and other manifestations of the nephrotic syndrome. The same disease in another patient, or at a different stage in the same patient, may cause marked proteinuria and other signs of the nephrotic syndrome. Glomerulonephritic dogs and cats may develop all the features of the nephrotic syndrome (proteinuria, hypoproteinemia, hypoalbuminemia and hypercholesterolemia) except edema. Even when present, the edema varies greatly in severity from individual to individual, and within the same individual. In fact, the clinical and biochemical manifestations may undergo partial or complete remission without treatment. Unfortunately, the likelihood of spontaneous remissions is unpredictable.

In addition to the biologic behavior of the underlying cause, the unpredictable variability of the natural clinical course of the

nephrotic syndrome is related to fluctuations in the levels of aldosterone, antidiuretic hormone, electrolytes, colloids and water within the body. Of these factors, the severity of the proteinuria and hypoalbuminemia is probably the most significant. As a generality, subcutaneous edema does not develop unless serum albumin concentration is less than 0.8 to 1.0 gram per 100 ml. Because of variations in the capacity of the body to compensate for increased protein loss by increased hepatic protein synthesis, and because of fluctuations in the concentrations of the hormones and electrolytes, however, not all patients with serum albumin concentrations of this magnitude develop edema.

With the progression of glomerular lesions and the onset of primary renal failure, the severity of proteinuria, hypoproteinemia and edema may decrease. This decrease occurs when reduction in glomerular perfusion with plasma is of such magnitude that it results in a significant reduction in the clearance of protein. In contrast to patients with remission of glomerular lesions, however, uremic nephrotic patients show a progressive increase in concentration of serum creatinine and urea nitrogen and a progressive loss of ability to concentrate or dilute urine.

## IMMUNE-MEDIATED GLOMERULONEPHROPATHY

Although the etiology of most forms of glomerulonephropathy is not completely understood, immunopathologic studies have convincingly demonstrated that at least two distinct humoral immunologic mechanisms play a major role in several types of glomerulonephropathy in man, dogs, cats, horses, other domestic animals and laboratory animals. There is little evidence that cellular immunity contributes significantly to the production of glomerulonephropathy, in contrast to renal transplant rejections, in which cellular immunity plays a prominent role.

**Immune-Complex Disease.** Immune-complex disease is characterized by the localization of soluble, circulating, non-glomerular antigen-antibody-complement complexes in glomerular capillary walls. Neither the antigen nor the antibody has any direct antigenic relationship to glomeruli. The size, solubility, complement-fixing capacity and *in-vivo* biologic activity of immune complexes are related to the concentration ratios of antigen and antibody (i.e., the ratio of one to the other). Complexes of antigen and antibody formed in the presence of a large excess of antigen are very small, do not bind large quantities of complement, circulate until they are catabolized or excreted and have a reduced capacity to induce immune injury. Complexes of antigen and antibody formed at equivalence (i.e., the point at which a maximum amount of antibody is bound to antigen as insoluble complexes) bind complement but are rapidly removed from the circulation by phagocytic cells of the reticuloendothelial system because they are large. They do not induce immune-mediated injury. In contrast, immune complexes formed in the presence of moderate antigen excess are of intermediate size and bind a relatively large quantity of complement. They circulate for relatively long periods of time because they are too small to be rapidly removed by phagocytic cells. If they become deposited in walls of blood vessels as a result of conditions associated with increased vascular permeability, they can initiate immunologically mediated tissue injury. Although the exact mechanism(s) that causes soluble immune complexes to become concentrated in glomerular capillaries is not well understood, it may be associated with the filtration function of glomeruli, overloading the phagocytic capacity of mesangial cells, and/or the liberation of vasoactive amines (such as histamine) as a result of an immune-mediated activation of blood platelets. Patients incapable of making a vigorous antibody response are most likely to develop pathogenic circulating immune complexes.

The activation of complement (an enzymatic system of plasma proteins) by immune complexes (or by the so-called alternate pathway of complement activation) is associated with several reactions, including the release of chemotactic substances, which attract polymorphonuclear leukocytes, and the phenomenon of immune adherence, which promotes the retention of PMN's in glomeruli. This mechanism is called neutrophil-dependent injury of the GBM. The PMN's may displace the endothelial cells lining the glomerular capillaries and approximate themselves along the GBM, presumably in an attempt to engulf immune complexes. If proteolytic enzymes (cathepsins, collagenase, elastase, etc.) and other lysosomal proteins are released from PMN's, the GBM and glomerular cells may be damaged. Glomerular damage results in nonselective renal clearance of plasma proteins and proteinuria. If the immune response is severe or prolonged, it may be associated with the formation and deposition of fibrin. The latter may interfere with resolution of the lesion and result in healing by replacement fibrosis. As mentioned previously, fibrin deposition in Bowman's space may stimulate the formation of epithelial crescents.

In neutrophil-dependent injury of the GBM, neutrophils are the effector of injury. Depletion of either complement or neutrophils from experimental animals will prevent the development of injury in this form of glomerulonephropathy, even though immune complexes are deposited in glomeruli. A neutrophil-independent form of immune-complex glomerulonephropathy has been observed in experimental animals in which removal of complement and neutrophils will not prevent the development of glomerular injury. Few neutrophils have been found in the glomeruli of dogs, cats and other species with naturally occurring immune-complex glomerulopathy associated with clinical signs. This observation suggests that neutrophil-independent injury of the GBM may occur, although the influence of neutrophils at a preclinical stage cannot be excluded. The mechanisms that cause neutrophil-independent glomerulonephritis have not been defined.

It has been hypothesized that the size of soluble immune complexes may influence their ability to traverse the GBM. The location of the soluble immune complexes with respect to the GBM may in turn influence the morphologic and functional results of their presence. Large, soluble immune complexes that are localized in the subendothelial portion of the capillary wall are exposed to the cellular defense mechanisms of the body and may stimulate an inflammatory and proliferative response following activation of complement. If this reponse significantly impairs glomerular perfusion, retention of substances normally filtered by the glomeruli will result. In addition, signs of inflammation may be detected via urinalysis (hematuria, pyuria, proteinuria). In one study of dogs in which immune complexes were concentrated on the subendothelial side of the GBM, renal failure, but not the nephrotic syndrome, was observed. Smaller, soluble immune complexes that have traversed the GBM and are concentrated on the subepithelial aspects of the glomerular capillary wall may be protected from circulating cells or tissue cells capable of degrading them. Although they may not stimulate an inflammatory or proliferative response, the fact that their presence is associated with proteinuria suggests that they may interfere with the filtration function of the GBM or visceral epithelial cells. Concentration of a significant quantity of immune complexes in both subepithelial and subendothelial locations would be expected to be associated with a combination of the alterations described above.

On the basis of the criterion that randomly distributed deposits of complement and immunoglobulin could be detected within, or adjacent to, the GBM by immunofluorescent and/or electron microscopy, immune-complex disease has been reported to account for approximately 80 per cent of immunologic glomerulonephropathy in man and is the only type of immunologic glomerulonephropathy encountered thus far in dogs and cats. This criterion does not provide conclusive evidence of the presence of immune-complex glomerulonephropathy, because definite proof requires demonstration of suspected antigen(s) in the glomerular immune-complex deposits, in addition to immunoglobulin and complement. Unfortunately, identification of antigens has been accomplished in only a few types of naturally occurring immune-complex glomerulonephropathy.

Acute poststreptococcal glomerulonephritis in man is an example of immune-complex disease. Attempts to produce acute glomerulonephritis in dogs by establishing an infection with various strains of hemolytic streptococci or by injecting streptococcal products have been unsuccessful.

A reversible mixed membranoproliferative glomerulonephropathy has been observed in dogs with pyometra. Good correlation existed between the severity of glomerular changes and the degree of reduction in glomerular filtration rate. Electron microscopic evaluation of kidneys obtained from affected dogs revealed slight to moderate swelling of endothelial and mesangial cells; irregular thickening of the GBM; and irregular deposits of electron-dense material on the subendothelial side of the GBM, within the GBM and within mesangial cells. Even though the kidneys were not examined by means of immunofluorescent microscopy, it was hypothesized that the glomerular lesions were caused by immune complexes. It was suggested that the antigen associated with immune-complex formation originated from the uterus, either as bacterial antigen or antigen from damaged uterine tissue. This hypothesis was supported by the finding that all dogs tested serologically had specific antibodies against strains of bacteria isolated from their uteri. In addition, the renal disease was functionally and structurally reversible following ovariohysterectomy. Recently, antigens of *Escherichia coli* have been observed to have an affinity for the parietal and epithelial surfaces of Bowman's capsule and tubular epithelium of dogs with pyometra.

Clinical, immunofluorescent and electron microscopic studies performed by other investigators and ourselves have revealed findings typical of immune-complex glomerulonephropathy in proteinuric dogs with *Dirofilaria immitis*. To date, however, the specific antigens (adult, microfilarial and/or infective larval) have not been identified.

Laboratory animals with a high incidence of naturally occurring immune-complex glomerulonephropathy often have chronic viral infections. Immune complexes have been observed in the glomeruli of dogs with experimentally induced and spontaneously occurring canine adenovirus (infectious canine hepatitis) infection. Canine adenovirus antigen has been identified in the glomerular immune deposits of some dogs. An unexpectedly high incidence of membranous glomerulonephropathy has also been observed in cats with spontaneously occurring and experimentally induced feline leukemia, a disease known to be caused by an RNA virus. Viral antigen-antibody complexes have been found in the glomeruli of some cats infected with feline leukemia virus.

Glomerulonephropathy associated with systemic lupus erythematosus in man is caused by immune complexes consisting of DNA (antigen), anti-DNA (antibody) and complement. It has not been determined whether the DNA antigen is native-host DNA, modified-host DNA or viral DNA. Chronic membranous glomerulonephritis is also a feature of canine SLE and may be associated with severe proteinuria and a nephrotic syndrome. Glomerulonephropathy may occur with or without involvement of other systems. Immunofluorescent and electron microscopic examination of renal biopsy samples reveals changes characteristic of immune-complex disease. Evaluation of spontaneously occurring and experimentally induced SLE in a breeding colony of dogs has revealed findings that incriminate an infectious agent (possibly a virus) in the pathophysiology of this disorder. Although membranous glomerulonephritis associated with canine SLE is usually progressive and irreversible, affected dogs may survive one to two years prior to succumbing to renal failure.

Several less well-defined types of naturally occurring glomerulonephropathy in dogs and cats have been described in which immunofluorescent and electron microscopic changes characteristic of immune-complex disease were observed. In one clinical study of 42 cases of canine glomerulonephropathy, 70 per cent of the cases had major extrarenal lesions, especially malignant neoplasms. We have observed immune-complex glomerulonephropathy in a dog with a prostatic sarcoma.

**Anti-GBM    Glomerulonephropathy.** Anti-GBM glomerulonephropathy is caused by the production of antibodies by the host that are directed against antigens of the glomerular basement membrane. In contrast to immune-complex glomerulonephropathy, the disease is not associated with circulating antigen-antibody complexes. Both neutrophil-dependent and neutrophil-independent types of anti-GBM disease may occur.

Anti-GBM glomerulonephritis accounts for approximately 3 to 5 per cent of all types of glomerulonephropathy in adult human beings. It has been experimentally induced in dogs on many occasions. The occurrence and incidence of naturally occurring anti-GBM glomerulonephritis in dogs and cats is unknown. Immunofluorescent and electron microscopic evaluation of kidney samples obtained from animals with naturally occurring renal disease has been performed so infrequently that meaningful generalities cannot be made.

**Immune-Mediated Tubular and Interstitial Disease.** In addition to producing glomerular injury, antibodies may also react directly with tubular basement membranes or deposit themselves in the tubular basement membranes, peritubular capillaries and interstitial tissue in the form of immune complexes and initiate a sequence of events that causes tubular and interstitial lesions.

## DIAGNOSIS

The presence of persistent proteinuria indicates the presence of generalized glomerular disease. Care must be used in interpretating the significance of proteinuria, however, since it may be of renal or nonrenal origin. A mild degree of proteinuria may occasionally be associated with fever or generalized passive congestion due to heart failure. Marked hematuria, regardless of cause, will be associated with moderate to severe proteinuria. Slight to large amounts of protein may appear in urine as a result of the presence of inflammatory exudate (hematuria, pyuria, proteinuria) from any location in the urinary tract, or as a result of contamination of urine with exudate from the genital tract. Proliferative glomerulonephropathy associated with exudation of inflammatory cells may result in a combination of proteinuria, pyuria and hematuria that is difficult to distinguish from inflammatory diseases of the lower urinary tract. Hypoproteinemia and hypoalbuminemia provide strong support for the conclusion that persistent proteinuria is of glomerular origin. Hypercholesterolemia is also a consistent finding in dogs with marked proteinuria of glomerular origin.

Since protein-losing glomerulopathies are not the only potential causes of ascites and pitting edema of subcutaneous tissue, other nonrenal causes of abnormal fluid accumulation (congestive heart failure, hepatic cirrhosis, malabsorption syndrome, etc.) should be considered.

Renal biopsies must be employed to establish the underlying cause of glomerular disease because clinical and laboratory findings are not sufficiently specific to allow a diagnosis other than glomerular disease. Light microscopy and the use of special stains usually will suffice to differentiate amyloidosis from other types of glomerular disease.

Both immune-complex disease and anti-GBM disease focus antigen-antibody reactions in glomeruli. Since both immunologic mechanisms have the potential to induce varying degrees of damage to glomeruli by activation of complement and other mediators of immune injury, they cannot be differentiated with certainty on the basis of clinical or laboratory findings, or by light microscopic examination of kidneys. Each, however, has characteristic immunofluorescent and ultrastructural patterns.

Immune-complex disease is characterized by the presence of randomly distributed accumulations of immune-complexes within and/or adjacent to the GBM when evaluated by means of immunofluorescent microscopy. Recent studies in man indicate that subepithelial deposits are primarily formed between visceral epithelial foot processes, explaining their characteristic interrupted but discrete appearance. The immune complexes appear as electron-dense deposits in subepithelial, intramembranous or subendothelial portions of the glomerular capillary wall when evaluated by means of electron microscopy.

Because anti-GBM antibodies combine with antigens distributed throughout the GBM, anti-GBM glomerulonephropathy is characterized by the presence of a smooth, diffuse, linear deposition of antibody and complement along the GBM when evaluated by means of immunofluorescent microscopy. In most cases, the accumulation of antibodies and complement cannot be observed by means of electron microscopy. In severe cases, however, a diffuse linear zone of rarefaction in the subendothelial portion of the glomerular capillary wall may be detected. It is suspected that this alteration is caused by separation of endothelial cells from the basement membrane by a large accumulation of antibodies and complement.

In either form of glomerulonephropathy, there may be irregular deposition of electron-dense and immunofluorescent material (containing immunoglobulins, complement, fibrinogen and plasma proteins) within glomerular capillary lumina, beneath capillary endothelium and in the mesangium.

## TREATMENT

**Immunosuppressant Drugs.** Experimental and clinical evidence implicating an immunologic basis for anti-GBM and immune-complex glomerulonephropathy and the success of corticosteroids and im-

munosuppressive drugs in controlling homograft rejections of renal transplants provide a logical basis for considering the use of various combinations of corticosteroids and immunosuppressants in the treatment of immunologic glomerulonephropathy. Drugs of this type have been used in the treatment of immune-mediated glomerular disease with the expectation that they will inhibit the production of pathogenic antibodies or suppress the inflammatory response initiated by antigen-antibody-complement reactions. However, there has been no documentation that naturally occurring immune-mediated glomerulonephropathy is consistently associated with hyperactivity of the immune system. In addition, inflammatory reactions are not always an integral part of the evolution of the disease process.

There are numerous reports concerning the value of corticosteroids and immunosuppressive drugs in the treatment of human beings with immunologic glomerulonephropathy. It is difficult to determine the results of most of these studies because they were performed without suitable controls, and because of the variability in the natural course of human glomerulonephropathy. The beneficial effect of corticosteroid and immunosuppressant therapy in human beings with immunologic glomerulonephropathy remains unsubstantiated. In general, the results of such therapy have been disappointing.

There is a paucity of available information concerning the natural history of different types of glomerular disease and the nephrotic syndrome in dogs and cats. Evaluation of several dogs with the nephrotic syndrome at the University of Minnesota has revealed an irregular and unpredictable pattern of clinical signs in some patients. Therefore, we are skeptical of reports that indicate that corticosteroid and immunosuppressant therapy was successful in inducing remission of clinical signs of the nephrotic syndrome in dogs with generalized glomerular disease. The conclusions of these investigators have been based on evaluation of a limited number of patients and apparently have not taken into account the possibility that clinical remission could have occurred without any form of therapy. Although corticosteroid therapy is frequently effective in suppressing hematologic and serologic manifestations of systemic lupus erythematosus in dogs, it appears to be ineffective in the treatment of lupus nephritis in dogs.

The widespread use of corticosteroid or immunosuppressant therapy in dogs with immunologically mediated glomerulonephropathy should be withheld until the natural course of the disease has been evaluated in a larger number of patients, and until the results of well-controlled clinical studies confirm or deny their value. This recommendation is based on the following: (1) corticosteroids and immunosuppressant drugs have the potential to inhibit beneficial as well as harmful immune and inflammatory responses; (2) these drugs may precipitate or aggravate renal failure by inducing gluconeogenesis; and (3) these drugs have the potential to perpetuate immunologic imbalances that favor the production of biologically active immune complexes. Too often the justification of empirical therapy is the hypothesis that some treatment is better than nothing at all. In one well-designed study of the long-term effect of corticosteroid therapy in human beings with membranous and proliferative glomerulonephritis, the death rate was higher in patients receiving corticosteroid therapy than in control groups. Similar results have been obtained in rats treated with immunosuppressant drugs (cyclophosphamide and 6-mercaptopurine) and methylprednisolone.

**Supportive and Symptomatic Therapy.** Therapy of dogs and cats with glomerulonephropathy is far from being hopeless. Some patients may undergo prolonged remission without the benefit of any form of therapy. Dogs with evidence of generalized glomerulonephropathy with and without the nephrotic syndrome have been effectively treated for more than two years with appropriate combinations of supportive and symptomatic therapy. The following recommendations concerning symptomatic and supportive therapy of different manifestations of generalized glomerular disease are intended as generalities only. The method used and the vigor with which it is pursued should be formulated according to the needs of each patient.

1. *Proteinuric, nonedematous, nonuremic:*
Provide unlimited access to water. If the protein loss is severe, formulate a diet with a sufficient quantity of high-quality protein to help compensate for protein loss in urine. Administer B-complex vitamins orally. Consider the use of anabolic agents such as Winstrol-V® (Winthrop), according to the manufacturer's recommended dosage.

2. *Proteinuric, nonedematous, uremic:*
Avoid stress-inducing factors, such as changes in home environment (hospitalization, board in kennels, etc.), and provide unlimited access to water. Administer anabolic agents. Cautiously supply additional high-quality protein in the diet to balance protein loss in urine. Do not provide excessive protein, since it will be deaminated, be metabolized for energy and increase the quantity of metabolic garbage to be excreted by failing kidneys (monitor BUN, serum creatinine and serum albumin concentration). Administer B-complex vitamins orally. Administer sodium chloride and sodium bicarbonate with caution, since the addition of excessive sodium may precipitate edema. (Consult the articles on management of renal failure for dosage recommendations.) Reduce the dosage or discontinue salt and bicarbonate therapy if significant edema develops. Oral calcium lactate may be used in lieu of sodium bicarbonate to combat metabolic acidosis.

3. *Proteinuric, edematous, nonuremic:*
Provide unlimited access to water. Provide a diet with a sufficient quantity of high-quality protein to help compensate for protein loss in urine. Avoid stress and administer anabolic agents. Administer B-complex vitamins orally. Some patients may tolerate a mild degree of edema without obvious harm. For moderate to severe edema, administer natriuretic diuretics such as furosemide (Lasix® [National]) or ethacrynic acid (Edecrin® [Merck]). These diuretics are so effective that removal of fluid by paracentesis is rarely necessary. Thoracocentesis should be considered only if pleural fluid is impairing respiration. Repeated paracentesis should be avoided if possible, since it will deplete the patient of fluids and metabolites. Prevent diuretic-induced fluid and electrolyte depletion by proper control of diuretic dosage and by replacement therapy with fluids and electrolytes when necessary. Intravenous administration of solutions containing protein is of potential value to patients in circulatory collapse caused by hypovolemia, or to initiate diuresis in a patient with refractory edema. It will produce only a transient effect and therefore is impractical for long-term therapy. Depending on the underlying cause of the nephrotic syndrome, control of edema may necessitate administration of low doses of oral diuretics for the life of the patient. Drug-induced hypokalemia has not been observed in nephrotic dogs receiving long-term therapy with low doses of furosemide at the University of Minnesota.

4. *Proteinuric, edematous, uremic:*
Avoid stress, administer anabolic agents and B-complex vitamins, and cautiously supply additional high-quality protein in the diet with the objective of minimizing urine protein loss. Do

not provide excessive protein, since some may be deaminated and metabolized for energy. Provide unlimited access to water unless the patient is vomiting, in which case fluids should be administered by the parenteral route. Administer sodium chloride and sodium bicarbonate with caution. Reduce the dosage or discontinue use of these drugs if the edema increases in severity. Oral calcium lactate may be provided in lieu of sodium bicarbonate to combat metabolic acidosis. Consider the use of furosemide or ethacrynic acid to control or eliminate the edema. Alternatively, aldosterone antagonists such as spironolactone (Aldactone®[Searle]) may be used to control edema. We have had no experience with the use of aldosterone-antagonizing agents.

## PROGNOSIS

Pending controlled studies that will elucidate the cause, pathogenesis, natural clinical course and therapeutic response of various types of glomerular disease, forecasts of the future course of events for glomerulonephritic patients will remain unpredictable. This statement must not be interpreted to indicate that the prognosis of glomerulonephropathy is uniformly unfavorable. Survival periods of more than two years have been noted in glomerulonephritic dogs with and without the nephrotic syndrome following supportive and symptomatic treatment at the University of Minnesota.

### SUPPLEMENTAL READING

Casey, H. W., and Splitter, G. A.: Membranous glomerulonephritis in dogs infected with Dirofilaria immitis. Vet. Pathol., 12:111–117, 1975.

Cochrane, G. G., and Koffler, D.: Immune complex disease in experimental animals and man. In Advances in Immunology.        Vol. 16. Dixon, F. J., and Kunkel, H. G. (eds.): New York, Academic Press, 1973.

Farquhar, M. G.: The primary glomerular filtration barrier—basement membrane or epithelial slits? Kidney Int., 8:197–211, 1975.

Farrow, B. R. H., Huxtable, C. R., and McGovern, V. J.: Nephrotic syndrome in the cat due to diffuse membranous glomerulonephritis. Pathology, 1:67–72, 1969.

Hardy, W. D.: Immunology of oncornaviruses. Vet. Clin. N. Am., 4:133–146, 1974.

Kurtz, J. M., Russell, S. W., Lee, J. C., Slauson, D. O., and Schechter, R. D.: Naturally occurring canine glomerulonephritis. Am. J. Path., 67:471–477, 1972.

Lewis, R. M., Andre-Schwartz, J., Harris, G. S., Hirsch, M. S., Black, P. H., and Schwartz, R. S.: Canine systemic lupus erythematosus. Transmission of serologic abnormalities by cell-free filtrates. J. Clin. Invest., 52:1893–1907, 1973.

Morrison, W. I., Nash, A. S., and Wright, N. G.: Glomerular deposition of immune complexes in dogs following natural infection with canine adenovirus. Vet. Rec., 96:522–524, 1975.

Murray, M., and Wright, H. G.: A morphologic study of canine glomerulonephritis. Lab. Invest., 30:213–221, 1974.

Obel, A., et al.: Light and electron microscopical studies of the renal lesions in dogs in pyometra. Acta Vet. Scand., 5:146–178, 1964.

Osborne, C. A., and Vernier, R. L.: Glomerulonephritis in the dog and cat: A comparative review. J. Am. Animal Hosp. Assn., 9:101–127, 1973.

Osborne, C. A., Stevens, J. B., McClean, R., and Vernier, R. L.: Membranous lupus glomerulonephritis in a dog. J. Am. Animal Hosp. Assn., 9:295–300, 1973.

Osborne, C. A., et al.: Natural remission of nephrotic syndrome in a dog with immune-complex glomerulopathy. J. Am. Vet. Med. Assn., in press.

Wilson, C. B., and Dixon, F. J.: Diagnosis of immunopathologic renal disease. Kidney Int., 5:389–401, 1974.

Wilson, C. B., and Dixon, F. J., Immunopathology and glomerulonephritis. Ann. Rev. Med., 25:83–98, 1974.

# CHRONIC INTERSTITIAL NEPHRITIS

DONALD G. LOW, D.V.M.
*Davis, California*

Chronic interstitial nephritis is a term used to describe focal or generalized fibrosis of renal interstitial tissue, which is usually accompanied by a marked infiltration of mononuclear cells and loss of functioning nephrons. Tubular and interstitial lesions tend to be more severe than glomer- ular lesions. In recent years, the terms chronic generalized nephritis and end-stage kidneys have often been substituted for generalized, advanced, chronic interstitial nephritis because they tend to convey more clearly the functional and morphologic states of the kidneys. No specific etiology is implied with such terms. In contrast, many veterinarians have associated chronic interstitial nephritis with canine leptospirosis. Few facts have been advanced to support the hypothesized leptospiral etiology of chronic interstitial nephritis, while, by contrast, other diseases, such as pyelonephritis, congenital and inherited renal diseases, and even glomerular diseases, have been clearly shown to lead to gross morphologic changes that, at termination, are difficult or impossible to distinguish from each other. All cause chronic interstitial fibrosis. Thus, the terms chronic generalized nephritis and end-stage kidney are preferred. When any of these diseases are progressive, a syndrome of polydipsia and polyuria commences after about 70 per cent of the nephrons are destroyed.

The clinician must also recognize that the renal lesion may be focal or of limited distribution within the kidneys and therefore may cause no detectable alteration of renal function. It is well known that loss of half of an animal's nephrons through nephrectomy produces no health problem for the animal, provided that the opposite kidney is normal. It should be equally apparent that the loss of half the nephrons through disease is well tolerated if the remaining half of the nephrons are normal. If the clinician approaches chronic renal disease from this viewpoint, he quickly appreciates the great difference between renal disease and renal failure. Any lesions found in the kidneys constitute disease, while failure does not have its clinical onset until 70 per cent or more of the nephrons are destroyed. While renal disease is quite common in older animals, renal failure is encountered much less frequently. For the majority of chronic progressive renal diseases, there is no therapy available that will halt or reverse the progress of the disease. The veterinary clinician, therefore, is often limited to managing the animal by providing the best possible environment for the surviving nephrons in order to minimize the work that they must perform.

For specific therapy, the reader is referred to the articles on "Medical Management of Polyuric Primary Renal Failure," "Intensive Diuresis in Polyuric Renal Failure" and "Peritoneal Dialysis." (See also "Prognosis of Renal Failure.")

# PROGNOSIS OF RENAL FAILURE

DELMAR R. FINCO, D.V.M.
*Athens, Georgia*

Regardless of the disease, the client seeks information regarding prognosis. An accurate prognosis provides a basis for logical decisions concerning the duration and intensity of therapy which a pet is to receive.

With regard to renal failure, it is helpful to categorize prognosis into short-term and long-term prognosis. Short-term prognosis is related to the clinician's success in combating signs of renal failure by symptomatic and supportive therapy during the first several days or weeks of illness, regardless of the underlying cause of disease. Long-term prognosis is related to one's ability to eliminate the cause of the disease, so that continued destruction of renal parenchyma does not occur.

## BASIS FOR PROGNOSIS

The prognosis of renal failure should not be based on a single piece of information, simply because no single observation has proved reliable as a prognostic indicator of renal failure. Formulation of an accurate prognosis of renal failure entails correlation of data obtained from history, physical examination and general or special laboratory examinations. These data should be used to answer the following questions: (1) What is the etiopathogenesis of the renal failure? (2) What is the degree of renal dysfunction? (3) What is the potential for reversibility of the lesions and for improvement in renal function?

## ETIOPATHOGENESIS OF RENAL FAILURE

Knowledge of the anatomic site of the abnormality is helpful in establishing a prognosis, since the kidney may be entirely normal in prerenal and postrenal causes of failure. With primary renal failure, knowledge concerning the cause of disease may be helpful inasmuch as the short-term and long-term effects of that disease on the kidneys may be known.

**Prerenal Failure.** Prerenal failure refers to abnormal renal function resulting from inadequate perfusion of the kidneys with blood. Causes include hypovolemia, shock, dehydration, adrenocortical insufficiency and circulatory impairment due to heart disease. If prerenal uremia is quickly and adequately treated, the prognosis is excellent, since no damage occurs to the kidneys. More prolonged or severe renal ischemia may result in varying degrees of tubular necrosis.

In some instances, prerenal uremia may be suspected because of identification of the prerenal factors previously listed. Generally, ability to form a concentrated urine (S. G. greater than 1.025) indicates prerenal rather than primary renal failure. Ability to produce a concentrated urine with primary renal failure is rare in the dog and cat but may be observed in cases of primary glomerular disease with glomerulotubular imbalance (consult the article on Glomerulonephropathy and the Nephrotic Syndrome). In some cases, history, physical examination and urinalysis are inadequate to differentiate prerenal from renal uremia. Renal biopsy is probably the best additional tool to use in this instance.

**Postrenal Failure.** Postrenal failure refers to abnormalities in urine outflow from the body. Common causes of postrenal uremia include urethral obstruction and rupture of the urinary bladder or proximal urethra. If outflow obstruction is corrected within a few days, the prognosis is excellent, since no secondary damage to the kidney occurs. More prolonged obstruction can result in hydronephrosis, which may be reversible. In contrast to the situation with obstruction, rupture of a segment of the urinary tract is not accompanied by back-up of urine in the kidneys, and therefore renal damage does not occur. In these instances, prognosis is dependent on repair of the leak and treatment of the uremia (short-term factors). Postrenal uremia due to obstruction is usually detectable by physical examination. Excretory urography may be required to diagnose urinary tract rupture or ureteral obstruction.

**Primary Renal Failure.** Primary renal failure refers to primary disease of the kidneys. Prognosis of primary renal uremia is variable, and thus the prognosis cannot be made with only the knowledge that renal failure is due to primary renal disease. When available, knowledge of the action of a specific microbial or chemical agent provides the clinician with information that can be of value in establishing the prognosis. For example, it is known that canine leptospirosis causes an acute interstitial nephritis that does not progress to a chronic form. This knowledge allows one to give a good long-term prognosis for leptospirosis, although the short-term prognosis is poor to fair, depending on the severity of disease and the response to antibiotic therapy. Renal amyloidosis is a slowly progressive and ultimately fatal disease. Knowledge that a patient has renal amyloidosis requires that a poor long-term prognosis be given, but the short-term prognosis is variable, depending on the stage of the disease in the individual patient. Unfortunately, the specific cause of primary renal disease is not always known. In these instances, the clinician must utilize all other information that is available in an effort to formulate a logical and accurate prognosis.

Identification of primary renal disease is accomplished by elimination of prerenal and postrenal factors as possible causes of renal failure. In addition, identification of specific functional deficiencies, such as inability to concentrate urine when dehydrated, or specific morphologic abnormalities, such as shrunken kidneys, support the diagnosis of primary renal failure.

## DEGREE OF RENAL DYSFUNCTION

The degree of renal dysfunction in renal failure can be estimated by certain common laboratory procedures, such as the blood urea nitrogen (BUN) or serum creatinine concentration. Serum creatinine concentration is influenced by fewer extrarenal factors than BUN. Dietary protein intake has a minor effect on BUN. The rate of protein catabolism may affect BUN but does not affect serum creatinine. However, both creatinine and urea are metabolized in significant amounts by enteric bacteria, and thus a nonrenal portal of exit from the body exists. In addition, laboratory analysis of creatinine is less precise than that for urea. A recent study revealed that only a general correlation existed between BUN and serum creatinine determinations on azotemic dogs and cats. From this study, no clear superiority of either BUN or serum creatinine was apparent. It was concluded that both tests should continue to be used as crude indications of renal function, but that neither should be used alone as a method of prognosis. This limitation exists because knowledge of the functional state of the kidney provides no information concerning the cause of the disease. Uremia could be prerenal, renal or postrenal, and BUN and serum creatinine concentrations do not distinguish the site of the lesion. Likewise the degree of dysfunction gives no information concerning the potential reversibility of the morphologic lesions in instances of renal uremia.

Methods of intensive supportive and symptomatic treatment make it possible to sustain life for short periods of time despite the presence of severe renal dysfunction. Because short-term prognosis is improved with these methods, long-term prognosis assumes more importance in the formulation of the overall prognosis. Long-term prognosis is more dependent on knowledge of the etiology and morphologic status of the kidney than on a single assessment of renal function.

While basing prognosis on a single determination of blood concentration of urea nitrogen or creatinine has no logical or theoretical basis, serial determinations of renal function may provide information. With serial determinations the clinician can judge the response of the kidney both to therapy and to renal compensatory and regerative processes that occur with the passage of time.

## POTENTIAL FOR REVERSIBILITY OF RENAL LESIONS

**Acute vs. Chronic Disease.** Reversibility of renal disease is dependent on the extent and severity of lesions and on the ability of the kidney to repair damage sustained. In general, there is potential for reversibility of kidney lesions and for improvement in kidney function in patients with acute renal failure. In acute disease, compensatory mechanisms have not been exhausted and parenchymal regeneration has not had an opportunity to occur. In contrast, the potential for reversibility of lesions is poor in chronic renal failure, since compensatory mechanisms have been exhausted and since the limits of parenchymal regeneration had occurred already. Although the long-term prognosis with chronic renal failure is poor, vigorous therapeutic procedures may reverse signs, so that a patient with chronic renal failure may live a comfortable existence for several months, despite the presence of progressive renal disease. The veterinarian should use all information available to differentiate acute from chronic renal disease inasmuch as these terms may be looked upon as being synonymous with potentially reversible and irreversible renal disease, respectively. Information helpful in making this differentiation is summarized below.

**History.** Duration of clinical signs may aid in differentiating acute from chronic renal failure. If a history of polydipsia and polyuria of several weeks' or several months' duration is obtained, and if the polydipsia and polyuria are due to renal failure, the veterinarian has accumulated evidence of chronic renal failure. If there is a history of ingestion of a nephrotoxic agent, such as ethylene glycol, or of exposure to a contagious disease with acute manifestations, the veterinarian has accumulated evidence of acute renal failure. However, the clinician should hesitate to make a judgment concerning acuteness of renal disease based on abruptness of onset of signs. In many instances, signs of uremia may be noted abruptly with chronic disease, because of either inadequate observation by the owner or insidious onset of chronic renal failure.

**Physical Examination.** Acute and chronic renal failure share many common clinical signs. These include depression, anorexia, vomiting, diarrhea, polydipsia, polyuria, oliguria and dehydration. Some signs are usually restricted to chronic renal failure and include mucosal ulcerations, progressive severe weight loss, mucosal pallor due to anemia and skeletal changes caused by renal secondary hyperparathyroidism. In the presence of these latter signs, the clinician has accumulated information consistent with chronic renal disease.

The kidneys should always be palpated, since determinations of kidney size may aid in differentiating acute from chronic renal failure. Knowledge that the kidney size is normal does not provide definitive information, since acute or chronic changes are possible in kidneys of normal size. Increase in kidney size may occur in association with acute renal disease, but it may also occur in association with hydronephrosis or with neoplasm. Decrease in kidney size is almost always associated with chronic generalized renal disease, and thus it represents a very significant finding.

**Radiography.** Radiography may aid in differentiating acute from chronic disease, by allowing estimation of kidney size in patients in which the kidneys are not palpable. In some instances, kidney size can be determined from survey radiographs. Excretory urography may aid in evaluating kidney size even in azotemic patients. Although excellent visualization of the kidneys with contrast agents is impaired in renal failure because of a decrease in renal blood flow and impaired ability of the kidneys to concentrate, visualization is frequently adequate for accurate determination of size. In addition to information on kidney size, radiography may be of value in assessing skeletal demineralization due to renal secondary hyperparathyroidism. Demineralization is not detectable in acute renal failure but may be observed in association with chronic renal failure.

**Laboratory Aids.** No test that measures renal function allows differentiation between acute and chronic renal disease. Contrary to other reports, determinations of serum creatinine, BUN or serum phosphorus are not of value in this regard. Findings on urinalysis are of limited value in differentiating between acute and chronic renal failure. Urine specific gravity may be fixed with either acute or chronic disease. Proteinuria is an unreliable indication of whether a process is acute or chronic. Examination of urine sediment may provide information indicating whether renal failure is associated with an inflammatory process. Unfortunately, inflammation may be acute or chronic, and so limited information is obtainable from this procedure. Casts may be detected in the urine in both acute and chronic renal disease, and their presence provides no definitive information as to whether the process is acute or chronic.

**Renal Biopsy.** Renal biopsy provides the only method for establishing the morphologic status of the kidney in the living patient. Knowledge of kidney morphology provides a basis for determining the reversibility of kidney lesions. Correlation of biopsy results with history, physical examination, radiography and laboratory findings allows the most precise prognosis of renal disease.

### SUPPLEMENTAL READING

Finco, D. R., and Duncan, J. R.: Evaluation of blood urea nitrogen and serum creatinine concentration as indicators of renal dysfunction. A study of III cases and a review of related literature. J. Am. Vet. Med. Assn., *168*:593–602, 1976.

Hall, J. W., *et al.*: Immediate and long-term prognosis in acute renal failure. Ann. Int. Med. *73*:515-521, 1970.

# MEDICAL MANAGEMENT OF OLIGURIC AND ANURIC PRIMARY RENAL FAILURE

DONALD G. LOW, D.V.M.
*Davis, California*

Treatment of oliguric and anuric primary renal failure in veterinary medicine demands accuracy in both diagnosis and prognosis if the therapeutic effort is to have any appreciable degree of success. The veterinary clinician may become aware of oliguric or anuric renal failure through history of reduced urine output reported by an owner, through establishing a history of ingestion of a nephrotoxic agent such as ethylene glycol or through learning of an injury that may have precipitated serious renal ischemia through prolonged hypotension. He may also learn of the problem through his own work-up of a case in which a urinalysis or a blood urea nitrogen or creatinine determination is included in the evaluation of the patient. This situation often prevails when a gastrointestinal upset is being investigated. The veterinarian may become cognizant of oliguric or anuric renal failure when he monitors renal function and urine output before, during and immediately following the administration of known nephrotoxic drugs, such as amphotericin B or thiacetarsamide sodium, or through the evaluation of renal function and urine output during and after extensive surgery and deep anesthesia. Although primary oliguric or anuric renal failure is most often of abrupt onset, it may occur as a terminal event in chronic progressive renal disease.

## DIAGNOSIS

Once the veterinarian is aware of oliguria or anuria in a patient, he must first eliminate prerenal and postrenal uremia from the problem list. Prerenal uremia can usually be discarded as a probable diagnosis if the animal is well hydrated and has adequate peripheral circulation. Under these conditions the clinician can usually safely assume that the kidneys are also perfused to a reasonable degree. Postrenal anuria can be eliminated in most cases by demonstrating an intact, patent urethra and urinary bladder in the normal anatomic position. In rare instances, bilateral obstruction or rupture of the ureters could be present and result in postrenal oliguria or anuria. Obstruction or injury to the ureter from a solitary kidney must also be considered.

When prerenal and postrenal factors causing oliguria and anuria have been eliminated, the clinician should turn his attention to the kidneys themselves. Blood urea nitrogen or creatinine concentrations should be monitored at least daily to evaluate the direction and rate of change of renal function. A complete blood count should be performed prior to therapy so that unaltered baseline data are available. Sodium, potassium, bicarbonate and blood pH must be measured at least daily. If urine flow is not reestablished early, it will be necessary to evaluate electrolytes and blood pH more frequently. An indwelling catheter should be placed in the bladder, and urine output should be carefully monitored. A complete urinalysis should be performed as part of the initial assessment of the patient and repeated as necessary. In acute renal failure (as in chronic) the specific gravity of the urine is expected to be between 1.008 and 1.020 but differs from the urinalysis of chronic renal failure, in that showers of casts and excessive numbers of red blood cells are often found, especially near the time of onset. Since the results of urinalyses vary markedly within a short period of time, one should not interpret the absence of casts and red blood cells as a reason to eliminate acute renal injury. Their presence, however, should direct the clinician's thoughts toward causes of acute renal failure.

When careful review of the history, physical examination and laboratory data and monitoring of urine output suggest that acute oliguric or anuric renal failure is present, renal biopsy is a high priority. Not only will the biopsy be useful in helping to establish the diagnosis, but it will be of great value in aiding the clinician to establish a prognosis. Since great effort is usually required to successfully treat a patient with anuric renal failure, the potential reversibility of the renal lesion must be established if the effort and expense are to be justified. The clinician must correlate all information from all sources if he is to be successful in

tered. The composition of the fluid used to repair a fluid deficit may vary depending upon the serum potassium concentration, the bicarbonate concentration and the blood pH. If the serum potassium concentration is elevated or if it is unknown, it is desirable to use isotonic saline intravenously as the rehydrating solution.

**Bicarbonate Requirement.** If the plasma bicarbonate concentration is known, the milliequivalents of bicarbonate necessary to adjust the blood pH can be calculated by the formula recommended by Finco: body weight in kg. $\times$ 0.6 $\times$ bicarbonate deficit. The bicarbonate deficit equals 25 minus the patient's plasma bicarbonate concentration. If the plasma bicarbonate and blood pH are unknown, a crude but useful estimate of bicarbonate requirements can be made from the severity of uremia present in the patient according to the following table from Osborne et al.:

| SEVERITY OF UREMIA | PROBABLE $HCO_3$ DEFICIT (mEq./LITER) | $HCO_3$ REQUIRED (mEq./kg. BODY WEIGHT) |
|---|---|---|
| Mild | 5 | 3 |
| Moderate | 10 | 6 |
| Severe | 15 | 9 |

establishing a patient's prognosis (see "Prognosis of Renal Failure"). The patient's owner must be fully informed about both diagnosis and prognosis, so that he can make the appropriate commitment to his pet.

## THERAPY

**Weight and Hydration.** As the initial step in therapy, the patient's weight and hydration should be carefully estimated, since these points will become the baselines for comparison during the course of the therapy. The patient should then be rehydrated. In oliguric and anuric renal failure, great emphasis must be placed on monitoring the patient's weight during therapy in order to avoid overhydration. The fluid deficit that is estimated to be present in the initial evaluation is replaced, and the patient is weighed as accurately as possible again. It is this second weight against which future gains or losses should be compared. Any gain in weight in an anorectic animal suggests overhydration; a slight loss of weight due to catabolism of body tissues is expected if proper fluid therapy is adminis-

Approximately one half the calculated bicarbonate deficit can be replaced during rehydration; the remaining portion should be administered over the next 24 to 48 hours.

**Diuresis.** After the patient is well hydrated, an effort to induce urine flow may be attempted using either mannitol or glucose as the osmotic diuretic (see article on "Intensive Diuresis in Polyuric Renal Failure"). Urine formation must be carefully monitored by means of an indwelling catheter. If urine formation is not initiated by a test dose of either mannitol or glucose, the clinician should give furosemide intravenously at a dose of 4 mg./kg. of body weight. The drug may be repeated at double dose after two hours if no urine flow has been established, but if this dose also fails to induce diuresis, this approach to therapy should be abandoned. Peritoneal dialysis remains as the only reasonable available alternative to sustain life until healing of the renal lesions can occur (see "Peritoneal Dialysis").

**Hyperkalemia.** Hyperkalemia is a common and serious complication of oliguric and anuric renal failure. When hyperkalemia is present, serious consideration should be given to moving the patient to a referral center (assuming that the client is interested) with adequate monitoring facilities and where extensive nursing support can be provided.

Hyperkalemia should be suspected in any oliguric or anuric patient with cardiac arrhythmias and muscle weakness. Electrocardiographic changes such as high amplitude peaked T waves and prolonged Q-T interval are associated with hyperkalemia. If hyperkalemia worsens, complete atrioventricular block and marked bradycardia may occur. Death due to hyperkalemia becomes a serious threat as the serum potassium concentration approaches 10 mEq./liter, while signs may appear at potassium concentrations as low as 7 mEq./liter. Whenever signs due to hyperkalemia are present, aggressive correctional therapy is indicated. Hypertonic glucose solution should be administered early in the course of treatment at the rate of 1 ml. of 10 per cent glucose per kg. of body weight intravenously. It has been shown that the administration of regular insulin does little to lower the serum potassium concentration beyond that accomplished through the use of glucose alone unless very large doses are used (Hiatt, 1971). Such doses should be avoided unless the capability of frequent monitoring of blood glucose concentrations will permit formulation of glucose or glucagon therapy to prevent life-threatening hypoglycemia. Acidosis aggravates the severity of hyperkalemia because the kidneys tend to conserve potassium and excrete hydrogen ion. Therefore the bicarbonate deficit should be repaired with intravenous sodium bicarbonate. If facilities to determine blood pH and bicarbonate concentration are not available, bicarbonate should be provided in accordance with the table above, using the upper limits of the dosage scale. Calcium gluconate or calcium lactate may be administered intravenously at a dose of 0.5 ml. per kg. of a 10 percent solution if cardiac arrhythmias persist. Peritoneal dialysis or hemodialysis must usually be instituted if longer-term survival is to be possible.

Because the use of intravenous glucose, calcium and bicarbonate provides only transient relief of hyperkalemia therapeutic measures that induce a more lasting response must be instituted. A potassium-binding resin, disodium polystyrene sulfonate (Kayexalate® [Winthrop]), may be administered orally at a dose of 50 grams per day in divided doses if emesis is not present, or by high enema at a dose of 50 grams in 100 ml. of water repeated every 3 to 4 hours, until the serum potassium concentration is below 5 mEq. per liter. Each gram of resin has the capacity to bond 1 mEq. of potassium.

## SUMMARY

By following these recommendations the clinician should have accomplished the following:

1. Eliminated prerenal uremia from the problem list.

2. Eliminated postrenal uremia from the problem list.

3. Established a diagnosis of intrinsic oliguric or anuric renal failure which may be either acute renal disease or an acute exacerbation of chronic renal disease.

4. Have reviewed all data from the history, physical examination and the laboratory in an effort to establish the etiology.

5. Have probably performed a renal biopsy, so that morphologic data may be compared with information from other sources.

6. Alleviated dehydration, acidosis and hyperkalemia.

7. Determined baseline urine with the aid of an indwelling urinary catheter, so that response to either osmotic diuretics or furosemide can be evaluated.

8. Considered the use of peritoneal dialysis, if intensive diuresis has been unsuccessful in initiating urine production.

Adequate hydration must be maintained, using care to avoid both overhydration and dehydration. A careful weight record should indicate a gradual loss of weight (approximately 0.5 per cent daily) if the patient is not eating. Fluid intake should equal measured urine output plus estimated insensible fluid loss plus fluids lost through vomiting or diarrhea. This figure should be compared to actual weight loss before administering the fluid. Insensible loss is usually 20 to 40 ml. per kg. per day, depending primarily upon the temperature and humidity of the environment. An effort should be made to provide some calories along with the fluid to minimize tissue breakdown with resultant increase in serum potassium, blood urea nitrogen, and nonvolatile metabolic acid concentration. Half-strength saline with 5

longer excrete in the urine, such as phosphorus and hydrogen ions. Substances normally conserved by the body, such as sodium, bicarbonate and water may be lost in excessive quantities in urine. In addition, substances normally produced by the kidney such as vitamin D and erythropoietin are produced in decreased quantities. Therapy designed to minimize the effects of deficits in these metabolites must therefore be instituted.

## URINARY SODIUM LOSS AND ACIDOSIS

During the course of chronic failure, excessive urinary sodium loss occurs because the kidney fails to conserve sodium. This phenomenon usually is not of clinical importance until the later stages of renal failure. Sodium loss results in decreased extracellular fluid volume which maintains a state of dehydration and reduced renal perfusion. Therefore, animals with chronic renal failure should not be placed on a restricted sodium diet but rather should receive normal or increased quantities of dietary sodium.

Administration of intravenous fluid therapy containing sodium may be helpful in reestablishing extracellular fluid volume during periods of dehydration or reduced dietary intake of sodium and water. Such episodes or crises are usually caused by anorexia or gastrointestinal loss of fluid and electrolytes. The objective of intravenous therapy is to maintain renal perfusion by repleting the lost electrolytes and fluids. Administration of excessive loads of sodium or water, termed osmotic therapy, is of questionable value. Such therapy probably fails to increase glomerular filtration rate over the chronic failure level once volume expansion has been achieved.

The point of onset of significant metabolic acidosis in chronic failure is quite variable. The majority of animals do not become acidotic until the late stages of failure, and therapy is not indicated until that point.

## DIETARY CONSIDERATIONS

During the past decade, significant advances have been made in the dietary management of renal disease. Considerable attention to protein, caloric, mineral and vitamin content of the diet may be beneficial to animals with renal failure. Since metabolites derived from dietary protein play an important role in the uremic syndrome, protein intake has received the most detailed attention. Despite these advances, considerable confusion concerning the rationale and implementation of dietary therapy for renal diseases still exists.

It is known that dietary protein contributes to blood urea concentration—the higher the protein intake, the higher the BUN. Although it is not urea per se which is responsible for the toxic signs of uremia, it may contribute to symptomatology. Protein intake should not be limited because of the urea moiety itself but because of decreased renal clearance of other nitrogenous metabolites.

Commercial diets currently available in veterinary medicine for use in patients with renal disease are not minimal protein diets. The quantity of protein that many of these diets deliver is not markedly different from some standard commercial diets. Data to support the use of these diets for either the prevention or the treatment of renal disease are not available.

In our experience, a minimal protein diet has been beneficial to chronically uremic animals. The formula consists of high carbohydrate, high fat and minimum protein-containing foods selected from table foods. A minimum of 60 calories per kg. of body weight per day is used. At least half the protein should be provided from cooked eggs, which provide protein of high biologic value. A strict counting of all protein should be followed, so that protein intake does not exceed 0.6 gm./kg. of body weight per day. Liberal salting of the animal's food will avoid the problem of daily sodium calculations and insure adequate sodium intake. This is important to maintain total body sodium balance, since many animals with chronic renal failure lose sodium in their urine.

The food products commonly used in this diet and their respective protein and caloric contents are shown in Table 1. In our experience, the most successful food items that uremic dogs will accept include a variety of pastries, noodles, butter, eggs, cream, gravy and ice cream. Based on the animal's weight, a diet providing the minimum requirements of protein and caloric intake is provided for the owner. After a trial period of at least three weeks, signs of depression,

**Table 1.**  *Food Used in Renal Failure*

| NAME | PROTEIN (GM.) | CALORIES |
|---|---|---|
| Bread, toast, 1 slice | 2.0 | 60 |
| Butter, margarine, 1 tsp. | — | 40 |
| Cake: cupcake, 1 | 2.6 | 130 |
| pound, 1 slice 2″ x 3″ x 5″ | 2.1 | 130 |
| sponge, 2″ slice | 3.2 | 120 |
| Candy: caramel, 1 oz. | 0.8 | 120 |
| chocolate, sweetened, 1 oz. | 2.0 | 140 |
| Carrots, 1 (5″ x 1″) | 0.6 | 20 |
| Corn flakes, 1 cup | 2.0 | 96 |
| Cream, light, 1 oz. | — | 50 |
| Cream cheese, 1 oz. | 2.6 | 106 |
| Doughnut, 1 | 2.1 | 130 |
| Egg, cooked, 1 | 7.0 | 120 |
| Gravy, 1 tbsp. | — | 80 |
| Ice cream, 1 oz. | 1.2 | 62 |
| Jelly, 1 tsp. | — | 60 |
| Macaroni and cheese, 1 cup | 17.8 | 460 |
| Milk, whole, 2 oz. | 2.0 | 40 |
| Pancakes, wheat, 4″ diameter | 1.8 | 60 |
| Rice, cooked, 1 cup | 4.2 | 200 |
| Soups: bouillon, consommé, 1 cup | 2.0 | 9 |
| chicken, 1 cup | 3.5 | 75 |
| Spaghetti, cooked, 1 cup | 7.4 | 220 |
| Sugar or honey, 1 tsp. | — | 20 |
| Sweet roll, 4″ x 1″, 50 gm. | 4.2 | 160 |

anorexia, vomiting and weakness should be reduced if dietary therapy is effective. The concentration of blood urea nitrogen may be reduced as a result of this diet, and therefore cannot be relied upon as a valid indicator of renal function.

There is no known benefit for recommending drastic dietary changes until the late stages of renal failure. Suggested criteria for instituting such a diet are as follows: stable BUN greater than 80 mg./100 ml., elevated serum inorganic phosphorus, plasma creatinine concentration greater than 2.5 mg./100 ml. or creatinine clearance less than 15 ml. per minute per square meter body surface area.

Determination of the dosage of dietary sodium depends on the kidney's ability to conserve and excrete sodium. As indicated above, most patients with chronic renal failure are relative sodium losers and therefore should receive normal or increased quantities of sodium. If edema or ascites is present, sodium restriction should be followed (consult the article on "Glomerulonephropathy and the Nephrotic Syndrome").

Animals suffering from chronic renal failure usually have elevated serum inorganic phosphorus, which represents a component of renal osteodystrophy. The low-protein diet described above represents a low-phosphorus intake and should reduce total body phosphorus. In addition, oral therapy using an aluminum hydroxide gel is helpful to bind phosphorus in the intestinal lumen and prevent its absorption. Many such products are on the market, and they must be given to effect to lower plasma inorganic phosphorus.

Dietary supplementation of calcium in the diet of chronic renal failure patients may be helpful in combating renal osteodystrophy. It has been shown that elevated oral calcium intake and vitamin D will reduce the severity of the intestinal defect for calcium absorption. If the serum calcium-phosphorus product approaches 70, additional therapy should be directed to lower the serum phosphorus before this therapy is begun. Calcium supplements are usually provided in the form of calcium carbonate (100 mg./kg. of body weight per day). Daily multivitamin capsules should be administered to insure adequate vitamin intake during the use of strict low protein diets.

Animals suffering from the nephrotic syndrome with urinary losses of protein greater than 1.0 gm. per square meter of body surface per day present a difficult problem. Hypoalbuminemia, hypercholesterolemia and edema frequently accompany the massive proteinemia. Protein restriction may further reduce plasma albumin levels and exacerbate edema. If glomerular filtration rate, as measured by creatinine clearance, is more than 10 ml./minute/square meter of body surface area, a standard protein and caloric diet is indicated. If glomerular filtration rate is markedly depressed, the dietary protein should be modified as for other patients with chronic renal failure. If edema or ascites is present, a restricted sodium intake should be provided (consult the article on "Glomerulonephropathy and the Nephrotic Syndrome").

[*Editor's Note:* The question of dietary protein levels in renal disease is under active investigation at present. It is generally agreed that high-protein diets are not a cause of renal disorders. However, as chronic renal insufficiency develops as a result of disease processes, severe restriction (with emphasis on high biologic value of the protein that is fed) produces an amelioration of many clinical signs. As the renal disease progresses, more and more drastic protein restriction becomes necessary to produce clinical improvement. Eventually the patient deteriorates to the point at which no dietary management is beneficial, electrolyte and toxic abnormalities develop and the patient succumbs.

Practical management of a feeding program for these patients is complicated by the fact that low-protein diets have poor palatability for dogs, and uremic patients usually are toxic and have notoriously poor appetites.]

---

# INTENSIVE DIURESIS IN POLYURIC RENAL FAILURE

DELMAR R. FINCO, D.V.M.
*Athens, Georgia*

*and* DONALD G. LOW, D.V.M.
*Davis, California*

Diuresis can be caused by water loss secondary to loss of an osmotic agent or by primary water loss. All diuretics used at present in dogs and cats act by causing urinary loss of osmotic agents with the exception of glucocorticoids, which seem to act as water diuretics. Osmotic agents cause diuresis by remaining in the lumen of renal tubules and preventing passive water reabsorption. Many diuretics, including furosemide, have diuretic action because of impairment of normal NaCl reabsorption by the kidney. Unabsorbed NaCl acts as the diuretic agent. Mannitol and glucose act directly as osmotic agents. Mannitol is restricted to the extracellular space but freely passes the glomerular filter. It is not reabsorbed by the renal tubules and thus is a potent diuretic agent. Glucose enters cells for metabolism but also freely passes the glomerular filter. Tubular reabsorption of glucose occurs, but the renal tubules have a limited quantitative capacity for glucose reabsorption. When a quantity of glucose in excess of tubular reabsorptive capacity is presented to the kidney, glucose remaining in the tubules prevents water reabsorption and diuresis ensues. Although more glucose than mannitol is required to induce diuresis, the same intensity of diuresis can be achieved with either compound.

In addition to effects on tubular reabsorption of water, some studies indicate that osmotic diuretics may affect systemic circulation or renal circulation and glomerular filtration. Studies reveal that furosemide has effects on pulmonary congestion unrelated to its diuretic properties. Glomerular filtration rate and renal blood flow are apparently increased moderately by furosemide and mannitol, although some conflicting data are reported on this point.

Osmotic diuretics have been used widely in human medicine for prophylaxis of renal shutdown during surgical procedures and after known exposure to nephrotoxic agents. They have also been used in anuric renal failure in attempts to induce urine flow. The efficacy of these agents for these conditions seems to be well established in man. Osmotic diuresis has also been advocated for use in the treatment of polyuric renal failure in the dog and cat. The subsequent discussion outlines rationale, desirable effects, potential complications and preferred methodology for this procedure.

## CHARACTERISTICS OF POLYURIC RENAL FAILURE

Most cases of renal failure in the dog and cat have a fixed urine specific gravity and polyuria. This indicates that at least two thirds of the nephrons are nonfunctional and that renal concentrating ability is lost (isosthenuria). If the progression of disease is slow, patients may have no signs other than polydipsia and polyuria for indefinite periods of time. With progression of disease, however, additional signs referrable to renal dysfunction eventually appear. Abrupt onset of depression, anorexia and vomiting herald the onset of a uremic crisis.

Patients in a uremic crisis are markedly

dehydrated because of polyuria, inadequate water intake and vomiting. The dehydration results in hypovolemia and impaired renal perfusion. Thus, a prerenal factor is superimposed on primary renal failure.

Although serum sodium concentration is usually normal, existing dehydration indicates an isotonic contraction of the extracellular space and a sodium deficit. There are probably deficits in chloride and potassium as well, although serum potassium concentration is usually normal. These deficits are probably due to losses associated with polyuria and vomiting. Hyperphosphatemia is characteristic of polyuric renal failure.

Acid-base status may range from normal to severe metabolic acidosis. Acidosis is caused by impaired renal excretion of hydrogen ions. Patients that are vomiting severely may lose hydrogen ions; acid-base status in these patients depends on whether hydrogen ion loss due to vomiting or hydrogen ion retention due to renal failure dominates.

Uremia is associated with retention of nitrogen wastes. Urea or creatinine is used as an index of this retention, but specific uremic toxins have not been identified. At present, even hemodialysis is an empirical form of therapy because of the lack of knowledge regarding uremic toxins. However, signs of uremia are fairly well correlated with BUN, and dietary approaches that decrease BUN seem to result in clinical improvement of the patient.

## OSMOTIC DIURESIS IN POLYURIC FAILURE

**Response of the Diseased Kidney to Diuretics.** Experimental evidence in man indicates that with both furosemide and mannitol, urine flow rate is enhanced even with severe renal failure. Thus, natural osmotic diuresis of renal failure can be augmented. Although diuresis may even be induced in dehydrated patients, it is to the disadvantage of the patient to do so because of accentuation of preexisting hypovolemia. Consequently, osmotic diuresis in the dog and cat should not be undertaken until dehydration has been corrected with a multiple electrolyte solution such as lactated Ringer's solution (see article on "Fluid Therapy").

**Benefits of Osmotic Diuresis.** The increase in renal blood flow and glomerular filtration rate that occurs with osmotic diuretics is small, but may be beneficial to the patient. More important are the immediate diuretic effects of osmotic agents. Diuresis is induced minutes after administration of the agent and persists until the agent is inactivated or excreted. In contrast, volume expansion by administration of electrolyte solutions does not initiate diuresis for hours after administration, and thus the same intensity of diuresis is not achieved.

Since the toxins of uremia are not defined, the benefit of diuresis can be judged only clinically or by the advantageous biochemical alterations that diuresis induces. Mannitol osmotic diuresis in chronic renal failure in humans produces significant increases in excretion of water and chloride and variable increases in urea excretion. Rehydration of dogs with multiple electrolyte solutions and subsequent diuresis cause a significant decrease in BUN and clinical improvement.

The apparent benefits of osmotic diuresis relate to inhibition of tubular reabsorption. Many compounds that pass though the renal glomeruli are subsequently partially or totally reabsorbed by the tubules. With osmotic diuresis, absorption is inhibited and loss occurs from the body. In essence, fluid with the composition of blood, minus cells and materials greater in MW than 70,000, can be removed from the body. Therefore, osmotic diuresis can act in the same manner as peritoneal dialysis without requiring the mechanical complexity of the latter procedure.

**Choice of the Diuretic Agent.** Major differences in potency do not exist, and thus other factors must be considered in making this choice.

Mannitol has no advantages over other agents but has the disadvantage of greater cost than glucose. Besides low cost, glucose is preferable to mannitol because glucose can be metabolized for energy. The patient in uremic crisis is in a catabolic state. Body fats and protein are being used to fulfill caloric needs, and protein catabolism accentuates the uremia.

Parenteral administration of 10 to 20 per cent glucose provides some calories to the patient in uremic crisis, in addition to inducing diuresis, and thus is protein-sparing. This nutritional advantage of glucose is extremely important.

Furosemide administration is technically simple but has significant disadvantages. It depends on chloride for diuretic action and results in considerably more NaCl loss than does glucose or mannitol. Since polyuric renal failure is a salt-losing disease, the potential exists for massive salt depletion. In addition, there is probably more likelihood of development of water deficits with use of furosemide than with glucose, since the glucose is given as an aqueous solution. Most importantly, furosemide has no effect on the negative caloric balance.

## MECHANICS—OSMOTIC DIURESIS

1. As previously indicated, restoration of fluid deficit with lactated Ringer's or a comparable solution is necessary prior to inducing diuresis (see article on "Fluid Therapy"). If clinical evidence of dehydration is not apparent, it is still advisable to give a quantity of fluid equal to 3 to 5 per cent of body weight. The fluid deficit should be administered intravenously over a period of about 1 hour.

2. After deficit therapy, weigh the animal accurately. This baseline weight is used to assess underhydration or overhydration during subsequent therapy.

3. Administer 20 per cent dextrose intravenously at a total dose of 25 to 65 ml./kg. and at a rate of 2 ml./min. for 10 to 15 minutes. Then reduce the infusion rate to 1 ml./min.

4. Catheterize the patient as soon as the IV infusion of glucose is begun, and empty the bladder.

5. Test newly formed urine (if any) for glucose.

6. If the test is positive, sufficient glucose to exceed the renal threshold has been administered, and anuria does not exist. Urine volume should increase if the procedure can safely be continued. A urine volume of 1 to 4 ml./min. should be obtained, depending on body size.

7. If adequate urine flow is not obtained by the time half the dose of glucose is given, the procedure must be discontinued, since overhydration and hyperosmolality will occur, and may be accompanied by pulmonary edema.

8. If adequate urine flow is obtained, all the osmotic agent is given. Lactated Ringer's (3 to 5 per cent of body weight) and glucose are repeated as above. Fluid input and urine output are measured so that reasonable balance is maintained. Two or 3 cycles of dextrose and lactated Ringer's solution are administered per 24 hours.

9. After 24 hours, the patient is reevaluated by (a) physical examination (b) BUN and (c) body weight.

10. If necessary, the entire procedure is repeated. Gain in weight indicates fluid retention and contraindicates lactated Ringer's prior to the osmotic agent. Loss of weight indicates fluid deficit, and lactated Ringer's should be administered in sufficient quantity to rectify the deficit.

11. Extreme weakness suggests potassium deficiency. If serum potassium concentration is less than 3.0 mEq./l. solutions containing 25 to 35 mEq./l. of potassium should be administered at a rate of 0.5 mEq./kg./hr. of potassium.

12. Initially, all fluids should be given intravenously. Lactated Ringer's to maintain hydration can be given subcutaneously if it is absorbed well. Generally, a response to therapy, as indicated by a decrease in BUN, will occur within 2 to 4 days. Failure to respond indicates severe functional impairment and dictates the use of supplementary techniques such as peritoneal dialysis.

13. If diuresis with dextrose fails, furosemide may be used at the recommended dosage to attempt to induce diuresis. If no urine forms after 1 hour, the dosage can be doubled. If this is not successful in inducing urine output, it can generally be assumed that the patient must be treated for anuria.

14. In instances in which clinical and laboratory response occurs, oral alimentation and medication are gradually resumed as the parenteral routes of therapy are abandoned. The oral medications (salt, bicarbonate, anabolic steroids, B vitamins) are continued indefinitely in chronic disease, or until renal function has improved sufficiently so that the patient can concentrate urine above 1.025 S.G. after acute polyuric disease.

### SUPPLEMENTAL READING

Gennari, F. J., and Fassirer, J. P.: Osmotic diuresis. New Engl. J. Med. 291:714-720, 1974.

Krishna, D. *et al.*: Renal and extrarenal hemodynamic effects of furosemide in congestive heart failure after acute myocardial infarction. New Engl. J. Med. 288:1087-1090, 1973.

Metaxis, P., *et al.*: Mannitol osmotic diuresis in patients with chronic renal failure. Am. J. Med. Sci. 259:175-181, 1970.

Shelp, W. D., and Rieselbach, R. E.: The effect of furosemide on residual nephrons of the chronically diseased kidney in man. Nephron 8:427-439, 1971.

# PERITONEAL DIALYSIS

I. M. GOURLEY, D.V.M.,
*and* H. R. PARKER, D.V.M.
*Davis, California*

If severely anuric or oliguric uremic patients are nonresponsive to an osmotic diuretic, an artificial substitute for renal function must be utilized (hemodialysis or peritoneal dialysis). The rationale for this treatment presupposes that if the animal can be kept alive for an extended period, repair of malfunctioning nephrons will allow return of complete or partial renal function sufficient to support life.

Hemodialysis for the treatment of uremic human patients is an accepted clinical procedure. In the small animal patient the technique is expensive and extremely demanding from a technical standpoint, requiring considerable expertise and close observation of the animal during and after extracorporeal dialysis. Consequently, hemodialysis is not yet practical for routine use by the small animal practitioner (Gourley *et al.*, 1973). Additionally, until there is a major immunologic breakthrough in tissue transplantation, use of the renal allograft for the treatment of end-stage renal disease should be held in abeyance (Gourley *et al.*, 1975).

In small animal practice, peritoneal dialysis has proved to be the method of choice for artificially providing kidney function. Peritoneal dialysis also can be used for the treatment of a variety of drug toxicities (e.g., barbiturates), the noxious agents being removed by the dialysis process.

## TERMINOLOGY

Dialysis is the transfer of water, ions and crystalloids through a permeable membrane as a result of diffusion.

Diffusion is the phenomenon by which a gas or substance in solution expands to fill the volume available because of motion of the particles. Molecules or ions of a substance in solution are in continuous random movement. Where solutes are abundant, they collide frequently and spread from areas of high concentration to low concentration until the concentration is uniform throughout the solution. Dispersion of ions

also is affected by their electrical charge whenever there is a difference in potential between two areas. Positively charged ions migrate to negatively charged ions, and conversely negatively charged ions migrate to positively charged ions.

Within the body, diffusion occurs within fluid compartments and from one compartment to another, provided that the barrier is permeable to the diffusing substances.

With peritoneal dialysis the abdominal cavity acts as a large compartment filled with a prescribed fluid (dialysate). Water and solutes diffuse across the peritoneal membrane to and from the extracellular space of the body and subsequently the intracellular space.

## GENERAL PHYSIOLOGICAL CONSIDERATIONS

During peritoneal dialysis, the equilibration of solutes between the plasma and dialysate is rapid for some solutes (i.e., urea), and slower for others (i.e., creatinine and phosphate). Therefore, repeated dialyses are required to reduce significantly the total levels of metabolic waste within the extracellular and intracellular spaces.

In a single dialysis period one can expect 90 per cent equilibration of urea and potassium after 40 minutes and 98 per cent equilibration after one hour. Because creatinine and phosphate are larger molecules, 2 hours are required for equilibration (80 per cent equilibration at one hour). (Parker *et al.*, 1972).

Following 5 to 7 dialyses of 40 to 60 minutes' duration, one can expect a significant reduction in plasma urea (e.g., a reduction in the BUN from 250 to 100 mg./100 ml.), creatinine (e.g., from 15 to 6.0 mg./100 ml.) and potassium (e.g., from 7.9 to 4.8 mEq./l.), and a significant improvement in acid-base balance (Parker *et al.*, 1972). A plasma increase (rebound) in the solutes occurs 2 to 3 hours after the last dialysis. This rebound represents equilibration of the solutes between the extracellular and intracellular

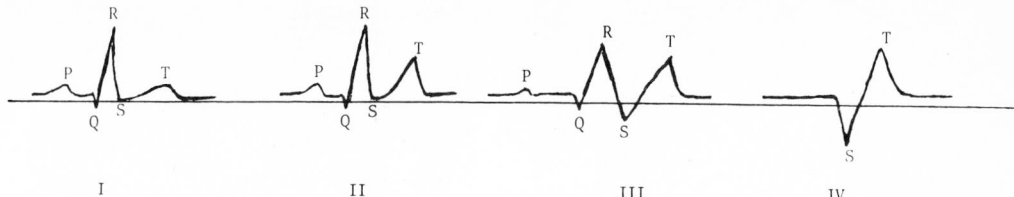

**Figure 1.** Electrocardiogram drawings depicting progressive electrical changes that indicate potassium toxicity and pending hyperkalemic fibrillation or cardiac arrest. *I*, Normal tracing. *II*, Increased vertical amplitude of T wave. *III*, Reduced amplitude of P wave, prolonged P/R interval and depressed ST segment with an increased T wave amplitude. *IV*, Atrial standstill and ventricular block with a depressed ST segment, which is followed shortly by fibrillation or arrest.

compartments of the body and is minimized only after several days of repeated dialyses, when the total body concentration of solutes is reduced (uremia controlled).

Use of the electrocardiogram provides information regarding the animal's potassium status, in that the electrical changes indicate pending hyperkalemic ventricular fibrillation or cardiac arrest. The first change with potassium toxicity is an increase in the T-wave vertical amplitude. Next, there is a depression or loss of the P wave (atrial standstill), a prolonged P-R interval, if the atria are functioning, and a depression of the ST segment. Finally intraventricular block occurs followed shortly by ventricular fibrillation or arrest (Fig. 1).

## METHODOLOGY

**All equipment must be sterilized and strict aseptic techniques must be followed during all phases of peritoneal dialysis.**

An ill animal being dialyzed usually lies quietly in lateral recumbency. If not, the patient can be restrained in a semistanding position by a canvas sling supported on a rack made of 3/4 inch electrical conduit (Parker *et al.*, 1972). Prewarmed (38 to 39° C.) dialysate fluid is infused into the peritoneal cavity at a rate of about 200 ml./ min. until the abdomen is noticeably distended. The fluid is allowed to remain in the abdominal cavity for 40 to 60 minutes. It is then withdrawn at the rate of about 60 to 70 ml./min., which requires about 15 minutes per liter of fluid. Initially, peritoneal dialysis should be repeated at least 5 to 7 times within a 24-hour time period. The frequency of the dialyses may be decreased as the uremia abates and the animal returns to a controlled physiologic state (Parker *et al.*, 1972).

Dialysate fluid is infused into and withdrawn from the peritoneal cavity (either manually or automatically) through a peritoneal catheter. A glass or plastic "Y" or "T" may also be used (Fig. 2). Infusions are made through one limb and withdrawals through the other. To assure asepsis, a closed system is preferred.

If the manual technique is utilized, the prewarmed dialysate fluid, contained in a suspended fluid bottle, is allowed to drain by gravity into the peritoneal cavity through plastic tubing attached by the "Y" or "T"

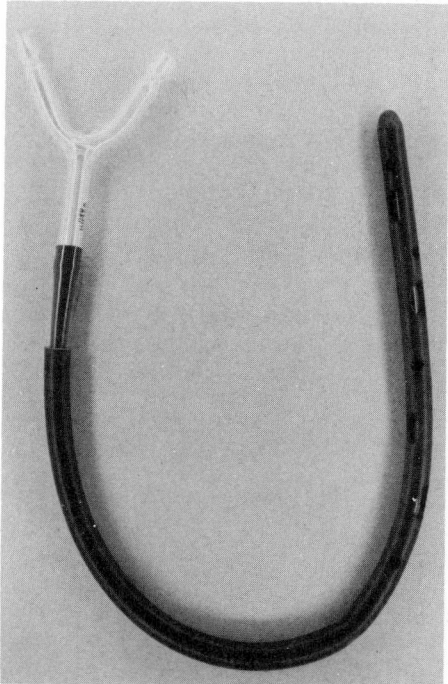

**Figure 2.** A fenestrated Bardex® catheter into which a smaller Bardex® catheter has been inserted intraluminally for about two thirds the length of the outer tube. This system functions well as an indwelling catheter for peritoneal dialysis. A glass or plastic "Y" or "T" insert into the larger catheter allows dialysate to be infused through one limb of the system and to be withdrawn from the other.

tube to the peritoneal catheter. When the abdomen is full, the infusion tube is clamped. After the appropriate time has elapsed, the other limb of the "Y" tube to the peritoneal catheter is opened and the fluid is allowed to drain from the abdomen into an empty graduated fluid container. Treatment is then repeated as necessary. Records of fluid volumes infused and removed should be kept.

When an automated system is used, a large volume of dialysate fluid is heated by suspending the fluid bottle in an elevated brass flask holder wrapped with a 36-inch length of thermostatically controlled heating tape. Polypropylene infusion tubing from the dialysate bottle is attached to the peritoneal catheter as for the manual technique. An electrically timed solenoid valve allows gravity flow of the warmed dialysate into the peritoneal cavity. As the peritoneal cavity is filled the inflow valve is closed by the electrical timer, and the fluid remains in the peritoneal cavity until the timer opens another solenoid valve enabling the dialysate to flow into a volumeter. As the volumeter fills with dialysate to a volume of dialysate approximately equal to that originally infused into the peritoneal cavity, the outflow solenoid valve is closed electrically and the inflow valve is opened, and the dialysis cycle is repeated (Fig. 3) (Parker *et al.*, 1972).

The main advantage of an automated system is reduction in labor required for chronic peritoneal dialysis.

With either system, peritoneal dialysis is discontinued with the return of kidney function, as determined by resumption of adequate and effective urine output.

## PERITONEAL CATHETERIZATION TECHNIQUE

Although several methods and types of peritoneal catheters for dialysis have been described for small animals, most fail because they become plugged with omentum, preventing adequate extraction of the dialysate from the peritoneal cavity.

A large-gauge Medicut® catheter* (Fig. 4) can be used satisfactorily in cats and toy breeds of dogs when relatively few dialyses are required and it is not desirable to place an indwelling catheter.

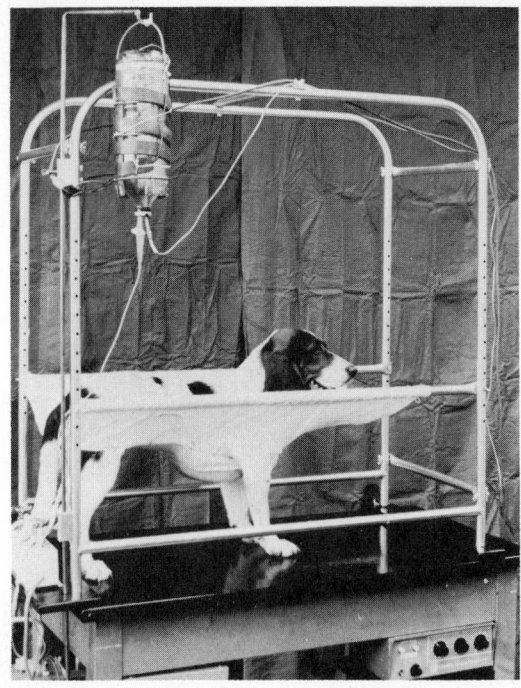

**Figure 3.**   Dog being restrained in a standing position by a canvas sling supported on a rack made of electrical conduit. Peritoneal dialysis is being administered by the automated system described in the text.

Generally, it is best to place an indwelling catheter. A Salem Sump Tube* or a Bardex® catheter** into which a smaller Bardex catheter or plastic tube has been inserted intraluminally for two thirds the length of the outer tube often functions well (Fig. 2).

In our experience the Parker catheter and technique (Parker *et al.*, 1972) has been the most effective for the withdrawal of dialysate from the peritoneal cavity (Fig. 5). The catheter is a segment of 1/8-inch ID Silastic® tubing† of variable length depending on the dog, with multiple fenestrations. To one end of the cannula a loop of No. 3 black braided silk is secured with cement.‡ Enough cement should be used to obliterate the end of the tube. A cuff of Dacron felt§ is cemented around the tube about two inches from the opposite open end.

With the use of local anesthesia a curved

---

*Medicut® catheter, Sherwood Industries Inc., St. Louis, Missouri 63103.

*Salem Sump Tube, Sherwood Industries Inc., St. Louis, Missouri 63103.

**Bardex® catheter, C. R. Bard Co., Murray Hill, New Jersey 07974.

†Silastic® brand medical grade tubing, Dow Corning Corp., Midland, Michigan.

‡Silastic® medical adhesive, silicone Type A, Dow Corning Corp., Midland, Michigan.

§Troy Mills, Inc., Troy, New Hampshire 03465.

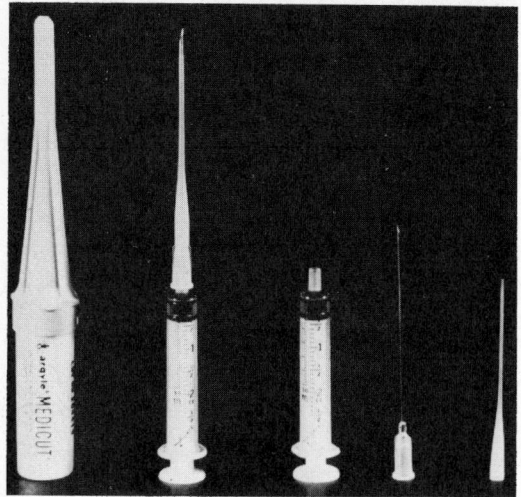

**Figure 4.** The Medicut® catheter, which can be used for peritoneal dialysis in cats and toy breeds of dogs when only a relatively few dialyses are required and it is desirable not to place an indwelling catheter.

metal open-ended "female" urinary catheter is inserted through a small incision in the right paralumbar fossa. Its tip is advanced along the ventral abdominal wall until it can be observed deflecting the left abdominal wall. With the lumen of the metal catheter as a guide, a 12- to 14-inch long 3/32-inch stainless steel rod needle armed with No. 3 black braided silk is passed transabdominally through the skin of the left abdominal wall. The guide tube and metal rod needle are removed, leaving the silk suture lying across the abdomen and within the peritoneal cavity.

The preplaced abdominal silk suture is tied to the silk loop of the peritoneal catheter, and the cannula is carefully pulled through the right skin incision into the transabdominal position and secured to the left abdominal wall by suturing the silk to the skin.

The silicone cannula extending from the right skin incision is pushed into the depth of the muscle incision bringing the Dacron cuff into contact with the peritoneum. This maneuver causes the cannula to deflect back under the bladder, removing it maximally from the omentum, and provides a good seal as fibrin infiltrates the Dacron cuff. The cannula on the right side is anchored further by 2 or 3 fixation sutures that pass through the skin and edge of the Dacron cuff. Care must be taken not to puncture the silicone tubing.

Between daily dialyses the cannula is flushed with sterile heparinized saline solution, plugged with a Luer-Lok plastic adapter. The abdomen is wrapped with appropriate bandage material.

Upon completion of peritoneal dialysis the cannula is removed by cutting the anchoring silk sutures on both sides of the abdomen.

## DIALYSATE FLUID

The composition of the dialysate fluid is critical and should approximate the normal solute composition of dog plasma with the exception of potassium.

Commercial solutions made for human patients can be used with fair success but are lower in both sodium and chloride ion concentrations (140 mEq./l. and 101 mEq./l.) as compared to normal dog plasma (sodium, 150 mEq./l., and chloride, 112 mEq./l.). For this reason it is best to add

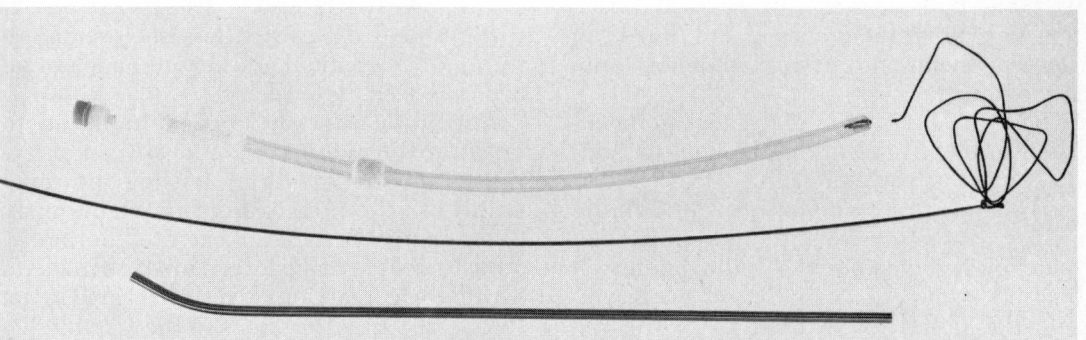

**Figure 5.** Parker indwelling cannula system for peritoneal dialysis. *Top,* Fenestrated Silastic® tube; *middle,* metal rod needle with suture material attached; *bottom,* the "female" urinary catheter. The technique for placement of the cannula is described in the text.

**Table 1.** *A. Composition of Stock Peritoneal Dialysis Solution*

| SALT | GRAMS/LITER | | CONCENTRATION mEq./l.) | | |
|---|---|---|---|---|---|
| NaCl | 6.57 | Sodium | 157.0 | Chloride | 117.5 |
| Na Acetate · 3H$_2$O | 6.10 | Calcium | 4.0 | Acetate | 45.0 |
| CaCl$_2$ anhydrous | 0.29 | Magnesium | 1.5 | | |
| MgCl$_2$ · H$_2$O | 0.15 | Totals: cations | 162.5 | anions | 162.5 |

Glucose or sorbitol as needed (see B below)      Osmolality = 305.0 mOsm./l.

### B. Add Glucose to Increase Osmolality

| | OSMOLALITY (mOsm./l.) | SPECIFIC GRAVITY* |
|---|---|---|
| Stock solution without glucose | 305.0 | 1.0051 |
| Stock solution with 1.0% glucose†‡ | 362.0 | 1.0081 |
| Stock solution with 2.0% glucose | 408.0 | 1.0100 |
| Stock solution with 3.0% glucose | 457.4 | 1.0118 |
| Stock solution with 4.0% glucose | 507.0 | 1.0129 |

*Specific gravity was determined with a TS meter (American Optical Co., Buffalo, New York).

†Add 20 ml. of sterile 50 per cent dextrose solution, etc., to previously sterilized stock solution immediately prior to use.

‡A similar solution can be made by adding 1.0 gm./l. NaCl to a commercial peritoneal dialysis solution (R-3100, McGaw Laboratories, Glendale, California).

From Parker *et al.*, 1972.

sodium chloride to commercial solutions (Table 1).

The plasma of uremic dogs is always hyperosmotic (BUN of 250 mg./100 ml. equals a plasma osmolality of between 350 and 400 mOsm./l.), owing to dehydration and elevated levels of urea, creatinine, phosphate and sulfate. If the osmolality of the dialysate is not adjusted to the approximate osmolality of the uremic animal's plasma, water will diffuse rapidly into the extracellular and intracellular spaces, causing overhydration (manifested mainly by pulmonary edema) and possibly death. Conversely, by utilizing a hyperosmolar dialysate fluid, water can be withdrawn from an overhydrated animal and thus is an effective therapeutic treatment for pulmonary edema.

The osmolality of the dialysate can be adjusted to that of the uremic animal by adding glucose or sorbitol (Table 1).

Plasma osmolality is not measured in the average laboratory because it requires an osmometer. Consequently, adjustments in dialysate osmolality usually are made empirically, based on evaluation of the patient's hydration and/or BUN.

Rapid changes in body weight are refer-

rable to water gain or loss (2 kg. body weight gain or loss equals about 500 ml. water). Comparison of values for total plasma protein and packed cell volume (PCV) provides an excellent index of the animal's hydration. If low, the animal is probably overhydrated; if high, it is probably dehydrated. If the plasma protein is normal and the PCV is low, the animal is anemic, which is common in uremic patients.

The use of solutions which deviate significantly in composition from those described in Table 1 is discouraged.

### REMARKS

Peritoneal dialysis requires close monitoring of the patient and maintenance of an accurate treatment record.

Antibiotic therapy is recommended to help prevent peritonitis and to treat infections concurrent with or causing the renal failure. In the renal patient in whom many of the antibiotics are not excreted normally, adjustments in drug dosage must be made to avoid toxic reactions. (Refer to article on "Adverse Drug Reactions in the Uremic Patient" for further details.)

Because dialysis removes significant

quantities of antibiotics, it is advisable to inject the antibiotic intraperitoneally at the termination of daily dialyses. Because of its low toxicity and broad spectrum of action, we have used 100 to 500 mg. of ampicillin* with no undesirable effects.

---

*Polycillin-N, Bristol Laboratories, Syracuse, New York 13201.

## SUPPLEMENTAL READING

Gourley, I. M., Parker, H. R., Bell, R. L., and Ishizaki, G.: Responses of nephrectomized dogs during hemodialysis. Am. J. Vet. Res., 34:1421–1425, 1973.

Gourley, I. M., Parker, H. R., Gribble, D. H., Conzelman, G. M., Jr., and Ishizaki, G.: Pathophysiological effects of renal allografts in the dog. Archives, ACVS, 4:22–34, 1975.

Parker, H. R., Gourley, I. M., and Bell, R. L.: Current developments in peritoneal and hemodialysis. Gaines 22nd Veterinary Symposium, Stillwater, Oklahoma, September 17, 1972, pp. 3–15.

---

# CURRENT STATUS OF HEMODIALYSIS AND RENAL TRANSPLANTATION

LARRY COWGILL, D.V.M.
*Davis, California*

*and* KENNETH C. BOVEE, D.V.M.
*Philadelphia, Pennsylvania*

## HEMODIALYSIS

Hemodialysis is a procedure that adjusts volume or solute composition of the extracellular fluid compartment by selectively regulating osmotic and diffusional gradients between the patient's blood and an artificial solution (the dialysate) across a semipermeable membrane. With hemodialysis it is possible to effect the net removal or addition of fluid and solute from the blood of uremic patients without loss of formed elements or plasma proteins, thus alleviating many of the biochemical and metabolic disturbances of uremia.

Today, hemodialysis is standard therapy for the management of end-stage renal disease and acute renal failure in man. Despite its clear and effective role in human medicine, hemodialysis has been virtually nonexistent as a therapeutic procedure in veterinary medicine and has received only occasional mention in veterinary literature (Butler, 1968, 1971; Cowgill and Bovee, 1975; Gourley et al, 1973; Parker et al, 1972). Early efforts in experimental dogs divulged many of the potential risks and complications of this complex and sophisticated procedure (Gourley et al., 1973); however, the availability of extracorporeal equipment and artificial kidneys more suitable for veterinary needs provides renewed enthusiasm for the development of veterinary hemodialysis (Cowgill and Bovee, 1975).

In principle, hemodialysis is identical to peritoneal dialysis except that an artificial membrane (cellulose or regenerated cellulose) replaces the peritoneal membrane, allowing a more direct and efficient transfer of solute and fluid between the blood and dialysate. A second distinction of hemodialysis is that the exchange process occurs outside the body and requires extracorporeal circulation of blood. During hemodialysis, products of uremia which are in high concentration in arterial blood pass by diffusion through the membranes of the artificial kidney into the dialysate flowing on the opposite side. These substances are cleared from the plasma before the dialyzed blood is returned to the patient's venous circulation. The normal chemical composition of the plasma is maintained or corrected, since normal solutes are present at physiologic concentrations in the dialysate solution, and rapid equilibration of the two fluids occurs. The distinct advantage of hemodialysis over peritoneal dialysis is its greater efficiency for fluid and solute removal. Treatment periods are therefore shorter, reducing patient fatigue and manipulation.

## INDICATIONS

The principal veterinary indication is acute reversible renal failure in patients whose fluid, electrolyte and metabolic disturbances are unresponsive or unmanageable by conservative supportive measures. By hemodialysis, such patients can be maintained in satisfactory health until renal function returns. A second specific indication for hemodialysis is the treatment of acute poisonings (e.g., barbiturate, some heavy metals) provided that the offending toxin is dialyzable. By this means, dialyzable toxins can be rapidly cleared from the body despite functional impairment to the normal excretory route.

The indications for maintenance hemodialysis in chronic progressive renal insufficiency are debatable. Although the challenge and potential is clear, economic and technical limitations will likely overshadow theoretical indications. Possible exceptions include patients with compensated renal insufficiency who periodically become decompensated as a result of environmental stresses, infection or dietary fluctuations. Another exception is patients with decompensated renal insufficiency who could be stabilized by proper dietary and medical management. In both groups, intermittent or limited courses of hemodialysis are indicated to establish a more physiologic baseline for continued conservative management. An additional specific indication is correction of severe fluid overloads associated with life-threatening pulmonary edema. For example, hemodialysis provides a rapid and direct approach for fluid removal from patients with congestive heart failure and renal hypoperfusion.

## EQUIPMENT

There are currently three major artificial kidney designs.

1. *Parallel plate dialyzers.* Plate dialyzers are constructed so that blood and dialysate flow alternately between layered sheets of cellulose membrane that are stretched over grooved frameworks.

2. *Coil dialyzers.* These units are formed from cellulose tubes that are wound around a central core, with mesh screen supports between successive wraps of the tubing forming a canister. The entire canister is immersed in the dialysate solution. Blood flows within the tubing while dialysate solution is pumped through the screen supports.

3. *Hollow fiber dialyzer.* This artificial kidney is the most recent design and is composed of thousands of capillary fiber membranes sealed in a plastic holder. As blood flows through the fibers, dialysate solution is circulated around them in a countercurrent direction within the holder.

Vascular access is generally gained through Teflon®-Silastic arteriovenous shunts which extend to the outside of the body, or surgically prepared subcutaneous arteriovenous fistulas. Since fistulas require time to heal before they become serviceable, they are unsuitable for most veterinary indications. Arteriovenous shunts can be quickly placed in the femoral vessels following light general or local anesthesia and used immediately if necessary. Properly placed and maintained shunts will function through an entire course of therapy and are most satisfactory for the intermittent vascular access that is required. In an extreme emergency, a simple cut down and vascular cannulation may be justified for limited dialysis treatments.

## EXPERIENCE AND EFFICACY

Present experience in veterinary hemodialysis has been limited to the treatment of experimental acute renal failure in subtotally or bilaterally nephrectomized dogs (Cowgill and Bovee, 1975; Gourley *et al.*, 1973). Our experience includes over fifty hemodialysis treatments with the Cordis-Dow hollow fiber artificial kidney (CDAK) (Cowgill and Bovee, 1975). Hemodialysis with the CDAK was found to be both an effective and an efficient means to control many of the metabolic disturbances of acute uremia. Plasma creatinine, urea nitrogen, phosphorus, potassium and osmolality were corrected to normal ranges following five hours of therapy. Similarly, electrocardiographic abnormalities typical of hyperkalemia were normalized within an hour following initiation of hemodialysis. Hydration was selectively regulated to correct volume deficits or volume overloads. Clinically, experimental patients remained alert, responsive and ambulatory. Subtotally nephrectomized dogs progressed from complete dependence on hemodialysis to the point at which continued treatments became unnecessary as renal function returned. Anephric dogs were maintained in satisfactory health for periods approaching one month on alternative-day hemodialysis. Although we have not maintained dogs for longer periods of time, extended treatments should be possible if necessary.

## COMPLICATIONS AND LIMITATIONS

Any procedure incorporating extracorporeal circulation of blood is subject to certain technical difficulties and patient risks. Hemodialysis is a clinically and technically demanding procedure requiring the constant presence of a highly skilled and well-trained attendant. Potential patient risks include hemorrhage, hypotension, hemolysis and embolization. With greater experience, refinement of techniques and stricter patient supervision, most of these risks have been eliminated or controlled. The cost of such therapy is not as yet well defined but should realistically conform to the cost of other forms of veterinary intensive care or specialized surgical procedures. Because of the need for highly specialized technical personnel, versatile clinical laboratory procedures, intensive care facilities, and the lack of appropriate case material, hemodialysis will likely be limited to a teaching or university setting.

## SUMMARY

In our experience, hemodialysis with the CDAK is an efficient and effective means for correcting the biochemical and metabolic disturbances of acute uremia in experimental dogs. It is a technically feasible procedure that awaits further trial and development in veterinary medicine. Hemodialysis should be considered as a new and valuable addition to the intensive care and supportive management of acute renal failure in dogs.

## RENAL TRANSPLANTATION

From the clinical point of view the application of renal transplantation should be the ultimate therapy for progressive irreversible renal failure. Considerable knowledge and experience exist concerning renal transplantation in the dog. The dog has been widely used as an experimental animal in the study of surgical problems related to transplantation, yet this knowledge has not been applied to clinical situations. The surgical problems of transplantation, including vascular accidents, acute renal failure, ureteral transplantation into the bladder, urinary reflux and infection can be managed by experienced persons. The central obstacle is the rejection reaction, which remains an incompletely solved problem.

The survival of allogeneic grafts is a function of genetically determined similarities between histocompatibility factors of the donor and recipient. In inbred strains of mice and other laboratory animals, one major histocompatibility locus and several minor loci have been shown to be present and to determine the survival of allogeneic grafts. The dog has been used as a model for studies of histocompatibility for marrow grafting and renal transplantation in both randomly bred and inbred animals. Serologic histocompatibility typing (Dausset *et al.*, 1971; Rapaport *et al.*, 1970) and mixed lymphocyte cultures (Rudolph *et al.*, 1969) have been carried out in the dog. Mixed lymphocyte culture was shown to correlate with serologic histocompatibility typing in littermates. Approximately 25 per cent of littermate pairs were nonreactive in lymphocyte culture, while all unrelated donor-recipient pairs showed incompatibility (Templeton and Thomas, 1971). These results indicate that dog leukocyte antigens are determined by a single genetic locus designated DL-A. However, transplantation between matched littermates does not achieve successful long-term transplantation results. It appears that additional important immunologic differences not detected by either serologic histocompatibility testing or mixed lymphocyte culture tests exist in the dog (Storb *et al.*, 1973).

More encouraging results have been demonstrated in a closely bred colony of beagles using mixed lymphocyte culture matching and unmodified recipients. The survival of the renal transplant was approximately 25 days as compared to 13 days for incompatible pairs. The average survival time for renal allografts in randomly selected dogs is generally 10 days (Rapaport *et al.*, 1970).

Long-term survival has been reported with the use of renal allografts and bone marrow allografts for which histocompatibility was determined and when total body radiation was given to the recipient. The use of immunosuppressive agents has been widely studied in the dog renal allograft model for the past 10 years. While some drugs have shown promise, the long-term survival rate has been quite poor and does not warrant a transplantation program based on this approach alone. It now appears that the clinical application of transplantation must await further information concerning histocompatibility testing and/or immunosuppressive therapy.

### SUPPLEMENTAL READING

Butler, H.C.: Advanced therapy for renal failure. Proc. 35th Annual Meeting, AAHA, 1968, pp. 174–182.
Butler, H. C.: Renal support systems and transplanta-tions. Proc. 38th Annual Meeting, AAHA, 1971, pp. 162–164.
Cowgill, L. D., and Bovee, K. C.: The feasibility and efficiency of hemodialysis in acutely uremic dogs. Proc. 42nd Annual Meeting, AAHA, 2:165, 1975.
Dausset, J., Rapaport, F. T., Cannon, F. D., and Ferrebee, J. W.: Histocompatibility studies in a closely bred colony of dogs. III. Genetic definition of the DL-A system of canine histocompatibility, with particular reference to the comparative immunogenicity of the major transplantable organs. J. Exp. Med., *134*:1222, 1971.
Gourley, I. M., Parker, H. R., Bell, R. L., and Ishizaki, G.: Responses of nephrectomized dogs during hemodialysis. Am. J. Vet. Res. *34*:1421–1425, 1973.
Parker, H. R., Gourley, I. M., and Bell, R. L.: Current developments in peritoneal and hemodialysis. Gaines 22nd Veterinary Symposium, Stillwater, Oklahoma, September 17, 1972, pp. 3–15.
Rapaport, F. T., Hanaoka, T., Shimada, T., Cannon, F. D., and Ferrebee, J. W.: Histocompatibility studies in a closely bred colony of dogs. I. Influence of leukocyte group antigens upon renal allograft survival in the unmodified host. J. Exp. Med., *131*:881, 1970.
Rudolph, R. H., Hered, B., Epstein, R. B., and Thomas, E. D.: Canine mixed leukocyte reactivity and transplantation antigens. Transplantation, 8:141, 1969.
Storb, R., Rudolph, H., Kolb, H. J., Graham, T. C., *et al.*: Marrow grafts between DL-A-matched canine littermates. Transplantation, *15*:92, 1973.
Templeton, J. W., and Thomas, E. D.: Evidence for a major histocompatibility in the dog. Transplantation, *11*:429, 1971.

# ADVERSE DRUG REACTIONS IN THE UREMIC PATIENT

CARL A. OSBORNE, D.V.M.
*and* JEFFREY S. KLAUSNER, D.V.M.
*St. Paul, Minnesota*

## INTRODUCTION

It is unfortunate that drugs used to prevent, control or eliminate disease also have the potential to induce disease. It is also unfortunate that the majority of pharmacokinetic and toxicity studies designed to minimize adverse drug reactions have been performed on normal animals, since most drugs are intended for use in patients with disease of one or more body systems.

The true prevalence of drug-induced renal disease in animals with normal renal function and the prevalence of adverse drug reactions in animals with varying degrees of renal insufficiency are unknown. This is undoubtedly related to the fact that many of these adverse reactions are unrecognized, while those that are recognized are not reported. In contrast to human medicine in which toxicity caused by the administration of a variety of drugs at normal therapeutic dosages recommended by the manufacturer has been well documented, there is an alarming paucity of information in the veterinary literature about the effects of various disease states on the pharmacologic action, metabolism and excretion of drugs.

Drugs are often administered to uremic patients without knowledge of the animals' normal metabolic pathways and without knowledge of whether or not the drugs' pharmacologic actions will be affected by the uremic state. Because of lack of an adequate explanation, many atypical symptoms that appear are ignored or attributed to an unusual manifestation of the underlying disorder. In some patients with renal failure, clinical deterioration is often attributed to progression of the underlying disease, without the possibility being considered that deterioration may be related, at least in part, to toxicity induced by the administration of drugs.

Since there are significant species differences in pathways of drug metabolism, determination of drug toxicity and major pathways of degradation and/or elimination of drugs from the body must be evaluated in the species in question before specific recommendations can be formulated. In the absence of such information in domestic animals, however, we are forced to use the alternative of formulating generalizations based on the laboratory animal and human analogue. The following generalities recommended for dogs and cats with renal insufficiency have been established on the basis of published reports of concepts related to drug toxicity associated with renal failure. Some of these generalities have not been substantiated by experimental and clinical investigations. It is emphasized that they are intended to be used as guidelines; they should not be interpreted as rigid facts.

## PATHOGENESIS

Because the kidneys are the major route of excretion of active and metabolized drugs from the body, and because of the inherent nephrotoxicity of some drugs, there is an increase in the frequency and severity of drug intolerance in patients with renal insufficiency. Some adverse effects of drugs which are generally of little clinical significance in the patient with normal renal function may become obvious in patients with renal insufficiency. Administration of inherently nephrotoxic drugs which are dependent on renal excretion for elimination from the body is especially hazardous. In man, a relationship exists between the rate of occurrence of adverse drug reactions and renal failure. In one study, the rate of adverse drug reactions in patients with serum urea nitrogen concentrations above 40 mg./dl. was 2 1/2 times higher than it was in patients with a BUN of below 20 mg./dl. (Smith *et al.*, 1966). Sedative and diuretic drugs produced adverse effects four times more often in patients with decreased renal function than in patients with normal renal function.

The pathogenesis of alterations in the pharmacodynamics of drugs in patients with renal insufficiency is complex (Reidenberg, 1971). One of the most significant abnormalities that predisposes a patient to adverse drug reactions is delayed excretion of bioactive parent drugs and/or their metabolites. The latter may occur as a result of altered glomerular filtration, tubular reabsorption or tubular secretion. As a result of decreased renal clearance, drugs normally eliminated from the body in urine increase in concentration. Continued administration of such drugs at dosages established for patients with normal renal function intensifies and/or prolongs their pharmacologic action.

Other abnormalities that predispose patients with renal failure to adverse drug reactions include abnormal protein binding of drugs. In uremic human beings, the percentage of drug binding to protein is decreased (Reidenberg, 1971). Thus a total serum diphenylhydantoin concentration in the normal therapeutic range could be toxic for a patient with renal failure, since the plasma and tissue concentrations of the unbound free bioactive drug would be abnormally elevated. The metabolites of a drug normally eliminated by the kidneys may also accumulate in a uremic patient. Although most drug metabolites are relatively nontoxic, they may displace the bioactive parent drug from its serum protein binding site.

Increased or decreased tissue sensitivity to drugs may also cause adverse drug reactions in uremic patients. For example, human beings and experimental animals with renal insufficiency have an increased sensitivity to barbiturates. The latter may be associated with an alteration in the plasma protein binding of the drug or alterations in the blood-brain barrier (Reidenberg, 1971). In contrast, uremic human beings have a decreased sensitivity to insulin. The latter is apparently related to a change in cellular sensitivity to insulin rather than the presence of insulin antagonists in uremic serum (Reidenberg, 1971).

Impaired rates of drug metabolism may

also be important. Alterations in metabolism may be associated with deficits or excesses in fluid, acid-base, electrolyte, endocrine and caloric balance. Delayed metabolism of drugs administered at usual dosages and maintenance intervals could result in adverse drug reactions.

## GENERAL RECOMMENDATIONS

**Overview.** The indications for drug therapy in patients with renal failure must be kept in perspective. The veterinary profession and the manufacturers and distributors of drugs have promulgated a concept of the effectiveness of drugs which is sometimes unrealistic. The public has responded by demonstrating its belief that most diseases and disorders can be resolved by the use of drugs. Not enough thought and emphasis have been placed on the fact that drugs can be harmful as well as helpful. The point to be emphasized is that no drug is completely safe. Too often, justification for use of empirical therapy is the hypothesis that some treatment is better than nothing at all.

Drugs should be advocated in the treatment of renal failure only when there is a known potential benefit to be gained from their use. One of the most frequent therapeutic errors in veterinary medicine is the routine use of antibiotics and corticosteroids for treatment of renal failure, irrespective of the underlying cause. As will be discussed, the indiscriminate use of both types of drugs may be harmful to a uremic patient.

**Objectives.** One must strive to maintain therapeutic blood or urine concentrations of a drug by formulating a dosage schedule that will not produce drug toxicity. The first step is to determine whether a significant quantity (> 30 per cent) of the drug is excreted by the kidneys. Drugs that are partly or completely metabolized or excreted by extrarenal organs such as the liver may require little adjustment in dosage. Examples of pharmacologic agents in this category include chloramphenicol, erythromycin, Lincocin® (lincomycin hydrochloride [Upjohn]), tylosin and novobiocin. Phenothiazine derivatives and short-acting barbiturates are also metabolized by the liver.

The next step is to determine whether a higher than normal therapeutic blood level of the active drug or its metabolites are likely to induce toxicity. For example, although penicillin is excreted primarily by the kidneys, it may be administered to patients with renal failure at usual dosages and maintenance intervals because it is relatively nontoxic, even at high blood concentrations. On the other hand, the toxicity induced by digoxin, a drug eliminated primarily as a result of glomerular filtration, is dose-related. Therefore the dosage of digoxin in patients with renal failure must be reduced.

One should also consider whether the uremic state will alter the in-vivo metabolism or therapeutic effect of the drug and whether the drug is inherently nephrotoxic. As a generality, the use of potentially nephrotoxic drugs (aminoglycoside antibiotics, amphotericin B, tetracyclines, etc.) should be avoided.

**Modification in Dosage.** Available information suggests that modification of drug dosage is not required until renal function declines to 30 per cent or less of normal. In our experience, reduction in renal function to this degree is usually associated with impaired ability to concentrate and dilute urine and with azotemia. **Caution!** A considerable degree of renal disease can be present before clinical and laboratory signs of renal failure develop. Such patients have a decreased renal reserve capacity and are more sensitive to the undesirable effects of nephrotoxic drugs and anesthesia than are patients with normal renal function.

In many instances, drug toxicity in patients with renal failure is dose-related. Clinical trials in man and experimental studies in laboratory animals have revealed that many drugs dependent on renal excretion for elimination from the body can be given with relative safety to patients in renal failure, provided that drug dosage is properly modified. When a reduced dosage is required to achieve a safe therapeutic blood level, the interval between the doses may be lengthened (constant dose, varying interval), or a reduced dose may be given at the recommended maintenance interval (varying dose, constant interval) (Aronson, 1975; Bennett *et al.*, 1970; Reidenberg, 1971).

Most nephrologists advocate the constant dose, varying interval method. The initial dose determines the drug concentration that will be achieved in the patient, while the rate of metabolism and excretion of the drug can be influenced by altering the time interval between maintenance doses. In order words, a normal therapeutic dose is given to achieve the clinically desired blood level. In order to maintain this therapeutic concentration, maintenance doses are given at varying intervals of time, depending on the prolongation of the biologic half-life of the drug induced by renal insufficiency. In order to implement this method, however, the biologic half-lives of various drugs at different degrees of renal insufficiency must be known. Ideally, quantitative clearance studies should be performed to evaluate the degree of renal insufficiency. Alternatively, the serum concentration of creatinine or urea nitrogen may be used as an index of glomerular filtration rate. Although a variety of tables pertaining to this information are available to physicians (Table 1) (Bennett *et al.*, 1970; Reidenberg, 1971), such information concerning domestic animals is not available. If we are to obtain these data in the future, veterinarians must inform pharmaceutical manufacturers and distributors of the urgent need for this information. A quantitative relationship between a routine test of kidney function and the speed of elimination of drugs must be determined experimentally in a representative sample of animals with renal disease.

A varying dose, varying interval method may also be used. It consists of giving a normal loading dose but reducing sub-

sequent dosage levels in addition to prolongation of time intervals between administrations of maintenance therapy.

Irrespective of the method used to modify dosage, each patient must be carefully monitored for side effects known to be associated with a particular drug. Early detection of signs arising from their use will permit the clinician to readjust their dosage or discontinue them before irreparable damage occurs. If the drug is inherently nephrotoxic, urinalyses should be periodically evaluated for the unexpected presence of red cells, white cells, protein and casts. Determinations of serial creatinine or BUN concentrations should also be performed. Serial serum creatinine or BUN concentrations should also be monitored to determine whether the dosage of non-nephrotoxic drugs that are excreted primarily by the kidneys requires further reduction.

## SPECIFIC RECOMMENDATIONS

In the absence of quantitative data about the serum half-life of the drug and quantitative data about renal function, establish the main route of excretion of the drug (Table 2). Use the working hypothesis that drugs primarily excreted by the kidneys will accumulate to a variable degree in patients with renal failure. Consider the use of drugs that are not dependent on the kidneys for metabolism or excretion (e.g., ampicillin, chloramphenicol, erythromycin, lincomy-

***Table 1.*** *Guide to Use of Drugs in Human Beings With Renal Insufficiency*

| | | | MAINTENANCE DOSE INTERVAL (HOURS) | | | |
|---|---|---|---|---|---|---|
| | | | | *Renal Failure* | | |
| DRUG | ROUTE OF EXCRETION | NORMAL HALF-LIFE (HOURS) | *Normal* | *Mild* | *Moderate* | *Severe* |
| Ampicillin | Renal and hepatic | 1.5 | 6 | 6 | 6 | 8–12 |
| Cephaloridine | Renal | 1.5 | 6 | 6 | 12 | 24–36 |
| Chloramphenicol | Hepatic and renal | 2.5 | 6 | Unchanged | Unchanged | Unchanged |
| Digitoxin | Hepatic and renal | 72–144 | 24 | 24 | 24–36 | 36–72 |
| Digoxin | Renal | 36 | 12 | 24 | 24–36 | 36–48 |
| Erythromycin | Hepatic | 1.5 | 6 | Unchanged | Unchanged | Unchanged |
| Furosemide | Hepatic | ? | 6 | Unchanged | Unchanged | Unchanged |
| Gentamicin | Renal | 2.5 | 8 | 8–12 | 12–24 | 48 |
| Kanamycin | Renal | 3–4 | 8 | 24 | 24–72 | 72–96 |
| Lincomycin | Hepatic and Renal | 4.5 | 6 | 6 | 6 | 8–12 |
| Nitrofurantoin | Renal | 0.5 | 8 | 8 | Avoid | Avoid |
| Penicillin G | Renal and Hepatic | 0.5 | 8 | 8 | 8 | 12 |
| Streptomycin | Renal | 2.5 | 12 | 24 | 24–72 | 72–96 |
| Tetracycline | Renal and Hepatic | 6–8 | 6 | 12 | 24–48 | 72 |

Modified from Bennett *et al.*: JAMA, *214*:1468–1475, 1970.

**Table 2.**   *Suggested Dosage and Potential Side Effects of Drugs in Dogs and Cats With Renal Insufficiency*

| DRUGS | ROUTE OF EXCRETION | NEPHROTOXIC | EXTRARENAL TOXICITY | DOSAGE |
|---|---|---|---|---|
| Amphotericin B | Unknown | Yes | Hepatic, renal | Normal |
| Ampicillin | Hepatic and renal | No | Gastrointestinal | Reduce |
| Cephaloridine | Renal | No | ? | Reduce(?) |
| Chloramphenicol | Hepatic and renal | No | Anorexia, diarrhea, bone marrow depression (esp. cats) | Normal |
| Digitoxin | Hepatic | No | Gastrointestinal, cardiac | Reduce(?) |
| Digoxin | Renal | No | Gastrointestinal, cardiac | Reduce |
| Doxycycline | Gastrointestinal (dog);?(cat) | ? | ? | Normal |
| Erythromycin | Hepatic and renal | No | Gastrointestinal, hepatic | Normal |
| Gentamicin | Renal | Yes | Ototoxic, gastrointestinal | Reduce |
| Kanamycin | Renal | Yes | Ototoxic | Reduce |
| Lincomycin | Hepatic | No | Gastrointestinal | Normal |
| Neomycin | Renal | Yes | Ototoxic | Reduce |
| Nitrofurans | Renal | No | Gastrointestinal, CNS | Avoid |
| Penicillin G | Renal and hepatic | No | Encephalopathy | Normal |
| Polymyxin B | Renal | Yes | CNS(?) | Avoid |
| Streptomycin | Renal | Yes | Ototoxic | Reduce |
| Sulfonamides | Renal | Yes | Gastrointestinal, CNS | Reduce |
| Tetracycline | Renal and Hepatic | Yes | Hepatotoxic | Avoid |
| Tylosin | Hepatic and renal | ? | ? | Normal (?) |
| Vancomycin | Renal | Yes | Ototoxic | Reduce |

cin, etc.) or that are infrequently associated with adverse drug reactions even when they accumulate as a result of renal insufficiency (e.g., penicillin G).

Although the excretion of penicillin G is prolonged in patients with renal failure, the infrequency with which this drug is associated with toxicity allows normal therapeutic dosages to be administered in the presence of uremia. Large doses of potassium penicillin G should be avoided in oliguric or anuric uremic patients, since these patients are predisposed to hyperkalemia. Potassium salts of penicillin G may be used in polyuric patients, however, since hyperkalemia is rarely associated with polyuric renal failure.

If potentially harmful adverse drug reactions are likely to occur as a result of retention of the drug secondary to renal insufficiency, seek an equally effective but less toxic substitute. Avoid the use of potentially nephrotoxic antibiotics whenever possible (Table 2). The inherent nephrotoxicity of aminoglycoside antibiotics (streptomycin, neomycin, gentamicin, vancomycin, kanamycin, tobramycin, etc.) is dose-related and therefore is especially noteworthy. If the use of potentially harmful drugs is absolutely imperative, do not allow potential toxicity to interfere with choice of an effective agent that has no substitute. Modify the dosage to minimize the possibility of adverse drug reactions and carefully evaluate the patient for renal or extrarenal signs of toxicity that are known to be associated with the drug (Table 2).

With the notable exception of doxycycline, the administration of tetracyclines to patients in renal failure may be detrimental for several reasons. Tetracyclines in high concentration apparently exert an inhibiting (or antianabolic) effect on hepatic enzyme systems in human beings and possibly in dogs (Czerwinski and Pederson, 1975; Sedwitz *et al.*, 1953; Shils, 1963). Impaired ability of the liver to synthesize amino acids into proteins results in the metabolism of the amino acids for energy. As a result the concentration of nitrogenous waste products that must be excreted by the kidneys is increased. While the normal kidney can excrete these metabolic by-products without difficulty, the functionally impaired kidney cannot. Several experimental studies and one clinical study in dogs indicate that tetracyclines may also produce renal lesions (Gourley, 1970; Obek *et al.*, 1974; Polec *et al.*, 1971). Experimental studies in dogs have revealed that mannitol has a protective effect on the azotemia produced by tetracyclines. (Polec *et al.*, 1971). The administration of outdated degraded tetracycline products containing citric acid may induce nephrotoxicity in man and dogs (Cluff *et al.*, 1975). Pending further investigations, it is recommended that tetracycline not be given to dogs or cats in renal failure.

Doxycycline is a unique tetracycline derivative with a broad spectrum of antibacterial activity that is excreted by the gastrointestinal tract in man and dogs (Schach Von Wittenau and Twomey, 1971). Clinical studies in anephric human patients have revealed that the half-life of doxycycline is not prolonged (Whelton *et al.*, 1974). It may be considered for the treatment of systemic infections in patients with renal insufficiency when a tetracycline compound is indicated.

It is again emphasized that prophylactic antibiotics should not be routinely used in the symptomatic and supportive treatment of renal failure. They are best reserved for use when there is evidence of infection. Because the host defense mechanisms of uremic patients are often impaired, the choice of antimicrobial agent should be based on the results of *in-vitro* antibiotic sensitivity tests. When possible, avoid the use of potentially nephrotoxic antibiotics (Table 2).

Selection of drugs for treatment of urinary tract infections because they are excreted in significant concentrations in urine should be carefully considered in patients with renal failure. Reduction in renal function may prevent the excretion of effective concentrations of the drug in urine. For example, the concentrations of sulfonamides, nalidixic acid and nitrofurans in the urine of human patients with renal failure are often too low to be of therapeutic value, and they may induce systemic toxicity (Reidenberg, 1971). Likewise, urinary acidifiers should not be given to patients with renal insufficiency. Since renal failure is typically associated with metabolic acidosis, administration of acidifiers will aggravate the severity of the acidosis and may cause death.

A variety of solutions have been recommended for use in the removal of urethral plugs from male cats, including sterilized saline, local anesthetic solutions, buffered acetic acid and solutions containing antibiotics. Caution in the use of these solutions is recommended, since accumulation of large quantities of acid, anesthetic or antibiotic solutions within an inflamed urinary bladder may result in absorption and systemic toxicity.

Except in instances of shock, the use of corticosteroids is not advocated for the supportive treatment of renal failure because these drugs stimulate the breakdown of protein into carbohydrate (gluconeogenesis) and thus increase the quantity of protein metabolic by-products that must be excreted by failing kidneys. Glucocorticoids may also aggravate the severity of skeletal demineralization associated with renal secondary hyperparathyroidism. We also are of the opinion that the widespread use of corticosteroids in the treatment of immunologically mediated glomerulonephropathy should be withheld until the natural course of the disease has been evaluated in a larger number of patients (see article on "Glomerulonephropathy and the Nephrotic Syndrome").

General anesthetics are usually associated with significant changes in hemodynamics when given at concentrations required for surgery. As a result, renal blood flow, glomerular filtration rate and the renal excretion of water and solutes are altered. Because the usual hazards associated with surgery and the postoperative period are often exaggerated in the presence of compromised renal function, the use of inhalant anesthetics is recommended. They are not dependent on renal excretion, they permit rapid change in depth of anesthesia and they allow rapid recovery following withdrawal.

Clinical experience has revealed that patients with renal failure are more sensitive to general anesthetics than are normal patients. Studies in human beings, rats and rabbits have revealed an increased sensitivity to standard doses of thiopental (Reidenberg, 1971; Richards *et al.*, 1973). We have used thiamylal sodium to induce anesthesia and halothane to maintain anesthesia for percutaneous renal biopsy in numerous dogs and cats. Since thiamylal (and other short-acting barbiturates) is primarily inactivated by the liver, it is considered to be an acceptable agent to induce anesthesia. Halothane is not inherently nephrotoxic. Although it does induce a reduction in renal blood flow as a result of hypotension, the hypotension is transient.

The association of methoxyflurane with nephrotoxicity has been extensively documented in man (Gottlieb and Trey, 1974). The syndrome is dose-related and is typically characterized by varying degrees of nephrogenic diabetes insipidus. It may be aggravated by obesity, concomitant administration of tetracycline and prolonged deep anesthesia. When this syndrome occurs in a patient with preexisting renal insufficiency, a uremic crisis that may lead to death can occur. This clinical syndrome is caused by nephrotoxic metabolites of methoxyflurane, including inorganic fluoride and oxalic acid. The renal lesions are characterized by the deposition of calcium oxalate crystals in the renal tubules and interstitial tissue and by chronic inflammation. Although clinical cases of methoxyflurane nephrotoxicity are apparently very uncommon in dogs and cats with normal renal function, the effects of this anesthetic in patients with renal failure have not been investigated. Prolonged deep anesthesia of dogs with normal renal function was reported to include an obligatory polyuria 12 to 24 hours following anesthesia (Stubbs *et al.*, 1971). The polyuria persisted for several days. Experimental administration of inorganic fluoride to normal dogs resulted in a dose-related impairment of ability to concentrate urine (Frascino, 1972). Simultaneous administration of tetracycline to normal dogs anesthetized with methoxyflurane increased the mortality rate compared to that of control dogs. (Stoelting and Gibbs, 1973). On the basis of these findings, it is recommended that methoxyflurane not be used to anesthetize patients with renal insufficiency.

Pending experimental and clinical investigations, ketamine should not be administered to uremic cats because the drug is dependent on the kidneys for its excretion in active form.

## SUMMARY

The best cure is prevention. Drugs should *not* be administered to patients with renal insufficiency with the philosophy that they may help but can be of no harm.

Adverse drug reactions will continue to occur as long as drugs are used for the diagnosis and treatment of renal disorders. Despite this fact, the frequency and severity of drug toxicity can be minimized by anticipation of potential problems, prudent selection of drugs, appropriate modification of dosage when necessary and careful monitoring of the patient for signs indicative of toxicity.

## SUPPLEMENTAL READING

Aronson, A. L.: The use, misuse, and abuse of antibacterial agents. Mod. Vet. Pract., 56:383–389, 1975.

Bennett, W. M., Singer, I., and Coggins, C. H.: A practical guide to drug usage in adult patients with impaired renal function. JAMA, 214:1468-1475, 1970.

Cluff, L. E., Caranasos, G. J., and Stewart, R. B.: Clinical Problems With Drugs. V. Major Problems in Internal Medicine. Philadelphia, W. B. Saunders Co., 1975.

Czerwinski, A. W., and Pederson, J. A.: Drug induced renal disease. Kidney, 8:20–23, 1975.

Frascino, J. A.: Effect of inorganic fluoride on the renal concentration mechanism. J. Lab. Clin. Med., 79:192–203, 1972.

Gottlieb, L. S., and Trey, C.: The effects of fluorinated anesthetics on the liver and kidneys. Ann. Rev. Med., 25:411–429, 1974.

Gourley, I. M.: Prevention and treatment of acute renal failure in the canine surgical patient. J. Am. Vet. Med. Assn., 157:1722–1728, 1970.

Obek, A., Petorak, I., Eroglu, L., and Gurkan, A.: Effects of tetracycline on the dog kidney. A functional and ultrastructural study. Israel J. Med. Sci., 10:765–771, 1974.

Polec, R. B., Yeh, S. D. J., and Shils, M. E.: Protective effect of ascorbic acid, isoascorbic acid, and mannitol against tetracycline-induced nephrotoxicity. J. Pharm. Exp. Ther., 178:152–158, 1971.

Reidenberg, M. M.: Renal Function and Drug Action. Philadelphia, W. B. Saunders Co., 1971.

Richards, R. K., Taylor, J. D., and Kueter, K. E.: Effect of nephrectomy on the duration of sleep following administration of thiopental and hexobarbital. J. Pharm. Exp. Ther., 108:461–473, 1953.

Schach Von Wittenau, M., and Twomey, T. M.: The disposition of doxycycline by man and dog. Chemotherapy, 16:217–228, 1971.

Sedwitz, J., Bateman, C., and Klopp, C. T.: Oxytetracycline toxicity studies in dogs. Antib. Chemother., 111:1015–1019, 1953.

Shils, M. E.: Renal disease and the metabolic effects of tetracycline. Ann. Int. Med., 58:389–408, 1963.

Smith, J. W., Seidl, L. G., and Cluff, L. E.: Studies on the epidemiology of adverse drug reactions. V. Clinical factors influencing susceptibility. Ann. Int. Med., 65:629–640, 1966.

Stoelting, R. K., and Gibbs, P. S.: Effect of tetracycline therapy on renal function after methoxyflurane anesthesia. Anesth. Analg., 52:431–436, 1973.

Stubbs, S., Fung, H., Wade, J., and Thomson, E.: The penthane controversy. High output renal failure following methoxyflurane (Penthrane) anesthesia in the dog. *In* Scientific Proceedings of Anesthesia and the Kidney. Dept. of Anesthesia, University of Manitoba, Winnipeg, Manitoba, Canada, 1971.

Whelton, A., Schach Von Wittenau, M., Twomey, T. M., Walker, W. G., and Bianehine, J. R.: Doxycycline pharmacokinetics in the absence of renal function. Kidney Int., 5:365–371, 1974.

Lower Urinary Tract

# NEUROGENIC URINARY INCONTINENCE

JOHN E. OLIVER, JR., D.V.M.
*Athens, Georgia*

*and* CARL A. OSBORNE, D.V.M.
*St. Paul, Minnesota*

Micturition is the physiologic process of storage and complete voiding of urine. Abnormalities of the nervous system may cause inappropriate voiding, inadequate storage of urine, incomplete voiding or absence of voiding. All these abnormalities may be considered as forms of incontinence, which is defined as the loss of voluntary control of micturition. Behavioral disorders resulting in inappropriate micturition and abnormalities of the urinary tract resulting in incontinence are discussed in other articles.

## ANATOMY AND PHYSIOLOGY OF MICTURITION

The neural organization of micturition is a complex integration of parasympathetic, sympathetic and somatic components involving all levels of the nervous system. A simplified description applicable to understanding most clinical problems is presented in Figure 1. Filling of the urinary bladder is accommodated by gradual stretching of smooth muscle called the detrusor. Sensory endings of the pelvic (parasympathetic) nerve detect changes in the amount of stretch. When capacity is reached, these afferent fibers discharge impulses to the sacral segments of the spinal cord (S-1, 2, 3). The signals are relayed through spinoreticular pathways to the pons (brain stem). Reflex integration occurs at this level, with a resultant efferent discharge down reticulospinal pathways to the sacral parasympathetic nucleus. Preganglionic parasympathetic neurons are activated, sending impulses through the pelvic nerve. Ganglia are located along the course of the pelvic nerve and in the bladder wall. Postganglionic neurons are acti-

vated, sending impulses to the detrusor muscle. Each muscle fiber in the detrusor does not receive direct innervation; rather, "pacemaker" fibers scattered through the detrusor are depolarized, with subsequent spread of excitation to adjoining muscle fibers through "tight junctions." Tight junctions are areas of fusion of the outer components of the cell membranes. The resulting wave of excitation causes contraction of the detrusor, which pulls the neck of the bladder open like a funnel and squeezes out urine. Simultaneously, inhibitory interneurons are activated in the sacral spinal cord which synapse on pudendal motor neurons. The pudendal neurons are silenced, resulting in a relaxation of the external urethral sphincter. When the bladder is empty, afferent discharge in the pelvic nerve subsides and is followed by cessation of discharge in the pelvic motor neurons. The detrusor muscle relaxes, the inhibitory interneurons no longer block pudendal motor activity and the external urethral sphincter returns to its normal state of contraction.

The external urethral sphincter (skeletal muscle) maintains a low level of tonus through spinal stretch reflexes. Sudden changes in intra-abdominal pressure (cough, sneeze) cause a rapid increase in tone in the sphincter and permit maintenance of urinary continence. Continence in the relaxed animal is maintained at the neck of the bladder ("internal sphincter") by the relaxation of the spiraling detrusor fibers.

The sympathetic nervous system has input to the bladder from spinal segments L-1 to 4, through the caudal mesenteric ganglion and the hypogastric nerve. Sympathetic neurons synapse on ganglia in the pelvic plexus and bladder wall as well as innervating blood vessels. The exact func-

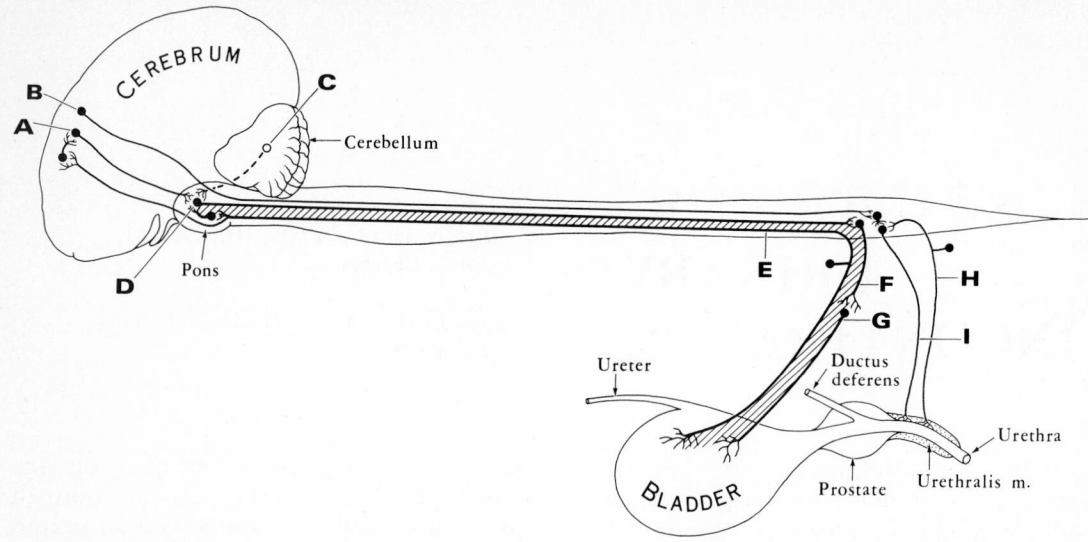

**Figure 1.** Anatomical organization of micturition: *A,* Cortical neurons for voluntary control of micturition. *B,* Cortical neurons for voluntary control of sphincters. *C,* Cerebellar neurons, which have inhibitory influence on micturition. *D,* Pontine reticular neurons, which are necessary for detrusor reflex. *E,* Afferent (sensory) pathway for detrusor reflex. *F,* Preganglionic pelvic (parasympathetic) neuron to detrusor. *G,* Postganglionic pelvic (parasympathetic) neuron to detrusor. *H,* Afferent (sensory) neuron from urethral sphincter, pudendal nerve. *I,* Efferent (motor) neuron to urethral sphincter, pudendal nerve.

### Table 1.  *Effects of Lesions of Neuromuscular System*

| LOCATION OF LESIONS | NORMAL FUNCTION | BLADDER | | |
| --- | --- | --- | --- | --- |
| | | *Voluntary Control* | *Sustained Detrusor Reflex* | *Tone* |
| Cerebral cortex to brain stem | Voluntary control to detrusor and sphincter | Absent | Normal | Normal |
| Cerebellum | Modulation (inhibition) of detrusor reflex | Normal, but increased frequency | Possible hyper-reflexia | Normal |
| Brain stem (pons) to sacral spinal cord | Sustained detrusor reflex | Absent | Lost early; small unsynchronized contractions late | Atonic early; possibly increased late |
| Partial lesions (reflex dyssynergia) | Sustained detrusor reflex | May be present | May be present | Normal to atonic |
| Sacral spinal cord or roots | LMN* to detrusor and sphincter | Absent | Absent | Atonic |
| Disruption of tight junctions of detrusor | Spread of excitation in detrusor | Absent | Absent | Atonic |

*LMN = lower motor neuron.

tion of the sympathetic input is not clear, since ablation of the hypogastric nerve does not significantly alter micturition. It is presumably inhibitory to micturition to some degree, perhaps having an effect on the storage capacity of the bladder. There are also excitatory fibers to smooth muscle, primarily in the trigonal region of the bladder. These fibers may be important in prevention of reflux in the ureters during micturition (DeGroat, 1975).

Voluntary control of micturition is mediated from the cerebral cortex to the pontine micturition center. Voluntary control of sphincters is derived from the cerebral cortex and is relayed to the sacral spinal cord nucleus of the pudendal nerve. Micturition can occur without cerebral cortex input, but there is no voluntary control.

The cerebellum has an inhibitory effect on the pontine neurons of micturition.

Abnormalities of micturition associated with lesions of the nervous system are outlined in Table 1.

## DIAGNOSIS OF URINARY INCONTINENCE

The minimum (or defined) data base recommended for evaluation of a patient with abnormal micturition is listed in Table 2. A thorough evaluation (as outlined) should reveal any additional problems as well as provide a diagnosis and prognosis. Specific points in the data base related to micturition are discussed below.

**History.** Evaluation of the onset and chronologic course of the problem will allow construction of a sign-time graph which is useful for determining the etiology of the disease (Oliver, 1972). The ability of the animal to control micturition voluntarily is an important differentiating feature (Table 3). In this context, voluntary control means that the animal is able to initiate voiding at appropriate times.

Associated problems such as paresis, fecal incontinence, pain, etc., are important criteria for differentiating neurogenic from

***Table 1.*** *Effects of Lesions of Neuromuscular System (Continued)*

| BLADDER | | | SPHINCTER | | |
|---------|---------------|-------------------|-------------------------------------|----------------------|----------------------------|
| Volume | Residual Urine | Voluntary Control | Reflexes (Perineal Bulboureth.) | Tone | Synergy with Detrusor |
| May be greater or smaller than normal | None | Absent | Normal to Hyper-reflexic | Normal to increased | Normal |
| Small | None | Normal | Normal | Normal | Normal |
| Large | Large | Absent | Normal to hyper-reflexic | Normal to increased | Absent |
| Large | Small to large | May be normal | Normal | Normal to increased | Absent |
| Large | Large | Absent | Absent | Flaccid | Absent |
| Large | Large | Normal | Normal | Normal | Normal (cannot evaluate, however) |

*Table 2.*   *Minimum Data Base for Diagnosis of Urinary Incontinence*

History
Physical Examination
  Includes: Observation of voiding and
           measurement of residual urine
Neurologic Examination
  Includes: Sphincter reflexes
Clinical Pathology
  Includes: CBC, urinalysis, BUN or creatinine
Radiology
  Includes: Survey abdomen and pelvis
           Contrast cystography, urethrography
           Intravenous pyelogram

non-neurogenic incontinence and in localizing lesions in neurogenic incontinence.

**Physical Examination.** Observation of voiding may help determine whether voluntary control is present, whether the detrusor reflex is present and whether the sphincter relaxes during voiding. Reflex dyssynergia (usually a result of partial spinal cord lesions) is characterized by voluntary initiation of voiding but is associated with a small urine stream that stops abruptly before the bladder is empty. Small spurts of urine may be produced intermittently as the animal strains to urinate against a closed sphincter. Absence of voiding or dribbling of urine when the urinary bladder is distended suggests absence of a detrusor reflex or obstruction of the urethra.

Palpation of the bladder before and after voiding will usually permit a flaccid atonic bladder to be differentiated from a small contracted bladder with thickened walls. Calculi or tumor masses may also be palpated. Manual expression of the bladder provides an evaluation of sphincter tone. Tone will be decreased when lesions are present in the sacral spinal cord, roots or pudendal nerve (lower motor neuron) and will be increased when lesions are present between the brain stem and L-7 (upper motor neuron).

Catheterization immediately after voiding allows an accurate measurement of residual urine, which should be less than 10 ml. in normal dogs. Most urethral obstructions can be localized when a catheter is passed through the urethal lumen.

**Neurologic Examination.** In addition to a complete neurologic examination for localization of abnormalities in the nervous system, it is imperative that reflexes through the sacral spinal cord also be evaluated. The tone of the external anal sphincter may be observed or palpated with a gloved finger. Reflex contraction of the sphincter can be elicited by squeezing the bulb of the penis or the vulva (bulbocavernosus reflex) or by pinprick or pinch of the perineum (perineal reflex). Both reflexes are dependent on the integrity of the pudendal nerve (afferents and efferents) and sacral segments of the spinal cord.

The history, physical examination and neurologic examination should provide adequate information to differentiate neurogenic from non-neurogenic disorders and to localize the site of the lesion in the nervous system when neurogenic disorders are present (Table 3).

**Electrophysiology.** Electrophysiologic tests have not been included in the minimum data base because they are not widely used at the present time. They will, however, provide more objective evidence of abnormalities detected during the general examination and may disclose subtle abnormalities which otherwise would not be recognized.

The cystometrogram (CMG) measures intravesical pressure during a micturition reflex. It provides information about bladder tone, bladder capacity and the detrusor reflex. The presence or absence of a detrusor reflex may be difficult to evaluate without a cystometrogram in some cases.

Electromyography of the skeletal sphincters may detect partial denervation, which is difficult to assess clinically.

**Laboratory Examination.** Hematology, blood chemistries and urinalyses provide information that may help one to detect non-neurogenic causes of abnormal micturition. They are essential if a meaningful prognosis is to be formulated. Disorders of micturition are frequently complicated by cystitis, ureteral reflux, pyelonephritis and/or uremia.

**Radiologic Examination.** Survey-radiographs provide information about kidney and bladder size, shape and position. Calculi or masses may be seen. A pneumocystogram, double contrast cystogram and/or urethrogram may be necessary to detect bladder and urethral masses or calculi. Intravenous urography (IVU) must be used to detect ureteral dilation caused by reflux.

*Table 3.  Algorithm for Diagnosis of Urinary Incontinence*

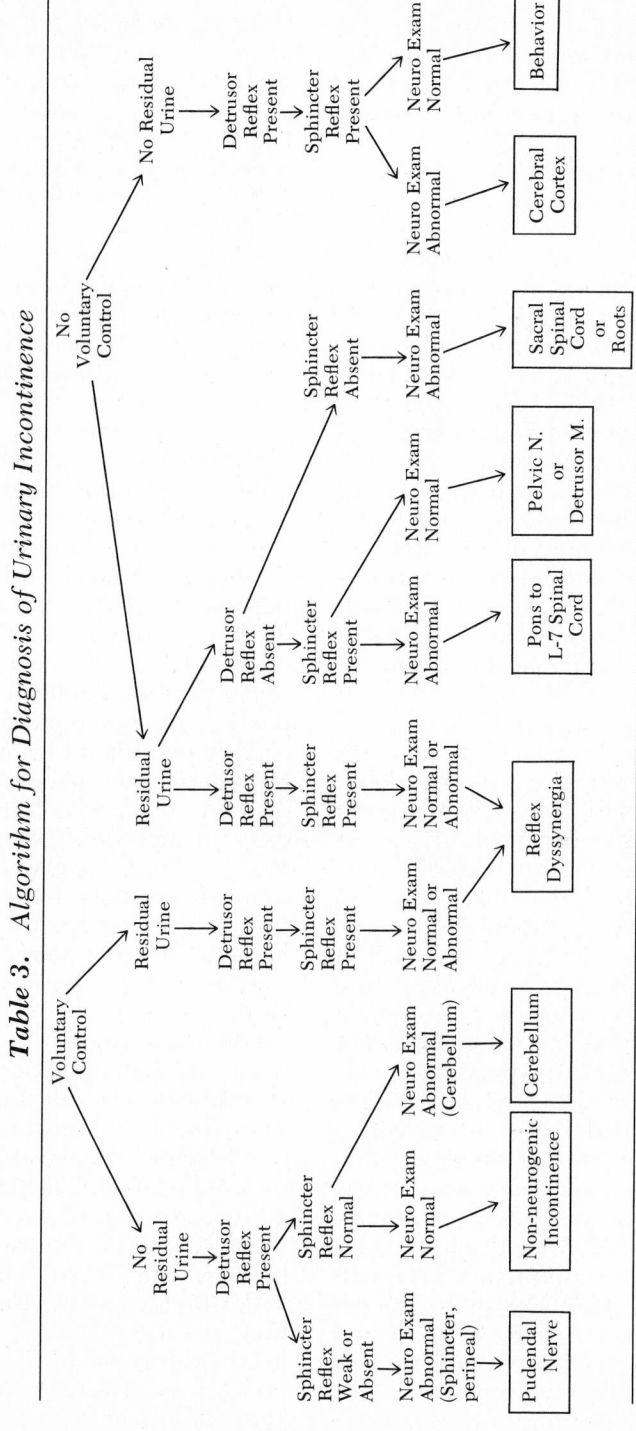

A voiding cystourethrogram is useful for assessing the coordinated function of the bladder and urethra.

## TREATMENT

Abnormalities of the nervous system causing disorders of micturition may be reversible or irreversible. Reversible lesions include spinal cord or peripheral nerve compressions (disks, trauma). Treatment should be directed toward correction of the primary cause of the disease (Hoerlein, 1971). Although management of the micturition problem may be only temporary in these cases, it may make the difference between success and failure.

Irreversible lesions include congenital defects and injuries or diseases associated with neuronal destruction. Management of these patients is dependent on the underlying problem. Behavior problems or cerebral cortex lesions that lead to inappropriate voiding (loss of house training, "marking" inside of house, etc.) may be managed by behavior modification or the use of anticonvulsants or tranquilizers, or the problem may be avoided by housing the pet outside. Such cases are often a diagnostic and therapeutic challenge.

Severe brain-stem or spinal cord lesions (above S-1) are characterized by detrusor areflexia and hypertonus of the sphincter. Most paraplegics fall into this category. Management of urinary bladder abnormalities in patients with reversible lesions of this type is critical if success is to be achieved. Management of patients with irreversible deficits of this type is often difficult and discouraging. Removal of urine by intermittent aseptic catheterization (t.i.d.) is imperative. If the sphincter is not excessively hypertonic (especially in females), expulsion of urine by manual expression of the bladder may be possible. The patient should be periodically catheterized following manual expression of the bladder to be certain that adequate emptying is being achieved. After the first 1 to 3 weeks, reflex bladder contractions may partially empty the bladder. Complete evacuation of the bladder is *rarely* accomplished by these segmental reflexes, and serious complications usually develop if assistance is not provided. If the animal appears to be voiding completely, this observation should be verified by catheterization immediately

after micturition. If a residual urine volume of more than 5 ml. is present, assistance must be continued.

Cystitis is a frequent complication of detrusor areflexia. Urinalyses, bacterial culture and antibiotic sensitivity tests are indicated to detect abnormalities at an early stage. Appropriate antibiotics should be administered (consult article on "Bacterial Infections of the Urinary Tract").

Partial lesions of the spinal cord may produce reflex dyssynergia (contraction of the bladder without relaxation of the sphincter). Limited trials with neuromuscular relaxants such as diazepam have given equivocal results to date. Partial rhizotomy of the sacral dorsal roots has been used with some success in man. Pudendal neurectomy will allow complete voiding but will also induce urinary incontinence.

Human beings with detrusor hyperreflexia caused by cerebellar or partial spinal cord lesions have been reported to respond to anticholinergic medication. Propantheline (Pro-Banthine®[Searle]) has been used at dosages from 7.5 to 30 mg. given t.i.d. in dogs.

Lesions of the sacral spinal cord or roots cause detrusor areflexia and sphincter areflexia. The same type of management as described for spinal cord lesions is suggested. Catheterization may not be required, since manual expression of the bladder is usually easy. Since nerve roots are peripheral nerves with the capability of regeneration, traumatic lesions at the lumbosacral junction that compress the cauda equina are much more likely to respond to decompression than similar lesions affecting the spinal cord.

Overdistention of the bladder which disrupts the tight junctions between smooth muscle fibers results in detrusor areflexia. Function will be restored in 1 to 2 weeks if the bladder is maintained in a decompressed state by the methods described above, provided that infection has not caused a proliferation of fibrous tissue in the bladder wall.

Prosthetic devices for control of micturition, such as bladder stimulators and artificial sphincters, have been used to a limited extent in experimental animals and in man. Frequent complications and prohibitive costs prevent their widespread use in veterinary medicine at the present time.

## SUPPLEMENTAL READING

DeGroat, W. C.: Nervous control of the urinary bladder of the cat. Brain Res. 87:201, 1975.

Hoerlein, B. F.: Canine Neurology. 2nd ed. Philadelphia, W. B. Saunders Co., 1971.

Oliver, J. E., Jr.: Neurologic examination, taking the history. Vet. Med./Small Animal Clin., 67:433, 1972.

Oliver, J. E., Jr.: Neurology of visceral function. Vet. Clin. N. Am. 4:517, 1974.

Oliver, J. E., Jr., and Young, W. O.: Air cystometry in dogs under xylazine-induced restraint. Am. J. Vet. Res., 34:1433, 1973.

Osborne, C. A., and Oliver, J. E., Jr.: Non-neurogenic urinary incontinence. In Kirk, R. W. (ed.): Current Veterinary Therapy VI. Philadelphia, W. B. Saunders Co., 1977.

---

# NON-NEUROGENIC URINARY INCONTINENCE

CARL A. OSBORNE, D.V.M.,
*St. Paul, Minnesota*

*and* JOHN E. OLIVER, D.V.M.,
*Athens, Georgia*

Urinary incontinence in dogs is a common clinical problem that may result from several fundamentally different disease mechanisms. Because formulation of specific treatment and an accurate forecast of the probable future course of the disease process are dependent on the underlying cause of urinary incontinence, every attempt should be made to establish a specific diagnosis. Consult the article entitled "Neurogenic Urinary Incontinence" for details concerning the etiopathogenesis, diagnosis and treatment of this form of incontinence. This article is concerned with ectopic ureters, patent urachus, estrogen-responsive urinary incontinence, obstructive (paradoxical) incontinence, urge incontinence and inappropriate micturition.

## ECTOPIC URETERS

### APPLIED ANATOMY AND PHYSIOLOGY

The ureters are primarily muscular tubes that actively transport urine produced in the kidney and stored in the renal pelvis to the urinary bladder. Urine that accumulates in the renal pelvis initiates peristaltic movement of pelvic and then ureteral smooth muscle. As a result, elongated boluses of urine are propelled through the ureteral lumen to the urinary bladder.

Anatomic ureterovesical sphincters are not present; however, the oblique course of the ureters through the bladder wall at the trigone forms a flap value that normally prevents retrograde flow of urine from the bladder. The ureterovesical valves protect the kidneys from abnormal retrograde pressure and from contamination with infected bladder urine.

### INCIDENCE

**Dogs.** Ureteral ectopia is a common cause of urinary incontinence in female dogs. In one survey of 54 dogs with ectopic ureters, Siberian huskies, West Highland white terriers, fox terriers and miniature and toy poodles had a higher risk for this anomaly than other breeds of dogs (Hayes, 1974). We have the clinical impression that black Labrador retrievers also have a higher than expected incidence of the disorder.

**Cats.** Only one case of ectopic ureter has been reported in the cat, suggesting that it is a very uncommon problem in this species (Reis, 1959).

**Sex.** Although the incidence of ectopic ureters in dogs is unknown, it has been more frequently recognized in females than in males. In a recent survey of the world literature, 35 of 36 reported cases were in females (Owen, 1973a). One investigator reported a female to male ratio of 21:1 (Hayes, 1974).

In the past, the consensus of opinion has

been that the frequency with which ectopic ureters are recognized in female dogs was associated with the almost invariable occurrence of urinary incontinence in females. The lack of urinary incontinence in male human beings with ectopic ureters has been used as additional support for this generality. Urinary incontinence does not occur in association with urethral termination of one or both ureters in man because all wolffian duct derivative structures are located proximal to the external urethral sphincter. When a ureter empties into the urethra, the urine flows back into the lumen of the urinary bladder because the proximal urethra is less resistant to urine flow than are the more distal portions.

Although the first reported case of an ectopic ureter in a male dog was not associated with urinary incontinence, two subsequent cases in male dogs in which ectopic ureters terminated in the urethra were associated with urinary incontinence (Osborne *et al.*, 1975).

**Age.** Since ureteral ectopia is a congenital anomaly, the incidence in young dogs is high. In one survey, 58 per cent of the female dogs with ectopic ureters were diagnosed before they were one year old (Hayes, 1974).

## ETIOLOGY

Termination of one or both ureters outside the urinary bladder occurs as a result of faulty differentiation of the mesonephric and metanephric ducts (Owen, 1973a). The underlying cause of faulty differentiation of these structures in the dog has not been established. Familial aggregations of ectopic ureters have been reported in black Labador retrievers (Holt and Kievit, 1971). The finding of certain breeds at high risk, coupled with the probable low risk of dogs of mixed breeding, suggests genetic involvement (Hayes, 1974). Ectopic ureters have been experimentally produced in the offspring of pregnant rats by altering their diet during certain stages of gestation.

## PATHOPHYSIOLOGY

**Location.** In female dogs, either or both ureters may terminate in the vagina, urethra, bladder neck or uterus. In a survey of the world literature, the vagina was the most common site of ureteral termination

(70 per cent), with the urethra (20 per cent), neck of the bladder (8 per cent) and uterus (3 per cent) being less common sites (Owen, 1973a). Although there is apparently no predisposition of either the right or left ureter, unilateral ectopia has been encountered far more frequently (approximately 80 per cent) than has bilateral ureteral ectopia (approximately 20 per cent) (Owen, 1973a).

**Associated Diseases.** Ectopic ureters are often associated with other congenital anomalies of the urinary system and with acquired diseases that develop as a sequel to ureteral ectopia.

MEGAURETER. Megaureter (ureteroectasia) characterized by dilation of the ureteral lumen and abnormal peristalsis is a very common finding. Megaureter was reported in 16 of 36 cases of ectopic ureters evaluated in one large survey (Owen, 1973a). Varying degrees of megaureter (2 to 10 times normal) were observed in all 20 ureters present in 17 dogs (16 with unilateral ectopia and 3 with bilateral ureteral ectopia) studied at the University of Minnesota. Some patients had concomitant dilation of the renal pelvis (pyelectasis).

The cause of megaureter has not been established. Although stricture of the ureter associated with hydroureter and hydronephrosis has been reported in a few patients, total obstruction to urine outflow would not be a plausible explanation because of the presence of urinary incontinence. In our series, anatomic obstruction of the ureters was observed in only one male dog with unilateral ureteral ectopia.

Megaureters might be related, at least in part, to the fact that the distal end of an ectopic ureter has no functional valve and permits reflux of urine. They may also be associated with urinary tract infection caused by *Escherichia coli* or *Pseudomonas* spp., organisms known to impair or inhibit ureteral peristalsis in the dog (Grana *et al.*, 1968). Developmental abnormalities of the ureters in human beings are known to be associated with decreased or absent peristaltic activity (Hutch and Tanagho, 1965; McLaughlin *et al.*, 1973). Impaired or inhibited peristalsis is associated with functional obstruction characterized by decreased emptying of affected ureters and resultant megaureter.

DECREASED RENAL SIZE. Reduction in renal size is often associated with an ectopic ureter. Although the observation that kidneys associated with ectopic ureters are sometimes smaller than normal is beyond question, the interpretation that reduction in size is always caused by congenital hypoplasia is erroneous. Since there is no functional sphincter at the distal end of an ectopic ureter, the potential for reflux predisposes the associated kidney to ascending bacterial infection. We have encountered small contracted kidneys in patients with ectopic ureters in which gross, microscopic and bacteriologic findings were typical of chronic generalized pyelonephritis.

DECREASED BLADDER SIZE. In one large survey of ectopic ureters in dogs, bilateral ectopic ureters were frequently associated with an abnormally small urinary bladder (Owen, 1973a). Many investigators have stated that such bladders are hypoplastic, implying that their reduction in size was also caused by embryologic maldevelopment.

We are of the opinion that reduction in the size of the urinary bladder in patients with bilateral ureteral ectopia may also be associated with disuse. Our conclusion is based on experimental studies in laboratory animals (Goss and Singleton, 1971) and dogs (Schmaelzle *et al.*, 1969) and clinical studies in dogs (Owen, 1973a, 1973b, 1973c) and man (Tanagho, 1974) which indicate that natural or surgically induced defunctionalization of the urinary bladder may be associated with a potentially reversible reduction in bladder capacity. Bilateral ureteral ectopia was observed in an incontinent 2-year-old female Siberian husky at the University of Minnesota. Both ureters terminated in the urethra. Despite the fact that neither ureter entered the urinary bladder, the dog could micturate in a normal fashion. The urinary bladder was normal in size. Apparently a significant quantity of urine expelled from the ureters into the urethra passed into the urinary bladder before being voided.

URETHRAL ABNORMALITIES. Dogs with ectopic ureters that terminate in the urethra may continue to have urinary incontinence following transplantation or extirpation of the affected ureter. Although less severe, urinary incontinence persisted in 4 of 5 female dogs with urethral ectopic ureters following surgical correction at the University of Minnesota. In contrast, all dogs (4) with vaginal ectopic ureters became continent following surgery.

MISCELLANEOUS. Other congenital anomalies that have been observed in dogs with ectopic ureters include agenesis of the urinary bladder and urethra, persistent hymen, an ectopic urethra and an abnormal cervix (Osborne *et al.*, 1972; Pearson and Gibbs, 1971).

## CLINICAL SIGNS

The clinical signs associated with ectopic ureters are dependent upon their site of termination and upon the presence or absence of other congenital or acquired abnormalities.

**Female Dogs.** In female dogs, ectopic ureters are usually associated with varying degrees of urinary incontinence. Affected dogs usually have a history of urinary incontinence since birth or weaning. Urine may drip from the vulva continuously or pool in the vagina and gravitate out of the vulva when body position is changed. Because the nerve supply and functional capacity of the urinary bladder are normal, the bladder does not become overdistended with urine. Patients with one ectopic ureter are typically able to micturate normally, since urine continues to pass into the urinary bladder through the unaffected ureter. Patients with bilateral ectopic ureters may be unable to micturate normally.

We have observed a progressive decrease in the severity of urinary incontinence in some female dogs which also had chronic generalized progressive disease of the associated kidney. The disease was thought to be caused by pyelonephritis. It is hypothesized that progressive destruction of the majority of functioning nephrons caused by ascending bacterial infection ultimately cause a progressive decrease in the total volume of urine produced by the kidney (even though remaining viable nephrons were producing an increased volume of urine).

**Male Dogs.** Only three cases of ectopic ureters have been reported in male dogs (Osborne *et al.*, 1975). In all cases, the left ureter terminated in the urethra. Two of the 3 cases had urinary incontinence which was surgically corrected.

## ENDOSCOPIC FINDINGS

Detection of abnormal openings in the vagina via endoscopy provides strong support for a diagnosis of ureteral ectopia. The opening of an ectopic ureter may be difficult to find, however. Satisfactory visualization of the entire mucosal surface of the vagina is dependent on the use of a vaginoscope that eliminates mucosal infoldings by distention of the vaginal wall. Glass (Pyrex) test tubes from which the bottoms have been removed and the ends fire-polished, pediatric proctoscopes, disposable plastic syringe cases from which a large rectangular section has been removed from the wall, and fiberoptic endoscopes are preferred over otoscopic cones and nasal speculums. Injection of air into the vaginal lumen may enhance visualization by causing distention of the vaginal wall.

Many female dogs with ectopic ureters have a persistent hymen. Visual inspection of the vagina of such patients often reveals a fleshy piece of tissue that is attached to the dorsal and ventral walls of the vagina. The lateral aspects of the structure often form slitlike openings with the vaginal wall and may be mistaken for ectopic ureteral orifices.

## Radiographic findings

Evaluation of the entire urinary tract by intravenous urography is indicated to confirm the presence of an ectopic ureter(s) and to determine if other abnormalities of the kidneys, ureters, urinary bladder or urethra are present. Although intravenous urography is an important diagnostic aid, visualization of the exact site of termination of the distal ureter may be difficult or impossible. Poor visualization may occur because of lack of sufficient contrast media in the lumen of the distal ureter. The latter may occur as a result of impaired ability of poorly functioning renal tissue to excrete a sufficient quantity of radiopaque media to opacify the ureter. This problem may be minimized by the use of high-dose urography (Osborne *et al.*, 1972). Accumulation of contrast media in the lumen of the urinary bladder may also interfere with visualization of the distal portion of the ureter.

As mentioned previously, ectopic ureters are frequently dilated and are often associated with dilation of the renal pelvis. The degree of megaureter detected by intravenous urography is dependent on the amount of radiopaque media in the ureter (and therefore the amount administered)

(McLaughlin *et al.*, 1973). The fact that there has been no uniformity in radiographic techniques performed in cases of ureteral ectopia reported in the literature may provide an explanation as to why megaureter has been a more consistent finding in cases evaluated by high-dose urography at the University of Minnesota than in other studies. When evaluated by high-dose urography, enlarged ureters are frequently filled with radiopaque media throughout their entire length and are often tortuous, and their diameter in some portions may be 2 to 10 times normal. In contrast, the entire length of normal ureters is rarely filled with radiopaque media because peristaltic contractions normally constrict the ureteral lumen.

When an abnormal orifice is detected in the vagina, or suspected to be in the urethra, catheterization of the orifice with a radiopaque catheter* followed by retrograde ureterography should be performed. This technique should not be used as a substitute for intravenous urography, since it may not reveal other abnormalities of the urinary system, including the presence of bilateral ureteral ectopia.

Retrograde urethrograms should be performed in male or female dogs suspected of having urethral ectopic ureters (consult article "Retrograde Contrast Urethrography").

Vaginography (colpography) may be of benefit in small female dogs which cannot be examined by endoscopy. To perform a vaginogram, inject a sufficient quantity of radiopaque contrast media through an inflated Foley catheter* to distend the vagina. The inflated balloon should be positioned just beyond the vulva to prevent loss of contrast material. If an ectopic ureteral orifice opens into the vagina, radiopaque media may reflux into it for a variable distance.

## Diagnosis

A history of urinary incontinence that has been present since birth or weaning in a dog (especially female) should stimulate a high index of suspicion of an ectopic ureter(s). Observation of an abnormal orifice in the vagina or failure to observe ureteral orifices at the trigone by cystoscopy pro-

---

*Available from American Cystoscope Makers, Inc., Pelham Manor, New York 10803.

vides supportive evidence. Additional support for the diagnosis may be obtained by injecting sterilized, colored dye into the urinary bladder. Normal colored urine should appear at the vulva or tip of the penis of patients with urinary incontinence caused by an ectopic ureter.

Radiographic detection of megaureter, especially when associated with pyelectasis and reduction in renal size, provides strong supportive diagnostic evidence. Retrograde ureterography provides definitive information concerning the ureter being studied.

In the event that endoscopic and radiographic studies fail to provide diagnostic information, the presence of an ectopic ureter may be confirmed by exploratory laparotomy. Lack of termination of one or both ureters at the trigone of the urinary bladder confirms the diagnosis. If the pathway of the distal ureter cannot be evaluated because of the pathway of the ureter through surrounding tissue, a cystotomy may be performed to determine if the ureteral orifices are in their normal location in the mucosal surface of the bladder. If a sufficient quantity of saline or other sterilized liquids is injected into the lumen of an ectopic ureter, it should bypass the bladder and immediately appear at the vulva or tip of the penis. The tip of a small catheter inserted into the lumen of an ectopic ureter should also pass through the vulva or external urethral orifice of the penis.

## TREATMENT

There is no effective medical treatment for urinary incontinence caused by an ectopic ureter.

Proper surgical management of a patient with urinary incontinence caused by ureteral ectopia is dependent on (a) the functional capacity of associated and contralateral kidneys; (b) the presence or absence of infection or other pathologic changes in the urinary tract (an attempt to eliminate or control infection of the urinary system with appropriate antimicrobial drugs should be made prior to surgery); (c) whether one or both ureters are ectopic; and (d) the site of termination of the anomalous ureter. Dogs with ureters that terminate in the urethra may continue to have urinary incontinence despite surgical correction of the affected ureter(s).

We have been successful with transplantation of the ureter when a submucosal anti-reflux tunnel has been made in the bladder (Archibald and Owen, 1974). Transplantation of the ureter into the urinary bladder is the procedure of choice if any of the following conditions exist: (a) normal function of the kidney drained by the ectopic ureter; (b) extravesical termination of both ureters or (c) reduced functional capacity of both kidneys. In the last situation, extirpation of a kidney may result in removal of a sufficient quantity of renal parenchyma to precipitate renal failure.

Nephrectomy and removal of as much of the anomalous ureter as possible should be performed when the kidney attached to the ectopic ureter is affected by generalized disease, or when intractable infection is present in the affected ureter or kidney (or both). When the ureter opens into the vagina, it should be resected to as low a level as can be conveniently reached by a lower abdominal incision. Care must be taken not to damage the vesicourethral sphincter by dissection of ectopic ureters that become buried in the wall of the urinary bladder. Tracing the ureter to its precise termination is not necessary, since, in our experience, the unresected distal portion rarely is a source of further trouble. If one or both ureters empty into the urethra, incomplete excision may result in the formation of a diverticulum, urinary stasis and persistent infection. Because of difficulties in operative exposure and the risk of damaging the vesicoureteral sphincter, however, it is usually preferable to perform an incomplete ureterectomy and await the results.

## PROGNOSIS

If surgical correction of a unilateral ectopic ureter that terminates in the vagina or uterus is feasible, a guarded to good prognosis should be offered. If one or both ectopic ureters terminate in the urethra, the owner should be advised that some degree of urinary incontinence may continue following surgical correction of the problem.

Transplantation of dilated ureters into the urinary bladder may be followed by varying degrees of vesicoureteral reflux. Vesicoureteral reflux in turn predisposes the patient to ascending infection of the kidney. A better long-term result may be obtained when the ureters have some degree of peristalsis and are not extremely dilated. We have obtained satisfactory results by transplanting dilated ureters without radiographic evidence of peristalsis into the urinary bladder in several patients, however.

## PATENT URACHUS

The urachus functions in the fetus to provide a channel of communication between the urinary bladder and the allantoic sac. The urachus is normally nonfunctional at birth.

### COMPLETELY PATENT URACHUS

If the urachal canal remains completely patent following birth, urine will be voided through the umbilicus. Urine scald dermatitis of the abdomen is common, as is secondary bacterial infection of the urinary bladder and umbilicus (omphalitis). Affected animals maintain the capacity to micturate normally.

The diagnosis may be confirmed by intravenous urography or retrograde cystography. Treatment consists of complete excision of the urachus and elimination of secondary bacterial infection with appropriate antibiotics.

### PARTIALLY PATENT URACHUS

The urachal canal may remain partially patent. If the patent portion of the urachal canal communicates with the bladder lumen, a blind diverticulum frequently is present. Urachal diverticula are frequently associated with recurrent cystitis. Diagnosis and treatment are the same as those described for a completely patent urachus.

Clinical signs are apparently uncommon in patients with a partially patent urachus that communicates with the umbilicus. Urachal cysts may form at any point between the umbilicus and urinary bladder as a result of persistence of secreting urachal epithelium in isolated stretches of patent lumen. Urachal cysts may become infected with bacteria, necessitating surgical excision.

## ESTROGEN-RESPONSIVE URINARY INCONTINENCE

Urinary incontinence may develop in ovariohysterectomized dogs after a variable period of time following surgery. Although the incidence of the problem is unknown, there is a general consensus of opinion that it is an uncommon sequela to ovariohysterectomy. In a survey of 30 cases at the University of Minnesota, there was no breed or age predisposition. The mean age at the time of onset of urinary incontinence was 8.45 years (range = 1 to 15 years).

### ETIOPATHOGENESIS

The etiology and pathophysiology of this syndrome have not been determined. The fact that affected dogs can micturate normally indicates that the nerve supply and detrusor muscle are not abnormal. One theory is that the uterine stump of affected animals becomes adhered to the bladder neck following ovariohysterectomy, and that subsequent retraction of the stump associated with senescence results in mechanical interference with physiologic sphincter activity. The hypothesis, however, does not provide an obvious explanation of the observation that administration of estrogens induces remission of urinary incontinence.

The fact that administration of low doses of estrogens to affected dogs is frequently associated with a remission of clinical signs, while withdrawal of estrogen therapy is associated with recurrence of urinary incontinence, has been interpreted by some to indicate that the disease is caused by hypoestrogenism. Similar observations have been made in women with stress incontinence (Musiani, 1972). It is thought that the mucosal lining of the trigone of women is dependent on estrogens, as is vesicourethral sphincter tone. The hypoestrogenism theory has not yet been substantiated inasmuch as the estrogen concentration of affected dogs has not been measured and compared to nonaffected ovariohysterectomized and normal dogs. This theory also does not offer an obvious explanation as to why urinary incontinence occurs only in a small percentage of ovariohysterectomized dogs.

## DIAGNOSIS

Estrogen-responsive urinary incontinence in ovariohysterectomized dogs is frequently an exclusion diagnosis that is established after other causes of urinary incontinence have been eliminated. Remission of urinary incontinence following therapy with estrogens is required to confirm the diagnosis.

## TREATMENT

Administration of low doses of estrogens usually results in remission of urinary incontinence. Diethylstilbestrol may be administered orally at a dose of 0.1 to 1.0 mg. per day for 3 to 5 days, followed by a maintenance dosage of approximately 1.0 mg. per week. Alternatively, 0.1 to 1.0 mg. of estradiol cypionate* may be parenterally administered at intervals of weeks to months. **Estrogens must not be administered in excessive quantities, since, in addition to inducing signs of estrus, they may cause severe thrombocytopenia, anemia and sometimes leukopenia.**

## OBSTRUCTIVE (PARADOXICAL) INCONTINENCE

### ETIOPATHOGENESIS

Paradoxical incontinence may occur in patients with partial obstruction of the urethra. It is most likely to be encountered in male dogs because of the long length of their urethras and because the os penis restricts the degree to which the urethra passing through its ventral groove can dilate. The obstructive lesion in the urethra (calculi, neoplasms, strictures, space-occupying masses in periurethral tissue) must be of such a nature that it prevents normal micturition but not so severe that it completely obstructs urine outflow. When the bladder becomes overdistended with urine, intravesical pressure exceeds the resistance imparted by the urethral lesion, and urinary incontinence results. Prolonged overdistention of the bladder may induce a variable degree of damage to structures in the bladder wall. If this occurs, the pathogenesis becomes complicated by neuromuscular

*ECP, The Upjohn Co., Kalamazoo, Michigan 49002.

deficit (consult article on "Neurogenic Urinary Incontinence"). The paradox of this syndrome is that urinary incontinence occurs in a patient with obstruction to urine outflow.

## DIAGNOSIS

Paradoxical incontinence should be suspected in patients with abnormal micturition characterized by voluntary or involuntary dribbling of urine and dysuria. The urinary bladder is usually overdistended with urine, and difficulty is encountered in expelling urine from the bladder by digital palpation. Insertion of a catheter through the urethral lumen may be difficult or impossible. Localization of the urethral lesion may be established with the aid of a catheter or by contrast urethrography (consult article on "Retrograde Contrast Urethrography"). The presence or absence of postrenal uremia should be determined by evaluating serum creatinine or urea nitrogen concentration.

## TREATMENT

**Specific.** Specific treatment is dependent on the nature of the underlying cause. Urethral calculi may be removed by urohydropropulsion (consult article on "Urohydropropulsion") or urethrotomy. A permanent urethrostomy proximal to the site of obstruction may be required for patients with irreversible urethral strictures. Neoplasms that have not metastasized should be surgically extirpated. In our experience, by the time transitional cell carcinomas of the urethra were of sufficient size to induce clinical signs, they were usually inoperable because of local invasion and metastases.

**Supportive.** The urinary bladder of patients with postrenal uremia should be decompressed as soon as possible by catheterization or, if necessary, cystocentesis. Abnormalities in fluid, acid-base and electrolyte balance associated with renal failure should also be corrected (consult articles on treatment of renal failure).

If the urinary bladder is hypotonic or atonic because of prolonged overdistention, the urinary bladder should be maintained in a nondistended state by manual compression, by intermittent aseptic catheterization or with the aid of an indwelling catheter. If neuromuscular structures have not been irreversibly damaged, normal bladder function may return (consult article on "Neurogenic Urinary Incontinence").

## URGE INCONTINENCE

Urge incontinence is defined as the involuntary loss of urine that occurs soon after the sensation of bladder fullness. It is characterized by inability to control micturition between the time of the urge to urinate and the ability to evacuate the bladder voluntarily. It is often caused by bacterial inflammation or trauma of the urinary bladder and urethral mucosa. (Consult articles on urinary tract infection for additional information about etiopathogenesis, diagnosis and treatment.)

Cystitis may develop in patients with small hyperactive neurogenic bladders as a result of retention of residual urine in the bladder lumen. In such patients, abnormal patterns of micturition may not be caused by bacterial inflammation. Diagnosis, prognosis and therapy are dependent on the underlying cause of neurogenic dysfunction (consult the article on "Neurogenic Urinary Incontinence").

## INAPPROPRIATE MICTURITION

Puppies, nervous adult dogs and animals with CNS lesions that cause psychomotor disturbances may have uncontrollable (or inappropriate) patterns of micturition. In some cases, inappropriate micturition may be confused with other causes of urinary incontinence. Inappropriate micturition associated with behavioral patterns is usually intermittent and is usually initiated by stress or fright. It may undergo remission as the animal matures or may be controlled by conditioning and training. The prognosis and therapy of psychomotor disturbances induced by CNS lesions is dependent on the biologic behavior of the underlying cause.

## SUPPLEMENTAL READING

Archibald, J., and Owen, R. R.: Urinary System. *In* Archibald, J. (ed.): Canine Surgery. 2nd ed. American Veterinary Publications, Inc., Santa Barbara, California, 1974.

Goss, R. J., and Singleton, S. D.: Disuse atrophy of the bladder after bilateral nephrectomy. Proc. Soc. Exp. Biol. Med., *138*:861–864, 1971.

Grana, L., Donnellan, W. L., and Swenson, O.: Effects of gram negative bacteria on ureteral structure and function. J. Urol., *99*:539–550, 1968.

Hayes, H. M.: Ectopic ureter in dogs. Epidemiologic features. Teratology, *10*:129–132, 1974.

Holt, J. C., and Kievit, T.: Correction of ectopic ureter. Aust. Vet. Practitioner, *1*:19–21, 1971.

Hutch, J. A., and Tanagho, E. A.: Etiology of nonocclusive ureteral dilatation. J. Urol., *93*:177–184, 1965.

McLaughlin, A. P., Pfister, R. C., Leadbetter, W. F., Salzstein, S. L., and Kessler, W. O.: The pathophysiology of primary megaloureter. J. Urol., *109*:805–811, 1973.

Musiani, U.: A partially successful attempt at medical treatment of urinary-stress incontinence in women. Urol. Int., *27*:405–410, 1972.

Osborne, C. A., Dieterich, H. F., Hanlon, G. F., and Anderson, L. D.: Urinary incontinence due to ectopic ureter in a male dog. J. Am. Vet. Med. Assn., *166*:911–914, 1975.

Osborne, C. A., Low, D. G., and Finco, D. R.: Canine and Feline Urology. Philadelphia, W. B. Saunders Co., 1972.

Owen, R. R.: Canine ureteral ectopia—A review. I. Embryology and etiology. J. Small Animal Pract., *14*:407–417, 1973a.

Owen, R. R.: Canine ureteral ectopia—A review. II. Incidence, diagnosis and treatment. J. Small Animal Pract., *14*:419–427, 1973b.

Owen, R. R.: Three case reports of ectopic ureters in bitches. Vet. Rec., *93*:2–10, 1973c.

Pearson, H., and Gibbs, C.: Urinary tract abnormalities in the dog. J. Small Animal Pract., *12*:67–84, 1971.

Reis, R. H.: Renal aplasia, ectopic ureter and vascular abnormalities in domestic cat. Anat. Rec., *135*:105–107, 1959.

Schmaelzle, J. F., Cass, A. S., and Hinman, F.: Effect of disuse and restoration of function on vesical capacity. J. Urol., *101*:700–705, 1969.

Tanagho, E. A.: Congenitally obstructed bladders: Fate after prolonged defunctionalization. J. Urol., *111*:102–109, 1974.

# CATHETER BIOPSY OF THE URETHRA, URINARY BLADDER AND PROSTATE GLAND

THOMAS MELHOFF, D.V.M.,
*and* CARL A. OSBORNE, D.V.M.
*St. Paul, Minnesota*

## INDICATIONS

Evaluation of the morphology of various types of cells (transitional epithelium, RBC, WBC, etc.) found in urine sediment is of proved value in the investigation of inflammatory and neoplastic diseases of the urogenital system. However, evaluation of the morphologic characteristics of individual cells found in urine is often more difficult than examination of cytologic preparations obtained from most other body organs and systems. This is partly associated with the fact that cells present in urine are subjected to osmotic and pH changes that are markedly different from their normal environment. In addition they may be exposed to toxic concentrations of enzymes and other metabolites excreted in urine. The problem may also be compounded by the fact that relatively few cells originating from the site of the lesion may be available for examination.

In human beings this problem has been circumvented by the use of cystoscopy and transurethral biopsy. Although cystoscopes may be used in large female dogs, the anatomy of male and small female dogs, and of domestic cats, prevents cystoscopic examination and biopsy of the bladder and urethra with the equipment currently available.

We have had varying degrees of success by using a flexible urinary catheter to obtain aspiration biopsy specimens from lesions in the bladder, urethra and/or prostate gland of dogs. The procedure may also be used in cats and other animals. The advantage of the catheter biopsy technique over conventional exfoliative cytology methods for urine sediment is the collection of a relatively large quantity of fresh cells from a specific site within the genitourinary tract in a fluid of similar composition to extracellular fluid. The major disadvantage of the technique is related to the fact that, although evaluation of the morphologic characteristics of a group of cells provides information, it does not always provide a diagnosis. Although a definitive diagnosis may be established on the basis of positive findings, tentative diagnoses cannot always be eliminated by exclusion on the basis of negative findings.

We have had the greatest success with this technique in confirming diagnoses of transitional cell carcinomas of the urethra and urinary bladder, thereby eliminating the need for diagnostic surgical procedures. It also has been of value in the evaluation of inflammatory and neoplastic lesions of the prostate gland. In addition to microscopic examination of cell population, aspirated tissue may be cultured for microorganisms.

We recommend this technique as an adjunct to the clinical evaluation of diseases of the lower urinary tract and prostate gland. Since it is easy to perform, of minimal discomfort to the patient and inexpensive, its use does not preclude further clinical investigations by radiography, punch biopsy, exploratory surgery, and so on.

## MATERIALS

A flexible urethral or ureteral catheter with openings (eyes) on the sides of the

1173

proximal end should be used. The size of the catheter, and thus its openings, should be as large as is consistent with atraumatic passage through the urethra in order to maximize the quantity of the biopsy sample.

Once the sample is obtained, it must be rapidly fixed in order to minimize artifactual changes caused by autolysis. If chunks of tissue are obtained with the catheter, they should immediately be transferred to a bottle of 10 per cent buffered formalin solution for processing by routine histologic techniques.

The liquid portion of the sample may be processed in a variety of ways. To insure proper handling of the specimen, we suggest consultation with the laboratory to which the sample is to be delivered before the sample is taken.

A few drops of the noncentrifuged sample may be placed on a microscope slide, fixed by air-drying and stained with new methylene blue, Wright's stain, etc. The same technique may be used for examination of sediment prepared from the sample (see below).

Concentration of cellular material may be achieved by routine methodology for the preparation of urine sediment (i.e., centrifugation at 1500 to 2000 rpm for 5 minutes). After removal of the supernatant, the sediment may be placed on several microscope slides and fixed by air-drying, proprietary cytologic fixatives* or Aqua-Net hair spray (Freeman, 1969). A nucleopore filter may be used to concentrate cells in lieu of centrifugation.

A cell block for routine histologic sectioning may be prepared by adding two drops of plasma and 2 drops of thrombin to the sediment (Constantian *et al.*, 1973). The clot that forms should be fixed in 10 per cent buffered formalin solution.

## TECHNIQUE

Localize the site of the lesion in the urinary bladder, urethra or prostate gland by palpation, catheterization or radiography (refer to the article on "Retrograde Contrast Urethrography"). Remove the urine from the bladder by catheterization. Insert the catheter through the urethra until the catheter openings are adjacent to the lesion. Correct positioning of the catheter may be facilitated by rectal or vaginal palpation or by radiography (using a radiopaque catheter).

Attach a 12-ml. syringe containing 3 to 10 ml. of an isotonic solution (i.e., physiologic saline solution or lactated Ringer's solution) to the catheter and inject all but 1 ml. of the solution into the urinary tract. Create negative pressure in the system by pulling the syringe plunger outward. The objective of this maneuver is to aspirate a small portion of the mucosal surface of the urinary tract into the openings of the catheter (Fig. 1). With the syringe plunger pulled out, move the catheter a short distance forward and backward. The aspiration portion of the procedure should be rapidly performed in order to minimize admixture of peripheral blood elements with the biopsy sample.

The negative pressure created with the syringe should gradually be released by allowing the plunger to return to its normal resting position. This should be accomplished before withdrawing the catheter in order to prevent contamination of the biopsy sample with cells located between the lesion and the external urethral orifice.

If material from the prostate gland is desired, the yield and representativeness of the sample may be improved by massaging the prostate gland per rectum during the biopsy procedure.

The biopsy sample may be removed from the catheter by injecting the remaining portion of isotonic solution through its lumen and harvesting the mixture in a test tube or small vial. Chunks of tissue should be removed with a wooden applicator stick and placed in 10 per cent buffered formalin solution. The remaining portion of the sample should be processed as described under the section on materials.

Postoperative antibiotics are indicated, since the integrity of the mucosal surface of the lower urinary tract is damaged by this procedure.

## INTERPRETATION

Knowledge of the normal histology and cytology of the urinary tract is prerequisite to meaningful interpretation of biopsy samples. Although examination of cytologic preparations by the clinician should be performed, consultation with a competent

---

*Cyto-Fixer®, Lab-Tek Plastics Co., Westmont, Ill.; Mucolexx®, Lerner Laboratories, Stamford, Connecticut; Spray-Cyte®, Clay-Adams, Inc., New York.

†Nucleopore Corp., 7035 Commerce Circle, Pleasanton, California.

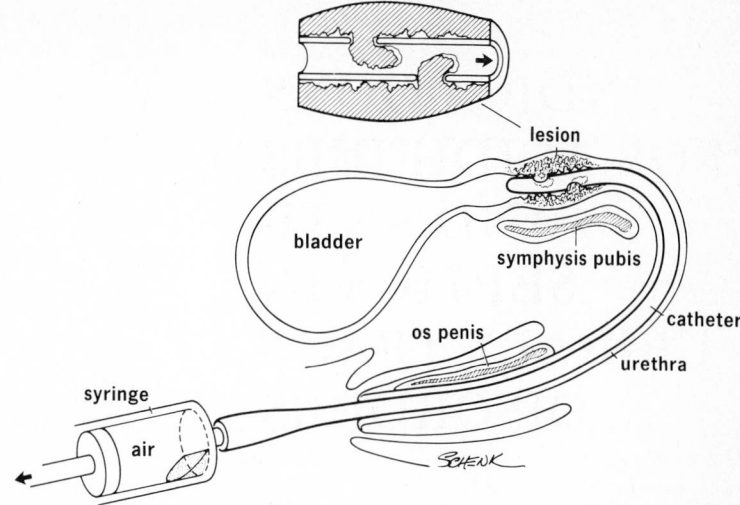

**Figure 1.** Schematic illustration of catheter biopsy of a urethral lesion in a male dog. A portion of the lesion has been aspirated into the lumen of the urinary catheter as a result of negative pressure created with a syringe. If a significant quantity of the lesion enters the lumen of the urethra (*insert*), a small plug of tissue may be harvested as the catheter is withdrawn.

pathologist, including confirmation of findings, is recommended.

A diagnosis of neoplasia following the examination of cytologic preparations is based on multiple criteria, including abnormal changes in individual cells and their nuclei and modification of cellular interrelationships (Table 1). Undifferentiated malignant cells derived from transitional cell carcinomas can usually be identified, provided that such cells are contained in the biopsy sample. Recognition of benign or well-differentiated malignant neoplasms on the basis of cytologic preparations may be difficult, however, since exfoliated cells may differ little from hyperplastic or even normal transitional epithelial cells.

Regardless of the type and degree of differentiation of the underlying tumor, secondary bacterial infection of neoplastic lesions may result in the collection of samples which are primarily composed of inflammatory cells and which contain relatively few neoplastic cells. Thus, a negative result does not exclude the presence of a neoplasm.

Because of difficulties that are sometimes encountered in evaluation of the significance of biopsy findings, the results should always be interpreted in association with other clinical, laboratory and radiographic findings.

### Table 1.  Abnormal Characteristics of Malignant Cells*

I. Structural alteration of cells and their nuclei
   A. Nuclear changes
      1. Disproportionate enlargement of the nucleus in relation to the cytoplasm
      2. Increase in chromatin content causing hyperchromasia
      3. Structural changes such as aberrant chromatin patterns, elongation, irregularity in outline, lobulation and budding, etc.
      4. Enlargement and/or increase in number of nucleoli
      5. Multinucleated cells, with atypical nuclei
      6. Increased mitotic activity; abnormal mitotic figures
      7. Marked thickening of nuclear membrane
   B. Cytoplasmic changes
      1. Changes in staining reaction
      2. Cytoplasmic inclusions such as pigment granules, leukocytes or cellular debris
      3. Atypical vacuolization
   C. Whole cell changes
      1. Increase in size
      2. Aberrant forms
II. Modification of cellular interrelationships
   A. Irregularity of pattern
   B. Anisocytosis and anisokaryosis
   C. Lack of distinct cell boundaries
   D. Dense crowding of cells and nuclei

*Modified from Prall *et al.*: Cancer, 29:1084–1089, 1972.

### SUPPLEMENTAL READING

Constantian, H. M., and DeGirdami, E. D.: Urothelial tumors detected by cytology: New cell block technique. J. Urol., *109*:304–307, 1973.

Freeman, J. A.: Hair spray: An inexpensive aerosol fixative for cytodiagnosis. Acta Cytol., *13*:416–419, 1969.

Osborne, C. A.: General principles of biopsy. Vet. Clin. N. Am., *4*:213–232, 1974.

Prall, R. H., *et al.*: Diagnostic cytology in urinary tract malignancy. Cancer, *29*:1084–1089, 1972.

Roszel, J. F.: Cytology of urine from dogs with botryoid sarcoma of the bladder. Acta Cytol., *16*:443–446, 1972.

Stevens, J. B., *et al.*: Biopsy sample management, staining and examination. Vet. Clin. N. Am., *4*:233–253, 1974.

# INDICATIONS FOR ACIDIFIERS AND ANTISEPTICS IN URINARY TRACT DISORDERS

ROBERT HARDY, D.V.M.
*St. Paul, Minnesota*

Urinary acidifiers and antiseptics have their greatest therapeutic application in the control or eradication of selected urinary tract diseases. These agents are readily available and relatively inexpensive. Clinicians should familiarize themselves with the indications and contraindications of these preparations, however, so that they may be rationally applied to clinical practice.

Two primary indications exist for the use of urinary acidifiers and urinary antiseptics: (1) they are very useful in controlling certain bacterial infections of the lower urinary tract, and (2) they are valuable as adjunctive prophylactic therapy for the aftercare of patients with urinary calculi.

## URINARY ACIDIFERS

Although the effectiveness with which urinary acidifiers alter urine pH varies with the drug in question, in general, two renal mechanisms are involved. The first is the formation and secretion of monosodium dihydrogen phosphate ($NaH_2PO_4$) into renal tubular fluid. This urinary acid dissociates readily in urine, effectively lowering the urine pH. The second method involves the renal excretion of intact metabolic acid residues, usually those resulting from degradation of organic compounds (i.e., mandelic, hippuric or gluconic acids).

The most frequently prescribed urinary acidifiers in veterinary medicine are DL-methionine, ammonium chloride, ascorbic acid, acid phosphate salts, mandelic acid and ethylenediamine dihydrochloride (Table 1). DL-*methionine* is an essential sulfur-containing amino acid that is oxidized within the body to sulfate. It is subsequently excreted into the urine as cystine sulfinic acid and acid sulfite. These two end products are strong organic acids capable of acidifying the urine to a pH as low as 5.0. Although toxic reactions are infrequent, adverse reactions reported in man include gastric irritation, behavioral alterations and aggravation of hepatic failure.

*Ammonium chloride* is classified as an acidifying diuretic. This drug is therapeutically effective for only short periods of time (5 to 6 days). Ammonium chloride is metabolized by the liver and converted to urea and a free hydrogen and chloride ion ($NH_4Cl \xrightarrow{liver} Urea + H^+ + Cl^-$). The excess hydrogen ions are initially excreted as sodium dihydrogen phosphate, which efficiently acidifies the urine. However, within several days, the kidney tubules adapt to the increased hydrogen load by producing ammonia ($NH_3$) as the covering cation for the hydrogen ($NH_3 + H^+ \rightarrow NH_4^+$). The ammonium ion ($NH_4^+$) is a weak acid compared to $NaH_2PO_4$. Once renal ammonia production equals ammonium ingestion, the acidifying effect on $NH_4Cl$ is neutralized. When given in high doses, ammonium chloride can produce a significant degree of metabolic acidosis.

*Ascorbic acid* is eliminated unchanged in the urine once its maximal renal tubular reabsorptive capacity is exceeded. Ascorbic acid has the potential to produce a dramatic lowering of urine pH but usually requires the administration of large doses at frequent intervals to maintain its acidifying effect. Because virtually all of the drug is excreted once its renal threshold is exceeded, ascorbic acid is virtually nontoxic.

*Acid phosphate salts* (ammonium, so-

1176

**Table 1.**  *Commonly Used Urinary Acidifiers and Dosage Recommendations*

| DRUG | DOSAGE (APPROXIMATE) | MANUFACTURER |
|---|---|---|
| Acid phosphates (pHos-pHaid®) | 250- or 500-mg. tablets; 1 to 2 tablets twice daily/7 to 15 kg. of body weight | Guardian Chem. Corp., Hauppauge, New York 11787 |
| Ammonium chloride | 200 mg./kg./day in divided dosages | Eli-Lilly & Co., Indianapolis, Indiana 46206 |
| Ascorbic acid | 200 to 500 mg. four times daily initially | Available as U.S.P. product from many sources |
| DL-Methionine (Odor-Trol®) | 200-mg. tablets; 1 tablet/7 kg. of body weight twice daily | Haver-Lockhart Labs., Shawnee, Kansas 66201 |
| Ethylenediamine dihydrochloride (Chlor-Ethamine®) | 100-mg. tablets; 1 tablet three times daily for cats | Pitman-Moore, Inc., Washington's Crossing, New Jersey 08560 |
| Mandelic acid (Mandelamine®) | 0.250-gm. tablets or suspension (250 mg./ teaspoon); 1 tablet/ 15 kg. of body weight four times daily | Warner-Chilcott Labs., Morris Plains, New Jersey 07950 |

dium and potassium) are infrequently used as urinary acidifiers in veterinary medicine. These drugs are weak urinary acidifiers and have had their greatest application in the prophylaxis of calcium phosphate and ammonium magnesium phosphate calculi. These drugs are considered to have *in-vivo* "calculolytic" activity independent of their effect on urine pH.

*Mandelic acid* is available at present only in combination with methenamine, a urinary antiseptic. Mandelic acid is a weak organic acid that has limited ability to lower urine pH but possesses antibacterial activity independent of its effect on urine acidity.

*Ethylenediamine dihydrochloride* (Chlor-Ethamine® [Pitman-Moore]) has been recommended for use as a urinary acidifier in cats subject to recurrent attacks of urolithiasis. Although the results of numerous uncontrolled clinical observations have been cited to substantiate this drug's usefulness in reducing the frequency of recurrences, it is questionable whether this effect is related in any way to alterations of urine pH. Our experience with this product indicates that its enteric coating produces highly variable degrees of absorption from the gastrointestinal tract.

## USE IN CONJUNCTION WITH ANTIBIOTICS

Urinary acidifiers are effective adjuncts to antibiotics in the treatment of bacterial cystitis. By lowering the urine pH, they render the environment of the urinary tract less conducive to bacterial growth. The degree of bacterial growth suppression depends on the pH obtained, the ability of the urine to contact the infectious agent and the susceptibility of the organism to pH changes. Acidic urine is bacteriostatic to a number of organisms (staphylococci, *Pseudomonas* spp., streptococci and *Proteus* spp.). Since infection can be controlled by prevention of bacterial growth, attaining bacteriostatic urine pH levels is clinically as effective as attaining those that are bactericidal. Conversely, within physiologic limits, alkalinization of urine does not significantly affect bacterial growth. Ascorbic acid has been found to be bactericidal for *Proteus* spp., *Escherichia coli*, *Alcaligenes faecalis*, *Staphylococcus albus* and *Streptococcus faecalis*, and bacteriostatic for *Pseudomonas aeruginosa* during *in-vitro* testing. The urine concentrations of ascorbic acid necessary to achieve such effects are easily attained by oral dosages. When the urine pH is maintained at 5.0 with DL-methionine, urine bacterial counts may be reduced a thousandfold.

In addition to their ability to suppress bacterial growth in the urinary tract, acidifiers enhance the pharmacologic activity of several urinary antiseptics and antibiotics. Lack of attention to the effective pH range of certain chemotherapeutic agents may lead to therapeutic failures. Urinary acidifiers are utilized in the treatment of chronic recurrent urinary tract infections in which long-term therapy is common. Often, they are used in conjunction with the urinary antiseptics discussed below. In general, acidifiers are nontoxic and may be used safely for long periods of time.

## USE IN CYSTITIS

Urinary acidifiers are of questionable value in the therapy of cystitis caused by urea-splitting bacteria (*Proteus* spp. and staphylococci). These bacteria degrade urea to ammonia, raising the urine pH. Success has been variable in controlling cystitis caused by urea-splitting bacteria with urinary acidifiers, because they may not be able to overcome the continuous production of urease and subsequently ammonia by such organisms. Such cases are best treated with antibiotics effective at an alkaline pH (gentamicin, kanamycin and streptomycin). Once infection is controlled, acidification and antibiotics effective in an acid environment may be utilized. Vigorous attempts to acidify the urine in treating cystitis caused by urea-splitting bacteria can result in serious metabolic acidosis, while producing no significant reduction in urine pH.

## USE IN THERAPY FOR URINARY CALCULI

Urinary acidifiers are considered valuable in the prophylactic therapy of certain types of urinary calculi. Urinary salts of calcium and magnesium (calcium phosphate, carbonate and ammonium magnesium phosphate) are more soluble in acid than in alkaline urine. The likelihood of such salts precipitating and forming calculi is reduced by maintaining an acid urine. In addition, since bacterial infection has been incriminated as a cause of phosphate urolith formation, and since acidification of the urine may control lower urinary tract infections, use of urinary acidifiers is indicated in treating certain types of urolithiasis. Alterations of urine pH alone should not be expected to provide complete control of uroliths, as multiple factors appear to be involved in their formation.

## CONTRAINDICATIONS

A number of contraindications to the use of urinary acidifiers exist. They should not be administered to any patient with a preexisting metabolic acidosis. Conditions commonly associated with an acidotic state include diabetes mellitus, renal failure, chronic diarrhea and hypoadrenocorticism. Urinary acidifiers also have no place in the immediate postobstructive therapy of cats with urolithiasis, since these animals are often uremic and acidotic. Urinary acidifiers should be utilized only after the uremic episode is over.

A number of antibiotics used to treat urinary tract infections are minimally effective in acid urine (streptomycin, kanamycin, gentamicin and neomycin) and, therefore, acidifiers may reduce or prevent their therapeutic effectiveness. Streptomycin, in particular, is 500 times more active at a pH of 8.5 than at 5.5. Several urinary calculi including xanthine, uric acid and cystine uroliths are more soluble in alkaline than in acid urine. Attempts to control the formation of these calculi include the administration of alkalinizing rather than acidifying agents.

A number of urinary acidifiers are known to be toxic to patients with hepatic failure. Ammonium chloride, DL-methionine and methenamine mandelate (Mandelamine® [Warner-Chilcott]) all may precipitate hepatic coma. The endogenous production of ammonia, and other by-products of the metabolism of these drugs, is thought to be the reason for their toxicity in patients with hepatic failure.

## DETERMINATION OF THERAPEUTIC EFFECTIVENESS

Individualization of drug dosage is necessary in every case. The dosage and frequency of administration are determined by patient response, unless toxic signs intervene. Urine pH is the primary criterion for determining therapeutic effect. The pH of the first voided morning urine has been recommended as the least likely to be altered by postprandial "alkaline tide" effects. In general, these drugs should be given frequently, i.e., 3 to 4 times daily, to maintain a consistent acid environment in the urinary tract. Urine sediment examination may be used in conjunction with pH as an index of clinical effectiveness. Both qualitative and quantitative assessment of acid-soluble urinary crystals serves as a crude index of drug adequacy. Particularly with struvite crystals in the cat, a marked decrease in quantity occurs when the urine pH is below 6.8.

The duration of therapy is highly variable. In the prophylactic therapy of recurrent feline urolithiasis, urinary acidifiers are often given for the life of the animal. The use of such drugs in cats that regularly eliminate an acid urine is questionable, however. In the dog, the benefits to be gained from long-term use of acidifiers in the control of acid-soluble calculi or chronic cystitis have yet to be determined. At present, available clinical data would tend to support the use of long-term therapy for these problems.

## URINARY ANTISEPTICS

This group of drugs includes a number of antibacterial agents that cannot be used to treat systemic infections. When sufficient quantities of these drugs are administered to attain effective plasma concentrations, systemic toxicity results. Such drugs are effective in combating urinary tract infections, however, since they are concentrated by the renal tubules and can back-diffuse into the renal parenchyma. Such drugs provide a form of local therapy, because only the kidney and bladder receive sufficient concentrations for antibacterial activity to occur. Some of the more commonly used urinary antiseptics are listed in Table 2.

*Methenamine* is a urinary tract antiseptic that derives its effect from its metabolism to formaldehyde. This drug decomposes in an acid environment to liberate formaldehyde and ammonia. Some ammonia production and intestinal loss may occur by the production of formaldehyde in the acid environment of the stomach. Thus, enteric-coated preparations are recommended. Because of this intestinal ammonia production, methenamine is contraindicated in hepatic failure. Except for this one contraindication, methenamine has virtually no systemic toxic effects, since no degradation occurs at the pH of blood. Since acid urine is critical for the antibacterial effect of this drug to develop, the urine pH should be maintained at 5.0 if possible. Methenamine is usually given in combination with mandelic acid (Mandelamine®) or hippuric acid (Hiprex® [Merrell-National]). Mandelic and hippuric acids have a bacteriostatic action in addition to their effect on pH. A more potent urinary acidifier may have to be given in conjunction with the previously mentioned weak organic acids to attain sufficient acidification. Methenamine alone is not contraindicated in renal failure, but the acids may be harmful. Methenamine is particularly useful in chronic cystitis caused by *E. coli* and other gram-negative urinary pathogens and has some effect on staphylococci. It is generally ineffective against *Proteus* spp., partially because of

**Table 2.** *Urinary Antiseptics and Dosage Recommendations*

| DRUG | DOSAGE (APPROXIMATE) | MANUFACTURER |
|---|---|---|
| Methenamine hippurate (Hiprex®) | 1.0-gm. tablets; ¼ tab/ 15 kg. body weight four times daily. Urine pH 5.0 or less | Merrell-National Labs., Division of Richardson-Merrell Inc., Cincinnati, Ohio 45215 |
| Methenamine mandelate (Mandelamine®) | 0.250-gm. tablet or suspension (0.250 gm/ teaspoon); 1 tablet/15 kg. body weight four times daily. Urine pH 5.0 or less. | Warner-Chilcott Labs., Morris Plains, New Jersey 07950 |
| Nalidixic acid* (NegGram®) | 250-mg. or 500-mg. capsules; 45 mg./kg./day divided into four equal doses. For prolonged usage, reduce dose to 30 mg./kg./day | Winthrop Labs., 90 Park Avenue, New York, New York 10016 |
| Nitrofurantoin (Furadantin®; Macrodantin®) | 50-mg. and 100-mg. tablets (Furadantin) or 25-mg capsules (Macrodantin); 4 mg./kg./day divided b.i.d. | Eaton Labs., Division of Norwich, Pharmacol Co., Norwich, New York 13815 |

*Use of nalidixic acid at dosages of 65 mg./kg./day in dogs and cats may result in convulsions. Even at the reduced dosage suggested, caution is advised. This drug has not been approved for veterinary use.

difficulties encountered with controlling urine pH in the presence of urease-producing bacteria.

*Nalidixic acid* (NegGram® [Winthrop]) is a synthetic antibacterial agent that is rapidly eliminated in the urine. Its use is limited exclusively to urinary tract infections. This drug is bactericidal to many common gram-negative urinary pathogens, including *E. coli*, *Klebsiella* spp., *Proteus* spp. and *Enterobacter*. Pseudomonas strains are singularly resistant. Rapid antibacterial resistance has been observed to occur with this agent. The plasma half-life is normally 8 hours in man but may be prolonged up to 24 hours in renal failure. This drug is usually administered for only one to two weeks. Nalidixic acid interferes with some urine glucose determinations, producing false positive reactions (Clinitest tablets*). At the present time, this drug is not approved for veterinary use in dogs or cats. When given at the recommended dosage for adults (65 mg./kg.), psychomotor seizures and grand mal convulsions may occur in cats and dogs. The use of a pediatric dosage (50 mg./kg./day) in four divided doses has been reported to be without these untoward reactions while remaining therapeutically effective (Bush, 1975).

*Nitrofurantoin* is a commonly used urinary tract antiseptic that is effective against many common urinary tract pathogens. Some of the more susceptible organisms include *E. coli*, *Klebsiella*, *Enterobacter*, staphylococci and streptococci. Occasional

*Proteus* and *Pseudomonas* strains are also susceptible. This drug is rapidly absorbed from the gastrointestinal tract and cleared from the plasma by the kidneys. Approximately 40 per cent is excreted unchanged in the urine. Nitrofurantoin is more effective in an acid urine (pH 5.5 or less). This drug is antagonistic to nalidixic acid. Nitrofurantoins are contraindicated in renal failure, since significant systemic toxicity can occur in the presence of impaired renal excretion (consult article on "Adverse Drug Reactions in the Uremic Patient").

Urinary antiseptics have their greatest clinical application in the therapy of chronic, antibiotic-resistant urinary tract infections. Drugs such as methenamine mandelate are particularly suited for long-term use when control is feasible but cure is unlikely.

## SUPPLEMENTAL READING

Bush, B. M.: Unexpected reaction to nalidixic acid. Vet. Rec., 96:255, 1975.

Goodman, L. S., and Gillman, H.: The Pharmacologic Basic of Therapeutics. 5th ed. The Macmillan Co., London, 1975.

Hardy, R. M., and Osborne, C. A.: The use and misuse of urinary acidifiers. Scientific Proceedings and Seminar Synopses of the 40th Annual Meeting of the American Animal Hospital Association, 1973.

Murphy, F. J., Zelman, S., and Mau, W.: Ascorbic acid as a urinary acidifying agent. 2. Its adjunctive role in chronic urinary infection. J. Urol., 94:300–305, 1965.

Short, E. C., and Hammond, P. B.: Ammonium chloride as a urinary acidifier. J. Am. Vet. Med. Assn., 144:864–867, 1964.

Yeaw, R. C.: The effect of pH on the growth of bacteria in urine. J. Urol., 44:669, 1940.

*Ames Laboratories.

---

# DISEASES OF THE URETHRA

RICHARD W. GREENE, D.V.M., *and* RICHARD C. SCOTT, D.V.M.
*New York, New York*

Diseases of the urethra seen in veterinary medicine include congenital anomalies, urethritis, tumors, obstruction, ruptures and prolapsed urethra. Since they are associated with other diseases of the urinary tract, a complete examination of the entire urinary system is necessary.

## CONGENITAL ANOMALIES

Congenital anomalies of the urethra occur infrequently in the dog and cat. They occur more often in males than females. Anomalies that have been reported include urethral agenesis, imperforate urethra and prepuce, hypospadias and epispadias, urethrorectal fistula and urethral diverticulum. Urethral abnormalities may also occur in association with hermaphroditism and pseudohermaphroditism. Since urethral anomalies may be associated with other abnormalities of the urinary tract, a complete examination should be performed prior to establishing a prognosis and formulating therapy.

## URETHRITIS

Urethritis is inflammation of the urethra. Bacterial urethritis may be associated with cystitis, prostatitis and vaginitis. While the etiologic agents causing bacterial urethritis are identical to those causing cystitis, prostatis and vaginitis, it is possible to have nonspecific urethritis in which no etiologic agents can be isolated.

Traumatic urethritis may occur as a result of excessive masturbation and licking, especially in the brachiocephalic breeds of dogs. It can also be caused by improper catheterization of the urethra of male or female dogs and cats during routine urine collection. Bite wounds of the penis may also cause traumatic urethritis. Inflammation resulting from trauma is frequently complicated by bacterial infection.

Urethritis can also be encountered following urethral obstruction in the dog and cat. (See articles on "Medical Management of the Feline Urologic Syndrome" and "Urohydropropulsion—Nonsurgical Removal of Urethral Calculi in Male Dogs.")

Clinical signs associated with urethritis include strangury and increased frequency of urination. If gross hematuria is present, it may be most prominent at the beginning of micturition. Dribbling of blood independent of micturition may also be encountered. If inflammation is severe and the urethral lumen becomes partially or completely occluded, severe strangury characterized by passage of urine may be observed. Complete inability to void urine as a result of uncomplicated urethritis is very uncommon.

### TREATMENT

If narrowing of the urethral lumen is severe enough to cause urine retention, it may be necessary to pass a Foley-type catheter (Imex Foley Catheter*) to decompress the urinary tract. In some instances it may be necessary to suture the catheter in place so that the animal can readily eliminate urine while medical therapy is administered. Because adverse reaction to the catheter in the urethra is unavoidable, it should be removed as soon as possible.

If urethral obstruction is due to calculi, surgical or nonsurgical removal of the obstruction is necessary in addition to medical therapy (refer to the article on "Urohydropropulsion").

Urethritis associated with masturbation may be controlled and prevented in some cases by castration.

Urethritis due to improper catheterization can be avoided if an attempt is made first to collect the urine by expressing the bladder and catching a midstream sample. If that fails, a sterile, well-lubricated catheter should be passed, using aseptic technique. The use of urinary antibiotics for 3 to 7 days following traumatic catheterization is a good prophylactic measure.

Antibacterial drug therapy is indicated in all types of urethritis. Ideally, bacterial culture and antibiotic sensitivity tests should be performed before instituting antibiotic therapy. We have had the best success with sulfisoxazole, chloramphenicol, gentamicin and nitrofurantoin. With the exception of gentamicin, these antibiotics should be used for at least 14 to 21 days. Gentamicin should be used for only 10 days, and then should be followed by one of the other antibiotics listed.

In some cases, antispasmodics (Jenotone® [Jen Sal†], 2 to 4 mg./kg. body weight administered IM or 1 tablet/12 kg. body weight PO; or Octin® [Knoll], 0.25 to 0.50 ml. administered IM or 1/2 to 1 tablet every 12 hours PO) and anti-inflammatory agents are helpful in relieving the spasms, inflammation and strangury that occur as a result of urethritis. These drugs should be continued for 2 to 3 days.

## TUMORS

Urethral tumors of dogs are uncommon; they are rare in cats. The most common

---

*Sterile disposable catheter, Iminmed Corp., New York, New York; E. R. Squibb and Sons, Inc., Princeton, New Jersey 08540.

†Jen Sal Laboratories, Kansas City, Missouri 64141.

presenting signs are progressive hematuria and dysuria. In severe cases, the patient may have great difficulty in voiding urine as a result of almost complete obliteration of the urethral lumen. Neoplasms of the urethra are discussed in greater detail in the article on "Urinary Tract Tumors."

Differentiation between urethritis and neoplasia of the urethra is sometimes difficult. A positive contrast urethrogram or an exploratory laparotomy and biopsy of the urethra may be the only means of differentiating these diseases. (Consult the articles on "Retrograde Contrast Urethrography" and "Catheter Biopsy of the Urethra, Urinary Bladder and Prostate Gland.")

## OBSTRUCTION OF THE URETHRA

Obstruction of the urethra most often occurs as a result of urolithiasis but may also be due to urethritis, tumors, strictures and foreign bodies.

The majority of urethral calculi are seen in the male and originate from the urinary bladder. Calculi may lodge at any point along the urethra, but the most frequent site is at the caudal end of the os penis, where the urethra passes through the ventral groove.

Strictures of the urethra may be congenital or may occur as a result of injury by uroliths, catheters or trauma. Chronic urethritis occurring as a postoperative complication of urethrostomy in the cat or dog, prostatectomy in the dog or urethral surgery for traumatic urethral rupture may be associated with strictures. Urethral strictures usually consist of fibrous scar tissue in the urethral wall. The stricture may be a narrow band or it may cover an area of several centimeters. On occasion, contraction of the scar is so severe that it almost completely occludes the urethral lumen. The force of the urinary stream may dilate the lumen of the urethra located proximal to the stricture.

Urethral obstruction should be suspected in patients with dysuria. Depending on the degree and duration of urethral obstruction, signs may vary from a sudden complete stoppage of urination to dribbling, hematuria and strangury. Obstruction due to stricture formation is usually a gradual process, while obstruction caused by urolith formation is typically acute. If complete obstruction persists for more than two days, signs of uremia develop.

Physical examination typically reveals varying degrees of distention of the urinary bladder. The site of the obstruction may be palpated in the urethra.

Catheterization of the urethra will usually reveal the site of obstruction. The texture of resistance noted during passage of the catheter may help to differentiate calculi from soft tissue strictures. Radiographs are usually required to determine the underlying cause. Most radiopaque uroliths can easily be identified by survey radiography. When radiolucent calculi or stricture due to scar formation is suspected, contrast radiographs of the urethra may be required to detect radiolucent calculi or soft tissue lesions.

### TREATMENT

Initial treatment of urethral obstruction should be aimed at reestablishing urine flow. If the underlying cause of the obstruction cannot be immediately removed, an indwelling catheter should be sutured to the prepuce while appropriate symptomatic and supportive therapy is administered.

Nonsurgical methods of relieving obstruction should always be attempted prior to considering surgery (see articles on "Urohydropropulsion—Nonsurgical Removal of Urethral Calculi in Male Dogs" and "Medical Management of the Feline Urologic Syndrome"). If nonsurgical methods fail, a urethrostomy or cystotomy should be performed.

Urethral strictures may be dilated with forceps or various sized, well-lubricated catheters, depending on their location. The purpose of this procedure is to dilate the scar tissue without producing additional urethral damage. Urethral dilation may have to be repeated several times to obtain the desired effect. Urinary antibiotics should be administered postoperatively. Corticosteroids have been recommended by some to inhibit scar formation. In most cases, however, surgery is necessary for the permanent repair of urethral strictures. Coexisting upper urinary tract infections should be treated with antibiotics.

## URETHRAL RUPTURE

Ruptures of the urethra may occur as a result of traumatic pelvic fractures or as a result of bite wounds to the perineal and penile urethra. Rupture may also occur following improper urethral catheterization or in conjunction with urethral blockage due to calculi. Foreign objects occasionally injure the urethra.

Signs associated with urinary rupture of the pelvic urethra are identical to those associated with rupture of the urinary bladder (see article on "Urinary Tract Emergencies"). Ruptures elsewhere in the urethra are usually manifested by swelling, pain and tenderness due to extravasation of urine into the surrounding tissue. Hematuria, dribbling of fresh blood from the urethra and strangury may be also present.

The integrity of the urethra should be considered in all patients with pelvic fractures. Radiographs taken after the introduction of contrast medium through a catheter will usually show contrast medium in the periurethral tissue if a rupture exists (see article on "Retrograde Contrast Urethrography"). Small tears may be difficult to diagnose.

## TREATMENT

Since the urethra has good capacity to regenerate following injury, small tears may heal spontaneously. An indwelling catheter should be placed in the urethra, sutured to the prepuce and left in place for 7 to 14 days. An Elizabethan collar should be used to prevent the patient from removing the catheter.

In cats with rupture of the penile urethra, a perineal urethrostomy may be necessary. If the rupture occurs in the abdominal urethra, an antepubic urethrostomy may be performed if primary repair cannot be obtained.

If the distal urethra is lacerated in a male dog, a urethrostomy can be performed to bypass the tear. If the laceration is in the pelvic urethra, laparotomy may be necessary to expose and repair the urethra. If a small laceration is present, it can be sutured with 3-0 chromic catgut. When the rupture is complete, anastomosis can be performed by placing an indwelling Foley catheter in the urethral lumen and approximating the tissues with chromic catgut.

The administration of appropriate fluid and antibiotic therapy is important following surgical intervention. Draining the laceration site is mandatory in order to remove the collected urine. If the rupture is in the external urethra, hot compresses should be applied to the area. Indwelling catheters should be removed in 10 to 14 days. Urethral stricture may occur as a postoperative complication.

## PROLAPSE OF THE URETHRA IN MALE DOGS

Although a prolapsed urethra is an infrequent finding in the dog, it occurs most often in the brachiocephalic breeds such as English bulldogs and Boston terriers.

Urethral prolapse is usually associated with excessive licking of the prepuce and hemorrhage from the preputial orifice. Examination of the penis reveals that the mucosa protrudes from the urethral orifice. The protruding portion of the mucosa can vary in length and color, from bright red to purple, depending on the extent of self-mutilation. Most cases of prolapse of the penile urethra result from excessive sexual excitement or masturbation. Excessive straining resulting from genitourinary tract infection or urethral calculi may also be a cause.

## TREATMENT

The prolapsed penile urethra should be reduced as soon as possible to prevent edema and irreversible damage. The prolapsed portion may reduce itself spontaneously; however, in most cases it will recur, and permanent cure is unlikely.

Two surgical procedures have been used to correct the prolapsed portion of the urethra. One method involves placing the dog under general anesthesia and manually reducing the prolapse with a male urinary catheter. While the catheter is held in place, a pursestring suture of nonabsorbable material is placed at the penile orifice. The catheter is then removed, and the suture is left in place for 5 days.

The second method is amputation of the prolapsed portion of the urethra while the animal is under general anesthesia. The mucosa is resutured to the penile tissue with 5-0 chromic catgut. This can be done either by placing stay sutures in the mucosa or by placing two straight intestinal needles perpendicular to one another through the penile tissue to prevent retraction of the mucosa into the urethral lumen following amputation. If any calculi, foreign bodies or congenital defects are present on the penis or prepuce, correction should be made at this time. Balanoposthitis, if present, should also be treated.

Whichever surgical technique is used, careful postoperative treatment is necessary for success of the operation. Failures are usually due to poor postoperative management.

## POSTOPERATIVE MANAGEMENT

If urethritis is present, either as a cause or a result of prolapse, therapeutic dosages of antibiotics should be administered for a minimum of 14 to 21 days. Sulfisoxazole, chloramphenicol, nitrofurantoin and gentamicin are the antibiotics that have been used most successfully. Gentamicin is reserved for resistant infections. Antispasmodics (Jenotone®), 4 mg./kg. of body weight administered IM, or 1 tablet/12 kg. body weight PO, and anti-inflammatory agents are helpful in relieving the spasms, inflammation and straining that occur as a result of urethritis. These drugs should be continued for 2 to 3 days postoperatively.

Tranquilizers or Elizabethan collars must be used to prevent continued self-mutilation. Estrogens such as estradiol (ECP) cyclopentylpropionate (0.25 to 1 mg. IM) or diethylstilbestrol pearls (1 mg. s.i.d. orally) can be administered to prevent bleeding from the surgical site caused by sexual excitement. In many cases, castration may be necessary, especially when masturbation was the initiating cause of the prolapse. The dog's cage should be covered to prevent his becoming excited and should be cleared of any material that would allow masturbation. Ointments (Panalog® [Squibb]) can be infused into the prepuce to reduce inflammation or infection of the prepuce or penis.

The dog may be released from the hospital on the fourth postoperative day, either wearing an Elizabethan collar or placed on tranquilizers. Urinary antibiotics should be dispensed, along with Panalog® for infusion into the prepuce twice daily. The animal should be reexamined in 7 to 10 days.

### SUPPLEMENTAL READING

Archibald J., and Owen, R.: Urinary system. In Archibald, J. (ed.): Canine Surgery. 2nd Archibald ed. American Veterinary Publications, Inc., Santa Barbara, California, 1974, pp. 673–701.

Campbell, M. F., and Harrison, J. H. (eds.): Urology. Volumes I, II and III. Philadelphia, W. B. Saunders Co., 1970.

Firestone, W. M.: Prolapse of the male urethra. J. Am. Vet. Med. Assn., 99:135, 1941.

Greene, R. W., and Scott, R. C.: Lower urinary tract disease. In Ettinger, S. J. (ed.): Textbook of Veterinary Internal Medicine. Philadelphia, W. B. Saunders Co., 1975.

Hobson, H. P., and Heller, R. A.: Surgical correction of prolapse of the male urethra. Vet. Med./Small Animal Clin., 66:1177–1179, 1971.

Sinibaldi, K. R., and Greene, R. W.: Surgical correction of prolapse of the male urethra in three English bulldogs. J. Am. Anim. Hosp. Assn., 9:450–453, 1973.

# MEDICAL MANAGEMENT OF THE FELINE UROLOGIC SYNDROME

DELMAR R. FINCO, D.V.M.
*Athens, Georgia*

"Feline urologic syndrome" (FUS) is a clinical diagnosis made on the basis of dysuria and hematuria in both sexes and of urethral obstruction in some male cats. It is a general term that appropriately identifies the clinical problem until a more specific diagnosis can be made. Unfortunately, the cause or causes of FUS have not been adequately identified. Surveys have revealed that most cats with dysuria and hematuria do not have significant bacteriuria. The viral theory of cause of FUS is attractive but unproved. The role of numerous other factors suspected or accused of causing FUS has not been intensively investigated.

At present, therapy of FUS is supportive and symptomatic and medical recommendations for prophylaxis are based on assumptions rather than on facts. For this reason, some aspects of therapy—particularly those concerned with long-term prophylaxis—are based on personal opinion.

## DYSURIA AND HEMATURIA WITHOUT URETHRAL OBSTRUCTION

Dysuria and hematuria suggest bladder and/or urethral inflammation. If urethral obstruction, obvious anatomic abnormalities and urolithiasis are ruled out by means of physical examination, either further diagnostic procedures or formulation of a plan of symptomatic therapy is in order. I prefer to perform quantitative bacterial cultures and antimicrobial sensitivity tests and urinalysis at this time. While awaiting culture results, the patient is discharged with therapy designed to (1) decrease smooth muscle spasm and discomfort, (2) minimize formation of crystals that may irritate the bladder and (3) resolve bacterial urinary tract infection (if present).

Parasympatholytic drugs (atropine, scopolamine, hyoscyamine) are used as antispasmodics at a dose of 0.25 mg. b.i.d. The owner is advised of side effects of these drugs, including mydriasis, constipation and decreased saliva secretion that causes licking.

About 1.0 gm. of salt is given each day to increase urine volume. Increased urine volume decreases the likelihood of crystal formation by decreasing the solvent:solute ratio of those salts likely to form crystals. Table salt may be mixed with food (1/4 tsp. equals about 1 gm.). Noncoated salt tablets may be administered orally but should be given after the cat eats in order to avoid gastric irritation and vomiting.

Studies have revealed that most cats with FUS have acid urine. In cases in which urine pH is above 6.8, it may be helpful to decrease urinary pH with urine acidifiers (see article on "Indications for Acidifiers and Antiseptics in Urinary Tract Disorders"). An initial dose of 100 mg. b.i.d. of D,L-methionine is given, but the dose should be adjusted to attain the urine pH desired.

Sulfonamides or chloramphenicol is ad-
ministered orally until results of quantitative urine cultures are available. If significant bacteriuria on an expressed sample is absent ($<10^3$ organisms/ml.), antibacterial therapy is discontinued. If significant bacteriuria is present ($>10^5$ organisms/ml.), sensitivity results are used to make appropriate choices of antibiotics. Detection of significant bacteriuria allows refinement of the FUS diagnosis to urinary tract infection, which can then be treated as outlined elsewhere (see articles on "Bacterial Infections of the Urinary Tract" and "Pyelonephritis").

Since the frequency of significant bacteriuria in cases of FUS is low, an alternative to initial urine culture may be the treatment of FUS for 10 to 14 days with antibiotics selected on an empirical basis. If signs do not resolve, urine culture should be performed (after antibiotics have been discontinued for 5 days) to determine whether significant bacteriuria exists. In the absence of significant bacteriuria, continued antibiotic therapy cannot be justified in chronic cases of dysuria and hematuria.

The client is informed that FUS may be chronic, and that the symptomatic therapy may not totally resolve the signs. Owners of male cats are warned about the signs and consequences of urethral obstruction. Persistence of signs for several weeks is justification for a contrast cystogram and urethrogram to determine whether anatomic defects of the bladder or urethra are present. The client is requested to provide adequate clean, cold water for the cat and to provide a balanced diet. No recommendations are made to the client concerning dry vs. canned foods.

## URETHRAL OBSTRUCTION

### PATHOPHYSIOLOGY

Urethral obstruction is a medical emergency. Observation of cats with induced feline urethral obstruction revealed that clinical signs are absent during the first 24 hours of obstruction, but become fulminating thereafter. However, the duration of time between blockage and signs of severe illness is variable. This variation may be related to bladder capacity and to the degree of trauma to the bladder mucosa. Severe bladder trauma occurs from distention and alterations in vascular perfusion. With damage, components of urine are reabsorbed into the blood, accentuating the severity of the condition. Obstruction lasting 72 hours is usually fatal unless emergency therapy is rendered.

The severity of alterations present in an obstructed cat at the time of entry will obviously depend on the astuteness of observation by the owner and his knowledge of the seriousness of the situation. As the public becomes familiar with FUS, more cases are presented before the physical condition of the cat has deteriorated severely. The alterations subsequently described for urethral obstruction in the cat typify the severe illness. Cases presented to the veterinarian can be expected to span the spectrum between normal and severe illness.

Ultimately, urethral obstruction causes dehydration (5 to 10 per cent), hyperkalemia, metabolic acidosis, hypocalcemia, hyperphosphatemia, mild hyponatremia, azotemia and hypothermia. Dehydration occurs because of lack of water intake and because of water loss from vomiting and insensible loss. Mild hyponatremia may be related to vomiting. Acidosis, hyperkalemia, azotemia and hyperphosphatemia are consequences of anuria. The moderate hypocalcemia is probably related to hyperphosphatemia.

## TREATMENT OF OBSTRUCTION

Therapy for urethral obstruction consists of the following: (1) removal of obstruction; (2) short-term maintenance of urethral patency; (3) correction of water, electrolyte and acid-base alterations; (4) body temperature and nutritional considerations; and (5) long-term prophylactic procedures. In the cat that is not extremely ill, treatment will usually be administered in the preceding order. In the moribund cat, however, it is probably advantageous to initiate (3) first and then proceed with (1) while parenteral fluids are being administered.

**Removal of Obstruction.** Principles to be followed in removal of obstruction include (1) use of clean procedures and sterile equipment and supplies, and (2) use of techniques that minimize trauma to the penis, urethra and urinary bladder.

Minimal physical or pharmacologic restraint of the cat should be used. The moribund cat may require no restraint; the alert, cantankerous cat may require general anesthesia. Inhalation anesthetics are preferred for general anesthesia.

Each clinician develops manipulative techniques that he or she prefers for relief of obstruction. I prefer to extrude the cat's penis and gently roll the tip between the finger and thumb in an attempt to dislodge debris in the tip. If this is not successful, the penis is gently washed with warm water, and a 3-1/2 French rubber catheter* coated with sterile lubricant is inserted into the urethra with a sterile forcep as saline is injected. If the obstruction is removed or forced back into the bladder, the catheter is inserted into the bladder and affixed to the prepuce as will be described later. If the obstruction cannot be removed or the rubber catheter cannot be passed beyond its eyelets, a polyethylene tomcat catheter* is used to back-flush. Since it is more rigid and has an opening on the end rather than side eyelets, it may be used successfully when the rubber catheter cannot. However, it is also likely to induce greater trauma and should therefore be used cautiously.

Many solutions have been advocated for back-flushing the urethra; however, no comparative studies of their efficacy exist. Theoretically, solutions with an acid pH should be advantageous for dissolving struvite crystals. However, nonbuffered acid solutions are probably irritating to tissues, and therefore buffered solutions should be used. One such solution (Walpole's solution, pH 5.2) has been advocated.

If obstruction cannot be removed by back-flushing, it is helpful to empty the bladder by cystocentesis. After preparation of the overlying skin, bladder puncture is made with a 22-gauge needle attached to a three-way valve and syringe. The bladder is emptied as thoroughly as possible, and back-flushing is resumed. Although there is some risk of bladder leakage or laceration from cystocentesis if the organ is friable, no superior alternatives exist for management of the problem.

During manipulations to remove obstruction, digital compression of the urinary bladder should be done gently and sparingly.

**Short-term Maintenance of Urethral Patency.** Recurrence of urethral obstruction within hours or a few days of removal of obstruction is common. Attempts to reinstitute urethral patency by repeated episodes of flushing and compression of the bladder

---

*Sherwood Medical Industries, Inc., St. Louis, Missouri 63103.

may lead to a vicious cycle of trauma, swelling and obstruction. For this reason, short-term use of indwelling urinary catheters is helpful in the management of the obstructed tomcat. Principles governing use of indwelling catheters in the cat are (1) use of a pliable rubber catheter to minimize trauma, (2) use of sterile technique in placement of the urinary catheter, (3) proper placement and adequate fixation of the catheter and (4) antibiotic therapy during and for at least 5 days following removal of the catheter.

A sterile, 3-1/2 French rubber catheter is used. This catheter is more difficult to pass than polyethylene catheters because of its flexibility, but it is better tolerated and less traumatic for the cat. The catheter tip is coated with sterile water-soluble lubricant and inserted in the urethra by manipulation with sterile forceps. An assistant slowly injects saline through the catheter as it is inserted; this apparently dilates the urethra and facilitates passage of the catheter. Once the catheter is passed to a point near the bladder, the assistant aspirates gently instead of injecting. As soon as urine can be aspirated, insertion of the catheter should be discontinued. Overinsertion of the catheter must be avoided, since it causes bladder trauma. Overinsertion may also lead to premature removal of the catheter by the cat, because bladder contraction can force the catheter out sufficiently far so that an external loop forms at the preputial orifice. The catheter is cut with 1/2 inch protruding from the penis. The end of the catheter is dried, retracted slightly, wrapped with 1/4-inch wide adhesive tape and sutured with two sutures to the prepuce (Fig. 1). Antibiotic ointment is placed in the preputial sheath. An Elizabethan collar is placed around the cat's neck to prevent automutilation. The catheter is usually left in place for 72 hours but may be removed sooner if gross evidence of hematuria disappears. Penicillin and streptomycin are administered IM during hospitalization. Oral antibacterial agents (sulfonamides, chloramphenicol) are given by the owner to maintain therapy for at least 5 days following removal of the catheter. Sterile techniques in placing the catheter and antibacterial therapy are essential, since indwelling urinary catheters are commonly associated with bacterial infection of the urinary tract. The cat is observed in the hospital for 24 hours after the catheter has been removed

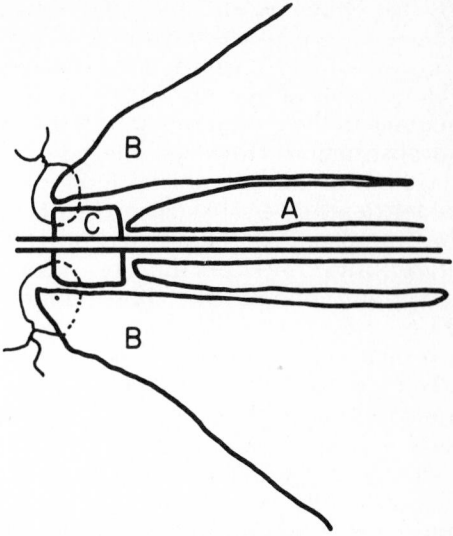

**Figure 1.** Schematic representation of an indwelling catheter properly placed and immobilized in the male cat. *A*, Penis. *B*, Prepuce. *C*, Adhesive tape wrapped around the catheter. The distal edge of the tape is sutured to the prepuce, so that only the tip of the catheter protrudes from the urethral orifice.

to determine whether urination can occur in a satisfactory manner.

**Correction of Water, Electrolyte and Acid-Base Alterations.** Of the alterations previously listed in this category, state of hydration, serum potassium concentration and acid-base status are the factors of greatest therapeutic importance.

Many cats are presented with FUS without significant imbalances, but others may have alterations that are life-threatening. Severe hyperkalemia is the most critical; it is accentuated by hemoconcentration associated with dehydration. It is imperative to manage the gravely ill cat with FUS on the assumption that hyperkalemia exists without waiting for laboratory confirmation. An electrocardiogram may indicate whether hyperkalemia is present, but the moribund cat may die if treatment is delayed. Consequently, treatment should be instituted immediately. A sample of blood taken at the time of venipuncture for fluid therapy can be used for laboratory analysis at a later date; its value will be explained later in this article. Once therapy has been initiated, an electrocardiogram can be obtained if desired.

Fortunately, a significant decrease in hyperkalemia can be achieved by relief of obstruction and administration of multiple electrolyte solution to correct water and acid-base deficiencies. Thus, all major imbalances (hyperkalemia, dehydration, acidosis) can be corrected by means of techniques used at present by most veterinarians in the management of feline urethral obstruction. However, the rate, route and volume of fluid administration is critical in order to achieve satisfactory results. The following scheme of therapy has proved effective both in experimental urethral obstruction and in cats with obstruction due to FUS.

Urethral obstruction is removed by methods previously described. The degree of dehydration is estimated (see article on "Fluid Therapy"), and intravenous administration of a warmed multiple electrolyte solution* is begun. The rate of flow is adjusted so that administration of the entire deficit is completed during one hour. At the completion of intravenous fluid administration, daily maintenance requirements (see "Fluid Therapy") are administered via subcutaneous injection. The state of hydration is subsequently evaluated by means of clinical examination and body weight determinations. Additional fluids are administered as needed. It is not uncommon for a cat to require 250 to 300 ml. of fluid/day following initial therapy. Fluid requirements after relief of obstruction may be large in the azotemic cat because an osmotic diuresis is associated with renal excretion of urea and other nitrogenous wastes. Renal damage associated with obstruction may also impair the cat's ability to concentrate urine. Failure to provide an adequate quantity of fluid following relief of obstruction is a common error in the management of urethral obstruction. If an error is to be made in the quantity of fluid to be administered, it should be made in the direction of giving more than is actually needed. The excess fluid will be excreted by the kidney and will provide additional solvent for removal of bladder debris.

Response to therapy is routinely evaluated by clinical observation and evaluation of BUN concentration. Evaluation of serum electrolytes and acid-base data will provide specific data concerning the status of the patient, but these tests may not always be available. Following removal of obstruction and administration of fluid therapy previously outlined, serum potassium and acid-base alterations were totally corrected in 24 hours in cats with experimental urethral obstruction. By contrast, in 24 hours BUN had decreased from 190 mg./dl. to 85 mg./dl. but was not normal until 48 to 72 hours. This suggests that monitoring BUN in cats with FUS may be used to determine whether hyperkalemia has persisted. If posttherapy BUN values are markedly decreased, it is likely that serum potassium concentration is normal.

Insulin and glucose are known to be effective in emergency treatment of hyperkalemia in other species, but the effect is dose-related. Although insulin and glucose have been used in the cat, simultaneous fluid therapy and relief of obstruction were also provided, and therefore no conclusions can be drawn concerning efficacy of the glucose-insulin therapy. Studies are needed to determine the effective dose of insulin for treatment of hyperkalemia in the cat.

**Body Temperature and Nutritional Considerations.** Cats with FUS that are extremely ill frequently have hypothermia. Therefore, fluids used to treat the cat should be warmed prior to administration. The hypothermic cat should be placed on a heating pad as soon as possible, and the temperature should be monitored until normothermia occurs. Normal body temperature is usually maintained by the cat 24 hours following relief of obstruction.

Studies with induced feline obstruction revealed that loss of body weight occurred that was not attributable to dehydration. This weight loss progressed for several days after relief of obstruction. It has not been established whether this weight loss is reversed by forced feeding or gavage, but close attention to the nutritional state of the cat with urethral obstruction is in order.

**Long-Term Prophylaxis of Urethral Obstruction.** Prevention of recurrence of urethral obstruction by medical manipulation is controversial. I restrict my recommendations to (1) use of salt orally for the life of the patient to induce water intake and increase urine output; (2) free access to clean, cold water; and (3) use of D,L-methionine as a urine acidifier in those cats in which acid urine is not produced. No dietary recommendations are made except to emphasize the need for a balanced diet.

Surgical procedures, predominantly perineal urethrostomy, are becoming more

---

*Lactated Ringer's solution, Multisol-R® (Abbott) or comparable products.

popular as prophylactic treatment for cats with FUS. Improvement in surgical techniques and the increased competency of the surgeon have apparently resulted in a decrease in the incidence of surgical complications. Since reports of long-term follow-up of surgical patients are not available at present, the long-term incidence of complications is unknown.

Surgery is contraindicated during the severe illness associated with urethral obstruction. Since some cats have but one episode of obstruction, and since the incidence of urethral obstruction decreases with age, conservative medical manage-ment seems logical during initial encounters with the problem. Surgery may be considered in instances of repeated obstruction or penile urethral stenosis. If surgery is recommended, the client should be advised that urethral obstruction, but not dysuria and hematuria, are remedied by the procedure.

### SUPPLEMENTAL READING

Finco, D. R., Kneller, S. K., and Crowell, W. A.: Diseases of the urinary system. *In* Catcott, E. J.: Feline Medicine and Surgery. 2nd ed. American Veterinary Publications, Inc., Santa Barbara, California, 1975.

# RETROGRADE CONTRAST URE-THROGRAPHY

GARY R. JOHNSTON, D.V.M.,
CARL R. JESSEN, D.V.M.,
*and* CARL A. OSBORNE, D.V.M.
*St. Paul, Minnesota*

## INDICATIONS

Radiographic evaluation of the urethra is an important diagnostic procedure for localizing diseases of the lower urinary tract of dogs and cats associated with dysuria, hematuria and partial or complete obstruction to urine outflow. We have found urethrography to be of value in the diagnosis of urethral neoplasms, calculi, strictures, trauma and anomalies. It has also been of value in the diagnosis of extraurethral diseases including disorders of the prostate gland and herniation of the urinary bladder.

## MATERIALS

**Catheters.** Urethral, ureteral and balloon catheters may be used (Fig. 1). Ureteral* and urethral** catheters (Nos. 3 to 10 French) are useful but will not prevent retrograde flow of contrast material out of the distal end of the urethra. In addition, a catheter adapter must be used with ureteral catheters to accommodate syringe tips.

Balloon catheters have the distinct advantage of preventing retrograde flow of contrast material out of the distal end of the urethra in male and female dogs and cats. Pediatric Foley catheters* have an inflata-ble balloon, are relatively inexpensive and can be sterilized by autoclaving. We have obtained excellent results with Swan-Ganz balloon catheters†. However, Swan-Ganz flow-directed balloon catheters are relatively expensive and should be resterilized with ethylene oxide gas.

Three-way directional valves‡ are recommended to aid in mixing and instilling contrast agents into the urethra.

**Positive Contrast Agents.** We have had success with organic iodinated compounds used for excretory urography (Hypaque-M, 75%® [Winthrop]; Renografin-76® [Squibb]; Conray® [Mallinckrodt]; etc.). To prevent backflow around the tips of nonballoon catheters these compounds should be mixed with sterile aqueous lubricants (K-Y Jelly®, [Johnson & Johnson], Lubafax® [Burroughs Wellcome], etc.) to increase their viscosity. In addition, increasing the viscosity of contrast agents will aid in distention of

---

*Available from American Cystoscope Makers, 609 East Channey St., Sullivan, Indiana 47882.

**Available from Sherwood Medical Industries, Inc., St. Louis, Missouri 63103.

†Available from Edwards Laboratories, 17221 Red Hill Avenue, Santa Ana, California 92705.

‡Available from Pharmaseal, Inc., Toa Alta, Puerto Rico 00758.

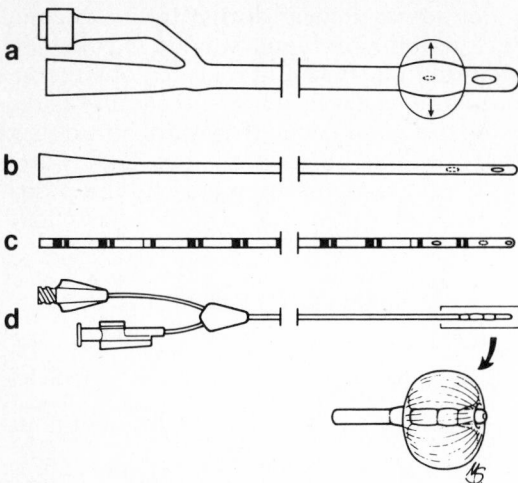

**Figure 1.** Drawings of catheters used for retrograde urethrography in dogs and cats: *a*, pediatric Foley catheter—air injected through the upper arm of the catheter will inflate the balloon (arrows); *b*, polypropylene urethral catheter with two eyes; *c*, whistle-tip ureteral catheter; and *d*, Swan Ganz flow-directed balloon catheter—air injected into the valve (lower arm) will inflate the balloon (*insert*).

the urethral lumen. Dilution of the contrast agents will prevent obliteration of small lesions by highly concentrated (radiodense) contrast materials. A final concentration of 50 to 150 mg. of iodide per milliliter of solution can be obtained following a 2 to 5 fold dilution of most commercially prepared radiopaque contrast agents.

These ingredients may be mixed in a sterilized container with a syringe plunger. Alternatively, they may be mixed by connecting the tips of two large-capacity syringes, one partially filled with contrast material and the other partially filled with diluent, with a three-way valve. Injection back and forth between syringes will provide adequate mixing. Care must be taken to prevent air bubbles from being trapped in the solution during the mixing process, since they may be mistaken for urethral filling defects following injection into the urethra. If a No. 3-1/2 French catheter is used, equal volumes of contrast material, aqueous lubricant and saline will provide a solution that is sufficiently viscous to accomplish the objectives outlined above but that can readily be injected through the lumen of the catheter. Equal volumes of contrast agent and aqueous lubricant are recommended for use with No. 7 French or larger catheters.

**Negative Contrast Agents.** Air, carbon dioxide or nitrous oxide may be used as negative contrast agents. Although air will provide satisfactory results, it may cause vascular emboli if the mucosa of the urinary tract is not intact. The high solubility coefficient of carbon dioxide and nitrous oxide prevents fatal embolism in instances of inadvertent escape into blood vessels. If negative contrast agents are used, exposure factors with reduced kvp. should be selected, e.g., kvp. reduced 10 per cent from optimal value.

## PROCEDURE

Proper patient preparation is prerequisite to optimal roentgenographic visualization of urethral lesions. The patient may be sedated or anesthetized following a cleansing enema. Overnight fasting and the use of purgatives are unnecessary, unless the kidneys, ureters and/or urinary bladder are also to be evaluated. Urine should be removed from the bladder by manual compression through the bladder wall, catheterization or, if necessary, cystocentesis. Positioning for the lateral projection includes extending the rear limbs forward as far as possible. A true ventral-dorsal projection is not as valuable as an oblique projection because of interposition of vertebrae between the urethra and film, and superimposition of the penile urethra over the membranous and prostatic urethra in male dogs.

Survey radiographs should be obtained prior to the administration of contrast agents in order to evaluate patient preparation and exposure factors. In addition, contrast material may obscure or alter the appearance of urethral lesions.

**Male Dog.** Balloon catheters are recommended. Position the tip of the catheter distal to the os penis and inject 1 to 2 ml. of lidocaine to anesthetize the area adjacent to the inflated balloon. Inflate the balloon and inject additional lidocaine to anesthetize the remaining portion of the urethra. Inject a sufficient quantity of diluted contrast solution (10 to 15 ml.) to fill and distend the urethra, and expose the film just prior to completion of the injection. Interpretation of the urethrogram will be difficult if the entire urethral lumen is not filled with contrast material. Exposure of additional views should be preceded by the injection of additional contrast material.

If urethral or ureteral catheters are used, the diameter should be as large as is consistent with atraumatic technique to minimize retrograde flow of contrast material. Position the tip of the catheter just distal to the os penis, occlude the external urethral orifice by applying digital compression around the catheter and repeat the procedure described above. The operator's hand should be removed from the x-ray beam just prior to exposure. Alternatively, the catheter tip may be positioned just proximal to the os penis to eliminate the need for digital occlusion of the external urethral orifice around the catheter. The latter technique has the disadvantage of impairing evaluation of the urethra distal to the tip of the catheter.

If a lesion of the prostatic urethra is suspected, the catheter may be guided to the level of the prostate gland with the aid of digital palpation through the rectal wall. The eyes (openings) of the catheter should be within the prostatic urethra. Following injection of diluted contrast material (approximately 5 to 10 ml.), the film should be exposed.

**Female Dog.** Balloon catheters (No. 8 French Foley or Nos. 5 to 7 French Swan-Ganz) are recommended to prevent backflow of contrast material around the catheter. The tip of the catheter should be positioned so that it is just inside the external urethral orifice when inflated. The procedure should be completed as described for male dogs.

**Male Cat.** A No. 3-1/2 French open-ended urethral catheter, or preferably a No. 4 French Swan-Ganz catheter, is recommended. The technique is basically the same as that described for male dogs. If a urethral catheter is used, position the tip just beyond the external urethral orifice and occlude the lumen of the urethra by applying digital pressure at the tip of the penis. Alternatively, the tip of the catheter may be advanced to the level of the proximal penile urethra to eliminate the need for digital occlusion of the urethral lumen at the tip of the penis. Following injection of 1 to 2 ml. of lidocaine, inject a sufficient quantity of contrast material to distend the urethral lumen (approximately 3 to 5 ml.), and expose the x-ray film.

If a Swan-Ganz catheter is used, anesthetize the urethra with lidocaine injected through an abscess cannula (or other suitable instrument). Insert the tip of the catheter into the urethral lumen until the balloon is just proximal to the external urethral orifice. Proceed as described above.

**Female Cat.** A No. 5 to 7 French Swan-Ganz catheter is recommended. The technique is basically the same as that described for female dogs. Following anesthesia with lidocaine and placement of the catheter, inject approximately 3 to 5 ml. of contrast material into the urethral lumen.

## INTERPRETATION

The mucosal surface of the urethra of male and female dogs and cats is normally smooth (Figs. 2 to 5).

**Male Dog.** The penile urethra normally has a uniform diameter (Fig. 2). The membranous urethra may vary in diameter from one portion to the next, depending on the volume of contrast solution in the urethral lumen. If the urethral mucosa has not been anesthetized with lidocaine, muscular spasms may constrict the lumen of the penile or membranous urethra. These constrictions may be mistaken for strictures on standard radiographs. Normal urethral spasms can usually be differentiated from strictures by repeating the procedure following the use of lidocaine, or by performing contrast urethrography with the aid of fluoroscopy or image intensification.

A slight decrease in the diameter of the urethra normally occurs just distal to the prostate gland. The diameter of the prostatic urethra is variable, being dependent on the degree of distention of the urinary bladder. If the bladder is distended, intravesical pressure will result in dilation of the prostatic urethra; if the bladder is empty, the lumen of the prostatic urethra will be smaller in diameter.

**Female Dog.** The urethra may vary in diameter and shape, depending on the quantity of contrast material injected (Fig. 3). Longitudinal folds in the mucosal surface are normal. If a balloon catheter is used, a slight dilation adjacent to the inflated balloon is commonly observed.

**Male Cat.** The proximal membranous (preprostatic) and distal membranous (postprostatic) urethra is usually uniform in shape and diameter (Fig. 4). Radiographic visualization of the bulbus urethrae was not achieved in male cats by the techniques described herein. Slight variations in diameter

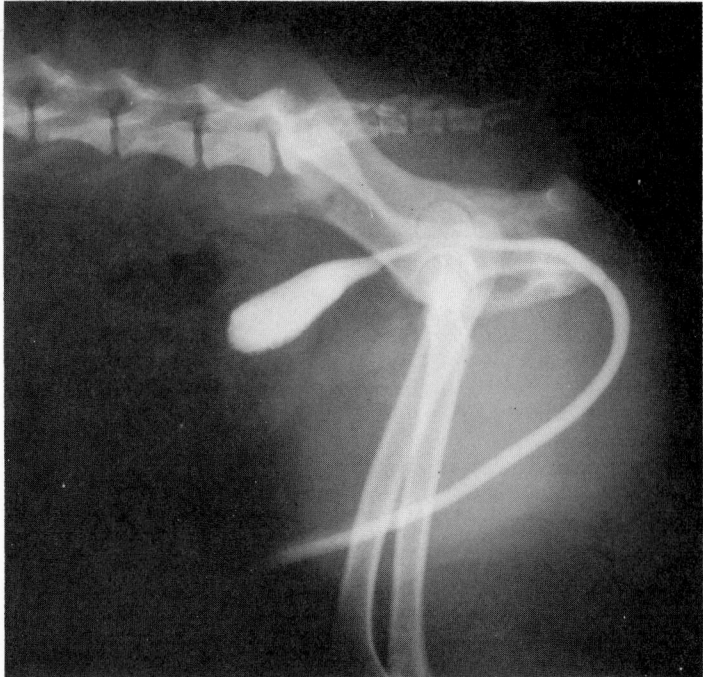

**Figure 2.** Normal retrograde urethrogram of an adult male dog. A Swan-Ganz catheter was used to prevent reflux of radiopaque contrast material out of the distal end of the urethra.

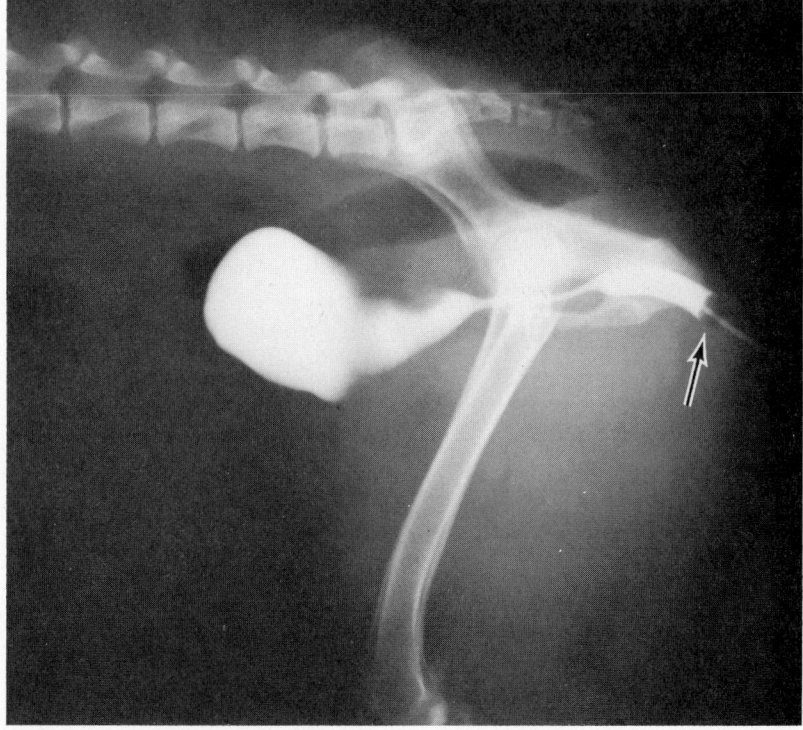

**Figure 3.** Normal retrograde urethrogram of an adult female dog. The inflated balloon of a Swan-Ganz catheter is visible in the urethra (arrow).

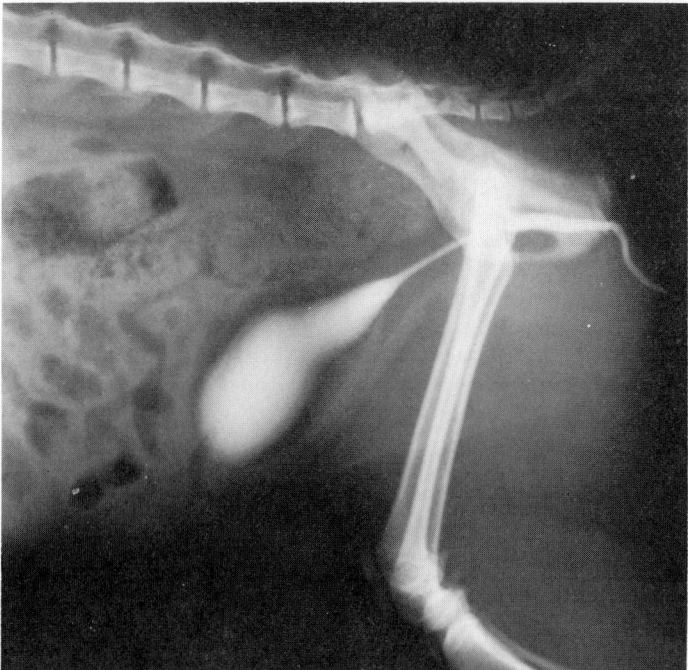

**Figure 4.** Normal retrograde urethrogram of an adult male cat. Retrograde flow of contrast material out the distal end of the urethra was prevented with a No. 4 French Swan-Ganz catheter.

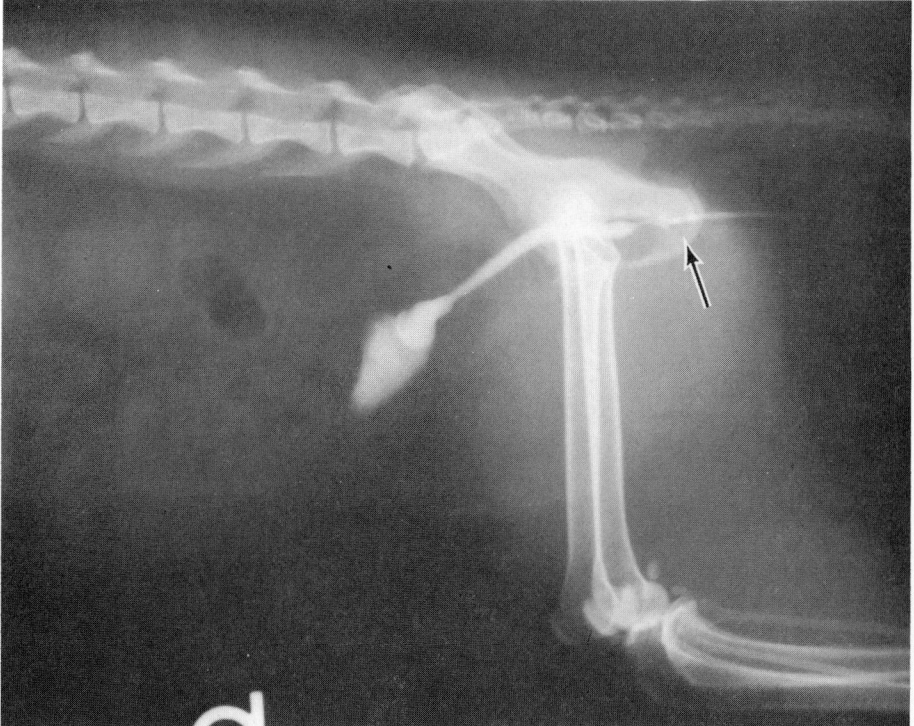

**Figure 5.** Normal retrograde urethrogram of an adult female cat. The balloon of a No. 4 French Swan-Ganz catheter is visible in the distal urethra (arrow).

from one portion of the urethra to the next may be observed if an insufficient quantity of local anesthetic has been injected, or if aqueous lubricant has not been mixed with the contrast material. A slight reduction in the diameter of the prostatic urethra is normal. The penile urethra is of maximum diameter at the level of the ischial arch, and gradually becomes smaller toward the external urethral orifice. Urethral spasms may occasionally be observed in the penile and distal membranous urethra.

**Female Cat.** The urethra may vary slightly in diameter and shape (Fig. 5). Longitudinal mucosal folds are normal.

**Abnormalities.** Urethral strictures are usually characterized by an abrupt reduction in the diameter of the urethral lumen and can always be detected at the same site on multiple radiographs. If strictures are caused by compression induced by extraurethral masses, the lesion causing the abnormality may be identified, and the contour of the mucosal surface is usually smooth. If strictures are caused by urethral neoplasms, calculi, traumatic wounds or surgical incisions, the mucosal surface is usually roughened and irregular.

One or more calculi may be observed anywhere along the urethra. Calculi that are radiopaque on survey radiographs may appear to be radiolucent when surrounded by contrast material.

Injection of contrast material into ruptured urethras will be followed by the escape of the material into the surrounding tissue.

Anomalies are often characterized by varying degrees of dilation and constriction of the urethral lumen. Ectopic termination of one or both ureters into the urethra can easily be detected by retrograde urethrography utilizing balloon catheters.

Soft tissue lesions localized with the aid of urethrography may be biopsied with the aid of a catheter (consult the article on "Catheter Biopsy of the Urethra, Urinary Bladder and Prostate Gland").

### SUPPLEMENTAL READING

Ackerman, N., Wingfield, W. A., and Corley, E. A.: Fatal air embolism associated with pneumourethrography and pneumocystography in a dog. J. Am. Vet. Med. Assn., *160*:1616–1618, 1972.

Morgan, J. P., Silverman, S., and Zontine, W. J.: Techniques of Veterinary Radiography. Davis, California, The Printer, 1975.

Park, R. D.: Urethrography. Vet. Clin. N. Am., *4*:883–887, 1974.

Ticer, J. W.: Radiographic Technique in Small Animal Practice. Philadelphia, W. B. Saunders Co., 1975.

Zontine, W. J.: The urethra. Mod. Vet. Prac., *56*:411–415, 1975.

# UROHYDRO-PROPULSION— NONSURGICAL REMOVAL OF URETHRAL CALCULI IN MALE DOGS

DONALD L. PIERMATTEI, D.V.M.
*Golden, Colorado*

*and* CARL A. OSBORNE, D.V.M.
*St. Paul, Minnesota*

Urethral calculi in male dogs invariably originate from the urinary bladder. Urethral uroliths may cause partial or complete obstruction to urine outflow at any point along the length of the urethra, but they do so most frequently at the caudal end of the os penis. At this site, the degree to which the cavernous urethra is capable of dilating is restricted by its passage through the ventral groove of the os penis.

## TECHNIQUE

### GENERAL CONSIDERATIONS

Regardless of the technique employed, care must be taken not to traumatize the urethra severely.

A liberal quantity of a mixture composed of one part sterilized aqueous lubricant (such as K-Y Jelly® [Johnson & Johnson], etc.) and 1 part sterilized water or saline should be injected through the flexible urethral catheter into the urethral lumen adjacent to the urolith(s). This maneuver will help to lubricate the calculi and the urethral mucosa, which is often inflamed and swollen.

If obstruction to urine outflow has been present for a sufficient period of time to cause a marked overdistention of the urinary bladder, it may be advisable to decompress the urinary outflow tract by attempting with care to pass a small-diameter (No. 3 French) catheter around the urolith. This will minimize the risk of rupturing the urinary bladder and may make the patient more cooperative by reducing the discomfort associated with urethral obstruction.

Depending on the disposition of the patient, sedation or general anesthesia may be required. Pharmacologic agents that are dependent on renal metabolism or renal excretion for inactivation and elimination from the body should be avoided. If an uncooperative patient is an anesthetic risk because of a uremic crisis, topical application of Anestacon* to the urethral mucosa, in combination with parenteral administration of low dosages of tranquilizers, may provide adequate patient restraint.

General anesthesia should be used whenever possible if calculi cannot be removed from the urethra of nonanesthetized patients by urohydropropulsion. We have encountered very few patients in which urethral calculi could not be removed following general anesthesia. Short-acting barbiturates (Surital® [Parke, Davis]) may be used, since they are primarily inactivated by the liver. Inhalant anesthetics such as halothane may also be considered, since they are not dependent on the kidneys for inactivation and excretion from the body. In addition, they permit rapid change in depth of anesthesia and allow rapid recovery following withdrawal.

*Two per cent lidocaine gel, Conal Pharmaceuticals Inc., Chicago, Illinois 60640.

### UROHYDROPROPULSION

Following lubrication of the calculi and urethral mucosa with an aqueous lubricant, an assistant should insert an index finger into the rectum and firmly occlude the lumen of the pelvic urethra by applying digital pressure against the ischium through the ventral wall of the rectum (Fig. 1). A bovine teat cannula (or suitable facsimile), with attached 35- to 60-ml. syringe loaded with sterilized saline, should then be inserted into the lumen of the penile urethra via the external urethral orifice. The penile urethra should be compressed around the shaft of the teat cannula by digital pressure. As a result of these maneuvers, a portion of the urethra from the external urethral orifice to the bony pelvis becomes a closed system (Fig. 1).

Saline should be injected into the urethra until a marked increase in the diameter of the pelvic urethra is perceived by the assistant (Fig. 1). Distention of the urethra to its maximum capacity must be achieved before a sufficient degree of pressure can be created within the urethral lumen to advance the calculi. At this point, the lumen of all portions of the isolated urethra, except that located in the ventral groove of the os penis, will be markedly dilated (Fig. 1). Dilation of the lumen of the segment of the urethra located in the ventral groove of the os penis is limited to that caused by stretching of the ventral portion of the urethral wall (Fig. 1).

**Antegrade Flush.** At this point in the maneuver, the teat cannula should be rapidly removed from the distal urethra. Simultaneously, digital pressure applied to the distal penile urethra should be rapidly released in order to permit rapid and forceful expulsion of saline out of the urethra (Fig. 1). Digital pressure applied to the pelvic urethra must be maintained. If the uroliths are small enough to pass through the distended portion of the urethra located in the ventral groove of the os penis, they will be carried with the saline toward the external urethral orifice. It is usually necessary to repeat the procedure several times in order to move the urolith(s) from the caudal end of the os penis to the external urethral orifice. The movement of the calculi within the urethral lumen may be monitored with the aid of a urethral catheter or, if necessary, by means of radiography.

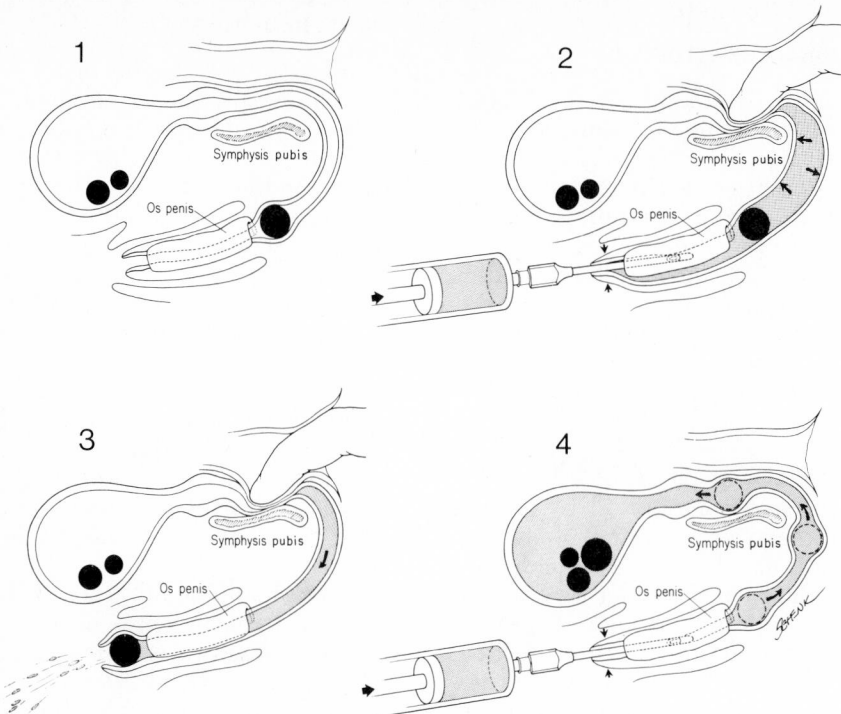

**Figure 1.**   Removal of urethral calculus by urohydropropulsion. *1*, Urethral calculus originating from urinary bladder lodged behind os penis. *2*, Dilation of urethral lumen by injecting fluid with pressure. Digital pressure applied to the external urethral orifice and the pubic urethra has created a closed system. *3*, Sudden release of digital pressure at the external urethral orifice and subsequent movement of fluid and calculus toward the external urethral orifice. *4*, Sudden release of digital pressure at the pubic urethra and subsequent movement of fluid and calculus toward the urinary bladder.

**Retrograde Flush.**   If the urethral calculi are too large to pass through the ventral groove of the os penis, the procedure should be modified. Instead of releasing digital pressure applied to the distal portion of the urethra, digital pressure applied to the pelvic urethra should be rapidly released (Fig. 1). Pressure should be maintained in the urethral lumen by forcing the syringe plunger forward until the assistant has released digital pressure applied through the rectal wall. This variation in technique will forcibly advance saline, and usually calculi, into the urinary bladder (Fig. 1). As was the situation with the antegrade flush, it may be necessary to repeat the procedure several times before the calculi reach the urinary bladder. The position of the urolith(s) may be monitored by means of palpation of the perineal and pelvic urethra, with the aid of a urethral catheter or by means of radiography.

Since urethral calculi invariably originate from the urinary bladder and are usually associated with cystoliths, all the calculi may be removed by cystotomy, eliminating the need for urethrotomy.

### SUPPLEMENTAL READING

Osborne, C. A., Low, D. G., and Finco, D. R.: Canine and Feline Urology. Philadelphia, W. B. Saunders Co., 1972.
Piermattei, D. L., and Osborne, C. A.: Nonsurgical removal of calculi from the urethra of male dogs. J. Am. Vet. Med. Assn., *159*:1755–1757, 1971.

Upper and Lower
Urinary Tract

# BACTERIAL INFECTIONS OF THE URINARY TRACT

JEFFREY S. KLAUSNER, D.V.M.,
*and* CARL A. OSBORNE, D.V.M.
*St. Paul, Minnesota*

## INTRODUCTION

Urinary tract infections (UTI) are associated with a variety of disorders that have in common the bacterial invasion of tissues composing the urinary system. The infection may be localized in the kidneys, ureters, bladder or urethra, or it may involve any combination of these structures. This article presents a general discussion of the etiopathogenesis, clinical findings, diagnosis and treatment of UTI. Consult other articles for details related to specific disease entities.

## ETIOLOGY

Both gram-positive and gram-negative bacteria have been isolated from dogs and cats with UTI (Table 1). Many of these organisms normally inhabit the large intestine. Although urinary tract infections are usually caused by a single species of bacteria, mixed infections may occu4 in a few instances.

**Table 1.** *Bacteria Frequently Isolated From Urine of Dogs and Cats With Urinary Tract Infections*

| GRAM-NEGATIVE | GRAM-POSITIVE |
|---|---|
| *Proteus* spp. | *Staphylococcus* spp. |
| *Escherichia coli* | *Streptococcus* spp. |
| *Pseudomonas aeruginosa* | |
| *Klebsiella* spp. | |
| *Pasteurella multocida* | |
| *Enterobacter* spp. | |

## PATHOPHYSIOLOGY

### NORMAL VS. ABNORMAL

In addition to polysystemic natural defense mechanisms, several characteristics of the urinary system make it inherently resistant to bacterial infection. Normal protective mechanisms include the anatomic structure of the urinary tract, frequent and complete voiding of urine, intrinsic antibacterial properties of the mucosa of the urinary tract and the antibacterial action of urine.

### ANATOMIC FEATURES

Urine in the kidneys, ureters and urinary bladder of normal dogs and cats is usually sterile. A resident population of bacteria is normally present in progressively increasing numbers from the proximal to the distal urethra. These organisms do not cause infections in normal animals. This is probably related, at least in part, to a functional high-pressure zone in the midurethra that prevents the migration of bacteria into the upper portion of the execretory pathway. Diseases that impair normal urethral pressures predispose the patient to infection.

In male dogs, the urinary tract is further protected from bacterial invasion by bactericidal prostatic secretions (Stamey *et al.*, 1968).

The specialized nature of the junction of the ureters with the urinary bladder also provides a protective effect. Although anatomic ureterovesical sphincters are not present, the oblique course of the ureters through the bladder wall at the trigone forms a flap valve, which normally prevents retrograde flow of urine from the bladder. Unidirectional flow of urine from the ureters into the bladder protects the kidneys from contamination with infected bladder urine. If the ureterovesical junction is damaged, vesicoureteral reflux will occur as soon as intraluminal bladder pressure exceeds intraluminal ureteral pressure. Secondary vesicoureteral reflux may occur in association with inflammation of the vesicoureteral junction, obstruction of the lower urinary tract, neurogenic disease of the bladder and ectopic ureters.

## MICTURITION

The mechanical washout induced by frequent and complete voiding of urine inhibits bacterial colonization of the urinary tract through the rapid elimination of organisms that reach the lumen of the urinary bladder. Diseases that decrease the frequency of normal micturition or that permit residual urine to remain in the urinary bladder following micturition (or both) predispose the patient to bacterial infection (Table 2). Once an infection is established, dysfunction in micturition may be further aggravated by bacteria (*Escherichia coli* and *Pseudomonas* spp.) that impair the contractility of smooth muscle (Grana *et al.*, 1968).

## MUCOSAL BARRIERS

The mucosa of the urinary bladder possesses intrinsic antibacterial properties. Although the exact mechanism(s) involved is unclear, it is apparently unrelated to serum antibody titers or phagocytosis (Norden *et al.*, 1968). Damage to the epithelial barrier caused by trauma (external force, calculi, catheterization, vigorous abdominal palpation, etc.) or neoplasia predispose the patient to secondary bacterial infection.

Urinary tract infections in dogs induce the production of specific local and systemic antibodies (Darwish *et al.*, 1968). The degree of benefit derived from the production of antibodies is unclear at the present time. Antibodies present in urine probably have minimal antibacterial activity because of the lack of complement activity and phagocytosis in the urine medium (Hanson *et al.*, 1975).

**Table 2.**   *Factors Predisposing to Urinary Tract Infection*

I.   Retention of urine
   A.   Mechanical obstruction to outflow
      1.   Urethral calculi, strictures, neoplasms
      2.   Herniated urinary bladder
      3.   Prostatic disease (uncommon)
   B.   Incomplete emptying of urinary bladder
      1.   Damaged innervation
         a.   Vertebral fractures, luxations, subluxations
         b.   Intervertebral disc disease
         c.   Vertebral osteomyelitis
         d.   Neoplasia
         e.   Vertebral or spinal cord anomalies
      2.   Anatomic defects
         a.   Vesicoureteral reflux
         b.   Diverticula
II.   Damage to epithelial barrier
   A.   Trauma
      1.   External force
      2.   Palpation
      3.   Catheterization
      4.   Calculi
   B.   Neoplasia
   C.   Excretion of cytotoxic drugs
III.   Altered urine volume or composition
   A.   Decreased urine volume
      1.   Decreased water consumption
      2.   Oliguric renal failure
   B.   Glucosuria (?)
IV.   Retrograde migration of bacteria
   A.   Congenital
      1.   Ectopic ureters
      2.   Urethral anomalies
      3.   Primary vesicoureteral reflux
   B.   Acquired
      1.   Urethral disease
      2.   Secondary vesicoureteral reflux
V.   Immunodeficiency
   A.   Disease
      1.   Congenital
      2.   Acquired
   B.   Immunosuppressant drugs

## ANTIBACTERIAL EFFECTS OF URINE

The antibacterial properties of urine are dependent on its composition. High concentrations of urea or organic acids, hyperosmolality and low pH inhibit bacterial growth (Mulholland *et al.*, 1969). Although the presence of glucose in urine has been incriminated as a predisposing cause of bacterial infection, cystitis has not been a frequent complication of diabetes mellitus in dogs or cats in our experience.

### ROUTES OF INFECTION

## ASCENDING ROUTE

Ascending migration of bacteria from the lower urinary and genital tracts is the most frequent route of infection. The intrinsic motility characteristic of some bacteria (*Proteus* spp., *Escherichia coli*, etc.) aids their retrograde migration through the excretory pathway. In man, there is a higher incidence of cystitis in females than in males. Uncontrolled clinical observations suggest a similar pattern in dogs. The latter may be related to the shorter length of the female urethra, through which bacteria must pass to reach the bladder.

## OTHER ROUTES

Potential routes of infection include extension from adjacent structures, dissemination of bacteria via blood vessels or lymphatics and descending migration from infected kidneys and ureters.

### UNCOMPLICATED VS. COMPLICATED INFECTION

Although some investigators have classified UTI as acute and chronic, this approach adds little to understanding the etiopathogenesis, diagnosis and treatment of this disorder because there is considerable overlap in cause, lesions and biologic behavior. Classifying UTI as complicated or uncomplicated is of much greater benefit to the clinician.

## UNCOMPLICATED INFECTION

Uncomplicated UTI occurs as a result of bacterial invasion of the urinary system without an obvious predisposing cause. The frequency with which it occurs in dogs and cats is unknown.

## COMPLICATED INFECTION

Complicated UTI occurs as a result of bacterial invasion of the urinary system secondary to identifiable diseases that interfere with the normal defense mechanisms of the body (Table 2). In such cases, the underlying cause must be removed or controlled if secondary bacterial infection is to be eliminated. Failure to do so often results in recurrent or persistent UTI.

## RECURRENT INFECTION

Recurrence of UTI following antibacterial therapy is common. Recurrences caused by the same organism that caused the initial infection are called relapses. Recurrences caused by a different organism are called reinfections. Recurrences may occur in uncomplicated or complicated cases of UTI and may be related to one or more of the following: failure to prescribe the proper antimicrobial agent, failure of the owner to administer the prescribed medication at the proper dosage and maintenance intervals, development of strains of bacteria that are resistant to antibacterial agents, failure to eliminate predisposing factors, and presence of deep-seated infections. Recurrences of UTI in human beings are usually caused by reinfection, unless a predisposing cause is present (Cattell, 1974).

## CLINICAL MANIFESTATIONS

Urinary tract infection may be symptomatic or asymptomatic. Clinical signs associated with UTI are variable, being dependent on the virulence of the causative organisms, the presence or absence of predisposing causes, the body's compensatory response to infection, the duration of infection and the site of infection. Of these factors, the site of the infection and the presence of predisposing causes probably are the most significant.

Signs characteristic of lower UTI include dysuria, frequent voiding of small quantities of urine and voiding of cloudy, foul-smelling or bloody urine. Abnormalities related to other body systems are usually absent in patients with uncomplicated infections. Their temperature, pulse and respirations are usually normal, they are alert and active and they usually have a normal appetite. Palpable abnormalities associated with uncomplicated lower UTI include any combination of the following (degree of change usually occurs in proportion to the severity and duration of infection): no detectable abnormalities, pain, spasm of the bladder musculature, an empty bladder or one that contains only a small quantity of urine, and thickening of the bladder wall. Palpable abnormalities associated with complicated lower UTI are dependent on the nature of the underlying cause (Table 2).

Signs characteristic of upper UTI are dependent on the degree of renal parenchymal involvement and the duration of the disease (consult the article on "Pyelonephritis"). Acute infections are uncommonly recognized in dogs and cats, but when present may be associated with fever, anorexia, depression and pain in the area of the kidneys, in addition to the typical signs of renal failure. Signs referrable to a predisposing cause may also be detected. Clinical signs associated with chronic generalized renal infection are similar to those associated with any cause of progressive, chronic, generalized renal disease.

## DIAGNOSIS

Information obtained from the history and physical examination may help to localize the source of clinical signs to the urinary system, but additional evaluation is required to localize the specific site of infection and to establish the underlying cause.

### URINALYSIS

Significant numbers of RBC, WBC and protein in urine are findings that suggest an active inflammatory lesion of the urinary tract. The detection of a significant number of bacteria in association with hematuria, pyuria and proteinuria indicates that the inflammatory lesion is active and has been *caused* or *complicated* by bacterial infection. The presence of more than 20 bacteria per high-power field in unstained sediment is suggestive of significant bacteriuria (i.e., greater than 100,000 organisms per milliliter of urine) (Kunin, 1972).

Urine pH will be alkaline if UTI is caused or complicated by urea-splitting bacteria. Urine pH may be acid, neutral or alkaline if the infection is caused by bacteria that do not produce urease. An alkaline urine pH in the absence of hematuria, pyuria, proteinuria and bacteriuria is usually a normal finding.

In order to localize the site of the inflammatory process, additional information is necessary. Signs of dysuria, increased frequency of micturition, thickening of the bladder wall, etc., indicate a disease process of the lower urinary tract. Involvement of the genital tract and urethra may be ruled out by careful collection of midstream urine samples or by collection of urine by catheterization or cystocentesis. Observation of WBC casts indicates renal tubular involvement in the inflammatory process;

absence of WBC casts does not exclude renal involvement in the inflammatory process. Additional procedures that may be of value in localizing the site of UTI include radiography and biopsy.

A direct immunofluorescent test capable of detecting bacteria coated with antibodies has been successfully used in man to distinguish between upper and lower UTI (Thomas *et al.*, 1974). Bacteria coated with antibodies are present in the urine of patients with upper UTI, but they rarely occur in patients with infections of the urinary bladder.

### URINE CULTURE

Urine should be collected for culture before antibacterial therapy is initiated. If antimicrobial therapy has already been instituted, it should be discontinued for approximately 5 days prior to urine culture in order to minimize the inhibition of *in-vitro* bacterial growth.

To be of value in diagnosis, prognosis and therapy, bacteriologic analyses must be performed on samples of urine that contain a representative sample of abnormal bacterial flora of the urinary tract. Urine for culture may be collected by obtaining a midstream sample during normal micturition, inducing micturition by applying digital pressure to the urinary bladder, catheterization or cystocentesis (Osborne *et al.*, 1972). Aseptic technique is mandatory if meaningful results are to be obtained. Only sterilized catheters and collection containers should be used, and the containers should have tight-fitting lids. Sterilized containers may be obtained by sterilizing paper cups in ethylene oxide gas or by sterilizing glass or metal drinking cups in an autoclave, or they may be purchased from commercial manufacturers.*

Because urine is a good culture medium at room temperature (bacterial counts may double every 45 minutes), it must be cultured within 30 minutes from the time of collection if significant results are to be obtained. If for any reason this is not possible, the samples should be immediately refrigerated. Refrigerated samples may be stored for several hours without significant additional growth of bacteria.

---

*Available from Falcon Co., 1950 Williams Drive, Oxnard, California 93030.

Although urine contained in the urinary bladder is normally sterile, urine that passes through the urethra and genital tract may become contaminated with resident bacteria normally present in these locations. The significance of bacteria in midstream urine samples, or those obtained by manual compression of the bladder may be difficult to interpret because they may represent pathogens or contaminants. Even catheterized samples may be contaminated as the catheter passes through the lower genital tract and urethral lumen. For this reason, urine culture techniques should include estimation of the numbers of bacteria present in each milliliter of urine (quantitative culture) in addition to identification of the bacterial organism(s) (qualitative culture).

The concept of significant bacteriuria was introduced to allow the diagnostician to distinguish between the harmless bacterial contaminants of urine and the pathogenic organisms causing infectious disease of the urinary system. This concept is based on the observation that a high bacterial count in a properly collected and cultured urine sample is indicative of UTI. In human beings, urine bacterial counts in excess of 100,000 organisms of a single species per milliliter of urine are considered to be significant (Kass, 1960). The isolation of 10,000 to 100,000 bacteria of a single species per milliliter in catheterized or midstream urine samples is interpreted as suspected bacterial infection. Urine from patients with suspected bacteriuria should be cultured a second time. If the same organism is isolated at a similar or higher concentration, the presence of bacterial infection is confirmed. The presence of less than 10,000 bacteria per milliliter in midstream or catheterized urine samples usually represents contaminants.

Although controlled experiments have not been performed, clinical studies of quantitative urine culture performed at the University Veterinary Hospital, University of Minnesota, utilizing the calibrated loop technique for quantitative culture have revealed that noncatheterized midstream urine samples and catheterized urine samples obtained from dogs with clinical, laboratory and radiographic evidence of urinary tract infection usually contained more than 100,000 bacteria per milliliter. Urine obtained from normal dogs was either sterile or contained less than 10,000 bacteria per milliliter of urine.

If the results of quantitative urine culture of noncatheterized midstream or catheterized urine samples are equivocal following serial cultures, collection of urine by cystocentesis should be considered. The presence of bacteria in urine aseptically collected by cystocentesis, even in low numbers, indicates the presence of UTI.

The most accurate results of quantitative bacterial culture of urine are obtained by dilution pour-plate methods and surface streaking of media plates with calibrated loops. Unfortunately these methods are relatively time-consuming and therefore have not been adopted as a routine procedure by most veterinarians. Recently several culture tests have been developed that permit rapid identification of significant bacteriuria. Clinical studies performed at the University of Minnesota revealed that Microstix®* reagent strips were of almost equal sensitivity as the calibrated loop technique in identifying significant bacteriuria in dogs and cats and in monitoring their response to antibacterial therapy (Klausner *et al.*, 1976). Encouraging results have also been obtained following preliminary evaluation of other commercially prepared screening tests† designed for quantitative urine culture. These tests should not be used as a substitute for standard laboratory procedures for bacterial culture, however, because they may be associated with false negative and false positive results, they may not permit identification of the type of bacteria causing UTI and they provide no information about the organism's *in-vitro* sensitivity to antimicrobial agents.

*In-vitro* antimicrobial sensitivity tests should be performed in conjunction with standard laboratory procedures for bacterial culture. The Kirby-Bauer method, a standardized disc diffusion technique, is recommended (Bauer *et al.*, 1959). Determination of the sensitivity of bacterial pathogens to antibacterial agents facilitates identification of infections associated with polyresistant bacteria and insures formulation of effective therapy.

---

*Microstix®, Ames Company, Elkart, Indiana 46514.

†Bacteriuria Screening Test, Baltimore Biologic Laboratory, Cockeysville, Maryland 21030; Culturia Test, Clinical Convenience Products, Inc., Madison, Wisconsin 53701.

## OTHER LABORATORY DATA

Leukocytosis, anemia, hypoproteinemia, etc., are rarely associated with bacterial infections of the lower urinary tract. If these abnormalities are detected, they should prompt a search for the presence of concomitant diseases of the kidneys, genital tract or other body systems.

## RADIOGRAPHY

Radiography is often indicated to detect diseases in which bacterial infection is not the only abnormality. Examples include urolithiasis, neoplasia, diverticula of the bladder wall, strictures of the urethra, etc. Radiographic detection of diffuse thickening of the bladder wall is suggestive of chronic cystitis but may also occur in association with diffuse neoplasia. Surgical biopsy may be required to differentiate the two diseases.

# TREATMENT

## SPECIFIC TREATMENT

The goals of therapy are the elimination of pathogenic bacteria from the urinary tract and the prevention of recurrent infection. The underlying cause(s) of complicated UTI must be eliminated or controlled if permanent eradication of bacterial pathogens is to be accomplished (consult other articles for details about urinary calculi, neoplasms, etc.).

Bacterial culture and determination of antibacterial sensitivity are advisable because many bacteria isolated from patients with UTI vary widely in their susceptibility to specific antimicrobial agents. *Pseudomonas aeruginosa, Proteus* spp., *Escherichia coli* and *Enterobacter* spp. are notable examples of urinary pathogens that are frequently associated with polyresistant strains (Hogle, 1970). When antibacterial agents are selected on the basis of antibacterial sensitivity tests, good immediate response is most likely to occur.

Although routine bacterial culture and antibiotic sensitivity testing of urine obtained from patients with acute cystitis is advisable, treatment without culture and sensitivity results is often dictated by economic and manpower considerations. If bacteriologic information is not available, a broad-spectrum antibiotic that attains high tissue and urine concentrations, and that is known to be effective in combating UTI caused by commonly isolated organisms, should be prescribed (Tables 1 and 3). For patients with chronic or recurrent UTI, culture and antibiotic sensitivity testing are essential if consistent response is to be obtained.

The effectiveness of bactericidal antibiotics (those that kill) as compared to that of bacteriostatic antibiotics (those that inhibit multiplication) has been the subject of considerable discussion and controversy. Although it would appear theoretically advantageous to kill rather than to inhibit the infecting organisms, this hypothesis has not been substantiated by data available in human medicine. Urinary tract infections often respond satisfactorily to agents that inhibit bacterial multiplication.

Avoid the use of antibiotic combinations, especially bacteriostatic and bactericidal combinations. If an antibiotic is clearly superior to others, and the patient can tolerate prolonged use without unwarranted risk, there is no logical reason to change. If it becomes necessary to use two or more drugs, they should be used serially (one at a time).

The dosage and interval between maintenance doses should conform to the recommendations of the manufacturer. Deep-seated and severe infections may require prolonged therapy with antibacterial agents that attain high tissue as well as high urine concentrations.

The duration of therapy should be tailored to the needs of the patient and therefore will vary with patient response to therapy. The absence of clinical signs is not itself a reliable index of successful eradication of infection. The duration of therapy should be based on the elimination of UTI

**Table 3.** *Antibacterial Agents Commonly Used to Treat Urinary Tract Infections*

| BROAD SPECTRUM | GRAM-NEGATIVE SPECTRUM | GRAM-POSITIVE SPECTRUM |
|---|---|---|
| Ampicillin | Gentamicin | Penicillins |
| Cephalosporins | Kanamycin | Tylosin |
| Chloramphenicol | Nitrofurantoin | |
| Hetacillin | Polymyxin-B* | |
| Sulfonamides | Streptomycin | |
| Tetracyclines | | |

*Especially *Pseudomonas* spp.

as detected by urine culture and urinalyses in addition to the amelioration of clinical signs. The following recommendations have been formulated as guidelines only; they should not be accepted as rigid facts.

The first episode of UTI should be treated for 2 to 3 weeks. It is recommended that chronic or recurrent urinary tract infection be treated for at least 4 to 6 weeks. Urine may be cultured with a commercially prepared screening test 3 to 5 days after the start of therapy (refer to earlier discussion of urine culture for details about screening tests for significant bacteriuria). Detection of significant bacterial growth in urine suggests that the antibacterial agent chosen for therapy is not effective and indicates the need for immediate reformulation of therapy (Stamey, 1972). Also perform a urine culture and urinalysis 3 to 4 days prior to the scheduled discontinuation of therapy (or sooner if necessary). Therapy may be discontinued if the urine is sterile and the urine sediment is normal. The results of urinalysis and urine culture should be evaluated 7 to 10 days following the discontinuation of therapy in order to detect recurrences at a subclinical stage.

If the results of posttherapy urinalyses and urine cultures are indicative of persistent or recurrent infection, continued therapy is essential. Persistent or recurrent UTI that does not respond to conventional antibacterial therapy is an absolute indication to evaluate the patient for a predisposing cause such as calculi, neoplasms, bladder diverticula, etc. Persistent or recurring infection should be handled by changing antibacterial agents, as suggested by sensitivity testing, until a satisfactory agent is found. Each product should be used for a sufficient period of time (at least 3 to 5 days) to evaluate its effectiveness.

In some patients with chronic UTI, eradication of pathogenic organisms or elimination of predisposing causes may be impossible. In such cases, it may be necessary to provide antibacterial therapy for the life of the patient. In our experience, ampicillin, nitrofurantoin and sulfisoxazole have usually been good choices for long-term therapy.

## ANCILLARY TREATMENT

**Urinary Acidifiers.** Urinary acidifiers have been advocated in the treatment of UTI because acid urine is somewhat bacteriostatic. Because the antimicrobial activity of urinary acidifiers is inferior to that of other products, however, they should be used only in conjunction with other modes of therapy. (For further details, consult the article on "Indications for Acidifiers and Antiseptics in Urinary Tract Disorders.")

Urinary acidifiers may also be used to enhance the pharmacologic activity of some antibiotics (penicillin, ampicillin, nitrofurantoins) and urinary antiseptics (methenamine).

Dosages of urinary acidifiers should be adjusted on the basis of response. Urine pH should be maintained at 6.5 or lower and should be monitored until it is established that acidification of urine is complete.

**Urinary Antiseptics.** Urinary antiseptics have been advocated as adjunctive therapy in the control of bacterial cystitis. (For further details, consult the article on "Indications for Acidifiers and Antiseptics in Urinary Tract Disorders".)

**Irrigation of the Bladder.** Although commonly used, this technique is of unproven and doubtful value. Intermittent irrigation of human urinary bladders with antibacterial solutions (neomycin, furacin, etc.) has provided only a transient antibacterial effect.

If this method of therapy is employed, only solutions which are known to be sterile should be injected into the bladder. The volume of solution should be sufficient to allow contact with all portions of the bladder mucosa. Caution in the use of solutions is recommended, since accumulation of large quantities of acid, anesthetic or antibiotic solutions within an inflamed urinary bladder may result in absorption and systemic toxicity.

**Increasing Urine Volume and Micturition.** The value of augmenting urine output by inducing polydipsia with oral salt is controversial. Increasing urine volume and urine output may enhance the elimination of bacteria and bacterial toxins. However, it may also reduce the antibacterial properties of urine and of the bladder mucosa and may decrease the concentration of antibacterial agents within the excretory pathway of the urinary system. Further evaluation is required before generalizations and specific recommendations can be established.

The patient should be provided with the opportunity to void urine frequently.

## SUMMARY OF THERAPEUTIC OBJECTIVES

1. Identify and eliminate predisposing (complicating) causes.

2. Identify causative bacteria by quantitative and qualitative culture techniques and choose antibacterial agents on the basis of antimicrobial sensitivity tests.

3. Treat aggressively with appropriate dosages of antibacterial agents. Alter urine pH to enhance antibacterial activity if necessary.

4. Continue antimicrobial therapy until there is clinical and laboratory evidence of response. Monitor the patient's response with bacterial cultures of urine and urinalyses.

5. Provide the patient with frequent opportunities to micturate.

## PROGNOSIS

If acute uncomplicated UTI is treated properly, a rapid remission of clinical signs usually occurs. The outcome of chronic uncomplicated UTI is more unpredictable (guarded). Although recurrences are common, cure is possible if proper therapy is administered for a sufficient period of time.

The prognosis for recovery from complicated UTI is dependent on the biologic behavior of the underlying cause. If the predisposing cause is eliminated, and adequate therapy for bacterial infection is provided, a favorable prognosis may be offered. If the predisposing cause is not or can not be eliminated, persistent infection or recurrences should be expected.

## SUPPLEMENTAL READING

Bauer, A. W., Perry, D. M., and Kirby, W. M.: Single-disc antibiotic-sensitivity testing of staphylococci. An analysis of technique and results. Arch. Intern. Med., *104*:208, 1959.

Cattell, W. R.: The management of urinary tract infection. Practitioner, *212*:27–36, 1974.

Darwish, M. E., Staubity, W. J., Scheuller, E. F., Rubin, M. I., and Neter, E.: Antibody response of dogs to experimental infection of bladder pouch. Invest. Urol., 6:66–71, 1968.

Grana, L., Donnellan, W. L., and Swenson, O.: Effects of Gram negative bacteria on ureteral structure and function. J. Urol., 99:539–550, 1968.

Hanson, L. A., *et al.*: Host-parasite relationship in urinary tract infections. Kidney Int., 8:28–34, 1975.

Hogle, R. M.: Antibacterial-agent sensitivity of bacteria isolated from dogs and cats. J. Am. Vet. Med. Assn., *156*:761–764, 1970.

Kass, E. H.: The role of asymptomatic bacteriuria in the pathogenesis of pyelonephritis. *In* Quinn, E. L., and Kass, E. H. (eds.): Biology of Pyelonephritis. Little, Brown and Co., Boston, 1960.

Klausner, J. S., Osborne, C. A., and Stevens, J. B.: Clinical evaluation of Microstix for detection of significant bacteriuria in the dog and cat. J. Vet. Res., 37:719–722, 1976.

Kunin, C. M.: Detection, Prevention and Management of Urinary Tract Infections. Philadelphia, Lea & Febiger, 1972.

Mulholland, S. G., Perry, J. R., and Gellinwake, J. Y.: The antibiotic properties of urine. Invest. Urol., 6:569–581, 1969.

Norden, C. W., Green, G. M., and Kass, E. H.: Antibacterial mechanisms of the urinary bladder. J. Clin. Invest., 47:2689, 1968.

Osborne, C. A., Low, D. G., and Finco, D. R.: Canine and Feline Urology. Philadelphia, W. B. Saunders Co., 1972.

Stamey, T. A.: Urinary Infections. Baltimore, The Williams and Wilkins Co., 1972.

Stamey, T. A., Fair, W. R., Timothy, M. M., and Chung, H. K.: Antibacterial nature of prostatic fluid. Nature, 218:444, 1968.

Thomas, V., Shelokov, A., and Forland, M.: Antibody-coated bacteria in the urine and the site of urinary-tract infection. New Engl. J. Med., 290:588–590, 1974.

---

# URINARY TRACT TUMORS

E. GREGORY MacEWEN, V.M.D.,
H. JAY HARVEY, D.V.M.,
*and* AMIYA K. PATNAIK, D.V.M.
*New York, New York*

Primary tumors of the urinary tract are uncommon, accounting for less than 0.5 per cent of the tumors seen in the dog and cat. Since there is no coordinated or systematic reporting and analysis of surgical biopsy data for canine and feline urinary tract tumors, the actual species and breed incidence of urinary tract tumors is unknown.

There is no known sex prevalence for these tumors, except for urethral carcinomas, which tend to occur more frequently in females. Most tumors are found in older animals (8 to 12 years of age), except for botryoid sarcomas, which occur in young dogs.

The etiology of urinary tract tumors is unknown, but bladder tumors have been experimentally induced in the dog with various dye compounds (e.g., naphthylamine). The clinical significance of this finding is unknown at this time.

The clinical manifestations of urinary tract tumors depend on the organ involved and the extent of disease, but most animals are presented because of one or more of the following signs: hematuria (gross or microscopic); palpable mass; strangury or incontinence. Dogs are rarely presented with signs directly attributable to renal failure.

Metastatic tumors in the kidney occur frequently and are usually found when there is metastatic spread to lungs and liver. Metastases rarely produce clinical signs, however, and are usually only apparent as incidental findings on postmortem examination. The most common metastatic tumors are mammary tumors, lymphosarcoma and hemangiosarcoma.

Very little information has been published on the incidence and histologic types of urinary tract tumors in dogs and cats. Thus, much of the data reported in this paper is the result of an analysis of 60 dogs with urinary tract tumors which underwent postmortem examination at The Animal Medical Center in the 10-year period from 1965 to 1975. All histopathology slides have been reviewed by one of the authors (AKP).

## RENAL TUMORS

### CLINICAL SIGNS

In our series of dogs and cats with primary renal tumors, most tumors were malignant. The most common tumor type was renal cell carcinoma or adenocarcinoma, which is a tumor derived from the tubular epithelium. Both types of tumors tend to occur in the right kidney more often (66 per cent) than in the left kidney and are rarely bilateral. Approximately one half the patients were presented not because of clinical signs related to renal disease (e.g., hematuria, polydipsia, etc.) but because of metastatic spread to other organs. These pa-

tients had a variety of clinical signs, including multiple subcutaneous masses, dyspnea from metastatic disease in the lungs, lethargy, weakness, anorexia and weight loss.

### DIAGNOSIS

A complete physical examination should be performed, and thoracic and abdominal radiographs should be taken. Further diagnostic studies, such as an intravenous pyelogram (IVP) and selective angiography may also be performed to delineate the extent of suspected renal masses.

Laboratory findings may include gross or microscopic hematuria. Anemia is usually present because of blood loss and, in some dogs, decreased erythropoietin levels. Polycythemia associated with renal adenocarcinoma has been reported in the dog but is rare, occurring in less than 5 per cent of cases. If metastasis to bones has occurred, the clinical pathologic findings may include hypercalcemia. An elevation in the blood urea nitrogen or creatinine should not occur unless 75 per cent of all kidney tissues has been destroyed.

Differential diagnoses include hydronephrosis, polycystic disease and feline infectious peritonitis without fluid accumulation. Thus, a biopsy and histologic examination are required for definitive diagnosis. An exploratory laparotomy is advised, as opposed to a closed percutaneous kidney biopsy, for the following reasons: (1) a more accurate biopsy can be obtained, (2) a nephrectomy can be performed for treatment and excision biopsy and (3) the remaining portion of the abdomen can be evaluated for possible metastatic disease. The most common types of tumors are renal carcinoma, transitional cell carcinoma of the pelvis, sarcomas and, in young animals (less than one year old), embryonal nephroma.

### TREATMENT AND PROGNOSIS

Prognosis depends on the histologic type of tumor and the extent of disease. Nephrectomy is the treatment of choice, provided that the remaining kidney is functioning normally. The affected kidney should be removed *en bloc* with its perirenal fat and adhering peritoneum. Total ureterectomy is indicated for tumors such as transitional cell carcinomas that originate in the renal pelvis. Ligation of renal vessels should be accomplished early in the procedure to minimize vascular dissemination of malignant cells. Excision and microscopic examination of regional lymph nodes may yield information of prognostic value. In our experience, most renal tumors have metastasized by the time a diagnosis is made. Regression of metastases following removal of primary renal tumors has been reported in humans but has not yet been reported in the dog.

Adjuvant therapy, chemotherapy or radiation therapy has not been adequately evaluated in the dog or cat. Radiation therapy would probably be detrimental because of the deep location and surrounding radiosensitive gut epithelium. Osborne (1974) reported that a partial regression was obtained after administering actinomycin D to a young dog with an embryonal nephroma. We attempted combined chemotherapy using cyclophosphamide (1 mg./kg. daily, orally), vincristine (0.0125 mg./kg. weekly, intravenously) and 5-fluorouracil (10 mg./kg. weekly, intravenously) in four dogs but did not obtain any disease regression.

In man, hormonal therapy has been advocated for disseminated renal carcinomas. We administered medroxyprogesterone (Provera® [Upjohn]) to one dog with a renal carcinoma, but the dog was euthanatized before an adequate evaluation of the effectiveness of therapy could be made.

There are few reports concerned with the histologic types or biologic behavior of renal tumors in the cat. In a recent review of 3145 postmortem examinations on cats over a 10-year period at The Animal Medical Center, one of the authors (AKP) found only two cases of renal cell carcinoma. Only one cat was treated; it survived 18 months after a nephrectomy.

## BLADDER TUMORS

Bladder tumors tend to occur in dogs with an average age of 9 to 10 years, although one type of bladder tumor, the botryoid rhabdomyosarcoma, tends to occur in young dogs (less than 18 months of age).

### CLINICAL SIGNS

The most common clinical signs of bladder tumors are hematuria, strangury and frequency of urination. Most dogs have a history of little or no response to prolonged antibiotic therapy for the cystitis. Physical examination may reveal a mass or thickening in the bladder.

### DIAGNOSIS

Radiographic evaluation of the bladder should include survey radiography and positive and negative contrast studies. Diffuse infiltrative tumors can produce a rough and thickened bladder wall, which is difficult to distinguish radiographically from chronic cystitis. An IVP can be performed to determine if obstruction is causing hydronephrosis or hydroureter. At least 20 to 25 per cent of our cases had some degree of hydroureter or hydronephrosis.

The final diagnosis can be made only on histologic examination of a biopsy sample. Urinary cytology is not that useful for establishing a firm diagnosis of malignancy (see article on "Catheter Biopsy of the Urethra Urinary Bladder and Prostate Gland"). In man, the cytologic findings agree with the histologic findings in about 50 per cent of the patients. In the animals seen at AMC, one third of the tumors were benign tumors (e.g., papillomas, leiomyomas and myxomas). About 90 per cent of the malignant tumors were of the transitional cell carcinoma type, while the remaining 10 per cent included leiomyosarcomas, hemangiosarcomas and the botryoid rhabdomyosarcomas.

The botryoid rhabdomyosarcoma is a tumor of embryonic myoblasts. It is reported most frequently in dogs 1 to 2 years old, in females and in St. Bernards, Dobermans, basset hounds and Great Danes. In most cases, the clinical signs (usually hematuria) have been present for up to 6 months. It is not uncommon to see hypertrophic pulmonary osteodystrophy associated with these tumors, even if there is no evidence of pulmonary metastasis. The tumors appear as friable, grapelike masses extending from the neck and trigone area into the lumen of the bladder. The prognosis is very poor, although we have not had the opportunity to attempt any therapy.

### TREATMENT AND PROGNOSIS

The type of treatment and prognosis of bladder tumors depend on the extent of the disease. Partial cystectomy is the treatment of choice when feasible. The regional lymph node should always be removed for histologic examination at the time of surgery to aid in the diagnosis and prognosis and to help determine the extent of disease. More radical extirpation may require ureteral transplantation, a technique of questionable practicality for household pets. Surgery has not been a very successful treatment for malignant tumors because of the usually advanced stage of disease at diagnosis and the infrequency with which discrete resectable tumors occur. We have found that about one third of the carcinomas have metastasized by the time the diagnosis is made. For nonresectable lesions, cryosurgery is another form of treatment that may be considered. Caution must be used in the application of the liquid nitrogen to prevent extensive necrosis of the surrounding normal tissue. We have not attempted cryosurgery on any of our clinical cases, but it has been used in man.

Chemotherapy has been attempted as an adjunct to surgery in the small number of cases with visible tumor remaining after surgery. The alkylating agents cyclophosphamide (2 mg./kg. daily, orally, or 10 mg./kg. weekly, intravenously) and thio-tepa (0.5 mg./kg. daily for 10 days, locally) were used. We were able to control the disease progression for a maximum of 6 months with minimal toxicity in 2 of 5 cases of bladder carcinoma after partial surgical excision. More studies are needed before the effectiveness of chemotherapy for bladder tumors can be adequately assessed. (Cancer chemotherapy is discussed fully in a separate article in this text.)

# URETHRAL TUMORS

## CLINICAL SIGNS AND DIAGNOSIS

Urethral tumors are rare and occur primarily in 10- to 11-year-old female dogs. In a recent review of 20 cases of urethral tumors, 18 were in females (Tarvin, 1976). Most dogs were presented with a history of strangury and hematuria. Digital palpation through the rectum may reveal a thickened and irregular urethra. Attempts to pass a urinary catheter may be unsuccessful because of stenosis. Radiographic procedures, such as a cystogram-pneumocystogram with a voiding urethrogram, may be used to define or demonstrate the extent of tumor involvement (see article on "Retrograde Contrast Urethrography"). In our series of cases, squamous cell carcinomas were most common, but a few sarcomas were also found.

## TREATMENT AND PROGNOSIS

Surgical excision is the treatment of choice. Tumors of the muscular layers, such as leiomyomas and leiomyosarcomas, may often be removed without entering the lumen of the urethra. The most useful surgical approach to the urethra in the female is by a posterior midline laparotomy combined, when necessary, with pubic symphysiotomy. Postoperative complications such as incontinence and stricture are more likely with extensive surgery. Localized or diffuse thickenings of the urethral wall should be biopsied before more radical surgery is performed in order to determine whether the lesion is neoplastic or granulomatous. The prognosis is very poor because the entire urethra is usually involved, making complete excision impossible. In addition, approximately one third of the patients had metastatic disease at the time of diagnosis (Tarvin, 1976). We have had no experience with treating these tumors with any form of chemotherapy.

Other therapeutic considerations include radiation therapy and cryosurgery. Cryosurgery needs to be investigated more extensively before generalities about its efficacy can be made.

## SUPPLEMENTAL READING

Kelly, D. F.: Rhabdomyosarcoma of the urinary bladder in dogs. Vet. Pathol., *10*:375–384, 1973.

Osborne, C. A.: Neoplasms of the urinary system. *In* Kirk, R. W. (ed.): Current Veterinary Therapy. Philadelphia, W. B. Saunders Co., 1974, pp. 878–883.

Osborne, C. A., Low, D. G., and Finco, D. R.: Canine and Feline Urology. Philadelphia, W. B. Saunders Co., 1972.

Osborne, C. A., Low, D. G., and Perman, V.: Neoplasms of the canine and feline urinary bladder. Clinical findings, diagnosis, and treatment. J. Am. Vet. Med. Assn., *152*:247, 1968.

Scott, R. C., and Patnaik, A. K.: Renal carcinoma with secondary polycythemia in the dog. J. Am. Anim. Hosp. Assn., 8:275–283, 1972.

Tarvin, G.: Primary canine urethral tumors. Surgical Residents' Seminar, The Animal Medical Center, New York, February, 1976.

# CYSTINE UROLITHIASIS

KENNETH C. BOVEE, D.V.M.
*Philadelphia, Pennsylvania*

Canine cystinuria is an inherited metabolic defect resulting in excessive excretion of the amino acid cystine. This inborn error of metabolism is caused by an anomaly of renal tubular transport of cystine and occasionally other amino acids. The only clinical consequence is the frequent formation of urinary calculi composed of almost pure cystine. Cystine calculi have been found only in the male dog, but cystinuria has been found in females in our laboratory.

This is not a rare condition; it represents approximately 10 per cent of all calculi in the dog. It occurs in many breeds and mongrels but appears to be most common in dachshunds. It is one of the most common causes of urethral obstruction in the male. The first episode of urethral obstruction due to cystine calculi usually occurs between the ages of 1-1/2 and 3 years. The fact that cystine calculi have not been found in the female may be explained by the wider urethral diameter allowing for the passage of small calculi.

Cystine is a nonessential sulfur-containing amino acid that is relatively insoluble in urine. It is normally present in the plasma in low concentrations and is associated with the metabolic pathway of methionine. Plasma levels of cystine in affected dogs are normal, indicating a faulty renal tubular reabsorption as the underlying basis for the cystinuria. The transport mechanism for cystine in the dog has recently been investigated (Bovee *et al.*, 1974). Cystine may be the primary and sole amino acid lost in the urine in some animals, or it may be accompanied by excessive loss of lysine or other dibasic amino acids. The mode of genetic transmission in the dog has not been completely established.

A male dog with cystine calculi may be seen at any stage of the familiar progression of cystic calculi, with intermittent hematuria and lower urinary tract obstruction. Bacterial cystitis seldom occurs in association with this calculus. These calculi are usually multiple and lodge in the urethra posterior to the os penis. They are small, round, smooth and yellow-brown in color. Diagnosis depends upon chemical identification of the cystine in the urine or the stone. The simple test for identification of cystine stones should be performed routinely, because these stones tend to recur, and specific treatment is beneficial.

Cystine calculi are more dense to x-rays than are the poorly visualized urate stones and are somewhat less dense than the more common triple phosphate calculi. Therefore, because of the number and size of calculi, the radiographic appearance may be of diagnostic significance.

Microscopic examination of the urinary sediment for cystine crystals may be a useful diagnostic procedure. These crystals are hexagonal and are best seen in highly concentrated acid urine.

Another method to detect the presence of cystine calculi is to determine the presence of excessive amounts of cystine in the urine. The chemical test utilizing the cyanide-nitroprusside reaction is a relatively sensitive test. Extreme care must be taken when handling and pipetting the sodium cyanide used in this test.

## TREATMENT

The initial step in treatment usually involves surgical removal of calculi from the urethra and bladder. The objective of medical therapy is to prevent the recurrence of calculi. In the absence of medical therapy, cystine calculi commonly recur within 6 to 12 months. In the case of an inborn error of metabolism, medical therapy must be continued throughout life.

The earlier conventional therapeutic approach for prevention of cystine involves (1) reducing urinary cystine excretion by the restriction of dietary protein precursors (feed a diet low in protein and particularly low in methionine content); (2) encouraging a high fluid intake, which dilutes the urine and decreases the urinary concentration of cystine; and (3) alkalinizing the urine to increase the solubility of cystine by increasing urinary pH. Results using one or a combination of these procedures have been generally disappointing. A low-methionine diet is quite unpalatable and therefore an impractical approach. Continuous alkalinizing therapy has some value in decreasing stone formation but is relatively inefficient. High water turnover and dilute urine can be accomplished by introducing a high-sodium diet. With the possible exception of a high fluid intake, none of these regimens seems necessary with the introduction of D-penicillamine (Cuprimine® [Merck]).

The chelating agent D-penicillamine reduces excess cystine excretion and cystinuria. The agent interacts with cystine to form a penicillamine-cysteine mixed disulfide that is more soluble than free cystine in the urine. This results in a decrease in free cystine excretion in the urine, and the likelihood of calculus formation is diminished.

The drug D-penicillamine is rapidly absorbed from the intestine and rapidly excreted via the kidney. The recommended dosage is 30 mg./kg. of body weight daily, divided into two doses (Frimpter *et al.*, 1967). This drug commonly causes nausea and vomiting and therefore must be mixed with food. In some cases, an anti-emetic drug is necessary to depress vomiting.

In man, toxic effects, including marrow depression, proteinuria, and hypersensitivity, have been reported. Similar toxic effects in the dog have not been reported; however, experience is limited and a careful study has not been conducted. Because of gastric irritation, the smallest dose tolerated by the dog is recommended in order to reduce the likelihood of serious intoxication. Hemograms and urinalyses should be periodically conducted. The drug also has an antipyridoxine effect.

In conclusion, the objective of therapy is to prevent recurrent stone formation. In our experience, D-penicillamine alone appears to be effective in attaining this objective. Owners should be advised not to breed these animals, thereby avoiding perpetuation of the disease.

### SUPPLEMENTAL READING

Bovee, K. C., Their, S. O., and Segal, S.: Renal clearance of amino acids in canine cystinuria. Metabolism, 23:51, 1974.

Frimpter, G. W., Thouin, P., and Ewalds, B.: Penicillamine in canine cystinuria. J. Am. Vet. Med. Assn., 151:1084, 1967.

---

# PHOSPHATE UROLITHIASIS

JEFFREY S. KLAUSNER, D.V.M., *and* CARL A. OSBORNE, D.V.M. St. Paul, Minnesota

Uroliths composed primarily of phosphate in combination with ammonium and magnesium or calcium are commonly called phosphate or triple phosphate calculi. They may be single or multiple, are typically yellow to white and are hard and radiopaque.

## INCIDENCE

Phosphate calculi are found more frequently in the urinary tract of dogs and cats than are other stone types. Although they have been encountered in most breeds of dogs, they have been observed most commonly in miniature schnauzers, corgis, dachshunds, Pekingese, cocker spaniels and Scottish terriers.

Studies in progress at the University of Minnesota indicate that phosphate urolithiasis in miniature schnauzers may be associated with an inherited predisposition. Ammonium magnesium phosphate calculi developed in 4 of 5 dogs of a test litter prior to 14 months of age.

Although dogs of any age (1 month to 15 years or older) may develop calculi, the mean age of occurrence is approximately 5 years. In one survey of reported cases of urolithiasis in dogs less than one year of age, 90 per cent had phosphate uroliths (Hardy *et al.*, 1972). Female dogs develop phosphate urolithiasis more frequently than do male dogs.

## ETIOPATHOGENESIS

Bacterial infection of the urinary tract, alkaline urine and genetic factors are thought to play a role in the development of phosphate uroliths. Other factors that have not been identified may also be important.

**Bacterial Infection.** Most dogs with phosphate urolithiasis also have infection of the urinary tract. Urease-producing bacteria, especially staphylococci, are commonly isolated. In contrast, bacterial infection of the urinary tract is not a consistent finding in patients with other types of uroliths (urate, cystine, oxalate). The association between phosphate calculi and urinary tract infection has also been exhaustively documented in human beings (Thompson and Stamey, 1973). The growth of calculi experimentally produced by implanting zinc foreign bodies in the urinary bladder was much greater in rats with bacterial urinary tract infection than in noninfected controls (Vermeulen and Goetz, 1954).

Bacteria can be frequently isolated from the center of phosphate uroliths, indicating that bacteria were present at the time when the stone began to develop. Bacteria have rarely been cultured from the center of nonphosphate calculi (Weaver, 1975).

A small percentage of dogs with phosphate urolithiasis have been observed to have sterile urine. In some of these cases, however, bacteria have been isolated from the center of the calculi. This observation indicates that bacterial infection of the urinary tract may undergo spontaneous remission after initiating calculi formation in some patients.

On occasion, both the center of calculi and urine obtained from dogs with phosphate urolithiasis have been sterile (Weaver, 1975). The significance of this observation, and its relationship to the hypothesis that phosphate calculi are caused by bacterial infection, is unknown.

The mechanism(s) by which bacteria initiate or augment the formation of phosphate uroliths has not been conclusively established. However, a large body of experimental and clinical evidence indicates that bacterial production of urease with subsequent formation of ammonium ions and alkalinization of urine is involved. Ammonium ions may also contribute to the formation of ammonium magnesium phosphate calculi. Other factors may also be involved, since infection with urease-producing bacteria is not invariably associated with the development of phosphate uroliths.

**Alkaline Urine.** Most, but not all, bacteria isolated from the urine of dogs with phosphate urolithiasis produce urease, an enzyme which degrades urea to ammonia. As a result, the pH of urine becomes alkaline. Ammonium magnesium phosphate and calcium phosphate salts are less soluble in alkaline urine than in acid urine. Other factors that may result in the formation of alkaline urine include the administration of alkalinizing drugs (sodium lactate, calcium lactate, sodium bicarbonate, etc.) and disorders associated with respiratory or metabolic alkalosis. If these factors maintain urine in an alkaline state, they may predispose patients to the formation of phosphate calculi.

**Genetic Factors.** A genetic predisposition to calculi may be present in some breeds of dogs. If infection of the urinary tract with urea-splitting bacteria plays an important role in the etiopathogenesis of phosphate calculi, a predisposition to infection associated with an inherited immunodeficiency state could be hypothesized. Although available data regarding phosphate urolithiasis in miniature schnauzers make this hypothesis attractive, meaningful generalizations cannot be made until it is established that urea-splitting bacteria definitely play a role in the formation of phosphate calculi, until the cellular and humoral immune systems of affected dogs have been evaluated and until the results of controlled breeding trials of affected and nonaffected dogs are known.

## CLINICAL FINDINGS

Clinical findings are dependent, at least in part, on the location of calculi in the urinary system.

Urethral calculi originate from the urinary bladder and may be associated with any combination of the following: frequent attempts to micturate, or inability to micturate; signs of renal failure that occur secondary to obstruction to urine outflow (postrenal uremia); and overdistention of the bladder with urine. Urethral calculi may be detected by means of palpation, catheterization or radiography.

Calculi in the urinary bladder are frequently associated with dysuria and hematuria. They may be detected by palpation or radiography. If the bladder is distended with urine, it may be impossible to palpate calculi until most of the urine is voided or removed.

Ureteral calculi are uncommonly encountered in the dog and cat, but they may occur. Ureteral calculi originate from the renal pelves. The infrequent occurrence of ureteral calculi is probably related to the relative infrequency with which renal calculi occur in these species. Ureteral uroliths may be associated with severe pain and/or obstruction to urine outflow and hydronephrosis. The presence of uroliths can be confirmed only by radiography or exploratory surgery.

Renal calculi account for approximately 10 per cent of the uroliths encountered in dogs. They may be associated with calculi elsewhere in the urinary tract. Renal uroliths may be associated with any combination of the following: renal pain caused by stimulation of pain receptors in the renal capsule; signs of uremia if bilateral renal involvement is present and 75 per cent or more of the renal parenchyma of both kidneys has been altered; and enlargement of affected kidneys as a result of obstruction to urine outflow and hydronephrosis. Renal calculi may be detected by radiography or exploratory surgery.

Abnormalities detected by urinalysis are usually consistent with inflammation (i.e., pyuria, hematuria and proteinuria). Bacteria can usually be detected in the urine sediment.

Significant numbers of bacteria (>100,000 organisms per milliliter of urine) can usually be cultured from the urine (consult the article on "Bacterial Infections of the Urinary Tract"). Bacteria may also be cultured from the center of phosphate calculi. Isolation of staphylococci should always alert one to the possible presence of phosphate urolithiasis.

Although radiopacity of calculi is dependent on their size and composition, phosphate calculi are typically radiopaque. Visualization of small calculi may require contrast radiography. Uroliths found in one portion of the urinary tract dictate radiographic evaluation of other portions for the presence of additional calculi. Two anatomic views at right angles to each other should always be obtained. Interposition of skeletal bone between uroliths and film is a common cause of failure to visualize calculi.

## DIAGNOSIS

The presence of uroliths is usually suspected on the basis of typical findings obtained by history and physical examination. Urinalyses, urine culture, and radiography may be required to eliminate the presence of urinary tract infection, diverticulae of the bladder, and neoplasia. Stone analysis is required to establish a diagnosis of phosphate urolithiasis once the calculus is removed from the patient. Bacterial culture of the center of calculi may also be of value.

Since therapy formulated to prevent recurrence of phosphate, urate, oxalate and cystine calculi is dependent on knowledge of the mineral composition of uroliths, analysis of uroliths by qualitative or quantitative methods is essential. Commercial kits* for qualitative stone analysis utilize chemical reagents to identify constituent radicals of calculi such as ammonium, carbonate, calcium, magnesium, phosphate, cystine, urate, etc. These kits are relatively inexpensive and simple to use. Since uroliths that are predominantly composed of one mineral type often contain traces of other minerals, it is important to sample representative areas of stones. The center of the urolith is especially important, since it is most likely to provide clues regarding the abnormality that initiated stone formation. Representative samples of uroliths may be obtained with a jeweler's saw.

Although somewhat more expensive, quantitative analyses† of uroliths provide more information about the type and quantity of compounds present (e.g., apatite, calcium oxalate dihydrate, struvite, etc.). They eliminate confusion caused by qualitative identification of traces of one mineral type in stones composed predominantly of another mineral type (i.e., identification of phosphates in urate calculi, etc.).

---

*Oxford Stone Analysis Set For Urinary Calculi, Oxford Laboratories, 1149 Chess Drive, Foster City, California 94404; Qualitative Urinary Calculi Analysis Kit, Alban Scientific, 901 South Grand Avenue, St. Louis, Missouri 63103.

†Available from Urolithiasis Laboratory, P.O. Box 25375, Houston, Texas 77005.

## TREATMENT

**Relief of Obstruction.** In patients with renal failure due to obstructive uropathy, every effort should be made to reestablish urine flow. Calculi lodged in the urethra of male dogs may be removed by urohydropropulsion (see the article on "Urohydropropulsion" for further details). A well-lubricated, small-diameter catheter may be used to bypass the calculi if urohydropropulsion is unsuccessful. Cystocentesis may provide immediate but temporary decompression of the obstructed urinary system. If all else fails, an emergency urethrotomy may be performed. If urine flow cannot be readily reestablished in uremic patients by use of the aforementioned techniques, alterations in fluid, electrolyte and acid-base balance should be minimized by appropriate fluid therapy and peritoneal dialysis.

**Removal of Calculi.** Removal of calculi is essential if the clinical signs caused by urolithiasis are to be eradicated. Surgery currently provides the most reliable method of removal of uroliths from the kidneys, ureters and urinary bladder and is recommended unless the patient is a poor anesthetic risk or has concomitant disease of another body system that is of greater significance. Calculi in the urethras of male dogs can usually be removed by urohydropropulsion.

The feasibility of medical therapy that will cause dissolution of phosphate calculi is being investigated. Therapeutic approaches currently being considered include prolonged acidification of urine, drugs that inhibit bacterial urease and administration of methylene blue.

Foreign body–induced ammonium magnesium phosphate cystic calculi will dissolve if rats are fed a diet that maintains an acid urine (Vermeulen *et al*, 1951). Although a variety of drugs are available to acidify the urine of dogs and cats, it may be difficult to keep the urine persistently acid. In addition, production of a large quantity of ammonium ions by urease-producing bacteria may prevent therapeutic acidification of urine until the infection is eradicated. Unfortunately, surgical removal of uroliths is usually required before the infection can be eliminated with antimicrobial agents.

Urease-inhibiting drugs, such as acetohydroxamic acid, prevent bacterial alkalinization of urine by blocking the degradation of urea to ammonia (Griffith and Musher, 1973). An acid urine pH can thus be maintained despite the presence of infection with urease-producing bacteria. Studies are in progress at the University of Minnesota to evaluate the efficacy and safety of acetohydroxamic acid in the dissolution and prevention of phosphate calculi in dogs.

Oral administration of methylene blue has been reported to produce inhibition and dissolution of artificial bladder stones in rats (Van't Riet *et al.*, 1964). The effect was attributed to ionic exchange between dye and crystals. Studies of the efficacy of methylene blue in the treatment of phosphate urolithiasis in human beings have produced conflicting results, but recent reports indicate that methylene blue is of little value in the dissolution of phosphate calculi (Smith, 1975).

## PREVENTION

Phosphate uroliths frequently recur following surgical removal (Weaver, 1970). Since the formation of phosphate calculi appears to be closely related to bacterial infection of the urinary tract, patients with bacteriuria should be vigorously treated with an antimicrobial agent selected on the basis of bacterial culture and antimicrobial sensitivity tests (for further details, refer to the article on "Bacterial Infections of the Urinary Tract"). Following eradication of urinary tract infection, urine cultures should be reevaluated at regular intervals in order to detect recurrences at a subclinical stage. Commercially manufactured screening tests for the detection of significant bacteriuria may be used (consult the article on "Bacterial Infections of the Urinary Tract").*

Acidification of urine by oral administration of a urinary acidifier is recommended. In addition to the fact that phosphate crystals are more soluble in an acid than an alkaline environment, acid urine is somewhat bacteriostatic. Dosages of urinary acidifiers should be adjusted on the basis of response;

---

*Microstix®, Ames Company, Elkhart, Indiana 46514; Bacteriuria Screening Test, Baltimore Biologic Laboratory, Cockeysville, Maryland 21030; Culturia Test, Clinical Convenience Products, Inc., Madison, Wisconsin 53701.

urine pH should be maintained at 6.5 or lower. Clients should be instructed to monitor the pH of urine periodically with commercially prepared pH strips and to adjust the dosage of acidifiers as necessary. (For further details, consult the article on "Indications for Acidifiers and Antiseptics in Urinary Tract Disorders.")

Increasing urine volume and urine output by oral administration of sodium chloride may interfere with the formation of calculi by decreasing the concentration of phosphate ions and other calculogenic material in urine. Polyuria may also enhance the elimination of bacteria and bacterial toxins. Induction of diuresis in rats was highly effective in preventing the formation of zinc foreign body cystic calculi (Grove *et al.*, 1950). Depending on the size of the patient, a dose of 0.5 to 10 grams of salt should be administered orally. A satisfactory increase in urine volume is indicated by a urine specific gravity below 1.025. We currently recommend that salt therapy be maintained for the life of the patient.

### SUPPLEMENTAL READING

Clark, W. T.: Staphylococcal infection of the urinary tract and its relation to urolithiasis in dogs. Vet. Rec., 95:204–206, 1974.

Finco, D. R., Rosin, E., and Johnson, K. H.: Canine urolithiasis, a review of 133 clinical and 23 necropsy cases. J. Am. Vet. Med. Assn., 157:1225–1228, 1970.
Goulden, B. E.: Clinical observations on the role of urinary infection in the etiology of canine urolithiasis. Vet. Rec., 83:509–514, 1968.
Griffith, D. P., and Musher, D. M.: Prevention of infected urinary stones by urease inhibition. Invest. Urol., 11:228–233, 1973.
Grove, W. J., et al.: Experimental urolithiasis. II. The influence of urine volume upon calculi experimentally produced upon foreign bodies. J. Urol., 64:549, 1950.
Hardy, R. M., et al.: Urolithiasis in immature dogs. Vet. Med./Small Animal Clin. 67:1205–1211, 1972.
Smith, M. J. V.: Methylene blue in renal calculi, results of five-year study. Urology, 6:676–679, 1975.
Thompson, R. B., and Stamey, T. A.: Bacteriology of infected stones. Urology, 2:627–633, 1973.
Van't Riet, B., et al.: Dye effects on inhibition and dissolution of urinary calculi. Invest. Urol., 1:446–456, 1964.
Vermeulen, C. W., and Goetz, R.: Experimental urolithiasis. IX. Influence of infection on stone growth in rats. J. Urol. 72:761, 1954.
Vermeulen, C. W., et al.: Experimental urolithiasis. III. Prevention and dissolution of calculi by alteration of urinary pH. J. Urol., 66:1–4, 1951.
Weaver, A. D.: Canine urolithiasis: incidence, chemical composition and outcome of 100 cases. J. Small Animal Pract., 11:83–92, 1970.
Weaver, A. D.: Relationship of bacterial infection in urine and calculi to canine urolithiasis. Vet. Rec., 97:48–50, 1975.
White, E. G.: Symposium on urolithiasis in the dog. I. Introduction and incidence. J. Small Animal Pract., 7:529–535, 1966.

# OXALATE UROLITHIASIS

RICHARD W. GREENE, D.V.M.
*New York, New York*

Oxalate urolithiasis, a frequent occurrence in man, is rarely seen in dogs in the United States. An incidence of up to 30 per cent has been reported in Europe, but most studies in the United States report a low incidence of oxalate calculi. In a recent study at The Animal Medical Center, oxalate stones represented 2.7 per cent of the calculi encountered in dogs. The mean age of dogs affected with oxalate stones in this study was 7.8 years, which was older than the mean age for other calculi groups represented (phosphate, cystine and urate). There was no breed predilection. Male dogs were more often affected than female dogs.

Oxalate calculi are usually radiopaque.

They are often single, hard, elliptical stones that have an irregular spiny surface. They are white to yellow in color and may be found in the kidneys, bladder or urethra. Oxalate is a metabolic end product of glyoxalate and ascorbate. As it is excreted in the urine, oxalate combines with calcium, forming an insoluble complex of calcium oxalate. Oxalate calculi usually form in acidic urine. Excretion patterns were unaffected in dogs with pH ranges of 5.9 to 8.0. The conditions favoring crystallization are unknown, making treatment very difficult.

Infection is not considered to be of etiologic importance in the formation of oxalate calculi. Inflammation and hemorrhage are often associated with oxalate urolithiasis because of trauma to the urinary tract caused by the spiny surfaces of these stones.

## TREATMENT

There is no definitive treatment for calcium oxalate calculi in the dog. Experimental work with new medication in man has been attempted, but until the "secret" of oxalate metabolism is discovered, surgical removal and forcing fluids by mouth is still the treatment of choice for both dogs and man. Urinary antibiotics should be administered postoperatively to eliminate urinary tract infection. Sodium chloride (1 to 10 gm. per day) should be added to the diet in divided doses to induce polyuria, thereby diluting the minerals and decreasing crystallization. Urinary acidifiers should be avoided, especially vitamin C, which seems to increase oxalate excretion in man. Diet does not seem to influence the formation of oxalate calculi.

### SUPPLEMENTAL READING

Brown, N. O.: Canine urolithiasis. Part II. Resident's paper, The Animal Medical Center, New York, April 30, 1975.
Cattell, W. R., et al.: The mechanism of renal excretion of oxalate in the dog. Clin. Sci., 22:43–52, 1962.
Goulden, B. E.: Clinical observations on the role of urinary infection in the aetiology of canine urolithiasis. Vet. Rec., 83:509–514, 1968.
National Academy of Sciences: Urolithiasis: Physical aspects. Washington, D.C., U.S. Government Printing Office, 1972.
White, E. G.: Urinary calculi in the dog with special reference to cystine stones. J. Comp. Pathol., 54:16–25, 1944.

# URATE UROLITHIASIS

DELMAR R. FINCO, D.V.M.
*Athens, Georgia*

## PATHOGENESIS

The definitive cause of urate urolithiasis is unknown. Urinary urate excretion is a predisposing cause, but not all urate excretors develop stones. Isolated cases of urate uroliths have been reported in the cat, but in small animal practice nearly all cases are found in the dog. The Dalmatian dog is predisposed to urate urolithiasis because of the mechanism of purine metabolism unique to this breed. Dalmatians do not convert all purines to allantoin, as do other dogs, and consequently both urates and allantoin appear in the urine. The site of the metabolic difference between Dalmatians and other dogs is the liver, not the kidney, as is sometimes reported. Both stone-forming and nonstone-forming Dalmatians have quantities of urate in the urine that exceed simple solubility. The urate exists in colloid suspension but can be flocculated by an increase in ammonium and hydrogen ion concentration of the urine. These observations have significant application in the prophylaxis of calculi.

Urate calculi in the Dalmatian are ammonium urate rather than uric acid as in man. This difference suggests that the pathogenesis of urate calculi formation may be different in the two species, and that therapeutic procedures successful in one species may not be successful in another.

## DIAGNOSIS

Not all calculi from Dalmatians are urate and not all urate calculi come from Dalmatians. Although it is an uncommon occurrence, Dalmatians may develop other uroliths, particularly phosphates. Urate uroliths have been identified in English bulldogs and in cats. Although typical visual descriptions have been given for the major stone types in dogs, gross appearance (size, shape, color, consistency) is not reliable for identifying chemical composition. Urate uroliths are generally radiolucent, but phosphate may be mixed with the urate, rendering it radiopaque. Analysis of the urolith is the only reliable method of determining the chemical composition. Commercial stone analysis kits* are available for qualitative chemical analysis. These kits provide data of satisfactory reliability at a cost of less than two dollars per analysis. Considering that most prophylactic procedures are specific for specific types of calculi, it is illogical not to have chemical analysis of calculi performed. The site of sampling of the calculus is important, because salts not significant in its initiation may be incorporated as it grows. The calculus should be split, and material from the center should be obtained for analysis.

Methods of diagnosis of urolithiasis are common knowledge, but a word of caution is necessary concerning evaluation of the patient. Regardless of the site at which calculi are found, the entire urinary tract should be radiographed. Both survey radiographs and negative and/or positive contrast radiography should be performed, since urate uroliths are not markedly radiodense.

Multiple sites of urolith deposition are common with urate urolithiasis, and knowledge of the distribution of the uroliths is essential for satisfactory management of the case.

## TREATMENT

Some pets with urate uroliths have urinary tract infection. Urinalysis and urine culture should be performed, and urinary tract infection should be treated if present (see articles on "Bacterial Infections of the Urinary Tract" and "Pyelonephritis"). Existing uroliths are usually treated surgically (urethrotomy, cystotomy, nephrolithotomy). Occasionally, diseases not related to urolithiasis may make surgery inadvisable. Conservative medical management should be undertaken in this situation. After surgical removal, a program of prophylaxis is explained to the owner, with emphasis placed on the high probability of recurrence if specific measures are not taken for the duration of the life of the pet.

The program of prophylaxis for urate urolithiasis is as follows:

1. Administration of allopurinol.† This compound interferes with the conversion both of hypoxanthine to xanthine and of xanthine to urate by competitive inhibition. Allopurinol administration results in a reduction in total purine excretion by mechanisms not entirely known. Of the total purine excreted, allopurinol results in xanthine and hypoxanthine excretion as well as some urate. Since the three compounds are independently soluble, chances of flocculation of the salts are decreased.

Allopurinol is administered at a dose of 30 mg./kg./day in divided doses t.i.d. for 1 month. The dose is then reduced to 10 mg./kg./day. The drug must be given constantly to achieve its effect, since the underlying metabolic trait of failure to convert urate to allantoin is not altered by the drug. In man, instances of dissolution of existing uroliths have been reported following use of allopurinol. Although several side effects of the drug have been reported in man, no reports of side effects exist from use of the drug in the dog.

2. Inducement of polyuria by administration of salt. Increased urine flow dilutes urate in the urine and decreases the chance of flocculation. Administration of salt orally to the patient is a satisfactory and economical way of inducing polyuria. For a 25-kg. dog, a dose of about 5 gm./day should be adequate, but urine volume or urine specific gravity should be determined in order to be assured of the desired effect. Urine specific gravity should be maintained at 1.035 or less.

3. Maintenance of urine pH between 6.5 and 7.0 by administering sodium bicarbonate orally. Since both hydrogen and ammonium ions enhance urate flocculation, decreasing the quantity of these ions in the urine may aid in preventing recurrence of urate uroliths. Ammonium secretion by the kidney is enhanced under conditions of increased hydrogen ion excretion by the kidney. Decreasing hydrogen ion excretion by administration of sodium bicarbonate is effective in minimizing ammonium excretion.

Sodium bicarbonate should be administered to effect (urine pH 6.5 to 7.0). A dose of 2 gm./day administered as tablets or as powder (1/2 tsp. baking soda is about 2 gm.) can be used as the initial dose.

4. Use of a low-purine diet. Some ingested purine is used for nucleic acid synthesis but most is metabolized to urate or allantoin and is excreted in the urine. De-

---

*Oxford Stone Analysis Kit, available from Scientific Products, Inc., in major cities.

†Zyloprim®, Burroughs Wellcome and Co., Inc., 3030 Cornwallis Road, Research Park, Triangle, North Carolina 27709.

creasing purine in the diet is a logical ancillary measure in the prevention of urate uroliths. Glandular organs (e.g., liver, kidneys) are particularly high in nucleic acids and should be avoided. A low-quality dog food that is high in vegetable sources of protein is a desirable diet for dogs predisposed to urate uroliths. Special all-vegetable diets may also be prescribed.

The prophylactic procedures outlined are usually effective in management of urate urolithiasis. If they are not, and urethral obstruction is a recurrent problem, consideration may be given to scrotal urethrostomy to alleviate recurrence of obstruction. The surgical procedure obviously does not decrease the rate of urolith formation.

### SUPPLEMENTAL READING

Finco, D. R.: Current status of canine urolithiasis. J. Am. Vet. Med. Assn., 158:327–335, 1970.

Porter, P.: Urinary calculi in the dog. II. Urate stones and purine metabolism. J. Comp. Pathol. Ther., 73:119–135, 1963.

Porter, P.: Physico-chemical factors involved in urate formation. Res. Vet. Sci., 4:580–602, 1963.

## Genital System

# GENITAL EMERGENCIES

MARC A. HALL, D.V.M.
*Ocoee, Florida*

*and* LARRY N. SWENBERG, D.V.M.
*Cincinnati, Ohio*

The following diseases have been classified as emergencies, since immediate care offers the best prognosis for functional recovery and, in some instances, is essential to the patient's survival.

## MALE

### PARAPHIMOSIS

This condition exists when an engorged or edematous penis cannot be retracted into the preputial cavity. It should be differentiated from paralysis of the retractor penis muscles, in which the unerect penis (though possibly edematous from trauma) protrudes from the preputial orifice. Paraphimosis is usually seen following coitus or masturbation when the glans penis has become engorged to a degree that the preputial orifice becomes trapped behind the glans and acts as a constricting ring. This aggravates venous congestion and sustains penile erection. Trauma induced by the dog's licking may further contribute to tissue edema.

Moderate phimosis may predispose a dog to paraphimosis. In some cases, poor distensibility of the preputial orifice creates a relative phimosis as an erection occurs. Occasionally, a sustained erection dries the penile tissues. As retraction begins, preputial hairs become adhered to the penis, invert the preputial orifice and produce a constricting ring of tissue. In addition, severe balanoposthitis, penile fractures and lacerations, foreign objects (such as rubber bands) and chronic priapism may cause paraphimosis. If untreated, the condition may result in urethral obstruction or ischemic necrosis of the penis. When the condition is of short duration, application of an obstetric lubricant or petroleum jelly to the penis and preputial orifice and eversion of preputial tissues or hair often allows the prepuce to be advanced forward over the penis. Applications of cold, hypertonic dextrose to the penis over a period of minutes may aid in reducing the edema.

If conservative measures fail, or if severe tissue damage exists, the dog should be anesthetized, the preputial hairs clipped and the tissues cleansed for surgery. Enlarging the preputial orifice by incising the ventral aspect of the prepuce for one to two inches provides adequate exposure of the penis and also facilitates its repositioning into the prepuce. Following evaluation of tissue viability, the penis should be debrided and the wounds should be closed with 3-0 to 5-0 chromic gut, or a similar absorbable synthetic suture material (Pol-dex® [Davis and Geck]). The preputial wound should be closed by suturing mucosa, subcutis and skin individually. If phimosis initiated the problem, a small wedge-shaped section of tissue should be removed from the ventral preputial orifice and the skin united to mucosa.

In cases in which swelling is severe or tissue viability is doubtful, an indwelling urinary catheter will assure unobstructed urination. Instillation of an antibiotic-steroid ointment into the prepuce and administration of systemic antibiotics and steroids will control inflammation and wound infection. In severely traumatized cases, penile-preputial adhesions can be avoided by daily extrusion of the penis combined with the instillation of an antibiotic-enzyme preparation (Elase® ointment [Parke, Davis]) into the preputial cavity.

**Prevention.** In breeding males, the problem may be prevented by trimming the preputial hair prior to mating and by maintaining preputial hygiene. When moderate phimosis exists, it should be surgically corrected. In males not used for breeding purposes, castration generally eliminates the copulatory effort leading to the problem.

## TRAUMA TO THE PENIS AND PREPUCE

Abrasions and lacerations of the prepuce and penis are common sequelae of automobile accidents, dog fights and fence jumping. Unless hemorrhage is severe, they rarely are complicated emergencies. Penile lacerations may be associated with significant hemorrhage, and the injury may involve the urethra.

Rupture of the penile urethra usually accompanies fracture of the os penis and should be suspected any time penile injury is accompanied by an adjacent fluctuant subcutaneous swelling. The clinician must determine whether this swelling is due to extravasation of urine, hematoma or abscess formation or to subcutaneous herniation of bowel.

Minor injuries to the penis and prepuce may be cleansed and treated with topical and systemic antibacterial agents and allowed to heal as open wounds. Licking should be controlled with an Elizabethan collar, and attention given to establishing adequate wound drainage when indicated. With larger wounds, arterial bleeding should be controlled by ligation. Hemorrhage associated with laceration of the cavernous tissues of the penis can best be controlled by debriding and suturing as described earlier. The vascular nature of the penile tissues combined with the excellent suturing characteristics of the tunica albuginea promotes first intention healing.

Following meticulous débridement, small lacerations of the penile urethra can generally be closed with a swedged-on, taperpoint needle on 4-0 or 5-0 chromic gut. Stinting the sutured area for 5 to 7 days with a pliable rubber catheter that fills the diameter of the urethra may reduce the incidence of postoperative stricture formation. If the penile urethra is ruptured but the tunics are intact, the passage of a urethral catheter along with concurrent drainage of subcutaneous urine may allow complete healing. The duration of stinting required is variable, depending on the extent of penile and urethral injury. Minor urethral tears usually heal in 5 to 7 days, whereas larger injuries that must heal with variable degrees of subepithelial fibrosis require 14 to 21 days of stinting to avoid stenosis following wound contracture. Positive contrast urethrography will aid in estimation of the magnitude of urethral damage. In cases in which injury to the penis and/or urethra is too extensive to allow functional recovery, a scrotal urethrostomy may be performed to salvage the patient.

## INJURY TO THE SCROTUM AND TESTICLES

Scrotal dermatitis of any etiology may progress to emergency proportions, owing to the dog's tendency to further traumatize these tissues by licking. The scrotum may become painful, erythematous and edematous and may exude serum. Immediate and aggressive therapy greatly reduces the patient's discomfort and convalescent period.

Analgesics or anesthetics are often required to allow even gentle cleaning of the scrotum. Steroid-antibiotic ointments should be applied three to four times daily until recovery is complete. Parenteral steroids greatly reduce the inflammatory reaction. If the lesions are deep or suppurative, parenteral antibiotics are indicated.

Collaring devices are often required to prevent self-inflicted trauma during healing. If attention is prompt, healing is generally uncomplicated. However, at times scrotal necrosis necessitates scrotal ablation and castration.

In cases of penetrating scrotal lacerations, all foreign material should be flushed from the scrotal sac using isotonic fluids and an aqueous antibiotic preparation. In cleansing the scrotum, surgical soaps are best removed with water, since mild tinctures of iodine or dilute alcohol often produce erythema of this tissue. Owing to their minimal tissue reactivity, fine nonabsorbable monofilament materials such as polypropylene or nylon should be used in scrotal skin. Special care should be used to avoid excessive suture tension. When drainage of the scrotal sac is indicated, Penrose drains should be placed to exit the skin just anterior to the scrotum at the site of a routine castration incision.

Owing to their tendency to result in sperm granulomas, lacerations or large puncture wounds invading the testicular parenchyma are best handled by unilateral or bilateral castration. This point should be stressed to owners of show or breeding stock if salvage therapy of testicular wounds is to be attempted. Wounds involving the common tunic only may be sutured with 5-0 gut and the scrotum closed as previously described.

## ORCHITIS

Acute bacterial orchitis may require emergency therapy. The owner's complaint usually centers on the dog's anorexia, his extreme reluctance to move and often his whining. On physical examination the dog may be febrile and the testicles may be firm, swollen and painful to palpation.

Fourteen to 21 days of broad-spectrum antibiotics are indicated to assure eradication of infection. A single dose of dexamethasone at 0.5 mg./kg. of body weight aids in rapidly reducing the inflammation and edema responsible for much of the damage incurred in testicular cellulitis. Should the dog remain febrile, or the testicles be soft when first examined, castration is indicated. In any case of orchitis, especially those accompanied by scrotal dermatitis, evaluation of serum for *Brucella* antibodies is indicated.

## TESTICULAR TORSION

Although uncommon in dogs and cats, testicular torsion usually requires immediate attention. The torsion usually involves a retained abdominal testicle that may be enlarged owing to neoplasia. Rotation of the testicle on its horizontal axis occludes venous drainage, causing severe engorgement and ultimate necrosis.

History usually reveals an older animal that has an acute onset of abdominal pain. Clinical signs include extreme resistance to abdominal palpation, restlessness, tenesmus, short cries of pain and occasionally vomiting.

A thorough physical examination will usually lead one to suspect testicular torsion. The cases we have seen have been unilaterally or bilaterally cryptorchid dogs over 5 years of age. On occasion one may feel an enlarged, painful mass in the area just caudal to the kidneys. Palpation may require the use of analgesics, provided that they are not contraindicated because of shock or cardiovascular disease.

Testicular torsion must be differentiated from other causes of acute abdominal pain, such as pancreatitis, peritonitis or intestinal obstruction. Definitive diagnosis will require exploratory laparotomy, but nonsurgical causes of acute abdominal pain should be ruled out prior to laparotomy to avoid unnecessary risk to the patient.

Treatment consists of surgical removal of the torsive testicle and removal of the opposite testicle if it is retained. This is best accomplished by a standard abdominal midline approach. Appropriate supportive therapy will vary with the status of the patient. Since in most cases pain is the major presenting complaint and vomiting is only periodic, intravenous fluids prior to and during surgery are usually adequate. Should shock exist, the patient must be stabilized prior to exploration of the abdomen. Histopathologic studies should be performed on the testicle, since many are neoplastic.

## PROSTATIC DISEASE

Trauma to the prostatic urethra may occur as a sequela of pelvic fractures and may result in urinary retention or urine peritonitis. Retrograde positive contrast urethrography will aid in localizing the injury. The urethral tear may be handled by simply stinting it with a large urethral catheter for 5 to 10 days, or stinting and suturing the urethra. Laceration of the prostatic parenchyma alone usually requires no specific therapy.

On occasion, prostatic hypertrophy may result in tenesmus sufficient to produce rectal prolapse or perineal herniation of bowel and, potentially, bladder. When constipation accompanies the hypertrophy, cleansing enemas are indicated. If a perineal hernia exists, the colonic cul-de-sac should be emptied of feces. If the bladder is in the hernial sac, an indwelling catheter is indicated to maintain urine flow until corrective surgery and castration can be performed. Anticholinergics should be administered. If the animal is not to be neutered, estrogens should be given to reduce the prostatic mass. If a rectal prolapse is also present, the prolapse should be re-placed following anesthesia and a pursestring suture should be placed around the anus.

Prostatitis with rupture of an infected cyst may result in fulminating peritonitis. A laparotomy in conjunction with supportive medical therapy should be performed. If the cyst is large and has a pedunculated base, it may be excised. Extensive paraprostatic abscesses are best handled initially by marsupialization of the abscess wall. With multiple small prostatic abscesses, marsupialization cannot be utilized. Here, aspiration of the abscesses and provision for good abdominal drainage in conjunction with intensive antibiotic and estrogen therapy (or castration) should be instituted. In all cases, treatment of the concurrent peritonitis necessitates liberal abdominal lavage, instillation of intraperitoneal antibiotics and provision for abdominal drainage. The intraperitoneal administration of systemic enzyme preparations (Varizyme® [Cyanamid]) will aid in the removal and prevention of fibrinous adhesions.

Owing to the chronic discharge of exudate associated with most marsupialized prostates, and the fact that not all prostatic abscesses are amenable to marsupialization, total prostatectomy seems an attractive alternative. However, owing to the inherent risk of renal shutdown associated with this procedure, dogs with preexistent peritonitis should be treated by the more conservative routes outlined until active infection is resolved and the patient is well stabilized. Total prostatectomy may then be performed with less risk.

# FEMALE

## DYSTOCIA

Dystocia can be defined as marked prolongation of the first or second stage of parturition, with resulting difficult or impossible delivery of viable offspring. Diagnosis is not always easy, since there is no clear division between normal and abnormal parturition.

Normal parturition includes three stages. Prior to or during stage one, the animal will become restless, will begin to segregate and will attempt to build a nest. Rectal temperature may drop to below 38° C. (100° F.), and a white mucoid vaginal discharge (cervical plug) may been seen. The animal will begin to pant, become anorexic and occasionally vomit late in stage one, which usually lasts 2 to 12 hours. When the allanto-chorion ruptures, the amnion, along with the fetus, pushes into the cervix and initiates stage two.

Active labor with abdominal contractions begins with stage two. One to two hours may pass prior to the first delivery, which may be followed quickly by the second delivery. A rest period of 30 to 90 minutes often occurs before the procedure is repeated, and this sequence continues until parturition is complete. Stage two may last up to 30 hours, depending on litter size and intervals between deliveries.

Stage three consists of expulsion of the placenta. The placenta passes either with the offspring or just prior to the succeeding delivery. If not passed with the last fetus, the final placenta should pass 10 to 15 minutes later.

Either maternal or fetal dystocias may occur. Maternal causes include primary and secondary uterine inertia, maternal pelvic abnormalities, psychologic disturbances, inguinal herniation or uterine torsion. Primary uterine inertia is associated with obesity, lack of exercise, uterine overload with a large litter, uterine infection or insufficient pituitrin levels to contract the uterus. It is more commonly seen in dogs, especially poodles, dachshunds, Yorkshire terriors, Chihuahuas and other breeds, that are overly protected. Secondary uterine inertia can be seen in all breeds owing to tiring of the uterine muscle from an obstruction within the birth canal, or prolonged parturition due to a large litter. Maternal pelvic abnormalities causing a narrowing of the birth canal are frequently associated with an old pelvic fracture with excessive callus formation or malaligned healing. Soft tissue obstructions such as neoplasms, abscesses or fibrous scars occur on occasion. Psychologic disturbances due to excitement, often caused by the owner, can result in frustration and confusion of the animal, with subsequent uterine inertia.

Fetal causes of dystocia include oversized fetuses, inadequate lubrication, malposition of a deformed fetus or death of the fetus with subsequent fetal emphysema. Oversized fetuses may occur in those animals that have a small litter (1 or 2 fetuses). Certain breeds having large heads and shoulders at birth, such as the English bull, pug and Boston terrier, often present problems as they pass through the birth canal. Deformed fetuses with congenital defects such as hydrocephalus, achondroplasia or supernumerary limbs may, on rare occasions, cause dystocia. Lateral or ventral malposition of the head and neck may cause dystocia but is uncommon in dogs and cats. Late death of the fetus *in utero* will lead to emphysema or fetal anasarca, with resultant dystocia.

Diagnosis of dystocia should be based on the history and physical examination. Information as to breeding dates, owner's first observation of stage two labor, intensity of contractions, environmental conditions and emotional stresses must be considered. Questions about previous deliveries and past medical history are also important. Previous injury or disease may influence the decision as to method of treatment.

Dystocia should be anticipated (1) if no deliveries occur within 4 to 6 hours after onset of stage two; (2) if more than 4 hours have elapsed after a delivery with no active labor, and more fetuses are known to be in the uterus; (3) if there are weak and/or infrequent labor contractions, with no offspring being delivered within 4 hours; (4) if signs of toxemia have developed; or (5) if a foul-smelling uterine discharge is present. A thorough physical examination including vaginal digital palpation must be performed prior to treatment. The perineum should be clipped and cleaned. Digital palpation with a sterilized glove should include (1) examination of the cervix to be sure it is completely dilated, (2) palpation of the pelvic inlet for adequate diameter to pass the fetuses and (3) determination of whether enough lubrication is present for passage of a fetus. When the examination is complete, the bladder should be emptied and an enema given to allow maximal space within the pelvic canal.

Treatment of dystocia usually follows one of the following four methods: (1) stimulation of uterine contractions with drugs, (2) manual manipulation of the fetuses with or without instrumentation, (3) cesarean section or (4) ovariohysterectomy. These methods may be used alone or in combination, depending on the case.

It has been our experience that maternal dystocias are the more common type seen, uterine inertia being the most common cause. Primary uterine inertias should be initially treated with pituitrin. An initial dose of 10 to 20 units of pituitrin should be given intramuscularly. Feathering the vagina may also stimulate labor. If no response is seen within 30 minutes, pituitrin should be repeated along with 2 to 10 cc. of a 10 per cent calcium gluconate solution intravenously. If three doses of pituitrin are given with no response, a cesarean section should be performed without further delay. Secondary uterine inertia should be treated in the same manner as primary uterine inertia unless there is an obstruction in the pelvic inlet. If a fetus is creating the obstruction and can be manually removed, the remaining litter can often be delivered normally. Obstruction caused by incomplete dilatation of the cervix reportedly responds to drug therapy. Diethylstilbestrol administered at a dosage of 0.5 mg./kg. of body weight (not to exceed 10 mg.) may be given intramuscularly prior to pituitrin to relax the cervix and sensitize the uterus to pituitrin. However, it is our opinion that diethylstilbestrol is of minimal value in dystocias, owing to the time required for the effects of the drug to occur. Complete dilatation of the cervix often requires only a little more time to occur naturally. If waiting jeopardizes the viability of a valuable pup, cesarean delivery is preferred to forcing labor against a poorly dilated cervix. Uterine inertia associated with psychlogic distress can often be solved by sedating the bitch lightly prior to pituitrin therapy.

Although not as common as maternal dystocia, fetal dystocia generally requires more rigorous therapy. In obstructed fetal dystocias the offending fetus may be removed by manual manipulation or instrumentation. Commonly used instruments include clamshell obstetric forceps, blunt spay hooks and sponge forceps. Because instruments may damage the uterine wall and/or the fetus, their use should be reserved for delivery of a dead or unwanted fetus, and then only when placement around the fetus can be visualized or palpated. Clamshell forceps have been advocated to bring the fetus into the pelvic canal, but abdominal and vaginal digital manipulation will usually provide the same result with less chance of damage to the fetus or dam. Sponge forceps are useful in the case of a dead fetus because of their holding and crushing ability. Crushing may reduce the size of the fetus enough to allow passage through the canal. When the dystocia is caused by abnormal presentation (usually head and/or limb deviation), a blunt spay hook may be used to correct the positioning while digitally retracting the fetus. Once the fetus is in the birth canal and can be grasped with gauze sponges, it can usually be delivered with gentle traction and manipulation. Lubrication of the birth canal prior to manipulation may be accomplished by forcing sterile lubricating gels (K-Y Jelly® [Johnson & Johnson]) around the body of the fetus into the birth canal.

Dams with dystocias that do not respond to drug therapy or manipulation are candidates for cesarean section. Selection of the proper anesthetic agent and supportive therapy must be based on careful evaluation of the dam. Lactated Ringer's solution should be administered intravenously to maintain adequate blood pressure and to assure an open vein, should other intravenous therapy be required during surgery.

Many different agents and combinations of agents have been used for cesarian delivery, including epidurals, inhalants, narcotics with local anesthetics, barbiturates, and muscle relaxants with local anesthetics. The ideal anesthetic for this procedure should provide adequate relaxation for the surgical procedure, be easily administered, have a wide margin of safety for fetuses and bitch and allow rapid recovery and nursing. We have found that the following two methods fulfill these criteria.

For routine cesarean sections in otherwise healthy bitches, we premedicate with atropine (0.1 mg./kg. of body weight) and administer an intravenous combination of oxymorphone (1 to 2 mg./5 kg. of body weight, but not to exceed 5 mg.) and acetylpromazine (0.5 to 1.5 mg. total, depending on the size of the bitch). In addition, a local anesthetic is injected into the midline. This combination is preferred, since it is uncomplicated, offers potent analgesia (oxymorphone is 10 times as potent as morphine), has minimal hypotensive affects and may be reversed rapidly with a narcotic antagonist (Narcan® [Endo], Lorfan® [Roche], Nalline® [Merck]) during or immediately following surgery. Even though narcotics will cross the placenta, most pups are active at the time of delivery. In the event of a depressed pup, the antagonist may be given in the umbilical vein, intramuscularly or subcutaneously. The incorporation of small amounts of acetylpromazine reduces or eliminates the hyperventilation often caused by oxymorphone and also potentiates the sedative effect of the latter. Undesirable sedation has not been a problem in the bitch or pups once the effect of oxymorphone is reversed. Since acetylpromazine potentiates the hypotensive effects of the narcotic, the precautionary use of intravenous fluids during surgery is recommended.

In dogs toxic from infection or emphysematous pups and in cats, we employ nitrous oxide and Fluothane® (Ayerst). The animal should be intubated and maintained on the lowest percentage of Fluothane possible (usually 1/2 to 1 per cent). Nitrous oxide must be terminated and blown off prior to allowing the patient to breathe room air.

In all cesarean sections we use a midline approach and employ standard cesarean procedures as outlined by Archibald in *Canine Surgery* (see Johnston reference). If not previously administered, Pituitrin is given intravenously prior to surgery to diminish uterine bleeding and aid in uterine involution. In the event of peritoneal soilage during surgery, the abdomen should be lavaged with warm isotonic saline. Abdominal drainage should be provided if necessary. In an infected uterus the bacteria should be cultured and the midline closed with a monofilament, nonabsorbable suture material. We recommend the administration of penicillin at 5000 units/kg. of body weight once a day in combination with kanamycin sulfate at 6 mg./kg. of body weight twice daily while waiting for culture results.

## ACUTE METRITIS

Acute metritis occurs frequently 3 to 4 days following whelping, owing to retention of placentas, uterine fluids or a fetus.

These disorders are frequently complicated by spontaneously occurring or iatrogenic ascending infection. Occasionally ascending infection follows estrus, artificial insemination or a natural mating. Organisms most commonly recovered are gram-negative bacilli.

(Consult the article on "Acute Metritis" for details about clinical findings commonly associated with acute metritis.)

Once acute metritis is diagnosed, the pups should be fed a commercial milk replacer. Radiography may permit visualization of a retained fetus, uterine fluid or extensive peritonitis. In cases with radiographic evidence of peritonitis, abdominal paracentesis and microscopic examination of recovered fluid will aid in detecting extension of infection to the peritoneum. Fluids from the uterus and abdomen should be cultured to assure proper choice of antibiotics.

Treatment of uncomplicated metritis consists of removing retained fetuses or placentas by instrumentation or surgery. Following this procedure, 10 to 20 units of Pituitrin should be given intramuscularly at 60-minute intervals for 3 doses to aid involution and expulsion of uterine fluid. For these purposes, parenteral ergonovine maleate (Ergonil® [Elanco]) may be used as an adjunct to Pituitrin therapy. Daily intrauterine infusion of antibiotics, parenteral enzymes (Varizyme® [Cyanamid]) and/or mucolytic agents (Alevaire® [Breon]) to liquefy and mobilize exudates is indicated if the uterus is crepitant or severely distended. If the cervix is inadequately dilated to allow drainage or infusion, diethylstilbestrol, 0.5 mg./kg. of body weight (25 mg. maximum), should be administered. Estrogens also increase the blood supply to the endometrium. Parenteral antibiotics should be administered for 10 to 14 days. Supportive intravenous fluids, B-complex vitamins and good nutrition assist recovery. If response to therapy is good, the bitch may be returned to her pups in 2 to 3 days.

In cases of acute metritis with peritonitis, exploratory surgery is indicated. In most of these cases venous thrombosis and uterine necrosis are so extensive that salvage of the uterus is precluded.

The treatment of choice includes extensive supportive therapy, ovariohysterectomy, abdominal lavage and peritoneal drainage.

## PYOMETRA

Initial therapy of toxic pyometra should be directed toward improving the patient's vital signs. The patient should be weighed, an indwelling catheter should be placed in the jugular vein, pretreatment blood samples should be collected and fluid therapy should be instituted to correct the metabolic acidosis and dehydration universal to toxic pyometra patients. Initially, the fluid of choice is lactated Ringer's solution enriched with sodium bicarbonate at 0.5 to 2 mEq./kg. of body weight as determined by the magnitude of the base deficit. This may be estimated in accordance with the severity of clinical signs of acidosis. Following initiation of fluid therapy, urine flow should be monitored with the aid of an indwelling catheter. At this point, an initial central venous pressure determination is prudent. The rate of fluid administration will vary with the degree of hypovolemia or endotoxic shock but should not exceed 80 ml./kg./hr. Rate and volume of fluid administered should be guided by periodic monitoring of the central venous pressure, body weight and urine flow rate. The patient's total requirements for fluids are calculated according to the formula presented in the article on "Fluid Therapy." Specific electrolyte deficits may be corrected following evaluation of laboratory results. Additional therapy includes broad-spectrum antibiotics given intravenously in conjunction with corticosteroids administered in therapeutic dosages for shock. If anuria exists following rehydration, attempts to induce diuresis with furosemide, mannitol or dextrose should be initiated. (Consult the article on "Canine Pyometra — A Polysystemic Disorder" for further details.)

Under no circumstances should a severely toxic pyometra patient be subjected to surgery. This maxim includes those patients with a ruptured uterus. Toxemia should be combated with massive corticosteroid, antibiotic and appropriate fluid-electrolyte therapy, and in the case of uterine perforation, abdominal drainage and lavage should be instituted. Once shock has been reversed, electrolyte and acid-base status normalized and adequate urine flow established, the patient is a candidate for surgical intervention.

Anesthetics that cause minimal hypotension and respiratory depression should be used. Premedication with atropine followed by Surital® (Parke, Davis) induction and maintenance by inhalation anesthesia is adequate for well-stabilized or compensated patients. If the patient is toxic, we prefer premedication with atropine and mask induction with 60 per cent nitrous oxide and 4 per cent Fluothane. Maintenance on ½ to 1 per cent Fluothane and 60 per cent nitrous oxide provides minimal side effects. To avoid potential apnea, nitrous oxide should be terminated during closure of the subcutis and the patient allowed to blow off this gas prior to breathing room air.

Because of prolonged healing time of many toxic patients, a nonabsorbable monofilament material such as stainless steel, polypropylene or nylon is preferred for closure of the abdomen. Continued supportive therapy as well as careful monitoring of urine output and body temperature is essential to the successful postoperative management of these patients.

## UTERINE PROLAPSE

Prolapse of the uterus through an open cervix may occur during or shortly after parturition. Prolapse may be complete, with one or both uterine horns everted through the vulva, or incomplete, with one horn partially everted into the vaginal canal. Tenesmus due to a retained placenta, dead fetus or metritis usually precedes the event and leads to eversion of the poorly involuted or atonic uterus. Complete prolapse may result in rupture of the broad ligament, intraabdominal hemorrhage and subsequent shock.

In cases of complete prolapse the diagnosis is obvious. If postpartum animals are straining (with or without vaginal discharge), digital palpation of the vaginal tract will allow differentiation between partial prolapse and metritis uncomplicated by prolapse. Treatment is aimed at replacing the uterus in normal anatomic position and preventing or eliminating uterine infection. General or epidural anesthesia is indicated to prevent straining and to facilitate abdominal palpation during replacement. With the animal's perineum elevated, partial prolapses should be digitally inverted while manual traction is applied through the abdominal wall. If necessary, a laparotomy should be performed to achieve complete inversion. Following replacement, 10 to 20 units of pituitrin should be given to stimulate uterine involution. Broad-spectrum antibiotics should also be given for 7 to 10 days. (Refer to the article on "Acute Metritis" for details about eliminating the preexisting infection that resulted in the prolapse.)

Complete prolapse usually necessitates more rigorous therapy. The prolapsed tissues must be examined for edema, necrosis or laceration following cleansing with warm, isotonic saline enriched with aqueous antibiotics. If the uterus is to be salvaged, necrotic areas should be debrided and lacerations sutured prior to replacement. Hypertonic glucose, saline or urea solutions may reduce the severity of edema. Following elevation of the perineum, the uterine horns should be inverted one at a time. After the uterine body is replaced, the horns should be retracted anteriorly by abdominal palpation. Intrauterine infusion of an aqueous antibiotic solution under slight pressure will assist complete inversion of the horns, after which pituitrin is administered. If anatomic replacement or tissue viability is questionable, a laparotomy should be considered. If uterine blood flow has not improved following replacement, ovariohysterectomy should be performed. If the uterus is too mutilated to allow replacement, ligation and amputation of the prolapsed portion of the uterus at the vulva will permit inversion. A laparotomy and complete ovariohysterectomy should then be performed. If the patient is in shock, administration of whole blood and/or polyionic fluids should precede exploratory surgery.

## UTERUS AND OVARIES

Torsions of the uterus and/or ovaries are uncommon problems in the dog and cat. Uterine torsion is seen during late pregnancy or parturition and involves rotation of a single horn or the uterine body. Ovarian torsion may accompany rotation of a uterine horn, or it may occur independently in a pendulous, neoplastic ovary.

Clinical signs of uterine torsion depend on the degree of rotation. Those over 180° are associated with rapid onset of abdominal pain, tenesmus, crying and restlessness, which may progress to severe weakness and signs of shock. Excluding tenesmus, symptoms of ovarian torsion are similar.

Definitive diagnosis is made by means of exploratory surgery after nonsurgical causes of an acute abdomen have been ruled out. Because of the risk of shock associated with torsions of this nature, definitive therapy should be instituted as soon as possible. Treatment of uterine torsion is aimed at derotation of the torsed segment and evacuation of the uterus. If tissues are viable, Pituitrin is given following derotation and again 60 minutes later to aid involution. If ischemic necrosis is extensive, ovariohysterectomy is indicated. If unilateral torsion and necrosis have occurred in a breeding animal, the affected horn and ovary may be excised. The prognosis should remain guarded until the animal is well stabilized following surgery. Antibiotics should be administered postoperatively for 7 to 10 days.

## VAGINA

Vaginal emergencies include traumatic lacerations of the vulva and vaginal wall or automutilation of vaginal prolapses. Cases we have observed have followed automobile accidents, trauma from instruments used during deliveries and forceful separation of dogs during mating. The animal with lacerations must be thoroughly examined for other possible injuries prior to surgical correction. If presented in shock following an accident, the animal must be stabilized and hemorrhage controlled prior to surgery. Since vaginal lacerations are generally near the exterior surfaces, they are readily repaired by standard surgical procedures. Extensive vaginal hyperplasia or patients with automutilation, necrosis and hemorrhage require surgical intervention. Exposure to deeper wounds is facilitated by episiotomy.

## MASTITIS

Septic mastitis usually occurs following parturition as a result of ascending infection but may result from penetrating wounds. Nonseptic mastitis may follow bruising of the glands, with resulting ischemic necrosis. This discussion is limited to acute fulminating mastitis; for further details, consult the article on "Non-neoplastic Diseases of the Mammary Glands of Dogs and Cats."

The owner may be made aware of the problem by observing that the pups become restless, cry frequently and begin to weaken from ingestion of the abnormal secretion or from lack of nursing. The patient is listless, febrile and anorexic; has hot, swollen, painful mammary glands; and hesitates to stay with the litter. Secretion from the involved glands is usually purulent and varies in color from cream to brown. If the mammary gland(s) is gangrenous, it is usually discolored (green to purple-black) and glistening on the surface.

Diagnosis of mastitis does not require complicated procedures. We routinely scan smears of material obtained from the teat canal or by needle aspiration of the inflamed gland stained with new methylene blue to assess bacterial and cellular components. We also perform bacterial culture and antibiotic sensitivity tests on this material. During treatment of infectious mastitis, the pups should be fed a commercial milk replacement. Until the culture results are available, broad-spectrum antibiotics should be administered, the infected glands should be hot-packed and necrotic tissue should be debrided. Frequent milking of the involved glands promotes removal of exudate and improves blood circulation. Since abscessation or the development of a gangrenous gland permits the absorption of toxins, abscesses should be lanced and drained as soon as possible. In the case of gangrenous mastitis, the gangrenous area should be debrided following administration of an analgesic such as oxymorphone or a general anesthetic. The debrided wound may be closed by suturing the skin over a Penrose drain, or it may be allowed to heal by second intention. We commonly apply enzymes such as chymotrypsin to the area in conjunction with an antibacterial ointment (Furacin® [Eaton]) for 48 to 72 hours. Satisfactory healing usually occurs if adequate drainage and/or debridement and antibiotic therapy have been provided.

## PUERPERAL TETANY

Puerperal tetany usually occurs in the bitch and queen within the first three weeks following parturition. Tetany may also occur later or in the immediate prepartum period, however.

The factor responsible for this syndrome is a reduction in the concentration of ionized calcium in extracellular fluids. As a consequence of the hypocalcemia, cell membrane potentials are altered, allowing spontaneous discharge of nerve fibers to produce tonic or tonoclonic contraction of skeletal muscles. The serum concentration of total calcium is generally less than 7 mg./dl. during tetany, although there is no consistent correlation between the development of tetany and the degree of hypocalcemia. Both the rate and magnitude of reduction in ionized calcium influence the onset and severity of tetany.

The underlying cause(s) of hypocalcemia is not well defined. A combination of calcium losses, including fetal ossification and lactation, along with inadequacies in osteoclastic activity and/or balanced calcium assimilation appears to be responsible for the disrupted homeostasis. The hypothesis that parathyroid inadequacy is largely responsible for the homeostatic defect is attractive, since it is unusual for most cats and larger breeds of dogs to experience puerperal tetany. Smaller, nervous dogs are especially prone to develop tetany.

In health, total plasma calcium consists of approximately 50 per cent ionized or biologically active calcium; the other fraction is un-ionized and protein-bound. Any factor initiating a shift toward the un-ionized form of calcium favors the development of tetany. One such factor is systemic alkalosis. Conceivably, a nervous bitch hyperventilating during sustained dystocia could develop a sufficient degree of respiratory alkalosis to reduce the concentration of ionized calcium. Here, tetany may occur even in the presence of marginally normal total serum calcium levels.

Although hypoglycemia and hypoproteinemia have been reported in cases of puerperal tetany, they play no role in the production of tetany. Hypoglycemia is a complication rather than a cause of tetany. Paradoxically, hypoproteinemia may actually delay development of tetany in patients with marginally low serum calcium levels by favoring the shift of un-ionized protein-bound calcium to ionized unbound calcium.

The role that stress plays in the development of puerperal tetany is nebulous. Although its precise role is undefined, stress could affect calcium homeostasis by reducing dietary calcium and vitamin D intake.

In summary, the precise mechanism by which the relative or absolute hypocalcemia develops is not well defined. It appears to be multifactorial and could involve any stage of calcium metabolism—intake, absorption and excretion as well as vitamin D and parathyroid-influenced osteoclastic activities.

Symptoms vary depending on the phase of the syndrome observed. Sequentially, most bitches exhibit nervousness or anxiety evidenced by pacing, whining and panting. Occasionally, hyperirritability is noted. Ataxia with an accompanying stiff-legged, seemingly painful gait follows, progressing rapidly to spastic lateral recumbency. Patients presented in tetany are often febrile, owing to the rigorous tonic or tonoclonic spasms. Occasionally the syndrome encompasses central nervous system disturbances characterized by epileptiform-like seizures, although consciousness is generally preserved. Auditory or tactile stimuli may incite either the tonic phase of the syndrome or seizure. Death may result as a complication of respiratory distress or hyperthermic cerebral edema. The duration of signs may span minutes to hours, depending on the severity of the problem.

The signs of puerperal tetany are not pathognomonic. They are only signs of hypocalcemia, which has multiple causes and multiple phases (pretetanic and tetanic). The tetanic phase includes spasms of peripheral origin, which appear similar to those of strychnine poisoning, and less often tonoclonic spasms of probable central origin, which appear similar to epileptiform seizures. Since the syndrome is associated with a wide array of symptoms depending on the phase observed, diagnosis depends heavily on a compatible history of a parturient or postpartum bitch with typical clinical symptoms. Once the diagnosis is made, it is rarely prudent to wait for laboratory confirmation of hypocalcemia before instituting therapy; however, in all cases, a pretreatment blood sample should be collected for analysis should the patient fail to respond as anticipated.

The goal of therapy is to reestablish and maintain normal blood calcium concentration. Since most patients are presented in tetany and often are hyperthermic, rapid remission of symptoms is desirable. This is readily accomplished by slow intravenous administration of 5 to 10 ml. of a 10 per cent calcium solution. Concurrent auscultation of the heart is recommended. If bradycardia or cardiac arrhythmias develop, infusion should be discontinued until normal heart rate and sinus rhythm return. When body temperature is about 41° C. (106° F.), the patient should also be cooled. Once relaxation is complete, intravenous calcium therapy should be discontinued. However, it is advantageous to administer an additional intramuscular dosage of one half the initial volume with an equal volume of physiologic saline to prevent immediate relapses. Occasionally, the administration of a therapeutic dosage of calcium will fail to produce relaxation. At that point the clinician must reassess the patient for factors such as respiratory alkalosis that would make her less responsive to calcium therapy. Complicating hypoglycemia should also be considered if there is mental dullness or tonoclonic types of seizures. Intravenous dextrose will correct hypoglycemia, and sedation will minimize hyperventilation. Response to calcium therapy should not be masked by anesthesia. This measure should be reserved for those patients suspected of puerperal tetany in whom further calcium administration is contraindicated and in whom there has been no response to intravenous dextrose or Valium® (Roche). The analysis of pretreatment blood samples should be performed as soon as possible as an aid to definitive diagnosis.

The final goal of therapy is maintenance of normal blood calcium concentration. This may be accomplished by removing the pups from the bitch for 24 hours, thus reducing ongoing calcium losses by lactation. Bitch's replacement milk (Esbilac® [Borden]) or similar formulas should be fed during this period. If older, the pups should be weaned. If the pups are young enough to benefit from further nursing, a regimen of alternate nursing and hand-feeding is appropriate for an additional day or two. Full nursing may then be reinstituted, provided that adequate dietary calcium therapy has been prescribed for the bitch.

In our experience, puerperal tetany has often been encountered in dogs receiving diets with marginal calcium-phosphorus ratios and total calcium levels. On a dry weight basis, diets of at least 1 per cent calcium with a calcium-phosphorus ratio of 1.4:1.0 have been recommended. We routinely institute calcium lactate or calcium gluconate therapy post partum in tetany-prone bitches at doses of 1 to 3 grams per day for 3 to 4 weeks, depending on the size of the bitch and litter, as well as the type of diet the dog was previously eating. In these ranges overdosage is unlikely, since excess calcium will not be absorbed unless vitamin D intake is inappropriately high. Because of the calorie demands of lactating bitches, their concern for diet palatability is generally reduced, and once stabilized from a tetanic episode, most bitches will accept commercial, well-balanced diets adequately.

Vitamin D therapy at dosages of 10,000 to 25,000 I.U. per day has been advocated to enhance intestinal absorption and bone resorption of calcium salts. Since most commercial dog foods are fortified with 5 to 10 times the dog's minimum daily requirement of vitamin D, and since many owners institute vitamin therapy on their own accord, caution should be exercised in prescribing this therapy. As a fat-soluble vitamin, it is not readily excreted when overdosed and has the potential to produce hypercalcemia and dystropic calcification, especially of the kidneys.

Corticosteroid therapy has been popularly employed as a method of reducing relapses. However, the immediate effect of steroids, especially in high therapeutic dosages, is to lower serum calcium concentration. Obviously their use is contraindicated prior to, or immediately following, reconstitution of serum concentration. Time is required for the catabolic effects of steroids to deplete bone protein matrix sufficiently to increase extracellular calcium concentration. The administration of 2.5 to 5 mg. of prednisolone may be instituted 24 to 48 hours after a tetanic episode. In our experience, if this drug is continued daily with gradual withdrawal, adverse reaction will not be a problem.

Balanced diets combined with routine postpartum calcium supplementation in tetany-prone bitches have been effective prophylactically in our experience. In resistant cases, modest steroid dosages may be instituted along with calcium a week prior to delivery and continued throughout lactation.

## SUPPLEMENTAL READING

DeHoff, W. D., Greene, R. W., and Greiner, T. P.: Surgical management of abdominal emergencies. Vet. Clin. N. Am., 2:141–153, 1972.

Johnston, D. E.: Male genital system. *In* Canine

Surgery. 1st Archibald ed. American Veterinary Publications, Inc., 114 Northwest St., Wheaton, Illinois.

Mara, J. P.: Pyometra. In Kirk, R. W. (ed.): Current Veterinary Therapy IV. Philadelphia, W. B. Saunders Co., 1971, pp. 762–764.

Osborne, C. A., Low, D. G., and Finco, D. R.: Canine and Feline Urology. Philadelphia, W. B. Saunders Co., 1972, pp. 249–253.

Roberts, S. J.: Causes of dystocia. In Veterinary Obstetrics and Genital Diseases. Published by the Author, Ithaca, New York, pp. 136–143, 1956. Distributed by Edwards Brothers Inc., Ann Arbor, Michigan.

Smith, K. W.: Female genital tract. In Canine Surgery. 1st Archibald ed. American Veterinary Publications, Inc., 114 Northwest St., Wheaton, Illinois.

Soma, L. R.: Anesthetic Management for Cesarean Section. In Veterinary Anesthesia. Baltimore, The Williams and Wilkins Co., 1971, pp. 303–309.

# ACUTE METRITIS

ROLF E. LARSEN, D.V.M.,
and JAMES W. WILSON, D.V.M.
St. Paul, Minnesota

Acute metritis is most often a disease of the immediate postpartum period. It commonly occurs as a sequela of dystocia and obstetric manipulations, abortion or retained placentas or fetuses. Less commonly, it occurs postestrum as a result of nonsterile artificial insemination or mating. It may also occur following an apparently normal whelping. In all cases, uterine involution is delayed, resulting in an enlarged flaccid uterus. Because the inflammatory process often involves all uterine layers, the uterus is usually thickened but very friable.

## CLINICAL SIGNS

Clinical signs usually begin one to three days following whelping and may be associated with any combination of the following: depression, fever, agalactia, anorexia, foul-smelling vaginal discharge and/or loss of maternal instincts. Physical examination may reveal an elevated temperature, increased heart rate or vaginal discharge, with consistency, color and odor varying from the normal brown, odorless lochia. An enlarged uterus can usually be delineated by abdominal palpation.

## LABORATORY FINDINGS

The presence of a retained fetus can usually be verified by palpation and radiographs. If placentas are retained, whelping history and the characteristics of the vaginal discharge are important diagnostic clues. Following normal whelpings, the dark green discharge characteristic of second stage labor will change to a blood-tinged mucoid discharge within 12 hours following complete passage of the membranes. If incomplete expulsion of placental material has occurred, the green discharge will persist for more than 12 hours after birth of the last fetus. When placentas are not expelled within 12 to 24 hours, acute metritis often results. Unless corrective measures are instituted during the early stages of this condition, necrosis of the uterine wall in the areas of placental attachment may result in severe peritonitis and even death. For this reason, owners should be encouraged to count placentas during whelping.

The hemogram usually reveals an immature leukocytosis; however, a normal count with hypersegmented neutrophils is not uncommon. Toxemia and/or dehydration, if present, may be associated with increases in packed cell volume, serum protein and BUN. If vaginal cytologic examination is performed, smears may contain clusters of endometrial cells with foamy cytoplasm, neutrophils, cellular debris, mucus and bacteria. Most stains used readily reveal organisms both inside and outside cells. Characterization of these organisms using Gram stains should aid in the choice of therapeutic regimen.

## PROGNOSIS

The prognosis of acute metritis is directly related to the condition of the bitch at the time of evaluation and the interval between onset of signs and institution of treatment. Because this condition can rapidly progress to severe toxicity and dehydration, any sign of the development of metritis is cause for immediate treatment. Early identification of acute metritis in most cases is dependent upon the owner. For this reason, one of the most important aspects of early diagnosis is education of the client about potential problems and signs that warrant immediate medical attention. Rectal temperatures should be taken for a week following parturition, preferably twice daily. Fever in excess of 103.0° F, signs of depression, decreased interest in caring for the pups or vaginal discharges with an offensive odor should prompt consultation with a veterinarian. Owners should be advised to clip the hair in the perineal region prior to whelping. This will facilitate cleansing the area during and after whelping and will enhance the owner's ability to observe passage of uterine contents.

## TREATMENT

Treatment of metritis uncomplicated by retained placentas consists of local and systemic antibacterial medication, stimulation of uterine drainage and supportive fluid therapy. When the bitch is examined, material for bacterial culture and determination of antibiotic sensitivity should be obtained from the region of the cervix. Intravenous or intramuscular loading doses of a broad-spectrum antibiotic should be initiated until the results of bacterial culture and antibiotic sensitivity tests are known. Intrauterine infusions of antibiotics will hasten recovery and may stimulate involution. Nitrofurazone or soluble tetracyclines are satisfactory for infusion in most cases until results of sensitivity testing are available.

Infusion of the uterus with a closing cervix is not always a simple task. A vaginoscope or speculum of at least 5 to 6 inches in length may be required, even in small bitches. In larger breeds, the cervix may lie 8 to 10 inches cranial to the vulva. A plastic insemination pipette with a smooth tip that can be manipulated through the vaginoscope is satisfactory for infusion of antibiotic solutions. The tip of the pipette should be placed against the folds at the external os. A distinct structure recognizable as the cervix is not visible, and the folds of the fornix should be gently probed with the infusion pipette until an opening that allows free passage of the antibacterial solution is found. The infusion should be made without actually attempting to pass the pipette into the uterus, which may be ex-

tremely fragile. Several attempts at proper placement of the pipette to insure passage of the liquid through the cervix are often necessary. If the uterine opening is visible, a soft rubber catheter may be passed into the body of the uterus for the infusion. In some bitches with a cervix that is not visibly open, ventral traction on the uterine body by external abdominal manipulation will align the cervix with the vagina and allow passage of a smooth-tipped catheter.

An intramuscular injection of oxytocin at a dosage of 1.0 unit/kg. of body weight should be given to stimulate myometrial activity; it may be repeated one to two hours following the initial injection. Poor response may indicate the need for ergonovine to stimulate myometrial contractions. Ergonovine may also reduce the severity of excessive uterine bleeding, owing to its ergot-like properties. Since ergonovine has a more intense effect on the myometrium than does oxytocin, it should not be used unless the response to oxytocin is inadequate. Both these drugs will act more forcefully on an estrogen-sensitized uterus. If estradiol or diethylstilbestrol is administered systemically to effect uterine sensitization, dosages should be at the low end of their suggested therapeutic range. Higher dosages reduce lactation and suppress bone marrow functions. An alternative method of administering the estrogenic compound is uterine infusion. Intrauterine infusions of Utonex® (Schering) are reported to give excellent results without causing potentially toxic high systemic levels.

Removal of the pups is indicated for optimal care of the bitch, but this decision must be tempered by an evaluation of the resources available for their care. If acute metritis is recognized and treated before the bitch becomes extremely toxic, the pups need only be withheld until a positive response occurs. It should be remembered that the use of estrogen will reduce or eliminate lactation. In some cases of reduced lactation due to treatment with estrogen, milk production may resume after a period of a few days to a week.

Surgical intervention may be warranted if severe signs are observed, if placental retention is suspected or if medical therapy is ineffective. The abdominal exposure should be adequate to allow easy visualization of both uterine horns, the uterine body and the cervix. The entire tract should be visually examined and palpated. Some cases of retained placenta may be associated with necrosis of the adjacent uterine wall. In such cases, the serosal surface often appears discolored. Crater-like deficits or swellings in the uterine wall may be palpated. Uterine necrosis, avascularity or laceration warrants complete ovariohysterectomy. If the uterus appears viable, surgical assisted manipulation and lavage are recommended. A catheter should be passed through the cervix into the uterus and directed into both horns. As each horn is lavaged, the surgeon should gently massage each horn in an attempt to break down accumulated debris. Postoperative care includes continuation of medical therapy.

## SUPPLEMENTAL READING

Arthur, G. H.: Wright's Veterinary Obstetrics. 3rd ed. Baltimore, The Williams and Wilkins Co., 1964.

Bloom, F.: Pathology of the Dog and Cat. Evanston, Illinois, American Veterinary Publications, Inc., 1954.

Christoph, H. J. Diseases of Dogs. Oxford, England, Pergamon Press, 1975.

Durfee, P. T.: Surgical treatment of postparturient metritis in the bitch. J. Am. Vet. Med. Assn., 153:40–42, 1968.

Kirk, R. W., McEntee, K., and Bentinck–Smith, J.: Diseases of the urogenital system. In Catcott, E. J. (ed.): Canine Medicine. Wheaton, Illinois, American Veterinary Publications, Inc., 1968.

Roberts, S. J.: Veterinary Obstetrics and Genital Diseases. Edwards Brothers, Inc. Ann Arbor, Michigan, 1971.

# CANINE PYOMETRA–A POLYSYSTEMIC DISORDER

ROBERT M. HARDY, D.V.M.,
and CARL A. OSBORNE, D.V.M.
St. Paul, Minnesota

Canine pyometra may be defined as an acute or chronic, polysystemic metestrual disease of the mature bitch. Pyometra is associated with a wide variety of clinical and pathologic manifestations related to both genital and extragenital lesions.

## ETIOPATHOGENESIS OF GENITAL LESIONS

The etiopathogenesis of genital lesions in canine pyometra is a complex process. Pyometra ultimately results from excessive and/or prolonged stimulation of the uterus by progesterone produced by retained and/or cystic corpora lutea. Progesterone initially produces cystic endometrial hyperplasia of the uterus. The uterine effects of progesterone are amplified by estrogen in many instances. Prolonged or repeated progesterone stimulation results in an acute inflammatory reaction that may be aggravated by secondary bacterial infection. A decrease in progesterone, following regression of the corpus luteum, is associated with resolution of the acute inflammatory reaction and plasma cell infiltration. Repeated cycles in dogs with functional closure of the cervix result in the development of chronic endometritis. Cervical patency is variable; closure of the cervix usually results in an exacerbation of clinical signs. Although bacteria do not initiate the disease process, their presence in advanced cases with severe endometrial and myometrial damage is often associated with bacteremia and/or septicemia.

Spontaneous recovery may occur following regression of the corpus luteum, relaxation of the cervix and discharge of the uterine contents. Such dogs usually have recurrent attacks at subsequent estrous cycles, however. The severity of recurrent attacks is dependent on the concentration of circulating progesterone, the degree of cervical patency and the severity of secondary bacterial infection.

## ETIOPATHOGENESIS OF RENAL MANIFESTATIONS

Renal involvement associated with pyometra may be related to prerenal azotemia, primary glomerular disease, reduction in tubular capacity to concentrate urine, concomitant renal disease(s) the etiology of which is unrelated to pyometra or combinations of these disorders.

If poor renal perfusion secondary to dehydration or shock develops in dogs or cats with pyometra, prerenal azotemia may develop. If the prerenal cause of poor renal perfusion is allowed to persist, varying degrees of ischemic tubular disease may develop. (Consult the article on "Glomerulonephropathy and the Nephrotic Syndrome" for specific details about prerenal azotemia.)

A mixed membranoproliferative glomerulonephropathy has been observed in dogs with pyometra. This lesion is probably caused by the deposition of immune complexes in glomerular capillary walls. We have not encountered glomerular lesions of sufficient severity to cause primary renal failure. The glomerulonephropathy associated with pyometra is apparently reversible following surgical removal of the uterus. (Consult the article on "Glomerulonephropathy and the Nephrotic Syndrome" for specific details.)

Impairment of tubular capacity to concentrate urine may be observed in dogs with pyometra. Obligatory polyuria and compensatory polydipsia in dogs with pyometra differ from the renal concentrating defect associated with generalized renal disease, in that dogs with pyometra have no impairment of their ability to dilute urine. Because solute can be removed from tubular filtrate in excess of water, the urine specific gravity may be significantly below ($< 1.007$) the specific gravity of glomerular filtrate (1.008 to 1.012). The inability of the kidneys to concentrate urine is related to a decrease in the capacity of the loops of Henle, distal tubules and collecting ducts to reabsorb water, in spite of adequate circulating levels of antidiuretic hormone, and to a decrease in the concentration of sodium in the renal medulla. Further studies must be performed to determine whether this tubular disorder is associated with an immunologic disturbance.

Although both primary renal failure and pyometra are frequently encountered in middle-aged and older dogs, the actual frequency with which pyometra occurs in association with unrelated renal diseases is unknown. Renal calculi, pyelonephritis and chronic generalized nephritis of undetermined etiology have been observed in dogs with pyometra at the University of Minnesota.

## PATHOPHYSIOLOGY OF DISEASE IN OTHER SYSTEMS

In addition to the genital and renal lesions described above, other body organs, including bone marrow, liver, spleen, adrenal glands and lungs, may be altered in canine pyometra. An increase in the myeloid-erythroid ratio due to hyperplasia of the myeloid elements is the most common bone marrow alteration. The tremendous demand for neutrophils produced by the inflamed endometrium frequently results in a massive outpouring of white blood cells into the peripheral circulation. A marked leukocytosis, which is frequently immature, occurs in many cases. In severely toxic animals, a decreased WBC count associated with immaturity and a mild to severe nonregenerative anemia may develop secondary to bone marrow depression. The most prominent change in the liver, spleen and adrenal glands is the presence of extramedullary myelopoiesis. This reflects the inability of the bone marrow to keep pace with the peripheral demand for neutrophils. Occasionally, unilateral or bilateral adrenal cortical collapse and medullary hemorrhage may develop. In animals that fail to respond postoperatively, the possibility of adrenal cortical collapse should be considered.

## CLINICAL FINDINGS

Pyometra usually occurs in dogs over 6 years of age. The severity of clinical signs in an individual patient is dependent upon the patency of the cervix, the stage of the estrous cycle, the presence or absence of secondary bacterial infection of the uterus, the duration of illness and the severity of the underlying uterine and extragenital lesions.

Signs of illness observed most often include depression, anorexia, vaginal discharge, vomiting, diarrhea, polydipsia, polyuria and nocturia. Signs less frequently observed by owners are abdominal distention and edema or enlargement of the vulva. The amount of vaginal discharge observed may be scanty or profuse and is dependent, in part, on the degree of cervical patency. The discharge is usually yellow-gray or brown in color and has a fetid odor. Dogs with pyometra in which the cervix is partially or completely closed accumulate large quantities of pus within the uterine lumen and tend to be more depressed and "toxic" appearing than dogs in which a patent cervix allows for uterine drainage. Although these signs are not pathognomonic of pyometra, their presence in nonspayed middle-aged bitches should be interpreted to suggest this disease until proved otherwise.

The onset of clinical signs usually follows estrus. Most clinical cases are examined within one to 12 weeks following the last observed estrus. The duration of clinical illness is variable. Of 79 clinical cases of pyometra of all degrees of severity evaluated at the University of Minnesota, the mean duration of illness was 12.7 days. Contrary to reports in the literature, there is no good evidence that pseudopregnancy, irregular heat cycles and/or lack of previous pregnancy predispose dogs to pyometra.

## PHYSICAL EXAMINATION

Abnormalities detected on physical examination of dogs with pyometra are variable but frequently include depression, dehydration, vaginal discharge and palpable uterine enlargement. The rectal temperature is usually normal. Subnormal temperatures may occur in severely toxic animals. Excess palpation may be hazardous, since the uterus may be friable and easily traumatized or ruptured. Rectally palpating the dog while the forequarters are elevated may be helpful in those dogs in which pyometra is suspected but in which the uterus is not palpable through the abdomen. Such a technique may permit palpation of an enlarged uterus at the pelvic inlet, just dorsal to the urinary bladder.

## LABORATORY FINDINGS

The hemogram is usually characterized by an absolute neutrophilia associated with varying degrees of immaturity. The total white blood cell counts usually range from 20,000 to 100,000/cu. mm. The higher counts are most often observed in cases in which uterine drainage is prevented by a closed cervix. Normal to subnormal white blood cell counts are rarely seen but, when present, are indicative of severe toxemia. Although surgical removal of the uterus re-

moves the demand for leukocytes, continued medullary and extramedullary myelopoiesis occurs for several days. As a result, postoperative white cell counts may exceed those observed preoperatively.

A normocytic, normochromic anemia is present in a significant number of cases. Of 101 pyometra cases surveyed by the authors, 25.7 per cent had a mild to severe anemia (PCV less than 36 per cent). Mild anemias may be masked in some cases because of clinical dehydration.

Moderate to marked hyperproteinemia occurs in most cases of pyometra. The plasma fibrinogen concentrations are usually within normal limits (500 to 700 mg./dl.). The serum albumin concentration tends to be mildly depressed, but the serum globulin concentrations are frequently elevated.

It is recommended that a complete urinalysis and determination of the serum concentration of blood urea nitrogen or creatinine be evaluated prior to surgery in all patients with pyometra. The presurgical BUN concentration was elevated (over 35 mg./dl.) in 17.7 per cent of 79 pyometra cases surveyed at the University of Minnesota.

It is difficult to assess presurgical renal function accurately without data obtained from a complete urinalysis. Since all dogs with pyometra have the potential to develop prerenal and/or primary renal failure, a complete urinalysis should always be evaluated in conjunction with the BUN concentration to determine the patient's renal functional status. Accurate formulation of preoperative, operative and postoperative fluid requirements depends on such knowledge.

Significant numbers of dogs with pyometra may have proteinuria in the absence of red cells and/or white cells. If large numbers of inflammatory cells are present in urine, it is difficult to assess accurately the origin of proteinuria. The presence of persistent proteinuria in the absence of RBC and WBC is indicative of glomerular disease (see article on "Glomerulonephropathy and the Nephrotic Syndrome"). Proteinuria occurring in association with significant numbers of RBC and WBC indicates the presence of an inflammatory lesion that may be located anywhere along the genitourinary tract. In some cases, proteinuria may occur as a result of contamination of urine with inflammatory exudate from the genital system. In order to eliminate as much genital tract contamination as possible, the vulva should be cleansed thoroughly prior to collection of a midstream urine sample. Alternatively, a urine specimen may be obtained by catheterization.

The cytologic examination of vaginal smears may be of diagnostic value in cases of pyometra with either an open or a closed cervix. Early metestrual vaginal smears normally contain many neutrophils and variable numbers of bacteria. By the 10th to 20th day of metestrus, most of the neutrophils and bacteria have been replaced by small, noncornified or large, flat epithelial cells with vacuolated cytoplasm. In contrast, vaginal smears from dogs with pyometra are characterized by excessively large numbers or masses of neutrophils and bacteria, which persist into late metestrus and anestrus.

## RADIOGRAPHY

In many cases of pyometra, radiography is not necessary to establish a diagnosis. Abdominal radiographs are valuable in such cases, however, to confirm the presence of an enlarged uterus and to evaluate the abdomen for concomitant diseases (abnormal kidney size, renal calculi, foreign bodies, peritonitis, etc.). All types of pathologic uteri, except uncomplicated cystic endometrial hyperplasia, should be visible on survey radiographs.

Affected uteri are characterized radiographically by the presence of a homogeneous tubular structure of fluid density in the posterior abdomen. In cases in which the intestines prevent adequate visualization of the uterus, abdominal compression techniques may be used to displace the intestines cranially. Contrast hysterography should not be routinely used, since it subjects the patient to unnecessary risks of uterine trauma or rupture. The only time that the normal uterus is radiographically visible is during the latter stages of pregnancy and for a variable time period following parturition.

## DIFFERENTIAL DIAGNOSIS

The presence of pyometra can be detected in most dogs without difficulty. Dogs with pyometra but without either physical or historical evidence of a vaginal discharge present the greatest diagnostic challenge. Other conditions characterized by polydipsia and polyuria, nonspecific and vague signs of illness and/or an enlarging abdomen must also be considered. Occasionally, a pregnant bitch will be encountered without a history of recent breeding. Prior to surgical removal, the uterus should be carefully palpated to confirm the diagnosis of pyometra and to eliminate the possibility of pregnancy.

A number of disease syndromes associated with polydipsia and polyuria may be confused with pyometra. Renal failure is particularly important because of the frequency with which the two diseases coexist. Other syndromes associated with polydipsia and polyuria that may be confused with pyometra include diabetes mellitus, hyperadrenocorticism and generalized hepatic disease.

## DIAGNOSIS

The diagnosis of pyometra can usually be made on the basis of clinical signs, laboratory data, radiography and microscopic examination of vaginal swabs. The detection of concomitant diseases, especially renal disease, requires a high index of suspicion. For this reason, urinalyses, hemograms and the serum concentration of creatinine or BUN should be evaluated in all suspected cases.

## THERAPY

**Surgical Treatment.** The most satisfactory treatment for the majority of patients with pyometra is ovariohysterectomy. Medical therapy should be considered only for valuable breeding bitches or dogs which are extremely poor surgical candidates. The use of supportive therapy (i.e., fluids, antibiotics, blood transfusions) may be required before, during and after surgery. Avoid any unnecessary therapeutic delays prior to surgery. Presurgical delay for prolonged supportive therapy is rarely associated with clinical improvement of the patient. In fact, patients often continue to deteriorate.

Surgery in pyometra cases complicated by renal failure presents special problems in terms of treatment and prognosis. Abnormalities causing poor renal perfusion in patients with prerenal uremia should be corrected prior to, during and following surgery to prevent or minimize the development of ischemic renal disease. Fluid deficits that are polyionic and isotonic in nature should be replaced by polyionic isotonic rehydrating solutions (lactated Ringer's solution).

Surgery may be successfully performed in patients with primary renal failure, provided that careful attention is paid to fluid and electrolyte balance and to the potential complications that may develop during the postoperative period. In those pyometra cases with impaired renal function, prophylactic renoprotective therapy should be employed. Adequate hydration must be maintained in order to insure sufficient renal perfusion during surgery.

The timely induction and maintenance of diuresis at surgery may effectively minimize or prevent renal failure in high-risk patients. The use of diuretics such as hypertonic dextrose (10 or 20 per cent), hypertonic mannitol (20 or 25 per cent), furosemide and ethacrynic acid, either singly or in combination, has provided the most consistent results. The effectiveness of these diuretics is related directly to their ability to induce and sustain diuresis. It is emphasized that diuretics are not effective substitutes for adequate hydration and electrolyte replacement. Diuretics may be detrimental to renal homeostatic defense mechanisms unless used in conjunction with adequate fluid and electrolyte replacement.

Either furosemide or ethacrynic acid may induce diuresis in some patients unresponsive to osmotic diuretics. These drugs may be administered either orally or intravenously at test dosages recommended by the manufacturers. If a significant diuresis is not achieved after a period of approximately 2 hours, the dosage should be doubled or tripled. The frequency with which furosemide or ethacrynic acid is administered depends on the objectives of therapy and patient response. Because of the potency of these drugs, the fluid and electrolyte balance of the patient should be monitored. Periodic replacement therapy with parenteral fluids may be required. If a significant diuresis does not develop, therapy with furosemide and ethacrynic acid should be discontinued.

Biopsy of the kidneys at the time of ovariohysterectomy may be indicated in patients with pyometra and concomitant primary renal failure. Visual inspection of the kidneys at the time of surgery and microscopic evaluation of a renal biopsy specimen may help to differentiate reversible lesions from irreversible ones. Detection of kidneys with significant gross renal lesions at the time of surgery is an indication for renal biopsy, since gross renal lesions are not a typical finding in pyometra nephritis.

Whether postoperative renal failure occurs more frequently in canine pyometra than in other major abdominal surgical procedures is unknown. Because of the large number of pyometra cases with some form of renal disease, the possibility for renal complications to develop during or following surgery may be greater in such animals. Careful presurgical, surgical and postsurgical attention to fluid and electrolyte needs of the patient is especially important to reduce the likelihood of development of such complications.

Leakage of uterine contents into the peritoneal cavity when the uterine stump is excised, or as a result of rupture of the diseased uterine wall, may also cause surgical complications. Both may result in varying degrees of peritonitis. In addition, leakage of exudate from the uterine stump predisposes the patient to formation of a postoperative stump granuloma. If peritoneal contamination occurs, the abdominal cavity should be flushed with warm lactated Ringer's solution, and water-soluble antibiotics should be placed into the peritoneal cavity prior to surgical repair of the abdominal wall.

**Medical Treatment.**  A number of nonsurgical methods for the treatment of canine pyometra are available. Although present evidence to support the use of such methods is limited, preliminary results appear encouraging. The objectives of medical therapy should include (1) restoration of reproductive capacity in valuable breeding animals, (2) drainage and lavage of the uterus, (3) elimination of secondary bacterial contaminants of the uterus and (4) removal of the source of progesterone production responsible for initiating the disease.

Hormones used to treat pyometra include estrogens, testosterone and oxytocin. Estrogens have been associated with varying degrees of success. They promote expulsion of uterine exudate by initiating cervical relaxation, increasing uterine muscular tone and increasing uterine contractility. Estrogens also increase the resistance of the uterus to bacterial infection. Estrogen may be given orally, as diethylstilbestrol, at a dose of 1 mg. twice daily for 7 days, followed by 1 mg. daily for 3 weeks. Although clinical improvement may occur following estrogen therapy, severe exacerbations necessitating surgical intervention often develop.

Testosterone has also been advocated for the medical treatment of pyometra. In one study, testosterone was administered at a dose of 25 mg. twice weekly to 10 dogs with pyometra. Clinical remission occurred in 7 dogs within 3 weeks. A severe exacerbation developed in one dog, necessitating ovariohysterectomy. The beneficial effects ascribed to testosterone therapy are thought to occur as a result of ovarian atrophy. Further clinical evaluation of this drug is required before meaningful generalizations can be made.

Both oxytocin and the ergot alkaloids have been used to stimulate expulsion of uterine exudate by increasing uterine motility. Because oxytocin is most effective in an estrogen-sensitized uterus and since pyometra is associated with a high level of progesterone activity, a priming period with estrogen should be considered prior to the use of this drug. Ergonovine maleate, one of the ergot alkaloids, is also more effective in an estrogen-primed uterus. Ergonovine maleate may be administered parenterally at a dose of 0.2 mg. twice daily for 10 days.

Under no circumstances should progesterone or related compounds be given to dogs with pyometra, since they will aggravate the disease. The use of progesterone to delay or prevent estrus may also result in the development of pyometra in some cases.

Several procedures have been developed to facilitate drainage of uterine exudate. Self-retaining catheters (male Foley No. 20) manually passed through an open cervix can be used to aspirate uterine contents. Following catheterization, instillation of mucolytic agents (Alevaire® [Breon]) into the uterus may be effective in decreasing the viscosity of inspissated uterine exudate. In animals with a closed cervix, catheters may be inserted following dilatation of the cervical lumen via a hysterotomy incision. In severely toxic animals, the uterus may be marsupialized through a small stab incision in the abdomen. This procedure provides drainage while supportive presurgical care is continued, and it is usually performed under local anesthesia.

Since the presence of persistent and/or cystic corpora lutea is a significant factor in the pathogenesis of canine pyometra, surgical removal of these structures has been advocated as part of a combined medical-surgical approach to pyometra treatment. The objective of this procedure is to promote regression of pathologic uterine changes by eliminating the major source of endogenous progesterone.

The use of systemic and intrauterine broad-spectrum antibiotics is important for the control of secondary bacterial infections. Antibiotic choices should be based on the results of culture and sensitivity testing of uterine exudate.

Medical therapy combining diethylstilbestrol, ergonovine maleate and systemic antibiotics, with or without surgical intervention to remove corpora lutea and establish uterine drainage, has been associated with encouraging early success. It is emphasized that medical therapy should be attempted only in valuable breeding animals in relatively good physical condition. The long-term reproductive health and fertility of animals receiving such therapy is currently unknown.

Although survival data on large numbers of pyometra cases are limited, most surveys indicate that an 80 per cent survival should be anticipated.

## SUPPLEMENTAL READING

Dow, C.: The cystic hyperplasia–pyometra complex in the bitch. J. Comp. Pathol., 69:237–250, 1959.

Ewing, G. D., Schecter, R. D., Whitney, R. C., and Wind, A. P.: The therapy of canine pyometra. J. Am. Anim. Hosp. Assn., 6:218, 1970.

Gourley, I. M.: Treatment of canine pyometra without ovariohysterectomy. *In* Bojrab, M. J. (ed.): Current Techniques in Small Animal Surgery. Philadelphia, Lea & Febiger, 1975.

Hardy, R. M., and Osborne, C. A.: Canine pyometra: pathophysiology, diagnosis and treatment of uterine and extra-uterine lesions. J. Am. Anim. Hosp. Assn., 10:245, 1974.

Sandholm, M., Vasenius, H., and Kivisto, A. K.: Pathogenesis of canine pyometra. J. Am. Vet. Med. Assn., 167:1006, 1975.

# CANINE VAGINITIS

PATRICIA SCHULTZ OLSON, D.V.M.
*St. Paul, Minnesota*

Vaginitis in the dog is being recognized with increased frequency. This may be related, at least in part, to the fact that breeders have become more conscientious about the potential dissemination of infectious agents by the transportation of breeding animals throughout the country. Client education has significantly increased the number of dogs examined by the veterinarian for reproductive disorders.

## CLINICAL FINDINGS

Any animal presented with a vaginal discharge and congested vaginal mucosa should be suspected of having vaginitis. The discharge should not be confused with normal proestral bleeding, the lochia immediately following parturition or abnormal uterine discharge. Proestral bleeding is a normal occurrence in the bitch and is usually associated with swelling of the vulva. Lochia, a greenish-colored material seen following parturition, rapidly diminishes in quantity within a few days after parturition and completely subsides within a few weeks. Uterine discharges may be associated with metritis or pyometra. In these cases the animal is often febrile and has signs of systemic illness. A thorough history, radiography, abdominal palpation and complete blood count will help differentiate vaginal from uterine discharges (refer to article on "Canine Pyometra–A Polysystemic Disorder").

Puppies often develop vaginitis prior to their first estrus. Although juvenile vaginitis is not normal, it usually requires no treatment and generally subsides following the first estrus. Cases of several weeks' duration may require treatment.

## DIAGNOSIS

A thorough vaginal examination should be performed using a sterilized vaginal endoscope, otoscopic cones for small breeds or young animals, fiberoptic equipment if available or a modified human anoscope (Pineda *et al.*, 1973). The anterior vagina should be evaluated for inflammation or other abnormalities. A well-lubricated, gloved finger may detect tumors, foreign bodies or malformations. A urine sample should be obtained by means of catheterization to rule out the possibility of concomitant cystitis.

Smears should be prepared by a direct impression of the vulval mucosa on a microscope slide, which is then stained with new methylene blue, and a cover-slip is applied. Deeper vaginal smears may be obtained by rubbing cotton-tipped applicators or glass rods against the vaginal mucosa and transferring cells to a glass slide for cytologic examination. Large numbers of leukocytes will usually be present on smears taken from a dog with clinical signs of vaginal infection. This finding must be interpreted with knowledge of the time of the animal's estrous cycle, since leukocytes are normally present in metestrual smears. Bacteria will be present in most vaginal smears, regardless of whether or not the dog suffers from clinical vaginitis.

Vaginal smears of any animal suspected of having vaginitis should be cultured. This can be done using a sterile culturette* or a sterilized cotton-tipped applicator, which is passed through the otoscope cone or vaginal speculum at the time of the vaginal examination. Both aerobic and anaerobic cultures can be prepared easily utilizing sheep blood agar plates and thioglycollate broth†. Aerobic microbes will generally grow both in enrichment broth and on blood agar plates. If growth of anaerobes in the thioglycollate broth is suspected, agar plates may be streaked with a sample from the

---

*Securline–MH-100 culture system, Precision Dynamics Corporation, 3031 Thornton Ave., Burbank, California 91504.

†Thioglycollate Medium®, BBL, Division of Becton-Dickinson Company, Cockeysville, Maryland 21030.

broth and incubated anaerobically. Once a potential pathogen is isolated, antibiotic sensitivity tests should be performed in order to formulate proper antimicrobial therapy.

## TREATMENT

Treatment for vaginitis is variable, being dependent on the cause of the infection, the stage of the estrous cycle and the antibiotic sensitivity results obtained by vaginal culture. In animals with primary bacterial vaginal infections, antibiotics may be infused directly into the vagina. Studies performed in other species indicate that intravaginal infusions may alter the estrous cycle (Mather *et al.*, 1976). Since no information is available at present to indicate which antibiotics are spermicidal to the canine spermatozoon, those antibiotics used for vaginal infusions must be chosen discriminately. Nitrofurazone (0.2 per cent Furacin® [Eaton]) has been used safely 48 hours prior to natural breedings or artificial insemination in the canine. One should always advise the owner not to breed the animal during the first estrus after a diagnosis of vaginitis has been made. Some breeders will not delay breeding, especially if the vaginitis is a recurring problem. In such cases rigorous treatment is recommended if the animal is to be freed of the infection prior to breeding. Bitches due to whelp within a few days also may be given antibiotic infusions in an attempt to reduce exposure of puppies to potentially pathogenic bacteria in the vaginal canal. Such intravaginal infusions are given during the last few days of gestation. Systemic antibiotics have been used in some dogs throughout their gestation, but the drugs should always be considered for their possible teratogenic effects.

In the nonpregnant animal that is not being bred, intravaginal infusions of antibiotics may be performed daily in conjunction with systemic antibiotic therapy. Diethylstilbestrol may be used in control of vaginal infections, but possible deleterious side effects of the drug should be considered (Jöchle, 1975).

In the treatment of secondary vaginitis, the inciting cause should be eliminated (neoplasia, foreign bodies, etc.) in addition to the recommendations described above.

## SUPPLEMENTAL READING

Jöchle, W.: Hormones in canine gynecology. A review. Theriogenology, Vol. 3, No. 4, April, 1975.

Mather, E. C., Hurtgen, J. P., and VanLeeuwen, W.: The effect of intrauterine manipulation and treatment on the equine estrous cycle. Proc. of the Eighth Int. Congress on Reproduction and Artificial Insemination. Cracow, Poland, 1976 (in publication).

Osbaldiston, G. W., Nuru, S., and Mosier, J. E.: Vaginal cytology and microflora of infertile bitches. J. Am. Anim. Hosp. Assn., 8:93–101, 1972.

Pineda, M. H., Kainer, R. A., and Faulkner, L. C.: Dorsal median postcervical fold in the canine vagina. Am. J. Vet. Res., 34:1487–1491, 1973.

Platt, A. M., and Simpson, R. B.: Bacterial flora of the canine vagina. Southwest Vet., 17:76–77, 1974.

# NON-NEOPLASTIC DISEASES OF THE MAMMARY GLANDS OF DOGS AND CATS

ARTHUR L. LAGE, D.V.M.
*South Weymouth, Massachusetts*

The majority of non-neoplastic diseases of the mammary glands of dogs and cats are listed in Table 1. The low incidence diseases of mammary tissue, such as tuberculosis, will not be discussed in this article.

The investigation of mammary lesions should be carried out with the same intensity and systematic approach (history, physical examination and laboratory aids) as with lesions involving any other body system. A careful physical examination of the mammary glands should be a part of every complete examination of both male and female patients. The discovery of mammary disease is often of greater significance to the patient than are unrelated symptoms that are of concern to the client. Following discovery of an asymptomatic mammary lesion during a general examination, persistence on the part of the clinician is usually required to obtain a diagnosis and to pursue proper therapy. The clinician should always view any lesion of a nonlactating mammary gland with suspicion and share his concern with the client. Persistence and thoroughness can be very rewarding, especially if the chance of cure of a malignant lesion is enhanced by early diagnosis and action. The history regarding mammary lesions should include questions about the entire reproductive system. Mammary discharges should be analyzed for clarity, color, smell and cytology. When indicated, bacterial culture and antibiotic sensitivity tests should be performed. The clinician should examine for mastodynia and classify its severity if present.

The majority of non-neoplastic mammary diseases of small animals consist of mastitis (septic and nonseptic) and cystic mammary disease. Treatment of most forms of mammary disease consists of variations of the same general form of therapy and will be discussed with each specific disease. Lesions of mammary tissue that do not respond to therapy should be excised totally, or biopsied to determine the need for further medical or surgical therapy.

## NONSEPTIC MASTITIS OF THE LACTATING MAMMARY GLAND

This disease occurs usually at the time of parturition to three weeks after weaning; the bulk of the cases occur one to four weeks after parturition. Most, but not all, cases of nonseptic mastitis occur in the lactating female. The patient is presented because of clinical signs and symptoms related to enlarged, sensitive breasts. Warm, enlarged, engorged, sensitive breasts are usually found on examination. Microscopic examination of the milk may reveal large numbers of white blood cells. Bacteria are conspicuously absent. Diagnosis is based on physical examination of the patient and

**Table 1.** *Common Non-Neoplastic Diseases of the Mammary Glands of Dogs and Cats*

I. Nonseptic mastitis
   A. Lactating mammary gland
   B. Nonlactating mammary gland
II. Septic mastitis
   A. Lactating mammary gland
   B. Nonlactating mammary gland
III. Galactorrhea of the nonpregnant female
IV. Gynecomastia
V. Cystic mammary disease (cystic mammary hyperplasia)

laboratory examination of the milk. Therapy consists of weaning the pups from the mother immediately and symptomatically treating the breasts by soaking them in warm water. It is usually better to stand the mother in warm water up to the middle of the lumbar vertebrae, rather than to use warm wet compresses. Floating the breasts in water provides nontraumatic massaging action and seems to provide better reduction in engorgement than do other forms of soaking. In cases in which only one breast is moderately involved, common sense will determine the value of immediate weaning. Often, however, weaning is a requirement for effective and rapid therapy. When engorgement is extreme and edema extends to the flank area and limbs, diuretic therapy should be added to the regimen. Furosemide (Lasix® [Hoechst]) has proved to be quite effective. Analgesics should be used when mastodynia is severe. Prophylactic antibiotic therapy should be used because of the good medium that inflamed, lactating mammae provide for bacterial growth. A broad-spectrum bactericidal antibiotic is recommended. There is some controversy in both human and veterinary medicine concerning the use of testosterone to reduce engorgement in the lactating mammary gland. The above modes of therapy should be used first. If no relief is provided after 48 hours, administer oral methyltestosterone at a dosage of 10 mg./25 kg. of body weight/day for 7 to 10 days.

In extreme cases, gangrenous, nonseptic mastitis of lactating breasts may result from inappropriate therapy or neglect. These cases require the medical and surgical management used for severe trauma cases, including shock therapy in some patients.

Galactostasis is a condition in which the mammary glands become hard (caked breast) and painful from engorgement with milk, and it is often associated with nonseptic mastitis. The enigmatic problem of whether to wean the babies or not should be based on the degree of accompanying nonseptic mastitis. When pain and warmth are moderate to extreme, the babies should be weaned, and the full spectrum of therapy previously discussed for nonseptic mastitis should be considered. If only one or two mammae are involved and if the accompanying nonseptic mastitis is mild, the encouragement of milk removal by the babies or by gentle pumping is recommended. Warm hydrotherapy by floating the breasts is often helpful.

## NONSEPTIC MASTITIS OF THE NONLACTATING MAMMARY GLAND

Nonseptic mastitis of the nonlactating mammary gland is usually caused by trauma. Contusions from external trauma, such as automobile accidents and malicious human attacks, constitute the greatest number of cases. Therapy consists of treating the local wound. In some cases, it may be necessary to excise a nipple.

## SEPTIC MASTITIS OF THE LACTATING MAMMARY GLAND

Septic mastitis of lactating mammae may result from introduction of bacteria through the nipple by nursing, by puncture wounds into the mammary tissue or by bacteremia or lymphogenous spread.

One or more of the mother's breasts are usually enlarged, painful and warm. On occasion a pointing abscess may develop. Systemic signs such as hyperthermia and pyrexia may be present, depending on the severity of the infection and the type of organism causing the disease. Examination of the milk will usually reveal large numbers of white blood cells and bacteria. Culture and sensitivity testing of the milk often reveal the presence of coliforms, streptococci and staphylococci.

Therapy consists of draining localized abscesses and treating the infection with warm soaks and bactericidal antibiotics. Treatment of nonabscessed glands consists of warm soaks, frequent appraisal of the mammae to check for abscess formation and administration of appropriate bactericidal antibiotics. The value of testosterone therapy is controversial (refer to the preceding section on nonseptic mastitis of the lactating mammary gland). Good environmental hygiene should be stressed. It is important that active therapy be continued for at least 7 to 10 days.

Regardless of the route of infection, babies must be weaned from the mother for the health of all. Babies should be examined and observed for several days for possible infection and, if necessary, should be treated with a bactericidal antibiotic.

## SEPTIC MASTITIS OF THE NONLACTATING MAMMARY GLAND

Septic mastitis of nonlactating mammary glands is usually caused by puncture wounds and lacerations from animal bites. Therapy is similar to that provided for septic wounds of the skin and subcutis anywhere on the body. In addition, warm soaks are recommended.

## GALACTORRHEA OF THE NONPREGNANT FEMALE

Milk production in nonpregnant females is almost exclusively observed in association with pseudocyesis. Effective treatment of pseudocyesis usually results in total remission of the galactorrhea when oral testosterone is part of the therapy. When discomfort is associated with galactorrhea, warm soaks are recommended.

Galactorrhea occasionally occurs as a side effect of drug therapy, especially tranquilizers; therefore, a proper history and physical examination are essential to determine the cause of unexpected milk production. Withdrawal of the offending drug should result in remission.

## GYNECOMASTIA

Enlargement of the mammary glands of males is usually associated with disorders characterized by a relative or an absolute increase in estrogen secretion or with undue susceptibility of mammary tissue to estrogens. Sertoli cell tumors are a common cause. Potential causes include hepatocellular failure, hyperthyroidism or thyrotoxicosis, bronchial carcinoma, hyperadrenocorticism, testicular atrophy and testicular neoplasia. On occasion, gynecomastia may occur following the administration of estrogenic substances.

There is usually a rather sudden increase in size of several or all mammae. The enlargement is usually progressive and may be associated with pain. Occasionally discharge from the nipple is observed.

Pseudogynecomastia is defined as enlargement of breasts due to deposition of adipose tissue. This condition may be mistaken for gynecomastia in obese animals. A good history and physical examination are needed in order to make the distinction.

Treatment of gynecomastia should be directed at the primary disease process.

## CYSTIC MAMMARY DISEASE (CYSTIC MAMMARY HYPERPLASIA)

Cystic mammary disease may occur as a result of any underlying endocrine imbalance involving the luteal phase of the cycle, or in patients with an apparently normally functioning pituitary-ovarian axis. Cystic mammary disease is frequently observed in patients with cystic endometrial hyperplasia; however, not all patients with cystic mammary disease have cystic uterine disease. A diagnosis can usually be established on the basis of the history, physical examination and microscopic examination of the excised mammary lesion. Because cysts frequently occur in neoplastic mammary tissue, establishing a diagnosis of cystic mammary disease without histopathologic confirmation is dangerous.

Since cystic mammary disease in the dog and cat is usually progressive, ovariohysterectomy is the best method of treatment. In cases associated with isolated cysts without disease of the remainder of the reproductive tract, excision of the cysts may be satisfactory.

Fibrocystic lesions and purely hyperplastic nodules have been reported. It has been suggested that endocrine imbalance (probably hyperestrogenism) is the cause.

Foreign body granulomas caused by mammary concretions have been observed by the author.

### SUPPLEMENTAL READING

Larson, B. L., and Smith, V. R.: Lactation. A Comprehensive Treatise: Volume I, The Mammary Gland/Development and Maintenance; Volume II, Biosynthesis of Milk/Diseases of the Mammary Gland and Lactation; Volume III, Nutrition and Biochemistry of Milk/Maintenance of Lactation. New York, Academic Press, 1974.

# PSEUDO-PREGNANCY

SHIRLEY D. JOHNSTON, D.V.M.
*St. Paul, Minnesota*

In the bitch, ovulation is followed by formation of a functional corpus luteum, which persists whether or not fertile mating has occurred. Pseudopregnancy, a syndrome of physiologic and behavioral changes in the nonpregnant metestrous female, has long been associated with progesterone activity of the persistent corpus luteum. However, metestrual serum progesterone concentrations have recently been reported to be the same in normal and clinically pseudopregnant bitches. This finding has led to use of the term "overt pseudopregnancy" for bitches in the luteal phase with signs of pseudopregnancy. The term "covert pseudopregnancy" has been used for normal bitches without clinical signs. The cause of pseudopregnancy (overt) in dogs is unknown.

Pseudopregnancy may occur after estrus in both young and aged bitches and may recur after subsequent heats. In the queen, which is an induced ovulator, pseudopregnancy is occasionally observed following nonfertile mating or stimulation of the vagina with a glass rod to induce ovulation and shorten estrus.

## CLINICAL SIGNS

Enlargement of the mammary glands 6 to 12 weeks after estrus is often the most noticeable sign and may be accompanied by the secretion of a clear to brownish liquid or of true milk. Mastitis may also occur. The bitch becomes restless, excitable and nervous, often nesting and mothering inanimate objects. Abdominal distention, self-nursing, vomiting, diarrhea, anorexia and polyphagia may occur. The queen rarely shows signs of pseudopregnancy. However, mammary engorgement and lactation, which subside by day 30 to 40, may occur. A diagnosis of pseudopregnancy may be established on the basis of the history and typical signs. Normal pregnancy and pyometra should be ruled out.

## TREATMENT

Overt pseudopregnancy will usually undergo remission without treatment. Until the cause of this syndrome is determined, hormone therapy will remain empirical at best and is probably unnecessary. In females which are extremely uncomfortable, light sedation followed by alternating hot and cold compresses applied to engorged mammary glands may be of value.

Hormones that have been reported to alleviate signs of false pregnancy in bitches include diethylstilbestrol (1 to 2 mg./kg. IM), testosterone (1 to 2 mg./kg. IM) and megestrol acetate (2 mg./kg. o.d. for 8 days *per os*). In the queen, diethylstilbestrol (0.5 mg./kg. IM) or testosterone (2 mg./kg. IM) given once, and repeated in one week if needed, has been reported to be effective.

Ovariohysterectomy is the only reliable prophylactic measure and may be recommended for females with recurrent, severe pseudopregnancy. There is evidence that recurrent false pregnancies do not predispose the bitch to other diseases of the reproductive organs, but overt pseudopregnancy often recurs after subsequent estrual cycles.

## SUPPLEMENTAL READING

Fidler, I. J., Brodey, R. S., Howson, A. E., and Cohen, D.: Relationship of estrous irregularity, pseudopregnancy and pregnancy to canine pyometra. J. Am. Vet. Med. Assn., *149*:1043–1046, 1966.

Hadley, J. C.: Unconjugated oestrogen and progesterone concentrations in the blood of bitches with false pregnancy and pyometra. Vet. Rec., *96*:545–547, 1975.

Smith, M. S., and McDonald, L. E.: Serum levels of luteinizing hormone and progesterone during the estrous cycle, pseudopregnancy and pregnancy in the dog. Endocrinology, *94*:404–412, 1974.

Stein, B. S.: Pseudocyesis. *In* Catcott, E. J. (ed.): Feline Medicine and Surgery. 2nd ed. Santa Barbara, California, American Veterinary Publications, Inc., 1975.

# PREGNANCY PREVENTION AND TERMINATION

THOMAS J. BURKE, D.V.M.
*Urbana, Illinois*

Prevention of pregnancy is most effectively achieved by physical prevention of copulation, by denying fertile males access to the bitch or queen or by obviating estrus. Recent pharmaceutical advances have placed the last within the realm of routine practice (see article on "Prevention of Estrus"). Strict confinement and ovariohysterectomy continue to be valid methods of pregnancy prevention. All methods require education of the owners about the basic reproductive physiology of their pets and the availability of current methods for curtailing the features undesirable to the owner.

Fertilization occurs in the oviducts. Nidation (implantation) occurs about the 18th to 20th day in the bitch and approximately the 14th day in the queen, in the estrogen-sensitized luteal-phase uterus.

In the postcoital bitch, diethylstilbestrol may promote passage of the zygotes through the oviduct, while preliminary research with mestranol suggests that it causes oviducal retention. In the queen, 0.25 mg. of estradiol cypionate administered IM 40 hours after coitus delayed oviducal passage of zygotes. Estrogen also counteracts the progesterone-induced receptibility of the endometrium. The period of time following ovulation requisite for these effects to produce death of the zygote is unknown, but it is probably less than 7 days in the bitch and 3 to 5 days in the queen.

Experimentally, induction of uterine disease may be accomplished by administration of either estrogen or progesterone. Concomitant estrogen-progesterone treatment produces pathologic or potentially pathologic uterine lesions more readily than either hormone does alone. Thus, the effect of estrogen on a luteal-phase endometrium may enhance the development of uterine disease. Estrogens also have been incriminated as a cause of aplastic anemia in the dog.

An owner inquiring about an "abortion shot" should be closely questioned about the mating. Lack of adequate knowledge about his pet's reproductive biology often is apparent at this time. A careful history that extracts only the owner's observations may obviate therapy. For example, many owners equate the presence of a male with mating, regardless of the stage of the estrous cycle of the female. When sufficient doubt exists as to the precise stage of the cycle, vaginal cytology should be employed to estimate the probability that mating occurred. Absence of sperm does not mean that mating has not occurred. Sperm are rarely seen, even in cases in which coitus was observed. If cytologic examination indicates estrus or early metestrus, the likelihood of successful copulation should be explained to the owner. At this time, the possible dangers of estrogen therapy for pregnancy prevention should be explained as well.

If the owner decides against treatment, an appointment can be scheduled for pregnancy diagnosis.

Mismating therapy consists of administration of an estrogen, estradiol cypionate (ECP® [Upjohn]), a dosage of 0.25 to 2 mg. IM. The owner should be advised that treatment may prolong the symptoms of estrus and that further treatments for subsequent matings are unnecessary and inadvisable. Prominent symptoms of uterine infection should be explained and a 30-day examination scheduled.

Diethylstilbestrol also has been recommended for mismating therapy at an initial dose of 1 to 2 mg./kg. IM, followed by a daily oral dose of 0.4 mg./kg. for 5 days.

Termination of an established pregnancy in the bitch may be accomplished by

1241

ovariectomy at any stage of gestation. Induction of luteolysis may thus be expected to induce abortion. Currently no safe medical treatment exists; but the results of research with prostaglandins may provide a safe and effective method.

Cats are far more difficult to treat, since most owners do not recognize that their pets are in estrus and the majority of matings are not observed. A careful history of the queen's behavioral pattern may provide information as to the stage of the cycle. Ovulation and rather rapid cessation of typical symptoms of estrus occur 24 to 48 hours after mating. Since the tom grasps the queen by the back of the neck with his teeth during coitus, patchy hair loss, fresh excoriations and punctures on the dorsum of the neck indicate recent copulation. Vaginal cytology may also be employed. Cellular changes are similar to those of the bitch. Sperm may be easily found within the first hour after coitus. The efficacy of estrogen therapy for mismating has not been thoroughly studied. Estradiol cypionate (0.25 mg. IM) has been used in a few cats within the first five days after cessation of estrual symptoms, and pregnancies did not result.

In the queen, prostaglandin (PG) $F_2$ $\alpha$THAM salt caused abortion or parturition after the 40th day of gestation when administered in two subcutaneous doses of 0.5 to 1.0 mg./kg. 24 hours apart. Abortifacient doses of $PGF_2\alpha$ are toxic in the bitch. $PGF_2\alpha$ has not been approved for clinical veterinary use in dogs and cats.

## SUPPLEMENTAL READING

Herron, M. A., and Sis, R. F.: Ovum transport in the cat and the effect of estrogen administration. Am. J. Vet. Res., 35:1277–1279, 1974.
Jackson, W. F.: Management of canine mismating with diethylstilbestrol. Calif. Vet., Nov.-Dec.:28–29, 1953.
Jöchle, W.: Hormones in canine gynecology. A review. Theriogenology, 3:152–165, 1975.
Jöchle, W., Lamond, D. R., and Anderson, A. C.: Mestranol as an abortifacient in the bitch. Theriogenology, 4:1–9, 1975.
Nachreiner, R. F., and Marple, D. N.: Termination of pregnancy in cats with prostaglandin $F_2\alpha$. Prostaglandins, 7:303–308, 1974.
Stein, B. S.: The genital system. In Catcott, E. J. (ed.): Feline Medicine and Surgery. 2nd ed. American Veterinary Publications, Santa Barbara, California, 1975, pp. 303–354.

# PREVENTION OF ESTRUS

LLOYD C. FAULKNER, D.V.M.
*Fort Collins, Colorado*

Estrus may be reversibly prevented as a convenience to an owner who wishes to preserve the pet's reproductive function. Contraceptives that reversibly prevent and delay estrus may be administered intermittently or continuously when the pet is not in proestrus or estrus. Agents that abbreviate proestrus and estrus when administered during these stages of the reproductive cycle are estrous suppressants; these agents postpone heat.

Contraceptive technologies that do not prevent estrus fail to maximally facilitate the responsible ownership of pets. Estrous bitches and queens, even when properly confined, attract males and thus create nuisances and hazards for owners and their neighbors.

In addition to efficacy in preventing estrus, contraceptive technology should be safe for the pet, present no hazards for humans and be readily available and acceptable to the owner. Pets are owned by people who commonly identify with their pets. The attitudes of owners toward contraception in their pets vary as widely as their attitudes toward human contraception. Prevention of estrus may not be acceptable to owners who derive vicarious satisfaction from sexuality in their pets.

Contraception is seriously overemphasized as a solution to a nationwide problem of free-roaming dogs and cats, including stray and straying pets. Sterile pets that are free to roam perpetuate the hazards to public health and most of the nuisances of uncontrolled, fertile pets. Responsible owners confine and control their pets to prevent their burdening the rest of society. Appropriate contraception facilitates responsible ownership and may reduce the millions of stray and straying pets that are killed annually to control their numbers.

*Ovariohysterectomy* is the standard of efficacy in preventing estrus and has the added advantage of removing genitalia which commonly become diseased. Conditions that maximize the safety of spaying, however, make the procedure costly and thus reduce its availability. Owners have a variety of attitudes toward ovariohysterectomy that diminish the acceptability of the procedure. These include the cost of surgery, the irreversibility of spaying, a belief that spaying causes obesity and lethargy, an anthropomorphic projection of fear of surgery (especially castration) and a vicarious aversion to depriving the pet of sexual pleasure. Regrettably, veterinary medicine has a dearth of concomitant investigational data to document the beneficial or adverse consequences of ovariectomy, ovariohysterectomy and hysterectomy in controlled studies. Reasoning is less assuring than hard evidence.

Progress in the development of alternatives to ovariohysterectomy to prevent estrus in dogs and cats is hampered by ignorance of the mechanisms of reproductive function in these species. Cows and sows are polyestrous throughout the year; regression of the corpus luteum (luteolysis) initiates the succeeding cycle. Mares and ewes are seasonally polyestrous; photoperiod and other environmental factors regulate seasonal function, but luteolysis initiates the succeeding estrous cycle within the breeding season. Luteolysis in bitches is followed by anestrus, which lasts for one to several months. Queens have distinctly seasonal peaks and nadirs of estrous activity. Queens ovulate reflexogenously in response to mating stimuli; if not stimulated to ovulate, queens resume estrous activity in about three weeks. The biologic clocks that regulate estrous cycles in bitches and queens are unknown.

The efficacy and widespread acceptance of *steroidal contraceptives* for humans have caused the pet-owning public and humane organizations to resent the fact that veterinary medicine has failed to develop suitable alternatives to costly surgical sterilization. Most laypersons are unaware that the bitch and queen are peculiarly susceptible to toxic side effects of the progestogenic and estrogenic steroids. Concerns for the cost of spaying and the senseless, inhumane slaughter of millions of neglected pets have overridden concern for the more fundamental problems of free-roaming pets and deliberate, profit-motivated breeding.

Veterinary experience with the *progestational steroids* in dogs and cats has precluded their widespread use in the United States, although they are used extensively in other countries. Estrus-preventing doses of steroids act by inhibiting the hypothalamo-hypophyseal axis in the secretion of gonadotropins, especially luteinizing hormone. Estrus-suppressing doses are also antiestrogenic. In appropriate doses, the progestins are highly effective in preventing estrus and ovulation in bitches and queens, but prolonged administration of estrus-inhibiting doses produces unacceptably high occurrences of endometrial hyperplasia and pyometritis.

Several progestational steroids have been tested for use in preventing estrus in dogs and cats. Megestrol acetate (Ovaban® [Schering]) has been approved by the Food and Drug Administration for suppression and postponement of estrus and blocking ovulation at a dosage of 2.2 mg./kg./day for 8 days at the onset of proestrus, or for delay of estrus at a dosage of 0.55 mg./kg./day for 32 days during anestrus. Megestrol acetate suppresses, but does not prevent, estrus when administered daily for 8 days in early proestrus. The bitch must be controlled until the signs of estrus, which are abbreviated by treatment, have disappeared. Administered in an 8- or 32-day schedule of treatment, megestrol acetate or similar progestin may not stimulate uterine disease and may, in fact, reduce the incidence of uterine disease when used to block ovulation. There is considerable evidence that spontaneous uterine disease is enhanced by the sequential, uterotropic effects of estrogenic and progestogenic ovarian steroids.

Pharmaceutical companies have hundreds of candidate steroids on the shelves of their research laboratories. These drugs are idle for use as estrous inhibitors for dogs and cats, because their manufacturers cannot justify the costs of research and development relative to the return on their investment. The unusual sensitivities of dogs and cats to toxic uterotropic effects of steroids discourage research and development of candidate steroids. Steroids with high ratios of androgenic:progestational activity inhibit the secretion of gonadotropins at doses that cause minimal androgenic effects. Dimethyl-19-nortestosterone (Mibolerone® [Upjohn]) has been used extensively in laboratory studies and field trials to prevent estrus in bitches and queens. Development of a steroid or nonsteroid which is a potent inhibitor of gonadotropic secretion without undesirable uterotropic or other side effects, and which could be delivered at a uniform rate for prolonged periods from an implant, would solve many problems for veterinary medicine.

It is unlikely, however, that any single technology will satisfy the various desires of the pet-loving public for effective, safe and inexpensive contraception for their animals. Humane organizations wish for a technology that permanently prevents estrus following a single administration that, hopefully, could be given by a technologist in the shelter or pound prior to adoption. Some owners desire a contraceptive which reversibly prevents estrus for six months to a year. Some owners are willing to administer an oral contraceptive daily. Too many owners do not control their animals adequately to administer a daily agent and will opt for permanent or long-term contraception.

The incorporation of a contraceptive agent in pet food is controversial. Medicated feed offers a simplified method of delivery for owners who are sufficiently motivated to use it effectively. The method raises serious questions, though, of the risks of human consumption and control of appropriate dosage.

The manufacturer of an *intravaginal contraceptive device* (Option One® [Agrophysics]) claims that the device prevents or suppresses estrus in a percentage of bitches, but the degree of estrous inhibition is unclear. The device must be fitted and placed in the bitch following examination to ascertain that the genital tract is free of disease and nongravid. Some experience in fitting and placing the device is required to minimize expulsion. The device is also contraindicated in several physiologic states, reducing its availability.

*Immunization against reproductive hormones* presents intriguing possibilities for the prevention of estrus. Pets could be actively or passively immunized against reproductive hormones to prevent estrus. Gonadotropins are immunogenic, and steroids can be rendered antigenic by coupling them to carrier proteins. Active immunization with gonadotropins has been used to cause gonadal atrophy and reproductive failure in dogs, but the adjuvant (Freund's complete) caused abscesses, and the duration of the response has been variable. Dogs immunized with a commercially available ovine gonadotropic preparation recovered after 20 to 30 weeks of reproductive failure.

Studies of hypothalamic gonadotropin releasers in dogs and cats have not been reported. Immunization against gonadotropin-releasing hormone (GnRH) offers distinct advantages, since the antigen is available as a pure, synthetic decapeptide. It is possible that once initiated, the immune system would continue to make antibodies against endogenous hormone.

Male sex steroids masculinize female fetuses when administered to pregnant females during critical periods of organogenesis. The masculinized females are sterile; the males are apparently unaffected. The ability to control this effect may allow breeders to supply a market for male and sterile female pets. The sterilized young may have other desirable or undesirable characteristics that remain to be determined.

For the immediate future, at least, ovariohysterectomy is the most practical approach to contraception as a partial solution to the problem of too many irresponsible owners of pets. The clinics are already built, equipped and staffed. Veterinarians must accept the fact that they have a vital role to play in contributing to the solution of a national problem. We must enjoin the cooperative efforts of veterinary practitioners, governmental agencies and humane agencies to make surgical sterilization available to all owners. Legitimate fees for surgery must be subsidized according to the owner's ability to pay. Responsible control of pets must be a condition of the program. Owners who fail to accept the demands of responsible ownership, including the prevention of estrus or other appropriate control of reproductive function, must be subject to effective sanctions. Many owners will be motivated only by adequate legislation and enforcement against irresponsible ownership.

## SUPPLEMENTAL READING

Burke, T. J., and Reynolds, H. A., Jr.: Megestrol acetate for estrus postponement in the bitch. J. Am. Vet. Med. Assn., 167:285–287, 1975.

Christie, D. W., and Bell, E. T.: The use of progestogens to control reproductive function in the bitch. Anim. Breed. Abstr., 38:1–21, 1970.

Faulkner, *et al*.: In Nieschlag, E.(ed.): Immunization with Hormones in Reproduction Research. Amsterdam, North-Holland, 1975, pp. 199–214.

Jöchle, W.: Pet population control: chemical methods. Canine Pract., *Sept.-Oct.*:8–18, 1974.

Sokolowski, J. H., and Zimbelman, R. G.: Canine reproduction: effects of multiple treatments of medroxyprogesterone acetate on reproductive organs of the bitch. Am. J. Vet. Res., 35:1285–1287, 1974.

---

# SEMEN COLLECTION AND ARTIFICIAL INSEMINATION OF DOGS

S. W. J. SEAGER, M.R.C.V.S.
*Houston, Texas*

The role of semen collection and artificial insemination in dog breeding is expanding, and veterinarians are frequently being asked to perform these services for purposes of fertility examination of the male and for artificial breeding. There are a number of reasons for the increased use of artificial insemination in dogs apart from the abnormal physical, anatomic and pathologic factors that prevent natural mating in both sexes:

1. Isolation of puppies at an early age, particularly if they are maintained in city apartments, deprives many of them of the necessary play and mounting patterns most should experience for later life, when they are expected to breed naturally.

2. Stricter leash laws plus the increase in traffic and resulting injuries are forcing people to keep their purebred dogs off the streets, thereby depriving many males of the casual sexual encounters that they had been exposed to in years past. This effectively prevents the natural sexual education that most young stud dogs acquire over a period of time.

3. Because of the time and patience required to learn this technique, many of the newer and younger dog breeders fail to acquire the art of obtaining natural breeding between a chosen sire and bitch. The result is that an increasing number of breeders turn to artificial insemination to achieve successful dog breeding. As more dog breeders have become aware of fertility problems in both sexes, semen evaluation of the stud dog has become an important clinical procedure.

Some small animal practitioners are hesitant to perform canine artificial inseminations. Perhaps one of the reasons for this is their infrequent opportunity to perform this clinical procedure. The techniques reported here are the result of considerable study devoted to the establishment of the best overall method of canine semen collection and insemination with regard to man-hours required, comfort of the animals, success in collection and optimal conception rates. These data are based on over 6000 ejaculations collected in a continuing study in this laboratory on dog reproduction and sperm preservation.

## COLLECTION OF THE EJACULATE

If veterinarians are going to perform this important service for breeders, they need to charge a realistic fee for the time spent and for the expertise involved in this procedure and should equip themselves for performing the service in a satisfactory manner. It is not satisfactory to collect dog semen with disposable gloves, kidney dishes, outer cases of disposable syringes or breakable

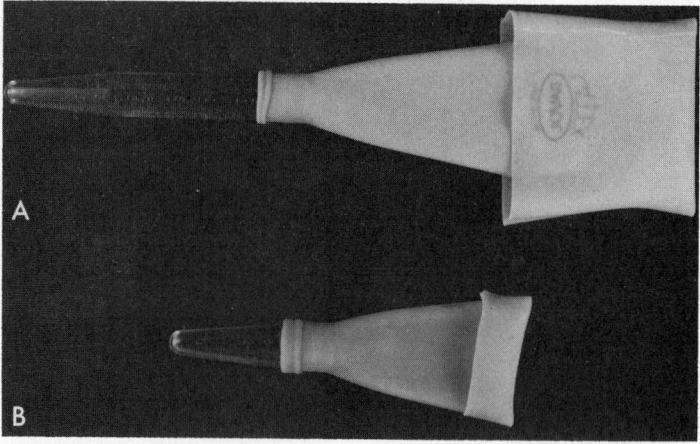

**Figure 1.** *A*, Artificial vagina used in canine semen collection consisting of a latex rubber cone and 15-ml. conical plastic centrifuge tube. *B*, A cutdown form of *A* used for small canines.

glassware. The most practical method of collecting dog semen is shown in Figure 1*A*. The apparatus consists of a rubber conical sheath (Continental Plastics, Darien, Wisconsin) and a plastic 15-ml. conical centrifuge tube. These can be utilized for 10- to 75-kg. dogs (Figs. 2 and 3). For smaller dogs, the equipment can be reduced in size, as shown in Figure 1*B*. Do not use a glass centrifuge tube for collection of dog semen. Since it can either be knocked from the veterinarian's hand or strike the floor or table leg during the collection process and break. The semen should not be used after such an occurrence, since the sample may be contaminated with glass particles or bacteria.

A variety of semen collection apparatus and methods have been recommended, including an artificial vagina and a glass or plastic funnel with centrifuge tube. The artificial vagina described by Harrop is not only expensive and cumbersome to use but also difficult to keep clean, and results are poor as compared to those of other methods. The funnel and centrifuge tube are unsatisfactory, in that hair and other debris can fall into the ejaculate. Careful attention is required in placing the funnel, since the dog's penis may strike the funnel during vigorous thrusts. Such contact with the penis against a hard, foreign object should be avoided, particularly if the dog is a shy breeder and

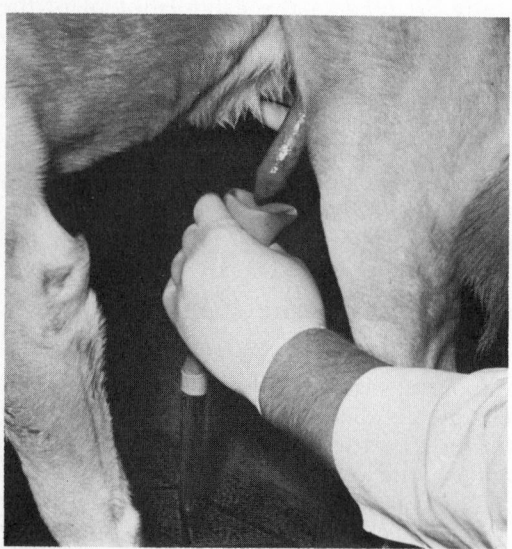

**Figure 2.** Placing the artificial vagina over the erect penis of a dog prior to ejaculation.

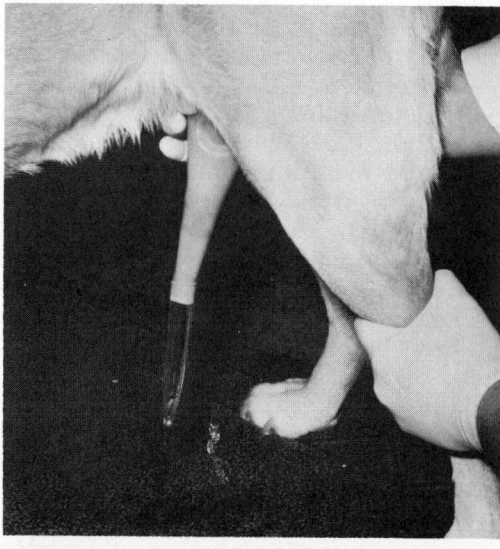

**Figure 3.** Placement of the artificial vagina over the erect penis as ejaculation commences.

one wishes to collect semen from him again. There is also a lack of soft contact for the dog's penis. The friction from the sheath assists in obtaining an ejaculate, especially from males lacking libido (Figs. 2 and 3).

**Collection Procedure.** It is important to provide the following for successful canine semen collections: (1) an isolated quiet room, with either nonslip flooring or a rubber mat for both the teaser bitch and the male; (2) a sturdy, anchored table leg or a wall ring, 12 inches from the floor, which is very useful to secure the teaser bitch for collection purposes; (3) only the necessary people in the room, with no interruptions during the collection procedures.

Secure the teaser bitch to the wall ring or table leg. Once secure, she can be held by an assistant kneeling on her right side with one hand under her chest (not her abdomen), supporting her and preventing her from sitting down during the mounting. Place the other hand over her muzzle to prevent possible injury to both handler and dog. A teaser bitch may not be required once the male has experienced the collection routine a few times and is familiar with it. In many cases a quiet bitch in any stage of her sexual cycle can be used as a teaser. We have found in most instances that a better collection will be obtained more frequently if a teaser bitch is used.

Veterinarians can perform many manipulative procedures without a dog's cooperation, such as the collection of blood, urine and spinal fluid. However, collecting an ejaculate from a dog by means of an artificial vagina does require the dog's cooperation. Therefore any attempt on your part to encourage his cooperation will provide rewarding results. If you have a dog from which it is difficult to collect semen, try to understand what is "turning him off." One must consider the dog's outlook on the whole process—whether he has been confined in a small examination room, possibly with a slippery floor, or with a somewhat objectionable snappy bitch, an apprehensive owner, a suspicious bitch owner and possibly an irritated veterinarian. With the canine's ability to detect body scents from human beings very quickly, just one or more of the above experiences may deter a young or shy dog from having any desire to mate naturally. The author has experienced a number of cases in which sexual response could not be elicited from the male when he was presented with a female in heat. These dogs were brought to a quiet room and, if small dogs, were put in a cage at waist level. They were quietly encouraged to relax, to accept the clinician's presence and to ejaculate. The dog owners and all extraneous distractions were kept from the room. These dogs underwent collection 4 to 5 times in this manner, and all subsequently achieved successful, natural matings.

It is important to maintain collection apparatus and insemination equipment dry and at approximate body temperature. Cold or wet equipment can discourage a dog from ejaculating and can also damage the spermatozoa. If a number of semen collections and evaluations are performed in a clinic, it is convenient to maintain a small thermocontrolled incubator at body temperature in which all collection, insemination and semen examination materials may be kept. The same incubator should not be utilized for growing bacterial or fungal cultures. Once the apparatus is removed from the incubator, it can be placed in a pocket or held in the hand to maintain it at approximate body temperature prior to use.

Everything should be prepared before the male is brought into the collection room. Assemble the sheath and centrifuge tube and don disposable gloves. Smear a *small* amount of lubricant (K-Y Jelly® [Johnson & Johnson]) inside the sheath to facilitate its removal after ejaculation has taken place. When the assistant has the teaser positioned, let the male enter the room. Recognition or conversation directed toward the male should be kept at a minimum, since this will distract some males. The male can be released to allow foreplay. The male will normally lick and smell the vulva prior to mounting. The male should not be allowed to urinate in the area. His attention should be directed toward mounting the bitch. The collector should kneel at the bitch's left shoulder and grasp the preputial sheath. After the male has mounted, the preputial sheath should be gently slipped back behind the bulbus glandis before full erection occurs. This is best accomplished by reaching between the male's rear legs with the right hand. Full erection is unlikely if the preputial sheath is not pulled back behind the bulbus glandis.

Once the penis reaches approximately 50 per cent of erection, do not attempt to push the prepuce behind the bulbus glandis, otherwise considerable pain and possible bleeding may result, and there is the possibility that the male may bite the collector. If erection occurs before the prepuce is pushed over the bulbus glandis, isolate the male from the female, which will result in subsidence of the erection. Start again, with the collector attempting to slide the prepuce back at an earlier stage in the collection procedure. It is important not to push the prepuce back too quickly during the collection procedure, since dogs resent this and seem to respond to the initial stimulation of the penis and glands penis through the preputial sheath. Once the penis has become erect, apply moderate downward pressure on the penis with the thumb and forefinger behind the bulbus glandis. Place the collection sheath gently over the penis at this time, about three fourths of the way up, as shown in Figure 2. Slight downward digital pressure on the base of the penis will cause full erection and ejaculation. Once the collection sheath is in place, the penis should be directed between the stud's legs, using a slight downward and backward pressure. Pulsations along the ventral surface of the penis will be felt during ejaculation. If the dog has urinated just prior to collection, the first two or three drops of ejaculate should not be collected, and the collection sheath should not be placed on the penis until these drops have been voided. In this laboratory, we have collected semen routinely from most studs on a three-times-per-week schedule with no apparent decrease in semen quantity or quality.

Dog semen is ejaculated in three fractions, the second being the sperm-rich fraction. Some dogs have a small first fraction (0.5 to 1 ml.). It is important to place the collection apparatus over the penis prior to the start of the second fraction. Once the clear third fraction of semen appears in the collection tube, the sheath should be *gently* removed from the swollen penis. Removal of the rubber sheath is facilitated by the lubricant, which was lightly smeared on the inside.

Occasionally, one dog may be more difficult to collect from than others. In this case, varying pressure applied between the thumb and forefinger, an up-and-down massaging motion on the penis, varying the pressure on the bulbus glandis and changing the grip from right to left hand may be necessary for successful collection. If pulsations can be felt and no ejaculate is visible, it is possible that the operator is constricting the base of the penis. Semen passage will be restricted until such pressure is released. To avoid this, release the hand grip occasionally during the collection procedure.

## ELECTROEJACULATION

This procedure has been reported in the dog, wolf and fox. In this laboratory, we have yet to fail to obtain an ejaculation from a dog by means of an artificial vagina and manual stimulation. Considering the ease and general acceptance of this method of collection in the domestic dog, electroejaculation is primarily of academic interest.

## ARTIFICIAL INSEMINATION

Prior to artificial insemination, examine the ejaculate for the following criteria: color, volume, pH, opacity, motility status, motility percentage, sperm count per ml., total sperm count and morphology. A written record should be kept of the semen examination for later referral and for sire evaluation. This detailed information will be useful in evaluating the dog's fertility. Such detail is not always necessary after the

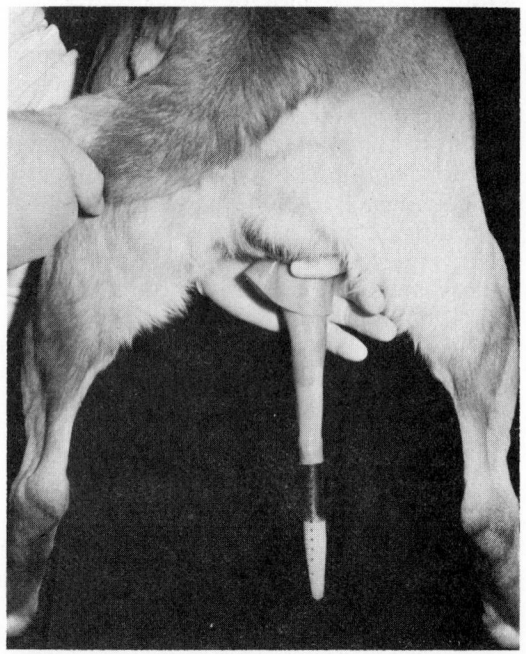

**Figure 4.**    Ejaculation into the artificial vagina; left-handhold on penis and artificial vagina.

first two or three ejaculates have been analyzed; however, *every* sample should be examined for motility, color and volume prior to insemination. There is little point in inseminating a bitch first, examining the small drop of semen remaining in the insemination rod for a fertility examination and finding the spermatozoa dead. It may be impossible to say that this particular semen is incapable of bringing about fertilization. Yet, the bitch has been legally bred, and a different male cannot be selected.

Insemination equipment includes an 18-inch plastic bovine insemination rod broken in half, a short rubber connector and a disposable syringe (Fig. 5). Disposable gloves should be worn for the collection of semen and insemination of dogs.

In order to achieve an optimal conception rate, as much care in the artificial insemination process needs to be taken as in the semen collection. The bitch can be tied closely to the ring in the wall or to a sturdy table leg and muzzled if there is any possibility that she will bite. The vulva should be washed with distilled water and blotted dry. Disinfectant or soap should not be used for this purpose. The assistant positions himself with his back to the wall and the dog's head and neck between his knees. He then

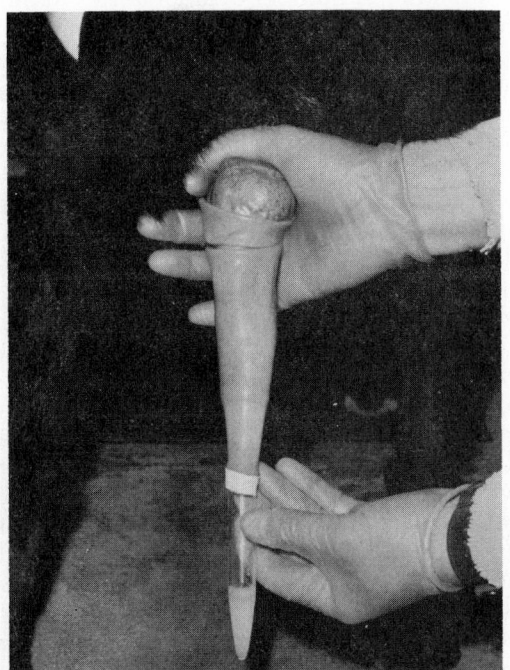

**Figure 5.** Ejaculation into the artificial vagina; change of handhold and grip to right hand.

elevates the bitch's hindquarters to an angle of about 60 degrees from the floor. If the bitch tries to get free, inward pressure applied with the knees will limit her movement. The bitch's hind legs are then gripped and rotated out slightly, at the same time holding the tail with one hand in order to expose the vulva. A small bitch can be inseminated in this elevated position on an examination table. These techniques have been established during the performance of over 1500 inseminations.

Before aspirating the fresh semen into the syringe, draw up 1 ml. of air into the syringe. Aspirate the semen slowly to prevent air bubbles from rising through the seminal fluid, since this may damage the sperm cells. Apply a small amount of lubricating jelly to the left index finger and insemination rod (K-Y Jelly® [Johnson & Johnson]). Gently insert the left index finger into the bitch's vagina and move it dorsally over the brim of the pelvis. In the toy breeds it may not be possible to insert the finger to this depth.

Insert the insemination rod alongside the index finger until it clears the pelvic brim. Tip the rod almost vertically and gently push it to the cervical os (Figs. 6 and 7). If any difficulty is encountered when inserting the rod to this depth, withdraw it one or two inches and redirect it at a slightly different angle. If resistance is still felt, instillation of a small amount of semen at this point will often allow insertion of the rod to the required depth. When the cervical os is reached (determined by moderate resistance and by achieving a depth of insertion of 8 to 9 inches in large breeds, 6 to 7 inches in medium-sized breeds and 4 to 6 inches in small breeds), slowly deposit the semen. Pinch off the rubber connector with the left thumb and forefinger and detach the syringe. Aspirate 1 ml. of air into the syringe and reattach the rubber connector to expel the remaining semen from the rod. Gently withdraw the insemination rod from the vagina.

Most of the literature recommends "feathering" of the vagina, inserting the finger into the vulva and keeping the bitch elevated for a time after insemination. There has been no published evaluation of these procedures and their relation to conception. Until proved contrary, our recommendation is that the bitch's hindquarters be maintained in the elevated position for 5

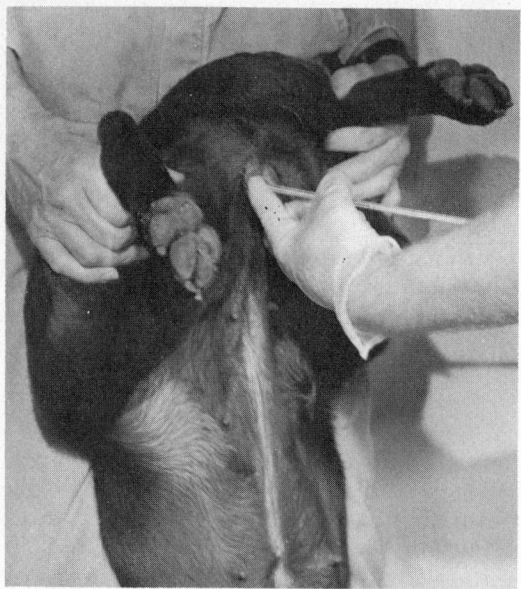

**Figure 6.** Insertion of lubricated index finger into posterior vagina; insemination rod is then inserted alongside index finger at angle shown.

minutes after insemination. Following the elevation period, gently return the bitch to her normal standing position. It is important not to pick her up by placing an arm under her abdomen, since this may cause the va-

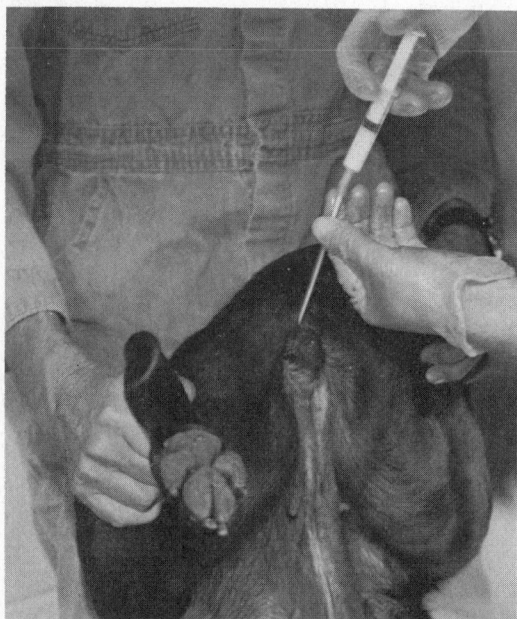

**Figure 7.** Rod is inserted vertically once it has passed pelvic brim; at this point, the semen is discharged gently into the anterior vagina at the os cervix; insemination rod, connector and syringe are demonstrated.

gina to tip, resulting in the possible loss of semen. If she must be carried, she should be cradled, with one arm around the chest and the other arm around the hindquarter, and placed in an isolated holding cage. Leave the bitch in the cage for approximately one half to one hour after insemination to let her rest quietly. This will help prevent semen loss.

Collection sheaths and tubes should be washed in detergent and rinsed thoroughly in distilled or deionized water to remove all soap residues. They can then be either air-dried or placed in a warm incubator. It is important that K-Y Jelly® be used sparingly in all cases, because too great a concentration of this lubricant can be spermicidal. Do not gas autoclave any rubber collection utensils because gas residues can remain spermicidal for many months.

## TIME OF INSEMINATION

Much has been written in relation to the onset of proestrus, estrus, vulval discharge, color and amount of discharge, vulval swelling and vaginal cytology in relation to the optimal time of insemination in the bitch. Although we have been following these procedures for nine years, we have not been able to identify an exact critical time for insemination. A number of laboratories in this country and other countries are defining the estrous cycle in the bitch by radioimmunoassay of serum hormone levels. In this laboratory we are correlating circulating hormonal levels by radioimmunoassay, pictorially recording the changes in the canine ovary by laparoscopy and identifying the clinical signs mentioned above. When these data become available, it may be possible to correlate more precisely the time of insemination with that of ovulation.

It is suggested that the bitch be inseminated (1) on the 10th and 12th days, counting day 1 as the first day of sanguineous vaginal discharge; or (2) on the 2nd and 4th days of true estrus; or (3) twice a day apart when the majority of the vaginal epithelial cells are mature. Reproductive history of previous heat cycles—their regularity and length—and how long standing-heat lasts should be evaluated. In some cases it may be advisable to inseminate a third time 48 hours later. The American Kennel Club regulations at the moment require that the bitch and the stud dog be on the same premises and that a veterinarian perform the collection and insemination and sign the breeding certificate attesting to this fact.

## SEMEN STORAGE

Harrop and Leonard have reported success in maintaining viable dog semen under refrigeration for as long as nine days. Foote and Kirk have reported 50 per cent motility after thawing semen from the frozen state. These investigators have made notable contributions to the technique of preserving dog semen. The author initiated a semen freezing program at the University of Oregon Medical School Department of Surgery in 1967 and published reports of the first pregnancy with frozen semen in 1969. In 1971, the American Kennel Club provided support for continuing this investigation of the use of frozen canine semen. Since this initial success, over 600 puppies have been born as a result of the utilization of frozen semen in this laboratory. Conception rates in some trials have been equal to those obtained by means of natural breeding. Semen has been stored for as long as eight years and shows little or no decline in motility. To date, the longest time period between storage and conception has been 36 months. Litter size, weights, sex ratios and postnatal mortality parallel those obtained in natural mating.

The American Kennel Club does not at this time approve for registration those progeny conceived as a result of insemination using frozen semen, but it is considered likely that they will accept registration of such offspring in the future. Utilization of frozen semen in dog breeding will provide an important and beneficial service to dog breeders in the United States and other countries.

## SUPPLEMENTAL READING

Asdell, S.: Dog Breeding. Boston, Little, Brown and Co., 1966.

Boucher, J. H., Foote, R. H., and Kirk, R. W.: The evaluation of semen quality in the dog and the effects of frequency of ejaculation upon the semen quality, libido and depletion of sperm reserves. Cornell Vet., 48:67–86, 1958.

Christenson, G. C., and Dougherty, R. W.: A simplified apparatus for obtaining semen from dogs by electrical stimulation. J. Am. Vet. Med. Assn., 127:50–52, 1955.

Foote, R. H.: The effects of electrolytes, sugars, glycerol and catalase on survival of dog sperm stored in buffered-yolk mediums. Am. J. Vet. Res., 25:32–36, 1964.

Hafez, E.: Reproduction and Breeding Techniques for Laboratory Animals. Philadelphia, Lea & Febiger, 1970.

Harrop, A.: The Semen of Animals and Artificial Insemination. London, Central Press Ltd., 1962.

Kirk, R.: Reproduction in the Dog. London, Brailliere, Tindall and Cox, 1959.

Laing, J. A.: Fertility and Infertility in the Domestic Animals. Baltimore, The Williams and Wilkins Co., 1970.

Seager, S.: Successful pregnancies utilizing frozen dog semen. Artif. Insem. Digest, 17:6, 1969.

Seager, S., Platz, C., and Fletcher, W.: Conception rates and related data using frozen dog semen. J. Reprod. Fert., 45:189–192, 1975.

Seager, S., Platz, C., and Hodge, W.: Successful pregnancy using frozen semen in the wolf. Int. Zoo Yearbook, 15:140–143, 1975.

# SEMEN COLLECTION, EVALUATION AND ARTIFICIAL INSEMINATION OF THE DOMESTIC CAT

S. W. J. SEAGER, M.R.C.V.S.
*Houston, Texas*

With the current increasing knowledge of reproductive physiology, breeders and veterinarians are becoming more aware of infertility problems in cats. In recent years, great strides have been made in the understanding of endocrinologic and neuroendocrinologic functions in cat reproduction as a result of the increased knowledge of physiology in general, the ability to estimate the number of circulating hormones by means of radioimmunoassay and the possibility of direct observation of the feline reproductive tract by means of laparoscopy. At this time semen collection in the cat is useful as a clinical procedure only for fertility examination. Information presented in this chapter is based on studies performed in our laboratory on semen collection, evaluation, freezing and insemination and on artificial induction of estrus in the domestic and wild Felidae.

If a tomcat is presented with a clinical history of having been bred to a number of queens without conception, several courses of action are possible. First, the male should be given a physical examination and his breeding history should be reviewed. Check that the testicles are present and are firm and free-moving within the scrotum. While a testicular biopsy is very useful in determining the reason for the absence of spermatozoa in the ejaculate, it is of little or no value in estimating the total sperm count, motility percentage, speed of progression of the spermatozoa or abnormal morphologic forms.

If a female in heat is available, she can be bred. The vagina can be either swabbed with a saline-moistened cotton-tipped applicator or injected with approximately 0.5 ml. of saline and back-flushed to obtain material for microscopic examination. This method is useful for checking the presence and motility of spermatozoa but will not give an accurate sperm count. It may be difficult to obtain a female in heat that is available for breeding when such a clinical test is desired.

Cat semen can also be collected by means of an artificial vagina or electroejaculation (Table 1). Semen collection by an artificial vagina is generally not practical in the veterinary hospital. The procedure requires an in-heat queen and tomcats that have been trained to ejaculate into an artificial vagina. This training takes two or three weeks on a daily basis. Approximately 3 out of 5 tomcats will give a satisfactory ejaculate within

**Table 1.** *Characteristics of Domestic Cat Semen\* Obtained by Means of Electroejaculation or Artificial Vagina*

| TOTAL SPERM COUNT ($\times 10^6$) | NORMAL VOLUME (ml.) | RANGE OF % MOTILE | SPEED OF PROGRES- SION\*\* |
|---|---|---|---|
| 15 to 130† | 0.10 to 0.50 | 60 to 95 | 4.5 to 5.0 |
| 15 to 130‡ | 0.02 to 0.12 | 60 to 95 | 4.5 to 5.0 |

\*Color: Normal color of feline semen is milky white.
Morphology: In general, from 2 to 10 per cent of flagella are coiled or bent.
\*\*Based on a scale of 0 to 5, 5 being optimum.
†In 200 ejaculates collected by means of electroejaculation.
‡In 34 ejaculates collected by means of artificial vagina.

1252

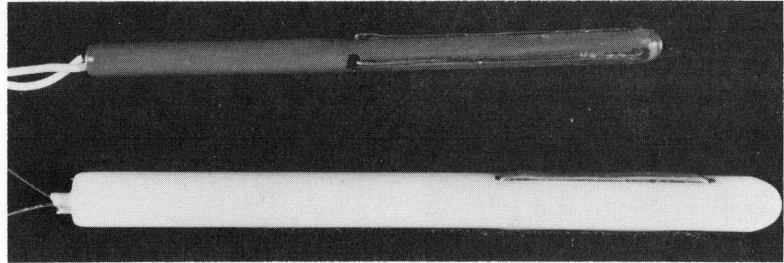

**Figure 1.**   Rectal probes made of acrylic material for electroejaculation in the domestic cat.

a reasonable period of time with such a collection procedure.

A practical alternative is electroejaculation. We have obtained over 200 ejaculates in the domestic cat and have found the following procedure to be satisfactory.

## METHODS AND MATERIALS FOR ELECTROEJACULATION

The male should be anesthetized with Ketaset® (Bristol), dosage 7 mg./kg., or CI744* (Parke, Davis). Acepromazine (Plegicil® [Ayerst]) can be used in combination with Ketaset®. Acepromazine dosage should not be greater than 2 mg./kg. Higher dosages have caused urine to be released in the ejaculate.

The electroejaculator† assembled in this laboratory is an isolated current sine-wave stimulator with the capability of a 0- to 50-volt range. This unit is connected directly to a 120-volt source. The ejaculator is an AC unit consisting of isolation transformer, variable transformer and appropriate meters for monitoring milliamps and voltage output.

The probes that have given the most satisfactory results in the cat are shown in Figure 1. A probe 1 cm. in diameter and 12 cm. long, with three raised, ventrally placed longitudinal stainless-steel or copper-alloy electrodes, approximately 5 cm. long, has given good results.

The well-lubricated (K-Y Jelly® [Johnson & Johnson]) probe is inserted into the rectum to a depth of approximately 6 to 7 cm. (see Figure 2). A surge-type electrical stimulus has provided better results than

has an on-off stimulus. After two or three stimulations of up to 4 volts, erection is normally obtained. The collection utensil is then placed over the penis, and with further mild stimulation, ejaculation is achieved (see Figures 3 and 4). Once fluid is no longer seen coming from the penis, stimula-

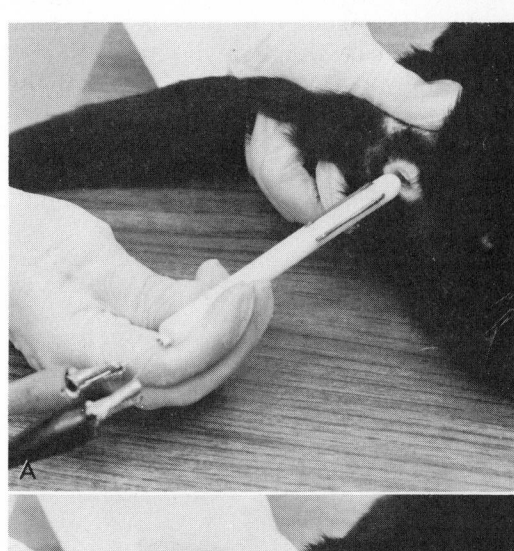

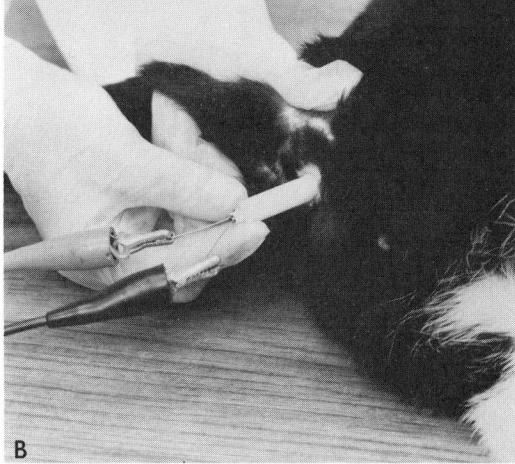

**Figure 2.**   Lubricated probe being inserted into male cat's rectum.

---

*CI744 is not commercially available at this time.

†Clinicians wishing to have a diagram of the electrical circuit, ejaculator assembling instructions and details of probe construction should contact the author.

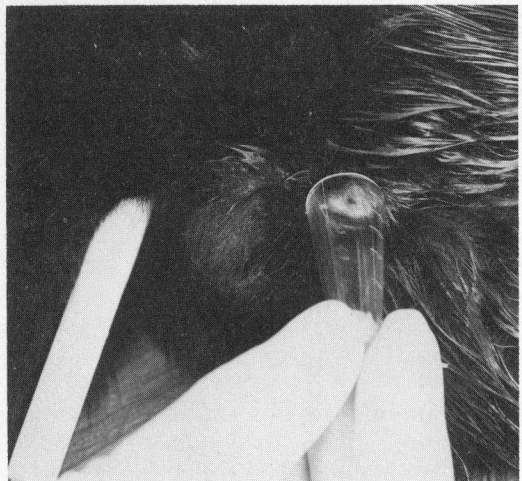

**Figure 3.** Utensil in place for collection of ejaculate.

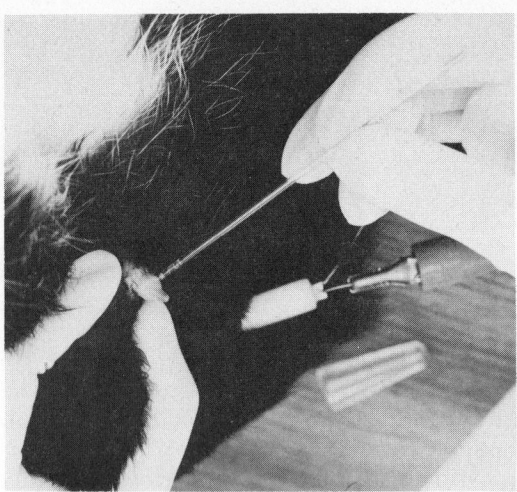

**Figure 5.** Capillary pipette being used to collect remaining drops of semen.

tion is stopped and the collection utensil is removed. Any semen residue is picked up with a capillary pipette and deposited with the remaining semen (Fig. 5). Once the ejaculate is obtained, it should be evaluated according to the following parameters: volume, sperm count, color, motility percentage, speed of progression and morphology (see Table 1).

### SEMEN FREEZING

We have induced pregnancy in domestic cats by utilizing frozen semen that has been collected by electroejaculation. The success of this technique is important to the future breeding in captivity of many endangered species of mammals, particularly wild Felidae. We have received requests regarding the use of frozen semen from cat breeders who wish to breed a certain male or female but who are reluctant to do so for fear of introducing new strains of upper respiratory disease viruses into their catteries. As is the case with breeders of valuable show dogs, cat breeders are reluctant to ship their animals by air to be bred in distant cities. A number of inquiries have been received in relation to the use of frozen semen in this context to avoid shipment of the animal. Perhaps when the techniques of semen freezing and insemination of the cat have been better refined, practitioners, particularly in predominantly feline practices, will be able to utilize frozen semen for cat breeding programs.

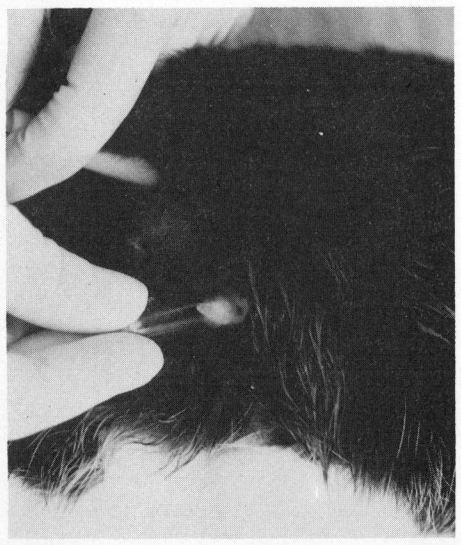

**Figure 4.** Utensil in place and erect penis.

### SUPPLEMENTAL READING

Scott, P. P.: Cats. *In* Hafez, E. S. F. (ed.): Reproduction and Breeding Techniques for Laboratory Animals. Philadelphia, Lea & Febiger, 1970, pp. 192–208.

Seager, S. W. J.: Semen collection and artificial insemination in large cats, wolves and bears. Am. Assn. Zoo Vet. Ann. Proc., 1974, pp. 29–35.

Seager, S. W. J., and Platz, C. C.: Electroejaculation of cats. *In* Klemm, W. R. (ed.): Electronics in Veterinary Medicine. 1976, pp. 410–418.

Sojka, N. J., Jennings, L. L., and Hamner, C. E.: Collection and utilization of cat semen for artificial insemination. J. Am. Vet. Med. Assn., *156*:1250–1251, 1970.

# CANINE ORCHITIS

DONALD H. LEIN, D.V.M.
*Ithaca, New York*

Orchitis and epididymitis occur with relative frequency in the dog but are quite rare in the cat. Usually the two structures are simultaneously affected—in orchiepididymitis, or epididymo-orchitis—and the surrounding tunica vaginalis testis are inflamed and adhesions—in periorchiepididymitis. Orchiepididymitis may be unilateral or bilateral, acute or chronic, suppurative or nonsuppurative, with varying degrees of fibrosis and degeneration. A febrile or systemic reaction may occur, but frequently the reaction remains local. The prostate gland and urinary tract may be involved. In bacterial orchiepididymitis, the tail of the epididymis is most frequently involved.

## ETIOLOGY

*Brucella canis* causes a primary orchiepididymitis. Because of its increasing diagnosis worldwide, its threat to public health and its venereal spread, with ensuing abortion in bitches, this organism should be the causative agent first considered in any case of canine orchiepididymitis. *Brucella abortus* has also been incriminated in orchiepididymitis and abortion in dogs. *Escherichia coli* and *Proteus vulgaris* are frequent causes, but other bacterial agents, such as the *Streptococcus* and *Staphylococcus* spp., and miscellaneous bacterial organisms can be involved. The bacterial agents frequently cause a suppurative process, with abscess formation, and involve the prostate gland and portions of the urinary tract, which may be the primary foci in retrograde infection of the epididymis and testis.

Mycoplasma agents have been isolated from three cases of unilateral orchiepididymitis by the author. In one of these dogs, hemolytic *Escherichia coli* was also isolated. Two of the dogs had abdominal-pelvic injuries prior to developing orchiepididymitis. One had a pelvic fracture as a result of an automobile accident; the other had undergone surgical resection of a portion of the ileum following recurrent ileitis. The third dog developed an unexplained unilateral hematocele in the vaginal cavity, with fibrinous adhesions between the visceral and parietal tunica vaginalis testis. All three cases exhibited extensive involvement of the tunica vaginalis testis, epididymis and testis, which indicates a possible extension from the peritoneal tunics surrounding the testis.

Canine distemper can cause orchiepididymitis in sexually mature dogs. A progressive fibrosing lesion of the epididymides and testicular degeneration will develop if the dog recovers from the acute disease. Distemper inclusion bodies are found in the epididymal epithelium and Sertoli cells of the testis. Infected males can spread the virus to susceptible females by venereal contact during coitus, with the development of endometritis and a blood-tinged vaginal discharge.

Puncture wounds or other traumatic wounds of the scrotum can cause orchiepididymitis by direct extension of microorganisms from the wounds. Mycotic infections or bacteria, such as in nocardiosis or actinobacillosis, are frequently the causative agents.

Sterile urine will produce an epididymo-orchitis when injected via the vas deferens. Dogs hit by automobiles or suffering other traumatic injuries may develop epididymitis if the urinary bladder is full at the time of trauma. Forceful introduction of the urine by retrograde action via the vas to the epididymis may take place.

Human tuberculosis in two dogs has been reported as a cause of granulomatous epididymitis.

## PATHOGENESIS

Infectious agents can enter the testis and epididymis by means of several routes. Bacterial agents such as *Escherichia coli* and *Proteus vulgaris* may enter via the vas by retrograde passage from existing urinary tract infections and/or prostatitis. *Brucella*

1255

spp. cause a persistent bacteremia, with hematogenous spread from the several points of entry into the body. Hematogenous or lymphatic spread of agents from existing sites of active inflammation in the body is another possible source of infectious agents. Agents can enter from the peritoneal cavity via the vaginal cavity and tunics or via traumatic puncture wounds to the scrotum.

Bacterial agents entering via the vas frequently cause acute suppurative epididymitis, especially in the tail of the epididymis, with possible extension throughout the epididymis, efferent tubules, rete testis and seminiferous tubules. Intraluminal abscesses are formed, with eventual breakdown of the epithelium and formation of large abscesses that may drain by fistulous tracts to the scrotal skin surface. Interstitial thickening caused by inflammatory cell infiltration and fibrosis quickly develops. The tunics covering the affected areas are inflamed, and adhesions form.

Inflammation is produced both by the infectious agent or irritant and by exposure of the immune system of the dog to the foreign spermatozoal antigens, resulting in an autoimmune reaction to spermatozoa, spermatogenic cells and possibly basement membranes of the seminiferous tubules. This has been well established in experimental *Brucella canis* infections in dogs and appears to result whenever the integrity of the seminiferous tubules, collecting tubules, rete testis, efferent tubules or epididymal ducts is destroyed or when an increased number of macrophages and leukocytes infiltrate the lumen and phagocytize spermatogenic cells and bacteria. Humoral and cell-mediated immune responses are both involved.

Testicular degeneration, resulting in poor quality semen with several defective spermatozoa or azoospermia, is caused by both thermal degeneration and autoimmune reactions, even in cases in which the inflammation is unilateral. The contralateral testis will show varying degrees of degeneration in the acute stage.

Chronic orchiepididymitis results in varying degrees of testicular degeneration and fibrosis and may lead to atrophy of the testicle. The epididymis usually becomes enlarged, hard and "woody." The scrotal contents are usually firmly adhered or "frozen" in position. Acute flare-ups and abscessation may occur. Inflammation of the spermatic cord may result in extensive vascular damage, leading to ischemic necrosis and loss or atrophy of the scrotal contents.

Insidious progressive nonsuppurative orchiepididymitis may be seen with agents such as *Brucella canis* and *Escherichia coli* and in canine distemper, with varying degrees of degeneration of the epididymis and testis and interstitial fibrosis with inflammatory cell infiltrates. Varying degrees of epididymal and testicular dysfunction occur. This condition may not be recognized for a long period of time by the average pet owner.

Extension of inflammation from the tunica vaginalis testis leads to severe periorchiepididymitis, adhesions and interstitial orchiepididymitis, usually along a well-demarcated progressive line of inflammation.

Sequelae of orchiepididymitis may include ductal and tubular blockage, spermatoceles and the formation of sperm granulomas.

## CLINICAL SIGNS

*Acute orchiepididymitis* may result in increased scrotal temperature, swelling and hyperemia, with pain elicited on palpation of the scrotum. The dog frequently resists examination of the scrotum, prefers to sit and may have referred posterior abdominal and pelvic pain. Libido and the desire for coitus may be depressed or lacking. The author has seen dogs seek a cool place to sit, such as outdoors on wet, cool or snow-covered grounds. Varying degrees of systemic involvement may be present.

The tail of the epididymis is usually enlarged, swollen and "doughy" to hard in consistency. The testis may be enlarged, lack resilience and be unusually firm. The testes are carried high, and frequently the dog will lick the edematous, congested scrotum. Scrotal dermatitis and "lick" granulomas may be produced and have been noted during the acute phase of *Brucella canis* infections. Some cases may result in abscessation, with drainage to the scrotal skin.

If suppurative prostatitis is present, a purulent or serosanguineous purulent discharge may be noted at the urethral opening of the penis, at the prepuce and on the hair around the preputial orifice. The dog will frequently clean the discharge from the penile area and a balanoposthitis may be present. Rectal palpation may reveal a febrile response, severe pain over the prostate, prostatic enlargement and abscessation, and massage per rectum may cause the discharge of purulent exudate from the penile urethra. During the acute phase, the semen contains varying numbers of leukocytes, usually polymorphonuclear leukocytes and a few macrophages. Concentration of spermatozoa may decrease, with increased numbers and types of primary and secondary sperm defects present. Primordial germ cells and syncytial giant cells from sloughed spermatogenic cells may be present. Increased agglutination of motile sperm may be present, usually in head-to-head agglutination.

Other signs of acute *Brucella canis* infection may include generalized lymph node enlargement and a persistent bacteremia, but the animal usually is afebrile. *Brucella canis* infections can be quite insidious. Detection may occur only after breeding. Poor conception or ensuing abortion in mated bitches may be the first clinical sign.

In *chronic orchiepididymitis* the testis may be completely atrophied or firm and fibrotic, with an irregular outline on palpation. The epididymis, especially the tail, is usually enlarged, firm and woody and is often irregular in outline. The scrotal contents usually adhere to the tunics and cannot be moved freely. Acute flare-ups may cause increased scrotal temperature and pain. Evidence of spermatoceles, sperm granulomas, fibrotic thick-walled abscesses, hydrocele, varicocele and funiculitis of the spermatic cord may be detected in the chronic process.

In unilateral involvement, the contralateral epididymis and testis may be quite normal or show varying degrees of degeneration. This is caused by sporadic acute attacks with thermal degeneration and/or autoimmune testicular degeneration. Semen from these dogs can vary from normal to reduced concentration, with varying percentages of primary and secondary spermatozoal defects and varying amounts of exudate and seminal fluids. This will also depend on the involvement of the prostate and urinary tract. Bilateral involvement may lead to azoospermia.

## DIAGNOSIS

A detailed history should be obtained prior to the physical examination. The history should include age, breeding dates and results, libido, previous fertility studies, treatments, fertility data on related animals or animals in a breeding colony, general health, treatment for other conditions, unusual signs, vaccination records and feeding and management practices.

If the history includes abortions, testicular abnormalities such as atrophy or epididymo-orchitis, poor semen quality, infertility or lymph node enlargement with or without the above signs, a possible *Brucella canis* infection should always be considered. The rapid slide agglutination test for *Brucella canis* (Pitman-Moore) should be run, since a *presumptive* diagnosis can be made in the office in a few minutes. "False" positive reactions have occasionally been found but not "false" negative reactions. If positive, a serum sample for tube agglutination test (titer in excess of 1:100 positive) as well as blood samples, seminal fluids, biopsy specimens of enlarged lymph nodes or bone marrow should be submitted for isolation of the organism and a definite diagnosis (see article on "Canine Brucellosis"). Remember that humans can become infected while handling infected specimens.

A physical examination of the scrotal contents and pelvic urogenital tract (by means of rectal digital palpation) and a general physical examination should be carried out to ascertain the degree and stage of involvement. Infectious diseases, such as canine distemper, should be presumptively diagnosed and recognized during this exam.

Samples of semen collected in sterile containers, seminal fluid collected from a sterile urinary catheter while massaging the pelvic genital tract and the affected epididymis, and urine samples collected in a sterile manner should be submitted to a diagnostic laboratory for culture and antibiotic sensitivity tests. Adequate restraint and sedation may be needed to examine and obtain specimens for submission. Heavy contamination with microorganisms from the prepuce may be reduced with broad-spectrum antibiotic and antifungal topical creams and/or by mild antiseptic solution treatment of the preputial cavity prior to sampling and collecting semen. Semen samples may be difficult to collect in the acute state, since pain and systemic involvement may drastically reduce libido. In the chronic state, libido is usually normal, and semen samples can usually be obtained.

Semen and seminal fluid should be examined cytologically for motility and concentration, evidence of microorganisms, inflammatory cell component and percentage of abnormal spermatozoa and spermatogenic cells. This will help ascertain the degree of degeneration and its possible etiology.

If a uni- or bilateral orchiectomy is performed, a portion of the affected organ should be submitted promptly in a sterile container to a diagnostic laboratory for possible isolation of microorganisms. The other portion should be fixed immediately in 10 per cent formalin solution, or Bouin's solution or other hard fixatives for examination of testicular morphology. Formalin creates shrinkage artifacts and renders interpretation of testicular morphology difficult, so Bouin's solution is preferred.

Sterile or negative cultural results from submitted specimens may indicate that antibiotic therapy was given prior to collection of specimens. However, other agents that require special media for growth, such as fastidious bacteria, mycoplasma or viral agents, may be involved. It is also possible that the etiologic agent is not a microorganism. Mixed isolates may be found and they can be etiologic or only contaminants. Draining scrotal abscesses should also be cultured and examined cytologically.

### DIFFERENTIAL DIAGNOSIS

The diagnosis must differentiate orchiepididymitis from the following: scrotal hernia; torsion of the testis; testicular tumors (especially a rapid-growing expansive seminoma); trauma of the testis and spermatic cord, with vascular damage and ischemic necrosis; scrotal dermatitis; congenital hydrocele; anomalies of the efferent tubules or epididymal duct that may lead to sperm stasis or spermatocele, formation of sperm granulomas or testicular degeneration; and scrotal skin tumors such as malignant mastocytoma, melanoma or squamous cell carcinoma.

A detailed history and a careful physical examination of the scrotal contents with digital rectal and abdominal palpation of the pelvic organs should be helpful in differentiating the above conditions from orchiepididymitis. Careful palpation of anatomic structures based on knowledge of their position, size and consistency in the normal state is essential. The tail and head of the epididymis, the vas deferens located on the medial aspect of the spermatic cord and the size of the spermatic cord when normal should all be observed. The lack of adhesions and pain in several of the above conditions is useful in differentiation.

Torsion of the testis or trauma with vascular damage and ischemic necrosis may be the most challenging condition to diagnose. Careful examination of the spermatic cord, epididymis, vas and testis along with other general physical signs (pulse, temperature and respiration rate) is helpful in making a differential diagnosis. For ease of examination, these patients should be sedated.

### TREATMENT

The majority of orchiepididymitis cases appear to be quite resistant to antibiotic or chemotherapeutic treatment. Surgical removal of the affected organs is usually the treatment of choice, especially if the patient is not a valuable breeding dog. Normal preinflammatory reproductive soundness is difficult to achieve, since the resulting inflammation, degenerative lesions and autoimmune reaction usually leave the animal with varying degrees of dysfunction and abnormal semen. If the condition is unilateral, confined to the epididymis, testis and their tunics without involving the prostate and urinary tract, immediate removal of the affected organs may save the contralateral gonad from thermal degeneration and render the animal sound for future breeding use. This is useful in the treatment of penetrating scrotal wounds that affect only one side.

Antibiotics or chemotherapeutic treatments are useful in treating systemic infections before and after surgery. Isolation of the etiologic agent and antibiotic sensitivity tests provide valuable information for sound therapy. If isolation of an agent is unsuccessful, broad-spectrum antibiotics should be used, since *Escherichia coli* and *Proteus* spp. are the most frequent agents involved. In the acute stage, hypothermic treatment of the scrotum may be beneficial. Therapy should be prolonged, since the prostate and urinary tract may be involved. Antibiotics and other chemotherapeutic agents can cause testicular degeneration, although most testes will regenerate satisfactorily after withdrawal of the drug. Before you use unfamiliar drugs on a valuable breeding dog, the manufacturer should be consulted for information about known testicular degenerative effects.

Evaluation of any treatment regimen must be followed by periodic bacteriologic examinations of seminal fluid and physical examination of the affected organs. Semen evaluation should be performed periodically. The goal of treatment is to eliminate the organism from the affected animal and return the animal to as near a normal reproductive function as possible. The owner must be made aware of the expense and time involved and that success by drug treatment alone cannot be assured. The prognosis for the return to normal reproductive use is usually poor. The prognosis for the life of the animal is good if there is no prolonged systemic involvement and if the affected portions can be removed surgically.

The dog infected with *Brucella canis* is difficult to treat, and the potential risk to humans and other dogs is of great concern. Several treatment schedules have been tried, but the poor response and potential danger of spread usually dictate against treatment. Most dogs are euthanatized when brucellosis is positively diagnosed. Treatment regimens using tetracycline hydrochloride or minocycline hydrochloride are described in the article on "Canine Brucellosis."

If prostatitis is present with orchiepididymitis, bilateral orchiectomy is beneficial to the treatment of this inflammation because it removes the source of testosterone needed for prostate function.

### CONTROL AND PREVENTION

Pretesting, preexamination and detailed histories of dogs prior to breeding are beneficial in preventing the spread of *Brucella canis* infection. Proper hygiene, good sanitation and management and sound vaccination and health programs as well as keen observation and good common sense are all helpful in controlling and preventing the above conditions.

# URINE SPRAYING IN CATS

BENJAMIN L. HART, D.V.M.
*Davis, California*

Urine spraying is the most frequent serious behavioral problem in cats. Spraying is routinely encountered in intact males and is occasionally encountered in males castrated either prepubertally (6 to 8 months) or postpubertally. Under some circumstances spayed and intact females may also spray. Dealing with this problem involves an understanding of the function of spraying and the factors that induce spraying, an interpretation of the medical history, formulation of a differential diagnosis and a determination of the most appropriate therapeutic approach.

### FUNCTION OF URINE SPRAYING

Urine spraying is a type of territorial marking engaged in by males after they reach sexual maturity. Objects in the immediate territory and home range are sprayed presumably as a mechanism for familiarizing the cat with its territory. The smell of his own urine is thought to make the cat more self-assured and confident, especially in regard to agonistic encounters with other males. Probably the most important immediate cause of spraying is an increase in anxiety or nervousness.

Cats probably do not intentionally mark the boundaries of their territory (as one would put up a fence) but rather tend to mark boundary areas because this is where anxiety-evoking encounters occur with other cats. Because of the offensive odor of male urine and its destructive effect on household objects, male cats are customarily castrated prior to puberty. Castration is also performed to prevent roaming and fighting.

During the breeding season the frequency of urine spraying increases. This may occur as a result of a seasonal increase in testosterone secretion and may also be related to increased agonistic interactions with other males and an increase in the general level of anxiety. Urine marks are undoubtedly useful in attracting sexually receptive females to the vicinity.

Urine spraying, like fighting and roaming, is a sexually dimorphic trait that normally occurs much more frequently in males than females. Spraying in intact females is normally restricted to the breeding season and is related to the attraction of male cats to the female's vicinity.

Although castration greatly reduces the occurrence of spraying, the neural pathways and neurons that mediate the behavior can still be activated by strong environmental stimuli. Problem spraying is usually limited to the small percentage of male cats in which castration does not prevent or eliminate spraying.

## WHY GONADECTOMIZED CATS SPRAY

Sometimes castrated males or spayed females kept as single pets start spraying for no apparent reason. However, in most instances environmental factors are related to the onset of spraying. These include changes in the animal's environment and other factors which increase its level of anxiety or nervousness. If, for example, the owner moves to a new house, there may be a transient period of spraying while the cat adapts to its new home. If new cats are introduced into a neighborhood or into the household of a nonspraying resident, the resident may start spraying. Sometimes the presence of sexually active males in the neighborhood may stimulate castrates to spray during the breeding season.

Crowding several cats together in one house increases the likelihood of spraying. Cats are not generally considered highly social animals, and when several cats are kept in the same house there are usually agonistic encounters of a continuing type between two or more of the animals. Because this raises the level of anxiety or nervousness, spraying may also occur.

## INTERPRETING THE MEDICAL HISTORY

**Distinguishing Spraying from Inappropriate Urination.** Most knowledgable cat owners recognize spraying, but there are some who may confuse inappropriate urination with territorial spraying. When presented with the possibility of spraying, first determine the type of urination in question. If urine is found 1 to 2 feet above ground level on vertical objects, then, of course, it is the result of spraying. Sometimes cats will urinate in inappropriate places such as on the owner's clothes, bed or even his lap, but the urine will be deposited on a horizontal surface from a squatting position. Another form of inappropriate urination is urination on the floor, sometimes right beside the litter box; this behavior may be a reflection of senility or an aversion to the cat box.

**The Question of Urinary Disorders.** Obtaining the medical history should involve a consideration of any concurrent or previous signs of urinary disorders. Urinary infections that cause an increase in urination may be confused with spraying. Although other clinicians have noted a correlation between cystitis or the presence of urinary calculi and spraying, we have not found a high incidence of urinary infections in cats that are actually spraying. If necessary, a urinalysis should be conducted to differentiate spraying from disease of the urinary tract.

Although spraying, or attempts to spray, is not one of the expected signs related to urethral obstruction, one should consider the possibility that an abnormal number of crystals or small calculi may cause sufficient discomfort to a male cat that he may adopt the least painful manner to expel them. It could be that by directing the penis backward and straightening the urethra, crystals or small calculi may be expelled with more force and more easily than in urination by the squatting fashion.

**Environmental Factors.** Once it is established that spraying is associated with a behavioral problem, it is useful to determine whether there are any environmental changes related to the onset of spraying. Did the spraying start with the onset of the breeding season? Have the owners recently moved to a new home? Do they know of any new male cats in the neighborhood? Has the cat recently become more nervous or anxious? How many other cats are kept in the same household?

Some of these factors may be transient, such as the onset of the breeding season or the owners' moving to a new home, and therefore once the spraying has been reduced or eliminated it may not recur. Other factors may tend continually to evoke spraying, and the owner should be aware that it may be difficult to obtain a long-term resolution to the problem. One of the most common situations associated with recurring spraying is an owner with a large number of cats who is reluctant to give up any.

**Androgenic Steroids.** The medical history may also give some indication of past treatment with some androgenic steroids. Preparations containing testosterone, which are given to stimulate metabolism, increase muscle tone or treat certain skin conditions in castrates, probably contain a sufficient amount of testosterone to evoke spraying. In some cases, spraying that is initially evoked by administration of an androgenic steroid may subsequently be maintained because of environmental stimuli.

## THERAPEUTIC APPROACHES

Of the suggestions here, you may find one or a combination of approaches useful. It is well to remind clients, however, that when dealing with the problem of spraying, we are not treating abnormal behavior but are attempting to alter a cat's normal response to certain social or environmental disturbances. Thus, no approach should be considered completely reliable.

**Punishment.** Most clients will have tried some form of punishment, such as yelling or throwing something at the cat, to stop spraying when they observe it. In some instances this approach has been effective and the cat will stop spraying inside the house (although it may continue to spray outside). Most cat owners, however, are aware of the futility of bringing the cat to the urine-soiled· spot and pointing it out or rubbing the cat's nose in it while slapping or hitting the animal for good measure.

**Castration.** If a sexually mature, intact male cat starts spraying, there is a good chance (approaching 90 per cent) that the spraying will be reduced or eliminated by castration. In most of these animals the spraying will be eliminated very soon after the animal has recovered from the operation. In some, however, the frequency of spraying is reduced gradually over a 2- to 3-month period following castration (Hart and Barrett, 1973).

Not all male cats that are castrated after they have started to spray will stop, however. Prepubertal castrates may start spraying several years after being castrated. The particular environmental factors involved may account for some of the individual variability in the response to castration. A male cat that is kept with several other cats would have a greater tendency to continue spraying than one who is the only cat kept in the household.

It may be useful to mention to clients that castration simply removes to a large degree the tendency for male cats to spray. It does not erase or eliminate the neural pathways in the brain that are involved in this relatively innate behavior. The same pool of neurons that respond to testosterone are also thought to be affected by olfactory, visual, auditory and other environmental stimuli.

**Administration of Long-acting Progestins.** Although less than 100 per cent effective, the single most useful approach in treating spraying behavior is the administration of a long-acting progestin such as medroxyprogesterone (Depo-Provera® [Upjohn]). The dose of medroxyprogesterone should be between 50 and 100 mg. for a normal-sized male cat and 50 mg. for a female. It should be administered subcutaneously or intramuscularly. Permanent remission of spraying may follow one injection, especially if environmental factors which evoked the behavior were transient in nature. When there is continual anxiety or nervousness on the part of the cat, or when there are other factors tending to stimulate the behavior, repeated injections at intervals of one to six months may be necessary to keep the behavior suppressed. Another progestin, megestrol acetate (Ovaban® [Schering]), has been used by some practitioners. Tablets are usually given to cats at the rate of 5 mg. daily for 3 to 8 days and then 5 mg. weekly.

Progesterone in oil (repository progesterone) is not recommended because blood levels are not maintained for a prolonged period. Some practitioners have found, however, that progesterone in oil at a dose of 10 mg./kg. does suppress spraying in some cats. It may be that the peaking effect of repository progesterone is beneficial in some cases. A combination of progesterone in oil and medroxyprogesterone may be effective when neither form alone is effective.

We have found that some forms of inappropriate urination (not spraying), such as on the owner's bed or clothes, may also be eliminated by administration of a progestin.

Medroxyprogesterone may be used in both intact and castrated male cats and in spayed females. Because this preparation may induce uterine complications, it should not be used in intact females during any stage of their estrous cycle. Even in spayed females and males, progestins are not without their risks. Several practitioners have reported enlargement of the mammary glands in some cats and the development of mammary carcinoma in females and males following repeated administration of medroxyprogesterone.

A rather common side effect of progestins is a pronounced increase in appetite. Some cats have a tendency to become calmer and more affectionate after treatment.

The mechanism by which progestins alter spraying is not understood. It may suppress the activity of neurons of the hypothalamus and elsewhere that are involved in the motivation of spraying, basically the converse of testosterone activation of these neurons. Estrogenic substances would not be expected to have similar suppressive effects.

**Psychosurgery.** When correction of a urinary disorder, administration of a long-acting progestin or alteration of the environment does not eliminate spraying, many cat owners request euthanasia. With this in mind, we have conducted a clinical experiment to determine the feasibility of brain surgery to eliminate spraying in castrated males and spayed females for which other approaches to control the behavior have not been successful. The approach is based on the use of a stereotaxic instrument with x-ray ventriculography to direct electrodes into the designated brain area. The site of electrode placement is based on a previous experimental study which showed that bilateral lesions of the medial preoptic-anterior hypothalamic area eliminated copulatory behavior in intact male cats (Hart *et al.*, 1973). It was reasoned that urine spraying, a basically masculine behavior, would also be affected by the same lesions. The results on a limited number of cases have been rewarding. Spraying has been eliminated, while the behavioral side effects have been relatively minor or at least tolerable. The most consistent side effect has been a pronounced increase in appetite.

This type of surgery can be performed only in properly equipped laboratories, and it is currently available on a referral basis. If we continue to have enough success with this approach, so that it is adopted by others, it may become more widely available.

### SUPPLEMENTAL READING

Hart, B. L.: Behavioral effects of long-acting progestins. Feline Pract., *4*:8–11, 1974.

Hart, B. L.: Spraying behavior. Feline Pract., 5:11–13, 1975.

Hart, B. L., and Barrett, R. E.: Effects of castration on fighting, roaming and urine spraying in adult male cats. J. Am. Vet. Med. Assn., *163*:290–292, 1973.

Hart, B. L., Haugen, C. M., and Peterson, D. M.: Effects of medial preoptic-anterior hypothalamic lesions on mating behavior of male cats. Brain Res., *54*:177–191, 1973.

Hernandez, F. J., Fernandez, B. B., and Gage, P. A.: Feline mammary carcinoma and progestogens. Feline Pract. 5:45–48, 1975.

# NEOPLASMS OF THE CANINE AND FELINE REPRODUCTIVE TRACTS

RALPH E. BARRETT, D.V.M.
*Pullman, Washington*

*and* GORDON H. THEILEN, D.V.M.
*Davis, California*

Many isolated case reports have identified numerous types of tumors affecting both the female and the male reproductive tracts (Tables 1 and 2). Feline genital tumors are rare; much less is known about their biologic behavior. There are almost no reports of genital neoplasia in male cats. The most frequently encountered tumors will be discussed in terms of clinical characteristics and therapeutic recommendations.

Data obtained from the history and physical examination of the genital tract may lead to suspicion of neoplasia; however, radiography, impression smear cytology, fine-needle aspiration biopsy and exploratory surgery and biopsy are usually necessary to make a definitive diagnosis. Laboratory and evaluation including a CBC, BUN, SGPT, urinalysis and thoracic and abdominal radiographs are indicated to detect metastases.

## TUMORS OF THE FEMALE REPRODUCTIVE TRACT

### OVARIAN TUMORS

Although many different ovarian tumors have been reported, they are infrequent in the bitch and rare in the queen. The granulosa-theca cell tumor and cystadenocarcinoma are the most common. There has been a tendency to differentiate primary ovarian tumors histologically into many different groups, but because of their rarity in the bitch and queen, these subclassifications have little meaning applicable to treatment and prognosis.

*Granulosa-theca cell tumors* constitute approximately 50 per cent of ovarian tumors in the bitch and queen. Mixed tumors of granulosa and theca cells are common, and they are therefore often grouped together. These tumors are usually unilateral, are nonmalignant and occur in older animals. Secretion of estrogen or progesterone frequently results in cystic endometrial hyperplasia, with a serosanguineous or mucopurulent vaginal discharge and prolonged estrus. Their gross appearance is smooth; their cut surface may be white or yellow, solid or cystic. About 10 to 20 per cent of granulosa cell tumors are malignant. Metastases to the omentum, lumbar lymph nodes, liver, spleen, kidney and lungs occur. If the tumor is large, or if metastasis has occurred, anorexia, vomiting, cachexia, palpable abdominal mass(es) and ascites may occur. Occasionally gynecomastia and bilaterally symmetrical alopecia develop.

*Cystadenomas and cystadenocarcinomas* probably arise from the surface epithelium of the ovary and epithelial cords in the underlying cortex. They may be unilateral or bilateral. Because they often produce steroids, they often are associated with cystic endometrial hyperplasia and bilaterally symmetrical alopecia. Ascites may develop, owing to lymphatic obstruction and/or secretion from the tumor. If these tumors remain in the bursa, they have a cauliflower appearance. Once large neoplasms escape from the bursa, typical papillae develop and often shed implants into the peritoneum. Papillary cystadenocarcinomas have been induced by prolonged administration of diethylstilbestrol. They regress following withdrawal of the hormone.

*Dysgerminomas* develop from germ cells and histologically resemble testicular seminomas. They constitute 6 to 12 per cent of canine ovarian tumors and 15 per cent of feline ovarian tumors. All are potentially malignant, but only about 20 per cent

1263

**Table 1.** *Reported Neoplasms of the Female Canine and Feline Reproductive Systems*

I. *Ovarian Tumors*

    A. Epithelial Origin:

        Cystadenoma* and cystadenocarcinoma*†, adenocarcinoma*

    B. Mesodermal Origin:

        Fibroma, leiomyoma*, polyps*

    C. Gonadal-stroma Origin:

        Granulosa cell*†, theca cell, luteoma, Sertoli cell type, mixed tumors (granulosa-theca cell)*

    D. Germ Cell Origin:
        Dysgerminoma*, teratoma*

    E. Metastatic Tumors:

        Pancreatic adenocarcinoma, uterine adenocarcinoma*, mammary adenocarcinoma, lymphosarcoma*, transmissible venereal tumor, reticulum cell sarcoma

    F. Non-neoplastic Proliferations:

        Follicular cysts, luteal cysts, cystic rete tubules, germinal inclusion cysts, paraovarian cysts

II. *Uterine Tumors*

    Leiomyoma*† (fibroleiomyoma, fibromyoma), leiomyosarcoma*, adenoma*, adenocarcinoma*, fibroma, fibrosarcoma, squamous cell carcinoma*, adenomyosis, lipoma, liposarcoma, lymphosarcoma*, polyp

III. *Vaginal and Vulvar Tumors*

    Leiomyoma†, leiomyosarcoma, lipoma, fibroma, neurofibroma, fibrosarcoma, transmissible venereal tumor, adenoma, lymphosarcoma

IV. *Tumors of the Female External Genitalia (Cutaneous)*

    Squamous cell carcinoma, sebaceous gland adenoma, histiocytoma, mast cell tumor and a variety of cutaneous neoplasms are possible

\*Reported in the feline.
†Most common tumor of the area.

metastasize. They are usually unilateral and well encapsulated and have a smooth surface and soft consistency. On cut surface they are white-gray and often have yellow areas of necrosis and areas of hemorrhage. They rarely cause clinical signs other than the presence of an abdominal mass. Signs of hyperestrogenism or hyperprogesteronism may be present in a small percentage of the affected bitches. Cells obtained from vaginal swabs may be characterized by the presence of keratinized pearls.

With few exceptions, *teratomas* (dermoid cysts) are benign unilateral tumors. They may become very large in size. Mineralization is a prominent radiographic component. Because of their large size, clinical signs are often associated with interference with other abdominal organs. Weight loss, intermittent intestinal obstruction with anorexia and vomiting are often present. Death due to rupture and hemoperitoneum has been reported.

In summary, dogs and cats with ovarian

**Table 2.** *Reported Neoplasms of the Male Canine Reproductive System*

I. *Preputial Tumors*

    A. Outside Prepuce:

        Mast cell tumor*, cornu cutaneum, papilloma, hemangioma, fibroma, sebaceous gland adenoma, lymphangioma, round cell sarcoma, hemangioendothelioma, fibrosarcoma, squamous cell carcinoma, reticulum cell sarcoma, circumanal gland tumor

    B. Preputial and Penile Tumors:

        Mast cell tumor*, transmissible venereal tumor*, papilloma, squamous cell carcinoma

II. *Prostatic Tumors*

    Adenocarcinoma*, adenoma, leiomyoma, leiomyosarcoma, metastatic carcinoma, sarcomas, lymphosarcoma

III. *Testicular Tumors*

    Sertoli cell tumor†, seminoma, interstitial cell tumor, teratoma, fibroma, lipoma, lymphosarcoma

IV. *Tumors of the Epididymis*

    Fibroma, spread of seminoma and Sertoli cell tumor

V. *Tumor of the Vas Deferens*

    Cystadenofibroma

VI. *Tumor of the Tunica Vaginalis*

    Leiomyoma

\*Most common tumor of the area.
†Reported in the feline.

tumors are most often presented with various combinations of cystic endometrial hyperplasia, vaginal discharge, bilaterally symmetrical alopecia and ascites. Nonspecific signs of anorexia, vomiting and cachexia are often present. Diagnosis is often made by abdominal palpation, exfoliative cytology of ascitic fluid or radiography. Final diagnosis is imperative for prognosis and is obtained by means of histopathologic evaluation. The treatment of choice is surgical extirpation. Most tumors are benign, and early detection and removal of malignant tumors may be curative. Once metastasis has occurred, the prognosis is poor. Chemotherapy has not been reported in veterinary patients; results of chemotherapy in women have been disappointing.

## TUMORS OF THE UTERUS, VAGINA AND VULVA

Both benign and malignant tumors of all histologic components of the uterus, vagina and vulva have been reported. In one study, 9 of 2361 canine tumors arose from the uterus. Clinical signs that may occur with uterine neoplasia include purulent vaginal discharge, a palpable abdominal mass, ascites, constipation, vomiting, weight loss and anorexia. Only 11 cases of uterine neoplasia have been reported in the cat; most were highly malignant adenocarcinomas. Leiomyomas are the most common tumor of the uterus of the bitch. The diagnostic and therapeutic approach is the same as that described for ovarian tumors. Early ovariohysterectomy is the treatment of choice.

Leiomyomas are also the most common neoplasm of the vagina and vulva; fibromas are second most common. They are most common in boxers and more frequent in nulliparous bitches. Although these masses may protrude from the vulva, owners are often unaware of their presence. Most originate in the vestibule (intraluminal) of the vulva. Leiomyomas are usually white to pink, pedunculated and pear-shaped. They may be associated with ovarian follicular cysts, estrogen-secreting tumors and cystic endometrial hyperplasia. Large intraluminal leiomyomas may obstruct the urethra and cause dysuria or edema of the labia of the vulva. Extraluminal leiomyomas (which are less common) may cause urinary retention, tenesmus, constipation and incontinence. These masses can often be palpated in the caudal portion of the abdomen.

Surgical extirpation following a dorsal episiotomy is the treatment of choice. Prognosis is good.

Leiomyosarcomas and fibrosarcomas are uncommon.

## TUMORS OF THE FEMALE AND MALE EXTERNAL GENITALIA

Of the numerous cutaneous and adnexal tumors that involve the female external genitalia, sebaceous gland adenomas and histiocytomas are most common. Surgical removal usually results in cure.

*Squamous cell carcinomas* may also develop in the skin of the vulva. These are usually rapidly growing, ulcerated, firm lesions. Treatment should consist of surgical excision followed by radiation therapy (3500 to 4500 rads given as 400 to 450 rads three times weekly). Orthovoltage x-ray therapy machines with a half-value layer of 2.20 mm. of aluminum and operated at 100 to 150 kvp. and 30 milliamperes frequently are used. The prognosis should always be guarded. Since these tumors are often only locally invasive, and are frequently radiosensitive, significant remissions may occur.

Many cutaneous tumors have been reported to occur on the outside of the prepuce of the dog (Table 2). Formulation of therapy should be based on the histological morphology of the neoplasm and the extent to which it involves adjacent tissues and if metastasis is present. *Mast cell tumors* are the most frequently reported tumor of the external genitalia. A diagnosis may readily be established by surgical or aspiration biopsy. Therapy may include surgical excision, irradiation, chemotherapy or combinations of these procedures. Mast cell tumors may be benign or extremely malignant. If the mast cells are malignant, surgery should be combined with radiation or chemotherapy. Radiation therapy similar to that described for squamous cell carcinomas is recommended. Chemotherapy utilizing cyclophosphamide (Cytoxan® [Mead Johnson]) at a dosage of 50 mg./m.² BSA orally every other day has been successful alone or in combination with prednisolone administered at a dosage of 20 mg./m.² BSA orally divided twice a day every other day. A third drug, vincristine sulfate (Oncovin® [Lilly]) administered at a dosage of 0.5 mg./m.² BSA IV once a week for 8 weeks can also be added to the regimen. Vinblastine (Velban® [Lilly]) may be superior to Oncovin®. Velban® is given at a dosage of 2 mg./m.² IV once a week for 8 weeks. Familiarity with the toxic effects of these drugs is imperative before they are used. Treatment should cease if the total WBC count falls below 3000/cu. mm., if the platelet count falls below 50,000/cu. mm., or if there is a significant rise in the concentration of BUN.

*Transmissible venereal tumors* (TVT) commonly involve the vulva, vagina, prepuce and penis of dogs in some areas of the United States and the world. Females and males are both susceptible. It is transmitted during coitus by cell transplantation. This tumor usually regresses spontaneously but on occasion may metastasize to regional lymph nodes, skin, spleen, liver, lungs, tonsils, brain and eye.

Clinical signs are usually associated with persistent dripping of frank blood or serosanguineous fluid from the prepuce or vulva. If the tumor is located near the urethral orifice, signs of dysuria may be present. The differential diagnosis includes foreign bodies, trauma, urethral prolapse, prostatic disease, estrus, cystitis and other tumors (especially mastocytomas and histiocytomas). The tumor's appearance ranges from early, small, hyperemic papules to more mature, large (3 to 6 cm.) cauliflower-like masses. While growing, the tumors typically appear bright red, owing to vascularization, but they become ulcerated and necrotic during regression. The tumor cells resemble large lymphoblasts or histiocytes when evaluated by exfoliative cytologic techniques.

Suspect C-type virus particles have been detected in TVT by electron microscopy, but all attempts to transmit the neoplasm by cell-free filtrates have failed. Karyotype studies have revealed that TVT cells always have a hypodiploid number of chromosomes, usually 58 to 60.

Treatment is often not necessary because TVT often spontaneously regress. If removal is necessary because of location or undesirable clinical signs, surgery is often curative. Persistent local lesions can be treated with radiation therapy as previously described. If metastasis has occurred, chemotherapy with vincristine, prednisolone and cyclophosphamide in conjunction with surgery and/or radiation therapy as described for mast cell tumors is indicated. Methotrexate administered orally at a dosage of 2.5 to 5.0 mg./m.² BSA daily for four days, and repeated weekly for 8 weeks, has also been successful. Chemotherapy has been more successful in male than in female dogs with TVT.

Tumors that do not regress probably occur in immunodeficient animals. Future immunotherapy regimens may be beneficial in these cases.

## TUMORS OF THE MALE REPRODUCTIVE TRACT

### TESTICULAR TUMORS

The three most common testicular neoplasms are Sertoli cell tumors (SCT), seminomas (SEM) and interstitial cell tumors (ICT). They occur with similar frequency, but ICT are infrequently associated with clinical signs. It is not known whether ectopic testicles have a higher incidence of neoplasia than descended testicles. Testicular tumors usually occur in dogs over 7 years of age. Since most testicular tumors usually do not metastasize, the treatment of choice is bilateral castration. If metastasis has occurred with SCT or SEM, surgical removal of distant lesions or local radiotherapy of accessible lesions may be tried. If extensive metastasis has occurred, the prognosis is grave. No chemotherapeutic agents have been reported to be of significant value in the treatment of metastatic tumors.

In the absence of clinical signs, a diagnosis is usually made by palpation during geriatric examinations. ICT are usually small and are not palpable. In contrast, SEM and SCT are often palpated as large, firm, nodular masses in part of the testicle, or they may obliterate the entire testicular architecture. Two or three tumor types are often present in an affected testicle. SEM and ICT often are associated with prostatic disease, perineal hernias or perianal gland adenomas and adenocarcinomas.

SEM and SCT can cause pain, owing to intrascrotal hemorrhage and edema, or signs of feminization. At present, the steroid imbalance responsible for feminization has not been identified. Signs of feminization may include (1) decreased libido, (2) attraction of other males, (3) posterior or generalized hyperpigmentation and alopecia, (4) atrophy of the nontumorous testicle, (5) penis atrophy, (6) pendulous prepuce, (7) "female-type" distribution of body fat, (8) gynecomastia, (9) enlarged nipples and (10) enlargement of the prostate due to squamous metaplasia or prostatitis. The latter may cause constipation or dysuria.

*Sertoli cell tumors* develop from the Sertoli (nurse) cells of the seminiferous tubules. They are usually unilateral, hard and lobulated and have a white or gray greasy surface that may contain golden specks. These may become very large and occur with greater frequency in ectopic testicles than do SEM or ICT. SCT are usually benign, but about 10 per cent metastasize to inguinal, iliac, sublumbar and abdominal lymph nodes, kidneys, liver, spleen, pancreas and lungs. Clinical signs of feminization are present in 25 per cent of dogs with SCT. These signs undergo remission 3 to 6 weeks after removal of a benign SCT. If signs persist following surgery, metastasis should be suspected.

*Seminomas* arise from the germinal epithelium of the seminiferous tubules. They are typically unilateral and have a soft, bulging, slightly lobulated, clay-colored and creamy cut surface. Although their morphologic appearance indicates that they are malignant, they are usually benign clinically. They may metastasize to regional abdominal lymph nodes. Occasionally, they invade the spermatic cord.

*Interstitial cell tumors* originate from Leydig cells between the seminiferous tubules. They are rarely diagnosed ante mortem, since they are of small size and usually do not produce hormones. They have a raised, soft, bulging cut surface of yellow-orange or brown color and frequently contain cysts with clear or bloody fluid. These are almost always benign, but rarely they metastasize to regional and abdominal lymph nodes, liver, spleen and lungs.

## TUMORS OF THE PROSTATE GLAND

The most common tumor of the canine prostate gland is the *adenocarcinoma*. In one study, the clinical signs associated with enlarged prostate glands were (listed in order of decreasing frequency) emaciation, rear-leg lameness, tenesmus, dysuria, polyuria and polydipsia, lumbar pain, urethral bleeding and hematuria at the beginning of urination. These tumors are highly malignant; when clinical signs develop, metastasis has usually occurred. They usually spread to the sublumbar lymph nodes, but metastasis to abdominal organs and lungs is also possible. Differential diagnoses of enlarged prostate glands include benign cystic hyperplasia, prostatic abscess, acute and chronic prostatitis, prostatic (congenital ductular) cyst and prostatic neoplasia. Neoplasia of the feline prostate has not been reported.

A diagnosis of prostatic neoplasia can be made by means of several procedures. Rectal palpation often reveals a firm, irregular, nodular enlargement of the prostate. It is usually asymmetrical and may adhere to the floor of the pelvis. Palpable sublumbar lymph nodes may also be detected. A pneumocystogram or retrograde urethrogram may help identify the extent of the mass. Aspiration of prostatic cells with a urethral catheter and exfoliative cytology may be necessary to confirm the diagnosis. Utilizing rectal palpation, the prostatic sample is obtained by placing the tip of an appropriate-sized catheter in the urethra at the posterior pole of the enlarged prostate. While an assistant aspirates prostatic material with a syringe attached to the catheter, prostatic cells are digitally "milked out" while palpating via the rectum. Biopsy samples may also be obtained by means of fine-needle aspiration biopsy per rectum. Routine cytologic stains are recommended for exfoliative cytology. If percutaneous biopsy sampling procedures are not diagnostic, exploratory laparotomy with prostatic biopsy and consideration of prostatectomy is indicated.

Castration and prostatectomy are recommended if metastasis has not occurred. Prostatic adenocarcinomas poorly respond to chemotherapy. In man, cryosurgery of the neoplastic prostate has been associated with elimination of the tumor and even regression of metastatic lesions in a few patients. It has been hypothesized that the remission may be associated with stimulation of the immune system.

### SUPPLEMENTAL READING

Brodey, R. S.: Neoplasms of the canine uterus, vagina, and vulva: A clinicopathologic survey of 90 cases. J. Am. Vet. Med. Assn., *151*:1294–1307, 1967.

Jubb, K. V. F., and Kennedy, P.: Pathology of Domestic Animals, Vol. 1, 2nd ed., Academic Press, New York and London. 1970, pp. 487–574.

Nielsen, S. W., and Lein, D. H.: Tumors of the testes. Bull. of WHO *50*:71–78, 1974.

Norris, H. J., Garner, F. M., and Taylor, H. B.: Pathology of feline ovarian neoplasms. J. Path. 97:138–143, 1969.

Taylor, P. A.: Prostatic adenocarcinoma in a dog and a summary of ten cases. Canadian Vet. J., *14*:162–166, 1973.

Section

# 13

# INFECTIOUS DISEASES

FREDRIC W. SCOTT, D.V.M.
*Consulting Editor*

# CANINE VACCINES AND IMMUNITY

RONALD D. SCHULTZ, Ph.D.,
MAX APPEL, D.V.M.,
LELAND E. CARMICHAEL,
D.V.M.
*Ithaca, New York*

*and* BRIAN FARROW, D.V.M.
*Sydney, Australia*

The purpose of a vaccination program is to prevent the development of overt clinical disease, by either preventing or limiting infection. The mechanisms by which the dog is protected from infection and disease after vaccination have been and are the subject of numerous past and current studies by microbiologists and immunologists. It is currently accepted that there are two arms of the specific host defense system: (1) the humoral (antibody) system consisting of B lymphocytes and the four immunoglobulin classes (IgG, IgM, IgA and IgE) and, to assist this system, K cells, phagocytic cells and effector molecules such as complement and properdin; and (2) the cell-mediated immune (CMI) system, consisting of T lymphocytes, a number of products called lymphokines and macrophages.

## FACTORS INFLUENCING HOST DEFENSE SYSTEM

Numerous factors can influence the host defense system and thus affect the immune response to vaccination. Factors to be considered in designing an effective vaccination program for the dog include the specific immunosuppressive or blocking effect of colostral antibody, the nature of the vaccine, the route of vaccination, the age of the dog, the general nutritional condition of the dog, concurrent infections and drug treatments. These factors will be discussed briefly with respect to the possible influence that each may have on the effectiveness of vaccination.

### COLOSTRUM

It is well known that approximately 95 per cent of immunoglobulin in the puppy comes from absorption of colostrum shortly after birth. Following absorption from the gut, specific colostral antibodies—particularly the IgG antibodies—have the ability to prevent vaccine antigens from reaching the lymphocytes, which are responsible for the genesis of active immunity. It is necessary therefore for this acquired antibody of colostral origin to reach low levels in pups before active immunization is possible. For puppies born to bitches immune to canine distemper (CD) and infectious canine hepatitis (CAV-1), this period of uncertain response to vaccination can be as long as 14 to 16 weeks after birth. A method of circumventing this blocking effect is the use of measles vaccine to protect against canine distemper. Also, vaccines that contain high titers of the vaccine viruses or bacterial antigens may be more effective in overcoming low levels of passive antibody than are vaccines with low titers. As will be mentioned later, these methods of overcoming the effects of colostral immunity are not absolute.

This situation presents an immunologic paradox, in that colostral antibody is extremely important for protection of the newborn pup against a multitude of potentially harmful antigens during the first few weeks of life; therefore, no consideration should be given to preventing the puppy from obtaining colostrum.

### NATURE OF THE VACCINE

Certain questions need to be considered to achieve the most effective vaccination program.

Is the vaccine virus a modified live or killed virus? If live virus vaccine is used, the vaccine should be handled according to directions supplied by the manufacturer so that it does not become inactive.

Does the bacterin contain adjuvant?

1271

If killed virus or bacterin is administered, is the agent present in a form and in a quantity that provides optimum antigenicity?

To achieve maximum success the entire dose of vaccine should be given as recommended and not divided and given to more than one dog.

## ROUTE OF VACCINATION

The directions specified by the manufacturer should be followed; for example, if a subcutaneous route is recommended, do not give the vaccine intramuscularly, and vice versa. Significant differences in host response to certain vaccines exist and are dependent on the route of administration of vaccine.

## AGE OF THE DOG

The age of the dog is important not only because of persistence of colostral antibody, but also because the relative hypothermia that exists during the first week or two of life can cause a state of CMI unresponsiveness. Optimum body temperatures between 38 and 39° C. are very critical for T cell as well as macrophage function in the dog. Body temperatures of less than 37° C. are not uncommon in the puppy during the first week or so of life, and this lower body temperature is capable of suppressing the CMI system, although humoral immunity (antibody production) does not appear to be affected to the same extent as CMI. Vaccination during this early period (i.e., less than 2 weeks of age) with live attenuated vaccines is not recommended.

There is also evidence to suggest that certain dogs in the later stages of life (i.e., 7 to 9 years of age) may have a decreased ability to produce antibody as well as a decreased CMI response. Annual revaccination during these later years therefore would be particularly important to maintain an active state of immunity.

## NUTRITIONAL STATE OF THE DOG

A severely debilitated dog may not respond adequately to vaccination. The general state of nutrition should meet minimal recommended standards to insure that nutritional factors do not interfere with immune responsiveness. If a debilitated dog is vaccinated, vaccination should be repeated when the dog's general condition has improved in order to insure adequate immunity. Also, some caution should be exercised when using modified live viruses in a severely debilitated animal.

## CONCURRENT INFECTIONS

It is important to insure that animals presented for vaccination are not already incubating the disease. This possibility frequently motivates owners to present their animals for vaccination and may lead to so-called "vaccination breakdowns." A detailed history as to possibility of exposure to infected animals combined with a thorough physical examination should be performed in every case presented for vaccination in order to minimize this possibility.

Other diseases may also be associated with immunosuppression and may potentially interfere with successful vaccination. For example, the general state of T-cell suppression present in cases of generalized demodectic mange may interfere with the response to vaccination or, at worst, may contraindicate use of live attenuated vaccines. Likewise, dogs infected with distemper virus develop a generalized T-cell suppression four days after infection, and vaccination with other antigens during this period may result in an inadequate immune response.

## DRUG TREATMENTS

Vaccines should not be given concurrently with immunosuppressive drug treatment (e.g., cyclophosphamide, azathioprine, methotrexate, corticosteroids). Corticosteroid treatment at therapeutic levels does not appear to influence antibody responses to vaccine viruses. However, primary vaccination with modified live virus vaccine cannot be highly recommended in dogs on steroid therapy. Attenuated virus should be harmless in a normal host but may produce clinical disease in an immunologically compromised host.

# MINIMAL DISEASE PREVENTION

The following basic recommendations are based on the Panel Report of the Symposium on Immunity to Selected Canine Infectious Diseases, the Rabies Subcommit-

*Table 1.* Vaccination Schedule

| VACCINE | TYPE OF VACCINE | AGE TO VACCINATE |
|---|---|---|
| Canine Distemper Virus (CDV) and/or | Modified live virus | First vaccination at 6 to 8 weeks of age; second vaccination at 12 to 16 weeks; revaccinate annually. |
| Measles Virus (MV) | Modified live virus | Vaccinate at 6 weeks of age, then vaccinate with CDV vaccine at 12 to 16 weeks. Do not use in bitches of breeding age. |
| Infectious Canine Hepatitis (ICH or CAV-1) | Modified live virus or inactivated vaccine | Vaccination schedule is same as for CDV vaccine and is commonly given with CDV in a combined vaccine. |
| Canine Herpesvirus | None available | |
| Rabies Virus | Modified live virus | First vaccination at 3 to 4 months of age; revaccinate at 1 year and at least every 3 years thereafter; if dog is over 4 months of age at first vaccination, revaccinate in 1 year, then once every 3 years. |
| | Inactivated virus | First vaccination at 3 to 4 months; second vaccination in 3 to 4 weeks; revaccinate annually. |
| Canine Parainfluenza Virus (CPI) | Modified live virus | Manufacturer recommendation: Give as combined vaccine with canine distemper and infectious canine hepatitis vaccines. |
| Canine Leptospirosis | Killed bacteria (bacterin) | First vaccination at 9 weeks; revaccinate when administering second CDV-ICH vaccine. Revaccinate annually. |
| Canine Brucellosis | None available | |

tee, Animal Health Committee, National Research Council, National Academy of Science and on recent research reports.

## RABIES

Two types of rabies vaccines are available: modified live virus and inactivated virus.

Live virus vaccines are of chicken embryo origin or cell culture origin. It is recommended that the first vaccination be administered at 3 or 4 months of age, again at one year and then at least once every three years after the vaccination at one year. If the first vaccination occurs after 4 months of age, the second vaccination is given one year later and then again at least every three years.

Inactivated virus vaccine is available with and without adjuvant. It is required that this vaccine be given more frequently than modified live virus because of a more rapid decline in immunity. If the first vaccination is undertaken at 3 months of age or older, the second vaccination should follow in 3 to 4 weeks, and annual revaccination is required thereafter.

## CANINE DISTEMPER VIRUS (SEE ARTICLE ON "CANINE DISTEMPER")

Modified live virus vaccines of chicken embryo or cell culture origin are recommended. In pups of unknown immune status and more than 3 months old, one dose of modified live virus vaccine should be given. If younger than 3 months old when first presented, two or more doses should be administered; the first dose should be given at weaning and the last dose at 12 to 16 weeks of age. Vaccination at 2-week intervals during this critical time of diminishing maternally acquired immunity more nearly approaches the ideal method. Annual revaccination is recommended. It is suggested that pregnant bitches not be vaccinated. This suggestion is made as a result of our lack of information with regard to the possible side effects of the virus on the fetus and not from any results indicating that vaccine virus can damage the canine fetus.

Vaccines are available that incorporate other viral and/or bacterial antigens with the canine distemper component, providing the advantages of protection against the component antigens with one injection. These vaccines incorporate modified CAV-1, modified canine parainfluenza virus and leptospira bacterins in various combinations. The use of measles virus vaccines to provide protection against canine distemper is discussed below.

Passive immunization of pups using antiserum or concentrated antiserum is not recommended, since it will delay subsequent active immunization and would seem to have less merit in most cases than do multiple doses of attenuated live virus vaccine.

## MEASLES VIRUS

Measles virus (MV) has been used with a variable degree of success for more than 10 years to protect young puppies from canine distemper. When first introduced, measles vaccine was given alone as the first vaccine to puppies 4 weeks of age or older. Recently a combination of CD and MV has become available commercially, and the manufacturers recommend that it be used at 6 weeks of age. The manufacturers claim that this combination protects a higher percentage of animals against distemper than when measles virus is given alone. Although it was originally thought that canine distemper antibody received from the colostrum did not interfere with MV vaccination, we have recently found that high levels (approximate titers of 1:300 to 1:500) can interfere with measles vaccination. Measles vaccination is not as sensitive to the blocking effects of colostral CDV antibody as is CD vaccine virus, and it is unlikely that any puppy 6 weeks of age would have enough CDV antibody to interfere with measles vaccination. This is unlike vaccination with CDV at this age, in which case 50 per cent or more of the puppies do not respond to CDV vaccine.

Measles vaccine can be used successfully to protect dogs from developing *disease* with CDV but will not protect against *infection* with CDV. Measles vaccination should be considered a temporary method to prevent canine distemper until canine distemper vaccine can be effectively administered. There are no indications for use of vaccines containing measles antigen in dogs over 16 weeks of age, and their use is contraindicated in breeding bitches.

## INFECTIOUS CANINE HEPATITIS (CAV-1) (SEE ARTICLE ON "CANINE ADENOVIRUS INFECTION")

Immunizing agents include inactivated virus or modified live virus (MLV) vaccine. Inactivated vaccines are safe and effective; however, they do not provide the long-term immunity found with live virus vaccines. Vaccination with live virus vaccine is not without its problems, since a small percentage of dogs receiving MLV vaccine will develop uveitis and corneal edema (blue eye). Although certain vaccine manufacturers advertise that their vaccine does not cause uveitis, we are not aware that a strain of CAV-1 virus exists that does not cause uveitis in a small percentage of dogs.

We have found that CAV-1 vaccine virus will cause disease when inoculated into term fetuses (58 days of age). This does not imply that vaccination of the bitch would cause disease in the fetus, but it would suggest that vaccines with attenuated CAV-1 virus not be given to pregnant bitches until more is known of their possible effects on fetuses.

CAV-1 vaccine may be given in combination with other viral and bacterial vaccine antigens. The use of suitably attenuated CAV-2 as an alternative to vaccinal CAV-1 strains has been recommended to avoid the ocular and renal lesions associated with CAV-1 and to provide protection against systemic CAV-1 infection. However, CAV-2 vaccines are currently not available. The necessity for annual revaccination against CAV-1 is questionable.

## CANINE PARAINFLUENZA VIRUS (CPI)

A modified live CPI virus vaccine in combination with CDV, with CAV-1 and with or without leptospira bacterin has recently become available commercially. The role of canine parainfluenza virus as a primary cause of contagious respiratory disease in the dog is well established. In addition, secondary infections with other viruses, bacteria and mycoplasmas may complicate the disease. When contagious respiratory disease as a result of CPI infection is a problem among dogs, incorporation of attenuated CPI virus in the vaccination program is indicated.

Direct inoculation of term fetuses with CPI virus (wild type) resulted in puppies that were weak at birth and survived for variable periods of time up to 9 days of age. As with CAV-1, these results do not necessarily indicate that CPI virus would infect the fetus during natural infection or after vaccination of the bitch; however, the results do suggest that pregnant bitches not be vaccinated until further research concerning this possibility has been performed.

## CANINE LEPTOSPIROSIS

If leptospirosis is endemic, vaccination with appropriate bacterin should be considered. Vaccination is recommended when the pup is 9 weeks of age or older. The second dose is given two to three weeks later, and a third is recommended after a similar period of time or when the final dose of CDV and CAV-1 is given. For effective immunity, revaccination should occur at least annually.

Anaphylactoid reactions have occurred as a result of vaccination with this bacterin, and provisions to treat such a patient should be readily available when giving this vaccine.

## CANINE BRUCELLOSIS

A vaccine against this disease is not available at the moment. Studies are in progress to determine the feasibility of vaccination to prevent canine brucellosis (see article on "Canine Brucellosis"). Although dogs that are infected with *Brucella canis* eventually become immune, the period necessary for immunity to develop is measured in terms of months. Methods to reduce the time needed for the dog to develop protective immunity are being considered and tested.

# FELINE IMMUNIZATION

FREDRIC W. SCOTT, D.V.M.
*Ithaca, New York*

Most of the basic parameters of immunization and the basic immune response outlined in the previous article ("Canine Vaccines and Immunity" by Schultz *et al.*) hold true for the cat as well as for the dog. The type of vaccine used, the route of vaccination, the effect of maternal antibody derived from colostrum and the age of the cat vaccinated can affect the immune response (or lack of it) that may occur in the cat following vaccination.

## NATURE OF THE VACCINE

Both inactivated and modified live virus (MLV) vaccines are available. The MLV vaccines especially must be handled and stored according to the instructions provided by the manufacturer in order to maintain potency. MLV vaccines should not be administered to pregnant cats.

## ROUTE OF VACCINATION

The route by which the vaccine is administered may affect the degree of protection provided. Feline panleukopenia (FPL) vaccine can be given IM or SC with equal effect. The MLV-FPL vaccines can also be given by the intranasal or aerosol route, but they will not result in immunization if administered by the oral route.

Rabies vaccine must be given by the IM route. Although extensive studies on the route of rabies vaccination in the cat have not been reported, studies in the dog have shown that the IM route is at least 100 times more effective than the SC route. The same should hold true for the cat.

The MLV respiratory vaccines appear to be more effective by the IM route than by the SC route. Additional studies are needed to clarify this point. Aerosol vaccination with respiratory vaccines may result in mild signs of illness.

## AGE OF THE CAT

The most frequent cause of vaccine failure with FPL vaccines is interference because of maternally derived immunity. These cats become susceptible later, after the passive immunity wanes. The level and duration of passive immunity following nursing are determined by the antibody titer of the queen at parturition, assuming that the kitten nurses. Although the majority of cats can be successfully immunized at 9 to 10 weeks of age, occasional kittens may not be susceptible to vaccination until 12 weeks of age. Therefore, if FPL vaccines are given at ages less than 12 weeks, they should be repeated at 4-week intervals until the cat is at least 12 weeks old.

Little is known about maternal antibody interference in feline viral rhinotracheitis (FVR) and feline calicivirus (FCV) disease vaccines. The same principles of colostral transfer, antibody half-life and vaccine virus neutralization should apply to these viruses as apply to FPL. Therefore, we can predict that there will be interference if the maternal titers are high enough. Generally the FVR and FCV titers are much lower than the FPL titer, and therefore the duration of interference (and passive protection) would be much shorter. It is doubtful that this will be longer than 5 to 6 weeks for the FVR and 7 to 8 weeks for the FCV. By 9 to 10 weeks of age, the vast majority of cats should be susceptible to FVR and FCV vaccination.

## FELINE PANLEUKOPENIA VACCINES

There are numerous excellent vaccines available for immunization of the cat against panleukopenia (Scott and Gillespie, 1971). If these are used correctly and at the proper age, cats should be completely protected against this very severe viral infection. It behooves veterinarians to immunize as many cats as possible within their practices.

The various vaccines available are listed in Table 1.

Several slightly different programs for the immunization of cats against panleukopenia have been presented during the past few years. The safest recommendation is to start the immunization program at an early age and vaccinate the kittens at frequent inter-

*Table 1.* Types of Feline Panleukopenia Vaccines

| BRAND NAME | SUPPLIER'S NAME | MODIFIED LIVE VIRUS | KILLED VIRUS | ORIGIN | | | | | DOSAGE (CC.) | ROUTE OF ADMINISTRATION |
|---|---|---|---|---|---|---|---|---|---|---|
| | | | | Feline Cell Line | Feline Tissue Culture | Ferret Tissue Culture | Feline Tissue | Mink Tissue | | |
| Delpan® | Dellen | — | Yes | Yes | — | — | — | — | 1 | SC or IM |
| Deltab® | Dellen | Yes | — | Yes | — | — | — | — | 1 | SC or IM |
| FDV | Burns-Biotec | — | Yes | — | Yes | — | — | — | 1 | SC |
| Feline Distemper | Abbott | — | Yes | — | Yes | — | — | — | 2 | SC |
| Feline Panleukopenia | Haver-Lockhart | Yes | — | — | Yes | — | — | — | 1 | SC or IM |
| Felipan® | Jensen-Salsbery | — | Yes | — | Yes | — | — | — | 1 | SC |
| Felocell® | Norden | Yes | — | Yes | — | — | — | — | 1 | SC or IM |
| Felocine® | Norden | — | Yes | Yes | — | — | — | — | 1 | SC or IM |
| Fel-O-Vax® | Fort Dodge | — | Yes | — | — | — | Yes | — | 2 | SC |
| Fevac TC | Fromm | — | Yes | — | Yes | — | — | — | 1 | SC |
| Leukogen-TC® | BioCeutics | Yes | — | Yes | — | — | — | — | 1 | SC or IM |
| Leukoid TC | Fromm | Yes | — | — | Yes | — | — | — | 1 | SC or IM |
| MEV® | Biol. Specialties | — | Yes | — | — | — | — | Yes | 1 | SC or IM |
| Panacine®L | Affiliated | Yes* | — | — | — | Yes | — | — | 1 | SC or IM |
| Panagen® | Pitman-Moore | — | Yes | — | Yes | — | — | — | 1 | SC or IM |
| Panavac® | Affiliated | — | Yes | — | Yes | — | — | — | 1 | SC or IM |
| Panleukovac® | Diamond | Yes | — | — | Yes | — | — | — | 1 | SC or IM |

*Liquid vaccine—does not need to be reconstituted.

Courtesy of Feline Practice, March, 1976.

vals until they are at least 16 weeks of age. This might prove beneficial in certain circumstances, such as in catteries or in colonies where kittens could be vaccinated at 6 weeks of age, followed by repeated vaccinations at 2-week intervals until the cats are 16 weeks old. However, most kittens presented to the practitioner must be immunized with a maximum of two or possibly three vaccinations. Therefore, the clinician must attempt to immunize the maximum number of cats with a reasonable number of vaccinations per cat.

Most recommendations indicate that the kittens should be vaccinated starting at 8, 9 or 10 weeks of age. A single vaccination will immunize the cats if they are susceptible at the time of vaccination. If interference occurred at the time of the first vaccination, chances are much greater that the cat will be susceptible to vaccination 4 weeks later instead of 7 to 10 days later. If the first vaccination was successful, the increase in titer following the second vaccination will be comparable whether it is given at 4 weeks or at 2 weeks, if inactivated vaccines are used. For MLV vaccines, the second vaccination would have no effect in a previously immunized kitten, owing to the high titer.

In reviewing the different programs for immunization of cats, the Panel for the Colloquium on Selected Feline Infectious Diseases (1970) preferred a 2-week interval rather than a 4-week interval, since not as many cats would be returned for revaccination 4 weeks later. After evaluating all the available information, the Panel recommends that two doses of inactivated vaccine be given at 2-week intervals, starting at 9 to 10 weeks of age. For maximum protection, especially in areas of high concentration of street virus, a third vaccination is recommended at 16 weeks. For the modified live virus vaccines, the first dose should be administered at 9 to 10 weeks of age, followed by a second dose of vaccine between 14 and 16 weeks of age. If the cat is older than 12 weeks at the time of the first vaccination with MLV vaccine, a repeat vaccination is not indicated.

With the advent of the respiratory vaccines for which there is good evidence for revaccination at a 3- to 4-week interval instead of 2 weeks, and since one should try to immunize the maximum number of cats with the least number of office visits, it now seems advisable to recommend the 4-week interval between vaccinations as outlined in Table 8.

## FELINE VIRAL RHINOTRACHEITIS VACCINES

As listed in Tables 2, 3, 4 and 5, the available FVR vaccines may be obtained as a single vaccine, in combination with calicivirus vaccine with FPL, or as a triple FPL-FVR-FCV vaccine (Scott, 1976). The FVR vaccines produce significant protection following vaccination and, as such, should be part of the routine vaccination program, as outlined in Table 8. Vaccinated cats develop a rapid anamnestic response when exposed to virulent virus, and local viral replication occurs. Some vaccinated cats may sneeze, and an occasional one may have watery eyes for 1 to 2 days. Severe systemic disease does not occur as it does in unvaccinated cats.

## FELINE CALICIVIRUS VACCINE

Until recently it was thought that multiple serotypes of FCV existed, in which case an effective vaccine would not be possible. Recent studies have shown that there is a single serotype of FCV with multiple strains. At least certain strains (including the one used in the available FCV vaccine) exhibit good protection against other strains of FCV. The same parameters apply to FCV vaccines as to the FVR vaccines, i.e., route of vaccination, anamnestic response when challenged, and good clinical protection against virulent virus exposure (but not protection against local viral replication) (Scott, 1976). These vaccines are produced in combination with FVR vaccine (Tables 3 and 4). Recommendations for these vaccines are the same as for FVR (Table 8).

## FELINE PNEUMONITIS (FPN) VACCINE

Although FPN is not as prevalent as FVR or FCV disease, it is evident that in some cat populations a severe, chronic respiratory disease is produced by the FPN agent, a chlamydia. According to recent studies, the one vaccine currently available (Table 6) appears to produce significant protection following a single IM vaccination (Strating, 1976). As with other respiratory vaccines, complete protection is not afforded, but clinical signs, if they do occur, are restricted to a very short course and are mild and local.

## Table 2.   *Types of Feline Viral Rhinotracheitis Vaccines*

| BRAND NAME | SUPPLIER'S NAME | MODIFIED LIVE | ORIGIN | DOSAGE (ML.) | ROUTE OF ADMINISTRATION |
|---|---|---|---|---|---|
| FVR® Vaccine | Pitman-Moore | Virus | Feline cell line | 1 | IM |
| Rhinocine | Affiliated | Virus | Cell culture | 1 | IM or SC |
| Rhinoid-TC® | Fromm | Virus | Feline tissue culture | 1 | IM |

Modified from Feline Practice, March, 1976.

## Table 3.   *Types of Feline Viral Rhinotracheitis-Calici Vaccines*

| BRAND NAME | SUPPLIER'S NAME | MODIFIED LIVE | ORIGIN | DOSAGE (ML.) | ROUTE OF ADMINISTRATION |
|---|---|---|---|---|---|
| Felomune-CVR® | Norden | Viruses | Cell culture | 0.5 | IN |
| FVR®-C | Pitman-Moore | Viruses | Cell culture | 1.0 | IM |

Modified from Feline Practice, March, 1976.

## Table 4.   *Types of Feline Viral Rhinotracheitis-Calici-Panleukopenia Vaccines*

| BRAND NAME | SUPPLIER'S NAME | MODIFIED LIVE | ORIGIN | DOSAGE (ML.) | ROUTE OF ADMINISTRATION |
|---|---|---|---|---|---|
| FVR® C-P | Pitman-Moore | Viruses* | Feline cell line and tissue culture | 1 | IM |

Courtesy of Feline Practice, March, 1976.
*FPL component inactivated.

## Table 5.   *Types of Feline Viral Rhinotracheitis-Panleukopenia Vaccines*

| BRAND NAME | SUPPLIER'S NAME | MODIFIED LIVE | ORIGIN | DOSAGE (ML.) | ROUTE OF ADMINISTRATION |
|---|---|---|---|---|---|
| Rhinocine-P | Affiliated | Yes* | Cell culture | 1 | IM or SC |
| Rhinocine-PL | Affiliated | Yes | Cell culture | 1 | IM or SC |

Modified from Feline Practice, March, 1976.
*FPL component inactivated.

## Table 6.   *Types of Feline Pneumonitis Vaccines*

| BRAND NAME | SUPPLIER'S NAME | MODIFIED LIVE | ORIGIN | DOSAGE (CC.) | ROUTE OF ADMINISTRATION |
|---|---|---|---|---|---|
| Pneumonitis | Fromm | Chlamydia | Chick embryo | 1 | SC or IM |

Courtesy of Feline Practice, March, 1976.

*Table 7.* *Types of Feline Rabies Vaccines*

| BRAND NAME | SUPPLIER'S NAME | MODIFIED LIVE VIRUS | KILLED VIRUS | ORIGIN | | | | DOSAGE (ML.) | ROUTE OF ADMINISTRATION |
|---|---|---|---|---|---|---|---|---|---|
| | | | | Canine Cell Line | Porcine Tissue Culture | Murine Tissue | Caprine Tissue | | |
| Endurall-R® | Norden | Yes | — | Yes | — | — | — | 1 | IM |
| Monorab® | Jensen-Salsbery | — | Yes | — | — | — | Yes | 2 | IM |
| SAD (ERA) Strain® | Jensen-Salsbery | Yes | — | — | Yes | — | — | 1 | IM |
| Trimune® | Fort Dodge | — | Yes | — | — | Yes | — | 1 | IM |

Courtesy of Feline Practice, March, 1976.

*Table 8.* *Feline Vaccine Recommendations*

| VACCINE | TYPE OF VACCINE | AGE AT FIRST VACCINATION (WEEKS) | AGE AT SECOND VACCINATION (WEEKS) | REVACCINATION | ROUTE OF ADMINISTRATION |
|---|---|---|---|---|---|
| Panleukopenia (FPL) | (1) Inactivated | 8 | 12 | Annual | SC or IM |
| | (2) MLV* | 8 | 12 | Annual | SC or IM |
| Viral Rhinotracheitis (FVR) | MLV | 8 (or earlier) | 12 | Annual | IM |
| Caliciviral Disease (FCV) | MLV | 8 (or earlier) | 12 | Annual | IM |
| Pneumonitis | MLV | 8 | — | Annual | SC or IM |
| Rabies | (1) Inactivated | 12 | — | Annual | IM |
| | (2) MLV | 12 | — | Annual | IM |

*Modified live virus.

Chronic disease (characteristic of natural infection in susceptible cats) apparently does not occur in vaccinated cats.

Although there are many basic parameters concerning immunity to FPN that are not known, it appears that if FPN is a problem in a particular area, the FPN vaccine should be part of the routine vaccination program. The age at which to vaccinate is not critical, since there appears to be little interference with maternal antibody by the time kittens would normally be old enough to be vaccinated. A single injection appears to afford adequate protection.

## RABIES VACCINES

The available rabies vaccines are listed in Table 7. The latest rabies vaccine recommendations are included in the 1976 Compendium of Animal Rabies Vaccines in the article on "Rabies" (page 1298).

### SUPPLEMENTAL READING

1976–77 Pratitioner's Guide to Feline Vaccines and Serums. Feline Pract., March, 1976, pp. 23–30.
Report of the Panel for the Colloquium on Selected Feline Infectious Diseases. J. Am. Vet. Med. Assn., *158*:835–843, 1971.
Scott, F. W.: Evaluation of an experimental vaccine against feline viral rhinotracheitis and feline calicivirus disease. Am. J. Vet. Res., in press, 1977.
Scott, F. W., and Gillespie, J. H.: Immunization for feline panleukopenia. Vet. Clin. N. Am., *1*:231–240, 1971.
Mitzel, J. R., and Strating, A.: Evaluation of a feline chlamydial pneumonitis vaccine in cats. Proc. Am. Soc. Microbiol., *76*:72, 1976.

# FELINE RESPIRATORY DISEASE COMPLEX

R. CHARLES POVEY, M.R.C.V.S.
*Guelph, Ontario*

The recent advent of vaccines for the protection of cats against the most significant of the agents responsible for the feline respiratory disease complex, namely, feline viral rhinotracheitis (FVR) virus and feline caliciviruses (FCV), has provided a new impetus to our interest in this complex. The availability of these vaccines should not obviate further research in this area, particularly in terms of the relationships between the infectious agents and other factors in this disease, the immune response in all its aspects and the epidemiology, especially the phenomenon of persistent "carrier" infections.

## ETIOLOGY

To assume that all the infectious agents responsible for respiratory disease in the cat have now been isolated would be a premature judgment. For instance, it is surprising that there is no feline adenovirus. It is clear, however, that the major part of the complex is induced by just two agents: feline viral rhinotracheitis (FVR) virus, also referred to as feline herpes virus I, and feline caliciviruses (FCV), formerly known as feline picornaviruses. The role of the chlamydial organism of feline pneumonitis is now thought to be of minor importance. Feline reoviruses have been isolated from the upper respiratory tract and experimentally produce mild signs, mainly conjunctivitis, but the practical importance of these viruses dose not appear to be great. A syncytium-forming virus has been cultured from cats with respiratory infections but does not produce disease experimentally. Some workers have advocated a primary role for mycoplasms, but this has not been confirmed experimentally. The roles of other bacteria such as *Pasteurella multocida, Bordetella bronchiseptica, Staphylococcus pyogenes* and *Streptococcus pyogenes* need to be evaluated with regard to their potential primary and secondary effects.

## EPIDEMIOLOGY

This complex is found worldwide and is usually endemic where cats are congregated in groups, e.g., breeding colonies, laboratory animal houses and boarding catteries. The source of the infection can be clinically ill animals, subclinically infected or reinfected cats, or persistently infected carriers. All three of these situations have occurred with both FVR and FCV infections.

Cats with clinical illness shed these viruses in ocular, nasal and oral discharges and, in the case of FCV, often feces, for periods of 1 to 3 weeks. Subclinical infections are seen with many strains of FCV that are of low pathogenicity, and subclinical reinfections in partially immune cats occur with FVR and FCV. In these latter cases, viral replication and shedding occur but usually for only one to several days.

In the carrier situation, there is a clear distinction between the behavior of FVR and FCV infections. With FVR, the virus becomes truly hidden, or latent, within as yet undefined cells, possibly in nerve ganglia, a site which is protected against the cat's immune system. Then from time to time there are replication and liberation of infectious virus from the sites of latency to be shed in ocular, nasal or oral discharges. Such sheddings not only have been experimentally induced by corticosteroid administration in some 80 per cent of cats that have clinically recovered from FVR but also have been shown to be associated with natural stress situations such as hospitalization, boarding and peak lactation. There is a lag period of approximately one week between the onset of the stress, natural or artificial, and the detection of reexcreted virus. This virus may be found in ocular, nasal or oropharyngeal secretions or in all three. The episode of shedding lasts from one to several days and then ceases for a period of weeks or months until it recurs. These reexcretions of FVR can occur without producing clinical signs, but often there are mild signs such as unilateral ocular discharge. Occasionally overt clinical disease is seen, particularly under corticosteroid stress. Although most cats that have experienced FVR infection remain chronically infected with the virus, it is believed that in all but a small proportion (perhaps only 10 per cent) there is no shedding under natural circumstances. Thus, only this 10 per cent should be considered epidemiologically important carriers.

Feline calicivirus carriers are both persistently infected with and continuous shedders of virus. The virus persists in predominantly epithelial locations, particularly of the tonsillar region despite moderate or high circulating antibody levels. The factors influencing development of the FCV carrier state are not known; however, the strain of virus as well as the immunologic competency of the cat is probably significant. Shedding by carriers can persist for a year or longer, but in many cases there is a sudden and permanent cessation of virus release, suggesting a change in either the virus or the host immune system. FCV carriers are generally free of clinical signs. Although many such cats are found to have chronic or recurrent gingivitis, a direct association with the FCV infection has not been proved.

Evidence is accumulating to suggest that transmission of the respiratory viruses occurs mainly via direct contact between a shedding and a recipient cat and that there is relatively little aerosol transmission, over distances of more than a few feet. The major risk in terms of indirect transmission comes from the hands of attendants, including owners, show judges or veterinarians. In the external environment, the herpesvirus of FVR is fragile, surviving less than 18 hours even under favorable conditions; FCV's, however, may survive for 8 to 10 days and apparently are quite resistant to the usual disinfectants.

Cats of all ages are susceptible, but newly weaned kittens are most severely affected. The incidence of antibodies in the population increases markedly with age.

## CLINICAL SIGNS

Ocular and nasal discharges accompanied by sneezing, a temperature of 40° C. (104° F.) or above, reduced appetite or anorexia and depression are the classic signs, but many variations are encountered, owing to differences in resistance of the cats, either in specific immunologic terms or in nonspecific ways such as general health, environment and nutrition. There are clinical pointers, however, which allow a reasonable degree of accuracy in differentiation of the etiologic agents, particularly FVR and

FCV. As mentioned before, these account for some 80 per cent of the cases, both occurring with similar frequency. Dual infections can also occur.

**Ocular Signs.** FVR is the most severe of the respiratory diseases, typically showing all the classic features referred to above and often including a pronounced conjunctivitis. Initial blepharospasm and epiphora progress to chemosis and profuse ocular discharge. In some cases there is corneal involvement with ulcerative keratitis even to the extent of descemetocele formation. FCV's show generally less ocular involvement, usually no more than epiphora and, very seldom, corneal involvement. Similarly, feline reovirus infection (FRI) is typically associated with lacrimation, photophobia and serous conjunctivitis. Chlamydia ("pneumonitis agent") conjunctivitis may be unilateral initially, spreading to the opposite eye within 5 to 7 days. The discharge rapidly becomes purulent, and without treatment the disease can become chronic, involving persistent conjunctival hyperemia with hyperplasia and follicle formation. There is little evidence that mycoplasms produce a primary conjunctivitis, but they have been associated with an initially unilateral serous to mucopurulent ocular exudate with less marked hyperemic changes. Bacterial activity secondary to a viral conjunctivitis produces purulent exudate with adhesion of the eyelids but often without chemosis or hyperemia of the conjunctiva.

**Nasal Signs.** Both FVR and FCV can produce sneezing with nasal discharge, which occurs with more regularity and severity in FVR. Reovirus and chlamydia are seldom associated with sneezing. Purulent nasal discharges indicate secondary bacterial activity. Ulceration of the external nares with hemorrhage is sometimes a feature of FCV infections. FVR in young kittens can cause osteodystrophy of the turbinate bones, and a major clinical problem is chronic or recurrent rhinitis or sinusitis in the cat that has recovered from FVR.

**Oral Signs.** The trademark of FCV infection is the large vesicle that rapidly ulcerates on the rostral dorsal margin of the tongue. Less common are multiple tongue ulcers or symmetrical erosions of the hard palate. As mentioned earlier, chronic gingivitis can be associated with FCV carriers, as can persistent pharyngitis, often with lymphoid hyperplasia, although no direct causal effect has been shown. FVR can also cause lingual ulceration, but the ulcers are typically several and small. In severe cases of FVR, multiple vesicles have been seen, particularly in the pharynx and occasionally extending even into the esophagus. Drooling of saliva can occur with FVR in the absence of any apparent oral lesion, although this might result from failure to swallow rather than from increased production of saliva.

**Tracheal Signs.** The tracheitis associated with FVR can result in a harsh, retching cough that is not a feature of the other respiratory infections.

**Pneumonic Signs.** Both FVR and FCV have been shown experimentally and naturally to be capable of producing primary pneumonia; indeed, interstitial pneumonitis is a frequent finding in experimental FCV infections and has been associated with sudden death in young kittens. Such primary pneumonias often go undetected clinically until a bacterial bronchopneumonia is superimposed. Chlamydia, reovirus and mycoplasms seldom, if ever, produce pneumonia in cats.

**Urogenital Signs.** Experimentally, FVR can produce genital lesions and abortion in queens in which the virus is directly implicated. Despite the fact that abortion is a frequent sequel to natural FVR infection in the pregnant cat, the virus has not been isolated from either genital tract or aborted material in such cases. FCV can be excreted in urine, and one isolate (Manx strain) has been associated equivocally with the feline urologic syndrome.

**Nervous Signs.** Rarely, FVR is associated with signs of generalized encephalitis, particularly in immunologically compromised, aged or terminally ill cats.

**Skin Signs.** There have been rare reports of skin ulceration with FVR infection and of paw erosions with FCV.

## DIAGNOSIS

The presence of the aforementioned clinical signs makes it possible for an etiologic diagnosis to be right more often than wrong. Supportive evidence can be obtained by examining conjunctival smears for the intracytoplasmic elementary bodies of *Chlamydia*, and on occasion intranuclear inclusions can be found with FVR.

*Table 1.  Characteristics of Upper Respiratory Infection of Cats*

| | RHINOTRACHEITIS (FVR) | CALICIVIRAL DISEASE (FCV) | REOVIRUS INFECTION (FRI) | PNEUMONITIS (FPN) | MYCOPLASMA AND OTHER INFECTIONS |
|---|---|---|---|---|---|
| Agent | Feline herpesvirus I | Feline caliciviruses (picornaviruses) numerous strains | Reovirus | Chlamydia psittaci (Miyagawanella felis; Bedsonia felis) | Mycoplasma spp., Staph. pyogenes, Strep. pyogenes, P. multocida, B. bronchiseptica and others |
| Inclusions | Intranuclear inclusions in respiratory epithelial cells, conjunctiva, etc. | None | Paranuclear cytoplasmic | Intracytoplasmic elementary bodies in conjunctival epithelial cells | None |
| Other hosts | None known | None known | None known | Mouse, hamster, guinea pig, rabbit | Some species specificity |
| Incubation (natural infection) | 2–10 days | 1–9 days | 4–19 days | 6–15 days | Usually secondary |
| Signs: Severity | Regularly more severe | Mild to moderate; subclinical infections common | Mild | Mild | Subclinical infections common |
| Ocular | Lacrimation, conjunctivitis, chemosis, occasionally keratitis | Lacrimation, sometimes conjunctivitis | Lacrimation | Conjunctivitis can be follicular | Conjunctivitis |
| Nasal | Serous or mucopurulent discharge, sneezing | Serous discharge, occasional sneezing; ulceration of external nares | Nasal discharge rare | Nasal discharge rare | None or purulent |

| | | | | | |
|---|---|---|---|---|---|
| Oral | Occasional small vesicles and ulcers in buccal epithelium | Frequent ulceration on anterior dorsal margin of tongue *and* hard palate, gingivitis | None | None | None |
| Other | Coughing, abortion, skin ulcers, CNS signs | Paw erosions | None | None | None |
| Course | 2–4 weeks | 7–10 days | 1–26 days | Often chronic or recurrent | May be chronic |
| Morbidity | High | High | 50 per cent | Variable | Variable |
| Mortality | High in kittens, aged or immunodepressed | Variable; may be moderate in young kittens | Very low | Very low | Very low |
| Carrier state | Latent phase with periodic excretion after stress | Continuous shedding until self-clearance | Probable | Yes | Yes |
| Immunity | Initially low and transient; can be boosted and become persistent | Some strains produce broad cross-protection clinically but allow reduced viral multiplication | Unknown | Weak, transient | Weak, transient |
| Maternal antibody | <9 weeks | <11 weeks | Unknown | Unknown | Unknown |
| Diagnosis | Demonstration of intranuclear inclusions in early conjunctival smears; tissue culture isolation; FA test | Tissue culture isolation, FA test | Tissue culture isolation, SN test, HA test | Conjunctival smears Giemsa-stained to show elementary bodies; CF test | Culture |
| Treatment | Symptomatic, supportive with antibiotics | Symptomatic, supportive with antibiotics | Symptomatic | Tetracyclines locally and systemically | Antibiotics |
| Prophylaxis | Live modified vaccine | Live modified vaccine | None | Live modified vaccine | None |

Modified from Panel Report, Colloquium on Feline Diseases. J. Am. Vet. Med. Assn., *158*:838–839, 1971.

Confirmation of FVR and FCV (which occasionally are present in combined infections) is best obtained by submitting a vigorously taken swab of the tonsillar region to a virology laboratory, making sure that the swab is transported in a fluid medium that is preferably buffered and that contains antibiotics. Both viruses grow readily in tissue culture within 24 to 48 hours.

## TREATMENT

In the absence of any thorough clinical trial of antiviral compounds, treatment should be as follows:

1. Clear airways by means of steam vaporizer, phenylephrine HC1 or mucolytic agents (e.g., Alevaire® [Breon]) given by nebulizer.

2. Counteract dehydration with lactated Ringer's solution subcutaneously or intraperitoneally (except in severe cases, when it should be given intravenously) or 5 per cent dextrose in 0.85 per cent saline at up to 60 ml./kg. body weight.

3. Combat bacteria with antibiotics such as ampicillin at 50 mg./kg./day for kittens for at least 5 days in 4 divided doses and chloramphenicol at 75 mg./kg./day for adults for no longer than 7 days in 3 divided doses.

4. Encourage healing and appetite with vitamins A (5000 I.U. daily for 10 days), B (particularly $B_{12}$ at 100 $\mu$g. daily) and C (up to 1 gram daily). Semiforce-feeding with raw liver strips in milk or baby foods is also helpful. Nursing should be conscientious.

## PROGNOSIS

In parallel with the immune response, recovery normally begins between 7 and 10 days after the onset of illness and proceeds rapidly in the absence of bacterial complications. In some animals the immune response is suppressed, typified by the severely depressed, rapidly dehydrating and debilitating FVR cases seen most often in purebred cats. In these cases, and in young kittens, the prognosis should be guarded. A number of cats that recover from acute upper respiratory disease are afflicted with chronic or recurrent rhinitis and occasionally sinusitis. The prognosis for permanent cure of these cases is poor. Sinus drainage, rhinectomy, antibiotics and autogenous bacterins provide only temporary remittance.

## PROPHYLAXIS

Chlamydial (pneumonitis) vaccine has been available for many years, but recently vaccines for the protection of cats against FVR and FCV disease have become available. In North America these are live modified virus vaccines marketed either as FVR alone or as FVR in combination with calicivirus and/or panleukopenia.* These vaccines are for intramuscular or intranasal administration. The intranasal vaccination is given as a single dose. For the intramuscular vaccines, two doses are recommended, at 9 and 12 or 12 and 15 weeks. Revaccination is recommended at 6 months to 1 year.

The development of these vaccines followed a reappraisal of two misconceptions concerning immunity to these diseases. First, immunity, in terms of clinical protection to challenge exposure, is much longer in duration with both FVR and FCV than was previously thought. Even with apparently low or undetectable antibody levels, there is rapid anamnestic response with boosting or antibody on challenge, which modifies the infection and makes it subclinical or at least milder than that following a primary exposure. Booster vaccinations should be given annually or prior to any special risk situation, such as boarding or hospitalization. Second, there have been many isolates of FCV, most of which vary somewhat in their antigenic make-up. However, it has been shown very recently that the relationship among virtually all the strains so far tested is sufficient to provide reasonable cross-protection.

Faced with an outbreak of feline respiratory disease or an endemic situation in a cattery, certain useful measures can be adopted. First, cats should be segregated into the smallest groups practicable, preferably individually, with solid partitions between cats or groups to prevent their direct contact. It is particularly important to separate kittens, who will be losing any maternal antibody from age 6 weeks onward, from

---

*FVR®-Vaccine, FVR®-C Vaccine and FVR®-P Vaccine, Pitman-Moore, Inc., Washington's Crossing, New Jersey 08560.

Felomune-CVR®, Norden Laboratories, Lincoln, Nebraska 68501.

Rhinoid-TC®, Fromm Laboratories, Grafton, Wisconsin.

adults, who may be carriers. Second, there is evidence that airborne transmission of FVR and FCV is not the most important route of spread and that it occurs only over a short distance, whereas indirect spread by means of fomites, particularly the hands of attendants, is important. Thus, a simple precaution is to disinfect the hands thor-oughly before handling each cat or, prefera-bly, to wear rubber gloves.

## SUPPLEMENTAL READING

Crandell, R. A.: Feline viral rhinotracheitis (FVR). Adv. Vet. Sci. Comp. Med., *17*:201–224, 1973.
Gillespie, J. H., and Scott, F. W.: Feline viral infec-tions. Adv. Vet. Sci. Comp. Med., *17*:163–200, 1973.

# CANINE RESPIRATORY DISEASE COMPLEX

MAX APPEL, D.V.M.
*and* DAVID BEMIS, Ph.D.
*Ithaca, New York*

Infectious respiratory disease in dogs that is not related to canine distemper is usually referred to as "kennel cough." This is a very common condition in dogs in any type of kennel or veterinary hospital or wherever dogs are housed together. Two main types of this clinical disease appear to be com-mon: One is a form of tracheobronchitis, with a dry cough but without pyrexia or anorexia. It is seen in dogs with a docu-mented history of vaccination against canine distemper and infectious canine hepatitis and is often seen in veterinary hospitals. It will be referred to in this article as the mild type of the canine respiratory syndrome. It occurs most often in the fall but can occur during any month of the year. Dogs can contract this condition year after year; however, if they are boarded in the same kennel more frequently during the year, they often become immune. The sec-ond clinical syndrome (severe type) in-cludes a productive cough and sometimes pyrexia, anorexia and bronchopneumonia in addition to tracheobronchitis. It is more common in pups in pet shops, in pound dogs and in SPCA dogs. It also occurs in veterinary hospitals and is not related to vaccination. The infectious respiratory dis-ease complex of dogs includes canine dis-temper, which will be only briefly men-tioned here, since it is described in an arti-cle later in this section.

## ETIOLOGY

Several viruses as well as mycoplasma and bacteria have been isolated from dogs with contagious respiratory disease.

1. *Canine distemper virus.* In pups with the severe respiratory syndrome, canine distemper virus is not uncommon, but in many cases is not present. In dogs with the mild syndrome, distemper is not involved.

2. *Simian virus 5 (SV$_5$)—a parainfluenza virus.* This virus is very common in both types of respiratory disease. In contrast to canine distemper virus, which causes a generalized virus infection, SV$_5$ infects only the surface epithelium of the upper and lower respiratory tract. Viremia and spread of virus to other organs is restricted by mac-rophages. The infection produces airborne virions and consequently spreads rapidly from dog to dog; after parenteral inocula-tion, it does not spread to the respiratory tract.

3. *Canine adenovirus type 2 (CAV-2).* CAV-2 is seen mostly in the severe type of respiratory syndrome and was originally designated Toronto A-26/61. It has been re-ferred to as infectious canine laryngo-tracheitis (ICL) virus. It is closely related serologically to canine adenovirus 1 (CAV-1), which causes infectious canine hepatitis (ICH). These viruses differ greatly in their pathogenicity. While CAV-1 causes a gen-

eralized disease, CAV-2 causes only local infection of the respiratory tract. Unlike CAV-1, CAV-2 does not replicate in endothelial cells and therefore does not produce ocular and renal lesions. CAV-2 has repeatedly been isolated from dogs with respiratory diseases, and respiratory disease has been produced with this virus in susceptible dogs. The virus alone produces a very mild disease, while complications with mycoplasma and bacteria cause a more severe tracheobronchitis. Like SV$_5$, replication of CAV-2 is restricted to the epithelium of the upper and lower respiratory tract. The virus spreads rapidly from dog to dog.

4. *Canine herpesvirus (CHV)*. In a few reports, canine herpesvirus has been recovered from dogs with respiratory disease, and some lung lesions have been reproduced experimentally in dogs older than 3 weeks of age. The role of canine herpesvirus in neonatal death of puppies is well documented. However, most investigators agree that canine herpesvirus does not play a significant role in respiratory diseases of dogs.

5. *Reovirus*. The role of reovirus type I in kennel cough appears to be similar to that of CHV. Reovirus I has been isolated from two dogs with pneumonia in which CDV was not ruled out. Mild lung lesions were found after experimental exposure; however, in all investigated outbreaks of the canine respiratory syndrome, the virus was not isolated and an increase in antibody titer was not found. Antibody to reovirus type III has been reported.

6. *Mycoplasma*. Dogs with or without respiratory disease are commonly infected with mycoplasma. It can be isolated from dogs with both types of the respiratory syndrome. Although mycoplasma infections increase the severity of viral respiratory infections in dogs, the induction of respiratory disease with mycoplasma alone has not been accomplished. In a recently investigated outbreak of kennel cough, SV$_5$ and mycoplasma were isolated from dogs with bronchopneumonia, pyrexia, anorexia and productive cough. These dogs were immune to CDV, CAV-1 and CAV-2 and were free of *Bordetella bronchiseptica*.

7. *Bacteria*. Although many bacterial organisms can be isolated from the nasopharynx of dogs, only *B. bronchiseptica* appears to play a major role in the canine respiratory disease syndrome of both types.

Until recently, it was believed that *B. bronchiseptica* was involved in the disease complex only secondarily to viral infection; however, it has now been determined that Bordetella alone does cause respiratory disease. If dogs are aerosolized with a mixture of organisms like *Streptococcus*, *Pasteurella*, *Staphylococcus* and *Bordetella* in equal doses, only *B. bronchiseptica* remains in the trachea and bronchial tree; the other organisms are cleared within 24 hours. Bordetella specifically attaches to the cilia of the bronchi and trachea and persists there for approximately three months. During this period of time bacterial titers gradually decrease. Cough is prevalent only in the early phase, with bacterial replications to high titers.

## EPIDEMIOLOGY

The epidemiology of canine distemper is discussed in that article.

*Parainfluenza (SV$_5$)* has a wide host range, including man, monkeys and rodents. It frequently has been recognized as a latent virus in cell cultures of monkey kidneys. Since SV$_5$ could be found only in monkeys that had contact with men, it was originally considered to be a human virus. Strain differences have been found between human and dog isolates. Whether there is transmission from dog to man, or vice versa, is not known. Infection along with signs of respiratory disease was experimentally produced in mice of all ages with a human isolate. Cats also were found to be susceptible to SV$_5$, and the virus has been isolated from cats with respiratory disease in a veterinary hospital. Cat-to-dog transmission and vice versa must be assumed. Rapid dog-to-dog transmission probably maintains the infection in a kennel, especially when new dogs are added continually. After exposure, dogs shed virus in respiratory secretions for only 8 or 9 days. The highest incidence of the mild type of the respiratory syndrome occurs in the fall, and it is not known whether the incidence of SV$_5$ infection is highest during this period or whether clinical signs are precipitated by weather conditions. Parainfluenza infections in humans follow a similar pattern. In pet shops, SV$_5$ can be isolated from diseased pups at any time of the year. Dogs in any age range not previously infected or vaccinated are susceptible to this virus. In a serum survey, approximately 30 per cent of dogs in the United States were found to have neutralizing antibody to $SV_5$. $SV_5$ was encountered in approximately 50 per cent of the kennel cough outbreaks investigated.

*CAV-2* is a virus very commonly found in young city pups and in pups in pet shops. This virus spreads rapidly from dog to dog, like $SV_5$, but transmission of this virus to other species has not been documented. A seasonal prevalence of this virus has not been found, because pups are constantly added to pet shops and litters of pups being born throughout the year maintain transmission of virus to susceptible pups in dense dog populations in cities. As with $SV_5$, CAV-2 is shed from infected dogs for only 8 or 9 days. Thereafter the virus becomes latent and can be isolated only by means of special procedures. CAV-2 was not found in CAV-1-vaccinated older dogs with kennel cough contracted in kennels or veterinary hospitals.

*Canine herpesvirus* appears to be restricted to the canine species. Although susceptible dogs of any age can become infected and then spread virus, transmission from dog to dog in kennels does not occur as frequently as with $SV_5$ and CAV-2. As with other herpesviruses, some carrier dogs may spread virus from time to time. Virus isolation attempts from most dogs are negative, although any dog infected with herpesvirus has become infected for its lifetime. If newborn pups from susceptible bitches become infected with this virus, mortality rates are very high. Conversely, pups 2 weeks of age or older usually do not show any clinical signs after being infected with this virus. They spread virus for approximately 10 days.

*Reovirus type I* has an extremely wide host range. Infected dogs shed virus for only several days and become immune to reinfection. The few reports of reovirus in canine respiratory disease do not elucidate the mode of transmission.

*Mycoplasma* is known to be present in many dogs with respiratory disease, but noncoughing dogs carry mycoplasma too. Once infected, a dog can spread mycoplasma for at least several weeks. The canine mycoplasma isolates appear to be species specific. Transmission from dog to dog occurs rapidly. In a survey made in young city dogs, over 80 per cent of all dogs were infected with mycoplasma.

The only species of *bacteria* known to contribute significantly to the respiratory disease problem is *B. bronchiseptica*. *B. bronchiseptica* is very common in rabbits and guinea pigs. It is pathogenic in pigs and has been isolated from other species, including man. A species specificity does not seem to exist, and the strains from different species cannot be separated serologically. Bordetella is potentially pathogenic for cats as well. Transmission, therefore, can occur from dog to dog as well as from many species to dogs, and vice versa. The number of organisms in the bronchial tree appears to be related to the observance of clinical disease. The mild type of the canine respiratory syndrome can be caused by *B. bronchiseptica* alone. In combination with one or more of the previously mentioned viruses, the disease syndrome may be more severe. Because *B. bronchiseptica* is shed by dogs for at least two months, the organism is probably consistently present in kennels. It survives for extended periods of time outside the host. A seasonal prevalence has not been found.

## CLINICAL SIGNS

The mild type of the canine respiratory syndrome is a type of tracheobronchitis, usually of a self-limiting nature. A dry, harsh, hacking cough is the most common sign. It may be followed by retching motions and sometimes vomiting. Partial obstruction of the air passages can cause harsh bronchovesicular sounds or dry rales. Palpation of the larynx or trachea may enhance coughing. Radiographic examination is usually normal in these cases. The clinical course of this syndrome usually ranges from one to three weeks. In some cases, pneumonitis or a more severe bronchopneumonia may follow the mild disease.

The severe type of the canine respiratory syndrome is of a different nature. Signs of depression, anorexia and elevated body temperature often accompany this condition. Rhinitis and conjunctivitis, which may be serous or mucopurulent, may or may not be seen. Tonsillitis is not uncommon. Coughing appears to be painful, and dogs may consequently be reluctant to cough. The cough is often productive. Severe bronchopneumonias are more often involved, and a low fatality rate is usually encountered in young pups. This type of disease is more severe because several agents are usually involved. In addition to SV₅, mycoplasma and *B. bronchiseptica* (which are seen in the mild form of canine respiratory syndrome), CAV-2 and sometimes distemper are involved in dogs in pet shops, SPCA kennels and pounds or in dogs kept under similar conditions. Respiratory signs may persist from one week to several weeks in surviving pups. Lesions eventually clear, although there may be persistent lesions in the lungs, owing to CAV-2, which causes proliferation of bronchial epithelium. *B. bronchiseptica* may persist for three months, but with few exceptions, lungs and respiratory tracts will be healed three months after exposure.

## DIAGNOSIS

Because virtually all acute contagious respiratory diseases in dogs that are not caused by distemper are called "kennel cough," the diagnosis is made according to clinical signs. If only a mild tracheobronchitis is involved, single agents like SV₅, CAV-2, *B. bronchiseptica* or mycoplasma may be present. In more severe cases, a mixture of agents may be expected. Pathognomonic signs for any single agent are not known. A differential diagnosis between agents involved can be made only by virus, mycoplasma or bacteria insolation, or by paired serum samples at the time of acute disease and again three weeks afterward. Virus isolations can be made in a variety of tissue cultures. Cytopathic effects, fluorescent antibody staining and serum neutralization tests are generally used to identify the virus involved. Mycoplasma and bacterial isolations should be made from the trachea or bronchi, because pharyngeal isolates may not be related to the disease. Besides, *B. bronchiseptica* is difficult to isolate from the pharynx. Sterile tracheal swabs taken at the time of bronchoscopic examination are suitable. Bronchial washings or tracheal aspirations can be used for such samples. Contamination from pharyngeal or tonsillar crypts should be avoided. Hematologic examination is very useful in order to rule out distemper. None of the other agents involved in the canine infectious respiratory syndrome produces any significant change in hematologic findings.

Respiratory diseases not caused by infectious agents would be ruled out. The infectious and contagious nature of the canine respiratory syndrome is usually evident in kennels. Single dogs with this condition presented to veterinarians usually have a history of boarding in a kennel or contact with other dogs with respiratory disease.

## TREATMENT

Elimination of the causative agent in canine respiratory disease is most desirable. Unfortunately, known antiviral drugs at present are not effective against the listed viruses. Mycoplasma and bacteria can be treated with antibiotics, although different isolates may be sensitive to different antibiotics. Antibiotics commonly used in the field are erythromycin, chloramphenicol, ampicillin, tetracycline, tylosin, kanamycin and gentamicin. In a recent study it was found that oral or parenteral inoculation of these antibiotics had no effect against *B. bronchiseptica* in the bronchial tree. The listed antibiotics were tested in dogs for three days, treatments were made every 12 hours and the doses ranged from 1½ to 3 times the recommended daily dose for dogs (see Kirk, *Current Veterinary Therapy V*, 1974). Twenty-four hours after the last treatment, bacterial titers in the trachea were determined. No difference in bacterial titers could be observed between treated and control animals.

Similar groups of animals received antibiotic treatment by aerosol. This was accomplished by the use of a face mask attached to a plastic Vaponefrin® nebulizer (Fisons). A suitable face mask can be made from plastic or Styrofoam drinking cups, or dogs can be placed in an oxygen chamber connected to a nebulizer. Aerosol mist was generated by a portable air compressor. A small compressor (as used in fish tanks, for example) is usually capable of reaching 10 lb. of pressure. Dogs were exposed to this mist for 10 minutes under 10 lb. of pressure, and treatment was repeated every 12 hours for three days. Doses of antibiotics used were as recommended for humans and were contained in 2½ ml. of normal saline. The doses were 333,000 I.U. polymyxin B, 250 mg. kanamycin or 50 mg. gentamicin.

Tracheal bacterial titers 24 hours after treatment were consistently 4 to 5 $\log_{10}$ lower in treated dogs than in controls. This effect was also observed after a single treatment with any of the above antibiotics. Bacterial titers after treatment remained low for 2 to 3 days. However, bacterial repopulation took place in the trachea, and in one week after treatment was stopped the levels reached those in the control dogs. Because clinical signs are related to bacterial titers in the bronchial tree, treatment should be continued until clinical signs disappear. One aerosol exposure every second day would be sufficient. Kanamycin and gentamicin usually are effective against *B. bronchiseptica* as well as against mycoplasma. Aerosolized antibiotics should be topically effective and should not be absorbed by the respiratory mucosa to minimize the systemic effects. Kanamycin, gentamicin and polymyxin B are poorly absorbed from the respiratory mucosa. This treatment should prove to be useful in both types of the canine respiratory syndrome, because *B. bronchiseptica* is frequently involved in both types.

Additional treatment of both types should be made according to clinical signs. If dry coughing is found, it should be depressed. Humidified air is very beneficial, and water vaporizers are commercially available. Drugs besides antibiotics can be added to the nebulizer. The use of bronchodilators is indicated to reduce irritation, bronchial swelling and constriction (isoproterenol, epinephrine, theophylline or aminophylline). Detergents (Alevaire® [Breon], Tergemist® [Abbott]), mucolytics (acetylcysteine, Mucomyst® [Mead Johnson]) and enzymes (pancreatic dornase) are indicated only if thick and tenacious secretions are present. Antitussives are indicated to control nonproductive coughing, because coughing itself may cause irritation. Antihistamines provide both bronchodilation and tranquilizing effect (diphenhydramine hydrochloride, pyrilamine maleate, chlorpheniramine maleate or promethazine hydrochloride). The use of steroids should be questioned, although immunosuppressive effects in dogs after steroid treatment appear to be limited. The more potent sedatives such as codeine and dihydrocodeine are indicated only in severe paroxysms of coughing and must be used with caution.

Good nursing care and good nutrition should always be provided. Dogs that develop bronchopneumonia require additional therapy, as discussed elsewhere in this text.

## PROGNOSIS

Prognosis in all dogs with kennel cough of the mild type is very good. Dogs recover within a few days or weeks without any persistent signs or lesions. However, pups in pet shops often develop bronchopneumonia, and prognosis in these cases should be guarded, depending on the state of the disease. Although mortality rate is low, some pups recover very slowly.

## PROPHYLAXIS

Attenuated live virus vaccines to control the viral agents involved in kennel cough are now available commercially. Unfortunately most pups being delivered to pet shops are not vaccinated before arrival. Vaccination at the time of arrival has only limited effect, because pups are exposed to virulent viruses simultaneously. Arrangements should be made to vaccinate pups at least 10 days prior to shipment or to exposure to virus. First vaccination of privately owned pups is best between 6 and 8 weeks of age. A combined measles-distemper vaccine is effective in controlling canine distemper. Parainfluenza $SV_5$ vaccine is now available commercially and should be given to pups of the same age range. When $SV_5$ vaccine is given intramuscularly, neutralizing antibodies develop which do not protect pups against aerosol infection of $SV_5$; however, an anamnestic immune response causes early clearance of virus, so that clinical signs do not appear. Adenovirus infections should be controlled. A CAV-2 vaccine has been developed but is not available and may not be licensed because of its oncogenic effect in hamsters. Because there is cross-protection between CAV-1 and CAV-2, CAV-1 vaccines can be effectively used to control CAV-2 infections. As with $SV_5$, dogs will become infected with virulent CAV-2 after intramuscular vaccination with CAV-1. An anamnestic immune response, again, restricts viral replication early, and spread of virus occurs only for 4 or 5 days instead of for 8 or 9 days. A safe prophylactic agent against mycoplasma infection is not available. Antibiotic aerosol therapy can be used in dogs known to be exposed to the agent. Vaccination attempts with *B. bronchiseptica* have failed until now, but additional tests are being made. As with mycoplasma, antibiotic aerosol may prevent the infection.

Prophylaxis by vaccination in older dogs should be continued. A satisfactory immune status against distemper, $SV_5$, CAV-1 and CAV-2 should be maintained by means of yearly booster vaccinations. In addition to vaccination, ventilation and disinfection of kennels are extremely important. Fifteen to 20 air changes per hour are recommended for ventilation. Commonly used disinfectants effective against bacteria and viruses are benzalkonium chloride (Roccal® [Winthrop]) and chlorhexidine (Nolvasan® [Fort Dodge]. Aerosol therapy with Nolvasan has been reported to be effective against kennel cough. We have tested its aerosol effect against *B. bronchiseptica* in dogs and have found it to be of limited value.

Isolation of individual animals into separate units would be very effective for controlling spread of infectious agents; however, this is often not feasible. Positive pressure ventilation through cages into a pipe exhaust system in the back of the cage is often used with success. Diseased animals should be kept in isolation units, although in most cases viral spread takes place before clinical disease occurs, and transmission continues in spite of isolation of diseased animals.

## PUBLIC HEALTH ASPECTS

Parainfluenza $SV_5$ spread from dogs to humans may be possible but has not been proved. Although antibody to CAV-1 has been found in humans, a possible cross-reaction with a human adenovirus has not been ruled out. Direct evidence for human CAV-1 or CAV-2 infection does not exist. Canine herpesvirus is restricted to dogs. Reoviruses are not species specific; therefore, spread from animal to man is possible. The pathogenicity of this agent in humans is not known. Mycoplasma species appear to be canine specific. *B. bronchiseptica* isolations have been made infrequently from humans with respiratory disease; however, they appear to be pathologically insignificant.

## SUPPLEMENTAL READING

Appel, M. J. G., Pickerill, P. H., Menegus, M., Percy, D. H., Parsonson, I. M., and Sheffy, B. E.: Current status of canine respiratory disease. Gaines Veterinary Symposium, Kansas, 1970, pp. 15–23.

Binn, L. N., Lazar, E. C., Rogul, M., Shepler, V. M., Swango, L. J., Claypoole, T., Hubbard, D. W., Asbill, S. G., and Alexander, A. D.: Upper respiratory disease in military dogs: bacterial, mycoplasma, and viral studies. Am. J. Vet. Res., 29:1809–1815, 1968.

Thompson, H., Wright, N. G., and Cornwell, H. J. C.: Contagious respiratory disease in dogs. Vet. Bull., 45:479–488, 1975.

---

# FELINE PANLEUKOPENIA

JACK H. CARLSON, D.V.M.
*Fort Collins, Colorado*

Feline panleukopenia (FPL) is a very serious, highly contagious disease of cats. It is also known as feline distemper and infectious enteritis. The virus infects all members of the family Felidae and the raccoon and coatimundi of the family Procyonidae. The same virus causes a highly fatal disease, mink enteritis. Besides causing the common form of enteritis and panleukopenia, the virus is also the etiologic agent in feline cerebellar ataxia and possibly other congenital defects.

## ETIOLOGY AND EPIDEMIOLOGY

FPL is a member of the parvovirus group. These are very small (18 to 22 nm.), nonenveloped, single-stranded DNA viruses. Distribution of the virus appears to be worldwide, with all tested isolates belonging to a single serotype.

Before the parvoviruses themselves can replicate, the host cell must undergo the DNA synthesis stage of mitosis. Because of this, cells or tissues having a high rate of proliferation are infected and destroyed. These include the lymphoid tissues, bone marrow and cryptal cells of the intestinal mucosa. The clinical, laboratory and pathologic manifestations of FPL can be directly or indirectly attributed to the destruction of these tissues.

Parvoviruses are probably the most resistant viruses known. FPL virus is resistant to the alcohol, phenol, heavy metal, quaternary ammonium and iodine or chlorine-based disinfectants in common use. Virus suspensions held at room temperature for over a year have shown little if any drop in infectivity. Only 0.2 per cent formalin and ethylene oxide gas disinfectants have been clearly shown to destroy the infectivity of FPL virus.

Heavy concentrations of virus are shed in the vomitus and feces of clinically ill cats, and recovered animals have been shown to shed small amounts of virus in urine and feces for up to a year. The lengthy shedding period and extreme resistance of the virus constitute a serious control problem for practitioners in their own hospitals.

While most cases of FPL are seen in young kittens, the virus can cause disease in susceptible cats of all ages. The typical epidemic outbreaks occurring in late summer are related to the significant build-up of the spring crop of kittens just losing their maternally derived antibody and becoming susceptible to the virus. Older cats are usually vaccinated or have recovered and are thus immune.

Mortality rates vary from 0 to 90 per cent in a given outbreak but probably average about 50 per cent. The resident microbial flora and concomitant disease (especially the very common, latent, upper respiratory viruses) probably play an important part in the variability of mortality rates. Virus strains may also differ in virulence.

Subclinical infections are apparently common. Up to 75 per cent of unvaccinated cats in the Ithaca, New York, area possessed neutralizing antibodies but lacked a history of clinical FPL. Once a clinical or subclinical infection has occurred, recovered cats are solidly immune for life.

## CLINICAL SIGNS

The typical case of FPL presents to the clinician showing signs of lethargy, anorexia and vomiting of a yellow fluid. Diarrhea is often present or develops later. The feces are yellowish, are soft to fluid and may be tinged with blood. The animal may act thirsty but will drink nothing. Temperatures are usually over 40° C. but may be subnormal. Severe dehydration is usually apparent, the skin being loose but leathery and failing to retract quickly when pinched. The mouth is dry, and vessels of the soft palate are large and blue.

Peripheral lymph nodes are usually normal. The mesenteric lymph nodes are often slightly enlarged and palpable. The gastrointestinal tract is palpably swollen and filled with excess gas and liquid. Abdominal palpation may be painful. Upper respiratory disease may also be evident, but its cause is usually reactivation of latent upper respiratory viruses such as the feline herpes- or caliciviruses (picornaviruses) induced by the stress of FPL. This complication is common enough to have resulted in the misnomer for FPL, feline distemper. Uncomplicated FPL does not present with upper respiratory disease.

FPL is a very acute, sometimes peracute disease. Death can occur within 12 hours from the onset of signs. It is not uncommon for a client to firmly believe that his cat has been poisoned in these cases. The typical acute course runs 3 to 5 days from the onset of signs. When death does occur, it is often preceded by severe depression, persistent vomiting, bloody diarrhea and cardiovascular collapse. Anemia and icterus are rarely present. Anemia if present is due to hemorrhage and will be of the regenerative type.

## DIAGNOSIS

Diagnosis of FPL is made when most of the clinical signs are present and are accompanied by a very low total leukocyte count, almost always below 2000/cu. mm. White blood counts of 0 to 500/cu. mm. are not uncommon.

The differential diagnosis should include intestinal foreign bodies, acute septicemia, acute toxoplasmosis, thallium poisoning and malignant lymphoma. The four latter conditions also can present with a leukopenia below 2000/cu. mm.

It is becoming increasingly apparent that a disease popularly called "chronic panleukopenia" is another disease entity altogether. This disease usually presents as a chronic, recurring diarrhea accompanied by a low WBC and a nonregenerative anemia. It is more common in older cats, many of which have been properly vaccinated against FPL. An acute form is occasionally observed which is characterized by severe, bloody diarrhea. Histopathologic appearances of the gut are nearly identical to those of FPL, making diagnosis extremely difficult. Limited studies have indicated that this syndrome may be an unusual manifestation of the feline leukemia virus.

The diagnosis of FPL can be confirmed by means of virus isolation, immunofluorescence, histopathologic and/or paired serologic laboratory techniques. Because FPL virus is so resistant, samples for virus isolation can be sent unfrozen by ordinary mail to a diagnostic laboratory. Spleen, intestine and feces provide excellent specimens.

Histopathologic diagnosis can be made on the basis of intestinal mucosal crypt and subsequent villus destruction. Specific intranuclear inclusions are present in cryptal lesions, but care must be taken to preserve them. Intestinal tissues should be fixed as soon after death as is possible in an acid fixative such as Bouin's or Zenker's solution. Formalin will not preserve the inclusions. Inclusions may not be present in intestinal lesions when death occurs several days after the onset of signs.

Paired serum samples, acute and convalescent, can demonstrate an increase in specific antibody by serum neutralization, hemagglutination inhibition or complement fixation techniques.

## TREATMENT

Treatment is primarily supportive, since specific antiviral agents are unavailable at present. Administration of fluids and electrolytes is the most critical need, since significant amounts of these are lost in the vomitus and diarrhea. Many different solutions have been used successfully for this purpose, lactated Ringer's solution being the most common. The fluids can be administered intravenously or subcutaneously. The intravenous route should be used when treating severely dehydrated animals. The precise electrolytes, types of fluids and their amounts of optimal replacement are not well established for FPL. The clinician must be alerted to the significant changes in the levels of blood pH

and electrolytes that can occur with persistent vomiting or diarrhea and should correct these as they may occur.

It is assumed by most workers that the severely damaged intestinal mucosa allows normal gut bacteria to penetrate and cause a secondary septicemia. For this reason, antibiotics are used prophylactically. Broad-spectrum antibiotics, the tetracyclines, choramphenicol or synergistic combinations such as penicillin and streptomycin are usually effective. Whatever the choice of antibiotic, it should be administered parenterally, since the absorption of a therapeutic dose through the damaged mucosa is unreliable. There is no reason to "sterilize" the gut with nonabsorbable oral antibiotics such as neomycin. Significant modification of the normal intestinal flora can cause serious problems in and of itself. Dosages for antibiotics that rely heavily on the kidney for their excretion may have to be recalculated if severe dehydration and shock are present, since renal function may be compromised. This is especially important for those antibiotics that may be toxic to the kidney. There is no evidence that prolonged antibiotic treatment is effective in preventing relapses. Once recovery begins, the damaged intestinal mucosa repairs itself quite rapidly, and there is no need for further antibiotic therapy.

There is no scientific evidence that specific antiserum therapy is beneficial once clinical signs have commenced. By this time, viral damage to the intestine has already occurred. Large amounts of serum or blood may be beneficial in that they restore fluids, electrolytes and plasma proteins that are lost through the damaged gut. If hemorrhage has been significant, blood transfusions are indicated.

Vomiting and diarrhea can be controlled to some extent by the use of antiemetic and antidiarrheal drugs. B-vitamins may be beneficial as supportive treatment. As soon as the animal will eat, it should be fed soft, easily digestible food such as baby food or a gruel of liquid and meat.

## PROGNOSIS

FPL is acute in nature. The severe signs usually last only 3 to 6 days. If the animal can be maintained for this period of time, the prognosis for recovery is good. There appears to be an indirect relationship between the WBC and the degree of clinical signs: the lower the WBC, the more severe the disease. The prognosis is much poorer for animals that vomit persistently.

The best indicator of impending recovery is an increase in the WBC. The WBC frequently rises to 50,000/cu. mm or greater within a few days after recovery begins. A very significant shift to the left is also noted with the increasing WBC. The appetite usually returns, and free serum neutralizing antibodies are present at about the same time as the WBC begins to rise. Experimentally, antibodies were demonstrated consistently 7 days after inoculation. This would correlate to about 3 to 4 days after the onset of clinical signs.

The question as to whether sequelae or relapses of FPL occur is controversial at present; many believe that they do. Misdiagnosis is always a problem. Chronic enteritis and/or colonic ulcers, often reported as sequelae to FPL, can be caused by indiscriminate antibiotic therapy. Chronic or recurrent FPL has not been reported experimentally nor have we observed it in our laboratory. Certainly this important point must be closely examined.

## PROPHYLAXIS

Three classes of FPL vaccines are commercially available. These are modified live virus (MLV), inactivated cell culture and inactivated tissue origin vaccine. Each has been proved efficacious. However, the vaccine must be administered after maternally derived antibody has disappeared, and this will depend on the level of immunity of the queen. The following table indicates when maternal immunity can be expected to disappear:

| TITER OF QUEEN* | | KITTEN SUSCEPTIBILITY AGE |
|---|---|---|
| High | 1:1000 to 1:10,000 | 12 to 16 weeks |
| Moderate | 1:100 to 1:1000 | 8 to 12 weeks |
| Low | 1:10 to 1:100 | 4 to 8 weeks |

*Serum neutralizing titers against 100 $TCID_{50}$.

A serum neutralizing titer of 1:30 or greater prevents infection by virulent street virus, 1:10 or greater blocks successful vaccination by both MLV and inactivated cell culture vaccines and any demonstrable titer neutralizes inactivated tissue origin vaccines. It is clear, then, that the animal must become susceptible to virulent virus before any vaccination can be successful. Queens that have recovered from clinical or subclinical FPL or that have been vaccinated with MLV vaccines usually have antibody levels in the high range.

A panel of the Colloquium on Selected Feline Infectious Diseases made the following recommendations to practitioners on the use of the available FPL vaccines:

| AGE IN WEEKS | MLV VACCINE | INACTIVATED VACCINE |
|---|---|---|
| First Vaccination | 9 to 10 | 9 to 10 |
| Second Vaccination | 14 to 16 | 11 to 12 |
| Third Vaccination | —— | 16 |

Properly vaccinated cats probably are immune for life, especially if vaccinated with MLV. This is yet unproved, and therefore the panel recommends a yearly booster.

Aerosol vaccination with MLV vaccine has been proved to be effective and may be especially valuable in controlling the disease in animal shelters. Aerosol vaccination of mink against canine distemper has been used effectively for years.

Pregnant animals must never be vaccinated with MLV vaccines. Inactivated vaccines should be used to vaccinate exotic cats, raccoons and coatimundi, because the pathogenicity of MLV vaccines for these animals is as yet undetermined.

Immune serum can be used in the face of an outbreak. One to 2 ml. subcutaneously provides temporary but effective immunity for 2 to 4 weeks. Of course, this would also block any vaccination attempt during this time.

## CONGENITAL DEFECTS

Clinical and subclinical disease of the dam at any stage of gestation may result in fetal death, resorption, mummification, abortion or congenital defects of the kitten. The fetus is especially vulnerable to the virus because most tissues have high cell proliferation rates. A well-described congenital defect caused by FPL virus is cerebellar ataxia. Cells of the cerebellum of the kitten proliferate rapidly just prior to and shortly after birth. Infection during this time destroys cells of the cerebellum and prevents its proper development. No abnormalities are observed until kittens reach

3 to 4 weeks of age, when balance and coordination normally develop. Ataxic kittens demonstrate incoordination, fine head tremors and hypermetria. The kittens appear otherwise normal. They are strong, healthy and vigorous. However, the ataxia is permanent.

Experimental infection of neonatal kittens demonstrated virus infection of many tissues that are not normally infected in older cats. It is conceivable that future studies may show other congenital defects to be caused by FPL. Recent evidence has indicated that certain retinopathies are caused by perinatal FPL infection.

## SUPPLEMENTAL READING

Carlson, J. H., Scott, F. W., and Duncan, J. R.: Feline panleukopenia. I. Pathogenesis in germfree and specific pathogen-free cats. Vet. Pathol., in press, 1977.

Carpenter, J. L.: Feline panleukopenia: Clinical signs and differential diagnosis. J. Am. Vet. Med. Assn., 158:857, 1971.

Csiza, C. K., deLaunta, A., Scott, F. W., and Gillespie, J. H.: Spontaneous feline ataxia. Cornell Vet., 62:300, 1972.

Feline Infectious Diseases Report. Proceedings of a Colloquium on Selected Feline Infectious Diseases J. Am. Vet. Med. Assn., 158:825–1137, 1971.

Scott, F. W., and Glauberg, A. F.: Aerosol vaccination against feline panleukopenia. J. Am. Vet. Med. Assn., 166:147, 1975.

# CANINE HERPESVIRUS INFECTION IN PUPPIES

LELAND E. CARMICHAEL, D.V.M.
*Ithaca, New York*

Canine herpesvirus (CHV) causes a fatal septicemic disease of infant puppies. The virus grows well in cultured dog cells, where typical cytopathic effects are observed. Fatal illness generally occurs in pups less than one month old; however, occasional cases have been observed in dogs as old as four months of age. Clinical features of the disease consist of the sudden death of apparently healthy puppies after a brief period of illness that usually lasts no more than 24 hours. Most commonly, pups are affected between the first and third weeks of life, with occasional fatal cases occurring after the third week. Herpesvirus infection has only rarely been found to be a cause of puppy deaths within the first three days of life. Generalized, nonfatal infection occurs in older pups but signs usually are not apparent. Signs are virtually absent in pups infected after weaning. The incubation period varies between 3 and 8 days in newborn puppies given virus intranasally.

Signs in older dogs inoculated with virus are limited to mild rhinitis or vaginitis. Recently, British investigators have associated a canine herpesvirus with abortions, stillbirths and infertility in a kennel of Alsatians. The virus recovered from the genital tracts of affected dogs was antigenically indistinguishable from canine herpesviruses isolated previously from neonatal pups; however, certain cultural differences were noted. Unfortunately, the genital isolate was not stored and is no longer available for study. Nevertheless, when vesicular lesions affecting the genital tract are observed, especially if recurrent infection is noted, attempts to isolate the virus should be made. There is no good evidence that the canine herpesvirus is associated with tracheobronchitis.

The disease is transmitted principally by means of contact between susceptible pups and infective oral or vaginal secretions, usually from the bitch. It also may be spread from an infected dog to susceptible newborn pups by kennel owners or contaminated objects. There is only one reported case of prenatal transmission; however, it is likely that such instances occur occasionally.

Pathologic changes are typical in affected pups. Lesions in inoculated and naturally affected puppies consist of disseminated focal necrosis and hemorrhages. Microscopic lesions are observed in all organs; however, macroscopic changes are readily seen, and these consist of focal necrosis and hemorrhages in the liver, intestinal tract, lungs and kidneys. Renal lesions are especially characteristic and appear as "speckled kidneys" (bright red spots on the gray background of necrotic cortical tissue). Lungs are usually diffusely pneumonic.

The differential lesions that distinguish this disease from canine hepatitis and toxoplasmosis are the focal areas of necrosis and hemorrhage, especially those that occur in the kidneys. Microscopic examination may reveal intranuclear "type A" inclusions in occasional cells at the periphery of necrotic foci, especially in the kidneys and liver. Inclusions are not numerous.

Inapparent infections are common in dogs. Although such infections occur without significant clinical signs, which are limited to mild serous rhinitis or vaginitis, the epizootiologic importance is apparent. Periodic recrudescence (shed) of the canine herpesvirus, similar to that reported in humans or cattle infected with herpes simplex or infectious bovine rhinotracheitis viruses, respectively, also has been observed in infected dogs. By use of immunosuppressant agents (corticosteroid drugs, antilymphocyte serum), viral recrudescense has been demonstrated as long as six months after primary intranasal infection. Despite persistent infections of the dog, bitches that had lost their pups because of the herpesvirus have not been reported to have suffered additional losses at subsequent whelpings.

Pups with maternal antibody are readily infected by CHV; however, there is no clinical illness, since the infection remains localized. Neutralizing antibodies develop after infection and have persisted at low levels for at least two years.

There is no vaccine available. Treatment is not successful.

### SUPPLEMENTAL READING

Carmichael, L. E.: Herpesvirus canis: aspects of pathogenesis and immune response. J. Am. Vet. Med. Assn., 156:1714, 1970.
Carmichael, L. E., Squire, R. A., and Krook, L.: Clinical and pathologic features of a fatal viral disease of newborn pups. Am. J. Vet. Res., 26:803, 1965.
Poste, G., and King, N.: Isolation of a herpesvirus from the canine genital tract: association with infertility, abortion and stillbirths. Vet. Rec., 88:229, 1971.
Wright, N. G., and Cornwell, H. J. C.: Experimental herpes virus infection in young puppies. Res. Vet. Sci., 9:295, 1968.

# RABIES

WILLIAM G. WINKLER, D.V.M.
*Atlanta, Georgia*

Rabies is a viral encephalitis, almost always fatal, that may affect any warm-blooded animal but is most common in carnivores and New World bats. In the United States, foxes, skunks and raccoons are the major wild carnivore hosts, though domestic dogs and cats remain a most important source of human exposure.

### ETIOLOGY

The rabies virus is a member of the rhabdovirus group. The "bullet"-shaped virion, approximately 75 x 180 nanometers, consists of a spiked outer envelope containing a helical RNA nucleocapsid. The virus is rapidly destroyed outside the body by desiccation, heat and ultraviolet light. It is easily inactivated with common disinfectants such as 70 per cent ethanol, 0.1 per cent quaternary ammonium compounds and organic iodine compounds.

### EPIDEMIOLOGY

Infection usually results from inoculation of virus-contaminated saliva into bite wounds. In recent years, other, much rarer means of transmission have been described, including oral transmission following ingestion of infected tissue and inhalation transmission, the latter being most often associated with virus of bat origin.

Once introduced into the body, rabies virus migrates along nerve pathways centripetally to the CNS and then centrifugally to the salivary glands. Highest concentrations of virus are in CNS tissue and salivary

**Table 1.** Compendium of Animal Rabies Vaccine in the United States—May, 1976*

| VACCINE | PRODUCED BY | MARKETED BY | FOR USE IN | DOSE(S) | ANIMAL'S AGE |
|---|---|---|---|---|---|
| **(A) MODIFIED LIVE VIRUS (MLV)** | | | | | |
| Chicken Embryo Origin Low Egg Passage, Flury Strain | AMERLAB | Amerlab (Rabies Vaccine®) | Dogs | 2 ml. | 3 months and 1 year |
| | FROMM | Fromm (Raboid®) | Dogs | 1 ml. | 3 months and 1 year |
| | | Haver-Lockhart (Rabies Vaccine®) | Dogs | 1 ml. | 3 months and 1 year |
| Canine Cell Line Origin High Egg Passage, Flury Strain | NORDEN | Norden (Endurall-R®) | Dogs | 1 ml. | 3 months and 1 year |
| | | | Cats | 1 ml. | 3 months |
| | | | Cattle | 2 doses of 1 ml. each 6 weeks apart | As required |
| Porcine Tissue Culture Origin High Cell Passage, SAD STRAIN | CONNAUGHT | Jensen-Salsbery (Rabies Vaccine®) | Dogs | 2 ml. | 3 months and 1 year |
| | | | Cats | 2 ml. | 3 months |
| | | | Cattle | 2 ml. | As required |
| | JENSEN-SALSBERY | Jensen-Salsbery (Rabies Vaccine®) | Horses | 2 ml. | As required |
| | | | Sheep | 2 ml. | As required |
| | | | Goats | 2 ml. | As required |
| Canine Tissue Culture Origin High Cell Passage, SAD STRAIN | PHILLIPS ROXANE | BioCeutics (Neurogen TC®) | Dogs | 1 ml. | 3 months |
| | | | Cats | 1 ml. | 3 months |
| Hamster Cell Line Origin High Cell Passage, Kissling Strain | AFFILIATED | Affiliated (Rabtect®) | Dogs | 1 ml. | 3 months |
| **(B) INACTIVATED VACCINES** | | | | | |
| Caprine Origin | BANDY | Bandy (Rabies Vaccine®) | Dogs | 2 ml. | 3 months |
| | | | Cats | 2 ml. | 3 months |
| | NATION | Jensen-Salsbery (Monorab®) | Dogs | 2 ml. | 3 months |
| | | | Cats | 2 ml. | 3 months |
| Murine Origin | ROLYNN | Fort Dodge (Trimune®) | Dogs | 1 ml. | 3 months and 1 year |
| | | | Cats | 1 ml. | 3 months |

All vaccines should be administered intramuscularly in the thigh muscles of the rear leg.

*Reprinted from Compendium of Animal Rabies Vaccines, U.S. Department of Health, Education, and Welfare, Public Health Service, Center for Disease Control, Atlanta, Georgia 30333.

glands, but terminally the virus may be found in any tissue, and all body fluids should be considered potentially infective.

The incubation period, influenced by virus strain, dose, inoculation site, host susceptibility and other factors, is extremely variable but is usually between 3 and 8 weeks. Any animal may shed virus in saliva prior to onset of frank illness, but dogs and cats almost invariably develop clinical signs within 5 days after onset of virus shedding.

## CLINICAL SIGNS

Clinical course of the disease in carnivores is variable but usually includes a stage of excitability and irritability ("furious" rabies) and a stage of paralysis ("dumb" rabies). An animal is said to have furious or dumb rabies depending on the stage observed to be most prominent.

In either case, prodromal signs include a slight rise in temperature and subtle per-

## REVISED NATIONAL RECOMMENDATIONS FOR ANIMAL RABIES VACCINATION

This is the second revision of the Compendium of Animal Rabies Vaccines. It is intended that in the future the Compendium shall be reviewed and revised at the beginning of each calendar year. The purpose of the Compendium is to provide information on rabies vaccines to practicing veterinarians, public health officials, and others concerned with rabies control. The Compendium should serve as the basis for animal rabies vaccination programs throughout the United States. Its universal adoption will be of benefit by providing the standardization of recommendations between jurisdictions which is necessary for a viable national rabies control program.

The Committee in reassessing the purposes of the Compendium concurred unanimously on the need to maintain an independent evaluation of all licensed vaccines to ensure that the public health considerations of animal rabies remain the paramount concern at all times. All rabies vaccines currently licensed by the U. S. Department of Agriculture are described in the Compendium; however, in two instances the Compendium recommendations for duration of immunity do not agree with the product labels. Based on available data and past experience with rabies biologics, the Committee recommends durations of immunity which do not agree with those that appear on the labels of one chick embryo, LEP Flury vaccine, and the hamster cell, Kissling strain, tissue culture vaccine.

**ROUTE OF INOCULATION**: The intramuscular (IM route of administration has been demonstrated to be far more effective than other routes and is recommended. The site of inoculation for IM administration is the rear leg thigh muscles.

**WILDLIFE VACCINATION**: No vaccine is licensed for use in wildlife in the United States, and data on efficacy and duration of immunity are generally lacking. In the event that it is necessary to vaccinate wild animals, only INACTIVATED vaccines should be used (some MLV vaccines may actually induce rabies in wild animals). In the absence of specific data, dosage should be based on the recommendations for vaccination of dogs; annual vaccination should be required.

**ACCIDENTAL HUMAN EXPOSURE TO VACCINE**: Accidental inoculation or other exposure may occur to individuals during the administration of animal rabies vaccines. Such exposures to INACTIVATED vaccines constitute no known rabies hazard. The Flury LEP and HEP strains and the SAD strain vaccines appear to constitute no known hazard, though this is based more on empirical observations than specific studies. However, available data on human exposures to any other modified live virus vaccines are inadequate. In the event of exposure to other MLV vaccines, public health officials should be contacted for specific recommendations.

Members of the CDC Compendium Committee for 1976 are W. G. Winkler, D.V.M., Chairman; M. K. Abelseth, D.V.M.; M. A. W. Hattwick, M.D.; and R. K. Sikes, D.V.M.

sonality changes. These usually last less than 48 hours.

In furious rabies, animals become hypersensitive to external stimuli and may bite any object that moves. Loud noises or bright lights may induce biting seizures. As the disease progresses with increasing loss of muscular control, the biting attacks become less effective and evolve into clonic and tonic convulsions. Animals often die during such seizures but may continue into the paralytic stage.

In paralytic rabies the loss of muscle control progresses to flaccid paralysis and ultimately prostration. Cranial nerves often show involvement early and produce the characteristic slack-jawed, hanging tongue appearance; often this is accompanied by altered phonation.

Hydrophobia is not a common feature of rabies in animals.

### DIAGNOSIS AND TREATMENT

Encephalitis with mandibular and lingual paralysis accompanied by behavioral changes may suggest rabies, but a definitive diagnosis requires demonstration of the virus in CNS tissue. Animals suspected of being rabid should be isolated in a secure facility, and health authorities should be notified (see Public Health Aspects).

There is no treatment for clinically rabid animals. Unvaccinated dogs or cats bitten by rabid animals should be destroyed or vaccinated and isolated for 6 months. Currently vaccinated animals should be revaccinated and quarantined for 90 days.

### PROPHYLAXIS

Effective vaccines are available; see Table 1 for current vaccine recommendations.

### PUBLIC HEALTH ASPECTS

All tissues and fluids from rabid animals should be considered to be infectious, and precautions should be taken to prevent contact with them. Animals suspected of being rabid should be isolated but not destroyed until health officials have been contacted to determine whether human exposure has occurred, since this would require laboratory examination of the animal tissue.

### SUPPLEMENTAL READING

Baer, G. M.: The Natural History of Rabies. New York, Academic Press, 1975.
Sikes, R. K.: Rabies. *In* Davis, J., Karstad, L., and Trainer, D. (eds.): Infectious Diseases of Wild Animals. Ames, Iowa, Iowa State University Press, 1970.
Sikes, R. K., *et al.*: Rabies vaccines, duration of immunity study in dogs. J. Am. Vet. Med. Assn., *159*:1491–1499, 1971.

# PSEUDORABIES IN DOGS AND CATS

D. P. GUSTAFSON, D. V. M.
*West Lafayette, Indiana*

In 1902, while investigating a fatal encephalopathy in an ox, Dr. Aladar Aujeszky of Budapest inoculated material from its brain into two puppies with fatal results. In the same report, a similar syndrome in a cat was briefly described. Thus, the first demonstration of the infectious nature of what was to be recognized as pseudorabies virus (PrV) was accomplished in dogs. The literature contains more than 50 reports of PrV infections in dogs and cats from both urban and rural communities on all but one of the continents of the world, the exception being Australia. The disease occurs more commonly in areas where swine are raised or consumed.

Pseudorabies, or Aujeszky's disease, is caused by a herpesvirus and is infectious for a broad spectrum of animal life. The disease in nature is apparently invariably fatal for dogs, cats, cattle, sheep, goats, deer, foxes, mink, badgers, opossum, rats and mice. Swine are much more resistant, yet in some outbreaks all very young swine die. Variations in virulence of PrV strains may be observed in swine, and there is resistance related to aging, which is not seen in other species. Successful experimental infections have been achieved in other mammals, including some subhuman primates, and in many species of birds. Natural infections of birds have not been reported.

## MODES OF INFECTION

Dogs and cats can be infected by a variety of routes, as has been demonstrated under laboratory conditions. The disease has been initiated by feeding infectious material and by subcutaneous, intramuscular, intracranial and intraocular routes. Since the oral route leads to infection, it might be assumed with good reason that infection could be established by inhalation of an aerosol of the virus. Under natural conditions an overwhelming number of reports find the source of virus to be virus-contaminated flesh of swine and sometimes of cattle or rats that was consumed by the affected dog or cat.

That rural dogs and cats might eat infected flesh available on farms and become infected seems clear. In urban areas, dogs and cats may be provided with raw pork from a refrigerated carcass. The source animal may be an asymptomatic carrier not identifiable upon ordinary inspection. A tragic infection in a kennel has been reported in Sweden. In a building that housed about 45 dogs, 14 dogs died of pseudorabies. Evidence presented strongly suggested that uncooked, infected pork from a packing house was the source of the virus. The construction of fences permitted contact between dogs. However, some dogs kept in, or adjacent to, pens where deaths had occurred survived and were serologically negative.

The number of PrV infections among swine has gradually been increasing in the United States since 1962, and as an expected corollary, the number of cases in other susceptible species has increased. Thus, the number of infections among dogs and cats has increased in a rather dramatic fashion but is essentially confined to rural areas.

In every instance in which the means of infection of cats has been described in the available literature and in experience, ingestion of virus-contaminated food has been noted. However, it must be recognized that other modes of access to the virus are possible, as has been indicated.

## THE DISEASE IN DOGS

Once a dog has become infected, the natural course of the disease proceeds to death in a short period of time. The incubation period has a range of about 2 to 10 days, with most cases between 3 and 6 days under natural conditions. Experimental intracerebral, subcutaneous or intramuscular exposures reduce the prodromal period and the course of the disease. As the dose of virus used to infect is increased, the duration of the disease is somewhat diminished. After signs of the disease appear, death occurs in a relatively short period of time—24 to 48 hours. Thus from infection to termination the natural disease usually lasts 5 to 8 days.

The syndrome runs a rather constant course, but there are exceptions. In a typical case, the dog goes through an excitement phase followed by dullness, coma and death. In the excitement phase, the dog is febrile and restless and may vomit bilious fluid. The saliva is usually copious and viscid. Clonic spasms of facial muscles, paralysis of an eyelid or the lower lip, incoordination of movement and difficult breathing often signal the onset of an intense pruritus somewhere about the head. The area is rubbed incessantly and becomes raw and often edematous. Vocal expressions of discomfort often accompany the progress of the syndrome, yet aggressive behavior toward objects or people has not been observed or reported. The course of the encephalopathy deepens into depression followed by coma and death. An exception to this syndrome would be the abbreviation or apparent absence of the excitement phase, in which case the disease course is also shortened.

The physiology of the pruritus has been studied. The itching is apparently caused by functional dissociation of the afferent nerve system between receptor and motor nerve elements. As a result of depression in cholinergic processes in the cerebral cortex by the virus and the toxic products that accompany it, the analyzing function of the cortex becomes altered, leading to a disturbance in esthesic perception.

## THE DISEASE IN CATS

The usual clinical syndrome in cats begins about 4 days after infection and generally parallels that in dogs but is less consistent than in the dog. The excitement phase is somewhat different in that cats first appear to be sluggish and then become agitated. Their movements suggest discomfort just prior to the onset of salivation, which in turn signals the approach of a variety of signs. At about this point the fur becomes matted with saliva and it appears that something is caught in the throat or that there is an obstruction in the esophagus. The cat resists being caught, and mewing is persistent. In many cases there is an intense pruritus localized on one side of the head and in such cases anisocoria is present. In a smaller number of cases pruritus and irritability are absent. The response to the pruritus is strong, and the area is often scratched raw. As the syndrome progresses, respiration becomes difficult and the pulse rate is increased, sometimes uncountable. The qualitative blood picture is normal, but because of dehydration the blood is concentrated. When the cat is picked up, it often immediately voids urine from a full bladder; males have been observed to have an erection of the penis. On palpation the intestines may be distended with gas. The signs soon diminish as the encephalopathy progresses to convulsive spasms, exhaustion and death. Cats usually die within 24 hours of the onset of symptoms. Less typically, the clinical signs are most difficult to interpret. In such instances the cats become feeble and salivate excessively, making frequent attempts to swallow. The head may be canted to one side, and the tail thrashes in a horizontal plane, but there are no signs of agitation, mewing or pruritus. Cats have been observed to live at least 36 hours after the onset of symptoms in such atypical cases.

## DIAGNOSIS

1. The clinical signs of the disease, especially when pruritus is pronounced, provide the basis for a presumptive diagnosis of pseudorabies. The course of the syndrome in both species is short and, once present, is fatal.

2. Laboratory diagnosis is made by means of fluorescent antibody tests. The tissue of choice for the test is the mesencephalon—that portion of the brain stem containing the gasserian ganglion of the trigeminal nerve. Almost as valuable is tonsillar tissue. Both contain high virus concentrations early, which persist until some time after death. The persistence of the virus after death is related to the speed of tissue denaturation, which is essentially a function of temperature. The lower the carcass temperature, the longer the virus will remain viable.

3. Diagnosis can also be made by isola-

tion of the virus in cell cultures. Extracts of tissues are inoculated into media bathing cell cultures. High-titered preparations will cause cytopathic effects in 18 hours, and very low-titered material must be held a maximum of 120 hours before it is discarded. The test is made specific for PrV through virus neutralization tests with reference antiserum.

4. Tissue extracts may be inoculated into a variety of laboratory animals for diagnosis on the basis of their response. Rabbits are highly sensitive to the virus and are commonly used. They are inoculated subcutaneously in the flank with tissue extracts suspected of containing PrV. Mice are less sensitive but are often used. These are inoculated intracranially with similar material. If the death of any laboratory animal is to be used to establish a diagnosis, familiarity with the syndrome, close observation and adequate control procedures are required.

## TREATMENT

There is no known treatment that will change the course of events once signs of the disease are present. However, to reduce expression of reaction to the virus, sedation is recommended.

## PROGNOSIS

Once the syndrome has begun, the prognosis in dogs and cats is death.

## PROPHYLAXIS

There are no prophylactic biologicals available in the United States from commercial sources. However, antiserum from swine is sometimes available from research organizations. While reports of the use of antiserum in cats and dogs has not been encouraging, it has been successfully used in swine and other animals. Timing is of the essence; it is essentially accurate to suggest that the latest that the antiserum can be administered within reason is 8 hours after exposure to the virus. Antiserum of at least 5 × $10^2$ titer against 100 $TCID_{50}$ of PrV should be given intraperitoneally. Finite doses for cats and dogs have not been established.

However, extrapolating from experience with swine, it seems likely that a minimum dose for a puppy would be 10 to 15 ml. and a maximum dose for a 30-kg. dog should be about 100 ml.

Antiviral chemicals that would have value in the same fashion as antiserum are in developmental phases but are unavailable.

## MANAGEMENT IN INFECTED ENVIRONMENTS

If an outbreak occurs on a farm in swine or other susceptible species, it would be wise to exclude dogs and cats from the virus-contaminated environment until the threat of transmission has passed. It is most important to prevent cats or dogs from eating virus-contaminated flesh or from being nipped by an infected animal, for the virus is very likely to be present in the oral fluids.

The virus is present in the tonsils and oral secretions of infected dogs and cats during the prodromal period as well as during the clinical course of the disease. While lateral spread among dogs or cats has not been widely recognized, it seems quite possible.

## PUBLIC HEALTH ASPECTS

The reports of human infections describe rather mild disease manifested by itching of a few days' duration. The descriptions of proof are not very convincing, but because some subhuman primates have been shown to be susceptible, caution is due. The threshold of infection for man seems high, since among those working in the laboratory or in the field with many strains of PrV, the record of seroconversion has remained constantly negative for 14 years.

### SUPPLEMENTAL READING

Gustafson, D. P.: Pseudorabies. *In* Dunne, H. W., and Leman, A. D. (eds.): Diseases of Swine, 4th ed. Ames, Iowa, Iowa State University Press, 1975, pp. 391–410.

Horvath, Z., and Papp, L.: Clinical manifestations of Aujeszky's disease in the cat. Acta Vet. Acad. Sci. Hung., *17*:49–54, 1967.

Hugoson, G., and Rockborn, G.: On the occurrence of pseudorabies in Sweden. II. An outbreak in dogs caused by feeding abattoir offal. Zbl. Vet. Med. B., *19*:641–645, 1972.

# CANINE ADENOVIRUS INFECTION

## (Infectious Canine Hepatitis, CAV-1)

LELAND E. CARMICHAEL,
D.V.M.
*Ithaca, New York*

Infectious canine hepatitis (ICH) is caused by one of the two canine adenoviruses recognized at present. The virus that causes the generalized disease and that is commonly known as ICH is now referred to as canine adenovirus type 1 (CAV-1). Aspects of the disease are fully discussed in the supplemental readings. The virus replicates in reticuloendothelial cells, vascular endothelium and parenchymal cells of the liver, producing characteristic intranuclear inclusions. There are many forms of the disease; however, the most common one is the mild or inapparent form that can be recognized only by means of an increase in specific (virus-neutralizing) antibody or the appearance, in recovered dogs, of acute anterior uveitis with corneal edema ("blue eye"). The most severe cases occur during the first few months of life; however, deaths have been reported in dogs as old as 13 years of age. During the first week after exposure, virus is present in all body tissues and can be isolated from the saliva and feces. Following clinical recovery, virus has been found to persist in kidneys and may be shed in the urine for several months.

Even though CAV-1 has not been shown to be transmitted by the airborne route, this virus has been recovered occasionally from lungs of dogs that showed the signs and lesions of acute respiratory disease. The significance of CAV-1 as a cause of severe respiratory illness is probably minor; however, the second canine adenoviral type, CAV-2 (prototype strain Toronto A-26/61), has been clearly associated with tracheobronchitis, especially when dogs had been assembled into groups and kept in close quarters. Infections with CAV-2, unlike CAV-1, are not generalized ones. Observations made by investigators in several laboratories have supported field observations that uncomplicated CAV-2 infection is very mild or clinically inapparent. Nonetheless, CAV-2 may lower pulmonary resistance to various additional agents, since field and laboratory cases of respiratory disease ("tracheobronchitis") associated with this virus also have commonly yielded bacterial and mycoplasmal organisms.

The two canine adenovirus types may be distinguished readily by various serologic tests; they also differ in pathogenicity, as noted above, and in other characteristics. Nevertheless, antigenic relatedness between CAV-1 and CAV-2 is very close, and CAV-2 protects dogs completely against inoculations with lethal doses of CAV-1. CAV-1 also protects against CAV-2. The use of suitable CAV-2 isolates as replacements for CAV-1 strains that have been shown to cause postvaccinal ocular and renal lesions is therefore feasible.

### TREATMENT

There is no specific therapy. Excellent vaccines have been available for more than a decade and have made cases of ICH relatively rare. Treatment is empirical. Antiserum given after the onset of signs is of no value; in fact, it may even be harmful.

Bacterial complications have not been a feature of severe ICH. Although antibiotics usually are given, there seems to be little justification for this practice, since the course of illness seems poorly correlated with attempts at therapy. Specific treatment for the corneal opacity usually is not required; however an ophthalmic atropine so-

1303

lution is helpful in reducing pain resulting from anterior uveitis. The role of corticosteroids is moot, since results have been variable.

## PROPHYLAXIS

The recommendations for prophylactic immunization differ little from those made in previous editions of this text. They are based on information presented at the Symposium on Immunity to Selected Canine Infectious Diseases in October, 1969. Since temporary protection by maternal antibody supplied to pups via the colostrum of immune mothers also neutralizes vaccine virus, vaccination is ineffective until the pup has lost essentially all maternally transmitted antibody. The age at which any pup will respond to vaccination cannot be stated, since it depends on the amount of maternal antibody transmitted. Only pups that nurse acquire significant amounts of protective antibody.

Approximately 50 per cent of randomly selected pups responded to ICH vaccination at 6 weeks of age, 75 per cent responded at 8 to 10 weeks and more than 95 per cent responded to vaccination at 12 weeks of age or older. Maternal antibody has occasionally persisted for as long as 16 weeks, but such cases are uncommon.

Materials available for immunization include concentrated and unconcentrated antiserum and vaccines that are either living or inactivated virus preparations.

**Antiserum.** Antiserum and globulin concentrates usually possess combined ICH, distemper and leptospiral antibodies. Although dosage rates have not been standardized, most antiserum preparations have adequate levels of antibody against CAV-1. Subcutaneous administration at recommended dosage levels provides temporary protection; however, the period of protection is variable and uncertain. Antiserum for protection against ICH is not recommended, since use of a modified live virus vaccine at intervals will accomplish the same goal without the problem of blocking active immunization. Sufficient antibody blocks immunization by both modified live virus vaccines and inactivated virus vaccines, despite a report to the contrary regarding effectiveness of inactivated CAV-1 vaccines in the presence of (maternally transferred) antibody.

**Inactivated Virus Vaccines.** These products are usually prepared from infected cell cultures, although formalin-inactivated suspensions of infected canine tissues have been used. Experiments have failed to confirm the claim that inactivated virus vaccines could be effectively given in the presence of passively transmitted antibody.

Inactivated vaccines are safe and effective. They do not provide the long-term immunity afforded by attenuated viral vaccines; however, they do not cause uveitis or corneal reactions ("blue eye"). Laboratory studies have not shown active immunity to last more than four months after two doses of inactivated (tissue culture origin, formalin-inactivated) vaccine. It is possible that longer protection is afforded by products containing adjuvants.

**Modified Live (Attenuated) Virus Vaccines.** Attenuated live virus vaccines are prepared from CAV-1 grown in swine or canine cell cultures. They have proved effective in reducing the incidence of clinical ICH; however, uveitis and corneal edema may occur one to two weeks after vaccination. Although extremely uncommon, permanent corneal damage, secondary glaucoma with buphthalmos and loss of vision have occurred as consequences of vaccination with attenuated virus vaccines. Eye reactions usually resolve spontaneously without treatment, other than palliative, within a few days (sometimes weeks) after the onset. The use of CAV-2 to eliminate ocular reactions is now being studied extensively. As noted above, cross-protection against CAV-1 by CAV-2 is complete.

**Recommended Vaccination Procedures.** Vaccination against ICH is recommended at the time of distemper immunization. Most veterinarians use multiple-component modified live virus vaccines. The duration of immunity to ICH is long; however, annual revaccination generally is recommended even though only a small proportion of immune dogs will lose their immunity within one year. This is usually done regardless of intent, since "boosters" for canine distemper usually contain modified CAV-1.

Pups older than 3 months of age should be given one dose of living attenuated virus vaccine or an inactivated product that contains an adjuvant. Two doses of an aqueous inactivated vaccine are required. If the pup is younger than 3 months of age, two or more doses should be given: one after the pup is weaned and the last at 12 to 16 weeks of age.

## SUPPLEMENTAL READING

Appel, M., *et al.*: Current status of canine respiratory disease. 20th Gaines Veterinary Symposium, Manhattan, Kansas, 1970, pp. 15–24.
Appel, M., *et al.*: Pathogenicity of low virulence strains of two canine adenovirus types. Am. J. Vet. Res., *34*:543–550, 1973.
Cabasso, V. J., and Wilner, B. I.: Adenoviruses in animals other than man. Adv. Vet. Sci. Comp. Med., *13*:160–219, 1969.
Carmichael, L. E., Medic, B. L. S., Bistner, S. I., and Aguirre, G. D.: Viral-antibody complexes in canine adenovirus type 1 (CAV-1) ocular lesions: Leukocyte chemotaxis and enzyme release. Cornell Vet., *65*:331–351, 1975.
Fastier, L. B., and Ott, R. L.: Infectious canine hepatitis. *In* Kirk, R. W. (ed.): Current Veterinary Therapy IV. Philadelphia, W. B. Saunders Co., 1971.
Symposium on immunity to selected canine infectious diseases. J. Am. Vet. Med. Assn., *156*:175–182, 1970.

# FELINE INFECTIOUS PERITONITIS

JACK M. GASKIN, D.V.M.
*Gainesville, Florida*

Feline infectious peritonitis (FIP) is a progressive, debilitating disease. Its mortality rate approaches 100 per cent. Although first described in 1963 as chronic fibrinous peritonitis, it was characterized as an infectious entity and was given the present name in 1966. FIP has been diagnosed in domestic cats in many places throughout the world; a few cases have been recognized in large exotic cats in zoos. At present no animals other than those in the family Felidae are known to be susceptible.

Many authorities believe that FIP has been increasing in incidence in the United States, notwithstanding more effective surveillance and reporting. Retrospective analysis has indicated that the earliest cases were seen in the Boston (Massachusetts), Davis (California) and New York City areas in 1953, 1954 and 1956, respectively. At present, FIP occurs throughout the United States and is most troublesome in catteries or multiple-cat households, in which it may spread insidiously and cause significant death loss.

## ETIOLOGY

Electron microscopic and ultrafiltration studies indicate that FIP is viral in origin. As yet the agent has not been isolated *in vitro*, but attempts at utilization of feline macrophage cultures may be successful, since ultrastructural studies of infected tissues have revealed virus particles associated with that particular cell type. One report has suggested that the virus closely resembles members of the coronavirus group and notably mouse hepatitis virus, which causes vasculitis, peritonitis and lymphoid necrosis in mice.

## EPIZOOTIOLOGY

Epizootiologic studies of FIP have not been conclusive. Experimental transmission has been achieved chiefly through parenteral inoculation of infective exudates, blood or tissue suspensions. In one instance, one of three kittens fed urine from an afflicted cat became sick. However, other studies have not uniformly demonstrated the infectivity of urine. The natural route or mechanism of transmission remains unknown.

The incubation period, as estimated from instances in which multiple cases have occurred on the same premises, may be as long as 4 to 5 months. However, the disease does not always spread readily to in-contact cats. One predisposing factor may be the immunosuppressive effect of infection with feline leukemia virus. It has been demonstrated that approximately 50 per cent of cats that died of infectious peritonitis were concurrently infected with leukemia virus.

Recently, the occurrence of FIP in a closed breeding colony has been described (Potkay *et al.*, 1974). In contrast to other reports that have indicated no seasonal incidence, most cases in this particular colony occurred in the fall and winter months, when there was an influx of house mice. Although this seasonal occurrence might have been related to the onset of cold weather and its stresses, the possible role of rodents as vectors of FIP could not be excluded. However, there have been instances of FIP developing in some (but not all) members of litters of kittens reared in isolation facilities in which no exposure to rodents has been possible.

The vast majority of cases of FIP occur in cats less than one year of age, although the disease has been recognized in cats as old as 18 years. Possibly, the agent of FIP is widespread and is encountered by many cats at a rather young age. It may produce subclinical infection in most cats but clinical signs and death in an unlucky few.

## CLINICAL SIGNS

FIP is a disease of many faces. Its primary manifestations may reflect involvement of different body systems, and both effusive and noneffusive forms occur. Classically, FIP is characterized by fibrinous peritoneal and/or pleural exudation, depression, fever, loss of weight and progressive debility. Clinical signs in the noneffusive form are generally referable to neurologic and/or ophthalmologic abnormalities reflecting meningoencephalitis and/or panophthalmitis, respectively.

Affected cats usually become sick insidiously, and initial signs such as intermittent anorexia, dehydration, listlessness and weight loss are nonspecific. In early cases, generalized abdominal sensitivity and enlarged mesenteric lymph nodes may sometimes be noted upon palpation. Usually afflicted cats are febrile, with body temperatures ranging from 103.0° to 105.0° F. (39.5° to 40.6° C.). If peritoneal effusion occurs, the abdomen may become conspicuously distended; this is often the reason affected cats are presented for examination. If peritoneal effusion is extensive enough to interfere with respiration, or if pleural effusion occurs, labored breathing may result. As the disease progresses, inappetence be-

comes complete, and emaciation and debility ensue. Jaundice is occasionally seen. Remarkably, many cats continue to purr and respond appreciatively to stroking up to the terminal stages of illness.

Cats with the noneffusive form also exhibit listlessness, anorexia, dehydration and fever. Involvement of the eyes may be manifested in the anterior ocular segment by chemosis, corneal edema, keratic precipitates, hyphema, floaters, aqueous flare, synechia and iridocyclitis. Posterior ocular signs include choroiditis and retinitis. Vasculitis results in exudation of cells and proteinaceous material that may partially obscure engorged and tortuous retinal vessels and lead to retinal detachment, with resultant blindness. Nervous manifestations include nystagmus, disorientation, incoordination, increased muscular rigidity, paresis, paralysis and seizures.

The course of FIP is progressive but considerably variable in duration. Although most cats die within 2 to 5 weeks, some have lingered beyond 3 months.

## DIAGNOSIS

The effusive form of FIP must be distinguished from other conditions associated with the accumulation of pleural or peritoneal fluids. Thoracic fluids may be produced by injuries, cardiac insufficiencies, empyema, chylothorax and neoplasia. Abdominal fluid accumulations occur with bacterial peritonitis, pansteatitis, toxoplasmosis, chylous ascites, congestive heart failure, liver disease, glomerulonephritis and neoplasia. Tuberculosis, although exceedingly rare in cats in the United States, may produce either pleuritis or peritonitis.

The exudate associated with FIP is very characteristic, and its analysis is a useful aid in differential diagnosis. The color generally varies from pale to dark yellow but may be greenish or bloody. The fluid is usually clear or only slightly cloudy and may contain occasional small white flecks of fibrin. The specific gravity usually exceeds 1.017, and some samples may clot upon exposure to air. Total white cell counts are often less than 1000/cu. mm., and differential counts vary with the stage of the disease. Neutrophils predominate in more acute cases, while mononuclear cells (lymphocytes, plasma cells, macrophages and mesothelial cells) are more numerous in chronic cases. The protein content of the exudate approximates that of serum, and the globulin fractions, especially gamma globulin, are elevated at the expense of albumin.

Hematologic analysis is of limited usefulness as a diagnostic tool in FIP. White blood cell counts may be normal, elevated or depressed. Generally there is a mild lymphopenia and a relative neutrophilia with a regenerative shift. Inclusion bodies have been reported to occur in approximately 1 per cent of circulating neutrophils of a low percentage of afflicted cats. Some cats develop a microcytic anemia, which becomes more severe when the course of the disease is prolonged. Total serum protein values are often elevated, and there is a decrease in the albumin/globulin ratio. In most cases there is a relative, and in some an absolute, hypergammaglobulinemia.

Early cases of the effusive form (i.e., before fluid exudate is obtainable) and many cases of the noneffusive form present a diagnostic challenge. Persistence of fever in spite of antibiotic therapy is suggestive, although this may also occur in such conditions as toxoplasmosis, pansteatitis and aleukemic lymphoma. Cats with the noneffusive form (and some with the effusive form) may develop a variety of nervous or ocular abnormalities. Taken in the context of the entire history and clinical picture, these may also be suggestive of a diagnosis of FIP.

The noneffusive form of FIP often involves the kidneys, which may be enlarged, nodular and readily palpable upon physical examination. Exploratory surgery may reveal raised granulomatous lesions on these as well as other abdominal viscera. An organ punch biopsy method for antemortem diagnosis of noneffusive FIP has recently been described (Abel and Johnson).

## TREATMENT

Feline infectious peritonitis is a frustrating disease. Although numerous treatment regimens have been applied, none has proved satisfactory. Only three patients have been reported to have responded to therapy. Tylosin, at 10 mg./kg., complemented with prednisolone, up to 0.25 mg./kg., both given orally twice daily, was utilized with supportive fluid and vitamin therapy as needed (Colgrove and Parker). Although a gradual reversal of clinical signs was reported over a treatment period of 40 to 80 days, application of this regimen in other cases has not been successful. Owners should be counseled that the prognosis is grave; at the owner's request, treatment should be instituted, and the patient should be made as comfortable as possible. Drainage of effusion should be attempted if the volume is sufficient to cause dyspnea or obvious discomfort. Antibacterial therapy, because of the debilitating nature of the disease, and corticosteroid therapy, to reduce inflammation, are indicated. Fluid therapy and enforced alimentation should be applied as needed.

## PROGNOSIS

Experience has demonstrated that nearly all cases of FIP end in death. If attempts at treatment fail to stabilize or improve the condition of an animal, euthanasia should be recommended. Death with dignity must certainly be a prerogative for that noble companion animal, the cat.

## PROPHYLAXIS

As yet, the etiologic agent of FIP has not been isolated and defined. Much remains to be discovered concerning the maintenance of the agent in nature and the means of transmission of the natural disease. Until such information is available, no specific recommendations can be made concerning the prevention or circumvention of this tragic disease. Experimental inactivated crude tissue vaccines, similar to those used in early work with feline panleukopenia, have failed to protect cats against FIP, although it must be recognized that the status of their antigenicity is not known and the constitution of a fair challenge with infective FIP material has not been established.

The virus that has been visualized in the tissues of experimentally infected cats by means of electron microscopy is an enveloped virus and should be susceptible to inactivation by drying and other adverse environmental influences. If this virus truly represents the agent of FIP, it is unlikely to survive for long outside the infected cat. Several investigators have commented that the disease transmits inefficiently and that proximity of infected and noninfected cats appears to have only slight bearing on the incidence of FIP. Some degree of natural immunity seems to be operative. Considering our present state of knowledge, it seems prudent to recommend isolation of inf cats and careful disinfection of quarters that may be contaminated. Hopefully, fruitful future research will provide some needed answers to the FIP dilemma.

## SUPPLEMENTAL READING

Abel, D. L., and Johnson, J. J.: Parenchymal FIP: Antemortem diagnosis by punch biopsy. Feline Pract., 5:44–50, 1975.
Campbell, L. H., and Reed, C.: Ocular signs associated with feline infectious peritonitis in two cats. Feline Pract., 5:32–35, 1975.
Colgrove, D. J., and Parker, A. J.: Feline infectious peritonitis. J. Small Animal Pract., 12:225–232, 1971.
Feldman, B. F.: Feline infectious peritonitis: A case report of a variant form. Feline Pract., 4:32–33 and 36–37, 1974.
Pedersen, N. C.: Feline infectious peritonitis: Something old, something new. Feline Pract., 6:42–51, 1976.
Potkay, S., Bacher, J. D., and Pitts, T. W.: Feline infectious peritonitis in a closed breeding colony. Lab Anim. Sci., 24:279–289, 1974.

# CANINE DISTEMPER

MAX APPEL, D.V.M.
*Ithaca, New York*

Canine distemper (CD) is an acute or subacute, contagious, febrile virus disease of dogs and other carnivores, with a worldwide distribution. Few dogs in isolated areas have not been exposed to the virus. Besides rabies, canine distemper is the only viral disease in dogs with a high percentage of fatalities. Since effective CD vaccines have become available, the disease has been well controlled in domestic and zoo carnivores; however, certain wildlife species and unvaccinated carnivores continue to spread the virus, which makes eradication virtually impossible.

## ETIOLOGY

Canine distemper is caused by a paramyxovirus, a large RNA virus closely related to measles and rinderpest viruses. All isolated CD viruses belong to one serotype. CDV is very sensitive to heat inactivation; however, it persists for several days at 4° C. and can remain viable for many years in a frozen state.

Although serologically indistinguishable, the different CD isolates vary in the duration and type of disease that they produce. Some strains cause a mild, transient disease in dogs; others cause an acute disease with a high mortality rate, with or without acute ~~phalitis~~; still others frequently cause ~~encephalitis~~ after a clinically mild ~~signs~~ of recovery from acute ~~response~~ in individual dogs

also varies greatly; however, experimental results with these strain differences have been consistent. All strains of virulent CDV have an immonosuppressive effect in dogs that has not been found after CD vaccination. Therefore, pneumonia and enteritis, caused by secondary bacterial and mycoplasma infections, toxoplasma, coccidia, etc., often complicate CD. *Bordetella bronchiseptica* is commonly involved. In spite of the earlier report by Carré in 1905 of the viral nature of canine distemper, *B. bronchiseptica* was believed to cause canine distemper until the situation was shown to be otherwise by Laidlaw and Dunkin in the late 1920's.

## EPIDEMIOLOGY

Canine distemper is a ubiquitous disease that produces a long-lasting active immunity. CD is enzootic throughout the world. In spite of very effective attenuated virus vaccines and extensive vaccination of dogs, CDV is still prevalent. Unvaccinated dogs and many wildlife species are susceptible to CDV and may carry and spread the disease. The natural host range includes all animals in the Canidae family (e.g., dingo, fox, coyote, wolf, jackal), the Mustelidae family (e.g., ferret, mink, skunk, badger, marten, weasel, otter) and the Procyonidae family, (e.g., raccoon, panda, kinkajou, coati). Experimentally, cats, pigs, monkeys, hamsters and mice became infected. All body excretions from infected animals contain virus, and it spreads rapidly from animal to animal by droplet infection and aerosols. During recovery, dogs may shed virus for several weeks, but once the dog is fully recovered, virus shedding ceases completely. Attenuated CD vaccine virus does not spread from dog to dog.

Incidence is highest in young dogs, but dogs of all ages may become infected. Young dogs become susceptible to CDV when they lose maternal antibody. Most puppies lose maternal antibody between 8 and 12 weeks of age. Young dogs between 3 and 6 months of age, therefore, are most often affected by the disease. Disease incidence decreases with age. Subclinical CD infections were estimated in 75 per cent of a dog population in Sweden by Rockborn.

In general, canine distemper induces life-long immunity. Attenuated live CD virus vaccines in most dogs induce long-range immunity as well. However, some dogs lose neutralizing antibody several months after vaccination, and there are reports of vaccinated dogs developing distemper later in life. Seasonal prevalence in the spring and fall has been observed by some investigators; however, some reports indicate year-round incidence. In most countries a constant supply of pups throughout the year maintains infection in the dog population.

## CLINICAL SIGNS

Canine distemper is an acute, febrile disease with fever beginning 3 to 6 days after exposure and lasting for only one or two days. The temperature curve is diphasic, the second rise occurring several days to several weeks after exposure, depending upon the strain. With the onset of the second temperature rise, conjunctivitis, rhinitis and gastrointestinal and respiratory signs may occur. Coryza, vomiting, diarrhea and coughing are seen in these dogs. Dogs with acute distemper are often anorectic and sometimes extremely dehydrated. Skin rashes that are sometimes seen are probably an allergic response to the virus infection. These signs are not seen in the mild transient form of CD. Lymphopenia occurs several days after exposure to all virulent strains and remains in acute disease, until death or recovery. It may not be found in cases of delayed encephalitis.

Nervous signs occur in dogs in either an acute or a more subacute form. Single signs suggesting local brain or cord lesions may occur, but more often multiple signs are observed. Convulsive seizures, incoordination, pacing, circling and psychic changes are most common in acute distemper. Disturbances in gait and posture, including ataxia, asynergy, paresis and others, can be seen. Rhythmic motor movements, usually called chorea, tic, tremor or myoclonus, are common neurologic signs during distemper or occur as a residual phenomenon. Optic nerve damage and retinal and retinochoroidal lesions can often be seen, with the majority of lesions in the peripheral and midperipheral nontapetal fundus. In some cases, optic neuritis is found initially as the sole clinical sign, later followed by progressive central nervous system lesions. Transient keratitis may be seen in CD. In some dogs with distemper encephalitis, hardening of footpads occurs. The frequent occurrence of this in Europe in the late 1940's prompted investigators to believe that this disease is caused by a different virus. Later, it was clearly shown that hard-pad disease is caused by distemper virus.

A disease syndrome in middle-aged to older dogs, so-called "old dog encephalitis" or subacute diffuse sclerosing encephalomyelitis, was postulated by Lincoln in 1971 to be caused by CDV. The disease is characterized by progressive motor and mental deterioration that is ultimately fatal. In a few of these cases viral antigen has been seen by means of fluorescent antibody and electron microscopy, but virus has not been isolated.

Clinical signs in foxes and mink are similar to signs in dogs. Canine distemper in foxes was often found to be complicated by *Salmonella*. Mortality in adult mink varies considerably, but kits have a mortality rate of close to 100 per cent, similar to ferrets.

## DIAGNOSIS

The general picture of canine distemper has changed since attenuated virus vaccines and antibiotics are now commonly used. Vaccines may have controlled CD viral strains that induce a rapid disease course better than they have controlled strains that cause delayed disease, because viral shedding continues for a long period of time in delayed cases. Use of antibiotics has reduced bronchopneumonia and enteritis due to secondary invaders. Less acute cases are seen, therefore, and in many dogs with subacute encephalitis, diagnosis is difficult. It can be attempted as follows:

**Clinical Signs.** Although none of the clinical signs mentioned in the previous section is pathognomonic for distemper, a combination of signs helps in the diagnosis of the disease. Presence of nervous manifestations in combination with elevated temperature and/or respiratory signs, diarrhea, catarrhal or mucopurulent discharges from eye and nose or hyperkeratosis of footpads is highly indicative of canine distemper. Differential white blood counts are most helpful, because in all acute cases and in many subacute cases of canine distemper lymphopenia is prevalent. Blood smears stained with new methylene blue can be rapidly evaluated. Eye examinations should be performed to detect the presence of retinopathies, optic neuritis or transient keratitis. Skin rashes may be seen in some animals.

**Fluorescent Antibody Test.** The direct or indirect FA test can be used for demonstration of distemper viral antigen. Because vaccine virus replicates only in lymphatic tissues in dogs, presence of viral antigen in surface epithelium is indicative of virulent virus. Imprints from mucous membranes are usually used for this test. Care should be taken to avoid a smearing effect in order to keep cells intact. Owing to nonspecific artifacts, diagnosis can be made only if viral antigen is clearly demonstrable within cells. Buffy coat cells and cells from CSF can also be used for this test. These tests are usually positive in acute distemper cases; however, in many subacute encephalitis cases, in which neutralizing antibody is present in dogs, either viral antigen has disappeared from peripheral cells and persists in the brain, or viral antigen is masked by distemper neutralizing antibody from the host. Viral antigen appeared to persist longer in footpads. The FA test of footpad biopsy specimens may be helpful.

**Inclusion Bodies.** Intracytoplasmic eosinophilic inclusion bodies in imprint preparations of conjunctival or vaginal tissues are considered pathognomonic for CD. In acute cases the FA test is superior to the inclusion body test, because it is more sensitive and more viral antigen is demonstrated; however, inclusion bodies tend to persist longer than demonstrable distemper viral antigen in cells and are less influenced by circulating neutralizing antibody.

**Virus Isolation.** For a long time secretions or tissue suspensions from infected dogs were inoculated into susceptible ferrets. When distemper virus was present in the inoculum, ferrets died from distemper between 10 and 14 days after inoculation. When the effect could be neutralized by pretreating the inoculum with specific CD antibody, the diagnosis was confirmed. Some distemper viral strains have a prolonged incubation period in ferrets; however, on a serologic basis no difference can be demonstrated. More recently, tissue culture systems have been employed for the isolation of virulent distemper virus. Canine macrophages are best suited for virulent distemper virus isolation. From 2 to 5 days after inoculation, giant cells appear in these cultures. Virus can be isolated from nasal or conjunctival swabs and from cerebrospinal fluid from dogs with acute distemper encephalitis. Special laboratory procedures are required for culturing these cells, and isolation attempts are negative from dogs with neutralizing antibody.

**Serology.** Serologic examination can be used for the diagnosis of canine distemper, but not in all cases. Paired serum samples are only useful in dogs that recover, because dogs dying from acute CD may never have antibody to CDV. The demonstration of CD antibody in cerebrospinal fluid is indicative of canine distemper. Vaccinated dogs and dogs that recover early from canine distemper do not have CD antibody in cerebrospinal fluid. Dogs dying from acute distemper and acute encephalitis may not have neutralizing antibody in serum or in cerebrospinal fluid. Dogs with subacute distemper encephalitis often have high serum antibody titers as well as neutralizing antibody in cerebrospinal fluid. However, simultaneous presence of albumin in CSF would indicate a nonspecific blood-brain barrier damage. Presence of complement-fixing antibody in serum is also indicative of a recent distemper infection. It persists only for several months after distemper in contrast to neutralizing antibody, which may persist for a lifetime.

**Serum Proteins.** A decrease in the serum albumin fraction and an increase in the alpha-2 fraction during initial and advanced stages of CD in dogs have been re-

virulent virus, hyperimmune serum can be used for this purpose up to 3 days post exposure. If serum with a titer of 1:3000 is used, 1 ml. is sufficient per 5 kg. of body weight to protect susceptible pups for 10 days against challenge virus. Because active intravenous immunization is effective for up to 4 days after exposure to virulent virus, it is the preferred choice.

Prophylaxis includes isolation of young pups from the dog population until the vaccine becomes effective.

## SUPPLEMENTAL READING

Appel, M., and Gillespie, J. H.: Canine Distemper Virus. Virology Monographs 11. New York and Wien, Springer Verlag, 1972.
Gorham, J. R.: Canine distemper. Adv. Vet. Sci., 6:287–351, 1960.
McGrath, J. T.: Distemper complex. In McGrath, J. T.: Neurologic Examination of the Dog. 2nd ed. Philadelphia, Lea & Febiger, 1960, pp. 127–136.
Wright, N. G., Cornwell, H. J. C., Thompson, H., and Lauder, I. M.: Canine distemper: Current concepts in laboratory and clinical diagnosis. Vet. Rec., 94:86–92, 1974.

# FELINE SALMONELLOSIS

JOHN F. TIMONEY, JR., M.R.C.V.S.
*Ithaca, New York*

Clinical salmonellosis is unusual in the cat, and few documented cases exist in the literature up to the present time. Surveys of salmonella carrier rates indicate that less than 2 per cent of cats in some studies and none at all in others are positive on rectal swab testing. Such low carrier rates are in marked contrast to the much higher rates often observed in other domestic species, including the dog. It would seem that the cat has a high natural resistance to infection by salmonellas and therefore seldom manifests clinical disease. Recent experience, however, indicates that this high resistance may be overcome by the stress of hospitalization and surgery or by grouping in laboratory holding facilities. Hospital-acquired (nosocomial) infections may result in epidemics of severe clinical salmonellosis with a high mortality in young cats.

## ETIOLOGY

*Salmonella typhimurium* is the serotype usually isolated from cats with the clinical disease, but other serotypes have occasionally been isolated from rectal swabs of healthy cats. The disease is difficult to reproduce experimentally even with fresh isolates taken from diseased cats, perhaps because of the difficulty of experimentally mimicking the stress that triggers the clinical disease observed in animal hospitals. The index cat may have had the clinical disease or have been a carrier when admitted, the stress of hospitalization converting the carrier state to the clinical disease; the outbreak then proceeds by cat-to-cat transmission. Other species suffering from salmonellosis may also be a source of infection for the cat.

## CLINICAL SIGNS

The disease is usually observed in cats less than a year old, about 5 days after admission to the hospital for such reasons as routine surgery, boarding or a medical problem unrelated to salmonellosis. In some cases the disease may appear as soon as 2 days after admission. The typical clinical picture is one of gastroenteritis with fever. There is lassitude, variation in appetite gradually leading to complete loss, fluctuation in temperature with peaks as high as 106° F. (41° C.), pallor of buccal mucous membranes, halitosis and loss of weight. Some cats drool excessively during the illness. Diarrhea and vomiting occur together in about 90 per cent of cases; in the others, there is either vomiting or diarrhea alone. The vomiting may be persistent, leading to dehydration and achlorhydria. Bile may be present in the vomitus. The feces may contain mucus and blood.

During an outbreak the morbidity may be 33 per cent and mortality can be in excess of 50 per cent. Nonfatal cases recover slowly.

Some cats experience a temporary recovery, are sent home and then suffer a sudden relapse and die within a few hours.

## LABORATORY FINDINGS

The outstanding change in the hemogram is a marked drop in WBC. Levels of WBC as low as 2500/cu. mm. may be observed in affected cats. Toxic changes are present in neutrophils. The marked leukopenia is apparently due to exhaustion of the bone marrow pool and is possibly an effect of endotoxin released from salmonellas during the process of digestion by phagocytic cells. As the animal recovers, the lymphocyte count begins to rise, followed by an increase in the neutrophil count. Serum protein is often decreased to levels as low as 3.5 g./100 ml. Percentage of MCHC may be reduced in some cases.

Bacteriologic culture of fecal specimens or rectal swabs during the earlier phase of the disease reveals large numbers of *S. typhimurium*. The organism is also present in large numbers in the mouths of affected cats, and oral swabs are positive. The heart-blood, spleen, liver and intestinal contents are positive when cultured at necropsy. Strains of *S. typhimurium* isolated from cases of feline salmonellosis often possess an R factor type antibiotic resistance to drugs such as kanamycin, ampicillin, tetracycline and streptomycin. Most strains, however, are sensitive to chloramphenicol.

Recovered cats may continue to shed salmonella in the feces for 4 weeks, but most cats have ceased to shed by about 10 days after recovery. Cats in contact with carrier animals may, themselves, become infected and shed the organism for about 7 days afterward without developing any clinical signs. Seroconversion is the rule in cats that recover, and Salmonella O and H titers in excess of 1:40 are found in sera 2 weeks after recovery. Seroconversion may or may not take place in infected cats that have not had clinical disease. Thus, serologic examination of cats to distinguish carrier animals is not reliable.

## PATHOLOGY

Necropsy of cats that die or are euthanatized *in extremis* reveals a wasted and dehydrated carcass, particularly if the animal has been ailing for some days. Mucous membranes are blanched, and the intestines exhibit a diffuse hemorrhagic enteritis, with contents tinged with blood and mucus. The parenchymatous organs may be normal but the liver frequently contains small necrotic foci about 2 mm. in diameter. The serous cavities may contain blood-tinged fluid.

## DIFFERENTIAL DIAGNOSIS

Feline salmonellosis, panleukopenia and *E. coli* enteritis have many clinical and laboratory features in common that may lead to confusion in diagnosis. Vaccination history, examination of hemogram, bacteriologic and viral examination of rectal and oral swabs will usually be very helpful in diagnosis. In the case of panleukopenia, the leukopenia is characterized by an almost complete absence of neutrophils, whereas in salmonellosis and *E. coli* enteritis some neutrophils remain. In the case of *E. coli* enteritis there is usually no vomiting.

## CONTROL CONSIDERATIONS

Feline salmonellosis is highly contagious in hospital environments, and strict isolation of suspected cats must be maintained. Separate instruments and utensils should be kept with each patient and sterilized after use. The index cat is usually either a clinical case admitted with a history of gastroenteritis or a carrier cat that develops clinical disease as a result of the stress of hospitalization or the debilitating effects of another illness. However, it is possible that contaminated feed or exposure to another animal species suffering from salmonellosis or to an attendant who is a carrier or is experiencing clinical salmonellosis may serve as a source of infection and should be considered during investigation of an outbreak. Since salmonellas appear to be shed in large numbers from the buccal cavity, the grooming habits of the cat cause the coat of the animal to become highly contaminated, and thus the attendant or owner caring for the animal may be dangerously exposed. Such persons should be advised of this hazard and should wear disposable gloves and protective aprons that can be removed after handling of the animal. The hands should be thoroughly washed and disinfected after sick cats or their litter and feed pans are handled.

## TREATMENT

An antibacterial agent should be administered parenterally and orally. Chloramphenicol and trimethoprim are excellent drugs for this purpose. Antibiotic sensitivity testing should be performed on isolates during the illness to check for development of new resistances. The amount of fluid lost through vomiting and diarrhea should be restored by means of oral or parenteral administration of electrolyte solutions. Such a solution should contain a high chloride level to replace losses of this ion during emesis. Dextrose (5 per cent) should also be provided to correct the endotoxin-mediated hypoglycemia. Ionosol G® (gastric) (Abbott) or Ringer's solution is a suitable solution for this purpose and is given at the rate of 20 to 40 ml./kg. body weight every 12 hours. In order to counteract endotoxin-mediated intestinal vasoconstriction, acetylpromazine should be given at 1.0 mg./kg. It should be remembered that adrenaline is contraindicated in treatment of endotoxic shock. Blood transfusion to replace white blood cells and hydrocortisone, 20 mg./kg., are also valuable aids in the correction of endotoxic shock. (See articles on "Fluid Therapy" and "Shock: Pathophysiology and Management.")

### SUPPLEMENTAL READING

Borland, E. D.: Salmonella infection in dogs, cats, tortoises and terrapins. Vet. Rec., 96:401–402, 1975.
Buxton, A., and Field, H. L.: Salmonella infection in farm livestock. Report of the 14th International Veterinary Congress, London, 2:270–280, 1969.
Timoney, J. F., Neibert, H. C., and Scott, F. W.: Feline salmonellosis: A nosocomial outbreak and experimental studies. Cornell Vet., in press, 1977.

# CANINE BRUCELLOSIS

LELAND E. CARMICHAEL, D.V.M.
*Ithaca, New York*

Brucellosis in dogs due to *Brucella canis* (*B. canis*) has been recognized since 1966, when widespread abortions were observed in colonies of beagles. Since that time, the disease has been diagnosed in various breeds, and its occurrence has been recorded on several continents. Although the disease is widespread in the United States, the reported incidence rates vary from approximately 1 to 6 per cent, depending on the area sampled and the type of diagnostic test employed.

The recent availability of a rapid slide test has made *presumptive* diagnosis of this disease relatively simple; however, the occasional occurrence of nonspecific agglutination when the stained antigen (Canine Brucellosis Diagnostic Test, [Pitman-Moore]) is mixed with a patient's serum emphasizes that the plate (slide) test should not be the only criterion applied in the diagnosis of this disease. False positive reactions have been observed with a small proportion of sera obtained from cases proved by extensive bacteriologic and serologic studies to be noninfected.

Since no treatment for the disease is certain, and the implications are very serious for dogs proved to be infected, vigorous attempts to establish a diagnosis by all available means should be made before an animal is declared infected. Unfortunately, there have been many instances when inadequate diagnostic procedures were applied and dogs were needlessly destroyed. Each individual case deserves extensive study. A basic knowledge of the general nature of brucellosis and the insidious nature of the disease in the dog, especially in the nonpregnant female and in apparently normal males, is important. Many fundamental questions about the *Brucella*-host interaction remain unanswered; however, the supplemental reading list includes useful references that should be consulted to amplify the brief description presented here.

## ETIOLOGY

The disease is caused by a small gram-negative coccobacillus that grows aerobically on enriched media, such as Albimi Brucella broth and agar or tryptose media. Growth is slow, requiring 48 to 72 hours for colonies to form. Unlike certain other *Brucella* spp., growth of *B. canis* is inhibited by $CO_2$. After several days' incubation, growth of translucent colonies becomes very mucoid (ropy in broth). Because of the mucoid ("rough") nature of the organism, it does not possess the smooth antigens of *B. abortus* or *B. melitensis*, and the usual brucellosis test antigens that are available for diagnosis of the disease in other domestic species are useless. *Brucella canis* cross-reacts extensively with *B. ovis*, rough variants of other *Brucella* species and additional bacterial species such as *Actinobacillus equuli*. Cross-reactions with unidentified microorganisms may give rise to nonspecific agglutinins and confuse the serodiagnosis. Biochemically, the canine brucella is similar to *B. suis*. Especially useful diagnostic characteristics, in addition to cultural and morphologic aspects, are dye inhibition reactions (no growth on basic fuchsin; growth in the presence of thionin) and the rapid production of urease by *B. canis*.

## EPIDEMIOLOGY

Since the initial recognition of the disease in commercial and private breeding kennels in 1966, the disease has been found to be widespread in the dog population throughout the United States. Accurate incidence rates are not available, since uniform test procedures have not been established; however, an "average incidence" appears to be about 1.5 per cent. Incidence rates of 5 to 6 per cent have been reported in the southern United States. The disease is not confined to the United States, for it now has been confirmed in Japan, Mexico, Germany, Czechoslovakia and, most recently, Brazil. Serologic evidence of the disease has been reported in Peru and Tunisia. Outbreaks in Czechoslovakia and Japan occurred after importation of infected dogs from the United States.

Transmission occurs principally by way of infectious vaginal discharges or mammary secretions following an abortion, and by the seminal fluids of infected males at the time of breeding. Spread via urine or other discharges is possible but is unproved and not likely. Males may shed organisms in semen for weeks or months after apparent recovery, presenting a formidable diagnostic challenge. Dogs are the only known natural host, although foxes were proved to be highly susceptible in experimental inoculations. As noted below, there have been human infections.

## CLINICAL SIGNS

Clinical signs in bitches include abortion after the 30th day of gestation, most commonly between the 45th and 55th day. Occasional litters may be born with some pups alive and some dead. Early embryonic deaths with termination of pregnancy may occur, suggesting to the owner that the bitch had failed to conceive. Generalized lymph node enlargement, principally due to reticular cell hyperplasia, is common in both sexes.

*Brucella canis* can be isolated readily from the blood or vaginal discharges of infected animals and from the fetal and placental tissues. Prolonged bacteremia, often lasting more than two years, is a notable feature of the canine disease. After several months' infection, bacteremia may be intermittent.

An important aspect of the disease in males is infertility. Between the second and fifth weeks after infection, abnormal sperm (30 to 80 per cent) are evident, with bent tails, swollen midpieces and distal protoplasmic droplets; by 20 weeks postexposure by the oral route, more than 90 per cent of the sperm may be abnormal, with severe reduction in motility. Neutrophils and monocytes are common in the ejaculate, and detached heads are evident. Clumps of spermatozoa with head-to-head agglutination are readily observed. Spermagglutinins have been found in both serum and seminal fluid samples from infected males. Brucella organisms may be isolated from ejaculated semen in abundance during the second month after infection; however, the number of organisms decreases rapidly after this time. Shedding is sporadic thereafter; however, organisms have been recovered from semen of infected dogs for as long as 60 weeks. The prostate gland is an abundant source of the organisms. In the male, epididymitis and orchitis, often followed by testicular atrophy, are common.

It is important to recognize that many infected animals appear normal, even though they may have bacteremia. There is no fever. Agglutinins appear in the serum approximately three weeks following oral infection and persist at high levels (titer value will depend on the particular test system employed) until recovery commences, typically one year or longer. Recovered animals are immune to reinfection.

## DIAGNOSIS

A diagnosis should not be made until adequate clinical, serologic and bacterial examinations are carried out. A history of abortions, infertility, testicular abnormalities (epididymitis, atrophy), poor semen quality or lymph node enlargement with or without these signs should lead to consideration of *B. canis* infection.

A rapid slide agglutination test that produces *presumptive* diagnostic information in a few minutes is now available (Pitman-Moore). This test is rapid and has proved to be highly accurate in identifying noninfected animals, for false negative reactions have not been observed. As noted above, false positive reactions have been found and the slide test should always be followed by additional examination. Several laboratories offer diagnostic assistance; however, there is no standardized procedure, and interpretation of tube agglutination test results varies.* Serum samples must be clear and not contaminated. It is not possible to interpret agglutination test results on sera from dogs that have received antibiotic treatment for brucellosis, unless an interval of at least four weeks has elapsed since cessation of treatment. One test requires incubation of serum dilutions and antigen for 48 hours at 52° C.; another test uses 2-mercaptoethanol. The latter gives slightly (about twofold) lower titers, but nonspecific reactions are reduced.

Serologic evidence of infection (generally indicated by tube agglutination test titers in excess of 1:200 or 2-mercaptoethanol titers

in excess of 1:100) should always be followed by attempts to isolate the organism by cultures of blood or by culture of lymph node or bone marrow biopsy specimens. Because of the serious prognosis, especially regarding use of an infected dog for breeding purposes, all available diagnostic aids should be employed.

## TREATMENT

There is no certain treatment; however, some success has been achieved experimentally. Evaluation of any treatment regimen must be followed by periodic bacteriologic and serologic tests, since early apparent success in treating the disease often has proved disappointing, even though a period of abacteremia may have occurred for a few weeks after cessation of a course of antibiotic therapy. The goal of treatment is to eliminate the organism from the infected animal—a difficult task for all brucella infections. Treatment may be considered in cases where it is made clear to the owner that the procedure is expensive in both cost and time and that success cannot be assured. Follow-up blood cultures and serologic tests are essential. These should be performed 6 to 8 weeks after cessation of any treatment.

Several treatment schedules have been tried, and most have been unsuccessful; however, the following have been claimed successful in some instances:

1. Tetracycline hydrochloride given orally (t.i.d.) for three weeks at 60 mg./kg. body weight/day. Treatment is discontinued for 3 to 4 weeks. A second course of tetracycline hydrochloride is then given, together with streptomycin (40 mg./kg/day, b.i.d.) with and without sulfadimethoxine (50 mg./kg., once daily).

2. Minocycline hydrochloride given orally (b.i.d.) for 14 days at 50 mg./kg. body weight/day. Simultaneous IM administration of streptomycin (20 mg./kg./day, b.i.d.) is given for the first 7 days and then discontinued. This treatment resulted in complete clearance of *B. canis* from the tissues of four of five treated female animals examined at necropsy six weeks after cessation of treatment. In the animal that did not show complete clearance, a few colonies of *B. canis* were isolated only from cultures of spleen.

Only intensive treatment schedules such as those described above have proved suc-

---

*The Diagnostic Laboratory, New York State College of Veterinary Medicine, Ithaca, New York 14853, offers a *B. canis* diagnostic service, where positive reactions in one laboratory are confirmed by additional tests in an independent facility. Diagnostic assistance also may be obtained from the Veterinary Services Diagnostic Laboratory, U.S.D.A., Ames, Iowa 50010. Instructions for shipping serum samples or blood for culture may be obtained from the Biologics Reagents Section, V.S.D.L., Ames, Iowa 50010.

cessful. Additional trials using newer antibiotics found inhibitory for *B. canis* in *in-vitro* tests are under study. Eradication of organisms from the prostate tissue of infected males has not been reported.

## CONTROL

Control and prophylactic measures should include the use of serum agglutination tests, blood cultures, isolation and removal of infected animals, good sanitation and common sense.

All females that have aborted or failed to conceive after successive matings, or males with genital disease, should be considered to be possibly infected with *B. canis*. Such dogs should be isolated immediately, and a serum sample should be taken and tested by the slide or tube agglutination test. Blood should be cultured. Dogs with positive blood cultures in a breeding kennel should be destroyed. Treatment may be considered for valuable pets and working dogs; however, owners should be advised of the cost and the uncertain outcome. Control within a breeding kennel consists of serologic testing and, if possible, blood cultures, with elimination of all positive animals. Repeated tests at monthly intervals should be performed on all dogs in a colony with infected animals. Animals found to be positive should be removed, and at least three negative monthly tests should be obtained on all dogs before a kennel can be considered negative. All dogs introduced into a kennel, especially if they are to be used for breeding, should be maintained in separate quarters until at least two negative tests, done at monthly intervals, are obtained. The entire kennel should be cleaned and disinfected daily. Roccal® (Winthrop) solu-tion and Wescodyne® (West Chemical) have proved to be bactericidal. Animal handlers should wear disposable gloves. Hands should be rinsed in disinfectant before each animal is examined for heat. Animals with titers that arouse suspicion should not be introduced into a kennel unless repeated tests indicate nonspecific agglutinins.

Bacterins are not available for prophylaxis.

## PUBLIC HEALTH ASPECTS

Human infections have been observed. At the present writing, 14 human cases have been reported. Six were laboratory workers. All have been relatively mild, and infected individuals responded well to tetracycline therapy. Headache, fatigue, enlarged regional lymph nodes without splenomegaly and mild fever were the principal signs. The owners of infected dogs should be informed of the public health risk but should not be alarmed, since man, like other non-canine species, appears relatively resistant.

### SUPPLEMENTAL READING

Carmichael, L. E., and Kenney, R. M.: Canine brucellosis: the clinical disease and immune response. J. Am. Vet. Med. Assn., 156:1726–1734, 1970.

Fredrickson, L. E., and Barton, C. E.: A serologic survey for canine brucellosis in a metropolitan area. J. Am. Vet. Med. Assn., 165:987–989, 1974.

Lewis, G. E.: Canine brucellosis. *In* Kirk, R. W., (ed.): Current Veterinary Therapy V. Philadelphia, W. B. Saunders Co., 1974, pp. 974–976.

Moore, J. A., and Gupta, B. N.: Epizootiology, diagnosis, and control of *Brucella canis*. J. Am. Vet. Med. Assn., 156:1737–1740, 1970.

Pickerill, P. A., and Carmichael, L. E.: Canine brucellosis: control programs in commercial kennels and effects on reproduction. J. Am. Vet. Med. Assn., 160:1607–1615, 1972.

# TOXOPLASMOSIS

J. K. FRENKEL, M.D.
*Kansas City, Kansas*

Recognition of the life cycle of *Toxoplasma* permits a broader understanding of how domestic animals and man develop toxoplasmosis, either as an infection or as disease. The essentials of the life cycle and transmission are shown in Figure 1.

## COCCIDIAN PHASE

*Toxoplasma* is an intestinal coccidian of cats, with oocysts measuring $10 \times 12$ microns which, like *Isospora*, develop two sporocysts, each containing four

POSTULATED TRANSMISSION OF TOXOPLASMOSIS

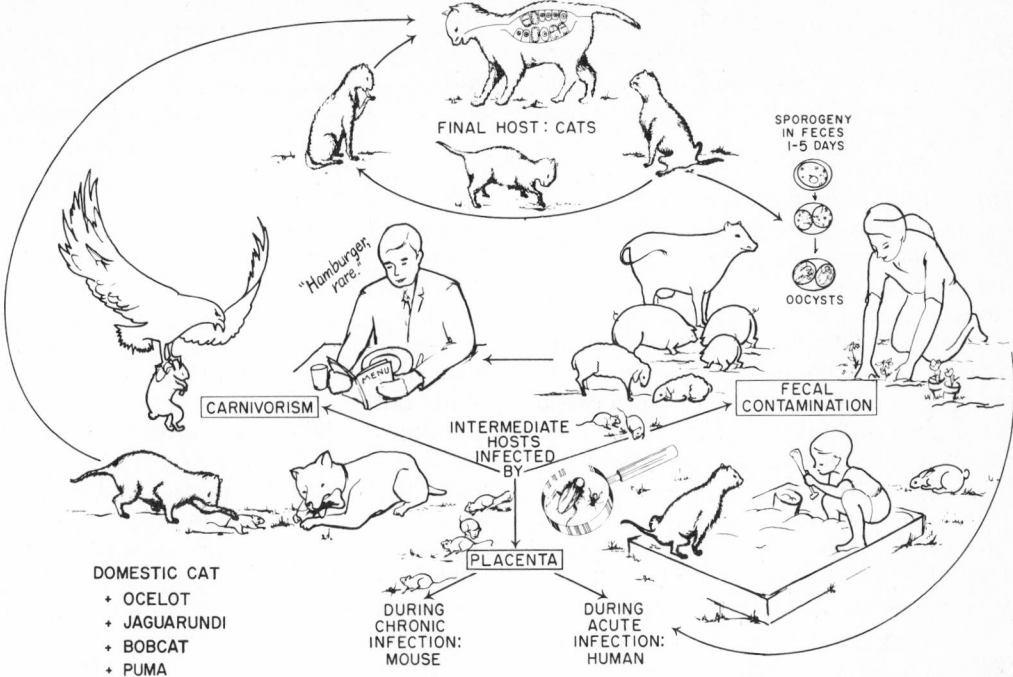

**Figure 1.**   Postulated life cycle of *Toxoplasma*. Cats and certain other felines are shown as final hosts, and other animals and humans as intermediate hosts. Flies and cockroaches can serve as transport hosts. At *right*, infection with oocysts is shown. At *left*, transmission by carnivorism is indicated. *Below*, the transplacental route of transmission is suggested. (Modified from Frenkel, J. K.: Toxoplasmosis. *In* Marcial-Rojas, R. A. (ed.): Pathology of Protozoal and Helminthic Diseases. Baltimore, The Williams & Wilkins Co., 1971, pp. 254–290. By permission of The Williams & Wilkins Co.)

sporozoites. Their size can be compared with two diameters of human red blood cells suspended in saline, and they are smaller than the common *Isospora felis* (40 × 30 microns) and *Isospora rivolta* (25 × 20 microns). Judging from studies available at present, only Felidae can reasonably be suspected of shedding *Toxoplasma* oocysts. There is no experimental support for the commonly held view that similarly sized coccidia of dogs and cats are identical. Although *Isospora* oocysts in cats that are shed unsporulated and measuring 10 × 12 μm. are not diagnostic, they should be presumed to be *Toxoplasma* until proved otherwise. The oocyst of *Hammondia hammondi* is of similar size and gives rise to muscle cysts in mice. Oocysts or sporocysts that are shed sporulated are likely to belong to a species of *Sarcocystis**.

*The author would be pleased to receive such oocysts for verification (University of Kansas Medical Center).

## STAGES

Acute infection generally leads to the formation of tachyzoites (rapidly multiplying forms), groups of which are found in many organs. As immunity develops, cysts are formed, containing bradyzoites (slowly multiplying forms) which become resting stages. Only in Felidae do oocysts and sporozoites develop.

## GENERALIZED TOXOPLASMOSIS

Generalized toxoplasmosis, involving extraintestinal tissues, is found in many birds and mammals, including cats. Infection occurs by ingestion of the oocyst, especially in herbivores; by ingestion of the cyst from infected meat; and occasionally transplacentally (Fig. 1).

## ASYMPTOMATIC INFECTION

*Toxoplasma* antibodies have been found in 40 to 60 per cent of cats in the Kansas-

Iowa area, in 24 per cent of dogs in the United States, in 6 to 56 per cent of sheep in the United States, in about 10 per cent of pigeons from the Capitol in Washington, D.C., in 10 per cent of wild rats in Birmingham, Alabama, and in a variable percentage of monkeys. Although we cannot be certain that all of these represent specific antibody and persisting infections, *Toxoplasma* has been recovered repeatedly from such animals, so that much credence should be given to such figures. In the human population of the United States, *Toxoplasma* antibody is acquired at a rate of 0.5 to 1 per cent per year of age. A greater prevalence is observed in France where meat is often eaten raw or slightly seared, and in moist tropical countries where cats are common and oocyst survival in the soil is good. The general prevalence is low in humans from dry and hot areas (Arizona) and in cold areas (Alaska); this should be similar in animals. However, in cats antibody rates are generally much higher than in humans when compared by age.

## LESIONS OF SYMPTOMATIC TOXOPLASMOSIS

Many organs are parasitized by *Toxoplasma*; when lesions become numerous, clinical signs and symptoms develop. Almost all infections are acquired via the gastrointestinal tract. In *acute* infection, the intestine may be significantly involved. In cats, enteroepithelial stages lead to gametocytes and oocysts, but the lesions are generally not serious. More advanced lesions may be seen in mice, puppies and marmosets in which tachyzoites may destroy epithelial cells, the lamina propria and submucosa. Clinically, diarrhea may be present. From the intestine, there is hematogenous and lymphogenous dissemination to many organs. The *liver* often contains focal necrotic lesions, occasionally leading to significant hepatitis with jaundice. The *lungs* are a favorite site for the multiplication of *Toxoplasma*, giving rise to interstitial and alveolar pneumonia which can become visible radiographically. The *lymph nodes*, especially those which drain the gut and the lungs, often show much proliferation of tachyzoites with tissue necrosis. There may be histologic *myocarditis* and *myositis* occasionally becoming clinically apparent. Ordinarily immunity is promptly acquired.

*Subacute* and *chronic* infections often involve the brain. At first, tachyzoites multiply in neurons, astrocytes and vascular structures, and lead to microglial nodules and occasionally infarcts, with signs of encephalitis. Retinitis is also found occasionally. In addition, *Toxoplasma* cysts develop, containing slowly multiplying bradyzoites which may persist for months and years. From time to time, a cyst ruptures and, in the presence of hypersensitivity, can give rise to significant tissue necrosis, although few if any *Toxoplasma* enter new cells. Lesions from cyst rupture are most likely to be symptomatic in the retina, brain and heart.

**Relapse.** When immunity wanes with passage of time or in consequence of treatment with corticosteroids, bradyzoites released by cyst rupture enter new cells and start to multiply as tachyzoites. This may lead to severe and often fatal encephalitis, pneumonia, myocarditis, retinochoroiditis and sometimes other lesions.

A variety of *signs and symptoms* have been reported, although asymptomatic infection is most common.

1. In *cats:* fever, bilirubinemia, mesenteric adenitis, dyspnea, diffuse pneumonia, leukopenia, anemia, iritis, retinitis, encephalitis and intestinal obstruction due to granuloma.
2. In *dogs:* pneumonia, hepatitis, encephalitis.
3. In *monkeys:* pneumonia, hepatitis, encephalitis.
4. In *pigs:* dyspnea, lymphadenitis, necrotizing enteritis, ataxia, paralysis, encephalitis and retinitis.
5. In *sheep:* dyspnea, pneumonia, encephalitis, abortion.
6. In *cattle:* dyspnea, cough, fever, encephalitic symptoms.
7. In *pigeons:* apathy, staggering gait, torticollis, encephalitis, chorioretinitis, conjunctivitis.
8. In *chickens:* encephalitis, circling gait, retinochoroiditis.
9. In *turkeys:* progressive encephalitis with emaciation.
10. In *chinchillas:* encephalitis.
11. In *silver foxes* and *mink:* pneumonia, encephalitis.
12. In *kangaroos:* rhinitis, apathy, dyspnea, paralysis, encephalitis.

In other animals, similar signs can be expected. Generalized disease and signs in the extraneural viscera are associated usually with acute infection, and nervous and ocular signs are associated with chronic infection.

## PUBLIC HEALTH PROBLEMS

**Cats.** After primary infection, cats and kittens may shed thousands to millions of *Toxoplasma* oocysts over a period of 10 to 14 days. After sporulation in one to five days, these oocysts are highly infectious to other animals and man. Antibodies are generally developed only toward the end of the period of oocyst production. Cats develop some immunity and, on reinfection, will shed few oocysts for a short period of time, or none at all. Oocysts in cat feces remain viable for a prolonged period of time, several months in moist soil, sand and water. They may persist in incompletely cleaned and disinfected litterpans for several months. Stray cats that live by hunting, especially of birds and small mammals, appear to be most important in the epidemiology of toxoplasmosis, since they contaminate the soil and sand piles, particularly around human habitations, with oocysts which may survive for a prolonged period of time. If a cat is found to shed oocysts measuring $10 \times 12$ microns, it is well to isolate it for a few days, and to carefully dispose of the feces until the oocysts cease to be present.

**Meat.** Infection of meat is variable, probably depending on animal maintenance practices, on contact with cats in barns and near watering places, and on the contamination of foodstuff with cat feces. Animals fed raw meat, such as dogs and other carnivorous pets, can acquire the infection. In addition, domestic and wild cats fed raw meat may develop the sexual stages, as mentioned above.

## DIAGNOSIS

Identification of oocysts in the feces of cats, a rising antibody titer and isolation of the organism are useful in making a clinical diagnosis.

1. *Fecal examination* in cats can be carried out by one of the usual flotation procedures, or by the following simplified method which can be followed by animal inoculation:

### MATERIAL NEEDED

| | |
|---|---|
| Plastic, paper or glass containers of 250 ml. | Rubber bulbs |
| | Containers to discard material and pipettes |
| Pipettes of 5 and 10 ml. | |
| Pasteur pipettes | |
| Wide-mouth centrifuge tubes of 50 ml. | Scissors |
| | Centrifuge |
| Bottles of 2 oz. | Slides and coverslips |
| Tongue depressors | Microscope |
| Gauze | |

### SOLUTIONS NEEDED

Sucrose, 1.15 specific gravity; 53 gm. cane sugar and 100 ml. water; with phenol 0.8 per cent wt./vol. (floating solution)

Sulfuric acid, 2 per cent vol./vol., 0.413 N (to preserve oocysts)

Sodium hydroxide, 3.3 per cent wt./vol., with 2 per cent phenol red (to neutralize oocyst suspension before injection into mice)

### METHODS

1. Collect the fecal specimen in a container, paper or plastic cup, or a beaker of 250 ml.; moisten with water and leave for an hour or two without agitation.
2. Discard the water; the feces should now be fairly soft.
3. If fat droplets are visible, thoroughly mix with tongue depressor 5 to 10 gm. feces in 50 ml. tapwater; centrifuge at 3000 to 6000 rpm for 10 minutes, and discard supernatant. If fat is not visible, proceed to step 4.
4. Emulsify 5 to 10 gm. of feces with a tongue depressor in about 60 ml. of sucrose solution.
5. Filter through three layers of gauze directly into centrifuge tubes of 50 ml., or use a funnel.
6. Balance tubes with sucrose solution; centrifuge at about 3000 rpm for 10 minutes.
7. With a Pasteur pipette, collect from the very surface of the solution about 0.5 to 1 ml.; put 1 drop on a slide and check it microscopically. Put the rest in a 2-oz. bottle containing 5 ml. of 2 per cent sulfuric acid to kill bacteria and to provide a better environment for oxygenation and for sporulation. The bottle can be capped after 30 minutes. Maintain at room temperature.
8. Three to five days should be allowed for sporulation. If the specimen is to be inoculated into mice, the sulfuric acid is neutralized with an equal amount of 3.3 per cent sodium hydroxide (NaOH) containing about 2 per cent of phenol red. After adding the major portion, add the remainder of NaOH drop-wise until the color changes from yellow to orange, which is the end point.
9. Since any oocysts present are now infectious, inject them carefully into mice, by the intraperitoneal route, applying 7 per cent of iodine in alcohol to the injection site, following withdrawal of the needle.
10. Follow the animals until death; bleed survivors after three weeks and have the sera serologically examined by the dye test, indirect fluorescent antibody test or agglutination tests. (See also isolation of *Toxoplasma*.)

2. *Serologic examination* should consist of two serum samples taken a week or more apart, which are compared in the same serologic test. The dye test is most versatile but requires human serum without antibody as accessory factor. The indirect fluorescent antibody test is sensitive and specific, but requires the appropriate antispecies serum free of antibody. The agglutination test requires large numbers of organisms but no additional serum. If antibody titers are found to rise by three to four tubes, this is presumptive evidence of concurrent toxoplasmosis. If antibody is absent in both tests, this excludes *Toxoplasma* as an etiologic agent in the observed disease; so does a stable antibody titer, if the symptoms are acute. However, retinochoroiditis is generally associated with a stable antibody titer. It should be noted that cats generally develop lower antibody titers than dogs, humans, etc., and that they develop antibody only towards the end of the period of oocyst production.

3. *Isolation of Toxoplasma* is best carried out by inoculating suspected material into mice. After intraperitoneal injection, exudate may be formed in which the crescentic tachyzoites may be seen after four to six days. If no organisms are found, such exudate, spleen, liver, lungs and lymph nodes can be subinoculated every four days into fresh mice to raise the level of organisms to one that is visible on smears and sections. Mice that die after 10 days should be examined for the presence of cysts in the brain; cysts are easily seen after about four weeks. The diagnosis should always be based on smears stained with Giemsa, or sections stained with hematoxylin, since the examination of fresh material often yields spurious results. Alternately, mice can be examined for antibody after three weeks.

### TREATMENT

Sulfadiazine and pyrimethamine (Daraprim® [Burroughs Wellcome]) interfere in sequential steps with the biosynthesis of dihydrofolate, and they act synergistically against *Toxoplasma*. Furthermore, the toxic side effects can be prevented and alleviated with yeast and folinic acid (Leucovorin® [Lederle]), the inhibited product, which mammals can use but *Toxoplasma* cannot. Hence, drugs and inhibitor can be given together.

*Sulfadiazine* is quickly excreted and the daily dose is given in four to six divided doses. For some animals, it can be incorporated into food or, as the sodium salt, into drinking water.

Sulfamerazine and sulfamethazine are also effective, and so are certain other sulfonamides dissolved in significant quantities in the intracellular fluid where *Toxoplasma* multiplies (e.g., sulfalene, sulfadoxine). However, other sulfonamides, such as sulfisoxazole and sulfadimetine, are not effective against *Toxoplasma*, since they are distributed almost entirely in the extracellular fluid space; sulfathalidine is not absorbed and so is not effective.

*Pyrimethamine* is slowly excreted and can be given once daily. A double loading dose can be given for the first three days of treatment.

As a general guide, Table 1 indicates the doses in food or water that can be administered, as may be most suitable (by mouth, in food or water, or intravenously) for a given animal species. These doses have been used mainly in mice, hamsters, cats and man. If it is known that the drugs are metabolized faster or slower by a given animal species, the doses should be modified accordingly. The shedding of oocysts by kittens can be nearly eliminated by treating with 120 mg./kg./day of sulfadiazine by itself, or by 60 mg./kg./day of sulfadiazine together with 0.5 mg./kg./day of pyrimethamine.

Treatment is directed at the symptoms of

*Table 1.* *Chemotherapy of Toxoplasmosis*

| DRUGS | DOSAGE |
|---|---|
| Sulfadiazine* (divided in four to six daily doses) | 60 mg./kg. animal/day |
| Pyrimethamine (Daraprim) | 0.5 to 1.0 mg./kg. animal/day |

| ANTAGONISTS† | DOSAGE |
|---|---|
| Folinic acid | 1 mg./kg. animal/day |
| Baker's yeast | 100 mg./kg. animal/day |

*Sulfamerazine, sulfamethazine, sulfalene and sulfadoxne may be substituted.

†Antagonists are used when the platelets or white blood count drops to one-half or one-quarter of what is normal for the species. Antagonists can be given together with the treatment, or prophylactically. Their need has not been established for most animals.

*If treatment with both drugs exceeds two weeks, platelet and white blood cell counts are advised.*

disease, until immunity is acquired and can control the infection. *The mere presence of antibody does not indicate disease or need of treatment.* The most life-threatening lesions requiring control are usually in brain and lungs. The enteric stages in cats usually produce little disease, since ulceration is rare, but they are also suppressed by the sulfadiazine-pyrimethamine treatment outlined. Several experimental coccidiostats were active against *Toxoplasma* in cell culture, and lasalocid was found to depress oocyst production in cats; however, they have not been shown to be effective against life-threatening lesions as is the sulfadiazine-pyrimethamine combination.

The treatment should be started as soon as diagnosis is probable, since a delay until diagnosis is confirmed may be fatal. All clinical symptoms of toxoplasmosis indicate deficient immunity, and the purpose of chemotherapy is to control further damage to the host until immunity is acquired. Young animals tend to be especially vulnerable and immunodeficient. Unless irreversible lesions are present when treatment is started, some clinical improvement is usually apparent in two to three days; if not, the diagnosis is doubtful. Chemotherapy should be continued beyond abatement of symptoms, and a duration of about two weeks is suggested. The drug combination is inhibitory but does not eradicate infection.

The chemotherapeutic regimen is toxic to the embryo and fetus; hence, pregnant animals should always be treated with the antagonists also. Retinochoroiditis as an isolated manifestation should be treated as outlined, and corticosteroids may be added without necessity to increase the drug dose. In immunosuppressed animals, the drug doses shown in able 1 can be used, since the drugs act independently of host immunity mechanisms. As the pharmacologic doses of corticosteroids commonly produce a relapse of chronic latent toxoplasmosis, chemotherapy could be given prophylactically; sulfadiazine alone has been found sufficient.

## PREVENTION

Animals are infected with *Toxoplasma* by the cyst stage from meat, the oocyst stage from cats and soil, or tachyzoites transplacentally. Preventive measures are specifically directed at each one. *Cysts* are present in the muscle and brain of chronically infected animals. Hence, carnivores should be fed with meat that has been heated thoroughly to over 150° F. (66° C.), or with dried or canned food. Hands should be washed after handling raw meat to remove cyst organisms from the skin. In zoos, large carnivores which eat raw meat are exposed to infection, and cooked meat should be substituted if possible.

"Indoor cats" should be restrained from hunting birds and mice, not only to prevent their becoming infected themselves, but to prevent their becoming a source of contamination to their owners. Litterpans should be cleaned daily before oocysts have sporulated and become infectious. Litterpans can be sterilized with boiling water or dry heat (150° F.). No practical chemical disinfectant is available. Feces should be disposed of in a toilet or burned, but not placed in garbage. Plastic gloves should be worn by persons particularly vulnerable, such as pregnant women.

"Outdoor cats" and wild felines which eat raw meat can become infected themselves and should be regarded as potentially infectious. This can be important in a zoo environment where cats may be caged near neotropical monkeys or kangaroos which, when they become infected, often die. Prevention of a zoo epidemic depends on control of the feces of such wild felines and of feral cats roaming the zoo. Brooms to clean cat cages which are used in other cages can be a vehicle of transmission of such oocysts. Also, cats may contaminate foodstuffs in bins or storage containers.

Flies, cockroaches and other coprophagous animals can serve as transport hosts of *Toxoplasma*. They must be controlled and access to food prevented.

Soil and sand contaminated by cat feces can remain infectious for many months. There is no practical manner of disinfection. Direct exposure to sun may, by heat and drying, accelerate attrition of oocysts. Exposure to 150° F. (66° C.) kills oocysts. Children's sandboxes should be covered when not in use. Handwashing is advised after contact with soil and sand, before eating and before touching mucous membranes.

If their food can be controlled, cats can be kept as relatively safe pets in regard to toxoplasmosis. Few people give up consistent pleasures for infrequent diseases. However, an infectious cat exposes not only its owner but neighbors as well. Stray cats present an important public health problem. Leash laws and fences, which provide a measure of protection against infection of children with larva migrans from dog ascarids, are not applicable to feral or stray cats, whose control by enforced legislation is essential if one wishes to curb the spread of toxoplasmosis in animals and man. Immune cats (those with antibody) are safer pets than nonimmunes, since on reinfection they shed few oocysts for short periods of time, or none at all. Development of a vaccine is in progress.

## SUPPLEMENTAL READING

Frenkel, J. K.: Toxoplasmosis: parasite life cycle, pathology, and immunology. In Hammond, D. M., and Long, P. L. (eds.): The Coccidia. Eimeria, Isospora, Toxoplasma, and Related Genera. Baltimore, University Park Press, 1973, pp. 343–410.

Frenkel, J. K., and Dubey, J. P.: Toxoplasmosis and its prevention in cats and man. J. Infect. Dis., 126:664–673, 1972.

Frenkel, J. K., Ruiz, A., and Chinchilla, M.: Soil survival of Toxoplasma oocysts in Kansas and Costa Rica. Am. J. Trop. Med. Hyg., 24:439–443, 1975.

Petrak, M., and Carpenter, J.: Feline toxoplasmosis. J. Am. Vet. Med. Assn., 146:728–734, 1965.

Siim, J., Biering-Sorenson, U., and Møller, T.: Toxoplasmosis in domestic animals. Adv. Vet. Sci. Comp. Med., 8:335–429, 1963.

# THE SYSTEMIC MYCOSES

DANNY W. SCOTT, D.V.M.
*Ithaca, New York*

The systemic mycoses of small animals (blastomycosis, coccidioidomycosis, cryptococcosis, histoplasmosis) are caused by fungi that are basically saprophytic and live in soil or organic debris. These diseases are not thought to be contagious. Infections are usually contracted via inhalation of infectious spores or mycelial fragments and rarely via skin penetration or ingestion. The organisms spread via the bloodstream, lymphatics and direct extension. The lesions caused by these infections are characterized by granulomatous inflammation, abscessation, ulceration, necrosis, fistulous tracts, fibrosis and nodule formation. Most infections develop slowly, and the course is chronic. Most of the diseases have a definite geographic distribution. The fungi involved in these infections (except cryptococcosis) are dimorphic, being mycelial at 25° C. and yeastlike at 37° C. These fungi (except *Cryptococcus neoformans*) reportedly cause disease much more commonly in dogs than in cats.

It is currently thought that cellular immunity is more important than humoral immunity in resistance to fungal infections. Most authorities believe that systemic mycoses become established more easily in debilitated, immunodeficient or immunosuppressed animals. Thus, a thorough search is indicated to rule out underlying immunosuppressive factors of endogenous or exogenous nature (malignancies, drug therapy, dysproteinemias, debilitation, etc.). Affected cats should be tested for feline leukemia virus infection, which is known to suppress cell-mediated immune responses. The deliberate impairment of immune responses (corticosteroid and anticancer therapy) has created another setting for infection by "opportunistic" fungi. It is safe speculation that systemic mycotic infection will continue to be an increasing cause of animal disease.

## NORTH AMERICAN BLASTOMYCOSIS (GILCHRIST'S DISEASE)

**Definition.** North American blastomycosis is a chronic systemic fungal disease, respiratory in origin, which frequently disseminates to the eyes and skin and occasionally to bone and other organs.

**Etiology and Epidemiology.** *Blastomyces dermatitidis* is a dimorphic fungus, appearing as a budding yeast (8 to 15 $\mu$, and rarely 30 $\mu$, in diameter) in tissues. The fungus is limited in geographic distribution to areas near the Great Lakes and the Mississippi and St. Lawrence River Valleys. The saprophytic source of the fungus in nature is not known.

**Clinical Signs.** Blastomycosis is a chronic wasting disease, affecting dogs more commonly than cats. The most frequent sites of infection are the lungs and the bronchial and mediastinal lymph nodes. Affected animals usually present with a chronic cough (dry or moist), persistent or phasic pyrexia (103° to 105°F.), poor appetite and weight loss. In one report, of 33 dogs experimentally infected via the natural airborne route, 32 (97 per cent) developed ocular lesions and 23 (70 per cent) developed skin lesions. Cutaneous involvement is characterized by subcutaneous pyogranulomas, abscesses and fistulas that originate as small papules. Skeletal involvement occurs in about 7 per cent of the cases and is characterized by lameness, soft tissue swelling, draining tracts and rarefying osteomyelitis.

## COCCIDIOIDOMYCOSIS (SAN JOAQUIN VALLEY FEVER)

**Definition.** Coccidioidomycosis is a chronic systemic fungal disease, usually respiratory in origin. In most cases, it is arrested in the lungs, but it may spread to virtually all organs or tissues.

**Etiology and Epidemiology.** *Coccidioides immitis* is a soilborne, dimorphic fungus, appearing as a nonbudding yeast in tissues. (Spherules are 20 to 100 $\mu$ in diameter and contain few to many endospores 2 to 5 $\mu$ in diameter.) The fungus is limited in geographic distribution to the southwest United States (Lower Sonoran Life Zones).

**Clinical Signs.** Coccidioidomycosis is a chronic wasting disease, affecting dogs more commonly than cats. The most frequent sites of infection are the lungs and the bronchial and mediastinal lymph nodes. Affected animals usually present with a chronic cough (dry), dyspnea, persistent or phasic pyrexia (103° to 105° F.), poor appetite and weight loss. The disseminated form of the disease appears to occur most commonly in boxers and Doberman pinschers, two months to two years of age, often three to five weeks after a primary respiratory disease. Bone lesions are often seen, characterized by lameness, soft tissue swelling, draining tracts and proliferative osteomyelitis. Bone lesions frequently begin in the epiphyseal areas, especially in the metacarpal and metatarsal bones.

## CRYPTOCOCCOSIS (TORULOSIS, EUROPEAN BLASTOMYCOSIS)

**Definition.** Cryptococcosis is a chronic systemic fungal infection, usually respiratory in origin, with a predilection for the central nervous system and the upper respiratory tract.

**Etiology and Epidemiology.** *Cryptococcus neoformans* is a soilborne fungus, occurring only in the yeast form, and appearing as a budding yeast (4 to 7 $\mu$ in diameter, with a thick polysaccharide capsule) in tissues. The fungus is ubiquitous in geographic distribution, and pigeon excreta are often sited as the source of infection. Pigeons are not infected naturally, but their excreta act as a good nutrient medium for the fungus. *C. neoformans* can live in pigeon excreta for two to five years and can be carried on the beaks and feet of pigeons.

**Clinical Signs.** Cryptococcosis affects the central nervous system and upper respiratory tract most commonly. Dogs and cats are affected with equal frequency. CNS signs are variable, depending on the area(s) of the brain involved. Upper respiratory tract involvement usually consists of chronic rhinitis and sinusitis, or nasopharyngeal granulomas. Cutaneous lesions are characterized by fluctuant, dome-shaped, frequently ulcerated granulomas, in which a grayish, gelatinous exudate is usually found.

## HISTOPLASMOSIS

**Definition.** Histoplasmosis is a chronic systemic fungal disease, usually respiratory in origin, with a marked predilection for reticuloendothelial tissue.

**Etiology and Epidemiology.** *Histoplasma capsulatum* is a soilborne, dimorphic fungus, appearing as a budding yeast (2 to 4 $\mu$ in diameter) in tissues. The fungus is limited in geographic distribution to areas near the Great Lakes, the Appalachian Mountains and the Mississippi, Ohio and St. Lawrence River Valleys. Soil contaminated by the dung of chickens, other birds and bats is especially rich in organisms.

**Clinical Signs.** Histoplasmosis is a chronic wasting disease, affecting dogs more commonly than cats. The most frequent sites of infection are the lungs and the bronchial and mediastinal lymph nodes. Affected animals usually present with a chronic cough (dry or moist), dyspnea, persistent or phasic pyrexia (103° to 106° F.), poor appetite and weight loss. An intestinal form is commonly seen and may be characterized by an intractable enterocolitis (often bloody), enlarged mesenteric lymph nodes, hepatosplenomegaly, jaundice, ascites, anemia, emaciation and pyrexia. A lymphoid form may be seen, in which generalized lymphadenopathy, pyrexia and anemia are seen.

## DIAGNOSIS OF THE SYSTEMIC MYCOSES

Historoclinical and laboratory findings vary with the organs and tissues affected. Moreover, historical, physical and most laboratory findings are suggestive and supportive, but not definitive.

Radiographic findings in the pulmonary forms of these diseases are quite suggestive and include hilar lymphadenopathy; peribronchial infiltrations; and a metastatic, nodular, interstitial lung pattern. Differential diagnosis would include neoplasia, actinomycosis and nocardiosis, and some bacterial pneumonias.

Routine hematologic and biochemical parameters are quite variable and undiagnostic. Many serologic antibody titer tests are available (precipitin, complement fixation, latex particle agglutination, agar gel immunodiffusion) but vary in reliability. Results may be negative in early or severe cases. Also, titers should usually be determined twice (10 to 14 days apart) in order to demonstrate a more diagnostic rise in titer.

Skin testing antigens (blastomycin, coccidioidin, cryptococcin, histoplasmin) are available for the demonstration of delayed-type hypersensitivity cutaneous reactions to the fungi. Test accuracy is hampered by (1) cross-reactions between the involved fungi, (2) anergy in disseminated cases and (3) positive reactions that indicate only exposure to the fungi (present or past). Most surveys indicate that 40 to 90 per cent of animals in endemic areas have positive skin test reactions.

Definitive diagnosis can only be made by isolation in culture or microscopic identification of the fungi. The fungi may be cultured on Sabouraud's, brain-heart infusion, blood or Littman's agars. Materials selected for culture and microscopy will vary with the tissues involved and might include sputum, feces, blood, urine, cerebrospinal fluid and cutaneous lesions. Direct smears and cultures of bronchial washings in the pulmonary forms of these diseases are positive in about 50 per cent of the cases. In such cases, pleural lavage with small amounts of physiologic saline followed by direct smears or cultures of the retrieved lavage fluid might be helpful. Biopsy and histopathologic examination of affected tissues is the most consistently diagnostic procedure. Histopathologic sections should be stained with specific fungal stains (periodic acid–Schiff, Gridley's, Bauer's, Gomori's methenamine silver), since the fungal elements are often difficult to differentiate from other cellular and tissue elements in routine hematoxylin-and-eosin–stained sections.

## TREATMENT AND PROGNOSIS OF THE SYSTEMIC MYCOSES

As is the case in so many diseases, the earlier the diagnosis can be made, and the more localized the infection, the greater are the chances for success. Prognosis also varies somewhat with the fungus involved. The primary respiratory forms of coccidioidomycosis and histoplasmosis are usually self-limiting and recover spontaneously or with symptomatic and supportive therapy. It is likely that about 90 per cent of these respiratory infections are terminated without specific antifungal therapy. However, the respiratory forms of blastomycosis and cryptococcosis are usually chronic and progressive, and the disseminated forms of all the systemic mycoses are usually fatal if not treated.

Therapy consists of combined surgical and chemotherapeutic techniques, when applicable. Amphotericin B (Fungizone® [Squibb]) is the drug of choice for the treatment of blastomycosis, coccidioidomycosis and histoplasmosis. The drug is a polyene antibiotic with fungistatic and fungicidal activity. Its mechanism of action involves binding with sterols in the cell membrane, resulting in leakage of potassium ions and other intracellular components and eventual lysis of sensitive fungi. Cerebrospinal fluid levels are poor, approximately 1/10 those of plasma. The drug should be reconstituted with 5 per cent dextrose in water, since solutions containing sodium chloride or preservatives inactivate it. Once reconstituted, amphotericin B may be kept for 7 days in a dark refrigerator.

The two main shortcomings of amphotericin B have been (1) the development of resistant strains of fungi and (2) toxic side effects. Toxic side effects reported in man are numerous and include hypersensitivity reactions, chills, fever, phlebitis, anemia, nausea, vomiting, anorexia, headache, nephrotoxicity, thrombocytopenia, grand mal seizures, cardiac arrest, ventricular fibrillation, hypokalemia and hepatic failure. The most common and significant toxic side effects in the dog and cat are (1) nephrotoxicity (distal tubular damage and vasoconstriction of renal arteries), (2) hypokalemia, (3) anemia (normocytic-normochromic) and (4) phlebitis. Acute toxicity to the kidney is strictly dose-dependent, but great variation exists between patients. From 80 to 100 per cent of humans treated with a therapeutic course of amphotericin B develop decreased renal function with azotemia. Many have permanent renal damage. Renal manifestations usually disappear when therapy is stopped, even though histologic lesions may persist.

Several therapeutic schedules have been recommended. Most regimens in man involve intravenous injections over a 45-minute to 6-hour interval with 500 ml. of 5 per cent dextrose in water. Rapid intravenous infusion or intraperitoneal injection techniques have been used most commonly in dogs. Because of the expense and logistic problems involved with dogs and cats (hospitalization, intravenous catheters, prolonged infusions) and the lack of convincing evidence in support of the efficacy and safety of any particular therapeutic regimen in dogs and cats, the rapid intravenous infusion technique is recommended. Recommended dosage is 0.5 to 1.0 mg./kg. dissolved in 5 to 10 ml. of 5 per cent dextrose, given three times per week by rapid intravenous injection. Dosages larger than 2.0 mg./kg. can result in hyperkalemia with associated cardiac arrhythmia and cardiac arrest. Pretreatment with small doses of phenothiazine tranquilizers or antihistamines may reduce nausea and vomiting, when these are seen. Blood urea nitrogen (BUN) should be monitored once or twice weekly, and complete blood count (CBC) every two weeks. Therapy must be discontinued temporarily if the BUN exceeds 75 mg. per 100 ml. Care must be taken to insure that an adequate potassium intake is maintained. Therapy with amphotericin B should be continued for four weeks *beyond clinical remission* to prevent relapses (average duration of treatment is two to four months).

5-Fluorocytosine (Ancoban® [Hoffman-LaRoche]) is a relatively new antifungal agent with both *in-vitro* and *in-vivo* activity against cryptococcosis, candidiasis, aspergillosis and chromomycosis. 5-FC is a fluoro-pyrimidine that inhibits nucleic acid synthesis in susceptible fungi but is not metabolized by mammalian cells. 5-FC has several characteristics which are advantageous for an antifungal therapeutic agent. It is administered orally and is well absorbed by the intestines, its distribution into body tissues is efficient and even, and it is relatively low in toxicity, being well tolerated over extended periods. Adverse reactions rarely reported in man include gastrointestinal disturbances, skin eruptions, leukopenia, thrombocytopenia and mild hepatotoxicity. The hepatotoxicities were completely reversed when therapy was discontinued.

Recommended dosage for 5-FC is 200 mg./kg. divided q.i.d. and given orally. Weekly CBC, BUN and serum glutamic-pyruvic transaminase (SGPT) determinations are also recommended. 5-FC may be used in patients with renal impairment (when amphotericin B is contraindicated) and in patients not responding to or relapsing following amphotericin B therapy. However, relapses and the development of resistant organisms frequently occur with 5-FC (up to 50 per cent of cases treated).

Other antifungal agents mentioned in the literature (stilbamidine, pentamidine, seromycin, hamycin) are not recommended, owing to toxicity, lack of efficacy or high percentage of relapses.

## PROPHYLAXIS AND PUBLIC HEALTH SIGNIFICANCE

The systemic mycoses are not thought to be contagious. The possibility of transmission from animal to animal or animal to man is extremely low. However, man is susceptible to these diseases, and proper care should be taken when handling these animals (wear gloves to protect wounds on hands, etc.). Proper sanitation, disposal of discharges (feces, urine, sputum, etc.) and cleansing of environment and fomites are essential.

The fact that infection occurs with fungi that are free-living forms in soil, in decaying vegetation and in bird excreta poses a difficult problem of control. Various plans for dust control, soil fungicides and vaccination programs have been reviewed but have lacked efficacy or practicality. Proper caution in, or avoidance of, high-risk areas is advised.

### SUPPLEMENTAL READING

Barrett, R. E., and Scott, D. W.: Treatment of feline cryptococcosis: Literature review and case report. J. Am. Anim. Hosp. Assn., *11*:511–518, 1975.

Beeson, P. B., and McDermott, W.: The mycoses. *In* Textbook of Medicine, 14th ed. Philadelphia, W. B. Saunders Co., 1975, pp. 442–455.
Bennett, J. E.: Chemotherapy of systemic mycoses. N. Engl. J. Med., *290*:30–32, 1974.
Butler, W. T., *et al.*: Electrocardiographic and electrolyte abnormalities caused by amphotericin B in dog and man. Proc. Soc. Exp. Biol. Med., *116*:857–863, 1964.
Furcolow, M. L., *et al.*: Supportive evidence by field testing and laboratory experiment for a new hypothesis of the ecology and pathogenicity of canine blastomycosis. Sabouraudia, *12*:22–32, 1974.
Jungerman, P. F., and Schwartzman, R. M.: Veterinary Medical Mycology. Philadelphia, Lea & Febiger, 1972.
Kaplan, W.: Epidemiology of the principal systemic mycoses of man and lower animals and the ecology of their etiologic agents. J. Am. Vet. Med. Assn., *163*:1043–1046, 1973.
Utz, J. P.: Chemotherapy of the systemic mycoses. Am. Family Phys., 7:108–114, 1973.

# NOCARDIOSIS AND ACTINOMYCOSIS

DANNY W. SCOTT, D.V.M.
*Ithaca, New York*

Infections with the actinomycetes (fungus-like bacteria), *Nocardia* spp. and *Actinomyces* spp., are occasionally seen in dogs and cats. Lesions caused by these organisms are characterized by abscessation, pyogranulomatous inflammation, draining tracts, ulceration, necrosis and fibrosis.

## NOCARDIOSIS

**Definition.** Nocardiosis is an uncommon acute or chronic pyogranulomatous infection, most often originating in the lung, with a marked tendency to spread to other tissues.

**Etiology and Epidemiology.** Nocardiosis in dogs and cats is caused by *Nocardia asteroides* (most) and *N. brasiliensis* (rare). *Nocardia* spp. are gram-positive, partially acid-fast, filamentous aerobes. They are common soil saprophytes and (except for *N. brasiliensis*) are worldwide in geographic distribution. Infections are contracted via inhalation, subcutaneous inoculation and ingestion. In man, *Nocardia* spp.

have a predilection for patients with depressed defense mechanisms (as a result of malignancy, dysproteinemia, debilitation or immunosuppressive drug therapy). Thus, a thorough search is indicated to rule out underlying immunosuppressive factors of an endogenous or exogenous nature.

**Clinical Signs.** *Nocardia* spp. produce a number of clinical syndromes in dogs and cats, and clinical signs vary depending on the tissues affected. A systemic form is seen in dogs in which the disease is indistinguishable from canine distemper (pyrexia, anorexia, emaciation, coughing, dyspnea, oculonasorrhea and neurologic signs). A primary respiratory form is seen in cats and dogs, characterized by pleural effusion and empyema (pyothorax). The cutaneous form of the disease is characterized by pyogranuloma formation, abscessation, ulceration and draining tracts. *Nocardia* spp. may also produce abscesses in the spleen, liver, kidney, omentum and central nervous system. Nocardial vertebral osteomyelitis has also been reported.

**Diagnosis.** Diagnostic aids depend on

the tissues involved. Radiography of the chest in the respiratory form may reveal hilar lymphadenopathy; pleural effusion; or a metastatic, nodular, interstitial lung pattern. Direct smears and cultures can be made from exudates or tissue aspirates. The typical thoracic exudate associated with nocardiosis is characterized by a "tomato soup–like" appearance and consistency. The so-called "sulfur granules" or "butter flecks" (mycelial clumps), so commonly found with actinomycosis, are uncommon in nocardiosis.

Histologic examination of biopsy specimens reveals pyogranulomatous inflammation. The organisms are not satisfactorily demonstrated in the usual hematoxylin-and-eosin–stained sections. Utilization of special stains (Brown and Brenn, Gomori's methenamine silver) allows satisfactory visualization of the organism. In general, *Nocardia* spp. can usually be distinguished from *Actinomyces* spp. by the absence of sulfur granules in exudates or tissues and the partial acid-fastness of the former.

**Treatment and Prognosis.** Recommended treatment of nocardiosis consists of combined surgical and chemotherapeutic measures. The drugs of choice are high doses of penicillin initially (100,000 units/kg./day intramuscularly) and long-term sulfonamides. Recommended sulfas include sulfadiazine (40 mg./kg. t.i.d. orally) or sulfadimethoxine (24 mg./kg. s.i.d. orally). Sulfa therapy should be continued for 4 weeks beyond clinical remission to avoid relapses (with average duration of therapy 2 to 4 months).

In cases of nocardial empyema, the use of chest tubes, daily pleural lavage with physiologic saline and intrathoracic infusions of penicillin and proteolytic enzymes have been very beneficial. Such therapy is continued until the thoracic fluid retrieved is clear and minimal in volume (average 9 to 11 days). Daily pleural lavage is advantageous in (1) facilitating the removal of exudate, tissue debris and toxic substances; (2) delivering a high level of specific antibiotic to the sites of infection; and (3) facilitating in concert with the use of proteolytic enzymes the liquefaction and removal of thick, tenacious exudate. This breaking down of loculated areas of infection and necrotic debris is instrumental in achieving a satisfactory therapeutic response and in eliminating nidi for future exacerbations.

Many encouraging reports have appeared recently in the medical literature on the successful treatment of nocardiosis in man with a combination of trimethoprim and sulfamethoxazole. This combination appears to be especially beneficial in patients with CNS involvement, in whom other sulfas apparently penetrate poorly in the cerebrospinal fluid.

The prognosis for recovery in nocardiosis has traditionally been poor. Clinically apparent nocardiosis is usually fatal if untreated. In man, with appropriate therapy, the recovery rate varies from 50 to 60 per cent (chest form) to 13 per cent (CNS involvement).

**Prophylaxis and Public Health Significance.** Nocardiosis is not thought to be a contagious disease. Thus, the possibility of animal to animal or animal to man transmission is extremely low. However, man can be infected with *Nocardia* spp., and proper care should be taken when handling these animals (wear gloves to protect wounds on hands; proper sanitation, disposal of discharges, etc.). The fact that infection occurs with free-living organisms in soil makes prophylaxis very difficult.

## ACTINOMYCOSIS

**Definition.** Actinomycosis is a chronic systemic disease characterized by pyogranulomatous and suppurative involvement of many tissues, especially skin, lungs and pleura, and spinal column.

**Etiology and Epidemiology.** Actinomycosis in dogs and cats is caused by *Actinomyces bovis* and, rarely, other *Actinomyces* spp. *Actinomyces* spp. are gram-positive, nonacid-fast, filamentous anaerobes. These organisms are opportunistic inhabitants of the oral cavity and bowel. Actinomycosis is worldwide in geographic distribution. Infections are usually produced by direct invasion of contiguous tissues, especially as a result of penetrating wounds, particularly the subcutaneous inoculation or inhalation of plant awns (foxtails, spear grass).

**Clinical Signs.** *Actinomyces* spp. produce a number of clinical syndromes in dogs and cats, clinical signs varying depending on the tissues affected. Clinical signs are often indistinguishable from nocardiosis, with pleural, cutaneous and vertebral osteomyelitis forms predominating. The vertebral osteomyelitis form usually involves the second and third lumbar vertebrae and is characterized by pyrexia, swelling and pain, and/or draining tracts in the lumbar region. Extension of the vertebral infection resulting in meningitis and meningomyelitis can occur.

**Diagnosis.** Diagnostic aids are as discussed for nocardiosis. The exudate in actinomycosis is thick and red-brown to coffee-colored and contains "sulfur granules" (mycelial clumps). In general, *Actinomyces* spp. can usually be distinguished from *Nocardia* spp. by the presence of sulfur granules in exudates or tissues, and the nonacid-fastness of the former. There is virtually always concurrent infection with other bacteria (especially *Bacteroides* spp.), and treatment must be directed at these organisms also.

**Treatment and Prognosis.** Recommended treatment of actinomycosis consists of combined surgical and chemotherapeutic measures. A careful search is in order for the underlying problems (plant awns, other foreign bodies, etc.), and, as mentioned above, treatment must be directed toward concurrent microbial invaders (by culture and sensitivity).

The drug of choice in actinomycosis is penicillin in high doses (100,000 units/kg./day IM, or 300,000 to 400,000 units/kg. 3 to 4 times daily, orally). Treatment should be continued for 4 weeks beyond clinical remission to avoid relapses (with average duration of therapy 2 to 4 months). In penicillin-allergic patients, tetracycline, chloramphenicol, erythromycin and lincomycin can be used.

[*Editor's Note*: Recently Clindamycin® (Upjohn) has been shown to be effective against *Actinomyces* spp. and shows promise in the treatment of actinomycosis in man. It may be useful in the disease in animals, too.]

The prognosis for recovery in actinomycosis varies depending upon the tissues involved. Clinically apparent actinomycosis is usually fatal if untreated. In man, with appropriate therapy, recovery rate varies from 90 per cent (cutaneous) to 40 per cent (chest form).

**Prophylaxis and Public Health Significance.** See discussion for nocardiosis.

### SUPPLEMENTAL READING

Beeson, P. B., and McDermott, W.: Actinomycosis and nocardiosis. *In* Textbook of Medicine. 14th ed. Philadelphia, W. B. Saunders Co., 1975, pp. 386–388.

Campbell, B., and Scott, D. W.: Successful management of nocardial empyema in a dog and cat. J. Am. Anim. Hosp. Assn. *11*:769–773, 1975.

Jungerman, P. F., and Schwartzman, R. M.: Veterinary Medical Mycology. Philadelphia, Lea & Febiger, 1972.

Maderazo, E. G., and Quintiliani, R.: Treatment of nocardial infection with trimethoprim and sulfamethoxazole. Am. J. Med., 57:671–675, 1974.

Utz, J. P.: Chemotherapy of the systemic mycoses. Am. Family Phys., 7:108–114, 1973.

# CANINE BABESIOSIS*

GEORGE E. LEWIS, JR., D.V.M.
*Urbana, Illinois*

*and* DAVID L. HUXSOLL, D.V.M.
*Kuala Lumpur, Malaysia*

Canine babesiosis is a tick-transmitted disease of wild and domestic dogs. Babesia organisms invade and multiply within the host erythrocytes. Characteristic clinical signs and symptoms include hemolytic anemia, presence of babesial parasites in host erythrocytes, pyrexia, bilirubinuria, lethargy and occasionally hemoglobinuria. Two different organisms, *Babesia canis* and *Babesia gibsoni*, are responsible for the vast majority of babesial infections reported to occur in domestic dogs throughout the world. Only *B. canis* infections are known to occur naturally in the United States. However, *B. gibsoni* will also be discussed

---

*The opinions or assertions contained herein are the private views of the authors and are not to be construed as official or as reflecting the views of the Department of the Army or the Department of Defense.

herein, for the continual movement and transportation of dogs across international boundaries provide the potential for establishment of *B. gibsoni* within the United States.

## ETIOLOGY

*Babesia canis* is the larger of the two canine babesias and is most often observed in the forms of characteristic pairs of teardrop- or pear-shaped parasites within infected red blood cells. Oval, round or ring-shaped bodies are also frequently observed. *Babesia canis* organisms measure 4.0 to 7.0 $\mu$ in length by 2.5 to 3.0 $\mu$ in width. Single large ovoid parasites appear early in infection and are soon followed by pairs of the typical pear-shaped mature *B. canis* organisms. There may be from 1 to 16 parasites within a single cell.

The smaller of the two babesias, *B. gibsoni*, usually appears within the host erythrocyte in delicate ring forms of 1.1 to 2.7 $\mu$ in diameter. Various other less common developmental forms of *B. gibsoni* have also been described. In smears of peripheral blood, stained by Giemsa or Wright's methods, both *Babesia* spp. appear to be vacuolated, to have a colorless to light bluish cytoplasm and to contain a not-so-obvious red nucleus. Virulence of strains of each of these two organisms is reported to vary considerably.

## EPIDEMIOLOGY

Both the canine babesias are transmitted from host to host by three-stage ticks. The brown dog tick *Rhipicephalus sanguineus* and *Haemaphysalis leachi* are both vectors of *B. canis*. The brown dog tick is considered the principal vector of *B. canis* in the United States. *Haemaphysalis bispinosa* is the principal vector of *B. gibsoni*. Both stage-to-stage (transstadial) and adult female-to-progeny (transovarial) transmission of *B. canis* and *B. gibsoni* have been reported in the vector ticks.

The larger of the two parasites, *B. canis*, is endemic throughout many of the tropical and subtropical areas of the world and has been reported in most of the southern and southwestern portions of the United States. *Babesia gibsoni* infections are not known to occur in the United States but have been reported from Africa, Asia and the Middle and Far East. Dogs infected with either species of babesia become carriers.

## CLINICAL SIGNS

The course of canine babesiosis may be acute and fulminating, subclinical or chronic. Mild infections frequently go undiagnosed. Infected dogs are often identified only after they have been subjected to the stress of hard work, a concurrent infectious disease or splenectomy and subsequently experience an exacerbation of parasitemia and clinical signs.

In general, young dogs are more susceptible and usually acquire a more severe infection.

The incubation period of *B. canis* in naturally acquired infections is thought to be from 10 days to 3 weeks. Incubation periods of 2 to 4 weeks have been reported for *B. gibsoni*. Parasites may appear in the blood before clinical signs are apparent. The initial clinical signs of infection are vague and usually consist of anorexia and intermittent elevations of body temperature. The major clinical manifestations of anemia, bilirubinuria and loss of condition soon become evident. The period of maximal parasitemia for *B. canis* varies from the average of 6 to 7 days after the first appearance of parasites in the blood to as late as 3 weeks. The degree of parasitemia may fluctuate from day to day, and a heavy parasitemia may, in the course of an hour or two, drop to a moderate or low level. With high parasitemia (occasionally 50 per cent or more of the erythrocytes contain one or more organisms), the blood appears thin and watery. On microscopic examination, marked anisocytosis, poikilocytosis, and hypochromasia are evident. Erythrophagocytosis by mononuclear cells of both normal and parasitized red cells is common. With severe anemia the red cell count may be $2.0 \times 10^6$/cu. mm. or less.

Various degrees of leukopenia, thrombocytopenia, reticulocytosis and bilirubinuria also occur in acute stages of babesiosis. Oral and conjunctival mucous membranes are pale and in later stages of severe babesiosis become white. Breathing becomes labored, and vomition is not uncommon. At this stage hemoglobinuria is usually evident. In such severe acute cases coma and death quickly ensue. However, most less severely infected dogs survive, but some degree of anemia may persist for several months.

In milder infections, which seem to be the most common form of babesiosis, the signs described above are less pronounced, and severe anemia, hemoglobinuria and high parasitemia are not obvious features. Temperature may remain high for several days or may fluctuate from day to day. Anemia is always present. Dogs recovered from babesiosis become carriers and clinically cannot be readily distinguished from normal, babesia-free dogs. Infected dogs may remain parasitemic for as long as 2 years or more.

The consistently high fever, hemoglobinuria and icterus often reported with acute *B. canis* infection are less conspicuous or absent in infections with *B. gibsoni*. Body temperature is extremely variable even during severe parasitemia in dogs infected with *B. gibsoni*.

## DIAGNOSIS

In endemic areas, a tick-infested, anemic and listless dog with consistent or intermittent fever may justify a tentative diagnosis of canine babesiosis. A thorough patient history should include information pertaining to the possible origination from, or travel into, *B. canis* and *B. gibsoni* endemic areas. Identification of babesia within host erythrocytes confirms the diagnosis. *Babesia canis* organisms are readily distinguishable from *B. gibsoni* on the basis of their larger size and characteristic pairs of teardrop-shaped parasites. For serologic diagnosis, a complement fixation test and an indirect fluorescent antibody test have recently been developed. Neither of these tests is readily available to practitioners.

Infections of *B. canis* and *B. gibsoni* may be complicated by concurrent infections with other hemotropic agents such as *Ehrlichia canis*, *Haemobartonella* and *Hepatozoon*. The canine *Babesiae* and *E. canis* often occur as mixed infections. In such cases *E. canis* is usually the less conspicuous agent and may remain undiagnosed. The anemia, leukopenia and thrombocytopenia initially invoked by *B. canis* infection are qualitatively similar to those produced by *E. canis* infection. Infection with either agent usually results in a carrier state. Blood smears in which babesia are detected should be thoroughly searched for *E. canis* morulae within the cytoplasm of mononuclear cells (see article on "Canine Ehrlichiosis").

## TREATMENT

Chemotherapeutics used for treatment of canine babesiosis are Berenil®, Phenamidine isethionate®, trypan blue, Acaprin®, Acriflavine® and pyrimethamine. Of these, Berenil® and Phenamidine® seem to be the most commonly used. Good clinical results have been reported with both drugs. A single deep intramuscular injection of Berenil® (Farbwerke Hoechst Ag. Frankfurt-am-Main, Germany) is recommended. In dogs, 7 mg./kg. body weight, administered in a 7 per cent aqueous solution, is considered the maximum dosage. Nervous signs occasionally accompany the administration of this drug. Phenamidine® (May and Baker, Ltd., Dagenham, England) solution should be administered by a single subcutaneous injection at the rate of 0.3 ml. for each kg. of body weight. A sensitization reaction, such as facial edema, may occur for a short time following administration.

Treatment of *B. gibsoni* infections, as compared to that of *B. canis* infections, with either of these drugs has often been less rewarding. Of the less commonly used drugs, trypan blue (an azo dye) and Acaprin® (a quinuronium derivative [Bayer, West Germany]) have been reported to be effective against *B. canis*. Trypan blue is injected intravenously in a 1.0 per cent solution at 2.2 mg./kg. body weight. Extravascular injection of trypan blue readily results in necrosis of surrounding tissues. Acaprin® has been reported to be efficacious when administered subcutaneously at a dosage rate of 0.25 mg./kg. of body weight. Rapid respiration, excessive salivation and nervousness may occur within 30 minutes.

Appropriate supportive therapy for severely anemic dogs should be provided in the form of whole blood transfusions, balanced electrolyte solution in 5 per cent dextrose and proper nutrition. The PCV is often the most reliable indicator of the course of the disease.

Prophylaxis is best accomplished by control and, when economically and ecologically feasible, eventual elimination of vector ticks from both dogs and their immediate environment. Clients taking dogs to endemic babesia areas should be advised to practice exacting tick control and daily grooming of their pet. The possible introduction of *B. gibsoni* into the United States in carrier dogs and ticks must be considered. Dogs used as blood donors should be carefully screened for evidence of canine babesiosis.

Human infections with *B. canis* have not been reported; however, 16 human cases of babesiosis have been described, indicating the zoonotic potential of certain babesia species (*B. bovis*, *B. divergens* and *B. microti*).

## SUPPLEMENTAL READING

Groves, M. G., and Yap, L. F.: *Babesia gibsoni* in a dog. J. Am. Vet. Med. Assn., 153:689–694, 1968.

Malherbe, W. D.: The manifestations and diagnosis of *Babesia* infections. Ann. N.Y. Acad. Sci., 64:128–146, 1956.

# CANINE EHRLICHIOSIS*†

GEORGE E. LEWIS, JR., D.V.M.
*Urbana, Illinois*

*and* DAVID L. HUXSOLL, D.V.M.
*Kuala Lumpur, Malaysia*

Canine ehrlichiosis is a tick-borne disease of dogs that results from infection with the rickettsial organism *Ehrlichia canis*. The infectious organism is transmitted from dog to dog by *Rhipicephalus sanguineus*, the brown dog tick. The disease may vary in severity from a relatively mild, acute, febrile syndrome to a severe, chronic and often fatal disease. Synonyms for canine ehrlichiosis include tropical canine pancytopenia, canine hemorrhagic fever, idiopathic hemorrhagic syndrome and tracker dog disease. Of these, only tropical canine pancytopenia has been widely accepted or used. Canine ehrlichiosis has been reported among dogs in North and South America, the Caribbean, Africa and the Middle East and throughout the Orient. The disease has been diagnosed in most areas of the United States.

## ETIOLOGY

The etiologic agent of canine ehrlichiosis, *E. canis*, is an obligate, intracellular parasite of canine mononuclear cells. Compact, grapelike clusters of this organism, termed morulae, develop within the cytoplasm of infected mononuclear cells, most often monocytes. Morulae may be seen in blood films prepared from infected dogs and stained with any of the Romanovsky type stains.

The isolation of a neutrophilic strain of *E. canis* from a dog in Arkansas has been reported. Morulae were found both in neutrophils and in eosinophils of dogs experimentally infected with this strain. This strain produced a relatively mild disease in the naturally infected dog from which the isolate was recovered, as well as in the experimentally infected dogs.

## EPIDEMIOLOGY

Vertebrate hosts for *E. canis* are restricted to members of the family Canidae. The fox, coyote and jackal have been experimentally infected. The disease also has been transmitted in the laboratory from foxes to dogs by ticks.

Many outbreaks or epizootics of canine ehrlichiosis have been associated with heavy tick infestations. The brown dog tick, *R. sanguineus*, is an efficient vector of *E. canis*, and transmission occurs transstadially (stage-to-stage of tick development) but not transovarially (from an adult female to her progeny).

Ticks may become infected as larvae and nymphs and then subsequently transmit *E.*

---

*The opinions or assertions contained herein are the private views of the authors and are not to be construed as official or as reflecting the views of the Department of the Army or the Department of Defense.

†In conducting the research described in this report, the investigators adhered to the *Guide for the Care and Use of Laboratory Animals*, as promulgated by the Committee on the Guide for Laboratory Animal Facilities and Care of the Institute of Laboratory Animals Resources, National Academy of Sciences— National Research Council.

*canis* to a susceptible dog during the feeding period of the next tick stage. Ticks may harbor infectious ehrlichiae for as long as 155 days after completion of engorgement and detachment as nymphs.

Once infected with *E. canis*, the dog remains a carrier until an effective therapeutic regimen is completed. Viable organisms are known to persist in the peripheral blood of dogs recovered from acute canine ehrlichiosis for more than 6 years. Also, the organisms seem to be constantly present in the peripheral venous blood of chronically infected dogs. In our laboratory, we have consistently been able to infect susceptible dogs with blood from chronic carriers.

Chronically infected dogs and/or wild canids, as well as infected ticks, probably serve as natural reservoirs of *E. canis*. Outbreaks seem to occur when susceptible dogs are taken into an endemic area or when *E. canis* is introduced into a population of susceptible dogs.

Infections of *E. canis* are often complicated by concurrent infections with other hemotropic agents such as *Babesia, Haemobartonella* or *Hepatozoon*. Mixed infections of *E. canis* and *Babesia canis* or *gibsoni* are common. In such cases the babesia is usually the most conspicuous agent, and *E. canis* may be overlooked.

Canine ehrlichiosis is most often reported in areas with tropical and subtropical climates where the vector tick populations are high. However, a wider global distribution of disease is expected when the vast distribution of *R. sanguineus* tick, found between 50° north latitude and 35° south, is considered. Indeed, the disease has been reported from many areas of the world with temperate climates, including many parts of the United States.

## CLINICAL SIGNS

Dogs infected with *E. canis* may be relatively asymptomatic or acutely ill, or they may develop an often fatal syndrome characterized by high fever, thrombocytopenia, leukopenia, anemia and hemorrhage. Ten to 20 days after attachment of infected ticks (or experimental inoculation with *E. canis*-infected blood) fever, serous nasal and ocular discharges, anorexia, depression, loss of weight, anemia, thrombocytopenia, increased erythrocyte sedimentation rate and lowered white cell counts become apparent. These signs of acute disease often persist for several weeks; however, their severity and duration are extremely variable, and all signs may not be evident. It is during this acute period that cytoplasmic morulae of *E. canis* can be demonstrated in mononuclear cells of stained peripheral blood films.

Hematologic changes are coincident with the appearance of other clinical signs. Between 10 and 20 days after exposure, dogs are maximally thrombocytopenic (10,000 to 36,000/cu. mm.) and leukopenic (3,100 to 7,000/cu. mm.), while the most severe anemia (RBC 2.0 to 3.6 × $10^6$/cu. mm.) occurs between the 20th and 28th day. The thrombocytopenia in acute ehrlichiosis is believed to result from increased destruction, consumption and/or sequestration of circulating platelets rather than decreased production. Lack of reticulocytosis and normal values for mean corpuscular volume are characteristic findings in acute disease and are suggestive of a reduced rate of erythrogenesis.

Experimental studies with beagles and German shepherds have shown that severity of chronic disease manifestations is often dependent upon the genetic stock and/or breed of dog infected rather than upon the strain of *E. canis* involved.

Most dogs survive the acute phase of disease that lasts 4 to 6 weeks. If untreated, these dogs remain chronically infected. Chronically infected dogs show few clinical signs, although hematologic values, particularly platelet counts, may remain moderately subnormal for many weeks following recovery from acute disease.

In certain breeds of dogs, particularly the German shepherd, the chronic phase may take one of two distinguishable clinical courses, referred to as mild chronic and severe chronic. The mild chronic disease in the German shepherd does not differ appreciably from the chronic disease observed in other breeds. In contrast, the severe chronic disease is often fatal. In those dogs that develop the latter syndrome, severe clinical signs appear 60 to 120 days post infection and include severe pancytopenia, depression, anorexia, emaciation and hemorrhage. Secondary bacterial infections are usually evident. In untreated dogs, death often occurs within several hours to a few days after the onset of hemorrhage. However, some dogs survive for months, showing only intermittent episodes of epistaxis. The severe chronic disease is thought to be primarily an aplastic anemia.

The possible injurious roles of circulating immune complexes, an ehrlichial endotoxin, antiplatelet substances and lymphocyte-mediated cytotoxicity as single or joint causes of the thrombocytopenia, and the occasional marrow aplasia of canine ehrlichiosis, have been incriminated and are currently being investigated.

## DIAGNOSIS

Canine ehrlichiosis is often reported to occur in the German shepherd and in German shepherd-like dogs. The disease also has been diagnosed in the beagle, Boston terrier, cocker spaniel, collie, poodle, Samoyed, springer spaniel and Scottish terrier breeds as well as in various hounds and mixed-breed dogs. Natural infections have been diagnosed in dogs from less than 1 to 13 years of age.

Canine ehrlichiosis is often difficult to diagnose clinically because the signs vary from those of the mild acute form to those of the severe, chronic, and fatal form of disease. However, high body temperature, leukopenia, anemia, thrombocytopenia, nasal and ocular discharges, epistaxis and weight loss should suggest a possible diagnosis of canine ehrlichiosis. Identification of the characteristic intracytoplasmic morulae in mononuclear cells in peripheral blood smears is conclusive. The number of infected cells that contain a morula may be less than 1 per cent, particularly during the chronic phase of disease, and are extremely difficult to find. A specific and sensitive indirect fluorescent antibody (IFA) test for detection of antibody to *E. canis* is available.* Using this test, serum antibodies to *E. canis* may be detected as early as 10 to 14 days after infection.

As long as a dog remains a carrier of *E. canis* an antibody titer will persist; however, after the organism is cleared by means of tetracycline therapy, the antibody titer gradually declines, usually over a period of 6 to 12 months, to nondetectable levels. Tetracycline-cleared dogs are susceptible to reinfection, even though they may maintain serologically demonstrable antibody to *E. canis*. The IFA test cannot be used to differentiate between primary infections and reinfections. Clinical and hematologic evaluations must be relied upon to identify reinfection, since a dog may remain serologically positive for many months following treatment.

It is not uncommon to encounter dogs with ehrlichiosis in nonendemic areas. Careful questioning of the owner often reveals that the affected dog has recently visited an endemic area.

Concurrent infections may also present a diagnostic problem. The thrombocytopenia, leukopenia and anemia initially invoked by *B. canis* infection are qualitatively similar to those produced by *E. canis* infection. In some instances, babesia infection may mask an underlying ehrlichia infection. In other cases, dogs have been diagnosed as having canine ehrlichiosis when the observed disease was due to babesia. Both agents have a relatively worldwide distribution and both are transmitted by *R. sanguineus*. Therefore, concurrent infections of *E. canis* and *B. canis* are not unexpected. In areas of the world where *B. gibsoni* is endemic, concurrent *E. canis* infections also should be considered. Blood smears in which babesia are detected should be thoroughly examined for the presence of *E. canis* morulae.

At necropsy, gross lesions in dogs with the severe chronic form of canine ehrlichiosis consist of generalized lymphadenopathy and hemorrhages in the subcutaneous tissues and major organs, particularly in the heart, lungs and gastrointestinal and urogenital tracts. These lesions are thought to reflect the terminal state of severe thrombocytopenia.

Histologically, there is an altered architecture of the lymphopoietic tissues, plasmacytosis and generalized perivascular lymphoid and plasma cell accumulations. These changes seem to reflect the continual stimulation of the reticuloendothelial system, to exaggeration, by the ever-present *E. canis* organisms. Bone marrow hypoplasia is evident in severe chronic cases.

Morulae can be found readily in impression smears of lung tissue from acute and often from chronically infected dogs. Tissues submitted for histopathologic examination should include lung, lymphatic tissue, brain and kidney, along with other routine specimens.

---

*Information regarding use of the IFA test for canine ehrlichiosis may be obtained by writing to Dr. M. Ristic, Department of Veterinary Pathology and Hygiene, University of Illinois, Urbana, Illinois 61801.

## TREATMENT

Tetracycline is the drug of choice for the treatment of canine ehrlichiosis. Dogs treated orally for 14 consecutive days with tetracycline hydrochloride at a dosage rate of 66 mg./kg. of body weight per day are cleared of the infection. Treatment during the acute phase of the disease results in remission of clinical and hematologic signs, usually within 14 days. However, dogs treated with tetracycline during the severe chronic phase of ehrlichiosis may respond poorly, with only gradual clinical improvement. Serum antibody to *E. canis* may be detected by the IFA test for as long as 12 months after tetracycline therapy. Appropriate supportive therapy should be provided, including whole blood transfusions, specific antibiotics to control secondary bacterial infections and proper nutrition as indicated by means of close monitoring of the patient.

## PROGNOSIS

Untreated dogs frequently recover clinically from acute disease, but all infected dogs remain carriers. As noted previously, many untreated dogs infected with *E. canis* undergo a second, severe exacerbation of canine ehrlichiosis and develop the severe chronic form of disease.

Dogs treated during the acute phase of disease, as well as those treated during the mild chronic phase, can be given a good prognosis. Those dogs treated during the severe chronic stage of disease should be given a guarded prognosis and closely monitored. It must be kept in mind that the presence of detectable antibody that develops during the course of *E. canis* infection does not seem to be associated with resistance to reinfection. Dogs that have received a therapeutic regimen of tetracycline are susceptible to reinfection.

## CONTROL AND PROPHYLAXIS

Control of canine ehrlichiosis in endemic areas should consist of vector tick control, treatment of clinically ill dogs infected with *E. canis*, serologic identification and treatment of carrier animals and prophylactic treatment of susceptible animals.

Continuous daily oral administration of tetracycline hydrochloride at 6.6 mg./kg. of body weight provides prophylaxis against initial infection with *E. canis*, as well as against reinfection. This treatment has been effective in preventing further spread of the disease and is believed to have been responsible for the control of several epizootics of canine ehrlichiosis.

If dogs are maintained on prophylactic medication long enough for infected ticks in the area to pass through one life cycle and for all infected adults to die out, *E. canis* may be eliminated from both the canine host and the vector ticks. The time required to effect such an *E. canis*-free environment has not been accurately determined; however, a minimum of one year should be considered. Clients taking dogs into ehrlichia endemic areas should be advised to practice exacting tick control and to include daily pet grooming and inspection for ticks. Dogs used as blood donors should be carefully screened for evidence of canine ehrlichiosis.

## PUBLIC HEALTH ASPECTS

Only members of the family Canidae are known to be naturally or experimentally susceptible to infection with *E. canis*. Attempts to infect small laboratory animals with infected dog blood, as well as attempts to infect nonhuman primates with *E. canis*-infected tissue culture, have been unsuccessful.

### SUPPLEMENTAL READING

Buhles, W. C., Jr., *et al.*: Tropical canine pancytopenia: Clinical, hematologic, and serologic responses of dogs to *Ehrlichia canis* infection, tetracycline therapy, and challenge inoculation. J. Infect. Dis., *130*:357–367, 1974.

Buhles, W. C., Jr., Huxsoll, D. L., and Hildebrandt, P. K.: Tropical canine pancytopenia: Role of aplastic anemia in the pathogenesis of severe disease. J. Comp. Pathol., 85:511–521, 1975.

Ewing, S. A.: Canine ehrlichiosis. Adv. Vet. Sci. Comp. Med., *13*:331–353, 1969.

Groves, M. G., *et al.*: Transmission of *Ehrlichia canis* to dogs by ticks (*Rhipicephalus sanguineus*). Am. J. Vet. Res., 36:937–940, 1975.

Hildebrandt, P. K., *et al.*: Pathology of canine ehrlichiosis (tropical canine pancytopenia). Am. J. Vet. Res., 34:1309–1320, 1973.

Huxsoll, D. L., *et al.*: Laboratory studies of tropical canine pancytopenia. Exp. Parasitol., *31*:53–59, 1972.

Walker, J. S., *et al.*: Clinical and clinico-pathologic findings in tropical canine pancytopenia. J. Am. Vet. Med. Assn., *157*:43–55, 1970.

# PET-
# ASSOCIATED
# ZOONOSES

JOHN S. REIF, D.V.M.
*Philadelphia, Pennsylvania*

There are over 150 diseases of vertebrate animals that are transmissible to man under natural conditions and are therefore classified as zoonoses. The intimate relationship that the household pet enjoys with his human associates makes transmission of zoonotic diseases a distinct possibility. The practitioner is frequently queried by his clients about the public health significance of animal disease. He serves as a reference for the medical profession and should play a leading role in establishing community policy on health issues that involve animals.

A complete discussion of the subject of pet-associated zoonoses is beyond the scope and format of this article. The interested reader is referred to a recent comprehensive textbook on this subject (Hubbert *et al.*, 1975). I urge practitioners to own this volume and/or a more concise reference source (Benenson, 1975). The purpose of this article is to present the salient features of the zoonoses transmitted from pets to man in the United States in table form and to discuss briefly some of the recent information concerning these diseases. The information presented is not intended to be completely comprehensive but to outline the major features of these infectious diseases. The list includes diseases of primates, laboratory animals and wildlife, since the practitioner is frequently called upon to examine these species or serve a consultative function.

## CANINE BRUCELLOSIS

Sixteen human infections with *B. canis* have been reported through 1974. Six of the cases resulted from accidental exposure of laboratory workers, 8 from exposure to infected dogs and 2 from an undetermined source. Because *B. canis* antibody does not react with the standard *B. abortus* antigen used in febrile agglutinin testing, the incidence of human *B. canis* infection may be higher than the number of reported infec- tions would indicate (CDC, Brucellosis Surveillance, Annual Summaries, 1973 and 1974).

The prevalence of canine antibodies against *B. canis* is surprisingly high (up to 10 per cent), especially in sexually active dogs that are allowed to roam freely (Fredrickson and Barton, 1974). The disease in man can be insidious and chronic and resembles that due to other strains of brucella. Transmission to man can occur by contact with blood, urine, tissues, semen and milk of infected dogs and especially by contact with infected vaginal discharges, stillborn fetuses and placental material following abortion. Dogs known to be infected should be isolated and handled carefully to prevent animal and human exposure.

## SALMONELLOSIS

Salmonellosis is a grossly underdiagnosed disease in the dog. A conservative estimate of the prevalence of salmonella-positive dogs in the United States is 10 per cent (Morse and Duncan, 1975). *S. typhimurium* is the serotype most frequently isolated; other frequent isolates include *S. anatum*, *S. derby*, *S. oranienburg*, *S. rubislaw*, *S. newport* and *S. montevideo*. Salmonellae appear to be a common contaminant of dehydrated dog foods, especially those containing meat meal.

Clinical canine salmonellosis is characterized by malaise, depression, fever, bloody fetid diarrhea, anorexia and dehydration. Less severe forms are difficult to diagnose. Stool culture should be performed to identify the pathogen.

Carriers of salmonella are often clinically normal but are occult fecal shedders. Shedding persists for an average of 6 weeks. A carrier state may persist for several months. The organism localizes in the ileocecal and other mesenteric lymph nodes.

Although the incidence of human infec-

*Bacterial and Spirochetal Zoonoses*

| DISEASE | ETIOLOGIC AGENT | ANIMALS INVOLVED | MECHANISM OF TRANSMISSION TO MAN | ADDITIONAL FEATURES |
|---|---|---|---|---|
| Brucellosis | *Brucella canis* | Dogs | Ingestion, contact | See text. |
| Leptospirosis | *Leptospira canicola* *L. icterohaemorrhagiae* Other serotypes | Dogs, cats, rodents, wildlife | Waterborne; direct contact through abraded skin, mucous membrane, ingestion | Contamination with infected urine. See text. |
| Rat Bite Fever | *Streptobacillus moniliformis* | Wild and laboratory rats, rarely other rodents | Oral and nasal secretions introduced by bite | Fever, chills, headache, muscle pain, rash, swollen joints within 10 days after bite. |
| Relapsing Fever | *Borrelia recurrentis* | Wild rodents (squirrel, prairie dog) | Tick bite | RARE; western U.S.—endemic form. |
| Salmonellosis | Many serotypes | Dogs, cats (?), turtles | Ingestion | See text. |
| Sylvatic Plague | *Yersinia pestis* | Wild rodents, rabbits, dogs (?) | Infected flea bites | Bubonic form results. Western and southwestern U.S. |
| Tuberculosis | *Mycobacterium tuberculosis*, *M. bovis* Atypical mycobacteria | Primates; dogs, cats | Airborne, ingestion | Primates highly susceptible; dogs and cats resistant. Zoos, urban areas. |
| Tularemia | *Francisella tularensis* | Rabbits, wild rodents | Animal bite, direct contact, ingestion, arthropod bite, waterborne, inhalation, especially handling tissues | Chills, fever; ulceroglandular, glandular, oculoglandular and pulmonary forms. |
| Wound Infections (Bacterial) | *Pasteurella multocida*, *P. pneumotropica* Streptococcus, tetanus | Dogs, cats, rodents | Bite, scratch | 30,000 people receive anti-rabies treatment in U.S./year; morbidity, psychic trauma. |

## Viral and Rickettsial Zoonoses

| DISEASE | ETIOLOGIC AGENT | ANIMALS INVOLVED | MECHANISM OF TRANSMISSION TO MAN | ADDITIONAL FEATURES |
|---|---|---|---|---|
| Psittacosis (Ornithosis) | *Chlamydia psittaci* | Psittacine birds, other birds | Airborne, desiccated droppings, direct contact | Healthy carriers shed intermittently under stress; fever, pneumonitis. |
| Rocky Mountain Spotted Fever | *Rickettsia rickettsii* | Dogs, rodents, rabbits | Tick bite, *Dermacentor variabilis* frequently implicated | Eastern, southern and western U.S.; fever, headache, rash. |
| Rabies | Rabies virus | Skunks, foxes, bats, raccoons, dogs, cats, primates | Bite wound, contact with saliva through abraded skin, scratch | See article on "Rabies." |
| Cat-scratch Disease | Unknown | Cats | Bite, scratch | Malaise, granulmmatous lymphadenitis, fever; rarely encephalitis, thrombocytopenia, conjunctivitis. |
| Lymphocytic Choriomeningitis | LCM virus | Mice, hamsters and guinea pigs; rarely dog or monkey | Probably by contaminated food or dust; virus in feces, urine and saliva | Recent outbreaks traced to pet hamsters and laboratory guinea pigs. |
| B-Virus Infection | *Herpesvirus simiae* | Primates (esp. rhesus and Old World species) | Bite wound, contact with saliva through abraded skin | Monkeys clinically normal. Encephalitis in man. |
| Monkeypox | Virus | Nonhuman primates | Contact | Vesiculopustular disease resembling smallpox; not seen in U.S. |
| Marburg Disease | Virus | African green monkeys | Contact with tissues of infected monkey | High fatality rate; one outbreak reported; not seen in U.S. |
| Infectious Hepatitis, Type A | Virus | Chimpanzees, other nonhuman primates | Contact exposure, fecal-oral route | Usually newly imported young chimps implicated. |

*Parasitic Zoonoses*

| DISEASE | ETIOLOGIC AGENT | ANIMALS INVOLVED | MECHANISM OF TRANSMISSION TO MAN | ADDITIONAL FEATURES |
|---|---|---|---|---|
| *A. PROTOZOAN DISEASES* | | | | |
| Balantidiasis | *Balantidium coli* | Nonhuman primates—especially chimpanzees | Ingestion | Dysentery. |
| Pneumocystis | *Pneumocystis carinii* | Dogs, cats, primates; importance unknown | Unknown | Pneumonia in ill, premature and immunodeficient infants |
| Toxoplasmosis | *Toxoplasma gondii* | Cats | Probably ingestion of oocysts from eating uncooked meat; cats? | See text and article on "Toxoplasmosis." |
| Chagas' Disease | *Trypanosoma cruzi* | Dogs, cats, primates, wildlife, rodents | Fecal material of triatomid bug | Mexico, Central and South America. RARE in U.S. |
| *B. CESTODE DISEASES* | | | | |
| Dog Tapeworm | *Dipylidium caninum* | Dogs, cats | Ingestion of dog or cat flea | RARE |
| Fish Tapeworm | *Diphyllobothrium latum* | Dogs | Ingestion of raw or partially cooked fish | RARE |
| Hydatidosis | *Echinococcus granulosus E. multilocularis* | Dogs | Ingestion of tapeworm eggs | Seen in sheep-raising areas. |
| Rat Tapeworm | *Hymenolepis diminuta* | Common in rats and mice; reported in hamsters | Ingestion of infected insects, fleas | Children; south and southwest U.S.; RARE |
| Dwarf Tapeworm | *Hymenolepis nana* | Rats and mice; rarely primates | No immediate host required; direct cycle, ingestion of eggs in feces | Children; south and southwest U.S.; common. G.I., neurologic and allergic symptoms. |

## C. NEMATODE DISEASES

| | | | | |
|---|---|---|---|---|
| Capillariasis | *Capillaria hepatica* | Rodents | Ingestion | Hepatitis, eosinophilia. |
| Dracunculiasis | *Dracunculus medinensis* | Dogs | Ingestion of infected cyclops | RARE |
| Filariasis | *Dirofilaria* spp. | Dogs | Bite of infected mosquitoes | See text. |
| Giant Kidney Worm | *Dioctophyma renale* | Dogs | Ingestion of infected fish | RARE |
| Cutaneous Larva Migrans | *Ancylostoma* spp. *Uncinaria* spp. | Dogs, cats | Infective larvae penetrate skin | See text. |
| Visceral Larva Migrans | *Toxocara* spp. *Toxascaris* spp. | Dogs, cats | Ingestion of ova | See text. |
| Strongyloidiasis | *Strongyloides stercoralis* | Dogs | Infective larvae penetrate skin; soil or fecal contact | Cutaneous, abdominal and pulmonary symptoms. Adults lodge in upper G.I. tract. |

## D. ARTHROPOD DISEASES

| | | | | |
|---|---|---|---|---|
| Scabies (Acariasis) | *Sarcoptes scabei* *Chylettiella* spp. | Dogs, cats | Contact with infected animals, contaminated clothing, fomites | Common in people exposed to canine scabies. Incidence increasing. |
| Tick Paralysis | *Dermacentor* *Amblyomma* Others | No requirement | Tick bite—usually scalp or neck | Most common in northwest and southeast U.S. Removal curative. |
| Flea Bite Dermatitis | *Ctenocephalides canis* and *felis* | Dogs, cats | Bite | Hypersensitivity may develop. |

tion acquired from dogs is unknown, numerous case reports suggest that transmission occurs frequently and rather easily by the fecal-oral route. Children, because of their habits and exposure to a contaminated environment, are frequently involved. Of the estimated 2 million cases of human salmonellosis that occur annually in the United States, several thousand are probably obtained from a family pet.

## LEPTOSPIROSIS

Leptospirosis is a disease in a state of changing epidemiologic patterns. It was previously considered an occupational disease of miners and abattoir, rice field, sugar cane, farm and sewer workers. The common denominator for these occupations was a wet environment and exposure to rats or other animal sources.

However, the potential for human infection from the pursuit of recreational activities is increasing. Numerous reports cite the prevalence of leptospiral antibodies in wildlife. Contact with infected dogs is responsible for approximately 30 per cent of human infections in the United States.

Furthermore, the scope of leptospiral serotypes isolated from dogs appears to be broadening. In addition to icterohaemorrhagiae and canicola, dogs also served as the probable source of human autumnalis, australis, hebdomadis and grippotyphosa infections in 1972–1974 (CDC, Leptospirosis Surveillance, Annual Summary, 1974).

Of special interest to practitioners is a recent report in which healthy immunized dogs acquired subclinical infections and shed *L. icterohaemorrhagiae* in their urine (Feigen *et al.*, 1973). These dogs were the presumed source of infection for a critically ill teenage girl and four others who lived in an upper middle class community. Leptospira bacterins may not protect against subclinical infections and renal shedding, although they will protect the dog from developing clinical leptospirosis. Vaccines are being developed that will prevent renal shedding of leptospira.

The clinical signs of leptospirosis in man are often nonspecific and include fever, headache, chills, vomiting, myalgia, conjunctivitis, stiff neck and backache as well as the more characteristic but seldom observed jaundice, hematuria and hemor-

rhage. The disease has a low index of suspicion among clinicians and is undoubtedly underdiagnosed.

## CAT-SCRATCH DISEASE

Cat-scratch disease (fever) is a subacute, self-limited infectious disease of presumably viral etiology (Carithers *et al.*, 1969). Typically, a papule develops at the site of a cat bite or scratch within 7 to 10 days, followed by regional granulomatous lymphadenitis. Malaise and fever often accompany the acute stage of the disease. The affected lymph nodes may suppurate. Regression occurs in 2 to 6 weeks. Complications are rare but include thrombocytopenia, rash, osteolysis, conjunctivitis and encephalitis.

The inciting event is recorded in about 90 per cent of cases as the bite, scratch or lick of a cat, usually a kitten. A skin test antigen prepared from lymph node aspirates has been used in hypersensitivity testing and shows a prevalence of presumed prior infection in 30 per cent of veterinarians and 4 per cent of the general population. In my experience, cats have been associated with several cases of cat-scratch disease in a single family. I would therefore warn clients regarding the possibility of further illness if a "carrier" cat is kept in the home.

## DIROFILARIA IMMITIS INFESTATION

Human pulmonary and cardiovascular dirofilariasis must be considered an "emerging zoonosis." Over 35 cases have been reported since 1961 (Gershwin *et al.*, 1974). Microfilariae, introduced into the circulation by the bite of an infected mosquito, may develop into immature parasites and lodge in a small pulmonary artery. An infarct surrounded by eosinophilic pneumonitis results. Rarely, microfilariae develop into adult worms in the cardiovascular system, but man is a "dead-end" host, and multiplication does not occur.

Clinical signs associated with pulmonary dirofilariasis have included cough and chest pain, rarely hemoptysis. The infestation is usually asymptomatic. The lesions are often discovered upon routine radiographic examination of the chest, where they appear as solitary pulmonary nodules or "coin lesions." Since such lesions cannot easily be differentiated from neoplasia, surgical resection follows, and pathologic examination reveals the nature of the disease. Individuals living in areas of the United States where canine dirofilariasis is endemic would appear to be at a low but definite risk for developing the disease.

## VISCERAL LARVA MIGRANS

Visceral larva migrans (VLM) was first introduced to describe a syndrome in young children characterized by eosinophilia, hepatomegaly, pulmonary infiltration, fever and hypergammaglobulinemia. The disease is seen predominantly in children in the 1 to 4 year age group, especially those having had the habit of pica. The disease is due to the migration of the second stage larvae of *Toxocara* spp. and is usually contracted by children eating dirt contaminated with embryonated ascarid eggs. While rarely fatal, the course tends to be chronic, and ocular involvement (endophthalmitis, retinal hemorrhage) and neurologic sequelae (meningoencephalitis) occur with some frequency (Mok, 1968).

Reliable estimates of the prevalence of this disease are not available, since a good serologic test has not been developed and liver biopsy remains the only definitive diagnostic method. However, the ubiquity of the parasite in the environment (e.g., city parks) and the unhygienic habits of children suggest that VLM is vastly underdiagnosed.

The veterinarian has a primary responsibility in prevention of VLM by (1) aggressive treatment of ascarids in puppies and kittens, (2) educating clients as to potential dangers of infected puppies and nursing bitches, (3) recommending sanitary methods of waste disposal and avoidance of exposure by children, (4) advising breeders and pet shops on methods of parasite control and (5) advocating measures that will minimize environmental contamination.

## CUTANEOUS LARVA MIGRANS

Cutaneous larva migrans (creeping eruption) is a dermatosis characterized by serpiginous intracutaneous lesions due to the migration of nematode larvae in the skin. Among the hookworm larvae, *Ancylostoma braziliense* is most commonly incriminated, although other species of *Ancylostoma* and *Uncinaria* may produce the disease. *Strongyloides stercoralis* causes similar lesions.

The larvae penetrate the skin after contact and migrate intracutaneously, producing intense pruritus and a narrow, slightly elevated linear erythematous lesion. The cutaneous phase may be followed by a pulmonary syndrome consisting of cough, wheezing and pulmonary and peripheral eosinophilia (Löfler's syndrome). The responsibility of the veterinarian in this disease is similar to that described for VLM.

## TOXOPLASMOSIS

Toxoplasmosis in man may be acquired by any of three means. Congenital infections leading to abortion, stillbirth or central nervous system and ocular abnormalities were recognized early. A second route of transmission is ingestion of raw or undercooked meat containing *Toxoplasma* cysts. Acquired toxoplasmosis most frequently leads to subclinical infection. If signs occur, they frequently consist of fever, malaise, muscle pain and cervical lymphadenopathy. Chorioretinitis may follow congenital or acquired toxoplasmosis. Less often, severe forms with visceral involvement produce hepatitis, myocarditis, pneumonitis or meningoencephalitis.

Interest in a third potential form of transmission, exposure to feces of cats, was awakened by the finding that Felidae shed infective oocysts in their feces after ingestion of infected mice (Frenkel and Dubey, 1972). Toxoplasma oocysts remain viable in the environment for several months under conditions of adequate moisture and temperatures between freezing and 45° C. There is rather good evidence that human infection can occur after exposure to cat feces, especially the seroconversion of laboratory personnel working with cat feces. However, the extent to which feline-to-human transmission occurs and the importance of the cat as a source of disease compared to the ingestion of *Toxoplasma*-infected meat remain rather unclear.

My recommendations for dealing with the zoonotic potential of toxoplasmosis are as follows: 1. Women of child-bearing age who contemplate pregnancy and who wish to keep a cat should have their antibody status determined by a physician. Those who possess a significant titer against toxoplasmosis are probably protected from reinfection.

2. Where susceptible individuals exist, including persons with immunodeficiency,

cats should be prevented from becoming exposed to the organism by avoiding the feeding of uncooked foods and preventing cannibalism.

3. After initial infection, cats shed oocysts in feces for approximately two weeks. To assess the absence of an active infection, three fecal examinations at 48-hour intervals should be performed and a careful search made for the small (10 to 12 $\mu$) oocysts.

4. To avoid exposure, the wearing of plastic gloves when handling litter and gardening is suggested. Litter pans should be cleaned daily with ammonia and emptied to circumvent the 48- to 72-hour period required for oocyst sporulation and infectivity. Keeping sandboxes covered and observing normal principles of sanitation and hygiene after handling a cat clearly make good sense.

5. Serologic testing of cats is of little use because of the evanescent nature of the antibody and the fact that cats with low levels of antibody may be reinfected. Based on some preliminary data from my laboratory, the most important factor in preventing human toxoplasmosis is avoiding the ingestion of raw or undercooked meat.

## DISEASE COMMON TO ANIMALS AND MAN

There are a number of diseases from which both animals and man suffer but which are not directly transmissible between species or members of the same species. These diseases arouse unnecessary fear and consternation when diagnosed. An understanding of their epidemiology is essential.

The systemic mycoses (histoplasmosis, blastomycosis, coccidioidomycosis) are environmental diseases acquired by inhalation of the fungus from contaminated soil. Rarely they may be acquired from laboratory cultures or indirectly from contact with a contaminated fomite. Histoplasmosis is not transmitted by birds, but avian and bat feces stimulate the growth of the organism in soil. The organism is dispersed in the air when the environment is disturbed by some activity such as demolishing or cleaning old farm buildings. Cryptococcus, a saprophytic yeast, is similarly potentiated in its growth by bird manure, especially of pigeons. Aspergillus is acquired by exposure of a susceptible host to the organism growing saprophytically in the environment.

## FELINE LEUKEMIA

Feline leukemia is a disease in which the zoonotic potential is still undetermined. A number of facts concerning its nature and epidemiologic behavior suggest that the feline leukemia virus (FeLV) be considered a potential human hazard until proved otherwise. The disease itself is the most common type of malignant neoplasm in the cat. Horizontal transmission of FeLV occurs readily in multiple-cat households and in the laboratory. FeLV can be detected in approximately 90 per cent of cats with feline lymphosarcoma. The C type RNA virus is present in abundant quantities in many tissues and body fluids, including salivary glands, suggesting the possibility that the agent may be spread by bite, scratch or aerosolization. FeLV and a similar agent which produces fibrosarcoma can be cultivated *in vitro* in human cell lines. Feline fibrosarcoma has been experimentally transmitted to kittens, puppies and at least one species of subhuman primate, the marmoset. While the FeLV is detected in only 0.1 per cent of healthy cats from leukemia-free households, antibody against a cell membrane associated antigen (FOCMA) may be present in up to 60 per cent of cats in an urban area, suggesting ubiquity of the agent and ease of transmission.

### SUPPLEMENTAL READING

Benenson, A. (ed.): Control of Communicable Diseases in Man. 12th ed. Washington, D.C., American Public Health Association, 1975.

Carithers, H. A., Carithers, C. M., and Edwards, K. O.: Cat scratch: Its natural history. JAMA, 207:312–316, 1969.

Feigin, R. D., *et al.*: Human leptospirosis from immunized dogs. Ann. Int. Med., 79:777–785, 1973.

Fredrickson, L., and Barton, C.: A serologic survey for canine brucellosis in a metropolitan area. J. Am. Vet. Med. Assn., 165:987–989, 1974.

Frenkel, J. K., and Dubey, J. P.: Toxoplasmosis and its prevention in cats and man. J. Infect. Dis., 126:664–673, 1972.

Gershwin, L. J., Gershwin, M. E., and Kritzman, J.: Human pulmonary dirofilariasis. Chest, 66:92–96, 1974.

Hubbert, W. T., McCulloch, W. P., and Schnurrenberger, P. R. (eds.): Diseases Transmitted from Animals to Man. 6th ed. Springfield, Ill., Charles C Thomas, 1975.

Mok, C. H.: Visceral larva mivrans—A discussion based on review of the literature. Clin. Pediat., 7:567–571, 1968.

Morse, E. V., and Duncan, M. A.: Canine salmonellosis: Prevalence epizootiology, signs and public health equipment. J. Am. Vet. Med. Assn., 167:817–820, 1975.

# AEROSOL THERAPY AND VACCINATION*

J. S. WALKER, D.V.M.,
*Greenport, New York*

*and* E. L. STEPHEN, D.V.M.
*Frederick, Maryland*

The scope of this article is limited to discussion of aerosol vaccination, aerosol administration of drugs for the therapy of pneumonias and details of the techniques involved. For information on aerosol therapy in its broadest context and its possible uses, see *Current Veterinary Therapy VI* (Bolton, 1977).

The aerosol administration of antimicrobial drugs and vaccines for the treatment of immunoprophylaxis of infectious respiratory diseases has had a history of interrupted attention and enthusiasm in veterinary and human medicine. Problems associated with aerosol therapy or vaccination have resulted in the past from drug-induced hypersensitivity, the use of ineffective drugs or vaccines and the application of inappropriate aerosol technology.

It has become evident from work in several countries that certain principles must be adhered to in order to achieve success with aerosol administration of vaccines and drugs. First, the drug or vaccine must be effective. Second, drugs or vaccines known to be allergenic by parenteral routes, e.g., the penicillins and neomycin, must not be used for aerosol therapy. As a general principle, drugs that cause hypersensitivity by parenteral routes will be many times more dangerous when administered as an aerosol. Third, the site of deposition of the drug or vaccine within the respiratory tract is dependent upon the particle size of the aerosol. Particles with a mass median diameter of ~8 $\mu$m. or larger will penetrate no further than the nasal passages and oropharynx. Optimum pulmonary deposition is achieved with aerosol particles between 1.5 and 4.0 $\mu$m. In this size range, approximately 40 to 50 per cent of the total retained dose will be deposited in the

lungs, 15 per cent in the trachea and large bronchi and 40 per cent in the nasopharynx. Data on the proportion of the presented dose that is retained in the respiratory tract using particles in this size range vary according to investigator, techniques used and material measured. We have adopted 50 per cent of the presented aerosol as a reasonable estimate for the effective retained dose in the respiratory tract. All dosage information presented is given as effective retained dose. It is emphasized that, even following parenteral administration, effective dose is largely unknown because of the question as to how much of the administered dose ultimately reaches effective sites in the treated subject. Fourth, the aerosol concentration is determined by the concentration of the drug in the spray suspension, air flow rates and the characteristics of the nebulizers. Estimates of presented dosages are determined from the respiratory minute volume of the treated animal and drug concentrations in the aerosol. The actual aerosol concentrations can be determined using standard aerosol sampling and assay techniques (Larson *et al.*, 1976). Last, aerosol therapy should be used only in conditions for which conventional parenteral therapy has failed or when current research shows that aerosol will afford a clear advantage.

## USES

Recent data on aerosol vaccination and the resultant immunity suggest certain generalizations. Aerosol vaccination with either inactivated or live vaccines produces optimum protection against respiratory pathogens. This results from stimulation and development of local immune systems, i.e., IgA and cell-mediated immunity in the respiratory tract, as well as systemic immunity, i.e., serum antibodies. If local immune mechanisms are operative at the time of exposure to the pathogen, the potential infec-

---

*The opinions or assertions contained herein are the private views of the authors and are not to be construed as official or as reflecting the views of the Department of the Army or the Department of Defense.

tion is generally aborted. If, however, only the humoral or systemic immune system is operative, the respiratory infection may be controlled, but the respiratory tissues are infected, resulting in a mild or subclinical infection. This, of course, is of epizootiologic as well as clinical importance. A recent, controlled study with feline panleukopenia virus demonstrated the feasibility of administering vaccines against feline infections by the aerosol route (Scott and Glauberg, 1975).

One of the major clinical problems is the management of pneumonias, particularly those of gram-negative etiology. Recent data indicate that the administration of aminoglycosides by aerosol has a distinct advantage over parenteral administration in these clinical circumstances. Mortality is significantly decreased and the period of convalescence is shortened following aerosol administration of the drugs when compared to parenteral administration. Also, nephrotoxicity is likely to be lessened following aerosol administration of the drugs, because kidney drug levels are lower than those following parenteral administration. Another drug being investigated abroad for aerosol administration is amphotericin B for the management of respiratory mycoses. Both the aminoglycosides and amphotericin B are poorly absorbed from the respiratory tract; hence, high pulmonary levels of the drug can be achieved for prolonged periods of time but are not toxic with aerosol administration to the host.

Other classes of drugs that appear to be promising candidates for aerosol administration are certain of the newer antivirals, specifically ribavirin*, used in the control of viral respiratory infections (Walker *et al.*, 1976).

## EQUIPMENT

In recommending equipment, we have especially considered cost, commercial availability and ease of operation. There are many systems and combinations of systems that can be used and are used in research situations, in which engineering talent is frequently available to deal with complex systems; however, these systems are not practical in the average clinical situation. Systems employing face masks and similar devices are not recommended except as discussed below. We feel that chambers ($O_2$-treatment cages) are a much better approach. Here the animal is not restrained or sedated, both of which are a risk and present a severe problem, i.e., clinical management, in the patient with a compromised respiratory system.

Two commercially available inexpensive nebulizers have been shown to produce particles of the desired size range for good pulmonary deposition; these are the DeVilbiss No. 40** and Vaponefrin®† (Larson *et al.*, 1976). The latter is in the form of a plastic disposable device, thus eliminating the need for resterilization. Both nebulizers require compressed air, supplied either by a precharged tank or by a small air compressor through a pressure regulator. The Vaponefrin® and DeVilbiss nebulizers should be operated at 10 and 20 psi, respectively.

An oxygen-type cage can be used and should be vented to the outside of the building after passage of the air through an "Airpure" absolute filter.‡ After each treatment the cage should be air-washed with clean, forced air, bypassing the nebulizer, for at least 10 minutes before opening the cage and removing the animal. This completes the administration of the total dose and minimizes the exposure of personnel handling the animal to residual aerosol of drug.

## AEROSOL VACCINATION

Experience with aerosol vaccines for immunoprophylaxis of respiratory diseases in small animals is so limited at the present time that no recommendations can be made as to dosage required, and thus, vaccine concentration needed, or conversely as to the time required to deliver the required dose by aerosol. However, as a general guide for future work, it should be kept in mind that the effective total dose retained by the animal when a DeVilbiss No. 40 is used in a 50-liter cage or the Vaponefrin® in

---

*Ribavirin (Virazole®) (for investigative work only), ICN Pharmaceuticals, Inc., 2727 Campus Drive, Irvine, California 92664.

---

**DeVilbiss No. 40, DeVilbiss Corp., Somerset, Pennsylvania.

†Vaponefrin® (plastic, standard), Fisons Corp., 2 Preston Court, Bedford, Massachusetts 01730.

‡"Airpure" absolute filter (size B, 7C70-L), Flanders Filters, Inc., Box 1219, Washington, North Carolina.

a 20-liter cage in 25 minutes will be approximately 1/10 that of the starting concentration of the vaccine solution. An example would be as follows: If the vaccine has $10^6$ particles/ml., then the approximate retained dose by a 2.5-kg. cat in a 20-liter box with a Vaponefrin® nebulizer for 25 minutes would be $10^5$. Only clinical experience and controlled experiments will determine what aerosol dose is required for effective protection against each respiratory disease in question. The above information is provided only as a rough guide for future studies.

## THERAPY

Two of the aminoglycosides currently recommended for treatment of bacterial pneumonia are gentamicin and kanamycin. A newer aminoglycoside, sisomicin*, may also prove effective. The dose for gentamicin should be 4 mg./kg./day and 8 to 12 mg./kg./day for kanamycin. Three or four days of therapy should resolve most pneumonias. The dose of ribavirin for the treatment of viral pneumonia, while experimental at the present time, should be 8 mg./kg./day for 4 to 5 days.

## SPECIFIC TECHNIQUES

In making the recommendations, several interacting variables were taken into consideration. These included (1) the performance characteristics of the two recommended nebulizers; (2) the fact that solution concentrations in the nebulizer increase during atomization; (3) the dissemination efficiencies of the nebulizers, including drug losses due to impaction on system surfaces; (4) the time required to reach maximum aerosol concentration in the treatment chamber; (5) changes in respiratory minute volumes, which vary as a function of the animal body weight to the 3/4 power (metabolic weight); (6) the size of the chamber and thus the volume of air to be displaced with drug-charged air; (7) the decrease in chamber drug concentration with time after the nebulizer is turned off; and so on. Hence, if the conditions specified below are changed to any marked degree, such as using another nebulizer, it will be neces-

*Sisomicin (for investigative use only), Schering Corp., Kenilworth, New Jersey 07033.

sary for the clinician to acquaint himself with all the factors involved or he will very likely lose control of the dosage delivered.

For animals weighing from 0.5 to 10 kg., the following is recommended for gentamicin therapy; for other drugs, see recommended dose and adjust concentrations as outlined below.

A. Nebulizer—Vaponefrin®, operating pressure 10 psi
B. Chamber—20-liter box
C. Spray concentration of drug—50 mg./ml. (5.0% solution)
D. Dosage—4 mg./kg./treatment period
E. Aerosol concentration—1.4 mg./liter
F. Minute volume—1.12 liters/min. (5-kg. animal)
G. Treatment-time —Total dose/aerosol concentration ×
   minute volume ×
   0.5 retention
   —20 mg./1.12 liters/min. ×
   1.4 mg./liter ×
   0.5 retention
   —25.5 min. plus 10 min. air-wash after nebulizer turned off
H. Dosage adjustment—Do this by adjusting spray concentration up to a limit of 10% solution, holding treatment-time constant. For 2 mg./kg./treatment period use 25 mg./ml. (2.5% solution) and for 8 mg./kg./treatment period use 100 mg./ml. (10% solution).
I. Treatment periods—Because of the high lung levels achieved and the slow clearance of the aminoglycosides from the lung treatment, once a day is all that is necessary.

For animals weighing from 10 to 20 kg., the following is recommended:

A. Nebulizer—DeVilbiss No. 40, operating pressure 20 psi
B. Chamber—50-liter box
C. Spray concentration of drug—100 mg./ml. (10% solution)
D. Dosage—4 mg./kg./treatment period
E. Aerosol concentration—1.8 mg./liter
F. Minute volume—2.62 liters/min. (15-kg. animal)
G. Treatment time—25.4 min. plus 10 min. air-wash after nebulizer turned off
H. Adjustment of dosage as discussed above, for smaller animal

*General Comments:* By simply using weight ranges, a slight discrepancy in dosage occurs at each end of the weight range. However, both extremes (under- or overdosing) are well within the therapeutic and safety limits of the drugs normally employed.

For treatment of animals larger than 20 kg., the chamber concept of treatment becomes less advantageous and even prohibitively expensive, owing to the amount of drug needed to charge the large volumes of air required by the large chambers. In such cases, the use of a face mask with attached nebulizer is likely to be the simplest and best approach. The operating conditions to be employed with such a system will vary greatly with the equipment used; no total system is commercially available at the present time on which to base specific recommendations. However, the same principles and requirements must be considered for mask systems as for chamber systems.

In the treatment of pneumonia of infectious origin, the single most important objective is a lowering and rapid elimination of the total biomass of the infectious organism. Once this is accomplished, the animal will very rapidly clear its respiratory passages. It has been found in well-controlled experiments that the total biomass of infecting organisms can be rapidly eliminated using effective drugs in aerosols even when occlusion of small bronchioles is present. Thus, the need for bronchial dilators, detergents, mucolytics, etc., is strictly empirical at this time and probably of little value in most cases of infectious pneumonia.

## SUPPLEMENTAL READING

Berendt, R. F., Long, G. G., and Walker, J. S.: Treatment of respiratory *Klebsiella pneumoniae* infection in mice with aerosols of kanamycin. Antimicrob. Agents Chemother., 8:585–590, 1975.

Bolton, G. R.: Aerosol therapy. *In* Kirk, R. W. (ed.): Current Veterinary Therapy VI. Philadelphia, W. B. Saunders Co., 1977, p. 12.

Fairchild, G. A.: Measurement of respiratory volume for virus retention studies in mice. Appl. Microbiol., 24:812–818, 1972.

Jemski, J. V., and Walker, J. S.: Aerosol vaccination of mice with a live, temperature-sensitive recombinant influenza virus (H3N2). Infect. Immun., 13:818–843, March 1976.

Larson, E. W., Young, H. W., and Walker, J. S.: Aerosol evaluations of the DeVilbiss No. 40 and Vaponefrin nebulizers. Appl. Environ. Microbiol., 31:150–151, 1976.

Scott, F. W., and Glauberg, A. F.: Aerosol vaccination against feline panleukopenia. J. Am. Vet. Med. Assn., 166:147–149, 1975.

Scott, G. H., and Sydiskis, R. J.: Responses of mice immunized with influenza virus by aerosol and parenteral routes. Infect. Immun., 13:696–711, March, 1976.

Walker, J. S., Stephen, E. L., and Spertzel, R. O.: The use of small-particle aerosols of antiviral compounds for the treatment of type A influenza pneumonia in animal models. J. Infect. Dis., 133:A140–149, June Suppl., 1976.

---

# ANTIVIRAL THERAPY

FREDRIC W. SCOTT, D.V.M.
*Ithaca, New York*

The availability of effective antiviral compounds to treat viral diseases would have tremendous application in veterinary as well as in human medicine. Considerable research is currently under way to find and evaluate such antiviral compounds. Unfortunately there are numerous factors that make the development of antivirals a very difficult field. This discussion will evaluate what is currently available to the small animal practitioner for use in antiviral therapy of small animal infectious diseases and will discuss some aspects of the field that are currently under investigation and what agents and methods may become available in the future.

## MECHANISMS OF VIRAL INFECTIONS

In order to appreciate the mechanism of antiviral therapy, one must understand the mechanism of viral replication. Viruses replicate within living cells and pass from cell to cell as relatively inert substances, each composed of a core of genetic nucleic acid surrounded by a protein or lipoprotein coat. Since viruses are inactive outside the cell, an extracellular antiviral compound would have to rely either on chemical or physical inactivation or on specific neutralization by means of immunoglobulins. Since physical and chemical inactivation usually would denature proteins of cells, as well as the lipoprotein coat of the virus, this method of antiviral therapy is for the most part too toxic to be practical.

The most effective way of eliminating virus, and the one used primarily in the natural recovery from infection, is through the use of specific immunoglobulins that neutralize the virus particle by forming antigen-antibody complexes, which are phagocytized and broken down by the body.

Most antiviral compounds are aimed at blocking the replication of the virus particle by preventing the virus from entering the cell, or in some way preventing replication of the virus within the cell.

## TOXICITY

The main problem in developing antiviral compounds has been their toxicity. Numerous available antivirals are effective in blocking viral replication, but their toxicity is so high, or their margin of safety is so narrow, that they are not safe for clinical use. Since most antivirals rely upon blocking either the nucleic acid replication or the protein synthesis of the viral particle within the cell, one can visualize that this mechanism of action would be very close to that involved in the normal physiology of the cell. Recently compounds have been developed that appear to be specific for blocking viral replication without interfering with cell metabolism. If these compounds prove to be relatively nontoxic and effective, they could have great value in medicine.

## INTERFERON

Interferon (IF) is one or more cell-derived proteins that act on other cells in many ways, including cell regulation and a broad-spectrum viral resistance. While there were great expectations regarding IF as the panacea antiviral, the problems of low titer and short duration of action have kept IF from being the cure-all for viral infections.

**Mechanisms of Interferon Action.** When a virus infects certain susceptible cells, in addition to the virus being replicated within that cell, the nucleus is stimulated to produce one or more proteins collectively called "interferon." IF passes out of the cell and in some way stimulates other cells of the same species to synthesize an antiviral protein that blocks the replication of virus within that sensitized cell. While the exact mechanism of protection is not known, there is evidence to suggest that the interferon-induced antiviral activity is due to an inability of ribosomes to initiate synthesis of protein from viral messenger RNA while allowing cell messenger RNA to be translated normally.

**Exogenous Interferon:** Until recently technology was not advanced sufficiently to produce high titer exogenous IF. Now human IF can be produced in leukocyte cultures in sufficient titer and quantity for clinical testing. To date, high-titer exogenous dog and cat interferons are not available, but technically it should be possible to produce them.

**Polynucleotide Inducers of Interferon.** Synthetic double-stranded RNA in the form of polyinosinic acid–polycytidilic acid (poly I–poly C) can be an effective inducer of IF in several animals. A complex, poly I–poly C – poly L–lysine (poly I-C-L), is under investigation and appears to have some merit. For example, the intravenous administration of poly I-C-L to cats at the dose of 3 to 5 mg./kg. results in serum IF being produced within 6 hours, but the IF is cleared from the serum within 24 to 36 hours.

**Virus Inducers of Interferon.** During natural infection with certain viruses, viral replication stimulates production of IF, which results in a degree of viral resistance in sensitized cells. This aids in reducing the severity of the disease until antibodies can be produced to eliminate the virus. Obviously there is a limit to the effectiveness of this resistance; otherwise, these viruses would not produce disease.

Certain viruses such as Newcastle disease virus (NDV) are good inducers of IF in several species even though they may not produce disease other than in their homologous species. At least one small animal clinician (Dr. A. W. Sears, Lancaster, California) is using exogenous cat IF for therapy of several feline infectious diseases (Sears, 1976). The exogenous cat IF is produced by intravenous inoculation of donor cats with attenuated NDV vaccine. The donor cats are euthanatized and bled out 12 hours after inoculation; the serum is harvested, contained in sterile vials and frozen until needed. Beneficial clinical results in several feline infectious diseases have been noted after the administration of 1 to 2 ml./cat of this IF-containing serum every 12 hours for 2 days. This interesting procedure may have merit and warrants further investigation and clinical trials. However, two problems may be encountered. First, the level of IF produced by this procedure may be relatively low. Second, as with blood donors, IF-donors should be tested for feline leukemia virus and *Haemobartonella*. Both these organisms are associated with the cellular elements of blood, but serum from infected cats should not be used to treat other cats.

## IDOXURIDINE

The topical application of idoxuridine (IDU, IUdR, 5-ido-2'-deoxyuridine, Stoxil®*) is effective against superficial infections of DNA viruses such as human or feline herpetic keratoconjunctivitis, for which it is the drug of choice.

This antiviral is an antimetabolite that is incorporated into the viral DNA in place of thymidine, which results in a deficient and unstable viral DNA. The antimetabolite action is also effective against cellular DNA and, hence, results in intolerable toxicity if given parenterally or orally. Stoxil® may be administered as either an ophthalmic ointment or drops. It has no effect upon bacterial or fungal corneal disease. There do not appear to be adverse effects if antibiotic ointment is used with Stoxil®. Topical corticosteroids normally are contraindicated in herpetic keratitis, since they may predispose to herpetic ulcers. However, studies on experimental herpes simplex keratitis in rabbits showed that the simultaneous ophthalmic use of IDU and topical corticosteroids did not prevent healing (Bistner *et al.*, 1971). IDU has no effect upon RNA virus.

## VIRAZOLE®†

Virazole® (ribavirin, I-β-D-ribofuranosyl-1,2, 4-triazole-3-carboxamide) is a synthetic nucleoside with promising clinical potential as a broad-spectrum antiviral. Virazole® appears to inhibit an early step in viral re-

plication involving the synthesis of viral nucleic acids, either DNA or RNA. Although not completely free of toxic reactions, Virazole® is sufficiently nontoxic to allow parenteral or aerosol administration. The antiviral has been licensed for human use in several countries, but in the United States it is available only for experimental use in animals not to be used for human consumption. The exact dose for dogs and cats has not been established, but the manufacturer suggests an experimental dose of 25 mg./kg. IM or SC b.i.d. until 2 days after the disappearance of symptoms. In view of studies in other animals this should be an effective and safe dose. Side effects with long-term high doses (100 to 200 mg./kg./day in rats and monkeys) have included vomiting, diarrhea and reversible anemia. Virazole® is contraindicated during pregnancy.

## DISODIUM PHOSPHONOACETATE (PAA)*

PAA is a highly promising, stable, nontoxic antiviral that appears to have considerable potential against several herpesviruses and possibly other DNA viruses. The DNA-dependent DNA polymerase (an enzyme necessary for DNA replication) is selectively inhibited by PAA. This inhibition appears to be specific for the viral enzyme with little effect on cellular DNA synthesis. In the cat, doses as high as 500 mg./kg./day SC or 5 per cent solution by aerosol were nontoxic.

Although the field of antiviral chemotherapy for small animal viral diseases is not as yet a routine procedure (with the exception of IDU therapy of herpes keratoconjunctivitis in the cat), there are interesting compounds being developed and evaluated that may provide an additional therapeutic tool for the treatment of these diseases.

### SUPPLEMENTAL READING

Bistner, S. I., Carlson, J. H., Shively, J. N., and Scott, F. W.: Ocular manifestations of feline herpesvirus infection. J. Am. Vet. Med. Assn., *159*:1223–1237, 1971.
Carter, W. A.: Selective inhibition of viral functions. Cleveland, Ohio, CRC Press, 1975.

---

*Smith Kline & French, 1500 Spring Garden Street, Philadelphia, Pennsylvania 19101.
†ICN Pharmaceuticals, Inc., 2727 Campus Drive, Irvine, California 92664.

---

*Abbott Laboratories, 14th and Sheridan Road, North Chicago, Illinois 60064.

# SHIPPING REGULATIONS FOR SMALL ANIMALS

## INTERSTATE REGULATIONS

The regulations regarding the entry of dogs and cats into the various states of the United States and Puerto Rico are summarized below (Table 1). The regulations summarized, insofar as they are known, are current to January 1977. No responsibility is accepted for their complete accuracy. For the exact requirements for each state, inquiry should be made to the State Veterinarian in the state of destination.

Under most circumstances, no animal that is affected with or has recently been exposed to any infectious, contagious or communicable disease or that originates from a rabies quarantine area shall be shipped or, in any manner, transported or moved into any state until written permission for such entry is first obtained from the State Veterinarian or chief animal health official of the state to which the animal is to be transported.

Common carriers will usually not accept dogs or cats for interstate movement without health certificates; thus it would seem advisable, even if not specifically required, that such certificates be issued by the accredited practicing veterinarian in the state of origin.

## INTERNATIONAL REGULATIONS

Travelers from the United States to foreign countries on vacations and duty assignments frequently desire to take their pets with them. Similarly, persons returning from abroad need to make arrangements for the reentry of their pets and for animals acquired in other countries. For both importations and exportations, there are usually health requirements with which one must comply.

## MOVEMENT INTO FOREIGN COUNTRIES

There are no United States regulations governing the movement of dogs and cats to any foreign country. The regulations that must be complied with are those of the receiving country. These regulations are many, varied and subject to change. If pets are to be moved to any foreign country except Canada, the owner should obtain from the nearest consulate of the country of destination that country's regulations governing the import of pets and procedural instructions, such as the number of copies to be furnished, an indication of whether the health certificate must be validated by the consulate or whether certified copies of the pedigree or photograph of the pet must accompany the health certificate.

Dogs from the United States may be imported into Canada through any Canadian customs port of entry when accompanied by a certificate signed by a veterinarian licensed in Canada or the United States. The certificate must show that the dog has been vaccinated against rabies during the preceding 12 months.

## IMPORTATION OR REENTRY OF DOGS INTO THE UNITED STATES

The entry of dogs into the United States from all foreign countries is under the jurisdiction of the Public Health Service of the United States Department of Health, Education, and Welfare. An excerpt from the United States Public Health Service regulations regarding importation of dogs is quoted:

Vaccination for rabies shall be accomplished with nerve tissue vaccine more than one month

1351

*Table 1.  Regulations for Shipping of Small Animals*

| STATE OF DESTINATION | RABIES VACCINATION | | TYPE (KV) | TIME LIMIT (MLV) | AGE EXEMPTION (MONTHS) | HEALTH CERTIFICATE REQUIRED |
|---|---|---|---|---|---|---|
| | Dogs | Cats | | | | |
| Alabama | Yes | No | Within 6 mo. of entry | | 3 | X |
| Alaska | Yes | No | Within 6 mo. of entry | | 4 | X |
| Arizona | Yes | No | KV (12 mo.); MLV (36 mo.) | | 4 | |
| Arkansas | Yes | No | Within 12 mo. of entry | | 3 | |
| California | Yes | No | Current rabies vac. | | 4 | X |
| Colorado | Yes | No | Within 12 mo. of entry | | 3 | |
| Connecticut | No | No | | | | X |
| Delaware | Yes | No | | | 4 | X |
| Florida | Yes | No | Within 6 mo. of entry | | | X |
| Georgia | Yes | No | Within 6 mo. of entry | | 3 | |
| Hawaii | No | No | 120 days quarantine | | | |
| Idaho | Yes | No | NT (6 mo.); CE (24 mo.) | | 4 | X |
| Illinois | Yes | No | KV (6 mo.); MLV (12 mo.) | | 4 | X |
| Indiana | Yes | Yes | Within 12 mo. of entry | | 3 | X |
| Iowa | Yes | No | KV (12 mo.); MLV (24 mo.) | | 3 | X |
| Kansas | Yes | No | Within 12 mo. of entry | | 3 | X |
| Kentucky | Yes | Yes | KV (12 mo.); MLV (24 mo.) | | 4 | X |
| Louisiana | Yes | No | NT (12 mo.); CE (24 mo.) | | 2 | X |
| Maine | No | No | | | | X |
| Maryland | Yes | No | Within 12 mo. of entry | | 4 | X |
| Massachusetts | Yes | No | Within 12 mo. of entry | | | X |
| Michigan | No | No | | | | X |
| Minnesota | Yes | No | KV (12 mo.); MLV (24 mo.) | | 6 | X |
| Mississippi | Yes | No | Within 6 mo. of entry | | 3 | X |
| Missouri | Yes | No | KV (12 mo.); MLV (24 mo.) | | 4 | X |
| Montana | Yes | No | MLV (24 mo.) | | 3 | X |
| Nebraska | Yes | No | KV (12 mo.); MLV (24 mo.) | | 4 | X |
| Nevada | Yes | No | NT (12 mo.); CE (24 mo.) | | 4 | X |
| New Hampshire | Yes | No | KV (12 mo.); MLV (36 mo.) | | 3 | X |
| New Jersey | No | No | | | | X |
| New Mexico | Yes | No | Within 12 mo. of entry | | 4 | X |
| New York | No | No | | | | X |
| North Carolina | Yes | No | Within 12 mo. of entry | | 4 | X |
| North Dakota | Yes | No | Within 36 mo. of entry | | 4 | X |
| Ohio | Yes | No | KV (12 mo.), CE (36 mo.) | | 6 | X |
| Oklahoma | Yes | No | NT (12 mo.); MLV (24 mo.) | | 4 | |
| Oregon | Yes | Yes | KV (6 mo.); MLV (24 mo.) | | 4 | X |
| Pennsylvania | No | No | | | | X |
| Puerto Rico | Yes | Yes | Within 6 mo. of entry | | 2 | |
| Rhode Island | Yes | No | KV (6 mo.); MLV (24 mo.) | | 4 | X |
| South Carolina | Yes | No | Within 12 mo.of entry | | 4 | X |
| South Dakota | Yes | Yes | Within 12 mo. of entry | | 3 | X |
| Tennessee | Yes | No | Within 12 mo. of entry | | No exemption | X |
| Texas | Yes | No | Within 6 mo. of entry | | No exemption | X |
| Utah | Yes | Yes | KV (12 mo.); MLV (24 mo.) | | 4 | X |
| Vermont | Yes | Yes | MLV (12 mo.) | | 4 | X |
| Virginia | Yes | No | Within 12 mo. of entry | | 4 | X |
| Washington | Yes | No | KV (12 mo.); MLV (24 mo.) | | 4 | X |
| West Virginia | Yes | Yes | Within 12 mo. of entry | | 6 | X |
| Wisconsin | Yes | No | KV (12 mo.); CE (36 mo.) | | 6 | X |
| Wyoming | Yes | No | Within 24 mo. of entry | | 4 | X |

NT, Nerve tissue; CE, chick embryo; KV, killed vaccine; MLV, modified vaccine.

but not more than 12 months before the dog's arrival, or with chicken embryo vaccine more than one month but not more than 36 months before arrival.

**SUPPLEMENTAL READING**

Traveling With Your Pet. New York, American Society for the Prevention of Cruelty to Animals, 1972.

# APPENDICES

## ROBERT W. KIRK, D.V.M.
### Consulting Editor

# A ROSTER OF NORMAL VALUES*

JOHN BENTINCK-SMITH, D.V.M.
*Ithaca, New York*

Variations in normal values due to age, sex, breed, diurnal periodicity and emotional stress at the time of sampling can be expected. The methodology will also affect the biologic parameters.

The values presented here are derived from the literature, standard texts, the Animal Medical Center (courtesy of Dr. Robert J. Wilkins) and our own data (New York State College of Veterinary Medicine). References are cited as footnotes within the tables and appear in full at the end of this Appendix.

More reliable interpretation is possible when control samples are processed at the same time and by the same methods. Values for the dog and cat are found below; values for birds, reptiles and exotic animals can be found on pages 726, 792, and in *Current Veterinary Therapy V*, p. 545 ("Clinical Laboratory Examination of Cage Birds" by J. L. Leonard), respectively.

## NORMAL BLOOD VALUES[22]

| ERYTHROCYTES | ADULT DOG | AVERAGE | ADULT CAT | AVERAGE |
|---|---|---|---|---|
| Erythrocytes (millions/$\mu$l.) | 5.5–8.5 | 6.8 | 5.5–10.0 | 7.5 |
| Hemoglobin (g./dl.) | 12.0–18.0 | 14.9 | 8.0–14.0 | 12.0 |
| Packed Cell Volume (vol. %) | 37.0–55.0 | 45.5 | 24.0–45.0 | 37.0 |
| Mean Corpuscular Volume (femtoliters) | 66.0–77.0 | 69.8 | 40.0–55.0 | 45.0 |
| Mean Corpuscular Hemoglobin (picograms) | 19.9–24.5 | 22.8 | 13.0–17.0 | 15.0 |
| Mean Corpuscular Hemoglobin Concentration (g./dl.) | | | | |
| Wintrobe | 31.0–34.0 | 33.0 | 31.0–35.0 | 33.0 |
| Microhematocrit | 32.0–36.0 | 34.0 | 30.0–36.0 | 33.2 |
| Reticulocytes (%) (excludes punctate retics.) | 0.0–1.5 | 0.8 | 0.2–1.6 | 0.6 |
| Resistance to hypotonic saline (% saline solution producing) | | | | |
| Minimum | 0.40–0.50 | 0.46 | 0.66–0.72 | 0.69 |
| initial and complete hemolysis | | | | |
| Maximum | 0.32–0.42 | 0.33 | 0.46–0.54 | 0.50 |
| Erythrocyte Sedimentation Rate | PCV 37 | 13 | PCV 35–40 | 7–27 |
| (mm. at 60 min.) | PCV 50 | 0 | | |
| RBC life span (days) | 100–120 | | 66–78 | |
| RBC diameter ($\mu$) | 6.7–7.2 | 7.0 | 5.5–6.3 | 5.8 |

| LEUKOCYTES | ADULT DOG | AVERAGE | ADULT CAT | AVERAGE |
|---|---|---|---|---|
| Leukocytes (no./$\mu$l.) | 6,000–17,000 | 11,500 | 5,500–19,500 | 12,500 |
| Neutrophils—Bands(%) | 0–3 | 0.8 | 0–3 | 0.5 |
| Neutrophils—Mature (%) | 60–77 | 70.0 | 35–75 | 59.0 |
| Lymphocyte (%) | 12–30 | 20.0 | 20–55 | 32.0 |
| Monocyte (%) | 3–10 | 5.2 | 1–4 | 3.0 |
| Eosinophil (%) | 2–10 | 4.0 | 2–12 | 5.5 |
| Basophil (%) | Rare | 0.0 | Rare | 0.0 |
| Neutrophils—Bands (no./$\mu$l.) | 0–300 | 70 | 0–300 | 100 |
| Neutrophils—Mature (no./$\mu$l.) | 3,000–11,500 | 7,000 | 2,500–12,500 | 7,500 |
| Lymphocytes (no./$\mu$l.) | 1,000–4,800 | 2,800 | 1,500–7,000 | 4,000 |
| Monocytes (no./$\mu$l.) | 150–1,350 | 750 | 0–850 | 350 |
| Eosinovhils (no./$\mu$l.) | 100–1,250 | 550 | 0–1,500 | 650 |
| Basophils | Rare | 0 | Rare | 0 |

*See reference 24.

## CANINE BLOOD PARAMETERS AT DIFFERENT AGES—AVERAGE VALUES[1]

| Age | millions/µl. RBC | Retic. % * | Nucl. RBC/ 100 WBC * | g./dl. Hb | Vol. % PCV | /dl. WBC | /dl. Neut. | /dl. Bands | /dl. Lymph. | /dl. Eos. |
|---|---|---|---|---|---|---|---|---|---|---|
| Birth | 5.75 | 7.1 | 1.8 | 16.70 | 50 | 16,500 | 1,300 | 400 | 2,500 | 600 |
| 2 weeks | 3.92 | 7.1 | 1.8 | 9.76 | 32 | 11,000 | 6,500 | 100 | 3,000 | 300 |
| 4 weeks | 4.20 | 7.1 | 1.8 | 9.60 | 33 | 13,000 | 8,600 | 0 | 4,000 | 40 |
| 6 weeks | 4.91 | 3.6 | 1.8 | 9.59 | 34 | 15,000 | 10,000 | 0 | 4,500 | 100 |
| 8 weeks | 5.13 | 3.9 | 0.3 | 11.00 | 37 | 18,000 | 11,000 | 234 | 6,000 | 270 |
| 12 weeks | 5.27 | 3.9 | Rare | 11.60 | 36 | 15,300 | 9,400 | 115 | 4,600 | 322 |

*See reference 10.

## FELINE BLOOD PARAMETERS AT DIFFERENT AGES[22]

| Age | millions/µl. RBC | g./dl. Hb | Vol. % PCV | /dl. WBC | /dl. Neut. | /dl. Lymph. |
|---|---|---|---|---|---|---|
| Birth | 4.95 | 12.2 | 44.7 | 7,500 | | |
| 2 weeks | 4.76 | 9.7 | 31.1 | 8,080 | | |
| 5 weeks | 5.84 | 8.4 | 29.9 | 8,550 | | |
| Average* | 4.80 | 7.5 | 26.2 | 11,770 | 4,600 | 6,970 |
| Range* | 3.90–5.70 | 6.6–8.4 | 21.0–33.5 | 7,500–14,500 | | 4,500–9,400 |
| 6 weeks | 6.75 | 9.0 | 35.4 | 8,420 | | |
| 8 weeks | 7.10 | 9.4 | 35.6 | 8,420 | | |
| Average* | 5.90 | 7.5 | 26.2 | 12,400 | 7,500 | 4,900 |
| Range* | 3.30–7.30 | 7.6–15.0 | 22–38 | 6,900–23,100 | | 1,925–10,100 |

*See reference 2.

## BASENJI DOGS[10]

| *Plasma Proteins (g./dl.)* | |
|---|---|
| 6–8 weeks | 5.33 ± 0.29 |
| 9–12 weeks | 5.87 ± 0.46 |
| 4–6 months | 6.6 ± 0.25 |
| 1–2 years | 7.03 ± 0.33 |

## CATS[22]

*Plasma Proteins (g./dl.)*

Lower values for younger animals
Adults 6–8

## EFFECT OF PREGNANCY AND LACTATION ON BLOOD PARAMETERS OF THE DOG[1]

| | GESTATION | | | | TERM | LACTATION | | |
|---|---|---|---|---|---|---|---|---|
| | 2 Weeks | 4 Weeks | 6 Weeks | 8 Weeks | 0 Weeks | 2 Weeks | 4 Weeks | 6 Weeks |
| RBC (millions/dl.) | 8.85 | 7.48 | 6.73 | 6.26 | 4.53 | 5.13 | 5.65 | 6.15 |
| PCV (Vol. %) | 53 | 47 | 44 | 37 | 32 | 34 | 38 | 42 |
| Hb (g./dl.) | 19.6 | 16.4 | 14.7 | 13.8 | 11.0 | 11.7 | 12.8 | 13.4 |
| Sedimentation Rate (mm. at 60 min.) | 0.6 | 11.0 | 31.0 | 14.0 | 12.0 | 14.0 | 14.0 | 13.0 |
| WBC (thousands/dl.) | 12.0 | 12.2 | 15.7 | 19.0 | 18.9 | 16.9 | 17.1 | 15.9 |

## EFFECT OF PREGNANCY AND LACTATION ON BLOOD PARAMETERS OF THE CAT[5]

| | GESTATION | | | | | TERM | LACTATION | |
| --- | --- | --- | --- | --- | --- | --- | --- | --- |
| | *1 Day Past Conception* | *2 Weeks* | *4 Weeks* | *6 Weeks* | *8 Weeks* | *0 Weeks* | *2 Weeks* | *4 Weeks* |
| RBC (millions/dl.) | 8.0 | 7.9 | 7.1 | 6.7 | 6.2 | 6.2 | 7.4 | 7.4 |
| PCV (Vol. %) | 36.1 | 37.0 | 33.0 | 32.0 | 28.0 | 29.0 | 33.0 | 33.0 |
| Hb (g./100 ml.) | 12.5 | 12.0 | 11.0 | 10.8 | 9.5 | 10.0 | 11.5 | 11.2 |
| Reticulocytes (%) (includes punctate retics.) | 9 | 11 | 9 | 10 | 20.1 | 15 | 9 | 6 |

| | ADULT DOG | AVERAGE | ADULT CAT | AVERAGE[22] |
| --- | --- | --- | --- | --- |
| Thrombocytes $\times$ $10^5/\mu$l. | 2–5 | 3–4 | 3–8 | 4.5 |
| Icterus Index | 2–5 units | | 2–5 units | |
| Plasma Fibrinogen (g./l.) | 2.0–4.0 | | 0.50–3.00 | |

## NORMAL BONE MARROW (Percentage)

| ERYTHROCYTIC CELLS | DOG[22] | CAT[18] |
| --- | --- | --- |
| Rubriblasts | 0.2 | 1.71 |
| Prorubricytes | 3.9 | |
| Rubricytes | 27.0 | 12.50 |
| Metarubricytes | 15.3 | 11.68 |
| Total Erythrocytic Cells | 46.4 | 25.89 |

| GRANULOCYTIC CELLS | | |
| --- | --- | --- |
| Myeloblasts | 0.0 | 1.74 |
| Progranulocytes | 1.3 | 0.88 |
| Neutrophilic Myelocytes | 9.0 | 9.76 |
| Eosinophilic Myelocytes | 0.0 | 1.47 |
| Neutrophilic Metamyelocytes | 7.5 | 7.32 |
| Eosinophilic Metamyelocytes | 2.4 | 1.52 |
| Band Neutrophils | 13.6 | 25.80 |
| Band Eosinophils | 0.9 | — |
| Neutrophils | 18.4 | 9.24 |
| Eosinophils | 0.3 | 0.81 |
| Basophils | 0.0 | 0.002 |
| Total Granulocytic Cells | 53.4 | 58.542 |
| M:E Ratio—Average | 1.15:1.0 | 2.47:1.0 |
| M:E Ratio—Range (Schalm) | 0.75–2.50:1.0 | 0.60–3.90:1.0 |

| OTHER CELLS | | |
| --- | --- | --- |
| Lymphocytes | 0.2 | 7.63 |
| Plasma Cells | 0 | 1.61 |
| Reticulum Cells | 0 | 0.13 |
| Mitotic Cells | 0 | 0.61 |
| Unclassified | 0 | 1.62 |
| Disintegrated Cells | 0 | 4.60 |

## BLOOD, PLASMA OR SERUM CHEMICAL CONSTITUENTS
### (B) = Blood, (P) = Plasma, (S) = Serum

Chemical constituents are liable to show markedly different values depending on the methodology employed.

| TECHNICON SMA 12/60 | ADULT DOG[25] | ADULT CAT[25] |
|---|---|---|
| Urea N (S) (mg./dl.) | 10–22 | 5–30 |
| Glucose (S) (mg./dl.) | 50–120 | 70–150 |
| Total Bilirubin (S) (mg./dl.) | 0–0.8 | 0–0.8 |
| Total Protein (S) (g./dl.) | 5.4–7.8 | 5.5–7.5 |
| Albumin (S) (g./dl.) | 2.2–3.4 | 2.2–3.5 |
| Alkaline Phosphatase (S) (mU./ml.) | 20–120 | 10–80 |
| Calcium (S) (mg./dl.) | 9.0–11.6 | 7.6–11.0 |
| Inorganic Phosphorus (S) (mg./dl.) | 3.7–6.0 | 3.0–6.0 |
| LDH (S) (mU./ml.) | 40–200 | 10–200 |
| SGOT (S) (mU./ml.) | 5–80 | 10–60 |
| SGPT (S) (mU./ml.) | 5–80 | 10–80 |
| Total $CO_2$ (S) (mEq./l.) | 17–25 | 16–25 |

| ELECTROPHORESIS | | |
|---|---|---|
| Albumin (S) (g./dl.) | 2.3–3.4 | 2.3–3.5 |
| Globulin (S) (g./dl.) | 3.0–4.7 | 2.6–5.0 |
| Alpha 1 (S) (g./dl.) | 0.3–0.8 | 0.3–0.5 |
| Alpha 2 (S) (g./dl.) | 0.5–1.3 | 0.4–1.0 |
| Beta (S) (g./dl.) | 0.7–1.8 | 0.6–1.9 |
| Gama (S) (g./dl.) | 0.4–1.0 | 0.5–1.5 |
| Albumin/Globulin Ratio, A/G (S) | 0.7–1.1 | 0.5–1.0 |

| OTHER CONSTITUENTS | | |
|---|---|---|
| Creatinine (S) (mg./dl.) | 1–2 | 1–2 |
| Uric Acid (S) (mg./dl.) | 0–1.5 | 0–1.9 |
| Lipase (S) (Sigma Tietz Units) | 0–1 | 0–1 |
| Amylase (S) (Somogyi Units) | 200–800 | 400–800 |
| (Harding Units) | 1600–2400 | |
| CPK (S) (International Units) | 0–70 | 10–60 |
| (mU./ml.) | 10–400 | 30–300 |
| Lactic Acid (S) (mg./dl.) | 3–15 | |
| Pyruvate (B) (mEq./l.) | 0.1–0.2 | |
| Total Cholesterol (S) (mg./dl.) | 125–250 | 75–150 |
| Cholesterol Esters (S) (mg./dl.) | 84–168 | 45–120 |
| Free Cholesterol (S) (mg./dl.) | 28–84 | 15–60 |
| Total Lipid (P) (mg./dl.) | 47–725 | 145–607 |
| Triglyceride (S) 24-hr. fast (mg./dl.)[19] | 47.2–63.4 | |
| Free Glycerol (S) 24-hr. fast (mg./dl.)[19] | 14.2–23.2 | |
| Bromsulfalein Retention Test (B) | <5% | |
| Iron (S) ($\mu$g./dl.) | 94–122 | 68–215 |
| Total Iron Binding Capacity (S) ($\mu$g./dl.) | 280–340 | 170–400 |
| Lead (B) (mcg./dl.) | 0–35 | 0–35 |

| ELECTROLYTES | ADULT DOG | ADULT CAT |
|---|---|---|
| Sodium (S) (mEq./l.) | 135–150 | 145–156 |
| Potassium (S) (mEq./l.) | 3.5–5.5 | 4.0–5.0 |
| Magnesium (S) (mEq./l.) | 1.4–2.4 | 2.2 |
| Chloride (S) (mEq./l.) | 99–110 | 108–120 |
| Sulfate (S) (mEq./l.) | 2.0 | |
| Osmolality (S) (mOsm./l.) | 280–305 | 280–305 |
| (S) (mOsm./kg.) | 280–310 | 280–310 |
| pH | 7.31–7.42 | 7.24–7.40 |

| BLOOD GASES (DOG) | | |
|---|---|---|
| $PO_2$ 85–95 mm. Hg (arterial) | standard temperature and pressure | |
| 40–60 mm. Hg (venous) | standard temperature and pressure | |
| $PCO_2$ 29–36 mm. Hg (arterial) | standard temperature and pressure | |
| 29–42 mm. Hg (venous) | standard temperature and pressure | |
| Base Excess (B) (mEq./l.) | ± 2.5 | ± 2.5 |
| Bicarbonate (P) (mEq./l.) | 17–24 | 17–24 |

## BLOOD, PLASMA OR SERUM CHEMICAL CONSTITUENTS
### (B) = Blood, (P) = Plasma, (S) = Serum

Chemical constituents are liable to show markedly different values depending on the methodology employed.

| ENDOCRINOLOGY | ADULT DOG | ADULT CAT |
|---|---|---|
| Insulin (S) (mcU./ml.)[25] | 0–30 | 0–50 |
| Cortisol (S) (mcg./dl.)[25] | 2–6 | 2–5 |

| | DOG | | | CAT | | |
|---|---|---|---|---|---|---|
| | *12 Weeks* | *1 Year* | *3–6 Years* | *10 Weeks* | *1 Year* | *>1 Year* |
| $T_3$ (% uptake)[3,12,13] | 44.7±0.94 | 44.2±1.26 | 43.1±2.7 | 55.6±2.37 | 58.3±2.40 | 57.7±1.88 |
| $T_4$ ($\mu$g./dl.)[3,12,13] | 3.24±0.51 | 2.25±0.35 | 1.49±0.46 | 2.82±0.73 | 2.43±0.55 | 2.12±0.69 |

| | | |
|---|---|---|
| $T_4$ Range ($\mu$g./dl.)[25] | 1.5–4.5 | 1.2–3.8 |
| Protein-bound Iodine ($\mu$g./dl.)[3,12,13] | 1.6–3.0 | |
| TSH Response to 5–10 Units I.M.[3,12,13]: | | |
| (a) At 72 hours—PBI increase of 3 $\mu$g./dl. (mean) | | |
| (b) At 12 hours—$T_4$ ($\mu$g./dl.) 3–4 fold increase | | |
| Thyroid Uptake Radioiodine ($^{131}$I%)[3,12,13] | 17–30 | |

| HEMOSTATIC PARAMETERS (No test should be interpreted without an accompanying normal control [see article on "Inherited Hemorrhagic Defects"].) | ADULT DOG | ADULT CAT |
|---|---|---|
| Bleeding Time | | |
| Dorsum of nose (min.) | 2–4 | 1–5[22] |
| Lip (sec.) | 85–110 | |
| Ear (min.) | 2.5–3 | |
| Abdomen (min.) | 1–2 | |
| Whole Blood Coagulation Time | | |
| Glass (Lee and White) (min.) | 6–7.5 | 8 min.[22] |
| Silicone (Lee and White) (min.) | 12–15 | |
| Capillary Tube (min.)[8] | 3–4 | 5.2±0.2[16] |
| Prothrombin Time (sec.)[8] | 6–10 | 8.6±0.5[16] |
| Puppies 1–4 hours old (sec.)[4] | 42.2 | |
| 6–12 hours old (sec.) | 49.1 | |
| 16–48 hours old (sec.) | 36.8 | |
| 48 hours old (sec.) | 24.5 | |
| Russell's Viper Venom Time (sec.)[20] | 11 | 9 |
| Partial Thromboplastin Time (sec.) | 15–25 | |
| Prothrombin Consumption (sec.)[20] | 20.5 | 20 |
| Fibrin Degradation Products ($\mu$g./ml.) | <10 | |

NORMAL RENAL FUNCTION AND URINE PARAMETERS

| *Urine*[17] | *Adult Dog* | *Adult Cat* |
|---|---|---|
| Specific Gravity | | |
| Minimum | 1.001 | 1.001 |
| Maximum | 1.060 | 1.080 |
| Usual Limits (normal water and food intake) | 1.018–1.050 | 1.018–1.050 |
| Volume (ml./kg. body weight/day) | 24–41 | 22–30 |
| Osmolality Urine | | |
| Usual Range | 500–1200 | |
| Maximal Limits | 2000–2400 | |
| Osmolality Plasma | 3000 | |

| *Urine Constituents*[25] (The following values are markedly affected by degree of concentration.) | *Adult Dog* | *Adult Cat* |
|---|---|---|
| Creatinine (mg./dl.) | 100–300 | 110–280 |
| Urea (g./dl.) | 1.0–2.5 | 1.0–3.0 |
| Protein (mg./dl.) | 0–30 | 0–20 |
| Amylase (Somogyi Units) | 50–150 | 30–120 |
| Sodium (mEq./l.) | 20–165 | |
| Potassium (mEq./l.) | 20–120 | |
| Calcium (mEq./l.) | 2–10 | |
| Inorganic Phosphorus (mEq./l.) | 50–180 | |

## BLOOD, PLASMA OR SERUM CHEMICAL CONSTITUENTS
### (B) = Blood, (P) = Plasma, (S) = Serum

Chemical constituents are liable to show markedly different values depending on the methodology employed.

| URINALYSIS—SEMIQUANTITATIVE VALUES | ADULT DOG | ADULT CAT |
|---|---|---|
| Protein | 0-trace | 0-trace |
| Glucose | 0 | 0 |
| Ketones | 0 | 0 |
| Bilirubin | 0 | 0 |
| 10–20% Dogs—high specific gravity | 1+ | |
| 5% Cats—high specific gravity | | 1+ |
| Urobilinogen (Ehrlich Unit) | 0-1 | 0-1 |
| (Wallace and Diamond) | <1:32 | <1:32 |

RENAL FUNCTION—DOG[6]

| | |
|---|---|
| Effective Renal Plasma Flow | $266\pm66$ ml./min./m² of body surface |
| | $13.5\pm3.3$ ml./min./kg. of body weight |
| Glomerular Filtration Rate | $84.4\pm19$ ml./min./m² of body surface |
| | 4 ml./min./kg. of body weight |

RENAL FUNCTION TESTS—DOG

| | |
|---|---|
| Phenolsulfonphthalein | |
| Excretion in urine at 20 min., 6-mg. dose[8] | 21-66% |
| Clearance (P) 1 mg./kg. at 60 min.[13] | $<80\mu$/ml. |
| T½ Clearance 5 mg./kg.[7] | 19.6 min. |
| Creatinine, Endogenous Clearance | $60\pm22$ ml./min./m² of body surface |
| | $2.98\pm0.96$ ml./min./kg. of body weight |

| CEREBROSPINAL FLUID[9] | ADULT DOG | ADULT CAT |
|---|---|---|
| Color | Clear, colorless | Clear, colorless |
| Pressure (mm. $H_2O$) | <170 | <100 |
| Cells/$\mu$l. | <5 lymphocytes | <5 lymphocytes |
| Protein (ml./dl.) | <25 | <20 |
| Glucose (mg./dl.) | 61-116 | 85 |

NORMAL SYNOVIAL FLUID—CARPAL, ELBOW, SHOULDER, HIP, STIFLE AND HOCK JOINTS[21]

| | ADULT DOG | |
|---|---|---|
| | *Range* | *Mean* |
| Amount ml. | 0.01–1.00 | 0.24 |
| pH | 7-7.8 | 7.33 |
| Leukocytes × 10³/$\mu$l. | 0-2.9 | 0.43 |
| Erythrocytes × 10³$\mu$l. | 0.320.0 | 12.15 |
| Neutrophils/$\mu$l. | 0-32 | 3.63 |
| Neutrophils(%)[15] | 10 | |
| Monocytes/$\mu$l. | 0-838 | 230.77 |
| Lymphocytes/$\mu$l. | 0-2436 | 245.6 |
| Clasmatocytes/$\mu$l. | 0–166 | 14.69 |
| Mononuclears(%)[15] | 90 | |
| Mucin Clot | Tight ropy clump | |
| | Clear supernate | |

## CANINE SEMEN[11]

Regular collection by hand manipulation with a teaser (125 ejaculates from small dogs, mostly beagles)[6].

| | Mean | Standard Deviation | Range |
|---|---|---|---|
| Volume (ml.) | 5 | 4.3 | 0.5-20.4 |
| % Motile Sperm | 75 | 7.5 | 30-90 |
| % Normal Sperm | 86 | 14.7 | 34-97 |
| pH | 6.72 | 0.19 | 6.49-7.10 |
| Concentration/cu. mm. ($10^3$) | 148 | 84.6 | 27.2-388.8 |
| Total Sperm per Ejaculate ($10^6$) | 528 | 321.0 | 94-1428 |

### FRACTIONATED EJACULATES (BASED ON 65 EJACULATES)

| | Mean | Range | pH |
|---|---|---|---|
| 1st Fraction | 0.8 ml. | 0.25-2.00 | 6.37 |
| 2nd Fraction | 0.6 ml. | 0.40-2.00 | 6.10 |
| 3rd Fraction | 0.4 ml. | 1.0-16.3 | 7.20 |

### PUREBRED LABRADOR RETRIEVERS, 18 TO 48 MONTHS OLD[23]

| | Mean | Range |
|---|---|---|
| Volume (ml.) | 2.2* | 0.5-6.5 |
| % Motile Sperm | 93 | 75-99 |
| % Unstained Sperm (Eosin Nigrosin) | 84 | 61-99 |
| Concentration/cu. mm. ($10^3$) | 564 | 103-708 |

*Only the first two fractions were collected, resulting in smaller volume and higher concentration of sperm/cu. mm. than would result if all the prostatic fluid (3rd fraction) were obtained.

### SUPPLEMENTAL READING AND REFERENCES

1. Andersen, A. C., and Gee, W.: Normal values in the beagle. Vet. Med., 53:135–138 and 156, 1958.
2. Anderson, L., Wilson, R., and Hay, D.: Haematological values in normal cats from four weeks to one year of age. Res. Vet. Sci., 12:579–583, 1971.
3. Baker, H. J.: Laboratory evaluation of thyroid function. In Kirk, R. W. (ed.): Current Veterinary Therapy IV. Philadelphia, W. B. Saunders Co., 1971.
4. Benjamin, M.: An Outline of Veterinary Clinical Pathology. 2nd ed. Ames, Iowa, Iowa State Press, 1961.
5. Berman, E.: Hemogram of the cat during pregnancy and lactation and after lactation. Am. J. Vet. Res., 35:457–460, 1974.
6. Boucher, J. H.: Evaluation of semen quality in the dog and the effects of frequency of ejaculation upon semen quality, libido, and restoration of sperm reserves. M.S . Thesis, Cornell University, Ithaca, N.Y., 1957.
7. Brobst, D. F., Carter, J. M., and Horron, M.: Plasma phenolsulfonphthalein determination as a measure of renal function in the dog. 17th Gaines Veterinary Symposium, University of Minnesota, 1967, p. 15.

8. Coles, E. H.: Veterinary Clinical Pathology. 2nd ed., Philadelphia, W. B. Saunders Co., 1974.
9. deLahunta, A.: New York State College of Veterinary Medicine, Cornell University, Ithaca, New York 14853. Personal communication.
10. Ewing, G. O., Schalm, O. W., and Smith, R. S.: Hematologic values of normal Basenji dogs. J. Am. Vet. Med. Assn., 161:1661, 1972.
11. Revisions and Corrections courtesy of Dr. R. H. Foote, Professor of Animal Physiology, Department of Animal Science, New York State College of Life Sciences, Cornell University, Ithaca, New York 14853.
12. Kallfelz, F. A.: Associate Professor of Clinical Nutrition, Department of Large Animal Medicine, Obstetrics and Surgery, New York State College of Veterinary Medicine, Ithaca, New York 14853. Personal communication.
13. Kallfelz, F. A., and Erali, R. P.: Thyroid function tests in domesticated animals. Am. J. Vet. Res., 34:1449, 1973.
14. Kaufman, C. F., and Kirk, R. W.: The sixty-minute plasma phenolsulfonphthalein concentration as a test of renal function in the dog. J.A.A.H.A., 9:66, 1973.
15. Miller, J. B., Perman, V., Osborne, C. A., Hammer, R. F., and Gambardella, P. C.: Synovial fluid analysis in canine arthritis. J.A.A.H.A., 10:392, 1974.
16. Osbaldiston, G. W., Stowe, E. C., and Griffith, P.

R.: Blood coagulation: comparative studies in dogs, cats, horses and cattle. Brit. Vet. J., *126*:512, 1970.

17. Osborne, C. A., Low, D. G., and Finco, D. R.: Canine and Feline Urology. Philadelphia, W. B. Saunders Co., 1972.

18. Penny, R. H. C., Carlisle, C. H., and Davidson, H. A.: The blood and marrow picture of the cat. Brit. Vet. J. *126*:459–462, 1970.

19. Rogers, U. A., Donovan, E. F., and Kociba, G. J.: Lipids and lipoproteins in normal dogs and dogs with secondary hyperlipoproteinemia. J. Am. Vet. Med. Assn., *166*:1092–1100, 1975.

20. Rowsell, H. C.: Blood coagulation and hemorrhagic disorders. *In* Medway, W., Prier, J. E., and Wilkinson, J. S. (eds.): Textbook of Veterinary Clinical Pathology. Baltimore, Williams & Wilkins Co., 1969, p. 247.

21. Sawyer, D. C.: Synovial fluid analysis of canine joints. J. Am. Vet. Med. Assn., *143*:609, 1963.

22. Schalm, O. W., Jain, N. C., and Carroll, E. J.: Veterinary Hematology. 3rd ed. Philadelphia, Lea & Febiger, 1975.

23. Seager, S. W. J., and Fletcher, W. S.: Collection, storage, and insemination of canine semen. Lab. Animal Sci., *22*:177–182, 1972.

24. Tasker, J. B.: Professor of Clinical Pathology, Department of Large Animal Medicine, Obstetrics, and Surgery, New York State College of Veterinary Medicine, Ithaca, New York 14853. Dr. Tasker was kind enough to review and correct this manuscript.

25. Wilkins, R. J.: Animal Medical Center, 510 East 62nd St., New York, New York 10021. Personal communication.

# TABLE OF STANDARDS FOR TAIL DOCKING

Compiled by
M. JOSEPHINE DEUBLER, V.M.D.
*Philadelphia, Pennsylvania*

**Table 1.** *Tail Docking**

| BREED | LENGTH AT LESS THAN ONE WEEK OF AGE |
|---|---|
| *Sporting Breeds* | |
| Brittany Spaniel | Leave 1 inch |
| Clumber Spaniel | Leave 1/4–1/3 |
| Cocker Spaniel | Leave 1/3 (about 3/4 inch) |
| English Cocker Spaniel | Leave 1/3 |
| English Springer Spaniel | Leave 1/3 |
| Field Spaniel | Leave 1/3 |
| German Shorthaired Pointer | Leave 2/5[s] |
| German Wirehaired Pointer | Leave 2/5[s] |
| Sussex Spaniel | Leave 1/3 |
| Vizsla | Leave 2/3[s] |
| Weimaraner | Leave 3/5 (about 1 1/2 inches) |
| Welsh Springer Spaniel | Leave 1/3–1/2 |
| Wirehaired Pointing Griffon | Leave 1/3[s] |
| *Working Breeds* | |
| Bouvier des Flandres | Leave 1/2–3/4 inch |
| Boxer | Leave 1/2–3/4 inch |
| Doberman Pinscher | Leave 3/4 inch (two vertebrae) |
| Giant Schnauzer | Leave 1 1/4 inches (three vertebrae) |
| Old English Sheepdog | If necessary—close to body (leave one vertebra) |
| Rottweiler | If necessary—close to body (leave one vertebra) |
| Schnauzer (Standard) | Leave 1 inch (two vertebrae) |
| Welsh Corgi (Pembroke) | Close to body (leave one vertebra) |
| *Terrier Breeds* | |
| Airedale Terrier | Leave 2/3–3/4‡ |
| Australian Terrier | Leave 2/5[s] |
| Fox Terrier (Smooth and Wirehaired) | Leave 2/3–3/4‡ |
| Irish Terrier | Leave 3/4[s] |
| Kerry Blue Terrier | Leave 1/2–2/3 |
| Lakeland Terrier | Leave 2/3‡ |
| Norwich Terrier | Leave 1/4–1/3 |
| Schnauzer (Miniature) | Leave about 3/4 inch—not more than 1 inch |
| Sealyham Terrier | Leave 1/3–1/2 |
| Soft-coated Wheaten Terrier | Leave 1/2 |
| Welsh Terrier | Leave 2/3‡ |

### *Table 1. Tail Docking\**—CONTINUED

| BREED | LENGTH AT LESS THAN ONE WEEK OF AGE |
|---|---|
| *Toy Breeds* | |
|     Affenpinscher | Close to body (leave $\frac{1}{8}$ inch) |
|     Brussels Griffon | Leave $\frac{1}{4}$–$\frac{1}{3}$ |
|     English Toy Spaniel | Leave $\frac{1}{3}$ |
|     Pinscher (Miniature) | Leave $\frac{1}{2}$ inch (two vertebrae) |
|     Poodle (Toy) | Leave $\frac{1}{2}$–$\frac{2}{3}$ (about 1 inch) |
|     Silky Terrier | Leave about $\frac{1}{3}$ (about $\frac{1}{2}$ inch) |
|     Yorkshire Terrier | Leave about $\frac{1}{3}$ (about $\frac{1}{2}$ inch) |
| *Nonsporting Breeds* | |
|     Poodle (Miniature) | Leave $\frac{1}{2}$–$\frac{2}{3}$ (about $1\frac{1}{8}$ inches) |
|     Poodle (Standard) | Leave $\frac{1}{2}$–$\frac{2}{3}$ (about $1\frac{1}{2}$ inches) |
| *Miscellaneous Breed (not registered by American Kennel Club)* | |
|     Cavalier King Charles Spaniel | Optional. Leave at least $\frac{2}{3}$. Always leave white tip in broken-colored dogs. |
|     Spinoni Italiani | Leave $\frac{3}{5}$ |

\* This list gives *approximate* guides for docking when done before puppy is one week old. If definite information was not given in the official breed standard, *opinions* were obtained from judges, breeders, veterinarians, and professional handlers.

An improperly docked tail may ruin a puppy for show purposes. If one is in doubt, consultation with an established breeder is suggested. There may be variations among puppies, and a knowledge of breed characteristics is important in determining the correct length to dock. M. Josephine Deubler

ˢ Taken from official breed standard.

‡ The tip of the docked tail should be approximately level with the top of the skull with the puppy in show position.

### IMPORTANT

Editor's note: The preceding data on tail docking were compiled from official standards published by the American Kennel Club or from information obtained directly from judges, veterinarians, breeders, and professional handlers. However, because of the ambiguous descriptions used in many standards, and because breed fashions change, veterinarians are cautioned to *use these figures as suggestions only!* Always obtain specific instructions from the owner as to length of dock!

# TABLES OF NORMAL PHYSIOLOGICAL DATA

## ELECTROCARDIOGRAPHY*

It is recognized that normal and abnormal electrocardiographic measurements overlap and that the criteria for the normal electrocardiogram serve only as a guide for the clinician. Deviations from normal in an individual electrocardiogram suggest but are not always diagnostic of heart disease. As additional statistical data become available for the electrocardiograms of dogs of each breed, body type, age and sex, the data herein may require revision, and "normal" may be more precisely defined. The *value of serial electrocardiograms* from an individual cannot be overemphasized, since serial changes best demonstrate electrocardiographic abnormalities.

### Criteria for the Normal Canine Electrocardiogram†

*Heart rate*—70 to 160 beats per minute for adult dogs; up to 180 beats per minute in toy breeds, and 220 beats per minute for puppies.

*Heart rhythm*—Normal sinus rhythm; sinus arrhythmia; and wandering sinoatrial pacemaker.

*P wave*—Up to 0.4 millivolt in amplitude; up to 0.04 second in duration; always positive in leads II and aVF; positive or isoelectric in lead I.

*P-R interval*—0.06 to 0.13 second duration.

*QRS complex*—Mean electric axis, frontal plane, 40 to 100 degrees.

Amplitude—Maximum amplitude of R wave 2.5 to 3.0 millivolts in leads II, III, and aVF. Complex positive in leads II, III, and aVF; negative in lead $V_{10}$.

Duration—To 0.05 second (0.06 second in large breeds).

*S-T segment and T wave*—S-T segment free of marked coving (repolarization changes).

S-T segment depression not greater than 0.2 millivolt in leads II and III and not greater than 0.3 millivolt in lead $CV_6LL$.

S-T segment elevation not greater than 0.15 millivolt in leads II and III.

T wave negative in leads $V_{10}$ and T wave positive in $CV_5RL$ (except in the Chihuahua).

T wave amplitude not greater than 25 per cent of amplitude of R wave.

### Criteria for the Normal Feline Electrocardiogram‡

*Heart rate*—240 beats per minute maximum.

*Heart rhythm*—Normal sinus rhythm or, infrequently, sinus arrhythmia.

*P wave*—Positive in leads II and AVF: may be isoelectric or positive in lead I; should not exceed 0.04 second in duration.

*P-R interval*—0.04 to 0.10 second duration (inversely related to the heart rate).

*QRS complex*—More variable than in the canine; the mean electric axis in the frontal plane is often insignificant. Often the QRS complex is nearly isoelectric in all frontal plane limb leads (so-called horizontal heart).

Amplitude—The amplitude of the R wave is usually low; marked amplitude of R waves (over 1.0 millivolt) in the frontal plane leads may suggest ventricular hypertrophy.

Duration—Less than 0.04 second.

*S-T segment and T wave*—S-T segment and T wave should be small and free of repolarization changes as well as marked depression of elevation.

*(From Ettinger, S. J.: Textbook of Veterinary Internal Medicine. Philadelphia. W. B. Saunders Company, 1975.)

---

*From Ettinger, S. J., and Suter, P. F.: *Canine Cardiology*. Philadelphia, W. B. Saunders Co., 1970.

†Derived from personal observations and from sources gratefully acknowledged in the bibliography and cited in the text of the chapter in *Canine Cardiology*.

‡From Ettinger, S. J.: *Textbook of Veterinary Internal Medicine*. Philadelphia. W. B. Saunders Co., 1975.

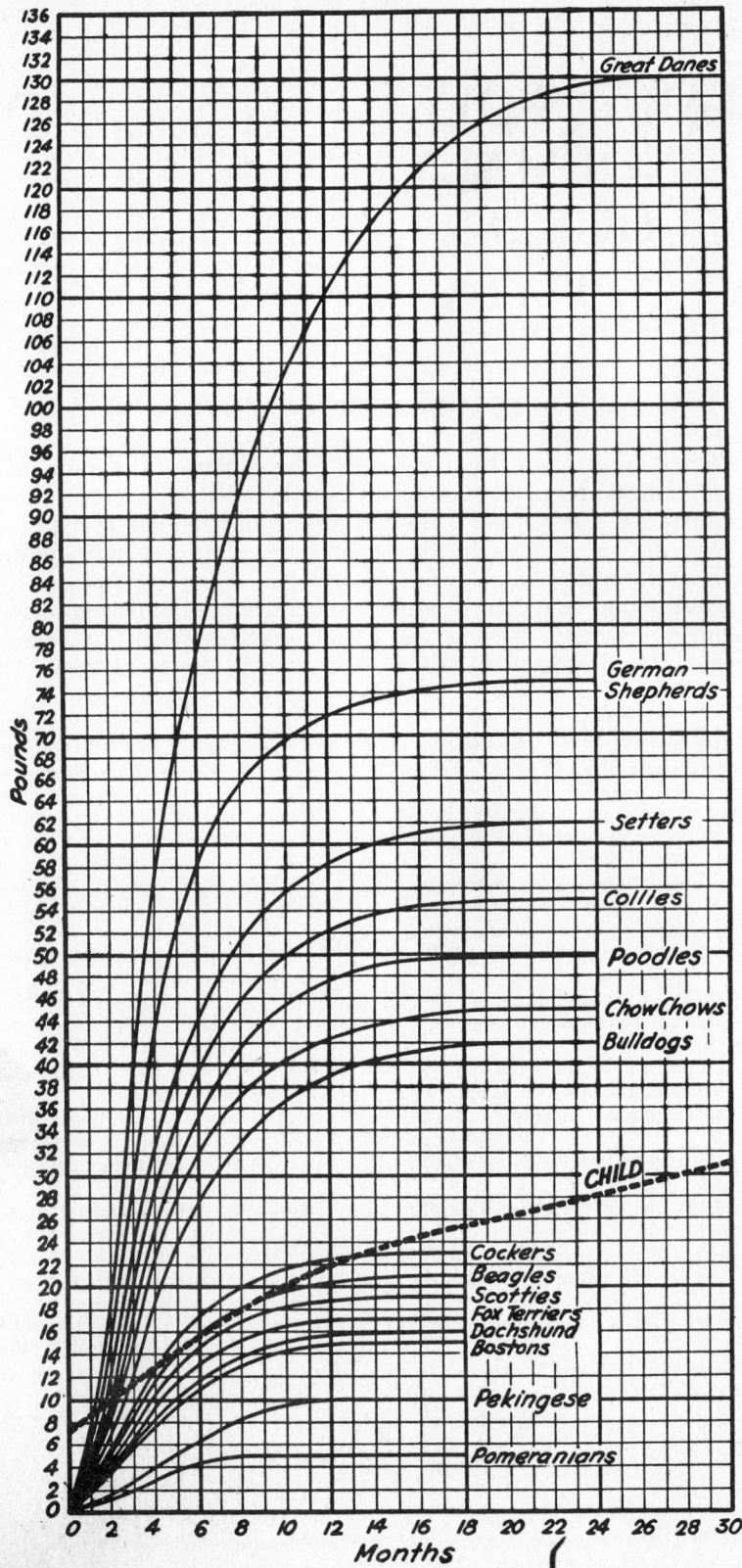

Fifteen breeds are marked. "Normal" rate-of-growth curves arrived at as indicated in charts of dachshunds, cocker spaniels, and German shepherds, compared with textbook growth-rate standard curve for human infant.

# FELINE GROWTH CHARTS

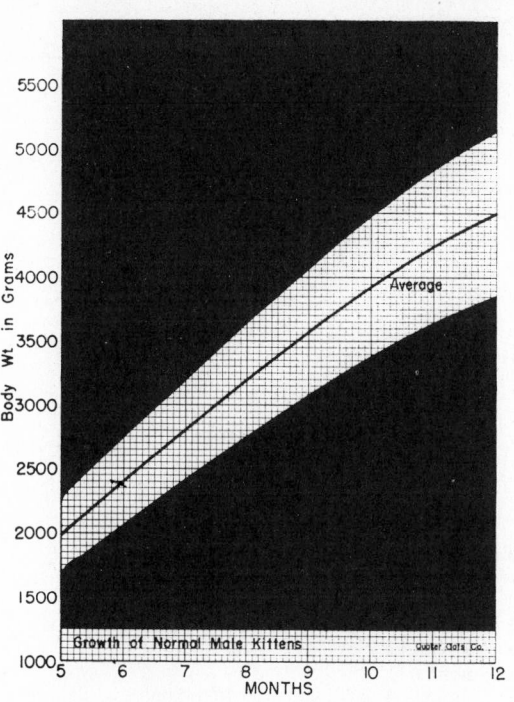

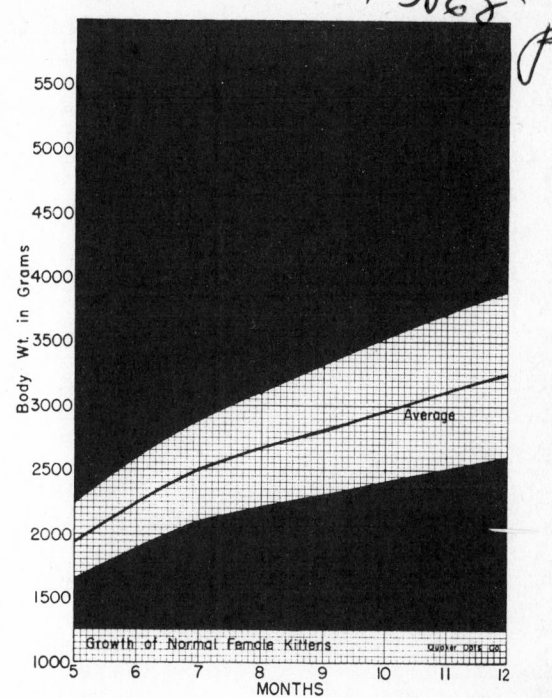

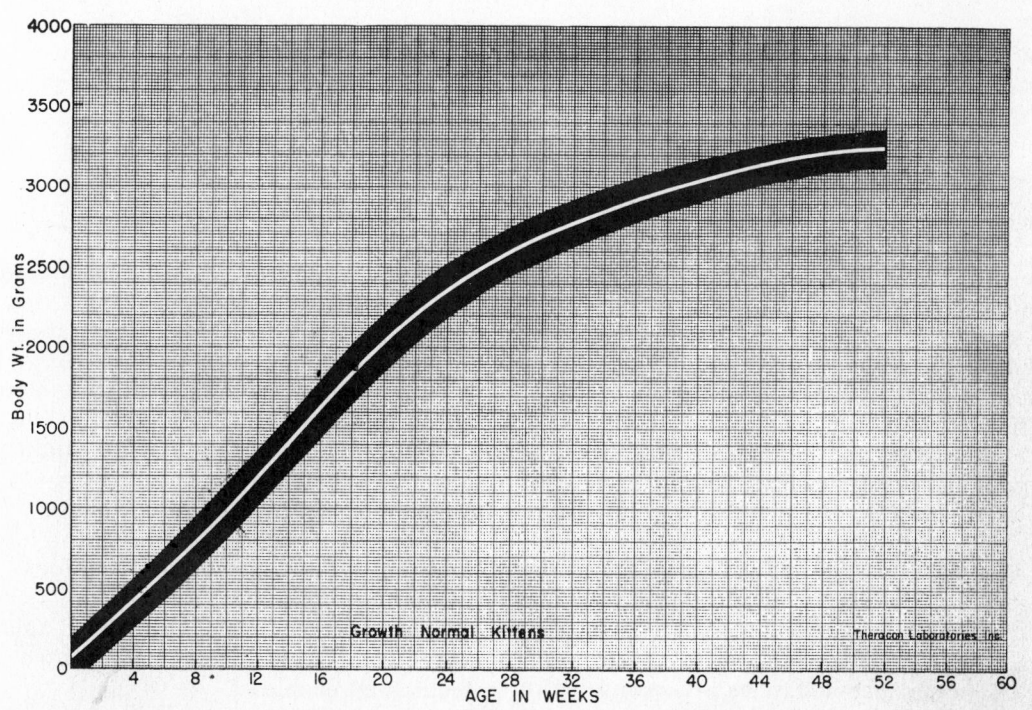

## TABLE OF DENTITION

| | I —Incisor | P —Premolar | |
| | C—Canine | M—Molar | |
| DOG | | | CAT |

*Dental Formulas*

| DOG | | CAT |
|---|---|---|
| $2(I \frac{3}{3} C \frac{1}{1} P \frac{3}{3}) = 28$ | Deciduous | $2(I \frac{3}{3} C \frac{1}{1} P \frac{3}{2}) = 26$ |
| $2(I \frac{3}{3} C \frac{1}{1} P \frac{4}{4} M \frac{2}{3}) = 42$ | Permanent | $2(I \frac{3}{3} C \frac{1}{1} P \frac{3}{2} M \frac{1}{1}) = 30$ |

*Eruption Dates*
Deciduous
(Vary widely)

| DOG | | | CAT |
|---|---|---|---|
| 4–5 weeks | I | 1 | 2–3 weeks |
| | I | 2 | |
| 5–6 weeks | I | 3 | 3–4 weeks |
| 3–4 weeks | C | 1 | 3–4 weeks |
| 4–5 weeks | P | 2 | upper—2 months; lower—none |
| | P | 3 | |
| 5–6 weeks | P | 4 | 4–5 weeks |

Generally teeth of large breeds erupt more rapidly than those of toy breeds.

Permanent

| DOG | | | CAT |
|---|---|---|---|
| 4–5 months | I | 1 | 3½–4 months |
| | I | 2 | |
| | I | 3 | 4–4½ months |
| 5–6 months | C | 1 | 5 months |
| 4–5 months | P | 1 | none |
| 5–6 months | P | 2 | upper—4½–5 months; lower—none |
| 5–6 months | P | 3 | 5–6 months |
| | P | 4 | |
| 4–5 months | M | 1 | 4–5 months |
| 5–6 months | M | 2 | None |
| 6–7 months | M | 3 | |

In some breeds, adult dogs lack the first and second premolars.
In many brachycephalic dogs, the last molars may be absent.

## DETERMINATION OF A DOG'S AGE FROM THE TEETH

By using the preceding Table of Dentition, one can tell the age of a dog quite accurately by eruption dates. Once the mouth is complete, determining the age becomes more difficult because much variation in wear and tooth health occurs as a result of diet and individual habit (such as bone and stone chewing). Some dogs develop tartar and alveolar periostitis much more readily than others. Abnormalities of occlusion can also give misleading results in the judgment of age by tooth wear. The following points may be helpful in judging the age of a dog.

One and one-half years: Cusps are worn off lower incisor I (middle).

Two and one-half years: Cusps are worn off lower incisor II (intermediate).

Three and one-half years: Cusps are worn off upper incisor I.

Four and one-half years: Cusps are worn off upper incisor II.

Five years: Cusps are worn slightly on lower incisor III (corner).

There is slight wear on the canines.

Six years: Cusps are worn off the lower incisors III (corners). The canines are becoming blunt.

Seven years and older: Individual animals vary widely; age determination from the teeth is unreliable.

*Table 1.* Nutrient Requirements of Dogs (Percentage or Amount per Kilogram of Food)

| | | TYPE OF DIET | | | |
|---|---|---|---|---|---|
| | | *Dry Basis* | *Dry Type* | *Semi-moist* | *Canned or Wet* |
| Moisture level (%): | | 0 | 10 | 25 | 75 |
| Dry-matter basis (%): | | 100 | 90 | 75 | 25 |
| *Nutrient* | | *Requirement* | | | |
| Protein | % | 22.0 | 20.0 | 16.5 | 5.5 |
| Fat | % | 5.5 | 5.0 | 4.0 | 2.0 |
| Linoleic or arachidonic acid | % | 1.6 | 1.4 | 1.2 | 0.4 |
| Minerals | | | | | |
| Calcium | % | 1.1 | 1.0 | 0.8 | 0.3 |
| Phosphorus | % | 0.9 | 0.8 | 0.7 | 0.25 |
| Potassium | % | 0.6 | 0.5 | 0.45 | 0.2 |
| Sodium chloride | % | 1.1 | 1.0 | 0.8 | 0.3 |
| Magnesium | % | 0.05 | 0.04 | 0.03 | 0.01 |
| Iron | mg. | 60.0 | 54.0 | 45.0 | 15.0 |
| Copper | mg. | 7.3 | 6.5 | 5.5 | 1.8 |
| Cobalt° | mg. | 2.4 | 2.2 | 1.8 | 0.61 |
| Manganese | mg. | 5.0 | 4.5 | 3.6 | 1.2 |
| Zinc | mg. | 20.0 | 18.0 | 15.0 | 5.0 |
| Iodine | mg. | 1.54 | 1.48 | 1.16 | 0.39 |
| Vitamins | | | | | |
| Vitamin A | mg. | 1.5† | 1.4 | 1.2 | 0.4 |
| Vitamin D | mg. | 0.007‡ | 0.006 | 0.005 | 0.002 |
| Vitamin E | mg. | 48.0 | 43.0 | 36.0 | 12.0 |
| Vitamin $B_{12}$ | mg. | 0.02 | 0.02 | 0.017 | 0.006 |
| Folic acid | mg. | 0.18 | 0.17 | 0.13 | 0.04 |
| Thiamine | mg. | 0.73 | 0.65 | 0.55 | 0.18 |
| Riboflavin | mg. | 2.2 | 1.9 | 1.6 | 0.5 |
| Pyridoxine | mg. | 1.0 | 0.9 | 0.75 | 0.25 |
| Pantothenic acid | mg. | 2.2 | 1.9 | 1.6 | 0.54 |
| Niacin | mg. | 10.6 | 10.0 | 7.5 | 2.5 |
| Choline | mg. | 1200.0 | 1100.0 | 900.0 | 300.0 |
| Vitamin K | mg. | 1.4 | 1.3 | 1.1 | 0.4 |

°The requirement for cobalt is related to the need for vitamin $B_{12}$. See text.

†This amount of crystalline A corresponds to 5000 IU/kg. of feed. (One mg. of vitamin A alcohol = 333 IU of vitamin A; 1 mg. of beta carotene = 1667 IU of vitamin A activity. For dogs, carotene is about one-half as valuable as vitamin A alcohol.)

‡This amount of pure vitamin D corresponds to 264 IU of vitamin D/kg. of feed.

Modified from *Nutrient Requirements of Dogs*, Publ. ISBN 0-309-02043-3, Committee on Animal Nutrition, Agricultural Board, National Academy of Sciences–National Research Council, Washington, D.C., 1972.

**Table 2.** *Nutrient Requirements of Dogs (Amounts per Kilogram of Body Weight per Day)*

| NUTRIENT | | ADULT MAINTENANCE | GROWING PUPPIES | NUTRIENT | | ADULT MAINTENANCE | GROWING PUPPIES |
|---|---|---|---|---|---|---|---|
| Protein | gm. | 4.4 | 8.8 | Vitamins | | | |
| Fat | gm. | 1.3 | 2.6 | Vitamin A | IU | 99.0 | 198.0 |
| Minerals | | | | Vitamin D | IU | 6.6 | 20.0 |
| Calcium | mg. | 200.0 | 400.0 | Vitamin E | | | |
| Phosphorus | mg. | 160.0 | 320.0 | ($\alpha$-tocopherol) | mg. | 2.0 | 2.2 |
| Potassium | mg. | 220.0 | 220.0 | Vitamin $B_{12}$ | $\mu$g. | 0.7 | 0.7 |
| Sodium chloride | mg. | 330.0 | 530.0 | Folic acid | $\mu$g. | 4.4 | 8.8 |
| Magnesium | mg. | 11.0 | 22.0 | Thiamine | $\mu$g. | 20.0 | 20.0 |
| Iron | mg. | 1.30 | 1.30 | Riboflavin | $\mu$g. | 44.0 | 88.0 |
| Copper | mg. | 0.17 | 0.17 | Pyridoxine | $\mu$g. | 22.0 | 55.0 |
| Cobalt | mg. | 0.055 | 0.055 | Pantothenic acid | $\mu$g. | 51.0 | 99.0 |
| Manganese | mg. | 0.110 | 0.22 | Niacin | $\mu$g. | 242.0 | 397.0 |
| Zinc | mg. | 0.110 | 0.22 | Choline | mg. | 25.0 | 55.0 |
| Iodine | mg. | 0.033 | 0.066 | Vitamin K | $\mu$g. | 33.0 | 66.0 |

Modified from *Nutrient Requirements of Dogs*, Publ. ISBN 0-309-02043-3, Committee on Animal Nutrition, Agricultural Board, National Academy of Sciences–National Research Council, Washington, D.C., 1972.


**Table 3.** *Estimated Daily Food Intakes Required by Dogs of Various Sizes*

| WEIGHT OF DOG | | REQUIREMENTS FOR MAINTENANCE | | | | REQUIREMENTS FOR GROWTH | | | |
|---|---|---|---|---|---|---|---|---|---|
| | | Air-Dry Food° | | Canned Dog Food† | | Air-Dry Food° | | Canned Dog Food† | |
| kg. | lb. | gm./kg. of Body Weight | kg./Dog | gm./kg. of Body Weight | kg./Dog | gm./kg. of Body Weight | kg./Dog | gm./kg. of Body Weight | kg./Dog |
| 2.3 | 5 | 40 | 0.09 | 134 | 0.31 | 80 | 0.18 | 268 | 0.62 |
| 4.5 | 10 | 33 | 0.15 | 113 | 0.51 | 66 | 0.30 | 225 | 1.01 |
| 6.8 | 15 | 28 | 0.19 | 95 | 0.65 | 56 | 0.38 | 212 | 1.44 |
| 9.1 | 20 | 27 | 0.25 | 90 | 0.82 | 54 | 0.49 | 178 | 1.62 |
| 13.6 | 30 | 25 | 0.34 | 88 | 1.17 | 50 | 0.68 | 172 | 2.33 |
| 22.7 | 50 | 25 | 0.57 | 84 | 1.91 | 50 | 1.13 | 167 | 3.79 |
| 31.8 | 70 | 25 | 0.79 | 84 | 2.67 | | | | |
| 49.8 | 110 | 24 | 1.20 | 83 | 4.13 | | | | |

°Air-dry foods contain 6 to 12 per cent of moisture. Calculations of the amounts of dry foods are based on energy supplied by food containing 90 per cent of dry matter, 77 per cent of protein plus carbohydrates, 5 per cent of fat, and 10 per cent of ash, fiber and other material. This supplies a calculated 1580 kcal./lb. (or 3480 kcal./kg.), of which 80 per cent is digestible. On this basis, digestible kcal. would be 1264/lb. (or 2784/kg.).

†Calculated on the basis of 25 per cent of dry matter and nutrient ratios the same as those stated in the preceding footnote. Total energy is calculated as 439 kcal./lb. and 966 kcal./kg. Available energy is calculated as 413 kcal. (85 per cent of the total)/lb. and 821 kcal./kg.

*Note:* The daily food intake for soft, moist diets depends on moisture level, acceptability and caloric content. Soft, moist products vary in moisture level.

From *Nutrient Requirements of Dogs*, Publ. ISBN 0-309-02043-3, Committee on Animal Nutrition, Agricultural Board, National Academy of Sciences–National Research Council, Washington, D.C., 1972.

*Table 4.    Protein, Calories and Sulfur Amino Acids in Some Common Food Products*

| PRODUCT° | ON A DRY BASIS | | | |
|---|---|---|---|---|
| | Dry Matter (%) | Protein (gm./100 gm. of food) | Kilo-calories/gm. | Total Sulfur Amino Acids in Each Gram of Protein (mg.) |
| Barley, grain | 89.0 | 13.0 | 3.3 | 34 |
| Carrot, roots, fresh | 12.9 | 6.6 | 3.5 | – |
| Corn, grits, cracked fine screened | 88.2 | 9.0 | 3.8 | 32 |
| Cattle, meat, lean | 37.5 | 75.0 | 4.4 | 43 |
| Oats, cereal byproduct, mx 4% fiber | 91.2 | 12.0 | 3.9 | 32 |
| Pea, seeds | 89.5 | 13.0 | 3.6 | 33 |
| Potato, tubers, fresh | 23.1 | 8.5 | 3.7 | 26 |
| Rice, groats, polished | 88.5 | 8.0 | 3.8 | 32 |
| Cattle, milk, skimmed dehy, mx 8% moisture | 94.3 | 36.0 | 3.6 | 37 |
| Soybean, flour, solv-extd fine sift, mx 3% fiber | 92.3 | 50.0 | 3.4 | 37 |
| Wheat, grain | 88.9 | 20.0 | 3.8 | 38 |
| Chicken, eggs wo shells, raw | 26.3 | 47.0 | 6.0 | 63 |
| Reference protein | – | 100.0 | 4.0 | 42 |

°NRC names.

From *Nutrient Requirements of Dogs*, Publ. ISBN 0-309-02043-3, Committee on Animal Nutrition, Agricultural Board, National Academy of Sciences–National Research Council, Washington, D.C., 1972.

my = 1/65 gr.
gm = 15.43 gr.

Warfarm
u ∅ M= Bozovido
mephyton 15 ml bid
7 day. (MSD)

# TABLE OF COMMON DRUGS: APPROXIMATE DOSES*

| NAME OF DRUG | DOGS | CATS |
|---|---|---|
| Acepromazine | 0.1 to 0.5 mg./kg. IV, IM or SC | 0.1 to 0.2 mg./kg. IM or SC |
| Acetazolamide | 10 mg./kg. q6h orally | Same |
| Acetylsalicylic acid (aspirin) | *Analgesic:* 10 mg./kg. q12h<br>*Antirheumatic:* (maximum) 40 mg./kg. q18h | 10 mg./kg. q52h<br>40 mg./kg. q72h |
| ACTH | 2 units/kg./day IM (therapeutic dose);<br>40 units/dog IM (response test);<br>post sample in 2 hours | Same |
| Aldactone (spirono-lactone) | 2 to 4 mg./kg. q12h | Same |
| Alevaire | 50 to 60 ml./hr. for 30 to 60 minutes q12h by nebulization | Same |
| Allopurinol (Zyloprim) | 10 mg./kg. q8h initially;<br>reduce to 2 to 3 mg. q8h for maintenance | None |
| Aminophylline | 10 mg./kg. IV slowly or same dose q8h IM or orally | Same |
| Ammonium chloride | 100 mg./kg. q12h orally | 20 mg./kg. q12h orally |
| Amocillin | 10 mg./kg. q12h | |
| Amphetamine | 4 mg./kg. IM or IV | Same |
| Amphotericin B | 0.25 to 0.50 mg./kg. IV or IP with 5% dextrose and water 2 to 3 times weekly | Same |
| Ampicillin | 20 mg./kg. q8h orally<br>6 mg./kg. q8h IM or IV | Same |
| Amprolium | 100 to 200 mg./kg./day in food or water for 7 to 10 days | None |
| Apomorphine | 40 μg./kg. IV | None |
| Aqua-B (vitamin B complex) | 0.5 to 2.0 ml. q24h IV, IM or SC | 0.5 to 1.0 ml. q24h IV, IM or SC |

*See Appendix Tables for Conversion of Weight to Body-Surface Area in Square Meters for Dogs, p. 1384.

| NAME OF DRUG | DOGS | CATS |
|---|---|---|
| Aqua MEPHYTON (vitamin $K_1$) | 5 to 20 mg. q12h IV, IM or SC | 1 to 5 mg. q12h IV, IM or SC |
| Arecoline hydrobromide | 1.5 mg./kg. orally after 12-hour fast | None |
| Ascorbic acid (vitamin C) | 100 to 500 mg./day maintenance; 100 to 500 mg. q8h urinary acidifier | 100 mg./day maintenance 100 mg. q8h urinary acififier |
| Atropine | 0.05 mg./kg. q6h SC, IM or IV; 1% topically in eye; 2 mg./kg. SC, IM or IV for organophosphate toxicity | Same (causes salivation if applied topically in the eye |
| Azulfidine | 60 mg./kg. q8h orally | None |
| BAL | 4 mg./kg. q4h IM until recovery | NONE! |
| Bethanechol | 5 to 25 mg. q8h orally | 2.5 to 5.0 mg. q8h orally |
| Bismuth (milk of) | 5 to 10 ml. q4h orally (May be increased 2 to 3 times if needed) | 2 to 5 ml. q4h orally |
| Bismuth (subnitrate, subgallate or subcarbonate) | 0.5 to 3.0 gm. q4h orally | Same |
| Blood | 20 ml./kg. or to effect IV (or IP) | Same |
| Brewers' yeast | 0.2 gm./kg. once daily orally | Same |
| Bunamidine (Scolaban) | 25 to 50 mg./kg. orally on empty stomach. Feed 3 hours later. Avoid excitement for 24 hours. | Same |
| Caffeine | 0.1 to 0.5 gm. IM | None |
| Calcium | Adult: 200 mg./kg. daily Pup: 400 mg./kg. daily | Adult: 100 mg./kg. daily Kitten: 200 mg./kg. daily |
| Calcium carbonate | 1 to 4 gm. daily | Same |
| Calcium EDTA | 25 mg./kg., diluted to 10 mg./ml. in 5% dextrose and water and given SC 4 times daily for 5 days | Same |
| Calcium gluconate (10% solution) | 10 to 30 ml. IV *slowly* | 5 to 15 ml. IV *slowly* |
| Calcium lactate | 0.5 to 2.0 gm. orally | 0.2 to 0.5 gm. orally |
| Canex | 0.3% rotenone in oil applied topically | Same |
| Canine distemper-hepatitis vaccine | 1 vial SC or IM at 8, 12 and 16 weeks of age and annual booster | None |
| Cardioquin | 10 to 20 mg./kg. q8-12h orally | Same |
| Cephalexin | 30 mg./kg. q12h orally | Same |
| Cephaloridine (Loridine) | 10 mg./kg. q12h IM or SC | Same |

| NAME OF DRUG | DOGS | CATS |
|---|---|---|
| Charcoal (activated) | 2 heaping tablespoonfuls in 200 ml. tap water orally for 15-kg. dog | 1 heaping teaspoonful in 60 ml. tap water orally |
| Cheracol—D | 5 ml. q4h orally | 3 ml. q4h orally |
| Chloramphenicol | 20 to 50 mg./kg. q8h orally; 10 mg./kg. q12h IM or IV | Same |
| Chlorethamine | 0.2 to 1.0 gm. q8h orally | 100 mg. q8h orally |
| Chlorpheniramine | 4 to 8 mg. q12h orally | 2 mg. q12h orally |
| Chlorpromazine (Thorazine) | 1.0 to 2.0 mg./kg. q12h IV or IM; 2.0 to 4.0 mg./kg. q8h orally; 0.5 mg./kg. IV as alpha blocker for shock; 0.5 mg./kg. for vomiting | Same |
| Chlorothiazide (Diuril) | 20 to 40 mg./kg. q12h orally | Same |
| Cod liver oil | 1 teaspoon/10 kg. once daily orally | Same |
| Codeine | 2 mg./kg. q6h SC for pain; 5 mg./dose q6h orally for cough | None |
| Colistimethate (Coly-Mycin) | 1 mg./kg. IM q6h | Same |
| Conofite | Apply topically daily for 4 weeks | Same |
| Coramine | ¼ to 1 ml./8 kg. SC, IM or IV | Same |
| Cyclophosphamide (Cytoxan) | 50 mg./m.$^2$ BSA orally every other day (See Tables of Weight Conversion) *For pemphigus:* Dogs <10 kg.—1.5 mg./kg. orally, once daily, 4 days/week Dogs 10 to 20 kg.—2.0 mg./kg. orally, once daily, 4 days/week Dogs >20 kg.—2.5 mg./kg. orally, once daily, 4 days/week | 12.5 mg./cat orally every other day |
| Cyclothiazide | 0.5 to 1.0 mg. once daily orally | None |
| Darbazine | 0.25 ml. q12h SC (up to 2 kg.); 0.5 to 1.0 ml. q12h SC (3 to 7 kg.); 2 to 3 ml. q12h SC (8 to 15 kg.); 3 to 4 ml. q12h SC (16 to 23 kg.); 4 to 5 ml. q12h SC (24 to 30 kg.); 6 ml. q12h SC (over 30 kg.) | Same |
| Daribiotic | 0.5 to 1.0 ml. q12h IM (for dose for small dog, see under Cat) | 0.25 ml. q12h IM |
| Delta albaplex | (For dose for small dog, see under Cat) 1 to 2 tablets/day orally (2 to 7 kg.); 2 to 4 tablets/day orally (8 to 15 kg.); 4 to 6 tablets/day orally (16 to 30 kg.); 6 to 8 tablets/day orally (over 30 kg.) | 0.25 ml. q12h; 1 tablet q12h |
| Desoxycorticosterone (acetate (DOCA) | 1 to 5 mg. q24h IM | 0.5 to 1.0 mg. q24h IM |
| Desoxycorticosterone pivalate | Each 25 mg. releases approximately 1 mg. DOCA/day for 1 month—given orally | Same |
| Dexamethasone (Azium) | 4 to 8 mg./kg. IV for shock 0.25 to 2.0 mg. once daily orally or IM | Same 0.1 to 0.5 mg. once daily orally or IM |

| NAME OF DRUG | DOGS | CATS |
|---|---|---|
| Dextran | 20 ml./kg. IV to effect | Same |
| Dextrose solutions (5% in water, saline or Ringer's) | 40 to 50 ml./kg. q24h IV, SC or IP | Same |
| D.F.P. (Floropryl) | 0.1% ointment for eyes, topically | Same |
| Diazepam (Valium) | 1 mg./kg. IV or orally, maximum 20 mg. | Same, maximum 5 mg. |
| Dichlorphenamide (Daranide) | For 15-kg. dog, give 50 mg. t.i.d. orally | 10 mg./animal t.i.d. orally |
| Dichlorvos (Task) | 25 to 30 mg./kg. orally (See manufacturer's recommendations) | None |
| Diethylcarbamazine (Caracide) | 30 to 60 mg./kg. orally (vermifuge), or 5 mg./kg./day (heartworm prevention) | 10 to 20 mg./kg. orally |
| Diethylstilbestrol | 0.1 to 1.0 mg./day orally, or 2 mg./kg. up to 25 mg. total IM (repositol) ONCE. Long-term dosage: 0.1 mg./2 kg. orally on alternate days | 0.05 to 0.10 mg./day orally (CAUTION); alternate-day dosage is best for maintenance |
| Digoxin | 0.1 to 0.2 mg./kg. in 4 equal doses over 48 hours (digitalization). Maintenance dose: $\frac{1}{6}$ of total digitalization dose or about 0.02 mg./kg. | Same |
| Dihydrocodeinone | 5 mg. q6h orally | None |
| Dimenhydrinate (Dramamine) | 25 to 50 mg. q8h orally | 12.5 mg. q8h orally |
| Diphenhydramine (Benadryl) | 4 mg./kg. q8h orally | Same |
| Diphenthane 70 | 200 mg./kg. orally after 12-hour fast; repeat in 3 weeks | Same |
| Diphenylhydantoin (Dilantin) | 6 mg./kg. q8-12h orally | None |
| Diphenylthiocarbazone | 60 mg./kg. q8h orally for 5 days *beyond* recovery | None |
| Dipyrone (Novin) | 0.5 ml./5 kg. IM, IV or SC | Same |
| Disophenol (D.N.P.) | 7 mg./kg. SC; repeat in 3 weeks | None |
| Dithiazanine (Dizan) | 4 to 6 mg./kg. once daily orally for 77 to 10 days (microfilariae) | 10 mg. once daily orally for 4 to 5 days (lungworm) |
| Domeboro's solution | 1 to 2 tablets/pint of water applied topically q8h | Same |
| Doxapram-V | 5 to 10 mg./kg. IV | Same |
| Doxylamine succinate | 1 to 2 mg./kg. q8h IM | Same |
| D-Penicillamine | 15 mg./kg. b.i.d. orally | None |
| Drocarbil (Nemural) | 4 mg./kg. orally after light meal; repeat in 3 weeks (with caution) | Same, with caution |
| Ephedrine | 5 to 15 mg. orally | 2 to 5 mg. orally |

| NAME OF DRUG | DOGS | CATS |
|---|---|---|
| Epinephrine (1:1000 solution) | 0.1 to 0.5 ml. SC, IM, IV or IC | 0.1 to 0.2 ml. SC, IM, IV or IC |
| Erythromycin | 10 mg./kg. q8h orally | Same |
| Estradiol (E.C.P.) cyclopentylpropionate | 0.25 to 2.00 mg. IM *once* | None |
| Ether | 0.5 to 4.0 ml. (Induce 8%; maintain 4% by inhalation) | Same |
| Ethoxzolamide (Cardrase) | 4 mg./kg. q12h orally | Same |
| Feline panleukopenia antiserum | None | 1 to 5 ml. SC (prevention), or 5 to 10 ml. SC (exposure) |
| Feline panleukopenia vaccine | None | 1 vial SC at 8, 12 and 16 weeks of age; annual booster |
| Ferrous sulfate | 100 to 300 mg./day orally | 50 to 100 mg./day orally |
| Flucytosine (Ancobon) | 50 mg./kg. q.i.d. orally | Same |
| Fludrocortisone acetate (Florinef) | 0.2 to 0.8 mg. once daily orally | 0.1 to 0.2 mg. once daily orally |
| Flumethasone | 0.0625 to 0.25 mg. daily IV, IM, SC or orally; 0.166 to 1.0 mg. IA or intralesional | One half dog dose |
| 9-Fluoroprednisolone (Predef) | 1 mg. once daily IM | 0.5 mg. once daily IM |
| Folic acid | 5 mg./day orally | 2.5 mg./day orally |
| Fulvidex | Topically in ear | Same |
| Furadex | 2 to 4 mg./kg. q8-12h orally | Same |
| Furosemide (Lasix) | 2 mg./kg. q12h IV, maximum total dose/dog=40 mg. 2 to 4 mg./kg. q8-12h orally | Same, maximum 5 mg. Same |
| Gentamicin | 4 mg./kg. q12h IM, then 4 mg./kg. q24h IM | Same |
| Glucagon | *Tolerance test:* 0.03 mg./kg. IV | None |
| Glycerin | 0.6 ml./kg. q8h orally | Same |
| Glycobiarsol (Milibis-V) | 200 mg./kg. once daily for 5 days; repeat in 3 months | None |
| Goodwinol | Topically for *Demodex*, once daily for 4 to 6 weeks | Same |
| Griseofulvin (microcrystalline) (Fulvicin) | 20 mg./kg./day once daily orally for 6 weeks, or 140 mg./kg./week once weekly orally for 6 weeks | Same |

| NAME OF DRUG | DOGS | CATS |
|---|---|---|
| Haloprogin | Apply topically daily | |
| Halothane | Induce 3%; maintain 0.5 to 1.0% by inhalation | Same |
| Heparin | 1 mg./kg. IV | Same |
| Hetacillin | 10 to 20 mg./kg. q12h orally | 50 to 100 mg. q12h orally |
| Hydrochlorothiazide (Hydrodiuril) | 2 to 4 mg./kg. q12h orally | Same |
| Hydrocortisone | 4 mg./kg. q12h orally | Same |
| Hydrocortisone sodium succinate | 20 to 40 mg./kg. IV for shock | Same |
| Hydrogen peroxide (3%) | 5 to 10 ml. q15min orally until emesis occurs | Same |
| Innovar-Vet | 1 ml./7 to 10 kg. IM, or 1 ml./12–30 kg. IV | None |
| Insulin (regular) | 2 units/kg. q2-6h IV (ketoacidosis), modified to effect | 3 to 5 units q6h SC, modified to effect |
| Insulin (intermediate) | 0.5 to 1.0 units/kg. q24h SC, modified as needed | 3 to 5 units q24h SC, modified as needed |
| Iron dextran | 10 mg./kg. IM weekly in divided doses | Same |
| Isometheptene (Octin) | 130 mg. q12h orally, or 50 to 100 mg. q12h IM | None |
| Isoproterenol (Isuprel) | 0.1 to 0.2 mg. q6h IM or SC; 15 to 30 mg. q4h orally; 1.0 mg. in 200 ml. 5% dextrose and water IV to effect; elixir=0.2 ml. q8h orally | Same |
| Jenotone | 2 mg./kg. q12h IM or SC | Same |
| Kanamycin | 6 mg./kg. q12h IM, or 10 mg./kg. q6h orally (not absorbed) | Same |
| Kaobiotic | 1 tablet/4 kg./day in 2 or 3 divided doses | Same |
| Kaopectate | 1 to 2 ml./kg. q2-6h orally | Same |
| Ketamine HCl (Vetalar) | None<br><br>BIRDS:<br>2 mg./kg. IM (may go to 100 mg./kg. in small species) | 10 to 30 mg./kg. (15 av.) IM or IV |
| Lactated Ringer's solution | 40 to 50 ml./kg./day IV, SC or IP | Same |
| Levallorphan | 1 to 2 mg. total IV to effect | None |
| Levamisole (L-tetramisole) | 10 mg./kg. once daily orally for 6 to 10 days (microfilariae) | 20 to 40 mg./kg. once daily orally, every other day for 5 to 6 treatments (lungworm) |

| NAME OF DRUG | DOGS | CATS |
|---|---|---|
| Lidocaine (without epinephrine) | 2 mg./kg. IV slowly over 2 to 4 minutes; follow with 1 mg./ml. of saline or 5% dextrose and water given at the rate of 25 to 40 mg. per 30 minutes | Same |
| Lime sulfur (1:16 to 1:40 solution) | Topically | Same |
| Lincomycin | 15 mg./kg. q8h orally, or 10 mg./kg. q12h IM | Same |
| Lindane | 0.025 to 0.1% aqueous solution topically | None |
| Lysodren (Mitotane) | (See Op' DDD) | |
| Mannitol hexanitrate | 15 to 30 mg. orally | Same |
| Mannitol (20% solution) | 1 to 2 ml./kg. q6h IV | Same |
| Maxidex | Topically in eyes q2-8h | Same |
| Maxitrol | Topically in eyes q2-8h | Same |
| Measles vaccine | 1 vial IM to dogs between 4 and 12 weeks of age | None |
| Meclizine (Bonine) | 4 mg./kg. once daily orally | Same |
| Megestrol acetate (Ovaban) | *For skin:* 1 mg./kg. daily orally | 0.5 mg./kg. daily orally for 2 weeks, then 2 times weekly if needed |
| | *To postpone estrus:* In proestrus—2 mg./kg. orally daily for 8 days In anestrus—0.5 mg./kg. orally daily for 32 days False pregnancy—2 mg./kg. orally daily for 8 days | None |
| Melatonin | 1 to 2 mg. SC once daily for 3 days; repeat monthly as needed | None |
| Mepazine (Pacatal) | 1.5 mg./kg. (antiemetic) | |
| Meperidine (Demerol) | 6 to 10 mg./kg. | 2 to 4 mg./kg. (Duration of effect only 1 to 2 hours in these species) |
| Mercuhydrin | 2 mg./kg. IM, SC or IV | Same |
| Metaraminol (Aramine) | 2 to 10 mg. SC or IM; 10 to 50 mg./500 ml. saline and infused IV to effect | |
| Methenamine mandelate | 10 mg./kg. q6h orally to effect | |
| Methetharimide | 12 mg./kg. IV | Same |
| Methicillin | 20 mg./kg. IM or IV q6h | Same |
| DL-Methionine | 0.2 to 1.0 gm. q8h orally | 0.2 gm. q8h orally |
| Methischol | 1 capsule/15 kg. q8h orally | 1 capsule q12h orally |

| NAME OF DRUG | DOGS | CATS |
|---|---|---|
| Methotrexate | 2.5 to 5.0 mg./m.² BSA once daily orally for 4 days; may repeat at 3-week intervals as needed (See Weight Conversion Tables) | None |
| Methoxamine (Vasoxyl) | 0.2 mg./kg. IV | |
| Methoxyflurane | Induce 1%; maintain 0.5% | Same |
| Methylprednisolone acetate | 1 mg./kg. once daily orally or once weekly (depo) IM; best maintenance dose is once orally every other morning | Same |
| Methyltestosterone | 0.5 mg./kg. once daily orally | Same |
| Metrazol | 10 mg./kg. IV, or 100 mg. orally | 6 mg./kg. IV |
| Metronidazole (Flagyl) | 60 mg./kg. once daily orally for 5 days | None |
| Metropectin | 2 to 4 tablets q8h orally | None |
| Metropine | 0.5 to 1.0 mg. q8h orally | None |
| Milk of magnesia | 5 to 30 ml. orally | 5 to 15 ml. orally |
| Mineral oil | 5 to 15 ml. orally | 2 to 6 ml. orally (careful!) |
| Mitotane (Lysodren) | (See Op'DDD) | |
| Mitox | Topically in ears once daily for 5 to 7 days, then once a week for 5 to 7 weeks | Same |
| Morphine | *Analgesic:* 1 to 2 mg./kg. IM or SC *Pulmonary Edema:* 0.2 mg./kg. IV; repeat as needed | 0.1 mg./kg. IM or SC (CAUTION) |
| Nafcillin sodium | 6 mg./kg. q6h orally or IM | Same |
| Nalorphine HCl (Nalline) | 5 to 20 mg. IV, IM or SC (1 mg./kg.) | Same |
| Naloxone HCl (Narcan) | Dose to effect, usually 0.2 to 0.4 mg. total dose | None |
| N-butyl chloride | 0.4 ml./kg. after 12-hour fast | None |
| Neo-Darbazine | Spansule #1: 1 capsule q12h orally (5 to 10 kg.) 2 capsules q12h orally (10 to 15 kg.) Spansule #3: 1 capsule q12h orally (15 to 30 kg.) 2 capsules q12h orally (over 30 kg.) | Same |
| Neomycin | 20 mg./kg. q6h orally (not absorbed), or 10 mg./kg. q12h IM or IV | Same |
| Neostigmine | 1 to 2 mg. IM as needed; 5 to 15 mg. orally as needed | |
| Niclosamide (Yomesan) | 150 mg./kg. orally; repeat in 3 weeks | Same |
| Nitrofurantoin | 4 mg./kg. q8h orally, or 3 mg./kg. q12h IM | Same |
| Nitrofurantoin sodium | 3 mg./kg. q12h IM (maximum 10 days) | |
| Nitrofurazone (0.2% ointment or solution) | Topically | Same |
| Novobiocin | 10 mg./kg. q8h orally | Same |

| NAME OF DRUG | DOGS | CATS |
|---|---|---|
| Nystatin | 100,000 units q6h orally | Same |
| Octin (Isometheptene) | 0.5 to 1.0 ml. IM; 1 tablet q8-12 orally | 0.25 to 0.50 ml. IM, or ½ to 1 tablet q12h orally |
| Op'DDD (Mitotane, Lysodren) | 50 mg./kg. once daily orally to effect (approximately 5 to 10 days), then once every 2 weeks | |
| Ouabain | 0.04 mg./kg. total dose IV; give ½ dose stat, then ⅛ dose q30min; maintenance = ¼ total dose q3h | Same |
| Oxacillin (Cloxacillin) | 10 mg./kg. orally q6h | Same |
| Oxymorphone (Numorphan) | 0.2 mg./kg. SC, IV or IM | 0.4 to 1.5 mg./cat SC, IM or IV |
| Oxytocin | 5 to 10 units IM or IV; repeat q15-30min | 0.5 to 3.0 units IM or IV |
| 2-PAM | 40 mg./kg. IV over 2-minute period q12h as needed (can be given IM or SC) | |
| Pancreatin | 2 to 10 tablets with food | 1 to 2 tablets with food |
| Paregoric | 3 to 5 ml. q6h orally | None |
| Penicillins | | |
| Pen G, Na or K | 20,000 units/kg. q4-6h IV or IM | |
| Pen G, Na or K | 40,000 units /kg. q6h orally (on empty stomach) | |
| Pen G, procaine | 40,000 units/kg. q24h IM | Same |
| Pen G and Pen benzathine | 40,000 units/kg. IM *once* — 1 cc / 18.2 lb. | |
| Pentazocine (Talwin) | 1 to 3 mg./kg. SC, IM or IV | Same |
| Pentobarbital | 30 mg./kg. IV to effect | Same |
| Phencyclidine (Sernylan) | WILD ANIMALS: Not recommended for routine use (1 to 2 mg./kg.) | |
| Phenobarbital | 2 mg./kg. q12h orally; 30 to 300 mg. IV to effect per day total dose | 4 mg./kg. q12h orally; 15 to 60 mg. IV per day total dose |
| Phenoxybenzamine (Dibenzyline) | 5 mg./kg. IV; use *carefully* | None |
| Phenylbutazone (Butazolidin) | → 20 mg / lb. body wt ÷ 3 doses  40 mg./kg. q8h orally | 10 to 14 mg./kg. q12h orally |
| Phenylephrine (Neo-Synephrine) | 0.15 mg./kg. IV | |
| Phthalofyne (Whipcide) | 180 mg./kg. orally after 24-hour fast; repeat in 3 months | None |
| Piperacetazine (Psymod) | 0.2 mg./kg. IV, IM, SC or orally; may repeat dose once if needed | Same |
| Piperazine | 100 to 200 mg./kg. orally; repeat in 3 weeks | Same |

| NAME OF DRUG | DOGS | CATS |
|---|---|---|
| Pitressin (ADH) | 10 units IV or IM (aqueous), or 0.5 to 1.0 ml. IM every other day (oil) | |
| Polymyxin B | 2 mg./kg. q12h IM | |
| Potassium chloride | 1 to 3 gm./day orally; IV maximum 10 mEq./hour and 40 mEq./day/dog | 0.2 gm./day orally |
| Prednisolone | 0.5 to 1.0 mg./kg. orally or IM b.i.d. Best maintenance dose is once orally every other morning | Same |
| Prednisone | 0.5 to 1.0 mg./kg. orally or IM b.i.d. Best maintenance dose is once orally every other morning | Same |
| Primidone | 25 mg./kg. orally b.i.d. | |
| Pro-Banthine | 7.5 to 30 mg. q8-12h orally | |
| Procainamide (Pronestyl) | 10 to 15 mg./kg. slowly IV; may repeat 2 to 4 hours as needed; ½ to 2 capsules q4-6h orally | Same |
| Promazine (Sparine) | 2 to 4 mg./kg. IM or IV | Same |
| Promethazine (Phenergan) | 2 mg./kg. once daily (antiemetic) orally or IM | Same |
| Propanolol | 0.2 mg./kg. slowly IV; 10 to 40 mg. q8h orally | 0.2 mg./kg. slowly IV; 5 to 10 mg. q8h orally |
| Propiopromazine (Tranvet) | 0.4 mg./kg. IV or IM | |
| Prussian blue | 0.4 gm./kg./day orally, subdivided into 3 doses | |
| Pyrimethamine | 2 mg./kg./day orally for 3 days, then 1 mg./kg. every other day | Same |
| Quadrinal | ¼ to ½ tablet q4-6h orally | ¼ tablet q4-6h orally |
| Quibron | 1 to 3 capsules q8h; elixir = 5 ml./15 kg. q8h orally | ½ capsule q8h; elixir= 2 ml. q8h orally |
| Quinacrine (Atabrine) | 50 to 100 mg. q12h orally for 3 days; repeat in 3 days | |
| Quinaglute | 10 to 20 mg./kg. q12h orally | Same |
| Quinidine | 10 to 20 mg./kg. q6-8h orally | Same |
| Rabies vaccine (C.E.O.) | 1 vial IM (per state regulations) | None |
| Rabies vaccine (T.C.O.) | 1 vial IM (per state regulations) | Same |
| Renzol | 1 tablet hr/10 kg. q8h orally | Same |
| Respireze | 1 tablet q6-8h (up to 12 kg.) orally; 2 tablets q6-8h (over 12 kg.) orally | None |
| Rheomacrodex | 100 to 500 ml. IV | 50 to 100 ml. IV |

1382 TABLE OF COMMON DRUGS: APPROXIMATE DOSES—*Continued*

| NAME OF DRUG | DOGS | CATS |
| --- | --- | --- |
| Riboflavin | 10 to 20 mg./day orally | 5 to 10 mg./day orally |
| Ringer's solution | 40 to 50 ml./kg./day IV, IP or SC | Same |
| Rompun | 1 to 4 mg./kg. SC, IM or IV | Same |
| Ronnel (Ectoral) | 35 mg./kg. orally b.i.d., or as 1 to 2% aqueous solution topically | None |
| Scopolamine | 0.01 to 0.02 mg./kg. SC, IM or IV | Same |
| Sodium bicarbonate | 2 mEq./kg. IV; 50 mg./kg. q8h orally | 2 mEq./kg. IV; 50 mg./kg. q8h orally |
| Sodium chloride (0.9% solution) | 40 to 50 ml./kg./day IV, IP or SC | Same |
| Sodium dioctyl sulfosuccinate | 100 to 300 mg. q12h orally | 100 mg. q12-24h orally |
| Sodium iodide (20% solution) | 1 ml./5 kg. q8-12h orally or IV | Same |
| Sodium levothyroxine | 0.1 to 0.6 mg. once daily orally, or 0.05 to 0.30 mg. b.i.d. orally | 0.05 to 0.10 mg. once daily orally |
| Sodium sulfate | 1 teaspoon/5 kg. orally | Same |
| Stanozolol (Winstrol-V) | ½ to 2 tablets q12h orally | ½ tablet q12h orally |
| Streptomycin or dihydrostreptomycin | 10 mg./kg. q8-12h IM | None |
| Styrid-Caricide | 1 ml./10 kg. once daily orally (heartworm prevention) | None |
| Sulfonamides Phthalylsulfathiazole | 100 mg./kg. q12h orally (not absorbed) | |
| Salicylazosulfapyridine | 60 mg./kg. q8h orally | Same |
| Sulfadimethoxyine | 20 mg./kg. q24h orally or IV | |
| Sulfamerazine or sulfamethazine | 50 mg./kg. q12h orally or IV | |
| Sulfisoxazole | 40 mg./kg. q8h orally | |
| Tannalbin | 1 to 3 gm. q8h orally | |
| Tansal (5% tannic acid, 5% salicylic acid and 70% alcohol) | Topically q8h | Same |
| Temaril-P | 1 capsule once daily orally (up to 5 kg.) 2 capsules once daily orally (5 to 10 kg.) 4 capsules once daily orally (10 to 20 kg.) 6 capsules once daily orally (over 20 kg.) | Same |
| Testosterone | 2 mg./kg. (up to 30 mg. total) once daily every 2 to 3 days orally; 2 mg./kg. (up to 30 mg. total) IM every 10 days (repositol) | Same |
| Tetracyclines | 16 mg./kg. q8h orally; 6 mg./kg. q12h IV or IM | Same |

| NAME OF DRUG | DOGS | CATS |
|---|---|---|
| Thenium closylate (Canopar) | ½ tablet b.i.d. orally up to 5-kg. dog; 1 tablet once daily for dogs larger than 5 kg.; repeat in 3 weeks | None |
| Thiabendazole | 50 to 100 mg./kg. once daily orally | None |
| Thiacetarsamide (caparsolate or filicide) | 0.2 mg./kg. IV b.i.d. for 2 days | 0.1 ml./kg . IV once on day 1; skip 1 day and repeat on day 3 |
| Thiamine | 10 to 100 mg./day orally | 5 to 30 mg./day orally |
| Thyroid (desiccated) | 10 mg./kg./day orally | Same |
| Toluene (methylbenzene) | 200 mg./kg. orally | Same |
| Tresaderm | Topically q12h | Same |
| Triacetyloleandomycin | 50 mg./kg. orally, divided q8h | |
| Triamcinolone (Vetalog) | 0.25 to 2.0 mg. once daily orally or IM | 0.1 mg. once daily orally or IM |
| Trifluomeprazine (Nortran) | 0.5 to 1.0 mg./kg. q12h orally | |
| Trimethobenzamide (Tigan) | 3 mg./kg. orally or IM (antiemetic) | Same |
| Trimethoprim and sulfadiazine (Tribrissen) | 30 mg./kg. q24h, or 15 mg./kg. q12h | Same |
| Tripelennamine | 1 mg./kg. q12h orally, or 1 ml./20 kg. IM | Same |
| Trisulfapyrimidine | 50 mg./kg. q12h orally | Same |
| TSH (Dermathycin) | 5 to 10 units IM or SC (response test); post sample in 10 hours | 5 units IM or SC |
| Tylosin | 10 mg./kg. q8h orally; 6 mg./kg. q12h IM or IV | Same |
| Vigoral | 1 to 3 tablets once daily orally | ½ to 1 tablet once daily orally |
| Vincristine | 0.5 mg./m.² BSA IV once a week as needed | 0.1 mg. IV once a week as needed |
| Viokase | 1 to 2 teaspoonfuls/lb. of food mixed 30 minutes before feeding | Same |
| Vi-Sorbin | 1 to 3 teaspoonfuls orally daily | ½ teaspoonful orally daily |
| Vitamins A | 400 units/kg./day orally for 10 days | Same |
| $B_{12}$ | 100 to 200 μg./day | 50 to 100 μg./day |
| D | 30 units/kg./day orally for 10 days | Same |
| E | 500 mg./day orally | 100 mg./day orally |
| K (menadione) | 2 mg./kg./day IM for 10 days | Same |

*Handwritten annotations:* AVM# 3-79 - 26.4 mg/kg or 12 mg/lb ÷ 2 doses q/2h ; Valium → diazepam

# TABLES FOR CONVERSION OF WEIGHT TO BODY-SURFACE AREA IN METERS FOR DOGS

| KG. | M.$^2$ | KG. | M.$^2$ |
|---|---|---|---|
| 0.5 | 0.06 | 26.0 | 0.88 |
| 1.0 | 0.10 | 27.0 | 0.90 |
| 2.0 | 0.15 | 28.0 | 0.92 |
| 3.0 | 0.20 | 29.0 | 0.94 |
| 4.0 | 0.25 | 30.0 | 0.96 |
| 5.0 | 0.29 | 31.0 | 0.99 |
| 6.0 | 0.33 | 32.0 | 1.01 |
| 7.0 | 0.36 | 33.0 | 1.03 |
| 8.0 | 0.40 | 34.0 | 1.05 |
| 9.0 | 0.43 | 35.0 | 1.07 |
| 10.0 | 0.46 | 36.0 | 1.09 |
| 11.0 | 0.49 | 37.0 | 1.11 |
| 12.0 | 0.52 | 38.0 | 1.13 |
| 13.0 | 0.55 | 39.0 | 1.15 |
| 14.0 | 0.58 | 40.0 | 1.17 |
| 15.0 | 0.60 | 41.0 | 1.19 |
| 16.0 | 0.63 | 42.0 | 1.21 |
| 17.0 | 0.66 | 43.0 | 1.23 |
| 18.0 | 0.69 | 44.0 | 1.25 |
| 19.0 | 0.71 | 45.0 | 1.26 |
| 20.0 | 0.74 | 46.0 | 1.28 |
| 21.0 | 0.76 | 47.0 | 1.30 |
| 22.0 | 0.78 | 48.0 | 1.32 |
| 23.0 | 0.81 | 49.0 | 1.34 |
| 24.0 | 0.83 | 50.0 | 1.36 |
| 25.0 | 0.85 | | |

(From Ettinger, S. J.: Textbook of Veterinary Internal Medicine. Philadelphia, W. B. Saunders Co., 1975.)

*Nomogram for the Estimation of Surface Area of the Dog**

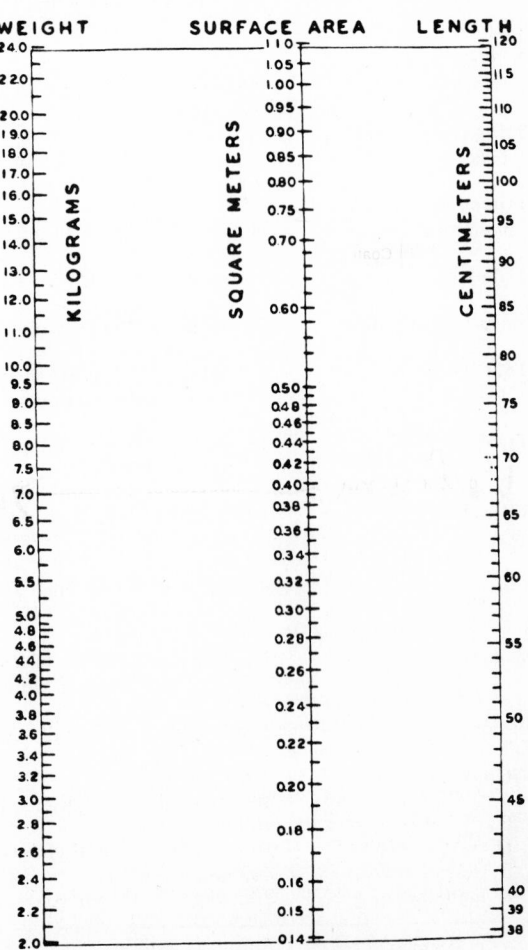

*Length = Nose to anus measured along abdomen.
From Smith, H. W.: Principles of Renal Physiology, 3rd ed. New York, Oxford University Press, 1957.

# TABLE OF SUSCEPTIBILITY OF VARIOUS EXOTIC ANIMALS TO CANINE AND FELINE DISTEMPER*

| FAMILY | SPECIES | Should Receive Canine Distemper Vaccine | Should Receive Feline Distemper Vaccine |
|---|---|---|---|
| Canidae[1] (Dogs) | Coyote | + | − |
| | Dingo | + | − |
| | Domestic | + | − |
| | Fox | + | − |
| | Jackal | + | − |
| | Wolf | + | − |
| | Cape Hunting Dog | + | − |
| | Racoon Dog | + | − |
| Procyonidae[2] | Bassariscus | + | − |
| | Coati | + | + |
| | Kinkajou | + | − |
| | Lesser Panda | + | + |
| | Racoon | + | + |
| Ursidae[1, 3] (Bears) | All Species | − | − |

| FAMILY | SPECIES | Should Receive Canine Distemper Vaccine | Should Receive Feline Distemper Vaccine |
|---|---|---|---|
| Mustelidae[2] | Ferret | + | − |
| | Fisher | + | + |
| | Grison | + | + |
| | Marten | + | + |
| | Mink | + | + |
| | Otter | + | + |
| | Sable | + | + |
| | Skunk | + | + |
| | Wolverine | + | + |
| | Badger | + | + |
| Viverridae | Binturong[2] | + | + |
| | Foussa | − | − |
| | Linsang | − | − |
| | Mongoose | − | − |
| | Civit | + | − |
| Hyaenidae[1] (Hyenas) | All Species | + | − |
| Felidae[1] (Cats) | All Species | − | + |

1. Dr. Paul S. Chaffee—Secty.-Treas., American Assn. Zoo Veterinarians—CANIDAE—Based on survey of Zoo veterinarians, all species of this family are susceptible to Canine Distemper and should be vaccinated. CANIDAE—MLV vaccines recommended, except in Lesser Panda, where killed vaccines should be used to be safe. HYAENIDAE —regular vaccination against canine distemper recommended as insurance although only a few cases actually reported. URSIDAE—several bears reported susceptible, but need for inoculation of this group is questionable.
2. Dr. Charles Sedgwick—Los Angeles Zoo—PROCYONIDAE—Coati, Lesser Panda and Raccoon should be immunized with both canine and feline vaccines. MUSTELIDAE—all species immunized with canine and feline vaccine. VIVERRIDAE—Binturong should be immunized with canine and feline vaccine.

  All species which have extreme susceptibility to canine and feline distemper viruses should receive the first injection prior to shipment.
3. Dr. Lynn Griner—San Diego Zoo—Reports 2 cases panleukopenia in young bear cubs. (Not verified by virus isolation.)

## RECOMMENDATIONS FOR IMMUNIZATION OF ZOO ANIMALS

Since very little documented data concerning duration of maternal antibodies, susceptibility to the virus, or the development of immune titers in the families or species of exotic zoo animals is available, recommendations concerning the size of the dose and number of injections are made with some reservations. We have conferred with zoo veterinarians who follow these common guidelines: The larger cats receive 2 or 3 doses of vaccine at one injection. All Felidae receive repeated injections at two week intervals until they are 3 months. Some give the first booster at 4 months, and follow with yearly boosters. If feline panleukopenia is diagnosed in a zoo population revaccination of the entire population is considered. (A similar plan is followed for canine distemper.)

*From *Norden News*. Lincoln, Nebr., Norden Laboratories, Spring, 1970.

# ROSTER OF SELECTED DRUGS AND UNUSUAL EQUIPMENT

## DRUGS

**Atropine sulfate** (various mfr.). 1% solution.

**Cetapred ophthalmic ointment** (Alcon).
**Chloroptic ophthalmic solution** (Allergan). 0.5% chloramphenicol.
**Chlortetracycline hydrochloride** (Aureomycin, Lederle). 250 mg. capsules in bottles of 16 and 100; recommended dosage for treatment of toxoplasmosis is 15 mg./lb. divided in 4 equal doses for 14 to 21 days, depending on response.
**Collyrium** (Wyeth). ½ oz. boric acid, ½ oz. sodium bicarbonate, ½ oz. sodium chloride, 2 oz. glycerin, 5 drops Roccal and distilled water to make 1 gal.
**Cyclophosphamide** (Cytoxan, Mead Johnson). Oral tablets: 50 mg., bottles of 100; recommended dosage for treatment of necrogranulomatous sclerouveitis is 2.5 mg./lb./day in 2 divided doses for 7 days, and 1.25 mg./lb./day in 2 divided doses thereafter.
**Cytoxan** (Mead Johnson).

**Folinic acid** (Calcium leucovorin, Lederle). 3 mg. of folinic acid-calcium salt in 1 ml. vials; recommended dosage to counteract folic acid inhibition in pyrimethamine therapy for toxoplasmosis is 1 mg. I.M. each day while on pyrimethamine.

**Garamycin ophthalmic ointment** (Schering).
**Gelfoam.** Upjohn Co., Kalamazoo, Mich.

**Isopto Alkaline ophthalmic solution** (Alcon).

**Maxitrol ophthalmic ointment** (Alcon).
**Maxitrol ophthalmic suspension** (Alcon).
**Mycitracin ophthalmic ointment** (Upjohn).

**Neo-Delta-Cortef** (Upjohn). Eye-ear drops, 0.25%, and ointment, 0.25 and 0.5%. Kalamazoo, Michigan

**Neosporin ophthalmic solution and ointment** (Burroughs Wellcome).

**opDDD** (Lysodren, Calbio). 500 mg. tablets, bottle of 100.
**Ophthaine** (proparacaine hydrochloride, Squibb). Ophthalmic solution.
**Ophthetic** (proparacaine hydrochloride, Allergan). Ophthalmic solution.

**Predmycin-P Liquifilm ophthalmic suspension** (Allergan).
**Prednisolone sodium phosphate** (Inflammase Forte, Smith Miller and Patch) or prednisolone acetate (1% Prednefrin Forte, Allergan). Ophthalmic solutions; the most potent commercially available topical corticosteroids; recommended, along with mydriatics and, in some cases, other medications, for all anterior uveitis syndromes.
**Pyrimethamine** (Daraprim, Burroughs, Wellcome). 25 mg. tablets in bottles of 30 and 100; recommended dosage for treatment of toxoplasmosis is 1 mg./lb. daily for 3 days, followed by 0.5 mg./lb. every other day for 10 to 21 days, depending on response.

**Ribavirin** (for investigative use only). ICN Pharmaceuticals, Inc., 2727 Campus Drive, Irvine, Calif.

**Sisomicin** (for investigative use only). Schering Corp., Bloomfield, N.J.
**Stoxil** (Idoxuridine, Smith, Kline and French).

**Triamcinolone acetonide** (Vetalog, Squibb). 5 ml. bottle of 6 mg./ml.; recommended dosage for administration retrobulbarly, under Tenon's capsule and subconjunctivally is 2 mg./injection site; repeat weekly when indicated.

**Urical** (Upjohn).

1386

## UNUSUAL EQUIPMENT

This list provides source information for special instruments and equipment described in the text.

**Adams Readacrit.** Clay-Adams Inc., New York, N.Y.

**"Airpure" absolute filter** (size B, 7C70-L). Flanders Filters Inc., Box 1219, Washington, N.C.

**Aerosol units.** See *Nebulizers.*

**Airshield Ethaire nonrebreathing valve and whistle.** Ethical Veterinary Supply Co., Long Island, N.Y.

**Aluminum, padded splints.** Aluminum and foam fence splint. Strips 16 inches × 2, 3 or 4 inches. American Hospital Supply, Evanston, Ill.

**AMBU self-inflating bag** (Air Shields Co.).

**Aspirator and compression pump.** Dia-Pump, model E.F., pressure and suction No. 08–000. Air Shields, Inc., Hatboro, Pa.

**Aural forceps** (Spreull's modification of Ormerod's aural forceps). Down Bros. and Meyer and Philips, Ltd., Surrey, England.

**Barkan Lamp.** Storz Eye Instruments, St. Louis, Mo.

**B.D. direct blood pressure.** Becton, Dickinson & Co., Rutherford, N.J.

**Beaver miniature knife.** Edward Weck & Co., Long Island City, N.Y.

**Bird Mark 7 respirator.** Bird Corp., Palm Springs, Calif.

**Blood parameter analyzer.** Model 95500. Beckman Instruments, Inc., Fullerton, Calif.

**Brecht infant feeder.** Davol Rubber Co., Providence, R.I.

**Bronchographic equipment.** C. L. Jackson standard bronchoscopes; laryngeal mirrors, sizes 00–6; Tucker flexible tip aspirating tubes, straight and curved tips, 50 cm.; Morrison specimen collector, nonspill, 10 cc.; Lukens specimen collector, 2 cc.; Thompson bronchial catheter, 20 F., for introducing contrast media.

Available from George P. Pilling & Sons, Ft. Washington, Pa.

**Butterfly needle.** Abbott Laboratories, North Chicago, Ill.

**Cataract cyroextractor, disposable.** Smith, Miller & Patch. New York, N.Y., or Alcon Labs., Ft. Worth, Texas.

**Catheters, intravenous.** Jelco Laboratories, Raritan, N.J.

**Cavitron.** The Dentist's Supply Co. of New York, York, Pa.

**Cope pleural biopsy needle.** Becton, Dickinson & Co., Rutherford, N.J.

**Cutdown catheter.** Becton, Dickinson & Co., Rutherford, N.J.

**Dental film supplies.** Kodak Ultraspeed Type 3; Bite-wing Morlite Code D.F. 42; Kodak Periapical Ultraspeed Morlite Code D.F. 58; Bite-wing tabs. Pittsburgh Specialty Co., Pittsburgh, Pa.

**Dentsply, Borden handpiece.** The Dentist's Supply Co. of New York, York, Pa.

**Dräger squeeze bag.** North American Dräger, Telford, Pa.

**Eye instruments, special.** Berens eye speculum, Grafe fixation forceps, Castroviejo needle holder, Scheie-Westcott scissors, Terson extracapsular forceps, Gill iris forceps, Kirby Hook extractor, 22 gauge lacrimal needle, Castroviejo cyclodialysis spatula. Storz Instrument Co., St. Louis, Mo.

**Eye loupe.** Edward Weck & Co., Long Island City, N.Y.

**Fixative for slides.** Spray-Cyte fixative for use in exfoliative cytology, 2 oz. Clay-Adams, Inc. New York, N.Y.

**Flexi-lum.** Flexible surgical light. Concept, Inc., Airport Station, St. Petersburg, Fla.

**Foley catheter.** Bard-Parker, Rutherford, N.J.

**Fungassay Dermatophyte Test Medium.** Pitman-Moore, Inc., Washington Crossing, N.J.

**Giemsa stain.** Fischer Scientific Co., Fair Lawn, N.J.

**Goldberg Refractometer.** American Optical Co., Buffalo, N.Y.

**Gram stain.** Fischer Scientific Co., Fair Lawn, N.J.

**Heating pad (water circulator).** Gorman-Rupp Industries Div., Bellville, Ohio.

**Humidifier.** Hankscraft cold stream vaporizer, Hankscraft, Inc., Reedsburg, Wis.

**Hydrion paper (pH).** Micro Essential Laboratories, Brooklyn, N.Y.

**Ictotest reagent tablets.** Test for urine bilirubin, bottles of 90 tablets. Ames Co., Inc., Elkhart, Ind.

**Infant feeding tube No. F815.** Sterilon Corp., Braintree, Mass.

**Insemination pipet.** Plastic blue tip Infuse-Ese. Alexander Shaw Corp., Wellesley Hills, Mass.

**Intracath.** Deseret Pharmaceutical Co., Sandy, Utah.

**Intramedic tubing.** PF–90/536 0.50 in. O.D. Clay-Adams, Inc., New York, N.Y.

**Jelco needle.** Johnson & Johnson, Raritan, N.J.

**Kimura spatula.** Edward Weck & Co., Long Island City, N.Y.

**Kirschner intensive care oxygen therapy unit.** Kirschner Scientific Co., Seattle, Wash.

**Lacrimal needle.** BD Lac No. 43. Becton, Dickinson & Co., Rutherford, N.J.

**Lactophenol cotton blue stain.** Fischer Scientific Co., Fair Lawn, N.J.

**Longdwell catheter.** Becton, Dickinson & Co., Rutherford, N.J.

**McMaster's fecal counting chamber kit.** H-L-4100. Haver-Lockhart, Kansas City, Mo.

**Microliter syringes.** 0.05 and 0.1 ml. capacity. Hamilton Co., Whittier, Calif.

**Nebulizers.** Croupette cool mist and oxygen tent, universal model, Air Shields, Inc., Hatboro, Pa. De Vilbiss No. 40 (5 cc.) and De Vilbiss No. 841 (300–1900 cc.), The De Vilbiss Company, Toledo, Ohio.

**New methylene blue stain.** Fischer Scientific Co., Fair Lawn, N.J.

**Non-rebreathing valve (Ethaire).** Ethical Veterinary Supply Co., Oceanside, N.Y.

**Ohaus animal subject box scale metric No. 730 and No. 701 weight.** Ohaus Scale Corp., Florham Park, N.J.

**Ophthalmic suture.** 4–0 silk, 6–0 silk, 7–0 silk, 4–0 chromic gut, 6–0 chromic gut. Ethicon, Sommerville, N.J.

**Otoscope (Spreull's).** EVSCO Pharmaceutical Co., Oceanside, N.Y.

**Pall Filter.** Pall Corporation, Glen Cove, Long Island, N.Y.

**pH meter.** Model 76004 expandomatic pH meter. Beckman Instruments, Inc., Fullerton, Calif.

**Polybite wing tabs.** Pulpdent Corp. of America, Boston, Mass.

**Polyglycolic acid suture, 3–0.** Dexon, Davis & Geck, Pearl River, N.Y.

**Premature infant feeding tubes.** Size 5 F., 15 inches. Becton, Dickinson & Co., Rutherford, N.J.

**Prosthetic canine eye.** L. O. Nezvesky, Ithaca, N.Y.

**Radon.** Sources: Nuclear Consultants Corp., St. Louis, Mo.; The Radium Chemical Co., Inc., New York, N.Y.; Radium Service Corp. of America, Kenilworth, Ill.

**Rochester bedside kit.** Rochester Products Co., Rochester, Minn.

**Rotosonic tooth scaler.** Ellman Roto-Pro Pfingst & Co., New York, N.Y.

**Schirmer tear test.** Iso-Sol brand, box of 50 sets. Crookes-Barnes Laboratories, Wayne, N.J.

**Scratch test kits.** Hollister-Stier Laboratories, Los Angeles, Calif.

**Silastic medical grade tubing.** Dow Corning Corp., Medical Products Div., Midland, Mich.

**Siliclad.** Clay-Adams, Inc., New York, N.Y.

**Tattoo instruments.** Nicholson Manufacturing, Inc., Denver, Colo.

**Taylor thermometers.** Taylor Instrument Co., Rochester, N.Y.

**Tech Lyte magnifier lamp.** Tech-Lyte, San Francisco, Calif.

**Temp-Pads.** Gaymar Ind., Buffalo, N.Y.

**Tes-Tape.** Urine sugar analysis paper, 100 test dispenser packages, 12 pkg./carton. Eli Lilly & Co., Indianapolis, Ind.

**Thermometer.** Nonconstrictive, continuous reading laboratory thermometer No. T21301002. Scientific Products Co.

**Thompson catheter.** George P. Pilling & Sons, Ft. Washington, Pa.

**Tooth extracting forceps.** Standard extracting forceps No. 10 or 11 or children's "300." Cleveland Dental Manufacturing Co., Cleveland, Ohio.

**Tooth root elevators.** Seldin root elevators, Nos. 2, 3 and 5. S. S. White Co., Philadelphia, Pa. Cleve-Dent exolever, curet tip, No. 301; gouge tip No. 304. Cleveland Dental Manufacturing Co., Cleveland, Ohio.

**Tooth scaler.** Scaler No. 2 (pick); No. 33 (hoe). Cleveland Dental Manufacturing Co., Cleveland, Ohio.

**Trylon Keyes cutaneous biopsy punch.** American Hospital Supply, Evanston, Illinois.

**Vaponefrin (plastic, standard).** Fisons Corp., Bedford, Mass.

**Venotomy sets.** Becton, Dickinson & Co., Rutherford, N.J.

**Vim-Silverman biopsy needle, (Franklin Modified).** V. Muller & Co., Chicago, Ill.

**Weber air turbine handpiece 200.** Weber Dental Manufacturing Co., Canton, Ohio.

**Whirlpool baths.** Ille electric turbine ejector and aerator, Model T.P. 100, cost approximately $225.00, Ille Electric Corp., Williamsport, Pa.; Hydrojet whirlpool bath, cost approximately $225.00, Boulevard Electronics Co., Chicago, Ill.

**Wood's lamp.** Burton Model No. 91312 U.V., Arista Surgical Co., New York, N.Y.

**Wright's stain.** Fischer Scientific Co., Fair Lawn, N.J.

# TABLE OF HOUSEHOLD MEASURES*

*From Kirk, R. W., and Bistner, S. I.: Handbook of Veterinary Procedures and Emergency Treatment. 2nd ed. Philadelphia, W. B. Saunders Co., 1975.

| MEASURE | APPROXIMATE EQUIVALENTS Metric | Apothecaries' |
|---|---|---|
| 1 drop | 1/20 ml. | 1 minim |
| 1 teaspoon | 5 ml. | 1+ dram |
| 1 dessertspoon | 8 ml. | 2 drams |
| 1 tablespoon | 15 ml. | ½ ounce |
| 1 wineglass | 60 ml. | 2 ounces |
| 1 glass | 250 ml. | 8 ounces |

# TABLE OF CONVERSION FACTORS*

*From Kirk, R. W., and Bistner, S. I.: Handbook of Veterinary Procedures and Emergency Treatment. 2nd ed. Philadelphia, W. B. Saunders Co., 1975.

| | | | |
|---|---|---|---|
| 1 milligram | = | 1/65 grain | (1/60) |
| 1 gram | = | 15.43 grains | (15) |
| 1 kilogram | = | 2.20 pounds | [avoirdupois] |
| | | 2.68 pounds | [Troy] |
| 1 milliliter | = | 16.23 minims | (15) |
| 1 liter | = | 1.06 quarts | (1 +) |
| | | 33.80 fluidounces | (34) |
| 1 grain | = | 0.065 gm. | (60 mg.) |
| 1 dram | = | 3.9 gm. | (4) |
| 1 ounce | = | 31.1 gm. | (30+) |
| 1 minim | = | 0.062 ml. | (0.06) |
| 1 fluid dram | = | 3.7 ml. | (4) |
| 1 fluidounce | = | 29.57 ml. | (30) |
| 1 pint | = | 473.2 ml. | (500 −) |
| 1 quart | = | 946.4 ml. | (1000 −) |

Figures in parentheses are commonly employed approximate values.

# TABLE OF APPROXIMATE CONVERSIONS —POUNDS TO KILOGRAMS*

*From Kirk, R. W., and Bistner, S. I.: Handbook of Veterinary Procedures and Emergency Treatment. 2nd ed. Philadelphia, W. B. Saunders Co., 1975.

| Pounds | Kilograms |
|---|---|
| 11 | 5 |
| 22 | 10 |
| 33 | 15 |
| 44 | 20 |
| 55 | 25 |
| 66 | 30 |
| 88 | 40 |
| 110 | 50 |
| 132 | 60 |
| 154 | 70 |
| 176 | 80 |
| 198 | 90 |
| 220 | 100 |
| 242 | 110 |

# TABLE OF CONVERSION FROM FAHRENHEIT TO CENTIGRADE THERMO-METRIC READINGS*

| Cent. Deg. | Fahr. Deg. | Cent. Deg. | Fahr. Deg. | Cent. Deg. | Fahr. Deg. | Cent. Deg. | Fahr. Deg. |
|---|---|---|---|---|---|---|---|
| −40 | −40.0 | −4 | 24.8 | 32 | 89.6 | 68 | 154.4 |
| −39 | −38.2 | −3 | 26.6 | 33 | 91.4 | 69 | 156.2 |
| −38 | −36.4 | −2 | 28.4 | 34 | 93.2 | 70 | 158.0 |
| −37 | −34.6 | −1 | 30.2 | 35 | 95.0 | 71 | 159.8 |
| −36 | −32.8 | 0 | 32.0 | 36 | 96.8 | 72 | 161.6 |
| −35 | −31.0 | +1 | 33.8 | 37 | 98.6 | 73 | 163.4 |
| −34 | −29.2 | 2 | 35.6 | 38 | 100.4 | 74 | 165.2 |
| −33 | −27.4 | 3 | 37.4 | 39 | 102.2 | 75 | 167.0 |
| −32 | −25.6 | 4 | 39.2 | 40 | 104.0 | 76 | 168.8 |
| −31 | −23.8 | 5 | 41.0 | 41 | 105.8 | 77 | 170.6 |
| −30 | −22.0 | 6 | 42.8 | 42 | 107.6 | 78 | 172.4 |
| −29 | −20.2 | 7 | 44.6 | 43 | 109.4 | 79 | 174.2 |
| −28 | −18.4 | 8 | 46.4 | 44 | 111.2 | 80 | 176.0 |
| −27 | −16.6 | 9 | 48.2 | 45 | 113.0 | 81 | 177.8 |
| −26 | −14.8 | 10 | 50.0 | 46 | 114.8 | 82 | 179.6 |
| −25 | −13.0 | 11 | 51.8 | 47 | 116.6 | 83 | 181.4 |
| −24 | −11.2 | 12 | 53.6 | 48 | 118.4 | 84 | 183.2 |
| −23 | −9.4 | 13 | 55.4 | 49 | 120.2 | 85 | 185.0 |
| −22 | −7.6 | 14 | 57.2 | 50 | 122.0 | 86 | 186.8 |
| −21 | −5.8 | 15 | 59.0 | 51 | 123.8 | 87 | 188.6 |
| −20 | −4.0 | 16 | 60.8 | 52 | 125.6 | 88 | 190.4 |
| −19 | −2.2 | 17 | 62.6 | 53 | 127.4 | 89 | 192.2 |
| −18 | −0.4 | 18 | 64.4 | 54 | 129.2 | 90 | 194.0 |
| −17 | +1.4 | 19 | 66.2 | 55 | 131.0 | 91 | 195.8 |
| −16 | 3.2 | 20 | 68.0 | 56 | 132.8 | 92 | 197.6 |
| −15 | 5.0 | 21 | 69.8 | 57 | 134.6 | 93 | 199.4 |
| −14 | 6.8 | 22 | 71.6 | 58 | 136.4 | 94 | 201.2 |
| −13 | 8.6 | 23 | 73.4 | 59 | 138.2 | 95 | 203.0 |
| −12 | 10.4 | 24 | 75.2 | 60 | 140.0 | 96 | 204.8 |
| −11 | 12.2 | 25 | 77.0 | 61 | 141.8 | 97 | 206.6 |
| −10 | 14.0 | 26 | 78.8 | 62 | 143.6 | 98 | 208.4 |
| −9 | 15.8 | 27 | 80.6 | 63 | 145.4 | 99 | 210.2 |
| −8 | 17.6 | 28 | 82.4 | 64 | 147.2 | 100 | 212.0 |
| −7 | 19.4 | 29 | 84.2 | 65 | 149.0 | 101 | 213.8 |
| −6 | 21.2 | 30 | 86.0 | 66 | 150.8 | 102 | 215.6 |
| −5 | 23.0 | 31 | 87.8 | 67 | 152.6 | 103 | 217.4 |
|  |  |  |  |  |  | 104 | 219.2 |

*From Catalogue 65, Hospital and Surgical Equipment. V. Mueller, Chicago.

# INDEX

- ECP - Upjohn → 2m Slabeth

(Fe m i nee - Tablets - Ethyl → Ethenal Estradiol
Pill os my Tablet

Humen's →
( Oes Estradiol Suppinate )
Sumlian

{ Anesthon
Returns Pleenta }  Cattle
mummfeed fetn
Persest Corpus
Pyometra .

Cattle

1.-
Heifers